KENDIG AND CHERNICK'S
Disorders OF THE
Respiratory Tract
IN Children EIGHTH EDITION

KENDIG AND CHERNICK'S
Disorders OF THE
Respiratory Tract
IN Children EIGHTH EDITION

Robert W. Wilmott, MD, FRCP
IMMUNO Professor and Chair
Department of Pediatrics
St. Louis University
Pediatrician in Chief
Cardinal Glennon Children's Hospital
St. Louis, Missouri

Thomas F. Boat, MD
Christian R. Holmes Professor
Vice President for Health Affairs
Dean of the College of Medicine
University of Cincinnati
Cincinnati, Ohio

Andrew Bush, MD, FRCP, FRCPCH
Professor of Paediatric Respirology
Imperial College
Consultant Paediatric Chest Physician
Royal Brompton Hospital
London, United Kingdom

Victor Chernick, MD, FRCPC
Professor Emeritus
Department of Pediatrics and Child Health
University of Manitoba
Winnipeg, Manitoba, Canada.

Robin R. Deterding, MD
Professor of Pediatrics
Department of Pediatrics
Director, Breathing Institute
Children's Hospital Colorado
University of Colorado
Aurora, Colorado

Felix Ratjen, MD, PhD, FRCPC
Head
Division of Respiratory Medicine
Sellers Chair of Cystic Fibrosis
Professor
University of Toronto
Hospital for Sick Children
Toronto, Ontario, Canada

ELSEVIER
SAUNDERS

ELSEVIER
SAUNDERS

1600 John F. Kennedy Blvd.
Ste 1800
Philadelphia, PA 19103-2899

KENDIG AND CHERNICK'S DISORDERS
OF THE RESPIRATORY TRACT IN CHILDREN   ISBN: 978-1-4377-1984-0

Notices

Knowledge and best practice in this field are constantly changing. As new research and experience broaden our understanding, changes in research methods, professional practices, or medical treatment may become necessary.

Practitioners and researchers must always rely on their own experience and knowledge in evaluating and using any information, methods, compounds, or experiments described herein. In using such information or methods they should be mindful of their own safety and the safety of others, including parties for whom they have a professional responsibility.

With respect to any drug or pharmaceutical products identified, readers are advised to check the most current information provided (i) on procedures featured or (ii) by the manufacturer of each product to be administered, to verify the recommended dose or formula, the method and duration of administration, and contraindications. It is the responsibility of practitioners, relying on their own experience and knowledge of their patients, to make diagnoses, to determine dosages and the best treatment for each individual patient, and to take all appropriate safety precautions.

To the fullest extent of the law, neither the Publisher nor the authors, contributors, or editors, assume any liability for any injury and/or damage to persons or property as a matter of products liability, negligence or otherwise, or from any use or operation of any methods, products, instructions, or ideas contained in the material herein.

Library of Congress Cataloging-in-Publication Data
Kendig and Chernick's disorders of the respiratory tract in children. – 8th ed. / [edited by] Robert W. Wilmott ... [et al.].
     p. ; cm.
  Disorders of the respiratory tract in children
  Rev. ed. of: Kendig's disorders of the respiratory tract in children. 7th ed. c2006.
  Includes bibliographical references and index.
  ISBN 978-1-4377-1984-0 (hardcover : alk. paper)
  I. Kendig, Edwin L., 1911- II. Wilmott, R. W. (Robert W.) III. Kendig's disorders of the respiratory tract in children. IV. Title: Disorders of the respiratory tract in children.
  [DNLM: 1. Respiratory Tract Diseases. 2. Child. 3. Infant. WS 280]
  618.92'2–dc23   2012000458

Content Strategist: Stefanie Jewell-Thomas
Content Development Specialist: Lisa Barnes
Publishing Services Manager: Catherine Jackson
Senior Project Manager: Carol O'Connell
Design Direction: Steve Stave

Printed in China
Last digit is the print number: 9 8 7 6 5 4 3 2 1

PREFACE

In editing this, the eighth edition of *Kendig and Chernick's Disorders of the Respiratory Tract in Children,* we are struck by how much has changed since the last edition. There have been remarkable new understandings of the basic mechanisms of lung disease in the last 7 years. We have recognized this by creating two new sections, each of which has a section editor: the section on Interstitial Lung Disease in Children edited by Robin Deterding and the Aerodigestive Section edited by Thomas Boat. Every chapter has been extensively updated and revised since the last edition, and there is an increased emphasis on the molecular mechanisms of disease and genetics. To save space we have limited the number of references in the paper version of the book, but the full reference lists are available in the online version.

There are now six editors who have enjoyed the collaboration on identification of authors, review of outlines, working with the individual chapter authors, and editing their work. With this edition we are joined by Robin Deterding of the University of Colorado and Felix Ratjen from the University of Toronto. Our plan is to add two new editors with each edition to establish a rotation that will allow some of us older ones to rotate off in the future. However, as you might have noticed, nobody has rotated off so far! However, we are delighted to recognize Dr. Victor Chernick's many years of contribution to the book with the change in its name.

There are 18 new chapters in this edition and 47 new authors have joined the team. Thirty-two authors have rotated off and we thank them all for their contributions. We particularly want to recognize Dr. Mary Ellen Wohl, who contributed several chapters to multiple editions of the book and who passed away in 2009.

Our goal in editing this book is to publish a comprehensive textbook of pediatric respiratory diseases for a wide audience: the established pediatric pulmonologist and intensivist, fellows in pediatric pulmonology or intensive care, pediatric practitioners, and residents. We also see this book as an important resource for pediatric radiologists, allergists, thoracic and cardiac surgeons, and others in the allied health specialties. We have covered both common and rare childhood diseases of the lungs and the basic science that relates to these conditions to allow for an understanding of pulmonary disease processes and their effect on pulmonary function. Edwin Kendig founded this book, which some say has become the bible of pediatric pulmonology, and we have strived to continue this tradition and this degree of authority and completeness.

The staff at Elsevier, especially Lisa Barnes and Judy Fletcher, have provided outstanding support for our work, and we are grateful for their organization, sound advice, attention to detail, and patience.

Finally, we must thank our families and partners for their patience during the writing of this book, which has been time consuming, and only their tolerance has made the work possible.

Robert W. Wilmott
Thomas F. Boat
Andrew Bush
Victor Chernick
Robin R. Deterding
Felix Ratjen

CONTRIBUTORS

Robin Michael Abel, BSc, MBBS, PhD, FRCS (Eng Paeds)
Consultant Paediatric and Neonatal Surgeon
Hammersmith Hospital, London, United Kingdom

Steven H. Abman, MD
Professor
Department of Pediatrics
University of Colorado School of Medicine
Director
Pediatric Heart Lung Center
Co-Director
Pulmonary Hypertension Program
Children's Hospital Colorado
Aurora, Colorado

Mutasim Abu-Hasan, MD
Associate Professor of Clinical Pediatrics
Pediatric Pulmonology and Allergy Division/
    Pediatrics
University of Florida
Gainesville, Florida

Najma N. Ahmed, MD, MSc, FRCP(C)
Assistant Professor
Department of Pediatrics
McGill University
Pediatric Gastroenterology
Department of Pediatrics
Montreal Children's Hospital
McGill University Health Center
Montreal, Quebec, Canada

Samina Ali, MDCM, FRCP(C), FAAP
Associate Professor
Pediatrics and Emergency Medicine
University of Alberta
Edmonton, Canada

Adrianne Alpern, MS
Graduate Researcher
Department of Psychology
University of Miami
Miami, Florida

Eric F.W.F. Alton, FMedSci
Professor of Gene Therapy and Respiratory Medicine
National Heart and Lung Institute
Imperial College London
Honorary Consultant Physician
Royal Brompton Hospital
London, United Kingdom

Daniel R. Ambruso, MD
Professor
Department of Pediatrics
University of Colorado School of Medicine
Anschutz Medical Campus
Pediatric Hematologist
Center for Cancer and Blood Disorders
Children's Hospital Colorado
Aurora, Colorado
Medical Director
Research and Education
Bonfils Blood Center
Denver, Colorado

M. Innes Asher, BSc, MBChB, FRACP
Paediatrics
Child and Youth Health
The University of Auckland
Auckland, New Zealand

Ian M. Balfour-Lynn, BSc, MD, MBBS, FRCP, FRCPCH, FRCS (Ed), DHMSA
Consultant in Paediatric Respiratory Medicine
Department of Paediatrics
Royal Brompton Hospital
London, United Kingdom

Peter J. Barnes, FRS, FMedSci
Professor
Imperial College London
London, United Kingdom

Robyn J. Barst, MD
Professor of Pediatrics
Department of Pediatric Cardiology
Columbia University College of Physicians
    and Surgeons
Attending Pediatrician
Department of Pediatric Cardiology
Morgan Stanley Children's Hospital of New York
    Presbyterian Medical Center
Director
Pulmonary Hypertension Center
New York Presbyterian Medical Center
New York, New York

Leslie L. Barton, MD
Professor Emerita
Pediatrics
University of Arizona College of Medicine
Tucson, Arizona

Deepika Bhatla, MD
Assistant Professor of Pediatrics
Saint Louis University
Bob Costas Cancer Center
Cardinal Glennon Children's Medical Center
St. Louis, Missouri

R. Paul Boesch, DO, MS
Asisstant Professor of Pediatrics
College of Medicine
University of Cincinnati
Asisstant Professor of Pediatrics
Division of Pulmonary Medicine and Aerodigestive
  and Sleep Center
Cincinnati Children's Hospital Medical Center
Cincinnati, Ohio

Matias Bruzoni, MD
Assistant Professor of Surgery and Pediatrics
Department of Surgery
Stanford University School of Medicine
Stanford, California

Andrew Bush, MD, FRCP, FRCPCH
Professor of Paediatric Respirology
Paediatric Respiratory Medicine
Imperial College and Royal Brompton
  Hospital
London, United Kingdom

Michael R. Bye, MD
Professor of Clinical Pediatrics
Pediatrics
Columbia University College of Physicians and Surgeons
Attending Physician
Pediatric Pulmonary Medicine
Morgan Stanley Children's Hospital of NY
  Presbyterian
New York, New York

Robert G. Castile, MD, MS
Professor of Pediatrics
Center for Perinatal Research
Nationwide Children's Hospital
Columbus, Ohio

Anne B. Chang, MBBS, FRACP, MPHTM, PhD
Professor
Child Health Division
Menzies School of Health Research
Darwin, Australia
Professor of Respiratory Medicine
Queensland Children's Medical Research Institute
Royal Children's Hospital
Brisbane, Australia

Michelle Chatwin, BSc, PhD
Clinical and Academic Department of Sleep
  and Breathing
Royal Brompton Hospital
London, United Kingdom

Chih-Mei Chen, MD
Institute of Epidemiology
Helmholtz Zentrum München
German Research Centre for Environmental Health
Institute of Epidemiology
Neuherberg, Germany

Lyn S. Chitty, PhD, MRCOG
Clinical Meolecular Genetics Unit
Institute of Child Health
Fetal Medicine Unit
University College Hospitals London
NHS Foundation Trust
London, England

Allan L. Coates, MDCM, B Eng (Elect)
Senior Scientist Emeritus
Research Institute
Division of Respiratory Medicine
Department of Pediatrics
The Hospital for Sick Children
Toronto, Ontario, Canada

Misty Colvin, MD
Medical Director
Pediatric and Adult Urgent Care
Northwest Medical Center
Tucson, Arizona

Dan M. Cooper, MD
Professor
Departments of Pediatrics and
  Bioengineering
GCRC Satellite Director
University of California, Irvine
Professor
Department of Pediatrics
UCI Medical Center
Professor
Department of Pediatrics
Children's Hospital of Orange County
Orange, California
Professor
Department of Pediatrics
Miller's Children's Hospital
Long Beach, California

Jonathan Corren, MD
Associate Clinical Professor
University of California, Los Angeles
Los Angeles, California

Robin T. Cotton, MD, FACS, FRCS(C)
Director
Pediatric Otolaryngology-Head and
  Neck Surgery
Cincinnati Children's Hospital
Professor, Otolaryngology
University of Cincinnati College of Medicine
Cincinnati, Ohio

James E. Crowe, Jr., MD
Professor of Pediatrics
Microbiology and Immunology
Vanderbilt University Medical Center
Director
Vanderbilt Vaccine Center
Nashville, Tennessee

Garry R. Cutting, MD
Professor
Institute of Genetic Medicine
Johns Hopkins School of Medicine
Baltimore, Maryland

Jane C. Davies, MB, ChB, MRCP, MRCPCH, MD
Reader in Paediatric Respiratory Medicine
    and Gene Therapy
Imperial College London
Honorary Consultant in Paediatric Respiratory
    Medicine
Royal Brompton Hospital
London, United Kingdom

Gwyneth Davies, MBChB
Clinical Research Fellow
Department of Gene Therapy
National Heart and Lung Institute
Imperial College
London, United Kingdom

Stephanie D. Davis, MD
Associate Professor of Pediatrics
Pediatrics, University of North Carolina at
    Chapel Hill
Chapel Hill, North Carolina

Alessandro de Alarcon, MD
Assistant Professor
Department of Pediatrics
University of Cinncinatti
Director, Center for Pediatric Voice Disorders
Cincinnati Children's Hospital
Cincinnati, Ohio

Marietta M. de Guzman, MD
Assistant Professor
Department of Pediatrics
Section of Rheumatology
Baylor College of Medicine
Pediatric Rheumatologist
Texas Children's Hospital
Houston, Texas

Michael R. DeBaun, MD
Professor of Pediatrics and Medicine
J.C. Peterson Chair in Pediatric Pulmonology
Director
Vanderbilt-Meharry Center for Excellence in Sickle
    Cell Disease
Vanderbilt University School of Medicine
Nashville, Tennessee

Sharon D. Dell, BEng, MD, FRCPC
Clinician Investigator
Division of Respiratory Medicine
Senior Associate Scientist
Child Health Evaluative Sciences
The Hospital for Sick Children
Assistant Professor
Department of Pediatrics
Faculty of Medicine
Unviersity of Toronto
Toronto, Canada

Robin R. Deterding, MD
Professor of Pediatrics
Department of Pediatrics
Director, Breathing Institute
Children's Hospital Colorado
University of Colorado
Aurora, Colorado

Gail H. Deutsch, MD
Associate Director
Seattle Children's Research Hospital Research
    Foundation
Seattle, Washington

Michelle Duggan, MB, MD, FFARCSI
Consultant Anaesthetist
Mayo General Hospital
Castlebar, Ireland

Peter R. Durie, MD, FRCP(C)
Professor
Department of Pediatrics
University of Toronto
Senior Scientist
Research Institute
Gastroenterologist
Department of Pediatrics
The Hospital for Sick Children
Ontario, Canada

Eamon Ellwood, DipTch, DipInfo Tech
Department of Pediatrics
Child and Youth Health
The University of Auckland
Auckland, New Zealand

Leland L. Fan, MD
Professor of Pediatrics
Pediatrics
Children's Hospital Colorado
University of Colorado
Aurora, Colorado

Marie Farmer, MD
Professeure Adjoint
Pédiatrie FMSS
Université de Sherbrooke
Neurologue Pediatre
Pédiatre
CHUS
Sherbrooke, Quebec, Canada

Albert Faro, MD
Associate Professor
Department of Pediatrics
Washington University
Physician Leader 7 East
St. Louis Children's Hospital
St. Louis, Missouri

Thomas W. Ferkol, MD
Professor
Pediatrics, and Cell Biology and Physiology
Washington University
St. Louis, Missouri

David E. Geller, MD
Associate Professor
Pediatrics
University of Central Florida
Director, Aerosol Laboratory and Cystic
    Fibrosis Center
Pediatric Pulmonology
Nemours Children's Clinic
Orlando, Florida

W. Paul Glezen, MD
Professor
Molecular Virology and Microbiology,
    and Pediatrics
Baylor College of Medicine
Houston, Texas

David Gozal, MD
Herbert T. Abelson Professor and Chair
Pediatrics
University of Chicago
Physician in Chief
Comer Children's Hospital
Chicago, Illinois

**Anne Greenough, MD(CANTAB), MBBS, DCH,
FRCP, FRCPCH**
Professor
Division of Asthma, Allergy and Lung Biology
MRC-Asthma UK Centre in Allergic Mechanisms
    of Asthma
London, United Kingdom

James S. Hagood, MD
Professor and Chief
Department of Pediatrics
Division of Respiratory Medicine
University of Californi, San Diego
La Jolla, California

Jürg Hammer, MD
Head
Division of Intensive Care and Pulmonology
Professor
University Children's Hospital Basel
Basel, Switzerland

Jonny Harcourt, FRCS
Consultant ENT Surgeon
Department of Paediatric ENT
Chelsea and Westminster Hospital
Consultant ENT Surgeon
ENT Department
Royal Brompton Hospital
London, United Kingdom

Ulrich Heininger, MD
Professor and Doctor
Division of Pediatric Infectious Diseases
University Children's Hospital
Basel, Switzerland

Marianna M. Henry, MD, MPH
Associate Professor of Pediatrics
Department of Pediatrics
University of North Carolina
Chapel Hill, North Carolina

Peter W. Heymann, MD
Head
Division of Pediatric Allergy
University of Virginia
Charlottesville, Virginia

Alan H. Jobe, MD, PhD
Professor of Pediatrics
University of cincinnati
Cincinnati, Ohio

Richard B. Johnston, Jr., MD
Associate Dean for Research Development
University of Colorado School of Medicine
Professor of Pediatrics
University of Colorado School of Medicine
    and National Jewish Health
Aurora, Colorado

**Sebastian L. Johnston, MBBS, PhD,
FRCP, FSB**
Professor of Respiratory Medicine
National Heart and Lung Institute
Imperial College London
Consultant Physician in Respiratory Medicine
    and Allergy
Imperial College Healthcare NHS Trust
Asthma UK Clinical Professor and Director
MRC and Asthma UK Centre in Allergic
    Mechanisms of Asthma
London, United Kingdom

Michael Kabesch, MD
Professor
Paediatric Pneumology
Allergy and Neonatology
Hannover Medical School
Hannover, Germany

Meyer Kattan, MD
Professor of Pediatrics
Columbia University College of Physicians
    and Surgeons
Director, Pediatric Pulmonary Division
New York Presbyterian-Morgan Stanley Children's
    Hospital
New York, New York

Brian P. Kavanagh, MD, FRCPC
Professor of Anesthesia, Physiology and Medicine
Department of Anesthesia
University of Toronto
Staff Physician
Critical Care Medicine
The Hospital for Sick Children
Toronto, Ontario, Canada

Lisa N. Kelchner, PhD, CCC-SLP, BRS-S
Clinical Research Speech Pathologist
Center for Pediatric Voice Disorders
Cincinnati Children's Hospital Medical Center
Cincinnati, Ohio

James S. Kemp, MD
Professor of Pediatrics
Department of Pediatrics
Washington University School of Medicine
Director of Sleep Laboratory
St. Louis Children's Hospital
St. Louis, Missouri

Andrew Kennedy, MD
Department of Pediatric and Adolescent Medicine
Princess Margaret Hospital
Perth, Australia

Carolyn M. Kercsmar, MD, MS
Director, Asthma Center; Pulmonary Medicine
Cincinnati Childrens Hospital Medical Center
Professor
Pediatrics
University of Cincinnati
Cincinnati, Ohio

Leila Kheirandish-Gozal, MD
Director of Clinical Sleep Research
Section of Pediatric Sleep Medicine
Associate Professor
Pediatrics
University of Chicago
Chicago, Illinois

Cara I. Kimberg, MD
Clinical Psychologist
St. Jude's Children's Research Hospital
Memphis, Tennessee

Paul S. Kingma, MD, PhD
Neonatal Director
Fetal Care Center of Cincinnati
Assistant Professor
University of Cincinnati Department of Pediatrics
Cincinnati Children's Hospital
Cincinnati, Ohio

Terry Paul Klassen, MD, MSc, FRCPC
Director
Alberta Research Center for Health Evidence
Department of Pediatrics
University of Alberta
Edmonton, Canada

Alan P. Knutsen, MD
Director, Pediatric Allergy and Immunology
Saint Louis University
Professor
Pediatrics
Saint Louis University
St. Louis, Missouri

Alik Kornecki, MD
Associate Professor
Pediatrics
University of Western Ontario
Consultant
Pediatric Critical Care
Children's Hospital
London Health Sciences Centre
London, Canada

Thomas M. Krummel, MD
Emile Holman Professor and Chair
Surgery
Stanford University School of Medicine
Susan B. Ford Surgeon-in-Chief
Lucile Packard Children's Hospital
Co-Director
Biodesign Innovation Program
Stanford University
Palo Alto, California

Geoffrey Kurland, MD
Professor
Pediatrics
Children's Hospital of Pittsburgh
Pittsburgh, Pennsylvania

Claire Langston, MD
Professor, Department of Pathology
    and Pediatrics
Baylor College of Medicine
Pathologist
Department of Pathology
Texas Children's Hospital
Houston, Texas

Ada Lee, MD
Attending
Department of Pediatrics
Pediatric Pulmonary Medicine
The Joseph M. Sanzari Children's Hospital
Hackensack University Medical Center
Hackensack, New Jersey

Margaret W. Leigh, MD
Professor and Vice-Chair
Pediatrics
University of North Carolina
Chapel Hill, North Carolina

Daniel J. Lesser, MD
Clinical Assistant Professor of Pediatrics
University of California, San Diego
Pediatric Respiratory Medicine
Rady Children's Hospital
San Diego, California

Sooky Lum, PhD
Portex Unit
Respiratory Physiology and Medicine
UCL, Institute of Child Health
London, United Kingdom

Anna M. Mandalakas, MD, MS
Associate Professor, Pediatrics
Retrovirology and Global Health
Baylor College of Medicine
Texas Children's Hospital
Director of Research, Global Tuberculosis and
    Mycobacteriology Program
Center for Global Health
Houston, Texas

Paulo J.C. Marostica, MD
Pediatric Emergency Section
Pediatric and Puericulture Department
Medical School of Universidade Federal do Rio Grande
    do Sul
Rio Grande do Sul, Brazil

Robert B. Mellins, MD
Professor Emeritus and Special Lecturer
Columbia University
Morgan Stanley Children's Hospital of
    New York
New York, New York

Peter H. Michelson, MD, MS
Associate Professor of Pediatrics
Department of Allergy, Immunology and Pulmonary
    Medicine
Washington University School of Medicine
St. Louis, Missouri

Claire Kane Miller, PhD
Program Director
Aerodigestive and Sleep Center
Cincinnati Children's Hospital
Field Service Assistant Professor
Department of Otolaryngology-Head and Neck
    Surgery
University of Cincinnati, College of Medicine
Clinical Speech Pathologist
Division of Speech Pathology
Cincinnati Children's Hospital
Adjunct Assistant Professor
Communication Sciences and Disorders
University of Cincinnati
Cincinnati, Ohio

Anthony D. Milner, MD, FRCP, DCH
Professor of Neonatology
Department of Pediatrics
United Medical and Dental School of Guy's
    and St. Thomas's Hospital
London, United Kingdom

Ayesha Mirza, MD
Assistant Professor
Infectious Diseases and Immunology
Pediatrics
University of Florida
Jacksonville, Florida

Miriam F. Moffatt, PhD
Professor of Respiratory Genetics
National Heart and Lung Institute
Imperial College
London, United Kingdom

Mark Montgomery, MD, FRCP(C)
Clinical Associate Professor
Department of Pediatrics
University of Calgary
Calgary, Canada

Gavin C. Morrisson, MRCP
Associate Professor
Pediatrics
University of Western Ontario
Consultant
Pediatric Critical Care
Children's Hospital
London Health Sciences Centre
London, Canada

Gary A. Mueller, MD
Department of Pediatrics
Wright State University School of Medicine
Children's Medical Center
Dayton, Ohio

Vadivelam Murthy, MD
Division of Asthma, Allergy, and Lung Biology,
    MRC and Asthma
United Kingdom Centre in Allergic Mechanisms of Asthma
King's College London
London, United Kingdom

Joseph J. Nania, MD
Consultant in Pediatric Infectious Diseases
Phoenix Children's Hospital, Scottsdale Healthcare
    and Banner Health Network
Phoenix, Arizona

**Manjith Narayanan, MD, DNB(Paediatrics),
MRCPCH, PhD**
Clinical Research Fellow
Child Health Division
Depatment of Infection, Immunity, and Inflammation
University of Leicester
Specialist Registrar
Department of Paediatrics
Leicester Royal Infirmary
Leicester, United Kingdom

Dan Nemet, MD, MHA
Professor of Pediatrics
Director, Child Health and Sports Center
Vice Chair of Pediatrics, Meir Medical Center
Sackler School of Medicine Tel Aviv University, Israel
Tel Aviv, Israel

Christopher Newth, MD, FRCPC, FRACP
Professor of Pediatrics
Anesthesiology and Critical Care Medicine
Children's Hospital Los Angeles
University of Southern California
Los Angeles, California

Andrew G. Nicholson, FRCPath, DM
Consultant Histopathologist specialising in thoracic
  pathology
Histopathology
Royal Brompton and Harefield NHS Foundation
  Trust
Professor of Respiratory Pathology
National Heart and Lung Division
Imperial College
London, United Kingdom

Terry L. Noah, MD
Professor
Pediatric Pulmonology
University of North Carolina
Chapel Hill, North Carolina

Lawrence M. Nogee, MD
Professor of Pediatrics
Pediatrics
Johsn Hopkins University School of Medicine
Baltimore, Maryland

Blakeslee Noyes, MD
Professor of Pediatrics
Department of Pediatrics
Saint Louis University School of Medicine
St. Louis, Missouri

Andrew Numa, MB, BS
Director
Intensive Care Unit
Sydney Children's Hospital
Senior Lecturer
Faculty of Medicine
University of New South Wales
Sydney, Australia

Hugh O'Brodovich, MD, FRCP(C)
Arline and Pete Harman Professor and Chairman
Department of Pediatrics
Stanford University
Stanford, California
Adalyn Jay Physician-in-Chief
Lucile Packard Children's Hospital
Palo Alto, California

Matthias Ochs, MD
Professor and Chair
Institute of Functional and Applied Anatomy
Hannover Medical School
Hannover, Germany

Øystein E. Olsen, PhD
Consultant Radiologist
Department of Radiology
Great Ormond Street Hospital for Children
  NHS Trust
London, United Kingdom

Catherine M. Owens, BSC, MBBS, MRCP, FRCR
Reader, Imaging Department
Consultant in Diagnostic Imaging
Cardiothoracic Imaging
University College London
London, United Kingdom

Howard B. Panitch, MD
Professor of Pediatrics
University of Pennsylvania School of Medicine
Director of Clinical Programs
Division of Pulmonary Medicine
The Children's Hospital of Philadelphia
Philadelphia, Pennsylvania

Nikolaos G. Papadopoulos, MD, PhD
Associate Professor
Allergy Department, Second Pediatric Clinic
University of Athens
Greece

Hans Pasterkamp, MD, FRCPC
Professor
Pediatrics and Child Health
University of Manitoba
Adjunct Professor
School of Medical Rehabilitation University
  of Manitoba
Winnipeg, Canada

Donald Payne, MD, FRACP, FRCPCH
Associate Professor
Paediatric and Adolescent Medicine
Princess Margaret Hospital
Associate Professor
School of Paediatrics and Child Health
University of Western Australia
Perth, Australia

Scott Pentiuk, MD, MeD
Assistant Professor of Pediatrics
Division of Gastroenterology, Hepatology,
  and Nutrition
Cincinnati Children's Hospital Medical Center
Cincinnati, Ohio

Thomas A.E. Platts-Mills, MD, PhD
Professor of Medicine
Division Chief
Asthma and Allergic Diseases Center
University of Virginia
Charlottesville, Virginia

Timothy A. Plerhoples, MD
Resident in Surgery
Department of Surgery
Stanford University School of Medicine
Stanford, California

Amy C. Plint, MD, MSc
Pediatrics
University of Ottawa
Emeregncy Medicine
Ottawa, Canada

Jean-Paul Praud, MD, PhD
Professor
Pediatrics
Universitè de Sherbrooke
Sherbrooke, Canada

Phil E. Putnam, MD
Professor
Department of Pediatrics
University of Cincinnati
Director, Endoscopy Services
Cincinnati Children's Hospital Medical Center
Cincinnati, Ohio

Alexandra L. Quittner, PhD
Professor
Psychology
University of Miami
Coral Gables, Florida

Shlomit Radom-Aizik, PhD
Director of Research
Pediatric Exercise Research Center
University of California, Irvine
Irvine School of Medicine
Irvine, California

Mobeen H. Rathore, MD, CPE, FAAP, FIDSA, FACPE
Professor and Associate Chairman
Pediatrics
University of Florida
Chief
Pediatric Infectious Diseases and Immunology
Wolfson Children's Hospital
Chief
General Academic Pediatric
University of Florida
Medical Director
Children's Medical Services
Department of Health
Jacksonville, Florida

Gregory J. Redding, MD
Professor
Pediatrics
University of Washington School of Medicine
Chief
Pulmonary and Sleep Medicine
Seattle Children's Hospital
Seattle, Washington

Erika Berman Rosenzweig, MD
Associate Professor of Clinical Pediatrics (in Medicine)
Pediatric Cardiology
Columbia University
College of Physicians and Surgeons
New York, New York

Marc Rothenberg, MD, PhD
Director
Allergy and Immunology
Cincinnati Children's Hospital Medical Center
Professor of Pediatrics
Allergy and Immunology
University of Cincinnati
Cincinnati, Ohio

Michael J. Rutter, MD
Associate Professor of Clinical Otolaryngology-Affiliated
Department of Otolaryngology
University of Cincinnati College of Medicine
Associate Professor
Pediatric Otolaryngology
Department of Otolaryngology
Cincinnati Children's Hospital Medical Center
Cincinnati, Ohio

Rayfel Schneider, MBBCh, FRCPC
Staff Rheumatologist
Paediatrics
The Hospital for Sick Children
Associate Professor
Paediatrics
University of Toronto
Toronto, Canada

L. Barry Seltz, MD
Assistant Professor of Pediatrics
Department of Pediatrics
Section of Hospital Medicine
University of Colorado School of Medicine
The Children's Hospital
Aurora, Colorado

Hye-Won Shin, PhD
Project Scientist
Department of Pediatrics
Institute for Clinical and Translational Sciences
University of California, Irvine
Irvine, California

Michael Silverman, MD
Emeritus Professor of Child Health
Institute for Lung Health
University of Leicester
Leicester, United Kingdom

Chrysanthi L. Skevaki, MD, PhD
Research Associate
Second Department of Pediatrics
University of Athens
Athens, Greece

Raymond G. Slavin, MD, MS
Professor of Internal Medicine
Saint Louis University School of Medicine
St. Louis, Missouri

Jonathan Spahr, MD
Assistant Professor of Pediatrics
Department of Pediatric Pulmonology
Children's Hospital of Pittsburgh
Pittsburgh, Pennsylvania

James M. Stark, MD, PhD
Associate Professor
Pediatrics
Wright State University
Associate Professor
Pediatrics
Dayton Children's Medical Center
Dayton, Ohio

Jeffrey R. Starke, MD
Professor of Pediatrics
Baylor College of Medicine
Infection Control Officer
Texas Children's Hospital
Chief of Pediatrics
Ben Taub General Hospital
Houston, Texas

Renato T. Stein, MD, MPH, PhD
Head
Pediatric Respirology
Department of Pediatrics
Pontificia Universidade Católica do RGS
Porto Alegre, Brazil

Janet Stocks, PhD, BSc, SRN
Professor
Portex Respiratory Unit
UCL, Institute of Child Health
London, United Kingdom

Dennis C. Stokes, MD, MPH
St. Jude Children's Research Hospital Professor
  of Pediatrics (Pediatric Pulmonology)
Department of Pediatrics
University of Tennessee Health Science Center
Chief, Program in Pediatric Pulmonary Medicine
Department of Pediatrics
Le Bonheur Children's Hospital
Chief, Program in Pediatric Pulmonary Medicine
St. Jude Children's Research Hospital
Memphis, Tennessee

Robert C. Strunk, MD
Strominger Professor of Pediatrics
Department of Pediatrics
Washington University School of Medicine
St. Louis, Missouri

Jennifer M.S. Sucre, MD
Resident
Department of Pediatrics
St. Louis Children's Hospital
Washington University
St. Louis, Missouri

Stuart Sweet, MD, PhD
Associate Professor
Pediatric Allergy, Immunology and Pulmonary Medicine
Washington University
St. Louis, Missouri

James Temprano, MD, MHA
Assistant Professor
Director, Allergy and Immunology
  Training Program
Department of Internal Medicine
Section of Allergy and Immunology
Saint Louis University
St. Louis, Missouri

Bradley T. Thach, MD
Department of Pediatrics
Washington University School of Medicine
Division of Newborn Medicine
St. Louis Children's Hospiital
St. Louis, Missouri

Bruce C. Trapnell, MD, MS
Professor
Internal Medicine University of Cincinnati
Adult Co-Director
Cincinnati Cystic Fibrosis Therapeutics Development
  Network Center
Pulmonary Medicine
Cincinnati Children's Hospital Medical Center
Director, Translational Pulmonary
  Medicine Research
Pulmonary Medicine
Cincinnati Children's Research Foundation
Cincinnati, Ohio

Athanassios Tsakris, MD, PhD, FRCPath
Professor
Department of Microbiology
Medical School, University of Athens
Athens, Greece

Jacob Twiss, BHB, MBChB, PhD, DipPaed, FRACP
Paediatric Respiratory and Sleep Medicine
Starship Children's Health
Auckland, New Zealand

Timothy Vece, MD
Pediatrics
Baylor College of Medicine
Houston, Texas

Ruth Wakeman, BSc (Hons) Physiotherapy, MSc
Advanced Pediatric Practice in Acute Care
Respiratory Practitioner/Physiotherapist
Department of Paediatrics
Royal Brompton and Harefield NHS
    Foundation Trust
London, UK

Colin Wallis, MD, MRCP, FRCPCH, FCP, DCH
Reader
Respiratory Unit
Institue of Child Health, University of London
Doctor
Respiratory Unit
Great Ormond Street Hospital
London, United Kingdom

Miles Weinberger, MD
Professor
Pediatric Allergy and Pulmonary Division
University of Iowa
Iowa City, Iowa

Daniel J. Weiner, MD
Children's Hospital of Pittsburgh of University
    of Pittsburgh Medical Center
Pittsburgh, Pennsylvania

Susan E. Wert, PhD
Associate Professor of Pediatrics
Division of Pulmonary Biology
Section of Neonatology, Perinatal, and Pulmonary
    Biology
Cincinnati Children's Hospital Medical Center
Cincinnati, Ohio

Jeffrey A. Whitsett, MD
Professor of Pediatrics
Pulmonary Biology
Cincinnati Children's Hospital Medical Center and the
    University of Cincinnati College of Medicine
Cincinnati, Ohio

J. Paul Willging, MD
Professor
Otolaryngology-Head and Neck Surgery
University of Cincinnati College of Medicine
Cincinnati Children's Hopsital Medical Center
Cincinnati, Ohio

Saffron A. Willis-Owen, PhD
Molecular Genetics
National Heart and Lung Institute
London, United Kingdom

Robert E. Wood, MD, PhD
Cincinnati Children's Hospital Medical Center
Division of Pulmonary Medicine
Cincinnati, Ohio

Jamie L. Wooldridge, MD
Associate Professor of Pediatric Pulmonology
Saint Louis University School of Medicine
Cardinal Glennon Children's Medical Center
St. Louis, Missouri

Peter F. Wright, MD
Professor of Pediatrics Pathology, Immunology,
    and Microbiology
Department of Pediatrics
Division of Pediatric infectious Diseases
Vanderbilt University School of Medicine
Vanderbilt Children's Hospital
Nashville, Tennessee

Sarah Wright, Grad Dip Phys
Physiotherapist
University of New Castle
New Castle, Australia

Carolyn Young, HDCR
Cardiorespiratory Unit
University College of London
Institute of Child Health
London, United Kingdom

Lisa R. Young, MD
Associate Professor of Pediatrics and Medicine
Department of Pediatrics and Department of Medicine
Vanderbilt University School of Medicine
Associate Professor; Director, Rare Lung Diseases
    Program
Division of Allergy, Immunology, and Pulmonary
    Medicine
Department of Pediatrics
Monroe Carell Jr. Children's Hospital at Vanderbilt
Associate Professor
Division of Allergy, Pulmonary, and Critical Care
    Medicine
Department of Medicine
Vanderbilt University Medical Center
Nashville, Tennessee

Heather J. Zar, MD, PhD
Chair of Department of Paediatrics and Child Health
Director of Paediatric Pulmonology Division
Red Cross War Memorial Childrens Hospital
University of Cape Town
Cape Town, South Africa

Pamela L. Zeitlin, MD, PhD
Professor
Pediatrics
Johns Hopkins School of Medicine
Baltimore, Maryland

CONTENTS

KENDIG AND CHERNICK'S
Disorders OF THE Respiratory Tract IN Children EIGHTH EDITION

General Basic Considerations

1 MOLECULAR DETERMINANTS OF LUNG MORPHOGENESIS

JEFFREY A. WHITSETT, MD, AND SUSAN E. WERT, PHD

■ OVERVIEW

The adult human lung consists of a gas exchange area of approximately $100\,m^2$ that provides oxygen delivery and carbon dioxide excretion required for cellular metabolism. In evolutionary terms, the lung represents a relatively late phylogenetic solution for the need to provide efficient gas exchange for terrestrial survival of organisms of increasing size, an observation that may account for the similarity of lung structure in vertebrates.[reviewed in 1,2] The respiratory system consists of mechanical bellows and conducting tubes that bring inhaled gases to a large gas exchange surface that is highly vascularized. Alveolar epithelial cells come into close apposition to pulmonary capillaries, providing efficient transport of gases from the alveolar space to the pulmonary circulation. The delivery of external gases to pulmonary tissue necessitates a complex organ system that (1) keeps the airway free of pathogens and debris, (2) maintains humidification of alveolar gases and precise hydration of the epithelial cell surface, (3) reduces collapsing forces inherent at air-liquid interfaces within the air spaces of the lung, and (4) supplies and regulates pulmonary blood flow to exchange oxygen and carbon dioxide efficiently. This chapter will provide a framework for understanding the molecular mechanisms that lead to the formation of the mammalian lung, focusing attention to processes contributing to cell proliferation and differentiation involved in organogenesis and postnatal respiratory adaptation. Where possible, the pathogenesis of congenital or postnatal lung disease will be considered in the context of the molecular determinants of pulmonary morphogenesis and function.

■ ORGANOGENESIS OF THE LUNG

Body Plan

Events critical to organogenesis of the lung begin with formation of anteroposterior and dorsoventral axes in the early embryo. The body plan is determined by genes that control cellular proliferation and differentiation and depends on complex interactions among many cell types. The fundamental principles determining embryonic organization have been elucidated in simpler organisms (e.g., *Drosophila melanogaster* and *Caenorhabditis elegans*) and applied to increasingly complex organisms (e.g., mouse and human) as the genes determining axial segmentation, organ formation, cellular proliferation, and differentiation have been identified. Segmentation and organ formation in the embryo are profoundly influenced by sets of master control genes that include various classes of transcription factors. Critical to formation of the axial body plan are the homeotic, or HOX, genes.[reviewed in 3–8] HOX genes are arrayed in clearly defined spatial patterns within clusters on several chromosomes. HOX gene expression in the developing embryo is determined in part by the position of the individual genes within these gene clusters, which are aligned along the chromosome in the same order as they are expressed along the anteroposterior axis. Complex organisms have more individual HOX genes within each locus and have more HOX gene loci than simpler organisms. HOX genes encode nuclear proteins that bind to DNA via a conserved homeodomain motif that modulates the transcription of specific sets of target genes. The temporal and spatial expression of these nuclear transcription factors, in turn, controls the expression of other HOX genes and their transcriptional targets during morphogenesis and cytodifferentiation.[reviewed in 9–14] Expression of HOX genes influences many downstream genes, such as transcription factors, growth factors, signaling peptides, and cell adhesion molecules,[13] that are critical to the formation of the primitive endoderm from which the respiratory epithelium is derived.[15]

Endoderm

The primitive endoderm develops very early in the process of embryogenesis (i.e., during gastrulation and prior to formation of the intraembryonic mesoderm, ectoderm, and notochord—3 weeks postconception in the human).[16] Specification of the definitive endoderm and the primitive foregut requires the activity of a number of nuclear transcription factors that regulate gene expression in the embryo, including (1) forkhead box A2, or FOXA2 (also known as hepatocyte nuclear factor 3-beta, or HNF-3β), (2) GATA-binding protein 6, or GATA6, (3) sex-determining region Y (SRY)-related HMG-box (SOX) 17, or SOX17, (4) SOX2, and (5) β-catenin.[17–24] Genetic ablation of these transcription factors disrupts formation of the primitive foregut endoderm and its developmental derivatives, including the trachea and the lung.[22,24–29] Some of these transcription factors are also expressed in the respiratory epithelium later in development when they play important roles in the regulation of cell differentiation and organ function.[reviewed in 30–34]

Lung Morphogenesis

Lung morphogenesis is initiated during the embryonic period of fetal development (3 to 4 weeks of gestation in the human) with the formation of a small saccular outgrowth of the ventral wall of the foregut endoderm, a process that is induced by expression of the signaling peptide, fibroblast growth factor 10 (FGF10), in the adjacent splanchnic mesoderm (Figure 1-1).[16] This region of the ventral foregut endoderm is delineated by epithelial cells expressing thyroid transcription factor 1, or TTF1 (also known as NKX2.1, T/EBP, or TITF1), which is the earliest known marker of the prospective respiratory epithelium.[35] Thereafter, lung development can be subdivided into five distinct periods of morphogenesis

based on the morphologic characteristics of the tissue (Table 1-1; Figure 1-2). While the timing of this process is highly species-specific, the anatomic events underlying lung morphogenesis are shared by all mammalian species. Details of human lung development are described in the following sections, as well as in several published reviews.[reviewed in 36–42]

The Embryonic Period (3 to 6 Weeks Postconception)

Relatively undifferentiated epithelial cells of the primitive foregut endoderm form tubules that invade the splanchnic mesoderm and undergo branching morphogenesis. This process requires highly controlled cell proliferation and migration of the epithelium to direct dichotomous branching of the respiratory tubules, which forms the main stem, lobar, and segmental bronchi of the primitive lung (see Table 1-1; Figure 1-2). Proximally, the trachea and esophagus also separate into two distinct structures at this time. The respiratory epithelium remains relatively undifferentiated and is lined by columnar epithelium. Experimental removal of mesenchymal tissue from the embryonic endoderm at this time arrests branching morphogenesis, demonstrating the critical role of mesenchyme in formation of the respiratory tract.[reviewed in 43] Interactions between epithelial and mesenchymal cells are mediated by a variety of signaling peptides and their associated receptors (signaling pathways), which regulate gene transcription in differentiating lung cells.[30–34,42,43] These epithelial-mesenchymal interactions involve both autocrine and paracrine signaling pathways that are critical

LUNG BUD FORMATION

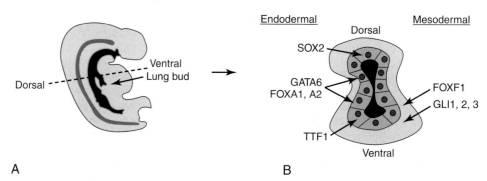

FIGURE 1-1. Lung bud formation. **A,** Lung development is initiated during the embryonic stage of gestation as a small, saccular outgrowth of the ventral foregut endoderm. **B,** Endodermal transcription factors critical for specification of the primitive respiratory tract include GATA6, FOXA1, and FOXA2, which are also expressed throughout the foregut endoderm. At this time, SOX2 expression is limited to the dorsal aspect (future esophagus) of the foregut endoderm, while TTF1 expression is limited to the ventral aspect (future trachea and lung) of the lung bud. Mesodermal transcription factors responsive to signaling peptides (e.g., SHH) released from the endoderm and critical for lung development include Gli1/2/3 and FOXF1. **C,** Expression of the signaling peptide, fibroblast growth factor 10 (FGF10), in the adjacent splanchnic mesoderm, induces outgrowth of the lung bud. FGF10 is secreted by mesenchymal cells and binds to its receptor, FGFR2, located on the endodermal cell surface, inducing formation of the lung bud.

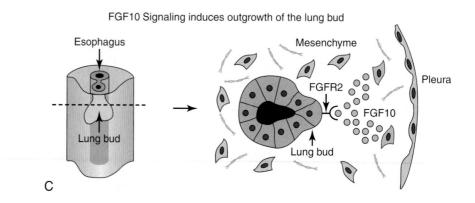

TABLE 1-1 MORPHOGENETIC PERIODS OF HUMAN LUNG DEVELOPMENT

PERIOD	AGE (WEEKS)	STRUCTURAL EVENTS
Embryonic	3 to 6	Lung buds; trachea, main stem, lobar, and segmental bronchi; trachea and esophagus separate
Pseudoglandular	6 to 16	Subsegmental bronchi, terminal bronchioles, and acinar tubules; mucous glands, cartilage, and smooth muscle
Canalicular	16 to 26	Respiratory bronchioles, acinus formation, and vascularization; type I and II cell differentiation
Saccular	26 to 36	Dilation and subdivision of alveolar saccules, increase of gas-exchange surface area, and surfactant synthesis
Alveolar	36 to maturity	Further growth and alveolarization of lung; increase of gas-exchange area and maturation of alveolar capillary network; increased surfactant synthesis

for lung morphogenesis (Figure 1-3). Paracrine signaling pathways that are important for initial formation of the lung bud and the expansion and branching of the primitive respiratory tubules include: (1) fibroblast growth factor (FGF10/FGFR2), (2) sonic hedgehog (SHH/PTCH1), (3) transforming growth factor-beta (TGFβ/TGFβR2), (4) bone morphogenetic protein B (BMP4/BMPR1b), (5) retinoic acid (RA/RARα, β, γ), (6) WNT (WNT2/2b, 7b, 5a and R-spondin with their receptors Frizzled and LRP5/6), and (7) the β-catenin signaling pathways.[30–34,42–45] Nuclear transcription factors active in the primitive respiratory epithelium during this period include: TTF1, FOXA2, GATA6, and SOX2. Likewise, nuclear transcription factors active in the mesenchyme at this time include: (1) the HOX family of transcription factors (HOXA5, B3, B4); (2) the SMAD family of transcription factors (SMAD2, 3, 4) that are downstream transducers of the TGFβ/BMP signaling pathway; (3) the LEF/TCF family of transcription factors, downstream transducers of β-catenin; (4) the GLI-KRUPPEL family of transcription factors (GLI1, 2, 3), downstream transducers of SHH signaling; (5) the hedgehog-interacting protein, HHIP1, that binds SHH; and (6) FOXF1, another SHH target.[30–34,40,43,44,47] Disruption of many of these transcription factors and signaling pathways in experimental animals causes impaired morphogenesis, resulting in laryngotracheal

MAJOR STAGES OF LUNG DEVELOPMENT

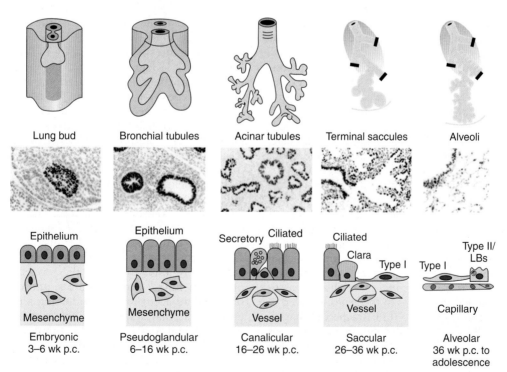

FIGURE 1-2. Major stages of lung development. The bronchi, bronchioles, and acinar tubules are formed by the process of branching morphogenesis during the pseudoglandular stage of lung development (6 to 16 weeks p.c.). Formation of the capillary bed and dilation/expansion of the acinar structures is initiated during the canalicular stage of lung development (16 to 26 weeks p.c.). Growth and subdivision of the terminal saccules and alveoli continue until early adolescence by septation of the distal respiratory structures to form additional alveoli. Cytodifferentiation of mature bronchial epithelial cells (secretory and ciliated cells) is initiated in the proximal conducting airways during the canalicular stage of lung development, while cytodifferentiation in the distal airways (ciliated and Clara cells) and alveoli (Type I and Type II cells) takes place later during the saccular (26 to 36 weeks p.c.) and alveolar (36 weeks p.c. to adolescence) stages of lung development. The alveolar stage of lung development extends into the postnatal period, during which millions of additional alveoli are formed and maturation of the microvasculature, or air-blood barrier, takes place, greatly increasing the surface area available for gas exchange.

RECIPROCAL SIGNALING IN LUNG MORPHOGENESIS

Paracrine signaling pathways

EPITHELIUM		MESENCHYME
SHH	$\longrightarrow$	PTCH1/GLI 1, 2, 3
FZ/β-catenin	$\longleftarrow$	WNT
FGFR2	$\longleftarrow$	FGF10
FGFR2	$\longleftarrow$	FGF7
FGF9	$\longrightarrow$	FGFR1
BMP4	$\longrightarrow$	BMPR1b
BMPR1a/b	$\longleftarrow$	BMP4/5
TGFβ2	$\longrightarrow$	TGFβR2
VEGF	$\longrightarrow$	VEGFR
PDGF	$\longrightarrow$	PDGFR

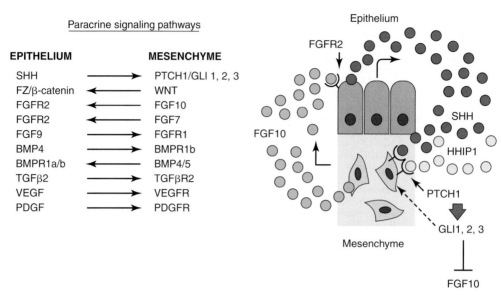

FIGURE 1-3. Reciprocal signaling in lung morphogenesis. Paracrine and autocrine interactions between the respiratory epithelium and the adjacent mesenchyme are mediated by signaling peptides and their respective receptors, influencing cellular behaviors (e.g., proliferation, migration, apoptosis, extracellular matrix deposition) that are critical to lung formation. For example, FGF10 is secreted by mesenchymal cells and binds to its receptor, FGFR10, on the surface of epithelial cells (paracrine signaling). SHH is secreted by epithelial cells and binds to its receptor, PTCH1, on mesenchymal cells (paracrine signaling), while HHIP1 is upregulated by SHH in mesenchymal cells, secreted, and binds back to receptors on cells in the mesenchyme (autocrine signaling). Binding of SHH to mesenchymal cells activates the transcription factors, GLI1, GLI2, and GLI3, which, in turn, inhibit FGF10 expression (negative feedback loop). In contrast, the binding of HHIP1 to mesenchymal cells attenuates or limits the ability of SHH to inhibit FGF10 signaling. Together, these complex, interacting, signaling pathways control branching morphogenesis of the lung, differentially influencing bronchial tubule elongation, arrest, and subdivision into new tubules.

malformations, tracheoesophageal fistulae, esophageal and tracheal stenosis, esophageal atresia, defects in pulmonary lobe formation, pulmonary hypoplasia, and/or pulmonary agenesis.[30–34,40,43–45]

Although formation of the larger, more proximal, conducting airways, including segmental and subsegmental bronchi, is completed by the 6th week postconception (p.c.), both epithelial and mesenchymal cells of the embryonic lung remain relatively undifferentiated. At this stage, trachea and bronchial tubules lack underlying cartilage, smooth muscle, or nerves, and the pulmonary and bronchial vessels are not well developed. Vascular connections with the right and left atria are established at the end of this period (6 to 7 weeks p.c.), creating the primitive pulmonary vascular bed.[39] Human developmental anomalies occurring during this period of morphogenesis include laryngeal, tracheal, and esophageal atresia, tracheoesophageal fistulae, tracheal and bronchial stenosis, tracheal and bronchial malacia, ectopic lobes, bronchogenic cysts, and pulmonary agenesis.[40,46] Some of these congenital anomalies are associated with documented mutations in the genes involved in early lung development, such as GLI3 (tracheoesophageal fistula found in Pallister-Hall syndrome), FGFR2 (various laryngeal, esophageal, tracheal, and pulmonary anomalies found in Pfeiffer, Apert, or Crouzon syndromes), and SOX2 (esophageal atresia and tracheoesophageal fistula found in anophthalmia-esophageal-genital, or AEG, syndrome).[40,46]

Pseudoglandular Period (6 to 16 Weeks' Postconception)
The pseudoglandular stage is so named because of the distinct glandular appearance of the lung from 6 to 16 weeks of gestation. During this period, the lung consists primarily of epithelial tubules surrounded by a relatively thick mesenchyme. Branching of the airways continues, and formation of the terminal bronchioles and primitive acinar structures is completed by the end of this period (see Table 1-1; Figure 1-2). During the pseudoglandular period, epithelial cell differentiation is increasingly apparent and deposition of cellular glycogen and expression of a number of genes expressed selectively in the distal respiratory epithelium is initiated. The surfactant proteins (SP), SP-B and SP-C, are first detected at 12 to 14 weeks of gestation.[48,49] Tracheobronchial glands begin to form in the proximal conducting airways; and the airway epithelium is increasingly complex, with basal, mucous, ciliated, and nonciliated secretory cells being detected.[36,38] Neuroepithelial cells, often forming clusters of cells, termed *neuroepithelial bodies* and expressing a variety of neuropeptides and transmitters (e.g., bombesin, calcitonin-related peptide, serotonin, and others), are increasingly apparent along the bronchial and bronchiolar epithelium.[50] Smooth muscle and cartilage are now observed adjacent to the conducting airways.[51] The pulmonary vascular system develops in close relationship to the bronchial and bronchiolar tubules between the 9th and 12th weeks of gestation. Bronchial arteries arise from the aorta and form along the epithelial tubules, and smooth muscle actin and myosin can be detected in the vascular structures.[39]

During this period, FGF10, BMP4, TGFβ, β-catenin, and the WNT signaling pathway continue to be important for branching morphogenesis, along with several other signaling peptides and growth factors, including: (1) members of the FGF family (FGF1, FGF2, FGF7,

FGF9, FGF18); (2) members of the TGFβ family, such as the SPROUTYs (SPRY2, SPRY4), which antagonize and limit FGF10 signaling, and LEFTY/NODAL, which regulate left-right patterning; (3) epithelial growth factor (EGF) and transforming growth factor alpha (TGFα), which stimulate cell proliferation and cytodifferentiation; (4) insulin-like growth factors (IGFI, IGFII), which facilitate signaling of other growth factors; (5) platelet-derived growth factors (PDGFA, PDGFB), which are mitogens and chemoattractants for mesenchymal cells; and (6) vascular endothelial growth factors (VEGFA, VEGFC), which regulate vascular and lymphatic growth and patterning.[30-34,40,42,43] Many of the nuclear transcription factors that were active during the embryonic period of morphogenesis continue to be important for lung development during the pseudoglandular period. Additional transcription factors important for specification and differentiation of the primitive lymphatics in the mesenchyme at this time include: (1) SOX18, (2) the paired-related homeobox gene, PRX1, (3) the divergent homeobox gene, HEX, and (4) the homeobox gene, PROX1.[40,42]

A variety of congenital defects may arise during the pseudoglandular stage of lung development, including bronchopulmonary sequestration, cystic adenomatoid malformations, cyst formation, acinar aplasia or dysplasia, alveolar capillary dysplasia with or without misalignment of the pulmonary veins, and congenital pulmonary lymphangiectasia.[40] The pleuroperitoneal cavity also closes early in the pseudoglandular period. Failure to close the pleural cavity, often accompanied by herniation of the abdominal contents into the chest (congenital diaphragmatic hernia), leads to pulmonary hypoplasia.

Canalicular Period (16 to 26 Weeks Postconception)

The canalicular period is characterized by formation of acinar structures in the distal tubules, luminal expansion of the tubules, thinning of the mesenchyme, and formation of the capillary bed, which comes into close apposition to the dilating acinar tubules (see Table 1-1; Figure 1-2). By the end of this period, the terminal bronchioles have divided to form two or more respiratory bronchioles, and each of these have divided into multiple acinar tubules, forming the primitive alveolar ducts and pulmonary acini. Epithelial cell differentiation becomes increasingly complex and is especially apparent in the distal regions of the lung parenchyma. Bronchiolar cells express differentiated features, such as cilia, and secretory cells synthesize Clara cell secretory protein, or CCSP (also known as CC10 or segretoglobin 1A1, SCGB1A1).[49,52-54] Cells lining the distal tubules assume cuboidal shapes and express increasing amounts of surfactant phospholipids[55] and the associated surfactant proteins, SP-A, SP-B, and SP-C.[48,49,56-60] Lamellar bodies, composed of surfactant phospholipids and proteins, are seen in association with rich glycogen stores in the cuboidal pre–type II cells lining the distal acinar tubules.[61-64] Some cells of the acinar tubules become squamous, acquiring features of typical type I alveolar epithelial cells. Thinning of the pulmonary mesenchyme continues; and the basal lamina of the epithelium and mesenchyme fuse. Capillaries surround the distal acinar tubules, which together will ultimately form the gas exchange region of the lung. By the end of the canalicular period in the human infant (26 to 28 weeks p.c.), gas exchange can be supported after birth, especially when surfactant is provided by administration of exogenous surfactants. Surfactant synthesis and mesenchymal thinning can be accelerated by glucocorticoids at this time,[60,65-67] which are administered to mothers to prevent respiratory distress syndrome (RDS) after premature birth.[68,69] Abnormalities of lung development occurring during the canalicular period include acinar dysplasia, alveolar capillary dysplasia, and pulmonary hypoplasia, the latter caused by (1) diaphragmatic hernia, (2) compression due to thoracic or abdominal masses, (3) prolonged rupture of membranes causing oligohydramnios, or (5) renal agenesis, in which amniotic fluid production is impaired. While postnatal gas exchange can be supported late in the canalicular stage, infants born during this period generally suffer severe complications related to decreased pulmonary surfactant, which causes RDS and bronchopulmonary dysplasia, the latter a complication secondary to the therapy for RDS.[70,71]

Saccular (26 to 36 Weeks' Postconception) and Alveolar Periods (36 Weeks' Postconception through Adolescence)

These periods of lung development are characterized by increased thinning of the respiratory epithelium and pulmonary mesenchyme, further growth of lung acini, and development of the distal capillary network (see Table 1-1; Figure 1-2). In the periphery of the acinus, maturation of type II epithelial cells occurs in association with increasing numbers of lamellar bodies, as well as increased synthesis of surfactant phospholipids,[55,61] the surfactant proteins, SP-A, SP-B, SP-C, and SP-D,[48,49,56-60,72] and the ATP-binding cassette transporter, ABCA3, a phospholipid transporter important for lamellar body biogenesis.[73] The acinar regions of the lung increase in surface area, and proliferation of type II cells continues. Type I cells, derived from differentiation of type II epithelial cells, line an ever-increasing proportion of the surface area of the distal lung. Capillaries become closely associated with the squamous type I cells, decreasing the diffusion distance for oxygen and carbon dioxide between the alveolar space and pulmonary capillaries. Basal laminae of the epithelium and stroma fuse; the stroma contains increasing amounts of extracellular matrix, including elastin and collagen; and the abundance of smooth muscle in the pulmonary vasculature increases prior to birth.[37] In the human lung, the alveolar period begins near the time of birth and continues through the first decade of life, during which the lung grows primarily by septation and proliferation of the alveoli,[74] and by elongation and luminal enlargement of the conducting airways. Pulmonary arteries enlarge and elongate in close relationship to the increased growth of the lung.[37] Pulmonary vascular resistance decreases, and considerable remodeling of the pulmonary vasculature and capillary bed continues during the postnatal period.[37] Lung growth remains active until early adolescence, when the entire complement of approximately 300 million alveoli has been formed.[74]

Signaling pathways that are critical for growth, differentiation, and maturation of the alveolar epithelium and capillary bed during these periods include the FGF, PDGF,

VEGF, RA, BMP, WNT, β-catenin, and NOTCH signaling pathways.[30-34,42,43] For example, FGF signaling is critical for alveologenesis during these periods. Targeted deletion of the FGF receptors, *Fgfr3* and *Fgfr4,* blocks alveologenesis in mice. Likewise, targeted deletion of *Pdgfa,* another growth factor critical for alveologenesis, interferes with myofibroblast proliferation and migration, resulting in complete failure of alveologenesis and postnatal alveolar simplification in mice.[30-34,42,43]

Nuclear transcription factors found earlier in lung development (i.e., FOXA2, TTF1, GATA6, and SOX2) continue to be important for maturation of the lung, influencing sacculation, alveolarization, vascularization, and cytodifferentiation of the peripheral lung. Transcription factors associated with cytodifferentiation during these periods include: (1) FOXJ1 (ciliated cells), (2) MASH1 (or HASH1) and HES1 (neuroendocrine cells), (3) FOXA3 and SPDEF (mucus cells), and (4) ETV5/ERM (alveolar type II cells).[32] Morphogenesis and cytodifferentiation are further influenced by additional transcription factors expressed in the developing respiratory epithelium at this time, including: (1) several ETS factors (ETV5/ERM, SPDEF, ELF3/5); (2) SOX genes (SOX-9, SOX11, SOX17); (3) nuclear factor of activated T cells/calcineurin-dependent 3, or NFATC3; (4) nuclear factor-1, or NF-1; (5) CCAAT/enhancer binding protein alpha, or CEBPα; and (6) Krüppel-like factor 5, or KLF5; as well as the transcription factors, GLI2/GLI3, SMAD3, FOXF1, POD1, and HOX (HOXA5, HOXB2 to B5), all of which are expressed in the mesenchyme.[30-34]

Control of Gene Transcription During Lung Morphogenesis
Numerous regulatory mechanisms influence cell commitment, proliferation, and terminal differentiation required for formation of the mammalian lung. These events must be precisely controlled in all organs to produce the complex body plan characteristic of higher organisms. In the mature lung, approximately 40 distinct cell types can be distinguished on the basis of morphologic and biochemical criteria.[75] Distinct pulmonary cell types arise primarily from subsets of endodermal and mesodermal progenitor cells. Pluripotent or multipotent cells receive precise temporal and spatial signals that commit them to differentiated pathways, which ultimately generate the heterogeneous cell types present in the mature organ. The information directing cell proliferation and differentiation during organogenesis is derived from the genetic code contained within the DNA of each cell in the organism. Unique subsets of messenger RNAs (mRNAs) are transcribed from DNA and direct the synthesis of a variety of proteins in specific cells, ultimately determining cell proliferation, differentiation, structure, function, and behavior for each cell type. Unique features of differentiating cells are controlled by the relative abundance of these mRNAs, which, in turn, determine the relative abundance of proteins synthesized by each cell. Cellular proteins influence morphologic, metabolic, and proliferative behaviors of cells, characteristics that traditionally have been used to assign cell phenotype by using morphologic and cytologic criteria. Gene expression in each cell is also determined by the structure of DNA-protein complexes that comprise the chromatin within the nucleus of each cell. Chromatin structure, in turn, influences the accessibility of individual genes to the transcriptional machinery. Diverse extracellular and intracellular signals also influence gene transcription, mRNA processing, mRNA stability and translation—processes that determine the relative abundance of proteins produced by each cell.

Only a small fraction of the genetic material present in the nucleus represents regions of DNA that direct the synthesis of mRNAs encoding proteins. There is an increasing awareness that sequences in the noncoding regions of genes influence DNA structure and contain promoter and enhancer elements (usually in flanking and intronic regions of each gene) that determine levels of transcription.[76] Nucleotide sequencing and identification of expressed complementary DNA (cDNA) sequences encoded within the human genome have provided insight into the amount of the genetic code used to synthesize the cellular proteins produced by each organ.[77] At present, nearly all of the expressed cDNAs have been identified and partially sequenced for most human organs. Analysis of these mRNAs reveals distinct, and often unique, subsets of genes that are expressed in each organ, as well as the relative abundance and types of proteins encoded by these mRNAs. Of interest, proteins bearing signaling and transcriptional regulatory information are among the most abundant of various classes of proteins in human cells. Organ complexity in higher organisms is derived, at least in part, by the increasingly complex array of signaling molecules that govern cell behavior. Regulatory mechanisms controlling transcription are listed in Figure 1-4.

Transcriptional Cascades/Hierarchies
Gene transcription is modulated primarily by the binding of transcription factors (or trans-acting factors) to DNA. Transcription factors are nuclear proteins that bind to regulatory motifs consisting of ordered nucleotides, or specific nucleotide sequences. The order of these specific nucleotide sequences determines recognition sites within the DNA (*cis*-acting elements) that are bound by these nuclear proteins. The binding of transcription factors to these *cis*-acting elements influences the activity of RNA polymerase II, which binds to sequences near the transcription start site of target genes, initiating mRNA synthesis.[76,78] Numerous families of transcription factors have been identified, and their activities are regulated by a variety of mechanisms, including posttranslational modification and interactions with other proteins or DNA, as well as by their ability to translocate or remain in the nucleus.[78] Transcription factors also activate the transcription of other downstream nuclear factors, which, in turn, influence the expression of additional trans-acting factors. The number and cell specificity of transcription factors have proven to be large and are represented by diverse families of proteins categorized on the basis of the structural motifs of their DNA binding or trans-activating domains.[76,78] These interacting cascades of factors comprise a network with vast capabilities to influence target gene expression. The HOX family of transcription factors (homeodomain,

CONTROL OF GENE EXPRESSION

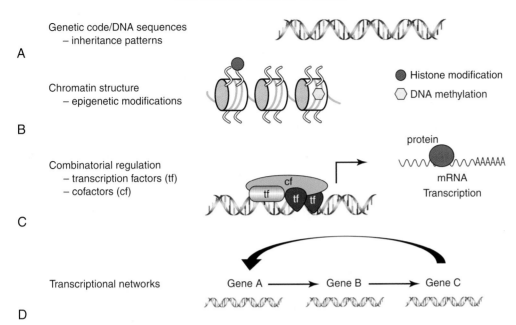

A

Genetic code/DNA sequences
– inheritance patterns

Chromatin structure
– epigenetic modifications

B

● Histone modification
⬡ DNA methylation

Combinatorial regulation
– transcription factors (tf)
– cofactors (cf)

C

protein

mRNA
Transcription

Transcriptional networks

Gene A ⟶ Gene B ⟶ Gene C

D

FIGURE 1-4. Control of gene expression. Diverse cellular mechanisms regulate varying levels of gene transcription that, in turn, control messenger RNA and protein synthesis governing cell differentiation and function during lung development. Inherited patterns of each individual's genetic code (**A**) are modified by epigenetic mechanisms that modify chromatin structure through methylation of DNA and/or modification of histone proteins (**B**). Binding of nuclear transcription factors to specific structural motifs (*cis*-acting elements) in DNA sequences is modified by associated cofactors and other transcription factors (**C**). Protein expression is often controlled by transcriptional networks, in which several genes are activated in series to induce or inhibit expression of downstream targets and/or other proteins (**D**).

helix-turn-helix-containing family of DNA-binding proteins) represents an example of such a regulatory motif. A series of HOX genes are located in arrays containing large numbers of distinct genes arranged 3' to 5' in distinct loci within human chromosomes.[7] HOX genes bind to and activate other downstream HOX gene family members that, in turn, bind to and activate the transcription of additional related and unrelated transcription factors, altering their activity and interactions at the transcriptional level.[10] Such cascades are now well characterized in organisms such as in *D. melanogaster*[74] and *C. elegans*.[79–81] Mammalian homologues exist for many of these genes, and their involvement in similar regulatory cascades influences gene expression and organogenesis in more complex organisms.[3–15] In the mammalian lung, TTF1 and FOX family members are involved in regulatory cascades that determine organogenesis and lung epithelial–specific gene expression. In addition, many other nuclear transcription factors, such as β-catenin, GATA6, POD1, FOXA2, NF1, FOXF1, GLI family members, ETS factors, N-MYC, CEBP family members, retinoic acid receptors (RAR), estrogen receptors, and glucocorticoid receptors, influence lung growth, cytodifferentiation, and function.[30–34]

Combinatorial Regulation of Gene Transcription and Expression

Advances in understanding mRNA expression profiles, genomics, chromatin structure, and mechanisms regulating gene expression are transforming current concepts regarding the molecular processes that control gene expression. Bioinformatics and advances in computational and systems biology are providing new insights into the remarkable interactions among genes that control other cellular processes. To influence gene expression, genes function in complex networks, which are dependent on each individual's inherited DNA sequences (genes) and on epigenetic mecha-

nisms independent of genetic constitution. Changes in chromatin structure (packaging of DNA, histones, and other associated proteins) influence the accessibility of DNA to the regulatory actions of various transcriptional complexes (proteins) and is dependent upon posttranslational modification of histone proteins by methylation or acetylation. The regulatory regions of target genes in eukaryotes are highly complex, containing numerous *cis*-acting elements that bind various nuclear transcription proteins to influence gene expression. Nuclear proteins may bind DNA as monomers or oligomers, or form homo- or hetero-oligomers with other transcriptional proteins. Furthermore, many transcriptional proteins are modified by posttranslational modifications that are induced by receptor occupancy or by phosphorylation and/or dephosphorylation events. Binding of transcription factors influences the structural organization of DNA (chromatin), making regulatory sites more or less accessible to other nuclear proteins, which, in turn, positively or negatively regulate gene expression. Numerous *cis*-acting elements and their cognate *trans*-acting proteins interact with the basal transcriptional apparatus to regulate mRNA synthesis. The precise stoichiometry and specificity of the occupancy of various DNA-binding sites also influence the transcription of specific target genes, either positively or negatively. This mode of regulation is characteristic of most eukaryotic cells, including those of the lung. For example, in pulmonary epithelial cells, a distinct set of transcription factors, including TTF1, GATA6, activator protein 1 (AP1), FOX family members, RARs, STAT3, NF1, and specificity protein 1 (SP1), act together to regulate expression of surfactant protein genes, which influence postnatal respiratory adaptation.[32,82–84]

Influence of Chromatin Structure on Gene Expression

The structure of chromatin is a critical determinant of the ability of target genes to respond to regulatory information influencing gene transcription. The abundance and organization of histones and other chromatin-associated proteins, including nuclear transcriptional proteins, influence the structure of DNA at genetic loci. The accessibility of regulatory regions within genes or groups of genes for binding and regulation by transcription factors is often dependent on chromatin structure. Changes in chromatin structure are likely determined by the process of cell differentiation during which target genes become available or unavailable to the regulatory influences of transcription factors.[85] Thus, the activity of a transcription factor at one time in development may be entirely distinct from that at another time. Chemical modification of DNA (e.g., methylation of cytosine) is also known to modify the ability of *cis*-active elements to bind and respond to regulatory influences. For example, cytosine-guanine (CG)–rich islands are found in transcriptionally active genes, and methylation of these regions may vary developmentally or in response to signals that influence gene transcription. Chromatin structure, in turn, is influenced by post-transcriptional modification of histones and other DNA-associated proteins by biochemical processes, including acetylation, methylation, demethylation, phosphorylation, ubiquitination, sumoylation, and ADP-ribosylation, which then influence the binding of transcriptional complexes and coactivator proteins that interact with the basal transcriptional machinery via polymerase II to alter gene transcription.[86]

Non-Transcriptional Mechanisms

While regulation of gene transcription is an important factor in organogenesis, numerous regulatory mechanisms, including control of RNA expression, mRNA stability, and protein synthesis and degradation are also known to provide further refinement in the abundance of mRNAs and proteins synthesized by a specific cell, which ultimately determine its structure and function.[87] For example, microRNAs (miRNAs) have been implicated recently in the regulation of proliferation, differentiation, and apoptosis of epithelial progenitor cells in the lung.[86] miRNAs are small (19 to 25 nucleotides), single-stranded, non-coding RNAs that regulate protein expression by binding to the 3' untranslated region of target mRNAs, which results in degradation or inhibition of protein translation in the cytoplasm. mi/RNAs are transcribed initially as very long primary transcripts (pri-miRNAs) that contain hundreds to thousands of nucleotides. This primary transcript is cleaved to release a much smaller 70 to 100 nucleotide fragment (pre-miRNA), which is then exported to the cytoplasm. Once in the cytoplasm, this fragment is further cleaved by an RNA polymerase II (DICER) to release a 19- to 25- nucleotide fragment, which is then incorporated into an miRNA-induced silencing complex (miRISC) that guides the miRNA to its target mRNA, where it binds to the mRNA affecting its translation and/or stability.[88] High expression levels of at least three members of the miR-17-92 cluster are present in the embryonic lung, but decline as lung development progresses.[89] Mice deficient in the miR-17-92 cluster exhibited hypoplasia of the lung,[90] while targeted deletion of DICER in the lung resulted in abnormal lung development with increased apoptosis and abnormal branching morphogenesis.[91] Overexpression of the miR-17-92 cluster during lung development resulted in the absence of normal terminal (alveolar) saccules, which were replaced with respiratory tubules lined by highly proliferative, undifferentiated epithelium, suggesting that downregulation of the miR-17-92 cluster is critical for normal cellular growth and differentiation.[92]

Receptor-Mediated Signal Transduction

Receptor-mediated signaling is well recognized as a fundamental mechanism for transducing extracellular information. Such signals are initiated by the occupancy of membrane-associated receptors capable of initiating additional signals (known as secondary messengers), such as cyclic adenosine monophosphate, calcium, and inositide phosphates, which influence the activity and function of intracellular proteins (e.g., kinases, phosphatases, proteases). These proteins, in turn, may alter the abundance of transcription factors, the activity of ion channels, or changes in membrane permeability, which subsequently modify cellular behaviors. Receptor-mediated signal transduction, induced by ligand-receptor binding, mediates endocrine, paracrine, and autocrine interactions on which cell differentiation and organogenesis depend. For example, signaling peptides and their receptors, such as FGF, SHH, WNT, BMP, VEGF, PDGF, and NOTCH have been implicated in organogenesis of many organs, including the lung.[30–34,42,43]

Gradients of Signaling Molecules and Localization of Receptor Molecules

Chemical gradients within tissues, and their interactions with membrane receptors located at distinct sites within the organ, can provide critical information during organogenesis. Polarized cells have basal, lateral, and apical surfaces with distinct subsets of signaling molecules (receptors) that allow the cell to respond in unique ways to focal concentrations of regulatory molecules. Secreted ligands (e.g., FGFs, TGFβ/BMPs, WNTs, SHH, and HHIP1) function in gradients that are further influenced by binding of the ligand to basement membranes or proteoglycans in the extracellular matrix.[30,33,34,43] Spatial information is established by gradients of these signaling molecules and by the presence and abundance of receptors at specific cellular sites. Such systems provide positional information to the cell, which influences its behavior (e.g., shape, movement, proliferation, differentiation, and polarized transport).

Transcriptional Mechanisms Controlling Gene Expression During Pulmonary Development

While knowledge of the determinants of gene regulation in lung development is rudimentary at present, a number of transcription factors and signaling networks that play critical roles in lung morphogenesis have been identified.[30–34,42,43] Lung morphogenesis depends on formation of definitive endoderm, which, in turn, receives signals from the splanchnic mesenchyme to initiate organogenesis along the foregut, forming thyroid, liver, pancreas, lung, and portions of the gastrointestinal tract.[17] The ventral plate of the endoderm in mammals forms under the direction of FOXA2, a transcription factor that is known to play a critical role in committing progenitor cells of the endoderm to form the primitive foregut.[17] FOXA2 is member of a large family of nuclear transcription factors, termed the *winged helix* family of transcription factors, that are involved in cell commitment, differentiation, and gene transcription in a variety of organs, such as the central nervous system and derivatives of the foregut endoderm, including the gastrointestinal tract, lung, and liver.[93] FOXA2 is required for the formation of foregut endoderm, from which the lung bud is derived, and plays a critical role in organogenesis of the lung. While FOXA2 plays a critical role in formation and commitment of progenitor cells to form the foregut endoderm, FOXA2 also influences the expression of specific genes in the respiratory epithelium later in development.[94–100] Conditional deletion of *Foxa2* after birth caused goblet cell metaplasia, airspace enlargement, and inflammation during the postnatal period,[101] while deletion of *Foxa2* prior to birth resulted in delayed pulmonary maturation, associated with decreased surfactant lipid and protein expression and the development of a respiratory distress-like syndrome.[100] Thus, FOXA2 plays a critical role in specification of foregut endoderm in the early embryo, and is used again in the perinatal and postnatal period to direct surfactant production, alveolarization, postnatal lung function, and homeostasis (Figure 1-5).

TTF1 (TITF1) is a 38-kd nuclear protein, containing a homeodomain DNA-binding motif, that is critical for formation of the lung and for regulation of a number of highly specific gene products produced only in the respiratory epithelium.[84,102,103] TTF1 is also expressed in the thyroid and in specific regions of the developing central nervous system.[35,102] In the lung, TTF1 is expressed in the respiratory epithelium of the primitive lung bud

(see Figure 1-2).[35,102,103] Ablation of *Titf1* in the mouse impaired lung morphogenesis, resulting in tracheoesophageal fistula and hypoplastic lungs lined by a poorly differentiated respiratory epithelium and lacking the distal, alveolar, gas exchange regions.[102,103,106,107] Substitution of a mutant *Titf1* gene, which lacked phosphorylation sites, restored lung development in the *Titf1* knockout mouse.[108] Expression of a number of genes, including those regulating surfactant homeostasis, fluid and electrolyte transport, host defense, and vasculogenesis, is regulated by TTF1 phosphorylation prior to birth. TTF1 regulates the expression of a number of genes in a highly specific manner in the respiratory epithelium, including surfactant proteins, SP-A, SP-B, and SP-C, and CCSP.[109–112] TTF1 functions in concert with other transcription factors, including FOXA2, GATA6, NF1, ERM, PARP2, SP1/SP3, TAZ, NFAT, and RARs to regulate lung-specific gene transcription.[32,113–123] TTF1 gene transcription itself is modulated by the activity of FOXA2, which binds to the promoter enhancer region of the TTF1 gene, thus creating a transcriptional network.[99] A combinatorial mode of regulation is evidenced by the apposition of clustered TTF1 *cis*-active elements and FOXA2 binding sites in target genes, such as the SP-B and CCSP genes.[96,116] The stoichiometry, timing, and distinct combinations of transcription factor binding, as well as posttranscriptional modification of TTF1 by phosphorylation, are involved in differential gene expression throughout lung development. TTF1 and other transcription factors are recruited to nuclear complexes at regulatory sites of target genes that influence respiratory epithelial cell differentiation, providing and translating spatial information required for the formation of the highly diverse epithelial cell types lining distinct regions of the respiratory tract (see Figure 1-5).

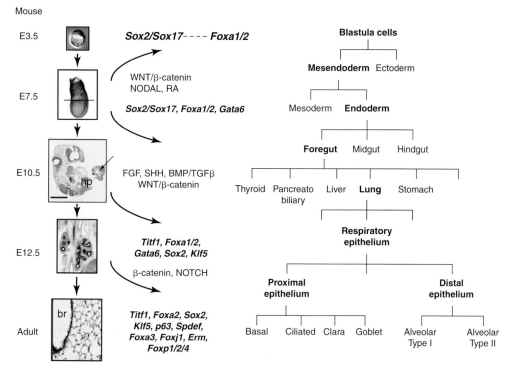

BLUEPRINT FOR LUNG EPITHELIAL CELL DEVELOPMENT

FIGURE 1-5. A blueprint for lung epithelial cell development. Cytodifferentiation of the respiratory epithelium is controlled by transcriptional networks of genes (highlighted) that are expressed throughout lung development, in conjunction with autocrine and paracrine signaling pathways that control structural morphogenesis of the lung. Additional transcription factors are induced or repressed later in development, and in the adult organ, to influence the differentiation of specific cell types.

Epithelial-Mesenchymal Interactions and Lung Morphogenesis

In vivo and *in vitro* experiments support the concept that branching morphogenesis and differentiation of the respiratory tract depends on reciprocal signaling between endodermally derived cells of the lung buds and the pulmonary mesenchyme or stroma.[30-34,43] This interdependency depends on autocrine and paracrine interactions that are mediated by the various signaling mechanisms governing cellular behavior (see Figure 1-3). Similarly, autocrine and paracrine interactions are known to be involved in cellular responses of the postnatal lung, generating signals that regulate cell proliferation and differentiation necessary for its repair and remodeling following injury. The splanchnic mesenchyme produces a number of signaling peptides critical for migration and proliferation of cells in the lung buds, including FGF10, FGF7, FGF9, BMP5, and WNT 2/2b, which activate receptors found on epithelial cells. In a complementary manner, epithelial cells produce WNT7b, WNT5a, SHH, BMP4, FGF9, VEGF, and PDGF that activate receptors and signaling pathways on target cells in the mesenchyme.[30,33,34,42,43]

Branching Morphogenesis, Vascularization, and Sacculation

Two distinct processes, branching and sacculation, are critical to morphogenesis of the mammalian lung. The major branches of the conducting airways of the human lung are completed by 16 weeks (p.c.) by a process of dichotomous branching, initiated by the bifurcation of the main stem bronchi early in the embryonic period of lung development. Epithelial-lined tubules of ever-decreasing diameter are formed from the proximal to distal region of the developing lung. Pulmonary arteries and veins form along the tubules and ultimately invade the acinar regions, where capillaries form between the arteries and veins, completing the pulmonary circulation.[37,42] The bronchial vasculature arises from the aorta, providing nutrient supply predominantly to bronchial and bronchiolar regions of the lung. In contrast, the alveolar regions are supplied by the pulmonary arterial system. Lymphatics and nerves form along the conducting airways, the latter being prominent in hilar, stromal and vascular tissues, but lacking in the alveolar regions of the lung.[124] A distinct period of lung sacculation and alveolarization begins in the late canalicular period (16 weeks p.c. and thereafter), which will result in the formation of the adult respiratory bronchiole, alveolar duct, and alveoli. During sacculation, a unique pattern of vascular supply forms the capillary network surrounding each terminal saccule, providing an ever-expanding gas exchange area that is completed in adolescence. Both vasculogenesis and angiogenesis contribute to formation of the pulmonary vascular system.[37,42] Signaling via SHH, VEGFA, FOXF1, NOTCH, Ephrins, and PDGF plays important roles in pulmonary vascular development.[30,33,34,42] For example, VEGFA and its receptors (VEGFR1, VEGFR2) are critical factors for vasculogenesis in many tissues. Targeted inactivation of *Vegf* and *Vefgfr1* in mice results in impaired angiogenesis,[125] while overexpression of the VEGFA 164 isoform disrupts pulmonary vascular endothelium in newborn conditional transgenic mice, causing pulmonary hemorrhage.[126] PROX1, a homeo domain transcription factor, is induced in a subset of venous endothelial cells during development and upregulates other lymphatic-specific genes, such as *VEGFR3* and *LYVE1*, which are critical for development of the lymphatic network in the lung.[124] Growth factors important for lymphatic development include VEGFC and its receptor, VEGFR3, as well as the angiopoietins, ANG1 and ANG2, and their receptors, TIE1 and TIE2.[124] Insufficiency or targeted deletion of these factors in mice impairs lymphatic vessel formation.[127,42]

Control of Lung Proliferation During Branching Morphogenesis

Dissection of the splanchnic mesenchyme from the lung buds arrests cell proliferation, branching, and differentiation of the pulmonary tubules *in vitro*.[43] Both *in vitro* and *in vivo* experiments strongly support the concept that the mesenchyme produces signaling peptides and growth factors critical to the formation of respiratory tubules.[43] In addition, lung growth is influenced by mechanical factors, including the size of the thoracic cavity and by stretch. For example, complete occlusion of the fetal trachea *in utero* enhances lung growth, while drainage of lung liquid or amniotic fluid causes pulmonary hypoplasia.[128,129] Regional control of proliferation is required for the process of dichotomous branching: division is enhanced at the lateral edges of the growing bud and inhibited at branch points.[130] Precise positional control of cell division is determined by polypeptides derived from the mesenchyme (e.g., growth factors or extracellular matrix molecules) that selectively decrease proliferation at clefts and increase cell proliferation at the edges of the bud. Proliferation in the respiratory tubule is dependent on a number of growth factors, including the FGF family of polypeptides. *In vitro*, FGF1 and FGF7 (also known as keratinocyte growth factor, KGF) partially replace the requirement of pulmonary mesenchyme for continued epithelial cell proliferation and budding.[131,132] FGF polypeptides are produced by the mesenchyme during lung development and bind to and activate a splice variant of FGFR2 (FGFR2IIIb) that is present on respiratory epithelial cells, completing a paracrine loop.[133,134] Blockade of FGFR2 signaling in the epithelium of the developing lung bud *in vivo*, using a dominant-negative FGF receptor mutant, completely blocked dichotomous branching of all conducting airway segments except the primary bronchi in mice.[135] FGF10 produced at localized regions of mesenchyme near the tips of the lung buds creates a chemoattractant gradient that activates the FGFR2IIIb receptor in epithelial cells of the lung buds, inducing cell migration, differentiation, and proliferation required for branching morphogenesis.[136] Deletion of *Fgf10* or *Fgfr2IIIb* in mice blocked lung bud formation, resulting in lung agenesis.[137,138] Increased expression of FGF10 or FGF7 in the fetal mouse lung caused severe pulmonary lesions with all of the histologic features of cystic adenomatoid malformations.[139,140] FGF7 is also mitogenic for mature respiratory epithelial cells *in vivo*, enhancing proliferation of bronchiolar and alveolar cells when administered intratracheally to the lungs of adult rats or by conditional targeted overexpression in mice.[141,142] Since FGF7 is produced during lung injury, it is likely that FGF signaling molecules mediate cell proliferation or migration to influence repair.[143] FGF7 and FGF1 increase expression of surfactant proteins *in vitro* and *in vivo*, suggesting that these factors enhance type II cell differentiation.[144,145] Signaling polypeptides known to influence branching morphogenesis and differentiation of the respiratory tract are listed in Box 1-1.

Role of Extracellular Matrix, Cell Adhesion, and Cell Shape

The pulmonary mesenchyme is relatively loosely packed, and there is little evidence that cell type is specified during the early embryonic period of lung development. However, with advancing gestation, increasing abundance of extracellular matrix molecules, including laminin, fibronectin, collagens, elastin, and proteoglycans, is readily detected in the mesenchyme adjacent to the developing epithelial structures.[146-152] Variability in the presence and abundance of various matrix molecules within the mesenchyme influences structural development, cytodifferentiation, and cell interactions *in vivo*. *In vitro*, inhibitors of collagen, elastin, and glycosaminoglycan synthesis, as well as antibodies to various extracellular and cell attachment molecules, alter cell proliferation and branching morphogenesis of the embryonic lung. Mesenchymal cells differentiate to form vascular elements (endothelium and smooth muscle) and distinct fibroblastic cells (myofibroblasts and lipofibroblasts), which all arise from the relatively undifferentiated progenitor cells of the splanchnic mesenchyme. While little is known regarding the factors influencing differentiation of the pulmonary mesenchyme, the development of pulmonary vasculature is dependent on VEGFs.[42] VEGFA is secreted by respiratory epithelial cells, stimulating pulmonary vasculogenesis via paracrine signaling to receptors that are expressed by progenitor cells in the mesenchyme.[153-156] PDGFA, another growth factor secreted by the respiratory epithelium, influences proliferation and differentiation of myofibroblasts in the developing lung by binding to the PDGF alpha receptor, and deletion of *Pdgfa* caused pulmonary malformation in transgenic mice.[157] The organization of both mesenchyme and epithelium is further modulated by cell adhesion molecules of various classes, including the cadherins, integrins, and polypeptides forming cell-cell junctions, which contribute to cellular organization and polarity of various tissues during pulmonary organogenesis. Furthermore, the surrounding extracellular matrix contains adhesion

molecules that interact with attachment sites at cell membranes, influencing cell shape and polarity.[147,149] Cell shape is determined, at least in part, by the organization of these cell attachment molecules to the cytoskeleton. Cell shape, polarity, and mobility are further influenced by cytoskeletal proteins that interact with the extracellular matrix, as well as neighboring cells. Recently, the planar cell polarity (PCP) pathway and its downstream effector, Rho kinase, have been shown to be critical for branching morphogenesis *in vivo* through their effects on cytoskeletal remodeling and organization, which influence apical-basal polarity within epithelia.[158,159] Mutations in the genes, *Celsr1* and *Vangl2* that are key components of the PCP pathway, disrupted the actin-myosin cytoskeleton during mouse lung development, resulting in hypoplastic lungs with fewer branches and terminal buds, thickened mesenchyme, and highly disorganized epithelia with narrow or absent lumina.[160]

Cell shape also influences intracellular routing of cellular proteins and secretory products, determining sites of secretion. *In vitro*, epithelial cells grown on extracellular matrix gels at an air-liquid interface form a highly polarized cuboidal epithelium that maintains cell differentiation and polarity of secretions *in vitro*. Loss of cell shape is associated with the loss of differentiated features, such as surfactant protein and lipid synthesis, demonstrating the profound influence of cell shape on gene expression and cell behavior.[161-163]

Autocrine-Paracrine Interactions in Lung Injury and Repair

As in lung morphogenesis, autocrine-paracrine signaling plays a critical role in the process of repair following lung injury. The repair processes in the postnatal lung, as in lung morphogenesis, require the precise control of cell proliferation and differentiation and, as such, are likely influenced by many of the signaling molecules and transcriptional mechanisms that mediate lung development. Events involved in lung repair may recapitulate events occurring during development, in which progenitor cells undergo proliferation and terminal differentiation after lung injury. While many of the mechanisms involved in lung repair and development may be shared, it is also clear that fetal and postnatal lung respond in distinct ways to autocrine-paracrine signals. Cells of the postnatal lung have undergone distinct phases of differentiation and may have different proliferative potentials, or respond in unique ways to the signals evoked by lung injury. For example, after acute or chronic injury, increased production of growth factors or cytokines may cause pulmonary fibrosis or pulmonary vascular remodeling in neonatal life, mediated by processes distinct from those occurring during normal lung morphogenesis.[164-169] The role of inflammation and the increasing activity of the immune system that accompanies postnatal development also distinguishes the pathogenesis of disease in fetal and postnatal lungs.

Host Defense Systems

Distinct innate and adaptive defense systems mediate various aspects of host responses in the lung. During the postnatal period, the numbers and types of immune cells present in the lung expand markedly.[170] Alveolar macrophages, dendritic cells, lymphocytes of various subtypes, polymorphonuclear cells, eosinophils and mast cells each have distinct roles in host defense. Immune cells mediate acute and chronic inflammatory responses accompanying lung injury or infection. Both the respiratory epithelium and inflammatory cells are capable of releasing and responding to a variety of polypeptides that induce the expression of genes involved in (1) cytoprotection (e.g., antioxidants, heat shock proteins); (2) adhesion, influencing the attraction and binding of inflammatory cells to epithelial and endothelial cells of the lung; (3) cell proliferation, apoptosis, and differentiation that follow injury or infection; and (4) innate host defense. An increasing array of cytokines and chemokines have now been identified that contribute to host defense following lung injury.[171,172]

The adaptive immune system includes both antibody and cell-mediated responses to antigenic stimuli. Adaptive immunity depends on the presentation of antigens by macrophages, dendritic cells, or the respiratory epithelium to mononuclear cells, triggering the expansion of immune lymphocytes and initiating antibody production and cytotoxic activity needed to remove infected cells from the lung. The lung contains active lymphocytes (natural killer cells, helper and cytotoxic T cells) that are present within the parenchyma and alveolus. Organized populations of mononuclear cells are also found in the lymphatic system along the conducting airways, termed the *bronchiolar-associated lymphocytes*. Cytokines and chemokines, including (1) interleukin (IL) 1, or IL1, (2) IL8, (3) tumor necrosis factor-α, or TNFα, (4) regulated on activation, normal T-expressed and secreted protein, or RANTES, (5) granulocyte-macrophage colony-stimulating factor, or GM-CSF, and (6) macrophage inflammatory protein-1α, or MIP-1α, are produced by cells in the lung and provide proliferative and/or differentiative signals to inflammatory cells that, in turn, amplify these signals by releasing additional cytokines or other inflammatory mediators within the lung.[172] Receptors for some of these signaling molecules have been identified in pulmonary epithelial cells. For example, GM-CSF plays a critical role in surfactant homeostasis. Genetic ablation of GM-CSF or GM-CSF-IL3/5β chain receptor in mice causes alveolar proteinosis associated with macrophage dysfunction and surfactant accumulation.[173-177] Pulmonary alveolar proteinosis in adult human patients is associated with high-affinity autoantibodies against GM-CSF that block receptor activation required for surfactant catabolism by alveolar macrophages.[178,179] Inherited defects in the GM-CSF receptor, including both the GM-CSF receptor alpha and beta chains, have been associated with alveolar proteinosis in children.[178,179] GM-CSF stimulates both differentiation and proliferation of Type II epithelial cells, as well as activating alveolar macrophages to increase surfactant catabolism. Thus, GM-CSF acts in an autocrine and paracrine fashion as a growth factor for both the respiratory epithelium and for alveolar macrophages. A number of additional growth factors, including FGFs, EGF, TGFα, PDGF, IGFs, TGFβ, and others, are released by lung cells following injury. These polypeptide growth factors likely play a critical role in stimulating proliferation of the respiratory epithelial cells required to repair the injured respiratory epithelium.[169,172] For example,

intratracheal administration of FGF7 causes marked proliferation of the adult respiratory epithelium and protects the lung from various injuries.[141]

Innate Defenses

The lung also has innate defense systems that function independently of those provided by the mesodermally derived immune system. The respiratory epithelium and other lung cells secrete a variety of polypeptides that serve defense functions, including bactericidal polypeptides (lysozyme and defensins), collectins (surfactant proteins, SP-A and SP-D), and other polypeptides that enhance macrophage activity involved in the clearance of bacteria and other pathogens. SP-A and SP-D, both members of the collectin family of mammalian lectins,[158] are secreted by the respiratory epithelium and bind to pathogenic organisms, enhancing their phagocytosis by alveolar macrophages.[180-183] Polypeptide factors with bactericidal activity, such as the defensins, are produced by various cells in response to inflammation within the lung, and are likely to play roles in host defense.[184] Thus, the immune system and accompanying production of chemokines and cytokines serve in an autocrine-paracrine fashion to modulate expression of genes mediating innate and immune-dependent defenses, as well as cell growth, critical to the repair of the parenchyma after injury. Uncontrolled proliferation of stromal cells leads to pulmonary fibrosis, just as uncontrolled growth of the respiratory epithelium produces pulmonary adenocarcinoma. Chronic inflammation, whether through inhaled particles, infection, or immune responses, may therefore establish ongoing proliferative cascades that lead to fibrosis and abnormal alveolar remodeling associated with chronic lung disease.[185]

Gene Mutations in Lung Development and Function

Knowledge of the role of specific genes in lung development and function is expanding rapidly, extending our understanding of the role of genetic mutations that cause lung malformation and disease. Mutations in the DNA code may alter the abundance and function of encoded polypeptides, causing changes in cell behavior that lead to lung malformation and dysfunction. While poorly understood at present, a congenital malformation, termed *acinar dysplasia*, is associated with decreased or absent levels of TTF1, FOXA2, and surfactant proteins; lungs from these infants are severely hypoplastic and lack peripheral airways at birth.[186] Such findings implicate the transcription factors TTF1 and FOXA2, or their upstream regulators, in acinar dysplasia. Mutations in TTF1 cause lung hypoplasia, hypothyroidism, and neurologic disorders.[187-195] Mutations in SOX9 influence the growth of the chest wall and cause lung hypoplasia in campomelic dwarfism,[196-200] while mutations in SOX2 have been associated with tracheoesophageal fistula, anophthalmia, microphthalmia, and central nervous system defects.[201] Similarly, defects in SHH and FGF signaling have been associated with lung and tracheobronchial malformations in human infants.[202,203] Mutations in the transcription factor FOXF1 have been causally linked to the lethal congenital malformation, alveolar capillary dysplasia with misalignment of the pulmonary veins.[204,205] Thus, it is increasingly apparent that mutations in genes influencing transcriptional and signaling networks that control lung morphogenesis cause pulmonary malformations in infants. Likewise, it is highly likely that allelic diversity in genes influencing lung morphogenesis will impact postnatal lung homeostasis and disease pathogenesis. Findings that SOX2 and TTF1 are frequently amplified in adults with squamous and non–small cell adenocarcinoma, respectively, links the processes controlling morphogenesis with those regulating epithelial cell proliferation and transformation in the respiratory tract.[206–208]

Postnatally, mutations in various genes critical to lung function, host defense, and inflammation are associated with genetic disease in humans. Hereditary disorders affecting lung function include: (1) cystic fibrosis, caused by mutations in the cystic fibrosis transmembrane conductance regulator protein; (2) emphysema, caused by mutations in α_1-antitrypsin; (3) lymphangioleiomyomatosis, caused by mutations in tuberous sclerosis complex 1 and 2; (4) alveolar proteinosis, caused by mutations in the GM-CSF receptor; and (5) respiratory distress, interstitial lung disease, and pulmonary fibrosis caused by mutations in the surfactant proteins, SP-B and SP-C, and in the phospholipid transporter, ABCA3.[209–214] In addition, mutations in polypeptides controlling neutrophil oxidant production lead to bacterial infections associated with chronic granulomatous disease.[215,216] The severity of disease associated with these monogenetic disorders is often strongly influenced by other inherited genes or environmental factors (e.g., smoking) that ameliorate or exacerbate underlying lung disease. The identification of "modifier genes" and the role of gene dosage in disease susceptibility will be critical in understanding the pathogenesis and clinical course of pulmonary disease in the future.

SUMMARY

The molecular and cellular mechanisms controlling lung morphogenesis and function provide a fundamental basis for understanding the pathogenesis and therapy of pulmonary diseases in children and adults. Future advances in pulmonary medicine will depend on the identification of genes and their encoded polypeptides that play critical roles in lung formation and function. Knowledge regarding the complex signaling pathways that govern lung cell behaviors during development and after injury will provide the basis for new diagnostic and therapeutic approaches that will influence clinical outcomes. Diagnosis of pulmonary disease will be facilitated by the identification of new gene mutations that cause abnormalities in lung development and function. Since many of the events underlying lung morphogenesis are likely to be involved in the pathogenesis of lung disease postnatally, elucidation of molecular pathways governing lung development will provide the knowledge to understand the cellular and molecular basis of lung diseases. Advances in recombinant DNA technology and the ability to synthesize bioactive polypeptides, and to add or delete genes via DNA transfer, are likely to influence the therapy of pulmonary disease in the future.

Suggested Reading

Cardoso WV, Lu J. Regulation of early lung morphogenesis: questions, facts and controversies. *Development.* 2006;133(9):1611–1624.

Crosby LM, Waters CM. Epithelial repair mechanisms in the lung. *Am J Physiol Lung Cell Mol Physiol.* 2010;298(6):L715–L731.

Galambos C, deMello DE. Molecular mechanisms of pulmonary vascular development. *Pediatr Dev Pathol.* 2007;10(1):1–17.

Maeda Y, Dave V, Whitsett JA. Transcriptional control of lung morphogenesis. *Physiol Rev.* 2007;87(1):219–244.

Morrisey EE, Hogan BL. Preparing for the first breath of life: genetic and cellular mechanisms in lung development. *Dev Cell.* 2010;18(1):8–23.

Nan-Sinkam SP, Hunter MG, Nuovo GJ, et al. Integrating the MicroRNome into the study of lung disease. *Am J Respir Crit Care Med.* 2009;179(1):4–10.

Riethoven JJ. Regulatory regions in DNA: promoters, enhancers, silencers and insulators. *Methods Mol Biol.* 2010;674:33–42.

Shannon JM, Hyatt BA. Epithelial-mesenchymal interactions in the developing lung. *Annu Rev Physiol.* 2004;66:625–645.

Warburton D, El-Hashash A, Carraro G, et al. *Lung organogenesis. Curr Top Dev Biol.* 2010;90:73–158.

Zorn AM, Wells JM. Vertebrate endoderm development and organ formation. *Annu Rev Cell Dev Biol.* 2009;25:221–251.

References

The complete reference list is available online at www.expertconsult.com

2 BASIC GENETICS AND EPIGENETICS OF CHILDHOOD LUNG DISEASE

Saffron A. Willis-Owen, PhD, and Miriam F. Moffatt, PhD

BACKGROUND

During childhood, long-term respiratory illnesses occur at a higher prevalence than all other chronic conditions combined.[1] Among the respiratory illnesses, asthma is the single most common acute disease of childhood affecting an estimated 300 million individuals worldwide.[2] The most common lethal inherited disease of childhood is cystic fibrosis, which occurs in approximately 1 in 3000 births in Northern European populations. Both diseases are considered to have significant heritable components underlying disease etiology.[3–6] Cystic fibrosis is inherited, with heritable factors accounting for 54% to 100% of inter-individual variation in disease presentation and severity.[3] Estimates indicate that asthma, on the other hand, is 36% to 79% heritable.[4–6] Despite consistent evidence of strong heritability and high levels of investment in the genetic characterization of these diseases, to date only a fraction of the total heritability of asthma has been accounted for, as compared with cystic fibrosis. The basis for this polarity lies in the type and number of underlying disease-causing factors.

Cystic fibrosis is a classic Mendelian disease. This means that its transmission follows a simple pattern of inheritance set forth by *Gregor Mendel* in the 1800s and is now recognized as characteristic of single-gene autosomal recessive disorders. Attempts to model the causation of asthma, on the other hand, indicate that the heritable proportion of disease risk is composed of multiple effects, each of moderate size (a so-called "complex" or "multifactorial" etiology). Cystic fibrosis and asthma have therefore required somewhat different approaches toward their genetic dissection, and this has influenced how successful disease gene identification has been.

In this chapter, we will outline the approaches taken to identify individual sources of disease heritability for respiratory illnesses of childhood, using cystic fibrosis and bronchial asthma as examples. In addition, we will also consider potential explanations for missing heritability (i.e., the proportion of heritability that remains unaccounted for by known genetic factors). We will highlight current shortfalls in research paradigms (e.g., genetic factors that are not amenable to detection via existing technologies and study designs), and we will discuss alternative sources of heritability inseparable from genetics during the early phase of heritability estimation (i.e., epigenetic inheritance and gene × environment interactions).

CYSTIC FIBROSIS: STRATEGIES FOR THE MAPPING OF A SINGLE GENE DISORDER

Cystic fibrosis (CF) follows a characteristic autosomal recessive pattern of inheritance, requiring two copies of a risk allele to be present for the expression of the disease phenotype. *De novo* mutation coupled with the inheritance of a single risk allele from one apparently disease-free (heterozygous carrier) parent are infrequent.[7] This relatively simple pattern of disease transmission can be considered indicative of single gene involvement and large-effect, highly penetrant alleles. These represent ideal conditions for the application of linkage mapping; a technique that traces allele and disease transmission in families. By using the patterns of allele sharing in individuals concordant for disease, it is possible to identify gross genomic intervals that contain disease-causing genetic lesions. This technique was successfully applied to CF across a series of experiments in the 1980s and resulted in the identification of a large contiguous interval located on the long arm of human chromosome 7 (7q31).[8–14] This locus was found to contain at least four transcribed sequences, three of which could be excluded following recombination mapping[15] and chromosome walking/jumping techniques.[16]

Recombination mapping directly compares the frequency and distribution of cross-over events within a defined interval between cases and controls, and chromosome walking uses each end of a DNA fragment to screen a library of DNA clones for the identification of adjoining sequences, the most distal elements of which become new probes. This technique allows the researcher to effectively "walk" along a DNA sequence of interest, while jumping impassable regions (e.g., those that are highly repetitive or rich in G and C nucleotides) by the omission of bases between defined intervals. Through a combination of DNA sequence analysis and interrogation of overlapping cDNA clones derived from cultured epithelial cell libraries with a genomic DNA segment obtained from the putative CF locus, Riordan and colleagues successfully cloned the fourth transcribed sequence in 1989.[16] The consensus region from the isolated overlapping cDNA clones revealed an Open Reading Frame (ORF) encoding a 1480 amino acid polypeptide (the *Cystic Fibrosis Transmembrane Conductance Regulator* or *CFTR*). Within the ORF, loss of a single phenylalanine residue at position 508 was observed in 68% of cystic fibrosis chromosomes as compared with 0% of disease-free controls. This mutation, now known as F508del, can be traced back at least 2300 years to Iron Age Europeans.[17] It is hypothesized to have persisted due to a heterozygote selective advantage possibly in terms of resistance to infectious pathogens such as the chloride-secreting diarrheas (*Vibrio cholerae* and *Escherichia coli*),[18] or alternatively as a reproductive advantage.[19,20]

CFTR represents the first human disease gene to be cloned exclusively through position-based methods, collectively termed *positional cloning*, without guidance from cytogenetic aberrations (i.e., rearrangements or deletions) as had been the case for previously cloned disease genes such as *Dystrophin (DMD)* in Duchenne muscular dystrophy.[21] The *CFTR* gene encodes an ABC protein that acts both as a chloride channel, regulating the flow of chloride anions and therefore water across cellular membranes. It also regulates the activity of several other substrate transporter pathways (e.g., chloride-coupled bicarbonate). These activities are required for normal fluid transport in the secretory epithelia of the lungs, gastrointestinal tract, pancreas, sweat glands, and testes; impairments lead to slowed epithelial surface fluid secretion, dehydration of epithelial surface materials, congestion, obstruction, and, ultimately, recurrent bacterial infections.

CYSTIC FIBROSIS: FINE-SCALE HETEROGENEITY IN DISEASE CAUSATION

Today almost 1900 disease-causing mutations have been documented in *CFTR (www.genet.sickkids.on.ca/cftr/StatisticsPage.html)*, although the majority of these are infrequent or specific to individual populations. F508del remains the most common mutation, with only five variants carrying frequencies above 1%.[22] *CFTR* mutations are now classified into five functional groups: (I) complete absence of *CFTR* protein production, (II) *CFTR* protein trafficking defects (with low or absent protein production), (III) defective regulation, (IV) defective chloride transport through *CFTR*, and (V) defective *CFTR* splicing with diminished production of wild-type *CFTR* (reviewed in [23]). These groupings have broad clinical implications, with mutation classes I to III associated with a more severe form of the disease and pancreatic insufficiency, the latter being a common feature of CF. With the exception of this crude heuristic, a marked variability in the clinical presentation and organ involvement of patients carrying identical *CFTR* alleles has been observed. As such, efforts are now focused on dissection of the genotype-phenotype relationship and the identification of factors capable of its modification.

Although environmental factors such as nutrition and exposure to infection undoubtedly influence clinical presentation and disease severity, evidence is also now accumulating in favor of a genetic contribution, suggesting that the condition may not in fact be a single gene disorder. Early experiments have shown that mice deficient for *CFTR* vary in disease severity (in particular the degree of intestinal obstruction), as a function of genetic background (i.e., strain).[16] Similar effects have also been documented in humans, although with varying degrees of replication. A number of potential genes with modifier effects have been proposed based on existing knowledge of CF disease biology (a candidate gene approach) and tested for association with various parameters of clinical presentation including disease severity, rate of pulmonary function decline, and survival. Many of these studies have relied, however, on small phenotypically and genetically diverse populations, thereby limiting the interpretation of the results. Two of the more consistent effects reported in the literature include *TGFβ1* (Transforming Growth Factor β1) and *MBL2* (Mannose binding lectin 2).

TGFβ1 is a pro-fibrotic cytokine involved in a variety of cellular processes such as growth, proliferation, differentiation, and apoptosis. Variants at the 5' terminus of this gene have been associated with lung disease severity in CF (determined through Forced Expiratory Volume in 1 second [FEV_1]) with odds ratios of around 2.2.[20] MBL2 is an antigen recognition molecule that is capable of binding a range of pathogens and symbionts including bacteria, fungi, viruses, and parasites, and it is involved in the complement-mediated (innate immune) host defense response. MBL2 protein deficiencies caused by prevalent mutations in both the promoter and exon 1 of the gene appear to moderate susceptibility to infectious diseases across a wide range of populations, in particular the critically ill, immunocompromised, and young (6 to 18 months).[24] Early research associated these low MBL-producing genotypes with poor lung function and survival in CF.[25,26] Recent research has implicated that the genotypes are involved in early bacterial infection,[27,28] providing a potential mechanism for MBL-deficiency–related pulmonary decline. Not all such experiments[29] support this observation, but this might be attributable to variation in sample size and consequently power of the studies.

NOVEL METHODS FOR THE IDENTIFICATION OF GENETIC MODIFIERS

Recent advances in technology have enabled a shift away from candidate gene, knowledge-driven approaches toward the identification of genetic modifiers. New high throughput techniques allow the simultaneous interrogation of all known genes in the human genome irrespective of their hypothesized role in disease. To date, only a handful of studies have applied such techniques to CF, and they focus predominantly on determining the global gene expression profile of the respiratory epithelium and its response to CF disease–causing mutations. Zabner and colleagues recently performed a systematic comparison between gene expression patterns of non-CF (wild type) and CF (F508del homozygous) primary human airway epithelial cell cultures under resting conditions.[30] Expression patterns were assayed across a total of 22,283 genes and examined for significant differences. Minimal changes were observed, with only 24 genes reaching a 1% False Discovery Rate (FDR) threshold; 18 were found to have increased expression in CF, and the remaining 6 genes had decreased expression. The 24 genes included *SLC12A4* (Solute Carrier family 12, member 4, a potassium and chloride transporter) and *IL21R* (Interleukin 21 Receptor, a type I cytokine receptor for interleukin 21), both genes of relevance to CF.

Data from these types of study provide potential clues into the biological pathways involved in CF and insights into the possible sources of inter-individual variability. The quality of data and the conclusions that can be drawn are, however, inextricably linked to the degree of stringency applied to the study design. Extraneous, uncontrolled sources of variation that originate from factors such as sample cell type composition, sample treatment prior to RNA extraction, and distribution of age, gender, and environmental exposures

TABLE 2-1 FACTORS PREVIOUSLY IDENTIFIED TO HAVE AN IMPACT ON GENE EXPRESSION DATA

VARIABLE	REFERENCES	SPECIES
Age	95, 96	Human, mouse, rat, dog
Sex	97–100	Human, drosophila, mouse, nematode
Ethnicity	101, 102	Human
Environment (lifestyle/geography)	103	Human
Diet	96, 104	Mouse, dog
Time of day	105–107	Human, rat, arabidopsis
Sample cellular composition	105	Human
Agonal factors (postmortem tissue)	108	Human
Method of sample preservation	109	Human
Platform	110–112	Human, mouse, rat
Cell culture conditions	113, 114	Human
Laboratory	111	Human

across sample groups can have profound effects on the transcriptional profile. This consequently can lead to anomalous differential expression results (Table 2-1).

ASTHMA

The term *asthma* is derived from the identical Greek word meaning "noisy breathing."[31] The disease manifests as periods of reversible airflow obstruction accompanied by bronchoconstriction and inflammation. Symptoms are variable but include wheeze, cough, chest tightness, and shortness of breath. While associated with normal life expectancy, unlike CF sufferers, asthma is still estimated to be responsible for approximately 1 in 250 deaths worldwide; and each death is viewed to be preventable.[2] Buoyed by the successes in Mendelian disease gene identification, genome-wide linkage methods were first applied to asthma in 1996[32] and were subsequently repeated across a variety of different population collections. These experiments led to the identification of numerous putative disease loci, only a proportion of which were found to replicate consistently between cohorts. While this failure to reproduce may reflect cryptic gene × environment interactions or ancestry-related variation in linkage disequilibrium (LD) patterns, the likelihood is that a proportion of the unreplicated linkage peaks actually represent false positives. Interestingly, a recent meta-analysis of genome-wide linkage studies for asthma involving more than 2000 families and 5000 affected individuals identified only one region—

chromosome 5 (141 to 169 centimorgans [cM])—that in all families attained genome-wide significance, and two regions—2p21-14 and 6p21—that attained significance only in families of European ancestry.[33]

Once identified, and replicated in more than one population, a small number of linkage intervals have been pursued by positional cloning (identification of underlying disease gene[s] by position-based methods). Relative to Mendelian diseases, this has proven to be an expensive and lengthy undertaking, typically requiring many successive rounds of fine-mapping in order to reduce the size of the linkage interval to a tractable number of genes. To date, six loci have been positionally cloned; *ADAM33* chromosome 20p13,[34] *DPP10* chromosome 2q14,[35] *PHF11* chromosome 13q14,[36] *NPSR1* (previously known as *GPRA*) chromosome 7p14,[37] *HLA-G* chromosome 6p21,[38] and *CYFIP2* chromosome 5q33.[39] The proteins encoded by these genes are engaged in a variety of distinct processes, including airway remodeling *(ADAM33)*, T-cell adhesion and differentiation *(CYFIP2)*, and transcriptional regulation *(PHF11)*.

Prior to these genes being identified, historical concepts of disease causation had been founded on simple observations such as efficacy of pharmacologic therapies (e.g., β2-adrenergic receptor agonists, see[40] for an excellent review). Positional cloning has consequently extended our knowledge of the biological systems underlying asthma, but the genes identified account for relatively little of the estimated 36% to 79% heritability of asthma, as the effect size of each locus is comparatively small. A recent meta-analysis of *ADAM33* variants and haplotypes found a maximum odds ratio of 1.46 (95% CI 1.21 to 1.76)[41], while a large German case-control study of *NPSR1* observed a maximum single-marker odds ratio of 1.40 (95% CI 1.04 to 1.88).[42] There are a number of potential explanations for why such a small amount of asthma heritability has been identified so far.

The Common Disease, Common Variant (CDCV) hypothesis, postulated in the late 1990s,[43] suggests that common diseases such as asthma and diabetes are caused by many prevalent alleles of small effect acting in concert to generate the disease phenotype. This model of causation provides a viable explanation for the shortfalls of linkage mapping. Linkage mapping possesses relatively low power in such scenarios being better designed for the identification of loci harboring recessive, highly penetrant effects, and situations of allelic heterogeneity in which multiple individually rare alleles co-localize to a common locus. A more appropriate technique for CDCV identification is genetic association. This approach directly compares allele frequencies between cases and controls, seeking sites at which allele frequency correlates with case status.

GENOME-WIDE ASSOCIATION

Genome-Wide Association (GWA) applies the power of genetic association across the entire genome simultaneously. The technique relies upon the prevalence of Single Nucleotide Polymorphisms (SNPs) occurring approximately once every 100 to 300 bases. Due to knowledge of linkage disequilibrium (LD) patterns in different populations available through the HapMap project *(http://*

snp.cshl.org/), it is possible to have near-complete coverage of common variation (minor allele frequency [MAF] ≥5%) via a SNP "tagging" method (Figure 2-1). Implementing the use of tag SNPs results in a reduction in the genotyping burden of high-density mapping experiments by defining a non-overlapping, fully informative marker set, omitting those markers the genotypes of which can be inferred from other proximal positions.

The first GWA scan for asthma was published in 2007.[44] It involved the genotyping of 317,000 genome-wide tag SNPs in a cohort of 2200 individuals, achieving approximately 79% coverage of common SNPs (MAF ≥5%), assuming an r^2 of 0.8 (where r^2 is a measure of the extent of LD between genotyped and un-genotyped markers). More than half of all markers that were significant at a 1% FDR threshold were located in a single locus on chromosome 17q21. This locus was found to possess *cis*-acting regulatory potential; in other words, it has the potential to moderate the activity of genes positioned in close proximity to it. Loci that operate on genes located distally, even on different chromosomes, are referred to as *trans-acting*. The 17q21 locus was initially observed to modulate the expression of *ORMDL3 (Orosomucoid-1-like `3);* an endoplasmic reticulum (ER)–based transmembrane protein involved in calcium signaling, cellular stress, and sphingolipid homeostasis.[45,46] The locus has since been shown to additionally regulate the expression of two other proximal genes—*ZPBP2* and *GSDMB*—in an allele-specific manner, achieving domain-wide *cis*-regulation through chromatin remodeling (specifically changes in insulator protein CTCF binding and nucleosome occupancy).[47] Contrary to a large proportion of early linkage and candidate gene association data, the relationship between 17q21 genotypes and asthma appears to be very robust, and a high level of replication across a diverse range of populations has been reported.[48–55] These studies have also shown that the 17q21 association may be driven by a subset of cases with early disease onset,[49] and both subject to environmental influences (early exposure to environmental tobacco smoke)[49] and capable of

calibrating environmental influence (amplifying the association between early respiratory infections and asthma).[56]

Since the publication of this first asthma GWA study in 2007, 14 additional screens have been published investigating not only the genetic etiology of asthma[57–62] but also a diverse array of related quantitative traits,[63–69] e.g. FEV$_1$. The most recent and largest of these screens included over 10,000 cases and 16,000 controls (all of whom were matched for ancestry), resulting in the generation of approximately 15 billion genotypes for analysis and the identification of 7 loci of genome-wide significance.[62] This represents an unprecedented leap forward in our understanding of disease biology, enabling the identification of more genes involved in the etiology of asthma within a single study than it has been possible to achieve in fourteen years of positional cloning. The results of all the GWA studies detailing the 33 loci identified are outlined in Table 2-2. With the exception of *DPP10*, none of the genes previously identified by the positional cloning approach for asthma have been found by the GWA studies. These positionally cloned genes have, however, replicated successfully across a number of prior focused experiments. This failure, therefore, by GWA to reaffirm their involvement is not necessarily an indication of error, but likely a reflection of differences in the types of effect amenable to detection via these two contrasting techniques as well as the phenotypes (traits) examined by the two methods.

A small number of the observed GWA effects confirm previously equivocal candidate genes, for example the alpha polypeptide of the Fc fragment of the high-affinity IgE receptor *(FCER1A)* association with total serum Immunoglobulin E (IgE). Others highlight distinct components of common biological pathways (e.g., *Interleukin [IL]33* and its receptor *IL1RL1)* or identify alternative members of previously implicated gene families to be of importance in disease etiology. An example of the latter is a GWA analysis of an FEV$_1$/FVC phenotype (the proportion of the forced vital capacity exhaled in the first second of expiration, which acts as an index of airway obstruction that controls for restrictive lung disease)

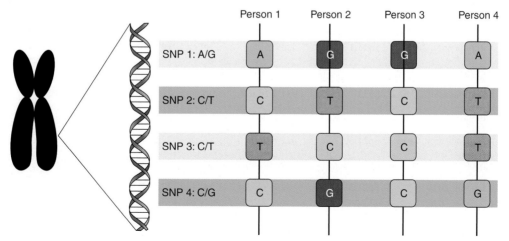

FIGURE 2-1. A haplotype tagging approach to SNP selection. Haplotypes are shown across four single nucleotide polymorphisms (SNPs) at a single chromosomal locus in four separate individuals (haplotypes are shown on the vertical). It can be seen that the allele at SNP 1 is perfectly predictive of the allele at SNP 3 (both SNP 1 and SNP 3 are highlighted in pale blue). An *A* allele at SNP 1 is always accompanied by a *T* allele at SNP 3 and the alternative allele *G* at SNP 1 is always accompanied by a *C* at SNP 3. A similar situation is seen for SNPs 2 and 4 (highlighted in green), where each is perfectly predictive of the other in terms of alleles present. The SNPs are therefore said to exhibit strong levels of linkage disequilibrium with one another, meaning that they are frequently co-inherited. Consequently, it is not necessary to genotype an individual for all four SNPs in this region. To gain complete genetic coverage, only two SNPs are required.

TABLE 2-2 SUMMARY OF GENOME-WIDE ASSOCIATION (GWA) FINDINGS FOR ASTHMA AND ITS RELATED TRAITS (AS OF OCTOBER 1, 2010)

PROPOSED GENE(S)	STUDY	CYTOGENETIC POSITION	PEAK MARKER	CHR	BP POSITION (HG19)	PEAK P-VALUE	PHENOTYPE
FCER1A	Weidinger et al. 2008	1q23	rs2251746	1	159,272,060	1.85×10^{-20}	IgE
DENND1B	Sleiman et al. 2010	1q31	rs2786098	1	197,325,908	8.55×10^{-9}	Asthma
CHI3L1	Ober et al. 2008	1q32.1	rs4950928	1	203,155,882	1.10×10^{-13}	Serum YKL-40 levels
IL1RL1	Gudbjartsson et al. 2009	2q12.3-q14.2	rs1420101	2	102,957,716	5.30×10^{-14}	Eosinophil count
IL18R1 / IL1RL1	Moffatt et al. 2010	2q12.1	rs3771166	2	102,986,222	3.4×10^{-9}	Asthma
DPP10	Mathias et al. 2010	2q12.3-q14.2	rs1435879	2	115,492,887	3.05×10^{-6}	Asthma
IKZF2	Gudbjartsson et al. 2009	2q13	rs12619285	2	213,824,045	5.40×10^{-10}	Eosinophil count
TNS1	Repapi et al. 2010	2q35	rs2571445	2	218,683,154	1.11×10^{-12}	FEV_1
GATA2	Gudbjartsson et al. 2009	3q21	rs4857855	3	128,260,550	8.60×10^{-17}	Eosinophil count
NPNT / INTS12 / FLJ20184 / GSTCD	Hancock et al. 2010	4q24	rs11727189	4	106,619,140	4.66×10^{-17}	FEV_1
GSTCD	Repapi et al. 2010	4q24	rs10516526	4	106,688,904	2.18×10^{-23}	FEV_1
HHIP	Repapi et al. 2010	4q31	rs12504628	4	145,436,324	6.48×10^{-13}	FEV_1 / FVC
HHIP	Hancock et al. 2010	4q31.21	rs1980057	4	145,485,738	3.21×10^{-20}	FEV_1 / FVC
PDE4D	Himes et al. 2009	5q12	rs1588265	5	59,369,794	4.30×10^{-7}	Asthma
IL5	Gudbjartsson et al. 2009	5q31	rs4143832	5	131,862,977	1.20×10^{-10}	Eosinophil count
RAD50 / IL13	Li et al. 2010	5q31.1	rs2244012	5	131,901,225	3.04×10^{-7}	Asthma
RAD50	Weidinger et al. 2008	5q31	rs2040704	5	131,973,177	4.46×10^{-8}	IgE
HTR4	Hancock et al. 2010	5q32	rs11168048	5	147,842,353	1.08×10^{-11}	FEV_1 / FVC
HTR4	Repapi et al. 2010	5q33.1	rs3995090	5	147,845,815	4.29×10^{-9}	FEV_1
ADAM19	Hancock et al. 2010	5q33.3	rs2277027	5	156,932,376	9.93×10^{-11}	FEV_1 / FVC
ADRA1B	Mathias et al. 2010	5q33	rs10515807	5	159,364,998	3.57×10^{-6}	Asthma
AGER	Repapi et al. 2010	6p21.32	rs2070600	6	32,151,443	3.07×10^{-15}	FEV_1 / FVC
AGER / PPT2	Hancock et al. 2010	6p21.32	rs2070600	6	32,151,443	3.15×10^{-14}	FEV_1 / FVC
HLA-DQ	Moffatt et al. 2010	6p21.32	rs9273349	6	32,625,869	7.0×10^{-14}	Asthma
HLA-DR/DQ	Li et al. 2010	6p21.3	rs1063355	6	32,627,714	9.55×10^{-6}	Asthma
GPR126	Hancock et al. 2010	6q24.1	rs3817928	6	142,750,516	1.17×10^{-9}	FEV_1 / FVC
-	Himes et al. 2009	8p12	rs11778371	8	27,319,905	8.10×10^{-7}	Asthma
IL33	Moffatt et al. 2010	9p24.1	rs1342326	9	6,190,076	9.2×10^{-10}	Asthma
TLE4	Hancock et al. 2009	9q21.31	rs23783823	9	82,039,362	7.10×10^{-6}	Asthma

TABLE 2-2 SUMMARY OF GENOME-WIDE ASSOCIATION (GWA) FINDINGS FOR ASTHMA AND ITS RELATED TRAITS (AS OF OCTOBER 1, 2010)—CONT'D

PROPOSED GENE(S)	STUDY	CYTOGENETIC POSITION	PEAK MARKER	CHR	BP POSITION (HG19)	PEAK P-VALUE	PHENOTYPE
STAT6	Weidinger et al. 2008	12q13.3	rs12368672	12	57,512,470	1.52×10^{-5}	IgE
SH2B3	Gudbjartsson et al. 2009	12q24	rs3184504	12	111,884,608	6.50×10^{-19}	Eosinophil count
SMAD3	Moffatt et al. 2010	15q22.33	rs744910	15	67,446,785	3.9×10^{-9}	Asthma
THSD4	Repapi et al. 2010	15q23	rs12899618	15	71,645,120	7.24×10^{-15}	FEV_1 / FVC
ORMDL3 / GSDMB	Moffatt et al. 2010	17q12	rs2305480	17	38,062,196	9.6×10^{-8}	Asthma
ORMDL3 (GSDMB, ZPBP2)	Moffatt et al. 2007	17q21	rs7216389	17	38,069,949	9.00×10^{-11}	Asthma
GSDMA / ORMDL3	Soranzo et al. 2009	17q21	rs17609240	17	38,110,689	9.40×10^{-9}	Total white blood cell count
GSDM1	Moffatt et al. 2010	17q21.1	rs3894194	17	38,121,993	4.6×10^{-9}	Asthma
PSMD3-CSF3	Okada et al. 2010	17q21.1	rs4794822	17	38,156,712	6.30×10^{-10}	Neutrophil count
PRNP	Mathias et al. 2010	20pter-p12	rs6052761	20	4,657,017	2.27×10^{-6}	Asthma
PLCB4	Okada et al. 2010	20p12	rs2072910	20	9,365,303	3.10×10^{-10}	Neutrophil count
IL2RB	Moffatt et al. 2010	22q12.3	rs2284033	22	37,534,034	1.2×10^{-8}	Asthma

CHR, Chromosome; bp, base pair; FEV1, forced expiratory volume in 1 second; FVC, forced vital capacity.

that identified a significant association with variants in the gene encoding *ADAM metallopeptidase domain 19 (ADAM19)*.[67] *ADAM19* is a member of the same gene family as *ADAM33*—a gene positionally cloned for asthma in 2002.[34] Both these genes are expressed in the human lung, with *ADAM19* localized to the apical part of the epithelium and *ADAM33* to the basal epithelial cells.[70] The genes have similar functional effects on integrin-mediated cell migration.[71] The remainder of the GWA findings for asthma relate to novel factors located in previously unsuspected genes or functional non-coding regions.

In some instances, more than one disease-specific screen has implicated the same locus. The 17q21 site including the gene *ORMDL3* has shown association not only for asthma but also total leukocyte cell count phenotypes. Interestingly, a GWA study for ulcerative colitis, a chronic disease involving inflammation of the gut epithelium, also found association with the chromosome 17q21 site.[72] The concordance between these GWA studies for the 17q21 locus indicates that the site may form an integral part of the inflammatory response, most notably within epithelial tissues. Consistent with this hypothesis, *ORMDL3* appears to be expressed across a broad range of immune tissues including peripheral blood leukocytes, bone marrow and lymph nodes, as well as

several epithelial disease-relevant tissues including the lung and colon.[72] Experimental modulation of *ORMDL3* expression in epithelial cells has been shown to produce downstream effects on the ER stress–induced unfolded protein response (UPR),[72] a mechanism of attenuating endogenous sources of cellular stress resulting from the accumulation of misfolded proteins in the ER, and a signaling pathway of relevance to the normal functioning of the mammalian immune system.[73]

As may be predicted by the CDCV theory, the asthma loci identified through GWA are characteristically of high frequency and low magnitude. The risk allele for the 17q21 marker most significantly associated with disease is present in 62% of asthmatics and 52% of non-asthmatics. Although genotypes at this site explain a large proportion of variance in gene expression phenotypes (29.5% of the variance in *ORMDL3* expression in lymphoblastoid cell lines),[44] the effect size for asthma is relatively small (an odds ratio of 1.45 in the original study[44] and 1.44 in a subsequent meta-analysis of nine populations[74]). Similarly, protective minor alleles in the asthma-associated gene *PDE4D* (*Phosphodiesterase 4D, cAMP-specific*, a modulator of smooth muscle contractility) yield an odds ratio of just 0.85 in Caucasian and Hispanic populations, and are present in approximately 28% of affected and 32% of unaffected individuals.[58] Consistent with these observations, the most highly powered GWA study of asthma to date recorded odds ratios ranging from just 0.76 to 1.26 for the seven disease loci identified. [62] Together these data suggest that GWA represents a productive tool for the identification of novel, common, low-magnitude effects involved in the etiology of multifactorial disease, but that collectively these factors are unlikely to account for the full heritability of asthma.

■ MISSING HERITABILITY

While GWA studies have led to the identification of numerous previously unrecognized factors involved in the etiology of asthma, these factors are of only moderate effect size, leaving a large proportion of disease heritability as yet unaccounted for. Clues as to the source(s) of this so-called "missing heritability" can be gleaned from direct comparisons between linkage and genome-wide association data. Several replicated linkage peaks show a complete absence of overlap with existing GWA data (e.g., the asthma susceptibility locus on human chromosome 19q13).[75–77] This is not only true of asthma, but also the majority of so-called complex traits. Simultaneous application of both linkage and GWA methods to large overlapping obesity cohorts recently demonstrated a complete lack of co-incidence between regions of linkage and association.[78] One reason for this may lie in the "common disease common variant" premise. GWA studies are typically powered to detect common effects of low magnitude. Coverage is calculated as the proportion of known variants (e.g., in the HapMap database) with a minor allele frequency above 5% captured at an r^2 of 0.8. Power rapidly declines when the degree of Linkage Disequilibrium (LD) between genotyped and un-genotyped variants decreases. Rare variants and situations of allelic heterogeneity are therefore not adequately captured by existing GWA strategies.

Allelic heterogeneity is a phenomenon whereby multiple disease-causing variants exist at the same locus. Sites harboring numerous individually rare, highly penetrant alleles of large effect are more amenable to detection via linkage (since these variants still lie within in the same region) rather than association (in which the signal may be diluted by alternative disease-causing variants exhibiting different levels of LD with the genotyped marker). There are now known cases of rare, highly penetrant alleles contributing to common diseases (e.g., the 16p11.2 deletions that occur in ~0.5% of children with severe early-onset obesity)[79] and well-described cases of allelic heterogeneity (e.g., the broad spectrum of disease-causing variants in the filaggrin [FLG] gene located within the 1q21 linkage peak for atopic dermatitis, a chronic inflammatory disease of the skin).[80]

The FLG gene has been shown to harbor an array of both prevalent and rare variants, including two loss-of-function alleles with odds ratios between 2.8 and 13.4[81] and a population attributable risk of around 11%.[82] The FLG mutations were identified via an exon resequencing strategy in a series of kindreds segregating for a related monogenic disease, Ichthyosis vulgaris, also known to exhibit linkage to chromosome 1q21.

Similar phenomena including situations of allelic heterogeneity and/or multiple rare allele genetic risk composition may as yet be found to contribute toward the pathophysiology of asthma. Indeed there is some evidence that the FLG loss of function alleles associate with asthma in the presence of AD. Recently developed "next generation" sequencing technologies that provide unprecedented depths and speeds of DNA sequence analysis will undoubtedly assist in answering this question (*www. illumina.com/technology/sequencing_technology.ilmn* and *www.genome-sequencing.com/*).

■ *HERITABLE* AND *GENETIC* ARE NOT INTERCHANGEABLE TERMS

Another potential explanation for the so-called "missing heritability" is the erroneous assumption that all sources of heritability must be genetic in origin. Estimates of heritability represent an amalgam of factors that can be transmitted down the germ line. Genetic sources of causation cannot be effectively separated from gene × environment interactions and epigenetic sources of heritability in standard twin study designs. As such, it remains feasible that residual heritability can be accounted for, at least in part by epigenetic factors and interactions between alleles and environments. The latter may vary between populations, depending on the prevailing environmental milieu and allele frequencies.

The term *epigenetic* refers to sources of inter-individual variation that can be transmitted down the germ line but is not due to change in the underlying DNA sequence. This includes DNA methylation; addition of a methyl group to the 5' carbon of cytosine residues, typically at CpG (Cytosine-phosphate-Guanine) dinucleotides, and various modifications of histones (e.g., methylation, acetylation, phosphorylation, ubiquitination, sumoylation, citrullination, and ADP-ribosylation); histones being the scaffold around which DNA is wound. Evidence suggests that these epigenetic marks may be environmentally malleable,[83] tissue specific,[83,84] subject to influences such as age[83–85] and sex,[84,85] and capable of maintenance across both the lifespan and across generations.

The role of DNA methylation in asthma has not yet been systematically explored in humans on a genome-wide basis. A number of small-scale focused studies have produced evidence consistent with environmentally determined patterns of DNA methylation. For example, a study following transplacental exposure to traffic-related polycyclic aromatic hydrocarbons identified individual loci at which the extent of methylation appears to associate with disease.[86] Likewise, a recent genome-wide survey of DNA methylation in a model organism (the mouse) revealed an array of sites at which the extent of DNA methylation was (a) subject to environmental influence, exhibiting a consistent relationship with the availability of methyl donors in the prenatal maternal diet, (b) correlated with gene transcription, (c) associated with various asthma-related traits in the offspring including airway hyperreactivity, serum IgE and lung lavage eosinophilia, and (d) demonstrated a trans-generational pattern of inheritance.[87]

Histone modifiers, in particular histone acetyltransferases (HAT) and deacetylases (HDAC), are also thought to play a role in the pathogenesis of asthma. HATs and HDACs are classes of enzyme that selectively add (acetylate) or remove (deacetylate) acetyl groups from conserved lysine amino acids in core histone proteins. Thus they dynamically control gene expression by altering the potential for histones to bind DNA. These antagonistic enzymes have been implicated in a variety of different processes from cell survival and proliferation to DNA repair and gene transcription.[88,89] Both their expression and activity have been found to differ in asthma[90] as well as chronic obstructive pulmonary disease (COPD),[91] another inflammatory disease of the lung.

Together these data suggest that epigenetic effects have the potential to contribute toward the etiology of asthma. Further systematic surveys will be required in order to specify the extent of this contribution; both in terms of the number and type of contributory loci, and proportion of phenotypic variance accounted for. Such approaches have already begun to be applied to a small number of alternative common, non-Mendelian diseases. A recent genome-wide scan for differential CpG methylation in diabetes mellitus, for example, identified a small number of both novel and known loci (i.e., loci overlapping with previously defined genetic susceptibility sites) that associate with presence or absence of diabetic nephropathy, which is a serious complication. The most significant of these sites achieved a P-value of 3.27×10^{-6}, and an odds ratio of just 1.88. This is an effect of comparable proportions to previously documented genetic factors.

ENVIRONMENTS: AN ADDITIONAL LAYER OF COMPLEXITY

Like epigenetic effects, current estimates of heritability also include interactions between genetic factors (G) and environments (E). These interactions are commonly referred to as Gene × Environment (G×E) interactions, but in reality they are not limited to genes but include sequence variants located in any portion of the genome (e.g., promoters, transcription factor binding sites, transcriptional enhancers). These sources of heritability have been extensively studied in asthma using a candidate gene approach. They have primarily focused on genes and variants already implicated in disease and identified through alternative techniques (positional cloning), or based on existing knowledge of gene or variant functionality (i.e., involvement in phenotypically relevant biological pathways such as pathogen detection or antimicrobial response). A small number of significant interactions have been observed. These include interactions between *TNF* genotypes and ozone exposure in childhood asthma and wheeze, and interactions between microbial exposure and variants in innate immunity genes (in particular *CD14* and the toll-like receptors *TLR4* and *TLR2*) in the determination of atopy phenotypes (e.g., serum IgE, eczema, and allergic sensitization) (reviewed by Vercelli[92]).

Since the majority of genes studied to date as potential sources of G×E in asthma were initially pursued following direct evidence of gene involvement, these results do not provide original information regarding new genetic risk factors. Instead they allow a redistribution of heritability between G and G×E. As yet there has been no systematic genome-wide association analysis of G×E in humans, although supplementary analyses of loci implicated by direct (G only) GWA indicate that a proportion of these sites may be subject to environmental moderation.[49] A recent unguided analysis of G×E effects in mice showed that, depending on the specific type of interaction occurring, a proportion of G×E effects may prove undetectable when G×E interaction is ignored.[93] As such, studies powered to detect effects of G alone may not be capable of identifying the full complement of latent G×E interactions. Consistent with this, a recent genome-wide G×E linkage analysis for asthma resulted in the identification of several previously unsuspected genomic sites, all of which proved undetectable in the same dataset when the interaction term (early life passive smoke exposure) was not included in the analysis.[94] (See Chapter 3 for a further discussion of G×E interactions in the context of the lung.)

IMPLICATIONS FOR THE HERITABILITY OF ASTHMA

Since the first genome-wide association of asthma was published three years ago, there has been a rapid and dramatic shift in our concepts of disease causation and the factors underlying it. Until recently, the most productive approach toward disease gene identification was positional cloning, a technique that interrogated the entire genome (using a relatively sparse marker set) for regions of disease and marker co-transmission in families. This approach was highly successful for Mendelian traits such as cystic fibrosis, but has been less productive in the field of multifactorial (complex) traits. The positional cloning technique did nonetheless result in the identification of six genes contributing toward the etiology of asthma. These genes, however, were only found to explain a relatively small proportion of the total disease heritability, leaving the source (or sources) of residual heritability unknown. Founded on the premise that common diseases are likely to be caused by common alleles, the research emphasis has now shifted from genome-wide linkage to genome-wide association, using dense haplotype tagging marker panels containing many hundreds of thousands of markers to effectively capture virtually all common variation in the human genome.

Since the first genome-wide association study for asthma in 2007, the approach has been applied to asthma or asthma-related traits a total of 14 times, and has led to the identification of more than 30 disease-relevant loci; almost all of which have been successfully resolved to individual genes (Figure 2-2). Like positionally cloned genes however, these loci appear to exert relatively small effects.

The origin(s) of missing heritability has become a topic of considerable interest and debate. In this chapter, we have discussed several possible sources, including rare

Section I

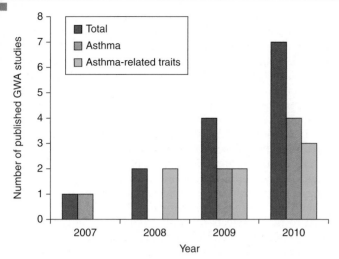

FIGURE 2-2. Publication of genome-wide association studies of asthma and related traits from 2007 to October 2010.

variants, situations of allelic heterogeneity, epigenetic effects, and G×E interactions. Systematic exploration of these sources is now required in order to determine their relative contribution to phenotypic variance, with the ultimate aim of specifying factors of sufficient size and penetrance to offer predictive or prognostic value in a clinical setting. Similar approaches (including GWA) may now usefully be applied to Mendelian traits such as cystic fibrosis in order to support the identification of cryptic modifier loci (altering disease progression or clinical presentation). Indeed the CF Modifier Gene Consortium has now completed a GWA study of CF, and the results will be available soon. Thus the genetic analysis of heritable chronic lung disease traits has come full circle, with techniques that were originally developed for exploration of multifactorial traits and diseases now being applied to single gene disorders for identification of new contributory factors including so-called gene modifiers.

Suggested Reading

Moffatt M, Gut I, Demenais F, et al. A large-scale genome-wide association study of asthma. *N Engl J Med.* 2010;363(13):1211–1221. This paper reports the findings of the largest GWA for asthma to date conducted by the GABRIEL Consortium *(www.gabriel-fp6.org/).*

Moffatt MF, Kabesch M, Liang L, et al. Genetic variants regulating ORMDL3 expression contribute to the risk of childhood asthma. *Nature.* 2007;448(7152):470–473. This paper reports the findings of the first GWA study for asthma.

O'Sullivan BP, Freedman SD. Cystic fibrosis. *Lancet.* 2009;373(9678):1891–1904. A comprehensive review of cystic fibrosis.

Vercelli D. Discovering susceptibility genes for asthma and allergy. *Nat Rev Immunol.* 2008;8(3):169–182. This review provides a comprehensive description of the genes discovered in asthma to date, and their biological functions.

Vercelli D. Gene-environment interactions in asthma and allergy: the end of the beginning? *Curr Opin Allergy Clin Immunol.* 2010;10(2):145–148. This review provides a detailed description of gene environment interactions in asthma.

References

The complete reference list is available online at www.expertconsult.com

3 GENE BY ENVIRONMENT INTERACTION IN RESPIRATORY DISEASES

CHIH-MEI CHEN, MD, AND MICHAEL KABESCH, MD

THE DEFINITION OF GENE BY ENVIRONMENT INTERACTION

In recent years, the term *gene by environment interaction* has become popular, but the meaning of the term varies considerably in different disciplines. When clinicians talk to statisticians and biologists, all may have their own view on gene by environment interactions. Gene by environment interactions need to be assessed by statisticians in large datasets, but they need to be proven experimentally in biological settings (e.g., by manipulating the presence of an environmental factor). Gene by environment interactions are only of clinical importance when they affect medicine and clinical practice. It is also important to note that the effect of gene by environment interaction may change with the age of the study subject. Environmental stimuli start to affect our health *in utero*. Throughout life, humans are exposed to different levels of environmental stimuli. Some exposures may have long-term effects (and the timing of the exposure is crucial for the effect size), while others may only cause strong short-term reactions (Figure 3–1).

In general, gene by environment interaction indicates some sort of interplay between genetic and environmental factors. The term may be misused in situations in which several independent risk factors (including genetic and environmental) contribute to the development or worsening of the diseases (so called *complex* or *multifactorial* diseases), while the dependence between these factors was not evaluated statistically or biologically.[1]

A statistical interaction is established only when the effect of one disease risk factor depends on another risk factor. A simple example is the interaction between the genetically determined expression of a detoxifying enzyme and the exposure to a toxic substance (environmental factor) on the occurrence of a disease. Disease will occur only when both factors are present. In epidemiology, the term *effect modification* is also commonly used to denote the existence of statistical interaction. When there is no interaction, the effects of each risk factor are consistent across the level of the other risk factor. Statistical interaction (or heterogeneity of effects) is usually defined as "departure from additivity of effects" as effects are not independent. In other words, the effect of a genetic risk factor is "multiplied" by the presence of an additional environmental risk factor. If the two risk factors are independent, they only "add up" but do not multiply. A simple example is shown in Table 3–1. It is helpful to draw such a table if one is to judge the presence of (claimed) gene by environment interaction. If combined effects are not multiplicative (but additive), gene by environment interaction is not present.

As indicated in an excellent review by Dempfle and colleagues,[1] interactions can be divided into removable and nonremovable types (Figure 3–2). An interaction is removable if a monotone transformation (e.g., taking logarithms or square roots of quantitative phenotypes) exists that removes the interaction. This implies that there is an additive relationship between the variables, just on a different scale. Therefore, nonremovable interactions are usually of greater interest. Nonremovable interaction effects are also called *crossover effects* or *qualitative interactions* (as opposed to *quantitative, removable interactions*).[1]

Confounding needs to be distinguished from interaction. *Confounding* refers to a mix of effects where a risk factor leads to a noncausative association. In gene by environment interactions, this relates to a correlation between genetic and environmental effects, which could be misinterpreted as interaction. This could be the case in a population with population stratification where unknowingly different ethnic groups are included in one study population and genetic as well as environmental factors depend on ethnicity.

Biological interaction is defined as the joint effect of two factors that act together in a direct physical or chemical reaction and the co-participation of two or more factors in the same casual mechanism of disease development.[1] In other words, genetic and environmental factors are acting directly on the same pathway. A gene by environment interaction can only be firmly ascertained when it is confirmed both statistically and biologically.[2] An observed statistical interaction does not necessarily imply interaction on the biological or mechanistic level.

In a statistical test, there is always the possibility of a false-positive finding or type I error (denoted as α). In studies of genetic effects on a specific health endpoint, it is common for numerous genetic loci to be considered simultaneously, especially in the case of genome-wide association studies. In these cases, statistical tests are used repeatedly, which results in multiple comparisons and an increase in type I errors. Nowadays, corrections for multiple testing are commonly applied in genetic studies, however there is still the possibility that the observed associations were random. Therefore, it is crucial to establish the biological plausibility and clinical relevance of the positive finding. *A priori* knowledge of biological interaction can facilitate the investigation of gene by environment interaction because correction of multiple testing strongly reduces the power. The power of statistical analysis also decreases with discrete outcomes. Therefore, unnecessary categorization or using cut-off values should be avoided.

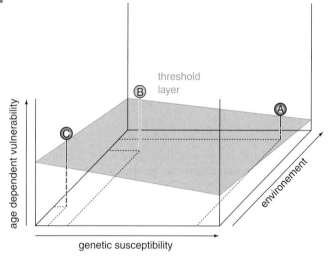

FIGURE 3–1. An asthma phenotype may result from an interaction between strong genetic and environmental effects independent of the timing of these effects *(A)*. However, contrary genetic predisposition and environmental factors may oppose each other, leading to no clinical expression of disease. Asthma may also result from strong environmental factors in the absence of a strong genetic predisposition *(B)*. Weak genetic susceptibility and relatively mild environmental risk may still lead to an asthma phenotype when risk occurs at a vulnerable time for disease development (e.g., the first year of life) *(C)*. (From Kabesch M. Gene by environment interactions and the development of asthma and allergy. *Toxicol Lett.* 2006;162(1):43–48. Used with permission.)

On the other hand, when an empirical gene by environment interaction is indicated (e.g., the association between exposure to certain carcinogens and the risk of disease development seems to be restricted to the subpopulation having the dysfunctional alleles), the observed

TABLE 3–1 RELATIVE RISKS (RR) FOR EXAMPLES OF ADDITIVE AND MULTIPLICATIVE MODELS OF ENVIRONMENTAL AND GENETIC RISK FACTOR INTERACTIONS

| | ENVIRONMENTAL RISK FACTOR | | GENETIC RISK FACTOR | |
| | *Additive Model* | | *Multiplicative Model* | |
	Absent	**Present**	**Absent**	**Present**
Absent	1	2	1	2
Present	1.5	2.5	1.5	3

(From Dempfle A, Scherag A, Hein R, et al., 2008. Gene-environment interactions for complex traits: definitions, methodological requirements and challenges. *Eur J Hum Genet.* 2008;16:1164–1172. Used with permission.)

interactions also need to be tested statistically to confirm whether the gene by environment interaction exists and the magnitude of it.

In this chapter, we will focus on asthma to illustrate how to investigate the effects of gene by environment interaction and how to interpret the clinical values, as most data on interactions in childhood respiratory diseases are available in that field.

GENE BY ENVIRONMENT INTERACTION IN ASTHMA

Asthma is a complex syndrome, and no standard method can be used to identify the disease with certainty. Based on a large-scale international study—the International Study

FIGURE 3–2. Examples of main and interaction effects. Phenotypic values depending on genotype G (two groups, e.g., under a dominant genetic model) and exposure E (also two groups, exposed *[yellow line]* and unexposed *[blue line]*). (**A**) Neither G nor E have a main effect and there is no interaction; (**B**) G has a main effect, E has no main effect, and there is no interaction; (**C**) E has a main effect, G has no main effect, and there is no interaction; (**D**) both G and E have main effects, and there is no interaction; (**E**) G and E have main effects, and there is an interaction (which can be removed by changing the phenotype scale, e.g., to a logarithmic scale); (**F**) G and E have main effects, and there is an interaction (which cannot be removed by any monotone transformation). (From Dempfle A, Scherag A, Hein R, et al. Gene-environment interactions for complex traits: definitions, methodological requirements and challenges. *Eur J Hum Genet.* 2008;16: 1164–1172. Used with permission.)

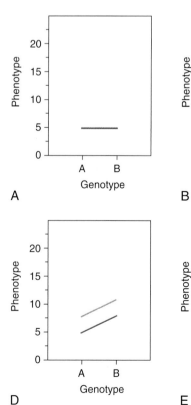

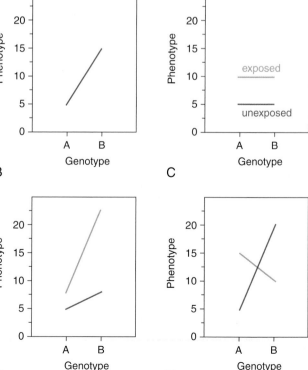

on Asthma and Allergy in Childhood (ISAAC)—the prevalence of asthma symptoms in 13- to 14-year-olds reached 31% in the United Kingdom and 17.5% in Germany in 2003.[3] Observational and interventional studies demonstrated that the development of asthma is a result of multiple genetic and environmental factors.[4,5] Family history is a long-established risk factor for asthma development with a positive predictive value ranging from 11% to 37% between different study populations, which underlines the importance of genetics in asthma etiology.[6] However, genetic variation does not fully explain asthma pathogenesis or epidemiologic findings. Numerous environmental factors have been examined in epidemiologic and experimental studies, including domestic and occupational chemical and microbiological exposure, diet, and lifestyle in general. However, no conclusive explanation was found for the development of asthma caused by environmental factors alone, and prevention strategies based on epidemiologic association findings are still lacking. Instead, genetic as well as environmental factors contribute to the complex disease as shown by segregation analyses.[7] In recent years, studies have attempted to investigate if gene by environment interaction effects truly exist in asthma, and thus better understand the development and course of the disease.

■ ENVIRONMENTAL TOBACCO SMOKE

Negative effects of environmental (passive) tobacco smoke (ETS) exposure on children's health are well documented. For asthma, ETS exposure is the single most prominent environmental risk factor for the development of childhood asthma worldwide.[8] Smoking during pregnancy and exposure to tobacco smoke in the home reduces children's lung function and increases the lifelong risk of asthma.[9] Tobacco smoke contains over 4000 chemical compounds, which include about 50 to 60 carcinogens, several mutagens, and many irritating or toxic substances. It has been noted that susceptibility to ETS exposure varies between individuals, thus a genetic component is suspected.

Genes may exist that increase the susceptibility to develop asthma specifically in the presence of tobacco smoke exposure.[10] Linkage studies that took smoking and passive smoking status into account differed significantly in their results from unstratified analyses. It was noted that some chromosomal regions that showed strong linkage with asthma and bronchial hyperresponsiveness (e.g., 1p, 3p, 5q, 9q) may harbour genes that exert their effects, mainly in combination with ETS exposure.[11,12] However, other linkage peaks for asthma or other allergic diseases seem not to be influenced by passive smoke exposure status. Thus, it may be speculated that a gene by environment interaction between passive smoking and genetic susceptibility may be causally involved in the development of asthma in some but not all children with asthma. Genes responsible for these linkage peaks in combination with ETS exposure have not yet been identified by positional cloning.

In addition to this systematic approach, specific candidate genes (selected by their putative function to be involved in a gene by environment interaction with ETS) have been investigated. Glutathione S-transferase genes (GST) are likely candidates as they contribute to biotransformation of xenobiotics and protection against oxidative stress.[13] GST enzymes, which are divided into classes such as alpha (A), mu (M), pi (P), and theta (T), may thus play a role in the detoxification of components found in passive (and active) smoke and also in the detoxification of other air pollutants. Conversely, genetic variations of GST can change an individual's susceptibility to carcinogens and toxins as well as affect the toxicity and efficacy of certain drugs. For GST classes T1 and M1, common gene deletions leading to a complete absence of the respective enzymes have been described. Approximately 50% of the Caucasian population show a deletion of GSTM1, and 15% to 20% show a deletion of GSTT1. In GSTP1, polymorphisms putatively influencing gene function and expression were detected.

It has been suggested that GSTM1-deficient children may have impaired lung growth in general.[14,15] The effect of genetic alterations in the GST system and smoke exposure on lung function seems not to be limited to childhood but may well extend into later life. Also, adult smokers with GSTT1 deficiency were shown to have a faster decline in lung function than those with functional GSTT1 enzymes.[16] In the same study, carriers of the GSTP1 allele 105Val showed lower lung function values, but an interaction between smoking and GSTP1 polymorphisms was not observed in this study or other studies.

In a study of more than 3000 children, the interaction of the genetically determined deficiency of the GST isoenzymes mu (GSTM1) and theta (GSTT1) with *in utero* and current ETS exposure was investigated specifically to assess gene by environment interaction models.[17] When ETS exposure was not included in the analysis, neither GSTM1 nor GSTT1 deficiency had an effect on the development of asthma. In children lacking GSTM1 who were exposed to current ETS, the risk for asthma and asthma symptoms was significantly elevated compared to GSTM1-positive individuals without ETS exposure. *In utero* smoke exposure in GSTT1-deficient children was associated with significant decrements in lung function compared to GSTT1-positive children who were not exposed to ETS. These findings indicate that environmental exposure to toxic substances is necessary to unravel the effect of genetically determined deficiencies in GST-dependent detoxification processes. Interaction models showed an overall trend for a positive interaction effect, above the expected multiplicative interaction between GSTM1 and GSTT1 deficiency or ETS exposure alone.

Experimental data support the observations from population genetics: In the lung tissue of GSTM1-deficient individuals, higher levels of aromatic DNA adducts have been found,[19] and cytogenetic damage to lung cells caused by smoke exposure increases with GSTM1 deficiency.[20] This indicates an increased damage to DNA and the destruction of tissue due to diminished GSTM1 function. Also, GSTT1-negative individuals showed significantly higher levels of DNA damage than GSTT1-positive individuals in experimental *in vitro* settings.[21] Furthermore, recent data indicate that GSTM1 may modify the adjuvant effect of diesel exhaust particles on allergic inflammation.[22] These observations may help to explain why

GST deficiency seems to exert a stronger effect on atopic asthma than on non-atopic asthma in population genetic studies.[17,23] Furthermore, a dosage effect for GSTT1 and GSTM1 alleles on the occurrence of atopic asthma was observed.[24] Studies have also investigated how polymorphisms of oxidative stress pathway–associated genes modify the effect of exposure to ETS on asthma; further evidence is needed to confirm the positive results observed in some of these studies.[25]

The modifying effects of genes involved in innate immune pathways on the association between ETS and asthma were also investigated because endotoxin is one component of cigarette smoke. Several genes were studied as potential effect modifiers, including *CD14, IL-10, IL-13,* and *IL-1 receptor antagonist (IL-1RA),* however, it is too early to draw any conclusions.[5,25]

AIR POLLUTION AND OXIDATIVE STRESS RESPONSE PATHWAYS

Previous studies showed that air pollutants, especially ozone and fine particles, are associated with the exacerbation of asthma symptoms.[26,27] A recent review assessing evidence from prospective cohort studies concluded that exposure to traffic exhaust contributes to the development of respiratory symptoms in healthy children.[28] Because oxidative stress was suggested as the major underlying mechanism of the toxic reactions induced by air pollutants,[29] studies have investigated modifications of the effect of exposures to air pollution by common polymorphisms with known functions related to the oxidative stress response. As noted earlier in the chapter, the most commonly studied genes include Glutathione S-transferase M1 (GSTM1) and Glutathione S-transferase P1 (GSTP1). GSTP1 polymorphisms are expressed in the respiratory tract and are also associated with an individual's susceptibility to oxidant defenses, xenobiotic metabolism, and detoxification of hydroperoxides. Studies from Mexico City showed that GSTM1 deficiency in children with a high level of ozone exposure increased the risk for asthma in an interactive manner.[30] In addition, it was reported that children who were homozygous for the GSTP1 Ile105 allele and were exposed to high levels of air pollution in China had a significantly higher risk of developing asthma.[31] While adverse effects of air pollutant exposures are mainly observed in individuals having a GSTM1-null genotype, evidence of the interaction effect between GSTP1 and exposures to air pollutants on respiratory diseases is not consistent.[25]

MICROBIAL EXPOSURES AND PATTERN RECOGNITION RECEPTOR

Microorganisms are ubiquitous in the environment, and there is a wide geographical variation of the quantities of different species and their compounds. Recent research has linked different levels of microbial exposures to asthma in support of the hygiene hypothesis. It was observed that children who were born in farm environments and continued to spend their early childhood in such environments had a lower risk of developing allergic respiratory diseases.[32,33] One of the major characteristics of the farm environment is the high level of microbial exposure. The effects of exposures to *endotoxin,* a constituent of the outer membrane of Gram-negative bacteria, were studied both in farm environments as well as inner-city homes. Studies investigating the effect of endotoxin exposure on asthma and allergy, however, do not always reproduce the protective effect observed in farm studies.[34] So far, it remains uncertain as to whether the protective effect observed in children from a farm environment was caused by exposure to one specific agent or exposures to an extensive variety of microbes.

Pattern recognition receptors identify pathogen-associated molecular patterns as part of the innate immune defense system. Toll-like receptors (TLRs), nucleotide-binding oligomerization domain (NOD)1 and NOD2, and CD14 are the most prominent examples of human pattern recognition receptors. CD14, a receptor molecule involved in the recognition of bacterial cell wall components (e.g., endotoxin) was the first to be studied in the context of environmental exposure. A promoter polymorphism was associated with serum levels of soluble CD14 protein in some studies and phenotypes of allergy in others. The CD14 polymorphism, which was identified in the promoter region of the gene, alters CD14 gene expression *in vitro.* Intriguingly, its effect seems to be dependent on the level of microbial exposure. This first was suggested by Donata Vercelli in her "endotoxin-switch theory"[35] and later was shown by association studies.[36,37] These data indicated that a polymorphism in the CD14 promoter modified IgE levels, depending on endotoxin load (which were measured in the children's mattresses as an indicator of microbial exposure). In farmer[36] and non-farmer[37] populations of children exposed to high levels of endotoxin, the polymorphic C allele is associated with lower IgE levels[36] and less allergy.[37] An opposite association is seen in individuals who are exposed to low endotoxin levels. However, the results are not consistent in the direction of the effect,[25,34] which may be caused by high variability of environment exposure levels and small sample sizes.

Genetic variations in TLRs may also predispose to allergies and asthma. In farm children (but not those growing up in rural environments without farm exposure), a polymorphism in the TLR2 promoter significantly modified the risk for developing allergic sensitization, hay fever, and asthma.[38] However, these data are derived from a subgroup analysis, and the prevalence of asthma and other atopic diseases is extremely low in farm children. Therefore, these data must be viewed as preliminary until they are replicated in an independent population with similar exposure characteristics showing the same direction of association.

GENOME-WIDE INTERACTION STUDIES (GWIS)

In 2007, the first genome-wide association study on asthma was published, and many more of these studies followed. In these studies, hundreds of thousands of common polymorphisms are genotyped per individual covering large areas of the genome. These data can be the basis for genome-wide interaction studies in which a systematic approach on gene by environment interaction analysis can be performed. A first study of this kind was published. It focused on genome by farming effect interaction,[39] and further studies on genome by smoking (active and passive smoke exposure) are in progress. In the first published GWIS, none of the previous suggested polymorphisms in candidate genes for genome by farming (or microbial) exposure interaction effects were found to be significant. However, a number of rare variants in genes so far unrelated to asthma were identified to show gene by environment interaction with farm exposure. Replication of GWIS as well as identification of biological plausibility for the statistical interactions need to be established before conclusions are possible.

EPIGENETICS: GENETIC AND ENVIRONMENTAL FACTORS

Epigenetics describes the fact that environmental factors can imprint on DNA without changing the nucleotide sequence of the genome by modifying the tertiary structure of DNA. A variety of molecular mechanisms are involved in epigenetic regulation, including posttranscriptional histone modifications, histone variants, ATP-dependent chromatin remodeling complexes, polycomb/trithorax protein complexes, small and other non-coding RNAs (siRNA and miRNAs), and DNA methylation. Epigenetic mechanisms seem to be important in cancer development, but very little is known about these effects in complex diseases such as asthma. Epigenetic studies in asthma are still at a very early stage. It would be surprising if epigenetic regulation was not involved in the development of asthma, which is driven by environmental as well as genetic susceptibility factors. However, existing epigenetic data is sparse, and to study epigenetics in asthma is a daunting task for the future.[40] Table 3–2 provides an overview on environmental factors related to asthma that may influence the mechanisms and genes involved in its development.

CONCLUSION

Based on previous research, there are reasons to believe that many genetic and environmental factors interact to cause asthma. However, genetic studies have generally ignored environmental factors, and environmental studies have generally ignored genetics. Thus, there are relatively few examples of specific gene by environment interactions in relation to asthma. Genetic studies assuming equal environmental exposure lead to false-negative findings when the effect of the specific gene is small. Environmental studies neglecting the effect of genetics lead to inconsistency. One of the major difficulties in gene-related research is the lack of statistical power, which can only be overcome by international collaborations. Furthermore, environmental exposure measurements need to be standardized. For example, exposures to air pollutants may be measured by personal monitoring or stationary monitoring, which are hardly comparable. Finally, for complex diseases, the power of detecting gene by environment interactions can also be enhanced by better-defined health endpoints, a challenge for such a vague entity as asthma.

Thus, while there is good reason to believe that gene by environment interactions play a role in asthma and other respiratory diseases in childhood, the evidence for such interactions is still slim and controversial. However, further investigations into gene by environment interactions are valuable as they could provide insight into mechanisms leading to asthma development and open the door for personalized medicine and true prevention of respiratory diseases in childhood.

TABLE 3–2 ENVIRONMENTAL FACTORS THAT HAVE BEEN REPORTED TO INFLUENCE ASTHMA AND EVIDENCE FOR CONSEQUENCES AT THE LEVEL OF EPIGENETIC MODIFICATIONS INDUCED BY THE SAME ENVIRONMENTAL FACTORS

ENVIRONMENTAL FACTOR	GENES PUTATIVELY INVOLVED IN GENE-ENVIRONMENT EFFECTS	EPIGENETIC MODIFICATIONS INDUCED BY THE ENVIRONMENTAL FACTOR	TARGET OF EPIGENETIC EFFECTS	TISSUE ANALYZED/DISEASE CONTEXT
Passive smoking	*IL1R*	DNA methylation	Global	Mouse lung tissue/lung cancer
In utero smoking	*GSTM1/GSTP1*	DNA methylation	Global + *AXL PTPRO*	Human buccal cells/effects of *in utero* tobacco smoke
Ozone/oxidative stress	*TNF*[41]	DNA methylation	Global	Murine melanocytes/cancer
Farm exposure	Innate immunity receptors	No data available	No data available	No data available
Endotoxin	*CD14*	Chromatin remodeling	*TNF/IL-1β*	Human promonocytic cells (THP-1), blood leukocytes/systemic inflammation

(From Kabesch M, Michel S, Tost J. Epigenetic mechanisms and the relationship to childhood asthma. *Eur Respir J.* 2010;36(4):950–961. Used with permission.)

Suggested Reading

Dempfle A, Scherag A, Hein R, et al. Gene-environment interactions for complex traits: definitions, methodological requirements and challenges. *Eur J Hum Genet*. 2008;16:1164–1172.

Ege M, Strachan DP, Cookson WO, et al. Gene-environment interaction for childhood asthma and exposure to farming in Central Europe. *J Allergy Clin Immunol*. 2010;127(1):138–144.

Kabesch M. Gene by environment interactions and the development of asthma and allergy. *Toxicol Lett*. 2006;162:43–48.

Kabesch M, Michel S, Tost J. Genetic mechanisms and the relationship to childhood asthma. *Eur Respir J*. 2010;36:950–961.

London SJ, Romieu I. Gene by environment interaction in asthma. *Annu Rev Public Health*. 2009;30:55–80.

Meyers DA, Postma DS, Stine OC, et al. Genome screen for asthma and bronchial hyperresponsiveness: interactions with passive smoke exposure. *J Allergy Clin Immunol*. 2005;115:1169–1175.

Vercelli D. Learning from discrepancies: CD14 polymorphisms, atopy and the endotoxin switch. *Clin Exp Allergy*. 2003;33:153–155.

References

The complete reference list is available online at www.expertconsult.com

4 THE SURFACTANT SYSTEM

PAUL KINGMA, MD, PhD, AND ALAN H. JOBE, MD, PhD

Pulmonary surfactant is a complex substance with multiple functions in the microenvironments of the alveoli and small airways.[1] The traditional functions of surfactant are biophysical activities to keep the lungs open, to decrease the work of breathing, and to prevent alveolar edema. Most of the components of surfactant also contribute to innate host defenses and injury responses of the lung. Surfactant deficiency states occur with prematurity and with severe lung injury syndromes. Recent studies in humans and in mice are defining an expanding number of genetic and metabolic abnormalities that disrupt surfactant and cause lung diseases that range from lethal respiratory failure at birth to chronic interstitial lung disease in later life. This chapter summarizes those aspects of surfactant biology that are relevant to children.

SURFACTANT COMPOSITION

Metabolism

Surfactant recovered from lungs by bronchoalveolar lavage contains about 80% phospholipids, about 8% protein, and about 8% neutral lipids, primarily cholesterol (Figure 4-1).[2] The phosphatidylcholine species of the phospholipids contribute about 70% by weight to surfactant. The phospholipids in surfactant are unique relative to the lipid composition of lung tissue or other organs. About 50% of the phosphatidylcholine species have two palmitic acids or other saturated fatty acids esterified to the glycerol-phosphorylcholine backbone, resulting in "saturated" phosphatidylcholine, which is the principal surface-active component of surfactant. About 8% of surfactant is the acidic phospholipid phosphatidylglycerol. Surfactant from the immature fetus contains relatively large amounts of phosphatidylinositol, which then decreases as phosphatidylglycerol appears with lung maturity.[3]

Four primary surfactant proteins have been identified: surfactant proteins A, B, C, and D.[4,5] Initial analyses of these proteins suggested that the hydrophilic surfactant protein A (SP-A) and surfactant protein D (SP-D) are primarily involved in pulmonary innate immunity, whereas the hydrophobic surfactant protein B (SP-B) and surfactant protein C (SP-C) facilitate surfactant lipid physiology. However, we now know that the surfactant proteins often cross these lines of functional classification.

SP-A and SP-D are members of the collectin family of innate defense proteins. Collectins are defined by four structural domains shared by all family members: a short amino-terminal cross-linking domain, a triple helical collagenous domain, a neck domain, and a carbohydrate recognition (CRD) domain.[4-8] Three neck domains combine and facilitate the formation of a collagen-like triple helix that then aggregates to form larger multimers of the collectin trimer. SP-A is a 24-kd monomer that further assembles to a bouquet of six trimers with a molecular size of 650 kd.[9-11] SP-A is encoded by two genes (Sftpa) located within a "collectin locus" on the long arm of chromosome 10 that also includes the genes for SP-D (Sftpd) and mannose binding protein.[12] In humans, SP-A synthesis begins during the second trimester of gestation and occurs primarily in the alveolar type II epithelial cells, Clara cells, and in cells of tracheobronchial glands. SP-A is required for the formation of tubular myelin and has several roles in pulmonary host defense.

SP-D is a 43-kd hydrophilic collectin with a monomer structure that is similar to SP-A, although the collagen domain of SP-D is much longer.[11,13] Structural studies demonstrate that SP-D trimers further combine into larger multimeric complexes through N-terminal interactions that are stabilized by disulfide bonds.[6,10,14] Although larger, more complex forms have been identified, SP-D exists predominately as a tetramer of trimeric subunits (dodecamer) assembled into a cruciform. SP-D is synthesized by type II cells and by Clara cells, as well as other epithelial cells. Like the other surfactant proteins, SP-D expression is developmentally regulated and induced by glucocorticoids and inflammation.[15] In addition to the complex roles of SP-D in pulmonary host defense, SP-D also influences surfactant structure and is required for surfactant reuptake and the regulation of pulmonary surfactant pool sizes.[16,17]

SP-B is a small hydrophobic protein that contributes about 2% to the surfactant mass.[1,4] The SP-B gene is on human chromosome 2 and is expressed in a highly cell-specific manner. The primary translation product is 40 kd, but the protein is clipped within the type II cell to become an 8-kd protein prior to associating with phospholipids during the formation of lamellar bodies. SP-B facilitates surface absorption of lipids into the expanding alveolar surface film and enhances their stability during the movements of the respiratory cycle. A genetic lack of SP-B causes a loss of normal lamellar bodies in type II cells, a lack of mature SP-C, and the appearance of incompletely processed SP-C in the airspaces.[18]

The SP-C gene is located on chromosome 8, and its primary translation product is a 22-kd protein that is processed to an extremely hydrophobic 35 amino acid peptide rich in valine, leucine, and isoleucine.[19] The SP-C gene is expressed in cells lining the developing airways from early gestation. With advancing lung maturation, SP-C gene expression becomes localized only to type II cells. SP-B and SP-C are packaged together into lamellar bodies and function cooperatively to optimize rapid adsorption and spreading of phospholipids. Surfactants prepared by organic solvent extraction of natural surfactants or from lung tissue contain SP-B and SP-C. Such surfactants are similar to natural surfactants when evaluated for *in vitro* surface properties or for function *in vivo*.

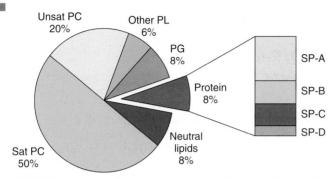

FIGURE 4-1. The composition of surfactant. Saturated phosphatidylcholines are the major components of alveolar surfactant. The proteins contribute about 8% to the weight of surfactant.

SURFACTANT METABOLISM AND SECRETION

The synthesis and secretion of surfactant by the type II cell is a complex sequence that results in the release of lamellar bodies to the alveolus by exocytosis.[20] Enzymes within the endoplasmic reticulum use glucose, phosphate, and fatty acids as substrates for phospholipid synthesis. The details of how the surfactant components condense with SP-B and SP-C to form the surfactant lipoprotein complex within lamellar bodies remain obscure. Ultrastructural abnormalities of type II cells in full-term infants with SP-B deficiency and ABCA3 deficiency indicate that these gene products are essential for lamellar body formation.[21] A basal rate of surfactant secretion occurs continuously, and surfactant secretion can be stimulated by β-agonists and purines, or by lung distention and hyperventilation.

The alveolar pool size of surfactant is about 4 mg/kg in the adult human.[22] The lung tissue of the adult human contains much more surfactant, and only about 7% of the surfactant lipids are in the secreted pool. The surfactant pool size per kilogram probably changes little with age after the newborn period. While no estimates exist for the full-term human, full-term animals have alveolar pool sizes of about 100 mg/kg, and this large pool decreases to adult values by about 1 week of age.[23] The alveolar surfactant pool size in the adult (and presumably young child) is small relative to other mammalian species (e.g., about 30 mg/kg in adult sheep), which may make the human lung more susceptible to surfactant deficiency with lung injury. Infants with respiratory distress syndrome (RDS) have alveolar surfactant pool sizes of less than 5 mg/kg.

The kinetics of surfactant metabolism have been extensively studied in adult, term, and preterm animal models.[24] In all species studied to date, including primates, the surfactant component synthesis to secretion interval is relatively long and the alveolar half-life of newly secreted surfactant is very long, on the order of 6 days in healthy newborn lambs.[25] The surfactant components are recycled back into type II cells, and recycling is more efficient in newborn than adult animals.[26] These observations have been validated by extensive studies in preterm and term humans using stable isotopes to label surfactant precursors or components.[27] A limitation of the studies is the need to have an endotracheal tube in place to allow repetitive sampling of lung fluid. Depending on the labeled precursor, the time from synthesis to peak secretion ranged from 2 to 3 days, and the half-life for clearance was 2 to 4 days in preterm infants. Similar values were measured for term infants. In general, preterm or term infants with lung disease have surfactant with smaller pool sizes, less synthesis and secretion, and shorter half-life values. These measurements include term infants with pneumonia, meconium aspiration syndrome, and congenital diaphragmatic hernia. There are no measurements of surfactant metabolism for older children. In one report in normal adults using sputum samples, peak labeling of surfactant phosphatidylcholine occurred about 2 days after the labeled precursor was given, and the subsequent half-life was about 7 days.[28] These studies demonstrate that replacement of endogenous surfactant pools is slow and alveolar pools turn over slowly.

ALVEOLAR LIFE CYCLE OF SURFACTANT

After secretion, surfactant goes through a series of form transitions in the airspace (Figure 4-2).[20] The lamellar bodies unravel to form the elegant structure called *tubular myelin*. This lipoprotein array has SP-A at the corners of the lattice and requires at least SP-A, SP-B, and the phospholipids for its unique structure.[29] Tubular myelin and other large surfactant lipoprotein structures are the reservoir in the fluid hypophase for the formation of the surface film within the alveolus and small airways. The hypophase is a very thin fluid layer covering the distal epithelium with a volume of about 0.5 mL/kg body weight that has a surfactant concentration of perhaps 10 mg/mL. New surfactant enters the surface film, and "used" surfactant leaves in the form of small vesicles. The surface-active tubular myelin contains SP-A, SP-B, and SP-C, while the biophysically inactive small vesicles that are recycled and catabolized contain very little protein. The total surfactant pool size is less than the amount of active surfactant because 30% to 50% of the alveolar phospholipids are in catabolic forms in the normal lung. Pulmonary edema and products of lung injury can accelerate form conversion and cause a depletion of the surface-active fraction of surfactant despite normal or high total surfactant pool sizes.[30] Surfactant is catabolized primarily by type II cells and alveolar macrophages. Granulocyte-macrophage colony-stimulating factor deficiency prevents alveolar macrophages from catabolizing surfactant and results in the clinical syndrome of alveolar proteinosis.[31] The important concept is that the alveolar pool of functional surfactant is maintained by dynamic metabolic processes that include secretion, reuptake, and resecretion balanced by catabolism.

SURFACTANT FUNCTION

Alveolar Stability

Alveoli are polygonal with flat surfaces and curvatures where the walls of adjacent alveoli intersect. Alveoli are interdependent in that their structure is determined by the shape and elasticity of neighboring alveolar walls.

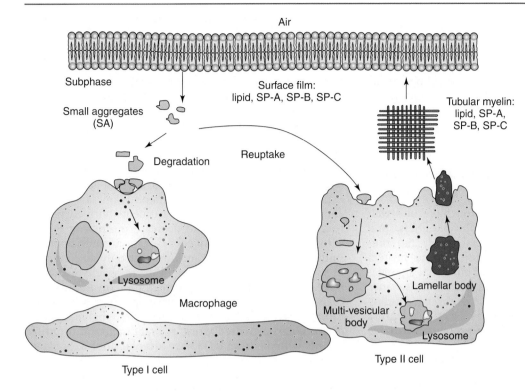

FIGURE 4-2. The alveolar life cycle of surfactant. Surfactant is secreted from lamellar bodies in type II cells. In the alveolar fluid lining layer, the surfactant transforms into tubular myelin and other surfactant protein–rich forms that facilitate surface adsorption. The lipids are catabolized as small vesicular forms by macrophages and type II cells and recycled by type II cells.

The forces acting on the pulmonary microstructure are chest wall elasticity, lung tissue elasticity, and surface tensions of the air-fluid interfaces of the small airways and alveoli. Although the surface tension of surfactant decreases with surface area compression and increases with surface area expansion, the surface area of an alveolus changes little with tidal breathing. The low surface tensions resulting from surfactant help to prevent alveolar collapse and keep interstitial fluid from flooding the alveoli. Surfactant also keeps small airways from filling with fluid and thus prevents the potentially ensuing luminal obstruction.[32] If alveoli collapse or fill with fluid, the shape of adjacent alveoli will change, which can result in distortion, overdistension, or collapse. When positive pressure is applied to a surfactant-deficient lung, the more normal alveoli will tend to overexpand and the alveoli with inadequate surfactant will collapse, generating a nonhomogeneously inflated lung.

Pressure-Volume Curves

The static effects of surfactant on a surfactant-deficient lung are evident from the pressure-volume curve of the preterm lung (Figure 4-3). Preterm surfactant-deficient rabbit lungs do not begin to inflate until pressures exceed 20 cm H_2O.[33] The pressure needed to open a lung unit is related to the radius of curvature and surface tension of the meniscus of fluid in the airspace leading to the lung unit. The units with larger radii and lower surface tensions will "pop" open first because, with partial expansion, the radius increases and the forces needed to finish opening the unit decrease. Surfactant decreases the opening pressure from greater than 20 to 15 cm H_2O, in this example, with preterm

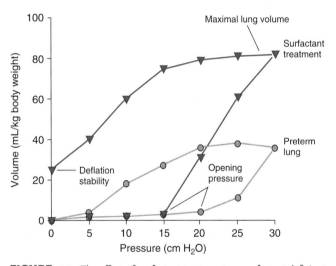

FIGURE 4-3. The effect of surfactant treatment on surfactant-deficient lungs. These idealized pressure-volume curves illustrate the effect of surfactant treatment with natural sheep surfactant on the opening pressure, the maximal lung volume, and the deflation stability of lungs from preterm rabbits. (Curves based on data from Rider ED, Jobe AH, Ikegami M, et al. Different ventilation strategies alter surfactant responses in preterm rabbits. *J Appl Physiol.* 1992;73:2089–2096.)

rabbit lungs. Because surfactant does not alter airway diameter, the decreased opening pressure results from surface adsorption of the surfactant to the fluid in the airways. The inflation is more uniform as more units open at lower pressures, resulting in less overdistension of the open units.

A particularly important effect of surfactant on the surfactant-deficient lung is the increase in maximal volume at maximal pressure. In this example, maximal volume at 30 cm H_2O is increased over two times with surfactant treatment. Surfactant also stabilizes the lung on deflation. The surfactant-deficient lung collapses at low transpulmonary pressures, whereas the surfactant-treated lung retains about 30% of the lung volume on deflation. This retained volume is similar to the total volume of the surfactant-deficient lung at 30 cm H_2O and demonstrates how surfactant treatments increase the functional residual capacity of the lung.

■ HOST DEFENSE FUNCTIONS OF SURFACTANT

SP-A and SP-D are pattern recognition molecules that bind a variety of polysaccharides, phospholipids, and glycolipids on the surface of bacterial, viral, and fungal pathogens.[4,5] SP-A and SP-D binding forms protein bridges between microbes that induce microbial aggregation and stimulate the recognition, uptake, and clearance of pathogens by host defense cells.[34,35] Although binding and aggregation of infectious microbes is a critical feature of SP-A and SP-D physiology, these proteins also have more complex roles in host defense.

SP-A and SP-D have been implicated in the stimulation and inhibition of several immune pathways. Both SP-A and SP-D bind CD14 and inhibit lipopolysaccharide-induced expression of pro-inflammatory cytokines through CD14 and toll-like receptor 4.[36–38] SP-A binds toll-like receptor 2 and inhibits pro-inflammatory cytokine release in response to peptidoglycan.[39] Gardai and colleagues proposed a model by which SP-A and SP-D might stimulate or inhibit inflammation through the competing actions of signal regulating protein α (SIRPα) and calreticulin/CD91.[40] Their model suggests that in the unbound state, the CRDs of SP-A or SP-D inhibit macrophage activation by binding to SIRPα, which inhibits activation of NFκB. In contrast, if the CRDs of SP-A or SP-D are occupied by a microbial ligand, binding to SIRPα is inhibited and instead the collectins bind to the macrophage-activating receptor, calreticulin/CD91, which turns on NFκB and subsequently induces pro-inflammatory mediator release and alveolar macrophage activation. SP-A also may contribute to adaptive immune responses. SP-A inhibits the maturation of dendritic cells in response to potent T-cell stimulators and enhances the endocytic ability of dendritic cells. In addition, SP-A downregulates lymphocyte activity and proliferation.[41]

The hydrophobic surfactant proteins SP-B and SP-C may also have host defense functions. Although SP-B can inhibit bacterial growth *in vitro*, overexpression of SP-B or reduced expression of SP-B in the lungs of mice does not alter bacterial clearance, suggesting that SP-B is not involved in innate host defense.[42] However, elevated levels of SP-B in the lungs of endotoxin-exposed mice decrease pulmonary inflammation.[43] Thus, SP-B may contribute to modulation of inflammation in the injured lung. SP-C binds lipopolysaccharide and blocks the production of tumor necrosis factor-α by macrophages.[44] However, possible roles for SP-C in bacterial clearance or lung inflammation *in vivo* have not been evaluated.

■ SURFACTANT DEFICIENCY

The Preterm Infant with Respiratory Distress Syndrome

RDS in preterm infants is a condition of surfactant deficiency that initially does not include lung injury, unless antenatal infection complicates the lung disease.[45] The surfactant system is normally mature by about 35 weeks' gestation, but early appearance of surfactant and lung maturation is observed in infants delivered prematurely. Early maturation is thought to occur in response to fetal stress resulting in increased fetal cortisol levels, or by exposure of the fetal lung to inflammation as a result of chorioamnionitis.[46] Maternal treatments with corticosteroids are routinely given to decrease the risk of RDS if delivery before 32 to 34 weeks gestation is anticipated.[47] Induced lung maturation includes not only an induction of surfactant but also thinning of the mesenchyme, which increases lung gas volumes. Unless preterm infants have early lung maturation, they develop progressive respiratory distress from birth characterized by tachypnea, grunting, an increased work of breathing, and cyanosis. Infants who die from RDS have alveolar pool sizes of surfactant of less than 5 mg/kg. Although similar in amount to the surfactant recovered from healthy adult humans, surfactant from the preterm infant has decreased function, probably because it contains less of the surfactant proteins that are critical for biophysical function.[48] The surfactant from the preterm infant also is more susceptible to inactivation by edema fluid, and the preterm lung is easily injured if a stable functional residual capacity (FRC) is not maintained, or if the lung is overstretched.

■ THE INJURED MATURE LUNG

Acute respiratory distress syndrome (ARDS) describes an overwhelming inflammatory reaction within the pulmonary parenchyma leading to global lung dysfunction.[49] ARDS is defined by acute onset, an oxygenation index less than 200 mm Hg, bilateral infiltrates on chest x-ray, and a pulmonary capillary wedge pressure of less than 18 mm Hg or absence of clinical evidence for left-sided heart failure (see Chapter 39). The etiology of ARDS is multifactorial and can occur in association with lung injury secondary to trauma, sepsis, aspiration, pneumonia, massive blood transfusions, or near drowning to name some associations. It is a common disease, affecting roughly 15% to 20% of all patients ventilated in the adult intensive care unit (ICU) and 1% to 4.5% of patients in the pediatric ICU. ARDS has a mortality rate of 25% to 50%.

Impairment of surfactant with ARDS can result from inhibition, degradation, or decreased production.[30,50,51] The proteinaceous pulmonary edema characteristic of ARDS can inactivate surfactant by dilution and by competition for the interface. Plasma proteins known to inhibit surfactant function include serum albumin, globulin, fibrinogen, and C-reactive protein. In addition to proteins, phospholipases (along with their products), fatty acids, and lipids inhibit surface activity. Epithelial cell injury by inflammatory mediators can decrease surfactant production and contribute to surfactant deficiency. Normally in the lung, about 50% of surfactant is present in the bioactive form that has a high SP-B and SP-C content. In ARDS, small vesicular forms increase and the pool of active surfactant is depleted.

The phospholipid content is decreased and the phospholipid composition is abnormal in bronchoalveolar lavage fluid (BALF) from patients with ARDS.[52] SP-A, SP-B, and SP-C are also decreased in BALF from patients with ARDS. The surfactant protein levels can remain low for at least 14 days after the onset of ARDS. Changes in surfactant composition including phospholipids, fatty acids, and proteins likely represent alveolar type II cell injury with altered metabolism, secretion, or recycling of components. SP-A and SP-B concentrations are also reduced in the lungs of patients at risk for ARDS, even before lung injury is clinically apparent. In contrast, SP-D levels in BALF were shown to remain normal, except in a subgroup of patients who later died. Decreased SP-D levels in BALF were 85.7% sensitive and 74% specific in predicting death with ARDS.[53]

GENETIC DEFICIENCIES OF SURFACTANT IN MICE AND HUMANS

Mice with targeted deletion of the *Sftpa* gene (*Sftpa*[−/−]) survive normally without changes in surfactant composition, function, secretion, and reuptake; however, there is no tubular myelin.[54] Although seemingly normal at baseline, significant defects are detected in pulmonary host defense in SP-A–deficient mice when they were subjected to a microbial challenge. Clearance of group B *Streptococcus, Haemophilus influenzae,* respiratory syncytial virus (RSV), and *Pseudomonas aeruginosa* is delayed in *Sftpa*[−/−] mice and the recognition and uptake of bacteria by alveolar macrophages are deficient.[55-57] Oxygen radical production and killing of engulfed microorganisms by *Sftpa*[−/−] macrophages are markedly reduced, while markers of lung inflammation are increased following infection in *Sftpa*[−/−] mice.[58]

Despite the considerable innate immune defects that are associated with SP-A deficiency in animal models, we have yet to find a human susceptibility to pulmonary infection that is caused by an *Sftpa* mutation. However, polymorphisms (genetic variants) in the human genes for SP-A, which affect their function, have been identified, and humans with these polymorphisms have increased susceptibility to infections with RSV and Mycobacterium tuberculosis.[59] Analyses suggest that SP-A polymorphisms may also affect infection severity since young children with RSV infection who are homozygous or heterozygous for asparagine at the amino acid position 9 are more likely to need intensive care, mechanical ventilation, or longer hospitalization.[50] Although there are no clear associations between *Sftpa* mutation and pulmonary infection, a recent study reported an association between familial pulmonary fibrosis and two heterozygous mutations in the *Sftpa* gene that caused SP-A misfolding and trapping of SP-A in the endoplasmic reticulum.[60] The extent to which these and other genetic variants will serve as clinically useful predictors of risk will require more analysis.

Mice with deletion of the *Sfptd* gene (*Sftpd*[−/−]) survive normally, but unlike SP-A–deficient mice that have relatively normal lungs at baseline, *Sftpd*[−/−] mice spontaneously develop pulmonary inflammation and airspace enlargement. In addition, *Sftpd*[−/−] mice accumulate increased numbers of apoptotic macrophages, and enlarged, foamy macrophages that release reactive oxygen species and metalloproteinases.[61,62] When *Sftpd*[−/−] mice are exposed to a microbial challenge, the uptake and clearance of viral pathogens including influenza A and RSV are deficient, whereas the clearance of group B *Streptococcus* and *Haemophilus influenzae* is unchanged.[63,64] However, oxygen radical release and production of the proinflammatory mediators are increased in *Sftpd*[−/−] mice when exposed to either viral or bacterial pathogens indicating that SP-D plays an anti-inflammatory role in the lung, independent of the clearance of pathogens.[58,63,64] SP-D deficiency has not been described in humans, but polymorphisms at amino acid position 11 are associated with increased risk of RSV infection.[65]

Gene-targeted mice lacking SP-B and infants with hereditary SP-B deficiency demonstrate the critical role of SP-B in surfactant function, homeostasis, and lung function.[66] Targeted disruption of the mouse SP-B gene causes respiratory failure at birth. Despite normal lung structure, the mice fail to inflate their lungs postnatally. Type II cells of SP-B–deficient mice have large multivesicular bodies but no lamellar bodies, and the proteolytic processing of pro-SP-C (the preprocessed form of SP-C) is disrupted.[4] Infants with SP-B deficiency die from respiratory distress in the early neonatal period with the same pathologic findings.[67] Mutations leading to partial SP-B function have been associated with chronic lung disease in infants. Because SP-B is required for both intracellular and extracellular aspects of surfactant homeostasis, SP-B deficiency has not been treated successfully with surfactant replacement therapy and survival is dependent on lung transplantation. It is important to note that mice and infants without the adenosine triphosphate–binding cassette transporter A3 (ABCA3) have type II cells without lamellar bodies and the same lethal respiratory failure phenotype as observed in SP-B deficiency.[68]

SP-C–deficient mice survive and have normal surfactant composition and amounts. However, surfactant isolated from SP-C–deficient mice forms less stable bubbles, demonstrating a role for SP-C in developing and maintaining lipid films.[69] SP-C mutations recently were identified in patients with familial and sporadic interstitial lung disease.[70] In these patients, *Sftpc* mutations alter the ability of the protein to fold correctly and result in the retention of SP-C in the endoplasmic reticulum and the subsequent development of endoplasmic reticulum stress, which, in turn, leads to pulmonary cell injury and death. Histological features of lung disease in these individuals include lungs with a thickened interstitium, infiltration with inflammatory cells and macrophages, fibrosis, and abnormalities of the respiratory epithelium.

Section I

SURFACTANT TREATMENT OF SURFACTANT DEFICIENCY

Respiratory Distress Syndrome

The respiratory morbidities of preterm infants with RDS have decreased strikingly in recent years because of the combined effects of antenatal corticosteroid treatments on lung maturation and more gentle approaches to mechanical ventilation.[71] The original randomized trials of surfactant for RDS evaluated treatments given after the disease was established, generally after 6 hours of age.[72] Other trials evaluated treatment of all high-risk infants soon after birth to prevent RDS. Subsequent trials demonstrated that treatments of the highest-risk infants (generally infants with birth weights less than 1 kg) as soon after birth as convenient, and before significant mechanical ventilation, will minimize lung injury. However, many very low birth weight infants can be transitioned to air breathing successfully using continuous positive airway pressure (CPAP), and the decision to treat with surfactant can be made after the initial stabilization at birth.[73,74] An advantage of allowing the infant to breathe spontaneously with CPAP used to recruit and maintain FRC is that hyperventilation and overdistention of the delicate preterm lung can be avoided. Larger infants who develop RDS are generally treated with oxygen and nasal CPAP until the inspired oxygen concentration approaches 40%. They then are treated with surfactant. Preterm infants will respond to surfactant treatments even if the treatment is delayed for several days.

Full-term infants with severe meconium aspiration or pneumonia also will respond to surfactant treatments with improved oxygenation.[75] Surfactant also can improve lung function in infants with the group B streptococcal sepsis/pneumonia syndrome.[76] Current practice is to treat most infants with severe respiratory failure with surfactant because there are no contraindications.

The surfactants that are commercially available for clinical use in infants are made from organic solvent extracts of animal lungs or alveolar lavages of animal lungs. While there are differences in composition, the clinical results do not demonstrate any compelling differences in clinical responses. All of the commercial surfactants lack SP-A, contain SP-C, and have variable amounts of SP-B. Surfactants that contain synthetic peptides or surfactant proteins are being developed for clinical use.

Acute Respiratory Distress Syndrome

ARDS is a significant therapeutic challenge for intensivists despite recent advances in the understanding of its pathophysiology and new treatment modalities. Surfactant content and composition are altered in ARDS, resulting in decreased surface activity, atelectasis, and decreased lung compliance.[51] The injury is generally not uniform throughout the lung, resulting in overinflation of more normal lung and atelectasis and filling of alveoli with fluid in other lung regions. The injured lung makes less surfactant, surfactant is inhibited by the highly proteinaceous edema and inflammatory fluid, and the fluid-filled alveoli are difficult to recruit to improve ventilation. Multiple animal models of ARDS respond very positively to surfactant treatments when combined with lung recruitment ventilation strategies. Unfortunately, multiple large randomized controlled trials using different surfactants have not shown clinical benefit in humans.[77,78] Recent trials have evaluated surfactant treatment of selective causes for ARDS, but again with no overall benefit.[79]

The experience in adult patients with ARDS differs strikingly with the clinical responses of preterm infants with RDS. Somewhere in between are the clinical responses of term infants with meconium aspiration and pneumonia who have modest but consistent clinical improvements that can decrease ECMO use and save lives.[80] Several small trials and clinical experiences have suggested that older infants and children with diseases such as acute RSV pneumonia respond to surfactant treatment. A trial by Willson and colleagues[81] demonstrated that, for a range of children from 1 to 21 years of age with various causes of ventilator dependent ARDS, surfactant treatments improved oxygenation and decreased mortality. Future studies of surfactant intervention for ARDS should be refined to better define which populations benefit from surfactant treatment. Future studies also can explore the potential for surfactant components to enhance host defense in diseases such as ARDS.

Suggested Reading

Carnielli VP, Zimmermann LJ, Hamvas A, et al. Pulmonary surfactant kinetics of the newborn infant: novel insights from studies with stable isotopes. *J Perinatol.* 2009;29(suppl 2):S29–S37 PMID: 19399007.

Davidson WJ, Dorscheid D, Spragg R, et al. Exogenous pulmonary surfactant for the treatment of adult patients with acute respiratory distress syndrome: results of a meta-analysis. *Crit Care.* 2006;10:R41 PMID: 16542488.

Jobe AH, Kallapur S, Moss TJM. Inflammation/infection: effects on the fetal/newborn lung. In: Bancalari E, ed. *The Newborn Lung: Neonatology Questions and Controversies.* Philadelphia: Saunders Elsevier; 2008:119–140.

Perez-Gil J, Weaver TE. Pulmonary surfactant pathophysiology: current models and open questions. *Physiology (Bethesda).* 2010;25:132–141 PMID: 20551227.

SUPPORT Study Group of the Eunice Kennedy Shriver NICHD Neonatal Research NetworkFiner NN, Carlo WA, et al. Early CPAP versus surfactant in extremely preterm infants. *N Engl J Med.* 2010;362:1970–1979 PMID: 20472939.

Whitsett JA, Wert SE, Weaver TE. Alveolar surfactant homeostasis and the pathogenesis of pulmonary disease. *Annu Rev Med.* 2010;61:105–119 PMID: 19824815.

Willson DF, Thomas NJ, Markovitz BP, et al. Effect of exogenous surfactant (calfactant) in pediatric acute lung injury: a randomized controlled trial. *JAMA.* 2005;293:470–476 PMID: 15671432.

References

The complete reference list is available online at www.expertconsult.com

5 THE STRUCTURAL AND PHYSIOLOGIC BASIS OF RESPIRATORY DISEASE

Matthias Ochs, MD, and Hugh O'Brodovich, MD, FRCP(C)

Knowledge of the normal development, structure, and physiologic function of the lungs is required to understand the pathophysiology that is seen in disease. Historically, the understanding of lung function was derived solely from clinical observation and postmortem histologic examination. The development of invasive and non-invasive techniques that were capable of assessing lung structure and function in living subjects greatly improved our understanding of lung physiology on an "organ basis." There has been an explosion of knowledge in cellular and molecular biology, which is covered in detail in other chapters. This chapter will focus on the normal structure of the lung and organ physiology.

NORMAL LUNG ANATOMY AND CELL FUNCTION

Knowledge of normal lung anatomy is one of the basic requirements for understanding lung function in health and disease. Because detailed descriptions of lung anatomy are available elsewhere,[1-3] this section will focus on selected aspects of gross and microscopic anatomy to enable the reader to understand the physiologic changes that occur in congenital and acquired lung disease.

The shape of the lung reveals three faces: the convex costal face opposed to the rib cage; the concave diaphragmatic face resting on the diaphragmatic dome, and the mediastinal face, where the right and left lung are oriented toward each other. The right and left lung are each embedded in a separate pleural cavity and are separated by the mediastinum. Except at the hilum (where airways, vessels, and nerves enter or leave the lung), the lung`s outer surface is covered by the visceral pleura, which also extends into the fissures, thereby demarcating the pulmonary lobes (Fig. 5-1).

AIRWAYS

The airways are composed of two functional compartments. A proximal conducting zone (the bronchial tree) continuously connects to a distal respiratory zone (the alveolar region), where gas exchange takes place. The basic structure of the airways is already present at birth, therefore neonates and adults share a common broncho-pulmonary anatomy (Figs. 5-2 and 5-3). When airways divide, they do so by dichotomous branching, over an average of 23 generations, although the number of times that branching occurs varies. This airway variability has physiologic implications; different pathways will have different resistances to air flow, and a heterogeneous dis-

tribution of gases or inhaled particles may occur. As the bronchi branch and decrease in size, they lose their cartilage and become bronchioles. Ultimately, a terminal bronchiole opens up into the alveoli-containing gas-exchanging area of the lung. In the human, the gas-exchanging area begins with several generations of respiratory bronchioles (i.e., bronchioles with alveoli attached to their wall) that connect to alveolar ducts whose "wall" completely consists of alveolar openings. The most distal alveolar ducts end in blind alveolar sacs. The unit of lung parenchyma distal to a terminal bronchiole (i.e., the unit in which all airways participate in gas exchange) is termed the *acinus*[4] (Fig. 5-4).

The airways are lined with a continuous epithelium that gradually changes from a ciliated pseudostratified columnar epithelium in the bronchi to a ciliated simple cuboidal epithelium in smaller bronchioles near the gas-exchanging units. At the transition into the alveolar region, the epithelium abruptly becomes squamous. At all levels, the epithelium is not made of a single cell type, but rather a mosaic of several cell types: lining cells and secretory cells, often with rarer cells with specialized functions interspersed (Fig. 5-5). Ciliated cells predominate throughout the bronchial and bronchiolar epithelium and are responsible for propelling mucus from the peripheral airways to the pharynx (Fig. 5-6). This mucociliary transport system is an important defense mechanism of the lungs. The mucous layer has two parts, a superficial gel layer with high viscosity and a deeper periciliary sol layer. The cilia form a dense, long carpet on top of the epithelial cells, and their coordinated to-and-fro action propels the gel mucous layer toward the oropharynx. Cilia are a derivative of the centrioles, and there are approximately 200 of them on the apex of each ciliated cell. The cilia are anchored within the cell with a basal body that is oriented in the direction of mucous movement. The shaft of the cilium has a central pair of single tubules that are connected via radial spokes to nine peripheral pairs of tubules. The tip of the cilium has tiny hooklets that probably help grab the gel component of the mucous layer and propel it forward. The cilium has a beat frequency of 8 to 20 Hz and is coordinated both with other cilia on that cell and concurrently with the cilia on adjacent cells to yield a synchronized wave flowing up the airway.[5] Primary ciliary dyskinesia (PCD) is a group of disorders that includes Kartagener's syndrome and the erroneously named *immotile cilia syndrome*. In PCD there are defects within the tubules, in their inner or outer dynein arms, or in the radial arms that result in a disorganized movement of the cilia that precludes normal mucociliary transport and results in chronic bronchitis and repeated pneumonias (see Chapter 71). Submucosal glands, which are present in large and small bronchi, are

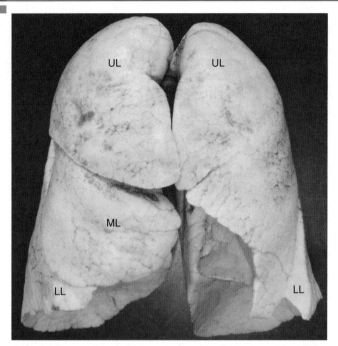

FIGURE 5-1. Dried human lung. The costal and diaphragmatic faces can be seen. The visceral pleura that covers the surface of the lungs extends into the fissures. The oblique fissure separates the upper lobe (UL) and lower lobe (LL) on both sides. The horizontal fissure separates the UL and middle lobe (ML) of the right lung.

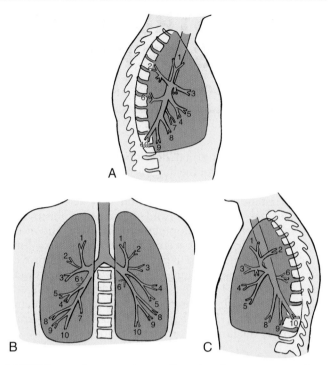

FIGURE 5-2. The nomenclature of bronchopulmonary anatomy, from a report by the Thoracic Society in 1950.[63] **A,** Right lateral view. **B,** Anterior view. **C,** Left lateral view. Segments: Right upper lobe: (1) apical, (2) posterior, (3) anterior. Right middle lobe: (4) lateral, (5) medial. Right lower lobe: (6) superior (apical), (7) medial basal, (8) anterior basal, (9) lateral basal, (10) posterior basal. Left upper lobe: (1) apical, (2) posterior, (3) anterior, (4) superior lingual, (5) inferior lingual. Left lower lobe: (6) superior (apical), (7) medial basal, (8) anterior basal, (9) lateral basal, (10) posterior basal. Note absence of medial basal segment (7) in the left lung. (Adapted from Negus V. *The Biology of Respiration.* Baltimore: Williams & Wilkins, 1955.)

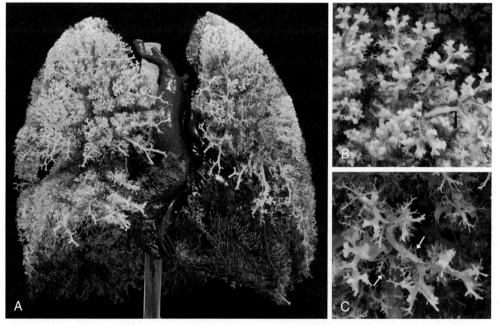

FIGURE 5-3. Resin cast of human lung airway and vascular trees. Airways are shown in yellow, pulmonary arteries in blue, and pulmonary veins in red. The chambers of the right heart and the pulmonary trunk (blue) as well as coronary arteries originating from the aorta (red) can also be seen **(A).** Higher magnifications show how pulmonary artery branches closely follow the airways, whereas branches of the pulmonary veins lie between bronchoarterial units **(B).** Small supernumerary arteries *(arrows)* take off at right angles **(C).**

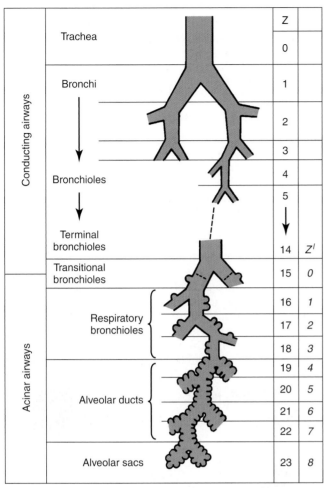

		Z	
Conducting airways	Trachea	0	
	Bronchi	1	
		2	
		3	
	Bronchioles	4	
		5	
	Terminal bronchioles	14	Z^I
Acinar airways	Transitional bronchioles	15	0
	Respiratory bronchioles	16	1
		17	2
		18	3
	Alveolar ducts	19	4
		20	5
		21	6
		22	7
	Alveolar sacs	23	8

FIGURE 5-4. Model of airway branching in the human lung over an average of 23 generations. The first 14 generations are purely conducting. Transitional airways lead into acinar airways, which contain alveoli and thus participate in gas exchange. (Modified from Weibel ER: Morphometry of the human lung. Heidelberg, Springer, 1963. From Ochs M, Weibel ER. Functional design of the human lung for gas exchange. In: *Fishman's Pulmonary Diseases and Disorders,* 4th ed. Fishman AP, Elias JA, Fishman JA, et al., eds. New York: McGraw-Hill, 2008, pp 23–69.)

the chief source of airway secretions and contain both serous and mucus cells. Goblet cells are seen in the trachea and bronchi (see Fig. 5-6). They produce mucin, a viscous mixture of acid glycoproteins that contributes to the mucous layer. Submucosal glands and goblet cells can increase in number in disorders such as chronic bronchitis, the result being mucous hypersecretion and increased sputum production. The basal cell, commonly seen within the pseudostratified columnar bronchial epithelium resting on the basement membrane but not reaching the lumen, is undifferentiated and acts as a precursor of ciliated or secretory cells (see Fig. 5-6).[6]

Whereas ciliated cells are still present in smaller bronchioles, goblet cells are gradually replaced by nonciliated bronchiolar epithelial cells (often termed Clara cells, although this eponym is debated[7]). These cells are characterized by their dome-shaped apex that protrudes into the airway lumen and by secretory granules. Their secretory products, which include the Clara cell secretory protein (CCSP), add to the bronchiolar lining layer. CCSP is thought to have immunomodulatory functions. In addition, these nonciliated bronchiolar epithelial cells are a site of Cytochrome P-450–dependent detoxification of xenobiotics, and they act as progenitor cells for the maintenance of the bronchiolar epithelium.[8]

There are several rarer cell types found within the airways; however, their functional significance is less well understood. The brush cell has a dense tuft of broad, short microvilli and is supposed to have sensory functions.[9] Neuroendocrine cells secrete mediators into subepithelial capillaries. Sometimes these cells are organized in clusters (neuroepithelial bodies) that are thought to have oxygen-sensing functions. Neuroepithelial bodies[10] are found more frequently within the fetal airways or in pediatric disorders characterized by chronic hypoxemia (e.g., bronchopulmonary dysplasia).

Histologically, the remainder of the airway consists of the submucosa, with its network of blood vessels and nerves, and a variable amount of smooth muscle and cartilage. Within the submucosa are mast cells containing

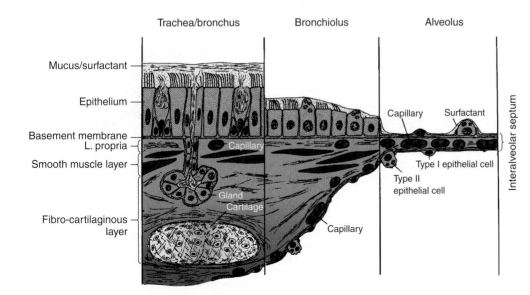

FIGURE 5-5. Schematic representation of wall structure along the airways. The epithelium is reduced from pseudostratified to cuboidal and then to squamous, but it retains its mosaic of lining and secretory cells. Only the trachea and bronchi contain cartilage as well as submucosal glands. Smooth muscle cells disappear in the alveoli. (From Ochs M, Weibel ER. Functional design of the human lung for gas exchange. In: *Fishman's Pulmonary Diseases and Disorders,* 4th ed. Fishman AP, Elias JA, Fishman JA, et al., eds. New York: McGraw-Hill, 2008, pp 23–69.)

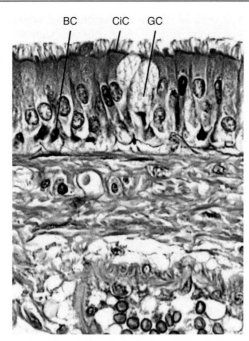

FIGURE 5-6. Light micrograph of the bronchial wall. The major cells types of the pseudostratified columnar respiratory epithelium can be seen: Ciliated cells (CiC), goblet cells (GC), and basal cells (BC). The mucosa's connective tissue layer (lamina propria), which contains blood vessels, can be seen underneath the epithelium. (Courtesy of G. Bargsten, Hannover.)

vasoactive peptides and amines, cells of the immune system (plasma cells, lymphocytes, and phagocytes), and submucosal glands. In the main stem bronchi, cartilage is present in C-shaped rings. However, as further branching of bronchi occurs, progressively less cartilage is present as plates. Cartilage adds structural rigidity to the airway and thus plays an important role in maintaining airway patency, especially during expiration. Congenital deficiency of airway cartilage and hence airway instability has been associated with bronchiectasis (Williams-Campbell syndrome) and congenital lobar hyperinflation (previously referred to as *congenital lobar emphysema*).

The smooth muscle content of the airway also varies with its anatomic location. In the largest airways, a muscle bundle connects the two ends of the C-shaped cartilage. As the amount of cartilage decreases, the smooth muscle assumes a helical orientation and gradually becomes thinner, ultimately reaching the alveolar ducts where the smooth muscle cells lie in the alveolar entrance rings. Muscle contraction increases airway rigidity in all airways.

Although it has been widely assumed that the airway muscles of newborn infants are inadequate for bronchoconstriction, this assumption is not correct. Even premature infants have smooth muscle, and although the amount may be statistically less than that seen in adults, it is likely enough to constrict the infant's much more compliant airways. Indeed, pulmonary function test results have demonstrated that airway resistance can be altered with bronchodilating drugs. The belief that infants have little or no smooth muscle in their airways is even less tenable in such disorders as Northway's old bronchopulmonary dysplasia[11] and left-to-right congenital heart disease, in which hypertrophy of the airway smooth muscle

has been demonstrated by morphometric measurement. Congenital deficiency of large-airway smooth muscle and elastic fibers is associated with marked dilation of the trachea and bronchi, which promotes retention of airway secretions and ultimately leads to recurrent pulmonary sepsis (Mounier-Kuhn syndrome).

ALVEOLAR REGION

Within the pulmonary lobule, defined as the smallest unit of lung structure marginated by connective tissue septae, one finds the lungs' region for gas exchange. The terminal respiratory (gas-exchanging) unit consists of the structures distal to the terminal bronchiole: the respiratory bronchioles (bronchioles with alveoli budding from their walls), alveolar ducts, and alveoli (Fig. 5-7).

As mentioned earlier in the chapter, the acinus is the portion of lung parenchyma distal to a terminal bronchiole (see Fig. 5-4). It is the basic functional unit of the lung. The acinus is approximately 6 to 10 mm in diameter in the adult lung. In the adult lung, these units have a total gas volume of 2000 to 4000 mL and a surface area of about 140 m^2 (Table 5-1),[12] yet all alveoli are within 5 mm of the closest terminal bronchiole. True alveoli are not spherical but more closely resemble hexagons with flat, sheet-like

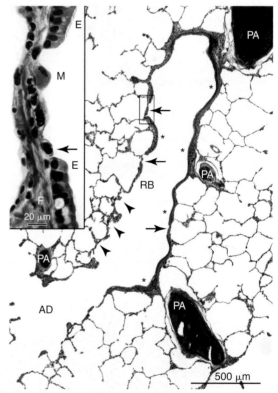

FIGURE 5-7. Light micrograph of respiratory bronchiole (RB) from human lung seen extending into alveolar ducts (AD). The wall is lined by typical bronchiolar cuboidal epithelium *(asterisks)*, which is interrupted by respiratory patches *(arrows)* and alveoli proper *(arrowheads)*. Note pulmonary artery branches (PA) following the respiratory bronchiole. Inset: Respiratory patch with capillary *(arrow)* and macrophage (M). The cuboidal ciliated epithelium (E) is replaced by thin squamous type I alveolar epithelial cells. Note thick fibrous layer (F) with smooth muscle cells. (From Ochs M, Weibel ER. Functional design of the human lung for gas exchange. In: *Fishman's Pulmonary Diseases and Disorders,* 4th ed. Fishman AP, Elias JA, Fishman JA, et al., eds. New York: McGraw-Hill, 2008, pp 23–69.)

TABLE 5-1 THE HUMAN LUNG IN NUMBERS

Alveolar number	480 million
Alveolar surface area	140 m²
Capillary volume	210 mL
Air-blood barrier thickness	2 μm

Data from Gehr P, Bachofen M, Weibel ER. The normal lung: Ultrastructure and morphometric estimation of diffusion capacity. *Resp Physiol.* 1978;32:121–140; Ochs M, Nyengaard JR, Jung A, et al. The number of alveoli in the human lung. *Am J Respir Crit Care Med.* 2004;169:120–124.

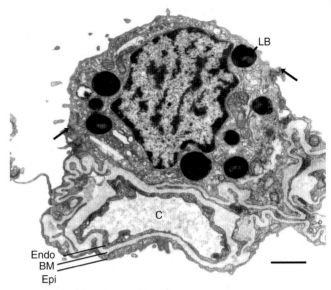

FIGURE 5-8. Electron micrograph of a human type II alveolar epithelial cell. The phospholipid-rich surfactant material is stored in lamellar bodies (LB) prior to secretion. On both sides, thin cell extensions of type I alveolar epithelial cells form tight junctions with the type II cell *(arrows).* A capillary (C) is seen underneath the type II cell. The thin side of the air-blood barrier is trilaminar and consists of the alveolar epithelium (Epi), fused basement membranes (BM) and the capillary endothelium (Endo). Scale bar = 1μm. (From Ochs M. A brief update on lung stereology. *J Microsc.* 2006;222:188–200.)

surfaces. The average alveolar diameter ranges from 200 to 300μm. Within the acini, interalveolar holes (termed *pores of Kohn*) are present in alveolar walls. Although they have been thought to provide channels for collateral ventilation, the fact that pores of Kohn are covered with surfactant[13] needs to be taken into consideration. Ultrastructural evidence suggests that they are used by alveolar macrophages to reach neighboring alveoli. In the newborn lung there are few, if any, pores of Kohn. This might contribute to the fact that relative to adult lung, infant lung is more predisposed to patchy atelectasis.

The alveoli are lined by two types of epithelial cells (Fig. 5-8). Type I alveolar epithelial cells are extremely broad, thin (0.1 to 0.5μm) cells that cover 95% of the alveolar surface. They are markedly differentiated cells that possess few organelles, and because they are so thin they provide a trivial barrier for gas exchange. Recent work has also demonstrated that these cells are capable of actively transporting Na⁺ with Cl⁻ and water following, and thus participate in the clearance of airspace fluid (see Chapter 38).[14] Type II epithelial cells are more numerous than type I cells, but because of their cuboidal shape they occupy only about 5% of the total alveolar surface area (Table 5-2). They are characterized histologically by microvilli and osmophilic inclusions termed *lamellar bodies,* which are storage sites for surfactant components (see Fig. 5-8).[15,16]

The type II alveolar epithelial cell maintains homeostasis within the alveolar space in several ways. First, it is the source of pulmonary surfactant and as such indicates maturity of the lung; surfactant decreases the surface tension at the alveolar air-liquid interface. Second, this cell is the precursor of the type I alveolar epithelial cell and thus plays a key role in the normal maintenance of the alveolar epithelium as well as in the repair process following lung injury. Third, it is capable of actively transporting ions against an electrochemical gradient and is involved in both fetal lung liquid secretion and in the postnatal reabsorption of fluid from the airspace following the development of alveolar pulmonary edema (see the discussion on fetal lung liquid secretion in "The Lung at Birth" later in the chapter). Two pediatric disorders associated with the type II alveolar epithelial cell are (1) its lack of maturity and surfactant secretion in respiratory distress syndrome (RDS) of preterm infants and (2) its decreased

TABLE 5-2 CELLULAR CHARACTERISTICS OF THE HUMAN LUNG

CELL TYPE	TOTAL CELLS (%)	CELL VOLUME (μm³)	APICAL SURFACE AREA (μm²)
Epithelium			
Alveolar type I	8	1764	5098
Alveolar type II	16	889	183
Endothelium	30	632	1353
Interstitial	36	637	
Alveolar macrophages	10	2492	

Data from Crapo JD, Barry BE, Gehr P, et al. Cell number and cell characteristics of the normal human lung. *Am Rev Respir Dis.* 1982;125:332–337.

lamellar body formation and surfactant secretion in surfactant dysfunction mutations (e.g., in genes encoding surfactant protein B or the lipid transporter ABCA3).

The cell junctions (zonulae occludentes) between type I and type II alveolar epithelial cells are very tight and thus restrict the movement of both macromolecules and small ions (e.g., sodium and chloride) (see Fig. 5-8). This tightness is an essential characteristic of the cells lining the alveolar space; it enables the active transport of ions. Also, these tight junctions provide a margin of safety for patients who are susceptible to pulmonary edema; significant interstitial pulmonary edema can be present without alveolar flooding, thus preserving gas exchange.

There is a thick side and a thin side to the alveolar air-blood barrier. Gas exchange is thought to occur predominantly on the thin side, where there are only the thin extensions of type I alveolar epithelial cells, fused basement membranes, and capillary endothelial cells (see Fig. 5-8). Capillaries undergo considerable stress (e.g., during exercise or lung hyperinflation) and must have great tensile strength. This strength is mainly imparted by type IV collagen located in the basement membrane. The thick side of the barrier consists of connective tissue, amorphous ground substance, and scattered fibroblasts. The thick side, in addition to providing structural support, acts as a site of fluid and solute exchange.[17]

PULMONARY VASCULAR SYSTEM

The lung receives blood from both ventricles. In the postnatal lung, the entire right ventricular output enters the lung via the pulmonary arteries, and blood ultimately reaches the gas-exchanging units by one of the pulmonary arterial branching systems. Arterial branches accompany the bronchial tree and divide with it, each branch accompanying the appropriate bronchial division (see Fig. 5-3B). In addition, supernumerary arteries take off at right angles and directly supply the gas-exchanging units (see Fig. 5-3C). The pulmonary capillary bed is the largest vascular bed in the body and covers a surface area of about 120 to 130 m². The network of capillaries is so dense that it may be thought of as a sheet of blood interrupted by small vertical supporting posts. The pulmonary veins that lie at the boundaries between lung units defined by bronchoarterial divisions return blood to the left atrium. By virtue of their larger numbers and thinner walls, the pulmonary veins provide a large reservoir for blood and help maintain a constant left ventricular output in the face of a variable pulmonary arterial flow.

The bronchial arteries (usually three originating directly or indirectly from the aorta, but variable in number)[18,19] provide a source of well-oxygenated systemic blood to the lung's tissues.[20] This blood supply nourishes the walls of the bronchi and proximal bronchioles, larger blood vessels, and nerves in addition to perfusing the lymph nodes and most of the visceral pleura. There are numerous communications between the bronchial arterial system and the remainder of the pulmonary vascular bed: a portion of the blood returns to the right atrium via bronchial veins, and a portion drains into the left atrium via pulmonary veins. Although normally the bronchial arteries receive

only 1% to 2% of the cardiac output, they hypertrophy in chronically infected lungs, and blood flow may easily increase by more than ten-fold. This is clinically important because virtually all hemoptysis originates from the bronchial vessels in disorders such as cystic fibrosis or other causes of suppurative bronchiectasis.

Histologically, the pulmonary arteries can be classified as elastic, muscular, partially muscular, or nonmuscular. The elastic pulmonary arteries are characterized by elastic fibers embedded in their muscular coat, whereas the smaller muscular arteries have a circular layer of smooth muscle cells bounded by internal and external elastic laminae. As arteries decrease further in size, only a spiral of smooth muscle remains (partially muscular arteries), which ultimately disappears so that vessels still larger than capillaries have no muscle in their walls (nonmuscular arteries). In the adult lung, elastic arteries are greater than 1000 μm in diameter, and muscular arteries are usually in the range of 250 μm. In the pediatric age group, histologic structure is not as easily determined from vessel size. During lung growth, a remodeling of the pulmonary vasculature occurs. Muscularization of the arteries lags behind multiplication of alveoli and appearance of new arteries. Therefore, the patient's age must be considered before histologic structure can be assumed from vessel size within the pulmonary acinus (Fig. 5-9). Notably, in the fetus and newborn the amount of pulmonary arterial smooth muscle is increased. This is functionally important because high pulmonary arterial resistance is a feature of the fetal circulation in association with a large right to left shunt via the ductus arteriosus.

The endothelium of the pulmonary vascular system is continuous and nonfenestrated. It is an intensely active cell layer and is not just serving a passive barrier function. The endothelial cell produces a glycocalyx that

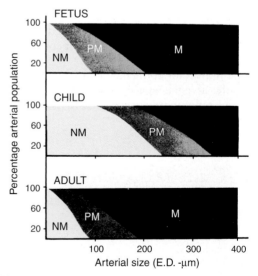

FIGURE 5-9. The populations of the three arterial types: muscular (M), partially muscular (PM), and nonmuscular (NM), in the fetus, child, and adult. The distribution of structure in size is similar in the fetus and the adult, whereas during childhood NM and PM structures are found in much larger arteries. *E.D.,* External diameter. (From Reid LM. The pulmonary circulation. Remodeling in growth and disease. *Am Rev Respir Dis.* 1979;119:531.)

interacts with blood-borne substances and blood cellular elements, thereby influencing such homeostatic functions as hemostasis. The endothelium produces von Willebrand factor, which is part of the factor VIII complex and is necessary for normal platelet function. Within endothelial cells, von Willebrand factor is stored in specific granules termed *Weibel-Palade bodies*.[21] Similarly, there are enzymes located on the surface and within the endothelial cell itself that are capable of synthesizing, altering, or degrading blood-borne vasoactive products. The individual cells are separated by gaps of approximately 3.5 nm in radius, which allow the free movement of water and small ions but restrict the movement of proteins. The cells and the basement membrane on which they sit carry different net surface charges, which affect the movement of anionic macromolecules such as proteins and thus affect lung water and solute exchange (see Chapter 38). The capacity of the pulmonary endothelium and its basement membrane to restrict fluid and protein movement is impressive. It has been estimated that in the adult human the amount of lung lymph flow is only 10 to 20 mL/hr despite a total blood flow of 300,000 mL/hr.

LYMPHATIC SYSTEM

There is an extensive interconnecting network of lymphatic vessels throughout the lung. The major function of this network is to collect the protein and water that has moved out of the pulmonary vascular space and to return it to the circulation, thus maintaining the lung at an appropriate degree of hydration. The lymphatic vessels travel alongside the blood vessels in the loose connective tissue of the pleura and bronchovascular spaces. It is likely that there are no lymphatics within the alveolar wall itself and that juxta-alveolar lymphatics represent the beginning of the pulmonary lymphatic system. Histologically, the lymphatic capillaries consist of thin, irregular endothelial cells that lack a basement membrane. Occasionally, there are large gaps between endothelial cells that allow direct communication with the interstitial space. Larger lymphatic vessels contain smooth muscle in their walls that undergoes rhythmic contraction. This muscular contraction plus the presence of funnel-shaped, monocuspid valves ensures an efficient unidirectional flow of lymph. In addition to helping maintain lung water balance, the lymphatic system is one of the pulmonary defense mechanisms. It aids in removal of particulate matter from the lung, and aggregates of lymph tissue near major airways contribute to the host's immune response.

INNERVATION OF THE LUNG

The lung is innervated by both components of the autonomic nervous system.[22] Parasympathetic nerves arise from the vagus nerve, and sympathetic nerves are derived from the upper thoracic and cervical ganglia of the sympathetic trunk. These branches congregate around the hila of the lung to form the pulmonary plexus. Myelinated and nonmyelinated fibers then enter the lung tissues and travel along with and innervate the airways and blood vessels.

Although the anatomic location of pulmonary nerves has been elucidated, their physiologic role in health and disease is incompletely understood. In general, the airways constrict in response to vagal stimulation and dilate in response to adrenergic stimulation. The postnatal pulmonary vasculature appears to be maximally dilated under normal conditions, and it is difficult to demonstrate any significant physiologic effect of either parasympathetic or sympathetic stimulation. The vascular response, however, is influenced by age and initial vascular tone. For example, in fetal lungs where there is an abundance of pulmonary vascular smooth muscle, vagal stimulation results in significant vasodilation, and sympathetic stimulation results in marked vasoconstriction.

Sensory nerves from the lungs are vagal in origin and arise from slowly and rapidly adapting receptors and from C-fiber receptors. The slowly adapting (stretch) receptors, located in the smooth muscle of the airway, are stimulated by an increase in lung volume or transpulmonary pressure. They induce several physiologic responses including inhibition of inspiration (Hering-Breuer reflex), bronchodilation, increased heart rate, and decreased systemic vascular resistance. The rapidly adapting vagal (irritant) receptors are activated by a wide variety of noxious stimuli, ranging from mechanical stimulation of the airways to anaphylactic reactions within the lung parenchyma. The rapidly adapting receptors induce hyperpnea, cough, and constriction of the airways and larynx. C-fiber receptors are the terminus of nonmyelinated vagal afferents. They include the J receptors that are located near the pulmonary capillaries and are stimulated by pulmonary congestion and edema; they evoke a sensation of dyspnea and induce rapid, shallow breathing along with laryngeal constriction during expiration.

In addition to the sympathetic and parasympathetic nervous systems, humans and several other species have a third nervous system within their lungs. The noncommittal name *nonadrenergic noncholinergic nervous system* has been chosen because its function and properties are not understood. Purines, substance P, and vasoactive intestinal polypeptide have been suggested as possible neurotransmitters for this system.

INTERSTITIUM

The interstitium plays several roles in lung function in addition to providing a structural framework that consists of insoluble proteins. The ground substance influences cell growth and differentiation and lung water and solute movement. The cells contained within the interstitial region of the lung not only play individual roles that result from their contractile or synthetic properties, but they also interact with other cells (e.g., the endothelium and epithelium) to alter the basic structure and function of the lung.

A continuous fiber scaffold is present in the interstitium, with an axial system (along the airways from the hilum to the alveolar ducts), a peripheral system (along the visceral pleura into interlobular septa), and a septal system (along the alveolar septa) (Fig. 5-10).[23] Most of the interstitial matrix of the lung is composed of type I

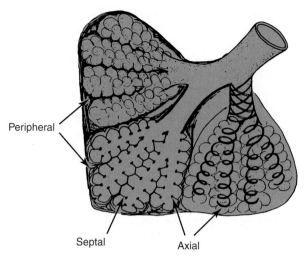

FIGURE 5-10. Schematic diagram of the fibrous support of the lung. (See text for detail.) (From Weibel ER, Bachofen H. How to stabilize the alveoli. Surfactant or fibers. *News Physiol Sci.* 1987;2:72–75.)

collagen which, along with the less common collagen subtypes, forms a structural fibrous framework within the lung. Elastin, a contractile insoluble protein, provides elasticity and support to the structures. Both elastin and collagen turn over very slowly under normal conditions. However, rapid remodeling with changes in these proteins sometimes occurs. In diseases such as α_1-antitrypsin deficiency (where neutrophil elastases degrade elastin) and pulmonary fibrosis (where there is increased amounts of collagen), there are marked qualitative and quantitative changes in these proteins. The remainder of the matrix is made up of proteoglycans and glycosaminoglycans. These carbohydrate-protein complexes can affect cell proliferation and differentiation in addition to their known effect on cell adhesion and attachment (e.g., laminin) and ability to diminish fluid movement (glycosaminoglycans).

Fibroblasts are capable of synthesizing components of the extracellular matrix (e.g., collagen, elastin, and glycosaminoglycans) and hence contribute significantly to the composition of the lung's interstitial space. They can be found within all of the interstitial regions of the lung, although their apparent structure may change, emphasizing the heterogeneity of this cell population.[24] For example, there are fibroblasts with contractile properties (myofibroblasts), some of which also contain lipid bodies in their cytoplasm (lipofibroblasts). Similarly, it is likely that morphologically similar fibroblasts are not similar in terms of proliferative capacity and ability to synthesize various types of collagen. Data suggest that fibrotic lung diseases are characterized by the loss of the normal heterogeneous fibroblast population and that there may be a selection for certain clones that promote inappropriate focal collagen deposition within the lung parenchyma.

Smooth muscle cells influence the bronchomotor and vasomotor tone within the conducting airways and blood vessels. They are also seen within the free edge of the alveolar septa together with elastic fibers, where they form an alveolar entrance ring that is capable of constricting or dilating. The smooth muscle cells form bundles connected by nexus or gap junctions that enable electrical coupling and synchronous contraction. The pericyte is another contractile interstitial cell that is found embedded in the endothelial basement membrane. It is believed to be a precursor cell that can differentiate into other cell types such as mature vascular smooth muscle cells.

There are a variety of interstitial cells that are concerned with innate and adaptive defense of the lung.[25] The interstitial macrophage and the alveolar macrophage are major effectors of the innate immune system, which they manage by ingesting particulate matter and removing it from the lung or by processing proteins or other antigens for presentation to adaptive immune cells. These macrophages are capable of secreting many compounds, including proteases and cytokines (substances capable of modulating the growth and function of other cells). B and T lymphocytes, including subsets such as T-regulatory cells (T-reg), are present in the lung and especially within the bronchus-associated lymphoid tissue (BALT), where they contribute to the humoral and cellular-mediated immune response. Further details on the innate and adaptive immune system are available in Chapter 7.

Although not within the interstitium per se, there are large numbers of intravascular cells such as granulocytes that adhere to the pulmonary endothelium. Indeed, next to the bone marrow and spleen, there are more granulocytes within the lung than in any other organ. These granulocytes can be released into the systemic circulation during such stimuli as exercise or the infusion of adrenalin, and this demargination is responsible for the concomitant blood leukocytosis. These leukocytes are also in a prime location for movement into the lung should an infection or inflammatory stimulus occur. There is much evidence to suggest that the pulmonary granulocyte contributes to the pulmonary dysfunction seen in acute lung injury or acute RDS. Leukocytes also contain proteases that are thought to play a role in the development of emphysema and in the lung destruction that occurs in cystic fibrosis.

GROWTH AND DEVELOPMENT OF THE LUNG

Prenatal Lung Growth

Lung development has been divided into various stages with names that reflect the respective histological appearance of the lung, the region of the lung that is most obviously developing, or both. The literature quotes different ranges for the different stages of human lung development. This concept is reinforced by the "overlap" between the different stages indicated in Figure 5-11. However, the available data contrasts with the mouse where at least the airway branching pattern is remarkably stereotypical in that all fetuses develop along the same timeline.[26] It may be that there are inadequate data for the human fetal lung to detect this stereotypical development during the longer gestation or that, as with all developmental profiles, each individual human fetus develops along its own timeline. Prenatal lung growth and development is discussed in greater detail in the literature[27, 28] and in Chapter 1.

The embryonic stage is the first stage of human fetal lung development and takes place from approximately

FETAL AND POSTNATAL LUNG DEVELOPMENT AND GROWTH

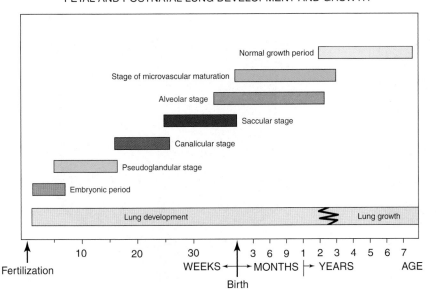

FIGURE 5-11. Various stages of lung development. The actual separation of individual stages is not discrete, and it overlaps. Note that the alveolar stage commences before normal term birth. (From Zeltner TB, Burri PH. The postnatal development and growth of the human lung. II. Morphology. *Respir Physiol.* 1987;67:269–282.)

3 to 6 weeks' gestational age (GA). The lung first appears as a ventral outpouching of the primitive gut. The primary bronchi elongate into the mesenchyme and divide into the two main bronchi. Another key event is that the main pulmonary artery arises from the sixth pharyngeal arch. Congenital abnormalities of the lung may occur during this stage (e.g. lung agenesis, tracheobronchial fistula).

The pseudoglandular stage occurs from approximately 6 to 16 weeks' GA. During this period, airway branching continues and the mesenchyme differentiates into cartilage, smooth muscle, and connective tissue around the epithelial tubes. By the end of the pseudoglandular period, all major conducting airways, including the terminal bronchioles, have formed. Arteries are evident alongside the conducting airways, and by the end of the pseudoglandular period all pre-acinar arterial branches have formed. Congenital abnormalities of the lung may occur during this stage (e.g., bronchopulmonary sequestration, cystic adenomatoid malformation, and congenital diaphragmatic hernia).

The canalicular stage occurs from approximately 16 to 26 weeks' GA, and during that time the respiratory bronchioles develop. By the end of this stage, each ends in a *terminal sac* (also termed a *saccule*). The glandular appearance is lost as the interstitium has less connective tissue and the lung develops a rich vascular supply that is closely associated with the respiratory bronchioles.

The saccular stage occurs from approximately 26 to 36 weeks' GA. During this period, significant capillary proliferation and thinning of the epithelium permits close contact between the airspace and the bloodstream, thus enabling gas exchange. Elastic fibers, which will be important in subsequent true alveolar development, begin to be laid down. At this time, cuboidal (type II) and thin (type I) epithelial cells begin to line the airspace.

The alveolar period commences at approximately 36 weeks' GA. Secondary septa form on the walls of the saccules and grow into the lumen forming the walls of true alveoli.

Distention of the lungs' airspaces by fetal lung liquid is essential for normal lung development. This fluid is neither a mere ultrafiltrate of plasma nor aspirated amniotic fluid. Rather it is generated by the epithelium's active secretion of chloride into the developing lung's lumen with sodium and water following passively (Fig. 5-12A). An inadequate amount of fetal lung liquid is associated with lung hypoplasia.

Congenital abnormalities of the lung may occur during the various stages.[28] In addition, factors such as oligohydramnios or decreased fetal breathing may interfere with the development of the distal lung unit, including the development of alveoli. In contrast, if there is obstruction to outflow of tracheal fluid, as occurs in laryngeal atresia, there is pulmonary hyperplasia.

THE LUNG AT BIRTH

Many dramatic changes must occur in the lungs during the transition from intrauterine to extrauterine life. The lung's epithelium must change from fluid secretion to fluid absorption, the distal lung units must fill with and retain inhaled air, and blood flow must increase approximately 20-fold.

At the time of birth, the lungs contain approximately 30 mL/kg of fetal lung liquid. Approximately ⅓ of this fluid is squeezed out during a vaginal delivery, but all of the fluid remains in the airspaces in an infant born by caesarian section. Thus, fetal lung liquid secretion must either greatly decrease or cease totally, and the fluid must be removed. Catecholamines released during labor can temporarily convert the fetal lung from a fluid-secreting organ to a fluid-absorbing organ[29] by initiating the active transport of sodium by the distal lung epithelium (see Fig. 5-12B). The clearance of fetal lung liquid from the newborn's airspaces takes many hours, and the increase in oxygen tension at the time of birth[30] is one key factor that permanently converts the lung epithelium into a sodium-absorbing mode.

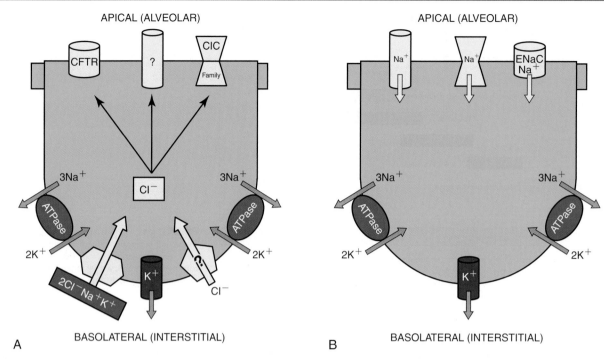

FIGURE 5-12. A, The polarized epithelium lining the fetal lung's lumen actively secretes Cl⁻, with Na⁺ and H_2O following, which creates in the fluid that distends the fetal lung. Cl⁻ enters on the basolateral side through membrane-bound protein transporters and is secreted out the apical membrane through different chloride channels, one of which is the chloride channel encoded by the cystic fibrosis transmembrane regulator (CFTR). The electrochemical gradient that drives the secretion is created by the basolateral Na⁺/K⁺ ATPase and K⁺ permeant ion channels. **B,** The polarized epithelium lining the perinatal and postnatal distal lung actively absorbs Na⁺, with Cl⁻ and H_2O following, which clears the fetal lung liquid that is present at birth. Na⁺ enters the cell down its electrochemical gradient through membrane-bound Na permeant ion channels located on the apical membrane. The basolateral Na⁺/K⁺ ATPase extrudes the intracellular Na⁺ across the basolateral membrane to the interstitial space. The electrochemical gradient that drives the absorption is created by the basolateral Na⁺/K⁺ ATPase and K⁺ permeant ion channels. A recent summary of research on luminal lung liquid and electrolyte transport is available.[65]

In utero, little blood flows through the lung despite a relatively high perfusion pressure. This is because of the abundance of pulmonary vascular smooth muscle and the vasoconstrictor effect of the low fetal partial pressure of oxygen (Po_2) (<30 mm Hg). Although during the last trimester, concomitant with surfactant production, blood flow increases to 7% of the cardiac output, it is only at birth that marked increases in the capacity and distensibility of the pulmonary vasculature occur. Several mechanisms are responsible for the changes in circulation. Inflation of the lung with air results in mechanical distention of the vessels, and improvement in oxygenation removes hypoxic vasoconstriction. In addition, the increase in partial pressure of oxygen in arterial blood (Pao_2) and changes in flow result in the release of mediators that contribute to the vasoconstriction of the ductus arteriosus[31] and umbilical vessels and dilation of the pulmonary vascular bed. After birth the vessels dilate, which allows the necessary blood flow to the lungs, and the measured wall/lumen ratio decreases. After about 10 days of extrauterine life, the lumina are wider, regardless of the gestational age of the baby.

POSTNATAL LUNG GROWTH

Postnatal lung growth continues throughout infancy and childhood and into the adolescent years. Throughout life, the average values of lung lobe weight expressed

as a percentage of total lung weight are approximately: right upper lobe 20%, right middle lobe 8%, right lower lobe 25%, left upper lobe 22%, and left lower lobe 25%. Throughout the pediatric years, the tracheal diameter approximately triples and the airways increase in their cross-sectional diameter (Fig. 5-13). Excised human lung

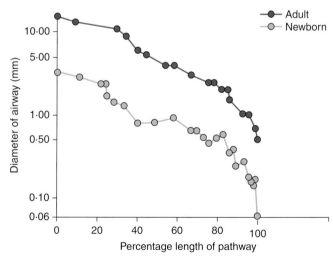

FIGURE 5-13. Diameter of the airway at different percentage points along the axial pathway in an adult lung and in the newborn lung. The pathway begins at the trachea, and the distal end of the terminal bronchiole corresponds to the 100% point. (Reproduced from Hislop A, Muir DC, Jacobsen M, et al. Postnatal growth and function of the pre-acinar airways. *Thorax.* 1972;27:265–274.)

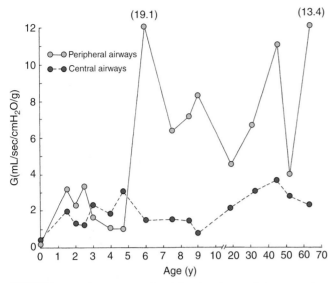

FIGURE 5-14. Comparison of peripheral and central airway conductance as a function of age in normal human lungs. The data are corrected for size by expressing the conductance as mL/sec/g of lung and for lung inflation by expressing all data at a transpulmonary pressure of 5 cm H₂O. (Replotted from Hogg JC, Williams J, Richardson JB, et al. Age as a factor in the distribution of lower-airway conductance and in the pathologic anatomy of obstructive lung disease. *N Engl J Med.* 1970;282:1283.)

studies suggest that this growth occurs until around 5 years of age and is associated with marked changes in the relative conductance of central versus more peripheral airways (Fig. 5-14).

Most postnatal lung growth involves the acinar area. New secondary septa continue to appear on the walls of the saccules and grow into the airspace, thus creating more true alveoli. Alveoli continue to increase in number through segmentation of these primitive alveoli and through transformation of terminal bronchioles into respiratory bronchioles, the latter being a process known as *alveolarization*. Alveolar dimensions and number both increase as the lungs and body grow with the internal surface area of the lung paralleling body mass (approximately 1 to 1.5 m²/kg of body weight). It is agreed that alveoli appear prior to birth, and various studies have suggested that there are approximately 20 to 150 million alveoli at birth. A morphometric study[32] of the lungs of 56 infants and children who died suddenly or after a brief illness indicates that there are approximately 200 to 300 million alveoli by the end of the second year of life, at which time alveolar multiplication slows markedly. After 2 years of age, boys have a larger number of alveoli and alveolar surface area than girls regardless of age and stature, and it is uncertain when alveolar multiplication ceases; however few, if any, new alveoli develop after 8 years of age.[32] Animal studies suggest that the adult lung can, under certain circumstances, develop a small number of new alveoli.[33] After alveolar multiplication stops, further growth of the airspace occurs through an increase in alveolar dimensions. In the mature adult lung, the final number of alveoli averages 480 million,[34] with individual subjects varying from 200 million to 800 million. The final number is related to total lung volume. An individual alveolus is

200 to 300 microns in diameter. As alveolar multiplication occurs, new blood vessels appear within the acinus. This explains the commensurate increase in the single breath diffusing capacity for carbon monoxide as the lungs grow.[35]

Prenatal (saccular) walls, as well as secondary septa that form postnatally during the alveolar period, contain a double-capillary network. The adult lung, however, contains a single capillary layer interwoven with a sheet of septal connective tissue. The phase of remodeling the septal capillary bilayer into a single layer (microvascular maturation) occurs from early after birth up to the age of about 2 to 3 years.

Healthy children grow along their lung function growth curve,[36,37] much like children grow along their own height curve. For example, if a healthy child is born with lung volumes at the 10th percentile, he or she will usually maintain this status throughout childhood.

When the structure and mechanical behavior of the young infant's and child's respiratory system are compared to those of the mature, but not the elderly, adult important differences emerge that are likely to influence the pattern of disease. Some of these differences, such as reduced lung recoil, are shared by the infant and elderly and likely influence the pattern of respiratory disease in both populations. The young lung lacks elastic recoil because elastin is still being created; as a result, airways are less well supported and there is greater airway closure; this favors inhomogeneity of gas exchange and the development of patchy atelectasis. The elderly have low lung recoil because they have lost elastin through the aging process, and there is greater loss of recoil when elastin degradation occurs by mechanisms promoting emphysema. The chest wall is relatively more compliant in the young child and stiffens with increasing age. As a result, the infant can develop paradoxical respiration. Respiratory muscle activation during inspiration can produce inward displacement of the rib cage, contributing to increased respiratory work for a given level of ventilation, particularly during rapid eye movement (REM) sleep. The deformability of the chest wall influences findings on physical examination. Chest wall–abdominal paradox may be normal in the premature infant during REM sleep but not in the older child or adult.

Postnatal lung growth can be impaired by restriction of the lung (e.g., in kyphoscoliosis) or augmented (e.g., in remaining lung postpneumonectomy). Lung capacities and flows continue to increase until late adolescence. Once adult life is achieved, then nonsmoking men and women have an annual decline in their FEV₁ of approximately 20 mL/year.[38] The rate of decline during adult life is increased when individuals smoke or have a history of repeated childhood respiratory disorders.

▰ VENTILATION AND MECHANICS OF BREATHING

The principal function of the lung is to perform gas exchange, that is, to enrich the blood with oxygen and cleanse it of carbon dioxide. An essential feature of normal gas exchange is that the volume and distribution of ventilation are appropriate. Ventilation of the lung depends on the adequacy of the respiratory pump (muscles and chest wall) and the mechanical properties of the airways and gas-exchanging units.

It is traditional and useful to consider mechanical events as belonging to two main categories: the static-elastic properties of the lungs and chest wall and the flow-resistive or dynamic aspects of moving air. Changes in one category may be associated with compensatory changes in the other. Thus, many diseases affect both static and dynamic behavior of the lungs. Often the principal derangement is in the elastic properties of the tissues or in the dimensions of the airways, and the treatment or alleviation of symptoms depends on distinguishing between them.

Before we discuss the mechanical aspects of lung function and gas exchange, it is important to review several basic physical laws concerning the behavior of gases and also the related abbreviations and symbols that will be used.

■ DEFINITIONS AND SYMBOLS

The principal variables for gases are as follows:
V = gas volume
$\dot{V}$ = volume of gas per unit time
P = pressure
F = fractional concentration in dry gas
R = respiratory exchange ratio, carbon dioxide/oxygen
f = frequency
D_L = diffusing capacity of lung

The designation of which volume or pressure is cited requires a small capital letter after the principal variable. Thus, V_{O_2} = volume of oxygen; P_B = barometric pressure.

I = inspired gas
E = expired gas
A = alveolar gas
T = tidal gas
D = dead space gas
B = barometric pressure

When both location of the gas and its species are to be indicated, the order is V_{IO_2}, which means the volume of inspired oxygen.

STPD = standard temperature, pressure, dry (0° C, 760 mm Hg)
BTPS = body temperature, pressure, saturated with water vapor
ATPS = ambient temperature, pressure, saturated with water vapor

The principal designations for blood are as follows:
S = percentage saturation of gas in blood
C = concentration of gas per 100 mL of blood
Q = volume of blood
$\dot{Q}$ = blood flow per minute
a = arterial
$\overline{V}$ = mixed venous
c = capillary

All sites of blood determinations are indicated by lowercase initials. Thus, Pa_{CO_2} = partial pressure of carbon dioxide in arterial blood; $P\overline{v}_{O_2}$ = partial pressure of oxygen in mixed venous blood; and Pc_{O_2} = partial pressure of oxygen in a capillary.

The measurement of pressures can be confusing because pressure can be expressed using different units. For example, atmospheric pressure at sea level can be expressed by many seemingly different, but similar, values: it is important to remember the following:

$$1\,atmosphere = 100\,kilopascals\,(kPa) = 760\,mm\,Hg = 760\,Torr$$

The unit Torr is named after Evangelista Torricelli, who discovered the principle of the barometer and used the height of a column of mercury to measure pressures; for general use, one can use the following equation:

$$1\,mm\,Hg = 1\,Torr$$

Both pleural space and ventilator pressures are typically described as cm H_2O since a water-filled manometer was the initial tool used to measure these pressures; it was very hard to measure these low pressures by looking at only millimeter changes in the height of a column of mercury. Care must be taken when reviewing the literature on pulmonary vascular pressures as they can be expressed in either mm Hg or cm H_2O. The conversion from cm H_2O to mm Hg is as follows:

$$1\,cm\,H_2O = 0.736\,mm\,Hg$$

Properties of Gases

Gases behave as an enormous number of tiny particles in constant motion. Their behavior is governed by the gas laws, which are essential to the understanding of pulmonary physiology.

Dalton's law states that the total pressure exerted by a gas mixture is equal to the sum of the pressures of the individual gases. The pressure exerted by each component is independent of the other gases in the mixture. For instance, at sea level, air saturated with water vapor at a temperature of 37° C has a total pressure equal to the atmospheric or barometric pressure with the partial pressures of the components as follows:

$$P_B = 760\,mm\,Hg = P_{H_2O}(47\,mm\,Hg) + P_{O_2}(149.2\,mm\,Hg) + P_{N_2}(563.5\,mm\,Hg) + P_{CO_2}(0.3\,mm\,Hg)$$

The gas in alveoli contains 5.6% carbon dioxide, BTPS. If P_B = 760 mm Hg, then,

$$PA_{CO_2} = 0.056(760 - 47) = 40\,mm\,Hg.$$

Boyle's law states that at a constant temperature, the volume of any gas varies inversely as the pressure to which the gas is subjected: PV = k. Because respiratory volume measurements may be made at different barometric pressures, it is important to know the barometric pressure and to convert to standard pressure, which is considered to be 760 mm Hg.

Charles' law states that if the pressure is constant, the volume of a gas increases in direct proportion to the absolute temperature. At absolute zero (−273°C), molecular motion ceases. With increasing temperature, molecular collisions increase, so that at constant pressure, volume must increase.

In all respiratory calculations, water vapor pressure must be taken into account. The partial pressure of water vapor increases with temperature but is independent of atmospheric pressure. At body temperature (37° C), fully saturated gas has a P_{H_2O} of 47 mm Hg.

Gases may exist in physical solution in a liquid, escape from the liquid, or return to it. At equilibrium, the partial pressure of a gas in a liquid medium exposed to a gas phase is equal in the two phases. Note that in blood the sum of the partial pressures of all the gases does not necessarily equal atmospheric pressure. For example, in venous blood, P_{O_2} has fallen from the 100 mm Hg of the arterial blood to 40 mm Hg, while P_{CO_2} has changed from 40 to 46 mm Hg. Thus, the sum of the partial pressures of O_2, CO_2, and N_2 in venous blood equals 655 mm Hg. This provides the physiologic reason why patients who experience a pneumothorax can eventually reabsorb their pneumothorax and do so more rapidly if they inhale gases with an $F_IO_2 > 0.21$.

ELASTIC RECOIL OF THE LUNG

The lung is an elastic structure that tends to decrease its size at all volumes. The elasticity of the lung depends on the structural components, the geometry of the terminal airspaces, and the presence of an air-liquid interface. When a lung is made airless and is then inflated with liquid, the elastic recoil pressure at large volumes is less than half that of a lung inflated to the same volume with air (Fig. 5-15). Thus, the most significant determinant of the elastic properties of the lung is the presence of an air-liquid interface.

The increase of elastic recoil in the presence of an air-liquid interface results from the forces of surface tension. What is surface tension? When molecules are aligned at an air-liquid interface, they lack opposing

molecules on one side. The intermolecular attractive forces are then unbalanced, and the resultant force tends to move molecules away from the interface. The effect is to reduce the area of the surface to a minimum. In the lungs, the forces at the air-liquid interface operate to reduce the internal surface area of the lung, and thus they augment elastic recoil. A remarkable property of the material at the alveolar interface, the alveolar lining layer containing pulmonary surfactant, is its ability to achieve a high surface tension at large lung volumes and a low surface tension at low volumes. Surfactant is a phospholipid-protein complex that when compressed forms insoluble, folded-surface films of low surface tension. The ability to achieve a low surface tension at low lung volumes tends to stabilize the airspaces and prevent their closure.

The exact method of lung stabilization and the concomitant role of surfactant in this stabilization can be debated. The classic interpretation is that without surfactant the smaller alveoli would tend to empty into the larger alveoli in accordance with the Laplace relationship, which relates the pressure across a surface (P) to surface tension (T) and radius (r) of curvature. For a spherical surface, P = 2T/r. The smaller the radius, the greater is the tendency to collapse. The difficulty with this hypothesis is that the individual lung units are drawn as independent but communicating bubbles or spheres (Fig. 5-16A). This is not representative of structure of the lung because the alveolar walls are planar, not spherical. In addition, the inside wall of one alveolus is the outside wall of the adjacent alveolus. This last explanation has been utilized to develop the interdependence model of lung stability, which indicates that surface and tissue forces interact to maintain the lungs' inherent structure, with the fibrous components playing an important role (see Fig. 5-16B).

The elastic recoil of the lung is responsible for the lung's tendency to pull away from the chest wall with the resultant subatmospheric pressure in the pleural space. Lung recoil can therefore be derived from measurement of the pleural pressure when no air flow is occurring and alveolar pressure is zero. (The pressure measurement is taken with the patient holding his or her breath for a brief period with the glottis open.)

The pressure within the esophagus can be used as an index for mean pleural pressure. This is a reasonable assumption as long as there is no paradoxical rib cage movement. However, it is not a reasonable assumption for premature infants, term infants in rapid eye movement (REM) sleep, and older infants with severe lung disease. For these infants, no average pleural pressure exists, and calculations of resistance and compliance will not be accurate using this method. When pleural pressure is estimated with an esophageal balloon, one must be careful to avoid artifacts resulting from the gravitational pressure of the mediastinum. For this reason, these measurements are best performed with the patient in the upright or lateral rather than the supine position. Once a series of pressure measurements has been made during brief breath-holds at different lung volumes, a pressure-volume curve of the lung can be constructed (Fig. 5-17).

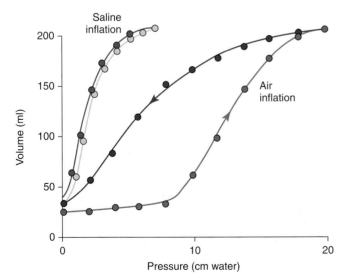

FIGURE 5-15. Comparison of pressure-volume curves of air-filled and saline-filled lungs (cat). Open circles, inflation, closed circles, deflation. Note that the saline-filled lung has a much higher compliance and also much less hysteresis than the air-filled lung. (From West JB. *Respiratory Physiology—The Essentials*, 8th ed. Baltimore: Williams & Wilkins, 2008.)

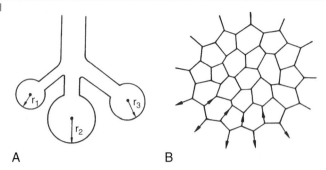

A   B

FIGURE 5-16. A, Classic model of the distal lung, in which individual alveoli would be controlled by Laplace's law: $P = 2\gamma/r$. Small alveoli would empty into large alveoli. **B,** Interdependence model of the lung, in which alveoli share common planar and not spherical walls. Any decrease in the size of one alveolus would be stabilized by the adjacent alveoli. (From Weibel ER, Bachofen H. How to stabilize the alveoli. Surfactant or fibers. *News Physiol Sci.* 1987; 2:72–75.)

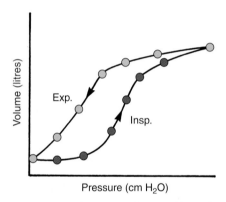

FIGURE 5-17. Pressure-volume curve of a normal lung. Pleural pressure and lung volume are simultaneously determined during brief breath-holds. Lung compliance is calculated from data obtained on the expiratory portion of the pressure-volume curve.

COMPLIANCE OF THE LUNG

The pressure-volume curve of the lung describes two measurements of the elastic properties of the lung: elastic recoil pressure and lung compliance. Elastic recoil pressure is the pressure generated at a given lung volume, whereas compliance is the slope of the pressure-volume curve, or the volume change per unit of pressure:

$$\text{Compliance} = \frac{\Delta\text{volume}}{\Delta\text{pressure}} = \frac{L}{cm\ H_2O}$$

Compliance depends on the initial lung volume from which the change in volume is measured and the ventilatory events immediately preceding the measurement as well as the properties of the lung itself. At large lung volumes, compliance is lower, because the lung is nearer its elastic limit. If the subject has breathed with a fixed tidal volume for some minutes, portions of the lung are not participating in ventilation, and compliance may be reduced. A few deep breaths, with return to the initial volume, will increase compliance. Thus, a careful description of associated events is required for correct interpretation of the measurement.

Changes in total lung compliance occur with age for two reasons; the lung's elastic recoil increases during childhood prior to declining during later adult life,[39] and the smaller the subject, the smaller is the change in volume for the same change in pressure. For example, $\Delta V/\Delta P$ is close to 6 mL/cm H_2O in infants, and is 125 to 190 mL/cm H_2O in adults. It is more relevant to a description of the elastic properties of the lung to express the compliance in relation to a unit of lung volume such as the functional residual capacity (FRC). When this is done, the compliance of the lung/FRC, or the specific compliance, changes much less. It is worth reemphasizing that total lung compliance is a function not only of the lung's tissue and surface tension characteristics but also of its volume. This is especially important to remember when compliance has been measured in newborn infants with RDS. The total compliance is a composite of the lung's elastic properties and the number of open lung units. In RDS, sudden changes in total measured compliance (if uncorrected for simultaneously measured lung gas volume) will predominantly, if not exclusively, reflect the opening and closing of individual lung units.

Lung compliance may also be measured during quiet breathing with pressure and volume being recorded at end-inspiration and end-expiration. The resultant value is the dynamic lung compliance. Although dynamic lung compliance does reflect the elastic properties of the normal lung, it is also influenced by the pressure required to move air within the airways. Therefore, dynamic lung compliance increases with increased respiratory rate and with increased airway resistance. Air flow is still occurring within the lung after it has ceased at the mouth, and pleural pressure reflects both the elastic recoil of the lung and the pressure required to overcome the increased airway resistance. Indeed, dynamic lung compliance can be used as a sensitive test of obstructive airway disease.

ELASTIC PROPERTIES OF THE CHEST WALL

The chest wall is also an elastic structure, but in contrast to the lung, it tends to push outward at low volumes and inward at high volumes. These phenomena are illustrated when air is introduced into the pleural space: the lung collapses and the chest wall springs outward.

Compliance of the chest wall can be measured by considering the pressure difference between the pleural space or esophagus and the atmosphere, per change in volume. Significant changes in thoracic compliance occur with age (Fig. 5-18). In the range of normal breathing, the thorax of the infant is nearly infinitely compliant. The pressures measured at different lung volumes are about the same across the lung as those measured across lung and thorax together. The functional significance of the high compliance of the neonatal thorax is observed when there is lung disease. The necessarily greater inspiratory effort and more negative pleural pressure can "suck" in the chest wall, resulting in less effective gas exchange and a higher work of breathing.

With advancing age, the thorax becomes relatively stiffer.[40] Changes in volume-pressure relations are profitably

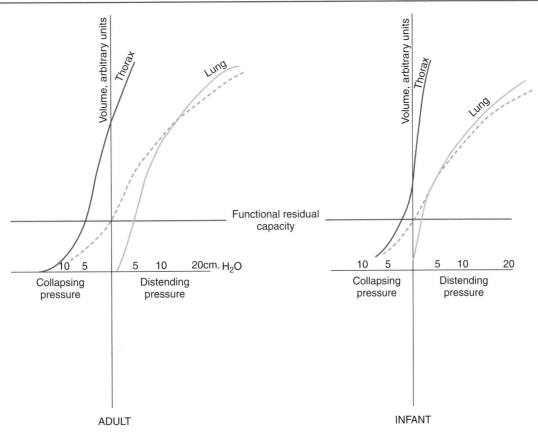

FIGURE 5-18. Pressure-volume relations of lungs and thorax in an adult and in an infant. The dashed line represents the characteristic of lungs and thorax together. Transpulmonary pressure at the resting portion (functional residual capacity) is less in the infant, and thoracic compliance is greater in the infant.

considered only if referred to a reliable unit, such as a unit of lung volume or a percentage of total lung capacity. Considered on a percentage basis, compliance of the thorax decreases with age. It remains unclear how much of this change is contributed by changes in tissue properties (e.g., increasing calcification of ribs and connective tissue changes) and how much is a disproportionate growth of the chest wall relative to the lung.

▬▬ LUNG VOLUMES

Definition

The partition of commonly used lung volumes can be understood by studying Figure 5-19. The spirogram on the left represents the volume of air breathed in and out by a normal subject. The first portion of the tracing illustrates normal breathing and is called the tidal volume (VT). The subject then makes a maximal inspiration followed by a maximum expiration: the volume of expired air is the vital capacity (VC). The volume of air that still remains in the lung after a maximal expiration is the residual volume (RV), whereas the volume of air remaining in the lung after a normal passive expiration is the FRC. The maximum amount of air that a subject can have in the lungs is called the total lung capacity (TLC). In healthy young subjects, TLC correlates best with the subject's sitting height.

The volumes and capacities of the lungs are determined by many factors, including muscle strength, static-elastic characteristics of the chest wall and lungs, airway status,

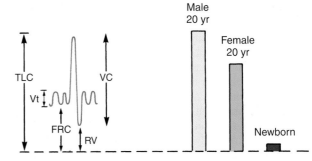

FIGURE 5-19. The lung volumes. The spirogram *(left)* demonstrates normal breathing followed by a maximal inspiratory effort and a maximal expiratory effort. *FRC,* Functional residual capacity; *RV,* residual volume; *TLC,* total lung capacity (6.0 L in an average male, 4.2 L in an average female, and 160 mL in an average 3-kg infant; see histograms on right); *VC,* vital capacity; *Vt,* tidal volume.

and patient age and cooperation. TLC is reached when the force generated by maximal voluntary contraction of the inspiratory muscles equals the inward recoil of the lung and chest wall. FRC occurs when the respiratory muscles are relaxed and no external forces are applied; it is therefore the volume at which the inward recoil of the lung is exactly balanced by the outward recoil of the chest wall (see Fig. 5-18).

Closing volume, the volume at which airways close in dependent regions of the lung, is not routinely measured but is important for our understanding of normal lung function (see: Distribution of Ventilation). Closing volume is graphically illustrated by the atelectasis observed in dependent regions of the infant lung in computed tomography scans of the chest.

In healthy children and young adults, end-expiratory lung volume during tidal volume breathing is equivalent to FRC. This is not the case in infants, who breathe at a lung volume higher than FRC. This higher volume seems to be a sensible solution to the infants' problem of having an airway closing volume that exceeds FRC. An infant maintains the expiratory lung volume higher than FRC by a combination of postinspiratory diaphragmatic activity, laryngeal adduction, and rapid respiratory rate, which minimizes the time for expiration.

The factors determining RV vary with age. In adolescents and young adults, RV occurs when the expiratory muscles cannot compress the chest wall further. In young children and older adults, RV is a function of the patency of small airways and the duration of expiratory effort.

Measurement

Tidal volume and VC can be determined by measuring the expired volume. The measurement of FRC and RV requires another approach. Because both volumes include the air in the lungs that the patient does not normally exhale, they must be measured indirectly. One method uses the principle of dilution of the unknown volume with a known concentration of a gas that is foreign to the lung and only sparingly absorbed, such as helium. The patient breathes from a container with a known volume and concentration of helium in oxygen-enriched air. After sufficient time has elapsed for the gas in the lung to mix and equilibrate with the gas in the container, the concentration of helium in the container is remeasured. Because initial volume × initial concentration of helium = final volume × final concentration of helium, the final volume, which includes gas in the lungs, can be calculated.

The multiple breath inert gas washout method[41] also can be used to calculate lung volumes such as FRC. In addition, it provides information regarding the lung clearance index (LCI) which is now recognized to be a sensitive indicator of peripheral airway dysfunction. It also has the advantage that it can be performed in uncooperative subjects such as infants and very young children[42] (see Chapters 11 and 12).

Neither the helium dilution nor multiple breath inert gas washout methods can measure gas behind closed airways ("trapped gas") or in regions of the lung that are poorly ventilated. There is, however, a method of measuring total gas volume within the thorax that depends on the change in volume that occurs with compression of the gas when breathing against an obstruction. Practically, this measurement requires the patient to be in a body plethysmograph and to pant against a closed shutter. The change in pressure can be measured in the mouthpiece; the change in volume can be recorded with a spirometer attached to the body plethysmograph:

$$V = P\Delta V / \Delta P$$

This method has the advantage of being able to be repeated several times per minute. It has the disadvantage of including some abdominal gas in the measurement.

There have also been concerns about the validity of the plethysmographic technique in patients with severe obstructive lung disease. This issue has not yet been resolved because the technique has been reported to overestimate the lung volume in adults but underestimate the lung volume in infants with obstructive lung disease.

Interpretation

Similar to body growth percentiles, there is a wide range of normal values for lung volumes. For example, the mean TLC for a child 140 cm tall is 3.2 L; however, the statistical range of normal (mean ± 2 SD) is 1.9 to 4.3 L. This range of normal values, when expressed as percentage predicted, is even greater for younger children or smaller lung volumes (such as RV). Owing to this wide range of normality, care must be exercised in the interpretation of lung volumes. Measurement of lung volumes is of greatest benefit when repeated over several months to assess the progress of a chronic respiratory illness and the efficacy of treatment. Healthy children grow along their lung function growth curve,[36,37] much like they grow along their growth percentiles.

The VC is one of the most valuable measurements that can be made in a functional assessment, because it is highly reproducible and has a relatively narrow range of normal values. It can be decreased by a wide variety of disease processes, including muscle weakness, loss of lung tissue, obstruction of the airway, and decreased compliance of the chest wall. VC is therefore not a useful tool to discriminate between types of lesions. Its chief role is to assign a value to the degree of impairment and to document changes that occur with therapy or time. In order to decide whether obstructive or restrictive lung disease is present, it is useful to measure expiratory flow rates (see Chapters 11 and 12) and to observe the pattern of abnormalities in the other lung volumes. In obstructive lung disease (e.g., asthma), the smallest lung volumes are affected first; RV increases owing to abnormally high airway resistance at low lung volumes, and as the disease progresses, the FRC increases. Although the increase in FRC (hyperinflation) may rarely be due to loss of lung recoil, the overdistention is usually compensating for partial lower airway obstruction. When the lung volume is increased, intrathoracic airways enlarge, and widespread partial obstruction may be partially relieved by the assumption of a larger resting lung volume. Whereas the total lung capacity is only rarely affected in obstructive disease (e.g., asthma) in children, TLC and VC are the first lung volumes to be affected in restrictive diseases of the chest wall (e.g., kyphoscoliosis) or lung (e.g., pulmonary fibrosis).

REGIONAL LUNG VOLUMES

During normal breathing, different areas of the lung have different regional lung volumes; the upper airspaces are inflated more than the lower airspaces. Because static-elastic properties are fairly constant throughout the lung, these different regional lung volumes result from the gradient of pleural pressure that exists from the top to the bottom of the lung. Although gravitational forces are thought to be largely responsible, the mechanisms

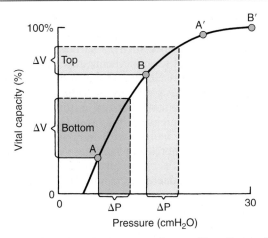

FIGURE 5-20. Pressure-volume curve of a normal lung *(heavy solid line)*. At functional residual capacity, distending pressure is less at the bottom than at the top; accordingly, alveoli at the bottom (A) are smaller (i.e., lower percentage regional vital capacity) than those at the top (B). When a given amount of distending pressure (ΔP) is applied to the lung, alveoli at the bottom increase their volume (ΔV) more than alveoli at the top, owing to the varying steepness of the pressure-volume curve. When fully expanded to total lung capacity (100% VC), alveoli at the bottom (A') are nearly the same size as alveoli at the top (B'), because both points lie on the flat portion of the curve. (From Murray JF. *The Normal Lung.* Philadelphia: Saunders, 1976.)

responsible for this pleural pressure gradient are incompletely understood. In the erect young adult lung, the pleural pressure is −8 cm H₂O at the apex and only −2 cm H₂O at the base. The significance of this phenomenon is that when a subject breathes in, the lowermost lung units will receive the majority of the inspired air (Fig. 5-20). This is advantageous because the majority of pulmonary blood flow also goes to the base of the lung, and thus blood flow and ventilation patterns are more closely matched.

▰ DYNAMIC (FLOW-RESISTIVE) PROPERTIES OF THE LUNG

Gas Flow Within Airways

The respiratory system must perform work to move gas into and out of the lungs. Because air moves into the lungs during inspiration and out of the lungs during expiration, and because the velocity of air flow increases from small airways to large airways, energy must be expended to accelerate the gas molecules. The respiratory system's resistance to acceleration (inertance) is minimal during quiet breathing and will not be considered further. However, inertance becomes quite significant during very high breathing rates, as occurs in high-frequency ventilation. During quiet breathing, frictional resistance to air flow accounts for one third of the work performed during quiet breathing. The magnitude of pressure loss due to friction is determined by the pattern of flow. Flow may be laminar (streamlined) or turbulent, and which pattern exists depends on the properties of the gas (viscosity, density), the velocity of air flow, and the radius of the airway. In general, there is laminar flow in the small peripheral airways and turbulent flow in the large central airways.

The laws governing the frictional resistance to flow of gases in tubes apply to pulmonary resistance. The equation for calculating the pressure gradient required to maintain a laminar flow of air through a tube is given by Poiseuille's law:

$$P = \dot{V}\left(\frac{8l\eta}{\pi r^4}\right)$$

where P = pressure, $\dot{V}$ = flow, l = length, r = radius of the tube, and n = the viscosity of the gas. The viscosity of air is 0.000181 poise at 20° C, or only 1% that of water. Because resistance = pressure/flow, it is clear that the most important determinant of resistance in small airways will be the radius of the tube, which is raised to the fourth power in the denominator of the equation.

The pressure required to maintain turbulent flow is influenced by airway diameter and gas density and is proportional to the square of the gas velocity. The effect of gas density on turbulent flow has both therapeutic implications. Children with viral laryngotracheobronchitis have marked narrowing of the subglottic area, which greatly increases the resistance to air flow. The pressure required to overcome this increased resistance in the large airways, and hence the work of breathing, can be decreased by administering a low-density gas mixture (70% helium, 30% oxygen).

Measurement of Resistance

Resistance (R) is calculated from the equation:

$$R = \frac{driving\ pressure}{airflow}$$

The pressure is measured at the two ends of the system—in the case of the lung, at the mouth and at the alveoli—and the corresponding flow is recorded. Measurement of alveolar pressure presents the greatest problem. Several methods have been used to measure alveolar pressure. The most common method employs a body plethysmograph. The subject sits in an airtight box and breathes through a tube connected to a pneumotachometer, an apparatus that measures air flow. When a shutter occludes the tube and air flow ceases, the mouth pressure is assumed to be equal to the alveolar pressure. Airway resistance can then be calculated because air flow, alveolar pressure, and ambient pressure are known.

Total pulmonary resistance can be measured in infants and children by the forced oscillation technique. This measurement includes airway resistance plus the tissue viscous resistance of the lung and chest wall. Nasal resistance is also included in the measurement if the infant is breathing through the nose. Although there are theoretical objections to this technique, it has several advantages. It does not require a body plethysmograph, estimates of pleural pressure, or patient cooperation, and it can be done quickly enough to be used on ill patients. A sinusoidal pressure applied at the upper airway changes the air flow, and the ratio of pressure change to flow change is used to calculate resistance. When the forced oscillations are applied at the so-called resonant frequency of the lung (believed to be 3 to 5 Hz), it is assumed that the force required to overcome elastic resistance of the lung and the force required to overcome inertance are equal and opposite, so that all of the force is dissipated in overcoming flow resistance. This technique has demonstrated that infants with bronchiolitis have about a two-fold increase in inspiratory pulmonary resistance and a three-fold increase in expiratory resistance.

Several new techniques have been developed that are capable of measuring lung function in infants and young children. Each has its advantages, underlying assumptions, and limitations, and these techniques are discussed in detail in Chapter 11.

Sites of Airway Resistance

The contribution of the upper airway to total airway resistance is substantial. The average nasal resistance of infants by indirect measurements is nearly half of the total respiratory resistance, as is the case in adults. It is hardly surprising that any compromise of the dimensions of the nasal airways in an infant who is a preferential nose breather will result in retractions and labored breathing. Likewise, even mild edema of the trachea or larynx will impose a significant increase in airway resistance.

In the adult lung, about 80% of the resistance to air flow resides in airways greater than 2 mm in diameter. The vast number of small peripheral airways provides a large cross-sectional area for flow and therefore contributes less than 20% to the airway resistance. Thus, these airways may be the sites of disease that may severely impair ventilation of distal airspaces without appreciably altering the total airway resistance. In the infant lung, however, small peripheral airways may contribute as much as 50% of the total airway resistance, and this proportion does not decrease until about 5 years of age. Thus, the infant and young child are particularly severely affected by diseases that affect the small airways (e.g., bronchiolitis).

Factors That Affect Airway Resistance

Airway resistance is determined by the diameter of the airways, the velocity of air flow, and the physical properties of the gas breathed. The diameter is determined by the balance between the forces tending to narrow the airways and the forces tending to widen them. One of the forces tending to narrow the airways is exerted by the contraction of bronchial smooth muscle. The neural regulation of bronchial smooth muscle tone is mediated by efferent impulses through autonomic nerves. Sympathetic impulses relax the airways, and the parasympathetic impulses constrict them. Bronchi constrict reflexly from irritating inhalants (e.g., sulfur dioxide and some dusts); by arterial hypoxemia and hypercapnia; by embolization of the vessels; by cold; and by some vasoactive mediators (e.g., acetylcholine, histamine, bradykinin, and leukotrienes). They dilate

in response to an increase in systemic blood pressure through baroreceptors in the carotid sinus and to beta sympathomimetic agents such as salbutamol (selective $beta_2$ agonist), isoproterenol ($beta_1$ and $beta_2$ agonist), and epinephrine (nonselective alpha and beta agonist). The large airways are probably in tonic contraction in health, because in unanesthetized adults, atropine or isoproterenol will decrease airway resistance.

Airway resistance changes with lung volume, but not in a linear manner. Increasing the lung volume to above FRC only minimally decreases airway resistance. In contrast, as lung volume decreases from FRC, resistance rises dramatically and approaches infinity at RV. Although alterations in bronchomotor tone play a role, it is the decrease in lung elastic recoil as lung volume declines that is the predominant mechanism for the change in airway resistance. The recoil of the lung provides a tethering or "guy wire" effect on the airways that tends to increase their diameter. Children of different ages will have different airway resistances owing to the different sizes of their lungs. Therefore, the measurement of airway resistance or its reciprocal (airway conductance) is usually corrected by dividing the airway conductance by the simultaneously measured lung volume. The resultant specific airway conductance is remarkably constant regardless of the subject's age or height.

Dynamic Airway Compression

During a forced expiration, both the pleural and the peribronchial pressures become positive and tend to narrow the airways; forces tending to keep airways open are the intraluminal pressure and the tethering action of the surrounding lung. During active expiration, however, the intraluminal pressure must decrease along the pathway of air flow from the alveoli to the mouth, where it becomes equal to atmospheric pressure. Therefore, at some point in the airway, intraluminal pressure must equal pleural pressure—the equal pressure point (EPP) (see Chapter 12 and Fig. 12-6). Downstream from the EPP, pleural pressure exceeds intraluminal pressure and thus is a force that tends to narrow the airways. Indeed, during periods of maximum expiratory flow, pleural pressure exceeds the critical closing pressure of the airways, which become narrowed to slits. Despite the cartilaginous support of the larger airways, the membranous portion of the wall of the trachea and large bronchi invaginates under pressure to occlude the airways. Maximum flow under this circumstance is therefore determined by the resistance of the airways located upstream from the EPP, and the driving pressure is the difference between the alveolar pressure and the pressure at the EPP. In disease states in which there is increased airway resistance, the EPP moves toward the alveoli because of the greater intraluminal pressure drop. Thus, small airways are compressed during forced expiration with severe flow limitation. With the measurement of pressure-flow and flow-volume curves during forced expiration, it is possible to calculate resistance upstream and downstream from the point of critical closure, or EPP. Increasing the lung volume increases the tethering action of the surrounding lung on the airways, and therefore close attention must be paid to the lung volume at which resistance measurements are made during these studies.

Work of Breathing

Work is defined as the force over distance or three-dimensionally as pressure during changes in volume. Thus, the work performed by the respiratory pump is defined by the volume changes of the lungs when the respiratory muscles generate a given pressure. The volume-pressure relationships of the respiratory system depend on properties of the lung and chest wall tissues or the ease with which the airways allow the passage of air. A substantial portion of the pressure generated by the respiratory muscles is applied to produce reversible rearrangements of the structure of the alveolar gas–liquid interface and the fibrous network of the lungs. Another large portion of the effort of the respiratory muscles is directed at producing rearrangements or interactions that are not reversible. The energy spent in such an effort is directly transformed into heat, which is then dissipated into the atmosphere or carried away by the circulating blood. The magnitudes of the work and the pressures derived from these processes generally bear a relationship to the rate of gas flow in and out of the lungs. In this regard, the respiratory system exhibits a resistive behavior for which the driving pressure determines the flow of air. Both the elastic and the resistive components of the work of breathing are usually increased in children with respiratory disease.

Respiratory work normally accounts for about 3% of an individual's total oxygen consumption. This work is increased in various diseases, and establishing a diagnosis and formulating a therapy in these patients is almost always simplified when the clinician distinguishes between conditions that affect primarily the elastic (restrictive respiratory disease) and resistive (obstructive respiratory disease) behaviors of the respiratory system.

■ DISTRIBUTION OF VENTILATION

The distribution of ventilation is influenced by several factors in the normal lung. The pleural pressure gradient results in a greater amount of the tidal volume going to the dependent areas of the lung (see Fig. 5-20). In addition, the rate at which an area of the lung fills and empties is related to both regional airway resistance and compliance. A decrease in an airway's lumen increases the time required for air to reach the alveoli; a region of low compliance receives less ventilation per unit of time than an area with high compliance. The product of resistance and compliance (the "time constant") is approximately the same in health for all ventilatory pathways. The unit of this product is time. Note the following:

$$Resistance = \frac{pressure}{flow} = \frac{cm\,H_2O}{L/sec}$$

and

$$Compliance = \frac{\Delta volume\,(L)}{\Delta pressure\,(cm\,H_2O)}$$

The product, then, is a unit of time, analogous to the time constant in an electrical system, which represents the time taken to accomplish 63% of the volume change.

As mentioned earlier in the chapter, peripheral airways contribute little to overall airway resistance after 5 years of age. However, in the presence of small airway disease, some areas of the lung have long-time constants but those of others are normal. This is particularly evident as the frequency of respiration increases. With increasing frequency, air goes to those areas of the lung with short time constants. These areas then become relatively overdistended, and a greater transpulmonary pressure is required to inspire the same volume of air because alveoli in these relatively normal areas are reaching their elastic limit. Thus, a decreased dynamic compliance with increasing frequency of respiration has been used as a test of small airway disease and indeed may be the only mechanical abnormality detectable in the early stages of diseases such as emphysema and cystic fibrosis.

Airway closure occurs in dependent areas of the lung at low lung volumes. The lung volume above RV at which closure occurs is called the *closing volume*. In infants, very young children, and older adults, airway closure occurs at FRC and therefore is present during normal tidal breathing.[39] This results in intermittent inadequate ventilation of the respective terminal lung units and leads to abnormal gas exchange, notably to a lower Pao_2 seen in these age groups.

■ PULMONARY CIRCULATION

Physiologic Classification of Pulmonary Vessels

The pulmonary circulation is the only vascular bed to receive the entire cardiac output. This unique characteristic enables the pulmonary vascular bed to perform a wide variety of homeostatic physiologic functions. It provides an enormously large (approximately 120 to 130 m^2) yet extremely thin surface for gas exchange, filters the circulating blood, controls the circulating concentrations of many vasoactive substances, and provides a large surface area for the absorption of lung liquid at birth. The nomenclature of the pulmonary vessels is at times confusing because the anatomic classification of the vessels often does not correspond to their physiologic role.

The anatomic and histologic characteristics of the pulmonary vasculature are described earlier in the chapter. It is important to understand that pulmonary vessels have been classified physiologically as extra-alveolar and alveolar vessels, fluid-exchanging vessels, and gas-exchanging vessels. When the outside of a vessel is exposed to alveolar pressure, it is classified as an alveolar vessel (capillaries within the middle of the alveolar septum), whereas extra-alveolar vessels (arteries, veins, and capillaries at the corner of alveolar septa) are intrapulmonary vessels that are subjected to a more negative pressure resulting from and approximating pleural pressure. The diameter of the extra-alveolar vessels is therefore greatly affected by lung volume, expanding as inspiration occurs. Although extra-alveolar vessels and alveolar vessels are subjected to different mechanical pressures, they are both classified as fluid-exchanging vessels because both leak water and protein and both can contribute to the production of pulmonary edema. The anatomic location of gas-exchanging vessels is unclear but is likely limited to the capillaries and smallest arterioles and venules.

PULMONARY VASCULAR PRESSURES

The pressure within the pulmonary circulation is remarkably low, considering that it receives the entire cardiac output (5 L/min in the adult human). Beginning a few months after birth, pulmonary arterial pressures are constant throughout life, with the average mean pulmonary arterial pressure being 15 mm Hg and the systolic and diastolic pressures being 22 mm Hg and 8 mm Hg, respectively. The pulmonary venous pressure is minimally higher than the left atrial pressure, which averages 5 mm Hg. The pressure within human lung capillaries is unknown, but work in isolated dog lungs suggests it is 8 to 10 mm Hg, approximately halfway between the mean arterial and venous pressures. These values refer to pressures at the level of the heart in the supine position; because of gravity, pulmonary arterial pressures will be near zero at the apex of the upright adult lung and close to 25 mm Hg at the base. Depending on their location, vessels have different pressures on their outside walls. As defined previously, the alveolar vessels are exposed to alveolar pressure, which fluctuates during the respiratory cycle but will average out close to zero. In contrast, the extra-alveolar vessels are exposed to a negative fluid pressure on their outer walls, estimated to be between −6 and −9 cm H₂O. The pressure on the outside of the pulmonary vessel is not a trivial matter, because the transmural pressure (inside pressure–outside pressure), rather than the intravascular pressure, is the pertinent hydrostatic pressure influencing vascular distention and the transvascular movement of water and protein (see Chapter 38).

PULMONARY VASCULAR RESISTANCE

The resistance to blood flow through the lungs can be calculated by dividing the pressure across the lungs by the pulmonary blood flow.

$$R = \frac{mean\ PA\ pressure - mean\ LA\ pressure}{pulmonary\ blood\ flow}$$

A decrease in resistance to blood flow can occur only through (1) an increase in the blood vessels' lumenal diameters or (2) an increase in the number of perfused vessels. Each of these will contribute to an increase in the cross-sectional diameter of the pulmonary vascular bed. The diameter of an already open pulmonary vessel can be increased by decreasing the muscular tone of the vessel wall (e.g., with a vasodilating agent) or by increasing the transmural pressure (e.g., through increased pulmonary arterial or left atrial pressure). Previously unperfused pulmonary vessels may be opened up ("recruited") when their transmural pressure exceeds their critical opening pressure. This occurs when intravascular pressures are raised or when a vasodilator has decreased the vessels'

critical opening pressure. An increase in cardiac output decreases the calculated pulmonary vascular resistance (PVR). This is important to remember when assessing vasodilating drugs; studies have been performed in which drugs were found to increase cardiac output substantially so that the calculated PVR falls. This decrease in resistance does not ensure that a particular drug has any direct vasodilating action at all, because the entire decrease in PVR may have resulted from its cardiac effects.

The interrelationship between lung volume and PVR is complex and is influenced by pulmonary blood volume, cardiac output, and initial lung volume. The principal reason for this complex relationship is that a change in lung volume has opposite effects on the resistances of the extra-alveolar and alveolar vessels. As the lung is inflated, the radial traction on the extra-alveolar vessels increases their diameter, whereas the same increase in lung volume increases the resistance to flow through the alveolar vessels (which constitutes 35% to 50% of the total PVR). It is reasonable to say, however, that PVR is at its minimum at FRC, and any change in lung volume (increase or decrease) will increase the PVR (Fig. 5-21).

Active changes in PVR can be mediated by neurogenic stimuli, vasoactive compounds, or chemical mediators. The normal adult pulmonary circulation appears to be maximally dilated, since no stimulus has been found that can further dilate the pulmonary vessels. In contrast, the neonatal lung or the vasoconstricted adult lung vasodilates in response to a variety of agents, including nitric oxide, acetylcholine, β-agonist drugs, bradykinin, prostaglandin E, and prostacyclin.

The pulmonary circulation can undergo significant vasoconstriction, which is surprising in view of the paucity of muscle in postnatal lung vessels. Hypoxia is the most common potent pulmonary vasoconstricting agent. Hypoxic vasoconstriction, which occurs when the alveolar Po₂ falls below 50 to 60 mm Hg, is a local response independent of neurohumoral stimuli. Although many suggestions have been made, the exact mechanism of

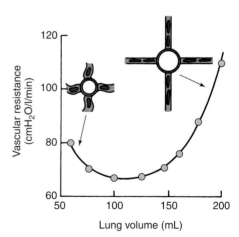

FIGURE 5-21. Effect of lung volume on pulmonary vascular resistance when the transmural pressure of the capillaries is held constant. At low lung volumes, resistance is high because the extra-alveolar vessels become narrow. At high volumes, the capillaries are stretched, and their caliber is reduced. (From West JB. *Respiratory Physiology—The Essentials.* Baltimore: Williams & Wilkins, 1974.)

hypoxia-induced vasoconstriction is unknown. Acidosis acts synergistically with hypoxia to constrict the pulmonary vessels; however, it is unlikely that CO_2 alone has any direct effect on the pulmonary circulation in humans. Stimulation of the pulmonary sympathetic nerves results in a weak vasoconstrictive response in the dog lung but little or no response in the normal human adult pulmonary circulation. Vasoactive substances (e.g., histamine, fibrinopeptides, prostaglandins of the F series, and leukotrienes) are capable of constricting the pulmonary vascular bed. It had been believed that vasoconstriction in the pulmonary circulation took place predominantly, if not exclusively, within the arterial section of the vascular bed. However, it has been demonstrated that other regions of the bed may narrow in response to stimuli. For example, hypoxia can constrict the pulmonary venules of newborn animals and might increase resistance within the capillary bed by inducing constriction of myofibroblasts that are located within the interstitium of the alveolar-capillary membrane. The fetal and neonatal pulmonary circulation contains a large amount of smooth muscle, which enhances the response to vasoconstrictive stimuli.

DISTRIBUTION OF BLOOD FLOW

Blood flow is uneven within the normal lung and is influenced by the vascular branching pattern and gravity that when standing results in more blood flow being directed to the dorsal caudal regions and less to the cephalad regions. Gravitational forces are largely responsible for the increasing flow from apex to base because the intravascular pressure of a given blood vessel is determined by the pulmonary arterial pressure immediately above the pulmonary valve and the blood vessel's vertical distance from the pulmonary valve. Thus, with increasing height above the heart, the pulmonary arterial pressure decreases and less perfusion occurs. The opposite occurs for vessels located in the lung bases, and together these gravitational effects are responsible for a pressure difference of approximately 23 mm Hg between apical and basal pulmonary arteries.

These regional differences in lung perfusion are best understood in terms of West's zones of perfusion (Fig. 5-22). West's zone I occurs when mean pulmonary arterial pressure is less than or equal to alveolar pressure, and as a result no blood flow occurs (except perhaps during systole). Zone I conditions are present in the apices of some upright adults and result in unperfused yet ventilated lung units (alveolar dead space). Moving down from the lung apices, pulmonary arterial pressure becomes greater than alveolar pressure, with the latter being greater than venous pressure. These are zone II conditions, and blood flow is determined by the difference between arterial and alveolar pressures and is not influenced by venous pressure; an appropriate analogy would be that of a vascular "waterfall," in which the flow rate is independent of the height of the falls. In zone III, left atrial pressure exceeds alveolar pressure, and flow is determined in the usual manner (i.e., by the arterial-venous pressure gradient).

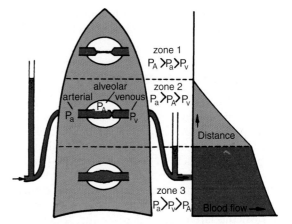

FIGURE 5-22. Model to explain the uneven distribution of blood flow in the lung based on the pressures affecting the capillaries. (From West JB, Dollery CT, Naimark A. Distribution of blood flow in isolated lung. Relation to vascular and alveolar pressures. *J Appl Physiol.* 1964;19:713.)

METHODS OF EVALUATING THE PULMONARY CIRCULATION

The chest radiograph is the most basic noninvasive and nonquantitative tool for determining the possible presence of pulmonary vascular disease. Prominence of the pulmonary outflow tract occurs when the elevated pressure distends the elastic main pulmonary arteries. Vascular markings may be increased or decreased; the former occurs when there is elevated pulmonary blood flow or volume without vascular remodeling, and the latter occurs when there is distal "pruning" of the vessel's image when vascular remodeling has occurred. Computerized axial tomography and magnetic resonance imaging provide greater detail of the right ventricle and pulmonary vessels.

Echocardiography is able not only to assess the structure and function of the right ventricle but also to provide a reasonable estimate of right ventricular pressure by assessing the small retrograde flow through the tricuspid valve that frequently occurs in significant pulmonary hypertension. Quantitative assessment of regional pulmonary blood flow can be made with intravenous injections of macroaggregates of albumin labeled with technetium[99m]. The macroaggregates occlude a very small portion of the pulmonary vascular bed. The amount of regional blood flow can be determined by imaging the lungs with a large field-of-view gamma camera and determining the count rate with a computer. The perfusion lung scintigram can be combined with a ventilation scintigram performed with either a radioactive gas (e.g., xenon 133 or krypton[81m]) or a radiolabeled (^{99m}Tc–diethylenetriamine-pentacetic acid) aerosol that is distributed like a gas.

Regional pulmonary angiography further delineates localized disturbance in blood flow, although the procedure requires cardiac catheterization. Direct measurements of pulmonary artery and pulmonary artery occlusion ("wedge") pressures add further information. Occasionally, drugs can be infused into the pulmonary artery to evaluate the potential reversibility of pulmonary hypertension.

Further details regarding the pathobiology and treatment of pulmonary hypertension are available elsewhere[43,44] and in Chapter 72.

MUSCLES OF RESPIRATION

The importance of the muscles of respiration derives from the fact that these muscles, like the myocardium, can fail under abnormal circumstances and can induce or contribute to an impending or existing ventilatory failure.

The principal muscle of respiration is the diaphragm, a thin musculotendinous sheet that separates the thoracic from the abdominal cavity. In adults its contraction causes descent of its dome and aids in elevation of the lower ribs, the latter referred to as the "bucket handle effect." Some work indicates that the diaphragm has two separate but related functions. The costal part of the diaphragm (largely innervated by C5) acts to stabilize and elevate the lower rib cage during contraction. The vertebral (crural) portion (largely innervated by C3), a much thicker muscle, descends with contraction and is largely responsible for the volume change that occurs.

Three anatomic characteristics of the infant's chest wall and diaphragm lead to decreased diaphragmatic efficiency and a lower fatigue threshold. First, the infant's chest wall is highly compliant,[40] so that when there is respiratory disease there is increased work. Second, the diaphragm is less effective as a result of its higher position within the chest and less apposition to the rib cage. Third, the infant's ribs are more horizontal, which lessens the bucket handle effect.[45]

Other skeletal muscles located in the chest or abdominal wall (e.g., the intercostals, scalenes, and abdominal muscles) can play an important role in ventilation. During normal breathing, most of the accessory muscles are silent. However, during abnormal conditions or disease states, these muscles are recruited to stabilize the chest or abdominal wall so that the diaphragm may be more efficient. In addition, it has been demonstrated that the external intercostal muscles contract in acute asthmatic attacks not only during inspiration but also during expiration; this contraction maintains a higher lung volume and hence increases airway diameter. When airways are occluded during inspiration, abdominal muscles contract powerfully during expiration, pushing the abdominal contents and diaphragm toward the thoracic cavity. This action lengthens diaphragmatic fibers and enhances the capability of the diaphragm to generate force during the subsequent inspiration (length-tension curve).

The upper airways must be kept patent during inspiration, and therefore the pharyngeal wall muscles, genioglossus, and arytenoid muscles are properly considered muscles of respiration. There is an increase in neural output to these muscles immediately before diaphragmatic contraction during inspiration. The newborn also contracts these muscles during expiration to provide an expiratory outflow resistance and thus keeps end-expiratory volume greater than the FRC.

Respiratory muscles, whether the diaphragm, upper airway, intercostal, or abdominal muscles, are not homogeneous muscles in terms of their cellular structure, blood supply, metabolism, and recruitment patterns. Adult mature skeletal muscles have a mixture of fibers, and respiratory muscles are no different. The adult diaphragm, for instance, is made of fast- and slow-twitch fibers. Slow-twitch fibers are oxidative, and fast-twitch fibers are either glycolytic or moderately oxidative. Slow-twitch fibers are fatigue resistant—they are recruited first during a motor act; they generate low tensions; and they usually have a higher capillary/fiber ratio than fast fibers. Fast-twitch fibers can be either fatigue resistant (fast, moderately oxidative) or fast fatiguing (fast glycolytic); they are recruited during motor acts that require large force output. Thus, during normal quiet breathing, it is presumed that only the slow-twitch fibers in the diaphragm are active. In contrast, at the height of an acute attack of croup, asthma, or bronchiolitis during which muscle contractions are strong, both fiber types can be active, with the fast fibers generating the bulk of the force.

Muscle fiber composition, innervation, and metabolism are different in early life. The process of muscle fiber differentiation and interaction with the central nervous system is a continuous process, starting *in utero* and continuing postnatally. For example, slow oxidative fibers increase *in utero* and postnatally, whereas fast glycolytic fibers decrease postnatally. Polyneuronal innervation transforms into one motoneuron = one muscle fiber—the adult type of innervation—postnatally. Whether the young infant's ability to resist muscle fatigue is jeopardized by premature muscle fiber composition, innervation, and metabolism is not known and deserves further investigation.

Respiratory muscle fatigue may arise from central drive fatigue, neural transmission fatigue, contractile fatigue, or a combination of these three phenomena. Many factors predispose respiratory muscles to fatigue. Factors that increase fuel consumption (e.g., increased loads with disease); limit fuel reserves (e.g., malnutrition); alter acid-base homeostasis (e.g., acidosis); modify the oxidative capacity, glycolytic capacity, or both of the muscle (e.g., decreased activity of the muscle and possible atrophy after prolonged artificial ventilation); and decrease the oxygen availability to the muscle (e.g., anemia, low cardiac output states, hypoxemia) all predispose the diaphragm to failure. Reactive oxygen species (free radicals) produced by the contracting diaphragm are also thought to play a role in causing fatigue, particularly in conditions of ischemia/reperfusion and sepsis. In addition, changes in the external milieu of the muscle cell (e.g., low phosphate levels or the presence of certain drugs such as anesthetics) can limit the contractile ability and lead to premature muscle fatigue.

Diaphragmatic muscle function can be assessed clinically by observing the movements of the abdominal wall. During normal inspiration and with the contraction of the diaphragm, the abdominal contents are pushed away from the thorax. Because the abdominal wall is normally compliant during inspiration, the abdominal wall moves out to accommodate the increased pressure from the contracting diaphragm. With diaphragmatic fatigue, weakness, or paralysis, it is possible to observe an inward motion of the abdominal wall. Through the action of other respiratory muscles (intercostals), a drop in pressure occurs in the thorax during inspiration.

Because of the "passive" behavior of the fatigued diaphragm, this pressure drop is transmitted to the abdomen, hence the movement of the abdominal contents toward the thoracic cavity.

The highly compliant chest wall in the newborn infant limits its expansion during inspiration. The chest wall becomes even more unstable during REM sleep, when intercostal muscle activity is inhibited and the rib cage is more prone to distortion. This creates an added load and the potential for diaphragmatic fatigue.

A patient's respiratory muscle strength can be measured using various techniques,[46] all of which are effort dependent. These include maximum inspiratory and expiratory pressures, sniff pressures, and indirectly by maximal cough flows. If the airway is occluded during normal breathing, the infant,[47] child, and adult diaphragm are all capable of generating airway pressures of greater than 100 cm H_2O during a maximal inspiratory effort. In the laboratory, respiratory muscle function can be assessed in more detail (e.g., using electromyographic measurements during repeated stimulation of the phrenic nerve). The measurement of transdiaphragmatic pressure (Pdi) by placing balloon catheters just above (esophageal) and below (gastric) the diaphragm can provide a surrogate measure for muscle strength and susceptibility for fatigue, the time tension index (TTI):

$$TTI = (P_{DI}/P_{DI_{max}}) * (T_I/T_{TOT})$$

P_{DI} = mean transdiaphragmatic pressure
$P_{DI_{max}}$ = maximal transdiaphragmatic pressure
T_I = inspiratory time
T_{TOT} = respiratory cycle time

In adults, when the TTI is less than 0.1, it is unlikely that diaphragmatic fatigue will occur.

A less invasive measure involves measuring inspiratory pressures at the mouth instead of across the diaphragm. In this situation,

$$TTI = (P_{I_{mouth}} / Pmax_{mouth}) * (T_I / T_{TOT})$$

The caveat for using mouth pressures is that it provides a measurement of force generation during the duty cycle by all respiratory muscles and not just the diaphragm. A TTI > 0.15 has been used to predict unsuccessful extubations in ventilated children.

To consider the main respiratory muscles—the diaphragm and the intercostal muscles—as the only respiratory muscles for breathing is insufficient, especially during stressful conditions or disease states. A number of muscles, such as the alae nasi, pharyngeal wall muscles, genioglossus, posterior cricoarytenoid, and thyroarytenoid, can play major roles in airway patency and hence in ventilatory output. Data indicate that upper airway muscles are strongly recruited during obstructive disease or during inspiratory occlusion, and that blood flow increases considerably to some of them (e.g., genioglossus). How prone these muscles are to fatigue under increased loads is unknown. How different these muscles are in terms of their structure, metabolism, and function in the neonate versus the adult is unclear and needs further research.

Because of the number of muscles involved, their location, and their function, the coordination of respiratory muscles becomes increasingly complex. The motor act of respiration should no longer be viewed as the result of one or two muscles contracting during inspiration and relaxing during expiration. At rest and even more so during disease states, the active coordination of various muscles becomes functionally very important. Defecation, sucking, and talking all involve the activation of several muscles that are shared by the respiratory apparatus for generating adequate ventilation. In some cases, obstructive apneas can actually be the result of muscle incoordination, with the diaphragm contracting when upper airway muscles that normally hold the airway open are relaxed.

GAS EXCHANGE

The vital process of gas exchange occurs in the terminal respiratory unit. The previous sections of this chapter deal with the problems of moving air and blood to and from these gas-exchanging units. This section focuses on the fate of gas once it is introduced into the lungs, how it is transferred from the alveolar space to the bloodstream, and how ventilation and perfusion are matched.

In Figure 5-23, the partial pressures of oxygen and carbon dioxide are depicted at various stages of the pathway from ambient air to the tissues. Because nitrogen is inert, changes in its partial pressure (P_{N_2}) in the gas phase depend on changes in the partial pressures of oxygen and carbon dioxide—gases that are utilized and excreted, respectively. In contrast, P_{N_2} in blood and tissue is identical because nitrogen is inert. The rather complex influences of dead space, alveolar ventilation, ventilation-perfusion relationships, and tissue metabolism on the partial pressures of oxygen and carbon dioxide are discussed in some detail, and frequent reference to Figure 5-23 is useful in clarifying some of the concepts.

ALVEOLAR VENTILATION

One component of the tidal volume (V_T) is the anatomic dead space, V_D (consisting of the nose, mouth, pharynx, larynx, trachea, bronchi, and bronchioles), where no significant exchange of oxygen and carbon dioxide with blood takes place. The other component of the V_T, V_A, undergoes gas exchange in the alveoli. Alveolar ventilation per minute is measured by the following equation:

$$V_A = V_T - V_D$$

In practice, V_D is difficult to measure, so the alveolar ventilation equation is used. Since all expired CO_2 comes from the alveolar gas,

$$V_{CO_2} = V_A \times \%CO_2/100 \text{ or}$$
$$V_A = V_{CO_2} \times 100/\%CO_2.$$

The $\%CO_2/100$ is the fractional concentration of CO_2 in the alveolar gas (FA_{CO_2}), which can be measure by

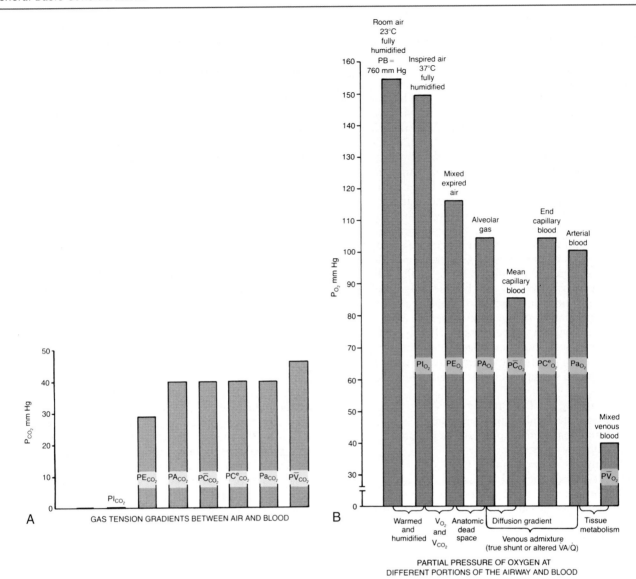

FIGURE 5-23. **A** and **B**, Partial pressures of oxygen and carbon dioxide in different portions of the airway and blood.

a rapid CO_2 analyzer. FA_{CO_2} can be converted to partial pressure of CO_2 by multiplying by $P_B - 47\,mm\,Hg$. Thus,

$$V_A = V_{CO_2}/PA_{CO_2}$$

In normal subjects, the P_{CO_2} in alveolar gas (PA_{CO_2}) is the same as the arterial P_{CO_2} (Pa_{CO_2}), which can be used to determine alveolar ventilation. Note the important relationship between alveolar ventilation and Pa_{CO_2}. When V_A is halved, then Pa_{CO_2} must double at a constant V_{CO_2}; when V_A is doubled, Pa_{CO_2} is halved at a constant V_{CO_2}.

DEAD SPACE

The volume of the conducting airways is called the anatomic dead space (VD_{anat}) and is approximately 25% of each tidal volume (V_T). Anatomic dead space in milliliters is roughly equal to the weight of the subject in pounds (for a 7-pound baby, 7 or 8 mL; for an

adult, 150 mL). In the normal premature infant, anatomic dead space is slightly higher than 30%. In practice, anatomic dead space is seldom measured but may be obtained by Fowler's method, which requires that a single breath of oxygen be inspired. On expiration, both the volume of expired gas and the percentage of nitrogen are measured. The first portion of the expired gas comes from the dead space and contains little or no nitrogen. As the breath is expired, the percentage of nitrogen increases until it "plateaus" at the alveolar concentration. By assuming that all the initial part of the breath comes from the anatomic dead space and all the latter portion from the alveoli, the anatomic dead space can be calculated. The same measurements can be made by monitoring the expired carbon dioxide concentration. In practice, anatomic dead space is difficult to define accurately, because it depends on lung volume (greater at large lung volumes when the airways are more distended) and on body position (smaller in supine position).

Physiologic dead space may be measured by making use of the argument originally developed by Bohr. Since all of the expired CO_2 (FE_{CO_2}) comes from the alveolar gas (FA_{CO_2}) and none from the dead space,

$$V_T \times FE_{CO_2} = V_A \times FA_{CO_2}.$$

And since $V_A = V_T - V_D$, then

$$V_T \times FE_{CO_2} = (V_T - V_D) \times FA_{CO_2}$$

and

$$V_D/V_T \cong FA_{CO_2} - FE_{CO_2}/FA_{CO_2}$$

And since the partial pressure of a gas is proportional to its fractioned concentration (F),

$$V_D/V_T = PA_{CO_2} - PE_{CO_2}/PA_{CO_2} \ (\text{Bohr equation})$$

Or, since alveolar P_{CO_2} and arterial P_{CO_2} are identical in normal subjects,

$$V_D/V_T = Pa_{CO_2} - PE_{CO_2}/Pa_{CO_2}$$

It is now quite clear that V_{Dphys} must be defined according to the gas being measured. Because oxygen is more diffusible in the gas phase than is carbon dioxide, physiologic dead space using oxygen or various inert gases is different from the CO_2 dead space. However, V_{Dphys} measurements using CO_2 are helpful in assessing patients because they reflect the portion of each breath that participates in gas exchange, particularly with respect to CO_2. An elevated V_{Dphys} indicates that areas of the lung are being underventilated in relationship to the amount of blood flowing through the region.

From the foregoing discussion, it is apparent that a V_T must be chosen that will allow adequate alveolar ventilation. For example, an adult might breathe 60 times per minute with a V_T of 100 mL for a minute ventilation of 6 L. Nevertheless, alveolar ventilation under these circumstances may be inadequate because primarily the dead space is ventilated. In selecting suitable volumes and rates for patients on respirators, it is useful to approximate normal values and to consider adequate alveolar ventilation rather than total ventilation. A discussion of high-frequency ventilation is beyond the scope of this chapter.

Alveolar Ventilation and Alveolar Gases

The amount of alveolar ventilation per minute must be adequate to keep the alveolar P_{O_2} and P_{CO_2} at values that will promote the escape of carbon dioxide from venous blood and the uptake of oxygen by pulmonary capillary blood. In health at sea level, this means that PA_{O_2} is approximately 105 to 110 mm Hg and PA_{CO_2} is 40 mm Hg (Fig. 5-23).

Arterial P_{O_2} is markedly affected by the presence of right-to-left shunts, and therefore it is not a good measurement of the adequacy of pulmonary ventilation. Pa_{CO_2} is minimally affected in the presence of shunts because $Pv-_{CO_2}$ is 46 mm Hg and Pa_{CO_2} is 40 mm Hg. If one third of the cardiac output is shunted, this raises Pa_{CO2} to only 42 mm Hg. Thus, the arterial P_{CO_2} is the optimum measurement of the adequacy of alveolar ventilation. When alveolar ventilation halves, Pa_{CO_2} doubles; when alveolar ventilation doubles, Pa_{CO_2} halves. Hyperventilation is defined as a Pa_{CO_2} less than 35 mm Hg, and hypoventilation as a Pa_{CO_2} greater than 45 mm Hg. Hypoventilation can occur as a result of respiratory center malfunction (e.g., congenital hypoventilation syndrome) or depression (e.g., anesthetics) or when there is profound disease involving the lung, chest wall, or respiratory muscles such that effective alveolar ventilation cannot be maintained. Inspired air has a fraction of inspired oxygen (FI_{O_2}) of 0.2093, and it is "diluted" in the alveoli by the FRC of air containing carbon dioxide and water vapor, so the partial pressure of oxygen in alveolar gas must be less than that of the inspired air (PI_{O_2}; see earlier discussion of Dalton's law). PA_{O_2} must be calculated from the alveolar air equation. When oxygen consumption equals carbon dioxide production, then,

$$PA_{O_2} = PI_{O_2} - PA_{CO_2}$$
$$PI_{O_2} = 0.2093 \times (PB - 47 \text{ mm Hg}) = 150 \text{ mm Hg}$$

If PA_{CO_2} is 40 mm Hg, then PA_{O_2} is 110 mm Hg. Usually the respiratory exchange ratio (R) is 0.8, or more oxygen is consumed than carbon dioxide eliminated, thereby decreasing PA_{O_2} slightly more than would be expected from the dilution of PA_{CO_2}. To account for changes in R, a useful form of the alveolar air equation for clinical purposes is

$$PA_{O_2} = PI_{O_2} - \frac{PA_{CO_2}}{R}$$

When PA_{CO_2} is 40 and R is 0.8, PA_{O_2} is 100 mm Hg. Note that breathing 40% oxygen raises PA_{O_2} to 235 mm Hg because FI_{O_2} is now 0.40. Note that this equation is less accurate during oxygen breathing when more arduous forms of the alveolar air equation may be used. However, this inaccuracy is seldom of importance in the clinical setting.

Because the partial pressures of alveolar gases must always equal the same total pressure, any increase in one must be associated with a decrease in the other. For example, if Pa_{CO_2} is 80 mm Hg and the patient is breathing room air (assuming an R of 0.8), the highest that PA_{O_2} can be is 50 mm Hg.

DIFFUSION

Principles

According to Henry's law of diffusion, the diffusion rate for gases in a liquid phase is directly proportional to their solubility coefficients. For example, in water,

$$\frac{solubility \ of \ CO_2}{solubility \ of \ O_2} = \frac{0.592}{0.0244} = \frac{24.3}{1}$$

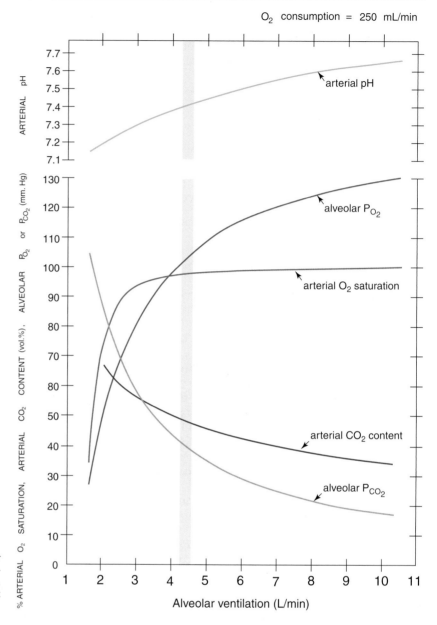

O$_2$ consumption = 250 mL/min

FIGURE 5-24. The effect of changing alveolar ventilation on alveolar gas and arterial blood oxygen, carbon dioxide, and pH. (From Comroe JH Jr, Forster RE II, Dubois AB, et al: *The Lung,* 2nd ed. Chicago: Year Book Medical, 1962.)

Therefore, carbon dioxide diffuses more than 24 times as fast as oxygen. The diffusion rate of a gas in the gas phase is inversely proportional to the square root of molecular weight (Graham's law). Therefore, in the gas phase,

$$\frac{rate\ for\ CO_2}{rate\ for\ O_2} = 0.85$$

That is, carbon dioxide diffuses slower in the gas phase than does oxygen. Combining Henry's and Graham's laws for a system with both a gas phase and a liquid phase (e.g., alveolus and blood): carbon dioxide diffuses 24.3 × 0.85 ≅ 20.7 times as fast as oxygen.

The barriers through which a gas must travel when diffusing from an alveolus to the blood include the alveolar epithelial lining, basement membrane, capillary endothelial lining, plasma, and red blood cell. As observed on electron micrographs of lung tissue, the thinnest part of the barrier is 0.2 μm but may be as much as three times this thickness.

Fick's law of diffusion, modified for gases, states:

$$Q/min = \frac{KS(P_1 - P_2)}{d}$$

The amount of gas (Q) diffusing through a membrane is directly proportional to the surface area available for diffusion (S), the pressure difference of the two gases on either side of the membrane, and a constant (K) that depends on the solubility coefficient of the gas and the characteristics of the particular membrane and liquid used, and is inversely proportional to the distance (d) through which the gas has to diffuse. In the lung of a given subject, exact values for K, S, and d are unknown. Therefore, for the lung, Bohr and Krogh suggested "diffusing capacity" (D$_L$). D$_L$ is simply the inverse of the total resistance to diffusion and can be expressed as the sum of the individual component resistances:

$$\frac{1}{DL} = \frac{1}{DM} + \frac{1}{\theta Vc}$$

where $1/DM$ is the resistance to diffusion of the gas across the alveolar-capillary membrane, plasma, and red blood cell membrane; θ is the reaction rate of the gas with hemoglobin; and Vc is the pulmonary capillary blood volume.

Measurement

Carbon monoxide and oxygen have been used to measure DL. Although the diffusing capacity of the lung for oxygen (DLO_2) has been measured, the process is both complicated and fraught with technical problems because the average capillary oxygen tension must be determined. For this reason, and because a defect in DLO_2 is rarely the cause of hypoxemia, it is not used in the clinical setting. Carbon monoxide (CO), however, has been used extensively in children to test diffusing capacity. The advantage of using CO is its remarkable affinity for hemoglobin, some 210 times that of oxygen, and therefore the capillary PCO is negligible and offers no backpressure for diffusion. To calculate the $DLCO$, one need know only the amount of CO taken up per unit time and the $PACO$.

Many techniques have been developed to measure the $DLCO$, but only two are discussed. The measurement of steady-state $DLCO$ is performed by having the patient breathe a gas mixture containing 0.1% CO for several minutes. Although this measurement requires only a little patient cooperation, its disadvantage is that the value obtained is strongly influenced by maldistribution of the inspired air; if the inhaled gas mixture is not distributed properly to all parts of the lung, the measured $DLCO$ will be decreased but not because of changes in DM, θ, or Vc.

The second technique, the measurement of single-breath $DLCO$, is less affected by airway disease. In this test, the subject takes a single large breath (from RV to TLC) of a CO-containing gas mixture. Following a 10-second breath-hold, the expired gases are collected so that $PACO$ can be determined.

The difference between these two techniques is exemplified by the patient with acute asthma, in whom the steady-state $DLCO$ value will be decreased, whereas the single-breath $DLCO$ value will be normal or increased. Another advantage of the single-breath $DLCO$ method results from the inclusion of helium in the inspired gas. This inert gas allows the $DLCO$ to be corrected for the alveolar volume in which it was distributed, a measurement known as KCO:

$$KCO = \frac{DLCO \text{ single breath}}{\text{alveolar volume}}$$

The KCO is the most useful parameter for comparing the DL of children of different ages and hence different lung volumes. In addition, the KCO helps differentiate among simple loss of lung units (atelectasis), a decrease in pulmonary blood volume (emphysema), and the (albeit rarely seen) true diffusion defect.

The $DLCO$ increases throughout childhood, is related to lung growth, and correlates best with subject height or body surface area. Clinically, a reduction in $DLCO$ may occur for many reasons, including surgical lung resection, diffuse lung disease (pulmonary fibrosis, cystic fibrosis), and emphysematous destruction of the alveolar-capillary membrane. In addition, anemia may decrease the $DLCO$, and equations to correct the $DLCO$ for anemia are available. Increases in $DLCO$ rarely occur and usually result from pulmonary vascular engorgement (increased Vc) or pulmonary hemorrhage (e.g., Goodpasture's syndrome and idiopathic pulmonary hemosiderosis).

It is important to note that with a nonexercising patient, impaired diffusion of oxygen from the alveolar air to the pulmonary capillary is rarely the cause of a low PaO_2. Diffusion limitation may occur during exercise in patients with interstitial lung disease. Hypoxemia in pulmonary diseases usually results from alveolar hypoventilation or an imbalance between ventilation and perfusion of lung units. Thus, low $DLCO$ values almost always reflect abnormalities in gas exchange rather than true diffusion defects.

SHUNT AND VENTILATION-PERFUSION RELATIONSHIPS

There are four pulmonary causes of arterial hypoxemia. We have already discussed two of these—alveolar hypoventilation and diffusion defects. The remaining two, intrapulmonary shunt and ventilation-perfusion defects, result from abnormalities in the distribution of the ventilation and perfusion of the gas-exchanging units.

Shunt refers to blood that reaches the systemic circulation without coming in direct contact with a ventilated area of the lung. Because this blood is deoxygenated, it lowers the PaO_2. There are several causes of shunt. In normal lungs, a small amount of shunt is present because the Thebesian veins and a portion of the bronchial vascular flow drain into the left side of the heart. Pathologic shunts result when abnormal vascular channels exist, as in cyanotic congenital heart disease or pulmonary arteriovenous fistula. Shunt, however, most commonly occurs in diseased lungs because alveoli are not ventilated but are still being perfused. This condition, known as intrapulmonary shunting, occurs in a variety of lung diseases, including pulmonary edema, atelectasis, and pneumonia.

A characteristic feature of shunt is that the resultant hypoxemia cannot be corrected by breathing pure oxygen, a reasonable consequence because, by definition, shunted blood does not pass ventilated lung units. One caveat is that when patients are placed on high oxygen concentrations, a very small increase in PaO_2 may occur because the blood-perfusing ventilated units will depart those units with higher amounts of dissolved oxygen. The characteristic that shunt is very poorly responsive to breathing pure oxygen can be a useful clinical tool; if PaO_2 is less than 500 mm Hg while the subject is breathing 100% oxygen, a significant shunt is present. If mixed venous (pulmonary arterial) blood is available for measurement

Section I

(or a mixed venous oxygen concentration is assumed), the amount of shunt can be calculated at any inspired oxygen concentration using the shunt equation:

Amount of oxygen in arterial blood =
amount of oxygen in blood that has
passed through pulmonary capillaries ($\dot{Q}c$) +
amount of oxygen in shunted blood ($\dot{Q}s$),

and

Amount of oxygen = content of oxygen per liter (Co_2) $\times$ blood flow ($\dot{Q}$).

Therefore,

$$Cao_2\ \dot{Q}t = Cco_2\ \dot{Q}c + C\overline{v}o_2\ \dot{Q}s$$

where $\dot{Q}t$ is total blood flow.

Since $\dot{Q}c = \dot{Q}t - \dot{Q}s$,

$$Cao_2\ \dot{Q}t = Cco_2\ \dot{Q}t - Cco_2 + \dot{Q}s + C\overline{v}o_2\ \dot{Q}s$$

and

$$\frac{\dot{Q}s}{\dot{Q}t} = \frac{Cco_2 - Cao_2}{Cco_2 - C\overline{v}o_2}$$

where $\dot{Q}s/\dot{Q}t$ is the fraction of the total cardiac output that is shunted.

The average ratio between alveolar ventilation and blood flow ($\dot{V}a/\dot{Q}$) is 0.8, but even in the normal lung may range from near zero (not ventilated) to infinity (not perfused). Nevertheless, the most common cause of arterial hypoxemia is a result of mismatch of ventilation and perfusion within the lung, which increases the normal scatter of $\dot{V}a/\dot{Q}$ values around the mean value. When a lung unit receives inadequate ventilation relative to its blood flow, $Paco_2$ rises (toward the mixed venous value of 46 mm Hg) and Pao_2 falls (toward the mixed venous value of about 40 mm Hg) and the oxygen content of the end-capillary blood falls. When this blood mixes with blood coming from normal $\dot{V}a/\dot{Q}$ regions of the lung, the result is a lowering of oxygen concentration and arterial hypoxemia (so-called *shunt-like effect*). In contrast to what occurs in a true shunt, administration of an enriched oxygen mixture will correct the hypoxemia due to ventilation-perfusion mismatch, by raising Pao_2 (Pn_2 must decrease in order to keep the sum of the partial pressures of gases equal to Pb). The increased Pao_2 results in an increased concentration of oxygen in the pulmonary capillary blood.

Whatever the absolute amount of regional ventilation and perfusion, the lung has intrinsic regularity mechanisms that are directed toward the preservation of normal $\dot{V}a/\dot{Q}$ ratios. When $\dot{V}a/\dot{Q}$ is high, the low carbon dioxide concentration results in local constriction of airways and tends to reduce the amount of ventilation to the area. When $\dot{V}a/\dot{Q}$ is low, the high alveolar carbon dioxide concentration results in local airway dilation and tends to increase ventilation to the area. Furthermore, a low $\dot{V}a/\dot{Q}$ with an associated low alveolar oxygen concentration causes regional pulmonary vasoconstriction and produces a redistribution of blood flow to healthier lung units. These effects on airways and vessels from changing gas tensions tend to preserve a normal $\dot{V}a/\dot{Q}$, but they are limited mechanisms, and derangements are common with pulmonary disease.

■ SYSTEMIC GAS TRANSPORT

Oxygen Transport

Once oxygen molecules have passed from the alveolus into the pulmonary capillary, they are transported in the blood in two ways. A small proportion of the oxygen exists as dissolved oxygen in the plasma and water of the red blood cell. For 100 mL of whole blood equilibrated with a Po_2 of 100 mm Hg, 0.3 mL of oxygen is present as dissolved oxygen. If this represented the total oxygen-carrying capacity of blood, cardiac output would have to be greater than 80 L/min to allow 250 mL of oxygen to be consumed per minute. During 100% oxygen breathing, Pao_2 is approximately 650 mm Hg, and 100 mL of blood contains 2.0 mL of dissolved oxygen; a cardiac output of about 12 L/min would be required if no hemoglobin were present and if the tissues could extract all of the oxygen.

Because 1 g of hemoglobin can combine with 1.39 mL of oxygen, between 40 and 70 times more oxygen is carried by hemoglobin than by the plasma, enabling the body to achieve a cardiac output at rest of 5.5 L/min with an oxygen uptake of 250 mL/min.

The potential usefulness of hyperbaric oxygen (i.e., oxygen under very high pressures) for a variety of clinical conditions is due to the fact that at a pressure of 3 atmospheres (absolute) (Pao_2 of about 1950 mm Hg), approximately 6.0 mL of oxygen is dissolved in 100 mL of whole blood, and this amount can meet the metabolic demands of the tissues under resting conditions, even when no hemoglobin is present.

The remarkable oxygen-carrying properties of blood depend not on the solubility of oxygen in plasma but on the unusual properties of hemoglobin. Figure 5-25 illustrates the oxyhemoglobin dissociation curve, showing that hemoglobin is nearly 95% saturated at a Po_2 of 80 mm Hg. The steep portion of the curve, up to about 50 mm Hg, permits large amounts of oxygen to be released from hemoglobin with small changes in Po_2. Under normal circumstances, 100% oxygen breathing will raise the amount of oxygen carried by the blood by only a small amount, because at a Po_2 of 100 mm Hg, hemoglobin is already 97.5% saturated. Even with air breathing, one is on the flat portion of the curve. The presence of a right-to-left shunt markedly affects Po_2 but may reduce the percentage saturation only minimally. For example, a 50% shunt with venous blood containing 15 mL of oxygen/100 mL will reduce the oxygen content of 100 mL of blood only from 20 mL to 17.5 mL. The blood is still 88% saturated, but Pao_2 is now 60 mm Hg instead of 100 mm Hg. Thus, the change in oxygen content is linearly related to

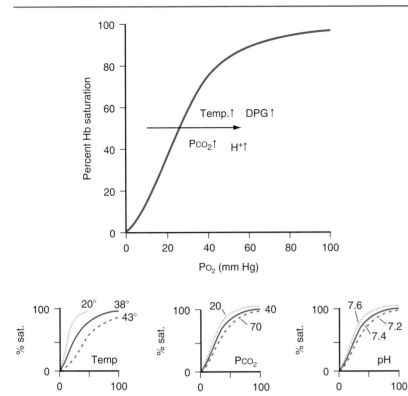

FIGURE 5-25. Oxyhemoglobin dissociation curves. The large graph shows a single dissociation curve, applicable when the pH of the blood is 7.40 and temperature is 38° C. The blood oxygen tension and saturation of patients with carbon dioxide retention, acidosis, alkalosis, fever, or hypothermia will not fit this curve because it shifts to the right or left when temperature, pH, or Pco_2 is changed. Effects on the oxyhemoglobin dissociation curve of change in temperature *(upper left)* and in Pco_2 and pH *(lower right)* are shown in the smaller graphs. A small change in blood pH occurs regularly in the body (i.e., when mixed venous blood passes through the pulmonary capillaries, Pco_2 decreases from 46 to 40 mm Hg, and pH increases from 7.37 to 7.40). During this time, blood changes from a pH of 7.37 dissociation curve to a pH of 7.40 dissociation curve. Note that increased 2,3-diphosphoglycerate also shifts the curve to the right. (From West JB: *Respiratory Physiology—The Essentials,* 5th ed. Baltimore: Lippincott Williams & Wilkins, 1995.)

the amount of right-to-left shunt, but the change in Po_2 is not, because the oxyhemoglobin dissociation curve is S shaped. It is also apparent that at levels greater than 60 mm Hg, Pao_2 is a more sensitive measure of blood oxygenation because neither percentage saturation nor oxygen content changes as much as Po_2 in this range. However, at Po_2 below about 60 mm Hg, relatively small changes of Po_2 produce large changes in saturation and content, and in this range the measurement of content may be more reliable than the measurement of Po_2.

The oxyhemoglobin dissociation curve is affected by changes in pH, Pco_2, and temperature. A decrease in pH, an increase in Pco_2 (Bohr effect), or an increase in temperature shifts the curve to the right, particularly in the 20 to 50 mm Hg range. Thus, for a given Po_2, the saturation percentage is less under acidotic or hyperpyrexic conditions. In the tissues, carbon dioxide is added to the blood, and this facilitates the removal of oxygen from the red blood cells. In the pulmonary capillaries, carbon dioxide diffuses out of the blood, facilitating oxygen uptake by hemoglobin. An increase in temperature has an effect similar to that of an increase in Pco_2 and thus facilitates oxygen removal from the blood by the tissues. Note that a patient who is pyrexic with carbon dioxide retention could not have a normal oxygen saturation during air breathing because of the Bohr and temperature effects on the oxyhemoglobin dissociation curve.

The erythrocyte concentration of 2,3-diphosphoglycerate (DPG) plays a major role in shifting oxyhemoglobin dissociation curves. DPG and hemoglobin are present in about equimolar concentrations in adult human red blood cells. There is strong binding between DPG and the β chain of hemoglobin, and this complex is highly resistant to

oxygenation. Shifts of the dissociation curve to the right associated with an increased DPG concentration (e.g., in anemia) facilitate the release of oxygen to the tissues. Because erythrocyte DPG concentration can change within a matter of hours, a regulatory role for DPG in maintaining optimal tissue oxygenation has been suggested.

The fetal oxyhemoglobin dissociation curve is to the left of the adult curve at a similar pH. Thus, at a given Po_2, fetal hemoglobin contains more oxygen than adult hemoglobin. This property ensures that an adequate amount of oxygen will reach fetal tissues, since the fetus *in utero* has a Pao_2 of about 20 to 25 mm Hg in the descending aorta. The different affinity of fetal hemoglobin for oxygen results from its interaction with DPG. Both fetal and adult red blood cells have similar intracellular concentrations of DPG, but fetal hemoglobin, which has a γ chain instead of a β chain, interacts less strongly with this molecule; therefore, the fetal oxyhemoglobin curve is to the left of the adult curve. Fetal hemoglobin disappears from the circulation shortly after birth, and less than 2% is present by a few months of age. Normal fetal development is not dependent on differences in maternal and fetal hemoglobins, because in some species they are identical.

Abnormal hemoglobins differ in their oxygen-carrying capacity. For example, hemoglobin M is oxidized by oxygen to methemoglobin, which does not release oxygen to the tissues; a large amount is incompatible with life. The formation of methemoglobin by agents such as nitrates, aniline, sulfonamides, acetanilid, phenylhydrazine, and primaquine may also be life threatening. Congenital deficiency of the enzyme hemoglobin reductase is also associated with large amounts of methemoglobin, and affected patients are cyanotic in room air. Similarly, sulfhemoglobin is unable to transport oxygen. Carbon monoxide has 210 times more affinity for hemoglobin than oxygen, so it is important to note that Po_2 may be normal in carbon monoxide poisoning but oxygen content will be reduced markedly.

Thus, a variety of factors may affect the position of the oxyhemoglobin dissociation curve. The position of the curve may be described by measuring the Po_2 at which there is 50% saturation, the so-called P_{50}. When the curve is shifted to the left, the P_{50} is low; when the curve is shifted to the right, the P_{50} is elevated. Although the P_{50} is the traditional method of describing the affinity of hemoglobin for oxygen (see Fig. 5-25), a more appropriate clinical measurement is the P_{90}. This is the Pao_2 at which the hemoglobin is 90% saturated and, as outlined in the following section, corresponds to the goal of oxygen therapy (Table 5-3).

Assessment of Blood Oxygenation

It is challenging to assess oxygenation at the bedside because the degree of visible cyanosis is influenced by many factors, including the patient's hemoglobin concentration and integrity of peripheral perfusion. Clinical cyanosis reflects the absolute concentration of deoxyhemoglobin (Hb), not the ratio of Hb to oxyhemoglobin (Hbo_2). Thus, the presence of anemia makes the clinical detection of a low Pao_2 more difficult, whereas cyanosis may be present in polycythemic patients even though the Pao_2 is only minimally decreased. It has been estimated that cyanosis will be seen when there is approximately 5 gm/dL of reduced hemoglobin (Hb) in the capillaries, which correlates with approximately 3 gm/dL in the arterial blood.[48]

TABLE 5-3 EFFECT OF TEMPERATURE AND ACUTE RESPIRATORY ACIDOSIS AND ALKALOSIS ON HEMOGLOBIN OXYGEN AFFINITY

TEMPERATURE*	P_{50}	P_{90}
28°C	16.5	35
32°C	20.5	44
40°C	32.0	68

RESPIRATORY ACIDOSIS AND ALKALOSIS†			
pH	PCO_2	P_{50}	P_{90}
7.56	20	22	48
7.48	30	24.5	52.5
7.40	40	27	58
7.32	50	29.5	63
7.26	60	31	67

*Pco_2 = 40 mm Hg, pH = 7.40
†Temperature = 37° C.
P_{50} and P_{90}: Po_2 at which 50% or 90% of the hemoglobin is saturated.
Data from Rebuck AS, Chapman KR. The P_{90} as a clinically relevant landmark on the oxyhemoglobin dissociation curve. *Am Rev Respir Dis*. 1988;137:962–963.

Hbo_2 can be assessed using oximeters. The pulse oximeter is most commonly used to noninvasively assess a patient's blood oxygenation. The pulse oximeter passes two different wavelengths of light—660 nm and 940 nm—through the patient's tissues. Hbo_2 absorbs the 660-nm wavelength, whereas Hb absorbs the 940-nm wavelength; the oximeter then determines the ratio of $Hbo_2/(Hbo_2 + Hb)$. The measurement is timed with the pulse of arterial blood and thus facilitates the measurement of an arterial-like Hb saturation value. Although appropriate in the majority of situations, it is important to remember the limitations of a pulse oximeter. It neither detects carboxyhemoglobin ($Hbco$) nor methemoglobin (metHb), and it will not work well if there is decreased perfusion or the patient has a dyshemoglobinemia. Technical issues, such as skin pigmentation, nail polish or motion artifacts, can also compromise the measurement. The Hb oxygen saturation of a blood sample can be directly analyzed using a co-oximeter, a device that uses multiple wavelengths of light to distinguish Hbo_2 from Hb, $Hbco$, and metHb. The use of a co-oximeter is mandatory when the clinician suspects carbon monoxide poisoning, as $Hbco$ is pink, or if metHb is suspected.

The Pao_2 of blood can be directly measured using the Clark oxygen electrode within a blood gas analyzer. Usually the hemoglobin saturation of a blood gas sample is calculated from the Pao_2 using assumptions for various parameters, such as the p50 of the patient's Hb, with correction for the patient's core body temperature.

Normal values for Hbo_2 during infancy, as measured by pulse oximetry, and Pao_2 from arterial blood samples, are illustrated in Figure 5-26.

Today the usual clinical practice is to measure SaO_2 with a pulse oximeter and to estimate $PaCO_2$ by measuring the PCO_2 of either a peripheral venous blood or arterialized blood sample. The latter refers to a blood sample that was obtained after the extremity was warmed and received topical medications to increase capillary blood flow and bring the sample's characteristics closer to those of arteriolar blood. In individuals who have adequate peripheral perfusion, it can be assumed that the $PaCO_2$ will be 6 mm Hg or less than the peripheral venous CO_2 gas tension ($PvCO_2$). If the estimated $PaCO_2$ is normal, or less than normal, then the clinician can be confident that the patient is not in hypercarbic respiratory failure. However, if the estimated $PaCO_2$ is elevated, then the clinician must obtain an arterial sample to directly measure the $PaCO_2$ because an elevated PCO_2 in an arterialized capillary or venous sample may indicate decreased peripheral perfusion. The PO_2 and calculated SaO_2 from an venous blood gas should be ignored.

Oxygen Delivery to Tissues

The cardiopulmonary unit not only must oxygenate the blood but also must transport oxygen to the systemic tissues in adequate amounts. The total oxygen delivery to the systemic tissues is determined by the Pao_2, the amount of saturated hemoglobin, and the left ventricular output (see the equation that follows). For an average adult with a Pao_2 of 100 mm Hg, a hemoglobin (Hb) concentration of 15 g/100 mL (97.5% saturation), and a cardiac output (C.O.) of 5 L/min, approximately 1000 mL of

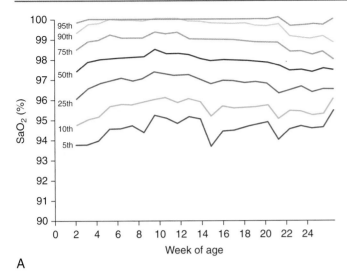

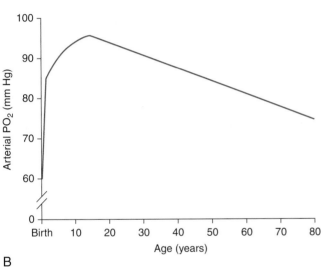

FIGURE 5-26. Median baseline Sao_2 (Spo_2) for healthy term infants who were studied at each postanatal week from 2 to 25 weeks after birth. Variations in Spo_2 with increasing age were not significant. Arterial Po_2 as a function of age from infancy to 80 years of age. The figure represents the data from numerous studies. (Median baseline Sao_2 reproduced with permission from Hunt CE, Corwin MJ, Lister G, et al. Longitudinal assessment of hemoglobin oxygen saturation in healthy infants during the first 6 months of age. Collaborative Home Infant Monitoring Evaluation (CHIME) Study Group. *J Pediatr.* 1999;135:580–586; Arterial Po_2 reproduced with permission from Murray JF. *The Normal Lung: A Basis for the Diagnosis and Treatment of Pulmonary Disease,* 2nd ed. Philadelphia: Saunders, 1986.)

oxygen is delivered to systemic tissues each minute. This large delivery of oxygen provides a significant margin of safety because, under normal circumstances, the systemic tissues use only one fourth of the available oxygen; mixed venous Po_2 is 40 mm Hg, and hemoglobin is 73% saturated. Mixed venous blood is by definition the blood within the main pulmonary artery but is often estimated from a central venous line.

The systemic oxygen transport equation is useful to emphasize a therapeutic principle: the three practical ways to improve oxygenation of peripheral tissues are to increase hemoglobin saturation, to increase hemoglobin concentration, and to augment cardiac output.

$$oxygen\ delivery = blood\ oxygen\ content \times cardiac\ output,$$

where

$$blood\ oxygen\ content\ /\ 100\ mL =\\ dissolved\ oxygen\ (0.003\ mL\ /\ 100\ mL\ blood \times\\ pao_2) + oxygen\ carried\ by\ hemoglobin\\ (1.39\ mL\ /\ g \times g\ Hb\ /\ 100\ mL)$$

OXYGEN THERAPY

Increased Inspired Mixtures

The concentration of oxygen in the inspired air should be increased when tissue oxygenation is inadequate. The response to an increased inspired oxygen concentration depends on which cause of hypoxia is present (Box 5-1). Most of the conditions characterized by hypoxemia respond well to added oxygen. For example, if airway disease results in a 30% decrease in ventilation to an acinus, this can be corrected by an appropriate increase in the concentration of oxygen in the inspired gas. In contrast, patients with shunts will only respond to a minimal degree because the shunted blood does not perfuse alveoli. The slight improvement in Pao_2 and Sao_2 that may be seen when patients with extensive intrapulmonary shunting inhale high concentrations of oxygen results from the additional amount of dissolved oxygen in the blood that perfuses ventilated alveoli. A direct attack on the underlying disorder in anemia, ischemia, and poisonings is clearly indicated; oxygen therapy may be a life-saving measure during the time required to treat the disease.

Oxygen therapy can be utilized to facilitate the removal of other gases loculated in body spaces, such as air in pneumothorax, pneumomediastinum, and ileus. High inspired oxygen mixtures effectively wash out body stores of nitrogen. With air breathing, the blood that perfuses the tissue

BOX 5-1   FOUR TYPES OF HYPOXIA AND SOME CAUSES

Hypoxemia (Low Po_2 and Low Oxygen Content)
Deficiency of oxygen in the atmosphere
Hypoventilation
Uneven distribution of alveolar gas and/or pulmonary blood flow
Diffusion impairment
Venous-to-arterial shunt

Deficient Hemoglobin (Normal Po_2 and Low Oxygen Content)
Anemia
Carbon monoxide poisoning

Ischemic Hypoxia (Normal Po_2 and Normal Oxygen Content)
General or localized circulatory insufficiency
Tissue edema
Abnormal tissue demands

Histotoxic Anoxia (Normal Po_2 and Normal Oxygen Content)
Poisoning of cellular enzymes so that they cannot use the available oxygen (e.g., cyanide poisoning)

spaces has an arterial oxygen tension of 100 mm Hg and a venous oxygen tension of 40 mm Hg. With oxygen breathing, although arterial tensions increase to 600 mm Hg, venous oxygen tensions do not increase above 50 to 60 mm Hg because of oxygen consumption and the shape of the dissociation curve. With air breathing, arterial and venous nitrogen tensions are the same, about 570 mm Hg. If the loculated gas were air at atmospheric pressure, the gradient for the movement of nitrogen to the blood would be very small. After nitrogen washout, with oxygen breathing, the lack of high elevation in venous oxygen tension permits movement of both nitrogen and oxygen from the pneumothorax into the blood. The increased pressure differences increase the rate of absorption of loculated air some 5- to 10-fold. This augmented clearance occurs while the extrapulmonary gas is predominately nitrogen.

Administration of Oxygen

There are several methods of delivering enriched oxygen gas mixtures to nonintubated patients. Known concentrations of oxygen can be piped into chambers that surround the infant's head, such as an oxygen tent or a head box. Usually, these chambers allow significant leakage of gases, so it is imperative that the O_2 concentration be measured inside the chamber near the patient's face. Another method is to run pure oxygen through nasal prongs or cannulae at specified flow rates. Although this method can be efficacious in improving the Pao_2, one must remember that it does not provide a constant FIo_2 during the breath, nor can the FIo_2 be accurately calculated or measured. The reason is that patients will "beat the system," because their inspiratory flow rates exceed the rate at which the pure oxygen is being piped toward their faces. A simple calculation illustrates the point. If a 70-kg man breathes at 30 breaths/min with an inspiratory/expiratory time ratio of 1:1, his duration of inspiration will be 1 second. Given a tidal volume of 0.5 L, his average inspiratory flow rate will be 0.5 L/sec or 30 L/min. Given that nasal prongs are usually set at 2 to 6 L/min for the average 70-kg man, it is immediately obvious that his initial portion of inspiration will be 100% oxygen but that the percentage will decrease quickly toward that of room air by the end of inspiration. This pattern is applicable not only to adults but also to younger children.

Thus, although one can "guestimate" what flow rate of oxygen the patient will require to normalize the blood oxygen tension, the actual FIo_2 will vary within and between breaths, especially if the patient changes the depth or pattern of breathing. In practice today in hospitalized children, oxygen flow rate is titrated by measurement of pulse oximetry.

Hazards of High Oxygen Mixtures

Hypoxemia in conditions associated with alveolar hypoventilation, such as chronic pulmonary disease and status asthmaticus, may be overcome by enriched oxygen mixtures without concomitant lessening of the hypercapnia. The patient may appear pink but become narcotized under the influence of carbon dioxide retention. In chronic respiratory acidosis, respiration may be maintained chiefly by the hypoxic drive. This is a condition that is rarely seen in pediatric patients but may occur in the terminally ill patient with cystic fibrosis.

With the institution of oxygen therapy, there is usually a small drop in minute ventilation as the hypoxic stimulus to breath is removed by the increase in Pao_2. Very rarely, a patient with chronic hypercarbic respiratory failure may cease breathing if excessive oxygen is given. It is therefore essential to measure the pH and $Paco_2$ in addition to the Pao_2 or saturation in these groups of patients. The goal of oxygen therapy is to give just enough oxygen to return the arterial oxygen saturation to the appropriate amount for the patient. The usual target is 90% in the infant, child, and adult. However, the target saturation may be less in the premature infant who is susceptible to retinopathy of prematurity or higher when there is significant pulmonary hypertension. When there is increased intracranial pressure, the clinician should utilize arterial blood samples to maintain the PaO_2 well above 100 mm Hg to ensure full saturation of hemoglobin and to further increase the oxygen content of blood by augmenting the amount of dissolved oxygen.

Excessive oxygenation of the blood can be dangerous. Human volunteers in pure oxygen at 1 atmosphere experience symptoms in about 24 hours, chiefly substernal pain and paresthesias. Laboratory animals exposed for longer periods die of pulmonary congestion and edema in 4 to 7 days. The toxicity of oxygen is directly proportional to its partial pressure. Symptoms occur within minutes under hyperbaric conditions and yet are not present after 1 month in pure oxygen at $\frac{1}{3}$ atmosphere. Some of the acute effects of oxygen are a slight decrease of minute ventilation and cardiac output and constriction of retinal and cerebral vessels and the ductus arteriosus. Retinal vasoconstriction does not seem to be a significant problem in mature retinas that are fully vascularized. In premature infants, however, the vasoconstriction may lead to ischemia. After the cessation of oxygen therapy, or with maturation of the infant, neovascularization of the retina occurs. The disorderly growth and scarring may cause retinal detachments and fibroplasia, which appears behind the lens; hence the names retrolental fibroplasia and retinopathy of prematurity.

As the care of premature infants with acute lung disease has improved, the survival rate has increased impressively. Regrettably, many of the survivors have chronic lung disease of prematurity or bronchopulmonary dysplasia (see Chapter 23). At the present time, it is difficult to determine the relative contributions of prematurity, ventilator-induced barotrauma, oxygen toxicity, and the preceding acute lung injury in the evolution of this serious disorder. It does seem prudent, however, to minimize the FIo_2 in these patients, given the damage that occurs in totally normal lungs exposed to very high concentrations of oxygen.

◼ CARBON DIOXIDE TRANSPORT AND ACID-BASE BALANCE

Buffering and Transport

Acids are normally produced in the body at the rates of 15 to 20 moles of carbonic acid and 80 mmol of fixed acids per day. For the cells to maintain their normal metabolic activity, the pH of the environment of the cells must be close to 7.40. The understanding of the regulation of hydrogen ion concentration requires knowledge of the buffering action of the chemical constituents of the blood and of the role of the lungs and kidneys in the excretion of acids from the body.

The most important constituents for acid-base regulation are the sodium bicarbonate and carbonic acid of the plasma, the potassium bicarbonate and carbonic acid of the cells, and hemoglobin.

The concentration of carbonic acid is determined by the partial pressure of carbon dioxide and the solubility coefficients of carbon dioxide in plasma and in red blood cell water. Carbonic acid in aqueous solution dissociates as follows:

$$CO_2 + H_2O \leftrightarrow H_2CO_3$$
$$H_2CO_3 \leftrightarrow H + HCO_3^-$$

The law of mass action describes this reaction:

$$\frac{[H^+][HCO_3^-]}{[H_2CO_3]} = K$$

In plasma, K has the value of $10^{-6.1}$. An equivalent form of this equation is

$$pH = pK + \log \frac{[HCO_3^-]}{H_2CO_3}$$

By definition,

$$pH = -\log[H^+]; pK = -\log K = 6.1 \text{ for plasma.}$$

Applied to plasma, in which dissolved carbon dioxide exists at a concentration 1000 times that of carbonic acid, the equation becomes

$$pH = 6.1 + \log \frac{[HCO_3^-]}{0.03 \, P_{CO_2}}$$

This form of the equation is known as the Henderson-Hasselbalch equation. A clinically useful form of this equation is as follows:

$$H^+ (nmol/L) = 24 \times \frac{P_{CO_2}}{HCO_3^-}$$

Thus, at a normal bicarbonate concentration of 24 mEq/L, when Pao_2 is 40 mm Hg, hydrogen ion concentration is 40 nM.

Just as oxygen has a highly specialized transport mechanism in the blood to ensure an adequate delivery to tissues under physiologic conditions, carbon dioxide produced by the tissues has a special transport system to carry it in the blood to the lung, where it is expired. The amount of carbon dioxide in blood is related to the Pco_2 in a manner shown in Figure 5-27. Unlike the relation of oxygen content to Po_2, the relation of carbon dioxide content to Pco_2 is nearly linear; therefore, doubling alveolar ventilation halves $Paco_2$. Oxygenated hemoglobin shifts the carbon dioxide dissociation curve to the right (Haldane effect), so that at a given Pco_2 there is a lower carbon dioxide content. This effect aids in the removal of carbon dioxide from the blood in the lung when venous blood becomes oxygenated. The average arterial carbon dioxide tension ($Paco_2$) in adults is 40 mm Hg and in infants is closer to 35 mm Hg; venous levels in both are normally 6 mm Hg higher. The small difference between arterial and venous Pco_2 is why the effect of venous admixture on arterial Pco_2 is very small.

Carbon dioxide is transported in the blood in three ways: dissolved in the blood, as bicarbonate, and as carbamino compound. At the tissue level, the processes involved in the uptake of carbon dioxide into the blood are as follows (Fig. 5-28):
1. Carbon dioxide diffuses into the blood from the tissue. Some carbon dioxide is dissolved in the plasma water in physical solution.
2. Carbon dioxide hydrates slowly in the plasma to form a small amount of carbonic acid.
3. Most of the carbon dioxide enters the red blood cells. A small amount is dissolved in the intracellular water. A fraction combines with hemoglobin to form a carbamino compound.
4. Because of the presence of carbonic anhydrase, a larger fraction in the red blood cell hydrates rapidly to form carbonic acid, which dissociates into H^+ plus HCO_3^-.
5. Bicarbonate diffuses into plasma because of the concentration gradient, and Cl^- ions enter the cell to restore electrical neutrality.

Hemoglobin is important in the transport of carbon dioxide because of two properties of the molecule. First, it is a good buffer, permitting blood to take up carbon dioxide with only a small change in pH. Second, hemoglobin is a stronger acid when oxygenated than when reduced; thus, when oxyhemoglobin is reduced, more cations are available to neutralize HCO_3^-. Carbon dioxide exists in two forms in the red blood cell because of this property of hemoglobin: as bicarbonate ion and as hemoglobin carbamate ($HbNHCOO^-$).

$$KHbO_2 + H_2CO_3 \leftrightarrow HHb + O_2\uparrow + KHCO_3$$
$$KHbO_2NH_2 + CO_2 \leftrightarrow HHb\dot{c} \, NHCOOK + O_2\uparrow$$

An enzyme in the red blood cell, carbonic anhydrase, accelerates the reaction $CO_2 + H_2O \leftrightarrow H^+ + HCO_3^-$ some 13,000 times. A concentration gradient between red cell and plasma causes the bicarbonate ion to leave the red cell. Because the red blood cell membrane is relatively impermeable to Na^+ and K^+, the chloride ion and water move into the red cell to restore electrical neutrality (chloride shift or Hamburger shift). Thus, although the larger portion of the buffering occurs within the red cell, the largest amount of carbon dioxide is in the plasma as HCO_3^- (Table 5-4). The shift of chloride and HCO_3^- was previously thought to be passive, that is, to occur by diffusion due to a concentration gradient. It is now known to be an active process dependent on a specific transport protein within the red blood cell membrane. This anion transport occurs rapidly, with a half-time of 50 msec.

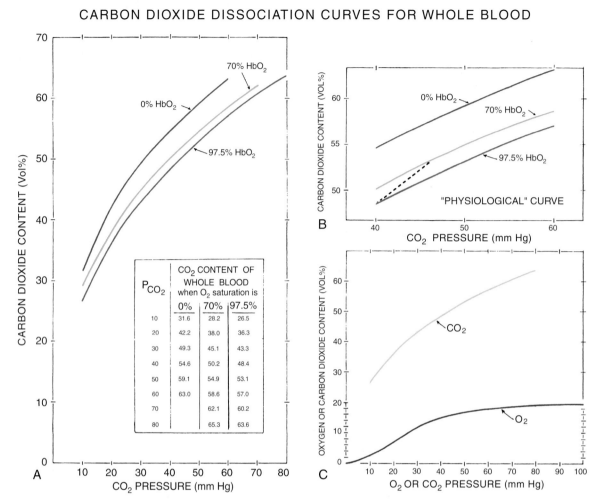

CARBON DIOXIDE DISSOCIATION CURVES FOR WHOLE BLOOD

P_{CO_2}	CO₂ CONTENT OF WHOLE BLOOD when O₂ saturation is		
	0%	70%	97.5%
10	31.6	28.2	26.5
20	42.2	38.0	36.3
30	49.3	45.1	43.3
40	54.6	50.2	48.4
50	59.1	54.9	53.1
60	63.0	58.6	57.0
70		62.1	60.2
80		65.3	63.6

FIGURE 5-27. Carbon dioxide dissociation curve. The large graph **(A)** shows the relationship between P_{CO_2} and carbon dioxide content of whole blood; this relationship varies with changes in saturation of hemoglobin with oxygen. Thus, P_{CO_2} of the blood influences oxygen saturation (Bohr effect), and oxygen saturation of the blood influences carbon dioxide content (Haldane effect). The oxygen–carbon dioxide diagram gives the correct figure for both carbon dioxide and oxygen at every P_{O_2} and P_{CO_2}. **B,** Greatly magnified portion of the large graph to show the change that occurs as mixed venous blood (70% oxyhemoglobin, P_{CO_2} 40 mm Hg). Dashed line is a hypothetical transition between the two curves. **C,** Oxygen and carbon dioxide dissociation curves plotted on same scale to show the important point that the oxygen curve has a steep and a flat portion and that the carbon dioxide curve does not. (From Comroe JH Jr. *The Lung,* 2nd ed. Chicago: Year Book Medical, 1963.)

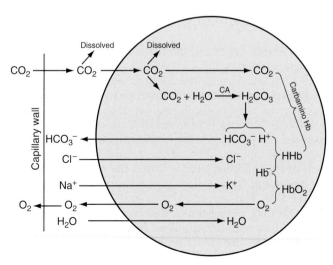

FIGURE 5-28. CO₂ transport in blood. (See text for further explanation.)

In the lung, a process the reverse of that just described takes place, because carbon dioxide diffuses out of the blood and into the alveoli. Diffusion of CO_2 is rapid, so the equilibrium between the P_{CO_2} of the pulmonary capillary and that of alveolar air is promptly achieved. About 30% of the CO_2 that is exchanged is given up from hemoglobin carbamate. When hemoglobin is oxygenated in the pulmonary capillary, chloride and water shift out of the red cell, and bicarbonate diffuses in to combine with hydrogen ion to form H_2CO_3, which in turn is dehydrated to form carbon dioxide. Carbon dioxide then diffuses out of the cell into the plasma and alveolar gas.

Although red blood cells from newborn infants have less carbonic anhydrase activity than adult cells, no defect in carbon dioxide transport is apparent. However, when breathing 100% oxygen, there is less reduced hemoglobin present in venous blood, and therefore less buffering

TABLE 5-4 CARBON DIOXIDE IN THE BLOOD

	ARTERIAL BLOOD		VENOUS BLOOD	
	M M/L BL	**%**	**M M/L BL**	**%**
Total	21.9		24.1	
Plasma dissolved CO_2	0.66	3	0.76	3
HCO_3^-	14.00	64	15.00	63
Cells dissolved CO_2	0.44	2	0.54	2
HCO_3^-	5.7	26	6.1	25
$HbNHCOO^-$	1.2	5	1.8	7

Note: Table gives normal values of various chemical forms of CO_2 in blood with an assumed hematocrit level of 46. Approximately twice as much CO_2 exists in the plasma as in the red blood cells, chiefly as HCO_3^-.

capacity for H^+ is present, leading to an increased Pco_2. This is an important consideration during hyperbaric oxygenation, when the venous blood may remain almost completely saturated with oxygen, H^+ is less well buffered, and tissue Pco_2 rises.

Acid-Base Balance

To understand acid–base balance within the body, it is important to differentiate between the processes that promote a change in acid–base state and the end result of all these primary and secondary processes. *Acidemia* and *alkalemia* refer to the final acid–base status within the blood (hence the suffix *-emia*). Two processes can promote the development of acidemia: metabolic acidosis (loss of HCO_3^- or gain of H^+) and respiratory acidosis (increase in Pco_2, which increases H^+ via carbonic acid). Two processes can promote the development of alkalemia: metabolic alkalosis (gain of HCO_3^- or loss of H^+) and respiratory alkalosis (decrease in Pco_2). Obviously, if there is a primary acidotic process, the body will try

to maintain homeostasis by promoting a secondary alkalotic process and vice versa. Therefore, to understand the patient's acid-base balance, one must first measure the pH of the blood, and if it is abnormal, determine what primary and secondary (compensatory) processes are involved. This is illustrated in Table 5-5; note, however, that the HCO_3^- shown in Table 5-5 is the standard HCO_3^- (i.e., corrected to a Pco_2 of 40 mm Hg; see later section entitled "Difference between Additions of CO_2 to Blood *In Vitro* and *In Vivo*").

Metabolic acidosis occurs in such conditions as diabetes (in which there is an accumulation of keto acids); renal failure, when the kidney is unable to excrete hydrogen ion; diarrhea from loss of base; and tissue hypoxia associated with lactic acid accumulation. When pH falls, respiration is stimulated so that Pco_2 will decrease and tend to compensate for the reduction in pH. This compensation is usually incomplete, and pH remains below 7.35. The pH, carbon dioxide content (HCO_3^- Pco_2), HCO_3^-, and Pco_2 are all reduced.

Metabolic alkalosis occurs most commonly after excessive loss of HCl due to vomiting (as in pyloric stenosis) or after an excessive citrate or bicarbonate load. The carbon dioxide content is elevated, and the Pco_2 will be normal or elevated, depending on the chronicity of the alkalosis.

Acute respiratory acidosis is secondary to respiratory insufficiency and accumulation of carbon dioxide within the body. The associated acidosis may be compensated for by renal adjustments that promote retention of HCO_3^-. Compensation may require several days. Patients in chronic respiratory acidosis who receive therapy that improves alveolar ventilation will have a decrease in their $Paco_2$, but their adjustment in bicarbonate will be much slower, resulting in a metabolic alkalosis of several days' duration. A simple rule is that if hypercarbic respiratory failure has occurred over many days, such that compensation has occurred, the clinician should slowly normalize the $Paco_2$ to avoid excessive metabolic alkalosis.

Acute respiratory alkalosis (e.g., secondary to fever, psychogenic hyperventilation, or a pontine lesion with

TABLE 5-5 BLOOD MEASUREMENTS IN VARIOUS ACID-BASE DISTURBANCES

	pH	PaCO₂ (mm Hg)	STANDARD HCO₃⁻ (mEq/L)	CO₂ CONTENT (mEq/L)
Metabolic acidosis	↓	↓	↓	↓
Acute respiratory acidosis	↓	↑	↔	Slight ↑
Compensated respiratory acidosis	(↔ or slight ↓)	↑	↑	↑
Metabolic alkalosis	↑	Slight ↑	↑	↑
Acute respiratory alkalosis	↑	↓	↔	Slight ↓
Compensated respiratory alkalosis	(↔ or slight ↑)	↓	↓	↓
Normal values	7.35–7.45	35–45	24–26	25–28

meningoencephalitis) is associated with high pH, low P_{CO_2}, and normal bicarbonate level. Renal compensation in time leads to excretion of bicarbonate and return of pH toward normal.

It is important to point out that the lung excretes some 300 mEq/kg of acid per day in the form of carbon dioxide, and the kidney excretes 1 to 2 mEq/kg/day. Thus, the lung plays a large role in the acid–base balance of the body, in fact providing rapid adjustment when necessary. The Henderson-Hasselbalch equation may be thought of as

$$pH \alpha \frac{kidney}{lung}$$

Difference Between Additions of CO₂ to Blood *In Vitro* and *In Vivo*

An appreciation of the difference between the so-called *in vitro* and *in vivo* CO_2 dissociation curves is necessary to clarify the confusion that has arisen regarding the interpretation of measurements of acid–base balance, particularly during acute respiratory acidosis (acute hypoventilation). When blood *in vitro* is equilibrated with increasing concentrations of CO_2, bicarbonate concentration also increases because of the hydration of carbon dioxide. If, for example, blood with a P_{CO_2} of 40 mm Hg and a bicarbonate concentration of 24 mEq/L were equilibrated with a P_{CO_2} of 100 mm Hg, the actual bicarbonate concentration would be measured as 34 mEq/L. In the commonly used Astrup nomogram, a correction for this increased bicarbonate due to CO_2 alone is made, and the standard bicarbonate (bicarbonate concentration at P_{CO_2} of 40 mm Hg) is considered to be 24 mEq/L, or a base excess of zero. With this correction, one can readily see that the metabolic (renal) component of acid-base balance is normal. However, confusion has arisen because the *in vitro* correction figures have been incorrectly applied to the situation *in vivo*. Unlike equilibration in the test tube, the additional bicarbonate generated during *in vivo* acute hypercapnia not only is distributed to water in red blood cells and plasma but also equilibrates with the interstitial fluid space; that is, bicarbonate ion equilibrates with extracellular water. If the interstitial fluid represents 70% of extracellular water, then 70% of the additional bicarbonate generated will be distributed to the interstitial fluid. Thus, an arterial sample taken from a patient with an acute elevation of P_{CO_2} to 100 mm Hg would have an actual bicarbonate concentration of 27 mEq/L. If 10 mEq/L were subtracted according to the *in vitro* correction, the standard bicarbonate would be reported as 17 mEq/L, or a base excess of −7, which would indicate the presence of metabolic as well as respiratory acidosis. This conclusion would be incorrect; actually, the bicarbonate concentration *in vivo* is appropriate for the P_{CO_2}. The situation is worse in the newborn infant because of the high hematocrit and large interstitial fluid space. Base excess values of as much as −10 mEq/L (standard bicarbonate 14 mEq/L) may be calculated despite the fact that the *in vivo* bicarbonate concentration is appropriate for the

particular P_{CO_2} and there is no metabolic component to the acidosis. Thus, the appropriate therapy is to increase alveolar ventilation and not to administer bicarbonate.

TISSUE RESPIRATION

Aerobic Metabolism

The ultimate function of the lung is to provide oxygen to meet the demands of the tissues and to excrete carbon dioxide, a by-product of metabolic activity. Thus, respiratory physiologists have been concerned with the assessment of respiration at the tissue level and the ability of the cardiopulmonary system to meet the metabolic demands of the body.

One method is to measure the amount of oxygen consumed by the body per minute ($\dot{V}_{O_2}$). This is equal to the amount necessary to maintain the life of the cells at rest, plus the amount necessary for oxidative combustion required to maintain a normal body temperature, as well as the amount used for the metabolic demands of work above the resting level. The basal metabolic rate is a summation of many component energy rates of individual organs and tissues and is defined as the amount of energy necessary to maintain the life of the cells at rest, under conditions in which there is no additional energy expenditure for temperature regulation or additional work.

In practice, $\dot{V}_{O_2}$ is measured after an overnight fast, the subject lying supine in a room at a comfortable temperature. This "basal" metabolic rate has a wide variability (±15% of predicted $\dot{V}_{O_2}$). Since absolutely basal conditions are difficult to ensure, the measurement of basal metabolic rate is not widely used at present.

The performance of the cardiopulmonary system can be more adequately assessed and compared with normal measurements under conditions of added work, such as exercise. During exercise, healthy subjects demonstrate an improvement in pulmonary gas exchange, cardiac output, and tissue oxygen extraction. Performance can be increased by physical fitness, and athletes are able to increase their cardiac output by six- or seven-fold. In children, the relationship between work capacity, ventilation, and oxygen consumption is the same as that in the adult. The maximal $\dot{V}_{O_2}$ that can be achieved increases throughout childhood, reaches its peak of 50 to 60 mL/min/kg between 10 and 15 years of age, and thereafter declines slowly with age.

At the tissue level, the ability of a given cell to receive an adequate oxygen supply depends on the amount of local blood flow, the distance of the cell from the perfusing capillary, and the difference between the partial pressures of oxygen in the capillary and in the cell. The critical mean capillary P_{O_2} appears to be in the region of 30 mm Hg for children and adults. Exercising muscle has 10 to 20 times the number of open capillaries as resting muscle does.

The body's response to exercise therefore is complex and depends on the amount of work, the rate at which the workload is increased, and the subject's state of health and degree of physical fitness. A detailed description of the physiologic response to exercise and its use in diagnosing cardiorespiratory disease is beyond the scope of this chapter, but exercise testing is now an essential tool in clinical medicine (see Chapter 13).

Anaerobic Metabolism

The adequacy of oxygen supply to the tissues has been assessed by measuring blood lactate, a product of anaerobic metabolism (Embden-Meyerhof pathway). When there is an insufficient oxygen supply to the tissues due to either insufficient blood flow or a decrease in blood oxygen content, lactic acid concentration within the tissues and blood increases. In the blood, this accumulation leads to metabolic acidosis.

During moderate to heavy muscular exercise, cardiac output cannot meet the demands of the muscles, and an oxygen debt is incurred, which is repaid on cessation of exercise. During this period, lactic acid accumulates, and therefore rigorous exercise is often associated with metabolic acidosis. There is an excellent correlation between the serum lactate level and the oxygen debt. Oxygen debt is not measurable at rest and is difficult to measure during exercise, but the adequacy of tissue oxygenation appears to be accurately reflected in the serum lactate level. In adult humans, blood lactate is less than 1 mEq/L but may increase to 10 to 12 mEq/L during very heavy exercise.

Relationship Between $\dot{V}o_2$ and $\dot{V}co_2$

In the normal subject in a steady state, the amount of carbon dioxide excreted by the lung per minute depends on the basal metabolic activity of the cells and the type of substrate being oxidized. The volume of carbon dioxide exhaled divided by the amount of oxygen consumed is known as the respiratory exchange ratio (R). For the body as a whole, the ratio is 1 if primarily carbohydrate is being metabolized, 0.7 if fat, and 0.8 if protein. Normally, the ratio is 0.8 at rest, approximately 1.0 during exercise, and greater than 1 at exhaustion when there is anaerobic metabolism. The respiratory exchange ratio may vary considerably with changes in alveolar ventilation and metabolism and therefore must be measured in the steady state (i.e., with a steady alveolar ventilation and a steady metabolic rate). For an individual organ, the metabolic respiratory quotient ($\dot{R}\dot{Q}$) is nearly constant but may vary from 0.4 to 1.5, depending on the balance of anabolism and catabolism in that organ. Thus, the measurement of R represents the result of many component-metabolizing organs and tissues. After birth, R decreases from nearly 1 to 0.7, indicating a loss of carbohydrate stores; when feeding has started, R approaches 0.8.

With breath-by-breath CO_2 and O_2 concentrations, R can be calculated on a breath-by-breath basis. Using this technique, it is possible to define more precisely the workload at which anaerobic metabolism begins (threshold for anaerobic metabolism). As lactic acid begins to accumulate in the blood, the carbon dioxide dissociation curve shifts to the right, and there is a sudden increase in expired CO_2. R therefore suddenly increases from about 1.0 to above 1.0. It has been shown that the threshold for anaerobic metabolism in both adults and children can be increased by training. This technique is particularly useful in children because it does not require blood sampling and can be readily applied to cooperative subjects with a variety of pulmonary and cardiac problems.

■ REGULATION OF RESPIRATION

The regulation of respiratory rhythm[49] and its control have been extensively studied over the past decades, including its abnormalities in diseases such as congenital hypoventilation syndrome[50] caused by Phox2b mutations, sudden infant death syndrome,[51] and sleep disorders.[52,53] A brief discussion is provided later in the chapter, but further details are available in the references cited[51-53] and in Chapters 76 and 77.

The study of the regulation of respiration centers around three main ideas: (1) the generation and maintenance of a respiratory rhythm, (2) the modulation of this rhythm by a number of sensory feedback loops and reflexes, and (3) the recruitment of respiratory muscles that can contract appropriately for gas exchange (Fig. 5-29).

The central nervous system, particularly the brainstem, has the inherent ability to function as the respiratory "sinus node," or the source of central pattern generation. The pacemaker neurons are located within the brainstem's preBötzinger Complex (preBötC) and are the main source of inspiratory rhythm. Each part of the respiratory cycle is controlled by distinct groups of neurons that interact dynamically with some stimulating, some inhibiting, and others having their effect dependent upon the phase of the respiratory cycle. The overall control of respiratory rhythm is influenced by many factors, including cortical behavioral influences; sleep state;

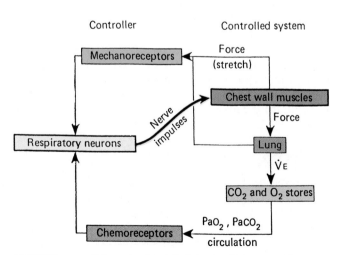

FIGURE 5-29. Schematic diagram of the respiratory control system. (From Fishman AP: *Pulmonary Diseases and Disorders.* New York: McGraw-Hill, 1980.)

peripheral and central chemoreceptors; and receptors within the lungs, joints, and muscles.

■ SENSORY FEEDBACK SYSTEM

The respiratory system is endowed with a wealth of afferent pathways to maintain control over several functional variables and adjust them at appropriate times. These pathways inform the central pattern generator about instantaneous changes that take place in, for example, the lungs, the respiratory musculature, the blood (acid-base), and the environment. The terms *sensory* and *afferent* refer not only to peripheral but also to central systems converging on the brainstem respiratory neurons.

Cutaneous or mucocutaneous stimulation of the area innervated by the trigeminal nerve (e.g., the face, nasal mucosa) decreases respiratory frequency and may lead to the generation of respiratory pauses. These respiratory effects become less important with age, their strengths are species-specific, and they depend on the state of consciousness. Because cortical inhibition of the trigeminal afferent impulses is more pronounced during REM sleep, trigeminal stimulation has a greater effect on respiration during quiet (non-REM) sleep.

The laryngeal receptor reflex is probably the most inhibitory reflex on respiration known. Sensory receptors are present in the epithelium of the epiglottis and upper larynx. Introduction into the larynx of small amounts of water or solutions with low concentrations of chloride will result in apnea. The duration and severity of the respiratory changes depend on the behavioral state and are exacerbated by the presence of anesthesia. They are also worse if the subject is anemic, hypoglycemic, or a premature infant. In the unanesthetized subject, the reflex effects are almost purely respiratory and are mediated by the superior laryngeal nerve, which joins the vagal trunk after the nodose ganglion.

Rapidly adapting, slowly adapting and J receptors (vagal) are present in the tracheobronchial tree and lung interstitial space and were described earlier in this chapter. These play an important role in informing the central nervous system about the status of lung volume, tension across airways, and lung interstitial pressure. Stretch receptors, when stimulated by lung inflation, prolong expiratory duration and delay the start of the next inspiration. J receptors are stimulated by lung edema, and they produce tachypnea with interspersed short periods of respiratory pauses.

O₂ and CO₂

The respiratory control system also receives information about O_2 and CO_2 tensions from sensory receptors located in specialized neural structures in blood vessels, airways, and the central nervous system.

Central chemoreceptors are located in the ventral lateral medulla, and increases in P_{CO_2} or H^+ concentration produce an increase in ventilation; conversely, a decrease in P_{CO_2} or H^+ concentration causes a depression of ventilation. This area is influenced primarily by the acid-base composition of CSF, and the delay in ventilatory response to changes in arterial P_{CO_2} and bicarbonate is due to the time required to change the CSF H^+ concentration. Carbon dioxide, which diffuses into the CSF in a few minutes, has a rapid effect on the central chemoreceptors. Changes in blood bicarbonate are much less rapidly reflected in the CSF (24 to 48 hours). Thus, with acute metabolic acidosis, arterial P_{CO_2} decreases along with CSF P_{CO_2}. Hyperventilation is produced by the H^+ stimulation of peripheral chemoreceptors, but this stimulus is inadequate to compensate fully for the metabolic acidosis because of inhibition from the decreased H^+ concentration in the CSF. After 24 hours, CSF bicarbonate decreases and restores CSF pH to normal. There is a further decrease in arterial P_{CO_2}, and arterial pH returns toward normal. From these observations, it has been suggested that the control of alveolar ventilation is a function of the central chemoreceptors, which are under the influence of CSF or brain interstitial fluid H^+, acting in association with the peripheral chemoreceptors, which are directly under the influence of the arterial blood.

The peripheral chemoreceptors are found in the human along the structures associated with the branchial arches. Two sets of chemoreceptors appear to be of greatest physiologic importance: (1) the carotid bodies, which are located at the division of the common carotid artery into its internal and external branches, and (2) the aortic bodies, which lie between the ascending aorta and the pulmonary artery. Afferent nerves from the carotid body join the glossopharyngeal (IX) nerve; those from the aortic bodies join the vagosympathetic trunk along with the recurrent laryngeal nerves.

The carotid and aortic bodies are responsive primarily to changes in the partial pressure of oxygen. At rest, they are tonically active, signifying that some ventilatory drive exists even at a Pa_{O_2} of 100 mm Hg. Inhalation of low oxygen mixtures is associated with a significant increase in ventilation when the Pa_{O_2} is less than 60 mm Hg. Potentiation of the hypoxic stimulus is achieved by an increase in Pa_{CO_2}. The response of the peripheral chemoreceptors to P_{CO_2} is rapid (within seconds), and ventilation increases monotonically with Pa_{CO_2}. The rate of the change in Pa_{CO_2} may be as important as the change. The peripheral chemoreceptors, also responsive to changes in arterial pH, increase ventilation in association with a decrease of 0.1 pH unit and produce a two- to threefold increase with a decrease of 0.4 pH unit. A variety of peripheral reflexes are known to influence respiration. Hyperpnea may be produced by stimulation of pain and temperature receptors or mechanoreceptors in limbs. Visceral reflexes (e.g., those that result from distention of gallbladder or traction on the gut) are usually associated with apnea. Afferent impulses from respiratory muscles (e.g., intercostals) may play a role in determining the optimum response of the muscles of ventilation to various respiratory stimuli. In newborn infants, an inspiratory gasp may be elicited by distention of the upper airways. This reflex is mediated by the vagus nerve and is known as the *Head reflex*. It has been suggested that this inspiratory gasp reflex is important in the initial inflation of the lungs at birth.

The Newborn Infant

A number of studies have demonstrated that the responsiveness to stimuli in newborn infants is different from that of older or mature adult subjects. Although the exact mechanisms for these differences have generally been elusive, the rapid maturational changes that occur in key control systems could serve as the bases for the different responses seen in early life. Like adults, infants increase ventilation in response to inspired carbon dioxide, and peripheral chemoreceptors are functional in newborn infants, as demonstrated by a slight decrease in $\dot{V}E$ with 100% oxygen breathing. The effect of hypoxia as a stimulant may differ in the first 12 hours of life; 12% oxygen in the first 12 hours of life fails to stimulate ventilation. In addition, it has been found that the newborn infant will increase ventilation only transiently in response to a hypoxic stimulus; ventilation rapidly falls below baseline. In adults, the increase in ventilation is maintained above basal levels, although it lessens with time.

The mechanisms responsible for this different response to hypoxia in the newborn are not well understood. The biphasic hypoxic response is likely multifactorial and may be due to one or more of the following: (1) reduction in dynamic lung compliance, (2) reduction in chemoreceptor activity during sustained (>1 to 2 min) hypoxia, (3) central neuronal depression due to either an actual drop in excitatory synaptic drive other than carotid input or changes in neuronal membrane properties reducing excitability, and (4) decrease in metabolic rate.

■ METABOLIC FUNCTIONS OF THE LUNG

The lungs have important nonrespiratory functions, including phagocytosis by alveolar macrophages, filtering of microemboli from blood, biosynthesis of surfactant components, and excretion of volatile substances. An equally important nonrespiratory function is the pharmacokinetic function of the pulmonary vascular bed: the release, degradation, and activation of vasoactive substances. The lung is ideally situated for regulating the circulating concentrations of vasoactive substances because it receives the entire cardiac output and possesses an enormous vascular surface area. As Table 5-6 illustrates, the pulmonary vascular bed not only handles a wide variety of compounds (amines, peptides, lipids), but also is highly selective in its metabolic activity. For example, norepinephrine is metabolized by the lung, whereas epinephrine, which differs from it only by a methyl group, is unaffected by passage through the pulmonary circulation.

The physiologic consequences of the metabolic functions of the lung can be illustrated by angiotensin-converting enzyme (ACE). A peptidase located on the surface of the endothelial cell, ACE is responsible for the degradation of bradykinin, a potent vasodilator and edematogenic peptide, and for the conversion of angiotensin I to angiotensin II, a potent vasoconstrictor. Angiotensin II production influences systemic blood pressure at all ages but is especially important during the neonatal period, because sympathetic innervation is incompletely developed.

TABLE 5-6 HANDLING OF BIOLOGICALLY ACTIVE COMPOUNDS BY THE LUNG

Metabolized at the endothelial surface without uptake	Bradykinin Angiotensin I Adenine nucleotides
Metabolized by the endothelial cell after uptake	Serotonin Norepinephrine Prostaglandins E and F
Unaffected by passage through the lung	Epinephrine Dopamine Angiotensin II Vasopressin PGA
Released by the lung	Prostaglandins (e.g., prostacyclin) Histamine SRS-A ECF-A Kallikrein

■ ACKNOWLEDGMENTS

In the previous seven editions of this chapter, the authors have included Mary Ellen Avery, Victor Chernick, Hugh O'Brodovich, Gabriel Haddad, and John West. This chapter has incorporated some information from the late Dr. Mary Ellen Wohl's chapter on Developmental Physiology of the Lung, which appeared in previous editions.

Suggested Reading

Normal Lung Anatomy and Cell Function

Crapo JD, Barry BE, Gehr P, et al. Cell number and cell characteristics of the normal human lung. *Am Rev Respir Dis.* 1982;125:332–337.

Crystal RG, West JB, Weibel ER, et al. *The Lung: Scientific Foundations.* 2nd ed. New York: Lippincott-Raven; 1997.

Gehr P, Bachofen M, Weibel ER. The normal lung: Ultrastructure and morphometric estimation of diffusion capacity. *Respir Physiol.* 1978;32:121–140.

Ochs M, Nyengaard JR, Jung A, et al. The number of alveoli in the human lung. *Am J Respir Crit Care Med.* 2004;169:120–124.

Parent RA. *Comparative biology of the normal lung.* Boca Raton: CRC Press; 1992.

Weibel ER. *The Pathway for Oxygen.* Cambridge: Harvard University Press; 1984.

Weibel ER. Lung cell biology. In: Fishman AP, Macklem PT, Mead J, eds. *The Handbook of Physiology. The Respiratory System.* Baltimore: Williams & Wilkins; 1985:47–91.

Weibel ER. Functional morphology of lung parenchyma. In: Fishman AP, Macklem PT, Mead J, eds. *Handbook of Physiology. The Respiratory System.* Baltimore: Williams & Wilkins; 1986:89–111.

Pulmonary Circulation

Rabinovitch M. Pathobiology of pulmonary hypertension. *Annu Rev Pathol.* 2007;2:369–399.

Growth and Development of the Lung

Metzger RJ, Krasnow MA. Genetic control of branching morphogenesis. *Science.* 1999;284:1635–1639.

Ochs M, Nyengaard JR, Jung A, et al. The number of alveoli in the human lung. *Am J Respir Crit Care Med.* 2004;169:120–124.

Whitsett JA, Wert SE, Trapnell BC. Genetic disorders influencing lung formation and function at birth. *Hum Mol Genet.* 2004;13(Spec No 2):R207–R215.

Lung Physiology

West JB. *Respiration Physiology—The Essentials.* 8th ed. Baltimore: Lippincott Williams & Wilkins; 2008.

Pulmonary Function Testing

ATS/ERS statement: raised volume forced expirations in infants: guidelines for current practice. *Am J Respir Crit Care Med*. 2005;172:1463–1471.

Beydon N, Davis SD, Lombardi E, et al. An official American Thoracic Society/European Respiratory Society Statement: pulmonary function testing in preschool children. *Am J Respir Crit Care Med*. 2007;175:1304–1345.

Loeb JS, Blower WC, Feldstein JF, et al. Acceptability and repeatability of spirometry in children using updated ATS/ERS criteria. *Pediatr Pulmonol*. 2008;43:1020–1024.

Miller MR, Hankinson J, Brusasco V, et al. Standardisation of spirometry. *Eur Respir J*. 2005;26:319–338.

Wanger J, Clausen JL, Coates A, et al. Standardisation of the measurement of lung volumes. *Eur Respir J*. 2005;26:511–522.

Respiratory Muscle Testing

ATS/ERS Statement on respiratory muscle testing. *Am J Respir Crit Care Med*. 2002;166:518–624.

Control of Breathing

The changing concept of sudden infant death syndrome. diagnostic coding shifts, controversies regarding the sleeping environment, and new variables to consider in reducing risk. *Pediatrics*. 2005;116:1245–1255.

Feldman JL, Del Negro CA. Looking for inspiration: new perspectives on respiratory rhythm. *Nat Rev Neurosci*. 2006;7:232–242.

Guilleminault C, Lee JH, Chan A. Pediatric obstructive sleep apnea syndrome. *Arch Pediatr Adolesc Med*. 2005;159:775–785.

Weese-Mayer DE, Berry-Kravis EM, Ceccherini I, et al. An official ATS clinical Policy Statement: Congenital central hypoventilation syndrome: genetic basis, diagnosis, and management. *Am J Respir Crit Care Med*. 2010;181:626–644.

References

The complete reference list is available online at www.expertconsult.com

6 BIOLOGY AND ASSESSMENT OF AIRWAY INFLAMMATION

Peter J. Barnes, FRS, FMedSci, and Andrew Bush, MD, FRCP, FRCPCH

INTRODUCTION

Inflammation is classically characterized by four cardinal signs: *calor* and *rubor* (due to vasodilatation), *tumor* (due to plasma exudation and edema), and *dolor* (due to sensitization and activation of sensory nerves. Inflammation is also characterized by infiltration with inflammatory cells, and these will differ depending on the type of inflammatory process. It is vital to recognize that inflammation is an important response that defends the body against invasion from microorganisms and the effects of external toxins. Failure of the components of the inflammatory response (e.g., neutrophil dysfunction, also known as Job's syndrome) has catastrophic consequences. Allergic inflammation is characterized by the fact that it is driven by exposure to allergens through IgE-dependent mechanisms, resulting in a characteristic pattern of inflammation.[1] The inflammatory response seen in allergic diseases is characterized by an infiltration with eosinophils and resembles the inflammatory process mounted in response to worm and other parasitic infections. The inflammatory response not only provides an acute defense against injury, but it is also involved in the healing and restoration of normal function after tissue damage from infection and toxins. In allergic disease, the inflammatory response is activated inappropriately and is harmful rather than beneficial. For some reason, allergens such as house dust mite and pollen proteins, activate eosinophilic inflammation, possibly as a result of their protease activity. Normally such an inflammatory response would kill the invading parasite (or the parasite would overwhelm the host) and the process would therefore be self-limiting, but in allergic disease the inciting stimulus persists and the normally acute inflammatory response turns into chronic inflammation, which may have structural consequences in the airways and skin. Cystic fibrosis (CF) bronchiectasis and persistent bacterial bronchitis are characterized by a neutrophilic pattern of inflammation, driven in part by chronic bacterial infection; the pathophysiology is covered in more detail in Chapters 26, 30, and 52. In this chapter, we place the most emphasis on allergic inflammation, as this underlies the most common noninfectious respiratory diseases of children.

ACUTE INFLAMMATION

Acute inflammation in the respiratory tract is an immediate defense reaction to inhaled allergens, pathogens, or noxious agents. Inhalation of an allergen (e.g., house dust mites) activates surface mast cells by an IgE-dependent mechanism. This releases multiple bronchoconstrictor mediators, resulting in rapid contraction of airway smooth muscle and wheezing. These mediators also result in plasma exudation and swelling of the airways and recruitment of inflammatory cells from the circulation—particularly eosinophils, neutrophils (transiently), and T-lymphocytes, mainly of the T helper 2 (Th2) type. This accounts for the late response that occurs 4 to 6 hours after allergen exposure and resolves within 24 hours, which should be regarded as an acute inflammatory reaction. The acute inflammatory response in the respiratory tract is usually accompanied by increased mucus secretion, which is a part of the defense system that protects the delicate mucosal surface of the airways. In CF, mucus secretion is a highly significant part of the airway pathology, in part mediated by the inflammatory response.

Chronic Inflammation

The normal consequence of an acute inflammatory process is complete resolution; for example, acute lobar pneumonia due to pneumococcal infection is characterized by a massive influx of neutrophils, with complete resolution and restoration of normal lung structure (unless the patient dies in the acute phase of the infection). Many inflammatory conditions of the respiratory tract are chronic and may persist for many years. This inflammation may persist even in the absence of causal mechanisms. This is well illustrated in patients with occupational asthma who continue to have asthma despite complete avoidance of sensitizing agents, and in adult patients with chronic obstructive pulmonary disease who have continued inflammation, even after stopping smoking for many years. The resolution of inflammation was previously thought to be a passive process, but it is now realized that there are important active control mechanisms. There are a number of potential mechanisms that are important in the normal resolution of inflammation. These include Interleukin-10 (IL-10),[2,3] CD200,[4,5] Annexin,[6] lung Kruppel-like factor (LKLF),[7] lipid mediators such as Resolvin E1 (RvE1) and Lipoxin A_4 (LXA$_4$), interferon (IFN)-γ, the IL-23 axis,[8,9] and Protectin D1 (PD1).[10] These mediators and regulators are discussed in more detail in the following paragraphs. The molecular and cellular mechanisms for the persistence of inflammation in the absence of its original causal mechanisms are not understood, but presumably involve some type of long-lived immunologic memory that drives the inflammatory process. Structural cells, such as airway epithelial cells that make up the airway wall, may also drive

Section I

the chronic inflammatory process. This is an important area of research, as understanding these mechanisms might lead to potentially curative therapies.

Structural Changes and Repair

The acute inflammatory response is usually followed by a repair process that restores the tissue to normal. This may involve proliferation of damaged cells (e.g., airway epithelial cells) and fibrosis to heal any breach in the mucosal surface. These repair processes may also become chronic in response to continued inflammation, resulting in structural changes in the airways that are referred to as *remodeling*.[11] However, it should be noted that the relationship between airway inflammation and remodeling is controversial; the conventional view—that inflammation leads to remodeling—has been challenged by human and animal work, which suggests that they may be parallel processes.[12–14] These structural changes in asthma and CF may result in irreversible narrowing of the airways, with a fixed obstruction to air flow. In asthma, several structural changes are found in the airway wall, including fibrosis, an increased amount of airway smooth muscle, and an increased number of blood vessels (angiogenesis). There is much debate about the importance of airway remodeling in asthma as it is not seen in all patients.

It may contribute to airway hyperresponsiveness (AHR) in asthma, but it may also have some beneficial effects in limiting airway closure.[15]

INFLAMMATORY CELLS

Many types of inflammatory cells are involved in airway inflammation, although the precise roles of each cell type and the interrelationship among cells is not yet clear (Figure 6-1). The inflammatory mechanisms in early wheeze, especially episodic (viral) wheeze, are little studied, but probably differ from those seen in multiple trigger wheeze (asthma). The evidence in episodic (viral) wheeze shows that the pattern is neutrophilic.[16–19] In children with asthma, the same kind of inflammation is seen in bronchial biopsies as in adults, which indicates that similar inflammatory mechanisms are likely.[13,20–24] Of note, the inflammatory pattern seen at bronchoscopy is the same in children with multiple trigger (asthmatic) wheeze, independent of their atopic status.[25] No single inflammatory cell accounts for the complex pathophysiology of asthma, although some cells predominate in allergic inflammation. The pattern of inflammation in CF is different, and it results in different pathophysiologic consequences and different responses to therapy. It should be noted also that inflammation may vary in different compartments

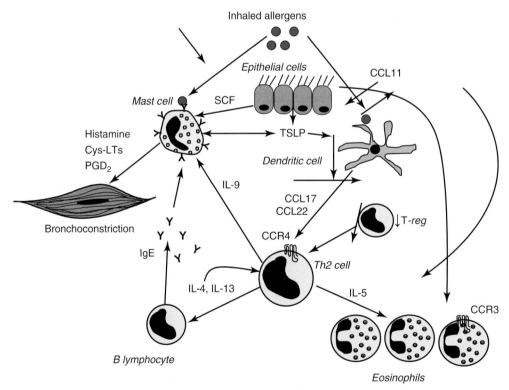

FIGURE 6-1. *Inflammation in asthma. Inhaled allergens activate sensitized mast cells by cross-linking surface-bound IgE molecules to release several bronchoconstrictor mediators, including cysteinyl-leukotrienes (cys-LT) and prostaglandin D$_2$ (PGD$_2$). Epithelial cells release stem-cell factor (SCF), which is important for maintaining mucosal mast cells at the airway surface. Allergens are processed by myeloid dendritic cells, which are conditioned by thymic stromal lymphopoietin (TSLP) secreted by epithelial cells and mast cells to release the chemokines CC-chemokine ligand 17 (CCL17) and CCL22, which act on CC-chemokine receptor 4 (CCR4) to attract T helper 2 (Th2) cells. Th2 cells have a central role in orchestrating the inflammatory response in allergy through the release of interleukin-4 (IL-4) and IL-13 (which stimulate B cells to synthesize IgE), IL-5 (which is necessary for eosinophilic inflammation) and IL-9 (which stimulates mast-cell proliferation). Epithelial cells release CCL11, which recruits eosinophils via CCR3. Patients with asthma may have a defect in regulatory T cells (T-reg), which may favor further Th2-cell proliferation.*

of the lung. In adults with asthma, transbronchial biopsy has shown evidence of very distal inflammation in the absence of proximal airway inflammation.[26–28] There is a dissociation between airway mucosal and airway luminal inflammatory patterns in asthma.[29] In CF, whereas the predominant inflammatory cell in the airway lumen is the neutrophil (as shown by sputum and bronchoalveolar lavage cytology), T-lymphocytes predominate in the proximal airway wall.[30]

Mast Cells

Mast cells are important in initiating the acute broncho-constrictor responses to allergens and probably to other indirect stimuli such as exercise and hyperventilation (via osmolality or thermal changes) and fog. Treatment of asthmatic patients with prednisone results in a decrease in the number of tryptase-positive mast cells. Furthermore, mast cell tryptase appears to play a role in airway remodeling, as this mast cell product stimulates human lung fibroblast proliferation. Mast cells also secrete cytokines, including IL-4 and eotaxin, which may be involved in maintaining the allergic inflammatory response, and tumor necrosis factor-α (TNF-α).[31] Mast cells are found in increased numbers in airway smooth muscle of asthmatic patients, and this appears to correlate with AHR, suggesting that mast cell mediators mediate AHR.[32]

However, there are questions about the role of mast cells in more chronic allergic inflammatory events, and it seems more probable that other cells, such as macrophages, eosinophils, and T-lymphocytes, are more important in the chronic inflammatory process and in AHR. Classically, mast cells are activated by allergens through an IgE-dependent mechanism. The importance of IgE in the pathophysiology of asthma has been highlighted by recent clinical studies with humanized anti-IgE antibodies, which inhibit IgE-mediated effects. Anti-IgE therapy is effective in patients, including children, with severe asthma who are not well controlled with high doses of corticosteroids, and it is particularly effective in reducing exacerbations.[33] The role of IgE in the treatment of severe asthma is discussed in Chapter 48.

Macrophages

Macrophages, which are derived from blood monocytes, traffic into the airways in inflammatory diseases under the direction of specific chemokines. In the airways, these monocytes differentiate into macrophages, which have the capacity to secrete many inflammatory proteins, chemotactic factors, lipid mediators, and proteinases. In asthma, they may be activated by allergen via low-affinity IgE receptors (Fc$_\varepsilon$RII). The enormous immunologic repertoire of macrophages allows these cells to produce more than 100 different products, including a large variety of cytokines that may orchestrate the inflammatory response. Macrophages have the capacity to initiate a particular type of inflammatory response via the release of a certain pattern of cytokines. Macrophages may both increase and decrease inflammation, depending on the stimulus. Alveolar macrophages normally have a *suppressive* effect on lymphocyte function, but this may be impaired in asthma after allergen exposure. In patients with asthma, there is a reduced secretion of IL-10 (an anti-inflammatory protein secreted by macrophages) in alveolar macrophages. Macrophages may therefore play an important anti-inflammatory role by preventing the development of allergic inflammation. There may be subtypes of macrophages that perform different inflammatory, anti-inflammatory, or phagocytic roles in airway disease, but at present it is difficult to differentiate these subtypes. There is evidence that alveolar macrophages show reduced phagocytosis of apoptotic cells and carbon particles in severe asthma so that inflammation does not resolve.[34,35]

Dendritic Cells

Dendritic cells are specialized macrophage-like cells that have a unique ability to induce a T-lymphocyte–mediated immune response and therefore play a critical role in the development of asthma.[36] There are three major lineages of dendritic cells: myeloid DCs (mDCs),[37] plasmacytoid DCs (pDCs),[38] and Langerhans cells (LCs).[39] Dendritic cells in the respiratory tract form a network that is localized to the epithelium, and they act as very effective antigen-presenting cells. It is likely that dendritic cells play an important role in the initiation of allergen-induced responses in asthma. Dendritic cells take up allergens, process them to peptides, and migrate to local lymph nodes where they present the allergenic peptides to uncommitted T-lymphocytes. With the aid of co-stimulatory molecules (e.g., B7.1, B7.2, and CD40), they program the production of allergen-specific T cells. Animal studies have demonstrated that myeloid dendritic cells are critical to the development of T helper type 2 (Th2) cells and eosinophilia.

Eosinophils

Eosinophilic infiltration is a characteristic feature of allergic inflammation. Allergen inhalation results in a marked increase in eosinophils in bronchoalveolar lavage fluid at the time of the late reaction, and there is a correlation between eosinophil counts in peripheral blood or bronchial lavage and AHR. Eosinophils are linked to the development of AHR through the release of basic proteins and oxygen-derived free radicals.[40] Several mechanisms are involved in *recruitment* of eosinophils into the airways. Eosinophils are derived from bone marrow precursors, and the signal for increased eosinophil production is presumably derived from the inflamed airway. Eosinophil recruitment initially involves adhesion of eosinophils to vascular endothelial cells in the airway circulation, their migration into the submucosa, and their subsequent activation. The role of individual adhesion molecules, cytokines, and mediators in orchestrating these responses has been extensively investigated. Adhesion of eosinophils involves the expression of specific glycoprotein molecules on the surface of eosinophils (integrins) and expression of such molecules as intercellular adhesion molecule-1 (ICAM-1) on vascular endothelial cells. The adhesion molecule very late antigen-4 (VLA4) expressed on eosinophils, which interacts with VCAM-1 and IL-4, increases its expression on endothelial cells. GM-CSF and IL-5 may be important for the survival of eosinophils in the airways and for "priming" eosinophils to exhibit enhanced responsiveness.

There are several mediators involved in the migration of eosinophils from the circulation to the surface of the airway. The most potent and selective agents appear to be chemokines (e.g., CCL5, CC11, CCL13, CCL24, and CCL26) that are expressed by epithelial cells. There appears to be a co-operative interaction between IL-5 and chemokines, so that both are necessary for the eosinophilic response in the airway. Once recruited to the airway, eosinophils require the presence of various growth factors, of which GM-CSF and IL-5 appear to be the most important. In the absence of these growth factors, eosinophils may undergo programmed cell death (apoptosis).

After humanized monoclonal antibody to IL-5 is administered to asthmatic patients, there is a profound and prolonged reduction in circulating eosinophils, and eosinophils recruited into the airway following allergen challenge.[41] However, there is no effect on the response to inhaled allergen and no reduction in AHR. Clinical studies with anti-IL-5–blocking antibody showed a similar profound reduction in circulating eosinophils, but no improvement in clinical measures of asthma control. A subsequent study attributed this to a failure to reduce mucosal eosinophilia.[42] Recent studies with highly selected patients with persistent sputum eosinophilia despite high doses of inhaled corticosteroids have shown a reduction in exacerbations.[43,44] These two studies underscore the importance of understanding the differing inflammatory process in subgroups of patients with asthma, rather than applying the same strategies to all patients.

Neutrophils

Neutrophils are the predominant inflammatory cells in patients with CF, and they appear to be involved in severe asthma, when increased numbers of neutrophils are found in the sputum and in bronchial biopsies (Figure 6-2).[45–47] Putative causes for airway neutrophilia are corticosteroid therapy, which inhibits neutrophil apoptosis, chronic infection with atypical organisms such as Chlamydia or Mycoplasma, exposure to passive smoking, and gastroesophageal reflux and aspiration. It is not certain whether these neutrophils play a pathophysiologic role. However, they may generate oxidative stress that could play an important role in the pathophysiology of severe asthma. There is an increase in sputum neutrophils in patients following loss of asthma control.[48]

T-Lymphocytes

T-lymphocytes play a very important role in coordinating the inflammatory response in asthma through the release of specific patterns of cytokines, resulting in the

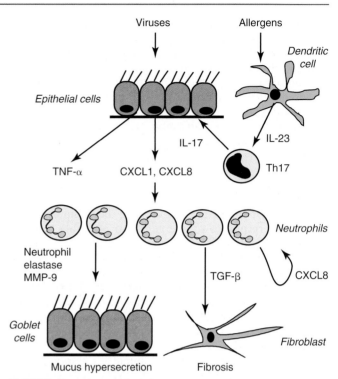

FIGURE 6-2. Neutrophilic inflammation in asthma. Viruses, such as rhinovirus, stimulate the release of CXCL8 and CXCL1 from airway epithelial cells. Allergens activate dendritic cells to release IL-23, which recruits helper T-cells that secrete IL-17 (Th17 cells) to release tumor necrosis factor-α (TNF-α), which amplifies inflammation, and CXCL1 and CXCL8, which recruit neutrophils into the airways. Neutrophils release more CXCL8 and also transforming growth factor-β (TGF-β), which activates fibroblasts to cause fibrosis, and neutrophil elastase and matrix metalloproteinase-9 (MMP-9), which stimulate mucus hypersecretion from goblet cells.

recruitment and survival of eosinophils and in the maintenance of mast cells in the airways.[49] T-lymphocytes are coded to express a distinctive pattern of cytokines, which are similar to that described in the murine T helper 2 (Th2) type of T-lymphocytes, which characteristically express IL-4, IL-5, IL-9, and IL-13 (Figure 6-3). This programming of T-lymphocytes is presumably due to antigen-presenting cells, such as dendritic cells, which may migrate from the epithelium to regional lymph nodes or which interact with lymphocytes resident in the airway mucosa. The naïve immune system is skewed to express the Th2 phenotype; data now indicate that children with atopy are more likely to retain this skewed phenotype than normal children. There is some evidence that early infections or exposure to endotoxins might promote Th1-mediated responses to predominate and that a lack of infection or a clean environment in childhood may favor Th2 cell expression and thus atopic diseases.[50] Indeed, the balance between Th1 cells and Th2 cells is thought to be determined by locally released cytokines, such as IL-12, which tip the balance in favor of Th1 cells, or IL-4 or IL-13, which favor the emergence of Th2 cells. Regulatory T cells (Tregs) suppress the immune response through the secretion of inhibitory cytokines (e.g., IL-10 and TGF-β) and play an important role in immune regulation with suppression of Th1 responses, and there is some evidence that Treg function may be defective in asthmatic patients.[51]

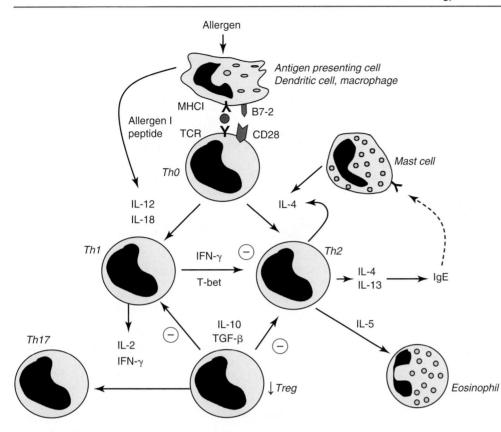

FIGURE 6-3. T lymphocytes in asthma. Asthmatic inflammation is characterized by a preponderance of T helper 2 (Th2) lymphocytes over T helper 1 (Th1) cells. Regulatory T cells (Treg) have an inhibitory effect, whereas T helper 17 (Th17) cells have a pro-inflammatory effect. *MHCI*, Class 1 major histocompatibility complex; *IL*, interleukin; *IFN-γ*, interferon gamma; *TGF-β*, transforming growth factor beta; *IgE*, immunoglobulin E; *Tho*, uncommitted T cell.

Th17 cells are CD4+ cells that predominantly release IL-17 and IL-22 and may be involved in neutrophilic inflammation in severe asthma and CF.[52] In contrast to Th1 and Th2 cells, Th17 cells are corticosteroid-resistant.

B-Lymphocytes

In allergic diseases B-lymphocytes secrete IgE, and the factors regulating IgE secretion are now much better understood.[53] IL-4 is crucial in switching B cells to IgE production, and CD40 on T cells is an important accessory molecule that signals through interaction with CD40-ligand on B cells. There is increasing evidence for local production of IgE, even in patients with intrinsic asthma.[54,55]

A subset of CD4+ T cells termed *invariant natural killer T (iNKT)* cells secrete IL-4 and IL-13, but their role in asthma is currently uncertain as there appears to be a discrepancy between the data from murine models of asthma and humans.[56]

Basophils

The role of basophils in asthma is uncertain, as these cells have previously been difficult to detect by immunocytochemistry. Using a basophil-specific marker, a small increase in basophils has been documented in the airways of asthmatic patients, with an increased number after allergen challenge. However, these cells are far outnumbered by eosinophils (approximately 10:1 ratio), and their functional role is unknown.[57] There is also an increase in the numbers of basophils, as well as mast cells, in induced sputum after allergen challenge.

Platelets

There is some evidence for the involvement of platelets in the pathophysiology of allergic diseases, since platelet activation may be observed and there is evidence for platelets in bronchial biopsies of asthmatic patients. After allergen challenge, there is a significant decrease in circulating platelets, and circulating platelets from patients with asthma show evidence of increased activation and release the chemokine CCL5.

STRUCTURAL CELLS AS SOURCES OF MEDIATORS

Structural cells of the airways, including epithelial cells, endothelial cells, fibroblasts, and even airway smooth muscle cells, may be an important source of inflammatory mediators, such as cytokines and lipid mediators in asthma and CF. Indeed, because structural cells far outnumber inflammatory cells in the airway, they may become the major source of mediators driving chronic airway inflammation. Epithelial cells may have a key role in translating inhaled environmental signals into an airway inflammatory response and are probably the major target cell for inhaled corticosteroids in asthma (Figure 6-4). Epithelial cells may also play an important role in CF in driving the neutrophilic inflammatory response through the release of CXCL1 and CXCL8. Through the release

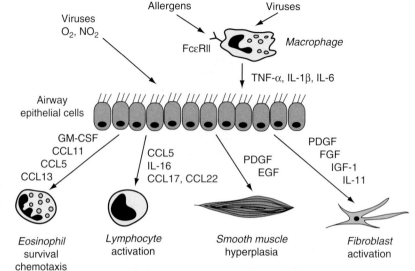

FIGURE 6-4. Airway epithelial cells in asthma. Airway epithelial cells may play an active role in asthmatic inflammation through the release of many inflammatory mediators, cytokines, chemokines, and growth factors. TNF-α, tumor necrosis factor alpha; IL, interleukin; CCL, C-C chemokine; PDGF, platelet-derived growth factor; EGF, epidermal growth factor; FGF, fibroblast growth factor; IGF, insulin-like growth factor.

of growth factors, airway epithelial cells may also be important in driving the structural changes that occur in chronic airway inflammation.[58] Epithelial cell integrity may also be an important factor in denying allergens exposure to the immune system; an increasing number of asthma susceptibility genes are expressed in the airway epithelium.[59–61]

INFLAMMATORY MEDIATORS

Many different mediators have been implicated in asthma, and they may have a variety of effects on the airway, which accounts for all of the pathological features of asthma[62] (Figure 6-5). Although less is known about the mediators of CF,[63] it is becoming clear that they differ from those implicated in asthma. Because each mediator has many effects, the role of individual mediators in the pathophysiology of airway inflammatory disease is not yet clear. The multiplicity and redundancy of effects of mediators make it unlikely that preventing the synthesis or action of a *single* mediator will have a major impact in the therapy of these diseases. However, some mediators

may play a more important role if they are upstream in the inflammatory process. The effects of single mediators can only be evaluated through the use of specific receptor antagonists or mediator synthesis inhibitors.

Lipid Mediators

The cysteinyl-leukotrienes, LTC_4, LTD_4, and LTE_4, are potent constrictors of human airways and may also increase AHR. Leukotriene antagonists have some bronchodilator and anti-inflammatory effects but are much less effective than inhaled corticosteroids in the management of childhood asthma.[64] Platelet-activating factor (PAF) is a potent inflammatory mediator that mimics many of the features of asthma, including eosinophil recruitment and activation and induction of AHR; yet even potent PAF antagonists, such as modipafant, do not control asthma symptoms, at least in chronic asthma. Prostaglandins (PG) have potent effects on airway function, and there is increased expression of the inducible form of cyclo-oxygenase (COX-2) in asthmatic airways; however inhibition of their synthesis with COX inhibitors, such as aspirin or ibuprofen, does not have an effect in most patients. Prostaglandin D_2 is a bronchoconstrictor prostaglandin produced predominantly by mast cells; it also activates a novel chemoattractant receptor termed *chemoattractant receptor of Th2 cells* (CRTh2) or *DP2-receptor*, which is expressed on Th2 cells and eosinophils and mediates chemotaxis of these cell types; it may provide a link between mast cell activation and allergic inflammation. Several oral $CRTh2/DP_2$ antagonists are now in clinical development.[65]

Cytokines

Cytokines are increasingly recognized to be important in chronic inflammation and to play a critical role in orchestrating the type of inflammatory response. They are the target for the development of new asthma therapies[66] (Figure 6-6). Many inflammatory cells (macrophages, mast cells, eosinophils, and lymphocytes) and airway

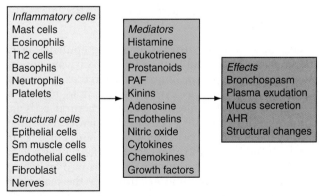

Inflammatory cells	Mediators	Effects
Mast cells	Histamine	Bronchospasm
Eosinophils	Leukotrienes	Plasma exudation
Th2 cells	Prostanoids	Mucus secretion
Basophils	PAF	AHR
Neutrophils	Kinins	Structural changes
Platelets	Adenosine	
	Endothelins	
Structural cells	Nitric oxide	
Epithelial cells	Cytokines	
Sm muscle cells	Chemokines	
Endothelial cells	Growth factors	
Fibroblast		
Nerves		

FIGURE 6-5. Multiple cells, mediators and effects. Many cells and mediators are involved in asthma and lead to several effects on the airways. Th2, T helper 2 cells; Sm, smooth; PAF, platelet-activating factor; AHR, airway hyperresponsiveness.

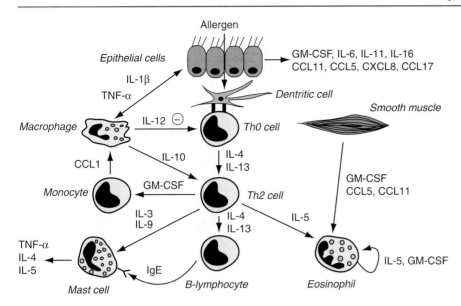

FIGURE 6-6. The cytokine network in asthma. Many inflammatory cytokines are released from inflammatory and structural cells in the airway and orchestrate and perpetuate the inflammatory response.

structural cells are capable of synthesizing and releasing cytokines. While inflammatory mediators like histamine and leukotrienes may be important in the acute and subacute inflammatory responses and in exacerbations of asthma, it is likely that cytokines play a dominant role in maintaining chronic inflammation in airway diseases. Research in this area is hampered by a lack of specific antagonists, although important observations have been made using specific neutralizing antibodies that have been developed as novel therapies.

The cytokines that appear to be of particular importance in asthma include the lymphokines secreted by T-lymphocytes. There is increased gene expression of IL-5 in lymphocytes in bronchial biopsies of patients with symptomatic asthma. However, as discussed earlier in the chapter, a blocking antibody to IL-5, while profoundly reducing circulating eosinophils, has no effects on the allergic response or on asthma control, except in a small subgroup of patients with steroid-resistant eosinophilic inflammation. IL-4 and IL-13 play a key role in the allergic inflammatory response since they determine the isotype switching in B cells that result in IgE formation. IL-4 (but not IL-13) is also involved in differentiation of Th2 cells and therefore may be critical in the initial development of atopy. Several antibodies that block IL-13 binding to the alpha chain of the IL-4 receptor, which is common to IL-4 and IL-13, are in development, but so far clinical results have been disappointing.

Other cytokines (e.g., IL-1β, IL-6, TNF-α, and GM-CSF) are released from a variety of cells, including macrophages and epithelial cells, and may be important in amplifying the inflammatory response. TNF-α may be an amplifying mediator in asthma and is produced in increased amounts in airways of patients with severe asthma. However, blocking TNF-α with a potent antibody had no clinical benefit in patients with severe asthma, and it also led to an increased risk of infections and cancers.[67] TNF-α and IL-1β both activate the pro-inflammatory transcription factors—nuclear factor-κB (NF-κB) and activator protein-1 (AP-1)—which then switch on many inflammatory genes in the asthmatic airway.

Thymic stromal lymphopoeitin (TSLP) shows a marked increase in expression in airway epithelium and mast cells of asthmatic patients.[68] TSLP appears to play a key role in programming airway dendritic cells to release CCL17 and CCL22 to attract Th2 cells (Figure 6-7).[69]

Other cytokines, such as interferon-γ (IFN-γ), IL-10, and IL-12, play a regulatory role and may inhibit the allergic inflammatory process (see the section that follows).

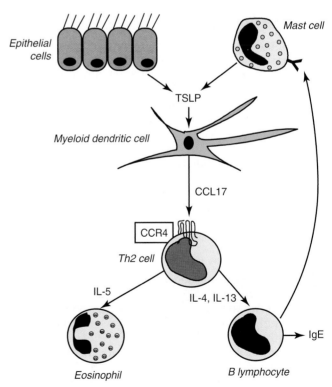

FIGURE 6-7. Thymic stromal lymphopoetin in asthma. TSLP is an upstream cytokine produced by airway epithelial cells and mast cells in asthma that acts on immature dendritic cells to mature and release CCL17, which attracts Th2 cells via CCR4. *Th2*, T helper 2; *CCL*, chemokine; *CCR*, chemokine receptor.

Chemokines

Many chemokines are involved in the recruitment of inflammatory cells in the airways.[26] Over 50 different chemokines are now recognized, and they activate more than 20 different surface receptors. Chemokine receptors belong to the seven transmembrane receptor superfamily of G-protein–coupled receptors; this makes it possible to find small molecule inhibitors, which has not been possible for classical cytokine receptors.[70] Some chemokines appear to be selective for single chemokines, whereas others are promiscuous and mediate the effects of several related chemokines. Chemokines appear to act in sequence in determining the final inflammatory response, and so inhibitors may be more or less effective depending on the kinetics of the response.

Several chemokines, including CCL5, CC11, CCL13, CCL24, and CCL26, activate a common receptor on eosinophils termed *CCR3*. Increased expression in the airways of asthmatic patients is correlated with increased AHR. CCR4 chemokines are selectively expressed on Th2 cells and are activated by the CCL17 and CCL22 chemokines. Epithelial cells of patients with asthma express CCL22, which may then recruit Th2 cells, resulting in coordinated eosinophilic inflammation.

CXC chemokines are involved in the recruitment of neutrophils. CXCL1 and CXCL8 play an important role in neutrophilic inflammation in severe asthma and CF.

Oxidative Stress

As in all inflammatory diseases, there is increased oxidative stress, as activated inflammatory cells, such as macrophages, neutrophils, and eosinophils produce reactive oxygen species. Evidence for increased oxidative stress in asthma and CF is provided by the increased concentrations of 8-isoprostane (a product of oxidized arachidonic acid) in exhaled breath condensates and increased ethane (a product of oxidative lipid peroxidation) in exhaled breath of asthmatic patients.[71,72] Increased oxidative stress is related to disease severity and may amplify the inflammatory response and reduce responsiveness to corticosteroids, particularly in severe disease and during exacerbations.

Nitric Oxide

Nitric oxide (NO) is produced by several cells in the airway by NO synthases. The inducible form of NO synthase (iNOS) shows increased expression, particularly in the airway epithelial cells and macrophages of asthmatic airways. Although the cellular source of NO within the lung is not known, inferences based on mathematical models suggest that it is the large airways that are the source of NO; in severe asthma there is evidence that small airways also produce it.[73] The combination of increased oxidative stress and NO may lead to the formation of the potent radical peroxynitrite that may cause tyrosine nitration of proteins in the airways.

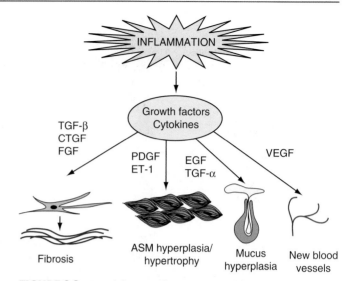

FIGURE 6-8. Growth factors and airway structural changes in asthma. *TGF,* transforming growth factor; *FGF,* fibroblast growth factor; *CTGF,* connective tissue growth factor; *EGF,* epidermal growth factor; *PDGF,* platelet-derived growth factor; *VEGF,* vascular-endothelial growth factor; *ET,* endothelin.

Growth Factors

Many growth factors are released from inflammatory cells and structural cells in airway diseases; these may play a critical role in the structural changes that occur in chronic inflammation, including fibrosis, airway smooth muscle thickening, angiogenesis, and mucous hyperplasia. While the role of individual mediators is not yet established, there is evidence for increased expression of transforming growth factor-β (a mediator associated with fibrosis), vascular-endothelial growth factor (a mediator associated with angiogenesis), and epidermal growth factor (a mediator that induces mucous hyperplasia and expression of mucin genes) (Figure 6-8).

▬ NEURAL MECHANISMS

Neural mechanisms may play an important role in the inflammatory response of airways. Neural reflexes may be activated by inflammatory signals, resulting in reflex bronchoconstriction, and airway nerves may release neurotransmitters, particularly neuropeptides, that have inflammatory effects.[74] There is a close interaction between nerves and inflammatory cells in allergic inflammation, as inflammatory mediators activate and modulate neurotransmission, whereas neurotransmitters may modulate the allergic inflammatory response. Inflammatory mediators may act on various prejunctional receptors on airway nerves to modulate the release of neurotransmitters. Inflammatory mediators may activate sensory nerves, resulting in reflex cholinergic bronchoconstriction or release of inflammatory neuropeptides (Figure 6-9). There is particular interest in the role of neural mechanisms in animal models and human disease caused by respiratory syncytial virus.[75–77]

Inflammatory products may also sensitize sensory nerve endings in the airway epithelium, so that the nerves become hyperalgesic. Hyperalgesia and pain *(dolor)* are

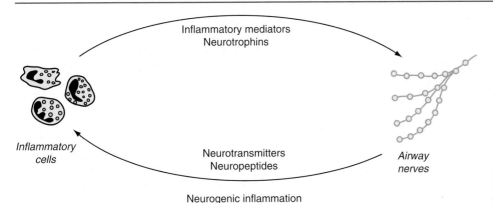

FIGURE 6-9. Two-way interaction between inflammation and neural control of the airways.

cardinal signs of inflammation, and in the asthmatic airway hyperalgesia may mediate cough and chest tightness, which are characteristic symptoms of asthma. The precise mechanisms are not yet certain, but mediators such as prostaglandins, certain cytokines, and neurotrophins may be important. Neurotrophins, which are released by various cell types in peripheral tissues, may cause proliferation and sensitization of airway sensory nerves.[78] Neurotrophins, such as nerve growth factor (NGF), may be released from inflammatory and structural cells in asthmatic airways and then stimulate the increased synthesis of neuropeptides (e.g., substance P) in airway sensory nerves, as well as sensitizing nerve endings in the airways. Thus, NGF is released from human airway epithelial cells after exposure to inflammatory stimuli. Neurotrophins may play an important role in mediating AHR in asthma.

Airway nerves may also release neurotransmitters that have inflammatory effects. Thus neuropeptides such as substance P (SP), neurokinin A, and calcitonin-gene–related peptide may be released from sensitized inflammatory nerves in the airways, increasing and extending the ongoing inflammatory response in asthma and other types of chronic inflammation.[79]

TRANSCRIPTION FACTORS

The chronic inflammation of asthma and CF is due to increased expression of multiple inflammatory proteins (i.e., cytokines, enzymes, receptors, adhesion molecules). In many cases, these inflammatory proteins are induced by transcription factors, DNA binding factors that increase the transcription of selected target genes (Figure 6-10). One transcription factor that may play a critical role in asthma is NF-κB, which can be activated by multiple stimuli, including protein kinase C activators, oxidants, and pro-inflammatory cytokines (such as IL-1β and TNF-α). There is evidence for increased activation of NF-κB in asthmatic airways, particularly in epithelial cells and macrophages. NF-κB regulates the expression of several key genes that are overexpressed in asthmatic and CF airways, including pro-inflammatory cytokines (IL-1β, TNF-α, GM-CSF), chemokines (IL-8, RANTES, MIP-1α, eotaxin), adhesion molecules (ICAM-1, VCAM-1), and inflammatory enzymes (cyclooxygenase-2, iNOS).[80] Many other transcription factors are involved in the abnormal expression of inflammatory genes in asthma, and there is growing evidence that there may be a common mechanism that involves activation of co-activator

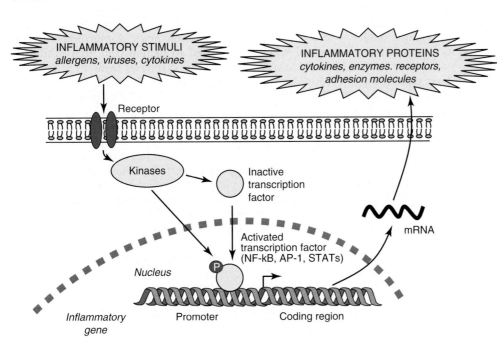

FIGURE 6-10. Pro-inflammatory transcription factors in asthma. Transcription factors play a key role in amplifying and perpetuating the inflammatory response in asthma. Transcription factors, including nuclear factor kappa-B (NFκB), activator protein-1 (AP-1), and signal transduction-activated transcription factors (STATs), are activated by inflammatory stimuli and increase the expression of multiple inflammatory genes.

molecules at the start site of transcription of these genes. They are activated by transcription factors that induce acetylation of core histones around which DNA is wound in the chromosome. Local unwinding of DNA opens up the chromatin structure and allows RNA polymerase and other transcription factors to bind, thus switching on gene transcription.[81]

Transcription factors play a critical role in determining the balance between Th1 and Th2 cells. The transcription factor GATA-3 determines the differentiation of Th2 cells and the expression of Th2 cytokines; it shows increased expression in asthmatic patients.[39] The differentiation of Th1 cells is regulated by the transcription factor T-bet. Deletion of the *T-bet* gene is associated with an asthma-like phenotype in mice, suggesting that it may play an important role in inhibiting the development of Th2 cells.

ANTI-INFLAMMATORY MECHANISMS

Although most emphasis has been placed on inflammatory mechanisms, there may be important anti-inflammatory mechanisms that may be defective in asthma, resulting in increased inflammatory responses in the airways.[82] Endogenous cortisol may be important as a regulator of the allergic inflammatory response, and nocturnal exacerbation of asthma may be related to the Circadian fall in plasma cortisol. The blockade of endogenous cortisol secretion by metyrapone results in an increase in the late response to allergen in the skin. Cortisol is converted to the inactive cortisone by the enzyme 11β-hydroxysteroid dehydrogenase, which is expressed in airway tissues. It is possible that this enzyme functions abnormally in asthma or may determine the severity of asthma.

Various cytokines have anti-inflammatory actions. IL-1 receptor antagonist (IL-1RA) inhibits the binding of IL-1 to its receptors and therefore has a potential anti-inflammatory capability in asthma. It is reported to be effective in an animal model of asthma. IL-12 and IFN-γ enhance Th1 cells and inhibit Th2 cells. IL-12 promotes the differentiation and thus the suppression of Th2 cells, resulting in a reduction in eosinophilic inflammation, and its expression may be reduced in asthmatic airways.

IL-10, which was originally described as cytokine synthesis inhibitory factor, inhibits the expression of multiple inflammatory cytokines (TNF-α, IL-1β, GM-CSF) and chemokines, as well as inflammatory enzymes (iNOS, COX-2). There is evidence that IL-10 secretion and gene transcription are defective in macrophages and monocytes from asthmatic patients; this may lead to enhancement of inflammatory effects in asthma and may be a determinant of asthma severity.[83] IL-10 secretion is lower in monocytes from patients with severe asthma compared to mild asthma, and there is an association between haplotypes associated with decreased production and severe asthma.

Another family of molecules of potential interest is the lung Kruppel-like transcription factor (LKLF) family proteins. LKLF plays a pivotal role in maintenance of T-lymphocyte quiescence;[7] this is of interest in view of our recent findings of increased T cells in the CF airway.[84] A recent manuscript showed that LKLF suppresses *P. aeruginosa*–induced activation of NFκB and subsequent IL-8 release from airway cells, but, in turn, its expression was inhibited by the pro-inflammatory cytokine TNF-α.[85] There was evidence that LKLF is abundantly present in normal small airway human tissue sections, but the signal lessens as inflammation worsens, and the presence of activated human neutrophils "switches off" LKLF in airway epithelial cells. This suggests a counterinflammatory role for LKLF in airway epithelium, and provides evidence for cytokine regulation of LKLF in a TNF-α–dependent fashion, suggesting that LKLF downregulation may be a mechanism by which the presence of neutrophil-secreted cytokines in the airway lumen contributes to the continuous activation of airway epithelium in CF lung disease.

Lipoxins (LX) are anti-inflammatory lipid mediators that modulate neutrophilic inflammation.[8] Reduced LXA$_4$ was first described in BALF from CF patients, and in a mouse model, exogenous LXA$_4$ was shown to abrogate inflammation and infection, and reduce disease severity.[86] Recent studies have further elucidated the regulation of this mediator.[9] Resolvin E1 (RvE1), which is a potent inhibitor of neutrophil transmigration across epithelial and endothelial barriers, has been shown to promote the resolution of airway inflammation by suppressing IL-23 and IL-6 production in the lung. This is of particular interest, given that IL-23 promotes the survival of TH-17 cells in the airway.[87] These cells secrete IL-17A, which has been linked to the pathogenesis of a number of inflammatory diseases[88] and which we have found in BALF from children with CF.[89] Furthermore, administration of antibodies to interferon (IFN)-γ leads to increased BALF leukocytosis, which was abrogated by co-administration of RvE.[90] So far there is little, if any, evidence for a role of this axis in CF or other pediatric inflammatory lung diseases.

The docosohexanoic acid Prostaglandin D (PD)1-derived mediator is one of the arachidonic acid–derived family of mediators that terminate inflammation, along with LXA$_4$ and its epimer aspirin-derived LXA$_4$, and RvE1 (above, derived from eicosopentanoic acid). A murine peritonitis model was recently used to demonstrate that inhibition of cyclo-oxygenase or lipoxygenases leads to a defect of resolution of inflammation, which could be rescued by RvE1, PD1, or an aspirin-triggered LPX$_4$ analog.[91] No airway data have been reported, but this is another potential mechanism of resolution of inflammation that merits further investigation.

Other mediators may also have anti-inflammatory and immunosuppressive effects. PGE$_2$ has inhibitory effects on macrophages, epithelial cells, and eosinophils, and exogenous PGE$_2$ inhibits allergen-induced airway responses. Its endogenous generation may account for the refractory period after exercise challenge. However, it is unlikely that endogenous PGE$_2$ is important in most asthmatics since non-selective cyclo-oxygenase inhibitors only worsen asthma in a minority of patients (aspirin-induced asthma). Several other lipid mediators, including lipoxins, resolvins and protectins, promote resolution of inflammation and may be reduced in asthma patients.[92]

NON-INVASIVE ASSESSMENT OF AIRWAY INFLAMMATION

Inflammation plays a key role in the pathophysiology of airway diseases, and suppression of this inflammation is a major aim of therapy. This implies that the degree of inflammation needs to be assessed during clinical management. Physiologic measurements, such as spirometry, measure the outcome of inflammation but only reflect inflammation indirectly. Furthermore, spirometry is a notoriously poor asthma endpoint in children,[93–95] and treatment with bronchodilators makes changes difficult to interpret. Direct measurement of inflammation by bronchial biopsy or bronchoalveolar lavage is valuable in research studies, but is clearly inappropriate for routine assessment and for repeated measurements, especially in children. This means that less invasive procedures need to be devised for assessing airway inflammation.

The characteristics of the ideal "inflammometer" are shown in Table 6-1. Unfortunately, no such instrument exists! There are two broad reasons for wishing to measure airway inflammation: to study the mechanisms of disease and as a clinical tool to monitor treatment in an individual. Unfortunately, the two are frequently confused. The finding that levels of a particular mediator are statistically significantly different between groups may lead to valuable pathophysiologic insights, but if the overlap between asthma and normal groups is considerable, measuring the mediator is likely to be completely useless as a monitoring tool in clinical practice. This is neatly illustrated by the use of measurements of exhaled and nasal NO in primary ciliary dyskinesia (PCD); exhaled nasal NO is lower in PCD than in normals, but the overlap means it cannot be used as a diagnostic tool; on the other hand, a low nasal NO almost completely differentiated PCD from normals.[96]

Induced Sputum

Sputum may be induced by nebulized hypertonic saline (3.5% or 7%) for analysis of inflammatory cells and mediators. This technique has been applied successfully to children; however, it is difficult to use in clinical practice, and up to 25% of children do not produce a useable sample.[97] In younger children, the figure is even higher. Furthermore, the technique of sputum induction may

induce wheezing in asthmatic patients, is time-consuming and uncomfortable, and may induce inflammation in the airways, making repeated measurements difficult. Sputum induction has proved to be a useful research technique in investigating airway inflammation in children. It measures proximal luminal inflammation, but relates poorly to airway wall pathology, and probably even more loosely to distal inflammatory changes. One study showed that the absence of eosinophils in induced sputum was predictive of a successful taper of inhaled steroids.[98] A second study[99] showed that a strategy of adjusting treatment to try to normalize induced sputum eosinophils measured every 3 months in children with very severe asthma was not beneficial compared with a standard strategy. A *post hoc* analysis did show a reduction in exacerbations in the month immediately following the measurement.[99] At the present time, there is insufficient evidence to recommend the routine use of induced sputum in clinical practice because of the technical issues involved in obtaining samples in children and the lack of studies showing improved outcome.

Exhaled Gases

There has been considerable recent progress in the measurement of exhaled gases that may reflect the inflammatory process in the airways.[100] This technique is technically simple and is feasible, even in young children. Repeated measurements are possible and also feasible in patients with severe disease.

Exhaled Nitric Oxide

Most progress has been made with NO, which can be detected in exhaled breath by chemiluminescence analyzers. The concentration of NO is increased in the exhaled breath of children (including infants) with asthma and decreases with inhaled corticosteroid therapy.[101] Using multiple flows, it is possible to partition exhaled NO into central and peripheral fractions; this provides information about inflammation in central and peripheral airways.[102] However, there are no data to show clinical utility in children. Exhaled NO is correlated with other markers of inflammation such as eosinophils in induced sputum and AHR in children; however, the relationship is not a particularly close one. The correlation between NO and airway eosinophilia is closest in steroid-naïve children (the group in whom it is least likely to be useful). Longitudinal studies[99] show that even in the same individual, the relationship between NO and sputum eosinophilia varies over time, with a high NO sometimes seen with a normal sputum eosinophil count, and vice versa.

There is some evidence that NO measurement may be useful in pediatric asthma. It may predict exacerbations in pollen-sensitive asthma,[103] and titrating an inhaled steroid dose to exhaled NO levels may improve outcomes without the use of an increased dose of medication.[104] In another study, a rise in exhaled NO predicted the need to reintroduce inhaled corticosteroids after weaning.[105] There is some suggestion in the cumulated literature that the role of NO may be to predict the risk of exacerbations of asthma, similar to persistent airway eosinophilia,

TABLE 6-1 CHARACTERISTICS OF THE IDEAL "INFLAMMOMETER"

Cheap
Easy to maintain and calibrate
Completely non-invasive
Easy to use, no co-operation needed
Directly measures all relevant aspects of inflammation
Provides rapid availability of answers
Evidence of beneficial clinical outcomes

but this has not yet been confirmed by a formal meta-analysis. Two recent studies showed no evidence of benefit in adding exhaled NO to standard monitoring.[106,107] This probably indicates that, if basic management is optimized, most children respond so well to low to moderate doses of asthma therapy that there is little scope for demonstrating additional benefit with NO measurements. Exhaled NO is paradoxically reduced in CF, which may reflect the high degree of oxidative stress and generation of superoxide anions that combine avidly with NO to form peroxynitrite, high concentrations of which are detectable in CF airways. It is also reduced in PCD, which is generally characterized by a less severe airway disease than CF; the mechanism of this reduction, and how it fits with the relative severity of airway disease, is still being studied.

Other Exhaled Gases

There are other exhaled volatile markers of inflammation, but these are less well characterized than NO. Exhaled carbon monoxide reflects the activation of heme oxygenase-1, an enzyme induced by stress. Concentrations of CO are increased in asthmatic children and children with CF; however, there is a large degree of overlap with values in normal children, and environmental factors interfere with the measurements, so it is less useful than exhaled NO. Ethane is formed by lipid peroxidation in response to oxidative stress, and levels are increased in asthma and CF, but this requires complex measurements by gas chromatography-mass spectrometry, so it is not practical in clinical studies.[108,109] Indeed, exhaled breath contains multiple hydrocarbons, and there is emerging evidence that these may show different patterns in different diseases, reflecting the different components of inflammation, so that each disease may have a unique "breathogram."[110,111] There are currently no studies to indicate that these measurements are useful in the routine clinical management of children.

Exhaled Breath Condensate

Exhaled breath condensate (EBC) is formed through condensation of cooled exhaled breath and has been analyzed for a variety of mediators, including hydrogen peroxide, lipid mediators, purines, and cytokines.[112,113] Measurement of pH has shown differences between diseases,[114] but it is difficult to interpret these data because the hydrogen ion concentration differences seem unphysiologically great and do not correlate with direct measurements of airway surface pH at bronchoscopy.[115] Differences in the patterns of mediators are found between asthma and CF, reflecting the different inflammatory mediators in the respiratory tract. Exhaled 8-isoprostane has been found to be a useful measurement of oxidative stress, with increased concentrations in severe asthma and CF. The concentrations of mediators in EBC are low, therefore sensitive assays are needed and great attention must be paid to the collection procedure and the avoidance of salivary contamination.

New approaches in the future will include metabonomic analysis, in which multiple metabolites are monitored, giving unique patterns for each disease.[116] EBC has never been demonstrated to be a useful clinical tool in pediatric chest disease.

Is AHR an Inflammatory Surrogate?

The first adult study to suggest that something more than standard monitoring improved asthma outcomes used AHR measurement over a 2-year period and demonstrated that a strategy aimed at normalizing AHR led to a greater use of inhaled corticosteroid and improved asthma outcomes.[117] There is one such pediatric study, which showed minor evidence of benefit using an AHR strategy.[118] This is not likely to be a clinically useful strategy; the measurements are time-consuming, and there is only a loose relationship between inflammation and AHR,[119] and between changes in AHR and changes in inflammation.[120,121]

Other Potential Undirect Inflammatory Markers

There have been some studies using blood or urine levels of various eosinophil proteins, but none suggesting that their routine measurement in clinical practice is useful. Elevations in these proteins may be due to extrapulmonary atopic disease, such as eczema or rhinoconjunctivitis, leading to a lack of specificity.

IS THERE A ROLE FOR INFLAMMOMETRY IN PEDIATRIC RESPIRATORY DISEASE?

Despite a profusion of research papers, no single set of guidelines is able to make an evidence-based recommendation that inflammometry should be a routine clinical tool. This may in part be due to a false perception that measurement of an inflammatory marker will mean perfect sensitivity and specificity, with no need to make any other measurement. It is interesting to compare the expectations of inflammatory markers, compared to what spirometry has delivered. No one would suggest abandoning spirometry, a routine measurement in every good asthma clinic, but spirometry is rarely diagnostic of asthma, correlates poorly with disease severity, and is a poor endpoint in clinical trials. We suggest that, as with spirometry, measurement of airway inflammation will find a role as part of the assessment process.

There is no one gold-standard diagnostic test for asthma. Many different physiologic measurements of airway caliber and responsiveness can be made; in general, they have poor sensitivity, but reasonable specificity for the diagnosis. Most clinicians would take the view that the more such tests are done, and the more that are negative, the more critically an alternative diagnosis should be sought. It may be that measurements of airway inflammation should be used in the same way.

In terms of monitoring asthma, it is clear that if the basics are right, most asthmatic children respond well to low-dose medications, and there is not likely to be a role for inflammometry. Whether it has a role in really severe asthma is discussed in Chapter 48. However, just as reports of severe symptoms of asthma in conjunction with no evidence of AHR should lead to a suspicion of overreporting, perhaps the same will be true for those with reports of severe symptoms and no evidence of inflammation.

In summary, currently there is no evidence that measurement of airway inflammation should be used routinely. There are hints of a possible role in the future, perhaps if it can be shown in children, as well as adults, that there are patients with discordance between inflammation and symptoms. Disappointingly, despite more than 10 years since the publication of the first proof-of-concept study that adult asthma is managed better by going beyond asking about symptoms and performing routine spirometry, more work is needed to determine which inflammatory markers should be measured, and in which children.

DIRECT MEASUREMENTS OF AIRWAY INFLAMMATION

There are far fewer bronchoscopic studies in children than in adults. This in part relates to ethics; any invasive procedure must be of direct benefit to the individual child. Neither parents nor children can consent to an invasive procedure that is of no direct benefit to the child. It has been shown that bronchoscopy, bronchoalveolar lavage, and endobronchial biopsy are safe in children with severe asthma when performed carefully by experienced personnel. It is ethical to take additional samples for research purposes at the time of a clinically indicated bronchoscopy, if the Institutional Review Board approves the procedure, the parents give informed consent, and the child gives age-appropriate assent.[122] The main problem with pediatric bronchoscopic studies is that they are invariably cross-sectional, because serial bronchoscopies are rarely, if ever, appropriate in children. Other problems include the general lack of milder asthmatics, since bronchoscopy is rarely indicated in these children, and the lack of true normal controls, since there is no non-respiratory indication for a bronchoscopy. This last issue is addressed by using children with upper airway disease, hemoptysis for which no cause is found, or chronic cough unrelated to asthma. None of these controls is completely suitable.

An alternative approach, also completely ethical with the previous caveats, is to do a blind non-bronchoscopic lavage and bronchial brushings in children who are intubated for routine pediatric surgery.[123,124] This is the only way that large numbers of normal or mildly asthmatic children can be studied.

THERAPEUTIC IMPLICATIONS

Inflammation is a key feature of asthma and CF so that anti-inflammatory treatments should play an important role in therapy. Inhaled corticosteroids have become the first-line therapy for asthma in children, as low doses are usually sufficient to control asthma. However, in severe asthma there is cellular and molecular resistance to the anti-inflammatory effects of corticosteroids[125] The inflammation in CF is also corticosteroid-resistant, and one should note that adverse effects have resulted from anti-inflammatory therapy. Better understanding of the inflammatory mechanisms involved in severe asthma and CF should lead to more effective therapies in the future.[126]

Corticosteroid Mechanisms

Corticosteroids have a broad spectrum of anti-inflammatory effects and switch off multiple activated inflammatory genes that have been activated by pro-inflammatory transcription factors (e.g., NFκB and AP-1[127]). Activation of these transcription factors recruits co-activator molecules that acetylate core histones, opening up the chromatin structure so that gene transcription is activated. Corticosteroids reverse this process partly by inhibiting the activity of co-activators but mainly by recruiting the nuclear enzyme histone deacetylase-2 (HDAC2) to the activated inflammatory gene complex to reverse histone acetylation and switch off gene transcription.

Mechanisms of Corticosteroid Resistance

In children, corticosteroid resistance may be the result of allergen exposure (at home or at school[128]) via IL-2– and IL-4–dependent mechanisms[129,130] or secondary to active and passive cigarette smoke exposure.[131–133] Obesity may also be a cause of steroid resistance.[134] Several molecular mechanisms of corticosteroid resistance have now been identified.[125] Neutrophilic inflammation is poorly responsive to corticosteroids as they increase neutrophil survival, and Th17-driven neutrophil inflammation, which is likely to be important in severe asthma and CF, is corticosteroid-resistant. An important mechanism of corticosteroid resistance that is secondary to oxidative stress is a reduction in HDAC2 activity and expression, resulting in amplified inflammation and reduced responsiveness to corticosteroids.[135] This reduction in HDAC is a combination of tyrosine nitration of the enzyme due to peroxynitrite formation and phosphorylation of the enzyme as a result of inhibiting phosphoinositide-3-kinase-δ.[136] Interestingly, this can be reversed by low concentrations of theophylline.

CONCLUSION

Airway inflammation is a critical component of many chronic airway diseases in children. The inflammatory response involves many different inflammatory cells that are recruited to and activated in the airways. Each of these cells releases multiple mediators, which then exert effects on the airway wall. In asthma, the major effects are bronchoconstriction and plasma exudation, whereas in CF the predominant response is mucus hypersecretion and airway wall destruction, ultimately leading to respiratory failure. Among the multiple mediators of inflammation, cytokines play an important role in orchestrating the inflammatory response and amplifying and perpetuating inflammation, whereas chemokines play a key role in selective recruitment of inflammatory cells to the airway. The molecular basis of inflammation is now understood better, with increased expression of multiple inflammatory genes, switched on by transcription factors such as NFκB and AP-1. Endogenous anti-inflammatory mechanisms counteract these effects, and there is some evidence that the mechanisms are defective in asthma, allowing inflammation to become more severe or to persist longer. Neural mechanisms and neurotrophins may also be involved in amplifying the inflammatory response. This complex inflammatory process should be monitored in the management of airway disease, and there are several new non-invasive approaches by breath analysis, including exhaled NO and exhaled breath condensate, that look promising in children. Corticosteroids are highly effective in suppressing inflammation in asthma, but they are poorly effective in severe asthma and are ineffective in CF as the result of several corticosteroid-resistance mechanisms.

Suggested Reading

Barnes PJ. Immunology of asthma and chronic obstructive pulmonary disease. *Nat Immunol Rev.* 2008;8:183–192.
Barnes PJ, Adcock IM. Glucocorticoid resistance in inflammatory diseases. *Lancet.* 2009;342:1905–1917.
Barnes PJ, Drazen JM, Rennard SI, et al, eds. *Asthma and COPD.* 2nd ed. Amsterdam: Elsevier; 2009.
Elizur A, Cannon CL, Ferkol TW. Airway inflammation in cystic fibrosis. *Chest.* 2008;133:489–495.
Hamid Q, Tulic M. Immunobiology of asthma. *Annu Rev Physiol.* 2009;71:489–507.
Pijnenburg MW, de Jongste JC. Exhaled nitric oxide in childhood asthma: a review. *Clin Exp Allergy.* 2008;38:246–259.

References

The complete reference list is available online at www.expertconsult.com

7 LUNG DEFENSES: INTRINSIC, INNATE, AND ADAPTIVE

JAMES M. STARK, MD, PHD, AND GARY A. MUELLER, MD

The practice of pediatric pulmonology often includes the child with "too many" respiratory infections. Considering the volume of air (and potential airborne pathogens) transiting the respiratory system daily, the question should actually be, "Why don't we get more infections?" The conducting airways branch 20 to 25 times between the trachea and the alveoli. The large surface area of the conducting airways and alveolar surfaces ($>70m^2$ in the adult) poses a great challenge for the lung defenses. These defenses have evolved to interact and protect the lung from potentially injurious or infectious agents. The anatomy of the lung, lung products, cell receptors (and subsequent signaling mechanisms), and host cellular responses all contribute to the normal lung defense, disease prevention, and injury repair. A defect in any of these defenses can result in an increased susceptibility to infection in the absence of classic immunodeficiencies. In this chapter, we will review several aspects of the lung defenses. First, we will consider the contribution of the airway anatomy, physiology, and secretory products in limiting access of pathogens to the respiratory tract (intrinsic defenses). We will then consider the roles of the various "pattern recognition" proteins and receptors that provide the first line of antimicrobial and inflammatory defenses against invading pathogens (innate defenses) and orchestrate subsequent cellular immunity and antibody development (adaptive defenses). Finally, once these responses are initiated, there has to be control to turn off the lung defenses and allow repair to occur. While there is a degree of redundancy in the function of the *intrinsic, innate,* and *adaptive* responses in the lung, defects in these defenses, which overwhelm the capacity of the defenses to protect the lung, or the inability to "turn off" inflammatory responses, can "tip the scale" and place the host at increased risk for infection, chronic inflammatory lung disease, and lung injury.

INTRINSIC LUNG DEFENSES

Aerodynamic Filtering

The anatomy of the airways and the dichotomous branching of the lower airways make important contributions to the defense of the lungs against infection. The initial barrier is the nose, which acts as an effective filter because of its unusual structure and surface area. Very large particles are filtered by the nasal hairs, and particles larger than $10\mu m$ impact on the surfaces of the turbinates and septum. Impaction is facilitated by the inertia of these large particles, as they have a high linear velocity and do not easily change direction to follow air flow. The tonsils and adenoids are strategically located to deal with larger soluble particles by specific local defenses. If the tonsils and adenoids are markedly enlarged, nasal resistance may be increased, resulting in mouth breathing and bypassing of the nasal anatomic defenses. Edema of the turbinates from viral infections or allergies may produce similar effects. Hydrophilic particles are enlarged by humidification of the inspired air, and this facilitates their impaction in the upper airways.

Particles between 2 and $10\mu m$ are removed from the air flow by impaction on the walls of the branching airways beyond the nose, and by sedimentation. Sedimentation occurs because the increasing cross-sectional area of the conducting airways leads to a decrease in the linear air flow velocity such that gravitational forces may act on the particles. Smaller particles (as small as $0.2\mu m$) may not sediment at all and are exhaled. Particles in the size range of 2 to $0.2\mu m$ generally penetrate the airways and can be deposited on the surfaces of the alveoli. Particles that are highly soluble are cleared from the lung in the lymphatic circulation. Particles in this size range include many bacteria, fungal spores, and larger (filamentous) viruses. Other physical factors may also be important in particle penetration. For example, an antigen such as *Alternaria* sp., which is $30\mu m$ long and $10\mu m$ wide, may penetrate deep into the lung because of its kite-like shape and efficient aerodynamic qualities. The electrostatic charges of particles may also affect lung penetration. Unipolar charged aerosols in high concentration may be deposited on the airway walls by electrostatic repulsion between the particles. Aerosol devices and metered-dose inhalers use particle size to direct deposition of the medication to different levels of the airway.

Humidification

Humidification begins at the nose and continues distally. Ultimately, inspired air is warmed to body temperature (37° C) and 100% relative humidity. As discussed later, adequate hydration of mucus is essential to its proper functioning. The upper airway receives some humidity from convection of warm, humidified alveolar gas. During exhalation, the temperature drops and condensation forms on the upper airways, keeping their surfaces wet. The isothermal saturation boundary (the point where air becomes body temperature) is at 100% relative humidity, and the humidity remains constant as gas continues to move distally. This point occurs somewhere below the carina and will shift, depending on ambient temperature, humidity, and volume and rate of air exchange. It will also shift distally when the upper airway is bypassed, such as by tracheostomy. It will never drop to the level of the respiratory bronchioles, so gas at functional residual capacity (FRC) is at stable temperature and humidity, and in equilibrium with the blood and alveolar tissue. These concepts become relevant during normal physiology (e.g., during bronchospasm in exercise or cold air) and under pathologic conditions, iatrogenic or otherwise (e.g., tracheostomy).[1]

Airway Reflexes

Sneezing, bronchoconstriction, and coughing are airway reflexes that act as nonspecific host defenses. Sneezing is a forceful expulsion of air that is triggered by receptors in the nose and nasal pharynx and is effective in clearing the upper pharynx and nose. The mechanisms are similar to coughing (described in the following paragraph). Bronchoconstriction may also prevent entry of particles into the distal airways by decreasing airway caliber and redirecting air flow away from the irritated airways. It leads to increased pulmonary resistance, decreasing air velocity in the peripheral airways, thereby increasing the likelihood of sedimentation.

Coughing is a forceful expulsion of air from the lungs that is under both voluntary and involuntary control. The anatomic type of sensory nerves involved in the human cough reflex has been difficult to delineate. There are at least nine sensory receptors in the bronchopulmonary system, and at least five involve the cough reflex.[2] It seems likely that the unmyelinated C fibers and the myelinated irritant receptors containing substance P and calcitonin-gene–related peptide (CGRP) are involved.[2] Cough receptors appear to be located within the epithelium of the pharynx, larynx, trachea, and the bifurcations of the major bronchi. These receptors can be stimulated by inflammatory mediators, chemical irritants, osmotic stimuli, and mechanical stimulation.[3] Respiratory sensations are elicited by central neural events as well as those just mentioned. Stimulation of respiratory afferents results in cognitive awareness of breathing and the urge to cough.[4]

The reflex of cough is initiated by stimulation of afferent fibers leading to the vagus nerve that connect to the cough center in the medulla oblongata and conscious awareness in the suprapontine brain. Some centrally-acting cough suppressants, such as opiates, have their effect in the medulla oblongata. Efferent fibers transmit stimuli along the vagus nerve and spinal cord to the larynx, diaphragm, and abdominal muscles to produce cough.[3] After the cough, a feedback loop occurs to determine if the cough satisfied the urge to cough. The limbic system is involved with this portion of the cough cycle, thus not all cough is purely reflexive. The cognitive urge to cough is an integration of respiratory afferents, respiratory motor system, affective state, attention, learning, and experience.[4]

The Mechanics of Cough and Abnormalities in the Cough Reflex

There are six important phases of cough that create high velocities in the upper airway. These flow rates are necessary to create shear rates required to clear mucus from the airway walls and to promote its expulsion through the larynx. The phases of coughing are summarized as follows:[5]

1. *Irritation phase*—cough triggered by stimulation of the irritant receptors in the tracheobronchial tree
2. *Inspiratory phase*—initiated by a deep breath, which is usually 1.5 to 2 times the tidal volume. Air enters the airway distal to secretions. The length-tension relationships of the respiratory muscles are increased and optimized for contraction, elastic recoil potential increases, and the bronchi dilate.
3. *Glottic closure*—necessary to build pressure for subsequent phases of cough
4. *Compression phase*—begins with closure of the larynx and is followed by contraction of the intercostal muscles and abdominal musculature, which rapidly leads to increased intrathoracic pressure. Esophageal pressures can reach levels as high as 300 cm H_2O or more in normal adults. This phase is fast, lasting approximately 200 msec.
5. *Expulsive phase*—initiated when the glottis opens and high air flows are achieved. Following the glottic opening, the airways may collapse by as much as 80% in tracheal cross-sectional area, which increases the linear velocity of exhaled gas, shearing mucus from the airway walls and moving it toward the mouth. Estimated velocities approach 25,000 cm/sec (¾ the speed of sound). The cough may be interrupted by a series of glottic closures, each with its own compressive and expulsive phases. These "spikes" in flow, or flow transients, can improve cough effectiveness by increasing the shear forces. In patients with significant airway malacia, the equal pressure point may be quite proximal and limit cough effectiveness. Efforts to move this point distally (e.g., positive expiratory pressure device at the mouth) should improve cough effectiveness.
6. *Relaxation phase*—characterized by a decrease in intrathoracic pressure associated with relaxation of the intercostal and abdominal muscles, and temporary bronchodilation.

Abnormalities of the cough mechanism can result in an ineffective cough. Cough receptors are not present in the alveoli or lung parenchyma, therefore coughing may be absent in children with extensive alveolar disease or pneumonic consolidation. It is possible that repeated stimulation of cough receptors will eventually lead to a decrease in their sensitivity. This mechanism may explain why cough is sometimes absent in children with gastroesophageal reflux and recurrent aspiration. A decrease in the sensitivity of the cough center occurs in obtunded patients and individuals under the influence of opiates. The efferent nerves can be affected by poliomyelitis or infantile botulism. Muscles of coughing can be affected by neuromuscular diseases such as spinal muscular atrophy or muscular dystrophy, leading to inadequate cough clearance of mucus from the airways and increased tendency toward atelectasis. Laryngeal disorders such as vocal cord paralysis, or the presence of a tracheostomy tube, prevent effective laryngeal closure so that the cough can lose its explosive quality and thereby airway clearance decreases. In patients with neuromuscular disorders, the use of cough-assist devices may be useful in enhancing airway clearance diminished by low muscular force.[5]

Mucus and Airway Surface Liquid

Respiratory mucus and mucociliary clearance are the major components of intrinsic lower respiratory defense. Mucus is a mixture of water, ions, glycoproteins (mucins), proteins, and lipids. Water is the predominate component (more than 90%) of normal mucus.[6] The airways between the larynx and the respiratory bronchioles are lined by ciliated columnar epithelium and covered by an airway surface liquid (ASL) layer that is 5 to 100 μm thick. With the advent of the capacity to measure airway surface liquid *in vivo* and the development of well-differentiated human airway epithelial cultures that exhibit mucus transport *in vitro*, it is has become possible to investigate the microanatomy of mucus transport in humans.[7] ASL consists of two distinct layers: the sol or periciliary liquid (PCL) layer adjacent to the epithelial surface, and the gel or surface mucus layer that appears to float on top of the sol layer. The periciliary liquid layer is a mucus-free zone at the cell surface approximately the height of the cilia. This layer is crucial because it provides a low-viscosity fluid in which the cilia can beat rapidly (8 to 20 Hz), moving the more viscous gel layer of mucus over it and shielding the epithelial surface from the overlying mucus layer.

Mucus provides several important airway defense functions. These are: (1) a covering sheet that entraps particulate matter and microorganisms; (2) a movable medium that can be propelled by cilia (the tips of cilia drive the gel layer over the sol layer toward the oropharynx); (3) a waterproofing layer that acts to reduce fluid loss through the airways; (4) a layer present to detoxify noxious inhaled irritants; and (5) a medium that transports essential secreted substances such as enzymes, defensins, collectins, antiproteases, and immunoglobulins (discussed later).

There are currently 21 human membrane-associated mucin (MUC) genes listed in Genbank.[6] MUC1, MUC4, MUC16, and seven others are constitutively expressed in the lung. These proteins function as epithelial membrane receptors, having extracellular, transmembrane, and cytoplasmic domains that participate in outside-in signal transduction. The intracellular cytoplasmic tail domain transmits signals through intracellular kinases. MUC1 and MUC4 dimerize and regulate the epidermal growth factor receptor (EGFR). These apical glycosylated proteins extend from 500 to 1500 nm above the cell surface and into the PCL. Thus they participate in the regulation of several biologic functions[8] and contribute to innate lung defenses (discussed later). Five human mucins are secreted and participate in the gel-forming extracellular mucus layer. These proteins polymerize via covalent disulfide linkages using cysteine-rich von Willebrand factor–like domains and other cysteine-rich regions. There are three others that are cysteine poor. MUC5AC and MUC5B are the predominant gel-forming mucins in the airway, with smaller contributions from MUC2, MUC8, and MUC19.[8] MUC5B is a secretory product of the submucosal glands, and MUC5AC is a product of the surface goblet cells. In addition, MUC7 is a secreted, non–gel-forming mucin found in airway secretions, originating from serous cells of the submucosal glands. The gel-forming mucins are very large macromolecule proteins that are heavily glycosylated, exhibiting extremely high molecular weights (thousands of kDA). They are highly water-absorbent and form tangled networks of polymers.[8,9] The branching oligosaccharide side chains contribute to the viscoelastic properties of normal mucus. Although cysteine accounts for less than 1% of the amino acid protein core, sulfhydryl bonds contribute to the polymerization of the glycoprotein and to the resulting viscous qualities of the mucus. Extensive cross-linking between long polymers can create disease states such as those seen in plastic bronchitis and fatal asthma. The diversity of the carbohydrate side chains of the mucin macromolecules creates, in effect, a library of carbohydrate sequences that can provide binding to an enormous repertoire of particles that land on the mucus layer.[8,9]

The properties of this mucin gel are the product of the mucin and water contents, concentrations of monovalent and divalent ions, and the pH of the ASL. The water content of ASL is controlled by regulating levels of ion transport in the PCL layer via the cystic fibrosis transmembrane regulator (CFTR), a calcium-activated (alternative) chloride channel, and the epithelial sodium channel (ENaC). These three ion channels control Na^+ reabsorption and Cl^- secretion by the respiratory epithelial cell, with passive movement of water across the epithelial membrane in response to ion transport. Dysregulation of both Na^+ and Cl^- contributes to the mucus and mucociliary transport abnormalities seen in cystic fibrosis.[7,10] Finally, in inflammatory states, large macromolecules such as DNA and polymerized actin from white cells, protoglycans, biofilms, and other combinations of bacteria and inflammatory cells can be present in large amounts and significantly increase the viscosity of the mucus.[8] In these inflammatory states, mucin proteins are relatively small contributors to the overall composition of the airway mucus.

Basal submucosal mucus secretion is regulated principally though the vagus nerve. However, in the inflammatory state several irritants and mediators contribute to mucin and mucus production. These include oxidants, proteases (including neutrophil elastase and *P. aeruginosa* proteases), components of activated complement, and a number of cytokines and chemokines (TNF-α, Platelet Activating Factor [PAF], IL-1β, interferons, and IL-8).[8,9] Tachykinin-mediated neural systems are present predominantly in the upper airways in humans, making it unlikely that these neural mechanisms regulate lung mucus production or transport. Autocrine/paracrine signaling occurs via 5′ nucleotides in the regulation of epithelial ion transport, ciliary beat frequency, and mucus secretion.[9] These data suggest that nucleotide release, both in response to ambient conditions and cough-induced shear stress, help regulate mucus clearance rates.

Ciliary beat frequency and the effectiveness of the ciliary beat are primary determinants of the mucus clearance rate. Movement of the ASL on airway surfaces involves two steps: First, the ciliary power stroke acts to move the mucus layer unidirectionally on the airway surface; second, the frictional interaction of the mucus layer with the PCL allows this underlying layer to travel along with the overlying mucus. Cilia also impart a vertical motion within the mucus layer, mixing particles, bacteria, and other pathogens into the mucus and facilitating their clearance. Ciliary dysfunction can therefore greatly diminish mucus clearance. The lubricating function of the PCL facilitates mucus movement along airway surfaces in response to coughing. In addition, deficiency or absence of the PCL allows adhesive interactions between the mobile mucins (MUC5AC and MUC5B) and the airway epithelial cell surface mucins (MUC1 and MUC4), effectively "tethering" the ASL to the epithelial surface and greatly reducing the efficiency of ciliary activity and of cough in mucus clearance.[10]

Therapy for Mucus Clearance Disorders

Mechanical: Cough clearance is the secondary defense when mucociliary clearance is impaired; an effective cough is essential as part of mucus clearance. The effectiveness of the cough depends on volume and flow of exhaled air and the biophysical properties of the mucus. Cough clearance can be achieved by a manually assisted cough or a mechanical insufflation-exsufflation device.[3] Mucus clearance or mobilization can be assisted in a number of ways such as traditional percussion and postural drainage, positive expiratory pressure devices, high-frequency chest wall oscillation, and intrapulmonary percussive ventilation.

Mucolytics: N-acetylcysteine cleaves disulfide bonds connecting mucin oligomers, reducing viscoelasticity. This may make excessively viscous mucus easier to clear by coughing, but it needs to retain enough viscoelasticity to respond to the shear forces applied by a cough. The severing of these bonds may also be disadvantageous, as they also neutralize pro-inflammatory mediators and inhibit biofilm formation.[5] Chronic inflammation produces mucus with breakdown products of white blood cells present in high quantities, namely DNA and F-actin. Dornase alfa (Pulmozyme) hydrolyzes DNA polymers, producing sputum that is less viscous, and is effective in cystic fibrosis; however, it has not been effective in other chronic inflammatory disorders (e.g., COPD, non-CF bronchiectasis, and asthma). Thymosin β 4 depolymerizes the F-actin network and can act synergistically with dornase alfa. This activity is under investigation for clinical use.[5]

Expectorants: These agents improve clearance by improving mucus hydration. Consumption of large volumes of water is ineffective, as are most traditional expectorants (e.g., guaifenesin). Hyperosmolar agents (e.g., 7% saline aerosol or dry powder mannitol) are in use or under investigation. These agents appear to draw fluid into the airway, not just the gel layer. Thus, they "unstick" the mucus from the epithelium. They also induce cough and are mucin secretagogues. The latter may help, as normal mucus mixed with the abnormal mucus of cystic fibrosis may be cleared more easily.[11]

Mucokinetics: These agents improve mucociliary beat frequency or power, improving clearance. The β-agonist bronchodilators are an example of this class. Bronchodilators may increase the volume and rate of air flow in some individuals, improving cough effectiveness.

Abhesives: The opposite of adhesives, abhesives decrease the tenacity of airway mucus and secretions. The expectorants noted previously are possible abhesives. Aerosolized surfactants can improve cough clearance under certain circumstances, such as chronic bronchitis.[12]

Mucoregulatory agents: These agents decrease mucus hypersecretion in inflamed airways. The macrolides are the best known of this class, producing immunomodulation via extracellular-regulated kinase pathways.[5] Anticholinergics reduce submucosal gland secretion by blocking signaling through muscarinic receptors. There is evidence that this action does not dry out tracheobronchial mucus, though anticholinergics do produce "dry mouth" if given systemically.[13]

Disorders of the Mucociliary System

Primary ciliary dyskinesia (PCD) is a genetic disease associated with defective ciliary structure and function, with resultant chronic oto-sino-pulmonary disease, male infertility, and (in about half of patients) *situs inversus*.[14] Cilia are complex structures composed of a highly organized array of microtubules and accessory elements, including inner and outer dynein arms, radial spokes, and nexin links (see Chapter 71). Ciliated epithelial cells have approximately 200 cilia per cell, and they move with intracellular and intercellular synchrony, sweeping mucus from the distal to the proximal airway. The beat frequency is 8 to 20 Hz, but it can accelerate with various stimuli (e.g., smoke, irritants, and β-agonist bronchodilators). Disruption of this structural organization has been associated with ciliary immotility or dysmotility. Electron microscopic ultrastructural analysis remains the current "gold standard" diagnostic test for PCD.[14] Videomicroscopy for ciliary beat frequency, beat pattern, and orientation are adjunctive tests. So far, mutations in eight genes have been associated with PCD in humans: DNAH5, DNAH11, DNAI1, DNAI2, and TXNDC3 mutations involve heavy, intermediate, and light chains of the outer dynein arm. KTU mutations alter a cytoplasmic protein needed for assembly of the dynein complex, and RSPH9 and RSPH4A mutations alter the radial spoke head. DNAI1 and DNAH5 make up 30% to 38% of all PCD, and 50% to 60% of PCD with outer dynein arm defects.[8]

Measurements of mucociliary clearance in patients with PCD have revealed no basal, cilia-dependent mucus clearance, although cough-dependent clearance is nearly normal. These patients maintain a nearly-normal mucus clearance rate by increasing the dependence on cough.[7] As a result, these patients exhibit milder airway disease than seen in cystic fibrosis and typically live into middle age and beyond. However, bronchiectasis and obstructive airway disease may still occur in preschool children.[15] Nitric oxide accelerates ciliary beat frequency in response to cyclic nucleotide challenge, though baseline ciliary beat frequency is not thought to be NO-regulated.[8] This would be consistent with the presumed need for increased mucociliary clearance with inflammatory stimuli.

Cystic fibrosis (CF) results from mutations in the respiratory epithelial inducible chloride channel (CFTR).[10] In people with cystic fibrosis, mucus transport appears to be significantly altered by depletion of an isotonic ASL as the result of mutations in *CFTR*. Under basal conditions, Na[+] absorption by the normal respiratory epithelium regulates ASL volume. When ASL volume is depleted, airway epithelial cells slow Na⁺ absorption and increase Cl⁻ secretion. By doing so, water stays in the ASL and volume increases. In CF, the airway epithelium has an accelerated basal rate of Na⁺ and volume absorption that results from the absence of tonic inhibitory effects of CFTR on the epithelial Na⁺ channel (ENaC). In addition, the CF epithelium lacks sufficient Cl⁻ transport through CFTR. These defects in Na⁺ and Cl⁻ transport result in volume depletion on the airway surfaces which, in turn, depletes the PCL, disrupts normal ciliary activity, and inhibits mucociliary clearance. Moreover, depletion of the PCL allows mucins in the mucus layer (MUC5AC and MUC5B) to contact mucins on the surface of the respiratory epithelium (MUC1 and MUC4), allowing molecular interactions that effectively "glue" the mucins together and further disrupt mucus clearance, and promote biofilm formation and infection. This dual effect of PCL depletion and mucin tethering may partially explain differences in severity of lung disease between patients with PCD and CF.[7] Primary ciliary dyskinesia (Chapter 71) and CF pulmonary disease (Chapter 52) will be discussed in greater detail but are presented here as examples of lung disease resulting from disruption of normal mucociliary clearance in the lung.

INNATE LUNG DEFENSES

Innate immunity is an ancient evolutionary system that provides multicellular organisms with the capability of immediate defense against a wide variety of pathogens (i.e., bacteria, fungi, viruses) without previous exposure. This system has many capabilities: It recognizes structures present on a wide variety of pathogens that are distinct from self. It provides early activation of host defenses and effector mechanisms that can destroy the pathogen within hours. It stimulates the production of inflammatory cytokines and chemokines that recruit and activate other immune cells. And it orchestrates the development of adaptive immune responses. The rapid inflammatory responses that follow exposure to infectious agents can be reproduced in the absence of traditional adaptive immune responses. Activation of cytokine expression within the lung can initiate a cascade of events resulting in cellular sequestration, recruitment, and activation at the site of infection. Some of these innate protein receptors can function in cellular adhesion and in recognition proteins such as complement components. Several families of pattern recognition receptors (PRRs) have been described that have the ability to recognize conserved patterns of molecular structures on pathogens (Pathogen Associated Molecular Patterns [PAMPs]) and to activate and orchestrate a cascade of intracellular pro-inflammatory signals in the cell bearing those receptors (either extracellularly or intracellularly). Secreted proteins contribute to innate lung defenses, including lectin-like proteins (collectin family) and antibiotic proteins secreted by a number of cell types within the lung. There are resident innate defensive cells that function as "first responders" to infection, producing mediators that "call in the troops" from the circulation. Finally, there are "early responders" recruited

from the circulation that fight infection in the absence of adaptive immune responses. Together, these defenses protect the lung during the early phases of microbial invasion, before adaptive responses can contribute to the host defense.

Complement

Several serum proteins reach the lung through transudation in response to inflammation, including the complement family and immunoglobulins. The complement system functions to coat foreign particles as opsonins for phagocytosis, to activate phagocytic cells by the local release of chemotactic agents (e.g., C5a), and to lyse cells through the activation of the late complement components C5, C6, C7, C8, and C9 (the membrane attack complex). Other important aspects of the complement pathway are the generation of anaphylatoxins (C3a and C5a) that cause the release of vasoactive mediators from mast cells, and the generation of C3b and C4 on cell surfaces where they interact with specific receptors on phagocytic cells.[16] The complement protein cascade is activated by three independent pathways: the classic pathway that is activated by antigen-antibody complexes (involving IgG or IgM), the alternative pathway that is activated by foreign carbohydrates (e.g., bacterial and fungal components), and the lectin pathway (activated by mannose-binding lectin and the ficolins[17]).

Complement deficiency is associated with recurrent infections, glomerulonephritis, or collagen vascular diseases such as systemic lupus erythematosus. Pneumonia has been described in association with C1 deficiency, although bacterial meningitis is a more common manifestation. Pneumonia complicated by empyema, pneumatoceles, and liver abscesses has been described as a consequence of C1r deficiency. Autoimmune disorders are associated with both C2 and C4 deficiency, although bacterial infections also occur in children with C2 deficiency (the most common complement deficiency). C3 deficiency (clinically the most severe and least common of the complement deficiencies) is associated with both autoimmune disorders and recurrent infections. C3 acts as an opsonizing agent and plays a role in both the classical and alternative pathways. C3 deficiency results in otitis media, pneumonia, sepsis, meningitis, and osteomyelitis, most commonly caused by *Streptococcus pneumoniae*, *Neisseria meningitidis*, *Klebsiella* sp., *Escherichia coli*, and *S. pyogenes*. C5 deficiency produces a complex defect due to the loss of chemotactic and anaphylatoxin activities; it leads to decreased lung clearance of *S. pneumoniae* but not *Staphylococcus aureus* in C5-deficient mice. The deficiencies late in the complement cascade (C5 to C9) impair serum bacteriocidal and cytolytic activities, resulting in increased susceptibility to systemic infection with encapsulated organisms such as *N. meningitidis* and *S. pneumoniae*; however pulmonary infections are relatively uncommon. Defects of the alternative pathway of complement activity are very uncommon. Properdin factor deficiency is usually associated with *N. meningitidis* infection, but it is also associated with pneumonia. Deficiency of factor H or I (regulatory proteins of both pathways) leads to autoimmune disorders and recurrent infections with *S. pneumoniae* and *Haemophilus influenzae*. Mannose-binding lectin (MBL) and ficolins function in pulmonary immunity by preventing hematogenous dissemination of respiratory pathogens. However, defects in MBL are also associated with infection by a number of respiratory pathogens.[18]

Most defects of complement synthesis are inherited as autosomal recessive disorders with the exception of properdin deficiency, which is an X-linked condition. Symptoms do not usually occur unless the child is homozygous for the deficiency, except in C2 and C4 deficiencies, in which the heterozygote may be symptomatic. Mutations in the gene or the promoter regions can lower levels of protein, or alter protein assembly, thereby resulting in a relative immune deficiency state.

Adhesion Proteins

Adhesion and migration of circulating inflammatory cells (or their progenitors) are integral to cell recruitment and activation response to injury. Three major families of adhesion molecules participate in these processes in the lung: the immunoglobulin superfamily, the integrins, and the selectins (Table 7-1).

The immunoglobulin superfamily is a group of polypeptide genes characterized by the presence of one or more regions homologous to the basic structural unit of the immunoglobulin gene. Immunoglobulins and the T cell receptors are the only members of this family that undergo somatic diversification for antigen recognition. These receptors can function as single peptide chains (e.g., intercellular adhesion molecule -1 [ICAM-1], CD4, LFA-3) or may need to be associated as polypeptides for activity (T cell receptors, immunoglobulins, MHC class I and II receptors, CD8). Several members of the immunoglobulin superfamily are involved in cell-cell adhesion, migration

of leukocytes from the vascular space, through the matrix, and into the airway.[19] Moreover, they are required for antigen presentation to T cells by dendritic cells and macrophages (see later in the chapter). These adhesive interactions can be simple, pairwise, or complex interactions involving multiple families of receptors as occurs in antigen presentation (the "immune synapse").

The integrins are a family of diverse molecules with a common structure that are involved in cell-substrate or cell-cell interactions. Members of this family are composed of two noncovalently associated polypeptide chains (α and β). In humans, there are 18 α and 8 β subunits that form 24 different heterodimers.[19] Subgroups of this family are defined by common, shared β chains. β1 integrins function primarily by interacting with matrix components (collagen, laminin, fibronectin).[20] β2 integrins (heterodimers of CD11a and CD18) are expressed almost exclusively on leukocytes, and mediate cell-cell adhesion[20] (see Table 7-1). LFA-1 is expressed by virtually all immune cells, with the exception of some tissue macrophages. Mac-1 and p150, 95 are found on macrophages, monocytes, granuloctyes, and some lymphocytes. Upon binding their extracellular ligands, integrins transmit signals from the outside that modulate and regulate various cellular functions. Lung epithelial cells express eight different integrin heterodimers (α2β1, α3β1, α6β4, α9β1, α5β1, αvβ5, αvβ6, αbβ8) that recognize extracellular matrix molecules. These integrins are critical for maintaining endothelial integrity, repair of damaged cells, and regulation of cell differentiation and proliferation.[21] The central role of the β2 integrins in inflammation is demonstrated in patients with leukocyte adhesion deficiency (LAD), an inherited syndrome characterized by recurrent or progressive bacterial skin and soft-tissue infections, diminished pus formation, and impaired wound healing. Despite systemic granulocytosis, granulocytes

TABLE 7-1   FAMILIES OF ADHESION MOLECULES IN THE LUNG

IMMUNOGLOBULIN SUPERFAMILY	INTEGRINS	SELECTINS
Members share the immunoglobulin domain structure.	Members consist of noncovalently-associated heterodimers of 2 chains: α and β	Consist of an extracellular signal sequence, a lectin-like domain, an epidermal growth factor–like domain, a number of short consensus repeats, and a membrane anchor
Only immunoglobulins and the T cell receptor undergo specific somatic diversification	Responsible for interactions between cells and between cells and matrix proteins (fibronectin, collagen)	Require Ca2+ for adhesion
Peptides can be paired or unpaired	Require divalent cations (Mg2+, Mn2+, Ca2+)	Recognize and adhere to carbohydrate moieties like lectins
Examples:	Examples:	Examples:
Immunoglobulins T cell receptor (CD3) MHC class I MHC Class II Intercellular adhesion molecule-1 (ICAM-1) (CD54) Intercellular adhesion molecule-2 (ICAM-2) Vascular cell adhesion molecule-1 (VCAM-1)	β2 integrins: LFA-1 (CD11a/CD18) Mac-1 (CD11a/CD18) p150, 95 (CD11c/CD18) β1 integrins: VLA-4 (α4β1, CD49d/CD29) VLA-5 (fibronectin receptor, CD49c/CD29)	E-selectin (ELAM-1) L-selectin (LECAM-1) P-selectin (GMP-140)

(pus) are absent in areas of infection, due to defective migration from vascular to extravascular sites.

The selectin family of adhesion molecules mediates adhesion between leukocytes and vascular endothelium.[19,22] Selectins are glycoproteins rich in glycosylation by O-linked and N-linked carbohydrates. Three structurally related molecules have been identified: E-selectin (ELAM-1), P-selectin, and L-selectin (LECAM-1). E-selectin is expressed on endothelial cells following stimulation by cytokines such as IL-1 or tumor necrosis factor, and supports neutrophil adhesion. L-selectin is expressed on all leukocytes and is shed by neutrophils following adhesion to endothelial cells. P-selectin mediates cellular adhesion of neutrophils and monocytes to activated platelets and endothelial cells. The N-terminal ends of these molecules are homologous and related to a number of calcium-dependent carbohydrate lectin molecules. The selectins also have similar lectin-binding ligands, which contain sialyl Lewis x (sLe^x) and sialyl Lewis a (sLe^a) antigens.

In addition to their role in orchestrating binding to cellular surfaces, adhesion proteins can function as pattern recognition binding receptors, working together with other cellular proteins to bind and internalize ligands.[21] Several human pathogens utilize integrins to invade host cells (*Yersinia enterocolitica* and *Y. pseudotuberculosis* bind to the integrin receptors directly); however, the majority of integrin-binding microorganisms bind indirectly using extracellular matrix binding proteins as a bridge to engage these receptors. For instance, *Staphylococcus aureus* binds to fibronectin and integrins during infection.[21] However, binding to the integrins can result in intracellular signaling

that may be important in innate immune responses to the pathogen. The β2 integrins (particularly Mac-1) function as receptors for complement components that serve as PRRs for certain pathogens. Finally, the integrins may function in concert with the toll-like receptors (see later in the chapter) to initiate intracellular signaling pathways that result in activation of the transcription factor NFκB, cell-cell interaction, and cytokine production.

Pattern-Recognition Receptors in Lung Innate Immunity

Toll-Like Receptors

The toll-like receptors (TLRs) are an ancient family of receptor proteins that have been evolutionarily conserved and expressed in plants, insects (drosophila), and animals (mouse, human). They have two functional regions. The extracellular domain (consisting of leucine-rich repeats and one or two cysteine-rich regions) recognizes an array of microbial components: sugars, proteins, lipids, DNA motifs, and double stranded RNA. The intracellular region contains a Toll/IL-1 receptor (TIR) domain. The TIR domain provides an intracellular scaffold that interacts with a number of "adapter" proteins to initiate and integrate well-defined signaling cascades, resulting in cellular activation and the production of several cytokines and chemokines.[23] Ten TLRs have been described in humans, and they are expressed by cell types involved in the first-line, innate immune defenses such as macrophages, neutrophils, and airway epithelial cells (Table 7-2). In addition, TLRs are expressed on macrophages, dendritic cells, and

TABLE 7-2 TOLL-LIKE RECEPTORS AND THEIR LIGANDS

TLR	CELLS EXPRESSING	LIGAND	SOURCE
TLR 1/TLR2	A, B, E, D, MC, MP, N, NK, PD, T	Triacylated lipoproteins	Bacteria
TLR2	A, D, MC, MP, N, T	Peptidoglycan, lipoteichoic acid Glycolipids, oxidized phospholipids Zymosan HSP60, HSP70, HSPGp96	Gram-positive bacteria Spirochetes Yeast Host
TLR3	A, D, NK, PD	dsRNA, mRNA	Viruses
TLR4	A, D, E, MC, MP, N, NK, PD	LPS, lipoteichoic acid Oxidized lipoproteins and phospholipids	Gram-negative bacteria RSV Host
TLR5	A, D, MP, N, T	Flagellin	Bacteria with flagella
TLR6/TLR2	A, B, D, E, MC, N	Diacylated lipoprotein Bacterial lipopeptides	Mycoplasma
TLR7	B, E, MP, N, PD	ssRNA	
TLR8	E, MP, N	ssRNA	
TLR9	D, E, N, PD, T	Unmethylated CpG DNA	Bacteria, viruses, insects Host
TLR10	B, E, N, PD, T	?	

A, Epithelial cell; *B*, B cell; *D*, dendritic cell; *E*, eosinophil; *HSP*, heat shock protein; *LPS*, lipopolysaccharide; *MC*, mast cell; *MP*, macrophage; *N*, neutrophil; *NK*, natural killer T cell; *PD*, plasmacytoid dendritic cell; *T*, T cell.

B and T lymphocytes, contributing to the development of adaptive immune responses.

Ligands have been identified for all but TLR10. The TLRs are located either at the cell surface (TLR1, TLR2, TLR4 to TLR6, TLR10) or in the lysosomal/endosomal membranes (TLR3, TLR7 to TLR9) (see Table 7-2). The individual TLR proteins have been found to associate as homodimers of identical protein chains and as heterodimers of different TLR proteins. The heterodimers exhibit different binding properties from those of parent chains, thereby extending the target repertoire of this relatively small family of proteins[23] (see Table 7-2). TLR1 to TLR2 and TLR2 to TLR6 heterodimers recognize lipotechoic acid and lipoproteins from gram-positive bacteria, and TLR4 recognizes the lipopolysaccharide of Gram-negative bacteria. TLR5 recognizes flagellin. TLR3, TLR7, and TLR8 recognize viral RNAs and their synthetic analogs. TLR9 is stimulated by bacterial unmethylated CpG DNA. The TLRs utilize a variety of co-receptor molecules to further extend the versatility of the receptors. For example, TLR2 and TLR4 interact with MD-2 (soluble extracellular protein) and CD14 in binding with LPS. Several additional immune recognition receptors are thought to cooperate with TLR in response to products of pathogens. Dectin-1 (a lectin-like receptor) is a major phagocytic receptor that recognizes β1,3-glucans thought to interact with TLR2 in binding and inflammatory response by macrophages or dendritic cells to zymosan. NOD2 is a cytosolic protein that recognizes muramyl dipeptide (a repeating structure in bacterial peptidoglycans) and is thought to amplify TLR-mediated signaling following LPS exposure. BCR binding to DNA-antigen complexes amplifies signaling in B cells following TLR9-DNA interactions. DC-SIGN is a lectin receptor that has been implicated in downregulating the induction of IL-12 by TLR. TLR interactions with FCγ receptors have also been suggested. Engagement and subsequent activation by TLR results in the expression of a variety of cytokines depending on the cell type activated. TNF-α, pro-IL-1β, and IL-6 are important pro-inflammatory mediators produced in response to TLR activation. In addition, a number of chemokines are produced that recruit other cell types to the site of infection. Activation of TLR has been implicated in the upregulation of microbial killing mechanisms, including production of NO. Differential TLR expression and signaling in different dendritic cell populations drive T cell differentiation into a T-helper type 1 (Th1) or T-helper type 2 (Th2) phenotype. Thus, TLR-TLR and TLR-adapter protein interactions determine the specificity and activation properties of the interactions of the TLR with their ligands and modify both innate and adaptive immune responses.[24]

Nod-Like Receptors

The nod-like receptor (NLR) family is a large family of intracellular receptors consisting of 23 reported members. They are located in the cytosol and regulate both inflammation and apoptosis (programmed cell death). These proteins are expressed in many cell types, including immune cells and epithelial cells.[24,25] Their general structure includes a central nucleotide-binding oligomerization (NOD) domain, and a C-terminal leucine-rich repeat (LRR) domain. The N-terminal effector region varies between the different proteins, resulting in activation of diverse downstream signaling pathways.[25] NOD1 and NOD2 (the best studied cytosolic NLR) are expressed in leukocytes and lung epithelial cells. NOD1 detects bacterial wall peptidoglycan containing meso-diaminopimelic acid (found primarily in the peptidoglycan cell wall of Gram-negative bacteria), whereas NOD2 recognizes muramyl dipeptide conserved in both Gram-positive and Gram-negative bacteria. These activate intracellular signaling cascades by activation of Rip2 kinase, leading to activation of NFκB and subsequent expression of pro-inflammatory cytokines, and reactive oxygen species production.[25] The NLRP (NLR family, pyrin domain containing) consists of 14 members characterized by a PYD domain. At least three members of this family (NLRP1-3) form multiprotein complexes called *inflammasomes*.[26] Inflammasomes consist of one or two NLRs, an adapter molecule ASC, and caspase 1. The inflammasomes respond to various microbial molecules and regulate caspase-1–mediated cell death and production of mature IL-1β and related cytokines (including IL-18) at a posttranslational level. NLRP3 is expressed in granulocytes, macrophages, monocytes, and dendritic cells. The NLRP3 inflammasome activators include microbial RNA, certain forms of DNA, bacterial pore-forming toxins, and MDP-1. This inflammasome mediates caspase-1–dependent processing of pro-IL-1β as well as pro-IL-18 to their mature forms and regulates caspase-1–dependent cell death. The NLR member NLRX1 (NLR family member X1) is the only NLR molecule localized in the mitochondrial membrane where it mediates production of reactive oxygen species upon bacterial infection.

In summary, the NLRs function as intracellular pattern recognition proteins involved in the recognition of conserved microbial components in addition to nonmicrobial signals such as silica and uric acid crystals. NLR signaling results in activation of NFκB, resulting in the induction of pro-inflammatory cytokines, chemokines, and antimicrobial molecules.[24]

RIG-Like receptors

The RNA helicases RIG-1 (retinoic acid inducible gene-1) and MDA5 (melanoma differentiation-associated gene 5) belong to the RIG-1–like receptor family of RIG-like receptors (RLRs).[25] Both helicases signal through the downstream adaptor MAVS (mitochondrial antiviral signaling), which mediates the IRF3/7-dependent production of antiviral type 1 interferons as well as the activation of NFκB-dependent induction of inflammatory cytokines.[25]

Cytosolic DNA Sensors

These molecules sense bacterial DNA within the host cytosol and are responsible for the production of Type I interferon responses.

Soluble Extracellular Pattern-Recognition Proteins

The soluble extracellular pattern-recognition proteins function like "innate antibodies."[27] Two families of proteins have been described: the collectins (collagenous lectins, including MBL, surfactant proteins SP-A and SP-D, and conglutinin) and the ficolins. These proteins recognize carbohydrate arrays on their targets via carbohydrate recognition domains (CRDs). Several members of the collectins and ficolins activate complement.[27]

Collectins

The collectins are members of a superfamily of collagenous, calcium-dependent (C-type) lectins. The family includes MBL, also known as mannose-binding protein, and surfactant-associated proteins A and D (SP-A and SP-D, respectively). As part of the innate immune system, the collectins have a key role as a first line of defense against invading microorganisms. Both SP-A and SP-D are secreted into the air spaces by alveolar type II cells and probably nonciliated bronchiolar cells. In the collectin monomeric subunit, there are four functional domains: the N-terminal cysteine-rich domain, a collagen domain, a coiled-coil neck domain, and a C-terminal C-type lectin domain (also known as a carbohydrate recognition domain, or CRD). Selective binding of collectins to specific complex carbohydrates is mediated by the CRD and requires calcium. Human SP-A is assembled as heterotrimers or homotrimers of two genetically different chain types, whereas SP-D is assembled as homotrimers. SP-A preferentially forms hexamers of trimeric units ($6 \times 3 = 18$ chains), whereas SP-D forms tetramers ($4 \times 3 = 12$ chains).[28] This amino-terminal association and cross-linking of the trimeric subunits permits bridging between spatially separated ligands via the C-terminal lectin domains, increasing binding affinity and specificity. SP-A and SP-D bind to a variety of polysaccharide, phospholipid, and glycolipid ligands. The three-dimensional trimeric and oligomeric structures give SP-A and SP-D additional orders of specificity for particulate antigens and invading pathogens. Multiple carbohydrate recognition domains in the collectin oligomer can simultaneously bind to different ligands on a single polysaccharide chain, increasing the binding avidity of the complex to greater levels than could be attained by binding to single ligands. SP-A and SP-D interact with a variety of Gram-negative and Gram-positive organisms, fungi, and several respiratory viruses including RSV, Influenza A virus, and CMV. SP-A and SP-D interact with the glycoconjugate and/or lipid moieties present on invading pathogens and receptors on host cells. Through these interactions, they provide a number of host defense functions.[29] They can *agglutinate* microorganisms by forming bridges between various carbohydrate ligands on the cell surface. MBL can lead to *activation of the complement cascade*, whereas SP-A can bind C1q, preventing the formation of active complement complex. Lung collectins can lead to opsonization through activation of complement and deposition of C3 (MBL), or can directly opsonize microorganisms (SP-A and SP-D). SP-A-mediated opsonization can lead to stimulation of phagocytosis and killing of pathogens. However, some organisms can increase their efficiency of infection by using SP-A as a Trojan horse to gain entry into cells. SP-A and SP-D can alter viral infectivity, presumably by blocking binding of virus to their surface receptors or by enhancing cellular uptake and killing. Finally, SP-A and SP-D can *alter the permeability* of bacterial and fungal cell membranes, resulting in enhanced cell killing.

A number of cell surface receptors have been described for SP-A and SP-D.[30] SP-210 (surfactant protein receptor 210 kDa) is the best characterized SP-A receptor. It is found on type II cells and alveolar macrophages. C1q receptors bind MBL and SP-A, although their presence/function in the lung is unclear. SP-A has been found to interact with CD14 and TLR4, implicating a role of SP-A in LPS-mediated cell responses. In addition, the SP-A-TLR4 interactions may be important in the uptake of RSV-F protein in the lung. Gp340 is an SP-D binding protein belonging to the family of scavenger receptors that may also bind SP-A. SP-D has also been shown to interact with CD14 and function in the modulation of LPS-elicited cytokine release.

MBL is a serum protein, although small amounts of this protein have been found in lung secretions.[18] It has been shown to bind to several important respiratory pathogens, promoting C4 deposition.

Ficolins

The ficolins are lectin recognition molecules that are structurally and functionally homologous to MBL.[18] Three ficolins have been described. Ficolin-1 (M-ficolin) is expressed in the lung, monocytes, and spleen. Ficolin-2 (L-ficolin) is a serum protein expressed in the liver. Ficolin 3 (H-ficolin) is expressed in liver but also by bronchial and type II alveolar epithelial cells. They share the collagenous structure of MBL, but the carbohydrate recognition domain of MBL is replaced by a fibrinogen-like domain. They assemble in large multimeric structures of several hundred kilodaltons and recognize molecular patterns such as acetylated compounds and sugars.[31] Like MBL, they activate complement through the lectin pathway.

Antimicrobial Peptides

Recent studies have confirmed Alexander Flemming's observations made almost 80 years ago that human airway secretions possess intrinsic microbiocidal and microbiostatic properties. These activities lay in several cationic polypeptide constituents: lysozyme, lactoferrin, secretory leukoprotease inhibitor (SLPI), and neutrophil and epithelial defensins. These antimicrobial proteins and peptides differ in their molecular specificity and mechanisms of action, acting as hydrolyzing enzymes, creating pores in the bacterial wall, or chelating iron. They would therefore be expected to act cooperatively and possibly synergistically against a broad spectrum of organisms, making it unlikely that these organisms would develop resistance to the group as a whole.

Lysozyme is the one of the most abundant antimicrobial proteins in the airways, with concentrations estimated at 0.1 to 1 mg/mL—levels sufficient to kill important pulmonary pathogens such as *S. aureus* and *P. aeruginosa*. Lysozyme damages the walls of bacteria and fungi by hydrolyzing β1-4 glycosidic bonds between N-acetylmuramic acid and N-acetylglucosamine, which are structural components of bacterial peptidoglycan and fungal chitin.[32] In humans, lysozyme is secreted predominantly by the serous cells of submucosal glands in the conducting airways, and, to a lesser extent, by airway epithelial cells and alveolar macrophages. It is also a component of both phagocytic and secretory granules of neutrophils. Its role in defending the human lungs from infection is still unclear, but recent studies in rodents suggest that it is an important component of the respiratory defenses.[32]

Lactoferrin is an iron-binding protein present in secretions such as tears, saliva, and bronchial secretions. It is present in ASL at concentrations similar to lysozyme (0.1 to 1 mg/mL). It is produced by the submucosal glands and neutrophils, and it has activity against both Grampositive and Gram-negative bacteria, and *Candida* species. The antimicrobial actions of lactoferrin result from chelation of iron, which is required by many bacteria for optimal growth, or by destabilization of bacterial membranes.[33] Some of the antimicrobial activities of lactoferrin are related to its ability to bind lipopolysaccharides (LPS) with high affinity. Indeed, recent *in vitro* studies indicate that lactoferrin is able to compete with the LPS-binding protein for LPS binding and prevent the transfer of LPS to CD14 present at the surface of monocytes.[33]

Antiproteases

There are two major protease inhibitors secreted at mucosal surfaces: secretory leukocyte protease inhibitor (SLPI) and elafin.[34] SLPI is an 11.9 kDA protein about 10-fold less abundant than lysozyme and lactoferrin in ASL. The N-terminal domain has modest activity against both Gram-positive and Gram-negative organisms. The C-terminal domain is an effective inhibitor of neutrophil elastase, cathepsin G, trypsin, chymotrypsin, tryptase, and chymase.[34] Elafin/Trappin-2 is a 9.9 kDA protein that has a narrower spectrum of inhibition, only inhibiting neutrophil elastase and proteinase 3. In addition to their antiprotease activity, the protease inhibitors have several other biologic activities in the lung, including anti-inflammatory effects on NFκB activity and antimicrobial activity against a number of organisms, including *Staphylococcus aureus* and *Pseudomonas aeruginosa*. In addition, SLPI may play a role in adaptive immunity through maintenance of mucosal tolerance.

Antimicrobial Peptides: Defensins and Cathelicidins

Human *defensins* are present in BAL fluid from noninflamed lungs at a concentration of about 100 ng/mL,[35] but these concentrations are increased in inflamed airways. Expression of defensins (peptides 3 to 5 kDa in size) is modulated locally by inflammation. Although 20 potentially expressed genes have been identified by the Human Genome Project, relatively few proteins have been isolated and characterized. Four human neutrophil peptides (HNP-1, HNP-2, HNP-3, and HNP-4) are located in neutrophil azurophilic granules (HNP-4 is less abundant than the other three).[35] Two other defensins (HD-5 and HD-6) are located in gastrointestinal epithelial cells. Four beta-defensin molecules have been described (hBD-1, hBD-2, hBD-3, and hBD-4), differing from the neutrophil defensins in the organization of their cysteines. Whereas hBD1 is expressed constitutively by epithelial cells, hBD2 to hBD4 are inducible. Whereas hBD-2 is highly expressed in the lung, hBD-3 is expressed in skin and tonsil and hBD-4 is expressed most highly in testis and stomach. In addition to their antimicrobial effects, defensins recruit inflammatory cells and promote innate and adaptive immune responses.[35]

Cathelicidins are members of a family of peptides with a conserved N-terminal region of 100 amino acid residues and a heterogeneous C-terminal region (10 to 40 amino acid residues). The human peptide (LL-37) displays LPS-binding activity and broad-spectrum microbiocidal activity. It is produced by neutrophils and respiratory epithelial cells and appears to have a similar role in lung immunity as the defensins.[35]

Cellular Defenses: At the Crossroads of Innate and Adaptive Immunity

Inflammatory Cells in the Lung

Our knowledge of the cellular constituents in the lung, their activation state, and their function have been considerably augmented in the last 20 years by the ability to safely perform flexible fiberoptic bronchoscopy and biopsy in both control subjects and clinical patients. Using bronchoalveolar lavage (BAL), the normal cellular constituents of the alveolar space have been determined in a number of studies in both adults and children. Macrophages are the major cellular component of BAL fluid, making up 81% to 95% of the cells obtained; the remainder are lymphocytes, neutrophils, and eosinophils, whose total cell numbers and percent composition vary greatly with disease state. Data obtained from BAL and biopsy studies provide direct evidence of the role of inflammatory cells, adhesion molecules, and cellular mediators in humans, and they confirm cell culture and animal studies.

The Respiratory Epithelium

The airway epithelium is more than a passive barrier to airway water loss or a passive fortification against bacterial and viral infection. Published data support the concepts of active participation of the airway epithelium in regulation of airway smooth muscle tone, the physical removal of inhaled substances through ciliary clearance, and secretion or transport of broad-spectrum antimicrobial substances. The respiratory epithelium is a functional interface between the pathogen and the innate or adaptive immune responses. These features make the airway epithelium a pivotal structure in respiratory physiology and pathology.

The respiratory epithelium participates in passive lung immunity in many different ways. The epithelium presents a physical barrier to viral and bacterial invasion, lining the respiratory tract from the nose to the alveoli with a wide range of cell types.[36] Ciliated epithelial cells are important in propelling mucus up the airway, thereby removing particulate material; injury to ciliated cells by agents such as oxidants can alter the ability to remove mucus from the airway. Tracheobronchial glands and goblet cells are important sources of airway mucus, which serves to nonspecifically trap particulates. The respiratory epithelium also functions in the regulation of water and ion movement into the airway mucus.[7] The respiratory epithelium acts as its own reservoir for injury repair, presumably using the basal cell layers as progenitor cells.[36] Finally, the respiratory epithelium serves to regulate airway smooth muscle tone through a number of mechanisms, thereby restricting ventilation to injured areas. These properties allow the respiratory epithelium to nonspecifically protect the lung from inhaled toxins or microorganisms.

Additionally, the respiratory epithelium performs more specific interactions with the innate and adaptive immune systems. Alveolar type II cells manufacture surfactant proteins A and D.[29,37] The respiratory epithelium can also be induced to produce a number of bioactive cytokines, including, IL-1, IL-6, IL-8, GM-CSF, and RANTES.[38] The respiratory epithelium can upregulate expression of a number of adhesion molecules that support interactions between the epithelial cell and inflammatory cells recruited to the lung, including neutrophils, eosinophils, and lymphocytes.[19,21] Epithelial cells metabolize arachidonic acid and produce a number of bioactive eicosanoids, either directly or through transcellular metabolism with airway inflammatory cells. Bacterial or viral binding to TLRs on the epithelial surface, or intracellular PRR such as the NOD receptors, can result in activation of NFκB or other transcription factors and signal cytokine production and expression of new cellular receptors on the epithelial surface, facilitating interaction with inflammatory cells with protective, or potentially injurious, consequences. The inflammation resulting from airway injury is thought to be responsible for the airway hyperresponsiveness and obstruction that accompanies a number of diseases, such as asthma.

Resident Cell Defenses: At the Interface of Innate and Adaptive Immunity

Three major groups of inflammatory cells reside primarily within the lung parenchyma itself: dendritic cells, macrophages, and mast cells. These cells are recruited from the circulation and expand locally from their bone marrow–derived precursors. The cells (particularly the macrophages and dendritic cells) are capable of migration; however, they reside primarily within the lung itself. Other inflammatory cells are recruited from the circulation in their mature form (i.e., neutrophils, eosinophils, and lymphocytes) and, once activated, are capable of their mature functions.

Dendritic Cells

Dendritic cells (DC) are the primary resident antigen presenting cell population in the lung and airway.[39] Activation of dendritic cells in response to *innate* stimuli is essential to initiate the *adaptive* response to lung-acquired antigens. In these processes, the phenotype and function of dendritic cells play an important role in initiating tolerance, memory, and polarized Th1 and Th2 differentiation. Antigen presentation to T cells is actively and tightly regulated *in vivo* by soluble factors produced by mature tissue macrophages. Therefore, the phenotype of the dendritic cells, the responses to innate stimuli and cytokines produced by macrophages, and the lung microenvironment play important roles in determining the subsequent host adaptive response to antigen.[39]

In humans, at least five different subsets of DC have been described. These subsets appear to have different functions within the lung. The majority of these DCs are derived from circulating blood monocytes, differentiating in the lung to produce the DC subsets. DCs have a rapid half-life in the conducting airways (about 2 days), whereas more distal lung DCs have a slower turnover rate. There are CD11b+ and CD11b– subsets, both of which express large amounts of CD11c on their surface. The biology and functions of these subsets of cells are complex. Resident, plasmacytoid, and alveolar DCs are found at the interface with the external environment (mucosal surfaces, skin). In these tissues, they have the ability to migrate to inflammatory foci, where they can take up antigen, process the antigen, and then emigrate through the lymphatics to the draining lymph nodes and associate with T cell–rich areas and initiate adaptive immune responses. This migration is accompanied by alterations in the repertoire of adhesion proteins and chemokine receptors on the DC surface.

As the initiator of T cell responses, DCs recognize and respond to danger signals, mature (alter their function), and initiate the adaptive immune response. DC receptors sample the environment and the "danger signals," resulting in activation of the DC to migrate and mature, process antigen for expression, and release cytokines to further modulate the immune response. TLR 1 to TLR 5 are expressed on DC and are downregulated during maturation. In addition, NOD receptors respond to injury/pathogen-related signals. These innate signals cause the maturation and activation of dendritic cells that result in the adaptive T cell and B cell responses.

Macrophages

Extensive literature supports the role of the macrophage as the central regulator of airway inflammation. Alveolar macrophages have four important attributes that contribute to their function: mobility, phagocytosis, receptor expression for signal recognition, and production and release of a number of bioactive mediators.[40] In the lung, they perform a variety of biologically significant functions: scavenging particulates, removing macromolecules, killing microorganisms, acting as accessory and regulatory cells for a number of immune functions, recruiting and activating other inflammatory cells, maintaining and repairing injured lung tissues, removing apoptotic cells, and modulating normal lung physiology. Many of these functions are "turned off" in the resting state but are upregulated with macrophage activation. The regulation of macrophage activation and turnover is undoubtedly important in pulmonary health or disease, because the activated functions of this cell can not only help to kill invading organisms and to recruit other inflammatory cells, but they can also contribute to pulmonary inflammation or fibrosis. Macrophages can cooperate with other cell types (dendritic cells and lymphocytes) by means of cell-cell interactions and cytokine signals to orchestrate development of cell-mediated immunity consisting of delayed-type hypersensitivity and cytotoxic T cells, and humoral immunity. Macrophages are present in the interstitium and at epithelial surfaces in the lung. They are far more abundant in the distal respiratory tract, particularly the alveolus, than in the tracheobronchial tree.

The macrophage population is usually constant in size, but this is the result of a dynamic steady state of cellular recruitment, cell division, and cell turnover. The turnover time for alveolar macrophages has been calculated to be 21 to 28 days in animal models. At the end of this period, cells exit from the lungs up the mucociliary escalator, although the mechanisms for this efflux are still unknown. Speculation also exists that a subpopulation of alveolar macrophages may cross the alveolar epithelium to return to the interstitium, or to migrate to regional lymph nodes. During acute inflammation, it is clear that monocyte influx is the major contributor to the expansion of the macrophage population, although local proliferation of resident macrophages contributes to a lesser degree. Following this acute inflammatory response, the number of alveolar macrophages returns to normal resting levels.

Ultrastructural analysis indicates that macrophages are metabolically active cells. They have well-developed vacuolar apparatus and a large number of mitochondria. The prominent cytoplasmic organelles in the alveolar macrophage are the secondary lysosomes and the Golgi apparatus. The alveolar macrophage is exposed to an aerobic environment, with a PO_2 of approximately 100 Torr, unlike the peritoneal macrophage that functions with a PO_2 of 5 Torr. Alveolar macrophages produce a number of oxygen metabolites, including O_2^- (superoxide anion), H_2O_2 (hydrogen peroxide), and OH^- (hydroxyl radical). These reactive oxygen intermediates play an important role in host antimicrobial defense: defects in ability to generate these oxygen products leads to high susceptibility to infections, as in chronic granulomatous disease (CGD). Uncontrolled production of these reactive oxygen intermediates may play a role in lung injury.

In order for macrophages to ingest microorganisms, receptor-mediated uptake is necessary. Three groups of receptors play important roles in opsonization: Fc (immunoglobulin) receptors, complement receptors, and the PRRs including the TLRs (Table 7-3). Three receptors for the Fc portion of immunoglobulin G (IgG) have been described on alveolar macrophages: FcγRI (a high-affinity Fc receptor for monomeric IgG), FcγRII (a low-affinity receptor for IgG and aggregated IgG), and FcγRIII (a low-affinity receptor for aggregated IgG). On human alveolar macrophages, FcγR for IgG subclasses IgG1 and IgG3 are present in greater numbers than receptors for IgG2 and IgG4. In addition, Fc receptors for IgE (FcεRII) and IgA have been described. The macrophage has access to any molecules recognized by these immunoglobulins through their Fc receptors. In addition, alveolar macrophages have membrane-bound, cytophilic IgG and IgA, which play a role in nonopsonic phagocytosis. Three complement receptors have been described on alveolar macrophages. The most important is CR1 (CD35), which mediates high-affinity binding to C3b and low-affinity binding to iC3b and C4b. CR3 (Mac-1) is the CD11b/CD18 member of the β2 integrin family, which binds iC3b with high affinity and C3dg and C3d with low affinity. CR4 (CD11c/CD18) binds iC3b. Surfactant protein A is thought to bind to macrophage complement receptors, thereby nonspecifically opsonizing microorganisms.

In addition to the reactive oxygen intermediates discussed earlier in the chapter, macrophages produce many intracellular and secreted products that are responsible for a number of their bactericidal and cell-activating activities (Table 7-4). Human alveolar macrophages have been shown to produce metabolites of arachidonic

TABLE 7-3 MACROPHAGE RECEPTORS INVOLVED IN CLEARANCE OF LUNG PATHOGENS.

"CLASSIC" MACROPHAGE OPSONIC RECEPTORS	PATTERN RECOGNITION RECEPTORS (PRR)	
Ig Receptors		
	Receptor	*Ligand*
Fcγ Receptors	CD36	Apoptotic cells
Fcγ RI	CD14	LBP/LPS
Fcγ RII	Mannose	Carbohydrates
Fcγ RIII	receptor	Sialic acid
FC RII	Sialadhesin	Glucans, RGD
FCα	Integrins	Apoptotic cells
	PS receptor	
Complement Receptors	**Toll-like Receptors (TLR)**	
CR1 (CD35)	TLR 2	pg, LTA, LPS
CR3 (mac-1; CD11b/CD18)	TLR 4	SP-A
CR4 (CD11c/CD/18)	TLR 9	CpG
	Scavenger Receptors (SR)	
	Receptor	*Ligand*
	SR-AI, SR-AII	LPS, LTA, CpG
	MARCO	Polyanion
	LOX-1	Phosphatidyl
	SR-PSOX	serine

CpG, Bacterial DNA containing unmethylated CpG; *Ig*, immunoglobulin; *LPS*, lipopolysaccharide; *LTA*, lipoteichoic acid; *pg*, peptidoglycan; *SP-A*, surfactant protein A.

acid by both the cyclooxygenase and lipoxygenase pathways, and mediators from both pathways play a role in the modulation of inflammatory reactions. Alveolar macrophages produce a large diverse array of enzymes that can be divided into three major groups: acid hydrolases, neutral hydrolases, and lysozymes (see Table 7-4). Acid hydrolases function primarily as intracellular digestive enzymes, but they can be secreted into the extracellular environment, where they display a number of actions (e.g., microbial killing, degradation of connective tissue, activation of complement components, and lysis of fibrin). Lysozyme is a major secretory product of macrophages, and it is bactericidal for many microorganisms (see earlier in the chapter). Finally, a number of cytokines and chemotactic factors are produced by alveolar macrophages (see Table 7-4). The pro-inflammatory cytokine IL-1 is one of the most important regulatory products of the macrophage. TGF-β also has many biologic functions, including chemoattraction for fibroblasts, and effects on the composition of the extracellular matrix. Through the generation of cytokines, the macrophage plays a central role in phagocyte recruitment and activation, wound healing, fibrosis, and modulation of actions of other innate and adaptive immune responses in the lung.

Macrophage products protect the lung from invading pathogens, yet overproduction of these products can lead to lung injury. Lung homeostasis depends on the regulation of these functions/products. In the quiescent state, the alveolar macrophage interacts with alveolar epithelial cells through the integrin αvβ6 on

TABLE 7-4 BIOACTIVE PRODUCTS OF LUNG IMMUNE CELLS

PRODUCT	MACROPHAGE	MAST CELLS	NEUTROPHIL	EOSINOPHIL
Granule Proteins and other bioactive protein products	Acid Hydrolases, Proteases, Lipases, Deoxyribonucleases, Glycosidase, Sulfatases, Phosphatases, Neutral Hydrolases, Plasminogen activator, Collagenase, Elastase, Lysozyme	Histamine, Heparin, Chondroitin sulfate E and A, Tryptase, Chymase, Carboxypeptidase, Cathepsin-G-like protease	Granulophysin (CD63), Acid β-glycerophosphatase, Azurocidin, α_1-antitrypsin, Myeloperoxidase, lysozyme, Cathepsins (A, D, E, F, G), β glucuronidase	MBP, EPO, ECP, EDN, Collagenase, Elastase, Histimanase, Phospholipase, Arylsulphatase
	Endothelin 1, Endothelin 3, Defensins, Plasmin Inhibitors, α_2-Macroglobulin		Defensins, elastase, $\beta2$ microglobulin, Lysozyme, Lactoferrin, histaminase	Substance P, Vasoactive Intestinal Pepetide (VIP)
Lipid mediators	PGE_2, $PGF_{2\alpha}$, TXA_2, LTB_4, $LT\,C_4$, 5-HETE, PAF	PGD_2, LTC_4, LTB_4, PAF	PAF LTB_4	PAF, TXB_2, PGE_2, 6-keto-$PGF_{1\alpha}$, LTC_4, 15-HETE
Reactive oxygen products	O_2^-, H_2O_2, OH		O_2^-, H_2O_2, HOCl	O_2^-, H_2O_2, HOCl, HOBr, OH
Reactive nitrogen products	NO, peroxynitrite		NO	
Cytokines and chemokines	IL-1α, IL-1β, TNF-α, TGF-β, PDGF, IL-6, IFN-α, IFN-β	TNF-α, GM-CSF, SCF, IL-3, IL-4, IL-5, IL-6, IL-10, IL-13, IL-14, IL-16, IFN-γ	IL-1β, TNF-α, GM-CSF, TGF-β, MIP-2	TGF-α, TGF-β, IL-1α, IL-2, IL-3, IL-4, IL-5, IL-6, IL-9, IL-10, IL-11, IL-12, IL-16, IFN-γ, GM-CSF
	IL-8, MIP-1α, MIP-1β, MIP-2, MCP-1	MIP-1α, T cell activation gene 3, lymphotactin, MCP-1 Interferon-γ	MIP-2, KC, IL-8, MIP-1α, MIP-1β, IFN-γ, CINC, GRO-α, IP-10	Eotaxin, IL-8, MIP-1α, MCP-1, MCP-3, MCP-4, RANTES

the epithelial surface, leading to localized activation of Transforming Growth Factor-β (TGF-β), which suppresses phagocytosis and cytokine production by the macrophage. TLR stimulation of macrophages leads to rapid loss of contact with the AEC, loss of $\alpha v\beta 6$ expression on the epithelial cells, and a decrease in TGF-β activation, thus allowing activation of the macrophages. As the infectious threat is removed, activated lymphocytes that have migrated to the lung will release interferon-γ, which stimulates production of matrix metalloproteinase 9 by macrophages, thus activating latent TGF-β and allowing macrophages to again adhere to the alveolar epithelial cell and turn off the inflammatory process.[40]

Macrophage function in the innate and adaptive response requires activation, and the type of response depends on the cytokines that stimulate the macrophage. The "classical" pathway for activation is driven by interferon-γ and enhances macrophage-dependent phagocytosis and microbial killing and MHC-dependent antigen presentation. Macrophages activated along this pathway are designated M1 macrophages based on their association with T helper type I (Th1) cell immune responses. This response is marked by production of IL-1β, IL-6, IL-12, TNF-α, and iNOS. The "alternative" pathway is triggered by macrophage exposure to IL-4 or IL-13, resulting in M2 macrophages. These macrophages express a distinct set of receptors and are associated with a Th2 lymphocyte response, which is implicated in the pathogenesis of allergy and asthma.[41]

Mast Cells

Mast cells have long been recognized as the major effector cells of allergic reactions, by virtue of their expression of high-affinity Fc receptors for immunoglobulin E (IgE) (FcεRI) and the vast array of mediators they produce. Mast cells are distributed in normal tissues throughout the body in close proximity to blood vessels and do not circulate in the blood. It has been postulated that they play a role in host defense against parasites, in wound healing, in immunoregulation, and in tumor angiogenesis. Although small in number, mast cells play an important role in health and disease.[42,43]

Human mast cells have been demonstrated to originate in the bone marrow from CD34+ c-Kit+CD13+ progenitor cells. Acquisition of IgE receptors appears to occur early in mast cell development. Once recruited from the circulation, mast cells acquire their mature phenotype in the tissue microenvironment. In interstitial spaces, a number of other cytokines influence the production of a number of serine proteases, which differ between mast cell phenotypes (mucosal versus serosal).[42,43]

Mast cells express a number of surface receptors that activate their biologic activities. IgE is the principal antibody responsible for type I type allergic responses in humans. The major receptor for IgE, the FcεRI (receptor for the Fc portion of IgE I), is present in large numbers on mature mast cells. Cross-linking of FcεRI results in mast cell triggering. The major biologic effect of FcεRI aggregation is the release of allergic mediators. In addition, FcεRI activation results in the production of a number of pro-inflammatory cytokines, including IL-4, IL-5, IL-6, IL-3, interferon γ, and TNF-α.[42] In addition to the FcεRI, mast cells express a number of TLRs, including TLR-1, TLR-2, TLR-4, and TLR-6. Expression of the TLR allows mast cells to recognize multiple potential pathogens and generate specific responses, including immediate inflammatory responses to limit infection, and regulation of adaptive immunity.[43]

Mast cell granules contain a large number of pre-formed mediators (see Table 7-4), which are released within minutes after cell activation. In addition, mast cells secrete several lipid mediators produced via both the cyclooxygenase (PGD_2) and lipoxygenase (LTC_4 and LTB_4) pathways of arachidonic acid metabolism. Mast cell proteases stimulate tissue remodeling, neuropeptide inactivation, and enhanced mucus secretion. Histamine stimulates smooth muscle cell contraction, vasodilatation, increased venular permeability, and mucus secretion. Histamine induces IL-16 production by CD8+ cells and airway epithelial cells. LTC_4, LTB_4, and PGD_2 affect venular permeability and can regulate the activation of immune cells. Finally, mast cells produce a diverse array of cytokines both constitutively (GM-CSF, TNF-α, and IL-6) and following mast cell activation (IL-1, IL-2, IL-3, IL-4, IL-5, IL-10, IL-13, IL-14, IL-16, and interferon γ).[43] IL-13 is critical to the development of allergic asthma.

It had been argued that mast cells represent a host system that evolved primarily to fight parasites. However, current research suggests that mast cells are more central to both innate and adaptive responses in the lung. Mast cells can phagocytose particles, present antigens, produce cytokines, and release vasoactive substances.[42,43] In addition, mast cells exhibit a wide array of adhesion and other receptors that enable them to react to both nonspecific and specific stimuli. Finally, the antigen-specific responses via IgE make mast cells part of the adaptive immune responses within the lung. Studies using mast cell knock-in and specific protease-deficient mice have demonstrated that mast cells can enhance host resistance and survival following bacterial infections. Mast cells can also perform functions such as antigen presentation and interactions with other immune cells via co-stimulatory molecules or secreted products that can enhance or suppress the development of innate or adaptive immune functions. They can limit infection, yet they may exacerbate Th2 or autoimmune disorders. They can help limit or turn off inflammation, but can exacerbate the responses to other stimulatory organisms or their products. They are therefore important as first regulators of homeostasis during innate or adaptive responses in the lung.[42]

Recruited Cellular Defenses

All pulmonary inflammatory cells are initially derived from bone marrow precursors recruited from the circulation. The cells discussed so far migrate to the lung in an "immature" form, and they mature or differentiate within the lung in response to local cytokines or through activation by pathogens. The cells discussed in the following section are recruited from the pulmonary circulation in their mature, active forms. In the process of recruitment, these cells move from a "quiescent" resting state to a state in which they are fully "activated" or "primed" for further cellular activities.

Neutrophils

Neutrophils are characterized by their multilobed nucleus and distinctive cytoplasmic granules that contain an arsenal of enzymes and proteins that contribute to neutrophil function. Neutrophils constitute about half the circulating white cell population, and their primary function is phagocytosis and killing of invading pathogens. In order for the neutrophil to accomplish this, it must respond to signals in the area of injury, adhere and transmigrate through the vascular endothelium, migrate to the area of infection, recognize the pathogen, phagocytose, and kill it. Interruption of any of these steps will leave the host susceptible to infections. Patients with leukocyte adhesion deficiency (LAD) are unable to recruit neutrophils into sites of inflammation, and, as a result, they sustain recurrent, life-threatening infections due to deficiency of the β2 integrins. In chronic granulomatous disease (CGD), the neutrophils lack components of the NADPH oxidase system, and affected neutrophils that have engulfed organisms cannot efficiently kill them. The processes of neutrophil recruitment and activation, followed by neutrophil removal (cell death, or apoptosis) after the resolution of the infectious process or injury, are closely regulated at several levels. Disruption of these regulatory processes can lead to acute or ongoing lung injury.

Neutrophils are short-lived cells; their life span from stem cell differentiation to removal in the tissues is 12 to 14 days. CD34+ myeloid progenitor cells in the bone marrow produce myeloblasts, which then differentiate through several recognizable morphologic stages into mature, nondividing polymorphonuclear neutrophils. It normally takes about 14 days for the neutrophil precursor to mature and be released into the blood.[44] Once in the circulation, neutrophil half-life is quite short (approximately 6 to 7 hours). The pulmonary capillary bed is unique in its ability to "concentrate" neutrophils. The term *margination* has been proposed to describe this increased concentration of neutrophils in *noninflamed* lungs. Margination is proposed to result from a discordance between the diameter of neutrophils (6 to 8 μm) and the capillary segments (2 to 15 μm). Morphometric and videomicroscopic studies have suggested that the neutrophil must change shape within 40% to 60% of these capillary segments to traverse the pulmonary circulation, increasing the pulmonary capillary transit time. This prolonged transit time is postulated to allow neutrophils time to sense and respond to the presence of inflammatory processes.[44]

In response to inflammatory stimuli, neutrophils further accumulate in preparation for migration *(sequestration)*. In much of the *systemic* circulation, neutrophil sequestration occurs in postcapillary venules in the form of rolling, and is mediated by selectins. In the lungs, the known adhesion molecules do not appear to mediate the initial events of sequestration. Rather, in the pulmonary capillary, inflammatory mediators alter the mechanical properties of the neutrophils, resulting in changes in deformability thought to be induced by polymerization of actin beneath the plasma membrane. This "stiffening" reduces the neutrophil deformability, lengthening the capillary transit times or stopping the movement of the neutrophil altogether in the sites of inflammation.[44]

Once sequestration has occurred, the neutrophils can adhere via selectin or CD11/CD18-ICAM-1 mechanisms used elsewhere in the circulation and migrate across the vascular endothelium into the lung.[44] In the process of migration into the lung, the neutrophils acquire an activated phenotype, resulting in a change in surface receptors compared to blood neutrophils.[45]

Once the neutrophil has migrated into the tissue, its primary purpose is to recognize, ingest, and destroy pathogens. Phagocytosis consists of two steps: (1) recognition and (2) internalization of the foreign material into the phagosome. Killing or neutralization then involves a secretory response. Materials may bind directly to the neutrophil, resulting in ingestion. However, as with macrophages, opsonization by serum proteins also occurs. Neutrophils exhibit both specific Fc-mediated binding and nonspecific binding using complement receptors CR1 and CR3, as used by macrophages. Intracellular killing is generally associated with the initiation of the respiratory burst. In addition, alternative mechanisms of killing exist, including secretion of granular proteins into the phagosome (see Table 7-4).

Secretion of granule contents from the neutrophil into its local environment is usually referred to as *degranulation*. In addition, the cell actively releases a number of other materials to the outside, including lipid mediators of inflammation (PAF, LTB$_4$). The signals initiating neutrophil degranulation and secretion are still unclear.[46] During inflammatory reactions, the earliest responses involve neutrophil emigration, with subsequent degranulation and secretion of granule contents. Degranulation involves the fusion of the granule membrane with either the developing or formed phagosome.

Eosinophils

Eosinophils are the second largest group of granulocytic cells in the circulation. They can be morphologically distinguished from neutrophils by their ability to be stained by negatively charged dyes, such as eosin. They are 8 μm in diameter and typically have two nuclear lobes. Their biologic function was unclear for most of the 20th century, but in the late 1960s and early 1970s the possibility was raised that eosinophils might be involved in immunity to parasites. This received experimental support in the mid 1970s in a report on eosinophil-dependent killing of schistosomula of *Schistosoma mansoni*. Current research has focused on the role of the eosinophil in pulmonary inflammation associated with asthma. Eosinophils and eosinophil products are present in the blood, sputum, and autopsy samples from patients with asthma, and there is a correlation between the presence of eosinophils and asthma severity. Eosinophils and their products are characteristic features of airway mucosa and bronchoalveolar lavage specimens following allergic antigen challenge in humans and animals. These lines of evidence indicate that eosinophilic infiltration in asthma may play a major role in the pathogenesis of the disease, and that prevention of eosinophil influx or release of eosinophil products may be major targets for asthma therapy.[47]

Eosinophils arise from bone marrow precursor cells. The migration of eosinophils from the bone marrow takes about 3.5 days after DNA synthesis has completed.

In the blood, the half-time of eosinophils is 18 hours. Like neutrophils, there appears to be a marginated pool of eosinophils, which are in dynamic equilibrium with the circulating pool. Eosinophils marginate and emigrate into the tissues through postcapillary venules, probably through interactions with a number of adhesion molecules similar to the margination of neutrophils in the pulmonary circulation. However, eosinophils, but not neutrophils, adhere to the ligand VCAM-1 on the endothelial surface and, once adherent, can be attracted by a specific array of chemotactic agents into the lung. The life span of eosinophils in the lung is unknown, although it is assumed that they survive for several days. *In vitro* studies demonstrate that eosinophils can survive for over a week in the presence of IL-3, GM-CSF, and IL-5.

Many of our concepts of the biologic roles of eosinophil have been derived from studies of their mediators and biologic functions (see Table 7-4). Eosinophil granules contain a number of unique proteins with extensive biologic activities that contribute to the role of the eosinophil in lung inflammation, including major basic protein (MBP), eosinophil peroxidase (EPO), eosinophil cationic protein (ECP), and eosinophil-derived neurotoxin (EDN). MBP accounts for over 50% of the eosinophil granule protein. MBP is a potent toxin for mammalian cells and parasites *in vitro*, and has been localized in tissues in hypersensitivity diseases and bronchial asthma. EPO is an abundant protein in the matrix of the human eosinophil granule, and differs from neutrophil myeloperoxidase structurally. Like myeloperoxidase, EPO catalyzes the oxidation of halides by H$_2$O$_2$ to form highly reactive intermediates, which have antibacterial and anti-helminth activities. ECP and EDN are closely related proteins, located in the granule matrix, and demonstrate neurotoxic properties. The cytotoxic action of ECP involves the formation of channels in cell membranes, like complement-membrane interactions. ECP is part of the family of pore-forming proteins that includes lymphocyte perforin. Collectively these eosinophil proteins have potent activity that implicates the role of the eosinophil in the control of parasitic diseases. However, these proteins also have activities that are associated with the pathogenesis of obstructive lung disorders. Other peptide products of eosinophils are elastase, histaminase, phospholipase and arylsulfatase (see Table 7-4).

Eosinophils produce two principal lipid mediators with biologic effects implicating them in asthma and allergic disease: PAF (platelet activating factor) and LTC$_4$ (see Table 7-4). PAF is capable of eliciting many of the characteristic features of the asthmatic airway. In a guinea pig model, PAF is one of the most potent inducers of airway microvascular leakage. It is also a potent bronchoconstrictor that can lead to airway hyperresponsiveness. Eosinophils also elaborate many products of arachidonic acid metabolism. They increase vascular permeability and enhance mucus production in animal and human models. Moreover, the sulfidopeptide leukotrienes have a major effect on airway smooth muscle contraction.

Activated eosinophils undergo a "respiratory burst" like that exhibited by neutrophils, and produce a similar repertoire of reactive oxygen intermediates following activation (see Table 7-4). Mechanisms of damage by eosinophil-produced oxidants are not well established, but peroxidation of lipids in the plasma membrane by O_2^- may be important. In the lung, oxygen radicals may cause increased vascular permeability and edema formation through effects on vascular endothelium, and they may cause increased smooth muscle contractility by effects on the airway epithelium.

Eosinophils have recently been demonstrated to produce a number of bioactive cytokines (see Table 7-4). The biological relevance and roles of these cytokines in eosinophil-effector cell interactions remains to be elucidated *in vivo*.

In summary, eosinophils synthesize a number of biologically active peptides that contribute to their ability to destroy parasites *in vivo*. However eosinophil products such as PAF, LTC₄, and reactive oxygen intermediates have the potential to disrupt the airways and they have physiologic activities that implicate the eosinophil as a primary effector cell in asthma, possibly to the extent of functioning as an antigen presenting cell to Th2 lymphocytes.[47]

Innate Lymphocyte Responses in the Lung: Natural Killer Cells, Natural Killer T Cells, and γδ T Cells

Although lymphocyte populations are generally regarded as part of adaptive immunity, several lymphocyte subsets function in innate responses including recognition and elimination of tumor cells and certain pathogens. They accomplish this through the use of limited sets of conserved recognition receptors. Three major lymphocyte populations will be considered in this context. Natural killer (NK) cells are bone marrow–derived lymphocytes that are distinct from either B cells or T cells. NK-T cells are T cells that express the NK cell marker, NK1, a highly restricted/limited repertoire of the CD3/T cell receptor (TCR) complex with specificity for antigens presented in association with CD1. These cells most closely resemble CD4 T cells in terms of cytokine production. Finally, γδ T cells have a limited diversity of TCRs that recognize self and bacterial/protozoan antigens. These innate lymphocytes are considered to be a first line of defense against tumors and infection, and in modulating inflammation in the lung.

NK cells are capable of lysing certain tumor cells without prior sensitization (thus the name *natural killer*). They were originally thought to primarily provide protection against tumor cells. Subsequently, they have been demonstrated to provide defense against viral infections. NK cells express several distinctive surface receptors that influence cell function: CD 56; killer cell immunoglobulin-like receptors (KIRs), which are inhibitory receptors that recognize specific major histocompatiblity complex (MHC) class I receptors; NK receptors NKR-P1, CD161, NKG2A-NKG2E, and CD94, which are inhibitory receptors; CD16 (FCγ RIII-FC receptor for target-bound IgG), which mediates antibody-dependent cell-mediated cytotoxicity; CD2; and the β2 integrins.[48]

NK cells develop in the bone marrow and require stem cell factor (c-kit ligand), IL-7, flt-3 ligand, IL-15, IL12, IL-18, and interferon-γ for maturation. NK cells only constitute a small population of cells (2.5% of splenic leukocytes). This population, however, can respond and expand quickly in response to infection, contributing significantly to innate defenses. One mechanism of early innate response is the presence of multiple activation receptors on the surface of individual NK cells. In addition, NK cells have constitutive expression of many cytokine receptors that allow them to be stimulated by pro-inflammatory cytokines early in the course of response to injury or infection. Stimulation of NK cells can lead to further production of cytokines (interferon γ, TNF-α, GM-CSF). Moreover, activated or infected macrophages and dendritic cells produce a number of cytokines that can stimulate NK cells to produce cytokines and chemokines. Interferon α/β enhances NK cell cytotoxicity. In addition, NK cells appear to play an important role in attenuation or resolution of immune responses through action on CD8 T cells or indirect control of DC.[48]

NK T cells are CD4 T cells that express a unique set of cellular receptors. These receptors include the NK receptors (including CD16) and a unique invariant TCR Vα24-Jα18/Vβ11, co-expression of the NK cell marker NK1.1, MHC restriction for the nonclassical class I molecule CD1d, and the ability to make large amounts of Th1 or Th2 cytokines. Ligands for this complex include glycolipids rather than peptide antigens in the context of the CD1d molecule. NK T cells appear to function primarily in regulating autoimmunity and malignancy. In addition, they appear to be important in the processing of lipids from mycobacteria.[49] This TCR is highly conserved in most animal species, suggesting it is a PRR. NKT cells can be activated directly by antigen interaction with receptors, or indirectly through exposure to cytokines (IL-12, IL-18) expressed by activated dendritic cells.[49]

γδ T lymphocytes are innate T lymphocyte populations that express the γδ T cell receptor with limited diversity. In humans, the Vγ2Vδ2 TCR is utilized by the majority of γδ T cells. These cells recognize small organic phosphate antigens from microbes. The population expands significantly in protozoan infections (e.g., malaria and toxoplasmosis) and mycobacterial infections.[50] Differential expression of interferon-γ and IL-4 influences the development of Th1 and Th2 responses, respectively.

Adaptive Lung Defenses

Most pathogens gain entry to the lung across mucosal surfaces. An important aspect of inflammatory and immune responses to the entry of respiratory pathogens is the ability to mount an appropriate, regulated immune response that can clear the infection rapidly and efficiently, yet not expose the surrounding tissues or the whole host to chronic inflammation. Innate immunity provides the first level of protection. Adaptive or specific immunity provides specific responses to antigens during acute infection and provides specific immune memory that protects against subsequent exposure. A number of cell types contribute to airway mucosal defense, as discussed earlier in the chapter. As part of the mucosal surface from the nasal airway to the conducting airways, the bronchial-associated lymphoid tissue (BALT) functions in the development of adaptive lung defense. The BALT is made up of intraepithelial lymphocytes, macrophages, dendritic cells, NK and NK T cells that recognize foreign substances, invading organisms or their exoproducts, and products of cell injury using the receptor systems described. The dendritic cells or macrophages interact with lymphocytes to create the cellular immune responses, or to signal antibody production. These cells migrate to local lymph nodes, tonsils, or adenoids; process antigens; generate cytokines; and generate the adaptive immune responses. While extensive reviews of humoral (B cell mediated) and cellular (T cell mediated) immunity, antigen presentation and cellular activation are well beyond the scope of this chapter, we will briefly discuss the roles of humoral and cellular immunity with respect to lung defense.

T Lymphocytes and Lung Defense

Several types of T lymphocytes (T cells) contribute to lung immunity and tissue pathology. Two major types of antigen receptors are used by T lymphocytes: the γδ TCR, and the αβ receptor (making up the CD4 and CD8 T cell populations). The αβ T cell mounts cytolytic responses to infected cells, synthesizes cytokines, and stimulates B cell responses. αβ T cells that express the receptor protein CD4 are termed *T helper (Th) cells.* CD4 T cells recognize antigens presented via the MHC class II antigen, and they provide effector function primarily by the release of cytokines. Th cells can be further differentiated phenotypically into Th1 and Th2 populations based on their profiles of cytokine production. Th1 cells differentiate in the presence of IL-12 and IL-18 and produce interferon-γ, IL-2, and TNF-α in response to antigen. These cells have been regarded as responsible for the delayed hypersensitivity response to viral or bacterial infection, stimulating local macrophage activation and neutrophil recruitment, and altering specific T cell responses. Th2 cells are driven to differentiate by the presence of IL-4, and in the presence of antigen they respond by making IL-4, IL-5, IL-10, and IL-13. These cytokines are responsible for driving B lymphocytes to make antibodies, and they lead to the recruitment and activation of basophils and eosinophils. The Th2 phenotype has been associated with an allergic/asthmatic phenotype in mouse models and human studies.[51]

αβ T cells that express CD8 are cytotoxic cells. In response to peptides presented by the MHC class I molecules, CD8 T cells function in target cell toxicity. CD8 T cell toxicity is mediated by the release of cellular granules containing perforin (perturbs the cell membrane) and granzymes (disrupt target cells by altering intracellular targets). In addition, CD8 T cells can initiate apoptosis in target cells by Fas-FasL interactions. CD8 cells reinforce viral defenses by rendering adjacent cells resistant to infection, presumably by release of interferons.

T cell responses are tightly regulated. Whereas responses are necessary to eliminate pathogens, uncontrolled responses can cause autoimmune inflammatory diseases.

B Lymphocytes

Humoral immunity is mediated by antibodies produced by B lymphocytes (B cells). Antibodies are proteins that function to eliminate or neutralize the antigens that specifically induce their production. The interaction of antigens with B lymphocytes triggers the production of specific antibodies and establishes the potential for a rapid release of large amounts of antibody upon future stimulation (immune memory).

As B cells differentiate, one of the first changes is the rearrangement of information coded in the variable (V), diversity (D), and joining (J) regions of the gene. Through genetic rearrangement, DNA for one discrete V region is opposed to that of specific D J regions. This rearrangement is responsible for the specific affinity (idiotype) of the antibodies produced by B cells. The commitment of B cells to make antibodies to certain antigens is established prior to exposure to those antigens.

Initially, B cells express IgM and IgD isotypes on the cell surface. Upon interaction of an antigen with membrane-bound IgM, the clone of B cells with the genetic information coding for the antigen-specific antibodies undergoes two changes: proliferation, which results in clonal expansion, and differentiation, which results in production of antibodies of different isotypes. In addition, the B cells begin to express MHC class II molecules on their cell surface, which allows them to interact with Th cells. This hypermutation and class switching of immunoglobulin genes, along with the generation of memory B cells and plasma-cell precursors, occurs in the germinal centers of secondary lymphoid follicles, in the presence of dendritic cells, Th cells, and macrophages. The organization of these structures provides an immune microenvironment that maximizes the generation of antibody responses by bringing all relevant cell types into close contact for cell-cell signaling; this was recently named the *immune synapse.* Depending on the type of antigen, the B cell response may be classified as T cell–dependent or T cell–independent. The T cell–independent pathogens can stimulate B cells without assistance from T cells. Examples of T cell–independent antigens include polysaccharides and polymerized flagellin, which provide numerous repeating epitopes. T cell–independent antigens do not induce the formation of germinal centers and therefore cannot induce the generation of memory B cells or somatic hypermutation that results in the production of high-affinity antibodies. The extent of class switching from IgM to other classes of antibodies is also severely limited in the absence of Th cell–generated cytokines. In general, protein antigens are T cell–dependent, and the peptide-MHC complexes on CD4 T cells provide the cytokine signals that initiate somatic hypermutation and immunoglobulin class switching.[52]

Humoral Immunity

Depending on the stage of development of the B lymphocyte, different immunoglobulin isotypes are produced. Prior to antigenic stimulation, the "naïve" B lymphocyte expresses IgM (and IgD) on its surface. Early in the antigenic response, IgM, IgG3, and IgG1 are produced by B lymphocytes. In the chronic response, the predominant isotypes produced are IgG2 and IgG4. In addition, IgA is important in the mucosal immune response. The relative concentrations of immunoglobulin isotypes present in the bronchoalveolar lavage fluid of healthy individuals are listed in Table 7-5.

TABLE 7-5 RELATIVE CONCENTRATION OF IMMUNOGLOBULINS IN SERUM AND BRONCHOALVEOLAR LAVAGE (BAL)*

	IgG1	IgG2	IgG3	IgG4	IgA	IgE
Serum	4.5	2.1	0.03	0.1	2	200
BAL	50	22	1.4	4	183	9

*Values for serum are in mg/mL; values for BAL are in µg/ml, except for IgE (where all values are ng/mL).

Immunoglobulin A

Secretory immunoglobulin A (IgA) is the predominant immunoglobulin isotype present in airway secretions. Secretory IgA is composed of two IgA molecules (dimeric IgA), a joining protein (J chain), and a secretory component. The dimeric IgA-J chain complex is produced by B lymphocytes in the submucosal tissues. The secretory component is produced by mucosal epithelial cells and acts as a receptor for dimeric IgA. After IgA binds to the secretory component, the entire complex undergoes endocytosis and is transported to the apical surface of the cell, where the secretory IgA complex is released into the mucosal environment. The secretory component serves to protect the secretory IgA complex from proteases present in the mucosal environment. Secretory IgA serves several functions, including neutralization of viruses and exotoxin, enhancement of lactoferrin and lactoperoxidase activities, and inhibition of microbial growth. Because dimeric IgA is able to bind two antigens simultaneously, it is capable of forming large antigen-antibody complexes. In this manner, IgA neutralizes microbes and facilitates their removal by mucociliary clearance, inhibits microbial binding to epithelial cells, and inhibits uptake of potential allergens.

In general, a serum IgA level of less than 7 mg/dL (0.07 g/L) is considered as selective IgA deficiency since this concentration is the lowest detectable limit established by most laboratories. When the serum IgA level is higher than 7 mg/dL but two standard deviations below normal for age, the condition may be referred to as *partial IgA deficiency*, which is quite common. The threshold of 4 years of age is used to avoid premature diagnosis of IgA deficiency, which may be transient in younger children due to delayed maturation of IgA production after birth.[53] Symptomatic individuals present with various manifestations including recurrent sinusitis, otitis media, pharyngitis, bronchitis, pneumonia, chronic diarrhea, and autoimmune syndromes. Individuals with associated IgE deficiency tend to have less serious pulmonary disease in contrast to individuals with normal or high IgE, who in addition to the above disorders suffer from allergic respiratory problems and pulmonary hemosiderosis.

In general, patients with selective IgA deficiency are treated symptomatically for respiratory, gastrointestinal, and allergic problems. Since most preparations of gamma globulin contain IgA, the use of gamma globulin increases the risk of anaphylaxis if the recipient has anti-IgA antibodies. Transfusion of blood products presents a similar problem for these individuals. In patients with a combined IgA and IgG deficiency who need immunoglobulin therapy or the transfusion of blood products, it is critical to either ensure that the recipient does not have IgA antibodies or use a preparation that does not contain IgA.[53]

Immunoglobulin G

Although concentrations of immunoglobulin G (IgG) in the airway are less than those of IgA, all IgG subclasses are detectable in respiratory secretions. As opposed to IgA, which is actively transported into the airway, IgG reaches the airway largely by transudation through the mucosa. IgG functions by opsonizing microbes for phagocytosis and killing, activating the complement cascade, and neutralizing many bacterial endotoxins and viruses.

IgG deficiency, as in X-linked agammaglobulinemia or common variable hypogammaglobulinemia, is associated with recurrent otitis media, sinusitis, bronchitis, and pneumonia. Recurrence of airway infections may result in chronic airway injury with bronchiectasis. The combination of altered opsonic activity and bronchiectasis results in chronic colonization with respiratory pathogens such as *Pseudomonas aeruginosa*.[54]

In patients suspected of IgG deficiency, quantification of IgG subclasses should be performed in addition to measurement of the antibody response to polysaccharide vaccines (*S. pneumoniae, H. influenzae*). IgG-deficient patients with recurrent respiratory tract infections often benefit from prophylactic antibiotics, intravenous gamma globulin therapy, and the use of airway clearance techniques. The identification of a selective IgG subclass deficiency, or combined subclass deficiency, is not predictive of the capacity to produce antibody to pneumococcal polysaccharide or tetanus toxoid antigen. However, failure to demonstrate an antibody response to pneumococcal polysaccharide or tetanus toxoid is an indication of a potentially serious problem. Children with deficiency of all IgG isotypes (e.g., Bruton's agammaglobulinemia) uniformly develop chronic airway infection and lung dysfunction unless treated aggressively.[54]

Immunoglobulin E

Immunoglobulin E (IgE) appears to participate in immunity to parasites. It binds to the parasites, and eosinophils then bind to the opsonized organisms via the IgE Fc receptors. Eosinophils are stimulated to release granular contents, resulting in lysis of the parasite. Isolated IgE deficiency has not been reported. IgE deficiency in combination with IgG4 deficiency has been described in a patient who suffered from recurrent otitis media and sinusitis. Job's syndrome (or hyper-IgE syndrome) is characterized by recurrent skin and lower respiratory tract infections, eczema, elevated IgE levels, and eosinophilia. Associated facial and bone abnormalities are common. Symptoms occur within the first month of life with severe eczema, mucocutaneous infections, sinusitis, and lower respiratory tract infections with *S. aureus* or *H. influenzae*. Development of empyema, lung abscess, and pneumatocele is common.[55]

Immunoglobulin M

Most immunoglobulin M (IgM) remains in the vascular space due to its high molecular weight. However, IgM does gain access to the airway by exudation or by active secretion via the secretory component. IgM is capable of agglutinating bacteria and activating the complement cascade. Therefore, despite the fact that low levels of IgM are detected in airway secretions, it plays a role in mucosal defense. Isolated IgM deficiency is not associated with recurrent respiratory infections. Individuals with IgM deficiency appear to have a specific defect in B lymphocyte maturation, but the B lymphocytes are capable of secreting other antibody isotypes.[54]

The Role of Programmed Cell Death and Removal of Dead Cells in Lung Health, Injury, and Repair

During the course of lung development, growth, and injury repair, dead and injured cells must be replaced in an orderly process in order to maintain lung function and to control lung inflammation. Acute lung injury (ALI) and adult respiratory distress syndrome are examples "explosive" lung inflammation and injury. However, chronic conditions such as cystic fibrosis lung disease and pulmonary fibrosis are slower-evolving processes. In both types of lung injury, there is evidence that the programs of cell death and removal of dead cells become disordered, leading to ongoing inflammation and lung injury. The lung cells have evolved orderly processes controlling the breakdown of cell contents (autophagy), controlled cell death (apoptosis), and removal of dead or dying cells (efferocytosis) to maintain lung function and homeostasis. While detailed description of these topics is beyond the scope of this chapter, a brief description of their role in lung injury and lung inflammatory responses is essential to the discussion of lung defense (Table 7-6).

Autophagy is an evolutionarily conserved process present in virtually all eukaryotic cells. Three types of autophagy are described: macroautophagy, microautophagy, and chaperone-mediated autophagy. We will focus on macroautophagy, hereafter referred to as simply autophagy.[56] Autophagy involves the sequestration of regions of the cytosol within double-membrane–bound compartments and the delivery of the contents of these compartments to the lysosome for degradation. While autophagy is important in the "recycling" of cellular components for reuse in a starvation state, there is recent evidence that autophagy is a component of innate immunity for the elimination of intracellular pathogens such as intracellular bacteria and viruses. Autophagy can be divided into three stages: initiation, execution, and maturation.[56] Initiation of autophagy is regulated by target of rapamycin (TOR) kinase that functions as an inhibitor. Other pathways involve activation

TABLE 7-6 AUTOPHAGY, APOPTOSIS, AND EFFEROCYTOSIS IN THE LUNG

PROCESS	PROTEIN/PROTEIN FAMILIES REQUIRED
Autophagy	
Initiation	TOR, class 3 phosphoinositide 3-kinases, trimeric G proteins
Execution	Autophagy genes (Atg) activation and complex formation Atg12, Atg7, Atg10, Atg5, Atg16 → Atg5-Atg12-Atg16 Complex present in autophagy isolation membrane
	Atg8, Atg4, Atg7, Atg3, phosphotidylethanolamine Atg8-phosphotidylethanolamine needed for association with autophagosome
Maturation	Lysosome-associated membrane protein 1 (LAMP1) and LAMP2
Apoptosis	
Extrinsic Pathway	TNF family of receptors (TNFR-1, FAS/CD95, Death receptor 3 (DR3, DR4, DR5, DR6) TNF-related apoptosis inducing ligand (TRAIL) Adaptor proteins, procaspase 8
Intrinsic Pathway	bcl2 family of proteins, cytochrome c Apoptosis protein activator factor 1 (APAF-1) Apoptosome = cytochrome c-APAF-1-procaspase 9, ATP
Common pathway	caspases 3, 6, 7
Alternate pathways	Fas/FasL, Perforin/granzyme (induced by CTL)
Efferocytosis	
"Eat me" signals	phosphatidyl serine, calreticulin, CD31
Receptors on phagocytic cells	Low-density lipoprotein receptor–related protein (LRP) MER receptor tyrosine kinase, αvβ3, αvβ5, scavenger receptors, CD44, CD14, complement receptors 3 and 4
	Adenosine triphosphate binding cassette proteins ABC-A1 and ABC-A7
Soluble factors	Cystic fibrosis transmembrane regulator (CFTR) collectins (SP-A, SP-D, MBL), C1q, ficolins, pentraxins

of trimeric G proteins and class III phosphoinositide 3-kinases. Execution of autophagy is mediated by a ubiquitination-like system that involves two key covalent conjugation pathways requiring the activation and complex formation by-products of the autophagy genes (Atg). The maturation step occurs by their fusion with endosomal vesicles forming interphagosomes that acquire lysosome-associated membrane protein 1 (LAMP1) and

LAMP2. These structures fuse with the lysosomes and acquire cathepsins and acid phosphatases to become autolysosomes[56] (see Table 7-6).

Apoptosis is a form of programmed cell death that is, for the most part, dependent on a family of proteins, the caspases. Apoptosis is characterized by cell shrinkage and formation of apoptotic bodies, generally keeping the cellular membranes intact. Apoptotic cells are characterized by caspase activation, DNA fragmentation, and externalization of phosphatidyl serine onto the cell surface. The caspases are proteases activated during apoptosis. Thirteen distinct human caspase genes have been identified. Seven are suggested to participate in apoptosis: the initiator caspases (caspase-2, caspase-8, caspase-9, and caspase-10) and the effector caspases (caspase-3, caspase-6, and caspase-7). These can be activated by themselves or by other proteases, resulting in a rapid chain reaction propagation of caspase activation. The initiator caspases can be activated by a series of polyprotein complexes, each activated in response to particular death signals.[57] Apoptosis can occur through convergent extrinsic or intrinsic pathways. The *extrinsic pathway* involves cell surface death receptors belonging to the Tumor necrosis factor-receptor (TNF-R) family including TNF-R1, Fas/CD95, Death Receptor 3 (DR3), DR4, DR5, and DR6. These receptors are characterized by an intracellular death domain (DD) that transmits the apoptotic signal. Binding of a death ligand to the death receptor induces activation of the death receptor, which recruits adaptor proteins through interaction between the DD of the death receptor and the DD of the adaptor proteins, This adaptor protein interacts with the apoptosis initiator enzyme procaspase 8, causing a complex of the death receptor, adaptor protein, and procaspase 8 (called the *death inducing signaling complex*), resulting in the auto-proteolytic cleavage of procaspase 8 to caspase 8. The intrinsic pathway is induced by the stimulation of the mitochondrial membrane and translocation of the bcl2 family of proteins within the mitochondrial membrane, altering mitochondrial membrane permeability. This increased permeability results in the release of cytochrome c and other factors into the cytoplasm, where it recruits a caspase adaptor molecule APAF1 and the apoptosis initiator enzyme procaspase 9. Cytochrome c, APAF1, procaspase 9, and ATP form a complex called the *apoptosome*, and procaspase 9 becomes activated to caspase 9. At this point, both intrinsic and extrinsic pathways converge into a common pathway, resulting in the activation of executioner caspases 3, 6, and 7.[57] In addition to the pathways of apoptosis discussed earlier in the chapter, cytotoxic T lymphocytes can induce apoptosis through the Fas ligand/Fas system and the perforin granzyme system (see Table 7-6).

Efferocytosis is the process of removal of apoptotic cells. This process is different from complement-induced or Fcγ-induced phagocytosis in that it involves both "professional phagocytes" (macrophages and dendritic cells) and other cell types, including epithelial cells and fibroblasts.[58] Apoptotic cells are recognized by fundamental membrane alterations that must occur (the "eat me" signals). These include externalization of phosphatidylserine and calreticulin onto the membrane surface. In addition, CD31 (platelet-endothelial cell adhesion molecule-1) functions as a co-ligand that enhances attachment (tethering) to the macrophages and engagement of the "eat-me" signals. An array of receptors has been shown to be associated with efferocytosis, including the low-density lipoprotein receptor–related protein (LRP, CD91), Mer receptor tyrosine kinase, αvβ3, αvβ3 integrins, scavenger receptors, CF44, CD14, and complement receptors 3 and 4.[58] Some receptors function primarily by holding the apoptotic cell and effector in close proximity, while other receptors are involved in transducing the effector signal. This results in cell activation and engulfment of the apoptotic target cell. The most immediate consequence of efferocytosis is the physical removal of apoptotic cells before membrane permeability begins, thereby helping to prevent release of internal toxic contents.[58] Efferocytosis appears to play a role in both innate and adaptive immune responses in the lung. Efferocytosis promotes resolution of innate immune responses by actively suppressing inflammatory mediator production through the action of TGF-β1, prostanoids, peroxidase proliferator–activated receptor (PPAR)-γ, and IL-10. Interaction with adaptive immunity is suggested by the association of autoimmune disease with the impaired removal of apoptotic cells.

Soluble innate pattern-recognition proteins serve to identify non-self or altered-self molecular patterns on the apoptotic cell surface.[59] The "eat me" signals on dying cell surfaces allow access to different lipids, intracellular glycoproteins, and nucleic acids at different stages of cell death. They replace the "don't eat me" signals such as CD31 and CD47 on live cells. During late stages of cell death, soluble components are released that serve as "find me" signals. Several soluble proteins in the lung recognize these signals on cell surfaces and serve to bridge the apoptotic cell with the phagocyte. These include many of the proteins discussed previously: the collectins (SP-A, SP-D, mannose-binding lectin, C1q), ficolins, pentraxins, soluble CD-14, IgM, and CR3. These molecules help identify the "eat me" signals on apoptotic cells and promote efferocytosis, thereby limiting inflammation.

■ SUMMARY

The lung is continuously exposed to potential pathogens. The multilayered defenses provided by the intrinsic, innate, and adaptive systems protect the lung from invasion, yet they are able to limit inflammatory responses and resolve lung inflammation after the pathogen has been eliminated. Although there is considerable overlap in the activities of these various defenses, defects can result either in recurrent infection or in persistent inflammation and lung injury.

Suggested Reading

Baker K, Beales PL. Making sense of cilia in disease: the human ciliopathies. *Am J Med Genet C Semin Med Genet.* 2009;151C:281–295.

Boucher RC. Airway surface dehydration in cystic fibrosis: pathogenesis and therapy. *Annu Rev Med.* 2007;58:157–170.

Litvack ML, Palaniyar N. Review: Soluble innate immune pattern-recognition proteins for clearing dying cells and cellular components: implications on exacerbating or resolving inflammation. *Innate Immun.* 2010;16:191–200.

Opitz B, van Laak V, Eitel J, et al. Innate immune recognition in infectious and noninfectious diseases of the lung. *Am J Respir Crit Care Med.* 2010;181:1294–1309.

Suzuki T, Chow CW, Downey GP. Role of innate immune cells and their products in lung immunopathology. *Int J Biochem Cell Biol.* 2008;40:1348–1361.

Tang PS, Mura M, Seth R, et al. Acute lung injury and cell death: how many ways can cells die? *Am J Physiol Lung Cell Mol Physiol.* 2008;294:L632–L641.

Ulanova M, Gravelle S, Barnes R. The role of epithelial integrin receptors in recognition of pulmonary pathogens. *J Innate Immun.* 2008;1:4–17.

Voynow JA, Rubin BK. Mucins, mucus, and sputum. *Chest.* 2009;135:505–512.

Wallis R, Mitchell DA, Schmid R, et al. Paths reunited: initiation of the classical and lectin pathways of complement activation. *Immunobiology.* 2010;215:1–11.

Yu J. Airway receptors and their reflex function. *Adv Exp Med Biol.* 2009;648:411–420.

References

The complete reference list is available online at www.expertconsult.com

II

General Clinical Considerations

8 THE HISTORY AND PHYSICAL EXAMINATION

Hans Pasterkamp, MD, FRCPC

At the beginning of the 21st century, the diagnosis of disease still requires a detailed medical history and a thorough physical examination. For the majority of patients in many areas of the world, additional information from laboratory tests and other data are of rather limited availability. Modern science and technology have changed the situation considerably in industrialized nations, but we are paying a high price. Cost containment in health care has become essential. Physicians need to be skillful in their history taking and physical examination techniques so they can collect a maximum amount of information before ordering expensive medical-technical investigations. The relevance of these skills in pediatric respiratory medicine is exemplified by clinical severity scores that are widely used in care maps for asthma, bronchiolitis, and croup in children, or in scores developed to manage patients suspected to have acute severe respiratory syndromes (e.g., during outbreaks of SARS, H1N1, and other forms or influenza).

The diagnosis of disease in children has to rely on the patient's history and on observations gathered during the physical examination, even more than in older patients. Young children cannot follow instructions and participate in formal physiologic testing, and physicians hesitate before subjecting their pediatric patients to invasive diagnostic procedures. Diseases of the respiratory tract are among the most common in children, and in the majority of cases they can be correctly identified from medical history data and physical findings alone. The following review of the medical history and physical examination in children with respiratory disease includes some observations that were made with the help of modern technology. These technologic aids do not lessen the value of subjective perceptions but rather emphasize how new methods may further our understanding, sharpen our senses, and thereby advance the art of medical diagnosis.

THE HISTORY

General Principles

The medical history should be taken in an environment with comfortable seating for all, a place for clothing and belongings, and some toys for younger children. Formula should be on hand to help quiet infants and toddlers. Privacy has to be assured, without the usual interruptions by phone calls and other distractions. If possible, the physician should see one child at a time because the presence of young siblings or other children in the room can be distracting. Data that should be recorded at the beginning include the patient's name and address, the parents' or guardians' home and work phone numbers, the name of the referring physician, and information on the kindergarten or school if this is relevant. In many cases, the history will be given by someone other than the patient, but the physician should still directly ask even young children about their complaints. When asking about the history of the present illness, the physician should encourage a clear and chronologic narrative account. Questions should be open-ended, and at intervals the physician should give a verbal summary to confirm and clarify the information. Past medical data and system review are usually obtained by answers to direct questions.

Structure of the Pediatric History

The physician should note the source of and the reason for referral. On occasion, the referral is made by someone other than the patient or the parents (e.g., a teacher, relative, or friend). The physician should identify the *chief complaint* and the *person most concerned about it*. The *illness at presentation* should be documented in detail regarding onset and duration, the environment and circumstances under which it developed, its manifestations and their treatments, and its impact on the patient and family. Symptoms should be defined by their qualitative and quantitative characteristics as well as by their timing, location, aggravating or alleviating factors, and associated manifestations. Relevant past medical and laboratory data should be included in the documentation of the present illness.

This general approach is also applicable when the emphasis is on a single organ system, such as the respiratory tract. The onset of disease may have been gradual (e.g., with some interstitial lung diseases) or sudden (e.g., with foreign body aspiration). The physician should ask about initial manifestations and who noticed them first. The age at first presentation is important because respiratory diseases that manifest soon after birth are more likely to have been inherited or to be related to congenital malformations. Depending on the duration of symptoms, the illness will be classified as *acute, subacute, chronic,* or *recurrent.* These definitions are arbitrary, but diseases of less than 3 weeks' duration are generally called *acute;* diseases between 3 weeks' and 3 months' duration are *subacute,* and those that persist longer than 3 months are *chronic.* If symptoms are clearly discontinuous, with documented intervals of well-being, the disease is *recurrent.* This distinction is important because many parents may perceive their child as being chronically ill, not realizing that young normal children may have six to eight respiratory infections per year, particularly during the first 2 years if the child is in a daycare setting or if he or she has older siblings.

Respiratory diseases are often affected by environmental factors. There should be a careful search for seasonal changes in symptoms to uncover possible allergic causes. Exposure to noxious inhaled agents, for example, from industrial pollution or more commonly from indoor pollution by cigarette smoke, can sustain or aggravate a patient's coughing and wheezing. Similarly, a wood-burning stove used for indoor heating may be a contributing factor. The physician should therefore obtain a detailed description of the patient's home environment. Are there household pets (e.g., dogs, cats, or hamsters) or birds (e.g., budgies, pigeons, or parrots)? What plants are in and around the house? Are there animal or vegetable fibers in the bedclothes or in the floor and window coverings (e.g., wool, feathers)? Are there systems in use for air conditioning and humidification? Is mold visible anywhere in the house?

There may be a relationship between respiratory symptoms and daily activities. Exercise is a common trigger factor for cough and wheezing in many patients with hyperreactive airways. A walk outside in cold air may have similar effects. Diurnal variation of symptoms may be apparent, and attention should be paid to changes that occur at night. These changes may also be related to airway cooling, or they may reflect conditions that are worse in the recumbent position, such as postnasal drip or gastroesophageal reflux. Food intake may bring on symptoms of respiratory distress when food is aspirated or when food allergies are present.

A large portion of children who present with respiratory symptoms are suffering from infection, most often viral. It is important to know whether other family members or persons in regular contact with the patient are also affected. When unusual infections are suspected, questions should be asked about recent travel to areas where exotic infective organisms may have been acquired. Drug abuse by parents or by older patients and others with high-risk lifestyles may lead the physician to consider the possibility of acquired immunodeficiency syndrome (AIDS).

Descriptions of respiratory disease manifestations may come from the parents or directly from an older child. Common symptoms are fever, cough and sputum production, wheezing or noisy breathing, dyspnea, and chest pain. Most of these are discussed in more detail later in the chapter.

The previous medical history will provide an impression of the general health status of the child. First, the birth history should be reviewed, including prenatal, natal, and neonatal events. The physician should inquire about the course of pregnancy, particularly whether the mother and fetus suffered from infections, metabolic disorders, or exposure to noxious agents (e.g., nicotine). The duration of pregnancy, possible multiple births, and circumstances leading to the onset of labor should be noted. Difficult labor and delivery may cause respiratory problems at birth (e.g., asphyxia and meconium aspiration), and the physician should ask about birth weight and Apgar scores. The physician should carefully review the neonatal course because many events during this period may affect the patient's respiratory status in later years. Were there any signs of neonatal respiratory distress (e.g., tachypnea, retractions, and cyanosis)? Treatment with oxygen or endotracheal intubation should be recorded. Some extrathoracic disorders provide valuable clues for diagnosis, such as the presence of eczema in atopic infants or neonatal conjunctivitis in a young patient with chlamydia pneumonia, particularly if there was a documented infection of the mother.

Much is learned from a detailed feeding history, which should include the amount, type, and schedule of food intake. The physician should ask whether the child was fed by breast or bottle. For the newborn and young infant, feeding is a substantial physical exercise and may lead to distress in the presence of respiratory disease, much as climbing stairs does in the older patient. The question of exercise tolerance in an infant is therefore asked by inquiring how long it takes the patient to finish a meal. To support the work of breathing, the caloric intake of infants with respiratory disease is often reduced despite an increased caloric need. This reduced caloric intake commonly results in a failure to thrive. Older patients with chronic respiratory disease and productive cough may suffer from a continuous exposure of their taste buds to mucopurulent secretions and may quite understandably lose their appetites, but medical treatment (e.g., with certain antibiotics) may have similar effects. Patients with food hypersensitivity may react with bronchospasm or even with interstitial lung disease on exposure to the allergen (e.g., to milk). Physical irritation and inflammation occur if food is aspirated into the respiratory tract. This happens frequently in patients with debilitating neurologic diseases and deficient protective reflexes of the upper airways but may also occur in neurologically intact children. A history of cough or choking during feeding should alert the physician to the possibility of pulmonary aspiration.

The physical development of children with chronic respiratory diseases may be retarded. Malnutrition in the presence of increased caloric requirements is common, but the effects of some long-term medical treatments (e.g., with steroids) should also be considered. Previous measurements of body growth should be obtained and plotted on standard nomograms. Psychosocial development may be affected if chronic lung diseases (e.g., asthma or cystic fibrosis) limit attendance and performance at school or if behavioral problems arise in children and adolescents subjected to chronic therapy. More severely affected patients may also be delayed in their sexual development.

Many diseases of the respiratory tract in children have a genetic component, either with a clear Mendelian mode of inheritance (e.g., autosomal recessive in cystic fibrosis, homozygous deficiency of α_1-antitrypsin, sex-linked recessive in chronic granulomatous disease, and autosomal dominant in familial interstitial fibrosis) or with a genetic contribution to the cause. Examples of familial aggregation of respiratory disease are chronic bronchitis and bronchiectasis or familial emphysema in patients with heterozygous α_1-antitrypsin deficiency, in which the susceptibility of the lung to the action of irritants (e.g., cigarette smoke) is increased. A mixed influence of genetic and environmental factors exists in polygenic diseases, such as asthma or allergic rhinitis.

When inquiring about the family history, the physician should review at least two generations on either side. The parents should be asked whether they are related by blood, and information should be obtained about any childhood deaths in the family. The health of the patient's siblings and also of brothers and sisters of both parents should be documented. Particular attention should be paid to histories of asthma, allergies and hay fever, chronic bronchitis, emphysema, tuberculosis, cystic fibrosis, and sudden unexpected infant death.

The physician should obtain a detailed report of prior tests and immunizations. Quite often this requires communication with other health care providers. Results of screening examinations (e.g., tuberculin and other skin tests, chest radiographs, and sweat chloride measurements) should be noted. Similarly, childhood illnesses, immunizations, and possible adverse immunization reactions should be documented. If the history is positive for allergic reactions, these have to be confirmed and defined. Previous hospital admissions and their indications should be listed, and the patient's current medications and their efficacy should be documented. If possible, the drug containers and prescriptions should be reviewed. The physician may use the opportunity to discuss the pharmacologic information and the technique of drug administration, particularly with inhaled bronchodilator medications.

One of the most important goals in taking a history is to become more aware of the particular psychological and social situation of the patient. It is impossible to judge current complaints or responses to medical interventions without an individual frame of reference for each patient. The physician should encourage the child and the parents to describe a typical day at home, daycare, kindergarten, or school. This will provide valuable information about the impact of the illness on daily routines, the financial implications, the existing or absent social support structures, and the coping strategies of the family. Compliance with medical treatment is rarely better than 50%, and physicians are generally unable to predict how well their patients follow and adhere to therapeutic regimens. Compliance can improve if the patient and the parents gain a better understanding of the disease and its treatment. It is important to recognize prior experiences that the family may have had with the health care system and to understand individual spiritual, religious, and health beliefs. Particularly in children with chronic respiratory ailments whose symptoms are not being controlled or prevented, the effort and unpleasantness (e.g., of chest physiotherapy) may limit the use of such interventions. The physician should also consider the social stigma associated with visible therapy, especially among peers of the adolescent patient.

A review of organ systems is usually the last part of the history and may actually be completed during the physical examination. Although the emphasis is on the respiratory system, questions about the general status of the child will be about appetite, sleep, level of activity, and prevailing mood. Important findings in the region of the head and neck are nasal obstruction and discharge, ear or sinus infection, conjunctival irritation, sore throat, and swallowing difficulty. The respiratory manifestations of coughing, noisy breathing, wheezing, and cyanosis are discussed in detail at the end of this chapter. Cardiovascular findings may include palpitations and dysrhythmia in hypoxic patients; there may be edema formation and peripheral swelling with cor pulmonale. Effects of respiratory disease on the gastrointestinal tract may appear with cough-induced vomiting and abdominal pain. There may be a direct involvement with diarrhea, cramps, and fatty stools in patients with cystic fibrosis. The physician should ask about hematuria and about skin manifestations, such as eczema or rashes, and about swellings and pain of lymph nodes or joints. Finally, neurologic symptoms (e.g., headache, lightheadedness, or paresthesia) may be related to respiratory disease and cough paroxysms or hyperventilation.

▄▄ THE PHYSICAL EXAMINATION

Traditionally, the physical examination is divided into inspection, palpation, auscultation, and percussion. The sequence of these steps may be varied depending on the circumstances, particularly in the assessment of the respiratory tract in children. The classic components of the physical examination and some modern aids and additions are discussed in the following sections.

Inspection

Much can be learned from simple observation, particularly during those precious moments of sleep in the young infant or toddler, who when awake can be a challenge even for the skilled examiner. First, the pattern of breathing should be observed. This includes the respiratory rate, rhythm, and effort. The respiratory rate decreases with age and shows its greatest variability in newborns and young infants (Fig. 8-1). The rate should be counted over at least 1 minute, ideally several times for the calculation

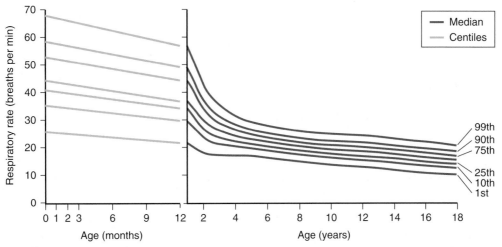

FIGURE 8-1. A and B, Mean values (solid line) ± 2 SD (dotted lines) of the normal respiratory rate at rest (during sleep in children younger than 3 years of age). There is no significant difference between the sexes, and regression lines represent data from both boys and girls. The respiratory rate decreases with age and shows the greatest normal variation during the first 2 years of life. (A, Data from Rusconi F, Castagneto M, Gagliardi L, et al. Reference values for respiratory rate in the first 3 years of life. *Pediatrics.* 1994;94:350. B, Data from Hooker EA, Danzl DF, Brueggmeyer M, et al. Respiratory rates in pediatric emergency patients. *J Emerg Med.* 1992;10:407.)

of average values. Because respiratory rates differ among sleep states and become even more variable during wakefulness, a note should be made describing the behavioral state of the patient. Observing abdominal movements or listening to breath sounds with the stethoscope placed before the mouth and nose may help in counting respirations in patients with very shallow thoracic excursions.

Longitudinal documentation of the respiratory rate during rest or sleep is important for the follow-up of patients with chronic lung diseases, even more so for those too young for standard pulmonary function tests. Abnormally high breathing frequencies or tachypnea can be seen in patients with decreased compliance of the respiratory apparatus and in those with metabolic acidosis. Other causes of tachypnea are fever (approximately 5 to 7 breaths per minute increase per degree above 37° C), anemia, exertion, intoxication (salicylates), and anxiety and psychogenic hyperventilation. The opposite, an abnormally slow respiratory rate or bradypnea, can occur in patients with metabolic alkalosis or central nervous system depression. The terms *hyperpnea* and *hypopnea* refer to abnormally deep or shallow respirations. At given respiratory rates, this determination is a subjective clinical judgment and is not easily quantified unless the pattern is obvious, such as the Kussmaul type of breathing in patients with diabetic ketoacidosis.

Significant changes in the rhythm of breathing occur during the first months of life. Respiratory pauses of less than 6 seconds are common in infants younger than 3 months of age. If these pauses occur in groups of three or more that are separated by less than 20 seconds of respiration, the pattern is referred to as *periodic breathing*. This pattern is very common in premature infants after the first days of life and may persist until 44 weeks postconceptional age. In full-term infants, periodic breathing is usually observed between 1 week and 2 months of age and is normally absent by 6 months of age. Apnea with cessation of air flow lasting more than 15 seconds is uncommon and may be accompanied by bradycardia and cyanosis. In preterm infants, a drop in oxygen saturation may be seen

up to 7 seconds after a respiratory pause when in room air and up to 9 seconds later when on supplemental oxygen.

Other abnormal patterns include *Cheyne-Stokes breathing*, which occurs as cycles of increasing and decreasing tidal volumes separated by apnea (e.g., in children with congestive heart failure and increased intracranial pressure). *Biot breathing* consists of irregular cycles of respiration at variable tidal volumes interrupted by apnea and is an ominous finding in patients with severe brain damage.

After noting the rate and rhythm of breathing, the physician should look for signs of increased respiratory effort. The older child will be able to communicate the subjective experience of difficult breathing, or dyspnea. Objective signs that reflect distressed breathing are chest wall retractions; visible use of accessory muscles and the alae nasi; orthopnea; and paradoxical respiratory movements. The more negative intrapleural pressure during inspiration against a high airway resistance leads to retraction of the pliable portions of the chest wall, including the intercostal and subcostal tissues and the supraclavicular and suprasternal fossae. Conversely, bulging of intercostal spaces may be seen when pleural pressure becomes greatly positive during a maximally forced expiration. Retractions are more easily visible in the newborn infant, in whom intercostal tissues are thinner and more compliant than in the older child.

Visible contraction of the sternocleidomastoid muscles and indrawing of supraclavicular fossae during inspiration are among the most reliable clinical signs of airway obstruction. In young infants, these muscular contractions may lead to head bobbing, which is best observed when the child rests with the head supported slightly at the suboccipital area. If no other signs of respiratory distress are present in an infant with head bobbing, however, central nervous system disorders, such as third ventricular cysts, should be considered. Older patients with chronic airway obstruction and extensive use of accessory muscles may appear to have a short neck because of hunched shoulders. Orthopnea exists when the patient is unable to tolerate a recumbent position.

Flaring of the alae nasi is a sensitive sign of respiratory distress and may be present when inspiration is abnormally short (e.g., under conditions of chest pain). Nasal flaring enlarges the anterior nasal passages and reduces upper and total airway resistance. It may also help to stabilize the upper airways by preventing large negative pharyngeal pressures during inspiration.

The normal movement of chest and abdominal walls is directed outward during inspiration. Inward motion of the chest wall during inspiration is called *paradoxical breathing*. This is seen when the thoracic cage loses its stability and becomes distorted by the action of the diaphragm. Classically, paradoxical breathing with a see-saw type of thoracoabdominal motion is seen in patients with paralysis of the intercostal muscles, but it is also commonly seen in premature and newborn infants who have a very compliant rib cage. Inspiratory indrawing of the lateral chest is known as *Hoover's sign* and can be observed in patients with obstructive airway disease. Paradoxical breathing also occurs during sleep in patients with upper airway obstruction. The development of paradoxical breathing in an awake, nonparalyzed patient beyond the newborn period usually indicates respiratory muscle fatigue and impending respiratory failure.

Following inspection of the breathing pattern, the examiner should pay attention to the symmetry of respiratory chest excursions. Unilateral diseases affecting lungs, pleura, chest wall, or diaphragm may all result in asymmetric breathing movements. Trauma to the rib cage may cause fractures and a "flail chest" that shows local paradoxical movement. Pain during respiration usually leads to "splinting" with flexion of the trunk toward and decreased respiratory movements of the affected side. The signs of hemidiaphragmatic paralysis may be subtle and are usually more noticeable in the lateral decubitus position with the paralyzed diaphragm placed up. This position tends to accentuate the paradoxical inward epigastric motion on the affected side.

Other methods to augment inspection of chest wall motion use optical markers. In practice, this technique is done by placing both hands on either side of the patient's lateral rib cage with the thumbs along the costal margins.

Divergence of the thumbs during expansion of the thorax supposedly aids in the visual perception of the range and symmetry of respiratory movements. This technique is of little use in children. A more accurate method of documenting the vectors of movement at different sites (but one that is not yet practical for bedside evaluation) is to place a grid of optical markers on the chest surface and film their positional changes during respiration relative to a steady reference frame. A similar concept is used in optical studies of chest deformities. Projection of raster lines onto the anterior chest surface allows stereographic measurement of deformities, such as pectus excavatum, and augments the visual image of the surface shape (Fig. 8-2). In practice and without such tools, however, the physician should inspect the chest at different angles of illumination to enhance the visual perception of chest wall deformities. Their location, size, symmetry, and change with respiratory or cardiac movements should be noted.

The physician should measure the dimensions of the chest. Chest size and shape are influenced by ethnic and geographic factors that should be taken into account when measurements are compared with normative data. Andean children who live at high altitudes, for example, have larger chest dimensions relative to stature than children in North America. The chest circumference is usually taken at the mamillary level during mid-inspiration. In practice, mean readings during inspiration and expiration should be noted (Fig. 8-3A). Premature infants have a greater head circumference than chest circumference, while these measurements are very similar at term (see Fig. 8-3B). Malnutrition can delay the time at which chest circumference begins to exceed head circumference.

Further objective documentation of the chest configuration may include measurements of thoracic depth (anteroposterior [AP] diameter) and width (transverse diameter). The thoracic index, or the ratio of AP over transverse diameter, is close to unity in infants and decreases during childhood. Measurements should be taken with a caliper at the level of the nipples in upright subjects. Normative values for young children are available but dated (Fig. 8-4). Most of the configurational change of the chest occurs during the first 2 years and is probably influenced by gravitational

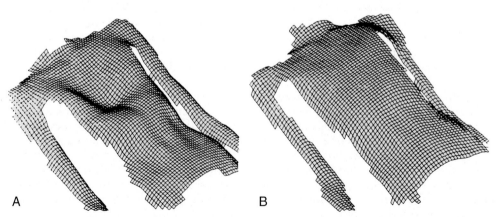

A   B

FIGURE 8-2. Optical markers augment the visual perception of chest wall deformities. In this example of rasterstereography, lines are projected onto the anterior thorax, and the surface image is computed as a regular network. The change of the funnel chest deformity before **(A)** and after surgery **(B)** is easily appreciated. In practice and at the bedside, the physician should inspect at different angles of illumination to enhance the visual perception of chest wall deformities. (From Hierholzer E, Schier F. Rasterstereography in the measurement and postoperative follow-up of anterior chest wall deformities. *Z Kinderchir.* 1986;41:267-271.)

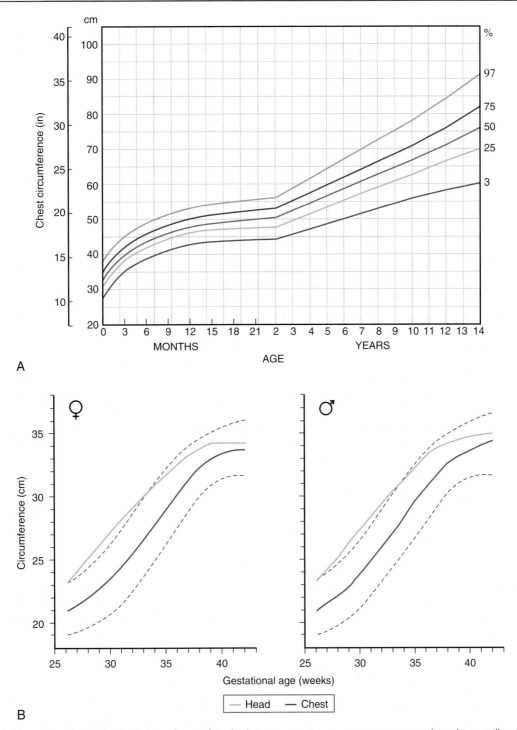

A

B

FIGURE 8-3. A, Normal distribution of chest circumference from birth to 14 years. Tape measurements are made at the mamillary level during mid-inspiration. Before plotting the values on the graph, one should add 1 cm for males and subtract 1 cm for females between 2 and 12 years of age. **B,** Normal distribution of chest circumference from 26 to 42 weeks of gestation. The dotted lines indicate the 10th and 90th percentiles, respectively. Note that chest circumference is close to head circumference at term. (**A,** From Feingold M, Bossert WH. Normal values for selected physical parameters. An aid to syndrome delineation. *Birth Defects.* 1974;10:14. **B,** Data from Britton JR, Britton HL, Jennett R, et al. Weight, length, head and chest circumference at birth in Phoenix, Arizona. *J Reprod Med.* 1993;38:215.)

forces after the upright position becomes common. Disease-related changes in thoracic dimensions occur either as potential causative factors (e.g., the elongated thorax with a stress distribution that favors spontaneous pneumothorax in lanky adolescents, particularly males who increase their thoracic height versus width more than

females) or as a secondary event (e.g., the barrel-shaped chest in patients with emphysema and chronic hyperinflation of the lung).

Inspection of the patient should also be directed to the extrathoracic regions. Many observations on the examination of the head and neck provide valuable clues to the

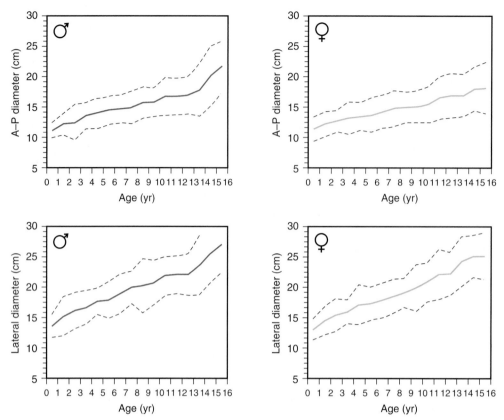

FIGURE 8-4. Mean values (solid line) ± SD (dashed lines) of the normal distribution of anteroposterior (AP) and lateral chest diameters in boys and girls. Caliper measurements are made at the mamillary level during mid-inspiration. (Data from Lucas WP, Pryor HB. Range and standard deviations of certain physical measurements in healthy children. *J Pediatr.* 1935;6:533-545.)

physical diagnosis. Bluish coloration of the lower eyelid ("allergic shiners"); a bilateral fold of skin just below the lower eyelid (Dennie lines); and a transverse crease from "allergic salutes," running at the junction of the cartilaginous and bony portion of the nose, may all be found in atopic individuals. The physician should always examine the nose and document bilateral patency by occluding each side while feeling and listening for air flow through the other nostril. Even without a speculum, one can assess the anterior half by raising the nose tip with one thumb and shining a light into the nasal passageways. Color and size of the mucosa should be noted. The frequency of asymptomatic nasal polyps seems to be high. Most polyps arise from the mucosa of the ostia, clefts, and recesses in the ostiomeatal complex and have the appearance of gelatinous tissue. Easily visible nasal polyps are common in patients with cystic fibrosis. Nasal polyposis may also be familial or associated with allergy, asthma, and aspirin intolerance.

The oropharynx should be inspected for its size and signs of malformation, such as cleft palate, and for signs of obstruction by enlarged tonsils. Evidence of chronic ear infections should be documented, and the areas over frontal and maxillary paranasal sinuses should be tested for tenderness. Inspection of the skin is important and may reveal the eczema of atopy. The finding of a scar that typically develops at the site of a successful bacillus Calmette-Guérin (BCG) vaccination may be relevant. In North American children, these scars are usually found over the left deltoid, but other sites, including buttocks and lower extremities,

are also used for BCG inoculation in different parts of the world. Common physical findings such as cyanosis, clubbing, and the cardiovascular signs of pulmonary disease are discussed in more detail at the end of this chapter.

Palpation

Palpation follows chest inspection to confirm observed abnormalities, such as swellings and deformations; to identify areas of tenderness or lymph nodal enlargement; to document the position of the trachea; to assess respiratory excursions; and to detect changes in the transmission of voice sounds through the chest. Chest palpation may offer the first physical contact with the patient, and it is very important for the physician to perform this procedure with warm hands.

Palpation should be done in an orderly sequence. Commonly, one begins with an examination of the head and neck. Cervical lymphadenopathy and tenderness over paranasal sinuses should be noted. Palpation of the oropharynx may be indicated to find malformations such as submucosal clefts or to identify causes of upper airway obstruction. The position of the trachea must be documented in every patient. This is a very important part of the physical chest examination because tracheal deviation most often indicates significant intrathoracic or extrathoracic abnormalities.

In the older child, the tracheal position is assessed by placing the index and ring fingers on both sternal attachments of the sternocleidomastoid muscles. The trachea is then felt between these landmarks with the middle finger on the suprasternal notch. In small children, palpation is done with one index finger sliding gently inward over the suprasternal notch. Looking for asymmetry, the physician should always make sure that the patient is in a straight position, and deformities (e.g., scoliosis) should be taken into account.

A very slight deviation of the trachea toward the right is normal. Marked deviations may indicate a pulling force toward the side of displacement (e.g., atelectasis) or a pushing force on the contralateral side (e.g., pneumothorax). The physician should note whether the displacement is fixed or whether there is a pendular movement of the trachea during inspiration and expiration that may suggest obstruction of a large bronchus. Posterior displacement of the trachea may occur with anterior mediastinal tumors or barrel chest deformities, whereas an easily palpable anteriorly displaced trachea is sometimes seen with mediastinitis. In patients with airway obstruction and respiratory distress, retractions of the suprasternal fossa may be seen, and a "tracheal tug" may be felt by the examiner.

Placing the hands on both sides of the lateral rib cage, the physician should feel for symmetry of chest expansion during regular and deep breathing maneuvers. Slight compression of the chest in the transverse and anteroposterior directions may help to localize pain from lesions of the bony structures. Voice-generated vibrations are best felt with the palms of both hands just below the base of the fingers placed over corresponding sites on the right and left hemithorax. Asymmetric transmission usually indicates unilateral intrathoracic abnormalities. The patient is asked to produce low-frequency vibrations of sufficient amplitude by saying "ninety-nine" in a loud voice. In young infants, crying may produce the vibrations that are felt as tactile fremitus over the chest wall. This fremitus is decreased if an accumulation of air or fluid in the pleural space reduces transmission. Small consolidations of the underlying lung will not diminish the tactile fremitus as long as the airways remain open, whereas collapse of the airways and atelectasis will reduce the transmission of vibratory energy if larger portions of the lung are affected.

Auscultation

Auscultation is arguably the most important part of the physical chest examination. The subjective perception of respiratory acoustic signs is influenced by the site and mode of sound production; by the modification of sound on its passage through the lung, chest wall, and stethoscope; and, finally, by the auditory system of the examiner. Knowledge about these factors is necessary to appreciate fully the wealth of information that is contained in the acoustic signs of the thorax.

Thoracic Acoustics

Observations on sound generation in airway models and electronic analyses of respiratory sounds suggest a predominant origin from complex turbulences within the central airways. The tracheal breath sound heard above the suprasternal notch is a relatively broad-spectrum noise, ranging in frequency from less than 100 Hz to greater than 2000 Hz. Resonances from the trachea and

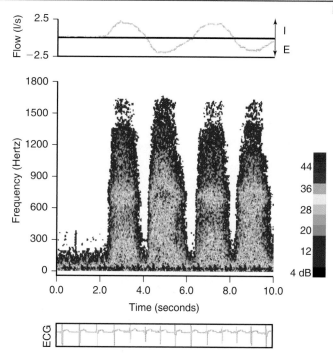

FIGURE 8-5. Digital respirosonogram of sounds recorded over the trachea of a healthy young man. Time is on the horizontal axis, frequency is on the vertical axis, and sound intensity is shown on a scale from red (loud) over orange and yellow (medium) to green, grey and black (low). Air flow is plotted at the top, with inspiration above and expiration below the zero line. The sonogram illustrates the broad range of tracheal sounds during both inspiration and expiration. There is a distinct pause between the respiratory phases. Expiration is louder than inspiration, and resonance is apparent around 700 Hz. In this example, the subject was holding his breath at the beginning. During this respiratory pause, heart sounds below 200 Hz are easily identified by their temporal relation to the simultaneously recorded electrocardiogram (ECG).

from supraglottic airways "color" the sound (Fig. 8-5). The lengthening of the trachea with growth during childhood causes lower tracheal resonance frequencies. A dominant source of tracheal breath sounds is turbulence from the jet flow at the glottic aperture. However, narrow segments of the supraglottic passages also contribute to sound generation. There is a very close relationship between air flow and tracheal sound intensity, particularly at high frequencies. In the presence of local narrowing (e.g., in children with subglottic stenosis), flow velocity at the stenotic site is increased, and so is the tracheal sound intensity. Relating tracheal sound levels to air flow measured at the mouth can provide information about changes during therapy. Auscultation over the trachea will provide some information under these circumstances, but objective acoustic measurements are required for accurate comparisons.

Basic "normal" lung sounds heard at the chest surface are lower in frequency than tracheal sounds because sound energy is lost during passage though the lungs, particularly at higher frequencies. However, lung sounds extend to frequencies higher than traditionally recognized. New observations on the effects of gas density indicate that lung sounds at frequencies above 400 Hz are mostly generated by flow turbulence. At lower frequencies, other mechanisms that are not directly related to air flow (e.g., muscle noise and thoracic cavity resonances) have prominent effects on lung

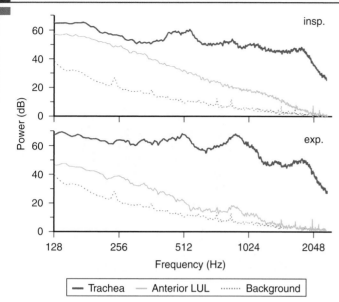

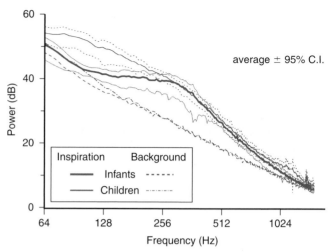

FIGURE 8-6. Average spectra of respiratory sounds at air flow of 1.5 ± 0.3 L/sec, recorded simultaneously at the suprasternal notch (trachea) and at the second intercostal space in the midclavicular line on the left (anterior left upper lobe [LUL]) of a healthy 12-year-old boy. The average sound spectrum during breath holding at resting end expiration (background) is plotted for comparison. Inspiratory lung sounds are louder than expiratory sounds, while the opposite is true for tracheal sounds. Lung sound intensity is clearly above background at frequencies as high as 1000 Hz. Expiratory lung sounds show some of the same spectral peaks that are present in tracheal sounds.

FIGURE 8-7. Average spectra of inspiratory lung sounds, recorded over the posterior basal segment of the right lung in healthy newborn infants (n = 10) and children (n = 9) at air flows of 15 mL/s/kg. The spectra of background noise at resting end expiration are plotted for comparison. Dotted lines mark the 95% confidence intervals (CIs). Note the similarity of spectral slopes in newborn infants and older children at frequencies above 300 Hz and the significantly reduced sound power at lower frequencies in newborns. (Data from Pasterkamp H, Powell RE, Sanchez I. Lung sound spectra at standardized air flow in normal infants, children, and adults. *Am J Respir Crit Care Med.* 1996;154:424-430.)

sounds, and gas density effects are less obvious. Inspiratory lung sounds show little contribution of noise generated at the glottis. Their origin is likely more peripheral (i.e., in the main and segmental bronchi). Expiratory lung sounds appear to have a central origin and are probably affected by flow convergence at airway bifurcations (Fig. 8-6).

Sound at different frequencies takes different pathways on the passage through the lung. Low-frequency sound waves propagate from central airways through the lung parenchyma to the chest wall. At higher frequencies, the airway walls become effectively more rigid and sound travels further down into the airways before it propagates through lung tissue. This information cannot be gathered on subjective auscultation but requires objective acoustic measurements. A trained ear, however, will recognize many of the findings that are related to these mechanisms. For example, lung sounds in healthy children and adults are not necessarily equal at corresponding sites over both lungs. In fact, expiratory sounds are typically louder at the right upper lobe compared with the left side. Similar asymmetry has been recognized when sound is introduced at the mouth and measured at the chest surface. A likely explanation for this asymmetry is the effect on sound propagation by the cardiovascular and mediastinal structures to the left of the trachea. Asymmetry of lung sounds is also noticeable in most healthy subjects during inspiration when one listens over the posterior lower chest. The left side tends to be louder here, probably because of the size and spatial orientation of the larger airways due to the heart.

Objective acoustic measurements have also helped to clarify the difference between lung sounds in newborn infants and in older children. The most obvious divergence occurs in lung sounds at low frequencies where newborn infants have much less intensity. This may be explained by thoracic and airway resonances at higher frequencies in newborn infants and perhaps also by their lower muscle mass. Lung sounds at higher frequencies are similar between newborn infants and older children (Fig. 8-7).

Adventitious respiratory sounds usually indicate respiratory disease. Wheezes are musical, continuous (typically longer than 100 msec) sounds that originate from oscillations in narrowed airways. The frequency of the oscillation depends on the mass and elasticity of the airway wall as well as on local air flow. Widespread narrowing of airways in asthma leads to various pitches, or polyphonic wheezing, whereas a fixed obstruction in a larger airway produces a single wheeze, or monophonic wheezing. Expiratory wheezing is related to flow limitation and can be produced by normal subjects during forced expiratory maneuvers. The situation is less clear for wheezing during inspiration, which is common in asthma but cannot be produced by healthy subjects unless it originates from the larynx (e.g., in vocal cord dysfunction). Very brief and localized inspiratory wheezes may be heard over areas of bronchiectasis.

Crackles are nonmusical, discontinuous (less than 20 msec duration) lung sounds. Crackle production requires the presence of air-fluid interfaces and occurs either by air movement through secretions or by sudden equalization of gas pressure. Another mechanism may be the release of tissue tension during sudden opening or closing of airways. Crackles are perceived as fine or coarse, depending on the duration and frequency of the brief and dampened vibrations created by these mechanisms. There may be a musical quality to the sound if a short oscillation occurs at the generation site. This has been called *tinkling crackle* or *squawk* and may appear during inspiration, typically in patients with interstitial lung diseases. Fine crackles during late inspiration are common in restrictive lung diseases and in the early stages of congestive heart failure, whereas coarse crackles during early inspiration and during expiration are frequently heard in chronic obstructive lung disease. Fine crackles are usually inaudible at the mouth, whereas the coarse crackles of widespread airway obstruction can be transmitted through the large airways and may be heard as clicks with the stethoscope held in front of the patient's open mouth. Some crackles over the anterior chest may occur in normal subjects who were breathing at low lung volumes, but they will disappear after a few deep breaths.

Several other abnormal respiratory sounds are not generated in intrathoracic airways. Pleural rubs originate from mechanical stretching of the pleura, which causes vibration of the chest wall and local pulmonary parenchyma. These sounds can occur during both inspiration and expiration. Their character is like that of creaking leather and is similar in some ways to pulmonary crackles. *Stridor* refers to a more or less musical sound that is produced by oscillations of critically narrowed extrathoracic airways. It is therefore most commonly heard during inspiration. Grunting is an expiratory sound, usually low-pitched and with musical qualities. It is produced in the larynx when vocal cord adduction is used to generate positive end-expiratory pressures, such as in premature infants with immature lungs and surfactant deficiency. Snoring originates from the flutter of tissues in the pharynx and has a less musical quality. It may be present during both inspiration and expiration.

There may also be cardiorespiratory sounds. These are believed to occur when cardiac movements cause regional flows of air in the surrounding lung. Because of its synchronicity with the heart beat, this sound may be mistaken for a cardiac murmur. It can be identified by its vesicular sound quality and its exaggeration during inspiration and in different body positions.

At the boundary between different tissues, reflection of sound may occur and sound transmission may decrease, depending on the matching or mismatching of the tissue impedances. Many of the acoustic signs of the chest are explained on the basis of impedance matching alone. The stethoscope is basically an impedance transformer that reduces sound reflection at a mismatched interface, namely, body surface to air. Because it is the only part of the sound transmission pathway that can be kept constant, it is best to always use the same stethoscope. The choice of a bell- or a diaphragm-type stethoscope depends on individual preference. Diaphragm chest pieces can be placed more easily and with less pressure on small chests with narrow intercostal spaces. Compared with bell-type stethoscopes, they tend to deemphasize frequencies below 100 Hz. Both the bell-type and the diaphragm stethoscopes show some attenuation at frequencies above 400 Hz.

Technique of Auscultation

Ideally, auscultation of the chest should be performed in a quiet room; however, with pediatric patients the usual setting may be anything but quiet. Fortunately, the human auditory system allows selective evaluation of acoustic signals even when they are masked by much louder surrounding noises. This psychoacoustic phenomenon,

known as the "cocktail party effect," at present cannot be reproduced by modern electronic techniques, which is but one of the reasons for the lasting popularity of the stethoscope.

This instrument, the most widely used in clinical medicine since its introduction almost 200 years ago, carries symbolic value for the health care profession, much like a modern staff of Aesculapius. Every child knows that doctors have stethoscopes. The physician should use this to advantage when assessing pediatric patients by encouraging children to listen themselves to their heartbeats and breathing sounds. Even infants may be fascinated as long as the stethoscope is shiny. Ice cold chest pieces, on the other hand, scare off most patients.

The patient should be in a straight position during auscultation because incurvature of the trunk may lead to artificial side differences of sound production and transmission. In newborns and young infants, a straight position may be best achieved when they are supine. Infants and toddlers will often be assessed while their parents hold them on their laps. Beginning auscultation on the back of these young patients will provoke less anxiety than a frontal approach. Older children can be examined in the sitting or standing position. The number of sites over the chest that are assessed during auscultation will be determined by the clinical situation. Ideally, all segments of the lung should be listened to, but this may not be possible, particularly in very young children.

Because the intensity of respiratory sounds is related to air flow, sufficiently deep respirations (with flow >0.5 L/sec) are needed for a good sound signal. An older patient will cooperate and breathe deeply through an open mouth. With infants and young children, however, one may have to rely on sounds made during sighs or deep inspirations in between crying. On the other hand, normal breath sounds can mask the presence of some adventitious sounds (e.g., fine crackles of low intensity). Asking the patient to take very slow, deep breaths with less air flow than is needed to generate normal breath sounds can help to unmask these adventitious sounds.

The physician should make note of the lung sound intensity over different areas of the chest in a qualitative way, keeping in mind that this intensity reflects both local sound generation and sound transmission characteristics of the thorax. It is therefore not correct to speak of local "air entry" when one actually refers to local breath sound intensity. Decreased breath sounds, for example, are common in asthma even when normal blood gases indicate that air entry has to be adequate. Obviously, a qualitative distinction between the absence or presence of local breath sounds will be easier than attempts at quantification. Also, when the stethoscope is placed over any given location, it is not known how large an area of the underlying lung is actually being assessed. In adult subjects, moving the chest piece of the stethoscope by 10 cm will position it to receive sound from entirely different lung units, but similar data for children are not available.

Assessment of regional ventilation by thoracic acoustic signs becomes more meaningful when two sites are compared simultaneously. Differential auscultation with special stethoscopes that employ two chest pieces or a single divided chest piece has not become popular in clinical practice. Comparative auscultation is absolutely essential for airway management in the emergency department and intensive care unit for assessment of endotracheal tube position or for identification of the side of a pneumothorax. Listening simultaneously to two homologous sites over both lungs may also help to detect local abnormalities. Atelectatic areas will transmit sound more slowly than inflated lung tissue, but the resulting phase shift is too small to be detectable on subjective auscultation. With local airway narrowing, however, the maximum sound intensity over the affected side may become sufficiently delayed to be perceived as "phase heterophony." In some cases, breath sounds may still be audible over the affected side after inspiratory efforts have ceased. This "post-effort" breath sound is a sign of incomplete airway obstruction.

There are special circumstances in which only the presence or absence of breath sounds is of interest (e.g., during transportation of critically ill patients in noisy vehicles and during resuscitation in the emergency department). Under these conditions, and when a firm attachment of the chest piece is important, a self-adhering stethoscope, based on negative suction pressure within the bell of the chest piece, may be applied. New techniques of adaptive electronic filtering are being used in stethoscopes that are optimized for use in very noisy environments.

Respiratory sounds should be documented according to their location and character. Normal projections of lobar borders to the surface of the chest are shown in Figure 8-8. These may be distorted by local pulmonary

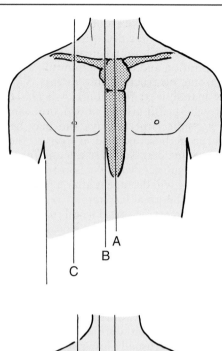
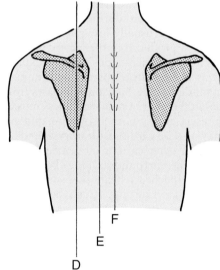

FIGURE 8-9. Vertical reference lines of the chest. The center line is indicated anteriorly by the suprasternal notch *(A)* and posteriorly by the spinous processes *(F)*. The sternal *(B)* and midclavicular *(C)* lines over the front, and the scapular *(D)* and paravertebral *(E)* lines over the back provide longitudinal landmarks of the thorax. From a lateral view, the midaxillary line is used for orientation. Horizontal reference points are the supraclavicular and infraclavicular fossae, Ludwig's angle (junction of the second rib at the sternum), the mammillae (normally at the fourth rib), and the epigastric angle. Posteriorly, the prominent spinous process of the seventh cervical vertebra and the supraspinous and infraspinous fossae of the scapulae provide markers for orientation.

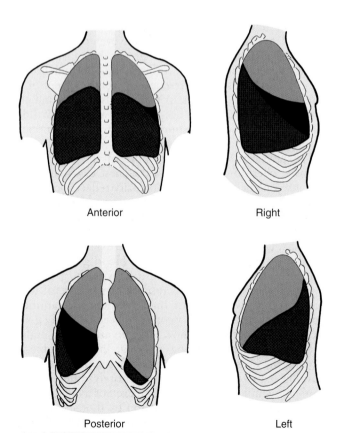

FIGURE 8-8. Projections of the pulmonary lobes on the chest surface. The upper lobes are pink, the right-middle lobe is black, and the lower lobes are red.

disease, and mapping of respiratory sounds should therefore be done with reference to external anatomic landmarks (Fig. 8-9). The examiner should be familiar with the segmental structure of the underlying lung.

Respiratory sound characteristics include the intensity (amplitude), pitch (predominant frequency), and timing during the respiratory cycle. Also, sounds will have a particular timbre (character) caused by the presence of resonances and overtones. Unfortunately, the terminology in use for the description of respiratory sounds is still confusing and imprecise. During a symposium on lung sounds in Tokyo in 1985, an attempt was made to achieve a global and uniform nomenclature for breath sounds. The resulting recommendations for classification of adventitious lung sounds are presented in Figure 8-10, and Table 8-1 summarizes the mechanisms and sites of generation, acoustic characteristics, and clinical relevance of the major categories of respiratory sounds.

A basic grouping into musical, continuous sounds of long duration and nonmusical, discontinuous sounds of short duration is made, with the former being referred to as *wheezes* and the latter as *crackles*. Furthermore, musical adventitious sounds or wheezes may be classified as high-pitched or low-pitched. Some use the term *rhonchus* for low-pitched wheezes (<200 Hz), whereas others describe the poorly characterized "secretion sounds," which share musical and nonmusical qualities, as *rhonchi*. Crackles are subclassified as fine or coarse. Regular breath sounds include tracheal/bronchial, bronchovesicular, and vesicular/normal sounds. Finally, other respiratory sounds should be specified, such as pleural rubs, expiratory grunting, and inspiratory stridor. Historical terms such as *rales* and *crepitations* should be abandoned, and flowery descriptions such as "raspy" or "blowing" breath sounds should not be used because these adjectives are even less well-defined than the suggested terms.

LUNG SOUND NOMENCLATURE

	English	French	German	Japanese	Portuguese	Spanish
Discontinuous						
Fine (high pitched, low amplitude, short duration)	Fine crackles	Ráles crepitants	Feines rasseln	捻髪音	Estertores finos	Estertores finos
Coarse (low pitched, high amplitude, long duration)	Coarse crackles	Ráles bulleux ou Sous-crepitants	Grobes rasseln	水泡音	Estertores grossos	Estertores gruesos
Continuous						
High pitched	Wheezes	Ráles sibilants	Pfeifen	ふえ（拪）音	Sibilos	Sibilancias
Low pitched	Rhonchus	Ráles ronflants	Brummen	いびき（拪）音	Roncos	Roncus

FIGURE 8-10. Recommendation from the 1985 International Symposium on Lung Sounds in Tokyo for a unified nomenclature of adventitious sounds. (Reproduced with permission from Cugell DW. Lung sound nomenclature. *Am Rev Respir Dis.* 1987;136:1016.)

TABLE 8-1 RESPIRATORY SOUNDS

	MECHANISMS	ORIGIN	ACOUSTICS	RELEVANCE
Basic Sounds				
Lung	Turbulent flow, vortices, other	Central (expiration), lobar to segmental airways (inspiration)	Low pass filtered noise (<100 to >1000 Hz)	Regional ventilation, airway caliber
Tracheal	Turbulent flow, flow impinging on airway walls	Pharynx, larynx, trachea, large airways	Noise with resonances (<100 to >3000 Hz)	Upper airway configuration
Adventitious Sounds				
Wheezes	Airway wall flutter, vortex shedding, other	Central and lower airways	Sinusoidal (<100 Hz to >1000 Hz, duration typically >80 msec)	Airway obstruction, flow limitation
Rhonchi	Rupture of fluid films, airway wall vibration	Larger airways	Series of rapidly dampened sinusoids (typically <300 Hz and duration <100 msec)	Secretions, abnormal airway collapsibility
Crackles	Airway wall stress-relaxation	Central and lower airways	Rapidly dampened wave deflections (duration typically <20 msec)	Airway closure, secretions

Modified from Pasterkamp H, Kraman SS, Wodicka GR. State of the art. Respiratory sounds—advances beyond the stethoscope. *Am J Respir Crit Care Med.* 1997;156:974-987.

Several auscultatory signs are based on the transmission of voice sounds. Speech sounds have a fundamental note of about 130 Hz in men and 230 Hz in women, with overtones from 400 Hz to 3500 Hz. Vowels are produced when particular pairs of overtones or formants are generated. On passage through the lung, the higher-frequency formants are filtered, and speech heard over the chest becomes a meaningless mumble. With consolidation and transmission of higher-frequency components, however, speech may become intelligible. This occurs with normal speech (bronchophony) and with whispered voice (pectoriloquy). There may be a change in vowels from *e* to *a* over areas of lung consolidation. The acoustic basis for these phenomena is the same as for bronchial breath sounds. The American Thoracic Society and the American College of Chest Physicians recommend the term *egophony* for all of these findings.

Percussion

Percussion is used to set tissues into vibration with an impulsive force so that their mechanical and acoustic response can be studied. If the vibrations are undamped and continue for a significant amount of time, the perceived sound will be resonant or "tympanic," whereas rapid attenuation of the vibrations will lead to a flat or "dull" percussion note. The former occurs when there is a large acoustic mismatch (e.g., tissue overlying an air-filled cavity), whereas the latter occurs when the underlying tissue is similar to the surface tissue and vibratory energy propagates away quickly. Structures that absorb energy when struck by a sound at their natural frequency continue vibrating after the initial sound is gone and are called *resonant*. The fundamental resonance of the thorax depends on body size and is about 125 Hz for adult males, between 150 and 175 Hz for adult females, and between 300 and 400 Hz for small children.

Chest percussion in children is performed by light tapping with the index or middle finger (the plexor) on the terminal phalanx of the other hand's middle finger (the pleximeter). The pleximeter should be placed firmly but not hard, and care should be taken that other fingers do not touch the chest wall, which may cause artificial damping of the percussion note. Percussion should be gentle, with quick perpendicular movements of the plexor originating from the wrist (Fig. 8-11). The patient should be relaxed during the examination because tension of the chest wall muscles may alter the percussion note. More importantly, chest deformities and scoliosis in particular will have a significant effect on percussory findings.

Symmetric sites over the anterior, lateral, and posterior surface of the chest should be compared in an orderly fashion. As with chest auscultation, findings should be reported with reference to standard external anatomic landmarks (see Fig. 8-9). The ribs and vertebral spinous processes are used for horizontal mapping. The level at which the tympanic lung resonance changes to a dull percussion note should be defined over the posterior chest during maximal inspiration and expiration to delineate the lung borders and their respiratory excursions.

Subjective assessment of percussion note differences includes both acoustic and tactile perception. Tympanic,

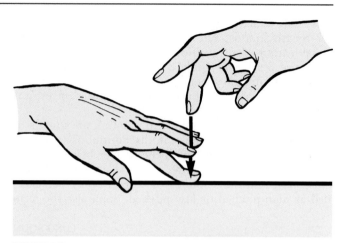

FIGURE 8-11. Percussion in children should be done with gentle perpendicular movements from the wrist and tapping of the plexor finger *(right)* on the terminal phalanx of the pleximeter finger *(left)*. The contact area of the pleximeter on the chest should be small, and other fingers should not touch the surface to avoid damping of the percussory vibrations.

lower-pitched percussion notes mean less-damped vibrations of longer duration, which are felt by the pleximeter finger. Dull sounds with higher frequencies correspond to vibrations that die away quickly. Dullness replaces the normal chest percussion note when fluid accumulates in the pleural space or when consolidation close to the chest wall occurs in the underlying pulmonary parenchyma. Similar to the vibrations generated by percussion, the vibrations from the patient's voice ("say 'ninety-nine'") will also not be felt under these circumstances. However, the tactile fremitus is equally absent over areas of pneumothorax, whereas the percussion note may have a hyperresonant quality.

Conventional percussion cannot detect small pulmonary lesions located deeply within the thorax. Auscultatory percussion has been proposed to overcome this limitation. This technique combines light percussion of the sternum with simultaneous auscultation over the posterior chest. A decrease in sound intensity is believed to indicate lung disease. The method is of little value, however, because even large intrathoracic lesions can remain undetected since percussion sounds either may be totally absorbed within the lung or may travel as transverse waves along the thoracic bones.

Taste and Smell

A complete physical examination extends beyond the perception of vision, hearing, and touch. Olfactory impressions should also be documented, even if they are subtle. Malodorous breath is easily noticed and may, particularly if chronic, indicate infection within the nasal or oral cavity (e.g., paranasal sinusitis), nasal foreign body, or dental abscess. Bad breath may also originate from intrathoracic infections, such as lung abscess or bronchiectasis, and it may also be noted in patients with gastroesophageal reflux. Nowadays physicians rarely use their taste buds to make a medical diagnosis. One particular disease of the respiratory tract in children, however, lends itself to gustatory diagnosis. Most often the discovery is made by the mother of a patient with cystic fibrosis who notices that the skin of her child tastes abnormally salty.

COMMON SIGNS AND SYMPTOMS OF CHEST DISEASE IN CHILDREN

There are several common complaints and presentations of children with chest diseases that deserve a more detailed description. In particular, cough and sputum production, noisy breathing, wheezing, cyanosis, digital clubbing, cardiovascular signs, and chest pain need to be discussed.

Cough and Sputum Production

Cough is not an illness by itself, but it is a cardinal manifestation in many chest diseases. Cough is probably the single most common complaint in children presenting to the physician. The act of coughing is a reflex aimed at removal of mucus and other material from the airways that follows the stimulation of cough or irritant receptors. These receptors are located anywhere between the pharynx and the terminal bronchioles. They send their afferent impulses via branches of the glossopharyngeal and vagus nerves to the cough center in the upper brainstem and pons. The efferent signals travel from the cough center via vagus, phrenic, and spinal motor nerves to the larynx and diaphragm as well as to the muscles of the chest wall, abdomen, and pelvic floor. Cortical influences allow the voluntary initiation or suppression of cough.

There are three phases of coughing: (1) deep inspiration; (2) closure of the glottis, relaxation of the diaphragm, and contraction of expiratory muscles; and (3) sudden opening of the glottis. During the second phase, intrathoracic pressures up to 300 mm Hg can be generated and may be transmitted to the vascular and cerebrospinal spaces. Air flow velocity during the third phase is highest in the central airways and may reach three fourths the speed of sound. This speed depends on the sudden opening of the glottis and influences the success of expectoration. Patients with glottic dysfunction and those with tracheostomies may therefore have a less effective cough.

Stimuli that cause coughing may originate centrally, such as in psychogenic cough, or they may be pulmonary, located either in the major airways or in the pulmonary parenchyma. Also, cough can be provoked by nonpulmonary causes, such as irritation of pleura, diaphragm, or pericardium and even through stimulation of Arnold's nerve (a branch of the vagus) by wax or foreign bodies in the external ear.

A detailed history should define the nature of the cough; whether it is dry, hacking, or brassy; and whether it is productive by sound and appearance. In young children, expectoration is unusual, but if observed, the quantity and quality of sputum should be noted. In particular, the physician should inquire about the color and odor of the expectorate and about the presence of blood in the sputum. The yellow-green color of purulent sputum results from the cellular breakdown of leukocytes and the liberation of myeloperoxidase from these cells. This finding indicates the retention of secretions and does not necessarily reflect an acute infection.

The timing of coughing is important, and its relationship to daily routines should be sought. Cough during or after feeding occurs with aspiration. Nighttime cough may be related to asthma or to postnasal drip, whereas productive cough early in the morning is typical for bronchiectasis. Cough following exercise or exposure to cold air points toward airway hyperreactivity. Seasonal worsening or coughing on exposure to potential allergens should be documented, as should the association of coughing and wheezing. The physician should ask about active and passive smoking, keeping in mind that, regrettably, there are quite a few children as young as 8 years of age who smoke regularly.

A detailed diary kept by the parents or the patient to note the frequency and timing of cough can be of value. Technology to record, quantify, and characterize cough is being developed. Some acoustic characteristics of cough are quite specific for certain diseases, such as the sound of a barking seal in viral croup or the whooping noise in pertussis. In patients with chronic cough, the physician should weigh the possible causes in view of their prevalence at different ages (Table 8-2). Also, complications of severe coughing paroxysms, such as pneumothorax, cough syncope, or nonsyncopal neurologic manifestations, should be considered. Regarding the last, the physician should inquire about lightheadedness, headache, visual disturbance, paresthesia, and tremor.

Noisy Breathing

Quite frequently a child is brought to the physician's attention because of abnormal breathing noises. This noise may be a nonmusical hiss, much like the one produced in normal subjects at increased rates of ventilation, or it may have the musical qualities of stridor and snoring. Also, bubbling and crackling noises may be heard, and the tactile perception may contribute to the impression of a "rattly" chest in these patients.

The physician should focus attention on the noise-generating structures of the extrathoracic airways that are located at points of anatomic narrowing (e.g., the nasal vestibule, the posterior nasal orifices, and the glottis). The most common cause of noisy breathing in toddlers and young children is nasopharyngeal obstruction; in young infants, laryngomalacia is a leading cause. It is

TABLE 8-2 CAUSES OF CHRONIC COUGH

INFANT	PRESCHOOL	SCHOOL AGE/ ADOLESCENCE
Congenital anomalies Tracheoesophageal fistula Neurologic impairment	Foreign body Infections Viral	Reactive Asthma Postnasal drip
Infections Viral (RSV, CMV) Chlamydia Bacterial (pertussis)	Mycoplasma Bacterial Reactive Asthma	Infections Mycoplasma Irritative Smoking
Cystic fibrosis	Cystic fibrosis Irritative Passive smoking	Air pollution Psychogenic

Data modified from Eigen H. The clinical evaluation of chronic cough. *Pediatr Clin North Am.* 1982;29:67.

uncertain to what degree sounds from large intrathoracic airways contribute to the noise of breathing. Placing the stethoscope within the airstream in front of the mouth, one hears predominantly those sounds that are produced locally in the mouth and larynx. Noisy breathing is a common finding in patients with asthma and bronchitis and does not necessarily reflect intrathoracic airway pathology because the upper airways are also frequently affected in these patients.

To clarify the causes of noisy breathing, the parents or patient should describe their own perceptions of the noise: Does it occur during inspiration, expiration, or both? Is it just an exaggeration of the normal breath sound noise, or does it have musical qualities? Did an episode of choking precede the onset of noisy breathing? Is the abnormal sound more prominent during certain activities, such as exercise? At what times of day or night and in which body positions is it most noticeable? The physician should also inquire about associated cough, sputum production, and dyspnea.

Children may suffer from partial obstruction of the upper airways during sleep; complete obstruction, which is found in adult patients with sleep apnea, is less common. Invariably, these children are heavy snorers at night, whereas normal children's snoring is largely confined to times of upper respiratory tract infection. Usually enlarged adenoids and tonsils cause the breathing disturbance. The physician should inquire about the typical signs and symptoms found in patients with increased work of breathing and abnormal sleep patterns at night (Box 8-1).

In the older child and adolescent, the physician should first inspect the nasal passageways and proceed to an examination of the oropharynx before auscultation of the neck and thorax. The acoustic signs should be checked while the patient breathes first with the mouth open, and then closed. In younger children, examination of the nose and mouth is unpopular and often results in agitation and crying. It is better to start with auscultation before inspection in these children. Noisy breathers should be examined when they are sitting or standing upright and when they are lying down because upper airway geometry is position dependent and may influence the respiratory sounds. The examiner should also note abnormal crying or speech in the patient, as this may point to laryngeal disease.

Wheezing

Wheezing is a common respiratory symptom and refers to musical, adventitious lung sounds that are often heard by the patient as well as the physician. Stridor is even more noticeable. Essentially, it is a very loud inspiratory wheeze originating from extrathoracic airways. When asking the patient or the parents about wheezing and stridor, one should keep in mind that the use of lung sound terminology among nonprofessionals is not better standardized than it is among health care providers. Therefore, the physician should inquire about musical, whistling noises during respiration, and, if necessary, demonstrate stridor or the forced expiratory wheeze that can be produced even by healthy individuals.

Most typically, wheezing is associated with hyperreactive airway disease, but any critical narrowing of the airways can produce wheezing. Box 8-2 lists conditions other than asthma that may be associated with wheezing and stridor. The wheezing that is typical in asthma originates from oscillations of airways at many sites. On

---

BOX 8-1 CLINICAL SYMPTOMS IN CHILDREN WITH HEAVY NOCTURNAL SNORING

Nighttime Manifestations
Profuse nocturnal sweating
Restless sleep
Abnormal movements during sleep
Special sleeping position
Enuresis

Problems with Growth and Nutrition
Anorexia
Weight < 3rd percentile
Nausea with or without vomiting

Behavioral and Learning Problems
Hyperactivity
Aggression
Social withdrawal

Minor Motor Problems
Lack of coordination
Clumsiness

Other Manifestations
Frequent upper airway infections
Frequent morning headaches
Excessive daytime somnolence

BOX 8-2 CAUSES OF WHEEZING AND STRIDOR OTHER THAN ASTHMA

Malformation
Cardiovascular anomalies (e.g., vascular ring)
Airway anomalies (e.g., web, cyst, hemangioma, malacia, stenosis)
Esophageal anomalies (e.g., enteric cyst)

Inflammation
Tracheitis
Bronchitis
Bronchiolitis
Bronchiectasis
Cystic fibrosis

Compression
Extrinsic
Esophageal foreign body
Lymphadenopathy
Malignancy
Intrinsic
Endobronchial foreign body
Tumor (rare)

Extrathoracic Disease
Laryngitis
Epiglottitis
Vocal cord paralysis
Retropharyngeal abscess
Peritonsillar abscess
Laryngomalacia
Polyps, adenoids

Other
Metabolic disturbances (e.g., hypocalcemia, hypokalemia)
Psychosomatic illness (e.g., emotional laryngeal wheezing, factitious asthma)

auscultation, one hears many different tones simultaneously, which is called *polyphonic wheezing*. Obstruction of a single airway can produce a single monophonic wheeze or, in the obstruction of extrathoracic airways, stridor. Both inspiratory and expiratory wheezes are present in the majority of asthmatic patients. The audible expiratory phase (expirium) is typically prolonged because of wheezing. Objectively measured expiratory time (expiration), however, is rarely prolonged except in very severe airway obstruction. Under these circumstances, air flow is minimal, and thus wheezing is absent. Respiration becomes ominously silent, and the patient may have carbon dioxide retention and cyanosis. In less severe cases, however, the proportion of inspiration and expiration occupied by wheezing correlates to some extent with the degree of air flow obstruction. Objective and reproducible wheeze quantification can be achieved by computer-assisted techniques, but in practice the quantification of wheezing severity is made by subjective assessment at the bedside.

Wheezes are often high-pitched and will therefore attenuate during their passage through lung tissue, particularly if the lungs are hyperinflated. Auscultation over the neck may give a better impression of respiratory sounds and should be included as a part of the routine physical examination. Tracheal auscultation to determine if and when there is wheezing after methacholine inhalation challenge has been advocated instead of spirometry in young children who are thought to have bronchial hyperreactivity. However, wheezing may be absent even if airways become significantly obstructed during bronchial provocation (Fig. 8-12). In our experience, wheezing heard at the chest but not necessarily at the trachea is very suggestive of airway narrowing and hyperresponsiveness. Listening to respiratory sounds over the neck may help to identify patients who are thought to be asthmatic but who generate the wheezing noises solely in the larynx. These are usually older children and adolescents who may have emotional problems and vocal cord dysfunction.

Cyanosis

Cyanosis refers to a blue color of the skin and mucous membranes due to excessive concentrations of reduced hemoglobin in capillary blood. The oxygen content of capillary blood is assumed to be midway between that of arterial and that of venous blood. Areas with a high blood flow and a small arteriovenous oxygen difference (e.g., the tongue and mucous membranes) will not become cyanotic as readily as those with a low blood flow and a large arteriovenous oxygen difference (e.g., the skin of cold hands and feet). A distinction is therefore made between peripheral cyanosis (acrocyanosis), which is confined to the skin of the extremities, and central cyanosis, which includes the tongue and mucous membranes. Circumoral cyanosis is not an expression of central cyanosis and is rarely pathologic. The absolute concentration of reduced hemoglobin in the capillaries that is necessary to produce cyanosis is between 4 and 6 g/100 mL of blood. This level is usually present when the concentration of reduced hemoglobin in arterial blood exceeds 3 g/100 mL. Clinical cyanosis will occur at different levels of arterial oxygen saturation, depending on the amount of total hemoglobin (Fig. 8-13).

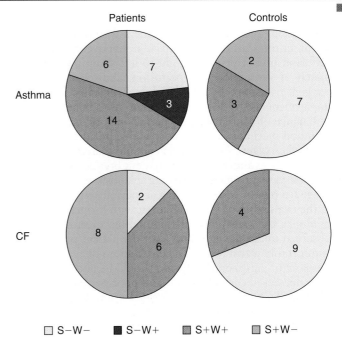

FIGURE 8-12. Summary of findings regarding wheeze as an indicator of significant flow obstruction during methacholine bronchial provocation in children. Negative responses (i.e., less than 20% decline in forced expiratory volume in 1 second [FEV] at a dose of 8 mg/mL [spirometry] and no wheeze [acoustic monitoring]) are indicated by a minus sign, and positive responses are indicated by a plus sign. Note the low sensitivity of wheeze as an indicator of air flow obstruction, particularly in children with cystic fibrosis. S, spirometry; W, wheezing. (Data from Sanchez I, Powell RE, Pasterkamp H: Wheezing and airflow obstruction during metacholine challenge in children with cystic fibrosis and in normal children. *Am Rev Respir Dis.* 1993;147:705, and Sanchez I, Avital A, Wong I, et al: Acoustic vs. spirometric assessment of bronchial responsiveness to metacholine in children. *Pediatr Pulmonol.* 1993;15:28.)

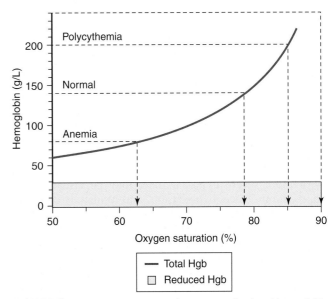

FIGURE 8-13. Cyanosis requires at least 30 g/L of reduced hemoglobin (Hgb) in arterial blood or 4 to 6 g/100 mL in capillary blood. The arterial oxygen saturation (SaO_2) at which cyanosis occurs is dependent on the amount of total Hgb. As illustrated, a child with 30 g/L of Hgb plus 110 g/L of oxyhemoglobin has an SaO_2 of 78%. In the anemic patient (i.e., total Hgb of 80 g/L with Hgb of 30 g/L), SaO_2 will drop much lower (to less than 65% in this example) before cyanosis occurs, whereas in the patient with polycythemia (i.e., total Hgb of 200 g/L), cyanosis appears at a higher SaO_2 (85%).

Physiologically, five mechanisms can cause arterial hemoglobin desaturation in the patient who breathes room air at normal altitude: (1) alveolar hypoventilation, (2) diffusion impairment, (3) right-to-left shunting, (4) mismatch of ventilation and perfusion, and (5) inadequate oxygen transport by hemoglobin. Clinically, diffusion impairment is of little importance as a single cause. Imbalance of ventilation and perfusion is by far the most common mechanism and is correctable by administration of 100% oxygen. The physician should therefore look for a change in cyanosis while the patient breathes oxygen.

Observer agreement regarding cyanosis was found to range from poor when assessing acrocyanosis to very good in the evaluation of young children with bronchiolitis. To minimize the variability of this finding, cyanosis is best observed under daylight and with the patient resting in a comfortably warm room. The distribution of cyanosis and the state of peripheral perfusion should be noted. Patients with decreased cardiac output and poor peripheral perfusion can be cyanotic despite normal arterial hemoglobin saturation. Some patients may become cyanotic only during exercise, a common response when restrictive lung disease reduces the pulmonary capillary bed and the transit time of erythrocytes becomes too short for full saturation during episodes of increased cardiac output. Congenital heart disease in infants may lead to differential cyanosis, which affects only the lower part of the body (e.g., in patients with preductal coarctation of the aorta). Less commonly, only the upper part of the body is cyanotic (e.g., in patients with transposition of the great arteries, patent ductus arteriosus, or pulmonary hypertension).

The clinical impression of cyanosis is usually confirmed by an arterial blood gas analysis or, more commonly, by pulse oximetry. Pulse oximetry, however, will not take into account the presence of abnormal hemoglobin. For example, in methemoglobinemia the oxygen-carrying capacity of blood is reduced and patients may appear lavender blue, but pulse oximetry may overestimate oxygen saturation in arterial blood (SaO_2). The blood of newborn infants, conversely, can be well saturated and not cyanotic at lower arterial oxygen tensions because of the different oxygen-binding curve of fetal hemoglobin. In the patient with hypoxemia who does not present with cyanosis (e.g., the anemic patient), the physician has to pay particular attention to other clinical signs and symptoms of hypoxia. These include tachypnea and tachycardia, exertional dyspnea, hypertension, headache, and behavioral changes. With more severe hypoxia, there may be visual disturbance, somnolence, hypotension, and ultimately coma. In addition, the patient may have an elevated level of carbon dioxide. Depending on how rapidly and to what extent the level of carbon dioxide has risen, the clinical signs of hypercarbia will largely reflect vascular dilatation. These signs include flushed, hot hands and feet; bounding pulses; confusion or drowsiness; muscular twitching; engorged retinal veins; and, in the most severe cases, papilledema and coma.

Digital Clubbing

Digital clubbing refers to a focal enlargement of the connective tissue in the terminal phalanges of fingers and toes, most noticeably on their dorsal surfaces. This sign was first described by Hippocrates, and the term *Hippocratic fingers* is used by some to denote simple digital clubbing. The pathogenesis of clubbing is still not entirely clear. Vascular endothelial growth factor (VEGF) from the continued impaction of shunted megakaryocytes and platelets in the digital vasculature, potentiated by hypoxia, is considered to drive the cellular and stromal changes in clubbing. Enhanced VEGF expression is a common finding in various diseases that are associated with digital clubbing. Aside from VEGF, platelet-derived growth factor may contribute to the stromal changes, including the maturation of new microvessels.

Clubbing of the digits may be idiopathic, acquired, or hereditary. Cystic fibrosis, bronchiectasis, and empyema are the most common pulmonary causes of acquired digital clubbing in children. Clubbing is also seen infrequently in extrinsic allergic vasculitis, pulmonary arteriovenous malformations, bronchiolitis obliterans, sarcoidosis, and chronic asthma. Box 8-3 shows a list of nonpulmonary diseases associated with clubbing. A systemic disorder of bones, joints, and soft tissues known as *hypertrophic osteoarthropathy* (HOA) includes digital clubbing. In the majority of cases, HOA is associated with bronchogenic carcinoma and other intrathoracic neoplasms, but the pediatrician may see HOA in patients with severe cystic fibrosis or chronic empyema and lung abscess. In addition to clubbing, these patients may have periosteal thickening; symmetric arthritis of ankles, knees, wrists, and elbows; neurovascular changes of hands and feet; and increased thickness of subcutaneous soft tissues in the distal portions of arms and legs. The primary idiopathic

---

BOX 8-3 NONPULMONARY DISEASES ASSOCIATED WITH CLUBBING

Cardiac
Cyanotic congenital heart disease
Subacute bacterial endocarditis
Chronic congestive heart failure

Hematologic
Thalassemia
Congenital methemoglobinemia (rare)

Gastrointestinal
Crohn's disease
Ulcerative colitis
Chronic dysentery, sprue
Polyposis coli
Severe gastrointestinal hemorrhage
Small bowel lymphoma
Liver cirrhosis (including α_1-antitrypsin deficiency)

Other
Thyroid deficiency (thyroid acropachy)
Chronic pyelonephritis (rare)
Toxic (e.g., arsenic, mercury, beryllium)
Lymphomatoid granulomatosis
Fabry's disease
Raynaud's disease, scleroderma

Unilateral Clubbing
Vascular disorders (e.g., subclavian arterial aneurysm, brachial arteriovenous fistula)
Subluxation of shoulder
Median nerve injury
Local trauma

or hereditary form of HOA—pachydermoperiostosis—appears with prominent furrowing of the forehead and scalp. Approximately half of the reported cases have a positive family history. Genetic studies suggest an autosomal-dominant inheritance with variable expression and a predilection for males.

Digital clubbing is not only an important indicator of pulmonary disease but also may reflect the progression or resolution of the causative process. Pulmonary abscess and empyema may lead to digital clubbing over the course of only a few weeks. In this case, clubbing will resolve if effective treatment is instituted before connective tissue changes become fixed. Interestingly, even long-standing finger clubbing seems to resolve in patients after successful heart and lung transplantation. In patients with cystic fibrosis, progression of finger clubbing suggests a suboptimal control of chest infections. It is therefore useful to quantify the degree of digital clubbing. Measurements have focused on the hyponychial (Lovibond) angle and on the phalangeal depth ratio (Fig. 8-14). Changes of the hyponychial angle are quantified on "shadowgrams" (projections of the finger's lateral profile onto a magnifying screen), whereas the phalangeal depth ratio is measured from plaster casts. Computerized analysis from digital photographs has provided information on the distribution of the hyponychial angle in healthy subjects and in patients with various diseases. Almost 80% of adult patients with cystic fibrosis have a hyponychial angle greater than 190 degrees, the upper limit of normal.

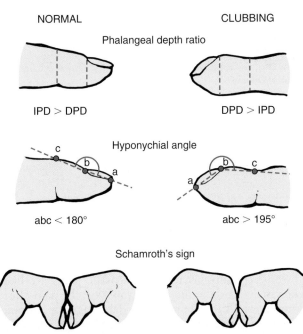

NORMAL   CLUBBING

Phalangeal depth ratio

IPD > DPD   DPD > IPD

Hyponychial angle

abc < 180°   abc > 195°

Schamroth's sign

FIGURE 8-14. Finger clubbing can be measured in different ways. The ratio of the distal phalangeal diameter (DPD) over the interphalangeal diameter (IPD), or the phalangeal depth ratio, is less than 1 in normal subjects but increases to greater than 1 with finger clubbing. The DPD/IPD can be measured with calipers or more accurately with finger casts. The hyponychial angle can be measured from lateral projections of the finger contour on a magnifying screen and is usually less than 180 degrees in normal subjects but greater than 195 degrees in patients with finger clubbing. For bedside clinical assessment, Schamroth's sign is useful. The dorsal surfaces of the terminal phalanges of similar fingers are placed together. With clubbing, the normal diamond-shaped aperture or "window" at the bases of the nail beds disappears, and a prominent distal angle forms between the end of the nails. In normal subjects this angle is minimal or nonexistent.

For routine clinical practice, the sign described by Schamroth, a cardiologist who developed finger clubbing during several attacks of infective endocarditis, is a most useful method of measuring finger clubbing (see Fig. 8-14). Another way is to place a plastic caliper with minimal pressure over the interphalangeal joint. If it is easy to slide the caliper from this joint across the nail fold, the distal phalangeal diameter to interphalangeal diameter ratio must be less than 1, and the patient has no clubbing.

Cardiovascular Signs

Pulmonary heart disease, or *cor pulmonale*, is a consequence of acute or chronic pulmonary hypertension and appears as right ventricular enlargement. The progression of chronic cor pulmonale to ultimate right ventricular failure is accompanied by certain physical signs. Initially, the right ventricular systolic pressure and muscle mass increase as pulmonary artery pressure rises. During this stage, cardiac auscultation may be normal or may reveal an increased pulmonary component of the second heart sound, caused by an increase in diastolic pulmonary arterial pressure. The physician should look for a parasternal right ventricular heave. As pulmonary hypertension progresses, there is an increase in right ventricular end-diastolic volume. Dilation of the main pulmonary artery and right ventricular outflow tract lead to systolic pulmonary ejection clicks and murmurs. Diastolic murmurs appear when pulmonary or tricuspid valves or both become insufficient. Third and fourth heart sounds at the left lower sternal border are signs of decreased right ventricular compliance. Most of these right-sided cardiovascular findings are accentuated during inspiration, which augments venous return. Finally, cardiac output falls while end-diastolic pressure and volume increase further in the failing right ventricle.

Clinical findings at this stage include hepatic engorgement, jugular venous distention, and peripheral edema. Occasionally, there may be cyanosis and intracardiac right-to-left shunting through a patent foramen ovale. The physician should exclude the possibility of congenital cardiac defects or acquired left-sided heart disease before making the diagnosis of cor pulmonale. Hyperinflation of the lungs should be taken into account as a cause of the attenuation of cardiovascular sounds and the lowering of the subcostal liver margin, which may be misinterpreted as hepatic enlargement.

Complete assessment of the cardiovascular system includes careful auscultation and palpation of the pulse to detect cardiac arrhythmia. This problem is common in patients with chronic lung disease and may appear as sinus or paroxysmal supraventricular tachycardia, atrial premature contractions, or ventricular ectopic beats. Causes include hypoxemia, acid-base imbalance, and enlargement of the right heart, but effects of common drugs such as aminophylline, beta sympathomimetics, or diuretics should not be overlooked.

During quiet spontaneous respiration, there is a phasic variation of arterial blood pressure. The widening of this normal respiratory variation is known as *pulsus paradoxus*. Increased respiratory resistance may exaggerate the normal inspiratory-expiratory difference in left ventricular stroke volume. This is mediated by effects of intrathoracic pressures on ventricular preload. Clinically, pulsus paradoxus is first assessed by palpation of the radial pulse and then is measured at the brachial artery with a sphygmomanometer as the difference in systolic pressure between inspiration and expiration. The pressure cuff is deflated from above systolic level, and the highest pressure during expiration at which systolic pulse sounds are heard is recorded. Similarly, the highest pressure at which every pulse is just audible throughout inspiration is also noted. In general, a drop of greater than 10 mm Hg during inspiration is taken as clinically significant, but only a severe paradox of greater than 24 mm Hg is a reliable indicator of severe asthma. The poor correlation between pulsus paradoxus and objective measurements of air flow obstruction may be explained by other factors that affect pleural pressure swings (e.g., the degree of pulmonary hyperinflation and the air flow rate). Furthermore, the accurate measurement of pulsus paradoxus is a challenge in tachypneic, tachycardic, and uncooperative young children. A work group on behalf of the British Thoracic Society Standards of Care Committee found pulsus paradoxus to be absent in one third of patients with the severest obstruction. In contrast to North American practice guidelines, it was therefore recommended that pulsus paradoxus be abandoned as an indicator of severity of asthma attack. In children, wheeze seems to be the clinical parameter of respiratory severity scores that correlates best with pulsus paradoxus, most likely because wheeze requires critical intrathoracic pressures. The application of pulse oximetry to view dynamic changes in the area under the plethysmographic waveform in relation to pulsus paradoxus shows some promise in improving the diagnostic value of this clinical sign.

Chest Pain

Chest pain is relatively common in older children and adolescents but may also present in younger children. The occurrence rate in an emergency department approaches 2.5 per 1000 patient visits, and chest pain accounts for an estimated 650,000 physician visits of patients between 10 and 21 years of age annually in the United States. Chest pain in children is most often benign and self-limited. Typical origins are musculoskeletal problems and idiopathic, dysfunctional, and psychogenic causes (Table 8-3). Younger children more frequently have underlying cardiorespiratory problems, whereas children older than 12 years of age are more likely to have psychogenic pain.

The history is most important in the assessment of these patients, who usually have few physical findings and rarely any laboratory data of diagnostic value. The physician should recognize a clinical profile suggestive of psychogenic pain but should also keep in mind that psychogenic and organic causes are not mutually exclusive. A substantial number of patients have a family history of chest pain. Parents of younger children should explain how they know that their child is in pain. It is important to determine whether sleep is affected, because organic pain is more likely than psychogenic pain to awaken the patient or to prevent the child from falling asleep. The duration of symptoms may be an indicator; acute,

TABLE 8-3 CAUSES OF CHEST PAIN IN CHILDREN

Thorax

Costochondritis
Tietze's syndrome
Muscular disease
Precordial catch
Trauma
Connective tissue disorders
Xiphoid-cartilage syndrome
Rib tip syndrome
Leukemia
Herpes zoster
Breast development or disease (e.g., gynecomastia, mastitis)

Lungs, Pleura, and Diaphragm

Asthma
Cystic fibrosis
Infection (e.g., bronchitis, pneumonia, epidemic pleurodynia)
Inhalation of irritants (e.g., chemical pneumonitis, smoking)
Stitch (associated with exercise)
Foreign body
Pneumothorax
Pleural disease (e.g., pleurisy, effusion)
Diaphragmatic irritation (e.g., subphrenic abscess, gastric distention)
Sickle cell anemia

Cardiovascular System

Structural lesions (e.g., mitral valve prolapse, idiopathic
  hypertrophic subaortic stenosis [IHSS], coronary disease)
Acquired cardiac disease (e.g., carditis, arteritis, tumor involvement)
Arrhythmia

Esophagus

Gastroesophageal reflux
Foreign body
Achalasia

Vertebral Column

Deformities (e.g., scoliosis)
Vertebral collapse

Psychogenic Causes

Anxiety
Hyperventilation
Unresolved grief
Identification with another person suffering chest pain

short-lasting pain is more likely to be organic than pain of many months of duration. Localized, sharp, and superficial pains suggest an origin in the chest wall, whereas diffuse, deep, substernal, and epigastric pains are likely to be visceral, originating in the thorax if the pain affects dermatomes T1 to T4 and in the diaphragm or abdomen if it affects dermatomes T5 to T8. The physician should inquire about cough or asthma, recent exercise or trauma, heart disease in the patient and the family, cigarette smoking, and emotional problems.

A close inspection and careful palpation of the chest and abdomen are essential. Common abnormal findings include chest wall tenderness, fever, or both. The physician should use pressure on the stethoscope to elicit local tenderness while the patient is distracted by the auscultation. Cardiac murmurs with or without a midsystolic click may be found in patients with mitral valve prolapsed, but this condition is rarely associated with chest pain, at least in children. More commonly, there are noncardiac causes of chest pain in children with mitral valve prolapse (e.g., orthopedic or gastroesophageal disorders). In general, the presence of systemic signs such as weight loss, anorexia, or syncopal attacks will direct the attention to organic causes of chest pain in children.

▊ CONCLUSION

In pediatric respiratory medicine, the most common clinical presentation is that of a child who coughs or wheezes, or both. Depending on the geographic location, the information gathered from the history and physical examination will carry different weight in the initial diagnostic approach. Pneumonia kills more children than any other disease. In countries with high morbidity and mortality from lower respiratory tract infections, assessment of children who cough will therefore initially focus on the possibility of pneumonia. A constellation of physical findings—particularly fever, tachypnea and retractions, nasal flaring in infants younger than 1 year of age, and history of poor feeding—increase the likelihood that the child has pneumonia. Any single clinical finding by itself, however, is not useful as a predictor.

Concurrent wheezing is more common in viral than in bacterial infections, and a history of preceding similar events and of improvement after bronchodilator inhalation can lead to different first steps in treatment. In most Western countries, the likelihood of pneumonia in a child who presents with cough with or without wheeze is lower, while asthma or prolonged symptoms after viral infections of the lower respiratory tract are common. Recurrent wheezing is particularly prevalent; up to 40% of children will present with wheezing during their first year of life but less than one third of these will have asthma when they reach school age. If the parents of a child younger than 3 years of age who only wheezes with colds do not have asthma or eczema and if the child does not have allergic rhinitis, the negative predictive value of this history is close to 90% with regard to having asthma by the age of school entry.

At school age, functional respiratory assessment by spirometry is generally possible. It is therefore surprising that only a minority of children with asthma symptoms will have lung functions tests. It would be comforting if this could be explained by a superiority of history and physical examination to detect abnormalities. However, the physician should recognize limitations of any component in the diagnostic workup. Only then can the value of a detailed history and a skillfully performed physical examination be appreciated.

Suggested Reading

General Reading

Britton JR, Britton HL, Jennett R, et al. Weight, length, head and chest circumference at birth in Phoenix, Arizona. *J Reprod Med.* 1993;38:215.
Carlo WA, Martin RJ, Bruce EN, et al. Alae nasi activation (nasal flaring) decreases nasal resistance in preterm infants. *Pediatrics.* 1983;72:338.
Carse EA, Wilkinson AR, Whyte PL, et al. Oxygen and carbon dioxide tensions, breathing and heart rate in normal infants during the first six months of life. *J Dev Physiol.* 1981;3:85.
Commey JO, Levison H. Physical signs in childhood asthma. *Pediatrics.* 1976;58:537.
DeGroodt EG, van Pelt W, Borsboom GJ, et al. Growth of lung and thorax dimensions during the pubertal growth spurt. *Eur Respir J.* 1988;1:102.
Edmonds ZV, Mower WR, Lovato LM, et al. The reliability of vital sign measurements. *Ann Emerg Med.* 2002;39:233.
Feingold M, Bossert WH. Normal values for selected physical parameters. *Birth Defects.* 1974;10:14.
Gadomski AM, Permutt T, Stanton B. Correcting respiratory rate for the presence of fever. *J Clin Epidemiol.* 1994;47:1043.
Gagliardi L, Rusconi F. Respiratory rate and body mass in the first three years of life. The working party on respiratory rate. *Arch Dis Child.* 1997;76:151.
Gilmartin JJ, Gibson GJ. Mechanisms of paradoxical rib cage motion in patients with chronic obstructive pulmonary disease. *Am Rev Respir Dis.* 1986;134:683.
Hierholzer E, Schier F. Rasterstereography in the measurement and postoperative follow-up of anterior chest wall deformities. *Z Kinderchir.* 1986;41:267.
Larsen PL, Tos M. Origin of nasal polyps. An endoscopic autopsy study. *Laryngoscope.* 2004;114:710.
Lees MH. Cyanosis of the newborn infant. *J Pediatr.* 1970;77:484.
McGee S. *Evidence Based Physical Diagnosis.* 2nd ed. St. Louis: Saunders Elsevier; 2007.
Peters RM, Peters BA, Benirschke SK, et al. Chest dimensions in young adults with spontaneous pneumothorax. *Ann Thorac Surg.* 1978;25:193.
Robotham JL. A physiological approach to hemidiaphragm paralysis. *Crit Care Med.* 1979;7:563.
Staats BA, Bonekat HW, Harris CD, et al. Chest wall motion in sleep apnoea. *Am Rev Respir Dis.* 1984;130:59.
Stinson S. The physical growth of high altitude Bolivian Aymara children. *Am J Phys Anthropol.* 1980;52:377.
Swartz MH. *Textbook of Physical Diagnosis. History and Examination.* 4th ed Philadelphia: WB Saunders; 2001.
Taylor JA, Del Beccaro M, Done S, et al. Establishing clinically relevant standards for tachypnea in febrile children younger than 2 years. *Arch Pediatr Adolesc Med.* 1995;149:283.
Usen S, Webert M. Clinical signs of hypoxaemia in children with acute lower respiratory infection. Indicators of oxygen therapy. *Int J Tuberc Lung Dis.* 2001;5:505.
Warwick WJ, Hansen L. Chest calipers for measurement of the thoracic index. *Clin Pediatr.* 1976;15:735.
Watkin SL, Spencer SA, Pryce A, et al. Temporal relationship between pauses in nasal airflow and desaturation in preterm infants. *Pediatr Pulmonol.* 1996;21:171.

Respiratory Sounds

Ackerman NB, Bell RE, deLemos RA. Differential pulmonary auscultation in neonates. *Clin Pediatr.* 1982;21:566.
Baughman RP, Loudon RG. Sound spectral analysis of voice transmitted sound. *Am Rev Respir Dis.* 1986;134:167.
Cugell DW. Lung sound nomenclature. *Am Rev Respir Dis.* 1987; 136:1016.
Forgacs P. *Lung Sounds.* London: Baillière Tindall; 1978.
Gavriely N, Palti Y, Alroy G, et al. Measurement and theory of wheezing breath sounds. *J Appl Physiol.* 1984;57:481.
Guilleminault C, Winkle R, Korobkin R, et al. Children and nocturnal snoring. Evaluation of the effects of sleep related respiratory resistive load and daytime functioning. *Eur J Pediatr.* 1982;139:165.
Hopkins RL. Differential auscultation of the acutely ill patient. *Ann Emerg Med.* 1985;14:589.
Kiyokawa H, Greenberg M, Shirota K, et al. Auditory detection of simulated crackles in breath sounds. *Chest.* 2001;119:1886.
Morrison RB. Post-effort breath sound. *Tex Med.* 1971;67:72.
Pasterkamp H, Kraman SS, Wodicka GR. Respiratory sounds. Advances beyond the stethoscope. *Am J Respir Crit Care Med.* 1997;156:974.
Wodicka GR, Shannon DC. Airway sound transmission analysis. In: Roberts JT, ed. *Clinical Management of the Airway.* Philadelphia: WB Saunders; 1994:87–97.
Yernault JC, Bohadana AB. Chest percussion. *Eur Respir J.* 1995;8:1756.

Pulsus Paradoxus

Arnold DH, Jenkins CA, Hartert TV. Noninvasive assessment of asthma severity using pulse oximeter plethysmograph estimate of pulsus paradoxus physiology. *BMC Pulm Med.* 2010;10:17–24.
Frey B, Freezer N. Diagnostic value and pathophysiologic basis of pulsus paradoxus in infants and children with respiratory disease. *Pediatr Pulmonol.* 2001;31:138.
Pearson MG, Spence DP, Ryland I, et al. Value of pulsus paradoxus in assessing acute severe asthma. British Thoracic Society Standards of Care Committee. *BMJ.* 1993;307:659.

Digital Clubbing

Atkinson S, Fox SB. Vascular endothelial growth factor (VEGF)-A and platelet-derived growth factor (PDGF) play a central role in the pathogenesis of digital clubbing. *J Pathol.* 2004;203:721.

Augarten A, Goldman R, Laufer J, et al. Reversal of digital clubbing after lung transplantation in cystic fibrosis patients. A clue to the pathogenesis of clubbing. *Pediatr Pulmonol.* 2002;34:378.

Bentley D, Moore A, Schwachman H. Finger clubbing. A quantitative survey by analysis of the shadowgraph. *Lancet.* 1976;2:164.

Husarik D, Vavricka SR, Mark M, et al. Assessment of digital clubbing in medical inpatients by digital photography and computerized analysis. *Swiss Med Wkly.* 2002;132:132.

Martinez-Lavin M. Exploring the cause of the most ancient clinical sign of medicine: finger clubbing. *Semin Arthritis Rheum.* 2007;36:380–385.

Nakamura CT, Ng GY, Paton JY, et al. Correlation between digital clubbing and pulmonary function in cystic fibrosis. *Pediatr Pulmonol.* 2002;33:332.

Schamroth L. Personal experience. *S Afr Med J.* 1976;50:297.

Van Ginderdeuren F, Van Cauwelaert K, Malfroot A. Influence of digital clubbing on oxygen saturation measurements by pulse-oximetry in cystic fibrosis patients. *J Cyst Fibros.* 2006;5:125–128.

Waring WW, Wilkinson RW, Wiebe RA, et al. Quantitation of digital clubbing in children. Measurements of casts of the index finger. *Am Rev Respir Dis.* 1971;104:166.

Cough and Wheezing

Altiner A, Wilm S, Däubener W, et al. Sputum colour for diagnosis of a bacterial infection in patients with acute cough. *Scand J Prim Health Care.* 2009;27:70–73.

Castro-Rodriguez JA. The Asthma Predictive Index: a very useful tool for predicting asthma in young children. *J Allergy Clin Immunol.* 2010;126:212–216.

Lalloo UG, Barnes PJ, Chung KF. Pathophysiology and clinical presentations of cough. *J Allergy Clin Immunol.* 1996;98(suppl):91.

Mountain RD, Sahn SA. Clinical features and outcome in patients with acute asthma presenting with hypercapnia. *Am Rev Respir Dis.* 1988;138:535.

Pasterkamp H. Acoustic markers of airway responses during inhalation challenge in children. *Pediatr Pulmonol Suppl.* 2004;26:175.

Rempel GR, Borton BL, Kumar R. Aspiration during swallowing in typically developing children of the First Nations and Inuit in Canada. *Pediatr Pulmonol.* 2006;41:912–915.

Shim CS, Williams MH. Relationship of wheezing to the severity of asthma. *Arch Intern Med.* 1983;143:890.

Stern RC, Horwitz SJ, Doershuk CF. Neurologic symptoms during coughing paroxysms in cystic fibrosis. *J Pediatr.* 1988;112:909.

Chest Pain

Owen TR. Chest pain in the adolescent. *Adolesc Med.* 2001;12:95.

Selbst SM, Ruddy R, Clark BJ. Chest pain in children. Follow-up of patients previously reported. *Clin Pediatr (Phila).* 1990;29:374–377.

Woolf PK, Gewitz MH, Berezin S, et al. Noncardiac chest pain in adolescents and children with mitral valve prolapse. *J Adolesc Health.* 1991;12:247.

Cyanosis

Salyer JW. Neonatal and pediatric pulse oximetry. *Respir Care.* 2003;48:386.

Wang EE, Law BJ, Stephens D, et al. Study of interobserver reliability in clinical assessment of RSV lower respiratory illness. A Pediatric Investigators Collaborative Network for Infections in Canada (PICNIC) study. *Pediatr Pulmonol.* 1996;22:23.

References

The complete reference list is available online at www.expertconsult.com

9 BRONCHOSCOPY AND BRONCHOALVEOLAR LAVAGE IN PEDIATRIC PATIENTS

ROBERT E. WOOD, MD, PHD, AND R. PAUL BOESCH, DO, MS

Visualization of the interior of the body is often the most effective and efficient way to evaluate a patient's problem. As an old Chinese proverb says, "A picture is worth a thousand words." Recent advances in endoscopic techniques and instrumentation have greatly enhanced the pulmonary specialist's ability to visualize the interior of the respiratory tract. This in turn has led to improvements in diagnosis and treatment.

Bronchoscopy—the visual examination of the airways—is usually performed for diagnostic purposes, but it is also useful for certain therapeutic maneuvers. Bronchoscopy may be performed with either rigid or flexible (fiberoptic) instruments, depending on the particular needs of the patient and the skills and instrumentation available to the bronchoscopist. In general, most things that can be done with a rigid bronchoscope can also be done with a flexible instrument, and vice versa. However, there are some notable exceptions. For example, a rigid instrument cannot be passed through an endotracheal tube, and a flexible instrument is quite unsuited for removal of aspirated foreign bodies from the lungs of children. For the most effective care of pediatric patients, both rigid and flexible instruments must be available, and there must be practitioners trained in the use of each type of instrument (although not necessarily the same person). In many patients, the combined use of both instruments may yield the most optimal result.

In addition to visualization, bronchoscopes also provide an effective means to obtain specimens from the lungs and airways. Tissue samples may be obtained by biopsy forceps, secretions may be aspirated from the airways, and bronchoalveolar lavage (BAL) yields samples of the fluid resident on the surfaces of the alveoli and distal airways. Bronchoscopy is primarily a clinical tool, but it is increasingly being used for investigational purposes as well. Although pediatric patients present special challenges (technical as well as ethical) to the investigative use of bronchoscopy, age alone is no contraindication to the use of bronchoscopy for research.[1]

Bronchoscopy involves the examination of at least part of the upper airway as well as the trachea and bronchi; this is especially true with (and an advantage of) flexible instruments. Rigid bronchoscopes are generally passed through the patient's mouth, while flexible bronchoscopes are generally passed through the patient's nose. Bronchoscopes may also be used to examine just the upper airway, although the high incidence of concurrent upper and lower airway lesions[2,3] makes it wise to examine both upper and lower airways unless there is a good reason not to do so.

INSTRUMENTATION

The rigid ("open tube") bronchoscope consists of a metal tube of appropriate diameter and length, which is passed into the trachea, and through which the operator may look and the patient may breathe. The instrument is not a simple metal tube; it is equipped to deliver anesthetic gases, and light to the distal tip.

The large open channel, through which instruments may be passed, is one of the major advantages of rigid bronchoscopes. However, visualization is challenging, especially when passing an instrument (such as biopsy forceps). A major advance in bronchoscopic technique came with the development of the glass rod telescope.[4] This device yields exceptionally fine optical performance, and various instruments such as biopsy and foreign body forceps have been designed specifically to work with the telescopes. Rigid bronchoscopes have holes in the side along the distal tip to allow ventilation of the contralateral lung when the bronchoscope is advanced into one main-stem bronchus.

The rigid bronchoscope must be an appropriate size for the patient. Therefore, a variety of instruments must be available to the pediatric bronchoscopist, ranging in diameters from 3 to 7 mm or larger and in length from 20 to 50 cm. There must be a full range of telescope lengths for the different length bronchoscopes. In addition, glass rod telescopes may be made with a prism on the distal end to facilitate observation of the upper lobes (typically 30, 70, or even 120 degrees).

Likewise, the auxiliary instruments (e.g., biopsy or foreign body forceps) must match the telescopes and bronchoscopes. A large variety of forceps and other devices has been developed for specialized purposes. Perhaps the most valuable are the "optical forceps," which are matched with a glass rod telescope and allow the bronchoscopist to operate the forceps under close and direct visualization.

The nomenclature of bronchoscope sizes can be confusing. In general, rigid instruments are defined by the diameter of the largest instrument that will pass through the bronchoscope, while flexible bronchoscopes are defined by their outer diameter. For example, a 3.5-mm flexible bronchoscope will easily pass through a "3.5-mm" rigid bronchoscope.

The flexible bronchoscope is essentially a solid instrument that is composed of thousands of glass fibers that carry the image and the light for illumination. The tip of the instrument can be deflected to guide it into the desired path or location. Most flexible bronchoscopes have a small suction channel through which secretions may be aspirated, fluids may be delivered to the airways, or small flexible instruments may be passed.

The typical pediatric flexible bronchoscopes are 3.5 or 2.8 mm in diameter, with a suction channel approximately 1.2 mm in diameter. Smaller instruments (2.2 mm) have no suction channel and therefore have somewhat limited utility when there are secretions or blood in the airways; they also cannot be used to obtain diagnostic specimens. Larger instruments, ranging from 4.5 to 6.5 mm in diameter, are used in adults. These instruments have suction channels ranging from 2.0 mm to 3.2 mm.

In contrast to the rigid bronchoscope, through which the patient breathes (either spontaneously or by positive pressure), the flexible bronchoscope forces the patient to breathe around the instrument. Therefore, the instrument must be small enough not only to fit into the airway but to allow the patient to breathe. Most full-term newborn infants can breathe around the 3.5-mm instrument (the 2.8-mm instrument can allow spontaneous breathing in infants as small as 1.5 kg), but great care must be taken to ensure the adequacy of ventilation during procedures.

Flexible bronchoscopes are quite limited in their ability to pass instruments through them. The most common instruments used with flexible bronchoscopes are flexible biopsy forceps and cytology or microbiology brushes. Small grasping forceps and folding retrieval baskets are also available but have limited usefulness, especially in pediatric patients. Suctioning is done directly with the bronchoscope, rather than by passing a device through the channel, as is the case with rigid bronchoscopes.

Flexible bronchoscopes are limited in their optical performance by the number of glass fibers that compose the image. While larger, adult-sized instruments now mostly utilize a video chip at the working tip (and thus generate an image with greater resolution), pediatric instruments, because of their small diameter, continue to rely on glass fibers to transmit the image. While the images obtained by flexible instruments are quite satisfactory for most clinical purposes, the glass rod telescope gives much greater resolution and image quality.

Care and Maintenance of Bronchoscopes

Bronchoscopy is not a sterile procedure, since the instruments pass through a nonsterile area (the nose and/or mouth). However, bronchoscopes and associated instruments must be cleaned and sterilized before use.[5] Transmission of infectious agents from patient to patient due to inadequate cleaning or sterilization procedures has been well documented.[6,7] In general, bronchoscopic equipment should be cleaned as soon as possible after use because dried blood and mucus are much more difficult to remove and will prevent adequate sterilization by any method.[8] At a minimum, the instruments should be flushed with water immediately after use, and, if possible, soaked in an enzymatic detergent until formal cleaning can be done.

Rigid bronchoscopes are cleaned by vigorous brushing with detergent, followed by rinsing; they may be sterilized by steam autoclaving. Glass rod telescopes and other associated components may not be exposed to steam, how-

ever, and must be sterilized with ethylene oxide or with liquid agents such as glutaraldehyde or peracetic acid.[9]

Flexible bronchoscopes are cleaned by careful scrubbing of the exterior with a soft cloth and enzymatic detergent. The suction channel must be cleaned by multiple passes of an appropriate cleaning brush. Thorough rinsing is followed by high-level disinfection[8,9] (with glutaraldehyde or peracetic acid) or sterilization (with ethylene oxide).

The lenses of rigid telescopes and flexible bronchoscopes must be carefully scrubbed and polished with a soft cloth during cleaning. Otherwise, small amounts of protein left on the lens will accumulate over time, making the image progressively less satisfactory.

Flexible bronchoscopes and glass rod telescopes are made of glass and are fragile (not to mention expensive). They must never be dropped or subjected to forces that will cause breakage. Flexible bronchoscopes should never be passed through a patient's mouth unless protected by a rigid bite block; an endotracheal tube will not protect the bronchoscope from severe damage by teeth.

The care with which instruments are cleaned and handled must match the care with which they are utilized in the patient's airway. Individuals who are responsible for cleaning and preparing the instruments must be well trained and supervised. The bronchoscopist must assume full responsibility for the care and cleaning of the instrument.

INDICATIONS FOR DIAGNOSTIC BRONCHOSCOPY

It is difficult to categorize the indications for diagnostic bronchoscopy without a great deal of overlap with other chapters. In a given situation, there may be more than one indication for bronchoscopy. In general, however, one may utilize a bronchoscope to define airway anatomy and/or airway dynamics and to obtain specimens for further diagnostic study. The diagnostic result of a particular procedure may include anatomic findings, definition of abnormal airway dynamics, or the results of microbiologic and microscopic evaluation of specimens obtained during the procedure. Bronchoscopy performed for diagnostic purposes may also have therapeutic benefit, such as the removal of a mucus plug causing atelectasis.

It should be noted that there is often great value in a normal bronchoscopic examination; the definitive exclusion of suspected problems (such as foreign body aspiration)[10] may be as important as a specific diagnostic finding. Bronchoscopy (rather than simple laryngoscopy) is often performed for patients in whom the suspected lesion is in the upper airway. Since effective laryngoscopy in children usually requires sedation and laryngeal anesthesia, it adds very little to the risk of the procedure to continue the examination into the lower airways. Unsuspected lesions in the lower airways are not uncommonly found.[2,3]

Airway obstruction is one of the most common general indications for diagnostic bronchoscopy and may involve the upper or lower airways, or both. The extent of anatomic obstruction, especially fixed obstruction in the subglottic space, is often much greater than would be suspected from clinical examination. If a patient is stridulous during the examination, the vibrating structures causing the noise will always be visible, if one is looking in the right place.

Imaging techniques (e.g., CT or MRI scans) can yield considerable diagnostic information about the lungs and even the airways. In some cases, such techniques may make bronchoscopy unnecessary. However, imaging studies are quite limited and cannot provide specimens or (in most cases) define abnormal airway dynamics. In general, radiologic studies should be performed prior to bronchoscopy, as it may be important to direct the focus of the bronchoscopy (e.g., BAL site) to a specific region of the lungs.

In general, there is only one indication for diagnostic bronchoscopy: when there may be information in the lungs or airways that is necessary to the care of the patient and is best obtained by bronchoscopy.

Care must be taken to ensure that airway dynamics are not altered by PPV, which will often prevent dynamic airway collapse. The depth of sedation may also influence the airway dynamics; if the patient is too deeply sedated, abnormal dynamics may not be visible, or muscle relaxation in the upper airway may lead to dynamic collapse that would not occur under ordinary circumstances such as natural sleep. The endoscopic findings must be correlated with the patient's history and the global clinical picture.

The choice between rigid and flexible instruments should be made with some care, if there is a choice available (Table 9-1). In many patients, the combined use of both rigid and flexible instruments can add immeasurably to the value of the procedures. Rigid instruments often distort the airway, while at the same time allowing better visualization of the anatomic details. This is especially true in the larynx and upper trachea. Rigid instruments lift the mandible and hyoid, and they allow a much better view of the posterior aspects of the larynx and cervical trachea. Flexible instruments do not distort the anatomy; they follow the natural curvature of the airway. However, they approach the larynx from behind and are therefore less capable of viewing details of the posterior aspects of the larynx, subglottic space, and cervical trachea (Fig. 9-1).

BRONCHOALVEOLAR LAVAGE

In many cases, bronchoscopic visualization alone is not sufficiently informative. BAL yields a specimen that can give representative data from the distal airways and alveolar surfaces, and it has become one of the more important aspects of diagnostic bronchoscopy.[11,12] BAL may be defined as the instillation into and recovery from the distal airways of a volume of saline that is sufficient to ensure that the fluid returned contains at least some fluid that

TABLE 9-1 INDICATIONS AND INSTRUMENTATION FOR DIAGNOSTIC BRONCHOSCOPY

INDICATION	RIGID INSTRUMENTS	FLEXIBLE INSTRUMENTS
Stridor	May alter airway dynamics	Preferred
Persistent wheeze (not responsive, or poorly responsive to bronchodilator therapy)		Preferred, especially to evaluate distal airway structure and dynamics
Atelectasis (persistent, recurrent, or massive)	May be needed to remove airway obstruction (e.g., foreign body)	
Localized hyperinflation		Preferred
Pneumonia 　Recurrent 　Persistent 　Patients who are unable to produce sputum 　Atypical or in unusual circumstances (e.g., immunocompromised patients)		Preferred (much better to obtain BAL specimens)
Hemoptysis	May be best if there is brisk bleeding	Preferred to evaluate distal airways
Foreign body aspiration 　Known 　Suspected	Mandatory for removal of foreign bodies	May be useful to examine for the possibility of foreign body; rarely useful for removal
Cough (persistent)		Preferred
Suspected aspiration	Preferred to evaluate posterior larynx and cervical trachea	Preferred to obtain BAL Combined use of both instruments very useful
Evaluation of patients with tracheostomies	Preferred to evaluate posterior larynx and subglottic space	Preferred to evaluate tube position and airway dynamics
Suspected mass or tumor	Preferred for laryngeal or tracheal lesions	Preferred for lesions in distal airways
Suspected airway anomalies		
Complications of artificial airways		

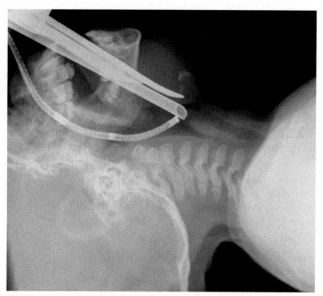

FIGURE 9-1. The rigid bronchoscope approaches the larynx directly, with mandibular lift. The flexible instrument approaches the larynx from behind, making it difficult to evaluate the subglottic space and posterior cervical trachea.

TABLE 9-2 INDICATIONS FOR BAL

Diagnosis of suspected infection
  Pulmonary infiltrates
  Dyspnea
  Hypoxia
  Tachypnea

Recurrent pulmonary infiltrates
Persistent pulmonary infiltrates
Interstitial infiltrates
Diffuse alveolar inflammation
Pulmonary hemorrhage
Alveolar proteinosis
Pulmonary histiocytosis
Suspected aspiration
Lung transplant
Hypereosinophilic lung diseases
Therapeutic removal of materials

was originally present on the alveolar surface. Both soluble and cellular constituents of the alveolar (and small airway) surface fluid are contained in the effluent. This epithelial surface fluid is diluted to an unknown but significant degree by the saline used in its collection. Therefore, the concentrations of substances measured in the BAL fluid do not give an accurate estimate of the concentration at the epithelial surface. Various methods have been employed to derive a reasonable measure of the dilution,[13] although none are free of problems because the epithelial fluid is not static. There is a constant flux of fluid and soluble constituents across the epithelial surface, and the duration and volume of the fluid employed for lavage may have substantial impact on the concentration of substances in the effluent.[14–16] Fortunately, for clinical purposes (and especially in pediatric patients), the information in most cases does not need to be quantitative. The primary value of BAL is to obtain a specimen from the distal airways that is relatively representative and can yield information about infectious or inflammatory processes. In general, BAL performs best in identifying that which does not belong in the airways, and interpretation of findings is highly influenced by the context in which the sample was obtained.

Indications for BAL

BAL is performed primarily for diagnostic purposes, although it can also be performed for therapeutic reasons. The main indications are listed in Table 9-2. BAL may be indicated for the diagnosis of infectious processes when a sputum specimen cannot be obtained or the results from sputum analysis are equivocal. In immunocompetent individuals, this may include the infant or young child who has cystic fibrosis[17,18] with pulmonary symptoms that require therapy. These children may be unable to produce sputum spontaneously, and cultures from the upper airway may either yield no pathogens when the bronchi are infected or yield pathogens when the lungs are sterile. BAL

cultures may identify atypical mycobacteria more reliably than sputum in patients with cystic fibrosis.[19] In immunocompromised individuals, the diagnosis of potential infections in the face of pulmonary infiltrates is valuable and often unattainable without BAL.[20–22] In both immunocompetent and immunocompromised individuals, BAL may help to distinguish infectious from non-infectious processes (such as occult hemorrhage) in the child with radiographic abnormalities. In general, however, if a satisfactory sputum specimen can be obtained, bronchoscopy solely to obtain cultures from the distal airways may not be indicated as a primary approach. It may, however, be indicated when therapy geared toward suspected pathogens based on a sputum sample fails to provide therapeutic benefit. BAL ideally should be performed (especially in immunocompromised patients) before antimicrobial therapy is started, but it may still be informative if there is a lack of clinical response or clinical deterioration.[23]

BAL is often indicated to distinguish infectious from non-infectious processes, such as alveolar hemorrhage (which may occur without frank hemoptysis), pulmonary alveolar proteinosis,[24] interstitial lung diseases,[25,26] or pulmonary infiltrates with eosinophilia.[27,28] BAL is also indicated in the evaluation of patients with suspected aspiration, both to obtain microbiologic specimens to guide antimicrobial therapy and to obtain evidence for the aspiration. Although a specific exogenous marker is not available, the presence of significant numbers of macrophages heavily laden with lipid may support a diagnosis of aspiration.[29] In patients who have undergone lung transplant, BAL is often used in conjunction with transbronchial biopsy to distinguish rejection from infection.[30] The finding of pepsin in the BAL of such patients may also indicate aspiration from GERD, which is a risk factor for non-alloimmune graft rejection.[31,32] BAL alone, however, is not sufficient to establish a diagnosis of transplant rejection.

In addition to diagnostic indications, BAL is occasionally indicated for the therapeutic removal of materials from the airway. This may include the removal of mucus plugs or blood clots, the removal of bronchial casts in plastic bronchitis, or whole lung lavage as a therapy in pulmonary alveolar proteinosis.[33,34] Additionally, BAL may be therapeutic for the removal of foreign lipoid material from the lung to prevent damage to the alveolar structures.

Techniques for BAL

BAL is most conveniently performed during flexible bronchoscopy. Care must be taken to avoid contamination of the lower airway specimen with upper airway secretions during passage of the bronchoscope through the upper airway (or by aspiration following topical laryngeal anesthesia). For routine procedures, it is helpful to gently suction away excessive nasal and oral secretions before inserting the bronchoscope and to continuously flush oxygen through the suction channel (flow approximately 2 L/min) while passing the bronchoscope through the upper airway. Excessive volumes of topical anesthetic should be avoided. Suction should not be performed through the bronchoscope until the tip of the instrument is deep within the lungs. In immunocompromised patients, or those in whom it is vital to minimize ambiguity in the results, it is useful to electively intubate the patient and pass the flexible bronchoscope through the endotracheal tube. The upper airway can then be examined after removing the endotracheal tube. In children who already have a tracheostomy tube in place, performing the BAL through the tracheostomy tube prior to examining the upper airway may lead to less contamination.

After the bronchoscope has been introduced into the lower airway, it should be gently wedged into the selected bronchus. Site selection is based on clinical, bronchoscopic, or radiographic findings and is extremely important. To minimize sampling error, BAL should be performed in the segment of known disease or in an anatomically dependent lobe in the setting of suspected chronic aspiration. Sometimes it is beneficial to perform BAL in multiple lobes. If there is diffuse disease, however, it is advantageous to wedge the bronchoscope into the lingula or right middle lobe bronchus. These bronchi are relatively long and horizontal; the tip of the bronchoscope is more likely to remain wedged into these bronchi during coughing than in a lower lobe bronchus. When the bronchoscope does not remain wedged, saline may spill into other bronchi, producing coughing and possibly respiratory distress.

With the bronchoscope wedged into the bronchus, sterile normal saline is instilled through the suction channel of the bronchoscope and immediately withdrawn. Enough air (1 to 2 mL) should be instilled after each aliquot to ensure clearance of the saline from the suction channel (the volume of the channel can be as high as 2 mL in bronchoscopes with larger suction channels). The fluid may be withdrawn by hand suction with a syringe, or it may be aspirated into a specimen trap. Although enough suction must be applied to overcome the resistance of the channel in the bronchoscope, too much negative pressure may cause the bronchus to collapse, thus preventing efflux of fluid and possibly causing trauma to the airway mucosa. Very short, frequent bursts of suctioning, or suctioning with only partial compression of the suction valve, helps maintain egress of fluid without completely collapsing small bronchi. Fluid return may also be impaired if the patient is not breathing spontaneously. In some patients (such as those with bronchomalacia), almost any amount of negative pressure will result in collapse of the bronchus, and fluid return may be challenging to achieve. In such situations, it may be necessary to instill additional volumes of saline in order to recover a representative specimen. The suction port of a flexible bronchoscope is offset from the optical axis of the instrument, so that if the bronchus into which the instrument is wedged is centered in the image, the suction port may be partially occluded by the bronchial wall. Positioning the bronchoscope so that the image of the bronchus is appropriately off-center may improve fluid return.

Some centers utilize saline that has been warmed to body temperature (37° C) to minimize bronchospasm and increase return,[35] although room temperature saline may be safely used with small-volume BAL. There is no consensus as to the number and volume of aliquots that should be used in BAL. In adult patients, it is common to utilize 3 aliquots of 100 mL or 5 aliquots of 50 mL.[11,12] Various protocols have been used in children. Some bronchoscopists use a standard volume of 10 to 20 mL in 2 to 4 aliquots regardless of body weight and age; others adjust the volume to the patient's FRC based on weight, or they adjust the volume based on weight using 3 mL/kg divided into 3 aliquots with a maximum of 20 mL/aliquot.[36,37] Given the great variability in alveolar surface area being sampled based on the child's size, the size of the bronchoscope, and the location of the wedge, no technique is truly capable of standardization. For clinical purposes, the precise volume is probably of little relevance, as the primary application in children is the detection of infectious agents and examination of the cellular constituents. There should be uniformity in technique within a given institution. For clinical research, consistent protocols may be helpful, but no technique will ensure that the dilution of specimens is truly uniform.

Generally, 40% to 60% of the instilled fluid will be recovered; the remainder of the fluid will be absorbed over a few hours. The first aliquot returned is relatively enriched in fluid from the surface of the conducting airways and may have a higher percentage of inflammatory cells.[38] Some bronchoscopists separate out this first aliquot for culture rather than pooling it with subsequent aliquots, although the bronchial surface fluid will be washed into the alveolar spaces by each aliquot, therefore "contaminating" the subsequent aliquots with bronchial contents. For routine purposes, the small differences in content from one aliquot to the next do not warrant different handling.

Performing a BAL usually prolongs the bronchoscopic procedure by 1 to 3 minutes, minimally increasing the risks of hypoxia, but it is well tolerated by most patients—even those who are critically ill. In patients with thrombocytopenia, BAL could theoretically increase the risk of bleeding, but it can be performed relatively safely in children with platelet counts >20,000 platelets/mL[39] and even fully heparinized for extracorporeal membrane oxygenation.[40] In cases of increased bleeding risk, it is essential to utilize deep sedation/anesthesia and paralysis (to prevent coughing on the scope) and avoid passage through the nose, and to take great care to minimize mechanical trauma to the bronchial mucosa. Some children develop transient fever after BAL, especially if their airways are significantly inflamed, but this is almost always transient and self-limited. A theoretical risk of spreading infection and causing iatrogenic pneumonia exists[6] but is rarely proven. The most problematic complication of BAL is not obtaining the correct information by not preparing for and adequately performing the procedure, or by failing to perform the appropriate analysis of the specimen.

Processing of BAL Specimens

BAL fluid should be processed promptly. To maintain cell viability, some centers keep the sample at 4° C prior to processing,[41] although this is most important if the sample will not be promptly processed by the laboratory and is not generally necessary. The sample should routinely be processed for microbiology and cytologic studies. Some research protocols call for filtering of the BAL fluid prior to processing (e.g., to remove mucus plugs). However, this procedure may alter the diagnostic value of the specimen, as cells and microorganisms may adhere to the filter, and there may be important information hidden within mucus plugs. The bronchoscopist should develop a routine technique for processing with the institutional laboratory service; pediatric specimens may require different processing and interpretation than specimens from adult patients.

Microbiologic studies are performed according to the clinical indications for the procedure. Because of the potential for contamination of BAL specimens by secretions from the oropharynx, semiquantitative culture techniques may help in the interpretation of results. In addition to cultures, other techniques such as special stains or polymerase chain reaction (PCR) may help to identify pathogens; the bronchoscopist should consult with the laboratory to determine what analyses may be available and the specific requirements for specimen volume and handling.

The basic cytologic analysis of a BAL specimen involves a cellular differential, which can be performed with simple stains such as Wright's or Giemsa stain. The specimen is centrifuged on to a slide;[42] most centers perform cytospins at 250 to 500 x g for 5 to 10 minutes.[41] Special stains are performed according to the clinical indications (for example lipid or iron stains, and methenamine-silver stains). Total cell counts may be performed, but they are of relatively limited value in interpretation because of the variable dilution of the specimen.[43] A differential cell count is generally more useful.

Although all BAL samples should be processed routinely for microbiologic studies and cytology, there is wide variability in practice as to the specific tests that are considered routine. This variability stems from differences in patient population, in institutional capabilities and preferences, and in advancing technologies. Table 9-3 lists some potential tests for BAL fluid.

TABLE 9-3 POTENTIAL BAL ASSAYS

Microbiologic Studies

Gram's stain
Cultures
  Bacterial (quantitative)
  Viral
  Fungal
  Mycobacterial
  Anaerobic
Stains
  Gomori-Grocott (methenamine-silver stain)
  Ziehl-Neelsen (acid-fast bacteria [AFB])
Immunoassays
  Chlamydia
  Mycoplasma
  Legionella
  Fungi
  Viruses
PCR
  Viruses
  Chlamydia
  Mycoplasma
In situ
  Viruses

Cytologic Studies

Total cell count
Stains for differential cytology
  Giemsa, Wright's, H&E
Flow cytometry
Trypan blue exclusion for cell viability
Lymphocyte subsets

Special Stains

Lipid Stains
  Oil Red O, Sudan IV
Iron Stain
  Prussian Blue
PAP Stains
  Periodic Acid Schiff

Electron Microscopy

Noncellular components

Surfactant proteins
  Cytokines

Interpretation of BAL Findings

The importance of context in the interpretation of BAL findings cannot be overstated. This includes the clinical characteristics of the patient as well as the location, timing, technique, and handling of the specimen, and the limitations of any tests performed. For instance, the density of a bacterial isolate that will be considered indicative of infection in the BAL from an immunocompromised patient may differ from that of an immunocompetent patient. In a child with chronic aspiration, sampling of a lobe known to be affected by bronchiectasis or a dependent lobe in a posterior lung base may provide the most representative sample. Similarly, BAL may not demonstrate evidence of aspiration in a child with swallowing dysfunction who has been fed solely by nasojejunal tube for the preceding month. Performing BAL in two different lobes in a patient with cystic fibrosis may improve the yield with respect to identification of all pathogens present.[44] To obtain the most accurate assessment, all aspects of clinical situation, timing, technique, and location of BAL must be considered both during the planning of bronchoscopy and at the time of interpretation.

In general, cell numbers in normal children will range between 100,000 and 250,000 cells/mL. Normal BAL fluid contains less than 5% neutrophils (usually 1% to 2%).[43,45,46] Patients with an active bacterial infection may have up to 95% neutrophils, and rarely less than 25%. Patients with a bacterial infection often have bacterial forms visible in the cytoplasm of neutrophils recovered in BAL.[47] This may be a useful measure to differentiate between infection and contamination of the specimen with oral secretions. Increased neutrophils can also be seen in chronic inflammatory states associated with aspiration, cystic fibrosis, ARDS, alveolitis, scleroderma, and asthma. Patients with an active or recent viral respiratory tract infection will also have neutrophilia. Normally, 80% to 90% of the nonepithelial cells in BAL are alveolar macrophages. Lymphocytes are the next most common cell type, composing 5% to 10% of the BAL cells in normal children. Although increased percentages of lymphocytes are not diagnostic of any specific disease, increased numbers are seen in sarcoidosis (20% to 50%), M. tuberculosis infection, interstitial lung disease, hypersensitivity pneumonitis, Pneumocystis jirovecii infection, and nontuberculous mycobacterial infection. Eosinophils are rare in normal subjects (0% to 1%); significant numbers suggest an allergic state, eosinophilic pneumonia, parasitic infection, interstitial lung disease, drug-induced lung disease, Pneumocystis carinii infection, or a foreign body reaction.[27,28] Greater than 25% may be seen in acute or chronic eosinophilic pneumonia, Loeffler syndrome, parasitic infections, Churg-Strauss syndrome, and idiopathic hypereosinophilic syndrome. Epithelial cells are common in BAL fluid but are not counted in the differential. Squamous cells from the upper airway (often covered in oral bacteria) and ciliated columnar cells from the lower airway can be seen.

Opinions vary as to what numbers of bacteria constitute adequate evidence of infection. In general, for common bacterial species such as Staphylococcus aureus, Haemophilus influenzae, and Streptococcus pneumoniae, concentrations of >100,000 organisms/mL of BAL fluid[48] in association with elevated neutrophils are adequate evidence of infection. In the absence of neutrophils (except in neutropenic patients), bacteria are more likely to represent contamination than infection. Density of bacteria in excess of 500,000 organisms/mL is common in clear-cut bacterial infection, as is the finding of intracellular bacteria. However, the interpretation of bacterial cultures is not always straightforward, especially if high densities of "oral flora" are recovered. Children with chronic aspiration of large volumes of oral secretions, for example, may routinely grow a mixture of organisms in association with mucus plugging and a large percentage of neutrophils, and therefore may warrant treatment for a polymicrobial infection. In pediatric patients, it is possible to obtain BAL specimens that are sterile, but the majority will have at least some oral flora even if there are no pathogens. In immunocompromised patients, the finding of pathogens that are not normally in the lung may be diagnostic, regardless of numbers. Pneumocystis jirovecii, Mycobacterium tuberculosis, Legionella pneumophila, Nocardia, Histoplasma, Blastomyces, Mycoplasma, influenza virus, and respiratory syncytial virus would likely represent true pathogens, whereas Herpes simplex virus, CMV, Aspergillus, atypical mycobacteria, and Candida may not be pathogens but merely contaminants or colonizing agents.

Viruses can be grown from BAL fluid, but it may take weeks, limiting the utility of this assay. Using PCR to detect viruses[49] can speed diagnosis and may be more sensitive, but the determination of whether or not a positive result represents an active viral pathogen is more challenging. Another indication of viral infection is the finding of viral cytopathic effect on stains. This is caused by nuclear inclusion bodies that on stain result in a halo or "Owl's eye" around the nucleus. This is not specific but can be helpful in suggesting that an isolated virus is truly a pathogen.

Fungi can be seen on stain, grown in culture, or detected by PCR.[49] Antifungal sensitivities may be determined on isolates grown in culture. A Gomori-Grocott (methenamine-silver) stain helps in the detection of fungi, especially Pneumocystis jirovecii, for which it can be diagnostic. Distinguishing contamination or colonization from true infection can be difficult, and always requires considering a laboratory result in the context of the patient's clinical condition. Mycobacteria must be cultured on special medium and may take up to 8 weeks to grow. With significant infection, the AFB smear may also be positive. Newer molecular methods such as nucleic acid probes[50] or DNA amplification[51] can speed detection.

Periodic Acid Schiff (PAS) staining is used to characterize the diffuse proteinaceous material in pulmonary alveolar proteinosis. The lamellar bodies that define the material as surfactant can be seen on electron microscopy.

Prussian blue stains detect iron in macrophages from pulmonary hemorrhage or hemosiderosis. Macrophages become positive for iron staining 36 to 72 hours after bleeding occurs, not immediately. If no further bleeding occurs, iron will largely clear in 12 to 14 days from the airways and in 2 to 4 weeks from the parenchyma. A small number of alveolar macrophages may continue to stain positive for up to 60 days.[52] It can be normal to have up to 3% of macrophages stain positive for iron.[53] A large percentage of hemosiderin-laden macrophages can be found in any of several disorders resulting from aspiration of blood, alveolar or airway bleeding, or compromise of the alveolar capillary membrane. These include conditions associated with capillaritis, cardiovascular disease, drug reactions, malignancies, post-transplantation, coagulopathy, necrotizing infections, diffuse alveolar damage, or idiopathic pulmonary hemosiderosis.

Oil Red O and Sudan IV will stain lipid if present in the phagosomes of alveolar macrophages. The lipid-laden macrophage index is the most commonly used BAL biomarker for the diagnosis of aspiration of food (from swallowing or gastroesophageal reflux).[29] This technique, however, is plagued by a lack of sensitivity and specificity, and cannot, as a standalone test, diagnose aspiration.[54-57] Despite the logic of utilizing a biomarker of aspiration found in the lungs, there is variability of results due to many factors. First, a lipid stain cannot differentiate the source of the lipid: aspiration from above versus reflux aspiration versus endogenous sources. Secondly, the segment in which a BAL is performed may not be one affected by the aspiration. Third, aspiration is an intermittent phenomenon and can vary in amount and frequency. Therefore, the timing of bronchoscopy may be significant. Also, lipid stains do not identify children who aspirate oral secretions but who are not being fed orally. Despite its flaws, the finding of heavy staining of lipid in alveolar macrophages, especially in the right clinical context, ought to prompt consideration of ongoing aspiration as a potential cause for respiratory symptoms.

Special Techniques

One extension of BAL is whole lung ("bronchopulmonary") lavage, used therapeutically in individuals with pulmonary alveolar proteinosis and a few other rare conditions. Alveolar proteinosis is less common in children than adults. Special techniques may be required for whole lung lavage;[33,34] it can be performed with partial cardiopulmonary bypass or by sequential single lung lavage.

Another special technique is nonbronchoscopic BAL. This involves blindly placing a catheter through an endotracheal or tracheostomy tube into a distal "wedged" position, instilling normal saline and then withdrawing that saline into a trap or syringe.[58] The suction catheter should have only one hole at the end. This is truly a blind procedure and is only likely to yield useful results in diffuse lung disease. Some groups have advocated the use of this technique routinely in neonates who are intubated with small endotracheal tubes.[36] However, the wide availability of a 2.8-mm flexible bronchoscope that can be used through endotracheal tubes as small as 3.5 mm has significantly decreased the need for nonbronchoscopic procedures.

Research Applications

A widely untapped arena for BAL is its use in clinical, translational, and basic science research.[1] In recent years, many new assays have been developed for the detection of inflammatory markers, the function of bronchoalveolar cells, and the detection of a wide array of noncellular BAL components. Some of these are used in clinical assays, such as the determination of lymphocyte subpopulations and the identification of surfactant proteins, but most are used strictly for research purposes. Limited reference data are available from children undergoing elective surgical procedures, as normal children do not ordinarily undergo flexible bronchoscopy with BAL. Development of collaborations and specimen banks may help to better define the normal population, thus allowing research to proceed more rapidly.

◼◼◼ THERAPEUTIC INDICATIONS FOR BRONCHOSCOPY

Therapeutic indications for bronchoscopy in infants and children primarily involve the restoration of airway patency. While the majority of such applications involve the use of a rigid bronchoscope, considerable therapeutic benefit can often be achieved with flexible instruments.

The removal of foreign bodies is one of the more common therapeutic applications of bronchoscopy in children. It is also one of the more difficult and potentially dangerous bronchoscopic procedures. Foreign body removal with a flexible bronchoscope should only be attempted under the most unusual circumstances. The devices that can be passed through a flexible instrument and used for foreign body retrieval are rudimentary at best, and airway management is difficult. Small, peripherally located foreign bodies[59] may best be reached with a flexible bronchoscope, but they may yet be difficult to remove.

Mass lesions in the airways can often be dealt with effectively with a bronchoscope. Granulation tissue is the most common such lesion and may result from foreign bodies, mycobacterial infection, or mechanical trauma associated with artificial airways. Less commonly, tumor masses may be found in children, usually a hemangioma or a bronchial carcinoid tumor.

Benign mass lesions can be resected, if appropriate, with either forceps or a laser. Malignant lesions, or lesions that extend through the bronchial wall, are usually best dealt with surgically rather than endoscopically, although endoscopic resection may be employed for temporary relief of obstruction in selected cases. In general, the use of endobronchial forceps is easier with rigid bronchoscopes; there is better potential for control of bleeding, and the forceps are larger and more readily manipulated than the small, flexible instruments that are used with flexible bronchoscopes. Laser applications may utilize either rigid or flexible instruments.[60,61] In the subglottic space and upper trachea, carbon dioxide lasers are often employed; these lasers require a direct line of sight between the laser and the lesion and are thus much more difficult to employ in the distal airways. Lasers within the near-infrared or visible light spectrum (e.g., neodymium:yttrium-aluminum-garnet [Nd:YAG], argon, KTP) can be operated through a flexible fiber as small as a few hundred microns in diameter. Therefore, these lasers are more appropriate for use in distal airway lesions, although the fibers are still relatively stiff and lesions in the upper lobes may be difficult to reach. Depending on the amount of laser energy delivered, tissue may be vaporized or merely desiccated. A potential risk of vaporization is that the heat produced may injure surrounding normal tissue; lasers should not be used exuberantly. Desiccation, rather than vaporization, of benign lesions may lead to less scarring afterwards.

Tracheal or bronchial stenosis, or severe localized tracheomalacia or bronchomalacia may be treated endoscopically. Depending on the nature of the lesion, the airway may be dilated[62] or lasered,[60,61] or a stent may be placed.[63] The effect of dilation or laser therapy may be temporary, however, and follow-up examinations (and repeated treatments) are almost always required. There is a variety of endobronchial stents that may be placed to ensure airway patency under certain conditions. However, none of these devices is truly appropriate for pediatric patients, and there is little experience with such devices in children, especially young infants. Great caution should be taken when considering stenting in pediatric patients. Stents are associated with numerous problems (e.g., mucus retention, formation of granulation tissue, and migration of the stent). In growing children, a stent has to be replaced periodically; otherwise, the child will develop iatrogenic stenosis. However, if the stent has become embedded in the airway mucosa, it may be nearly impossible to remove safely.[64] Nevertheless, in highly selected patients, stenting may be the only way to achieve and maintain airway patency.

Mucus plugs or blood clots in the airways causing atelectasis will usually yield to endoscopic treatment. Localized trauma from endotracheal suctioning is a common cause of mucus plugs. Children with small (usually organic) foreign bodies, cystic fibrosis, asthma, or allergic bronchopulmonary aspergillosis may also develop central mucus plugs. In some cases, mucus plugs must be removed with forceps, much as though they were a foreign body. Most mucus plugs, however, will yield to suctioning through a flexible bronchoscope. By touching the tip of the flexible bronchoscope to the proximal surface of the mucus plug and applying constant suction, plugs much larger than the diameter of the suction channel can often be removed, even in pieces. Local lavage with saline or a mucolytic agent (1% N-acetylcysteine or dornase alfa) can also be helpful to dislodge a mucus plug.

Alveolar filling disorders such as alveolar proteinosis or lipid aspiration are treated by bronchopulmonary lavage. While this may be accomplished after a fashion, directly through a bronchoscope, it is more effective to utilize large volumes of saline and to lavage relatively large areas of the lung at one time. In adults, a double-lumen endotracheal tube is used[65]; this is not feasible in smaller patients. A flexible bronchoscope can be used to position a single-lumen cuffed endobronchial catheter through which an entire lung can be lavaged with large volumes, while ventilation is maintained with a nasopharyngeal tube.[33] Segmental lavage can also be performed with a flexible bronchoscope.[34]

Flexible bronchoscopes are valuable in the management of tracheostomy and endotracheal tubes. The difficult or complicated intubation can be readily accomplished by passing the endotracheal tube over a flexible bronchoscope.[66] Problems with tube positioning or tube patency can be resolved quickly with a flexible instrument.

Bronchoscopy can be used in the management of intractable air leaks.[67] A systematic search for the bronchus leading to the air leak can be made with a Fogarty catheter, which is inflated in a bronchus while observing the air leak from the chest tube. Alternatively, saline instillation may be used to observe the consistent disappearance of the saline into the bronchus leading to the air leak. When the site of the leak is defined, fibrin glue or Gelfoam can be packed into the bronchus that leads to the site of the air leak. More proximal leaks, as from the stump of a resected bronchus, can be treated directly by application of tissue adhesive.[68]

CONTRAINDICATIONS TO BRONCHOSCOPY

Bronchoscopy should not be performed in the absence of a suitable indication, appropriate equipment, and personnel who are skilled in its use. Otherwise, there are no absolute contraindications to bronchoscopy. However, if the same diagnostic information can be obtained by a less expensive, less invasive, or potentially less hazardous technique, then bronchoscopy is not indicated.

Relative contraindications to bronchoscopy include any factor that will increase the risk. Specific risk factors should be treated and, if possible, alleviated prior to bronchoscopy. Cardiovascular instability, bleeding diatheses (i.e., thrombocytopenia or hypoprothrombinemia), severe bronchospasm, and hypoxemia are primary examples. Some conditions that increase the risk are themselves indications for bronchoscopy, such as severe airway obstruction. In these cases, the procedure is performed with both diagnostic and therapeutic intent, and it can be life-saving. Appropriate modifications must be made in the techniques chosen for anesthesia and monitoring when there are additional risk factors.

ANESTHESIA FOR BRONCHOSCOPY

Safe and effective bronchoscopy requires that the patient be safe, comfortable, and reasonably still during the procedure. Adequate oxygenation and ventilation must be maintained, and the patient must be carefully and continuously monitored. Depending on the individual child's situation and the procedure planned, these criteria can be met with either light general anesthesia or with sedation (usually performed by the intravenous administration of a narcotic and/or a benzodiazepine[69] and administered by the bronchoscopist). Sedation and general anesthesia are merely points on a continuum between the fully awake state and surgical anesthesia; it matters little how the desired safe state is achieved. Furthermore, "conscious sedation," in which reflexes are preserved and the patient may respond to verbal instructions, is not appropriate for most pediatric procedures. Deep sedation and light "general anesthesia" are virtually indistinguishable. An advantage of general anesthesia is that an anesthesiologist takes full responsibility for monitoring the patient, thus allowing the bronchoscopist to concentrate on the endoscopy. Additionally, the drugs used by anesthesiologists have a more rapid onset and recovery than the typical narcotic/benzodiazepine combination. Current practice guidelines for sedation[70] mandate the presence of a trained individual whose sole responsibility is to monitor the patient, although this person does not have to be an anesthesiologist. Our current practice at Cincinnati Children's Hospital is to utilize an anesthesiologist, and the child is sedated with general anesthetic agents (inhaled or given intravenously) to a point that maintains spontaneous breathing but ensures safety and comfort.

Sedation and anesthesia diminish or abolish protective reflexes. To reduce the risk for aspiration of gastric contents, patients should be given nothing by mouth for several hours prior to the procedure. Clear liquids may be given up to 2 hours before the procedure.[71,72] It is prudent to aspirate the stomach with a catheter before proceeding with the bronchoscopy. Young infants may become dehydrated or hypoglycemic if kept NPO for too long, and intravenous fluid may be necessary prior to a procedure.

General anesthesia should be employed in any situation in which intravenous sedation is not suitable. Children who have undergone numerous invasive procedures are often difficult to sedate, and there should be a low threshold for switching to general anesthesia. Likewise, children who have a history of difficult sedation are poor candidates for repeated attempts at sedation. Unstable upper airway obstruction is a prime indication for general anesthesia because sedation may result in significant hypoxemia or a sudden need for an artificial airway. In this case, the use of a very–short-acting agent (e.g., propofol) or an inhalational agent may reduce the risk, while the usual agents used for intravenous sedation increase the risk. General anesthesia should be considered for complicated and/or prolonged procedures (e.g., the extraction of extensive mucus plugs) or for laser procedures.

When general anesthesia is utilized for diagnostic bronchoscopy, careful attention must be given to airway dynamics. If the patient does not breathe spontaneously, then the usual airway dynamics are reversed; airway pressure during inspiration exceeds that during expiration. This may result in diagnostic confusion in patients with tracheomalacia and/or bronchomalacia. During therapeutic procedures, PPV is often utilized.

Flexible bronchoscopes are small enough that the patient can usually breathe around them. Spontaneous breathing is the rule for most flexible procedures. However, in some circumstances it may be necessary to provide for PPV. This is simple if the patient is intubated with an endotracheal tube that is large enough to accommodate the flexible bronchoscope. However, this approach may present problems in very small children. Ventilation may be assisted via a mask (through which the flexible bronchoscope is passed), a laryngeal mask airway, or a nasopharyngeal tube.[73] The introduction of 2.8-mm flexible bronchoscopes dramatically extended downward the size of endotracheal tubes through which a flexible bronchoscope can be passed while maintaining PPV (3.5 mm endotracheal tubes versus 5.0 mm with the 3.5 mm instrument).

Many techniques are suitable for effective general anesthesia during bronchoscopy. Traditional inhalational agents (e.g., halothane) are being replaced by newer, short-acting agents (e.g. sevoflurane and propofol). The safety record of general anesthesia in recent years has removed many of the earlier objections to its use, and pediatric patients should not be deprived of its benefits when appropriate.

Like general anesthesia, sedation may be produced by a variety of agents and techniques.[69] Important principles of sedation include careful preparation of the patient; the use of fractional doses of short-acting agents with titration of total dose to the needed effect; appropriate monitoring before, during, and after the procedure; and careful selection of agents.

In general, the drugs chosen for sedation should be matched to the specific needs of the child and the procedure. For totally noninvasive procedures such as MRI, purely sedative agents (e.g., chloral hydrate)[74] or a barbiturate, may be used.[75] However, invasive procedures that involve any discomfort (and this would include bronchoscopy) are best performed with an analgesic agent (e.g., a narcotic) as well as an amnesic agent (e.g., a benzodiazepine), or with properly applied general anesthesia.

Sedative agents have a variety of physiologic effects in addition to reducing the level of consciousness. The most important of these is depression of respiratory drive, which may last longer than the sedation. Children who have undergone sedation for procedures may be at greater risk after the procedure is completed than during the procedure itself. This is because there is no longer the stimulation of the procedure, and staff awareness and alertness may be diminished. Effective monitoring must be continued until all the effects of sedation have resolved.[70]

Pharmacologic agents to reverse the effect of narcotics and benzodiazepines are available, and some physicians utilize these agents routinely at the completion of procedures.[76] This is not necessarily a good idea, however, as their effect is considerably shorter than the respiratory depression induced by the sedative agents. Furthermore, patients awakened abruptly from sedation are often disturbed and may become combative. Monitoring must be continued whether or not a reversal agent has been given; indeed, it may be argued that monitoring must be continued longer after reversal than without it. On the other hand, such agents should always be readily available in the event of serious respiratory depression.

No matter how it is administered, sedation involves more than giving drugs. Children are often very responsive to suggestion, whether positive or negative and whether intentional or inadvertent. Simple distraction or more formal methods of focusing attention on something other than the procedure[77,78] may be surprisingly effective in children, especially in the 3- to 8-year age group. Even infants respond to tone of voice and the atmosphere around them. Careful preparation of the child and the parents, focusing on positive aspects and creating positive expectation, can be powerful adjuncts to pharmacologic sedation. On the other hand, negative suggestion can make even the most powerful drugs less effective. A screaming, upset child will require much higher doses of virtually any agent to achieve effective sedation, and that child's recovery will be prolonged. For this reason, presedation with oral drugs (e.g., chloral hydrate or midazolam) and careful attention to atmosphere and language can often facilitate deeper sedation with minimal doses of other agents.

During the process of sedation or induction of anesthesia, many children experience a phase of disinhibition or excitement, during which their behavior may be difficult to control. This should be expected and not be interpreted as an adverse or allergic reaction to the drug used. In fractional dosing for sedation, a sufficient dose should be given initially to get beyond the disinhibition phase; if very small doses are given initially, disinhibition may be prolonged, and the total sedative dose required may be significantly increased.

TECHNIQUES FOR BRONCHOSCOPY

Facilities for Bronchoscopy

It is important that bronchoscopy be performed in a suitable facility. Because of the need for general anesthesia, rigid bronchoscopy is almost always performed in an operating room. The relative ease with which flexible bronchoscopy can be performed makes it tempting to use the instrument in unconventional places such as at the bedside or in an emergency room. While there are clearly circumstances in which such practice is justified, bronchoscopy is a serious procedure with the potential for lethal complications, and it should be performed only by physicians who are well trained and with full preparation for all contingencies. Therefore, a fully equipped and staffed endoscopy suite or operating room is the most appropriate venue. With suitable preparation, bronchoscopy (rigid or flexible) can be performed at the bedside in an intensive care unit, but this may still place the bronchoscopist at a disadvantage in terms of access to equipment and supplies in the event of difficulties. If bronchoscopy is performed in an intensive care unit, the bronchoscopist must take along everything that possibly will be needed and have it readily at hand.

Rigid Bronchoscopy

The appropriate rigid bronchoscope (length and diameter) is chosen for the patient. Under a satisfactory level of general anesthesia, the patient is positioned supine with the shoulders supported and the head slightly extended. The larynx is exposed with a laryngoscope, and the tip of the bronchoscope is gently advanced through the glottis and into the trachea. With the proximal end of the bronchoscope closed with a lens cap or with a telescope in place, the side port is attached to the anesthesia circuit and the patient can be ventilated with positive pressure.

The bronchoscope is manipulated to visualize the tracheal and bronchial anatomy; the head and neck may be turned to help direct the bronchoscope into the main-stem bronchi. Telescopes greatly facilitate inspection and can be used in conjunction with a video camera. Angulated telescopes make it much easier to visualize the upper lobe segments. The telescope must be removed and cleaned if the lens becomes covered with secretions; suctioning is performed with a suction pipe or a suction catheter. During suctioning, ventilation may be momentarily interrupted. It is also possible to work for extended periods with an open proximal end, while maintaining ventilation with a Venturi jet injector.[79]

When instrumentation is required (e.g., the removal of a foreign body), the instruments may be passed through the open channel of the bronchoscope. Unfortunately, this significantly impairs the view of the operative site, as the instruments obstruct the line of vision. Optical forceps, which incorporate the glass rod telescope and allow direct visualization of the operative site, are in most cases the preferred instrument for biopsy and for foreign body extraction. Very small flexible forceps can also be passed through a side arm and alongside the telescope, but the tip of these instruments may be difficult to control.

At Cincinnati Children's Hospital, the vast majority of rigid bronchoscopic procedures (including foreign body removal) are performed using only the glass rod telescopes; the open tube sheath is employed in special circumstances. This technique requires that the patient breathe spontaneously, so anesthetic technique is critical; however it is much easier to evaluate airway dynamics.

Because the overall size of the instruments is smaller, mechanical complications are less frequent.

Flexible Bronchoscopy

Most diagnostic procedures can be performed in pediatric patients with the standard 2.8-mm or 3.5-mm pediatric flexible instrument. In older children, a larger instrument may be used (especially if a larger suction channel is needed), while in very small infants it may be appropriate to use a 2.2-mm ultrathin bronchoscope. The patient is properly prepared for the procedure and is positioned supine with the head and neck in a neutral position. In special circumstances, it is possible to perform flexible bronchoscopy in a sitting or other position.

Flexible bronchoscopes are usually inserted transnasally. This avoids the potential for the patient to bite (and thus destroy) the instrument and also affords a view of the nasal and nasopharyngeal anatomy. Another advantage of this approach is that the bronchoscope does not contact the tongue; the tongue is a very powerful muscle and can readily move the bronchoscope in ways contrary to the intent of the bronchoscopist. A flexible bronchoscope may also be inserted orally if desired, always with a suitable bite block, even with the patient under general anesthesia, or through an artificial airway such as an endotracheal tube (with a bite block) or tracheostomy tube.

The tip of the flexible bronchoscope can be flexed or extended in a single plane; movement to one side or another is accomplished by rotation. The instrument is directed to the site of interest by advancing the shaft while controlling the angulation and rotation at the tip. This combination of three simultaneous movements requires good hand-eye coordination on the part of the bronchoscopist. In contrast to glass rod telescopes, the image rotates as the instrument is rotated; this may produce disorientation on the part of the operator who is unaccustomed to using flexible instruments. As the instrument is advanced through the airway, secretions may be removed by suctioning, and topical anesthetic can be applied (also through the suction channel).

The patient must be able to breathe around the instrument. Most infants who are 3 kg or larger can breathe satisfactorily around the standard 3.5-mm pediatric flexible bronchoscope (infants larger than about 1.5 kg can usually breathe around the 2.8-mm instrument). Smaller infants will not be able to do so, and their procedures must be performed with an ultrathin instrument or with apneic technique. If the patient is intubated, the bronchoscope must be small enough to readily pass through the tube (Table 9-4).

Flexible bronchoscopes are much smaller than rigid instruments (although the glass rod telescopes are equally small if used alone) and can be advanced much farther into the distal airways. Depending on the instrument used and the size of the patient, airways as small as 2 mm and as far as 14 to 16 generations from the carina may be inspected.

The instruments that can be passed through a flexible bronchoscope are quite limited because of the small diameter of the suction channel (1.2 mm in pediatric instruments, 2.0 to 3.2 mm in "adult" instruments). The most common of these instruments are cup or "alligator" biopsy forceps,

TABLE 9-4 ARTIFICIAL AIRWAYS AND FLEXIBLE BRONCHOSCOPES USED IN PEDIATRIC PATIENTS

INSTRUMENT DIAMETER	SMALLEST TUBE THAT CAN BE USED*	SMALLEST TUBE FOR ASSISTED VENTILATION	SMALLEST TUBE FOR SPONTANEOUS VENTILATION
2.2 mm	2.5 mm	3.0 mm	3.5 mm
2.8 mm	3.0 mm	3.5 mm	4.0 mm
3.5 mm	4.5 mm	5.0 mm	5.5 mm
4.7 mm	5.5 mm	6.0 mm	6.5 mm

*For intubation only

brushes, grasping forceps, expandable basket retrieval devices, angioplasty balloon catheters (for dilation of stenoses), microcautery electrodes, and laser fibers.

Special Procedures

Transbronchial biopsies can be obtained through flexible or rigid bronchoscopes for the investigation of localized or diffuse lung disease.[80–82] The forceps are passed through the bronchoscope into the selected bronchus and are advanced to the desired depth, opened, advanced, closed, and withdrawn. This is best done with fluoroscopic guidance, both to reduce the risk of complications (e.g., penetration of the pleura) and to maximize success in obtaining adequate specimens from the desired area. Such specimens are very small, even with the largest available instruments, but they are useful in the diagnosis and management of selected lung diseases. Because of the small size of the specimens and the nature of pediatric lung disease, as well as for technical reasons, transbronchial biopsy is performed much less frequently in children than in adults (primarily in lung transplant recipients). Complications of transbronchial biopsy include bleeding (which may be massive), pneumothorax, and perforation of other organs.

Biopsy of endobronchial lesions is more straightforward and can yield useful diagnostic information. Such lesions are less common in pediatric patients than in adult patients (where malignant lesions are much more frequent). Small biopsy specimens can be obtained with flexible forceps via a flexible bronchoscope, under direct vision. Because of the very small size of such specimens and the risk of bleeding, biopsy of endobronchial lesions may be best done with a rigid instrument; this allows the use of larger forceps and perhaps better control of hemorrhage should it occur. Endobronchial lesions in pediatric patients are most often granulation tissue, but tumors (e.g., hemangiomas or carcinoid tumors) may also be found. These bleed rather vigorously when biopsied.

In adults (and, by extension, adolescents—although the indications are much less common), needle aspiration samples can be taken from lymph nodes or tumor masses that are adjacent to the trachea or main bronchi, using blind or ultrasound guided technique. Great caution must be taken to ensure that what is biopsied is not a blood vessel.

Bronchial brushing is performed to obtain specimens of bronchial epithelial cells for a variety of studies (e.g., morphologic, physiologic, and molecular). Flexible cytology brushes are passed through the bronchoscope, and the bronchial surface is gently abraded to obtain the specimen. One potential problem with brushing is the loss of much of the specimen (or contamination of the specimen) when the brush is withdrawn through the bronchoscope. To minimize this problem, many cytology brushes are packaged with an outer sheath and have very short bristles. The sheath is passed through the bronchoscope, the brush is extended to collect the specimen, and then the brush is withdrawn into the sheath. With conventional technique, up to several hundred thousand epithelial cells can be obtained in this fashion.

Brushes are also used to obtain specimens for microbiologic diagnosis. One potential advantage of bronchoscopy is that specimens can be obtained from the lower airways without contamination by mouth flora. Unfortunately, however, there is a significant risk of such contamination by passage of the bronchoscope through the nose and/or mouth on the way to the distal airways. Specimens obtained by simple aspiration through the bronchoscope often show evidence of oral flora. To surmount this problem, a protected microbiology specimen brush has been developed.[83] This brush is protected by two concentric sheaths; the outer sheath is plugged with wax to prevent secretions in the bronchoscope channel from contaminating the brush. This specimen collection system functions very well to avoid contamination of the brush specimen by secretions present in the suction channel of the bronchoscope. Unfortunately, however, it does not guarantee freedom from contamination by upper airway flora. If any oral secretions are aspirated into the trachea and bronchi during the preparation for the procedure and insertion of the bronchoscope, then the site from which the specimen is collected will be contaminated, and it makes relatively little difference what technique is used to obtain the specimen. Topical laryngeal anesthesia almost always results in contamination of the trachea and at least central bronchi to some extent with oral flora.

Foreign body extraction should be performed with a rigid bronchoscope.[84,85] When the foreign body is a manufactured object, it is helpful to practice on an identical object to ensure that the forceps chosen will allow a firm grasp of the object. There is a great variety of forceps available for use with different types of foreign bodies. It may be helpful to pass a balloon catheter beyond the foreign body and then use the inflated balloon to pull the object proximally.[86] Foreign body extraction may be complicated by the presence of inspissated secretions or granulation tissue. Foreign bodies such as nuts, which may fragment, may be present in multiple sites, and a very thorough examination of all bronchi should be made after removing a foreign body. In rare circumstances, such as a straight pin lodged in the periphery of the lung, a flexible bronchoscope may be better than a rigid instrument for foreign body removal.

Laser applications in bronchoscopy[87] (other than for subglottic or high tracheal lesions) are relatively uncommon in pediatric patients. However, in selected circumstances,[61] a laser can be used to ablate tissue in a very controlled, hemorrhage-free manner. A quartz laser fiber can be passed through a rigid or flexible bronchoscope to direct the laser energy very precisely. Lesions as small as 0.5 mm can be created, but care must be taken to ensure that the energy delivered does not create enough steam to injure surrounding normal tissue.

Balloon dilation of bronchial or tracheal stenoses is a useful technique that can eliminate the need for thoracotomy in some patients. An angioplasty balloon catheter is used; these devices can be inflated at very high pressure (up to 15 atmospheres). A catheter with a predetermined inflated diameter is positioned in the desired location under direct vision. The balloon is then inflated, and a pressure of several atmospheres is maintained for 30 to 60 seconds before deflating the balloon. In most cases such catheters cannot easily be passed through the suction channel of a pediatric flexible bronchoscope, but a flexible instrument can be used to guide the positioning of a catheter that has been passed alongside the bronchoscope (either through an endotracheal tube or a rigid bronchoscope).

Bronchoscopic intubation is a technique that facilitates difficult or complicated intubations,[66,88,89] and it should virtually always be successful if the right instruments are available and the operator is skilled in their use. A flexible bronchoscope is passed through a suitable endotracheal tube, and the bronchoscope is then passed into the trachea (usually through the nose, but an oral approach may be used instead). With the tip of the bronchoscope held just above the carina, the endotracheal tube is advanced over the flexible bronchoscope until its tip is seen through the bronchoscope. The bronchoscope must be held so that its shaft is straight while the endotracheal tube is advanced over it; otherwise, damage to the bronchoscope may result. The bronchoscope is withdrawn, the patient is ventilated, and then the bronchoscope is inserted again to verify the position of the endotracheal tube and to ensure that the anatomy and patency of the distal airways are adequate.

COMPLICATIONS OF BRONCHOSCOPY

Every procedure has the potential for complications, ranging from trivial to lethal. Bronchoscopy is no exception, although lethal complications in pediatric patients are rare. The risk of complications is a function of inherent risk factors in the patient (e.g., disease state, severity of disease, age), the procedure performed, the skill and experience of the bronchoscopist and bronchoscopy team, and the patient's preparation for the procedure.

In general, the risk is greater with rigid bronchoscopy than with flexible bronchoscopy. This is because foreign body extraction is perhaps the most challenging, difficult, and risky bronchoscopic procedure commonly performed in pediatric patients, and it is always done with a rigid instrument. In addition, the relatively large diameter and rigid nature of the bronchoscope make it more likely to traumatize the mucosa of the subglottic space or airways. However, flexible bronchoscopy is not immune to serious complications, and at least one death has been reported in association with a flexible bronchoscopy in a pediatric patient.[90] Disaster lurks around the corner for the unwise or unwary.[2,91]

Mechanical complications of bronchoscopy result from direct trauma to the airway. Pneumothorax or pneumomediastinum, subglottic edema, and hemorrhage are the most common. Such complications are more likely when auxiliary instruments such as biopsy forceps are used. The greatest risk is incurred during the extraction of foreign bodies and in the performance of transbronchial biopsy. The risk of mechanical complications can be reduced by careful selection of instruments and procedures.

Physiologic complications of bronchoscopy include hypoxia, hypercapnia, hypotension, laryngospasm, bronchospasm, cardiac arrhythmias, and aspiration. There is a constant risk of hypoventilation during bronchoscopy due to anesthesia or airway obstruction. Smaller patients are at greater risk of airway obstruction. All bronchoscopes (rigid as well as flexible) produce some degree of airway obstruction. Vagal stimulation due to inadequate topical anesthesia or catecholamine release due to inadequate sedation/anesthesia may result in cardiac arrhythmia. Laryngospasm or bronchospasm are usually due to inadequate topical anesthesia. Seizures can result from lidocaine toxicity. The risk of physiologic complications can be reduced by careful attention to patient preparation and to anesthetic and monitoring techniques.

Bacteriologic complications of bronchoscopy include the introduction of infectious agents into the lung from the patient's upper airway, or from another patient if the instruments are not adequately cleaned and sterilized. Infection in one part of a patient's lung can be spread to other areas. Although the risk appears to be low, it is possible that bacterial endocarditis could occur in susceptible patients following bronchoscopy; appropriate antimicrobial prophylaxis should be considered for the patient at risk. However, if a BAL specimen is to be obtained for culture, the prophylactic antibiotics should not be administered until after the BAL specimen is obtained. Bronchoscopy can also result in the spread of infectious agents from the patient to the personnel performing the bronchoscopy; sensible precautions should be taken to protect personnel. Older patients known to have cavitary tuberculosis, for example, represent a very high risk to the bronchoscopy team, and bronchoscopy should be delayed in most cases until appropriate therapy has been given for a sufficient time to greatly reduce this risk.

There are also cognitive risks of bronchoscopy: the failure to obtain useful information or making the wrong diagnosis. Other than death of the patient, the most serious risk of diagnostic bronchoscopy is to perform the procedure and obtain the wrong diagnostic result. Even failure to perform bronchoscopy when it is the best or only way to obtain information necessary for the patient's care could be considered an error or complication. The bronchoscopist must be aware of the many pitfalls that await the unwary.[89] Video recording the procedure allows later review of the observations and sometimes leads to a revision of the diagnosis. To augment teaching, consultative reports, and even research data acquisition, serious consideration should be given to recording all procedures.

Cognitive risks are reduced by adequate training and experience on the part of the bronchoscopist and support staff. There is no simple guideline as to the requirements for training of a bronchoscopist; obviously, inherent aptitude varies greatly from individual to individual. In order to safely and effectively perform procedures, the bronchoscopist must develop both manual skills and an effective knowledge of anatomy, pathology, indications for bronchoscopy, and techniques for anesthesia/sedation. A formal, comprehensive training program should be a prerequisite, but there is no substitute for good judgment and experience. Most authorities suggest that a minimum of 50 to 100 procedures performed with a suitable mentor are required before an individual should be certified to do bronchoscopy independently.[92,93]

Complications of bronchoscopy may include more than adverse effects on the patient or personnel. Failure to utilize a bite block when a flexible bronchoscope is passed through a patient's mouth, for example, can result in destruction of the instrument. Flexible bronchoscopes currently cost in excess of $20,000 (USD). The smaller the bronchoscope, the more fragile the instrument. Flexible bronchoscopes are often damaged during passage through endotracheal tubes. Biopsy forceps can also perforate the suction channel, thus decommissioning the instrument.

Economic Aspects of Bronchoscopy

Bronchoscopy is not a simple, inexpensive procedure. Total cost will depend on institutional variables as well as the nature and extent of the procedure performed. Specific costs include support for equipment and procedure rooms, consumable supplies, laboratory charges for processing of diagnostic specimens, monitoring of the sedated patient before and after the procedure, record keeping, support of ancillary staff, and professional fees.

When general anesthesia is used instead of sedation performed by the bronchoscopist, costs are generally higher, but this should not be a significant factor in decision making if the services of an anesthesiologist significantly enhance the safety of the patient.[94]

Although definitive studies of cost-effectiveness in pediatric practice have not been reported, bronchoscopy is often a cost-saving procedure. For example, the early identification of a specific infectious agent in the immunocompromised patient with pneumonia can mean that more expensive multiple antimicrobial therapies can be avoided (thus also reducing potential risk of complications of such treatment). Young patients with cystic fibrosis who are admitted to hospital for intensive therapy are sometimes discovered at bronchoscopy to have no evidence of bacterial infection; evidence may be found instead for other causes of the persisting symptoms (such as gastroesophageal reflux with microaspiration). The definitive identification of causes of pulmonary symptoms such as stridor can reduce "doctor shopping" and multiple expensive diagnostic evaluations. The cost associated with missed diagnoses (when bronchoscopy is not performed) may be enormous.

References

The complete reference list is available online at www.expertconsult.com

10 DIAGNOSTIC IMAGING OF THE RESPIRATORY TRACT

Carolyn Young, HDCR, Øystein E. Olsen, PhD, and Catherine M. Owens, BSc, MBBS, MRCP, FRCR

Pediatric chest radiology is a complex subject, and the clinical sections of this book cover a full understanding of all relevant pathologies with which it aids diagnosis. This chapter gives a brief overview of the imaging modalities used to help achieve an accurate and timely diagnosis, thus enabling prompt treatment of the many varied pathologic entities encountered within the pediatric thorax. The dedicated reader may wish to consult more specialized and comprehensive texts.[1–3]

The utility of imaging modalities is often uncertain because of: (1) an increasing number of available techniques and (2) the presence of numerous rare disease entities in children. Nevertheless, modern clinical practice is highly dependent on radiology.

We will discuss areas of specific concern within the pediatric age group, in particular: (1) radiation protection; (2) technical challenges (e.g., motion and breathing artifacts); (3) developing anatomy and pathophysiology; and (4) to a certain degree, different interpretation of images compared with images obtained in adults.

PLAIN RADIOGRAPHY

The plain chest radiograph remains the basis for the evaluation of the chest in childhood. In the neonate, satisfactory films can be obtained in incubators using modern mobile x-ray apparatus. The baby lies on the cassette, and the film is exposed. Although one can make automatic triggering of the exposure, an experienced radiographer will usually be able to judge the end of inspiration. An adequate inspiration occurs with the right hemidiaphragm at the level of the eighth rib posteriorly. Films in expiration frequently show a sharp rightward kink in the trachea and varying degrees of opacification of the lung fields, with apparent enlargement of the heart. Films should be well-collimated, with the baby positioned as straight as possible. Lordotic films should be avoided, especially if the size of the heart is of particular interest. Monitoring equipment should be removed to the extent that is safe clinically.

Computed radiography is particularly useful in intensive care, and the facility of data manipulation (e.g., edge enhancement) improves visualization of supportive apparatus, such as tubes and lines.

Children older than 5 years of age can usually cooperate sufficiently to stand for a posteroanterior film in the same way as adults. In younger children, some form of chest stand is needed in which an assistant, preferably the caregiver, can hold the child in front of a cassette while standing behind a suspended protective lead apron. With proper collimation, the dose to the caregiver is small, and this position allows straighter positioning of the child than a position to the side. The difference between a posteroanterior projection and an anteroposterior projection in the small child is usually negligible. High-kilovoltage technique, with added filtration and the use of a grid, allows evaluation of the trachea and major bronchi, which is important in stridor.

SPECIFIC FEATURES OF THE CHEST RADIOGRAPH IN CHILDREN

The Thymus

The normal thymus (Fig. 10-1) is a frequent cause of widening of the anterior mediastinum during the first years of life. The lateral margin often shows an undulation, the thymic wave, which corresponds to the indentations of the ribs on the inner surface of the thoracic cage. Particularly on the right, the thymus may have a triangular, sail-like configuration. The thymus may involute in times of stress, and steroids can induce a decrease in size. At times, the differentiation of a physiologic thymus from pathology in the anterior mediastinum can be difficult. Ultrasound examination will usually differentiate cystic lesions from the homogeneous normal thymic tissue. Occasionally, the normal thymus can act as a significant space-occupying structure in the superior mediastinum, and in such cases, differentiation may be helped by either ultrasound or magnetic resonance imaging (MRI), which shows homogeneous echogenicity/signal within a normal thymus. On MRI, a normal thymus has intermediate signal on T2-weighted images (similar to the spleen and lymph nodes) and shows minimal uniform enhancement on T1-weighted images after intravenous contrast medium injection (Fig. 10-2).

The Cardiothoracic Ratio

In toddlers, the cardiothoracic ratio can at times exceed 0.5, and care should be exercised in overdiagnosis of cardiomegaly, particularly if the film may be expiratory.

Kink of the Trachea to the Right

Kinking of the trachea to the right is a frequent feature of a chest film taken at less than full inspiration. This is a physiologic buckling and does not represent a mass lesion.

Soft Tissue

Soft tissue may be prominent in children, and the anterior axillary fold that crosses the chest wall can mimic pneumothorax. Similarly, skin folds can cast confusing shadows at times. Plaits of hair over the upper chest can mimic pulmonary infiltrations in the upper lobes.

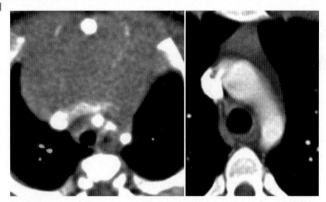

FIGURE 10-1. Axial contrast-enhanced computed tomography shows the considerable difference in thymic size in a 3-month-old child compared with a 10-year-old child.

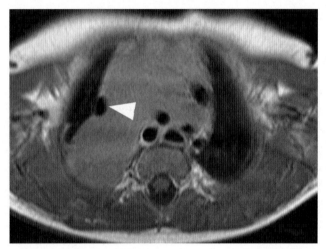

FIGURE 10-2. Chest radiograph *(not shown)* in a 3-month-old child showed an unusual upper mediastinal contour. Magnetic resonance imaging (T1-weighted spin echo after intravenous injection of gadolinium chelate) shows normal signal and no abnormal contrast enhancement from a normal, but large thymus, extending posterior to the right brachiocephalic vein *(arrowhead)*. There is no sign of vascular or airway compression.

Pleural Fluid

Whereas in adults an early sign of pleural effusion is blunting of the costophrenic angles, in children it is more common to see separation of the lung from the chest wall, with reasonable preservation of the clarity of the costophrenic angles and accentuation of the lung fissures. In the supine position, an apical rim of soft tissue density is seen, and if a moderate to large unilateral effusion is present, the affected hemithorax has a diffuse increase in density, with preservation of vascular markings simulating ground-glass parenchymal opacification. This is due to pleural fluid collecting in the dorsal (dependent) pleura.

▬▬ SYSTEMATIC REVIEW OF THE CHEST RADIOGRAPH

Without a systematic analytical approach to the pediatric chest radiograph, the possibility of missing relevant radiologic information is high. To combat this, knowledge of the various pitfalls in interpretation, anatomic variants, and pathologic processes relevant to the specific age group are vital. This is particularly important when there is one very conspicuous abnormal imaging finding, which can result in cessation of more intense scrutiny of the remainder of the film. Image review should therefore follow a strict systematic order, including checking the putative identity of the radiograph, and should include the following.

General Degree of Lung Inflation

Flattening of the diaphragm or diaphragmatic domes below the level of the eighth posterior ribs, elongation of the mediastinum, and widening of the intercostal spaces are all signs of pulmonary overinflation. Intercostal bulging of the pleura or lung parenchyma may be a sign of high ventilator pressures in an intubated child.

Generalized pulmonary underinflation is usually due to radiographic exposure during expiration, but it may be a real finding confirming small lung volumes (as in cases of idiopathic respiratory distress syndrome, in which the lung parenchyma is noncompliant, or in bilateral pulmonary hypoplasia) or associated with lobar collapse.

One should also consider elevation of the diaphragm, with consequential lung compression due to bowel distention, pneumoperitoneum, or the presence of a large abdominal mass. Hence, the periphery of the radiograph (e.g., the area under the diaphragm) should always be carefully and routinely inspected as part of a systematic review.

Asymmetrical Lung Volume

In the absence of pneumothorax, mediastinal shift toward a lung with uniformly increased density compared with the contralateral lung is a sign of differential inflation of the two lungs. This may be caused by overinflation of the more lucent lung (e.g., due to a ball-valve mechanism in the central airways), in which case the ipsilateral hemidiaphragm would be flattened (Fig. 10-3).

Alternatively, it may be caused by volume loss in the denser lung, in which case the diaphragm of the denser hemithorax would be elevated. This may be a sign of unilateral pulmonary hypoplasia, aplasia, or agenesis (Figs. 10-4 to 10-6), in which case the mediastinum is shifted toward the hemithorax containing the small lung, and ipsilateral elevation of the hemidiaphragm is seen. Combined overinflation of one lung and volume loss of the other can sometimes be seen secondary to mass lesions that affect the central airways (Fig. 10-7).

Other causes of asymmetrical lung volumes include diaphragmatic paresis/paralysis and a large abdominal mass lesion that causes elevation of the ipsilateral hemidiaphragm. The diaphragm may also be apparently elevated secondary to a subpulmonic fluid collection. In congenital diaphragmatic hernia, the multicystic appearance of bowel content may or may not be obvious within the thorax (Fig. 10-8). If seen, it may sometimes be difficult to distinguish from congenital cystic adenomatoid malformation (Table 10-1).

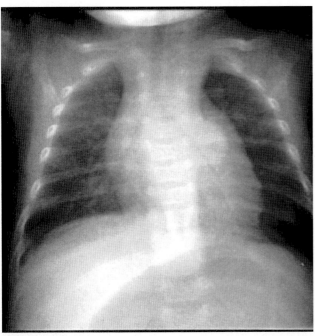

FIGURE 10-3. Chest radiograph in a young child shows a semicircular left convex distortion of the left mediastinal outline due to a bronchogenic cyst and secondary overinflation of the left lower lobe.

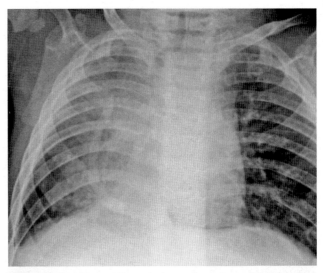

FIGURE 10-5. Chest radiograph shows a hypoplastic right lung with an abnormal vascular structure running toward the diaphragmatic level medially. This represents systemic venous drainage of the right lung. The shape of the abnormal vein resembles a Turkish scimitar (bowed sword), hence, the denotation scimitar syndrome (see Figures 10-39 and 10-41).

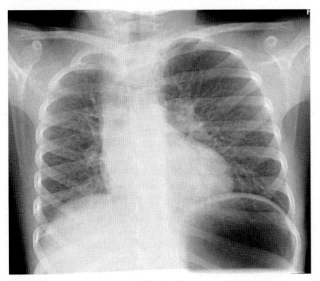

FIGURE 10-4. In a 10-year-old girl who presented with shortness of breath, this chest radiograph shows a small right hemithorax (rib crowding, diaphragmatic elevation, compensatory large left lung), but no lung opacification. This was later diagnosed as an interrupted right pulmonary artery (see Figures 10-40 and 10-60).

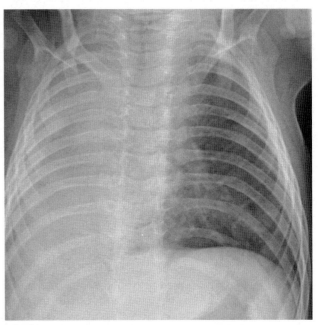

FIGURE 10-6. The right hemithorax is opacified by the mediastinal structures that are shifted to the right. However, there is no overexpansion of the left lung or pleura. On computed tomography, the right lung was absent (see Figure 10-42).

Lobar Overinflation

Lobar overinflation may have a similar appearance to whole-lung overinflation. However, there is usually evidence of lobar confinement because one can identify the lobar outline as it herniates across the midline, and the remaining ipsilateral pulmonary lobes show compressive atelectasis or collapse (Fig. 10-9). The left-upper, right-middle, or left-lower lobe is usually affected by congenital lobar overinflation. A lateral radiograph may be helpful in deciding which lobe is involved, although computed tomography (CT) of the chest is required in most cases to clarify

the anatomy and identify a potential underlying causative abnormality. This could be an extrinsic lesion causing partial bronchial compression (e.g., mediastinal bronchogenic cyst) or a mass within the bronchial lumen causing a ball-valve effect (e.g., endobronchial granuloma or adenoma).

Mediastinal Distortion

Mediastinal distortion may occur secondary to a mediastinal mass. Therefore, the normal outline of the mediastinum should always be reviewed. On the left, this

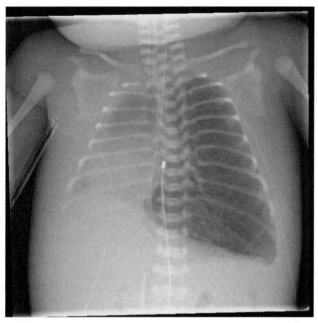

FIGURE 10-7. Chest radiograph of a neonate with respiratory distress syndrome shows an overexpanded left lung (inverted left hemidiaphragm, intercostal bulging of the left lung) as well as a small right hemithorax (elevated right hemidiaphragm, crowding of the right ribs). Both were secondary to a central bronchogenic cyst (see Figure 10-38), although this is not apparent on the chest x-ray but is seen subsequently on CT scan.

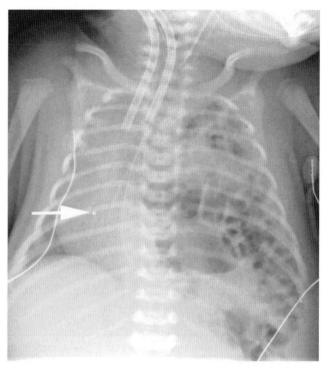

FIGURE 10-8. An infant with antenatally diagnosed left congenital diaphragmatic hernia. Chest radiograph shows disruption of the lateral left diaphragmatic outline, bowel in the left hemithorax, and mediastinal shift to the right. Note venous-arterial extracorporeal membrane oxygenation with a metal marker on the tip of the venous cannula (arrow). The endotracheal tube is too high.

constitutes the thymus, aortic arch, pulmonary outflow tract, pulmonary hilum, and left heart border; on the right, it constitutes the thymus, azygos vein, hilum, and the right heart border. In young children, the outline of the superior structures may be obscured by a normal thymus (discussed earlier), which should never obscure the posterior paraspinal lines because the thymus lies in the anterior mediastinum. Any distortion of the airways (e.g., narrowing, deviation, or splaying of the main bronchi) suggests extrinsic mass effect or functional/structural abnormalities of the airways (Fig. 10-10).

Mass lesions disrupting the paraspinal lines or involving the apices of the chest are most likely localized in the posterior mediastinum, and the list of differential diagnostic possibilities includes congenital abnormalities (lateral meningocele, neurenteric cyst, duplication cyst), neoplasm (neurogenic tumor), and infection (spondylodiscitis). Rib or vertebral body erosion suggests an aggressive lesion, such as infection or malignancy (e.g., neuroblastoma).

Any abnormal appearance of the thymus (discussed earlier), such as inappropriate size or shape or evidence of associated airway compression, suggests an anterior mediastinal mass lesion. Diagnostic differentials include rebound thymic hyperplasia, germ cell tumor, T-cell lymphoma, and thymoma.

Any other mass lesion in the mediastinum usually originates from the middle mediastinum. In the young child, the diagnosis is likely to be a congenital abnormality (e.g., bronchogenic cyst). In the older child, the diagnosis is likely to be enlarged lymph nodes, which may be reactive or due to malignant disease (lymphoproliferative disease, which is rarely metastatic); sarcoidosis (rare, usually paratracheal); or idiopathic hyperplasia.

Lung atelectasis (discussed earlier) should be considered when there is loss of the upper mediastinal outline, even without apparent lung opacification.

TABLE 10-1 DIFFERENTIAL DIAGNOSES IN ASYMMETRICAL LUNG VOLUME

	Increased Ipsilateral Density	Decreased Ipsilateral Density	Normal Density
Small lung	Atelectasis	Swyer-James syndrome	Hypoplasia
	Central airway obstruction	(Macleod's syndrome)	Interrupted pulmonary artery
	Congenital venolobar syndrome		
	Diaphragmatic elevation/paresis		
Large lung		Primary/secondary congenital overinflation	
		Central airway obstruction with ball-valve effect	

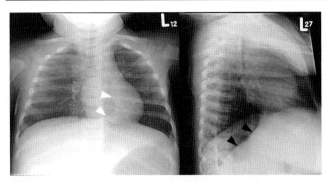

FIGURE 10-9. The lateral view is not part of a routine chest radiograph. In this case, the anteroposterior view shows probable lobar overexpansion of the right lung *(white arrowheads)*, but it is not clear which lobe is involved. The lateral view is helpful, showing depression of the posterior diaphragm *(black arrowheads)* and thereby clarifying right lower lobe involvement, which is uncommon in lobar overinflation (congenital lobar emphysema).

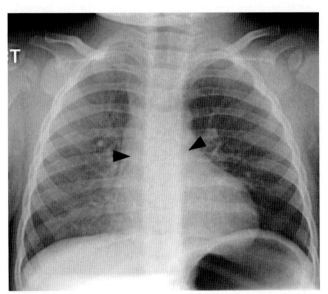

FIGURE 10-10. A 2-year-old boy presents with pyrexia. Chest radiograph shows displacement of the left main and lower lobe bronchi by a subcarinal mass *(between arrowheads)* and associated reduced radiopacity of the left lung due to air trapping. The mass was later proven to be lymphadenopathy caused by *Mycobacterium avium-intracellulare*.

Hilar Expansion

Unlike in adults, where bronchogenic carcinoma is a common cause of hilar adenopathy, in children, hilar enlargement is not unusual with infections. However, prominent hila may also be seen due to enlargement of the pulmonary arteries and, in infants, due to a bronchogenic cyst (see Fig. 10-3). Distinguishing vascular from nodal enlargement can be difficult, but pulmonary arterial enlargement should result in a concave lateral hilar outline, whereas soft tissue masses are said to cause a convex lateral hilar margin, with a noticeable increase in soft tissue density at the enlarged hilum.

False impressions of hilar enlargement occur when the child is rotated on the film cassette: a hilum that is pointing away from the detector becomes more distinct from the heart shadow and consequently appears more prominent. A repeat exposure may be necessary in some difficult inconclusive cases, and CT/MR imaging may be performed if there is doubt.

Peribronchial markings should not be prominent in children, unlike in adults. More distinct markings in the perihilar regions, particularly with coexisting general overinflation, often represent bronchial inflammation (e.g., asthma or infection). Other conditions included in the differential diagnosis will be discussed in the section on high-resolution computed tomography (HRCT). Patchy perihilar opacification, with air bronchograms, is usually due to radiographic summation of peribronchial thickening, but it may be difficult to distinguish from airspace opacification (consolidation).

Lung Opacities

The plain radiograph usually allows distinction between *atelectasis,* which is defined as parenchymal opacification with loss of volume, and *consolidation,* which is opacification without volume loss and with the outline of gas-filled bronchi (air bronchograms) (Fig. 10-11). Opacities in the lungs can be localized according to the neighboring structure that is obscured (silhouette sign). Loss of the upper mediastinal outline is consequent on upper lobe opacification, loss of the heart borders is caused by right middle lobe or lingular opacification, and loss of diaphragmatic definition is caused by lower lobe pathology.

There are several important signs of volume loss. First, the entire hemithorax may appear shrunken, with ipsilateral mediastinal shift, diaphragmatic elevation, and crowding of the ribs. Second, adjacent noncollapsed lung may show compensatory overinflation and appear hypertranslucent due to dilution of vascular shadows. Third,

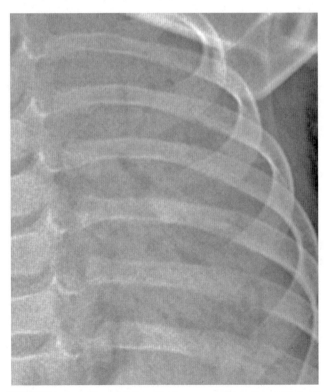

FIGURE 10-11. Consolidation. The lung parenchyma is opacified with obvious air bronchograms, but there are no vascular markings.

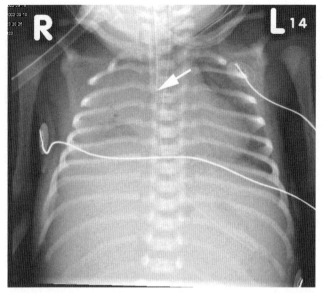

FIGURE 10-12. The tip of the endotracheal tube is in the proximal right main stem bronchus *(arrow)*. There is associated atelectasis of the right upper lobe (loss of definition of the right upper mediastinal border, opacification of the left upper hemithorax, elevation of the right hemidiaphragm, and crowding of the right ribs).

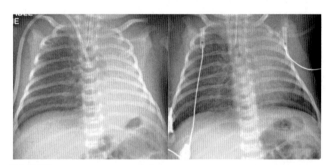

FIGURE 10-13. A neonate in the intensive care unit with increasing oxygen requirement. Chest radiograph *(left)* shows loss of the left cardiomediastinal and diaphragmatic outlines, opacification of the left hemithorax without air bronchograms, and mediastinal shift to the left. These findings strongly suggest left lung collapse, and, at bronchoscopy, a mucous plug was removed from the left main stem bronchus. Immediately afterward *(right)*, there is considerably improved aeration of the left lower lobe (diaphragm now seen), but persistent collapse of the left upper lobe (persisting mediastinal blurring and shift).

the hilum may be displaced, either cranially or caudally, toward the atelectasis (Fig. 10-12).

It is important to recognize these signs, even with no apparent lung opacity, particularly in upper lobe atelectasis, where the affected segments, or the whole lobe, may be collapsed against the mediastinum and therefore difficult to identify.

The clinical and radiographic history of atelectasis may give important clues as to the causative pathology. Acute atelectasis may be caused by a dislodged endotracheal tube, an aspirated foreign body, or mucous plugging (Fig. 10-13) and may therefore require further nonradiologic investigation and intervention. Chronic atelectasis is more likely caused by extrinsic airway obstruction (e.g., bronchogenic cyst, mediastinal lymphadenopathy, neoplasms) or chronic infection (e.g., tuberculosis) and may therefore require CT/MR imaging. In a febrile infant with respiratory distress

and multifocal segmental atelectasis that changes location over the course of hours, one may suspect infection with respiratory syncytial virus, causing bronchiolitis.

Consolidation has many causes, as in adults, and is due to any process that replaces air in the terminal airspaces with fluid, mucus, or cellular material. The clinical history, the distribution of abnormality, and the presence of associated calcification, lymphadenopathy, or pleural effusion may assist in interpretation of the specific cause (Figs. 10-14 and 10-15). Typically, pulmonary edema causes bilateral patchy consolidation in a perihilar distribution as well as pleural fluid (discussed earlier), although there may be lateral predominance.

Ground-glass change, a description initially confined to HRCT, also is used now to describe radiographic lung opacification with partial preservation of vascular markings, with or without air bronchograms (Fig. 10-16). This sign is nonspecific and may be caused by interstitial or partial airspace opacification processes. In the neonatal setting, it is often used in the description of respiratory distress syndrome (Fig. 10-17), usually combined with

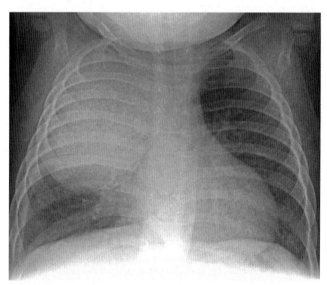

FIGURE 10-14. In a 1-year-old girl with cough, chest radiograph shows a calcified mass in the right upper and mid zones. Also seen is pleural fluid, which was caused by infection with *Mycobacterium tuberculosis* (see Figure 10-57).

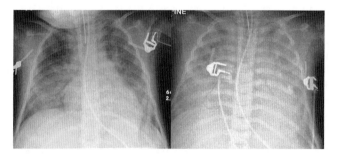

FIGURE 10-15. A 3-year-old boy who was treated in the intensive care unit after a traffic accident had increasing difficulty with oxygenation. Chest radiograph on admission *(left)* shows patchy areas of consolidation. Hemorrhagic fluids returned via the endotracheal tube. The second day *(right)*, there was almost complete whiteout of both lungs, with air bronchograms and loss of the cardiomediastinal and diaphragmatic outlines. The findings confirm extensive pulmonary hemorrhage.

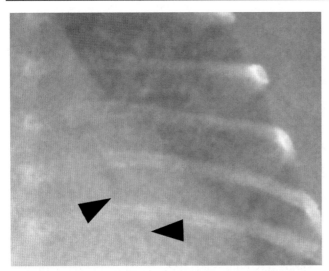

FIGURE 10-16. Ground-glass change. There is moderately increased opacity of the lung with air bronchograms *(arrowheads)*, but preservation of vascular markings.

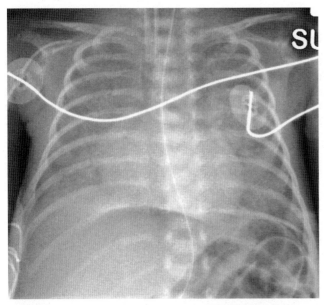

FIGURE 10-17. In a 3-week-old infant born at 32 weeks' gestation on ventilator support, there is bilateral diffuse ground-glass change (opacification, blurring of the cardiomediastinal and diaphragmatic outlines, preserved vascular markings), in keeping with respiratory distress syndrome. Note the lucency overlying the liver, outlining the right hemidiaphragm as well as bowel wall in the upper left quadrant. This is diagnostic of pneumoperitoneum. The child had bowel perforation secondary to necrotizing enterocolitis.

generally decreased lung volumes. Pleural fluid may give a similar appearance (discussed earlier).

Focal and Multifocal Lung Densities

Focal and multifocal lung densities often require additional CT/MR imaging for their definitive underlying cause to be elucidated, except in cases with clear clinical evidence of infectious pneumonia. In children, pneumonic consolidation often has a more distinct, rounded appearance (round pneumonia), which should be recognized and followed with plain radiographs only. In equivocal cases,

CT/MR imaging is necessary for further characterization of the lesion. Differential diagnosis of a solitary parenchymal lesion includes congenital malformation, such as sequestration (usually in the posterobasal left lower lobe), microcystic congenital cystic adenomatoid malformation, and vascular malformation. A lung abscess may have no apparent gas-fluid level.

Multifocal lesions may represent infectious processes (e.g., fungus, tuberculosis, papillomatosis) (Fig. 10-18), granulomatous disease, Langerhans cell histiocytosis, other inflammatory disease (Figs. 10-19 and 10-20),

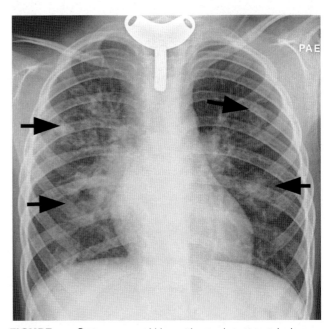

FIGURE 10-18. In a 13-year-old boy with a tracheostomy tube because of laryngeal papillomatosis, chest radiograph shows multiple nodular processes, some of which are cavitating, caused by parenchymal dissemination of the papillomatosis (arrows; see Figure 10-43).

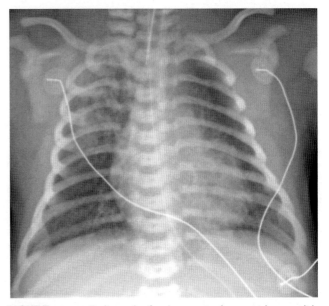

FIGURE 10-19. Radiograph of male neonate shows patchy consolidation in the right upper zone and behind the heart on the left, with overinflated lungs. This picture is commonly seen in meconium aspiration.

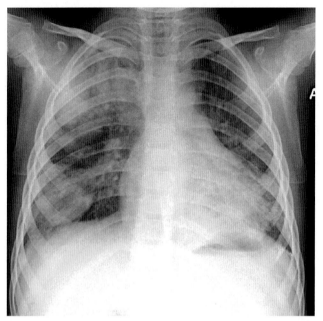

FIGURE 10-20. A 6-year-old boy presented with difficulty breathing. Inflammatory markers were increased. Chest radiograph shows areas of opacification in the right upper and mid zones and the left mid zone that represent vasculitic lesions (see Figure 10-54). On plain film, this is indistinguishable from multifocal pneumonia.

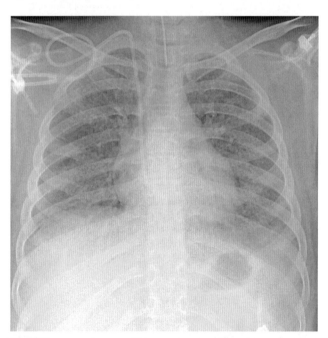

FIGURE 10-21. A 4-year-old boy undergoing chemotherapy had acute respiratory failure. Chest radiograph shows globally increased density of both lungs in a granular pattern, with preservation of vascular markings. This was due to diffuse interstitial pneumonitis caused by bleomycin (see Figure 10-46).

diffuse interstitial lung disease (Fig. 10-21), or metastases (e.g., nephroblastoma, hepatoblastoma, malignant germ cell tumor, sarcoma).

Some lung lesions tend to be predominantly cystic in radiographic terms (containing a gas-filled cavity). Pneumatoceles usually follow pneumonia, classically caused by infection with *Staphylococcus aureus*, occasionally by *Klebsiella*.

Multifocal multicystic parenchymal lesions may be congenital cystic adenomatoid malformation, Langerhans' cell histiocytosis nodules at the cavitating stage, Wegener's granulomatosis, disseminated laryngeal papillomatosis (see Fig. 10-18), or necrotizing vasculitis (see Fig. 10-20).

Pulmonary Interstitial Emphysema

Pulmonary interstitial emphysema is a complication that occurs when high ventilatory pressures are used to ventilate stiff lungs. It appears as lacelike lucencies in a linear pattern radiating from the pulmonary hilum to the surface of the lung, and it may be further complicated by pneumothorax or pneumomediastinum (Figs. 10-22 to 10-24). In some cases, this may be difficult to distinguish radiologically from ventilator-induced central bronchial dilation. There are rare reported cases of apparent spontaneous pulmonary interstitial emphysema in term babies who have never been ventilated. The differential diagnosis includes congenital or acquired cystic lung disease.

Lung Abscess

A lung abscess is a cavitated lesion that normally contains both fluid and gas. The consequent gas-fluid level is easily recognized, but it may be missed unless the x-ray beam is tangential (i.e., horizontal) to the gas-fluid interface. With a diverging beam, the fluid level appears more blurred and meniscoid (Fig. 10-25).

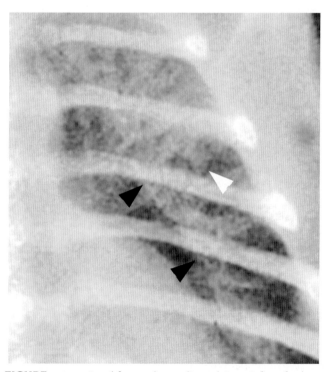

FIGURE 10-22. Detail from a chest radiograph in an infant after long-standing ventilatory support shows monotonous tubular lucencies *(white arrowhead)* suggestive of pulmonary interstitial emphysema. The mediastinal border is seen very crisply, with a medial lung edge *(black arrowheads)* due to anterior pneumothorax.

Diffuse Interstitial Lung Disease

We will discuss diffuse interstitial lung disease in more detail later in the chapter in the section on HRCT. More advanced interstitial processes may be appreciated radiographically as peribronchial thickening, ground-glass change, or interstitial nodules (Figs. 10-21 and 10-26).

Pneumothorax

In young children, the appearance of pneumothorax differs from the typical adult appearance. The variation is due to differences in lung parenchymal elasticity. In children, there is often no peripheral lucent zone on supine radiographs, which is the typical appearance in adults, because in the child, gas collects anteriorly in the anterior pleural reflection (Figs. 10-27 and 10-28). Increased clarity of the cardiac outline may be the only finding, and it should be assessed carefully. If there is clinical doubt, a lateral shoot-through or decubitus x-ray should be performed. These are more sensitive for detecting small-volume pneumothoraces.

Skeletal Abnormalities Associated with Respiratory Disorders

On conventional radiographs, undermineralization of the skeleton can be diagnosed confidently only in severe cases. Associated with prematurity, this metabolic bone condition is commonly seen in infants with idiopathic respiratory distress syndrome. Bone mineral loss is also a feature of a multitude of constitutional disorders and may be seen secondary to systemic corticosteroid therapy.

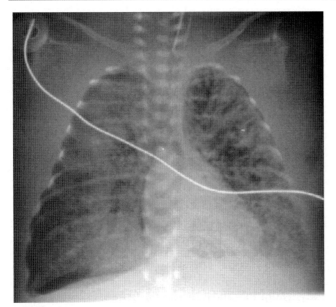

FIGURE 10-23. A 6-week-old girl born at 30 weeks' gestation was very difficult to ventilate. Chest radiograph shows overexpanded lungs that are seen bulging out intercostally, with the diaphragm flattened. Concurrently, there is increased opacification of the lungs, which is presumed to be due to respiratory distress syndrome. Linearly arranged bubbly lucencies can be seen radiating from the hila, suggesting pulmonary interstitial emphysema secondary to high-pressure ventilation. There is also a pneumothorax seen at the base of the right lung.

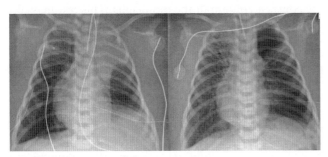

FIGURE 10-24. A 6-week-old girl was ventilated with high-pressure settings (chest radiographs show a flattened diaphragm and splayed ribs). After an acute exacerbation *(left)*, the radiograph showed collapse of the left upper lobe (opacification without air bronchograms, increased interlobar fissure, and elevated diaphragm). The next day *(right)*, the left upper lobe had re-expanded, but a left pneumothorax is seen. Linear bubbly lucencies can be seen from the hili to the lung edges, suggesting pulmonary interstitial emphysema.

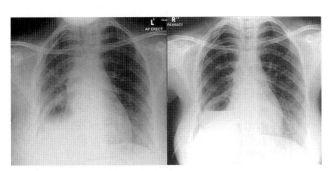

FIGURE 10-25. Two chest radiographs obtained in the same patient on the same day. The right is a true erect exposure showing the gas-fluid level of an abscess within the right lung, whereas the left is semierect and does not show the gas-fluid level of the abscess.

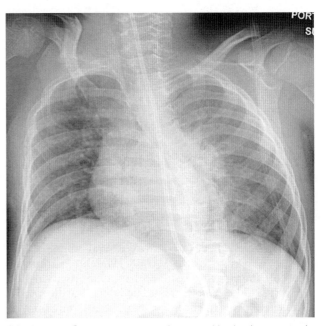

FIGURE 10-26. Chest radiograph of a 9-year-old girl with gastroesophageal reflux and chronic aspiration shows bilateral perihilar bronchial wall thickening, particularly in the upper zones (see Fig. 10-53). Apparent rotation is caused by scoliosis.

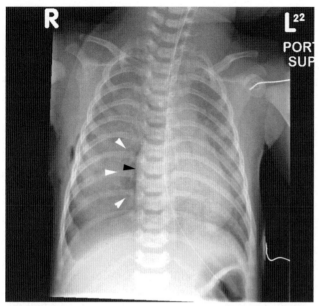

FIGURE 10-27. An anterior pneumothorax as seen typically in infants. The white arrowheads show the lateral boundary of the lucency. Gas adjacent to the right heart border causes a crisp outline *(black arrowhead)*.

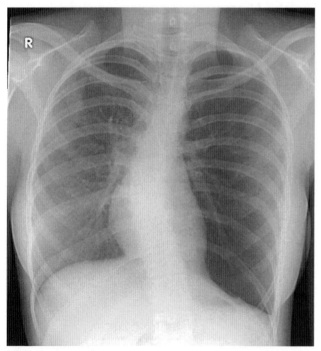

FIGURE 10-28. Chest radiograph of a 12-year-old girl shows a hyperlucent left hemothorax, inversion of the left hemidiaphragm, and a very crisp cardiodiaphragmatic outline. This is suggestive of anterior tension pneumothorax. Scoliosis is noted.

Scoliosis may be caused by vertebral abnormalities, which may be part of the VATER (Vertebral, Anorectal, Tracheo-Esophageal, Renal/Radial malformations) or VACTERL (like VATER, but including Cardiovascular malformations) sequences, or, more commonly, may be caused by neuromuscular disorders. In addition, it may be secondary to chest conditions, such as hypoplastic lung, atelectasis, or empyema, in which case the resultant spinal curvature is concave toward the side of the abnormality.

Both focal and multifocal osseous lesions may be associated findings in conditions that also involve the lungs. Well-defined lytic ("punched out") lesions in the ribs or scapulae and collapse of vertebral bodies are features of Langerhans' cell histiocytosis. More ill-defined lesions are seen in primary neoplasms (e.g., Askin's tumor), lymphoma, infection (e.g., tuberculosis), or infection associated with chronic granulomatous disease. Erosion of posterior rib elements, with splaying, is seen with thoracic paraspinal neuroblastoma.

FLUOROSCOPIC TECHNIQUES

Limitation of radiation exposure is vital in childhood, but a quick fluoroscopic screening examination of the chest (using pulsed rather than continuous fluoroscopy) can frequently prove extremely useful, particularly when evaluating differing lung radiolucencies in suspected foreign body aspiration and generally in stridor.[4] With obstructive overinflation, the affected lung will show little volume change with respiration, and the mediastinum will swing contralaterally on expiration. Fluoroscopic lateral views may also be valuable for dynamic evaluation of tracheomalacia, where the trachea may be seen to collapse during expiration.

Barium swallow is still the primary study in patients with suspected vascular ring, which abnormally indents the contrast column in the esophagus. This test may also be valuable for assessing extrinsic masses. Laryngeal cleft and tracheoesophageal fistula can be excluded with a good-quality single-contrast study when a water-soluble contrast medium with a high iodine concentration is delivered under pressure via a nasal tube to the esophagus. The child is kept prone and screened with a horizontal beam to facilitate visualization of contrast leakage into the trachea or bronchi.

Thin-section CT has almost eliminated the need for bronchography in children; however, the technique still is used in functional studies for assessing the dynamics of intermittent airway obstruction (Fig. 10-29). With this technique, the mucosa of the trachea and the first to third generations of bronchi are coated with water-soluble contrast medium, which is instilled with a repeated small-bolus technique via a fine tube at the subglottic level in the intubated child.[5]

SPIRAL COMPUTED TOMOGRAPHY

Computed tomography is an invaluable technique in many pediatric chest diseases.[6] However, it is vital to assess the diagnostic benefit versus the radiation risk to the patient. CT is currently the most sensitive way of imaging the lungs due to its high spatial resolution. High-speed scanning allows for superb depiction of even small vessels after delivery of an intravenous bolus of iodinated contrast medium. In the younger child (younger than 5 years of age), sedation or general anesthesia may be required, although this need has reduced with the introduction of multi–detector row, or multislice, CT (MDCT) scanners with faster acquisition times.

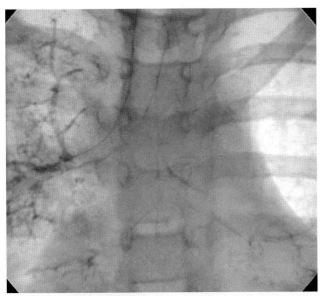

FIGURE 10-29. Bronchogram in a girl with stridor shows a long stenosis of the distal trachea, with an abnormal origin of the right upper lobe bronchus from the trachea (see Figs. 10-36 and 10-37). (Image courtesy of Dr. D. Roebuck, London.)

Unlike HRCT, spiral CT acquires volumetric data on the whole chest, usually after intravenous injection of contrast medium, which allows detailed anatomic depiction of the mediastinal and pulmonary vasculature and distinction between vascularized and cystic/necrotic mass lesions.

Spiral CT potentially shows the thoracic anatomy in a multiplanar manner and has increased sensitivity over a conventional chest radiograph. CT is ideal for visualizing chest/pleural lesions and can detect extension of mediastinal masses through the chest wall. The trachea and major bronchi are well visualized, and extrinsic and intrinsic airway masses are easily diagnosed. The increased sensitivity of chest CT versus chest x-ray for the detection of pulmonary nodules has been studied extensively.

There are many advantages of conventional CT over plain chest x-ray; however, cardiac and respiratory motion artifacts may significantly degrade image quality. The paucity of mediastinal fat in children compared with adults may preclude detection of small mediastinal lesions. Spiral CT and ultrafast electron beam CT are particularly useful for investigating the major intrathoracic airways, and cardiovascular and mediastinal abnormalities. The advantage of quick scan times in children is particularly useful, reducing the need for sedation and giving excellent vascular opacification with relatively lower contrast volumes.

ISOTROPIC COMPUTED TOMOGRAPHY

Modern day MDCT scanners, with increasing number of detector rows (acquires up to 320 simultaneous sections per tube rotation) and sub-second tube rotation speeds, have further enhanced performance, delivering faster scan time (improved temporal resolution) with a wider scan range. When this is combined with the use of smaller detector elements (down to 0.5 mm), this enables acquisition of isotropic volumetric datasets (where the slice thickness is equal to the pixel dimensions), resulting in improved spatial resolution in the cranio-caudal/longitudinal axis, with reduced partial volume artifacts. It is now possible to acquire high-resolution thoracic CT in spiral mode in children, without breath holding and with minimal motion artifact due to faster scanning time.

Isotropic imaging requires the reconstruction of overlapping thin section datasets that are susceptible to image noise. To overcome this, using post-processing software, the data are manipulated into arbitrary cross-sectional planes and presented as two-dimensional or three-dimensional displays that have the same partial resolution as that of the original acquired dataset. The ability to view volumetric data in any plane enhances the interpretation and assessment of the bronchial tree and is crucial in defining pulmonary nodules, thus allowing better differentiation between organ interfaces that are parallel to the scan plane to aid diagnostic accuracy.

The main advantages of MDCT over conventional single-detector CT are decreased acquisition time (increased temporal resolution) and the ability to acquire isotropic data (increased spatial resolution). The term *isotropic* implies that image resolution in all three dimensions is almost equal, so that *post hoc* image reconstruction in all planes is possible without the loss of structural detail. These benefits have dramatically expanded the application of CT in the evaluation of cardiovascular and airway diseases. MDCT is now commonly used in place of conventional angiography because the images are acquired more safely, without the need for arterial puncture, and often without the need for general anesthesia or sedation because acquisition times are very rapid (2 to 8 seconds). The additional benefit over angiography is that superb anatomic images of the mediastinum and lung parenchyma are acquired in the same data set, without additional radiation. The overall dose in MDCT is significantly lower than that in conventional angiography. Thus, MDCT can aid in the diagnosis of pulmonary embolus, arteriovenous malformation, aneurysm, and dissection. However, conventional angiography has the advantage of allowing therapeutic intervention in the same procedure, unlike MDCT. Images of the airway acquired simultaneously can ascertain the presence of airway stenosis and narrowing as well as show the cause of possible extrinsic compression.

DATA PROCESSING

Depending on the clinical application, the acquired volumetric data can be reformatted and displayed as a two-dimensional image using multi-planar reconstruction (MPR) and multi-planar volume reconstructions, known as *maximum intensity projection* (MIP) or *minimum intensity projection* (MinIP). The techniques used to display three-dimensional images include shaded-surface display (SSD), volume-rendering technique (VRT), and perspective rendering (e.g., virtual bronchoscopy [VB]).

Multi-Planar Reconstruction

MPRs are two-dimensional tomographic sections that are interpolated along an arbitrary imaging plane. This allows the operator to manipulate and view axial images in the different planes (i.e., the coronal, sagittal, or arbitrary angulated planes) or in a single tomographic curved plane along the axis of a structure of interest (e.g., a bronchus or a tortuous vessel).[7,8] Slice thickness of the MPR is operator-dependent, and increasing the thickness will improve the signal-to-noise ratio. MPR enhances the perception of the image; provides additional diagnostic value in demonstrating the presence of small focal lesions, defining the vertical extent of a bronchial stenosis (Fig. 10-30); and is used in the presurgical assessment of vascular rings and the tracheobronchial tree.[9]

Multi-Planar Volume Reconstructions: Maximum Intensity Projection and Minimum Intensity Projection

MIP is a rendering tool used to extract contrast-enhanced anatomic structures of higher attenuation values than adjacent structures as in CT angiography (Fig. 10-31). The data are displayed in volume slabs to avoid obstruction from overlying vessels or bony structures. These thicker slabs are useful in depicting the peripheral airway, detecting and localizing micro-nodular or micro-tubular patterns, and analyzing mild forms of uneven attenuation of the lungs.[10] On the other hand, MinIP displays structures with the lowest attenuation values used in demonstrating the central airway and air trapping in the lungs (Fig. 10-32).

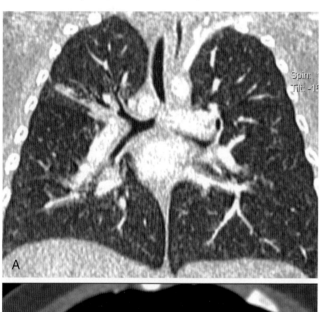

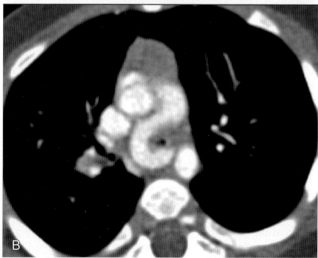

FIGURE 10-30. Coronal MPR **(A)** and axial MIP **(B)** images in a 5-month-old child presenting with stridor. There is tracheal stenosis caused by the presence of a pulmonary sling with almost complete occlusion of the distal trachea with marked narrowing of the LMB origin related to the aberrant left pulmonary artery, which has an anomalous origin from the right pulmonary artery, passing behind the trachea and in front of the esophagus. Cartilaginous rings were not identified in this examination. The coronal MRP image **(A)** has been postprocessed on a high-resolution (bony) algorithm more suitable for viewing lung parenchyma but giving a more "noisy" (i.e., grainy) image.

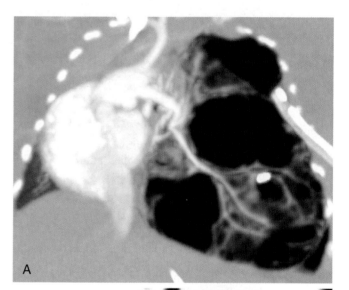

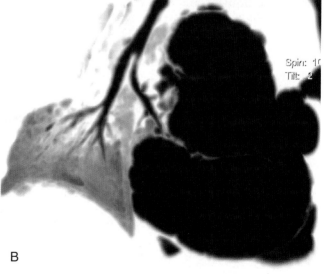

FIGURE 10-31. Multi-loculated air-filled cystic mass in a 4-day-old neonate with an antenatally diagnosed congenital thoracic malformation treated with antenatal drainage; see catheter on CXR **(C). A,** MIP image, where data with maximum intensity (contrast) is aggregated thus enhancing the blood supply. A branch pulmonary artery can be seen supplying the left lower lobe. **B,** MinIP, where data with lowest intensity (air) is combined to highlight the tracheobronchial tree emphasizing the very dilated cystic acinar units in the lung parenchyma and the abnormal ptosed and narrowed LMB.

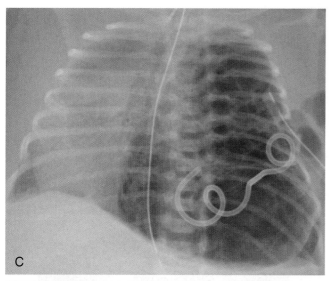

FIGURE 10-31.—Cont'd The chest radiography in **(C)** shows the enlarged hyperlucent left lung with herniation across the midline causing compression and shift of the mediastinum and right lung (which is atelectatic). Note the coiled left intrathoracic pigtail drain that was placed antenatally.

Shaded-Surface Display

Shaded-surface display (SSD) is a surface-rendering technique that uses a threshold-base algorithm to generate a three-dimensional image. There are limitations to this postprocessing technique (e.g., loss of data in the thresholding process), hence this technique has been superseded by volume-rendering techniques (VRTs).

Volume-Rendering Technique

VRT is a processing technique (used for interpreting CT angiography, CT bronchoscopy, and orthopedic imaging datasets) that utilizes all acquired volumetric data without being subject to information loss. This is in order to display an image in a three-dimensional format so that the image can be further manipulated and viewed in different orientations (Fig. 10-33). VRTs are used to depict structural and vascular anatomy (Fig. 10-34) and their relationship to adjacent structures and to displaying structures that course parallel or oblique to the transverse plane (and also those that develop or extend into multiple planes).[7,8] Applying a transparency filter highlights the

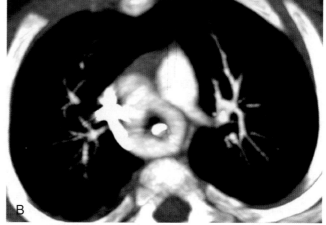

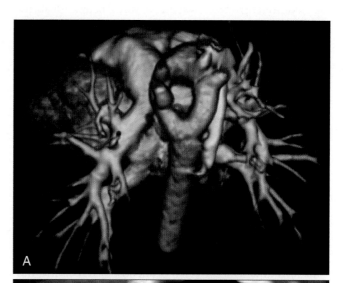

FIGURE 10-32. A 5-year-old child with segmental LUL overinflation. The coronal thin MinIP **(A)** shows a well-defined anterior segmental area of regional air trapping in relation to segmental overinflation. A thin axial section **(B)** shows the lung parenchyma anatomy in the most favorable setting. Note the clarity of the definition of the bronchial wall and adjacent pulmonary artery branch within the hyperlucent segment of the LUL.

FIGURE 10-33. A 3-month-old child with a double aortic arch viewed as a volume-rendered image **(A)** and as an axial MIP image **(B).** Note the almost identical caliber of the "balanced" R and L arches (the more common finding is of a cephalad and larger dominant right aortic arch. A nasogastric tube can be seen adjacent to the trachea.

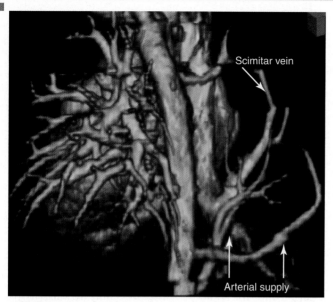

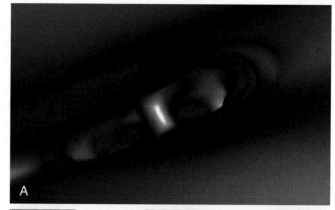

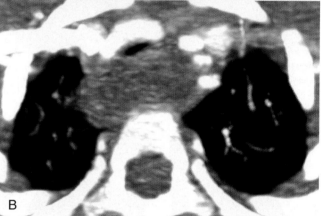

FIGURE 10-34. VRT image of a 4-year-old child. A scimitar vein is seen joining the supra-hepatic portion of the IVC inferior to the right atrium. The systemic artery arises from the descending aorta and supplies the right lung.

FIGURE 10-35. This 2-year-old child presented with tracheal stenosis. The virtual bronchoscopy demonstrates a dramatic AP narrowing of the trachea at the level of the carina that is compressed by an enlarged esophagus posteriorly (diagnosed as achalasia of the esophageal cardia on barium study), as seen in (B).

tracheobronchial tree, which, in turn, better illustrates short focal areas of narrowing, the craniocaudal length of a tracheobronchial stenosis, and other tracheobronchial anomalies. The mediastinal vasculature is best displayed as color-coded opacifications used for evaluating complex congenital cardiovascular anomalies.

Virtual Bronchoscopy

Virtual bronchoscopy (VB) is a perspective surface-rendering technique that takes advantage of the natural contrast between the airway and the surrounding tissues,[9] mimicking a bronchoscopic view of the intraluminal surface of the air-containing tracheobronchial tree (Fig. 10-35). VB provides an additional viewing dimension; the operator can navigate in real time along the lumen of the airway, where bronchial surfaces can be visualized, and even across obstructions that an endoscope cannot traverse.[7,11] This technique is used when bronchoscopy is contraindicated or when tracheal stenosis cannot be otherwise evaluated.[12] Although dynamic VB can technically be used, virtual bronchography is more valuable.

■ REVIEW OF FINDINGS

The interpretation of findings requires systematic review of all anatomic structures and areas, including those shown in Table 10-2 and Figs. 10-36 to 10-44).

Depiction of the parenchymal anatomy and abnormality with spiral CT is inferior to that depicted with HRCT. On the other hand, the spiral scan covers the whole volume of the lungs; therefore, it is more sensitive for demonstrating solitary lesions, such as metastasis or a fungal lesion.

Computed tomography performs poorly in differentiating between pleural effusion and empyema.[13] Pleural thickening and enhancement are often present in reactive effusions. Plain radiography, followed by ultrasound, is the investigation of choice because ultrasound has the ability to visualize the fibrinous septations of an infectious process. However, CT is useful in distinguishing between empyema and lung abscess. Empyema shows a wide pleural base (see Fig. 10-44), whereas a lung abscess is usually seen partially separated from the pleura, with a wedge of lung on either side in the imaging plane.

■ PITFALLS

Technical factors may confound interpretation. Some artifacts may impede detection of significant lesions. In young children, there is invariably some degree of dependent lung opacification. When the distinction between atelectatic lung and nodular change is difficult, it may be helpful to repeat a few slices of the scan with the child in the prone position. Streak artifacts may be seen and are caused by high-concentration contrast medium in the innominate vein at the site of delivery. This may degrade the imaging of structures in the upper mediastinum. The peridiaphragmatic areas are also difficult to assess because lesions are difficult to depict separately from the diaphragm in the transaxial plane. Whenever possible, therefore, multiplanar reconstructions in the coronal and sagittal planes should be reviewed.

TABLE 10-2 MAIN REVIEW AREAS FOR SPIRAL COMPUTED TOMOGRAPHY OF THE CHEST

STRUCTURE/AREA	ABNORMALITIES
Airways	Extrinsic compression (see Figs. 10-36 and 10-37) Caliber change
Vessels	Vascular rings Aberrant vessels
Anterior mediastinum	Thymic enlargement, nodularity, heterogeneous enhancement
Middle mediastinum	Enlarged lymph nodes Bronchopulmonary foregut malformations (see Fig. 10-38) Cardiac abnormalities
Posterior mediastinum	Benign lesions: Duplication cyst, meningocele, ganglioneuroma, abscess, extramedullary hematopoiesis Malignant lesions: Neuroblastoma
Hila	Enlarged lymph nodes
Lung parenchyma	Lung/lobar aplasia, agenesis, hypoplasia, overinflation (see Figures 10-39 to 10-42) Focal lesions: Nodules, consolidation, atelectasis (see Fig. 10-43)
Pleura	Transudate, exudates, pus, hemorrhage, lymph (see Fig. 10-44)
Chest wall and spine	Osseous or soft-tissue lesions: Infection, benign and malignant tumors Abnormal configuration: Scoliosis, pectus deformities
Upper abdomen	Lesions of the liver, spleen, adrenal glands, and upper poles of kidneys Retroperitoneal, peritoneal, and abdominal wall lesions

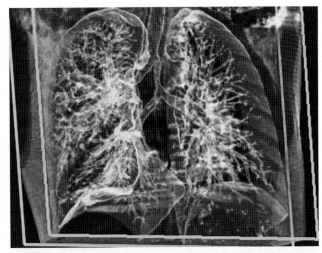

FIGURE 10-37. Volume-rendering of computed tomography volume data in the same child as in Figs. 10-29 and 10-36 shows the anatomy of both the central and peripheral airways, with distal tracheal stenosis.

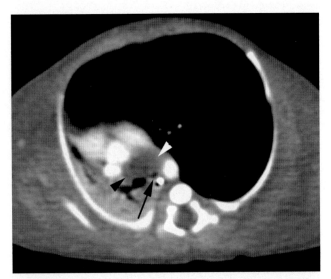

FIGURE 10-38. Contrast-enhanced spiral computed tomography shows a precarinal bronchogenic cyst *(arrowheads)*, with associated narrowing of the left main stem bronchus *(arrow)*, a hyperinflated left lung, and a collapsed right lung (see Fig. 10-7).

On the other hand, some artifacts mimic pathology. Tachypnea or motion will inevitably blur the final image, and this phenomenon is easily confused with ground-glass change. Apparent bronchiectasis in the lingula and right middle lobe may sometimes be an artifact due to motion in which a single airway branch is represented twice in the image. Small parenchymal nodules (<5 mm) usually represent benign processes, even in children with known malignant disease. Therefore, one should not automatically interpret such findings as lung metastases.[14]

■ DOSE

Dose considerations are particularly important in pediatric imaging. CT delivers the largest radiation burden of all imaging modalities. Therefore, its indications should be restricted and the dose kept as low as reasonably achievable.[15,16]

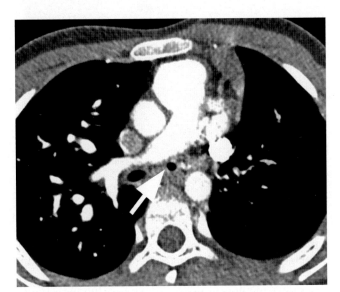

FIGURE 10-36. On arterial phase computed tomography of the same girl as in Fig. 10-29, there is narrowing of the trachea *(arrow)* where it passes between the right pulmonary artery and the descending aorta. This is an intrinsic defect due to complete cartilaginous rings.

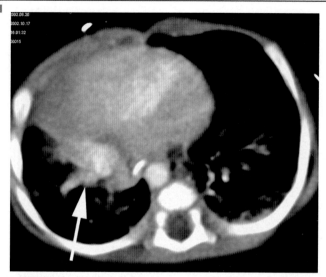

FIGURE 10-39. Contrast-enhanced spiral computed tomography shows systemic venous drainage of the hypoplastic right lung into the right atrium (*arrow; see Figs. 10-5 and 10-41*).

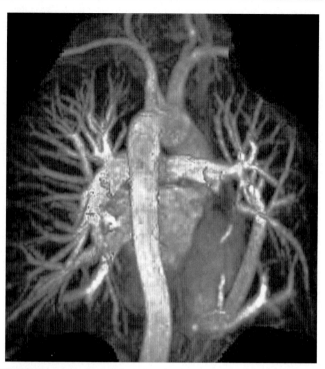

FIGURE 10-41. Three-dimensional magnetic resonance imaging scan shows the infra-atrial drainage of a scimitar vein (*arrow,* posterior view; see Fig. 10-5 and 10-39).

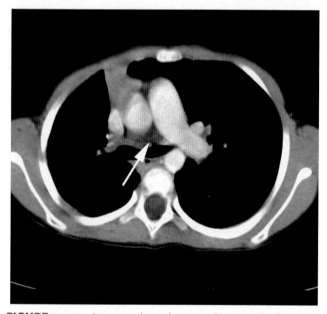

FIGURE 10-40. Contrast-enhanced computed tomography throughout the mediastinum shows a small right lung and no enhancement in the normal site of the right pulmonary artery *(arrow)*. Because the right pulmonary artery is absent, the right lung must receive a systemic supply; however the collaterals cannot be seen (see Figs. 10-4 and 10-60).

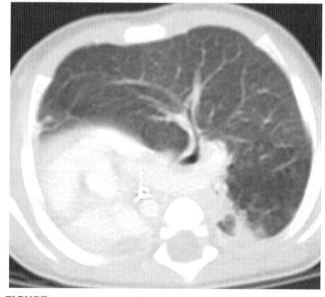

FIGURE 10-42. Contrast-enhanced computed tomography shows agenesis of the right lung and compensatory increased volume of the left lung, which appears structurally normal (see Fig. 10-6).

Pediatric scanning parameters should be optimized and adjusted according to patient size, based on body weight or diameter or the region of interest. Reducing the tube current and/or tube potential (kV) will reduce the radiation dose; this is because the dose is directly proportional to the tube current and is exponentially related to kVp, so that a reduction in kV from 120 to 100 can further reduce the dose by 30% to 70%.[17,18] In fact, it is preferable (in angiographic chest imaging) to use a lower kV as it enhances the CT attenuation of iodinated contrast, thus increasing the contrast-to-noise ratio in the perfused structures and improving overall image quality while minimizing dose.

It is widely accepted that dose reduction is associated with an increase in image noise. However, air in the chest acts as a high contrast medium so has a higher tolerance of image noise level, thus enabling lower scanning parameters to be set.

Another method of dose reduction is the use of automatic exposure control (AEC) that is now a common application in MDCT. The aim of AEC is to modulate the tube current according to patient specific attenuation that

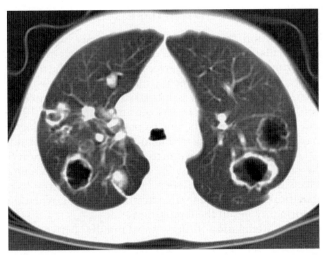

FIGURE 10-43. Chest computed tomography of an 8-year-old girl with laryngotracheal papillomatosis shows multiple peripheral nodules and cavities with posterior dominance, in keeping with pulmonary dissemination (see Fig. 10-18).

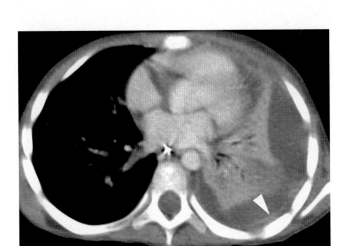

FIGURE 10-44. Contrast-enhanced computed tomography confirms the ultrasound finding of consolidated lung (note air bronchograms) and pleural fluid. There is mild pleural thickening and enhancement that is nonspecific *(arrowhead)*. Computed tomography did not show calcification. Acid-fast bacilli were cultured from the pleural fluid. This case shows the currently nonspecific role of computed tomography in imaging of pleural fluid (see Fig. 10-45).

ultimately reduces dose without degrading image quality.[19] However, this technique still requires adjustment of parameters to patient size to ensure dose optimization. Three basic methods of tube current modulations are used in AEC, with different manufacturers adopting different methodology, or a combination of the three that includes (1) patient-size modulation, (2) z-axis modulation, and (3) rotational or angular modulation.

Scanner detector configuration and use of beam-shaping filters affect dose efficiency. Scanners that use a matrix array detector configuration (equal width of all detector rows) are less dose-efficient than those using adaptive array detectors (outer rows wider than inner rows), with greater beam utilization and reduced penumbra.

Depending on the collimation (e.g., slice thickness of 0.6 or 1.2 mm with a 64-slice scanner), tube current, and length of the scan, the absorbed dose varies in equivalence to between 25 and 50 chest radiographs for a 2-month-old infant. In pediatric applications, the tube current should be substantially reduced, and image quality can usually be dropped (lower signal-to-noise ratio) without loss of relevant diagnostic information. Some suggested settings and dose calculations are shown in Table 10-3.

■ HIGH-RESOLUTION COMPUTED TOMOGRAPHY

HRCT is the modality of choice in suspected interstitial lung disease. It allows a detailed structural assessment of secondary pulmonary lobules and intrapulmonary interstitium, thereby aiding the diagnostic workup. HRCT usually allows a confident radiologic diagnosis in cases of alveolar proteinosis, pulmonary lymphangiectasia, and idiopathic pulmonary hemosiderosis.[20] It can be used to guide lung biopsy and thoracoscopic procedures, by targeting areas of active disease. HRCT allows early detection of diffuse pulmonary parenchymal disease to the level of the secondary pulmonary lobule, and is useful in the characterization of opportunistic infection in the immunocompromised patient. Serial imaging may be useful in monitoring disease activity.

The recommended technique in children with diffuse pulmonary disease includes HRCT slices of approximately 1- to 2-mm thickness at 1- to 2-cm intervals from the lung apices to the lung bases (depending on the size

TABLE 10-3 SUGGESTED PEDIATRIC CHEST PROTOCOL WITH ESTIMATED EFFECTIVE DOSE FROM CLINICAL DATA (AND EQUIVALENT NUMBER OF CHEST RADIOGRAPHS), BASED ON A TUBE COLLIMATION OF 0.6 MM ON THE SIEMENS 32-DETECTOR-ROW SCANNER

BODY WEIGHT (KG)	TUBE KILOVOLTAGE (KV)	TUBE CURRENT (MAS)	CTDIVOL (MGY)	EFFECTIVE DOSE (MSV)	
<9	80	60	0.81	0.8	
<15	100	30	1.13	1.1	(×32 CXR)
<25	100	38	2.04	1.7	
<35	100	45	2.08	2.1	(×36 CXR)
>35	100	60	4.70	3.5	

of the thorax). A high-resolution image construction algorithm is mandatory. If possible, CT slices should be obtained at full inspiration to diminish vascular crowding, particularly in the dependent areas of the lung, where atelectasis is more common in children than in adults.

Knowledge of the anatomic basis for HRCT is a prerequisite for understanding abnormal features. Supplying arterial and bronchiolar branches pass in the core of the secondary pulmonary lobule, and draining veins and lymphatics pass in the connective tissue between lobules, the interlobular septa. The subpleural interstitium connects to the interlobular septa, constituting the peripheral fiber system. Extending from the hila, the bronchovascular interstitium extends centripetally.

■ DOSE

Adjustment of the radiation dose to the size of the child is crucial for radiation protection. The dose can be substantially reduced from a standard adult dose without loss of diagnostic information. Suggested settings and calculated doses are shown in Table 10-4.

■ CONTROLLED VENTILATION TECHNIQUE

A method for noninvasive controlled ventilation in sedated children may be particularly useful in HRCT. Positive pressure is applied at a facemask, and the pressure applied is adjusted by changing the setting of a pressure pop-off valve. Respiratory pauses are induced by means of a step increase in ventilation combined with rapid lung inflation at a pressure of 25 cm water, given synchronously with spontaneous tidal inspiration. Lung inflations are repeated approximately three to six times until a respiratory pause occurs. Inspiratory or expiratory scans then can be acquired with minimized motion artifact.[21]

■ INTERPRETATION

Interpretation of HRCT images is based on the presence and distribution of certain findings (e.g., septal thickening, ground-glass change, nodular change), which may represent a variety of histopathologic processes.

Regional or Generalized Increased Density

Consolidation (Fig. 10-45) and atelectasis may appear alike on plain radiographs, as discussed earlier. On HRCT, subsegmental atelectasis may be recognized by the traction it exerts on adjacent bronchi (traction bronchiectasis).

Ground-glass change is increased pulmonary attenuation, with preservation of vascular markings (Figs. 10-46 and 10-47). This may be due to partial airspace filling or may represent dense intralobular septal thickening that is too subtle to be resolved due to the inherent resolution of the HRCT scanner. Thus, the concept of partial volume effects comes into play when HRCT images show hazy opacification resembling airspace opacification when the abnormality lies in the interstitium.

Lung attenuation differs substantially between full inspiration and expiration. Diffuse, global ground-glass change may therefore be difficult to distinguish from a normal expiratory phase in the lungs. The posterior tracheal membrane is a helpful indicator because it is posteriorly convex on inspiration and horizontal or slightly anteriorly convex on expiration.

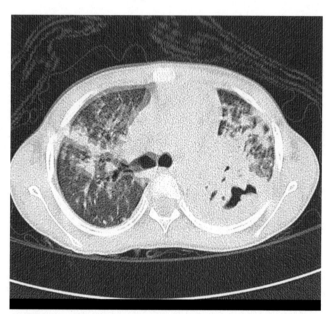

FIGURE 10-45. High-resolution computed tomography at a higher level in the same child as in Fig. 10-44 additionally shows cavitation within the left upper lobe consolidation. This was later proven to be due to *Mycobacterium tuberculosis*. Abundant motion artifacts are noted.

TABLE 10-4 SUGGESTED PEDIATRIC HIGH-RESOLUTION CHEST PROTOCOL WITH CALCULATED COMPUTED TOMOGRAPHY DOSE INDEX (AND ESTIMATED ABSORBED DOSE WITH DOSE EQUIVALENT NUMBER OF CHEST RADIOGRAPHS), BASED ON A TUBE COLLIMATION OF 1.0 MM ON THE SIEMENS 32-DETECTOR-ROW SCANNER

BODY WEIGHT (KG)	TUBE KILOVOLTAGE (KV)	TUBE CURRENT (MAS)	CTDIVOL (MGY)	EFFECTIVE DOSE (MSV)	
<15	100	20	0.12	0.3	(×8 CXR)
<25	100	30	0.25	0.3	
<35	100	35	0.29	0.35	
>35	100	42	0.35	0.4	(×16 CXR)

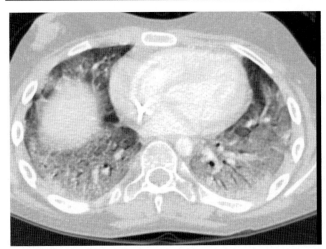

FIGURE 10-46. High-resolution computed tomography in a 4-year-old child undergoing chemotherapy shows widespread ground-glass change whose cause cannot be determined. However, in this setting, it is suggestive of drug-induced pneumonitis, in this case, probably bleomycin (see Fig. 10-21).

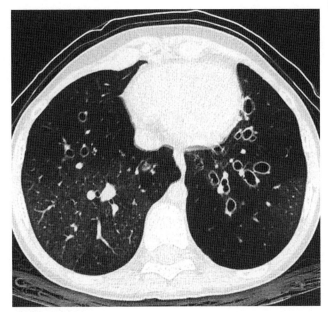

FIGURE 10-48. High-resolution computed tomography slice shows bronchial dilation with mild bronchial wall thickening (large airway disease), as well as almost globally hypoattenuating lung parenchyma and associated hypovascularity (small airway disease) in a 9-year-old boy with bronchiectasis.

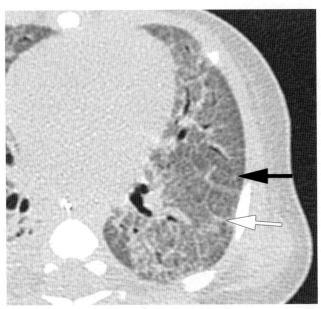

FIGURE 10-47. Detail from high-resolution computed tomography in a 3-month-old boy with neonatal onset of chILD shows homogeneous ground-glass change, interlobular septal thickening (*white arrow*), and discrete centrilobular nodules (*black arrow*).

Regional or Generalized Decreased Density

Circulating blood accounts for most of the normal parenchymal radiopacity. Consequently, decreased radiodensity is most commonly caused by abnormally reduced perfusion due to reflex vasoconstriction in small airway disease. This can be regional (mosaic attenuation) or global (Fig. 10-48).

Differentiation between mosaic attenuation and regional ground-glass change is often difficult. In this case, acquisition of expiratory scans to document air trapping associated with small airway disease can be useful (Figs. 10-49 and 10-50). In uncooperative children, if breathing cannot be controlled voluntarily (normally younger than 5

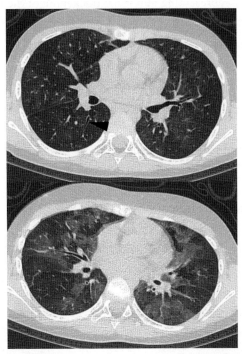

FIGURE 10-49. In an 11-year-old girl who received a bone marrow transplant, on inspiration (*top*), there are global attenuation differences seen in a mosaic pattern, as well as bronchial dilation (*arrowhead*). The mosaic pattern is accentuated on expiration (*bottom*), suggesting air trapping within low-attenuating segments.

years of age), a few slices can be acquired in alternating decubitus positions. The dependent lung simulates expiration as the dependent hemithorax is splinted and its motion restricted, causing underaeration of the dependent lung and hyperaeration of the nondependent lung, effectively providing an expiration view of the dependent lung and an inspiration view of the nondependent lung.[22]

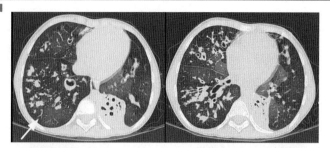

FIGURE 10-50. High-resolution computed tomography in an adolescent girl with end-stage cystic fibrosis shows mosaic attenuation, dilation, and wall thickening of the bronchi; mucus within the bronchi; and terminal branches with tree-in-bud sign *(arrow)*. On expiration *(right)*, there is accentuation of the mosaic pattern, confirming small airway obstruction.

This is useful in practice for the detection of air trapping in the dependent lung. In small airway disease, the contrast between underperfused and more normal tissue increases on expiration due to air trapping, enforcing the mosaic appearance.

Septal Thickening

Intralobular interstitial thickening appears as fine weblike outlines, representing abnormal thickening of the lobular connective tissue or lobular bronchovascular interstitium due to inflammation or edema. If it is coarser, it resembles ground-glass change (discussed earlier).

Interlobular septal thickening is best appreciated in the subpleural lung, where it outlines the secondary lobules. It may be the result of interstitial edema, hemorrhage, fibrosis, cellular infiltration, or lymphangiectasia (Figs. 10-47 and 10-51). Diseases that affect the peripheral acini of two adjacent lobules may give the same appearance.

Peribronchovascular thickening is prominence of the bronchial walls or pulmonary arteries, usually with conspicuous centrilobular arteries. In the more extreme forms, this is caused by cellular infiltration (tends to appear nodular) or edema (smooth).

Interlobular septal thickening superimposed on ground-glass change is termed the *crazy paving pattern,* which typically is seen in childhood-type pulmonary alveolar proteinosis.

Nodules

Centrilobular nodules are nodular densities that are located centrally in the secondary pulmonary lobule. They represent small infiltrates associated with bronchioles and alveolar ducts (e.g., infection, hypersensitivity pneumonitis). Centrilobular nodules (Figs. 10-47 and 10-52) may coexist with peribronchial inflammation and impaction of fluid, cells, or mucus in the centrilobular bronchioles (see Fig. 10-50). The nodular branching patterns cause the characteristic tree-in-bud finding. This is a sign in infectious bronchitis/bronchiolitis, bronchiectasis, and tuberculosis. Perilymphatic nodules are small infiltrates associated with the visceral pleura, interlobular septa, and bronchovascular bundles (e.g., sarcoidosis). Random nodules are small infiltrates with no predominant anatomic association, typically seen in hematogenously spread disease (e.g., metastatic disease, miliary tuberculosis).

Bronchial Change

Bronchiectasis is dilation of the bronchus. The commonly used cutoff point for normal/abnormal equals the diameter of the adjacent artery. In early phases of cystic fibrosis, small airway disease represented by mosaic attenuation may be the only finding evident on HRCT. With advancing disease, the typical pattern is seen: bronchial dilation accompanied by bronchial wall thickening, mucus impaction, and architectural distortion (see Fig. 10-50). Bronchial dilation with minimal bronchial wall change

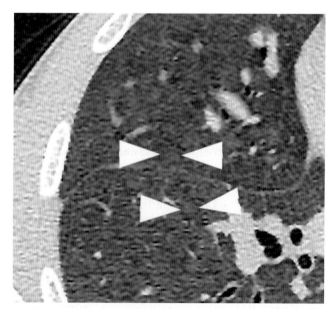

FIGURE 10-52. In an 8-year-old girl with intermittent hemoptysis, high-resolution computed tomography shows centrilobular ground-glass nodules *(arrowheads)* and mild fissural thickening. This is suggestive of idiopathic pulmonary hemosiderosis, which was confirmed histologically.

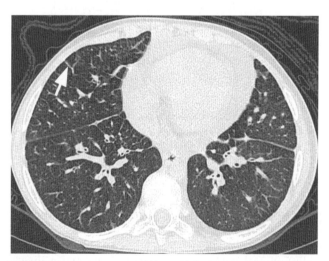

FIGURE 10-51. In a 13-year-old boy with known enteric lymphangiectasia, high-resolution computed tomography shows thickening of the oblique fissures, interlobular septal thickening *(arrow)*, and peribronchovascular thickening. This suggests mild pulmonary involvement.

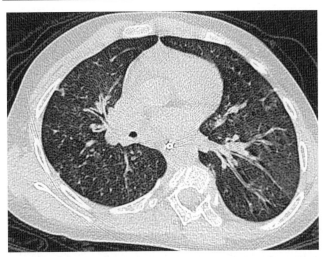

FIGURE 10-53. High-resolution computed tomography confirms bronchial wall thickening and shows small foci of subpleural interlobular septal thickening in a 9-year-old girl with gastroesophageal reflux and chronic aspiration (see Fig. 10-26).

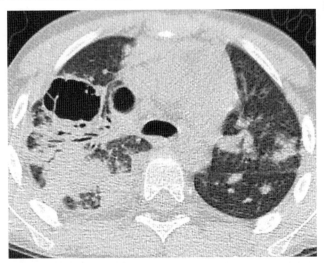

FIGURE 10-54. High-resolution computed tomography shows architectural distortion with large nodular change, air cyst, traction bronchiectasis, and pleural thickening in the right lung, and nodular change in the left. Histopathology verified nonspecific necrotizing vasculitis (see Fig. 10-20).

and coexisting severe small airway disease usually points toward constrictive bronchiolitis (see Fig. 10-48). Bronchial wall thickening without dilation, often with patchy consolidation, is often seen in chronic aspiration (Fig. 10-53). It is sometimes difficult to distinguish between bronchial distention secondary to high ventilator pressure and genuine bronchial dilation. There is much controversy regarding reversibility of bronchiectasis, so serial imaging is the gold standard for irreversibility (i.e., fixed dilatation and wall thickening).

A paper by Gaillard and colleagues[23] advised caution with diagnosing "bronchiectasis," as reversibility of radiologic findings can be seen in children. They suggest that serial imaging be required to confirm irreversibility before using the term *bronchiectasis* in children. They add that, as diagnostic criteria are derived from adult studies that have not been validated in children, cautious interpretation be made of CT findings. Their study included 22 children over a 6-year period who had at least two lung CT scans, with a median scan interval of 21 months (range 2 to 43 months). Bronchial dilation resolved completely in six children, and there was improvement in a further eight patients. Hence, labeling children with an irreversible lifelong condition requires caution on the part of the radiologist.

Architectural Distortion

Fibrosis and altered elasticity of the tissues permanently alters the structure of the lung parenchyma. This is seen as reduced parenchymal attenuation, cysts, deviation of vessels, bronchi and interlobular septa, and traction bronchiectasis (see Fig. 10-50). Cyst formation may also be caused by cystic resolution of pneumonia, forming a pneumatocele, or necrotic change of a preexisting parenchymal nodule (e.g., degeneration of granulomatous change in Langerhans' cell histiocytosis, vasculitis, or Wegener's granulomatosis) (Fig. 10-54). Seen in end-stage disease, honeycombing is the result of clusters of

thick-walled air cysts, representing structurally distorted, dilated respiratory bronchioles lined by fibrotic tissues, collapsed alveoli, and vessels.

ANGIOGRAPHY

In noncardiac chest pathology, angiography is most commonly used for mediastinal vasculature and cystic congenital lung malformations. Magnetic resonance angiography is a useful noninvasive technique with no radiation burden.

Interventional techniques, such as embolization of bronchial arteries, are performed in cases of severe hemorrhage/hemoptysis in cystic fibrosis. Therapeutic embolization of feeding vessels to intralobar or extralobar sequestrations or to pulmonary arteriovenous malformations can be performed using metallic coils, thereby avoiding thoracotomy.

MAGNETIC RESONANCE IMAGING

The importance of nonionizing radiation techniques in pediatrics cannot be overemphasized, and MRI is a highly desirable diagnostic tool for use in children, although drawbacks include the increased use of sedation or general anesthesia, because of the prolonged scan times, and usually closed imaging systems.

The multiplanar imaging capabilities of electrocardiogram-gated MRI and magnetic resonance angiography make these important methods for evaluating cardiac lesions; anomalies of the mediastinal vessels; and masses, such as bronchopulmonary foregut malformations, chest wall masses, bone marrow infiltrations, tracheobronchial abnormalities, and neurogenic masses. The multiplanar capability of MRI, combined with its superb soft-tissue contrast resolution, allow for diagnosis that is more specific. Ongoing refinements, with improved gating techniques and shorter scan times, are under continuous development and continue to enhance the role of MRI in evaluating the pulmonary hila, lung parenchyma, heart, and diaphragm.

Although MRI is well established in cardiac imaging, experience with lung MRI is still limited. The main technical problems are: (1) low proton density in the lungs and hence a very weak signal return (echo) from the lung parenchyma and (2) pulse and motion artifacts from the heart, from the great vessels, and from breathing, causing significant image degradation. Breathing hyperpolarized helium allows detection of signal from within the airspaces. Unfortunately, the gas has a short half-life and is not readily available in most imaging centers.

MRI achieves tissue contrast first by adjusting the train of excitation, refocusing radiofrequency pulses, and switching magnetic field gradients. A T1-weighted MRI sequence takes advantage of the relatively fast realignment with the main magnetic field of fat molecules, so that fat appears bright on the acquired images. Such images are generally useful for studying anatomy. T2-weighted MRI sequences play on the relatively slow realignment of water molecules with the main magnetic field. Because water appears bright on these images, they are particularly helpful in detecting fluid collections and edema. These fundamental MRI techniques provide good depiction of structural change in cystic fibrosis.[24]

A second facility for creating image contrast, or enhancing inherent tissue imaging contrast, is the administration of intravenous MRI contrast medium, which is usually gadolinium chelate. This is typically combined with a T1-weighted pulse sequence and gives superb images of vascular structures, even the most peripheral vessels potentially. Additionally, contrast media are useful for detecting vascular enhancement in inflammatory or neoplastic lesions (Figs. 10-55 to 10-57). Ultrafast pulse sequences with three-dimensional acquisition of volumetric MRI data are diag-

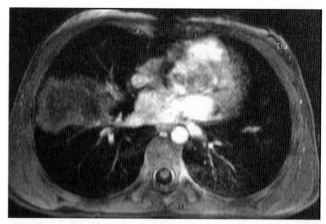

FIGURE 10-56. A 12-year-old boy who received a heart-lung transplant had a right-sided density on chest radiographs. Magnetic resonance imaging (T1-weighted gradient echo, breath-hold, gadolinium-enhanced) shows an enhancing mass lesion in close relation to the right oblique fissure. Histopathologically, this was diagnosed as (posttransplant) lymphoproliferative disease.

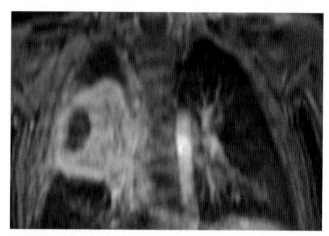

FIGURE 10-57. Contrast-enhanced magnetic resonance imaging scan (gradient echo) in a 1-year-old boy with cough and pyrexia shows enhancement in the right upper lobe, except in a presumed necrotic focus, and mediastinal enhancement. Mycobacterium tuberculosis was later confirmed microbiologically (see Fig. 10-14).

nostically promising and can be implemented on most modern scanners. Although the diagnostic accuracy is still largely unknown, MRI potentially may be used for imaging parenchymal lung lesions,[25] and high accuracy compared with CT has been demonstrated for nodules of 3 mm or larger in size.[26] Quantification of regional pulmonary perfusion is promising in assessment of small airway disease. This can be achieved with time-resolved measurements, following an intravenous bolus of gadolinium. Although not widely used, the technique is available on most modern MRI systems, and there is good agreement with function tests.[27] A noncontrast technique, arterial spin labeling, is promising judged by early feasibility studies.[28] The potential advantage of the latter is that no injection is required and measurements may be repeated as necessary. A combined noncontrast ventilation/perfusion technique has recently been described, however this is not yet in the clinical domain.[29]

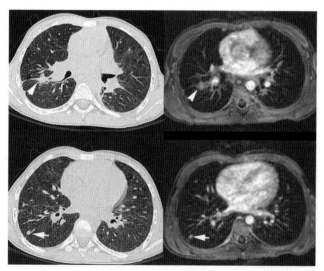

FIGURE 10-55. In a 12-year-old boy with chronic granulomatous disease, high-resolution computed tomography *(left)* and contrast-enhanced three-dimensional gradient echo magnetic resonance imaging *(right)* acquired on the same day show corresponding findings of spiculated, enhancing lesions near the right hilum *(arrowheads)* and subpleurally in the right lower lobe *(arrows)*.

ENDOBRONCHIAL ULTRASONOGRAPHY

A recent paper published by Steinfort and colleagues[30] advocates that endobronchial ultrasound (EBUS) should be used in pediatric patients. The technique of endoscopic ultrasound has been used for the gastrointestinal tract for many years and recently has significantly advanced bronchoscopic techniques in adult respiratory medicine. The use of image guidance with ultrasound allows more accurate localization and sampling of peripheral pulmonary lesions, as well as mediastinal and hilar masses. This results in a greater diagnostic yield with reduced procedural complication rates in clinical practice, so it would appear that EBUS performance characteristics in adult populations are equivalent to surgical procedures that were previously considered the gold standard. However, when compared to surgical approaches, there has been a dramatic reduction in morbidity and mortality among adult patients requiring invasive diagnostic procedures.

Steinfort and colleagues illustrate and advocate the various types of EBUS in clinical use, the methods of usage, and the clinical indications for each procedure, highlighting the potential role for EBUS in pediatric pulmonology.[30]

Radial probe EBUS is used in the investigation of peripheral lung lesions (e.g., suspected invasive pulmonary aspergillosis) and could be adopted in children to achieve accurate biopsy of such lesions.

Linear probe EBUS allows minimally invasive biopsy of mediastinal and hilar lesions. It has potentially greater performance characteristics than current biopsy techniques, with no significant complications reported to date. It may be useful in the diagnosis of lymphoma, or neurogenic tumors, and many other diseases resulting in mediastinal or hilar lymphadenopathy.

Certainly EBUS is a minimally invasive technique allowing tissue sampling of peripheral lung lesions, or mediastinal/hilar masses, with high diagnostic accuracy, and a significantly lower morbidity and mortality than alternative approaches. Hence, the indications for and the usage of EBUS in pediatric patients appear to be promising and will surely increase in the future.

ULTRASONOGRAPHY

Ultrasound is particularly important in pediatric practice because it obviates the need for ionizing radiation. The real-time and portable application of ultrasound makes it even more useful, especially in intensive care units. Because air is highly reflective, the applications of chest ultrasound are limited; however, ultrasound is useful in patients with complete radiographic opacification of a hemithorax because it can distinguish between pleural fluid, consolidation, atelectasis, and parenchymal masses (Fig. 10-58). It also allows characterization of pleural fluid collections as simple, complicated, or fibroadhesive, which is important information for planning thoracocentesis or thoracotomy. It also can be used to study a prominent thymus and thereby obviate unnecessary CT scanning.[31]

Doppler ultrasound with color flow, and power Doppler, aid in the evaluation of vascular status and patency and abnormal vascular anatomy. Ultrasound is useful in the

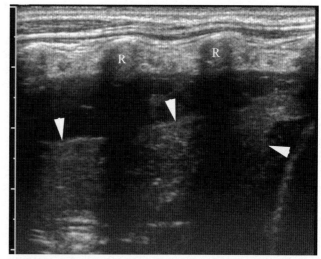

FIGURE 10-58. Coronal ultrasound image of the left hemithorax shows consolidated lung *(arrowheads)* surrounded by fluid, which is mainly anechoic, but with some echogenic strands. Note the acoustic shadows from the ribs (R). Acid-fast bacilli were cultured from the pleural fluid.

diagnosis of bronchopulmonary foregut malformations, particularly intralobar and extralobar sequestrations in which the systemic arterial supply to the lesion can be traced with color Doppler in real time, thus both verifying the diagnosis and acting as a road map for the surgeon (Fig. 10-59).

Ultrasound has a role in assessing spontaneous diaphragmatic movement, and can be easily performed at the bedside. The skilled operator will be able to assess paresis and paradoxical movement and evaluate the differential diagnoses of upper abdominal mass and subpulmonary collection, although the accuracy of assessing diaphragmatic function per se compared with phrenic nerve stimulation is unknown.

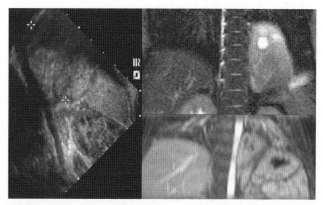

FIGURE 10-59. A neonate with an antenatally diagnosed chest mass was scanned with ultrasound *(left)*, which showed a nonaerated, noncalcified mass lesion (between calipers) paraspinally, immediately above the left hemidiaphragm. The magnetic resonance images also show a cyst *(upper right,* inversion recovery), seen as high signal, and confirm the close relation to the aorta and the intrathoracic position of the mass *(lower right,* contrast-enhanced gradient echo), where the diaphragm *(dark line)* is seen separating the lesion from the stomach (intermediate signal ellipsoid). There was no change in size over time, and the systemic supply from the aorta to this sequestration was later verified. The differential diagnosis for a paraspinal mass in this age group would include neuroblastoma.

RADIONUCLIDE IMAGING

Nuclear medicine techniques are used to help delineate cardiac function, right-to-left pulmonary arteriovenous malformations, pulmonary embolism, inflammatory lung disease, and lung ventilation/perfusion (Fig. 10-60). While nuclear medicine has been the sole means of functional assessment of the heart and lung, the technique is gradually being replaced by CT for assessment of pulmonary embolism and small airway disease and by MRI for combined assessment of cardiac morphology and function.

Positron emission tomography (PET) is a promising modality. It uses biologically interesting radionuclides (e.g., carbon 11, oxygen 15, nitrogen 13) to mark biochemical substrates (e.g., glucose). PET is therefore a modality for metabolic rather than structural studies, and in patients with malignant disease, PET uses the relatively high glucose metabolism in malignant cells for imaging.

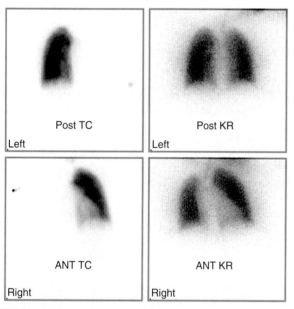

FIGURE 10-60. A ventilation/perfusion isotope study in a patient with absent right pulmonary artery on computed tomography confirms interrupted pulmonary arterial supply to the right lung *(left)*. The hypoplastic right lung has preserved ventilation *(right;* see Figs. 10-4 and 10-40).

Combined with CT, anatomic and functional data can be fused into one image. The clinical efficacy of the technique is being explored.

In a recent study by Klein and colleagues[32] the authors demonstrated foci of enhanced activity on FDG PET scans in CF patients, but not controls, with higher focal activity occurring during CF exacerbation and infection. These foci cleared with antibiotic therapy. Co-registered CT images assisted localization of the PET foci and showed corresponding CT scan findings with many additional features on CT not observed on PET scans. The authors suggest that further studies are needed to validate their results and to determine whether FDG-PET/CT can predict the nature and severity of disease in CF patients.

CONCLUSION

The approaches to radiologic evaluation of the child cannot be extrapolated from adult imaging. Particular awareness of the issues of radiation protection, developmental anatomy and physiology, and the range of pediatric disorders is crucial. As with every test, the key is first to pose a focused question and then to select the best way of answering it, usually in consultation with expert colleagues.

Suggested Reading

Frush DP, Donnelly LF, Rosen NS. Computed tomography and radiation risks. What pediatric health care providers should know. *Pediatrics.* 2003;112:951–957.

Lucaya J, Strife JL. *Pediatric Chest Imaging. Chest Imaging in Infants and Children.* Berlin: Springer-Verlag; 2002.

Puderbach M, Eichinger M, Gahr J, et al. Proton MRI appearance of cystic fibrosis: comparison to CT. *Eur Radiol.* 2007;17:716–724.

Siegel MJ. *Pediatric Body CT.* Philadelphia: Lippincott Williams & Wilkins; 1999.

Siegel MJ, Schmidt B, Bradley D, et al. Radiation dose and image quality in pediatric CT: effect of technical factors and phantom size and shape. *Radiology.* 2004;233:515–522.

References

The complete reference list is available online at www.expertconsult.com

11 PULMONARY FUNCTION TESTS IN INFANTS AND PRESCHOOL CHILDREN

Janet Stocks, PhD, BSc, SRN, and Sooky Lum, PhD

Pulmonary function tests (PFTs) are an integral component of clinical management in school-age children and adults with lung disease. However, until recently, assessment of pulmonary function in infants and preschool children has been restricted to specialized research establishments because of a lack of suitable equipment and difficulties in undertaking these measurements in small, potentially uncooperative subjects. The realization that insult to the developing lung may have lifelong effects (with much of the burden of respiratory disease in later life having its origins prenatally or during the first years of life) has now focused attention on the need to develop sensitive methods of assessing respiratory function in infants and preschool children. As discussed in this chapter, assessment of respiratory function in the very young has major implications for our understanding of respiratory health and disease, not only during childhood, but also throughout life. Such tests can provide objective outcome measures to identify early determinants of respiratory function, distinguish changes due to disease from those related to growth and development, and evaluate the effects of new diagnostic and therapeutic advances.

HISTORICAL BACKGROUND

The first recorded attempts to measure lung function in infants were made over 100 years ago, but relatively little progress was made thereafter until the 1960s, when many tests originally developed for assessing adults (including plethysmography and esophageal manometry) were adapted for use in infants. During the 1980s, new tests were developed specifically for infants, including occlusion techniques for assessing passive respiratory mechanics and the "squeeze" or rapid thoracoabdominal compression (RTC) technique for measuring partial forced expiratory maneuvers. During this period, the first commercially available equipment designed for use in infants became available. With the release of more automated and computerized systems, infant PFTs were no longer restricted to specialized physiology laboratories and were used in a wider range of settings, including neonatal intensive care units. As the diversity of users and applications increased, so did the need for international standardization of equipment and techniques, a challenge that led to the formation of the European Respiratory Society/American Thoracic Society (ERS/ATS) Task Force on infant lung function in 1991. This task force has been responsible for a large number of initiatives over the last 20 years, including recommendations for both users and manufacturers of infant lung function equipment.[1,2]

Accurate evaluation of respiratory function in preschool children (approximately 3 to 6 years of age)[3] is equally important if we are distinguish the various phenotypes of early childhood wheezing, identify early evidence of lung disease in those with chronic disease such as cystic fibrosis (CF), monitor resolution of lung disease in those born prematurely or requiring intensive care in the neonatal period, and guide clinical management by providing objective outcome measures with which to assess efficacy of therapeutic interventions. However, until the start of the current millennium, the preschool years (when the child is too old to sedate yet too young to cooperate with conventional PFTs) were generally considered to be the "dark ages" of pediatric pulmonology. This situation has now changed. With specially trained operators, adaptation of techniques, and a suitable environment, at least 50% of children 3 years of age and the majority of children older than 4 years of age can successfully perform a wide range of PFTs. Techniques that have now been adapted for the preschool age group include spirometry, the forced oscillation technique (FOT), the interrupter resistance (R_{int}) technique, plethysmographic assessments of specific airway resistance (sR_{aw}), and measures of functional residual capacity (FRC) and gas-mixing efficiency using gas dilution and multiple breath inert gas washout (MBW) techniques. Recommendations regarding the use of these techniques have been published by an ATS-ERS Task Force.[3]

OVERVIEW

This chapter provides an overview of the following:
- Differences in assessing pulmonary function in infants and young children compared with older subjects
- PFTs that are feasible in infants and young children
- Limitations of these tests, an appreciation of which is essential not only for the prospective user, but for those referring very young children for such tests or who are reviewing the ever-increasing literature in this field
- Use of infant and preschool PFTs as outcome measures in clinical and epidemiologic research
- Difficulties in interpreting results from this age group, unless suitable controls or repeatability data are available
- Key areas for future clinical and research applications

This chapter focuses on the widely available PFTs for children 0 to 6 years of age, with only brief mention of specialized applications that are limited to a few research centers. Similarly, due to the complexity of the subject, only brief mention is made of applications in the intensive care unit. For simplicity, the term *infant PFTs* is used to refer to all measurements obtained in sleeping infants and young children (generally younger than 2 years of age), whereas *preschool PFTs* is used to refer to tests used in awake young children (generally 3 to 6 years of age). Limited success has been obtained in children 2 to 3 years of age, but the failure rate is higher due to the more limited coordination or cooperation. Most operators therefore prefer to defer testing in the awake child until after the third birthday.

Detailed descriptions of the theory, equipment, data collection, analysis, and quality control relating to individual techniques have been described previously and will not be provided. Instead, the emphasis of this chapter is on the application and interpretation of these tests and their potential role in pediatric pulmonology. In addition to suggestions for further reading, more extensive references are provided in the online version, these being generally limited to key publications during the last few years.

■ DIFFERENCES IN ASSESSING LUNG FUNCTION IN INFANTS AND PRESCHOOL CHILDREN

Infants and Toddlers Younger Than 2 Years of Age

In addition to the marked developmental changes in respiratory physiology that occur during the first years of life, which affect both the measurement and interpretation of results, the major differences in undertaking infant PFTs relate to sleep state, sedation, ethical issues, posture, and the need to miniaturize and adapt equipment for measurements in small subjects who tend to be preferential nose breathers and who cannot be asked to undertake special breathing maneuvers.

■ DEVELOPMENTAL CHANGES PERTINENT TO INFANT PFTS[4]

Influence of the Upper Airways

Infants are preferential nose breathers, with nasal resistance representing approximately 50% of total airway resistance (R_{aw}). Changes in lower R_{aw} as a result of disease or therapeutic interventions may therefore be masked, especially if there has been a recent upper respiratory tract infection (URTI). It is recommended that infant PFTs be postponed for at least 3 weeks after the onset of any respiratory infection. Because the nose also acts as an efficient filter, less aerosolized material (whether delivered as a challenge or a therapeutic intervention) may reach the lung than in a mouth-breathing adult. The upper airways also play an important role in modulating expiratory flow and lung volume.

Compliance of the Chest Wall and Dynamic Elevation of End-Expiratory Level

During infancy, although lung recoil is similar to that found in older subjects, the highly compliant chest wall results in minimal outward elastic recoil. During passive

expiration, the lungs therefore recoil to a much lower volume in relation to total lung capacity (TLC) than in older subjects. The potential difficulties imposed by the resultant instability of functional residual capacity (FRC) and tendency for small airway closure during tidal breathing are, however, at least partially compensated for by dynamic elevation of end-expiratory level during the first 6 months of life. The expiratory time constant (τ_{rs}) is the time (in seconds) taken for the lungs to passively deflate to 63% of its original volume. 95% of lung emptying is complete within 3 time constants, hence dynamic hyperinflation will occur if the duration of expiration is less than 3 expiratory time constants. This is most likely to occur in the presence of either a short expiratory time (rapid respiratory rate) or a long time constant (elevated expiratory resistance) such that the infant breathes in before reaching the passively determined resting lung volume. The τ_{rs} is the product of respiratory compliance (C_{rs}) and respiratory resistance (R_{rs}), so in a healthy 4-kg neonate (with a C_{rs} of 40 mL · cm H_2O^{-1} and an R_{rs} of 40 cm H_2O · L^{-1} · sec) the τ_{rs} would be 0.16 seconds, and lung emptying would be virtually complete within 0.48 seconds. However, if the resistance rises to 80 cm H_2O· L^{-1} · sec in the presence of airway disease, the τ_{rs} will double, requiring expiratory time to be at least 0.96 seconds for complete lung emptying (i.e., a respiratory rate of less than 30 per minute in the presence of an inspiratory/expiratory ratio of 1:1). In contrast, in an infant with respiratory distress syndrome (RDS) in whom compliance is very low (e.g., <10 mL · cm H_2O^{-1}), the high elastic recoil and short τ_{rs} will result in rapid lung emptying and potential atelectasis.

Awareness of the impact of underlying differences in respiratory pathophysiology on the expiratory τ_{rs} is vital if appropriate ventilator settings are to be selected in young children requiring intensive care, but is also relevant to the spontaneously breathing child. During the first months of life, infants modulate both expiratory time and flow to maintain an adequate FRC. This is mediated through tonic and phasic vagal stretch receptors that are exquisitely sensitive to changes in resting lung volume. In contrast to adults, the Hering-Breuer inflation reflex is physiologically active over the tidal range during the first year of life. The instantaneous change in breathing rate and pattern in response to small changes in resting lung volume can be seen during the application of continuous negative or positive pressure, as well as after an apneic pause. In addition to changes in respiratory rate, infants often use post-inspiratory diaphragmatic and laryngeal activity to slow (or brake) expiratory flow. The latter is particularly noticeable in those with RDS, who may exhibit audible grunting. Intubation removes this defense mechanism and can lead to rapid deterioration unless compensated for by an appropriate level of positive end-expiratory pressure.

The ability to modulate expiratory flow and timing and hence resting lung volume may be physiologically beneficial to the infant, but it can complicate attempts to assess respiratory function. Whereas the active Hering-Breuer inflation reflex facilitates assessment of passive respiratory mechanics in infants (discussed later in the chapter), the variability of end-expiratory level may impede assessment and interpretation not only of lung volumes, but also of respiratory mechanics and forced expiratory flow (FEF), which are highly volume-dependent. Developmental changes in respiratory rate and mechanics may all have significant effects on the interpretation of longitudinal changes in various indices, such as timed forced expired volumes.[5]

SLEEP STATE, SEDATION, AND DURATION OF THE TESTING PROCEDURE

Although attempts have been made to assess lung function in awake infants, measurements are normally made during sleep, which facilitates positioning of the facemask, brief airway occlusions (for passive respiratory mechanics and plethysmography), and application of thoracoabdominal pressure during forced expiratory maneuvers. A representative and stable end-expiratory level is essential for reproducible measures of resting lung volume or respiratory mechanics and can normally only be achieved if the child is in quiet, rather than rapid eye movement, sleep. Since the duration of quiet sleep epochs is inversely proportional to postmenstrual age (PMA = gestational + postnatal age) and may last <10 minutes in a preterm infant, this can present a real challenge when undertaking measurements in very young or immature infants. As the infant adapts to extrauterine respiration during the first 48 hours after delivery, reliable testing is similarly difficult because of the instability of breathing patterns and lung mechanics during this period.

Studies in Unsedated Infants

Unless clinically indicated, sedation is generally contraindicated for PFTs in newborn infants.[6] Successful measurements using a full range of tests can usually be achieved during natural sleep after a feeding in all infants up to at least 44 weeks PMA. Tests based on tidal breathing recordings (including FOT and MBW) may be applicable in the unsedated infant up to 4 months' postnatal life, whereas forced expiratory maneuvers and plethysmography generally require sedation, certainly beyond 3 months of age. As discussed later in the chapter, unsedated studies are more readily acceptable to both parents and some ethics committees, but they limit the range of investigations that can be undertaken and extend the duration of testing. Success rates depend on the age of the infant and type of procedure, but are generally around 60% in both home-based and hospital studies of unsedated infants, compared with approximately 90% for most studies of sedated infants.

Studies in Sedated Infants

Some research ethics committees are reluctant to give approval for healthy infants to be recruited for research studies requiring sedation, while others consider it unethical to sedate vulnerable infants with respiratory disease unless results can be interpreted properly.[7] Sedation is usually achieved using oral chloral hydrate in doses of 50 to 100 mg/kg. The hospital-specific protocol for sedation should always be followed. With the exception of a small proportion of "high-risk" children (e.g., those with known or suspected upper airway obstruction in whom sedation is generally contraindicated due to the risk of exacerbating symptoms[6]), chloral hydrate has been shown to have an excellent safety record and has been administered to thousands of infants worldwide without adverse side effects.[7] Nevertheless, the bitter taste of chloral hydrate is rarely appreciated by the recipients, who may object loudly, making this the most stressful aspect of infant PFTs for parents. Furthermore, its action can be unpredictable, with time taken to fall asleep after administration ranging from 15 minutes to more than 2 hours. The duration of subsequent induced sleep can be equally variable, such that the investigators rarely have longer than 45 minutes in which to collect PF data. Consequently, important decisions are required regarding which tests are most appropriate on any particular occasion. Given the time required to obtain fully informed parental consent and for the infant to fall asleep, parents may need to spend 3 to 4 hours in the infant PFT laboratory. This may limit their ability or willingness to attend for repeat measurements at intervals of less than 6 months. Caution with respect to repeated sedation also limits the frequency with which serial PFTs can be performed, potentially limiting their clinical usefulness in individual infants.

SAFETY ISSUES AND POSTURE

For all studies involving infants, strict safety precautions must be followed. Resuscitation equipment, including suction, must be available. Two skilled operators who are fully trained in basic life support (one of whom has prime responsibility for monitoring the well-being of the infant) must be present. Pulse oximetry is used for continuous monitoring throughout the testing session.

Most infant PFTs are obtained in the supine position, which will influence not only diaphragmatic position and efficiency of the respiratory musculature, but also the FRC, lung mechanics, and distribution of ventilation. One must take into account such changes when interpreting longitudinal changes that span into later childhood. The neck and shoulders should be supported in the midline in slight extension, with the position stabilized by a neck roll or head ring to optimize upper airway patency throughout the procedures. Extreme care should be taken to avoid any depression of the jaw during placement of the facemask.

EQUIPMENT REQUIREMENTS

One of the greatest difficulties in assessing respiratory function in infancy and early childhood has been that of obtaining suitable equipment. Until recently, the lack of commercially available, well-validated systems meant that most research establishments used their own custom-built equipment and software. This impeded training, meaningful comparison of results between different centers, and attempts to establish multicenter trials with infant PFTs as outcome measures. Recent technologic advances and close collaboration between members of the ERS-ATS Task Force[1] has now resulted in a new generation of commercially available infant PFT devices.[8-10] Users and potential purchasers of such equipment must ensure not only that it meets the basic requirements specified by the ERS-ATS Task Force (including the ease with which it can be cleaned between every subject), but that results are interpreted in relation to appropriate equipment-specific reference equations or healthy controls studied with identical equipment.[7,9] The selected device also must be appropriate for the intended measurement conditions and body size because commercially available equipment is rarely validated for use in infants receiving assisted ventilation, those born preterm, or those with a body weight below 3 to 4 kg. Given the time-consuming nature of these investigations and the impossibility of repeating measurements in the event of equipment failure, attention to detail with respect to calibration, regular maintenance of equipment, and a good supply of spare parts are even more essential when assessing infants than when testing older subjects.

LEAKS AND DEAD SPACE

An oronasal mask is generally required when undertaking infant PFTs which, even when using the smallest appropriate size with judicious use of therapeutic putty, may significantly increase equipment dead space. This is likely to increase tidal volume (VT) and may elevate the end-expiratory level. Furthermore, difficulties in estimating the true effective dead space of the mask (i.e., that which is not occupied by the child's face during use) may lead to increased variability within and between subjects and centers when calculating FRC or indices of ventilation inhomogeneity. Air leaks around the facemask are one of the most common sources of error when undertaking infant PFTs, yet they can be difficult to identify. Such leaks are most likely to occur during tests that require airway occlusions or administration of positive airway pressure (e.g., plethysmographic lung volumes, occlusion techniques, and the raised volume technique), but they also invalidate all other assessments. Many centers use therapeutic putty to create an airtight seal between the face and the mask (Fig. 11-1), whereas others depend on

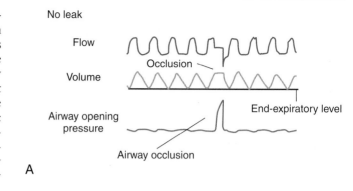

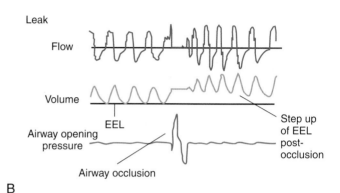

FIGURE 11-2. Occlusion test to check for leaks around the facemask. Time-based recording of flow, volume, and pressure at the airway opening during spontaneous tidal breathing. **A,** When there is no leak through or around the facemask, there will be a period a zero flow during a brief airway occlusion; a stable end-expiratory level, as seen from a tidal volume trace, will be maintained after release of the occlusion. **B,** In contrast, if air escapes around the side of the mask during such an occlusion, there will be a step-up of the end-expiratory level (EEL), as shown here. (Copyright © Janet Stocks.)

an air-filled cushioned mask, particularly in very young and unsedated infants. Whatever the approach, operators must be vigilant at all times to avoid serious errors caused by air leakage. Warning signs include low VT (values <6 mL/kg being rare when an infant is breathing through a mask), drift of the VT signal (wherein expiratory volume is less than that inspired), or failure of the end-expiratory level to return to baseline after a brief airway occlusion (Fig. 11-2).

PRESCHOOL CHILDREN

Assessment of preschool children presents a number of special challenges. Such children may not have the necessary coordination or concentration to perform the physiologic maneuvers required for conventional PFTs. They also have a short attention span and are easily distracted and thus need to be engaged and encouraged by the operator to participate in the test. Although measurement conditions for testing preschool children are broadly similar to those required for older subjects, every effort should be made to make the environment as child-friendly (and safe!) as possible. This includes provision of suitable furniture, games, and wall coverings as well as adaptation of the normal lung function terminology, with terms such as

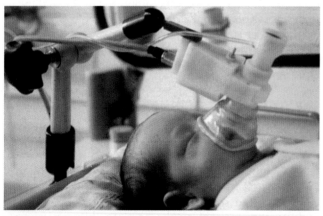

FIGURE 11-1. Infant lung function tests using a facemask and a pneumotachometer. Note the use of a ring of silicone putty to create an airtight seal during the recordings. (Copyright © Carefusion.)

blowing games and puffing playrooms replacing the more familiar spirometry and lung function lab.

To this end, the most important acquisition for any preschool setup is personnel with suitable temperaments (including a love of children, infinite patience and stamina, and a good sense of humor). Adaptability, meticulous attention to detail, and a thorough background in respiratory physiology are also essential requirements because appropriate criteria for acceptable tests in the preschool child may differ markedly from those established for older subjects.[3] The criterion for a successful preschool PFT session should be not so much that valid results have been obtained, but that the child (and their parents) wants to return for subsequent visits. Because young children tire easily, visits should be timed to maximize success (i.e., morning or early afternoon, without coinciding with times of regular naps). The emotional and developmental stage of the child will be an important determinant of success when undertaking preschool PFTs, especially when more active cooperation is required, such as for spirometry. The child's medical history may also be highly relevant. Those delivered extremely prematurely or with extended neonatal hospitalization may display considerable antipathy toward hospital environments in general as well as orofacial aversion. Such children will need particular understanding. It may be helpful to send the parents home with equipment such as a mask, tubing, or mouthpieces with which to familiarize the child before subsequent appointments are arranged.

The need to gain the child's confidence, provide the necessary coaching, and offer opportunities for rest when required mean that plenty of time should be set aside for this age group, particularly those younger than 4 years of age or who are attending for the first time. The use of computer games and appropriate incentives to help the child understand what is required during special maneuvers (e.g., forced expirations) can be extremely helpful, whereas encouragement to sit quietly during more prolonged periods of data collection (e.g., when using the MBW technique to assess gas-mixing efficiency) can be provided by having the mother read a favorite book to the child or allowing the child to watch a favorite video. The choice of such videos, however, must be considered carefully since those that lead to overt laughter, breath-holding, or vocal participation are not conducive to high-quality PFTs!

Commercial equipment is available for most preschool PFTs, albeit not specifically designed for this age group.[3] The potential effects of using equipment developed for older and larger individuals, particularly with respect to dead space, resistance, and resolution needs to be considered.

ANTHROPOMETRY AND BACKGROUND DETAILS

Given the rapid rate of somatic growth during infancy and early childhood, accurate measurements of height and weight using a calibrated stadiometer and scales are essential. Two trained operators are required to obtain valid measurements in infants, and these procedures can

be equally challenging in lively preschoolers. For accurate interpretation of lung function tests, it is also helpful to record data on environmental, genetic, and socio-economic factors that are likely to affect lung growth, including sex; ethnic group; family history of asthma and atopy; cigarette smoke exposure, both prenatal and postnatal; allergen exposure, including pets; relevant current and past medical history; and medication use. Validation of current maternal smoking report using cotinine analysis of infant urine or maternal saliva is also helpful. There remains an urgent need to assess the effect of ethnicity on various lung function parameters in infants and young children.[11,12]

METHODS OF ASSESSING PULMONARY FUNCTION IN INFANTS AND YOUNG CHILDREN

Although there may be a need to measure lung volumes, compliance, and surface area in order to assess impact of some congenital cardiac defects or potential alveolar hypoplasia associated with "new" BPD,[13] the emphasis placed on the assessment of airway function during early life, using techniques to assess resistance and forced expired maneuvers, reflects the fact that most respiratory problems in young children beyond the neonatal period are dominated by transient or persistent wheezing disorders. There is increasing awareness that airway obstruction may be determined not only by the caliber of the airways, but also by the compliance of the airway wall and the elastic recoil of the surrounding parenchyma, leading to the search for suitable outcomes that will reflect these characteristics and hence improve the interpretation of results.

An ideal lung function test for infants and young children will meet the following criteria:

- Acceptable both to the child and the parents
- Applicable to any age and arousal state
- Independent of subject cooperation
- Simple and involves no risk
- Reproducible
- Sensitive enough to distinguish between health and disease
- Able to reflect the clinical situation or provide accurate and specific information about lung structure and function
- Cheap

No such test currently exists, and even if it did, no single test is ever likely to provide all of the necessary information for a clinical or research study. Nevertheless, there are a wide variety of techniques now available for measuring lung volume, respiratory mechanics, ventilation inhomogeneity, and the control of breathing. As summarized in Table 11-1, some of these tests can be applied to both age groups, whereas others are applicable only in sleeping infants or relatively cooperative preschool children.

When designing a protocol for either clinical or research studies, it is vital to consider not only which combination of PFTs is most appropriate, but also the order in which these should be performed. The very first step is to formulate a clear question, which in turn will allow clarity

TABLE 11-1 FEASIBILITY OF VARIOUS PULMONARY FUNCTION TESTS IN CHILDREN OF DIFFERENT AGES *

Measurement Conditions	INFANTS AND TODDLERS 0 TO 2 YEARS Sleeping With or Without Sedation	PRESCHOOL CHILDREN 3 TO 6 YEARS Awake with Some Active Cooperation
Technique		
Tidal breathing parameters	✓	✓
Plethysmographic FRC	✓	X (occasional applications only)
Plethysmographic TLC, RV, and so on	Specialized laboratory only	X
FRC by gas dilution or multiple breath washout (MBW)	✓	✓
Gas-mixing efficiency by MBW	✓	✓
Plethysmographic R_{aw}	If heated rebreathing system available	X
Plethysmographic sR_{aw}	(✓)	✓
Occlusion Technique Respiratory mechanics (R_{rs}, C_{rs}, time constant)	✓	X
Interrupter Technique (Rint)	(✓) not yet validated	✓
Forced Oscillation (Zrs)	✓	✓
Forced expiratory maneuvers using tidal or raised-volume RTC	✓	X
Voluntary forced expiratory maneuvers, i.e., spirometry	X	✓

*The suggested age range provides a rough indication only, and feasibility will depend on the developmental as well as the chronologic age of the child. Some tests, such as specific airway resistance or interrupter resistance, may be feasible in children between 2 and 3 years of age, but the success rate is generally much lower than in those older than 3 years of age.
C_{rs}, compliance of the total respiratory system; *FRC*, functional residual capacity; R_{aw}, airway resistance; R_{int}, interrupter resistance; R_{rs}, respiratory resistance; *RV*, residual volume; *RVRTC*, raised volume rapid thoracoabdominal compression; sR_{aw}, specific airway resistance; *TLC*, total lung capacity; Z_{rs}, impedance of the respiratory system.

of thought about what is the best technique. Given the potential effect of lung inflations or deep inspirations on underlying respiratory mechanics, it is generally advisable to perform tests based on tidal breathing recordings before any forced expiratory maneuvers. When considering what is feasible within any given test occasion, both the age and clinical status of the subject and the expertise of the operators must be taken in to account. When setting up new facilities for either infant or preschool PFTs, it is wise to commence with a relatively simple baseline protocol that can be successfully completed in the majority of subjects, and then to gradually introduce new techniques or interventions as expertise and confidence develop.

ASSESSMENT OF LUNG VOLUME AND VENTILATION

Why Measure Lung Volumes?

As in older subjects, measurement of lung volume is essential for accurate interpretation of respiratory mechanics, as well as for defining normal lung growth. It must, however, be remembered that only FRC can be measured in infants

and preschool children, and it rarely provides information on the number and size of alveoli or the surface area available for gas exchange (which may be critical when investigating the effects of prenatal and postnatal insults on subsequent lung growth).[13] Furthermore, the ability of the lung to expand rapidly to fill available space after surgical repair (e.g., congenital diaphragmatic hernia) may limit the clinical value of measuring lung volume in young children with congenital lung hypoplasia. Reduced FRC due to restrictive lung disease may be found in young children with rare lung conditions (e.g., interstitial lung disease or hypoplasia), but this pattern is more common in children with disorders that affect the chest wall (e.g., scoliosis, pectus excavatum, or myopathy) or in those with surfactant deficiency or atelectasis due to conditions such as RDS. The most common abnormality of lung volume during infancy is that associated with airway obstruction, wherein both hyperinflation (due to dynamic elevation of lung volume in the presence of elevated R_{aw} and a long τ_{rs}) and gas trapping (due to peripheral airway closure) result in elevated FRC values in wheezy infants and those with diseases such as CF. As discussed later in the chapter, the ability to detect such hyperinflation will depend on both the underlying pathophysiology and the measurement technique selected. One of the greatest potential uses for lung volume measurements in infants and children is with respect to optimizing ventilatory support in those receiving intensive care. As discussed later, despite growing interest and research activity in this field, considerable technologic difficulties must be overcome before such measures are likely to influence the clinical management of individual children.

TIDAL BREATHING PARAMETERS

Accurate measurement of tidal breathing is fundamental to most infant and preschool PFTs. The potential advantages of noninvasive monitoring of lung function during natural sleep have resulted in persistent efforts to analyze tidal breathing parameters, either from changes in flow and volume at the airway opening or from body surface measurements. Although superficially appearing to be one of the simplest investigations to undertake, such measurements and their interpretation are in fact highly complex. Tidal breathing parameters have been used for the following:

- To determine V_T and breathing frequency
- To determine minute ventilation
- To investigate the control of breathing
- To establish regularity of breathing patterns prior to assessments of lung volume and mechanics
- As an integral part of sleep staging
- When measuring exhaled nitric oxide
- As an indirect measure of airway mechanics
- To trigger equipment

Patterns of tidal flow-volume loops can yield potentially important information about the likely site of obstruction (Fig. 11-3). Peripheral airway narrowing generally produces a concave pattern of the expiratory flow-volume loop, with peak tidal flow occurring early in expiration. This pattern probably reflects a reduction in postinspiratory diaphragmatic or laryngeal braking in the presence of a prolonged τ_{rs} due to elevated R_{aw}. Flattening of the expiratory limb is suggestive of a fixed extrathoracic airway obstruction, whereas marked convexity of the volume axis may reflect physiologic braking of expiratory flow. A pattern of inspiratory fluttering may be associated with laryngomalacia, whereas stiff lungs (low compliance and high elastic recoil) may be reflected by a relatively small V_T, with high peak flow and rapid lung emptying. Considerable caution is required when interpreting such loops due to marked natural physiologic variability within and between children, particularly during early infancy. Attempts to quantify such patterns have resulted in numeric descriptors of the tidal flow pattern, such as the time to peak tidal expiratory flow as a ratio of total expiratory time (t_{PTEF}:t_E) (Fig. 11-4). This index, which is sometimes referred to as the *tidal breathing ratio,* may be reduced in the presence of airway obstruction and has been shown to be a valuable outcome measure in various epidemiologic studies investigating early determinants of airway function.[14,15] However, this measurement is only distantly related to airway function and, as with most

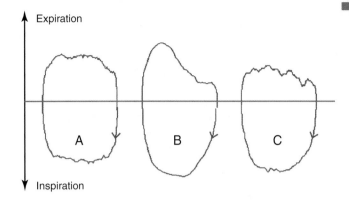

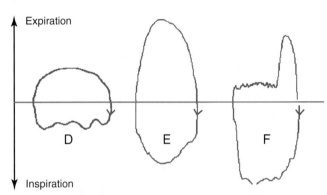

FIGURE 11-3. Patterns of tidal flow-volume loops. Normal *(A)*; flow limitation or airway obstruction *(B)*; laryngeal braking or fixed intrathoracic obstruction *(C)*; fixed extrathoracic obstruction *(D)*; reduced compliance (i.e., rapid lung emptying due to stiff lungs or increased elastic recoil) *(E)*. Marked expiratory grunting may occur in the presence of decreased functional residual capacity or stiff lungs to increase the expiratory time constant *(F)*. (Copyright © Janet Stocks.)

tidal breathing parameters, conveys mixed information on the interaction between control of breathing and airway mechanics, thereby requiring cautious interpretation, especially within individual infants and children. It has not been found to be discriminative in infants with CF or recovering from BPD.[16,17] A wide range of methods have been developed to study the control of breathing in infants,[16,18] but these tend to be restricted to specialized centers. Assessments of V_T, respiratory rate and minute ventilation have also been used as secondary outcomes when assessing the effects of factors such as preterm birth and exposure to maternal smoking or pollution.[19–21]

Equipment and Procedure

In addition to developmental changes and those related to disease processes, patterns of tidal breathing will vary within and between individuals according to posture, sleep state, and the physical properties of the equipment, making it vital to standardize measurement conditions before meaningful interpretations can be made. Various types of flow meters, including pneumotachometers (PNTs) and, more recently, ultrasonic flowmeters

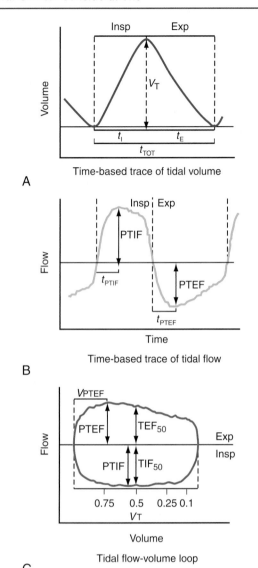

A

Time-based trace of tidal volume

B

Time-based trace of tidal flow

C

Tidal flow-volume loop

FIGURE 11-4. A–C, Tidal breathing parameters. In addition to tidal volume (V_T) and respiratory rate, the following parameters are often calculated from recordings of tidal breathing: tidal expiratory (Exp) and inspiratory (Insp) flow when 50% V_T remains in the lung (TEF50 and TIF50, respectively); inspiratory time (t_i); expiratory time (t_E); total breath time (t_{TOT}); peak tidal inspiratory flow (PTIF); peak tidal expiratory flow (PTEF); time to peak expiratory flow (tPTEF); time to peak inspiratory flow (tPTIF); volume expired before PTEF is attained (VPTEF); and tidal breathing ratio (tPTEF:t_E). (Copyright © Janet Stocks.)

(USFM) have been used to measure tidal flow in infants and preschool children. It is essential that the device selected is appropriate with respect to resolution, deadspace, and equipment resistance for the age and size of the child to be studied. Accuracy and comparability of tidal breathing parameters is also influenced by technical factors such as the sampling rate and resolution of the equipment and the algorithms used for breath detection, adjustment to body temperature, pressure, saturated (BTPS) conditions, and compensation for any volume drift. A minimum recording period of at least 30 to 60 seconds (minimum of 20 breaths) has been recommended when reporting tidal breathing parameters in infants.

Common factors that distort tidal breathing measurements in infants include air leaks around the mask or mouthpiece, upper airway artifacts (head position) that lead to snoring or extrathoracic airway obstruction, secretions, and laryngeal braking. Sighs can significantly influence control of breathing and tidal waveform analysis, particularly in preterm and newborn infants.

Calculation and Reporting of Results

Tidal flow and volume waveforms can be described using time-based V_T or tidal flow signals and the flow-volume loop. Apart from V_T and respiratory rate, the most commonly reported parameters are illustrated in Figure 11-4. Various tidal breathing indices, including the degree of thoracoabdominal asynchrony, can also be assessed using respiratory inductance plethysmography or similar body surface measurements.[22]

Advantages and Limitations

Accurate recordings of tidal breathing patterns are frequently essential when interpreting other lung function tests in infants and young children. The greatest advantage of undertaking detailed analysis of tidal breathing per se is undoubtedly the noninvasive nature of these recordings. However, it is extremely difficult to record a true baseline for tidal breathing when using any system that requires facial attachments due to the added deadspace, and attempts to use body surface measurements have met with limited success, except in large epidemiologic studies. In health, the pattern of tidal breathing is highly variable, and although assessments have been performed in awake, newborn infants, repeatable measures normally require that infants be in quiet sleep, when they are also likely to tolerate more direct and discriminative measures of pulmonary function. Similarly, once preschool children have settled and established a regular pattern of breathing, measurements of sR_{aw} or ventilation inhomogeneity, which are likely to be more informative, can be performed almost as easily as those of tidal breathing.

Initial reports in the 1980s regarding the potential value of t_{PTEF}:t_E in predicting subsequent wheezing in previously healthy infants[14] led to a plethora of studies that used this simple index as an outcome variable. Indeed, when used in large epidemiologic studies of young infants, t_{PTEF}:t_E has proved to be a useful outcome measure when studying the effects of maternal smoking in pregnancy or identifying those at increased risk of subsequent wheezing disorders. The clinical usefulness of this approach is however severely limited within individuals by the marked within- and between-subject variability of breathing patterns. Even within epidemiologic studies, the discriminative ability of t_{PTEF}:t_E diminishes with increasing age and has not been found to be a useful outcome in young children with CF.[17] This illustrates the important, yet often forgotten, principle that techniques that are eminently suited to studying large groups to derive information of potential mechanistic importance may be too variable to use in the clinical management of individuals.

Future Directions

Despite the problems discussed in the previous sections, the potential for noninvasive outcomes that can be measured in unsedated infants has inspired several groups to continue the search for improved methods of collecting and analyzing tidal breathing data. In addition to Fast Fourier transform (FFT) of the recorded signals to quantify the harmonic content of the entire tidal flow waveform (rather than depending on indices derived from a limited number of points), there is increasing interest in the use of more refined body surface measurements to record tidal breathing.

Electrical impedance tomography (EIT) permits visualization of the spatial distribution of ventilation and hence any functional regional inhomogeneity.[23-26] Briefly, EIT takes advantage of differences in conductance of electricity by different biological tissues. The resistivity of lung tissue is approximately five times greater than that of most other soft tissues in the thorax, and it increases considerably when air moves into the alveoli during inspiration so that the electrical current must flow around them. High-frequency, low-amplitude currents are passed between pairs of electrodes on the body, and the potentials between all of the other pairs of electrodes are simultaneously measured (Fig. 11-5). The ratio of the potentials to the applied current are transfer impedances, with the EIT images being reconstructed from a set of transfer impedance measurements. Serial measurements using EIT in ventilated infants have been able to identify the redistribution of lung ventilation and changes in the magnitude of regional ventilation in response to alterations in ventilator settings, surfactant instillation, and changes in posture. Several EIT systems have been described for thoracic imaging, although none is yet available commercially and analytic methods are still being developed.[27] Provided further adaptations of hardware and software can be implemented to improve practical handling and facilitate stable and undisturbed measurements in the intensive care unit, this noninvasive method could become a useful bedside monitoring tool of regional lung ventilation in critically ill infants, with important implications for optimizing lung volume and minimizing lung injury.

Optoelectronic plethysmography (OEP), which allows the assessment of tidal volume changes by measuring chest wall surface motion after applying a series of light-reflective markers, has recently been applied to newborns. Preliminary results suggest an acceptable degree of agreement with simultaneous short-term (2-minute duration) measurements obtained using pneumotachography. An alternative completely noncontact approach based on similar principles is currently being validated in several centers.[28]

This method, known as structured light plethysmography (SLP), also measures changes in lung volume by detecting chest and abdominal wall movements during breathing. Rather than attaching light-reflective markers, a structured light pattern is projected onto the chest and abdominal wall, and two overhead digital cameras record the movement of the pattern as the child breathes; it is then processed to calculate the internal volume of the chest and abdomen and any changes in lung volume during breathing (Fig. 11-6). In additional to standard lung function parameters, SLP also provides information about regional changes in air movement and allows comparisons of the relative contributions of thoracic and abdominal wall movements. Although further developmental work is required before these technique are ready for clinical application, they offer exciting possibilities for future noninvasive monitoring of tidal breathing and alterations in regional ventilation or lung volume, either at baseline or in response to short-term interventions.

Exciting new tools are also being used to explore the complexity of developmental changes in the control of breathing.[16,29,30] These tools offer a step forward from the current, more subjective nature of clinical observation in this field. It has also been shown that noninvasive assessments of intercostal and diaphragmatic muscle activity, using transcutaneous electrodes[31] or magnetic stimulation

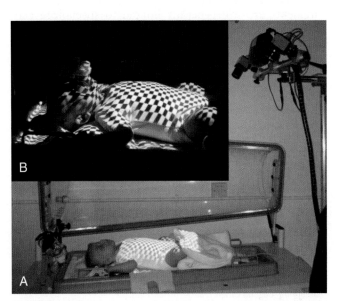

FIGURE 11-6. Assessment of tidal breathing using structured light plethysmography (SLP). **A,** Quantitative assessments of tidal breathing during quiet sleep using SLP. **B,** Recordings can be validated by undertaking simultaneous assessments using a pneumotach, but unlike respiratory inductance plethysmography, calibration does not require any measure of air flow during calibration. (Copyright © Janet Stocks.)

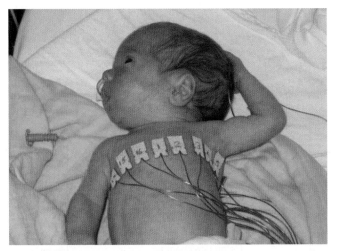

FIGURE 11-5. Placement of electrodes for monitoring changes in lung volume using electrical impedance tomography (EIT) in a preterm infant.

of phrenic nerves,[32] are feasible even in naturally sleeping infants. In addition to providing a more comprehensive picture of pulmonary mechanics and their interdependence on respiratory control, this could contribute to future studies of EMG-triggered mechanical ventilation.

Despite recognized difficulties in accurately interpreting measures of exhaled nitric oxide as a noninvasive marker of airway inflammation in infants due to the influence of nasal breathing and the marked flow dependency of such measures, bedside equipment for evaluation of such markers is now available for use in infants and preschool children, and their potential utility in both clinical and epidemiologic research studies has been described.[21,33–38] A detailed description of these measurements in older children is provided in Chapter 12.

PLETHYSMOGRAPHIC ASSESSMENT OF LUNG VOLUMES

Infants

The principles of plethysmography (which assesses total thoracic gas volume, including any gas trapped behind closed airways) are identical for infants and older subjects. Infants are not able to cooperate in the special breathing maneuvers required to reach either residual volume (RV) or total lung capacity (TLC). Consequently, until recently, the only lung volume that could be routinely measured in spontaneously breathing infants was FRC. Introduction of the raised volume technique in the mid-1990s, whereby a bias flow or pump is used to inflate the sleeping infant's lungs toward TLC before a small jacket (which is previously wrapped around the chest and abdomen) is inflated to force expiration means that quasi-values of TLC, expiratory reserve volume (ERV), and residual volume (RV) can now be calculated.[39] While commercial equipment is available to undertake such measurements,[8] these measurements are still generally limited to specialized centers, and FRC remains the most common measure of lung function in this age group.

Assessments of plethysmographic FRC in infants (Fig. 11-7)[39,40] have been widely used in both clinical and epidemiologic research.[8,39,41–46] A few centers still retain

their own custom-built equipment, but the majority of measurements are now made using a commercially available device.[8,41,47]

It is generally recommended that airway occlusions are performed at end inspiration in infants, with subsequent subtraction of the inspired VT when calculating for FRC. This is less disturbing to the infant, causes less glottic closure, and facilitates improved equilibration of pressures throughout the respiratory system when compared with end-expiratory occlusions. Critical quality control issues during data collection and analysis have been reported[40] and include the need to ensure adequate thermal equilibration of the box before commencement of data recording, a stable end-expiratory level before and after the occlusion, absence of any air leak, and no phase lag (i.e., no looping on the X-Y plot) between the box and mouth pressure signals during the occlusion (Fig. 11-8). The shutter is usually closed for 6 to 10 seconds, or until at least two complete respiratory efforts have been made. The maneuver should be repeated until three to five technically satisfactory occlusions have been performed, with the result reported as the mean (SD) of technically satisfactory maneuvers. Such data can usually be obtained within 5 minutes. The coefficient of variation (100 × [SD/mean]) from three to five runs is generally less than 4% (range: 1% to 10%).

Advantages and Limitations

The major advantages of infant plethysmography include the following:
- The rapidity and reproducibility with which measurements can be attained.
- The fact that all gas within the lungs, including that in nonventilating or slowly ventilating areas, is measured. Paired measurements of FRC using gas dilution and plethysmographic techniques may be useful in detecting gas trapping, although since plethysmography may overestimate FRC, and gas dilution techniques underestimate it, considerable errors may result.

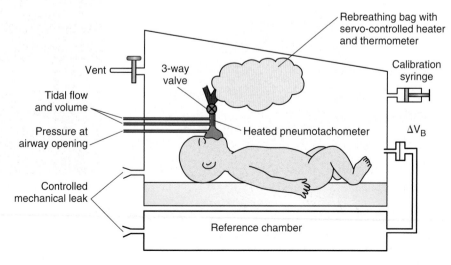

FIGURE 11-7. Infant plethysmography. Measurements of plethysmographic functional residual capacity are made while the infant sleeps within the plethysmograph and makes respiratory efforts against a closed shutter. Provision of a heated rebreathing bag or other means of compensating for changes in the temperature and humidity of respired gas allows simultaneous assessment of airway resistance. ΔVB, changes in box volume. (Adapted from Stocks J, Sly PD, Tepper RS, et al. Infant Respiratory Function Testing. New York: John Wiley & Sons, 1996, pp 1-577.)

Time-based recording

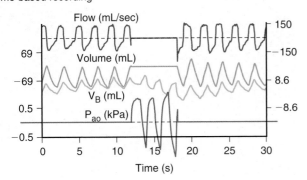

A

X-Y plot of box volume vs P$_{ao}$ during airway occlusion

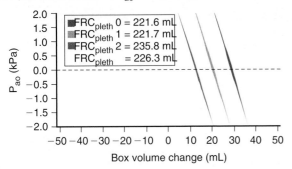

B

FIGURE 11-8. Criteria for technically acceptable measurements of plethysmographic functional residual capacity (FRC$_{pleth}$). **A,** Time-based trace of flow, tidal volume, box volume, and pressure at the airway opening before, during, and after shutter closure for measurement. As can be seen from the tidal volume trace, the shutter was closed at end inspiration. The infant made three respiratory efforts against the occlusion before shutter release. Note zero flow during the occlusion and stability of the tidal volume trace postocclusion, indicating absence of any leak. **B,** X-Y plot of pressure changes at the airway opening (Pao) versus changes in box volume, which are used to calculate FRC. The slopes represent the three respiratory efforts against the shutter during a single occlusion, with FRC for that occlusion being reported as the mean of these efforts. Note the good phase relationship (no looping) between changes in box volume and Pao. *kPa,* kilopascals; *VB,* box volume signal. (Copyright © Janet Stocks.)

The major disadvantages of infant plethysmography include the following:
- The equipment is expensive, relatively bulky, and not suitable for bedside assessments.
- Commercially available plethysmographs have not been validated for infants <3 kg.
- As in adults, overestimation of FRC may occur when there is severe airway obstruction.
- Historic reference data is not appropriate for current commercially available equipment,[47] and equipment-specific equations have yet to be developed. The use of contemporary controls studied with the same equipment is therefore required for accurate interpretation of results.[7,9]

Preschool Children

Although there has been considerable success in obtaining plethysmographic measurements of specific resistance in preschool children (discussed later), very young

children rarely tolerate panting against a closed shutter. Although a recent study did suggest that it is feasible to measure FRC using plethysmography in this age group,[48] such measurements are generally limited to those that can be obtained using one of the gas dilution or washout techniques until 5 or 6 years of age.

▬ GAS DILUTION OR WASHOUT TECHNIQUES TO ASSESS LUNG VOLUMES

Gas dilution techniques measure the lung volume that readily communicates with the central airways during tidal breathing. Apart from the differing measurement conditions discussed earlier and the need to miniaturize equipment, methods of assessing FRC by gas dilution or washout are much the same in infants and preschool children as in older subjects. Details of equipment specifications and techniques for performing these measurements in infants have been published.[41,49,50] Although closed-circuit helium dilution was widely used in the past, most assessments are now obtained using either the bias flow nitrogen washout technique[51] or multiple-breath inert gas washout (MBW)[10,19,50,52,53] (Fig. 11-9). The latter measures breath-to-breath changes in the concentration of an inert gas during the washout process and provides information on both lung volume and ventilation inhomogeneity. Equipment designed for older subjects can often be adapted for use in preschool children, provided care is taken to minimize equipment dead space.

With the exception of a few highly specialized applications,[51] assessments of lung volumes by gas dilution or washout are generally confined to those of FRC in infants and young children. Attempts to derive values for static lung volumes over an extended volume range in preschool children by combining measures of FRC by gas dilution with spirometric assessments of forced expiration are unlikely to be reliable due to the irregularity of

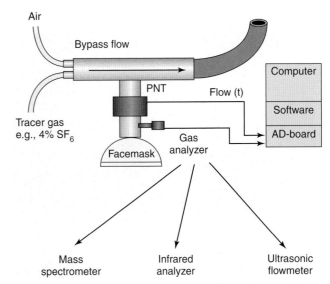

FIGURE 11-9. Multiple-breath inert gas washout. Schematic diagram of equipment used for measuring functional residual capacity and ventilation inhomogeneity using this technique. AD-board, analog to digital; *PNT,* pneumotachometer; *SF6,* sulfur-hexafluoride. (Copyright © Janet Stocks.)

tidal breathing in this age group. Similarly, the coordination required to perform a single-breath washout, which could potentially provide such information, generally precludes the use of this approach in those younger than 6 years of age.

Multiple-Breath Inert Gas Washout

The MBW test was introduced in the 1950s for measuring FRC and assessing overall ventilation inhomogeneity. It is generally performed during tidal breathing. The original test was the N_2 MBW test, using 100% O_2 for the washout. Although this is a valuable and simple technique for use in preschool and older children, use of 100% O_2 may alter tidal breathing patterns in young infants and is therefore less suitable in this age group, particularly if measures of ventilation inhomogeneity are also required. A wide range of alternative nonresident inert gases, including helium, argon, and sulfur-hexafluoride (SF_6), may be used as the tracer gas, with a range of appropriate devices, such as the catharometer, emission spectrometer, ultrasonic flowmeter (Fig. 11-10), or respiratory mass spectrometer (Fig. 11-11), being used to measure instantaneous gas concentrations.[54]

Methodological Considerations

The MBW technique simply requires the child to breathe tidally through a facemask or mouthpiece attached to a flowmeter and gas analyzer and is therefore eminently suitable for both infants and preschool children. When using an inert tracer gas, the subject initially re-breathes a gas mixture containing a fixed percentage of the tracer (e.g., 4% SF_6) via a bias flow, set to exceed the peak inspiratory flow. Wash-in continues until gas concentrations have equilibrated throughout the lung, as indicated by identical concentrations of the tracer gas throughout inspiration and expiration. The gas supply is

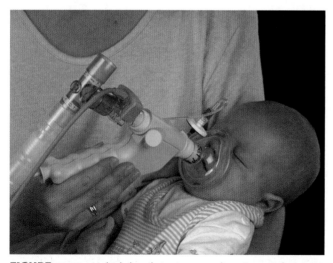

FIGURE 11-10. Multiple-breath inert gas washout in an infant using an ultrasonic flowmeter. (From Hammer J, Eber E: *Paediatric Pulmonary Function Testing. Progress in Respiratory Research*, Vol. 33. Basel: S. Karger AG, 2005. Permission granted by S. Karger AG, Basel.)

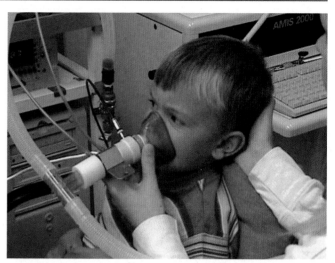

FIGURE 11-11. Multiple-breath inert gas washout in a preschool child using a mass spectrometer. Similar measurements can be made in sleeping infants. (Copyright © Janet Stocks.)

then disconnected during expiration so that the washout can commence, with the subject breathing room air until the end-tidal SF_6 concentration is less than 0.1% (i.e., 1/40th of the starting concentration) (Fig. 11-12). Flow and gas concentration are measured continuously during inspiration and expiration, and the exhaled tracer gas volume is determined by integrating the product of flow and the tracer gas concentration over time. FRC is calculated by dividing the BTPS-corrected volume of exhaled tracer gas by its concentration in the lungs just before washout. As in older subjects, values are corrected for apparatus dead space and volume inspired above the representative end-expiratory level at the time of switching. FRC should be calculated from at least two (ideally, three) technically acceptable measurements that are within 10% of each other.

A mask is usually used for data collection in both infants and preschool children[55] (see Figs. 11-10 and 11-11). Measurements in infants should be undertaken during periods of quiet sleep, whereas those in preschoolers are performed while the child is seated and awake. Cooperation in preschoolers is enhanced by allowing them to watch a favorite video or listen to a story during the recordings. Care is required to maintain a leak-free seal and to ensure that the child does not dribble into the equipment. Given suitable measurement conditions, technically satisfactory measurements of both FRC and indices of ventilation inhomogeneity using MBW can be obtained in approximately 80% of children between 3 and 5 years of age (increasing from approximately 65% at 3 years to more than 90% by 5 years).[56]

With their rapid respiratory rate and higher ratio of V_T/FRC, wash-in and washouts are generally much faster in infants and preschool children than in older subjects. Both phases of the technique are generally completed within 1 to 2 minutes in healthy infants and within 5 minutes in those with airway disease. Consequently, it is usually possible to complete three technically successful runs within 20 minutes. With the exception of

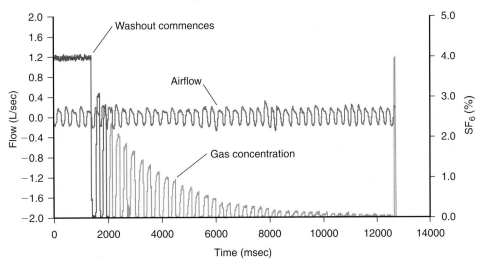

FIGURE 11-12. Time-based trace of air flow and inert gas concentration during multiple-breath washout of an inert gas. Washout commences once the concentration of inert gas in the lungs has equilibrated with that inspired during the wash-in phase, and continues until the tracer gas is cleared from the lungs, which in this example took approximately 110 seconds. SF6, sulfur-hexafluoride. (Copyright © Janet Stocks.)

measurements in unsedated neonates, in whom both measurement error and physiologic variability are likely to be slightly greater,[52] the coefficient of variation for repeat within-occasion measures is approximately 5% (range, 2% to 15%). The ultrasonic flowmeter, which simultaneously measures tidal flow and tracer gas concentration (see Fig. 11-10), provides a promising alternative to respiratory mass spectrometry during MBW.[23,57-60] There is increasing interest in using nitrogen rather than SF₆ in conjunction with ultrasonic flow technology during MBW in preschool and older children, which would decrease costs and increase applicability.

The accuracy of recordings is dependent on the following:
- Accurate calibration
- Stability of the breathing pattern before the child is switched into the circuit
- Absence of leaks
- Wash-in and washout continuing long enough to reach equilibrium

A potential cause of increased variability of results is the occurrence of sighs. These may mobilize gas in slowly ventilating or closed areas of the lungs, especially in subjects with marked ventilation inhomogeneity. The occurrence of such sighs should always be noted, and additional runs should be performed if necessary.

Advantages and Disadvantages

Disadvantages of the MBW and gas dilution techniques include the following:
- They only measure the readily ventilated gas volume, not gas trapped behind closed airways.
- They may require prolonged washout in those with severe, particularly obstructive disease.
- There has been a paucity of commercially available, well-validated equipment, although this situation should be resolved within the next few years.

Advantages of the MBW technique include the following:
- It is suitable for bedside measurements.
- It can be undertaken at all ages, including unsedated newborn or preterm infants.
- It provides simultaneous assessments of gas-mixing indices as a measure of ventilation inhomogeneity.

▄ GAS-MIXING EFFICIENCY

Although initially described many years ago, the use of MBW to assess gas-mixing efficiency or ventilation inhomogeneity was only used intermittently in infants and young children until the last decade, reflecting the complexity of data analysis and lack of commercially available equipment. During recent years, technologic advances, combined with an increasing awareness that conventional measures of airway function may not detect early changes in peripheral airway function until lung disease is well established, have led to a resurgence of interest in this field. Since measurements of ventilation efficiency are performed during spontaneous tidal breathing, they are applicable to subjects of all ages.

Theoretical Background

The human lung is constructed for optimal mixing of fresh inspired air with the resident gas in the lungs. How well this works will determine the gas-mixing efficiency. Poor gas mixing is a consequence of increased ventilation inhomogeneity and is reflected both by the time and/or relative ventilation required to clear a tracer gas from the lungs and by the magnitude of the phase III slope (alveolar plateau) of inert gas concentration during expiration.

A large number of parameters that reflect overall ventilation inhomogeneity can be calculated from the MBW. Higher values signify increased inhomogeneity.[54,61,62]

- The lung clearance index (LCI) is the most commonly quoted measurement and represents the number of "lung turnovers" required to complete the washout (where a "turnover" represents the expired volume equivalent to the subject's FRC, such that the LCI = cumulative expired volume/FRC).
- The mixing ratio is calculated from the ratio between the actual and the estimated ideal number of breaths needed to lower the end-tidal tracer gas concentration to 1/40th of the starting value. The ideal number of breaths is proportional to the ratio between the FRC and alveolar VT (i.e., VT minus equipment and airway dead space).
- Inhomogeneity of ventilation distribution may also be expressed by moment analysis of the washout curve.[19,23] The zeroth moment is the area under the washout curve (end-tidal gas concentration plotted against lung volume turnover). The first and second moments give more weight to the latter part of the washout curve

by multiplying the end-tidal gas concentration by the turnover (first moment) or the turnover squared (second moment). The ratios between the first and zeroth moments and between the second and zeroth moments are usually calculated over the first eight turnovers, with higher ratios indicating that a greater portion of the lungs is slowly ventilated (Fig. 11-13). Some of the other available indices have specific advantages, but indices such as the LCI and the mixing ratio are robust and relatively intuitive for patients and parents as well as medical personnel to understand. An ATS-ERS Task Force on MBW has been established to provide guidelines on how best to standardize data collection and analysis and improve interpretation of results.

Increases in LCI or other indices of gas-mixing efficiency result from differences in specific ventilation between parallel lung units. This can result from asymmetrical narrowing of the airway lumen at branch points throughout the airway tree, which in turn may be caused

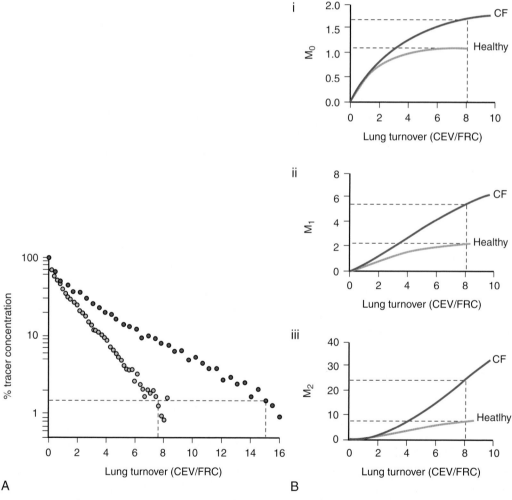

FIGURE 11-13. Calculation of indices of ventilation. **A,** Calculation of lung clearance index (LCI). Representative traces from multiple-breath sulfur-hexa-fluoride washout (MBWSF$_6$) in a healthy infant *(green circles)* and one with cystic fibrosis (CF) *(blue circles)*, demonstrating the prolonged tail. Dotted lines show the number of turnovers required to reduce the tracer gas to 2% of the initial tracer concentration (equivalent to the LCI), which in this example was 7.7 for the healthy child and 15 for the child with CF. **B,** The concept of moments. The graph shows moments derived from MBW SF6 in a healthy infant and one with CF. The horizontal dotted lines indicate values for moments at eight lung turnovers. i, The zeroth moment (M0) obtained from the area under the tracer concentration versus turnover; ii, the first moment (M1) derived from the area under the curve described by panel i; iii, the second moment (M2) derived from the area under the curve described by panel ii. As the moment number increases, there is increased weighting toward the end of the washout trace. *CEV,* cumulative expired volume; *FRC,* functional residual capacity. (Copyright © Janet Stocks.)

by inflammation, scarring, or obstruction by mucus, or may be secondary to changes in airway tone. Additionally, inhomogeneity may result from parenchymal changes in the subtended lung units, resulting in changes in compliance and differing time constants for filling and emptying. It should be noted that completely obstructed lung units give no signal; thus a child with a mucus plug totally blocking a main bronchus may have a normal LCI.

Gas mixing in the lungs takes place through two mechanisms. Convective gas transport (bulk flow) predominates in the conducting airways (i.e., the central airways down to and including the terminal bronchioles), whereas diffusion (molecular diffusion, or Brownian movement) predominates in the intra-acinar airways. The quasi-stationary diffusion-convection front is a transition zone where diffusive gas transport and convective gas transport are of similar magnitude. This occurs in the region of the entrance to the acinus and in its proximal portion. Poor gas mixing that occurs in the vicinity of this area as a result of interaction between convective and diffusive gas mixing is termed either *acinar-* or *diffusion-convection-dependent inhomogeneity* (S_{acin} or DCDI). Proximal to this front, inhomogeneity results from convective flow inhomogeneity, secondary to differences in specific ventilation between parallel lung units that fill and empty sequentially. This inhomogeneity of more proximal origin is termed either *conductive-* or *convection-dependent inhomogeneity* (S_{cond} or CDI).[54]

Equipment and Procedure

Equipment and procedures for assessing ventilation inhomogeneity are identical to those described earlier for measurements of lung volume by MBW. The use of this technique in preschool and school-age children has been well described,[3,54,63] whereas guidelines for more standardized measurements in infants are currently in progress.[23,60] Recent studies have reported technically successful results in more than 80% of 3- to 5-year-old children.[56,64]

Advantages and Limitations

As with most PFTs, errors will occur when using the MBW if there is too large an external dead space in relation to VT, if there are any leaks from the circuit, if there are faulty calibrations, or if there is a highly irregular breathing pattern. In addition, when using this technique, particular care must be taken to ensure the following:
- Correct alignment of signals from the gas analyzer and flowmeter during data collection
- Appropriate correction of the PNT signal for variations in the dynamic viscosity of the gas sample
- Switching into and out of the tracer gas mixture at the appropriate phase of respiration

Some of these problems could be minimized by increasing automation and online quality control feedback. There is an urgent need to establish recommendations with respect to data collection and analysis and to develop and validate commercially available equipment to facilitate more widespread use of this technique. Due to the

potential effect of sighs or deep inhalations, MBW should be performed toward the beginning of any test protocol and certainly before any technique that requires lung inflation or forced expiratory maneuvers. With the exception of unsedated preterm infants, within-subject repeatability on the same occasion is good. Preliminary data on within-subject, between-occasion repeatability and the ability of LCI to detect changes in response to acute interventions in school-age children have recently become available, but they still need to be established for younger children.

Clinical Applications

In health, gas-mixing efficiency appears to remain remarkably stable throughout the first 18 years of life[65] (Fig. 11-14), thereby enabling the effects of disease to be distinguished from those of growth and development with greater confidence than when dealing with most parameters of lung function, which are highly dependent on age and body size. Nevertheless, recent studies have indicated that the upper limit of normal is somewhat higher in infants.[10,53] There may also be subtle differences in the predicted normal range according to the equipment used.[59]

During a longitudinal study of healthy preschool children, LCI remained stable over a mean interval of 3.7 years, with a mean (95% CI) within-subject change of 0.0 (–0.2, 0.2), and a 95% range of –1.3 (95% CI; –1.65, –0.95) and 1.3 (0.95, 1.65).[64]

Indices of ventilation inhomogeneity are increased in children and adults with CF, asthma, chronic obstructive pulmonary disease, and post-transplant bronchiolitis obliterans, and in infants and preschool children with bronchopulmonary dysplasia (BPD) and CF (Fig. 11-15). In older subjects, an increased LCI is usually reflected by a longer washout time. This is not necessarily true in infants and young children with lung disease, who may simply increase their minute ventilation (increased respiratory rate and VT) to compensate for less efficient gas mixing. The LCI is a much more sensitive method of detecting early changes in lung function in young children with CF

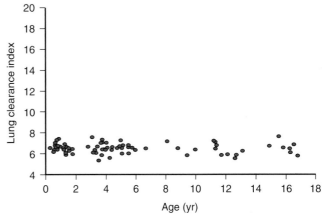

FIGURE 11-14. Lung clearance index (LCI) in healthy children from birth to 18 years of age. Note the relative stability of the LCI throughout childhood, making it one of the few parameters of lung function that is not dependent on age or body size. (Unpublished data, Institute of Child Health, London, 2004; Copyright © Janet Stocks.)

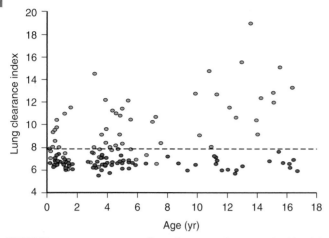

FIGURE 11-15. Comparison of lung clearance index (LCI) in healthy children and those with cystic fibrosis (CF). Collated data from studies performed at the Institute of Child Health, London, 2002–2004. The dashed horizontal line shows the 95% upper limit of normal (i.e., LCI, 7.8) derived from healthy children (*blue circles*). Elevated LCI values were observed in many infants and preschool children with CF (*green circles*) and in virtually all of those older than 7 years of age. (Copyright © Janet Stocks.)

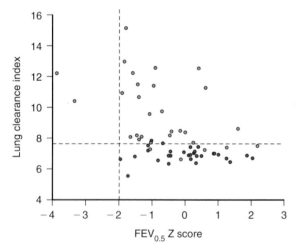

FIGURE 11-16. Lung clearance index (LCI) versus forced expired volume in 0.5 second (FEV0.5) in healthy preschool children and those with cystic fibrosis (CF). LCI is plotted against FEV0.5 Z scores in 30 healthy preschool children (*blue circles*; mean [SD] age, 4.1 [0.9] years) and 30 children of similar age with CF (*green circles*). Results from all of the healthy children fell within normal limits (*dotted lines*; i.e.,<7.8 for LCI and Z score greater than −1.96 for FEV0.5). An abnormally low FEV0.5 was observed in only two of the children with CF, whereas 22 of 30 children with CF had an abnormal LCI. (Copyright © Janet Stocks.)

than conventional spirometry (Fig. 11-16), measurements during the preschool years being highly predictive of lung function some 4 to 6 years.[64] Similarly, S_{cond} was found to be the most sensitive indicator of abnormal pulmonary function in preschool wheezers.[66]

■ RESPIRATORY MECHANICS: RESISTANCE AND COMPLIANCE

Introduction

Assessments of respiratory mechanics can provide an indication of lung and chest wall stiffness and of airway caliber or obstruction, and hence of the effort that is required

to ventilate the lungs (work of breathing). Compliance is calculated as the change in lung volume per unit change in pressure, that is:

$$C = \Delta V / \Delta P,$$

where resistance is calculated as the pressure required to drive flow

$$R = \Delta P / \Delta Flow.$$

Hence, to assess respiratory mechanics it is necessary to record changes in pressure and flow, with volume usually obtained by integrating flow ($V = Flow \times time$). While flow and volume are usually measured using some type of flowmeter at the airway opening during assessments of respiratory mechanics, pressure changes can be measured in a variety of ways, which will determine exactly which outcome is measured. Thus if R_{aw} is to be measured in isolation, then a measure of pressure changes between the alveoli and airway opening (such as can be obtained during plethysmography) is required. In contrast, during the occlusion techniques, the sum of pressure changes across the chest wall, lungs, and airways are measured such that the resistance and compliance of the total respiratory system are assessed.

Since compliance increases as the lungs grow (whereas resistance decreases), results are often standardized for lung size by expressing them as specific compliance (sC = C/FRC) or specific resistance (sR = R × FRC). Assessments of respiratory mechanics are sometimes expressed as elastance (where E = P/V, i.e. the reciprocal of compliance) or conductance (where G = Flow/P, i.e. the reciprocal of resistance).

The frequency with which respiratory compliance has been measured in infants reflects not only the relative ease with which such measurements can be performed in early life but the fact that, in contrast to older subjects, changes in the elastic properties of the lung often dominate the underlying pathophysiology of lung disease in newborn infants. Most of these techniques can be performed during tidal breathing and require minimal cooperation from the child, other than breathing through a facemask or mouthpiece. Esophageal manometry, which is used to assess pulmonary or lung mechanics (Airways + lung tissue) was once commonplace during assessments of infant lung function, but has generally been replaced by assessment of passive total respiratory mechanics using the occlusion techniques. The exception to this is in ventilated or preterm infants, who may already have a nasogastric tube in situ for feeding purposes. Catheter tip transducers may be used instead of esophageal balloons or water-filled catheters to record changes in transpulmonary pressure.

■ PLETHYSMOGRAPHIC ASSESSMENTS OF AIRWAY RESISTANCE

Whole-body plethysmography is a well-established method for measuring lung volume and airway resistance (R_{aw}) in adults and older children, and it has been successfully adapted for measurements in both sleeping infants[40] and awake preschool children.[67] Measurements of R_{aw} have been used to study normal airway growth and development in relation to lung volume during the first year of life and have demonstrated tracking of airway function during this period.[45] They have also been used to discriminate between healthy infants and those with respiratory disease or a history of wheezing.[44,45,68] Plethysmographic measurements of sR_{aw} (i.e., $R_{aw} \times FRC$) are becoming an increasingly popular method of assessing both baseline airway function and bronchial responsiveness in preschool children with and without respiratory disease. Because resistance decreases as lung volume increases with growth, values of sR_{aw} remain relatively independent of changes in body size. This should facilitate attempts to distinguish changes in airway function due to disease from those resulting from growth and development, especially during early life, when somatic growth is so rapid. sR_{aw} has been used as an outcome measure in cross-sectional and longitudinal studies of healthy young children[69,70] as well as those with CF[56,71] and asthma.[66,72,73] It has also been widely used to assess bronchial responsiveness and to document the effect of anti-asthmatic therapies in preschool children.[66,72-75]

Methodological and Theoretical Considerations

The principles of plethysmographic assessment of R_{aw} measurements are identical for infants and preschool children and for older subjects.[40,67] The subject sits, or in the case of an infant, lies, inside a relatively airtight chamber, the whole-body plethysmograph, while changes in air flow are recorded at the airway opening using a PNT attached to a mouthpiece or mask. R_{aw} can be calculated by relating changes in plethysmographic pressure (which are inversely proportional to changes in alveolar pressure) to changes in flow throughout the breathing cycle (Fig. 11-17). For reliable assessments of R_{aw}, changes in box pressure must only reflect changes in alveolar pressure

required to drive flow, not those arising from changes in the temperature and humidity of the respired gas. In the past, this was achieved by breathing heated, humidified air at BTPS conditions or panting during assessments of R_{aw}, whereas most modern plethysmographs rely on electronic compensation of the resultant phase lag between box pressure and air flow signals.

Changes in plethysmographic pressure during spontaneous breathing are calibrated in terms of alveolar pressure changes by using the relationship between the changes in plethysmographic (box) pressure and that recorded at the airway opening during an airway occlusion. The latter is assumed to represent changes in alveolar pressure during periods of no air flow, such as those that occur during respiratory efforts against a closed shutter during plethysmographic assessments of FRC (discussed earlier). Although most sleeping infants will continue to make respiratory efforts against the shutter during a 6- to 10-second airway occlusion, this procedure is too demanding for most awake young children, thereby precluding direct measurements in preschool children. Measurements of sR_{aw}, which is the product of FRC and R_{aw} ($sR_{aw} = FRC \times R_{aw}$), can be obtained, however, by using a single-step procedure without needing to breathe against a closed shutter, making this an ideal test for preschool children.[67,69]

Equipment and Procedure

Infants

Since infants cannot be requested to pant, infant plethysmographs have traditionally used a heated rebreathing system to provide respired gas under BTPS conditions (see Fig. 11-7). This is an effective method, but is technically difficult, thereby limiting the use of infant plethysmography to specialized laboratories. Recent concerns about potential infection risks, buildup of CO_2 during rebreathing, and the need to make the technique more widely available prompted a search for alternative solutions. Regrettably, initial attempts to apply electronic thermal compensation to infant data have proved disappointing, suggesting that more sophisticated algorithms may be required to cope with the added complexities of undertaking these measurements during nose breathing.[76]

The equipment and technique used for undertaking plethysmographic assessments of R_{aw} have been described previously.[1,40] Commercially available equipment that meets most of the ERS-ATS recommendations for plethysmographic measurements of lung volume in infants is now available, but none has a validated method of measuring R_{aw}, with such measurements currently limited to departments who have retained their own custom-built equipment.

As with older subjects, it is important for thermal equilibrium to be established after the box has been closed and before recordings are started. Once breathing is quiet and regular, the infant is switched from breathing air directly from the plethysmograph to a rebreathing system containing warmed, humidified air under BTPS conditions. Simultaneous changes in air flow and box pressure are then recorded. Technically acceptable loops are

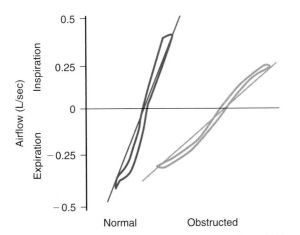

FIGURE 11-17. Specific airway resistance loops from a healthy child and one with airway obstruction. Changes in box volume are proportional to changes in alveolar pressure, reflecting the greater effort required to effect air flow *(flatter slope)* in the presence of airway obstruction. (Copyright © Janet Stocks.)

those in which there is minimal phase lag between these two signals at moments of zero flow (i.e., end inspiration and end expiration). Full details of the derivation of the equations used during the calculation of R_{aw} have been described previously.[40]

Preschool Children

As discussed earlier in the chapter, sR_{aw} can be obtained simply by measuring changes in air flow relative to changes in plethysmographic volume without simultaneous measurement of FRC (see Fig. 11-17). The same plethysmograph used in older subjects can be used for measuring sR_{aw} in preschool children. Measurements can be carried out using either a mouthpiece and nose clips (as in older subjects) or a specially adapted facemask fitted with a flexible, noncompressible mouthpiece that prevents nose breathing and provides a stable airway opening.[67] Before the child is asked to enter the plethysmograph, all procedures must be demonstrated and explained. If the child is hesitant to enter the plethysmograph or to stay inside once the door is closed, measurements can be performed with the child sitting on an adult's lap, provided care is taken to adjust for the extra occupied volume within the box when calculating results. Once the child is confident and comfortable, the plethysmograph door can be closed. Measurements should not be initiated for at least 1 minute after closure to allow thermal equilibration within the box. Once there is minimal drift of the box signal and the child is breathing regularly with a stable breathing pattern, measurements can begin. If measurements are made with an accompanying adult, the adult should breathe normally until the child's respiration has stabilized and then perform a deep inspiration followed by a slow expiration so that a constant low expiratory flow is generated during a 15- to 20-second period of data collection. Technical acceptability is based primarily on the respiratory rate, regularity of the breathing pattern, and absence of distortions due to leak, movement, or talking (Fig. 11-18).

During measurements, the child should sit upright with the neck slightly extended. Although it has been recommended that respiratory rate is maintained between 30 and 45 breaths per minute,[1,67] recent work suggests that sR_{aw} is more dependent on within-subject changes in flow than respiratory rate. Encouraging the child to adopt a regular, comfortable, and natural breathing rhythm without elevation of end expiratory level or undue turbulence will minimize intersubject and intrasubject variability.[69]

Reporting of Results

Resistance changes throughout the breathing cycle are due to a combination of factors, including the flow and volume dependency of R_{aw}. Hence, there is no single value that represents resistance. Most plethysmographs include numerous methods of calculating R_{aw} and sR_{aw}, which can be confusing when comparing results from different centers. It has been suggested that the most robust outcomes to report in preschool children are either "effective specific airway resistance (sR_{eff})," which is calculated by the regression of $\Delta V_{pleth}/\Delta Flow$ throughout the entire breath, or total specific airways resistance (R_{tot}), which is calculated from the slope of the line connecting the point of maximum

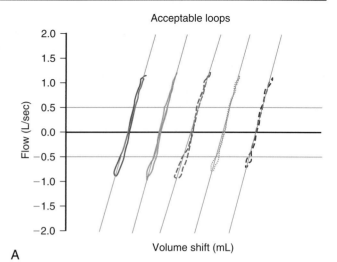

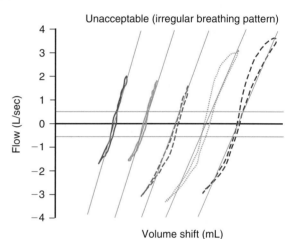

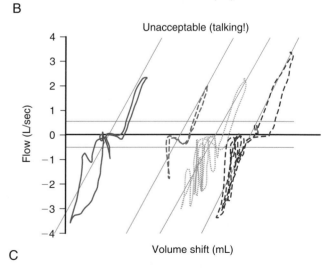

FIGURE 11-18. Specific resistance measurements and quality control criteria. **A,** A regular reproducible breathing pattern with a good phase relationship *(closed loops).* **B,** In contrast, a variable respiratory rate and pattern resulted in highly variable values for specific airway resistance. **C,** The subject started to talk to the operator, thereby invalidating the recordings. (Copyright © Janet Stocks.)

ΔV_{pleth} swings during inspiration and expiration.[69] Assessment of R_{aw} at fixed flows, (e.g., 0.5 L/s), as is commonly reported in adults, is not recommended in young children due to its strong inverse correlation with age. Reference values vary according to which parameter is selected, with values of sR_{tot} generally exceeding those of sR_{eff}. It should be noted that the "default" predicted values for sR_{aw} commonly displayed on many modern plethysmographs are still based on data collected under BTPS conditions and are inappropriate for measurements derived after electronic compensation.[69]

Recent attempts to collate available sR_{aw} data from young children identified marked variation in methodology and analysis between centers, which necessitated exclusion of some data.[69] Errors in factory settings of software may also contribute to intercenter differences in sR_{aw}.[77] Nevertheless, preliminary reference equations and recommendations for recording and reporting both sR_{eff} and sR_{tot} have been developed for White European children from 1908 measurements that were obtained under similar conditions (Fig. 11-19).[69]

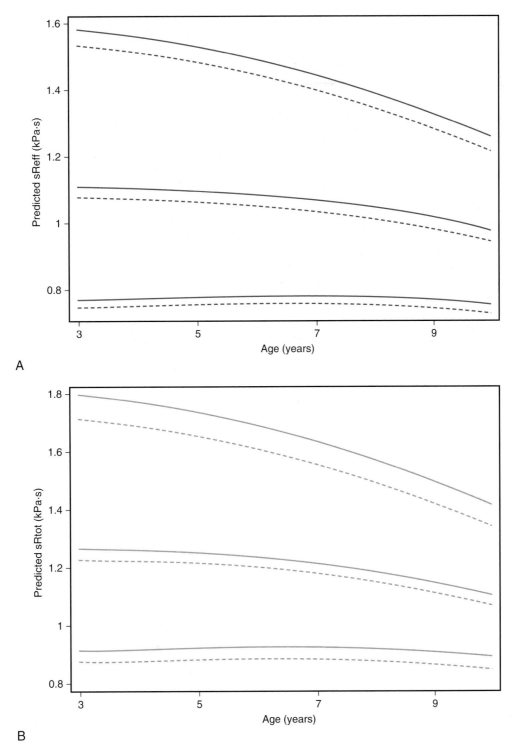

FIGURE 11-19. Predicted values of sR_{aw} (kpa.s) with upper and lower limits of normal, **(A)** sR_{eff} and **(B)** sR_{tot} for children aged 2 to 11 years of age. Solid lines represent equations for boys, whereas dotted lines represent equations for girls. (Reproduced from: Kirkby J, Stanojevic S, Welsh L, et al. Reference equations for specific airway resistance in children: the Asthma UK initiative. *Eur Respir J.* 2010;36:622-629, with permission from the European Respiratory Society.)

Advantages and Limitations

The major advantages of plethysmographic R_{aw} are that they represent a direct reflection of airway caliber that can be obtained during tidal breathing using identical techniques and equipment from preschool children to adults. Although infant plethysmography provides valuable data in specialized centers, it remains limited by the lack of any validated method of obtaining reliable results without reliance on a heated rebreathing bag and the potential dominance of the upper airway in these nose-breathing subjects. Improvements in commercially available software, including computer animation and data storage, are required to facilitate both data collection and quality control in this age group. There remains an urgent need to develop a standard protocol for data collection, criteria for quality assurance, and methods for reporting results.[69] This in turn would facilitate development of more reliable and appropriate reference data from healthy children, including those from diverse ethnic backgrounds.

■ PASSIVE RESPIRATORY MECHANICS

Measurements of passive respiratory mechanics (compliance, resistance, and τ_{rs}) are potentially possible if a state of relaxation can be induced in the respiratory system. This is feasible only in highly trained adults during spontaneous breathing and hence is not applicable to preschool children. However, in contrast to older subjects, the vagally mediated Hering-Breuer inflation reflex is active within the tidal range throughout the first year of life, which has allowed widespread assessment of passive mechanics in infants. Although significant changes in R_{rs} have been reported among infants with airway disease,[78] the major role of these measurements is probably with respect to assessing compliance in conditions in which there is likely to be restrictive pulmonary changes (e.g., respiratory distress syndrome, chronic lung disease of infancy, pulmonary hypoplasia, interstitial lung disease, and cardiac disease with pulmonary overperfusion.)[68,79–83]

The occlusion technique for measuring passive respiratory mechanics is based on the ability to invoke this reflex by performing brief intermittent airway occlusions during spontaneous tidal breathing. Activation of vagally mediated pulmonary stretch receptors when the airway is occluded above FRC leads to inhibition of inspiration and prolongation of expiratory time (Fig. 11-20). Provided there is no respiratory muscle activity and rapid equilibration of pressures across the respiratory system during occlusion (as shown by the presence of a pressure plateau), alveolar pressure and hence elastic recoil of the respiratory system can be measured at the airway opening. By relating this recoil pressure to the volume above the passively determined end-expiratory volume at which the airway occlusion was performed or to the air flow occurring on release of the occlusion, the compliance and resistance of the respiratory system can be measured. The major limitation of this technique, as with all methods that depend on intermittent airway occlusions, is that pressures may not equilibrate rapidly enough in the presence of substantial airway obstruction or a rapid respiratory rate to allow accurate measurements at the airway opening. Full details of data collection and analysis and quality control criteria have been published, together with discussions of the relative advantages and limitations of this technique.[81,84]

Methodological and Theoretical Considerations

Various adaptations of the occlusion technique have been developed since it was first described in the late 1970s. The most commonly used approach for which commercially available equipment is available is the single-breath, or single-occlusion, technique (Fig. 11-21).

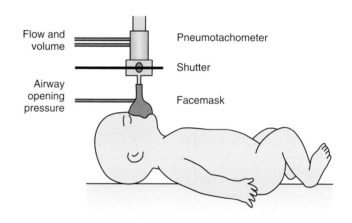

FIGURE 11-21. Occlusion technique. Schematic diagram of equipment used for passive mechanics using the occlusion technique in infants. (Copyright © Janet Stocks.)

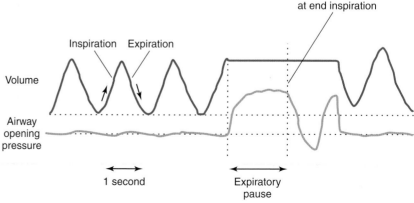

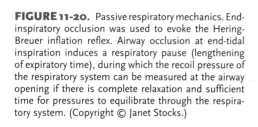

FIGURE 11-20. Passive respiratory mechanics. End-inspiratory occlusion was used to evoke the Hering-Breuer inflation reflex. Airway occlusion at end-tidal inspiration induces a respiratory pause (lengthening of expiratory time), during which the recoil pressure of the respiratory system can be measured at the airway opening if there is complete relaxation and sufficient time for pressures to equilibrate through the respiratory system. (Copyright © Janet Stocks.)

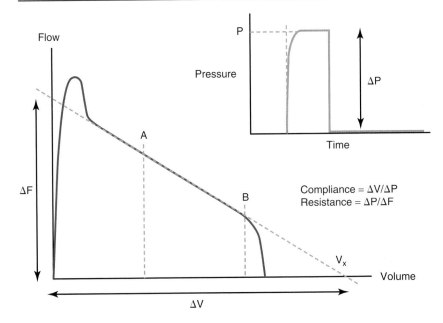

FIGURE 11-22. Assessment of passive respiratory mechanics using the single-breath occlusion technique. The volume of air in the lung above the passively determined end-expiratory level (i.e., ΔV) is calculated by extrapolating the linear portion of the descending flow-volume curve to zero flow (i.e., V_x). During periods of no air flow (i.e., airway occlusion) and in the presence of complete respiratory muscle relaxation, as seen by the attainment of a pressure plateau, pressures equilibrate and the elastic recoil pressure of the respiratory system can be measured at the airway opening (ΔP). Respiratory system compliance can then be calculated as $\Delta V / \Delta P$. Similarly, by relating ΔP to ΔF, respiratory resistance is calculated. (Copyright © Janet Stocks.)

When using this technique, resistance, compliance, and the passive τ_{rs} of the respiratory system can be calculated from a single airway occlusion (Fig. 11-22). Since time constant = volume/flow, τ_{rs} can simply be derived from flow-volume relationship during a passive expiration, which frequently follows the release of a brief airway occlusion. Compliance of the total respiratory system (C_{rs}) is calculated by relating the volume above the passively determined lung volume at the moment of airway occlusion to the elastic recoil pressure measured during occlusion. Because infants frequently dynamically elevate FRC and may breathe in slightly earlier than usual after occlusion, it is necessary to extrapolate the linear portion of the flow-volume plot to zero flow to estimate the appropriate volume change when calculating C_{rs}. Since $\tau = R_{rs} \times C_{rs}$, respiratory resistance (R_{rs}) can simply be derived as C_{rs}/τ.

The optimal duration of airway occlusion is a compromise between ensuring sufficient time for pressure equilibration to occur, while making the occlusion brief enough to allow passive expiration after its release. A minimum occlusion time of 400 msec and a maximum occlusion time of 1.5 seconds in which to attain a pressure plateau lasting at least 100 msec has been recommended.[84] Results are usually expressed as the mean of three to five valid measurements.

Advantages and Limitations

The advantages of the single-occlusion technique are that the equipment is relatively simple and inexpensive (consisting of a flowmeter and a shutter with which to effect the airway occlusion, attached to a facemask) and that measurements can easily be made at the bedside. As with all infant PFTs, attainment of a stable respiratory pattern and a leak-free seal around the mask are essential for successful data collection. Valid measurements depend on the following three fundamental assumptions:

- Complete relaxation of the respiratory system during both the occlusion and the subsequent expiration.
- Pressure at the facemask equilibrates rapidly and hence represents alveolar pressure.
- The lung can be treated as a single compartment model, with a single value of τ.

With persistence, these conditions can be achieved in the majority of healthy infants during quiet sleep, but they are more difficult to satisfy in infants with severe airway disease, in whom pressure equilibration may not occur rapidly enough and in whom the respiratory system can rarely be described by a single time constant. It should also be remembered that results from the single-occlusion technique reflect the combined mechanics of the entire respiratory system (chest wall, lungs, and airway), which may reduce the ability to detect subtle changes in lung function in those with respiratory disease.

INTERRUPTER TECHNIQUE

Occlusion techniques for assessing passive respiratory mechanics are not applicable in awake preschool children because these children will not relax the respiratory muscles during or after release of the airway occlusion, thereby precluding reliable assessment of either elastic recoil pressure or the passive respiratory time constant. Nonetheless, resistance of the respiratory system can be assessed in this age group by using the interrupter technique (R_{int}), which relies on much shorter interruptions to air flow than those used during occlusion techniques (Fig. 11-23).

The measurement of R_{int} has become an increasingly popular lung function test for preschool children over the past decade since equipment for its measurement is commercially available and the technique only requires passive cooperation. The technique is safe, quick, noninvasive, available, inexpensive, applicable in field studies[85] and delivers results that are clinically relevant and which seem suitable for assessing bronchodilator responses.[86–90] An ATS/ERS consensus statement was published in 2007,

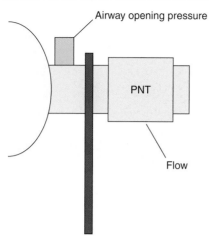

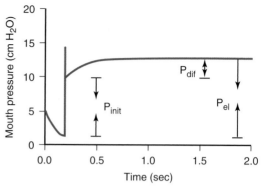

FIGURE 11-23. Schematic diagram of equipment used for the interrupter technique. *PNT*, pneumotachometer. (Copyright © Janet Stocks.)

FIGURE 11-24. Schematic changes in mouth or mask pressure during the interrupter technique. Schematic description of the pressure-time curve showing mouth pressure changes after a sudden interruption of air flow at mid expiration. *P_{init}*, rapid initial change in mouth pressure (P_m); *P_{dif}*, secondary slower change in P_m; *P_{el}*, final plateau representing the pressure due to the elastic recoil of the respiratory system. (Copyright © Janet Stocks.)

largely based on personal experience, in an attempt to make the procedure more uniform and facilitate comparisons between centers.[3]

Theoretical and Methodological Considerations

Theoretically, when air flow at the mouth is suddenly interrupted, there will be a rapid initial change in mouth pressure (P_{init}) followed by a slower change (P_{dif}) up to a plateau (P_{el}) (Fig. 11-24). P_{init} is virtually instantaneous and reflects the pressure difference due to R_{aw} at the time of interruption. During tidal breathing in preschool children, P_{init} and thus R_{int} include a component of lung tissue and chest wall resistance, as well as R_{aw}. P_{dif} is due to the visco-elastic properties of the respiratory tissues and reflects stress adaptation (relaxation or recovery) within the tissues of the lung and chest wall, plus gas redistribution (pendelluft) between pulmonary units with different pressures at the time of interruption. The final plateau represents the pressure due to elastic recoil of the respiratory system and may take several seconds to be reached, especially in the presence of airway obstruction. The total time of interruption should be less than 100 msec, to ensure that its duration is too short to be noticed by the child. Consequently, a final pressure plateau is rarely observed with the interrupter technique.

When these measurements are performed, there is a series of rapid oscillations in pressure between the rapid and the slow change in P_m after air flow interruption (Fig. 11-25). This is due to the inertia and compressibility of the air column in the airways. These oscillations may be more or less damped depending on the time constant of the total system (including the chest wall, lungs, upper airways, and equipment), but their presence often makes it difficult to determine P_{init} accurately. Several methods have been proposed to extrapolate P_{init}. The greater the component of P_{dif} that is incorporated into the R_{int} measurement, the higher R_{int} will be with respect to pure R_{aw} and the more it will approach the resistance of the total respiratory system. Even when P_m is linearly back-extrapolated to the beginning of the interruption, it is still partially dependent on the final part of the pressure-time curve. Therefore, it does not represent pure R_{aw}.

An ATS-ERS Task Force has published preliminary recommendations[3] which, in addition to technical specifications, stress that measurements should be made with the child sitting upright, breathing through a mouthpiece and filter, wearing a nose clip, and supporting the cheeks. Reference equations derived from over 1000 young children (ages 3 to 13 years) have recently been collated to provide sex-specific reference equations for R_{int} (Fig. 11-26).[91]

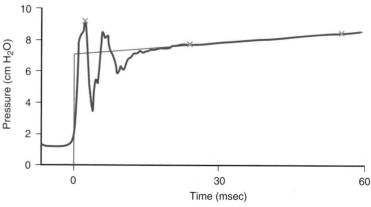

FIGURE 11-25. Technically acceptable interruption for assessing interrupter resistance. Actual pressure-time trace showing mouth pressure (P_m) during a 100-msec interruption. The straight line represents the linear back-extrapolation of P_m to the beginning of the interruption (To Δ when P_m reaches 25% of the difference between the first peak and the baseline value) using pressures measured 30 msec and 70 msec later. (Copyright © Janet Stocks.)

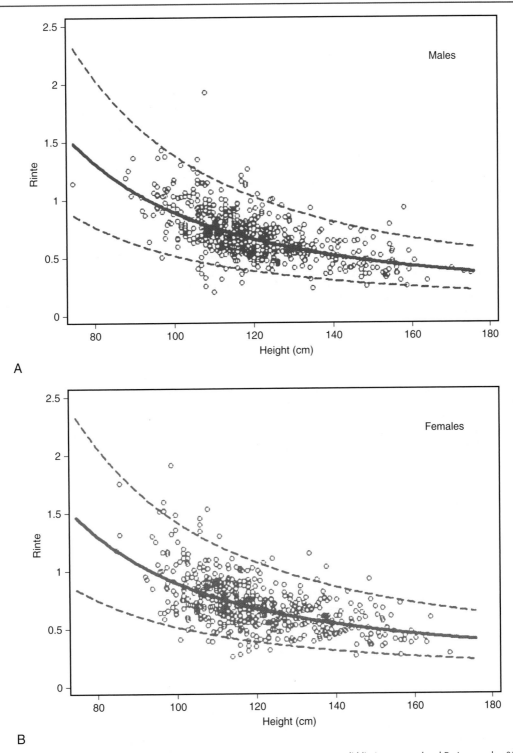

A

B

FIGURE 11-26. Sex-specific reference equations for expiratory interrupter resistance (Rinte; *solid line*) expressed as kPa.L^{-1}.s and 95% prediction limits *(dashed lines)* for **(A)** males and **(B)** females.

Advantages and Limitations

The major advantages of the interrupter technique are its portability and the simplicity of data collection, making it potentially ideal for use in fieldwork. The major limitation is that it is dependent on rapid equilibration between mouth pressure and alveolar pressure after interruption. Ventilation inhomogeneity or severe bronchial obstruction, as well as compliance of the cheeks and

upper airways, may delay this equilibration, such that alveolar pressure and hence R_{int} will be underestimated. Supporting the child's cheeks during R_{int} measurements is an effective means of reducing upper airway compliance when bronchial obstruction is mild to moderate, but it will not prevent underestimation of R_{int} in the presence of severe bronchial obstruction. This has led to some concerns about using R_{int} as an outcome measure in challenge tests. Furthermore, there is still some controversy about the best way to calculate and report results, particularly with respect to how to calculate pressure at the moment of interruption.[3]

Further studies are required to determine the best algorithm to calculate P_m during the interruption and to establish the cutoff value for a decrease in R_{int} beyond which bronchodilator response should be considered clinically significant within an individual. The role of R_{int} as the primary outcome in challenge tests and the usefulness of the interrupter technique in comparison with other techniques for lung function testing in preschool children remain to be determined.[87,88,92,93] When assessing bronchial responsiveness, knowledge of both within-occasion repeatability and the likely magnitude of response to such interventions in healthy children of similar age remains vital for meaningful interpretation of results.[3,94,95]

In contrast to its widespread use in preschool children, the application of R_{int} in infants is still in the early stages, and information on repeatability and guidelines for its use are still evolving.[96,97]

Forced Oscillation Technique

Respiratory impedance (Z_{rs}) describes the spectral (frequency domain) relationship between pressure and air flow throughout the respiratory cycle, providing a global measure of resistive, elastic (viscous), and inertial forces and the opportunity to investigate the frequency dependence of respiratory mechanics. R_{rs} is measured using the Forced Oscillation Technique (FOT) by superimposing small-amplitude pressure oscillations on the respiratory system and measuring the resultant oscillatory flow. Detailed descriptions of data collection and analysis, together with guidelines for the application and interpretation of FOT for both adult and pediatric populations, have been published.[3,98] As with the interrupter technique, FOT can be applied during spontaneous tidal breathing and requires no special maneuvers. It can also be used to define impedance of the lungs in infants and older subjects, but since this requires an esophageal catheter to measure transpulmonary pressure, measurements in preschool children are generally limited to respiratory system impedance, with trans-respiratory pressure changes being measured at the mouth (P_m).

FOT has been used to assess baseline lung function and airway responsiveness in preschool children with asthma, wheezing, CF, and prior BPD.[73,86,99–106] Several specialized applications of the technique at high and low frequencies have been made in infants to investigate the nature and severity of underlying pathophysiology, although these tend to be restricted to specialized research laboratories.[23,107,108]

Methodological and Theoretical Considerations

In most clinical setups, pressure and flow are measured at the mouth (P_m), with pressure oscillations that are generated by a loudspeaker being applied either at the airway

opening (the standard and most commonly used technique) or around the head (the head generator technique) [Fig. 11-27]. Data are usually collected over periods of 8 to 16 seconds, with up to five technically satisfactory sets being recorded for each child. FFT is used to convert the time-based flow and pressure signals recorded during the application of the sinusoidal oscillations to the frequency domain, that is, to a number of different sine waves with different frequencies, amplitudes, and phases (Fig. 11-28). Respiratory impedance (Z_{rs}) is calculated by distinguishing the changes in pressure and flow caused by the applied oscillations from those occurring during tidal breathing. Impedance can then be divided into the components of the P_m signal that are in phase with flow, which represent resistance of the respiratory system (R_{rs}, also known as the 'real' part) and the out-of-phase signal, reactance (X_{rs}, elastance and inertance), sometimes referred to as the "imaginary" part.

The excitation signal may be a single sine wave as shown in Figure 11-28 or, more commonly, a multifrequency signal, the classic approach being use of pseudorandom noise (PRN) in which computer-driven forced pressure oscillations that represent a mixture of different frequencies (usually harmonics of 2 Hz in the range 2 to 48 Hz) are applied in a single burst. Although the use of a single sine wave may be ideal to track variations in Z_{rs} within a breath, with time or with changing breathing patterns, application of PRN allows the frequency response of the respiratory system to be described and is therefore often preferable.

Time discrete, impulse oscillation (IOS) is an adaptation of PRN that works by superimposing many frequencies and adding them together to generate a so-called "rectangular pulse." IOS is performed by applying this rectangular pulse signal to the airways with a pressure step wave every 200 msecs through a loudspeaker/pulse generator to the airway opening via a mouthpiece. The superimposed pressure oscillations during normal spontaneous breathing are composed of several frequencies, allowing assessment of R_{rs} and X_{rs} at several frequencies simultaneously by Fast Fourier analysis. Since all frequencies are applied in just one rectangular pulse, the measurement time is reduced while maintaining a very low noise-signal ratio. Commercially available equipment suitable for measuring Z_{rs} in preschool children is available both for the IOS and PRN FOT techniques.

When using standard FOT, most of the clinically relevant information has been reported from measurements at relatively low frequencies (5 to 8 Hz). The lower limit of frequencies depends on the subject's breathing rate, since it may be difficult to obtain reliable data at less than 6 Hz in small children with breathing rates between 0.5 and 1 Hz (i.e., 30 to 60 breaths per minute). The upper limit is dictated by possible artifacts related to compliance of the cheeks and pharyngeal wall, which may result in considerable upper airway wall vibration if respiratory impedance is measured at high frequencies, especially in small children. The use of cheek support is recommended to minimize such artifacts. The head generator technique was designed to minimize upper airway wall motion, but it requires more cumbersome equipment than the standard technique and is now rarely used.

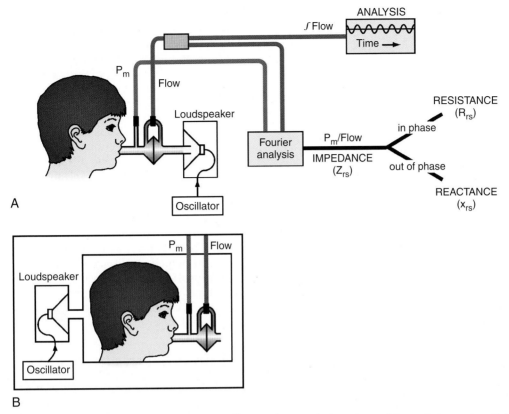

FIGURE 11-27. A, Schematic diagram of circuitry for the forced oscillation technique. The impedance of the respiratory system (Z_{rs}) can be measured by superimposing small-amplitude pressure oscillations on the respiratory system and measuring the resultant oscillatory flow. **B,** Pressure oscillations are applied either at the airway opening using a standard generator or around the entire head (head generator). The latter method is more cumbersome, but may reduce artifacts due to the compliance of the upper airway, which may be particularly important in young children. P_m, mouth pressure; R_{rs}, respiratory resistance; X_{rs}, respiratory reactance (i.e., elastance and inertance). (Copyright © Janet Stocks.)

Advantages and Limitations

While application of FOT requires minimal cooperation from the subject, data collection and analysis can be technically challenging, and further work is required to establish international guidelines regarding quality control in young children and standardize methods of reporting results.[101,109] A number of publications have reported reference ranges for FOT using a variety of techniques[3,110–112] all of which show an inverse relationship between R_{rs} with height. Nevertheless, there are marked differences between these equations, including much higher values obtained when using a modified facemask rather than a mouthpiece, reflecting the wide range of techniques used. Although data collected using FOT and IOS are similar, the results obtained using these techniques are not interchangeable.

Currently the wide degree of variability between healthy children of similar age or body size limits the extent to which this technique can be used to assess either the presence or the severity of airway disease within individuals. It may, however, be a valuable tool for detecting changes within individuals on the same occasion, particularly when assessing bronchial responsiveness.[73,86,99–105,113]

■ CHEST WALL MECHANICS

A relatively neglected area of investigation, but one that has received more attention recently, is that relating to chest wall mechanics and the respiratory muscles.[31,114,115]

Dysfunction of the respiratory muscles may not only result in disease, but also render an infant or child unable to compensate for the effects of such disease, with subsequent respiratory failure.[115,116] Information regarding the strength of the respiratory muscles may be potentially useful in a number of clinical situations, including whether to wean an infant from the ventilator and the assessment of recovery from acute infections. Methods of assessing respiratory muscle strength include determination of maximal inspired and expired pressure during respiratory efforts against brief airway occlusion.[117] Simple assessment of respiratory muscle strength does not, however, reflect either endurance or susceptibility to fatigue, and the marked within- and between-subject variability of this measure may limit its clinical usefulness. Consequently, work is being undertaken to evaluate the discriminative ability of alternative indices, such as the tension-time index of the respiratory muscles. Although still to be evaluated in infants and young children, the latter has several advantages in that it is noninvasive, does not require placement of gastric or esophageal pressure transducers, and assesses muscle fatigue in all of the respiratory muscles, not simply the diaphragm. Noninvasive respiratory EMG measurements alone or in combination with lung function might provide a more comprehensive picture of pulmonary mechanics in future studies.[31]

Diaphragmatic function can also be assessed using nonvolitional tests, such as phrenic nerve stimulation. A recent modification, using magnetic rather than electrical

Time-based recording of flow and pressure

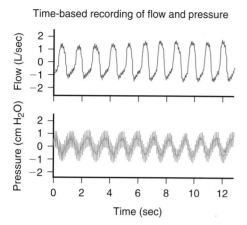

Signals transformed to the frequency domain

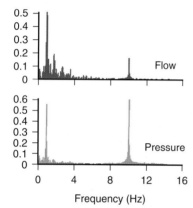

FIGURE 11-28. Time-based and Fast Fourier transform (FFT) recordings during FFT. During application of sinusoidal oscillations, the resultant pressure and flow signals are fed into a Fourier analyzer, averaged over the measurement period (usually 8 to 16 seconds), and the component of mouth pressure (P_m) and flow caused by the applied oscillations are distinguished from changes due to tidal breathing. Respiratory impedance is then calculated over a range of frequencies. Impedance is further divided into the components of the P_m signal that are in phase with flow, which represent the resistance of the respiratory system (also known as the real part), and the out-of-phase signal, or reactance, which is also sometimes referred to as the imaginary part. (From Stocks J, Sly PD, Tepper RS, et al. Infant Respiratory Function Testing. New York: John Wiley & Sons, 1996, pp 1-577.)

stimulation, has increased the potential clinical applicability of this technique and has been adapted for use in infants. By placing suitable catheters in the lower third of the esophagus and stomach, trans-diaphragmatic pressure changes can be measured after magnetic stimulation of the left and right phrenic nerves.[118]

■ FORCED EXPIRATORY MANEUVERS

Beyond the neonatal period, most respiratory disorders are characterized by airway obstruction and narrowing, which result in increased work of breathing due to increased airway resistance and hence reduced air flow. Reductions in airway caliber may occur not only due to obstruction associated with secretions, inflammation, airway wall thickening, or increased bronchial smooth muscle tone but as a result of reduced lung or chest wall elasticity, a lack of alveolar tethering, or increased airway wall compliance, all of which are associated with

reduced flows and volumes during forced expiratory maneuvers. Spirometry, whereby the subject inspires to TLC and exhales forcefully to RV, is the most frequently used method for measuring airway function in older children and has been used extensively to assess the nature and severity of airway disease and response to therapeutic interventions (see Chapter 12 for explanation of flow limitation, achievement of which is essential when undertaking spirometric assessments). Detailed criteria for standardized data collection and interpretation have been published by the ATS and ERS,[119] but even school-age children may have difficulty meeting some of the conventional quality control criteria. Despite earlier convictions that reliable spirometric measurements could not be routinely obtained in children younger than 6 years of age, the majority of preschool children are able to perform satisfactory maneuvers, provided suitable modifications are implemented, as discussed in the following sections.

By substituting voluntary effort with externally applied pressure to the chest and abdomen to force expiration, it has also been possible to adapt these measurements for sleeping infants.

■ ASSESSMENTS IN INFANTS

Partial Forced Expiratory Maneuvers

Infants cannot be instructed to perform forced expiratory maneuvers, but partial expiratory flow volume (PEFV) curves can be produced by wrapping a jacket around the chest and abdomen, and inflating this at the end of tidal inspiration to force expiration. The resultant changes in air flow (and hence volume) are recorded through a flowmeter attached to a facemask, through which the child breathes (Fig. 11-29). This technique is usually referred to as the "squeeze," or tidal rapid thoracoabdominal compression (RTC), technique. V'_{maxFRC}, which measures FEF at low lung volumes (i.e., similar to FEF_{75} in older children), is the most commonly reported parameter derived from this technique (Fig. 11-30). Guidelines regarding data collection and analysis for tidal RTC have been published,[120] as have sex-specific collated reference data.[121] The validity of such reference equations for interpreting data collected with the new generation of commercially available infant lung function equipment, however, has recently been questioned (Fig. 11-31).[9] The tidal RTC technique has been used widely in clinical and epidemiologic research studies, reductions in V'_{maxFRC} being identified in babies born to mothers who smoke during pregnancy and in those with airway disease.[122,123] Interpretation of results may, however, be confounded by several factors, as discussed in the following sections.

Methodological Considerations

To ensure that accurate and reproducible V'_{maxFRC} data are obtained, it is essential that:
- Any leaks around the facemask are eliminated
- A stable and representative end-expiratory level is established before forcing expiration
- Flow limitation is achieved.

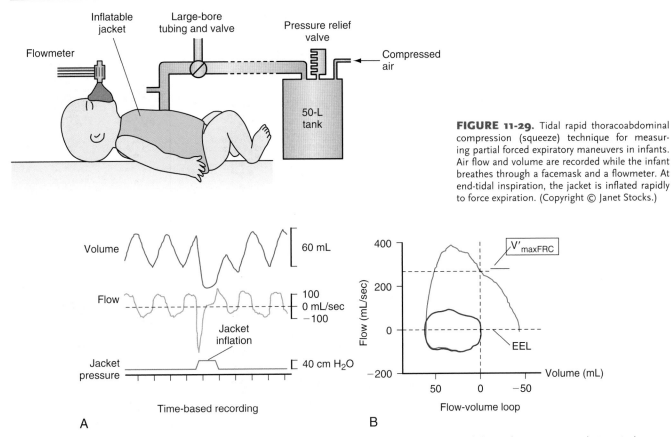

FIGURE 11-29. Tidal rapid thoracoabdominal compression (squeeze) technique for measuring partial forced expiratory maneuvers in infants. Air flow and volume are recorded while the infant breathes through a facemask and a flowmeter. At end-tidal inspiration, the jacket is inflated rapidly to force expiration. (Copyright © Janet Stocks.)

FIGURE 11-30. **A** and **B,** Partial expiratory flow volume maneuvers derived from the tidal rapid thoracoabdominal compression technique. Jacket pressure commences at approximately 30 cm H_2O and is increased in increments of 5 to 10 cm H_2O until further increases elicit no further increase in forced expiratory flow at functional residual capacity (i.e., when maximum flow at FRC [V'_{maxFRC}] is attained). *EEL,* end-expiratory level. (Copyright © Janet Stocks.)

An initial jacket pressure of 20 to 30 cm H_2O is usually applied at the end of tidal inspiration, with the aim of transmitting approximately 10 to 15 cm H_2O to the pleural space. Jacket pressure is subsequently increased in increments of 5 to 10 cm H_2O until further increases do not elicit any further increase in flow at FRC. The "optimal" jacket pressure varies considerably from child to child (i.e., 20 to 120 cm H_2O), depending not only on jacket efficiency, but also on the underlying respiratory mechanics. Infants with airway disease require far lower pressures to achieve flow limitation than healthy subjects. Measurements are repeated until three to five technically acceptable and reproducible maneuvers at optimal jacket pressure have been obtained. Because minor fluctuations in end-expiratory level can have marked effects on V'_{maxFRC}, it is recommended that V'_{maxFRC} be reported as the mean of the three highest technically acceptable results.

Advantages and Limitations

Measures of forced flow and volume reflect the integrated output of lung and airway mechanics and, as such, cannot be used to locate airway obstruction at any particular airway generation or anatomic location. Nevertheless, since V'_{maxFRC} is measured at low lung volumes, it is believed to reflect primarily airway caliber upstream (i.e., distal) to the airway segment subjected to flow limitation. This

makes it a useful measure of intrathoracic airway function in infants, in whom nasal resistance composes such a large portion of total resistance. However, since the caliber of the intrathoracic airways is determined not only by their anatomic dimensions, but by the distending pressures surrounding them, full interpretation of results may require simultaneous measurement of lung volume and elastic recoil of the respiratory system, which are rarely available. Nevertheless, this technique provides a useful forcing function that can provide a valuable measure of airway function in infants. As in older subjects, both the shape of the loop and the numeric values derived contribute to the interpretation of results (Fig. 11-32).

Forced Expiratory Maneuvers From Raised Lung Volume

Despite the popularity of the tidal RTC, its value when assessing either baseline airway function or bronchial responsiveness may be limited by the dependence of reported values of V'_{maxFRC} on resting lung volume, which may not be stable in infants, particularly in the presence of disease or following interventions. The tidal RTC technique has therefore been modified to allow measurements over an extended volume range using what has become known as the *raised volume rapid thoracic compression* (RVRTC) technique (Fig. 11-33).[2] Similar to spirometric assessments in older subjects, the RVRTC allows

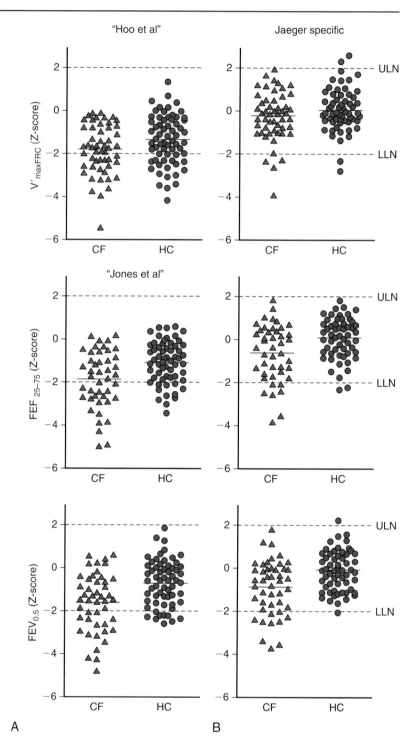

FIGURE 11-31. Comparison of FEFV data from healthy infants (HC) and those with CF; **(A)** before and **(B)** after adjustment for equipment. The solid lines denote the mean value for the group, and the upper and lower limit of the normal range (ULN and LLN, as defined by ±1.96 Z-scores) are shown. Reliance on published reference would have resulted in 17 (38%) CF infants and 9 (15%) HC being classified as having "abnormal" FEV0.5 (<−1.96 Z-scores). After adjusting for equipment, 41% (7/17) of CF infants with abnormal results were shown to have been misclassified. Similarly, for forced expiratory flows, 20 (45%) and 25 (49%) CF infants were identified as having diminished FEF25-75 and V'maxFRC, respectively, when using the unadjusted published references, of which 65% (13/20) and 80% (20/25) would have been misclassified. (Copyright © Janet Stocks.)

the infant's lungs to be inflated toward TLC before rapid inflation of the jacket initiates forced expiration from this elevated lung volume, with the maneuver ending when the infant reaches RV (Fig. 11-34). During initial attempts to apply this technique, infants frequently inspired before reaching RV. Application of three to five augmented breaths to induce a respiratory pause before forcing expiration subsequently overcame this problem.

As with most infant lung function tests, the clinical utility of RVRTC in the individual infant has yet to be established. However, this technique has been used to improve the understanding of lung and airway growth in the healthy

infant, and several studies have indicated that RVRTC may be more discriminative than tidal RTC for distinguishing the effects of respiratory disease on airway function. In clinical research studies, RVRTC has the potential to quantify the degree of airway obstruction,[38,43,124] monitor changes in airway mechanics over time,[124-127] and evaluate bronchial responsiveness (Fig. 11-35).[34,128-132] With the exception of one recent study,[8] the RVRTC has been found to be highly discriminative in identifying early airway disease in infants with CF.[53,127,133-137] In contrast to studies in older subjects, indices derived from the RVRTC are as discriminative in identifying abnormalities in lung function

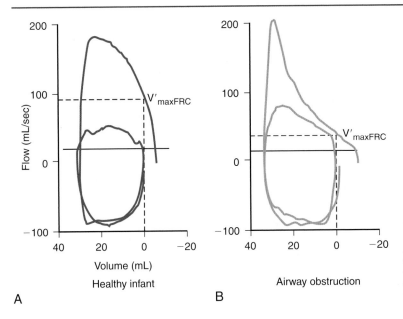

A   Healthy infant

B   Airway obstruction

FIGURE 11-32. Comparison of partial flow-volume loops in health and disease. **A,** In a healthy newborn infant, maximal flow at FRC (V'_{maxFRC}) is 92 mL/sec. **B,** In an infant of similar age and weight, but with evidence of airway obstruction, much lower flows are recorded and the descending portion of the expiratory flow-volume loop has a characteristically scooped-out shape (concave to the volume axis). (Copyright © Janet Stocks.)

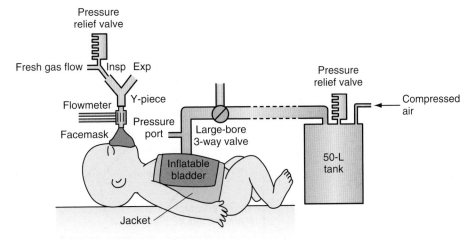

FIGURE 11-33. Forced expiratory maneuvers from increased lung volume. Using a system of valves or bias flow, the infant's lungs are inflated toward total lung capacity using a preset standardized inflation pressure (usually 30 cm H_2O) before an external forcing function is applied. The latter is achieved by rapid inflation of a jacket wrapped around the thorax and abdomen. This allows forced measurement of expiratory flow and volume over a wide volume range, as in older subjects. Jacket pressure is increased incrementally until further increases elicit no further increase in forced expiratory flow and volume. *Exp*, expiration; *Insp*, inspiration. (Copyright © Janet Stocks.)

in infants with CF as when using the LCI from multiple breath washout, although since the two techniques do not necessarily identify the same subjects, the use of both techniques is recommended in this population.[53]

Methodological Considerations

The airway pressure used to augment inspiration is most commonly 30 cm H_2O, although some centers initially used 20 cm H_2O. Optimal jacket pressure can either be estimated during prior assessments of V'_{maxFRC} or by gradually increasing jacket pressure while administering sequential lung inflations.[2] The procedure is repeated until at least two technically satisfactory and repeatable maneuvers have been recorded with values generally being reported from the best curve (i.e., that with the highest product of forced vital capacity (FVC) and either forced expiratory volume in 0.5 second ($FEV_{0.5}$) or forced expiratory flow

at 75% of expired FVC ($FEF_{75\%}$). Figure 11-36 shows the relationship between a partial and raised volume forced expiratory maneuver recorded from the same infant at the same jacket pressure. Although there is insufficient evidence to produce firm guidelines, an ATS-ERS Task Force has recently produced a consensus statement that provides preliminary recommendations pertaining to equipment, study procedures, and reporting of data for the RVRTC, based on what is perceived to be current best practice.[2]

Analysis and Reporting of Results

The values that are most commonly reported from RVRTC include the following:
- FVC-Forced vital capacity from the applied inflation pressure (e.g., FVC_{30})
- $FEV_{0.4/0.5/0.75}$-Forced expired volume at 0.4; 0.5 or 0.75 seconds

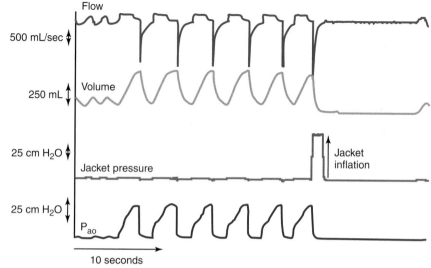

A   Time-based trace

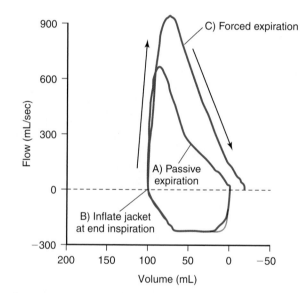

B   Flow-volume curve

FIGURE 11-34. Forced expiratory maneuvers using the raised volume technique. **A,** Time-based trace. After an initial period of tidal breathing, a preset, standardized intermittent positive pressure of 30 cm H$_2$O is applied at the airway opening to inflate the lungs toward total lung capacity. The jacket is inflated at the end of the sixth augmented breath to force expiration from increased lung volume. **B,** Flow-volume curve obtained during passive and forced expiration from increased lung volume. (Copyright © Janet Stocks.)

- FEF$_{50\%/75\%/85\%}$-Forced expiratory flow at 50%, 75%, or 85% of expired FVC
- FEF$_{25\%-75\%}$-Forced expiratory flow between 25% and 75% of expired FVC

It should be noted that despite common use of the term FVC for the total volume expired during the raised volume technique, this does not necessarily equate to measures in older subjects, because infants have been observed to take a sigh at the end of an inflation to 30 cm H$_2$O, demonstrating that TLC has not actually been attained. Calculations of FEV$_1$, and to a lesser extent, FEV$_{0.75}$ are rarely feasible in young infants, except in the presence of marked airway obstruction, due to the rapid lung emptying and short forced expiratory time (FET) that occurs during early life.[138,139] There is a marked negative age dependency of FEV$_t$/FVC ratios during infancy and early childhood,[140,141] and, in contrast to data from older subjects, such ratios discriminate poorly between infants with respiratory disease or impaired lung development compared with

control subjects.[126,127] Although measures of timed forced expired volumes (FEV$_t$) are more reproducible than forced flows and have been found to be discriminative in both clinical and epidemiologic studies,* the latter may be equally sensitive when studying wheezy infants during both baseline measurements and assessments of bronchial responsiveness.

Preliminary collation of RVRTC data from healthy infants (3–149 weeks) studied in the United States, London, and Brazil, all of whom were measured using similar handmade equipment and techniques, show an encouraging degree of overlap. However, more recent data collected with the new generation of commercially available equipment shows more diversity and suggests that establishment of equipment-specific normative data or availability of a contemporary control group may be essential for appropriate interpretation of such results (see Fig. 11-31).[7,9]

---

*References 34, 43, 53, 125, 127, 129, 135, 137, and 142–145.

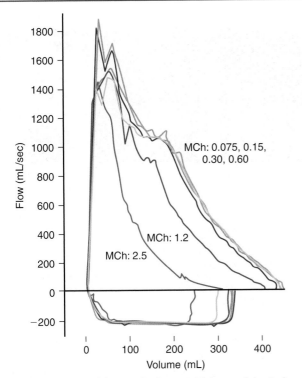

FIGURE 11-35. Use of the raised-volume rapid thoracoabdominal compression technique to assess bronchial responsiveness in an infant. After baseline values for forced expired flow and volume were established using this technique, the maneuver was repeated after incremental doses of methacholine (MCh). Highly repeatable measurements were obtained with the first four doses, followed by a significant bronchoconstrictor response at higher doses. Note changes in the shape of the forced expiratory flow volume (FEFV) curve as well as reduction in flows. (Courtesy of R. Tepper, Indianapolis.)

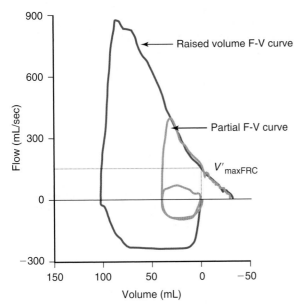

FIGURE 11-36. Overlay of tidal and increased volume forced expiratory flow volume (FEFV) curves from the same infant, illustrating the relative size of tidal and augmented breaths before forced expiration. *F-V*, flow-volume curve; V'_{maxFRC}, maximal flow at FRC. (Copyright © Janet Stocks.)

Advantages and Limitations

As in older children and adults, $FEF_\%$ can only be reliably reported if a valid assessment of FVC is available. Underestimation of FVC (with concomitant overestimation of $FEF_\%$) will occur if the child breathes in before RV has been reached. By contrast, underestimation of FVC because of failure to deliver the specified inflation pressure or because of accumulation of gas in the stomach, with upward displacement of the diaphragm, will result in underestimation of both FEV_t and $FEF_\%$. Failure to reach flow limitation by using too low a jacket pressure may have minimal effect on FVC, but will underestimate both FEV_t and particularly flow. However, the choice of optimal jacket pressure remains debatable because the use of a high enough pressure to achieve flow limitation at high lung volumes may result in negative flow dependency at low lung volumes, particularly in infants prone to airway narrowing and closure.

The raised volume technique is technically more demanding than partial flow-volume maneuvers. Extensive training and dedicated personnel who can ensure precision with respect to timing and inflation pressures are essential to assure accurate results. Leaks around the facemask occur more easily during positive pressure inflations. Some children, particularly those with severe airway disease, will not relax sufficiently or will consistently inspire before RV is reached, thereby invalidating calculations of both FVC and $FEF_\%$. Repeated inflations may result in accumulation of gas in the stomach, which will be uncomfortable for the child and invalidate the results. The lung inflations required during RVRTC may also affect subsequent measures of lung function,[146,147] such that important decisions need to be made regarding the order of tests within a protocol. Finally, considerable caution is required in infants who are oxygen-dependent, in whom repeated lung inflations might lead to prolonged apnea.

Potential advantages of RVRTC include the following:
- Forced expiratory flow volume (FEFV) outcomes are measured from a reproducible lung volume
- Flows can be assessed over an extended volume range from near TLC to RV.
- Flow limitation should be easier to achieve.
- Longitudinal assessments of similar outcomes are possible from infancy to adulthood.

Preschool Spirometry

Data Collection

With appropriate training and encouragement (Fig. 11-37), 60% to 80% of children between 3 and 6 years of age can achieve acceptable spirometry results, although more than the maximum of eight maneuvers recommended by the ATS may be necessary to achieve, this due to the initial training required.[3,5,148,149] These measurements should generally be performed at the end of a test protocol, due to the potential and unpredictable effects of deep inhalation and forced expiration on other measures of respiratory function. Young children need to be taught what is meant by taking a big breath in or blowing out as hard and fast as possible (see video 11-3, online supplement). A variety of blowing games involving straws, bubbles, party whistles, and so forth can facilitate this process, as can

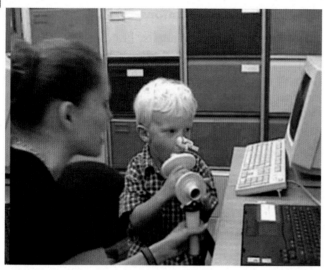

FIGURE 11-37. Preschool spirometry. Most preschool children older than 3 years of age will tolerate nose clips, although this is not imperative for acceptable results. As with all preschool tests, it is vital to establish a good relationship between the technician and the child. Judicious use of computerized incentives may improve both individual performance and success rates. (Copyright © Janet Stocks.)

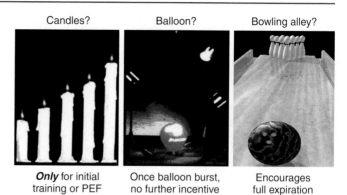

Candles?   Balloon?   Bowling alley?

Only for initial training or PEF   Once balloon burst, no further incentive   Encourages full expiration

FIGURE 11-38. Choice of computerized incentive for preschool spirometry. Effective use of computerized incentive spirometry is dependent on selecting the appropriate game. Several of the choices, including the birthday cake candles, provide no incentive for the child to continue blowing once peak expired flow (PEF) has been achieved, whereas others may be too complex for the child (or, on occasion, the operator) to understand! Whichever game is selected, it is essential that appropriate targets be set and a sufficient number of trials be allowed to ensure that the child reaches true potential. (Copyright © Janet Stocks.)

demonstrations from the operator and the use of carefully selected computer incentives. If such incentives are used, computerized games such as blowing out the candles must be used only to teach the child how to achieve peak expired flow because they provide no incentive for the child to continue blowing out to RV, and consequently may result in underestimation of FVC (Fig. 11-38). Considerable investigator input is required when setting computerized targets. If too low, the child may not make maximum efforts, but if too high, the child will become discouraged.

Preschool spirometry is usually performed with the subject seated. Most preschool children tolerate nose clips quite happily, although their use does not appear to be mandatory for acceptable recordings.[150] As with older subjects, acceptable curves are those with a rapid rise to peak flow, smooth expiration, and no evidence of early inspiration (Fig. 11-39). It can be difficult to judge the quality of the results during data collection, and all loops should therefore be saved for review once

the test has ended. Most young children appear to enjoy spirometry and will happily make repeated efforts to achieve their target. Although many of the curves may need to be rejected (Fig. 11-40), three technically satisfactory curves (discussed later) can usually be obtained with persistence.

Reporting of Results
Values that should be recorded when undertaking preschool spirometry include the following:
- FVC, $FEV_{0.75}$, FEV_1, (provided FET exceeds 0.75 and 1 seconds, respectively), from which timed-expired volumes as fractions of FVC (e.g., $FEV_{0.75}$/FVC, and FEV_1/FVC) can be calculated. $FEV_{0.5}$, $FEF_{25\%}$, $FEF_{50\%}$, $FEF_{75\%}$, and $FEF_{25\%-75\%}$ may also be reported but are unlikely to provide additional clinically relevant information.
- Duration of forced expiration (FET)
- Back-extrapolated volume at the start of expiration (both as an absolute volume and as percent FVC)
- Absolute and percent differences between key parameters from the two "best" maneuvers (e.g., ΔFVC, $\Delta FEV_{0.5}$, ΔFEV_1, $\Delta FEV_{0.75}$, $\Delta FEF_{25\%-75\%}$)

FIGURE 11-39. Technically acceptable spirometry data from a 3-year-old child. As with older subjects, acceptable curves are those with rapid rise to peak flow (PEF), smooth expiration, and no evidence of early inspiration on the flow-volume curve, as shown on the left, and with the volume-time trace *(right)* approaching a plateau. (Copyright © Janet Stocks.)

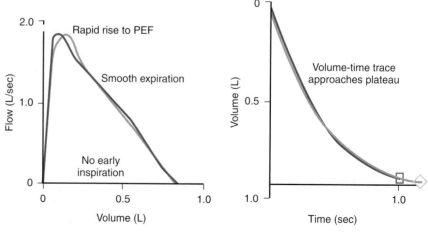

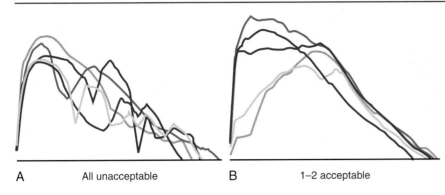

FIGURE 11-40. A and **B,** Technically unacceptable spirometry data. During initial attempts, this child was unable to produce any acceptable data, whereas during the second set of five maneuvers, one acceptable curve with a second of borderline quality was achieved, with reproducible overlay during the second half of forced expiration. (Copyright © Janet Stocks.)

Quality Control

Preliminary recommendations regarding quality control for preschool children, including criteria for the start and end of testing, have been published.[3,148] Some examples of acceptable and unacceptable curves are shown in Figures 11-39 and 11-40. The main differences with respect to criteria used for adults are the following:

- Visual inspection is usually adequate to detect a slow start to the forced expiration, with the majority of children younger than 6 years of age being able to achieve a volume of back-extrapolation to the start of testing of less than 80 mL or less than 10% (Fig. 11-41).
- Technically acceptable data should not be judged by the duration of the effort because young children's lungs may empty extremely quickly (i.e., in <1 second).
- The ability to produce FEV_1 is age-dependent in both health and disease. Consequently, $FEV_{0.5}$ and $FEV_{0.75}$ should be calculated and reported in addition to FEV_1 for all children younger than 6 years of age. For many 2- to 4-year-old children, only the shorter timed volumes will be reportable.

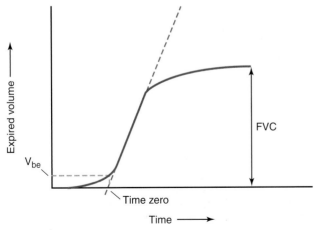

FIGURE 11-41. Start-of-test quality control criteria for preschool spirometry. Start-of-test quality control criteria for adults and older children specify a back-extrapolated volume (V_{be}) at the beginning of expiration that is less than 5% of forced vital capacity (FVC). This is not attainable by the majority of preschool children, whereas most can achieve a volume of back-extrapolation at the start of the test of less than 80 mL or less than 10%. (Reproduced from Aurora P, Stocks J, Oliver C, et al. Quality control for spirometry in preschool children with and without lung disease. *Am J Respir Crit Care Med.* 2004;169:1152-1159, with permission from the American Thoracic Society publisher; Copyright © Janet Stocks.)

- Further investigation of the discriminative ability of different spirometric parameters is an important area for future research.[5] Recent work suggests that $FEV_{0.75}$ may be a more suitable parameter when undertaking longitudinal studies that continue into early school age.[64]
- Evaluation of the end of the test by visual inspection is more difficult in preschool children, in whom there may be a relatively abrupt cessation of expiration. Modification of commercially available software to allow more objective evaluation of the change in the rate of lung emptying toward the end of expiration is required.
- Where incomplete expiration due to early inspiration is identified, timed expired volume may still be reportable, even though FVC and FEF cannot be reported from such maneuvers.
- Repeatability can be assessed as for adults, but criteria of 100 mL or 10% of best effort for ΔFVC and ΔFEV_t between the two highest technically acceptable maneuvers may be more appropriate in this age group.

Interpretation of Results

It remains to be proven whether spirometric measures obtained during the preschool years are sensitive enough to influence clinical or research practice (discussed later). The rapidity with which FEFV parameters increase during early childhood is illustrated in Figure 11-42, which shows collated data for $FEV_{0.5}$ obtained using the RVRTC technique during infancy and spirometry in children between 3 and 9 years of age. There have been numerous publications reporting normative spirometry data from healthy preschool children, some of which differ markedly from each other, which could significantly bias interpretation of results from children with respiratory disease.[151,152] A recent international initiative collated spirometry data from healthy young Caucasian children 3 to 7 years of age (n = 3,777) from 15 centers across 11 countries and linked these with existing data from older subjects to provide a continuous reference with a smooth transition into adolescence and adulthood. These reference ranges improve existing pediatric equations for white children by considering the between-subject variability to define a more appropriate age-dependent lower limit of normal, but urgently need to be extended to other ethnic groups, a challenge that has been taken by the ERS Global Lungs Initiative Task Force (see www.lungfunction. org for details).

Caution needs to be exercised when interpreting longitudinal changes in FEFV outcomes, especially those commencing in infancy due to marked changes in measurement

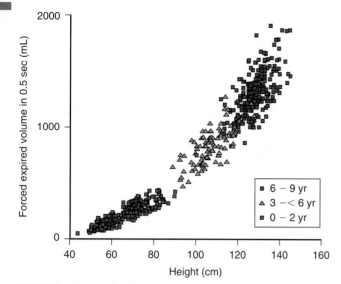

FIGURE 11-42. Collated measurements of forced expired volume in 0.5 second (FEV0.5) from birth to 9 years of age. Measures of FEV0.5 were collected in 413 healthy children (219 boys, 194 girls; 86% white) on 595 test occasions, using the raised volume rapid thoracoabdominal compression technique in supine, sedated infants and young children up to 2 years of age and using spirometry in awake, seated children from 3 years of age onward. The main determinant of FEV0.5 was height at the time of testing, which showed a strong curvilinear relationship (r2 = 0.97).

reflect more central airway function than the same measure when recorded during infancy, due to the reduced rate of lung emptying with growth (Fig. 11-43). Consequently, longitudinal measurements of $FEV_{0.5}$ or $FEV_{0.75}$ in the same subject are unlikely to provide physiologic information from the same airway generations over time. Although FEV_1 is routinely measured in older subjects, as discussed in Chapter 12, the underlying physiology of this parameter is complex.

There are limited data on within-subject, between-occasion repeatability of spirometry data in preschool children with which to interpret the clinical significance of change following interventions. A recent study in 45 asthmatic children and 22 healthy controls (mean age 5.1 years, range 3 to 7 years) found that while there was no significant group change in baseline spirometry values after an interval of 1 to 3 weeks, there was considerable within-subject between-test variability, which was greater in asthmatics (mean change [95% Limits of Agreement]: 0.1 [-1.7;1.6] $FEV_{0.75}$ Z-scores in asthmatics vs. 0.2 [-1.1; 0.7]) Z-scores in health.[72] During a longitudinal follow-up study of 45 healthy preschool children recruited as a control group for those with CF, there was no significant group change in FEV_1 Z-scores after a mean interval of 3.7 years, but there was considerable within-subject between-occasion variability, with changes in FEV_1 Z-scores ranging from −1.8 to 1.4 in individual subjects, values that must be borne in mind when interpreting the significance of clinical changes over time in those with respiratory disease.[64]

conditions (e.g., sleeping, supine infant breathing through mask subjected to external RTC versus upright, awake child making maximal voluntary efforts through a mouthpiece). In addition, during the preschool years, $FEV_{0.5}$ may

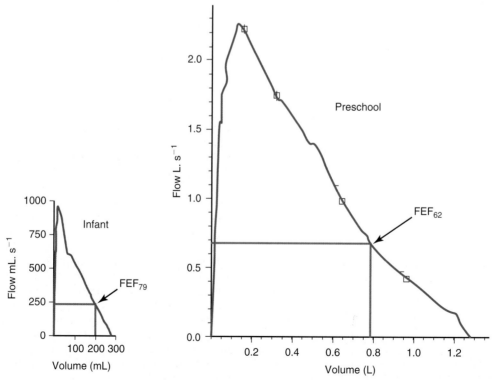

FIGURE 11-43. Developmental changes in the rate of lung emptying: position of the $FEV_{0.5}$ on the FEFV curve. In this example, $FEV_{0.5}$ during infancy is recorded when 79% of FVC has been expired, whereas 3 years later, only 62% of FVC has been expired in the first 0.5 seconds of the forced expiration. (Reproduced from Lum S and Stocks J: Chapter 4, Forced expiratory manoeuvres in European Respiratory Monograph. *Paediatric Lung Function.* 2010;47: 46-65, with permission from the European Respiratory Society.)

ASSESSMENT OF BRONCHIAL RESPONSIVENESS

Assessing whether airway function improves after the use of bronchodilator drugs is probably one of the most important clinical investigations performed in older children and adults and is recognized as having an increasing role when assessing preschool children.* The response to bronchoconstrictors in preschool children is less frequently examined, and such measurements do not play such a central role in clinical management. Nevertheless, demonstrating a lack of any evidence of bronchial hyperresponsiveness (BHR) may be useful in excluding a diagnosis of asthma, and a range of tests have been used to assess BHR in preschool children.[75,88,161-165]

The clinical role of assessing bronchial responsiveness during infancy is less clearly defined due to the difficulty in both performing and interpreting these tests at this age. While there is convincing evidence that the airways are fully innervated and capable of responding to a range of challenges during fetal and early postnatal life,[4,130] the effectiveness of bronchodilators in wheezy infants remains controversial. This reflects the fact that, in many infants who wheeze, the reduction in baseline airway function is not due to reversible bronchoconstriction, but is the result of transient conditions associated with diminished airway patency. Lack of information regarding within test repeatability also limits interpretation. A large number of studies have, nonetheless, been undertaken to assess bronchial responsiveness in infants, primarily using partial or raised volume FEFV maneuvers to evaluate response.[43,128,129,163,166-168]

Bronchial hyperresponsiveness in early life has been found to be a risk factor for subsequent symptoms of asthma in some, but not all, reported studies, and several studies have emphasized that bronchial responsiveness is likely to be more discriminative than baseline respiratory function in the assessment of preschool children and young school-age children with persistent wheeze. Important issues to address in the assessment of airway responsiveness include the technique used to assess the change in airway function, the agent used, the dosage and delivery efficacy of aerosol, quantification of the airway response, and the potential clinical utility of the information obtained.[3,169]

Methodological Issues

Choice of Tests

The most commonly used test to assess airway response in older subjects is spirometry, although plethysmography is also a popular choice. In infants, the vast majority of studies have used partial, or more recently, raised volume flow-volume curves. In contrast, although spirometry has also been used in preschool children, this is a demanding test, and its use in intervention studies is usually reserved for slightly older children. The most commonly used tests for assessing bronchial responsiveness in preschool children

have been the interrupter technique, FOT, and plethysmographic assessments of specific resistance, although some investigators have used more indirect methods (particularly during bronchial challenge), including transcutaneous oxygen tension,[163,170] auscultation (wheeze),[164] or tidal breathing parameters[171] to assess responsiveness. The most important distinction is between techniques that require deep inflation to total lung capacity and those that are obtained during tidal breathing or at volumes close to FRC. Deep inflation can modify airway responses,[172] and the difference in response before and after such maneuvers is sometimes used to localize the site of response in older subjects.

Technical problems related to the choice of method can influence the interpretation of airway responsiveness in early life. Thus, although the tidal RTC technique has been frequently used in infants during both bronchodilator and challenge tests, changes in FRC that may be induced by the intervention, but are not routinely measured during the procedure, may result in paradoxical changes in V'_{maxFRC} and an underestimation of airway responsiveness. Although the use of RVRTC should minimize problems associated with referencing flows to FRC, measured FVC can be underestimated secondary to accumulation of gas in the stomach from repeated maneuvers as well as by inspiration before RV is reached during forced expiration. Furthermore, the effect of repeated lung inflations on baseline respiratory mechanics and responsiveness has yet to be established in infants.

Similarly, even though resistance is a more direct measure of airway caliber than maximal expiratory flow, a measured decrease in resistance may include reductions in extrathoracic resistance due, for example, to changes in the vocal cords or the pharyngeal airway. When tests such as the single-occlusion or interrupter techniques are used, bronchoconstriction after administration of a challenge may increase ventilation inhomogeneity or increase the time needed to reach pressure equilibration, resulting in a potentially dangerous underestimation of the change in resistance. When such tests are used, it is therefore recommended that transcutaneous oxygen tension be monitored, in addition to oxygen saturation. Given that marked reductions in airway function may occur during any challenge test, safety is of paramount importance. When such tests are performed in infants and preschool children, two fully trained operators, at least one of whom must be a nurse or physician, should always be present.

Choice of Provocative Stimulus

As in older subjects, many pharmacologic and physical stimuli have been used in challenge tests for infants and young children. Histamine and methacholine are the most commonly used agents that act directly on smooth muscle. Methacholine has been favored in most epidemiologic studies. Adenosine monophosphate and hypertonic saline cause bronchoconstriction via the release of mediators and have been used to provide a more indirect, and possibly more physiologic stimulus. Exercise testing

---

*References 3, 72, 73, 75, 87, 88, 92, 93, 99, 100, 104, 113, and 153–160.

is obviously not appropriate for infants and does not appear to have been adapted for use in preschool children. The use of cold or dry air challenges is gaining popularity in this age range. As in older subjects, inhalation of a β_2-adrenergic agonist drug, such as salbutamol (albuterol) or terbutaline, is routinely used both to reverse the effects of challenge tests and to assess bronchodilator response.

Administration of an Inhaled Agent

The method chosen to administer the inhaled pharmacologic agent will be influenced by the need for portability, the age and clinical status of the child, and the purpose of the assessment (clinical or research). The aerosol dose delivered to the airways will depend on the device used to generate the aerosol, the method of delivering the aerosol, and the location of aerosol deposition. Aerosol output varies according to the type and operating conditions of each nebulizer and the physical properties of the liquid to be aerosolized. The quantity of aerosol inhaled will depend on the size of the inhaled volume, whether inhalation is via the nasal or oral route, and whether the child is asleep, quietly awake, or crying, because different inspiratory flow patterns will accompany each of these states (see Chapter 18).[4] Whichever delivery system is used, an appropriate bronchodilator should be prepared before the first dose of challenge agent is administered.

Aerosols are generally delivered to infants during tidal breathing, whereas older, cooperative subjects often take deep inspirations to maximize aerosol delivery throughout the lung. Deep inspirations can also be used to deliver aerosols to sleeping infants, using techniques similar to those employed in ventilated subjects, or during RVRTC. The potential effect of deep inhalations on the lung function parameters being measured must be considered when choosing the mode of delivery. The effectiveness of the response to the generated aerosol will depend on the site of aerosol deposition. Only a small fraction of the pharmaceutical agent aerosolized by the nebulizer or metered-dose inhaler actually deposits within the airways.

There is currently no standardized dosage or method for delivery for the evaluation of bronchodilator responsiveness in infants and young children. Selection of dosage has varied among that used clinically, that demonstrated to reverse the acute effects of a bronchoconstricting agent (e.g., methacholine or histamine), and that required within an individual to effect an increase in heart rate.

Evaluation of Response

There is currently no consensus on how to evaluate whether an infant or young child has demonstrated an improvement in airway function after the administration of a bronchodilator. Different approaches include: (1) comparison of the best pretest and posttest values, (2) comparison of the pre-mean and post-mean values from several replicates, and (3) definition of a specific pre-to-post change for the individual, based on the variability of the measurement in the population.[3,87,99,100,159] The importance of assessing within-subject variability between occasions, in the absence of any intervention, if such tests are to be interpreted in a meaningful fashion, has been stressed.[3]

As in older subjects, constructing a dose-response curve that quantifies the dose of agonist required to produce a specified reduction from baseline airway function has been used to summarize the degree of airway reactivity in infants and young children. When FEF is used to assess airway responsiveness in infants, the provocative concentration of the agonist needed to produce a 30% reduction from baseline (PC$_{30}$) in V'$_{maxFRC}$, or FEF$_{25\%}$, is often used. The magnitude of this decrease has been found to exceed the intra-subject within-test variability of the measurement, and it is frequently associated with a change in the shape of the flow-volume curve from convex to concave (Fig. 11-35).[130] An alternative approach, based on the magnitude of response to a fixed intervention in relation to within-subject variability, is required when single-step tests, such as cold or dry air challenges, are used.

Age-Related Changes in Hyperresponsiveness

In infants, heightened responsiveness may result not only from anatomically small airways or increased smooth muscle tone, but also from relatively thicker airway walls, decreased chest wall recoil, reduced airway tethering, or increased airway wall compliance. Together with the difficulties in estimating the dose of agonist that will actually be delivered to the lung in infants and young children, such factors make it virtually impossible to interpret apparent changes in bronchial reactivity during the first few years of life. Any comparisons between results obtained in infancy and in later life, especially those derived from longitudinal studies, must consider not only all of the factors discussed earlier, but also the posture in which measurements are obtained.

As discussed earlier in the chapter, failure of infants and young children to respond to inhaled bronchodilators may be partially attributed to difficulties in delivering adequate amounts of aerosolized drugs in this age group, but may also reflect differences in the underlying pathology, with wheezing in younger children being due to factors such as congenitally small airways, airway wall edema, or secretions rather than to bronchial smooth muscle shortening. Whereas increased airway responsiveness is evident in most asthmatic adults and older wheezy children, this is not routinely the case in wheezy infants or preschool children. The degree of bronchodilator response appears to be age-related, and it is often (although not always) minimal or absent before 18 months of age, but well established by 6 to 8 years of age.

Future Directions

With increasing awareness of the importance of assessing the reversibility of a reduction in baseline airway function to improve the discriminative ability of currently available tests for preschool children, it is essential for international guidelines and standardized protocols for undertaking such tests to be developed as rapidly as possible, together with an assessment of which tests are most appropriate under specified conditions and for specific populations of young children. Some preliminary recommendations have been published recently.[3]

The usefulness of assessing airway responsiveness must be approached in relation to how the information obtained will be used. Several research studies have demonstrated significant responses to bronchodilators and apparently increased bronchial reactivity even in healthy infants and young children, and what determines a clinically significant bronchodilator response for an individual child has yet to be clearly defined. It is unlikely that assessment of airway reactivity will play a role in the clinical management of individual infants.

APPLICATIONS OF PFTS IN INFANTS AND PRESCHOOL CHILDREN

Epidemiologic Research into Early Determinants of Respiratory Function

In recent years, there has been increasing use of PFTs to provide objective outcome measures in population-based studies of respiratory health and disease during early life. The sex of an infant has a marked effect on airway function, as reflected by lower maximal expiratory flows in boys compared with girls at any given height, both during infancy and in later childhood. This may contribute to the increased prevalence of wheezing in boys at all ages to puberty. Sex-specific reference data should therefore be used when predicting normal ranges of airway function.[69,91,121,140] Although less is known about the effect of ethnic group on lung function during early life, both nasal and R_{aw} have been shown to be lower in Afro-Caribbean than in white infants, which impacts on patterns of tidal breathing. Preliminary data suggest that ethnic differences in spirometric values, long recognized among older children and adults, may also be detectable in preschool children.[11,12,148]

There is powerful evidence of the adverse effects of maternal smoking on infant lung function. This effect is apparent at least 7 weeks before the expected date of delivery and is independent of postnatal exposure, as demonstrated by studies that have assessed lung function in healthy infants before discharge from the neonatal unit. A review of the literature found conclusive evidence that smoking during pregnancy is associated with a reduction in FEF (by, on average, approximately 20%), as well as increases in both airway and total resistance.[173] There is also substantial evidence regarding the adverse effect of maternal smoking during pregnancy on postnatal control of breathing, particularly with respect to a blunted response to hypoxia, hypercapnia, and arousal stimuli.[174–176] In infants born to atopic mothers, exhaled nitric oxide levels are increased shortly after birth in those exposed to maternal smoking, whereas the reverse appears to be true among those delivered to nonatopic mothers.[177]

Specific vulnerability to passive tobacco smoke exposure may, however, vary markedly between individuals according to genotype. Glutathione S-transferase (GST) may increase the risk of asthma and wheezing among those exposed to intrauterine tobacco smoke because it functions in pathways that are possibly involved in asthma pathogenesis (e.g., xenobiotic metabolism and antioxidant defenses). A recent study showed that GST genes may be especially important during fetal development as they may modify, through efficient detoxification, the effects of in utero maternal smoking on airway responsiveness and V'_{maxFRC} in infants.[166] Similarly, in an earlier study of school-age children, the long-term effects of in utero exposure to maternal smoking on lung function and on asthma and wheezing were largely restricted to children with GST null genotype.[178] Such studies underline the complex relationship between genetic and environmental factors on the development of airway disease and the importance of taking gene by environment interactions into account in future epidemiologic studies.

Although maternal smoking during pregnancy remains the most significant and avoidable source of exposure to tobacco products in early life and is likely to be largely responsible for diminished airway function in the first few years of life, continuing postnatal exposure to tobacco smoke from either parent will increase the risk of respiratory infection, wheezing illnesses, and diminished lung function throughout childhood. Furthermore, maternal smoking has been shown to be a risk factor for allergic sensitization and asthma only in children with a genetic predisposition.[179] The effect of parental smoking has an equally adverse effect on infants with lung disease,[127,142] thereby necessitating careful recording of such exposures if the results of either clinical or research studies are to be interpreted correctly, as well as to provide appropriate health education for the parents.

A family history of atopy, particularly maternal asthma, has been shown to be associated with diminished airway function and increased airway responsiveness during both infancy and the preschool years.[20,167,180,181] Similarly, after adjustment for all known confounders, including age, sex, and current body size, $FEV_{0.4}$ was found to be significantly lower in infants born small for gestational age than in appropriately grown control subjects, with a similar tendency noted for FEF.[182] These changes persisted throughout the first year of life.[126] Higher levels of NO_2 during pregnancy were also found to be related to elevated exhaled nitric oxide levels and associated with higher minute ventilation and tidal flows in newborns.[21] Many of these epidemiologic studies have highlighted the complex interactions among birth weight, socioeconomic status, family history of atopy, parental smoking, and airway function in infants, and they have emphasized the need for large numbers of infants to be recruited to studies such as these if meaningful conclusions are to be reached.

INFANT LUNG FUNCTION AS A PREDICTOR OF SUBSEQUENT RESPIRATORY MORBIDITY

The Tucson Children's Respiratory Study was the first longitudinal assessment of the natural history of asthma that included infant PFTs. More than 1200 children were enrolled at birth. Eight hundred of these were still participating at 13 years of age,[183] although only 10% of these subjects had had lung function measured in the first few months of life. This study was the first to provide evidence that diminished airway function precedes wheezing illness, in that $t_{PTEF}:t_E$ was significantly lower in boys (although not in girls) who subsequently wheezed with a lower respiratory illness in the first year of life.[14] Although there was no significant difference in V'_{maxFRC} between those who did and did not wheeze when follow-up was limited to the first year of life, subsequent follow-up revealed a diminution of V'_{maxFRC} shortly after birth in those who wheezed during the first year and who had had at least one additional wheezing lower respiratory infection by 3 years of age.[183] This cohort has now been followed up to young adulthood, with clear evidence of "tracking of lung function," with those in the lowest quartile for lung function at birth maintaining this position through to young adulthood.[184]

Similar findings were reported from the East Boston study (which also used V'_{maxFRC} as an outcome measure) and in the East London study, which found elevated premorbid values of R_{aw} in those who subsequently wheezed in the first year.[45] In contrast, the Perth longitudinal study suggested that reduced airway function in early life was associated with persistent wheeze at 11 years, but not with transient wheeze.[167] Discrepancies between results may reflect differences in techniques, methods of statistical analysis, population, and environment as well as the fact that, although a large number of children may be recruited to longitudinal studies during infancy, the number in whom repeated lung function measures can be made on all test occasions throughout childhood may be relatively small due to the inherent difficulties in conducting such studies. Nevertheless, despite the wide range of techniques used, all of these studies have provided evidence of diminished premorbid lung function shortly after birth among those with subsequent wheezing illness.

Although one of the major aims of these epidemiologic studies, namely, to predict which infants who wheeze are likely to progress to asthma in later life, has not yet been realized, considerable knowledge has been gleaned regarding the range of different wheezing phenotypes. It is now generally acknowledged that those with very early onset of wheeze (in the first year of life), whose mothers smoke, and in whom there is no family history of asthma or atopy have a relatively low risk of persistent asthma. In contrast, those in whom the onset of wheeze occurs later or in the absence of significant exposure to prenatal or postnatal tobacco smoke, where there is a maternal history of asthma, persistent personal atopy (eczema and allergy, initially to food, especially egg, and later to inhalants), and increased bronchial responsiveness (with or without diminished flow) in infancy, have a much higher risk of subsequent asthma. Interesting data are also beginning to emerge from large epidemiologic studies of "high-risk" preschool children (i.e., those with a family history of atopy or a history of persistent wheezing), many of which are designed to follow up large cohorts of young children into school age, which may shed further light on these associations.* Recent evidence suggests that IgE antibody responses reflect several different atopic vulnerabilities that differ in their relation with asthma presence and severity.[186,187]

_____
*References 66, 85, 142, 163, 180, and 185.

Although the extent to which tracking of lung function (i.e., the extent to which those with low initial levels of airway function for their age or body size subsequently retain this position) occurs in school-age children is debatable, serial measurements of lung function have revealed considerable tracking during early life. This has been demonstrated in healthy term[126] and preterm[188] infants, in infants and young children with CF,[64,127,134,189] and between infancy and school age in those with BPD.[190]

APPLICATIONS DURING CLINICAL RESEARCH STUDIES

Difficulties in Assessing Lung Function in Infants and Young Children with Respiratory Disease

Despite numerous attempts to monitor changes in lung function as a means of identifying early onset of pulmonary disease during the first year of life, the natural course of pulmonary involvement in infants with respiratory disorders remains relatively poorly understood. As discussed earlier, problems encountered include the following:

- The need for sedation
- Difficulties in repeating measurements frequently enough
- Lack of appropriate reference data and information regarding within- and between-subject variability, especially in the presence of disease
- Confounding of measurements by developmental changes in respiratory physiology
- Many of the assumptions underlying lung function tests in early life, particularly those involving brief airway occlusions, (e.g., requirements for a single time constant and/or rapid pressure equilibration during periods of no flow) are not valid in the presence of respiratory disease.

Such problems are compounded if attempts are made to undertake measurements in the intensive care unit.[191,192] Additional factors include the following:

- The relative invasiveness of some of these techniques in clinically unstable infants
- Insensitivity of the test to changes in respiratory mechanics within individuals, due, for example, to the relative magnitude of resistance of the endotracheal tube
- Use of inappropriate tests to investigate the underlying pathophysiology
- Inaccuracies in displayed values of V_T[193]
- Confounding of results due to interactions between the ventilator and spontaneous breathing activity
- Leaks around the endotracheal tube
- The heterogeneous nature of the population with respect to maturity, body size, and clinical severity
- The multitude of possible treatment modalities to which ventilated infants and young children may be exposed
- Inappropriate adjustment of lung function results for body size

Clinical Research Studies

Despite these problems, many studies describe the application of infant lung function tests in clinical research, with the tidal RTC technique for measuring V'_{maxFRC}

remaining one of the most commonly used methods for assessing airway function in this age group.[145] In the past, far fewer publications reported the use of PFTs as outcome measures in preschool children due to the paucity of suitable tests, but this situation is changing rapidly, with many cross-sectional and longitudinal studies now being undertaken in this age group.*

As discussed earlier, baseline airway function has been shown to be reduced in both infants and preschool children with recurrent wheeze, although in some studies, significant differences between such populations are evident only when bronchial responsiveness is compared.[153,199] Longitudinal studies in which preschool lung function is related to wheezing phenotypes are underway to assess the sensitivity and specificity of these tests in predicting subsequent outcome and discriminating those with airway disease from healthy control subjects.[66] Serial measurements of lung function from infancy into the preschool or school-age years in recurrently wheezy children are also beginning to emerge.[14,161,186,194,200–206]

The application and interpretation of PFTs in infants and children with CF have been summarized recently,[†] with most studies reporting diminished lung and airway function in symptomatic infants and young children. It has been shown that airway function is reduced at an early stage in infants with CF, even in the absence of symptoms or clinically recognized previous lower respiratory illness, and that this does not catch up during infancy and early childhood.[64,127,134] More recently, evidence of infection, inflammation, and abnormal chest computed tomography findings have been reported to be present at 3 months of age in a significant portion of infants with CF diagnosed by newborn screening.[212] Preliminary findings from the London CF collaborative study of newborn screened infants also indicate diminished lung function in approximately 50% of such infants before 3 months of age.[137] These findings have important potential implications for early interventions in CF.

Although several reports have suggested that RVRTC may be a more sensitive means of discriminating changes in lung function in infants with respiratory disease than either tidal breathing parameters[17] or V'_{maxFRC},[124,213] it should be remembered that this technique is more complex to apply.[2]

A variety of techniques, including spirometry,[56,134,189,198] plethysmography,[56,71] FOT,[71,103,104] interrupter resistance,[71,86,214] and MBW,[53,56,61,63,64] have been used to assess pulmonary function in preschool children with CF, with some of these studies being longitudinal and beginning in infancy or early childhood. All have shown significant group differences between children with CF and healthy control subjects, although most show considerable overlap between the groups, with results from many young children with CF falling within the normal range. The exception is with respect to results obtained with MBW, wherein abnormal results are found in the majority of young children with CF, despite normal results for other measures of lung function[64] (Fig. 11-16). However, during infancy the RVRTC has been shown to be as discriminative as the MBW in detecting abnormal lung function in those with CF.[53]

Relatively few studies have been designed wherein results from infant or preschool lung function tests have been used to assess response to therapeutic interventions, such as antibiotics or corticosteroids. As discussed earlier, interpretation of such studies is often limited by lack of knowledge regarding the natural disease process and within-subject repeatability of the measurements, as well as by the relatively small sample size and the heterogeneous nature of both disease severity and individual response to therapy. Further, randomized controlled trials using standardized equipment and protocols are necessary to determine the true role of lung function tests during early life in evaluating such interventions. However, the complexities associated with multicenter studies of either preschool and particularly infant lung function should not be underestimated.[8,19,69,77]

Applications During and After Intensive Care

Numerous studies have attempted to use parameters derived from infant lung function tests to assess the effects of preterm delivery, neonatal lung disease, and ventilatory support.* The most commonly used approaches in recent years have been assessments of passive respiratory mechanics and lung volumes.

The only "static" volume that is routinely measured in infants during mechanical ventilation has been that at end expiration, with or without positive end-expiratory pressure,[220] although determination of lung volume over an extended volume range, using the negative deflation technique, has also been described in a few specialized centers.[146] During recent years, there has been increasing use of EIT in the ICU.[23–26] A critical review of the most common techniques currently applied in pediatric intensive care, together with its usefulness and shortcomings, has recently been published.[192] It has been suggested that the major benefit of pulmonary function testing in intensive care is related to objective assessments of scientific investigations rather than of direct benefit to clinical management. Although some studies have suggested that early measurements of respiratory mechanics may be predictive of subsequent BPD, this has not been confirmed in any randomized controlled studies, probably due to the enormous numbers of subjects that would be required to achieve sufficient power of study.

Preterm delivery, even in the absence of any initial respiratory disease, has been shown to have an adverse effect on subsequent lung growth and development, which persists and may even worsen throughout the first year of life.[125,143,188,217,221]

Most studies in infants with BPD or chronic lung disease of infancy (CLDI) have suggested that lung volumes are low early in infancy, but subsequently become normal or elevated. This has been attributed to the fact that, over time, pulmonary fibrosis may become less important relative to airway disease and lung volume may increase disproportionately with growth. Studies of infants with BPD/CLDI have also reported reduced compliance, increased resistance, and decreased flow during the first

---

*References 3, 48, 56, 64, 66, 72, 77, 86–88, 99, 103, 104, 134, 155, 156, and 194–198.
†References 61, 78, 86, 133, 136, and 207–211.

*References 10, 16, 19, 23, 24, 41, 43,44, 80, 81, 105, 125, 144, 188, and 215–219.

year of life.[43,222] Recently, using a modified single-breath hold technique for assessing pulmonary diffusing capacity, Balinotti and colleagues found that clinically stable infants and toddlers with CLDI have reduced pulmonary diffusing capacity but similar alveolar volume when compared with healthy term controls.[13] A review series on lung function testing in infants and young children with CLDI has been published[223] summarizing available data and critically discussing the potential role of lung function testing in these children with acute respiratory disorders and CLDI. The series includes a review on lung and chest wall mechanics,[81] tidal breathing and respiratory control,[16] functional residual capacity,[41] forced expiratory maneuvers,[145] and global and regional ventilation inhomogeneity.[23] Follow-up to school age has shown that these changes may persist throughout early childhood.[190,222,224,225] Lung function tests have also been used as objective outcome measures to assess the effect of different types of ventilatory support, including extracorporeal membrane oxygenation and high-frequency oscillation, during the neonatal period on subsequent lung growth and development.[44,122,123,221,226]

Interpretation of Lung Function Results in Infants and Young Children and Their Role in Clinical Management

As in older subjects, the clinical usefulness of any lung function test within an individual infant or preschool child will always be enhanced if serial measures rather than a single assessment can be undertaken. However, during infancy the frequency with which PFTs can be repeated is limited by the need for sedation and the time-consuming nature of the tests that may place considerable burden on parents who are already struggling to cope with a child with lung disease. When requesting such PFTs, it is essential that the choice of tests is based on the question to be answered, clinical reasoning, and knowledge of the suspected underlying pathophysiology, rather than simply on the equipment that happens to be available in any given center. Given the marked influence of factors such as preterm delivery, intrauterine growth retardation, sex, ethnic group, and maternal smoking during pregnancy, it is important to take a careful history from the parents when performing such tests in infants and young children with respiratory problems.

What Is Normal?

In order to identify the nature and severity of any underlying pathophysiology in an individual, it is essential to have a clear idea of what range of values to expect in a healthy child of similar age, sex, body size, and ethnic group.[152] Therefore, reliable interpretation of pulmonary function results relies on the availability of appropriate reference data to help distinguish between health and disease. The use of inappropriate reference equations and misinterpretation, even when potentially appropriate equations are used, can lead to serious errors in both underdiagnosis and overdiagnosis, with its associated burden in terms

of financial and human costs. It is important to remember that lung function results from healthy children and those with respiratory symptoms or disease often overlap to such an extent that a result within the normal range does not exclude disease. Similarly, while abnormal lung function results are often associated with symptoms and disease, they may simply be "atypical" and must always be interpreted in the light of all other clinically relevant information.

Clinicians in respiratory medicine have become familiar with the concept of expressing lung function as percent predicted, ([observed/predicted] *100), where the predicted value is derived from reference equations. The median predicted value is 100%, and any deviation from 100% indicates an offset from the predicted value. Conventionally the variability between healthy subjects is taken to be a standard deviation (SD) of 10%. On this basis, the normal predicted range would be from 80% to 120%. However, it has been clearly demonstrated that this is not the case and that between-subject variability differs markedly according to age of the subject and lung function outcome.[140,152,227] Thus, in a 3-year-old the SD for FEV_1 is close to 17%, whereas that for FEF_{25-75} is 27% such the "normal range" for these measures extends from 67% to 133% for FEV_1 and 46% to 154% for FEF_{25-75}. If this age- and outcome-dependent variability is ignored, many children will be flagged incorrectly as "abnormal."[140]

A better approach to reporting lung function measures is to express results as Z-scores (or Standard Deviation Score [SD]) scores). The Z-score is a mathematical combination of the percent predicted and the between-subject variability to give a single number that accounts for age- and height-related lung function variability expected within comparable healthy individuals.[152] The upper and lower limits of normal (ULN and LLN) are conventionally defined as Z-score of ±1.64, a range that encompasses 90% of healthy subjects. However, due to increased uncertainty regarding reliability of reference ranges for infants and young children and the fact that multiple PFTs are often used in the assessment, these limits may be set at ±1.96 Z-scores to encompass 95% of the healthy population. Unlike percent predicted, where each outcome has a different cutoff, the same cutoff of −1.64 or 1.96 Z-scores applies across both sexes and all ages, ethnic groups, and pulmonary function indices. Z-scores are useful for tracking changes in lung function with growth or treatment, as they allow comparison of lung function results obtained with different techniques. An increasing number of clinical research studies are now reporting infant and preschool lung function as Z-scores.[8,64,122,142,190,228]

Regardless of whether Z-scores or % predicted are used to express results, the age-specific normal range should always be included in the lung function report. Particular caution is required when interpreting results that lie close to the somewhat arbitrary "cutoffs" between health and suspected disease, especially when results are limited to a single test occasion. As with all tests, PFTs should be seen as only one part of the whole clinical picture.

As mentioned earlier, marked biases between predicted values can occur due to alterations in equipment and protocol,[9] differences in population characteristics, the statistical methods applied, or simply as a result of sampling error due to too small a sample of healthy children being studied.[229]

When selecting reference data with which to interpret clinical lung function results from an infant or young child, it is essential to check how appropriate these data are with respect to the following:

- Whether the same equipment, technique, and methods of analysis were used
- Whether a comparable and sufficiently large population was studied, with even distribution of age and body size
- Whether original raw data are available for inspection of quality control applied
- Whether appropriate statistical techniques were used

There is an urgent need for greater national and international consensus as to which reference equations should be used in infants and young children, a task that should be made easier, at least for preschool children, by international efforts to collate available data in this age range.[69,91,140,152]

The need for sedation and the duration of studies limit the number of healthy infants who can be studied at any one center. While international collaborative efforts led to the publication of sex-specific reference data for V'$_{maxFRC}$ during infancy that proved appropriate at the time for custom-built equipment,[121] the development of commercially available devices for infants appears to have introduced some bias,[7-9,47,230] necessitating the development of equipment-specific equations for infant PFTs before clinical studies in individual infants can be interpreted properly.

Can Lung Function Tests Be Used in the Clinical Management of Individual Infants and Preschool Children?

Although there is little doubt about the potential value of infant lung function tests as a means of providing objective outcome measures in clinical or epidemiologic research studies, their potential usefulness with respect to influencing clinical management within an individual infant remains debatable.[231-233] The clinical usefulness of any technique depends not only on its ability to measure parameters that are relevant to the underlying pathophysiology and to discriminate between health and disease, but also on within-subject repeatability both within and between test occasions. As discussed earlier, although highly reproducible measurements of lung function can be made in infants during the same test occasion, little is known about within-subject, between-test repeatability. The dearth of appropriate reference data also limits the extent to which disease severity can be assessed except in departments that regularly test healthy infants using identical techniques. Despite these limitations, a recent informal ATS survey identified a large number of centers around the world that reported undertaking infant lung function tests, including assessment of bronchodilator responsiveness, to "assist in clinical management." This situation urgently needs rational discussion and debate to ascertain the extent to which appropriate clinical decisions can actually be made under such circumstances.

In contrast, given the increasing success with which preschool children can be studied, the gradual establishment of more appropriate reference equations for many techniques in this age group and the determined efforts to establish within- and between-occasion repeatability in both health and disease in order to identify what constitutes a clinically significant change within an individual (as a result of disease progression or response to treatment), the potential use of PFTs to aid clinical management looks increasingly feasible in preschool children with respiratory problems, as in their older counterparts.

Future Directions

If appropriate equipment were to be miniaturized or incorporated into the ventilatory circuit so that continuous online monitoring of relevant parameters could be undertaken, one major area in which infant lung function tests could influence clinical management lies in the neonatal and pediatric intensive care unit. Given the current rate of technological development, this is certainly feasible but will demand a major commitment by all concerned, plus the recognition that many tests used to date are either too complex or insensitive to provide reliable and relevant information to guide treatment. Techniques that should be targeted include those that measure both absolute values and changes in lung volume, tissue mechanics, and distribution of ventilation, with results being carefully integrated with other relevant outputs. Meaningful interpretation and use of such data will also require an improved knowledge of respiratory physiology among pediatricians and intensive care physicians. Another area in which there may be a role for lung function tests during early life is with respect to longitudinal measurements from birth through the preschool years in high-risk groups (e.g., those with persistent wheezing, CF, and chronic lung disease of infancy), particularly if those at higher risk or with early signs of lung disease can be identified to allow more aggressive treatment and thus maximize lung health and prevent permanent damage, without exposing those who will not benefit to potentially harmful side effects during rapid lung growth and development.

◼ SUMMARY AND CONCLUSIONS

There has been remarkable progress in the field of infant and preschool lung function testing during the last decade. Commercially available equipment and international recommendations are now available for the most commonly used tests of infant lung function. Forced expiratory maneuvers can be performed over the full lung volume range throughout infancy and the preschool years, whereas noninvasive assessments of gas-mixing efficiency that are applicable from birth to old age offer the possibility of detecting (and hence potentially treating) early changes in airway function in children with respiratory disease. This field has also moved to a situation where testing of preschool children from at least 3 years of age is seen to be increasingly feasible, using a wide variety of tests under both laboratory and field conditions.

Lung function testing in infants and young children will, nevertheless, always present a challenge, and it is therefore essential that the purpose of any test is clearly defined at the outset and that dedicated operators with the necessary expertise and patience are available to undertake and interpret such measurements. Despite its vital role in clinical and epidemiologic research, given the need for sedation, the specialized equipment, and the difficulty in repeating measurements at frequent enough intervals, it is unlikely that lung function testing will ever gain a routine place in the clinical assessment of infants with respiratory disease. In contrast, provided standardized protocols can be developed that incorporate appropriate quality control criteria for young children, together with reliable reference data and information regarding the relative sensitivity and specificity of the various tests in differentiating healthy children from those with respiratory disease, lung function tests for preschool children could soon assume a role similar to that of tests used for their school-age counterparts. To achieve this goal, continuing international collaboration will be required, together with input from manufacturers to ensure that the available equipment and software is optimized for this very important age group.

Suggested Reading

Beydon N, Davis SD, Lombardi E, et al. An official American Thoracic Society/European Respiratory Society statement: pulmonary function testing in preschool children. *Am J Respir Crit Care Med.* 2007;175: 1304–1345.

Frey U. Clinical applications of infant lung function testing: does it contribute to clinical decision making? *Paediatr Respir Rev.* 2001;2:126–130.

Gappa M, Pillow JJ, Allen J, et al. Lung function tests in neonates and infants with chronic lung disease: lung and chest-wall mechanics. *Pediatr Pulmonol.* 2006;41:291–317.

Hammer J, Eber E. *Paediatric pulmonary Function Testing.* Basel: Karger; 2005.

Kirkby J, Stanojevic S, Welsh L, et al. Reference equations for specific airway resistance in children: the asthma UK initiative. *Eur Respir J.* 2010;36:622–629.

Lum S, Stocks J. Forced expiratory manoeuvres. In: Merkus P, Frey U, eds. *European Respiratory Monograph: Paediatric lung function.* ERS Journals Ltd; 2010:46–65.

Lum S, Stocks J, Castile R, et al. ATS/ERS Statement: Raised volume forced expirations in infants: Guidelines for current practice. *Am J Respir Crit Care Med.* 2005;172:1463–1471.

Merkus PJ, Stocks J, Beydon N, et al. Reference ranges for interrupter resistance technique: the Asthma UK Initiative. *Eur Respir J.* 2010;36:157–163.

Oostveen E, MacLeod D, Lorino H, et al. The forced oscillation technique in clinical practice: methodology, recommendations and future developments. *Eur Respir J.* 2003;22:1026–1041.

Robinson PD, Goldman MD, Gustafsson PM. Inert gas washout: theoretical background and clinical utility in respiratory disease. *Respiration.* 2009;78:339–355.

Stanojevic S, Wade A, Cole TJ, et al. Spirometry centile charts for young Caucasian children: the Asthma UK Collaborative Initiative. *Am J Respir Crit Care Med.* 2009;180:547–552.

Stocks J, Coates A, Bush A. Lung function in infants and young children with chronic lung disease of infancy: The next steps? *Pediatr Pulmonol.* 2007;42:3–9.

Stocks J, Godfrey S, Beardsmore C, et al. Standards for infant respiratory function testing: Plethysmographic measurements of lung volume and airway resistance. *Eur Respir J.* 2001;17:302–312.

Stocks J, Modi N, Tepper R. Need for healthy controls when assessing lung function in infants with respiratory disease. *Am J Respir Crit Care Med.* 2010;182:1340–1342.

References

The complete reference list is available online at www. expertconsult.com

12 PULMONARY FUNCTION TESTING IN CHILDREN

ROBERT G. CASTILE, MD, MS, AND STEPHANIE D. DAVIS, MD

The most frequently performed test of pulmonary function in children and adults is forced expiratory spirometry. Because spirometry permits the assessment of only those volumes of air that can be voluntarily exchanged, additional techniques have been devised that allow the measurement of all of the gas contained in the lungs. Measurements of lung volume and forced expiratory flow form the foundation of pulmonary function testing in children. This chapter also includes a description of other tests that are often performed in the pediatric pulmonary function laboratory: maximal respiratory pressures, diffusing capacity of the lung, resistance of the respiratory system and airways, multiple breath washout, and exhaled nitric oxide.

INDICATIONS FOR TESTING

Tests of pulmonary function in children enable clinicians to: (1) detect mechanical dysfunction of the respiratory system;(2) quantify the degree of dysfunction detected;(3) define the nature of the dysfunction as obstructive, restrictive, or mixed;(4) track disease over time; and (5) evaluate the effect of acute and long-term therapeutic interventions. Lung function tests also serve as outcome measures in clinical trials. These and other indications for performing pulmonary function tests in children are summarized in Box 12-1.

LABORATORY ENVIRONMENT

Testing should be done in a room that is not used for other procedures that may cause distress in children. Parents may be present during testing to support the child emotionally, but the child must focus his or her attention on the pulmonary function technician. The technician should be experienced in both pulmonary function testing and working with children. Most children are able to perform voluntary tidal breathing and rudimentary forced expiratory maneuvers by 3 years of age. A child who is able to perform respiratory maneuvers (taking a deep breath and blowing out forcefully) in the office in response to an examiner's verbal requests is likely to perform even better with the visual feedback provided by real-time monitoring of the flow-volume curve. With practice, most children can voluntarily perform respiratory maneuvers well enough to provide useful physiologic information by 4 to 5 years of age.[1]

LUNG VOLUMES

The earliest spirometric measurements of lung volume and its expirable subdivisions were made by Hutchinson in 1846.[2] Figure 12-1 shows a volume-time plot of a vital capacity maneuver. This diagram shows all of the major subdivisions of lung volume. The maneuver begins with normal tidal breathing. The subject then inhales to maximally fill the lungs. This is followed by a maximal expiratory effort and then a return to normal tidal breathing. Tidal volume (VT) is the volume of air either inspired or expired with each normal tidal breath. The amount of air inspired from the resting expiratory level to full inflation is the inspiratory capacity (IC). Inspiratory reserve volume (IRV) includes all of the extra volume that can be inspired above the tidal range (IC – VT). Expiratory reserve volume (ERV) is the volume below the tidal end-expiratory level that can be forcefully expired from the lungs. Vital capacity (VC) is the maximal amount of air that can be expelled from the lungs after maximal inspiratory effort. VC represents the total voluntarily exchangeable lung volume. Even when the maximal amount of air has been expired from the lungs, some volume remains. The volume of air remaining in the lungs after maximal expiratory effort is the residual volume (RV). The maximal amount of air that can be contained in the lungs at the end of maximal inspiration, total lung capacity (TLC), is the sum of RV and VC. Functional residual capacity (FRC) is the amount of air in the lungs at the end of normal tidal expiration. It represents the sum of ERV, which is expirable, and RV, which is not expirable. These various components of TLC are referred to as *fractional lung volumes*. All of these volumes, except RV, TLC, and FRC, can be measured with a spirometer.

Residual volume can be determined by measuring FRC and subtracting ERV. FRC can be measured by gas dilution techniques or by using a whole-body plethysmograph. Gas dilution techniques measure the communicating gas volume in the thorax. The plethysmographic method measures all gas contained in the thorax. Each method is subject to different errors in the presence of disease, particularly airflow obstruction.

GAS DILUTION TECHNIQUES

Helium Dilution

Although it was recognized in the early 19th century that the nonexpirable volume of the lungs could be measured by gas dilution techniques,[3] it was not until the 1930s that these methods were applied clinically.[4] In the helium dilution method, the patient's lung volume is part of a closed-circuit spirometer system containing air and a known concentration of the inert gas helium (~10%). The concentration of helium in the original closed system is diluted in direct proportion to the helium-free volume added to the circuit by the air from the patient's lungs.

BOX 12-1 USES OF PULMONARY FUNCTION STUDIES IN CHILDREN

To establish pulmonary mechanical abnormality in children with respiratory symptoms

To quantify the degree of pulmonary dysfunction

To define the nature of pulmonary dysfunction (obstructive, restrictive, or mixed obstructive and restrictive)

To aid in defining the site of airway obstruction as central or peripheral

To differentiate fixed from variable and intrathoracic from extrathoracic central airway obstruction

To follow the course of pulmonary disease processes

To assess the effect of therapeutic interventions and guide changes in therapy

To detect increased airway responsiveness

To evaluate the potential risk of diagnostic and therapeutic procedures involving anesthesia

To monitor for pulmonary side effects of chemotherapy or radiation therapy

To aid in prediction of the prognosis and quantify pulmonary disability

To investigate the effect of acute and chronic disease processes on lung growth

To serve as measures of outcome in clinical trials

Specifically, the patient breathes into a closed circuit that contains a water-sealed spirometer, a helium analyzer, a blower fan for circulating gas throughout the system, a carbon dioxide absorber, and a regulated oxygen source to compensate for oxygen consumed during the measurements (Fig. 12-2). The patient's end-expiratory tidal breathing level is monitored using the spirometer, and oxygen is added to the system to maintain a constant volume. The patient continues to breathe while connected to the system until there is complete equilibration between the gas in the spirometer system and the air in the patient's lungs. Equilibration is considered to have occurred when the helium concentration has fallen to a new steady-state level. FRC is determined based on the premise that the product of the initial helium concentration (C_i) and the volume of the system (V_{sys}) must equal the product of the final helium concentration (C_f) and the volume of the system after the child's lung volume (FRC) has been added.

$$C_i \times V_{sys} = C_f (V_{sys} + FRC)$$

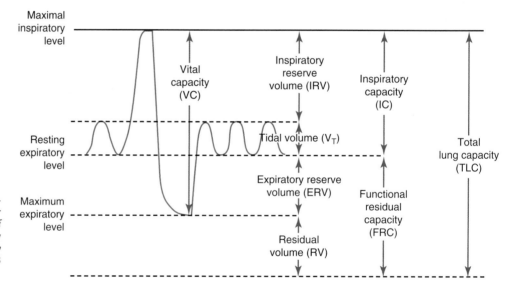

FIGURE 12-1. Tidal breathing followed by a vital capacity maneuver demonstrating the subdivisions of lung volume. (Modified from Murray JF, Nadel JA. *Textbook of Respiratory Medicine*, 2nd ed. Philadelphia: WB Saunders, 1994, p 801.)

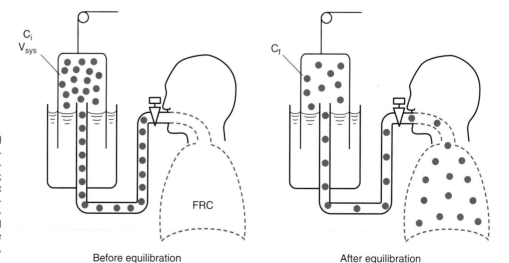

FIGURE 12-2. Helium dilution method for measuring functional residual capacity (FRC). C_f = final helium concentration; C_i = initial helium concentration; V_{sys} = system volume. Dots represent helium molecules, which, after equilibration, decrease in concentration in proportion to the subject's FRC. (Modified from West JB. *Respiratory Physiology. The Essentials*. Baltimore: Williams & Wilkins, 1974, p 15.)

Before equilibration   After equilibration

Then FRC can be calculated from the known volume of the spirometer circuit and the initial and final helium concentrations in the circuit using the following formula:

$$FRC = V_{sys}(C_i - C_f)/C_f$$

FRC measured using the helium dilution method is abbreviated as FRC_{helium}.

Nitrogen Washout

Nitrogen is present in the lung in a known concentration (~80%). During the nitrogen washout technique for measuring FRC, nitrogen is washed from the child's lungs using a one-way bias flow of 100% oxygen by the mouth. The total amount of nitrogen washed from the lungs provides a measure of the patient's resting FRC. Although the specific methods used in clinical practice vary in their details, volume is again measured in terms of gas dilution. FRC represents the unknown volume. The nitrogen concentration of the air in the lungs is measured during exhalation. The total volume of gas expired during the washout and the concentration of nitrogen in the washout volume can be measured. As with the helium dilution method, the product of FRC and the nitrogen concentration in the lungs must equal the product of the total washout volume and the nitrogen concentration of the washout gas. FRC then equals the product of the washout volume and the nitrogen concentration of the washout volume divided by the nitrogen concentration of the air in the lungs.

In the open-circuit method (Fig. 12-3), 100% oxygen is inspired through a bias flow or one-way nonrebreathing system, and a mixture of nitrogen and oxygen is exhaled. The patient continues to breathe 100% oxygen until all of the nitrogen has been washed from the lungs. The amount of nitrogen exhaled is quantified by collecting the total volume of gas expired, the washout volume (V_{wo}), and measuring its nitrogen concentration (C_{wo}). FRC can then be calculated by dividing the volume of nitrogen exhaled ($C_{wo} \times V_{wo}$) by the concentration of nitrogen in the lungs (C_L):

$$FRC = (C_{wo} \times V_{wo})/C_L$$

Alternatively, the nitrogen concentration in the expiratory limb of the circuit can be continuously integrated to obtain an index of the total amount of nitrogen exhaled. This integrated nitrogen system is calibrated using known volumes of air. FRC is calculated by dividing the integrated nitrogen value obtained from the patient washout by the nitrogen value obtained for the known calibration volume. This method assumes the mean nitrogen concentration in the lung to be equal to that of air. In practice, nitrogen continues to wash out from the blood and body tissues at a slow, nearly constant rate after all of the nitrogen has been washed from the lungs. At this point, the test is complete. The rate of nitrogen washout from blood and tissues, measured at the end of lung washout, can be used to correct the washout FRC for nitrogen coming from the body. In practice, this small difference is often negligible. FRC measured using the nitrogen washout method is abbreviated as $FRC_{nitrogen}$. The results obtained with the open-circuit nitrogen washout method are comparable to those obtained with the closed-circuit helium dilution method.[5] It should be noted that both of these methods may underestimate FRC because they measure only volumes of air that communicate with the mouth during tidal breathing. Gas dilution methods do not measure volumes of air behind closed airways (trapped gas) and can underestimate volumes in severely obstructed, nearly closed areas (i.e., those with very long time constants).

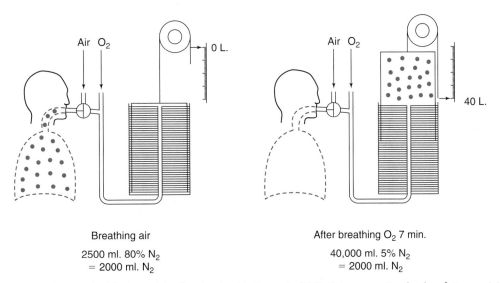

FIGURE 12-3. Nitrogen washout method for determining functional residual capacity (FRC). Dots represent molecules of nitrogen. Initially, all molecules are in the lungs as 80% nitrogen *(left)*. During 100% oxygen breathing, the nitrogen molecules are washed out of the lung and collected in the spirometer *(right)*. FRC is calculated from the total washout volume in the spirometer and the nitrogen concentration of the expired gas. In the example given, the expired volume is 40 L and the nitrogen concentration is 5%. Thus, the total amount of nitrogen expired is 2000 mL, which represents 80% of the patient's FRC. The patient's full FRC is, thus, 2500 mL. (Modified from Comroe JH, Forster RE, DuBois AB, et al. *The Lung. Clinical Physiology and Pulmonary Function Tests*, 2nd ed. Chicago: Year Book, 1974, p 14.)

◼ PLETHYSMOGRAPHY

The plethysmographic technique for measuring thoracic gas volume (TGV) was introduced by Dubois and colleagues in 1956[6] and depends on the principle of Boyle's law (pressure × volume = constant). Air is compliant; it can be compressed or expanded. The compliance of a volume of gas, such as the volume of air in the thorax, increases or decreases in proportion to the volume of that gas. The thorax is more compressible or compliant with more air present. Less air leads to a stiffer thoracic cavity. Thus, the quantity of air in the thorax can be measured by determining its stiffness or compliance. The compliance of gas is measured in terms of the volume change that occurs in relation to a given pressure change.

To measure the pressure-volume relationship of the air contained in the thorax, the child sits with nose clip in place in a closed box called a *whole-body plethysmograph* (Fig. 12-4). The child breathes through a mouthpiece, and a shutter is closed at end-expiration. The child is then asked to pant (make positive and negative pressures against the closed shutter at a frequency of about 1 per second). The pressure changes are measured at the mouth, and it is assumed that they are transferred uniformly throughout the thoracic cavity. These pressure changes expand and compress the gas contained in the thorax. Prior to beginning, the panting maneuver should be practiced with the door of the box open. To prevent pressure changes in the oral cavity, the child should be instructed to support the cheeks with his or her hands during panting.

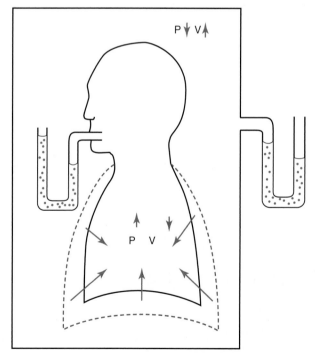

FIGURE 12-4. Plethysmographic method for measuring functional residual capacity. When the subject makes an expiratory effort against a closed airway, intrathoracic pressure *(P)* increases and lung volume *(V)* decreases. The increase in box volume results in a decrease in box pressure that allows the change in lung volume to be quantified. Lung volume is obtained from the ratio of the change in lung volume to the change in mouth pressure from Boyle's law. (Modified with permission from West JB. *Respiratory Physiology. The Essentials.* Baltimore: Williams & Wilkins, 1974, p 16.)

The plethysmograph, or body box, allows measurement of the changes in TGV that occur in relation to the changes in intrathoracic pressure produced by the subject. When the positive intrathoracic pressures produced by the subject's expiratory efforts against the closed shutter compress and thereby cause a decrease in TGV, pressure in the closed plethysmograph becomes more negative. When the subject makes an inspiratory effort, the TGV and the box pressure increase. These changes in box pressure occur in direct proportion to the volume changes that occur in the thorax. The box itself can be calibrated (also using Boyle's law) such that the relationship of change in pressure to change in volume in the box surrounding the child is known. If, for example, 100 mL of air is injected into the box using a syringe and the box pressure increases by 1.0 cm H_2O, then for every 0.1 cm H_2O change in box pressure, box volume (whether occurring via injection of air into the box or as a result of volume change within the child's thorax) has changed by 10 mL. In this manner, changes in TGV (as reflected by changes in box pressure) can be related to changes in mouth pressure, and the compliance of the air contained in the thorax can be determined. The magnitude of the ratio of the change in box pressure (ΔP_{box}) to the change in mouth pressure (ΔP_m) provides a measure of the volume of air contained in the thorax by the following formula:

$$TGV = (\Delta V/\Delta P_m) \times (P_{baro} - 47) \times (1.36 \text{ cm } H_2O/\text{mm Hg}),$$

where P_{baro} = barometric pressure in millimeters of mercury, ΔV is measured as P_{box} calibrated in terms of volume in milliliters, ΔP_m is measured in centimeters of water, and the factor 1.36 converts barometric pressure from millimeters of mercury to centimeters of water.

Plethysmography measures the volume of air contained in the lungs when breathing is occluded. TGV is the gas volume in the lungs at the time of occlusion. If the shutter is closed at end-tidal expiration, then TGV equals FRC. Measurements of FRC can also be made with plethysmographs that measure volume change directly using a spirometer or obtain volume as the integral of flow from a pneumotachometer placed in the wall of the box. By convention, FRC measured plethysmographically is abbreviated as FRC_{pleth}. Plethysmography measures all gas within the lungs and airways including gas that does not communicate with the mouth. Thus air trapped behind closed airways and noncommunicating structures (e.g., intraparenchymal cysts) is measured by plethysmography. In the presence of severe airflow obstruction, changes in mouth pressure may substantially underestimate changes in alveolar pressure and result in an overestimation of FRC_{pleth}.[7]

A plethysmograph can also be used to measure airway resistance (R_{aw}).[8] R_{aw} is the ratio of change in alveolar pressure (ΔP_{alv}) to change in flow ($\Delta V'$) measured at the airway opening ($R_{aw} = \Delta P_{alv}/\Delta V'$). Resistance is, in effect, the pressure change required to produce a flow of 1 L/second into or out of the lungs. The inverse of this ratio ($\Delta V'/\Delta P_{alv}$) is termed the *airway conductance* (abbreviated G_{aw}) and represents the flow in and out of the lungs produced by a positive or negative change in P_{alv} of 1 cm H_2O. R_{aw} is measured with the subject sitting in the plethysmograph wearing a nose clip and breathing through a flowmeter that vents within the confines of the box. As the subject is breathing into and from the box, the total volume of the lung-plethysmograph system remains unchanged. When the subject breathes, changes in P_{alv} are generated to overcome the resistance of the airways and move air in and out of the lungs. These small changes in P_{alv} compress and rarify the gas in the lungs. These small changes in alveolar volume produce pressure changes in the box (P_{box}) that are opposite in direction and proportional to the changes in P_{alv}. Although much smaller in magnitude, these changes in P_{box} due to compression of gas in the lungs are identical to those that occur during the previously described TGV maneuver. In practice, R_{aw} is measured with the subject panting rapidly with very shallow changes in volume. Panting serves to open the glottis and minimize artifacts due to heating/cooling and humidification/dehumidification of the inspired and expired air. With the subject panting, the ratio of $\Delta V'$ and ΔP_{box} is measured. Then, with the subject still panting, a shutter is closed to block breathing (just as in the TGV maneuver) and the ratio of ΔP_m and ΔP_{box} is measured. With the airway opening closed, ΔP_m equals ΔP_{alv}. Measuring the relationship of ΔP_m ($=\Delta P_{alv}$) to ΔP_{box} during the larger changes in lung volume that occur during the occlusion permits changes in P_{alv} to be known in terms of changes in P_{box}. R_{aw} can then be determined by dividing the ratio of $\Delta P_{alv}/\Delta P_{box}$ measured with the shutter closed by the ratio of $\Delta V'/\Delta P_{box}$ measured with the shutter open:

$$R_{aw} = (\Delta P_{alv}/\Delta P_{box})/(\Delta V'/\Delta P_{box}) = \Delta P_{alv}/\Delta V'$$

R_{aw} must be adjusted for the resistance of the flowmeter and connecting tubing. If the box is calibrated for volume as described earlier in this section, TGV during the occlusion can be calculated. As conductance and resistance vary with the lung volume level at which they

were measured, G_{aw} and R_{aw} are frequently adjusted by the measured TGV. These adjusted measures are termed *specific* G_{aw} or R_{aw} (G_{aw}/TGV and $R_{aw} \times TGV$, respectively).

FORCED EXPIRATORY SPIROMETRY

Historical Background

It was not until approximately 100 years after Hutchinson[2] first published spirometric measurements of lung volumes in 1846 that forced expiratory spirometry was recognized as a valuable tool for assessing lung function in patients with respiratory disease.[9] In the early 1950s, measurements of timed forced expiratory volumes (e.g., forced expiratory volume expired in 1 second, or FEV_1) were recognized as useful measures of lung function.[10] By the mid-1950s, measurements of mid-expiratory forced flow were noted to be highly reproducible (within a given individual), sensitive measures of early airway dysfunction.[11] In the late 1950s, Fry, Hyatt, and colleagues introduced the concept of the maximal expiratory flow-volume curve and demonstrated, with the use of isovolume pressure-flow plots, that forced expiratory flows were limited.[12-14] As a direct result of these physiologic insights, forced expiratory spirometry rapidly became the most widely used test of pulmonary function in both adults and children.

FLOW LIMITATION

In 1958, Hyatt and colleagues[14] demonstrated that expiratory flows were limited throughout most of the forced expiratory maneuver. They measured intrathoracic pressures with an esophageal catheter and plotted them against expiratory flows measured at the mouth at specific (iso) lung volumes. These isovolume pressure-flow curves (Fig. 12-5) demonstrated clearly that expiratory

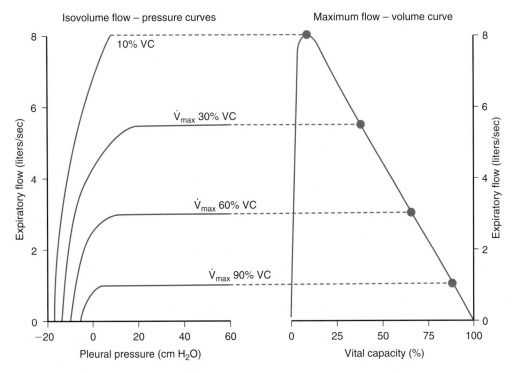

FIGURE 12-5. From a series of isovolume flow-pressure curves at varying percentages of expired vital capacity (VC) *(left)*, it is possible to construct a maximal expiratory flow-volume curve *(right)*. A similar flow-volume curve can be obtained by simply plotting expired flow against volume using an X-Y recorder during a single forced expiratory vital capacity maneuver. $\dot{V}_{max}$, maximal expiratory flow. (Modified with permission from Murray JF. *The Normal Lung.* Philadelphia: WB Saunders, 1976, p 102.)

flows become limited or effort-independent at relatively modest positive intrathoracic pressures. Figure 12-5 demonstrates that flows over most of the descending portion of the maximal flow-volume curve are limited. The transpulmonary pressures required to achieve flow limitation increase somewhat at higher lung volumes. In 1985, Pedersen and associates[15] demonstrated that even peak flow can be flow-limited with sufficient effort.

In 1967, Mead and colleagues[16] introduced the concept of an airway *equal pressure point* (EPP) (Fig. 12-6). They pointed out that, during forced expiration, the driving pressure forcing flow from the lungs was the sum of the pressure actively applied to the pleural space plus the lung recoil pressure. As the actively generated increase in pleural pressure is applied to both the alveoli and the airway walls, it is only the lung recoil pressure at any lung volume that allows pressure inside the airways to be higher than pressure outside the airways. During forced expiration, flow-related frictional and convective accelerative intrabronchial pressure losses occur. At some point along the airways from the alveoli to the mouth, flow-related pressure losses will equal the elastic recoil pressure, and the difference between intrabronchial and extrabronchial pressures will be zero. This point along the path of flow is the EPP. Distal from this point, further intrabronchial

airway pressure losses result in lower pressures within the airways than around them and leads to dynamic compression of downstream airways. This model provided insight into the mechanical factors that control airway dynamics during forced expiration, but did not explain the mechanism of flow limitation.

In 1977, Dawson and Elliott[17] pointed out that elastic tubes cannot carry a fluid or gas at a mean velocity greater than the speed at which pressures will propagate along the tube; that is, the mean rate at which gas molecules can flow through a flexible tube cannot exceed the speed at which the pressure driving the flow is propagated along the tube. This velocity of pressure propagation along the tube is referred to as the tube wave speed. The pertinent wave speed of pressure propagation in elastic tubes equals the inverse square root of the quotient of the tube wall specific compliance and gas density. The equation is

$$P_{ws} = (\rho dA/dPA)^{-1/2}$$

where P_{ws} is pressure wave speed, A is airway area, ρ is gas density, and dA/dP is airway compliance. During flow limitation, this wave speed, by definition, equals the speed of gas molecules flowing in the tube. Thus, bulk flow, limited by this mechanism, is the product of the tube wave speed and the cross-sectional area of the tube at the point of limitation. This point of limitation is referred to as the *choke point*. The bulk flow at wave speed is then the product of the speed limit of the gas molecules flowing in the tube (i.e., P_{ws}) and the cross-sectional area of the tube (A). Thus, the equation for the flow at wave speed is

$$V'_{ws} = (\rho dA/dPA)^{-1/2} \times A$$

where V'_{ws} is flow at wave speed limitation. Minimal algebraic rearrangement reveals that maximal flows at choke points are determined by gas density, airway-specific compliance, and airway area, as follows:

$$V'_{ws} = (\rho)^{-1/2} \times (dA/dPA)^{-1/2} \times A$$

Forced expiratory flows limited by this mechanism vary in inverse proportion to the square root of gas density and airway-specific compliance and will be directly proportional to the airway cross-sectional area at the site or sites of flow limitation. Increased airway wall compliance, such as occurs in bronchiectasis, will lower wave speed limits and forced expiratory flows. Reductions in the airway cross-sectional area, such as those occurring secondary to bronchospasm, will also decrease forced expiratory flows. Breathing a gas with lower density, such as helium-oxygen, permits higher maximal flows.

Figure 12-7 illustrates pressure wave speed (P_{ws}) flow limitation in a rigid tube (see Fig. 12-7A) and a compliant tube (see Fig. 12-7B). The blue circles represent air molecules, each with a cloud of negatively charged electrons surrounding a proton and neutron core. In Figure 12-7A, pushing another air molecule "instantaneously" into the tube will result in expulsion of the last molecule in the line from the end of the tube. This does not, however, happen instantaneously. When the electron cloud of the first molecule moves forward, it "pushes" on the

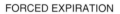

FORCED EXPIRATION

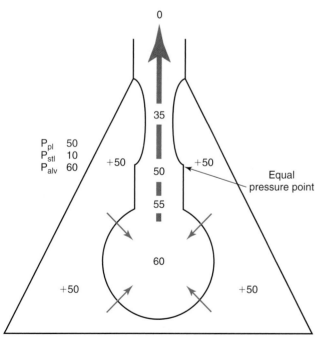

FIGURE 12-6. Schematic representation of the equal pressure point concept. Pleural pressure (P_{pl}), static elastic recoil pressure of the lung (P_{stl}), and alveolar pressure (P_{alv}) are expressed in centimeters of water. Pleural, alveolar, and airway pressures for a typical forced expiratory maneuver are shown. During forced expiration, muscular effort results in an increase in pleural pressure. The alveolar pressure driving flow is the sum of applied pleural pressure and lung elastic recoil pressure. As pressure is dissipated along the airways during airflow (60-55-50- ... 0), there must be a point at which the pressures inside and outside the airway wall are equal (equal pressure point). Downstream from this point, the airways are compressed because lateral pressure in the lumen of the airway is lower than the pressure surrounding the airway wall. (Modified with permission from Murray JF. *The Normal Lung.* Philadelphia: WB Saunders, 1976, p 103.)

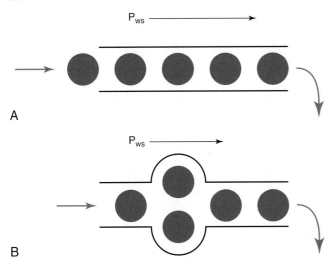

FIGURE 12-7. Pressure wave speed (P_{ws}) flow limitation in **(A)** a rigid tube and **(B)** a compliant tube. Blue circles represent air molecules. Flows are limited by the speed at which pressure is propagated along the tube (i.e., P_{ws}). In tube A, the speed of pressure propagation depends only on the compliance of the air in the tube. Thus, an increase in pressure driving flow proceeds from one end of the tube to the other at the speed of sound. In tube B, the speed of pressure propagation depends not only on the compliance of the air in the tube, but also on that of the walls of the tube. Because the walls of the tube are far more compliant than the air in the tube, P_{ws} and thus maximal possible flow velocities are much slower in tube B (see text).

second negatively charged field. The second molecule then "springs" forward to influence the third, and so on until the last molecule moves out of the tube. This process of pushing together and springing forward is a pressure wave, and in air, pressure waves move at a finite speed, the speed of sound. The last air molecule in the line will not move out of the tube instantaneously, but rather in the time that it takes the pressure wave to move down the tube. The compressibility (i.e., compliance) of the gas in the tube controls the rate at which pressure is propagated. Thus, P_{ws} sets the limit on how quickly the molecules can flow through the tube. In Figure 12-7B, both the air in the tube and the walls of the tube are compliant and the compliance of the tube wall far exceeds that of the gas. When the first molecule is forced into the tube, the rate at which the pressure wave moves down the tube is slower than in the case of the rigid tube because the walls of the compliant tube stretch to absorb pressure and then rebound to return pressure to the tube. This markedly slows the rate at which the pressure wave moves down the tube. Again, P_{ws} sets the limit on how fast the last molecule in the line can be expelled, making the maximal velocities at which the air molecules can flow in the compliant tube much lower than for the rigid tube. In the lung, compliance of the airway wall plays a central role in determining the maximal velocities at which air molecules can flow. With the speed limits set by the wave speed, the airway cross-sectional area determines how many molecules can pass at that maximum velocity.

The elastic properties of the airway and its cross-sectional area thus interact to determine wave speed limits. Flow limitation occurs along airways where the product of airway elastance (i.e., stiffness—the inverse of compliance) and airway cross-sectional area is minimal. The site at

which flow limitation occurs is thus dependent on the geometry of the bronchial tree and the manner in which changes in lung volume and flow-related pressure distributions affect that geometry. Flow limitation at wave speed is most likely to occur downstream of EPPs, where airways are dynamically narrowed and flow velocities are increased. Flow limitation (choking) occurs at points where the gas molecule velocities flowing through these airway narrowings are equivalent to the speed of pressure propagation.

At high lung volumes, the level of the bronchial tree with the smallest total cross-sectional area is in the trachea. In smaller airways, the airway cross-sectional area depends heavily on the elastic properties of the lung parenchyma. The total small airway cross-sectional area is large at high lung volumes and decreases steadily as forced expiration proceeds to lower lung volumes. Peripheral airway resistance thus increases steadily with decreasing lung volume. Both increases in resistive losses and declining lung elastic recoil pressures diminish intra-airway pressures as exhalation proceeds. As a result, the EPP and the location (or locations) where airways are dynamically compressed move toward the alveoli as lung volume decreases. Thus, the site of flow limitation, or choking, during a forced expiratory maneuver occurs initially in the trachea or central airways in normal subjects and moves progressively upstream toward the alveoli as forced exhalation proceeds.

As the site of flow limitation moves from the central to more upstream airways, the number of sites of choking must increase in an exponential manner. Only when all airways at a given level of the bronchial tree are choked will flow be limited at that level. Mead[18] realized that the manner in which global sites of flow limitation move from central to more peripheral airways must be complex. Figure 12-8 shows initial flow limitation in the trachea at high lung volumes. As lung volumes decrease and the wave speed limits of the airways upstream diminish, choking is likely to occur in some upstream segments. Based on the complex nature of the bronchial tree, Mead speculated that it would be unlikely for all segments at a given level in the bronchial tree to reach their wave speed limits simultaneously.[18] Thus, he postulated that a sequential choking of airways upstream of the initial site of flow limitation occurred. Upstream movement of the global site of flow limitation would occur only when all upstream pathways were choked. According to this model, movement of the choke point in central and medium-sized airways was confirmed physiologically by McNamara and colleagues in 1987.[19] These sudden jumps of the global site of flow limitation that occur when the last remaining upstream airway chokes result in sudden decreases in flow, or "bumps" in the configuration of the flow-volume curve. This process probably repeats multiple times as forced expiration proceeds and the global site of flow limitation moves upstream from central to peripheral airways, with the number of sites of flow limitation increasing as lung volume decreases. Thus, in a general way, the flows measured during forced expiration reflect the functional anatomy of more central airways at high lung volumes and that of more peripheral airways at lower lung volumes.

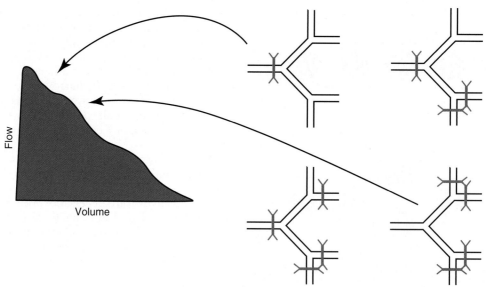

FIGURE 12-8. Movement of the global site of low limitation from the trachea to more peripheral airways. Flow limitation is shown occurring initially in the trachea at high lung volumes *(upper left)*. As lung volume decreases, segmental airways upstream from the controlling tracheal site of flow limitation become "choked" *(upper right)*. Eventually, only a single upstream pathway remains "unchoked" *(lower left)*. When the final pathway "chokes" *(lower right)*, the global site of flow limitation moves upstream, and this is accompanied by a sudden fall in maximal flow or a "bump" in the configuration of the maximal expiratory flow-volume curve. (Modified from Mead J. Expiratory flow limitation. a physiologist's point of view. *Fed Proc.* 1980;39:2771-2775.)

As forced expiration proceeds from maximal inspiration, choke points multiply and cascade irregularly from central to peripheral airways. Flows measured at the mouth, however, reflect only the stepwise movement of global sites of flow limitation as these sites move from one level in the bronchial tree (where flow has become limited in all contributing pathways) to the next. In subsequent work published in 1994, McNamara and colleagues[20] reported that this interdependent pattern of airway emptying inherently tends to hide airway nonhomogeneities. Because the global site of flow limitation does not move upstream until the upstream segment with the highest flow or wave speed has become flow-limited, the behavior of more slowly emptying segments is hidden or silent. This phenomenon may explain why even extensive degrees of nonhomogeneity located in the small airways are not reflected as marked changes in forced expiratory flows measured at the mouth. Thus, spirometry is a suboptimal tool for the early detection of nonhomogeneously distributed distal airway disease.

At low lung volumes, flow may not be limited by the wave speed mechanism, but rather by viscous flow limitation. In very small airways, viscosity-related pressure losses may result in decreases in the cross-sectional area and an effective limitation of flow at lower limits than those imposed by wave speed.[21] This possible change in the mechanism of flow limitation at low lung volume has no apparent clinical significance.

◼ EQUIPMENT

Forced expiratory maneuvers in children are quantified using either a spirometer (dry rolling seal or water seal) or a pneumotachometer to measure flow and then integrating the flow signal to obtain volume. Most current devices provide immediate feedback on performance

by plotting the maximal expiratory flow-volume curve. Devices that provide a continuous real-time plot of flow versus volume are the most useful in monitoring the efforts of children.

Equipment used for testing children should be capable of accurately measuring small volumes and low flows. Volume measurements should be accurate to within 30 mL or ± 3%. Flow measurements should be accurate to 0.1 L/sec or ± 5%.[22] Lemen and associates [23] assessed the frequency content of forced expiratory maneuvers in children and recommended that equipment have a flat dynamic response through 12 Hz for flow and 6 Hz for volume to record flow and volume accurately during maximal expiratory maneuvers. Calibration should be performed daily to ensure the accuracy of measurements. Equipment for testing children should permit adjustment of mouthpiece size. Guidelines for testing children were first published by Taussig and colleagues.[22] Equipment and test performance standards for spirometry were updated by a joint American Thoracic Society/European Respiratory Society (ATS/ERS) Task Force in 2005.[24]

◼ TESTING PROCEDURE

To perform a full maximal expiratory flow-volume maneuver, children must be able to do three things: (1) blow out forcefully, (2) take a deep breath to full inflation, and (3) continue to blow out forcefully until no more air can be exhaled. These three elements are most easily learned in that order. Most children who blow using a mouthpiece quickly learn how to increase their effort in relation to the positive feedback of producing larger and larger flow-volume curves. Going to full inflation is also learned relatively easily, because taking deeper breaths also produces higher and wider flow-volume curves on the monitor. The third element is the most difficult to learn, because it provides little inherent sensory feedback, thus requiring the child to follow the technician's instructions attentively. Only after the first two steps are mastered should a concerted effort be made to get the child to "continue blowing until the technician tells you to stop." To avoid injury due to syncope, the forced expiratory maneuver is usually performed while sitting. However, if the child performs better standing, one may perform the procedure in this position. The head should be in a neutral, erect position. The inspiration to TLC should be rapid (<2 seconds), and the child should be coached to not pause or close the glottis prior to the forced expiratory maneuver, as slow preceding inspirations and end inspiratory pauses have been reported to produce reductions in FEV_1 and forced vital capacity (FVC).[24-27] A nose clip is recommended but not essential, because the velum closes voluntarily during forced expiratory maneuvers, thus preventing losses through the nose.[28] The nose clip can be omitted when it is a source of distraction for a child or a cause for concern.

Adequacy of performance is best judged by monitoring the expiratory flow-volume and volume-time relationships. According to current ATS/ERS recommendations, acceptable maneuvers should continue for at least 3 seconds in children younger than 10 years of age and 6 seconds in children older than 10 years of age.[24] Volume at the end of the maneuver should be unchanging (<25 mL) for at least 1 second.[24] Some younger children are able to forcefully empty their lungs completely in less than 3 seconds and will electively discontinue the maneuver prior to achieving ATS/ERS criteria. Results from these electively aborted efforts can provide useful clinical information. The level of effort is usually adequate to produce flow limitation if there is an initial rapid rise to a sharp peak in flow and the effort is smoothly sustained over the entire FVC. Adequate testing requires the collection of three maximal expiratory flow-volume curves that appear similar in configuration with FVCs matching within 5% or 150 mL (100 ml for FVC ≤1 L), whichever is less.[24] Recent data in children using these updated guidelines report an 85% success rate by 10 years of age, with failure to reach an unchanging volume-time plateau being the most common reason for lack of acceptability.[29] Occasional patients demonstrate steady declines in FEV_1 and/or FVC with repeated FVC maneuvers. This may be due to fatigue, disinterest, or bronchospasm (spirometry-induced broncoconstriction). In the latter situation, inhaled albuterol may reverse the observed declines in function and be helpful in identifying airway hyperresponsiveness. Curves often have small details or "bumps" in configuration. These details should be similar on all curves if they are uniformly flow-limited. In children whose forced expiratory efforts appear suboptimal, the upper limit of forced flows can roughly be determined by asking the child to take a deep breath and then cough repeatedly until the lungs are empty. This maneuver produces repeated cough transients, followed by short, flow-limited segments (Fig. 12-9). This technique is useful in children of all ages for determining maximal flow limits.

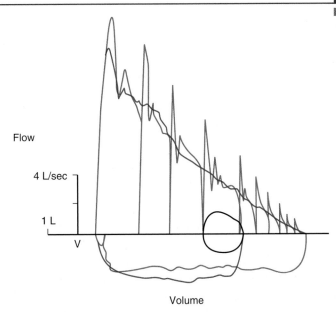

FIGURE 12-9. Repetitive coughing maneuver demonstrating maximal expiratory flow limits. From tidal end-expiration, the subject took a deep inspiration to total lung capacity (TLC) and then performed a maximal forced expiratory maneuver (in blue). From residual volume (RV), the subject took another deep breath to TLC and coughed repeatedly to RV (in red).

■ CALCULATION OF RESULTS

Forced expiratory maneuvers may be expressed as either volume-time spirograms or maximal expiratory flow-volume curves. Figure 12-10 shows volume-time spirograms from a normal child (see Fig. 12-10A) and from a child with moderate obstruction (see Fig. 12-10B). FEV_1, FVC, and forced expiratory flow between 25% and 75% of expired vital capacity (FEF_{25-75}) can be readily determined from spirograms. FEV_1 (see Fig. 12-10A) represents the volume of air expired in the first second of the forced expiratory maneuver. Ideally, the initiation of the forced exhalation should occur abruptly, without delay. In many children, however, the onset of forced expiration is gradual, making the exact point in time when expiration had its onset, and thus FEV_1, difficult to determine. For this reason, the back-extrapolation method is used.[24] To designate a time of onset for the maneuver, a line drawn through the steepest portion of the spirogram is back-extrapolated through the time axis (see Fig. 12-10A, solid red line). The FVC (see Fig. 12-10A) is the entire volume of gas expired during the maneuver. FEF_{25-75} (see Fig. 12-10B) is obtained by connecting the points between 25% and 75% of expired FVC with a straight line. The slope of this line represents a crude estimate of the rate of change of volume in relation to time (i.e., flow) during the midportion of the forced expiratory maneuver.

Instantaneous maximal flows at specific lung volumes are measured from the maximal expiratory flow-volume plot. Figure 12-11 shows both maximal inspiratory and maximal expiratory flow-volume efforts from a normal child. This combination of maximal inspiratory and expiratory efforts is referred to as the *maximal flow-volume loop*. Instantaneous expiratory flows (FEFs) at 25%, 50%, and 75% of expired FVC are shown. These are standardly referred to as FEF_{25}, FEF_{50}, and FEF_{75}, respectively. The highest flow recorded is the peak flow, or FEF_{max}.

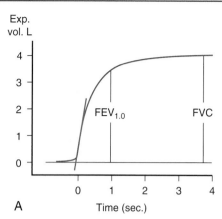

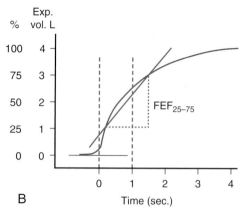

A   B

FIGURE 12-10. Volume-time spirograms from a normal child **(A)** and a child with obstructive airway disease **(B).** On the normal spirogram, zero time is determined by extrapolating the steepest part of the curve through the time axis. Forced expiratory volume in 1 second (FEV) and forced vital capacity (FVC) are measured directly from the tracings. Forced expiratory flow between 25% and 75% of expired vital capacity (FEF₂₅₋₇₅) is calculated by determining the slope of the line drawn connecting points on the spirogram at 25% to 75% of expiratory vital capacity. (Modified from Chernick V, Kendig EL. *Kendig's Disorders of the Respiratory Tract in Children,* 5th ed. Philadelphia, WB Saunders, 1990, p 150.)

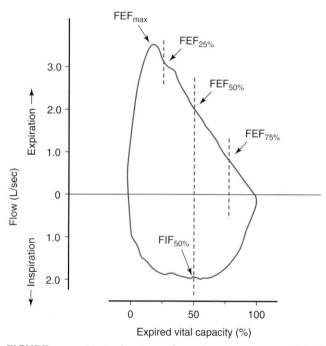

FIGURE 12-11. Maximal expiratory flow-volume loop in a normal child demonstrating instantaneous expiratory and inspiratory forced expiratory flow measurements. (Modified from Chernick V, Kendig EL. *Kendig's Disorders of the Respiratory Tract in Children,* 5th ed. Philadelphia: WB Saunders, 1990, p 151.)

Expired flows and volumes are standardly corrected to conditions of body temperature saturated with water. The final results are calculated from a minimum of three acceptable forced expiratory efforts (see the previous section entitled Testing Procedure). The highest FVC and FEV_1 values from any of the three efforts are accepted as the final results. FEF_{25-75} and instantaneous flow values (e.g., FEF_{50} and FEF_{75}) are calculated from the single curve with the highest sum of FEV_1 and FVC. This is necessary because early termination of forced expiratory maneuvers can result in significantly higher measurements of FEF_{25-75} and instantaneous flows. The FEV_1/FVC ratio should be calculated from FEV_1 and FVC values obtained from a single effort.

Peak flow, or FEF_{max}, is often measured independently with a peak flowmeter and reported separately from the results of forced spirometry. Peak flow is measured by instructing the subject to take the deepest possible breath and then blow out as quickly and as forcefully as possible. There is no need to sustain the effort through the complete FVC. Usually, the best effort of five attempts is recorded.

Maximal inspiratory flows are not limited and are effort-dependent. This measurement is useful in distinguishing the nature of central airway obstructive lesions and should be performed whenever a central airway problem is suspected. To ensure maximal effort, this measurement should not be done immediately before or after a maximal expiratory effort. The patient should first be asked to push all of the air out of the lungs and then to inspire as rapidly as possible to full capacity. This should be done several times, until a consistent inspiratory flow-volume pattern is established. The curve shape shown in Figure 12-11 is typical of a normal maximal inspiratory effort. Only the forced inspiratory flow at 50% of vital capacity (FIF_{50}) is typically measured from these inspiratory curves. In normal individuals, FIF_{50} is approximately equal to FEF_{50}.

ASSESSING AIRWAY RESPONSIVENESS

There is no consensus regarding drug, dose, or route of administration to be used for assessing airway responsiveness in the clinical laboratory. Airway responsiveness is, however, most frequently assessed by administration of a bronchodilator. Albuterol has become the primary drug used to assess bronchial responsiveness in the pulmonary function laboratory. Ideally, the patient should not have taken short-acting β agonists or anticholinergic bronchodilators for 4 hours and sustained-release β agonists or methylxanthines for 12 hours before testing. Inhaled corticosteroids need not be discontinued. Resting heart rate should be recorded. After baseline spirometric measurements are obtained, albuterol is administered using either a nebulizer or a metered-dose inhaler with a spacer. The nebulized dose of albuterol is usually 2.5 mg in 3 mL normal saline. A nose clip should be worn during albuterol nebulization, but is not necessary when using a metered-dose system.[30] Albuterol can be delivered more rapidly using a metered-dose inhaler and a spacer (Figure 12-12). Good technique is essential when using the metered-dose inhaler and spacer. The patient first exhales, then places the spacer tubing in the mouth, inhales to TLC, and holds his or her breath for 5 to 10 seconds. The metered-dose inhaler is triggered just as inspiration begins. A dose of 4 puffs (360 μg) given in intervals of ~30 seconds has been recommended for testing to ensure adequate delivery.[24] A ≥10% increase in heart rate that is sustained for 2 minutes is helpful in confirming effective albuterol delivery in children. Post-albuterol spirometry is initiated at 15 minutes after drug delivery for albuterol and 30 minutes for anticholinergic agents such as ipratropium bromide.[24] Forced expiratory maneuvers should then be repeated every 1 to 2 minutes until three acceptable tests are recorded. Although the onset of action of albuterol occurs in 5 to 15 minutes, this drug has the disadvantage of having a peak response that occurs 30 to 60 minutes after delivery. Frequently, flows continue to increase with subsequent maneuvers. Spirometry should be repeated until a plateau in FEV_1 is observed. For purposes of interpretation, it is helpful to record the time after albuterol administration when the best measurement was obtained. When post-bronchodilator testing is terminated in less than 30 minutes, changes in lung function indices may be underestimated. The dose and route of albuterol administration, the change in heart rate, and pretest medication history should also be recorded and considered when interpreting the measured response.

Airway responsiveness can also be assessed by measuring changes in pulmonary function that occur after airway challenges that produce bronchoconstriction. These challenges include inhalation of methacholine, histamine, leukotrienes, and prostaglandins that directly stimulate airway smooth muscle cell receptors. Other challenges include exercise, hyperventilation of subfreezing dry, cold air, various specific antigens, ultrasonic nebulized distilled water, and inhaled hypertonic saline that indirectly trigger bronchoconstriction by a variety of mechanisms. Methacholine inhalation is the most common clinical method used for bronchoconstrictor challenge testing. Increasing concentrations of methacholine from 0.0625 to 16 mg/mL are given by nebulization in a stepwise progression. Pulmonary function is measured at baseline and after each increasing dose of methacholine, until FEV_1 decreases by 20% or the maximum dose (16 mg/mL) is reached. Results are expressed in terms of the dose concentration of methacholine that produces a 20% decline in FEV_1 (provocative concentration, PC_{20}) as calculated from the relationship between FEV_1 and the logarithm of methacholine dose concentration. This method is reviewed in detail in the 1999 ATS Guidelines on Methacholine and Exercise Challenge Testing.[31] Lower provocative doses are indicative of greater degrees of airway reactivity. Effective, abbreviated, single-concentration methacholine challenge screening protocols have also been described.[32–34]

Bronchial provocation tests should be done with caution, and all bronchoconstriction that is induced should be reversed at the end of the test with bronchodilators. All patients who are considered for clinical assessment of airway reactivity with bronchoconstrictor stimuli should be assessed using bronchodilators before being scheduled for bronchoconstrictor challenge testing. Patients in whom increased airway reactivity has been clearly demonstrated using bronchodilators or in whom the diagnosis of asthma has been clearly established do not need to undergo clinical bronchoconstrictor challenge testing. Patients whose baseline FEV_1 is less than 80% at presentation for testing may be at increased risk for the development of severe bronchospasm during bronchoconstrictor challenge. For methacholine challenge testing, a baseline FEV_1 <60% is considered a relative contraindication to testing and <50% an absolute reason for not proceeding.[31] These strategies should limit bronchoconstrictor challenge testing for patients with respiratory symptoms for which a specific etiology has not been found and should minimize the risk of severe episodes of bronchoconstriction during testing. Evaluations of airway responsiveness should be performed in laboratories with experience in airway challenge testing and should be conducted by highly trained personnel who are capable of assessing and managing patient responses.

INTERPRETATION OF RESULTS

Before an attempt is made to interpret pulmonary function test results in physiologic terms, the quality of the measurements should be assessed. Tests should be evaluated in terms of patient effort, reproducibility, and freedom from artifacts. Less than optimal measurements should be interpreted with caution. After the measurements are evaluated for quality, the interpreter's job is to discern whether the results are normal or abnormal.

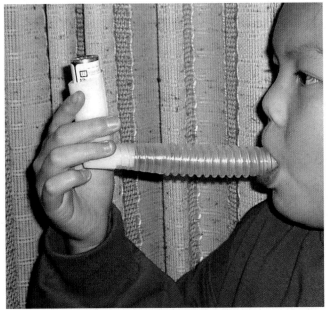

FIGURE 12-12. Child receiving metered-dose inhaled albuterol using a disposable spacer. The spacer is a 6-inch length of commercially available, corrugated ventilator tubing with a smooth internal surface.

If abnormality exists, the type and degree of abnormality must be established. Discerning abnormality from normality involves the comparison of test results with reference standards.

REFERENCE STANDARDS

Reference values serve two main purposes. First, they provide a large number of pulmonary function measurements made on children without respiratory disease with which individual patient measurements can be compared. Second, they provide the interpreter with an expectation of how lung function should change over time with normal growth. Growth-related changes in pulmonary function test results correlate best with height. Height should be measured accurately using a stadiometer. Age also contributes significantly to between-subject variations in pulmonary function. This effect is most pronounced during the transition from childhood to adolescence related to variation in the timing of the pubertal growth. The patterns of change in pulmonary function with growth are also significantly affected by gender and race. Most reference values provide independent prediction equations for males and females.

The largest single series of spirometric measurements in normal children was published by Wang and associates in 1993.[35] This longitudinal study, which involved six representative cities in the United States, reported more than 80,000 measurements in approximately 12,000 Caucasian and African-American children from 6 to 18 years of age. Spirometry was performed while seated without nose clips. Figure 12-13 shows smoothed percentile plots (in blue) for the growth of FEV_1 for Caucasian boys based on the longitudinal data of Wang and colleagues.[35] Similar plots and reference equations based on height and age for boys and girls and for African-American and Caucasian children for FVC, FEV_1, FEF_{25-75}, and FEV_1/FVC are available in that publication.[35] Both flow and volume measurements made in normal children grow along percentile curves. Children with large FEV_1 measurements relative to the mean, for example, continue to maintain those levels into adult life. In children, the change in pulmonary function over time provides the most sensitive measure of respiratory disease. Children who demonstrate decreasing levels of lung function in terms of percent predicted or percentile values can be presumed to have respiratory disease, even if all their measured lung function values fall within two standard deviations of the mean for the reference population.

In 2000, Hankinson and colleagues[36] published equations based on height and age for spirometry derived from measurements made cross-sectionally on 4634 normal Caucasian, African-American, and Mexican-American adults and 2795 children ranging from 8 to 80 years of age. Maneuvers were performed standing with nose clips in place. These data have the advantage of encompassing both children and adults and including Mexican Americans but are suboptimal for very young children. Predicted normal values derived from these data are somewhat higher during the transition from childhood to adolescence (10 to 15 years of age) than those predicted using measurements by Wang and associates.[35] In 2005, a subcommittee of

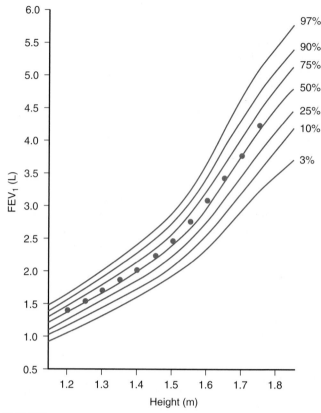

FIGURE 12-13. Smoothed percentiles of forced expiratory volume expired in 1 second (FEV_1) by height for Caucasian boys without respiratory disease from six cities in the United States. The red dots represent predicted values for boys calculated from the compiled normative relationships of Stanojevic and colleagues *(www.growinglungs.org.uk)* using the U.S. Centers for Disease Control and Prevention 50th percentile height and age growth chart data for boys *(www.cdc.gov/growthcharts)*. (From Wang X, Dockery DW, Wypij D, et al. Pulmonary function between 6 and 18 years of age. *Pediatr Pulmonol.* 1993;15:75-88.)

the Cystic Fibrosis Foundation Registry Committee recommended use of the normative equations of Wang and colleagues[35] in children beginning at 6 years of age with transition to the equations of Hankinson and associates[36] at 18 years of age in males and 16 years in females (Margaret Rosenfeld, personal communication). To provide more accurate reference ranges from 4 years through the transition into adulthood, Stanojevic and associates[37] combined the data of Hankinson and colleagues[36] from Caucasian subjects with three other published series of pediatric normative spirometry results from Caucasian children.[38-42] Using sophisticated methods similar to those used to create growth charts for height and weight, they developed smoothly changing reference curves based upon height and age closely matching those published by Wang and associates,[35] including the transition period from childhood to adolescence (see Fig. 12-13). Subsequently, these authors have added preschool spirometry to their data set, extending the range of predicted values down to 3 years of age (available at www.growinglungs.org.uk). Normative reference data for fractional lung volumes in children are dated and far more limited than those available for spirometry. For plethysmographic volumes, the prediction equations most commonly used are those of Zapletal and colleagues[41] or Rosenthal and associates,[42] and for helium dilution, those of Cook and Haman[43] or Weng and Levison.[44] Composite reference equations were published by Polgar and Weng in 1979.[45] Reference values for lung volumes were summarized in 1995 by Stocks and Quanjer.[46]

For the purpose of distinguishing abnormal from normal findings, test results are most commonly examined as percents of the predicted mean values. The 2005 ATS/ERS Task Force statement[47] on interpretation of lung function tests recommends setting the lower limit of the normal range at the 5th percentile. In practice, 80% of predicted has been used in children as the approximate lower limit of normal for FEV_1 and FVC. The data of both Wang and colleagues[35] and Hankinson and associates[36] suggest this to be a reasonable rule of thumb. However, the results of Stanojevic and colleagues[37] demonstrate clearly that, in children younger than 10 years, between-subject variability increases as age decreases, reducing the lower limit of normal to ~75% of predicted at age 4 to 5 years. Expressing pulmonary function results in terms of Z-scores (predicted minus measured divided by standard deviation of predicted) has intrinsic value in that it identifies the patient's position in the predicted normal distribution without reference to or the need to recall the lower limit for each different measure. In this schema, the 5th percentile is equivalent to −1.64 standard deviations (Z-score). The equations of Stanojevic and associates[37] provide age-specific standard deviations that permit expression of results in Z-scores and precise discrimination of the normal range. For FEF_{25-75}, the data of Wang and colleagues[35] suggest that, as a rule of thumb, values <67% of the predicted can be considered below the normal range; however, when interpreting results, one should keep in mind the increasing variability of this measure in younger children. Normality or abnormality of a given result cannot be determined completely by an arbitrary cutoff level. Because the normal range of most measures of lung function is wide, not knowing a child's initial or predisease level of lung function can also present problems. For example, children who have had disease-related decreases in lung function from one standard deviation above to one standard deviation below the mean value will be judged "normal" if their prediseases level of function is not known. All results must be interpreted in light of the patient's clinical history.

Measurements of volumes including FVC, FEV_1, TLC, RV, and FRC are lower in relation to standing height in African-American children than in Caucasian children.[47-50] This difference is diminished by about 40% to 50% if lung function is compared in terms of sitting rather than standing height.[50,51] It is common practice to reduce predicted values for FVC, FEV_1, and TLC in African Americans by 12% and for FRC and RV by 7% to account for these race-related differences in pulmonary function.[47,52] This approach is, however, less than optimal, because race-related differences vary with age and height.[36,48] The use of race-specific prediction equations is the best way to account for racial differences in FVC and FEV_1 in children.[35,36] Adequate reference measurements comparing differences in fractional lung volumes between African-American and Caucasian children are

not available. Until more data become available, it would seem reasonable to predict TLC in African-American children by reducing the predicted values derived from Caucasian reference populations by 12%.[47] When controlled for height, measurements of FVC and FEV_1 in normal Hispanic and Native American children differ little from those of Caucasian children.[36,51-55] Differences in pulmonary function between Asian and Caucasian populations have been reported,[56-58] and for the most part these differences fall between those reported for African-American and Caucasian children. The 2005 ATS/ERS Task Force report on interpretation of lung function tests[47] suggests using a correction factor of 0.94 to adjust Caucasian predicted values for Asians.

Some of the variation in studies reporting racial differences in pulmonary function may relate in part to the fact that race, as self-identified, does not take into account the admixture of world populations. Recently, Kumar and associates[59] reported an inverse relationship between the percentage of genetic markers of African ancestry and both FVC and FEV_1 (i.e., subjects with less genetic markers had higher measures of function). One must consider this source of variation when interpreting pulmonary function results from patients of differing self-identified races and ethnicities. Reference values should be chosen that match the characteristics of the population being tested and should not be extrapolated beyond the age and height limits of the population studied.[47,60,61]

In patients with neuromuscular weakness and spinal deformities, arm span is often used to estimate height and calculate predicted values of pulmonary function.[62] For children whose arm span is difficult to determine accurately, FEV_1 and FVC can be predicted based on measurements of ulnar length.[63]

TYPE OF PULMONARY DYSFUNCTION

Abnormalities of pulmonary function can be restrictive, obstructive, or a mixture of both. Restrictive disorders are characterized by a decrease in lung volumes. This decrease may be caused by one of many mechanisms. Lung volume excursion may be decreased by chest wall deformity or increased chest wall stiffness, as in scoliosis. Respiratory muscle weakness may also reduce lung volume excursion. Increased elastic recoil of the lungs caused by an interstitial inflammatory process or fibrosis may also reduce lung volumes. Alveolar filling processes, such as lobar pneumonia, also reduce lung volume and, in that light, represent restrictive processes. Other space-occupying processes in the thoracic cavity, (e.g., large bullae or congenital cysts) or processes that fill the pleural space, (e.g., effusions) are restrictive. Any pulmonary process that reduces the amount of air filling the alveoli is restrictive.

Obstructive processes are characterized by reductions in airflow that may occur at any level of the bronchial tree and may be due to intrinsic narrowing or extrinsic compression. Reductions in airflow may also occur in relation to decreases in the integrity of the structure of airway walls, as in bronchiectasis, or in relation to global decreases in lung elastic recoil, as in emphysema. When small airways are narrowed, they frequently close at low lung volumes, and this process results not only in reduced flow but also in reduced FVC. Any process that causes a reduction in airway cross-sectional area at any level in the bronchial tree is obstructive.

Classically, restrictive and obstructive disorders have been distinguished by examining the ratio of airflow to lung volume. Airflow in restrictive disorders is usually reduced in proportion to reductions in lung volume. Thus, the ratio of FEV_1 to FVC, which is approximately 85% in normal individuals, remains unchanged or is increased (>80%) in restrictive disorders. In obstructive disorders, airflow is reduced proportionally more than lung volume, and thus FEV_1/FVC decreases. Restrictive and obstructive processes can also be distinguished visually by examining the shape of maximal expiratory flow-volume curves (Fig. 12-14). Patients with restrictive disorders have maximal expiratory flow-volume curves that are similar in shape to those of normal individuals, but smaller in terms of both flow and volume. The equal reduction of airflow and lung volume results in a flow-volume configuration that approximates a miniature of a normal curve configuration. In patients with increased elastic recoil, flow may actually increase slightly in proportion to lung volume. This relative increase in flow in relation to lung volume may produce a somewhat "bulging" appearance of the curve and an elevated FEV_1/FVC ratio. Obstructive processes produce a "scooped," or "sagging," appearance to the flow-volume curve. This scooped configuration occurs in relation to nonhomogenous airway emptying. With mild obstructive disease, this scooped appearance begins at low lung volumes. As obstructive diseases progress, the scooped configuration involves more and more of the descending portion of the curve.

Reductions in FVC in patients with obstruction occur at low lung volumes as affected airways close and trap gas. Dramatic reductions in FVC are not seen until the level of airway obstruction becomes fairly severe. Declines in FVC secondary to airway closure and gas trapping are accompanied by increases in the RV/TLC ratio. Reductions in

lung volume in restrictive processes may occur at either high or low lung volumes. Patients with neuromuscular disorders (e.g., Duchenne muscular dystrophy) may not have enough inspiratory respiratory muscle strength to fully inflate the lungs or adequate expiratory respiratory strength to push to RV.[64] Similarly, thoracic deformities that limit chest wall mobility (e.g., scoliosis) may prevent patients from either fully reaching TLC or completely emptying the air from the lungs at end-expiration. Classically, RV/TLC ratios remain unchanged in restrictive disorders, but they may be either increased or decreased, depending on the etiology of the restriction.

Mixed restrictive and obstructive processes are difficult to distinguish using forced expiratory spirometry alone. When reductions in the magnitude of forced expiratory flow appear disproportionately large in relation to reductions in the FEV_1/FVC ratio or in relation to the degree of scooping seen on the maximal expiratory flow-volume curve, mixed obstructive and restrictive dysfunction should be suspected. The presence of a restrictive component can be confirmed by measurement of TLC, which will always be reduced in restrictive processes. Both plethysmographic and gas-dilution measurements provide adequate measures of TLC in patients with pure restrictive disease. In patients with obstructive disease and air trapping, gas-dilution methods underestimate FRC and TLC because they do not measure gas in noncommunicating, closed portions of the lungs. However, plethysmographic measurements may artificially overestimate lung volume in patients with airway obstruction.[65]

One can recognize central airway obstruction involving the larynx and trachea because it produces distinctive changes in the configuration of maximal expiratory flow-volume loops (Fig. 12-15). Fixed central airway obstruction results in reductions in forced expiratory and forced inspiratory flow at high and mid lung volumes. If a lesion (e.g., a solid mass) produces an orifice-like reduction in central airway size, the flow produced through this orifice will remain approximately constant in relation to effort, producing a maximal flow-volume loop that is flattened on both inspiration and expiration (see Fig.12-15A). Central airway obstructive lesions may also be variable. Variable extrathoracic lesions produce significantly greater reductions in inspiratory than in expiratory forced flows (see Fig. 12-15B). Isolated diaphragmatic weakness may also produce this configuration. Variable intrathoracic lesions result in reductions in forced flows that are substantially greater during expiration than during inspiration (see Fig. 12-15C). Because the flows produced are at least partly effort-dependent, it is important to encourage the subject to make reproducible and maximal efforts, particularly while performing the maximal inspiratory maneuver. Normal values for maximal inspiratory flow at 50% of VC have been reported for children.[66]

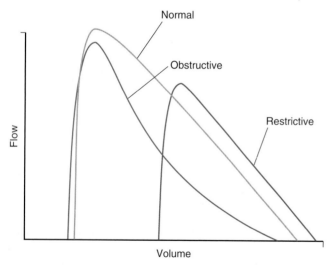

FIGURE 12-14. Changes in the maximal expiratory flow-volume curve configuration occurring with mild to moderate restrictive *(blue)* or obstructive *(red)* respiratory dysfunction. (Data from Baum GL, Wolinsky E. *Textbook of Pulmonary Diseases*, 5th ed. Boston: Little, Brown, 1994, pp 115-116.)

DEGREE OF PULMONARY DYSFUNCTION

The degree of pulmonary dysfunction must necessarily be interpreted in relation to clinical experience. As noted in the earlier discussion of reference standards, values ≥80%

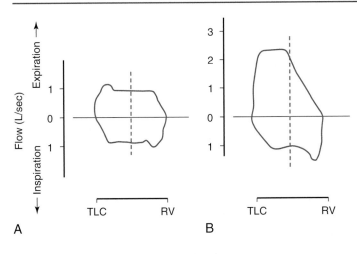

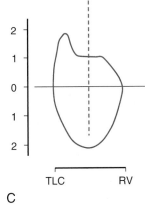

FIGURE 12-15. Maximal flow-volume curve loop configurations in central airway obstruction. **A**, Fixed central airway obstruction; **B**, variable extrathoracic central airway obstruction; **C**, variable intrathoracic central airway obstruction. *RV*, Residual volume; *TLC*, total lung capacity. (Modified from Chernick V, Kendig EL. *Kendig's Disorders of the Respiratory Tract in Children*, 5th ed. Philadelphia: WB Saunders, 1990, p 151.)

of predicted for FEV$_1$ are commonly considered to be within the normal range. Using FEV$_1$ in percent of mean predicted value, a rough and arbitrary guide to the degree of obstructive dysfunction is as follows: Normal function is 80% of predicted and above; mild dysfunction is 60% to 79% of predicted; moderate dysfunction is 40% to 59% of predicted; and severe dysfunction is below 40% of predicted. For pulmonary processes characterized as restrictive, the same limits are useful approximations of the degree of deficit using the percent predicted value of FVC rather than FEV$_1$ to assess the degree of dysfunction. When available, the percent predicted value for TLC provides the best estimate of the degree of volume restriction.

This simplistic approach to estimating the degree of pulmonary dysfunction provides only a rough guide. Pulmonary function measurements must be interpreted individually and should guide patient management only in relation to the overall assessment of clinical status. A patient whose percent predicted FEV$_1$ is 80% of predicted may have mild or even moderate dysfunction if the pre-disease FEV$_1$ was 100% or 120% of predicted. Another individual whose FEV$_1$ is 80% may simply have relatively small lungs and be entirely normal. If this latter individual experiences a decrease in FEV$_1$ to 59% of predicted, he or she may have only mild airway obstruction.

Patients with progressive obstructive airway disease demonstrate progressive changes in the configuration of the flow-volume curve that correlate roughly with the degree of dysfunction (Fig. 12-16). With the exception of the purely central airway abnormalities discussed earlier, reductions in forced expiratory flows in patients with obstructive processes are first seen at low lung volumes. These reductions in flow occur first at low lung volumes because the portions of the lungs supplied by the affected airways empty more slowly and, thus, are still emptying at a low rate when most of the other unaffected airways have completed the emptying process. As more airways or larger airways controlling greater and greater portions of the lung volume become involved in the process, the reduction in flows and the scooping configuration of the maximal expiratory flow-volume curve begins at higher and higher lung volumes. A maximal expiratory flow-volume curve with a peak flow that is near normal but with a scooping configuration over its entire

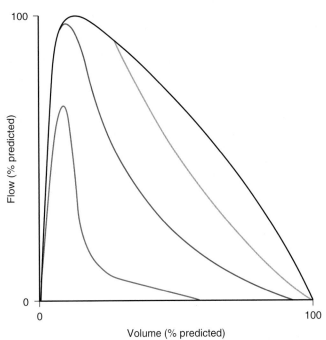

FIGURE 12-16. Typical changes in the maximal expiratory flow-volume curve configuration related to progressive obstructive pulmonary dysfunction. Curves are plotted superimposed at total lung capacity. The outer curve is representative of a normal configuration *(black)*. Curves with progressively lower flows have configurations typical of mild *(green)*, moderate *(blue)*, and severe *(red)* dysfunction, respectively. (Modified from Rudolph AM, Kamei RK. *Rudolph's Fundamentals of Pediatrics*. Norwalk, Conn: Appleton & Lange, 1994, p 543.)

descending portion is typical of moderate dysfunction, with the obstructive process affecting approximately half of the air flowing from the lungs.

However, the scooped configuration of the flow-volume curve does not indicate the site of obstruction. Either severe obstruction of a single main stem bronchus or narrowing of approximately 50% of the small or medium airways could, for example, produce similarly scooped maximal expiratory flow-volume curves, typical of moderate obstruction. Nonhomogeneous emptying occurring at any level of the bronchial tree will produce scooping of the flow-volume curve. The site of nonhomogeneous obstruction may, however, be suspected clinically. Low flows at low lung volumes (scooping of the lower part of the maximal expiratory flow-volume curve) are often considered indicative of early small airway obstructive disease. Although this is most often the case clinically, a similar flow-volume curve configuration also could be observed in a patient with postpneumonic bronchiectasis involving a single segmental bronchus. This single involved segment of the lung will empty slowly and nonhomogeneously in relation to the remainder of the lung and will result in low flows at the end of forced expiration. Diffuse obstruction of the small airways involving an equivalent portion of the lung volume would produce a maximal expiratory flow-volume curve with a virtually identical configuration. Thus, interpretations involving the site of airway obstruction, with the exception of the typical central airway changes discussed earlier, should be made with appropriate caution.

As noted earlier in the section entitled Flow Limitation, spirometry may not detect early nonhomogeneously distributed distal airway obstructive abnormalities. Measures of lung function may remain within the normal range in the presence of substantial obstructive disease, particularly in patients whose initial function is in the high normal range. However, as obstructive airway disease progresses and levels of function fall below the normal range, FVC, FEV_1, and FEF_{25-75} decline at different rates (Fig. 12-17). FEF_{25-75} and other measures of instantaneous flow (FEF_{50} and FEF_{75}) decline early in the course of progressive obstructive disease and are generally considered early indicators of airway dysfunction. FVC tends not to be affected until later in the course of obstructive airway disease, at which time it declines rapidly. FVC declines initially in relation to air trapping due to closure of the airways at end-expiration. Reductions in FVC

accelerate later in the course of disease as more airways close and diffuse fibrotic changes begin to add a restrictive component to the obstructive process. FEV_1 declines almost linearly in relation to disease progression and, thus, tends to be the best long-term measure of the degree of obstruction. In restrictive disorders, measures of airway function decline in concert with reductions in lung volume, making volume measurements (e.g., FVC or, if available, TLC) the best long-term measures of the degree of dysfunction.

■■ ASSESSING CHANGES IN DEGREE OF PULMONARY DYSFUNCTION

Levels of change in measurements of pulmonary function that are indicative of clear changes in clinical condition are difficult to state in absolute terms. There is some general agreement regarding levels of change in function that are indicative of increased airway reactivity. An increase in FEV_1 or FVC of 12% or 200 mL after the administration of a bronchodilator is considered a positive response.[47] Other studies done in various settings in adults and children have suggested that levels of change in FEV_1 as low as 8% and as high as 25% indicate a positive response to bronchodilators.[47,67] Changes in FEF_{25-75} and instantaneous flows should be considered only secondarily when evaluating bronchodilator response. For these measures, increases of 35% to 50% are generally considered indicative of a positive response.

There is also general agreement about the level of change in pulmonary function that constitutes a positive response to a bronchoconstrictor challenge. A decrease in FEV1 of ≥10% following exercise is considered abnormal and >15% is considered diagnostic for exercise-induced bronchospasm.[31] For the more commonly performed methacholine bronchoconstrictor challenge, a 20% decline in FEV_1 is considered indicative of increased airway reactivity.[31] Results must always be interpreted in light of the baseline level of obstruction and the quality of the forced expiratory efforts. If the PC_{20} is ≥16 mg/mL, it can be concluded with a reasonable degree of certainty that the patient does not have asthma. A PC_{20} of <1 mg/mL strongly supports a clinical diagnosis of asthma. PC_{20} levels between 1 and 16 mg/mL may or may not support a clinical diagnosis of asthma and need to be interpreted in relation to the patient's past and recent history of symptoms, symptoms during testing, and post-testing degree of reversibility following a bronchodilator.[31,68]

There is less agreement regarding the degree of change in pulmonary function that constitutes a significant improvement or decline over time in relation to therapeutic interventions or disease progression. Changes in lung function of one standard deviation or more than 10% have been suggested as constituting a significant intrasubject change in lung function.[69] In 1990, Pattishall[70] reported that a 10% or 15% change in FVC or FEV_1 was considered significant in most pediatric laboratories. Intrasubject variability (and, thus, the degree of change in function representing a significant change) varies, depending on the pulmonary function parameter measured, the interval between tests, and the type of patient tested. In healthy

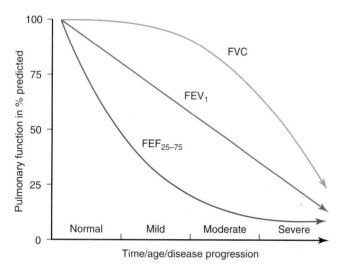

FIGURE 12-17. Course of pulmonary function test results in chronic obstructive pulmonary disease. Forced expiratory flow between 25% and 75% of expired vital capacity (FEF_{25-75}) *(blue)* declines early in the course of progressive obstructive lung disease. Forced vital capacity (FVC) *(green)* remains nearly normal and then declines rapidly late in the course of the disease. Forced expiratory volume expired in 1 second (FEV_1) *(red)* declines almost linearly as disease progresses.

subjects, changes in FEV_1 and FVC of 5% within a day, 11% to 12% from week to week, and 15% from year to year were generally considered significant by participants in the 1991 ATS Workshop on Lung Function Testing.[71] These critical limits approximately double in patients with chronic respiratory disease or when more variable measures of function, such as FEF_{25-75} or instantaneous flow, FEF_{50} and FEF_{75}, are being used. Intrasubject variability in adults and children with chronic respiratory disease is significantly higher than that in normal individuals.[72,73] It is thus difficult to make general statements regarding the degree of change in lung function that constitutes a significant change in clinical status. In the final analysis, serial changes in pulmonary function must be interpreted in light of the individual patient's overall clinical situation.

OTHER TESTS OF FUNCTION

Maximal Respiratory Pressure

Respiratory muscle strength can be assessed by measuring maximal inspiratory and maximal expiratory pressures. These measurements are useful for assessing and following patients with respiratory muscle weakness due to neuromuscular problems, such as spinal cord injury, Guillain-Barré syndrome, diaphragmatic paralysis, muscular dystrophy, myasthenia gravis, and steroid myopathy. In fact, recent data in children with Duchenne muscular dystrophy indicate that maximal respiratory pressures are more sensitive than spirometric indices at detecting the onset of early pulmonary impairment.[74] Measurements of respiratory pressure in humans were first recorded by Hutchinson in 1846.[2] Formal measurements of average maximal inspiratory and expiratory pressures in normal children and adults were reported in 1964.[75] In 1969, Black and Hyatt[76] described a simple handheld device for assessing maximal respiratory pressures in the clinical setting, and they provided normal reference values for men and women.

Maximal respiratory pressure measurements are made by having the child make forceful inspiratory (Müeller maneuver) or expiratory (Valsalva maneuver) efforts into a system that is effectively closed except for a small air leak. The maximal pressures generated during brief 1- to 2-second efforts are recorded. The device used to measure these pressures is a short, cylindrical metal or acrylic (Plexiglas) tube (diameter ~3 cm; length ~12 cm) with a firm rubber mouthpiece that can be handheld and pressed tightly against the lips (Fig. 12-18). The tube should have a 1- to 2-mm hole to permit a small air leak. This ensures that the pressures generated by the subject have not been made with the cheeks alone. A subject with a closed glottis can generate substantial negative pressure by sucking with the buccal muscles alone. The volume flowing in through the small hole fills the oral cavity rapidly. This makes it impossible to maintain high negative pressure for 2 seconds, and indicates that the glottis is closed. With the glottis open, the volume change occurring over 2 seconds due to the air leak is small relative to that of the lungs and upper airways, and it has minimal effect on the measured pressures. The small air leak serves a similar

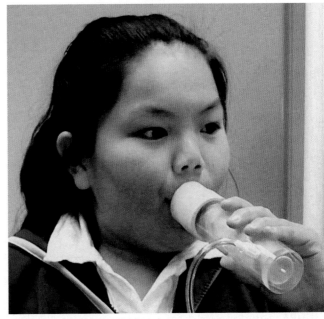

FIGURE 12-18. Child performing a maximal inspiratory pressure maneuver. This handheld device consists of an acrylic (Plexiglas) cylinder with a 1.5-mm hole (air leak) at the distal end and a pressure port connected by clear tubing to a pressure transducer. The rubber mouthpiece is pressed firmly to the face, with the lips inside the device. Visual feedback is provided by a pressure-time plot on a computer monitor (*not pictured*).

function during expiratory maneuvers. Pressures are measured with the mouthpiece pressed firmly to the face, with the lips inside as if blowing a bugle. This is most important for the measurement of expiratory pressures, which can exceed $200\,cm\,H_2O$. If pressures are measured with a scuba-type mouthpiece (lips around the mouthpiece), the maximal pressures generated are limited by the ability of the buccal muscles to tighten around the mouthpiece and prevent leaks. Individuals with normal muscle strength cannot prevent leaks at pressures above 120 to $150\,cm$ H_2O. In patients with generalized muscle weakness, leaks may occur at even lower positive pressures. In patients with muscle weakness and limited buccal strength, measurements made with a facemask can provide an estimate of respiratory muscle strength.[77]

In the past, pressures have been assessed by observing maximal needle excursions on mechanical aneroid pressure gauges. More recently, pressure changes within the tube have been measured using analog transducers and have been recorded digitally. Pressures are measured with the child seated. Nose clips are generally placed but are not absolutely necessary. The force generated by muscles varies in relation to muscle fiber length (i.e., length-tension characteristic). Figure 12-19 shows that the maximal inspiratory and expiratory pressures that can be generated are a function of VC.[32] For the respiratory system, the optimal length for force generated by the expiratory muscles (muscles of the chest wall and abdomen) occurs near TLC and by the inspiratory muscles (primarily the diaphragm) near RV. For this reason, patients are asked to take a deep breath to near TLC before pressing the mouthpiece to the lips and making a forced expiratory effort, and then to breathe out maximally before making a forced inspiratory effort. Maximal pressures measured

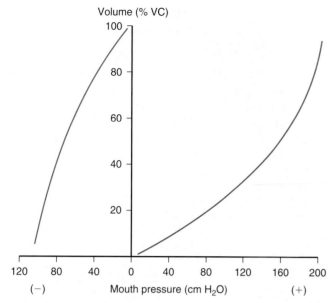

FIGURE 12-19. Plot of mouth pressure versus vital capacity (VC) showing how maximal inspiratory (*left*) and maximal expiratory (*right*) pressures change with lung volume. Inspiratory pressures are maximally negative near residual volume. Expiratory pressures are maximally positive near total lung capacity. (From Hyatt R, Scanlon P, Nakamura M. *Interpretation of Pulmonary Function Tests. A Practical Guide.* Philadelphia: Lippincott, 1997. By permission of Mayo Foundation for Medical Education and Research.)

at mid lung volumes are generally lower and more variable. Inspiratory and expiratory maneuvers should be repeated at least five times because recorded pressures usually increase and plateau with repeated efforts. The highest pressure obtained from two to three serial measurements matching within 20% is recorded as maximal respiratory pressure.

Using this method, normal men can produce maximal expiratory pressures of $233 \pm 84\,cm\ H_2O$ and maximal inspiratory pressures of $-124 \pm 44\,cm\ H_2O$.[32] Normal women can produce maximal expiratory and inspiratory pressures of $152 \pm 54\,cm\ H_2O$ and $-87 \pm 32\,cm\ H_2O$, respectively.[32] Maximal pressures measured with the lips surrounding the mouthpiece are approximately 30% to 40% lower than those measured with the lips inside the mouthpiece, and they may not reflect true respiratory muscle strength. Maximal pressures in girls are similar to those measured in women. Pressures in boys are 80 to $100\,cm\ H_2O$ lower than those in men. These values increase to adult levels in adolescence,[78] but the rate of increase is not affected by the growth spurt during puberty.[79]

Although maximal respiratory pressures are variable between patients, they are very useful for assessing changes in respiratory muscle strength in individual patients, once they have become familiar with the measurement. Normal values for measurements of maximal pressures made at FRC have been published, making comparative assessments of respiratory strength possible in children who have difficultly performing maneuvers near TLC and RV.[80] The reference standards used to compare results should correspond to the method used to measure pressures. Tables summarizing normal

reference standards for adults and children for all methods are available in the ATS-ERS Statement on Respiratory Muscle Testing.[81] Enthusiastic coaching by the technician is essential to ensure optimal results in children. In practice, a child who can generate a maximal expiratory pressure of $100\,cm\ H_2O$ or more and a maximal inspiratory pressure of $-80\,cm\ H_2O$ or less is unlikely to demonstrate clinically significant respiratory muscle weakness. Children who are unable to produce maximal expiratory pressures greater than $40\,cm\ H_2O$ with maximal effort are likely to have impaired ability to cough.

■ DIFFUSING CAPACITY FOR CARBON MONOXIDE

The diffusing capacity for carbon monoxide ($D_{L}CO$) provides information about the rate at which oxygen is transferred from the lung to the pulmonary capillary bed. Oxygen travels from the alveoli to the red blood cells in the pulmonary capillaries by passive diffusion. The transfer of oxygen depends on the difference in oxygen tension between the alveolus and pulmonary capillary blood as well as the area and thickness of the alveolar-capillary interface. Carbon monoxide follows the same pathway from the alveolus to the red blood cell, where it binds with hemoglobin. The transfer of carbon monoxide across the alveolar-capillary membrane is diffusion-limited. The transfer of carbon monoxide is limited, not by pulmonary blood flow, but rather by the rate of diffusion across the alveolar-capillary and the red blood cell membranes. Carbon monoxide transfer is limited only by the rate of diffusion because the concentration of carbon monoxide in the lung during testing is low and the number of hemoglobin-binding sites is so high that they do not become saturated. Therefore, $D_{L}CO$ is a measure of the impedance to gas flow across the alveolar-capillary interface.

The simplest and most widely used technique for measuring $D_{L}CO$ is the single-breath method. This method, first described by Krogh in 1915,[82] was subsequently developed as a clinical test of lung function by Forster and colleagues in 1954.[83] To perform this test, the child first breathes out to RV and then takes a deep breath (>90% to 95% of VC) from a spirometer containing a mixture of 0.3% carbon monoxide, a tracer gas (e.g., 10% helium, 0.3% neon, or 0.3% methane), 21% oxygen, and the balance nitrogen. The breath is held at near full inspiration for 10 seconds, and the child then exhales completely. Concentrations of carbon monoxide and the tracer gas are measured in the alveolar fraction of the expired gas. The concentration of carbon monoxide reaching the alveoli at the beginning of the breath hold is lower than the inspired concentration (0.3%), because it is diluted by the volume in the lungs at the beginning of the maneuver (i.e., RV). The change in the concentration of the tracer gas is used to calculate mean alveolar carbon monoxide concentration at the start of the breath hold. It also provides a measure of alveolar volume by gas dilution. The volume of carbon monoxide taken up in 10 seconds is the product of the alveolar volume and the difference between the estimated starting concentration and the measured expired concentration of alveolar carbon monoxide. Diffusing capacity is the volume of carbon monoxide transferred from alveolar gas to blood in milliliters per minute divided by the difference between mean alveolar-capillary carbon monoxide pressure and mean pulmonary capillary carbon monoxide pressure. Mean capillary carbon monoxide pressure is assumed to be zero because carbon monoxide binds tightly to hemoglobin in the red blood cell. DLCO values should be adjusted in accordance with ATS recommendations[84] based on the patient's hemoglobin values because low or high values can affect results. For children younger than 15 years of age (and all women),

Adjusted DLCO = measured DLCO ×
$$(9.38 + \text{hemoglobin})/(1.7 \times \text{hemoglobin}).$$

For men and boys 15 years of age and older,

Adjusted DLCO = measured DLCO ×
$$(10.22 + \text{hemoglobin})/(1.7 \times \text{hemoglobin}).$$

In North America, DLCO is expressed in milliliters per minute per millimeter of mercury. In Europe, the same measurement is referred to as the transfer factor, and it is expressed in millimoles per minute per kilopascal. Further details can be found in the 2005 ATS/ERS document on this technique.[84]

The DLCO value varies directly with lung size. Normal reference equations for adults predict DLCO based on height, sex, and age.[84] Published equations differ substantially in their predictions. In adults, the average normal single-breath DLCO is approximately 20 to 30 mL/min/mm Hg, is somewhat higher in men than in women, and declines with advancing age.[32] Normal reference values for children are limited.[42,85,86] Values in elementary school–age children range from 10 to 15 mL/min/mm Hg and increase with height until they reach adult levels in late adolescence. If predicted results consistently do not match the clinical situation, the reference equations and the details of testing should be re-evaluated. In young children with a VC of <1.5 to 2.0 L, methodologic modifications may be necessary to ensure the accuracy of measurement. This may also be true for older children who have restrictive disease and similarly small volumes.

Most conditions for which DLCO is clinically useful result in decreases in carbon monoxide transfer. DLCO is valuable in adults for assessing the degree and progression of emphysema, and it may be helpful in distinguishing emphysema (low DLCO) from chronic obstructive pulmonary disease due predominantly to bronchiectasis (normal DLCO). DLCO is also low in interstitial lung disorders, including sarcoidosis, collagen vascular diseases (lupus erythematosus, scleroderma), hypersensitivity pneumonitis, histiocytosis X, and drug-induced lung disease (amiodarone, bleomycin, methotrexate). DLCO may be reduced in congestive heart failure, alveolar proteinosis, bronchial obstruction, bronchiolitis obliterans, pulmonary vascular obstruction (obliterative pulmonary vasculitis, pulmonary embolus), and chronic liver disease (hepatorenal syndrome).[87] DLCO monitoring in patients who undergo lung transplantation may aid in the early detection of bronchiolitis obliterans. DLCO is helpful clinically when it detects abnormality in the face of otherwise normal spirometry findings and fractional lung volumes. DLCO may be reduced before the development of hypoxemia at rest or with exertion in patients with pulmonary vascular disorders, such as primary pulmonary hypertension, recurrent pulmonary emboli, or obliterative vasculopathy. DLCO should also be measured in patients with unexplained dyspnea.

Although intended to be a measure of the size and thickness of the alveolar-capillary membrane, DLCO is affected by many factors that can complicate the interpretation of results. DLCO is increased in conditions that increase pulmonary blood flow and thus alveolar-capillary volume and surface area. In patients with left-to-right intracardiac shunts, DLCO may be elevated related to increases in pulmonary capillary blood volume although alveolar-capillary membrane function remains normal. DLCO increases by approximately two-fold during exercise because of recruitment of pulmonary capillaries and the related increase in the alveolar-capillary membrane surface area. DLCO may be elevated in patients with asthma or obesity, again probably because of increased pulmonary blood volume, but these increases are not of any clinical significance. DLCO is decreased in patients with anemia and increased in polycythemia. Therefore, hemoglobin levels should be considered when interpreting results. Severe anemia or anemia that develops in the course of chemotherapy should not be interpreted as lung disease. Pulmonary hemorrhage may result in acute increases in DLCO related to the binding of carbon monoxide to hemoglobin in the airspaces and the airways. DLCO has been used to monitor the extent of intra-alveolar hemorrhage in Goodpasture's syndrome. Smoking in adults and adolescents can produce carboxyhemoglobin levels as high as 10% to 12%. Each 1% increase in the level of carboxyhemoglobin results in approximately a 1% decrease in DLCO because of the reduction in the alveolar-to-capillary pressure gradient for carbon monoxide. The Valsalva maneuver reduces pulmonary blood volume and therefore reduces carbon monoxide uptake. The Müeller maneuver, supine posture, and altitude produce increases in DLCO. Alveolar hypoxia and alveolar hypercarbia in patients with compensated respiratory failure reduce the alveolar-to-capillary gradient for oxygen, enhance the gradient for carbon monoxide, and increase DLCO. These latter influences are modest or are not relevant in the normal clinical setting and, therefore, do not affect the interpretation of results.

The interpretation of results is also confounded by disease-related factors that affect the distribution of ventilation and pulmonary blood flow. DLCO is measured only in areas of the lung into which both gas and blood flow. Uneven distribution of ventilation and perfusion reduces the effective area for alveolar-capillary gas exchange. Therefore, results in patients with airway obstruction must be interpreted with caution. Global DLCO decreases if carbon monoxide does not reach an area of the lung or reaches an area in lower concentration. As with other dilutional methods, alveolar volume may be underestimated in patients with airway obstruction. Nonhomogeneous lung emptying can obscure the normal sharp demarcation between anatomic dead space and alveolar gas, resulting in a sample that does not reflect mean alveolar carbon monoxide concentration. D$_{LCO}$ is generally decreased if pulmonary capillaries are obstructed. However, this may not be the case in pulmonary hypertension of precapillary origin. Large pulmonary emboli reduce perfusion to regions of the lung, but global changes in pulmonary vascular pressures may increase perfusion to other regions, blunting expected reductions in D$_{LCO}$. Intuition would suggest that pneumonectomy should reduce D$_{LCO}$ by half. This is usually not the case, however, because when all of the cardiac output flows through a single lung, recruitment of pulmonary capillaries increases the surface area for gas exchange and results in a less than 50% reduction in D$_{LCO}$. Interpretation of results requires careful consideration of multiple factors, including other measures of lung function, possible test-related and disease-related confounders, and the patient's clinical situation. D$_{LCO}$ should not be obtained routinely, but rather ordered for specific clinical indications.

MEASURES OF RESISTANCE

Interrupter Resistance

The interrupter technique for measuring resistance (Rint) was first described by von Neergaard and Wirz in 1927[88] and then further validated by Mead and Whittenberger in 1954.[89] Rint uses a shutter device to briefly interrupt airflow during normal tidal breathing and is thus easily performed in school-age children. Rint can be measured during inspiration or expiration, but measurement during expiration is generally recommended. The test is performed with the child sitting comfortably with nose clips in place and the head in an erect posture. The child breathes tidally through a mouthpiece, and a shutter is closed rapidly (<10 milliseconds) and briefly (about 100 milliseconds). This interruption of airflow leads to an initial rapid rise in mouth pressure followed by oscillations and an eventual slow rise in pressure (see Figure 11-25). The initial rapid rise occurs in relation to the sudden change in resistance within the airways. The final slow rise is related to parenchymal visco-elastic properties of the lung and redistribution of gas between the airways with differing time constants.[1,90,91] Applying hand pressure over the cheeks is recommended to avoid the influence of upper airway compliance on resistance measurements. A minimum of five acceptable measurements should be collected, and these are reported as the median value. Technically acceptable maneuvers should have no leak and should demonstrate an initial rapid rise followed by a slower smooth rise to a plateau. The child should not vocalize or swallow during the measurement.[1,90]

Rint is calculated as the ratio of the pressure change measured at the mouth during the interruption and the airflow recorded immediately before the interruption. Assumptions include that equilibration occurs between the airway opening and the alveoli during the brief interruption and that the respiratory system represents a single compartment that is linear.[90] In patients with significant airway obstruction, Rint may be underestimated due to

lack of complete equilibration of pressure between the airway opening and the alveoli.[92] Rint measurements reflect the resistance of the entire respiratory system (airways resistance, lung tissue resistance, and chest wall resistance), which explains why Rint measurements in normal subjects are higher than measures of resistance made using esophageal catheters.[89]

There are a number of papers reporting normative data for Rint, but one should use caution when choosing reference values because the technique and equipment may vary across laboratories. For Rint, reference values have been reported for children[93–96] using relatively large sample sizes. A recent publication reported normative Rint results from 1090 children between 3 and 13 years of age calculated using linear back extrapolation.[95] These data points were obtained from published and unpublished sources from different laboratories and currently provide the largest set of normative Rint values in children. For Rint, within-occasion repeatability has been reported to be 20% to 36% or within about 0.25 kPa/L/s. This suggests that a decrease after bronchodilator must be >35% or >1.25 Z-score to be considered significant.[97–99] Long-term variability has been reported to be 32% to 38% for healthy children and 20% to 52% for children with cough and/or wheeze.[97–99]

Rint has also been used in a number of studies to discriminate disease from health. Rint has been shown to discriminate subjects with cystic fibrosis and asthma from healthy controls.[100,101] Children with smoking parents have also been shown to have increased Rint.[102] The simplicity of this technique makes this lung function measurement particularly attractive for large trials in young children. However, in children who can perform spirometry, Rint offers an advantage only in the tiny minority in whom repeated forced expiratory efforts fail to produce adequate results.

FORCED OSCILLATION

Initially described more than 50 years ago,[103] the forced oscillation technique (FOT) is measured during tidal breathing, requires little active participation, and thus can easily be performed in children. External pressure oscillations are delivered at the airway opening, and flow and pressure changes are measured to obtain the impedance (Z_{rs}), resistance (R_{rs}), and reactance (X_{rs}) of the respiratory system. Z_{rs} represents the ratio of the maximum (peak to peak) changes in pressure and flow measured at the mouth resulting from the applied oscillatory pressure signal. The oscillatory pressure and flow signals produced by the forced oscillatory input pressure signal (i.e., the forcing function) are out of phase at most frequencies, and the degree to which pressure and flow are out of phase varies with frequency. Z_{rs} can thus be described at each frequency as having two components: a real or pressure-flow in-phase component (R_{rs}) and an imaginary or out-of-phase component (X_{rs}). The real component (R_{rs}) depends on the resistive behavior of the respiratory system, and the reactive component (X_{rs}) depends on the elastic and inertive behaviors of the respiratory system. Airway resistance is the main component of R_{rs} at most frequencies utilized for the FOT.[90,104]

Historically single, multiple, and mixed spectra of sinusoidal pressure oscillations have been applied to the airways to measure respiratory system resistance. Most commercial FOT devices utilize input signals composed of a wide spectrum of frequencies (e.g., 4-48 Hz). In routine clinical settings, the usual indices reported are within the frequency range of approximately 4 to 16 Hz. Over this range of frequencies, R_{rs} is relatively frequency-independent, while X_{rs} typically transitions from negative to positive values and crosses zero as frequency increases. The resonant frequency is defined as the frequency at which X_{rs} equals zero and represents equilibrium of the elastic and inertive elements. When X_{rs} is negative, the elastic elements dominate.[104]

To perform the technique, the child tidal breathes through a facemask or mouthpiece while sitting upright. To minimize the effects of oscillation of the upper airway and cheeks, the patient's cheeks are supported from behind by the technician's hands (Fig. 12-20). Pressure oscillations are commonly delivered within a frequency range of 4 to 50 Hertz. Three to five acceptable maneuvers are collected, and the mean results are reported. Resistance and reactance should be reported with reference to frequency in Hertz. Guidelines have been published describing proper procedure for children.[1,90,104]

Normative data have been reported from a number of laboratories[105–107] and provide reference values. Resistance in children declines with age, and no difference between genders has been reported. Short-term intrasubject coefficients of variation for R_{rs} range from 5% to 14%.[104,108] Day to day and weekly reproducibilities have been reported to be 16% and 17%, respectively.[108,109]

FOT has been used to diagnose airway obstruction and assess bronchodilator responsiveness in asthma.[110,111] Measures of X_{rs} have been reported to improve in children with cystic fibrosis following treatment for a pulmonary exacerbation,[112] and indices of R_{rs} and X_{rs} are reported to be abnormal in children with a history of chronic lung disease.[113] More work is needed to better define the clinical utility of the FOT in children.

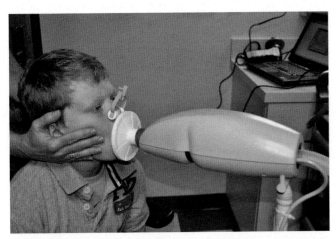

FIGURE 12-20. Child performing a forced oscillation maneuver. To minimize the effects of oscillation of the upper airway and cheeks, the child's cheeks are supported from behind by the technician's hands.

PLETHYSMOGRAPHIC AIRWAY RESISTANCE

Details regarding the technique and the procedure to measure airway resistance by whole body plethysmography[7,114] are described earlier in the chapter in the section entitled "Plethysmography."

Normative data have been published for R_{aw} and specific R_{aw} (sR_{aw}) in children.[115,116] A recent initiative published reference measurements for sR_{aw} on 2872 children compiled from five centers.[116] Methodological differences were noted between some centers, emphasizing the importance of quality control and choosing proper reference values when performing clinical and research protocols. For sR_{aw}, few data are available assessing repeatability. For shorter-term repeatability, the within-subject coefficient of variation has been reported to be 8% to 11% in healthy subjects and the intraclass (within occasion) correlation has been reported to be 0.86 in healthy subjects.[117,118] The short-term coefficient of variation for asthmatic children has been reported to be 9.3%.[119]

sR_{aw} is increased in patients with asthma and cystic fibrosis.[120,121] A recent study demonstrated that sR_{aw} correlated with FEF_{50} and was only weakly associated with FEV_1.[121] These studies suggest that sR_{aw} may be useful for detecting early flow limitation.

MULTIPLE BREATH WASHOUT

This tidal breathing technique evaluates nonhomogeneity of ventilation and has increased in popularity over the past decade.[122] This measurement is especially useful in children with peripheral airway obstruction where standard measures of lung function do not detect the presence of early disease.[123,124] In diseases of the airway that affect the distal bronchi, overall airway resistance is often not abnormal. Thus, a technique using inert gases that mix in these airways and have minimal solubility in the blood is ideal for detecting abnormalities of gas exchange or mixing.

To perform the technique, the child breathes in an inert gas (i.e., nitrogen, sulfur hexafluoride, or helium) until equilibration occurs. Most of the recently published studies in children have been performed using sulfur hexafluoride as the inert gas. Once the gas has equilibrated, the inert gas is disconnected and washed out. During the washout phase, the child tidal breathes into the system until the gas reaches 1/40th of its concentration at equilibration. The inert gas concentrations may be measured using a mass spectrometer, infrared gas analyzer, sidestream ultrasonic flow sensor, or nitrogen analyzer.[125,126] Guidelines for performing this technique have been developed for preschool children[1] and are being developed for school-age children. The technique has the potential to span all age ranges, making it especially attractive for children with chronic diseases where tracking progression is important.

The most common lung function index measured using this technique is the lung clearance index (LCI), which is the ratio of the cumulative expired washout volume and FRC. Typically, the mean of three LCI measurements is reported. The cumulative expired volume reflects the sum of the tidal volumes required to reduce the concentration to 1/40th of the concentration of the inert gas prior to washout.

Cumulative expired volume =
number of tidal breaths × (tidal volume − dead space volume)

In children with nonhomogeneous obstructive disease, the LCI is elevated and thus washout takes longer and requires more tidal breaths compared to normal children. FRC is typically calculated during the washout phase, although with some closed systems FRC is calculated during wash-in.[122,125]

Few studies documenting LCI levels in normal children have been published. More normative investigations are needed.[124] As noted in Chapter 11, LCI values have a higher upper limit of normality during infancy, but otherwise do not change with growth, making this measure attractive as a clinical and research tool. LCI has been shown to be increased in patients with cystic fibrosis compared to healthy controls[123,124] and to correlate with CT scores.[127] Recently, LCI was reported to improve after treatment with DNase[128] and hypertonic saline[129] in school-age children with cystic fibrosis. More studies evaluating how LCI is altered following therapeutic interventions will be critical to establishing the clinical utility of this tool.

EXHALED NITRIC OXIDE

Over the past decade, exhaled nitric oxide has emerged as a measurement useful in the clinical management of children with chronic airway disorders. This subject is discussed in detail in Chapter 6. Nitric oxide (NO) is a proinflammatory mediator that is produced when the amino acid arginine is converted to citrulline and NO. NO synthases catalyze this conversion and occur in different isoforms including a constitutive isoform and an inducible isoform. The inducible form is present in the airway epithelium within epithelial cells, type II pneumocytes, neutrophils, macrophages, vascular smooth muscle cells, and fibroblasts. The functions of NO within the airway include bronchodilator and immunomodulatory effects and regulation of ciliary beat frequency.[130]

Fractional exhaled NO (F_ENO) is associated with eosinophilic airway inflammation and has been demonstrated to decline following steroid treatment. These two findings have led to increasing use of this measurement in the management of asthmatics and in children with chronic respiratory symptoms, especially those with eosinophilic airway inflammation. Measurement of F_ENO levels facilitate management in children presenting with chronic respiratory symptoms by acting as a surrogate marker for eosinophilic lower airway inflammation. Documentation of normal F_ENO levels, for example, can provide evidence that steroids are not likely to be helpful.[131]

Procedural recommendations from the ATS/ERS describing the measurement of F_ENO in adults and children have been published.[132,133] NO is measured in parts per billion (ppb) using chemiluminescence and infrared technologies. Both single-breath online measurements and the offline method with a constant flow rate are described in these documents. In offline measurements, the gas is collected in a separate receptacle for later analysis. It is important for the operator to understand that NO contamination may occur from the atmosphere, the nose, or the gastrointestinal tract. The esophageal sphincter usually prevents gastrointestinal tract contamination. Ambient NO measures should be performed for quality control purposes. For both the online and offline methods, breath holding should be avoided to prevent NO accumulation within the oropharynx. Patients should refrain from food and drink for 1 hour prior to the testing since nitrate-containing products may affect results. Measurements should be avoided during respiratory infections because F_ENO can be elevated in these illnesses. F_ENO measures should be performed prior to spirometry since drops in NO levels have been reported after these maneuvers.[133]

To perform the single-breath online measurement, the child is seated, inhales to TLC, and then exhales immediately through an orifice while maintaining a constant flow rate. Recommendations from the ATS/ERS international committee are (1) a flow rate of 50 mL/second during exhalation, (2) a NO plateau for a minimum of 2 seconds, (3) inspired NO gas concentrations of <5 ppb, and (4) an expiratory pressure of 5 to 20 cm H_2O to assure closure of the velum and prevention of contamination from the nose. A constant flow rate is important because F_ENO concentrations correlate inversely with flow rates. The flow rate at which the measurement is made should be recorded. The procedure is repeated two to three times, and the mean of these levels is reported. The technician should wait 30 seconds in between measurements.[133]

Additional recommendations for the offline method are the following: (1) an expiratory pressure of 5 cm H_2O to avoid nasal NO contamination and (2) the receptacle for collecting F_ENO, typically a balloon, should be equal to or larger than the child's VC. Commercial systems are available. Performing the technique is relatively straightforward and thus easily applicable in school-age children.[133]

Normative F_ENO levels in children have been reported to be between 5 and 25 ppb.[130,134–137] F_ENO levels increase with age[134] secondary to growth related to increases in airway surface area, relative changes in expiratory flow rates, and repeated infections leading to changes in levels of the inducible form of NO synthase.[131] Reproducibility has been reported to be high for F_ENO measures, with an intraclass correlation of >0.9[134] and within-subject repeatability measures within 1.6 ppb.[134]

In a number of studies,[138] F_ENO measurements have been shown to aid in the diagnosis of asthma, especially when other clinical parameters are not diagnostic. Measurement of F_ENO levels is useful diagnostically for identifying atopic asthmatic children with clinical symptoms, but normal spirometry. F_ENO levels may also be helpful for predicting steroid responsiveness and for monitoring therapeutic responses.[139,140] Lack of a F_ENO response to steroids may indicate poor adherence to treatment. F_ENO has also been noted to be elevated in atopic children without asthma.[134] Clinical use of F_ENO measurements for other respiratory diseases has not become routine, but investigators have reported diminished levels in cystic fibrosis and primary ciliary dyskinesia. However, in primary ciliary dyskinesia, nasal NO measurements, not F_ENO, have been reported as a potential screening tool for this disease.[141] Elevated $F_E NO$ levels have been reported in liver cirrhosis, hepatopulmonary syndrome, bronchiolitis obliterans, and during viral respiratory illnesses.[131]

Suggested Reading

American Thoracic Society/European Respiratory Society. ATS/ERS Statement on Respiratory Muscle Testing. *Am J Respir Crit Care Med.* 2002;166:518–624.

ATS/ERS Recommendations for Standardized Procedures for the Online and Offline Measurement of Exhaled Lower Respiratory Nitric Oxide and Nasal Nitric Oxide, 2005. *Am J Respir Crit Care Med.* 2005;171:912–930.

Hyatt R, Scanlon P, Nakamura M. *Interpretation of pulmonary function tests. A practical guide.* 3rd ed. Philadelphia: Lippincott-Raven; 2009:3.

Macintyre N, Crapo RO, Viegi G, et al. Standardisation of the single-breath determination of carbon monoxide uptake in the lung. *Eur Respir J.* 2005;26:720–735.

Miller MR, Hankinson J, Brusasco V, et al. ATS/ERS Task Force. Standardisation of spirometry. *Eur Respir J.* 2005;26:319–338.

Oostveen E, MacLeod D, Lorino H, et al, on behalf of the ERS Task Force on Respiratory Impedance Measurements. The forced oscillation technique in clinical practice: methodology, recommendations and future developments. *Eur Respir J.* 2003;22:1026–1041.

Pellegrino R, Viegi G, Brusasco V, et al. Interpretative strategies for lung function tests. *Eur Respir J.* 2005;26:948–968.

Stanojevic S, Wade A, Stocks J. Reference values for lung function: past, present and future. *Eur Respir J.* 2010;36:12–19.

Wanger J, Clausen JL, Coates A, et al. ATS/ERS Task Force. Standardisation of the measurement of lung volumes. *Eur Respir J.* 2005;26:511–522.

References

The complete reference list is available online at www.expertconsult.com

13 EXERCISE AND LUNG FUNCTION IN CHILD HEALTH AND DISEASE

DAN M. COOPER, MD, SHLOMIT RADOM-AIZIK, PHD,
HYE-WON SHIN, PHD, AND DAN NEMET, MD, MHA

THE BIOLOGIC RELEVANCE OF EXERCISE IN THE GROWING CHILD

While the idea that "exercise is good for children" seems axiomatic, translating this vague notion into specific, biological mechanisms that actually could be used to influence health has proven difficult. Never before has the need for such research been so great. We find ourselves in the midst of an emerging epidemic of pediatric obesity, type 2 diabetes, and the metabolic syndrome, all, in large measure, ominous consequences of unprecedented levels of physical *inactivity* in children.[114,168] The parallel epidemic of childhood asthma seems equally intractable, disproportionately affects lower socioeconomic strata children,[228] and is itself linked to physical inactivity and obesity.[124,178,244,264] At the same time, therapeutic advances result in increasing numbers of childhood survivors of a wide range of conditions including premature birth, congenital heart disease, lung disease (e.g., cystic fibrosis [CF]), pediatric arthritis, sickle cell disease, and cancer. In these children, fitness is impaired, and physical activity is beneficial[84,136,256,262,267] only if the "exercise dose" does not exacerbate underlying inflammatory, metabolic, or physiologic abnormalities. Identifying optimal levels of exercise must be based on a better understanding of the mechanisms that link exercise with health and disease in the growing child; this concept drives this current review.

For both healthy children and those with chronic diseases, the ability to engage in play, exercise, and other physical activities is an essential component of daily life. For the pediatrician, precise assessment of the cardiorespiratory and metabolic responses to exercise can be a valuable tool in diagnosing disease, assessing its impact, and recommending specific programs of physical activity. As noted in other chapters, analysis of static pulmonary function can yield important information about the capability of the respiratory system in children. However, testing the mechanical properties of the lung at rest does not reveal the consequences of disease on metabolic function when the organism is stressed. To accomplish this, respiration in its fullest sense must be assessed. By measuring gas exchange at the mouth (oxygen uptake [$\dot{V}O_2$], carbon dioxide output [$\dot{V}CO_2$], and ventilation [$\dot{V}E$]) and the heart rate responses to exercise-induced increases in metabolism, one can evaluate the relationship between respiration of the cells and respiration of the whole organism.

A striking new paradigm has emerged in which the health and possibly disease effects of exercise and physical activity can be viewed as a balance between proinflammatory and anti-inflammatory, catabolic and anabolic activity (Fig. 13-1). We now know that exercise can lead to a substantial perturbation of cellular homeostasis including a profound metabolic acidosis, markedly altered oxygen, and substrate flux in tissue and mitochondria, and, on occasion, frank tissue injury. Even in healthy adults and children, exercise results in what appears to be a "danger" type activation of innate immune responses[58,147,175,214] that involves increased levels of circulating cytokines (e.g., interleukin-6 [IL-6]), leukocytosis, alterations in both gene expression and epigenetic control elements in circulating leukocytes (Fig.13-2),[189–192] and leukocyte adhesion molecules that have been associated with lung diseases such as asthma and CF.[66,222] An intriguing question is: Given the profound inflammatory response that occurs with exercise, why doesn't everyone wheeze with physical activity?

In contrast, the salient features of the healthy adaptation to repeated exercise are both anti-inflammatory and anabolic consisting of increased muscle mass, angiogenesis and arteriogenesis, increased bone strength, and the formation of new mitochondria. In the years to come, an exercise test in a child may be used not only to gauge cardiorespiratory capacity, but also to gain insight into the broader stress, immunologic, and inflammatory state of that individual and its implication for physical performance.

PHYSICAL ACTIVITY AND GROWTH IN CHILDREN—EARLY DEVELOPMENTAL FACTORS

The widely held but largely intuitive notion that vigorous physical activity occurs more frequently in children and adolescents than in adults is increasingly supported by scientific investigation.[23,54,133] Exercise in children is not merely play, but, rather, contributes to long-term processes of growth, development, and risk factors for adult disease. Indeed, as demonstrated by Borer and colleagues,[40] in some species sedentary behavior is associated with reduced growth and growth hormone (GH) pulsatility (e.g., Fig. 13-3). In children, levels of habitual physical activity are increasingly shown to influence the development of bone mineralization and lean body mass (the latter a surrogate for muscle mass).[31]

There is now a growing body of data supporting the idea that there exist "critical periods" of development during which a variety of stimuli can alter the overall programming of developmental processes.[46,51,181] Closely tied to the concept of a critical periods of growth and development is the theme of *pediatric origins of adult disease.*

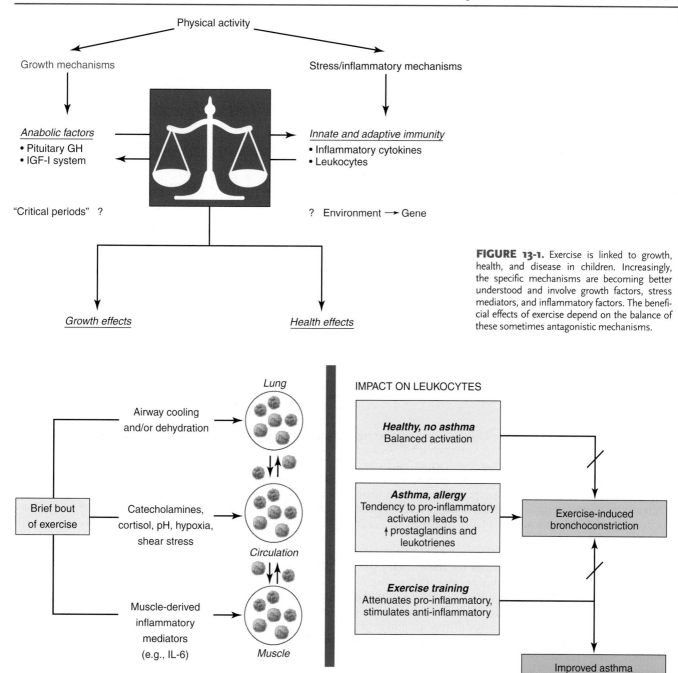

FIGURE 13-1. Exercise is linked to growth, health, and disease in children. Increasingly, the specific mechanisms are becoming better understood and involve growth factors, stress mediators, and inflammatory factors. The beneficial effects of exercise depend on the balance of these sometimes antagonistic mechanisms.

FIGURE 13-2. Why doesn't everyone wheeze with exercise? A hypothetical model of EIB and its inhibition by exercise training. Neutrophils and monocytes readily exchange among the circulation, muscle, and lung. Exercise leads to activated cells, but the activation is balanced between proinflammatory and anti-inflammatory mediator productions. In asthmatic syndromes, neutrophils and monocytes are abnormally stimulated by exercise, leading to excessive production of mediators that, in combination with factors like airway cooling and dehydration, can stimulate bronchoconstriction. It is hypothesized that exercise training stabilizes the activation of neutrophils and monocytes and attenuates EIB in susceptible individuals. The exercise-training associated leukocyte stabilization may also improve asthma control in general.

It is now clear that physical activity profoundly influences the development of bone, muscle, and fat tissue even in fetal and early life.[78,159,132,203,204,266] Our own recently published data show that increased physical activity in neonatal rats led to increased muscle mass and reduced levels of circulating inflammatory cytokines in adulthood.[44] Levin and coworkers[129] selectively bred rats to manifest a diet-induced, early-onset obesity (DIO) phenotype. These investigators found that "...early-onset exercise ameliorates, while early-onset caloric restriction accentuates, the development of obesity in genetically predisposed rats."

The pioneering work of Roberts and coworkers,[202] among the first investigators to use doubly labeled water (DLW) to assess total energy expenditure (TEE) in newborns, is also illustrative. These investigators found that low-energy expenditure was specifically related to reduced physical activity in full-term babies born to

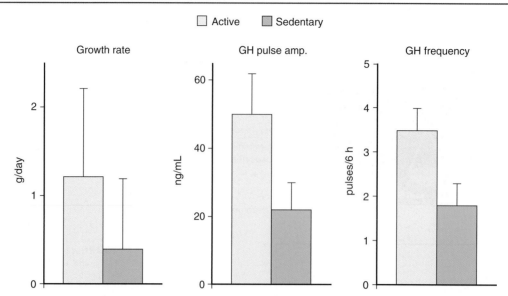

FIGURE 13-3. Effect of exercise on GH pulse amplitude and somatic growth in the hamster. Active hamsters (those who had running wheels) grew more rapidly. The increased growth rate was accompanied by greater GH pulse amplitude and frequency. In children and adolescents, more physically active individuals have greater muscle mass and circulating levels of IGF-I, a growth factor known to be involved in the adaptation to exercise and stimulated by GH. (Data redrawn from Borer KT, Nicoski DR, Owens V. Alteration of pulsatile growth hormone secretion by growth-inducing exercise: involvement of endogenous opiates and somatostatin. *Endocrinol.* 1986;118:844-850.)

overweight mothers. The low TEE was an important correlate of rapid weight gain in infants who became overweight. They concluded that "the most appropriate approach to preventing obesity in susceptible infants may be to increase their energy expenditure, rather than decrease their energy intake. Further research is required to investigate the applicability of our findings to other groups of infants."

In an American Heart Association (AHA) Scientific Statement focused on the guidelines for the primary preventions of atherosclerotic cardiovascular disease beginning in childhood,[118] the data are summarized and the authors conclude, "The existing evidence indicates that primary prevention of atherosclerotic disease should begin in childhood." In a more recent AHA statement focused on children with specific cardiac lesions, Pemberton and colleagues[177] noted, "Development of guidelines and consensus statements to encourage regular physical activity outside of competitive sports will require research to determine the type, duration, and intensity of activity in which an individual with a particular cardiac lesion can participate safely."

Finally, as levels of physical activity progressively decline in children,[237] it is reasonable to speculate that sarcopenia, the debilitating loss of muscle mass observed in the elderly,[206] will ultimately be found to have roots in inadequate muscle development during childhood, a sad echo of our current understanding of osteoporosis. There are now promising new indications that epigenetic mechanisms, increasingly seen as determinants of the lifelong effects of brief physiologic perturbations[105] in skeletal muscle, may play a role in the long-term effects of childhood exercise on adult "physical activity phenotypes."[150]

■ A BIOLOGIC APPROACH TOWARD EXERCISE TESTING IN CHILDREN

The progressive exercise protocol in which power on a cycle ergometer or treadmill is increased until the subject reaches his or her maximal level of tolerance (e.g., Bruce Protocol, Godfrey Protocol, Ramp Protocol) remains the cornerstone of most exercise tests in children and adults.[60,93,111,232] However, despite much discussion and debate about protocols and the advantages and disadvantages of treadmills and ergometers, there has yet to emerge a common, standardized approach for testing fitness and exercise capacity in children.[99,265] Other obstacles to multicenter trials that involve exercise and fitness outcomes in children include the lack of common terminologies, common calibration procedures, and approaches for data harmonization. Steps are underway to overcome these barriers, and it is hoped that much progress will have been made by the next edition of this review.

Most pediatric exercise tests last between 10 and 15 minutes, and usually about the last half of the test is performed at work rates that are above the subject's lactate or anaerobic threshold (LAT). Our understanding of the maturation and development of the cardiorespiratory system in children has been greatly enhanced by investigations into maximal and supramaximal physiologic responses to exercise in children and adolescents. It is becoming increasingly apparent, however, that peak or maximal exercise tests are not representative of patterns of physical activity actually encountered in the lives of children.

While sustained heavy exercise rarely occurs in children, traditional exercise testing focuses largely on the peak or maximal oxygen uptake ($\dot{V}O_{2max}$), which can only be measured from sustained exercise precisely in the high-intensity range. $\dot{V}O_{2max}$ probably occurs only in the confines of the exercise laboratory, and a "true" $\dot{V}O_{2max}$ (i.e., a plateau or decrease in $\dot{V}O_2$ while the work rate continues to increase) is observed in only about 28% of children and adolescents.[61] Because of this, cardiopulmonary exercise testing in children includes a growing variety of less effort-dependent protocols such as the physical work capacity (PWC) at a specified HR. In the PWC testing paradigm,[73,75,242] the subject performs a progressive exercise test in which the main variable is the work rate achieved at a specified submaximal HR (usually around 150 to 170 bpm). The PWC has been used in a number of studies of exercise and pediatric lung diseases such as asthma and CF.[29,170] Other submaximal approaches to exercise testing that are more amenable to field studies (e.g., the 20-meter shuttle run and the 6-minute walk/run test) have also been used to assess fitness in children with a variety of lung diseases and pulmonary hypertension.[2,86,122,128,131]

Normal results of maximal exercise tests are obtained from studies done in large samples of healthy children. These values are profoundly effort dependent, and, healthy subjects are routinely cajoled and prodded to continue exercising in the high-intensity range in order to achieve data of optimal quality. In contrast, patients with known or even suspected abnormalities are not encouraged as vigorously as are healthy subjects. Lactic acidosis and respiratory or cardiac insufficiency can accompany high work rates, and this causes reasonable concern regarding the safety of high-intensity exercise testing in individuals with heart or lung disease. As a consequence of such *de facto* differences in testing strategies, published "normal" maximal values may not be appropriate for children with suspected impairments.

REAL PATTERNS OF PHYSICAL ACTIVITY IN CHILDREN

To better understand how formal exercise testing in children relates to actual patterns of physical activity observed in children under natural conditions, a direct observation system that quantifies the duration, intensity, frequency, and interval duration of children's physical activities was developed.[23,38] We used this system to assess the level and tempo of energy expenditure under free-ranging, natural conditions experienced by 15 children 6 to 10 years of age in southern California. Observations were recorded every 3 seconds during 4-hour time blocks from 8:00 AM to 8:00 PM. Using indirect calorimetry, calibration studies in the laboratory determined $\dot{V}O_2$ (mL/min/kg) during each coded activity, and activities were categorized by intensity (low, medium, or high). Subjects were found to engage in low-intensity activities 77.1% of the time and high intensity activities 3.1% of the time (Fig. 13-4). The median duration of low- and medium-intensity activities was 6 seconds; the median duration of high-intensity activities was only 3 seconds, with 95% lasting less than 15 seconds. However, different types of high-intensity activities were often strung together. Thus, it appears that under natural

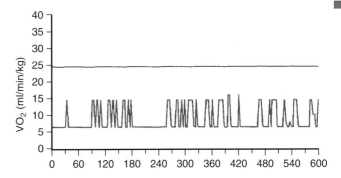

A

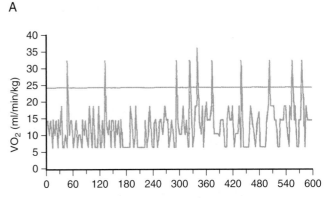

B

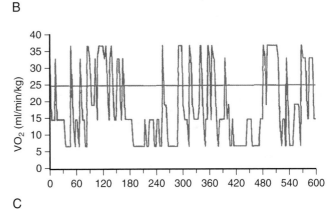

C

FIGURE 13-4. Profiles of estimated children's $\dot{V}O_2$ during 10-minute periods. The data were derived from direct observations of children. The solid line represents the anaerobic or lactate threshold (LAT). **A,** Profile of a girl's $\dot{V}O_2$ during a representative 10-minute period of relatively low activity. **B,** Profile of a girl's $\dot{V}O_2$ during a representative 10-minute period of relatively moderate activity; 5% of observations are above LAT. **C,** Profile of a boy's $\dot{V}O_2$ during a 10-minute period of relatively intense activity; 26.5% of observations are above LAT. (Data from Bailey RC, Olson J, Pepper SL, et al. The level and tempo of children's physical activities: An observational study. *Med Sci Sports Exerc.* 1995;27:1033-1041.)

conditions of daily living, children engage in short bursts of intense physical activity interspersed with varying intervals of low and moderate intensity.

THE CARDIORESPIRATORY RESPONSE TO EXERCISE

Consider, for example, the important acts of fleeing from a predator or, in more modern terms, running to avoid an oncoming car. When sudden and large increases in metabolic demand are imposed by physical activity, the whole organism can successfully function only by means of an integrated response among several organ systems. At the very onset of exercise, before there has been sufficient time for an in increase in environmental oxygen uptake, the healthy human must have sufficient stores of oxygen, high-energy phosphates, nonaerobic metabolic capability, and supplies of substrate to perform significant amounts of physical activity. As exercise proceeds, cardiac output increases and blood flow is diverted to the working muscles without compromising the critical flow of oxygen and glucose to the brain.

Ventilation and pulmonary blood flow must increase to precisely match the energy demand of the working muscles so that homeostasis for $PaCO_2$ and pH are maintained. There must be sufficient increase in substrate availability (i.e., glucose, fat, protein), but without depleting the peripheral blood glucose stores. And finally, the heat produced during exercise must be dissipated so that homeostasis for body temperature is maintained. In summary, as diagrammed in the late 1960s by Wasserman[252] events at the cellular level are closely linked to events in the heart and lungs (Fig. 13-5).

Maturation of Cardiorespiratory Responses to Exercise

The acute physiologic adjustments to physical activity in children are not simply scaled-down versions of those observed in adults. Maturation of cardiorespiratory, neurologic, and peripheral metabolic processes occur throughout childhood. These changes influence cardiorespiratory responses to physical activity rather profoundly, and they must be understood in order to properly interpret exercise tests.

Breathing increases during exercise. The stimulus for the exercise hyperpnea is, to a large extent, the increased production of CO_2 at the cells.[182,257] Thus, during progressive exercise in adults, the relationship between $\dot{V}E$ and $\dot{V}CO_2$ is significantly closer than the relationship between $\dot{V}E$ and $\dot{V}O_2$.[252] The concentration of CO_2 in the arterial blood measured as the $PaCO_2$ is held constant throughout most of progressive exercise despite large increases

in metabolically produced CO_2. The control of breathing during exercise in adults has been reviewed elsewhere[249,251] and includes central and peripheral chemoreceptors. In addition, mechanoreceptors in the exercising muscles may also play a role as suggested by Gozal and colleagues [95] from studies done in patients with congenital central hypoventilation syndrome. There is evidence that respiratory control does mature during childhood,[226] but much work needs to be done to fully understand the interaction between nervous system maturation and the control of breathing during exercise.

The robust nature of $PaCO_2$ homeostasis is reflected in healthy subjects at higher work intensities when additional CO_2 is liberated from the chemical combination of lactic acid (produced from anaerobic metabolism) and the ubiquitous buffer, bicarbonate. During this phase of isocapnic buffering,[259] $PaCO_2$ and pH remain constant as $\dot{V}E$ increases in proportion to $\dot{V}CO_2$. Only at very high work intensities, when the pH begins to fall and the peripheral chemoreceptors are additionally stimulated, does hyperventilation occur and $PaCO_2$ fall ("respiratory compensation point").[260]

The ability to rapidly increase the metabolic rate is sustainable only if substantial cellular accumulation of metabolically produced CO_2 is prevented, otherwise, pH falls rapidly and ATP-based energy metabolism pathways cannot operate. Redistribution of CO_2 from cells is facilitated by several mechanisms including: dissolution in body fluids and tissues; binding with hemoglobin; and, most importantly, rapid conversion to HCO_3^- with hemoglobin serving as a buffer for increased H^+. There is evidence suggesting that the linkage between $\dot{V}CO_2$ and $\dot{V}E$ undergoes a process of maturation during growth; that is, there is a difference between children and adults in the ventilatory response to changes in metabolic rate. These differences can be readily seen from a variety of exercise protocols.

Progressive exercise provides a relatively simple way to gauge the coupling of ventilation with $\dot{V}CO_2$ (Fig.13-6). The alveolar gas equation suggests that the relationship

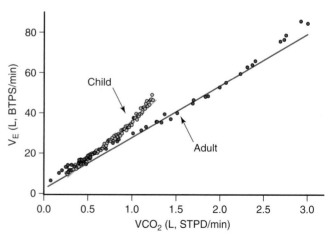

FIGURE 13-6. The relationship between $\dot{V}E$-$\dot{V}CO_2$ during a progressive exercise test in a 9-year-old girl and a young adult. Since $\dot{V}E$ is driven by $\dot{V}CO_2$, these data tend to have a high signal-to-noise ratio. The slope of the $\dot{V}E$-$\dot{V}CO_2$ relationship is easily calculated using standard linear regression techniques. These slopes tend to be higher in children compared with adults, indicating a generally higher ratio of dead space to tidal volume.

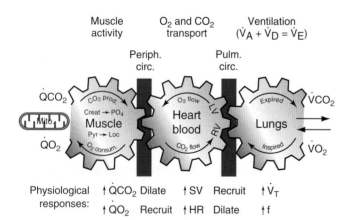

FIGURE 13-5. The physiologic mechanisms that link respiration at the cellular and whole-body levels made famous by Karlman Wasserman in this depiction of interlocking gears.

is determined by the CO_2 "set-point" (i.e., the level at which $PaCO_2$ is regulated) and the ratio of dead space to tidal volume (VD/VT):

$$\dot{V}_E = \left(863 \times PaCO_2^{-1} \times \left(1 - VD/VT\right)^{-1}\right) \times \dot{V}CO_2$$

As shown in Figure 13-6, there is a linear relationship between $\dot{V}_E$ and $\dot{V}CO_2$ for most of the progressive test.[57] Factors such as elevated $PaCO_2$ will tend to lower the magnitude of the slope, while a high VD/VT will render the slope steeper.

We and others have found it helpful to quantify the relationship between $\dot{V}_E$ and $\dot{V}CO_2$ by calculating the slope of the best fit line through the linear portion of the relationship (see Fig.13-6). Normal values have now been established for this parameter.[97,142,143] The slope of the relationship ($\Delta\dot{V}_E /\Delta\dot{V}CO_2$) decreases with increasing size among children and teenagers. Younger children need to breathe more than adults for a given increase in metabolic rate (i.e., $\Delta\dot{V}CO_2$). It has not been determined whether this results from lower CO_2 stores in children associated with apparently lower $PaCO_2$ and lower hematocrit (i.e., less hemoglobin buffering capacity and consequently, less CO_2 "stored" in the blood).[15,28,169]

Additional data demonstrate substantial differences between children and adults in the $\dot{V}_E$ and $\dot{V}CO_2$ responses to, and recovery from, 1 minute of high-intensity exercise[14](Fig. 13-7). We used these short exercise protocols because they more closely mimic patterns of activity actually observed in real life in children. Adults took longer than children did to recover from exercise, and $\tau\dot{V}CO_2$ (τ = the recovery time constant, the time required to reach about 63% of the end-exercise to pre-exercise steady-state values) and $\tau\dot{V}E$ increased with work intensity in adults, but not in children. These results are consistent with the hypothesis of a reduced anaerobic capability in children (see later in the chapter). If high-intensity exercise in children results in a smaller increase

in lactic acid concentrations, then less CO_2 will be produced from bicarbonate buffering of hydrogen ion.

$PaCO_2$ seems to be controlled at lower levels in children compared with adults.[41,42,226] These observations were corroborated indirectly by the measurements of end-tidal PCO_2 ($P_{ET}CO_2$) made in our 1-minute exercise studies showing that pre-exercise and peak-exercise values were significantly lower in children compared with adults, and more directly in a study of arterial $PaCO_2$ in children by Ohuchi and coworkers.[169] A lower CO_2 set-point may also explain, in part, the greater slopes of the $\dot{V}_E$-$\dot{V}CO_2$ relationship that we and others[158] observed in progressive exercise tests: If alveolar PCO_2 is lower, then greater $\dot{V}_E$ is needed to excrete a given amount of CO_2. Both the magnitude of the $\dot{V}_E$-$\dot{V}CO_2$ slopes and the growth-related decrease in them were quite similar to findings we obtained in a previous study of ventilatory responses in children and young adults.[57]

The coupling of $\dot{V}CO_2$ and $\dot{V}_E$ is closer in children than in adults. The rise in $P_{ET}CO_2$ with exercise seen in both children and adults indicates that $\dot{V}CO_2$ increased more rapidly than $\dot{V}_E$, but the exercise-induced jump in $P_{ET}CO_2$ was much smaller in children (from 37.8 ± 0.4 to 40.1 ± 0.3 mm Hg) compared to adults (from 40.5 ± 0.2 to 49.9 ± 0.4 mm Hg), suggesting that $\dot{V}_E$ kept pace with $\dot{V}CO_2$ better in children than in adults during exercise and early in recovery. Ratel and colleagues explored the implications of this closer coupling on acid-base balance during exercise in children.[195] Qualitatively similar observations have been made during recovery from exercise. While recovery $\tau\dot{V}_E$ was significantly longer than $\tau\dot{V}CO_2$ in adults following one-minute of high-intensity exercise, the recovery times for $\dot{V}_E$ and $\dot{V}CO_2$ were indistinguishable in the children. Although $P_{ET}CO_2$ is only an indirect estimate of alveolar or arterial PCO_2, the patterns in $P_{ET}CO_2$ appropriately reflected the disparity in the time constants of $\dot{V}_E$ and $\dot{V}CO_2$ in high-intensity exercise: in children, end-recovery PETCO$_2$ was virtually the same as

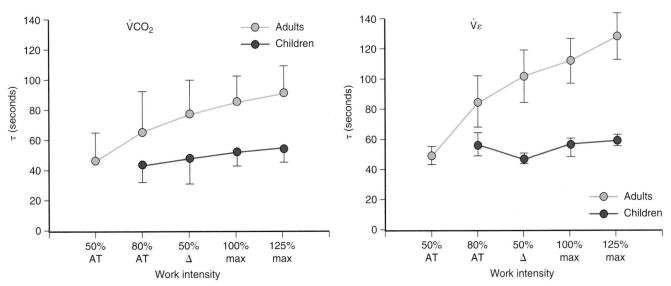

FIGURE 13-7. Recovery time constants (τ) for $\dot{V}CO_2$ *(left panel)* and $\dot{V}E$ *(right panel)*. Data are presented as mean $\pm$ SD. Recovery times were significantly shorter in children compared with adults. In adults, $\tau\dot{V}CO_2$ increased with increasing work intensity from 50% AT to 80% AT ($p < 0.01$) and from 80% AT to 50% Δ. ($p < 0.05$). For above-AT exercise, the $\dot{V}CO_2$ time constant at 50% Δ was significantly lower than 125% max. Note significantly shorter $\tau\dot{V}CO_2$ than $\tau\dot{V}E$ in the high-intensity range for adults ($p < 0.001$). In children, no significant differences were found between $\tau\dot{V}CO_2$ and $\tau\dot{V}E$. (Data from Armon et al.)

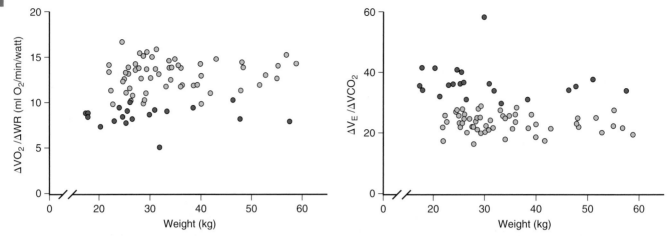

FIGURE 13-8. Dynamic variables in progressive exercise tests in CF subjects *(blue circles)* and controls *(green circles)* as a function of body weight. $\Delta VO_2/\Delta WR$ data are shown in the *left panel*, and $\Delta VE/\Delta VCO_2$ in the *right panel*. Both variables were significantly abnormal in CF subjects. (Data from Moser C, Tirakitsoontorn P, Nussbaum E, et al. Muscle size and cardiorespiratory response to exercise in cystic fibrosis. *Am J Respir Crit Care Med.* 2000;162:1823-1827.)

pre-exercise, while in adults, a persistent hyperventilation manifested itself as significantly lower $P_{ET}CO_2$. Increasingly, investigators are using exercise tests to gauge how disease states (e.g., CF, bronchopulmonary dysplasia, or status post Fontan correction for single ventricle congenital heart anomalies)[72,155,183,198,209] alter the relationship between CO_2 production and ventilatory control[156] (Fig. 13-8).

Bar-Or and coworkers were among the first to note maturational differences in exercise capacity (for reviews see [24,106]), even when appropriately scaled to body size. These investigators devised a protocol specifically for testing supramaximal, predominantly anaerobic exercise (the Wingate test). Even differences between 8- and 11-year-old boys were observed, with the younger subjects able to produce only 70% of the (size-adjusted) power generated by the older subjects. Much research still needs to be done to better elucidate the early-onset flow oxygen utilization in tests like the Wingate, as technologies

such as near-infrared spectroscopy have demonstrated substantial oxygen utilization, even in tests originally felt to be primarily anaerobic.[163]

As yet, unexplained maturational differences in oxygen uptake responses to exercise have also been observed. Several lines of evidence suggest that the lower *anaerobic* capacity of children is associated with increased oxygen utilization during submaximal work. For example, we found significantly greater cumulative O_2 cost of exercise in children at virtually all work rates from a series of 1-minute exercise bouts (Fig. 13-9).[268] These observations have been expanded upon and updated by Hebestreit and colleagues,[100] who studied children at even higher work rates than those used in our studies and those by Fawkner and Armstrong.[80–82] Finally, larger oxygen dependence of exercise in children is also seen in progressive exercise tests in which both the $\Delta \dot{V}O_2/\Delta WR$[60] and the ratio of $\dot{V}O_2max$ to maximal WR[268] were higher in younger subjects compared with

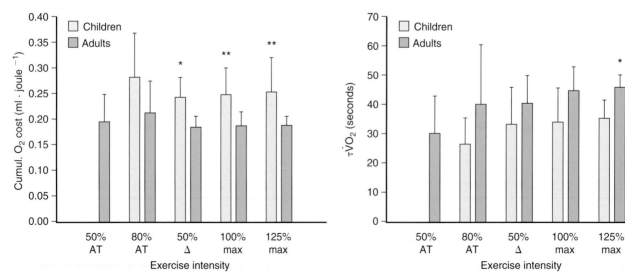

FIGURE 13-9. Oxygen cost *(left panel)* and response time (τ) *(right panel)* to brief exercise in children and adults. Oxygen cost is greater and response time is shorter in children compared with adults (see text).

older subjects. While the mechanisms of these differences between children and adults remain unclear, recent work from Kaczor and coworkers[113] point toward lower levels of the key enzyme lactate dehydrogenase in the muscles of children. This might explain the generally lower lactate production in response to exercise in children compared with adults.

The apparent differences between children and adults in gas exchange and other metabolic responses to exercise suggested hypotheses focused on ATP and energy metabolism differences at the level of the exercising muscle itself. There is increasing evidence suggesting maturation of energy metabolism during growth. The oxygen cost of high-intensity exercise, normalized to the actual work done (O_2/joule), is higher in children, suggesting less dependence on anaerobic metabolism.[268] As noted, after vigorous exercise, blood and muscle lactate concentrations are lower and serum pH higher in children than in adults.[173] Finally, the increase (slope) in $\dot{V}O_2$ during constant work rate high-intensity exercise is smaller in children than in adults.[13] Because the slope of $\dot{V}O_2$ during high-intensity exercise is correlated with serum lactate levels,[205] the smaller slopes in children further support the idea that lactate levels in response to high-intensity exercise are truly smaller in children. No definitive mechanism has been established for the growth-related differences in the adaptive response to high-intensity exercise. One problem has been the lack of noninvasive methods to study muscle metabolism.

The use of ^{31}P-nuclear magnetic resonance spectroscopy (^{31}P-MRS) now provides a safe way of monitoring intracellular Pi, phosphocreatine (PCr), and pH[48] that is acceptable for studies in children. These variables, in turn, allow the assessment of muscle oxidative metabolism and intramuscular glycolytic activity. We hypothesized that the growth-related changes in whole-body $\dot{V}O_2$ and O_2 cost of exercise observed during high-intensity exercise depend on a lower ATP supply by anaerobic metabolism in children. This could result either from changes in the mechanism of glycolysis in muscles or from a different pattern of fiber-type recruitment. We therefore expected a maturation of the kinetics of high-energy phosphate metabolites in muscle tissue during exercise. This hypothesis was tested by examining Pi, PCr, P-ATP, and pH kinetics in calf muscles during progressive incremental exercise. Results obtained from children were compared with those from adults. As shown in Figures 13-10 and 13-11, there were marked differences in Pi/PCr and pH between the children we studied. Ours was a small sample size study consisting of 10 prepubertal children (8 boys) whose mean age was 9.3 years old. The expense and availability for research of MR facilities has limited progress in this field.

There have been a handful of more recent investigations into potential maturational changes in ATP dynamics in response to exercise in children. Ratel and colleagues,[197] for example, studied seven boys (mean age 11.7 years old, Tanner approximately 1.5 [early pubertal]) and noted that the rate constant of PCr recovery and the maximum rate of aerobic ATP production were about two-fold higher in young boys than in men. They concluded that their results "…illustrated a greater mitochondrial oxidative capacity in the forearm flexor muscles of young children. This larger ATP regeneration capacity through aerobic mechanisms in children could be one of the factors accounting for their greater resistance to fatigue during high-intensity intermittent exercise."

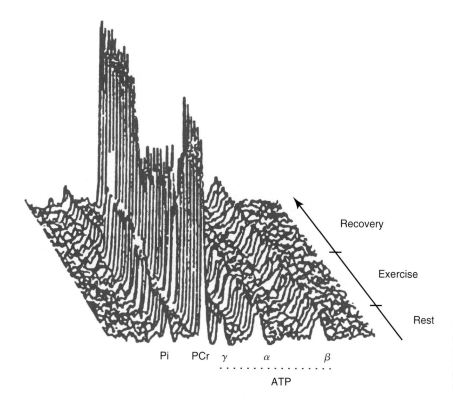

Recovery

Exercise

Rest

Pi   PCr   γ   α   β

ATP

FIGURE 13-10. ^{31}P-MRS spectra from right calf of an 8yr-old boy at rest, during incremental exercise, and recovery. (Data from Zanconato S, Reidy G, Cooper DM. Calf muscle cross sectional area and maximal oxygen uptake in children and adults. *Am J Physiol.* 1994; 267:R720–R725.)

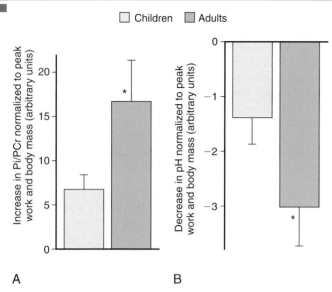

FIGURE 13-11. Effect of exercise on intramuscular increase in Pi/PCr **(A)** and decrease in pH **(B)** in children and adults. Exercise leads to significantly ($p < 0.05$) smaller changes in ATP-related kinetics, consistent with lower lactates observed during heavy exercise in children. (Data adapted from Zanconato et al.)

Interestingly, Willcocks and colleagues[263] used magnetic resonance spectroscopy (MRS) to study quadriceps exercise in five girls and six boys who were 13 ± 1 years old (clearly at more advanced pubertal status than our study or that of Ratel and coworkers). Willcocks and colleagues concluded that,

"The time constant for the PCr response was not significantly different in boys, girls, men, or women. [However] the mean response time for muscle tissue deoxygenation was significantly faster in children than adults. The results of this study show that the control of oxidative metabolism at the onset of high intensity exercise is adult-like in 13-year-olds…, but that matching of oxygen delivery to extraction is more precise in adults."

Clearly, this is an area of fundamental developmental physiology in need of further work. As noted compellingly in a recent review by Ratel and coworkers,[196] "Although it has been stated that children experience a larger increase in peak anaerobic power than in peak oxygen uptake during growth, experimental data derived from *in vitro* and *in vivo* muscle measurements, blood samplings, and oxygen uptake dynamics do not provide a consensus regarding the corresponding metabolic profile. Time-dependent changes in muscle oxidative capacity and anaerobic metabolism with respect to growth and maturation still remain a matter of debate. More specifically, it still remains unclear whether a metabolic specificity exists before puberty (i.e., whether a larger contribution of aerobic or anaerobic processes to energy production is present before puberty). Comparative analyses between children and adults must be performed under carefully standardized conditions. Accurate quantitative investigations of rates of aerobic and anaerobic ATP production should eventually allow us to determine whether prepubertal children have fully efficient or immature glycolytic activity and whether any adaptive oxidative changes occur during maturation."

USEFUL VARIABLES OF EXERCISE TESTING IN CHILDREN

In Table 13-1, the gas exchange and heart rate variables of exercise testing in children are briefly outlined. The gas exchange response to progressive, cycle ergometer exercise in a healthy 7-year-old boy tested in our laboratory is shown in Figure 13-12. Following a period of unloaded pedaling (0 watt), the work rate increases in a linear manner. This protocol is known as a *ramp work rate input*[258] and is one of several types of progressive exercise tests that can be used in children. Gas exchange is collected breath-by-breath and displayed on-line. Note that the increase in $\dot{V}O_2$ does not immediately follow the onset of exercise. The response time of $\dot{V}O_2$ (RT) is determined by the cellular, circulatory, and respiratory adaptations to the increase in energy demand in the muscle tissue. Following this, $\dot{V}O_2$ typically increases in a linear manner with increasing work rate. However, the $\dot{V}O_2$ response may either "bend up" or "bend down," depending on the magnitude of change of the work rate input.[98] In the data shown in Figure 13-12, note that there was a plateau in $\dot{V}O_2$ at the end of exercise despite a continuing increase in the work rate. The appearance of a plateau classically defines the $\dot{V}O_{2max}$. It is important to distinguish the $\dot{V}O_{2max}$ (i.e., where a plateau or reduction in $\dot{V}O_2$ occurs despite an increasing work rate) from the peak $\dot{V}O_2$ (i.e., the highest $\dot{V}O_2$ achieved by a particular subject).

From cross-sectional population studies, the $\dot{V}O_{2max}$ changes in roughly direct proportion with body weight.[16,60] This is at odds with the empirically observed "¾ power law" (which is demonstrated most commonly in Kleiber's "mouse-to-elephant" curve)[120] and with the so-called "surface area law." The surface area law stemmed from the belief that for mammals, all metabolic rates were determined by the rate of heat loss and heat production. Since heat loss was determined largely by the ratio of surface area to body mass, and since for spheres and cylinders (geometrically close to the shape of animals) the ratio of surface area to body mass scaled to the ⅔ power of body mass, it was concluded that metabolic rate must be proportional to body mass to the ⅔ power, which states that in mammals metabolic rates ($\dot{V}O_{2max}$ can be considered a metabolic rate) must scale to the ⅔ power of body mass.[96]

The finding of a direct relationship between $\dot{V}O_{2max}$ and body weight in children (i.e., a scaling factor of 1) suggests that the mechanism that links structure and function during the growth process within a species is different from the processes that determine the relationship between metabolic rates and body size in mature animals of different species. More recently, this idea was supported by a series of investigations of the relationship between $\dot{V}O_{2max}$ and muscle size in which the latter was measured using magnetic resonance imaging of muscle cross-sectional area in children and adults.[269]

Although $\dot{V}CO_2$ increases with progressive exercise, its pattern is not identical to that of $\dot{V}O_2$. Note in Figure 13-12 that the respiratory exchange ratio measured at the mouth (R, the ratio of $\dot{V}CO_2$ to $\dot{V}O_2$) is constant at the beginning of exercise but begins to increase well before maximal exercise, indicating that $\dot{V}CO_2$ is increasing at a faster rate than $\dot{V}O_2$. The mechanism for the increase in R is the

TABLE 13-1 CARDIORESPIRATORY AND METABOLIC VARIABLES OBTAINED FROM EXERCISE TESTING

EXERCISE VARIABLE	PHYSIOLOGIC IMPORTANCE
Maximal oxygen uptake ($\dot{V}O_{2\,max}$, peak $\dot{V}O_2$)	A plateau or decrease in $\dot{V}O_2$ despite a continuing increase in work rate. Care must be taken to distinguish the peak $\dot{V}O_2$ (the largest $\dot{V}O_2$ achieved by the subject) from the true $\dot{V}O_{2\,max}$.
Anaerobic, lactate, or ventilatory threshold (AT, LT, VAT)	The point during progressive exercise when lactate concentration begins to increase in the blood. The usual gas exchange manifestations of the AT are hyperventilation with respect to $\dot{V}O_2$ (increase in $\dot{V}_E/\dot{V}O_2$ and end-tidal PO_2), which occurs when $\dot{V}_E/\dot{V}CO_2$ and end-tidal PCO_2 are constant.
Work efficiency, or the O_2 cost of exercise (roughly, the inverse of efficiency; O_2 cost)	These variables are determined from the relationship of $\dot{V}O_2$ to the work rate.
Response time of gas exchange adaptations to exercise (mean response time, time constant—RT, MRT, τ)	The mathematically derived descriptor of the time required for $\dot{V}O_2$, $\dot{V}_E$, and $\dot{V}CO_2$ to achieve a steady state in response to or in recovery from a work rate input.
Ventilatory response to exercise ($\Delta\dot{V}_E/\Delta\dot{V}CO_2$)	Slope of the linear portion of the relationship between $\dot{V}_E/\dot{V}CO_2$ during progressive exercise. (Note that the ventilatory equivalent of CO_2 is the ratio $\dot{V}_E/\dot{V}CO_2$ and is not the same as the slope.)
Respiratory compensation point (RCP)	The point during heavy exercise when hyperventilation for $\dot{V}CO_2$ occurs. Presumably, at these heavy work loads, bicarbonate is no longer able to adequately buffer the lactic acid produced during high-intensity exercise, and pH changes. This stimulates the peripheral chemoreceptors.
O_2 pulse	The ratio $\dot{V}O_2/HR$. This ratio represents the amount of O_2 extracted per heart beat, which is not the same as the slope of the $\dot{V}O_2$-HR relationship during progressive exercise.
$\dot{V}O_2$-HR slope ($\Delta\dot{V}O_2/\Delta HR$)	This ratio represents the slope of the linear portion of the relationship between $\dot{V}O_2$ and HR during progressive exercise.

increased production of lactic acid, most likely consequent to anaerobic metabolism occurring at the muscle cells.[253] The buffering of the hydrogen ions releases additional CO_2. Since ventilation is stimulated by the flow of CO_2 to the respiratory centers, $\dot{V}E$ increases as well. Thus, as shown in Figure 13-12, the ratio of $\dot{V}E$ to $\dot{V}O_2$ increases. The hyperventilation for $\dot{V}O_2$ results in an increase in the end-tidal PO_2 ($P_{ET}O_2$). But since $\dot{V}E$ and $\dot{V}CO_2$ increase proportionately, the ratio of these two variables remains constant. This *constellation* of findings—an increase in R, $\dot{V}_E/\dot{V}O_2$, and $P_{ET}O_2$ while the $\dot{V}E/\dot{V}CO_2$ and $P_{ET}CO_2$ remain constant—constitutes the noninvasive measurement of the anaerobic or lactate threshold (LAT).

Studies of the lactate or anaerobic threshold have been made in large numbers of children using both treadmill and cycle ergometer exercise.[60,199] While the LAT in adults occurs at a metabolic rate (expressed as the $\dot{V}O_2$) equivalent to 40% to 60% of the subject's maximal $\dot{V}O_2$, this ratio is higher in children. Since the ratio of the LAT to $\dot{V}O_{2max}$ can be increased consequent to training programs,[65] one possible explanation is that children are generally "fitter" than adults. This, however, has not yet been substantiated.

A number of theories has been proposed to explain the phenomenon of increasing blood lactate concentrations during progressive exercise.[117,248] Most prominent are: (1) oxygen lack at the muscle tissue level resulting in anaerobic metabolism and an increase in lactate production relative to uptake; (2) a reduction in lactate uptake independent of oxygen availability; and (3) an oxygen-independent increase in lactate production due to increased "shuttling" of lactate associated with exercise.[43] Although the mechanisms of the LAT have not been entirely determined, its role as a physiologic marker

distinguishing between low-intensity and high-intensity exercise is gaining use.[53,230]

The speed with which the work rate increases during progressive exercise testing can influence the gas exchange response. In choosing the appropriate increment time and magnitude (or slope in the case of a ramp type input), several factors must be considered. First is the response time and delays known to occur in the gas exchange response. Because these times are different for $\dot{V}O_2$ and $\dot{V}CO_2$, care must be taken to ensure that observed changes in variables such as R (the ratio of $\dot{V}CO_2/\dot{V}O_2$) do not result from these dynamic delays. If, for example, the slope is too steep for the capabilities of the subject being tested, then an increase in R may be observed that is not related to the production of lactic acid, but results from differences in the dynamics of the gas exchange responses. In general, about 10 to 15 minutes of duration for a progressive exercise test in healthy children and adults is optimal.

For children 6 to 8 years of age, a ramp slope of 5 watts/min is used. For older children, 10 to 30 watt/min ramp slopes are used. The selection of the magnitude of the work rate input often involves an "educated guess" on the part of the investigator and requires some experience in assessing the capability of a particular child. A variety of maximal type exercise protocols suitable for studies in children have been reviewed by Washington and colleagues.[250]

ALTERNATIVES TO MAXIMAL TESTING

Although the clinical utility of *maximal* values can be questioned, much useful information is available from progressive exercise protocols. Gas exchange and HR responses

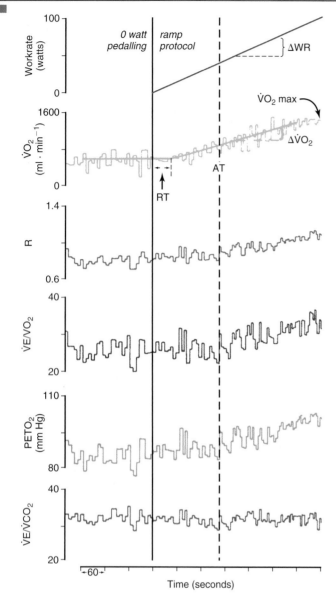

FIGURE 13-12. Breath-by-breath gas exchange response to exercise in a 7-year-old boy. The protocol used was a "ramp" type progressive work rate test in which the child exercised to the limit of his tolerance. The AT indicates the anaerobic or lactate threshold.

the final, single, data point at peak or maximal power. As noted above, there are a variety of approaches to exercise testing that rely on submaximal values. In a recent and intriguing study, for example, Isasi and coworkers[108] found that fitness measured by the PWC170 was inversely correlated with resting levels of serum C-reactive protein— a known circulating indicator of inflammation. This supports the relationship between fitness and stress/inflammatory factors alluded to above.

The time course of the onset and recovery of gas exchange and HR in response to exercise may also prove in the years to come to be clinically useful in exercise testing in children. Investigations into the underlying mechanisms of these responses (e.g., the concepts of oxygen deficit and debt[141]) compose an important chapter of modern exercise physiology. In the 1970s, computing and other technological advances permitted breath-to-breath measurement of gas exchange, and facilitated much more precise kinetic analysis and modeling of the gas exchange responses than had been previously possible.[33,253] One of the first attempts to gauge children's kinetic responses to exercise in a clinical setting was made in 1974, even before breath-by-breath measurements were widely available. Drakonakis and Halloran[71] measured oxygen uptake recovery from exercise in children with a variety of congenital heart lesions by (laboriously) collecting consecutive 1-minute samples of expired gas in balloons. The investigators found that children with cyanotic lesions showed markedly slowed recovery times following an exercise input.

Analysis of gas exchange and HR kinetic responses to exercise can be used to gain insight into cardiac, respiratory, and metabolic function,[89,218,241] for example, the use of this approach in children who have undergone Fontan surgical correction of congenital heart lesions,[241] Figs. 13-13 and 13-14). Since the pioneering work of Macek and coworkers,[138] research into kinetic exercise responses in children has steadily advanced and will increasingly become part of standard exercise testing in children.[80,152]

continuously change during progressive tests, and often the relationships between these changing variables (referred to as *dynamic* relationships) can be quantified using straightforward analytic techniques. As noted, the LAT in children and young adults can be determined noninvasively from the dynamic responses of gas exchange during progressive exercise. Simple linear regression analysis of HR and $\dot{V}O_2$ can provide noninvasive indicators of cardiac function.[60] The slope of the regression changes systematically with maturation and with diseases (e.g., heart failure). Similarly, linear regression analysis of $\dot{V}E$ and $\dot{V}CO_2$ can be used to assess respiratory efficiency and control during exercise, and are abnormal in patients with diseases ranging from cystic fibrosis[155] to heart failure.[12] The real clinical value of progressive exercise testing for children may prove to be in the rich cardiorespiratory data obtained *during* the submaximal phases rather than from

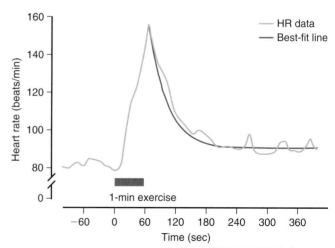

FIGURE 13-13. Heart rate (HR) response before, during, and after 1 min of exercise in a 14-year old Fontan group subject. The recovery kinetics were quantified using a single exponential, as shown.

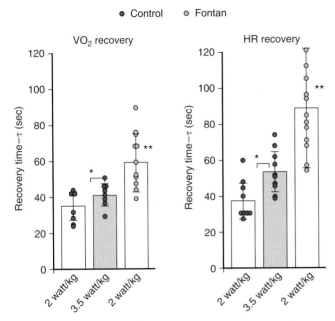

FIGURE 13-14. HR and $\dot{V}O_2$ recovery times for control and Fontan group subjects. In control subjects, recovery times were longer after the higher work rate protocols (*p < 0.05). In Fontan group subjects, recovery times were prolonged compared with the same absolute (2 W/kg) and relative (3.5 W/kg) protocols in control subjects (**p < 0.001).

THE PROBLEM OF SIZE

The evaluation and diagnosis of disease using exercise testing requires knowledge of adaptive mechanisms at both the cellular and organ-system's level. In children, interpretation of these adaptations is confounded by the rapid change in body size and development that characterizes the growth process. For example, how can one appropriately compare the $\dot{V}O_{2max}$ achieved by a 6-year-old child to that achieved by an 18-year-old? Should an obese 6-year-old child who weighs as much as a normal 12 year-old be expected to have the same $\dot{V}O_{2max}$ as the older child?

The consequences of a particular strategy to normalize data among differently sized subjects is not inconsequential. For example, when body weight was used to compare exercise responses in lean and obese children, the obese children demonstrated *low* anaerobic thresholds per kilogram of body weight.[200] Based on this type of observation, it has been suggested that obese children are unfit and less physically active than leaner children. The problem here is that the LAT (like $\dot{V}O_{2max}$) is determined in large part by the active muscle mass. Body weight is only partially determined by muscle mass, and in the case of the obese child, the proportion of muscle mass to body weight is decreased.

Thus, normalization to body weight in the case of obese children might lead the clinician to conclude that these subjects were less fit than nonobese children. But, by contrast, if the normalization is made to body height, lean body mass, or by strategies which minimize the size-dependence of the particular exercise parameter, then the degree of abnormality in the obese child is significantly reduced.[59] This determination is important–if the obese child is deemed "inactive," then the therapeutic approach ought to include programs of exercise. Such programs are expensive, require behavioral changes, and necessitate extensive supervision. For the obese child who is as physically active as leaner children, additional increases in physical activity may prove to be an impossible task.

In many areas of pediatrics, body surface area (BSA) has been used for drug dosages, energy expenditure, and so on. The use of BSA stems from the so-called "surface area law," which, as noted, was a popular concept in comparative physiology in the nineteenth century.[96] Much controversy surrounds the idea that metabolic rates in homeothermic animals are determined by the rate of heat loss, in turn dependent on the ratio of surface area to body mass. Moreover, the BSA is a *derived* value based on the actually measured height and weight and then calculated using a set of assumptions that have not been rigorously tested.

As in the case of obesity, simple ratios of metabolic rates to body weight may lead to incorrect clinical conclusions unless the investigator clearly examines the underlying assumptions (e.g., to what extent does body mass actually reflect muscle mass). On the other hand, height and weight are simple-to-obtain and highly accurate assessments of body size. Moreover, the correlation between height and weight in children is much higher than in adults,[60] probably because obesity in children is less prevalent than in adults (although obesity is increasing at an alarming rate in American children),[224] and direct measurements of body size probably introduce less uncertainty than *calculated* values like body surface area.

Many investigators have attempted to measure lean body mass as an estimate of muscle mass, and several techniques have been developed including: (cumbersome) underwater weighing, skinfold thickness calipers, computerized tomography, magnetic resonance imaging, and dual x-ray absorptiometry.[94,135,184,212,225] Each of these techniques has advantages and disadvantages, and the choice of methodology ultimately depends not only on scientific factors (e.g., which component of lean body mass must be measured) but also on issues of expense, exposure to ionizing radiation, time required to complete the particular test, and the availability of facilities and personnel capable of performing the measurement accurately. Given the wide array of choices and the lack of a single "gold standard" for normalization, it behooves each investigator and clinician to precisely define how normalization was accomplished and the rationale for using any particular approach. The interested reader may gain more in-depth understanding of the problem of size and scaling by consulting sources in the reference list.*

METHODS OF ASSESSING EXERCISE RESPONSES IN CHILDREN

Sophisticated exercise systems that allow breath-to-breath measurement of gas exchange are commercially available, but these packages are invariably designed for adults. As a consequence, "off-the-shelf" exercise system

*References 56, 76, 101, 151, 233, 238.

components—ranging from the dimensions of the cycle ergometer to the deadspace of breathing valves—are often inappropriate for children and increase the noise-to-signal ratio of the data obtained. Greater demand for exercise testing in children will eventually encourage manufacturers to market systems designed specifically for children.

Existing and new technologies need to be applied imaginatively to develop strategies for testing exercise in individuals with physical disabilities and for young children between 1 and 6 years of age. These populations are often ignored in research because they are difficult to study. This is unfortunate because exercise testing in these children could provide important clinical as well as basic biologic information about the fundamental interaction of respiration and growth and development in both health and disease (see, for example [231,236]).

A variety of methodologies can be used successfully to measure cardiorespiratory or metabolic responses in children. The two most common testing devices are the cycle ergometer and the treadmill. With cycle ergometry, the work rate input is determined by the load on the cycle's flywheel, and the subject pedals at a constant rate. In treadmill exercise, external work rate is increased by various combinations of increasing treadmill speed and incline. Consequently, the fundamental difference between these two input devices is that with the cycle ergometer the work rate (power) input is known precisely, while with treadmill exercise the external work rate can only be estimated. Hence, when one is attempting to relate gas exchange responses to specific work rates, the cycle ergometer is easier to use. Moreover, in studies of the transition between one level of exercise and another, the transition in work rate on the cycle ergometer is brought about simply by changing the load on the flywheel, while on the treadmill changing work rate involves adjustments of the incline or treadmill speed. These changes often evoke an anxiety response and may change the muscle groups involved in the exercise.

There are certain disadvantages to cycle ergometer exercise. The child is asked to maintain a constant pedaling rate; this is difficult for younger children who are unfamiliar with bicycles, particularly at low work rates. Variability in pedaling rate with a constant external load will result in variability in work rate. This can be compensated for by specially designed ergometers in which the external load is adjusted to the pedaling rate to maintain a constant work rate. In addition, not every child is adept at bicycle riding, and the investigator must always be aware that cardiorespiratory responses are "task-specific." In other words, a trained swimmer may be quite fit yet perform poorly on a cycle ergometer.

Special skills are required on the part of the clinician to achieve successful exercise testing in children. Younger subjects easily succumb to the barrage of sensory input in the laboratory and have difficulty focusing on the exercise task at hand. They will come off the mouthpiece, vary pedaling rate, or change running speed on the treadmill. In addition, siblings often accompany the subject to be tested, and this can provide additional distraction. In our laboratory, we have attempted to deal with these problems in a systematic manner. First, there are always at least two trained individuals conducting the test; the

role of one is to stay with the subject at all times. Usually, gentle, continuous verbal encouragement will help the child focus on the task at hand. We have also found that the use of videos and computer games are very helpful in occupying a sibling or the subject during breaks in the testing period. Finally, we have now published extensively using a cycle ergometer–based exercise protocol in which the child exercises for 2-minute constant work rate bouts with a 1-minute rest interspersed. Even with heavy exercise, we have found that this protocol is enjoyable for most children and permits us to precisely quantify the work done when gauging physiologic or immunologic results for exercise.[190]

Gas exchange analysis systems are of two general types: continuous-measurement (breath-by-breath) and discrete measurement (requiring mixing chambers of the exhaled gas). Both systems can yield useful and accurate information on cardiorespiratory responses to exercise. For investigations of the dynamic or kinetic responses of gas exchange to various work rate inputs, breath-to-breath systems offer the advantage of providing sufficiently high density of data to permit subsequent mathematical analysis (e.g., curve fitting) that would be otherwise unavailable. Commercial systems are available that can be adapted to the needs of children (e.g., reduced system deadspace, smaller crank radius for pedaling, adjustable seats). And while the mass spectrometer is still advantageous as a gas analyzer (rapid response, small sampling volume), advances in discrete gas analyzer technology have made these devices quite suitable for most systems designed for breath-by-breath analysis.

SAFETY OF EXERCISE TESTING IN CHILDREN

There is mounting evidence that clinical exercise testing is safe in children, even in children suffering from chronic heart or lung disease. Several investigators have examined the safety of maximal exercise testing in children. Alpert and coworkers[4] reviewed 1730 studies performed in their laboratory over a 9-year period in which children performed cycle ergometry testing to fatigue. Included in their sample was a large number of children with congenital heart disease. There were no deaths, and the total complication rate was 1.79%. Complications included chest pain, dizziness or syncope, and decreased blood pressure. Hazardous arrhythmias occurred in only 0.46% of subjects. These data echo observations in children with various heart abnormalities summarized recently by Rhodes and colleagues.[201] In general, patients with certain conditions (e.g., acute myocardial or pericardial inflammatory disease, severe outflow tract obstruction for which surgical intervention is clearly indicated, severe aortic dilation) should not be tested.[171]

Cardiopulmonary exercise testing raises as yet unanswered safety questions in children with a history of asthma or allergy. Vigorous exercise can trigger a transient bronchial narrowing and a reduction in pulmonary function variables in healthy individuals even with no history of asthma or allergies.[6] This exercise-induced acute airway hyperresponsiveness (AHR) is observed not uncommonly in elite athletes.[207,208] The mechanism of exercise-induced AHR in the absence of known allergy or asthma is not fully understood. Even in children with suspected allergies and asthma, exercise challenges (ranging from sophisticated in-laboratory procedures to having the child run up and down stairways in the pediatrician's office building) are common. Anecdotally, these procedures seem safe. Indeed, in the authors' laboratory we have performed hundreds of such challenges in children with suspected asthma and have had no major complications, other than, of course, inducing wheezing or pulmonary function evidence of bronchoconstriction. We have followed the safety guidelines for exercise challenge outlined by the ATS[63] that includes ready availability of "rescue" medications, use of pulse oximetry, and the presence of appropriately trained staff of nurses, physicians, and therapists.

NORMAL VALUES

In all aspects of pulmonary function testing and exercise assessment, the clinician is faced with the problem of choosing normal values. As noted above, there are a number of large-series investigations of normal values for both pulmonary function testing and exercise results in children. But variations in methodology and in the racial and socioeconomic composition of population groups necessitate validation of normal values for any particular laboratory. For example, we compared the maximal $\dot{V}O_2$ obtained in our laboratory in 1984 with values obtained by Astrand in Sweden in the 1950s. While the results for boys in our study ranging from 6 to 18 years of age were indistinguishable from the Swedish boys, the girls in our community demonstrated significantly lower values than did their Swedish counterparts.[16,60] A relentless reduction in physical activity has become apparent worldwide over the past 2 to 3 decades[237] and represents a worrisome trend for the health of our nation in the years to come. Ideally, each laboratory should develop its own set of normal values. At the very least, a sample of local healthy children can be tested to help choose an appropriate set of normal values. Some recent relatively large-sample normative values for children are included in the references.[134,187,234,245]

EXERCISE-INDUCED ASTHMA AND OTHER TESTS FOR BRONCHIAL REACTIVITY IN ASTHMATIC CHILDREN

Despite much recent progress in understanding asthma pathophysiology and the development of new therapies, the health care use associated with asthma and the associated disruptions to family and community life have not decreased substantially.[50] The link between physical activity and asthma is strong, but it remains enigmatic. Physical activity is a "double-edged sword" for the child with asthma. On the one hand, exercise is a common trigger of wheezing, occurring in as many as 80% of affected children in some studies.[7,64] On the other hand, exercise and fitness training seem to benefit asthma control in many affected children.[79,87,188]

As succinctly stated by Lucas and Platts-Mills,[137] "It is our belief that an exercise prescription should be part of the treatment for all cases of asthma. The real question is whether prolonged physical activity and, in particular, outdoor play of children plays a role in prophylaxis against persistent wheezing. If so, the decrease in physical activity might have played a major role in recent increases in asthma prevalence and severity." As recently noted by Voelkel and Spiegel:[247]

"In spite of numerous attempts to control asthma by treatment with bronchodilators, steroids, antigen-directed desensitization, and IgE-directed therapy, use of leukotriene receptor blockers and mast cell release inhibitors, a true control of the asthma syndrome with its multiple manifestations (exercise-induced, nocturnal, steroid-resistant, etc.), has so far eluded us. The reason is that . . . the disease . . . is perhaps much more an integrated system problem than only a bronchial problem."

Critical exercise-asthma treatment issues remain enigmatic and poorly studied, ranging from rare but tragic instances of death due to exercise induced bronchoconstriction (EIB) in asthmatic youth[70,123] to the lack of clinically validated paradigms of "return to play" following an exercise-associated asthma attack.[3] Despite the accepted clinical goal of ensuring that children with asthma fully participate in all types of exercise, physical fitness and participation in physical activity have been shown repeatedly to be impaired in children with asthma.[124,244,264] Participation in school physical education among children with asthma is reduced by as much as 40%.[119,153] Moreover, Conn and coworkers[55] recently discovered excessive use of electronic media in children with asthma, particularly in those with activity limitation. Whether these findings result from the *perception* of disability[36] or from poorly managed exercise-associated wheezing is not known. Whatever the causes, reduced participation in physical activity is an ominous finding in a child with asthma.

There is emerging data suggesting that exercise is beneficial for asthma in terms of disease control and pathogenesis. A growing number of animal studies (such as those by Pastva and colleagues[172] and Hewitt and coworkers[102,103] examined how brief exercise and exercise-training modulated subsequent lung inflammatory responses to ovalbumin (OVA) challenge in OVA-sensitized rats. These studies demonstrated a generally moderating effect of exercise on subsequent lung inflammatory responses to acute allergen challenges, specifically by decreasing NF-κB nuclear translocation and IκB-α phosphorylation, thereby diminishing key pro-inflammatory (and possible neuroadrenergic) control pathways. In children, studies of the benefits of exercise and physical activity have yielded mixed results,[162] perhaps due to a number of barriers to such research. However, a recent study from Bonsignore and coworkers[39] concluded that exercise training in combination with anti-inflammatory therapy might synergize to attenuate airway response to methacholine challenge in asthmatic children.

It is increasingly recognized that poorly controlled asthma in children can set the stage for lung disease in adulthood,[88] thus efforts to improve fitness and asthma control in children and adolescents—a "critical period" of growth and development[115]—are bound to have effects on health that last a lifetime. As noted by Ploeger and colleagues:[185]

To optimize exercise prescriptions and recommendations for patients with a chronic inflammatory disease, more research is needed to define the nature of physical activity that confers health benefits without exacerbating underlying inflammatory stress associated with disease pathology.

The upper limit of postexercise fall in FEV_1 (mean ± 2 SD) in normal children was found to be 6% to 8%.[20] In asthmatic children, the severity of exercise induced asthma (EIA) may be influenced by the severity of asthma[85] and by pre-exposure to allergens.[157] Moreover, the severity, duration, and type of exercise may influence the severity of EIA. Running, as compared to swimming under the same inspired air conditions and work intensity, will result in much more EIA.[26] There also exists the well-described phenomenon of refractoriness to EIA[254] (Fig. 13-15). It is also important to note that the recovery from EIA differs in younger children compared with older children. For example, Hofstra and coworkers[104] demonstrated that 7- to 10-year-olds with EIA improved FEV_1 by a mean of 1.60%/min following the challenge, but improvement in 11- to 12-year-olds was significantly prolonged (0.54%/min).

The mechanism of EIA remains enigmatic. As noted, exercise has been demonstrated to be a vigorous stimulant of the stress/inflammatory immune system (see Fig. 13-15[210]) involving increased levels of circulating IL-6 and intracellular adhesion molecules, many of which are involved in the pathophysiology of bronchoconstriction.[161,174] Moreover, hypoxia, such as can occur in the peripheral and pulmonary circulation during exercise, further stimulates IL-6 and pronounced systemic leukocytosis.[176] Hypoxia also stimulates endothelium to produce a variety of neutrophil attractants leading to neutrophil sequestration and activation.[154] Indeed, given the robust stress/inflammatory response in healthy children, one might wonder why all children do not wheeze when they exercise.

Many heated debates in the 1980s and 1990s focused not so much on mechanisms of asthma and EIB *per se*, but on EIB triggers. For example, the role of airway cooling and dehydration (caused by increased ventilation during exercise) as a "cause" of EIB was, at the time, viewed by some as being at odds with the idea of EIB/asthma as a disease involving abnormal responses of inflammatory cells.[91,149] Exercise alters *local* airway homeostasis (e.g., heat exchange, hydration) similarly in asthmatics and controls, but EIB occurs in susceptible individuals[90] who often have *systemic* signs of altered immunity ranging from food allergy[32] to eczema.[45] In the past 15 years, remarkable new insights into the inflammatory and immune cell consequences of exercise have been made.[62,145] We are now in a position to explore new hypotheses of EIB that incorporate a variety of mechanisms including: environmental factors (e.g., immune activation by exposure to air pollution), inherently abnormal innate immune cells, and any of a variety of specific triggers (including, among others, exercise-associated airway dehydration)—all intriguing and testable potential mechanisms of EIB in asthma.

The effect of climate on EIA has been extensively studied. Breathing warm and humid air during exercise almost completely abolishes EIA, while breathing dry and cold air increases its severity.[25,107,255] Respiratory heat loss (RHL) from the airway mucosa during exercise was suggested by Deal and colleagues[68] as the trigger for bronchoconstriction, and they showed that exercise and hyperventilation with similar RHL will result in similar bronchoconstriction. However, respiratory heat loss cannot entirely account for the triggering stimulus for EIA, as some asthmatic patients will develop EIA while breathing warm humid air at body temperature and humidity, which will not result in RHL.[9,10,35] Also, Noviski and coworkers[166] exercised a group of asthmatic children at two levels of exercise while the respiratory heat and water loss was kept constant by altering the inspired air conditions. They found that the harder exercise with a mean $\dot{V}O_2$ of approximately 1.6 times greater than $\dot{V}O_2$ of the less strenuous exercise resulted in EIA that was greater by almost 1.7 times.

Anderson recently reviewed the interaction of indirect challenges to elicit bronchial hyperreactivity and compared exercise with other triggers.[8] She suggested that changes in osmolarity of the fluid lining the airways during exercise are the triggering stimulus for EIA. It has also been suggested that EIA and hyperventilation-induced asthma (HIA) are the result of cooling and rewarming of the airway mucosa causing hyperemia and bronchial obstruction.[22,90]

Mediator release from circulating leukocytes and/or the airway mast cells was suggested as the intermediary pathway involved in EIA, HIA, and osmotic-induced asthma (OIA). Neutrophil chemotactic factor and histamine have been found to rise in blood after exercise,[125-127] as have intracellular adhesion molecules[11] and other inflammatory cytokines known to play a role in asthma even in healthy children.[47,160,161] Recent data point toward the neutrophil as playing a particularly important early mechanistic role in triggering bronchospasm.[121,213] Pre-exercise treatment with sodium cromoglycate (which has been shown to prevent mediator release from mast cells *in vitro*) prevented EIA.[167] Terfenadine, a H_1 histamine antagonist, has been shown to reduce the severity of EIA, HIA, and OIA.[83,261] The leukotriene LTD_4 may be one of the mediators released during exercise,[140] but leukotriene-blocking

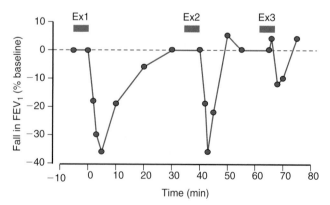

FIGURE 13-15. Refractoriness in exercise-induced bronchoconstriction. Note the lack of a robust drop in FEV, in this 11-year-old girl following the third of three exercise challenges. (Data from Weiler-Ravell D, Godfrey S. Do exercise- and antigen-induced asthma utilize the same pathways? Antigen provocation in patients rendered refractory to exercise-induced asthma. *J Allergy Clin Immunol*. 1981;67:391-397.)

agents have only mixed success in blocking EIA.[37] As noted by McConnell and colleagues,[148]

> Incidence of new diagnoses of asthma is associated with heavy exercise in communities with high concentrations of ozone, thus, air pollution and outdoor exercise could contribute to the development of asthma in children.

Given recent research in the ways in which exposure to air pollutants can influence asthma and lung inflammation,[1,69] the association between ozone, exercise, and asthma further supports the idea that immune/inflammatory dysregulation may play a role in EIA.

We recently developed an animal model of EIB.[121] Brown-Norway rats that had been sensitized, via ovalbumin (OVA) injection, showed a modest degree of airway hyperreactivity (assessed by breath sounds) in response to a seemingly unrelated trigger: brief exercise. The rapid onset of the change in breath sounds following the exercise challenge was similar to EIB observed clinically in humans. Exercise, even in the absence of prior sensitization to OVA, led to increased lung IFN-γ without an increase in immune cell infiltration, suggesting that that resident leukocytes or macrophages were responsible. This model may prove useful in better understanding, and, ultimately preventing, EIB, a serious and sometimes life-threatening consequence of asthma in humans.[34,70]

■ EXERCISE AND OTHER TESTS FOR BRONCHIAL REACTIVITY

Bronchial hyperreactivity to methacholine (MCH) or histamine is a characteristic feature of asthma [52,112,239] but is also present in patients with other types of chronic obstructive lung diseases.* Avital and colleagues[20] compared bronchial reactivity to exercise, MCH, and adenosine 5'-monophosphate (which probably acts by increasing the release of mediators from mast cells) in children with asthma, in children with pediatric chronic obstructive pulmonary disease (PCOPD, including CF, bronchiolitis obliterans, primary ciliary dyskinesia, and bronchiectasis), and in healthy controls. While the asthmatics responded to all three challenges, the PCOPD patients responded only to MCH, whereas the controls did not respond to any of the three challenges. MCH could distinguish both asthma and PCOPD from controls, but could not distinguish asthma from PCOPD. Exercise and adenosine 5'-monophosphate (AMP) not only distinguished asthma from controls, but could also distinguish asthma from PCOPD. In a recent study involving 135 children and young adults with mild to moderate asthma, Avital and coworkers[17] compared the response to MCH, AMP, and exercise challenges, evaluating the relationship between asthma severity and response to these challenges. These investigators found that the sensitivity of MCH challenge in detecting bronchial reactivity was 98%, that of AMP challenge was 95.5%, and that of exercise was 65%. Logistic regression analysis and receiver operating characteristic (ROC) curves of the three challenges showed that MCH was the best discriminator between

severity groups. Therefore, it seems that exercise and AMP are specific stimuli for asthma and that AMP is more sensitive than exercise in the detection of bronchial hyperreactivity in asthmatic patients. In known asthmatics, MCH is the best challenge to predict the severity of the disease.

The diagnosis of asthma in preschool children may be difficult, as these children usually cannot reliably perform spirometric measurement of lung function. There are promising new approaches including digitized assessment of recorded breath sounds that may, in years to come, prove useful for assessing EIB in younger children.[92] The response to inhaled MCH or AMP can be measured in young children by auscultation, an increase in respiratory rate, or desaturation.[18] In the proper hands, challenge testing is virtually free of complications.[227]

Children should avoid physical activity for at least 3 hours before exercise testing because they may show an attenuated response due to refractoriness. Medications that can influence the pulmonary response to exercise should be stopped prior to the test: 6 and 12 hours for short- and long-acting beta-adrenergic drugs, respectively; 8 hours for anticholinergic drugs; and 24 hours for cromolyn sodium. Caffeine-containing drinks or food should also be avoided before the test. Corticosteroids can be continued without any change as their immediate effect on EIA is probably not significant. Baseline pulmonary function (FEV$_1$) should be at least 65% of the predicted value.[221]

The exercise test can be performed by using either a bicycle ergometer or a treadmill. Our standard test for demonstrating EIA is either a 6- to 8-minute run on a treadmill at a speed of 3 to 5 mph, with a slope of 10% or, alternatively, cycle ergometer exercise calculated to achieve about 70% of the child's predicted $\dot{V}O_{2max}$. This will result in an oxygen consumption of about 60% to 80% of $\dot{V}O_{2max}$ and a heart rate of 170 to 180 bpm.[74] Lung function is measured before exercise and repeated until satisfactory reproducibility is demonstrated. Measurements are performed in duplicate after exercise (recording the best value) at 1, 3, 5, 10, and 15 minutes after exercise. It is becoming increasingly apparent that the onset of EIB and its recovery is more rapid in younger children compared with adults,[246] and these observations should be taken into account when measuring PFTs after the exercise challenge. Lung function is assessed by FEV$_1$ using a spirometer, but peak flow measurements can also be used, especially in young children, as they are easier to perform. The asthmatic response is expressed by the percent fall in lung function from baseline. A 10% or greater fall in FEV$_1$ or PEF is considered a positive response. Bronchodilators should be prepared before the exercise test, as some children may respond with a severe asthmatic attack.

■ EXERCISE AND EXHALED NO

Nitric oxide (NO) performs many important functions (e.g., smooth muscle relaxation and host defense) and can be detected in the exhaled breath of humans (eNO). There is mounting evidence demonstrating that exhaled NO could serve as a noninvasive marker of lung inflammation, especially for, but not limited to, asthma.[27] However, until fairly recently the majority of eNO studies were

---

*References 19, 21, 186, 193, 194, and 223.

structured to define disease-specific NO modifications, and thus the potential significance of NO alteration related to exercise-induced inflammatory or immune responses was minimized. Utilizing eNO could allow us to understand endogenous exercise-associated immune responses since inflammatory cytokines have been reported to modulate endogenous NO in airway cell culture models.[110,229]

Given the nature of complex NO exchange dynamics (i.e., eNO originates from both airway and alveolar compartments and is thus highly dependent on the exhalation flow rate)[219,243] and the multisystem physiologic responses to exercise, it is not surprising that there are inconsistencies in the reports of the impact of exercise on exhaled NO. After exercise, exhaled NO concentration has been reported to be increased,[30] unchanged,[109] or decreased.[49,144,146,179,240] Scollo and colleagues[211] reported no significant change in exhaled NO concentration up to 18 minutes after an exercise challenge in children. However, De Gouw and colleagues[67] extended exhaled NO monitoring for 30 minutes in healthy adults and observed a small decrease in exhaled NO concentration shortly after the exercise (<5 minutes) and an increase >20 minutes after exercise. Shin and coworkers[215,216] demonstrated that exercise intensity could possibly modulate NO exchange in the healthy humans. They quantified several flow-independent parameters characteristic of NO exchange in response to moderate- to high-intensity exercise in healthy controls. This group observed no significant changes in eNO at flow rates of 50 mL/s and 250 mL/s regardless of exercise intensity. However, high-intensity exercise resulted in significant acute changes in NO parameters 3 minutes postexercise that returned to baseline values at 60 minutes postexercise. These results suggest that endogenously produced NO following exercise may be useful to probe metabolic and structural features of the airways using the flow-independent NO parameters.

Much research effort has focused on utilizing eNO as a noninvasive marker of asthma in both adults and children.[5,27,165] Changes in eNO during and after exercise in asthmatics are well recognized,[30,49,180] and, more recently, alterations in eNO have been reported to play a role in the pathogenesis of both exercise-induced and thermally-induced bronchoconstriction in children and adults.[67,116,211,235]

The precise diagnostic role of eNO in EIB has yet to be determined. Some studies suggest that eNO can be used as a surrogate predictor of EIB. ElHalawani and colleagues[77] showed that the mean baseline eNO was 41 ppb in an EIB group and 25.6 ppb in the group without EIB among the subjects having a decrease in FEV_1 of >15% following exercise. The subjects with <12 ppb of baseline eNO did not develop bronchial hyperresponsiveness to exercise. In addition, Shin[217] and Silkoff[220] separately reported that the flow-independent NO parameter $D_{aw}NO$ (airway nitric oxide diffusion capacity) was significantly elevated in subjects with asthma, regardless of steroid treatment. Silkoff's study demonstrated that the highest values of $D_{aw}NO$ were associated with the best pulmonary function and least bronchial reactivity. Shin and colleagues [217]further evaluated the relationship between NO parameters and spirometry indices in EIB. They concluded that $D_{aw}NO$ was not altered following exercise challenge, and spirometry was decoupled with NO exchange dynamics in EIB. Their study suggested that $D_{aw}NO$ can be served as a sophisticated maker of EIB as well as steroid-independent asthma characteristic.

For children, the association between EIB and eNO has been investigated by various groups, but the outcomes remain inconsistent. Several investigators demonstrated that baseline eNO positively correlated with EIB in asthmatic children.[130,139,164] While eNO can be predictive of EIB in young wheezing children, its ability to predict exacerbation following exercise is low, even among asthmatic children having highly elevated baseline eNO. Recently, Bonsignore and coworkers[39] showed that exercise training in mild stable asthmatic children improved exercise capacities with reduced episodes of exacerbation without altering eNO. Clearly, additional work is needed to determine whether a minimally invasive test based on the presence of a specific gas in the exhaled breath can find a useful role in the management of EIA in children.

SUMMARY

The pediatrician attempting to assess the health status of his or her patients frequently asks the question, "How is the child doing?" With exercise testing, a precise answer to this question often can be obtained. We have attempted to demonstrate that the cardiorespiratory response to exercise is a function of metabolism and growth and development as well as an index of the functional capabilities of the heart and lungs. Hopefully, child health care professionals will avail themselves of this resource. Finally, much more research has yet to be done before we fully understand the optimal role of physical activity in the life of healthy children or in those suffering from chronic diseases.

References

The complete reference list is available online at www.expertconsult.com

14 INTEGRATING PATIENT-REPORTED OUTCOMES INTO RESEARCH AND CLINICAL PRACTICE

ALEXANDRA L. QUITTNER, PHD, ADRIANNE N. ALPERN, MS, AND CARA I. KIMBERG, MD

Patient-centered care, which is based on a collaborative relationship between a health care professional and his or her patient, was named one of the six "aims for improvement" by the Institute of Medicine in 2001.[1] The goal of this aim was to create a medical community in which patients' perceptions, beliefs, and preferences were considered during routine care and medical decision making.[2] This requires the development of patient-reported outcomes (PROs). PROs reflect patients' perceptions of the impact of their disease on daily functioning and the frequency and severity of their symptoms. In December 2009, the Food and Drug Administration (FDA) recognized the importance of PROs for evaluating the efficacy of new medications and laid out a framework for PRO development.[1] This guidance reflects a change in health outcomes research and is consistent with a patient-centered model of care. This chapter will focus on the reliability, validity, and utility of PROs for children with respiratory diseases in the context of both research and clinical practice.

DEFINITION OF A PRO

A PRO is any measure of a patient's health status that reflects how a person functions, feels, or survives, as reported by the patient himself or herself.[3] Health-related quality of life (HRQOL) measures are one type of PRO that typically includes several domains of functioning.[4] These tools capture the aspects of functioning known only to the patient, including his or her symptoms, behaviors, and daily functioning (e.g., frequency of cough, physical limitations, worries about the future). PROs can be used for several purposes: (1) as primary or secondary outcomes in clinical trials, (2) to evaluate pharmaceutical, surgical, or behavioral interventions, (3) to assess the effect of a disease on multiple aspects of patient functioning, and (4) to develop individualized treatment plans.[5-8]

To date, 14% of registered clinical trials include a PRO as either a primary or secondary endpoint, and this number is expected to increase as new PROs are developed.[9] This trend has been attributed to advances in medicine, which have increased the number of available treatments for chronic diseases, as well as their complexity, time commitment, and side-effects. Thus, adherence to these treatment regimens has become more challenging, potentially affecting patients' management of, and adaptation to, their disease. Recently, Aztreonam for Inhalation was approved on the basis of a PRO (Cystic Fibrosis Questionnaire-Revised Respiratory Symptom Scale; CFQ-R).[10] This is the first time a respiratory drug has been approved using a PRO, highlighting the importance of the patient's perspective.[11]

DEVELOPMENT AND UTILIZATION OF PROS

To be utilized in a drug registration trial, a PRO must meet strict psychometric criteria (e.g., reliability, validity, responsivity). A conceptual framework, which links the relevant concepts (e.g., respiratory symptoms) of the PRO to the label claim, must also be hypothesized and tested, followed by calculation of several types of reliability and validity (Table 14-1).

PROs must be sensitive to change on an individual and group level, and to interpret the magnitude of this change, the minimal important difference (MID) score must be identified.[12] The MID reflects the smallest, clinically meaningful change that a patient can reliably detect.[13,14] The MID can be established using patient input, using a Global Rating of Change question or statistical distribution methods (e.g., ½ SD of change, 1 standard error of measurement). The minimal change identified using these methods should converge around a similar value.

HEALTH-RELATED QUALITY OF LIFE MEASURES

HRQOL measures are one of the most frequently used types of PROs. The World Health Organization provided the first definition of health more than 50 years ago: "a state of complete physical, mental, and social well-being, and not merely the absence of disease or infirmity."[15] Accordingly, HRQOL measures are typically multidimensional instruments that evaluate four core domains: (1) disease state and physical symptoms, (2) functional status (e.g., performing daily activities), (3) psychological and emotional functioning, and (4) social functioning. Patient perceptions of HRQOL are expected to vary across different domains of functioning. HRQOL instruments can track the natural progression of a disease, evaluate responsivity to pharmacologic or behavioral interventions, and facilitate shared medical decision making. For example, if a patient starts a new treatment for asthma, an HRQOL measure can assess its effectiveness in reducing asthma symptoms, such as wheezing. The tool can also be used to evaluate whether this treatment has become onerous for the patient, if a scale measuring treatment burden is included.[16]

TABLE 14-1 PSYCHOMETRIC CRITERIA FOR A PATIENT-REPORTED OUTCOME (PRO)

	DEFINITION
Reliability	
• Test-retest	Stability of patient report when no change has occurred
• Internal consistency	Relationship among items that compose a scale
• Interrater	Agreement between two raters on the construct or rating choices
Validity	
• Content	Key concepts and items are represented on the instrument
• Discriminant	Instrument discriminates between sample characteristics (disease severity, gender) or groups receiving different interventions
• Convergent	Measure correlates with health-related variables in expected directions; instrument correlates with other measures that are similar
• Predictive	Instrument predicts changes in health status

HRQOL instruments can be divided into two categories: generic and disease-specific, each with its own unique set of advantages and disadvantages. Generic HRQOL measures are composed of general items that are relevant to populations with and without a chronic illness. Examples of generic HRQOL measures include the Pediatric Quality of Life Inventory, the Child Health and Illness Profile, and the Youth Quality of Life Instrument. Generic HRQOL measures can be utilized across patient populations to compare the impact of a disease on different patient groups.[17] These instruments correlate with disease severity and distinguish between healthy and chronically ill populations.[18] However, these measures are not specific to the symptoms and challenges of a particular disease and, therefore, are not sensitive to change or useful in generating treatment recommendations.

In contrast, disease-specific HRQOL instruments are designed to reflect the unique symptoms and challenges of a particular patient population. For example, a hallmark symptom of CF is excess mucus production. This symptom would not appear on a generic measure or one focused on a different respiratory condition, such as asthma. Thus, inclusion of items that are highly relevant to a specific population leads to greater sensitivity to treatment effects and is more informative for clinical care. This is the rationale for using disease-specific instruments for the purposes of drug registration trials.[17]

DEVELOPMENTAL CONSIDERATIONS

Developing HRQOL measures for children poses unique challenges, ranging from cognitive limitations to the shifting importance of peers, school, and parents over the course of development. Comprehending and responding to items requires several cognitive skills, such as focused attention, receptive and expressive language, and a conceptual understanding of the illness. All of these skills emerge gradually and at different points across development. Further, the relevance and importance of a given domain is likely to change over the course of childhood and adolescence.[4] For example, social functioning is integral to adolescents' overall quality of life, but is less relevant for preschoolers. Accordingly, measures created within a developmental framework are more accurate and valid than measures downwardly extended from adult instruments. This ensures that the most relevant areas of functioning are measured in a cognitively appropriate manner for a particular age group.[19]

HRQOL measures for children must undergo rigorous testing to ensure that individuals within the target age range understand the vocabulary and concepts contained in the questionnaire. Research shows that children between 2 and 6 years of age have a more limited understanding of medical terms and concepts.[21,22] Children in this age group are able to report on observable areas of health (e.g., symptoms and levels of pain) using a pictorial format. They may, however, have more difficulty reporting on their emotional and social functioning. By school age, children demonstrate a better understanding of the interplay between their health status and daily functioning.[23] In fact, several studies have found that school age children are able to provide reliable reports of their symptoms and functioning.[24–26]

Changes in cognitive and attentional capacity across development underscore the importance of response options and mode of administration when eliciting information from children. The number and types of response options must be developmentally appropriate for the specific age range. While adult measures typically utilize 5- to 7-point Likert scales (which are equal interval, defined ratings across a continuum of responses), little research has been conducted on the ability of young children to discriminate between response choices.[26] Therefore, developers of pediatric measures often use fewer response options or include a visual analog scale.[18,27,28] Specifically, many instruments use illustrations to attach meaning to the endpoints of the scale (e.g., "a whole lot," "not at all") or to define each response option.[29]

To reduce errors based on reading difficulties and distractibility, an interviewer can administer measures to children. The interviewer can redirect the child and make the experience more interactional and rewarding (e.g., concrete rewards, such as stickers, can help maintain their focus). During the interaction, the interviewer should avoid asking leading questions that may influence the child's responses. In addition, because young children tend to select response options at endpoints rather than using the full range of responses,[25,30] a forced choice format is a useful alternative (Fig. 14-1). Research shows that children as young as 4 years of age can make forced choices.[31] Finally, use of technology (e.g., computer-based, Internet) may facilitate the accurate completion of HRQOL measures for children; colors, animations, and other features can make the process more gamelike and

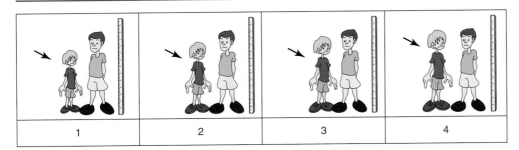

FIGURE 14-1. Example of CFQ-R response choices for the preschool version. The interviewer asks "Do you think you are short?" Children are asked to first choose between the extreme choices (1 and 4), and then to discriminate between the extreme and less extreme choice (e.g., 1 and 2, "Do you think you are really really short, or a bit short?").

engaging. Similarly, completing a measure may be more rewarding for children when cartoon illustrations are incorporated into each question.[32,33]

USE OF PROXY RESPONDENTS

Proxy respondents, such as parents, also may be useful depending on the age of the child (e.g., infants), his or her level of disease severity, and possible cognitive limitations related to the disease process.[34,35] Proxy-reports of HRQOL may also provide different information than the child's self-report. Parent reports tend to correlate better with child reports for observable phenomena, such as physical functioning and symptom frequency (e.g., climbing stairs, coughing). Potential discrepancies between parent and child reports are important to consider because they could affect: (1) the focus of a clinic visit, (2) medical decision making, and (3) health care utilization.[36]

Literature on the relationship between proxy and patient reports is somewhat inconsistent. Some findings suggest that children endorse more emotional distress, somatic complaints, and physical difficulties than their parents do.[24,37,38] In contrast, Britto and colleagues found that adolescents with CF rated their HRQOL better than their parents did across domains measuring general health, behavior, and physical functioning.[39] Note that discrepancies in research findings may also occur if different types of instruments are compared (e.g., generic versus disease-specific). Although proxy measures for health care providers have been developed, their validity is limited because providers spend less time with their patients and observe them across fewer contexts.

CLINICAL UTILITY

The use of HRQOL measures in routine practice facilitates the systematic, efficient collection of information about patients' perceptions of their daily functioning. This information can serve several purposes, such as promoting communication between the patient and provider, identifying frequently overlooked problems, monitoring disease progression, and tailoring interventions to key aspects of a patient's daily life.[4,40] Accordingly, both quality of life and health outcomes may improve as a result of integrating information from HRQOL measures into routine care. To date, the most established benefit of this integration is enhanced communication between patients and health care providers.[41,42]

First, HRQOL measures can provide a systematic way to facilitate discussion between the patient and provider. Depending on the patient, he or she may report some

symptoms (e.g., frequent cough) but disclose others only when directly asked (e.g., fatigue or absences from school or work). Research shows that both patients and physicians find HRQOL assessments helpful in defining patient concerns and enhancing communication, which has important implications for health outcomes.[40] Numerous studies have found that discussions of both physical and psychosocial issues during medical visits lead to improved treatment adherence, higher patient satisfaction, and fewer symptoms.[43-45] A second benefit is the identification of frequently overlooked problems that are important to the patient (e.g., depression, treatment burden).[46] This is particularly critical in the management of chronic respiratory diseases, since multiple domains of functioning are typically affected and treatment regimens are both time- and energy-intensive.[47,48] For example, patients with CF may spend 2 to 4 hours per day doing prescribed treatments, which may cause social isolation and depression.[49] In addition, physiologic measures, such as lung function, correlate only modestly with patient reports of symptom frequency, changes in daily activities, or emotional functioning.[50] Thus, HRQOL data may alert providers to these critical issues using a standardized methodology (Fig. 14-2). Note that most of this research has been conducted with adults, highlighting a need for this research with pediatric populations.

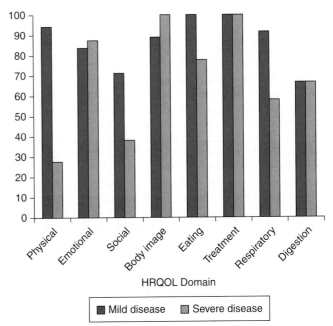

FIGURE 14-2. Example CFQ-R profile for two children, one with mild disease (FEV$_1$% predicted = 107) and one with severe disease (FEV$_1$% predicted = 41).

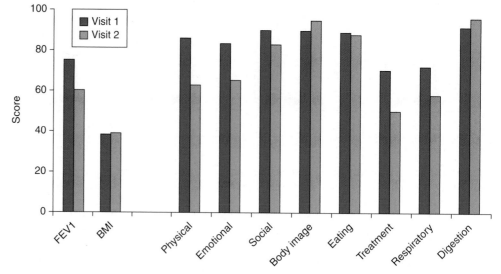

FIGURE 14-3. Example of HRQOL assessments at two clinic visits, one year apart, as measured by the CFQ-R. Domain scores are on a 0 to 100 point scale, with higher values indicating better HRQOL. This individual experienced a decline in FEV_1 and corresponding declines in some domains of functioning, such as respiratory symptoms and treatment burden.

When given at regular intervals, HRQOL measures can monitor disease course, both in terms of natural progression of disease and response to drug or behavioral interventions (Fig. 14-3). Monitoring disease progression can lead to early identification of new concerns (e.g., weight loss), as well as the exacerbation of existing challenges (e.g., increased fatigue). In addition, HRQOL assessment can evaluate the patient's responsivity to a new treatment. Because HRQOL instruments are multidimensional, they allow for differentiation of the benefits of a new medication (e.g., improvement in respiratory symptoms) from its side effects (e.g., increased treatment burden). It is also possible that patients with the same lung function score may report very different levels of functioning in the physical, social, or emotional domains. Data from HRQOL measures may assist the provider in targeting interventions to address these concerns (see Fig. 14-2).

HRQOL feedback has also been shown to impact clinical decision making in arthritis, epilepsy, and cancer (e.g., medication changes, referrals).[51-54] To date, these studies have not been performed in patients with respiratory conditions. In the future, profiles of individual functioning could also be used to predict how an individual will respond to a given treatment and which treatment is most likely to maximize benefits and minimize cost (e.g., decreased fatigue, financial costs).

Studies testing the feasibility of integrating HRQOL and physiologic measures in routine care for respiratory disorders are at the beginning stages but demonstrate considerable promise. For example, adult patients with CF are using home spirometers that are linked to their pulmonary center, along with daily symptom diaries. Utilizing these measures together may allow the CF team to identify the early signs of exacerbation and either suggest that the patient come in for a clinic visit or take antibiotics at home. A study by Santana and colleagues demonstrated that administration of HRQOL was feasible in a lung transplant clinic and did not prolong clinic visits.[55] Results indicated improved communication

between patients and health care providers; additionally, the inclusion of HRQOL data influenced patient management with respect to medication changes, number of referrals, and tests ordered. While there were no linkages between the patients' HRQOL scores and health outcomes, the authors used a generic measure that may not have been sensitive to the specific concerns of this population.

Another group of researchers evaluated the feasibility of using computer-administered HRQOL measures in the waiting rooms of primary care practices.[56] Nearly all health care practitioners (94%) and most adult patients (86%) supported the continued use of these measures in the future, as the instruments were found to facilitate communication and track patients' functioning. In order to increase their utilization in health care settings, HRQOL measures need to have both Web- and computer-based applications. These formats allow for quick administration and scoring, with an option to print the profile scores immediately before the patient-provider discussion.

■ SUMMARY

As the medical community progresses toward a patient-centered model of care, it is important for health care professionals to understand the role of PROs in both research and clinical care. PROs, including HRQOL assessment, can track disease progression, evaluate the effects of pharmacologic or behavioral interventions, and guide treatment decisions. However, the validity of the findings is largely dependent on the attributes of the PRO instrument itself, including its content, reliability, and validity. The following section reviews the available disease-specific HRQOL measures for several pediatric respiratory disorders (i.e., asthma, CF, sleep apnea, and vocal cord dysfunction). Specifically, this section provides an overview of the available instruments followed by a summary of the measures' strengths and weaknesses. Based on the information available to date, we have recommended the best instrument for each respiratory condition.

■ REVIEW OF DISEASE-SPECIFIC RESPIRATORY HRQOL MEASURES

Asthma Measures

Thirteen disease-specific HRQOL measures for children with asthma are available, which vary with respect to their psychometric properties, clinical utility, and responsiveness to change. (Table 14-2). While many measures demonstrate good internal consistency and test-retest reliability, responsivity to pharmacologic or behavioral interventions has been demonstrated less extensively. Only the PAQLQ has an established MID, enhancing its clinical utility in assessing meaningful change.

Asthma measures vary with respect to informant type, target age range, and practical utility (e.g., language translations, respondent burden). While several measures have corresponding child and parent versions, few include self-report versions for children younger than 6 years of age. Translations into multiple languages exist for three measures (CAQ, DISABKIDS-Asthma Module, and PAQLQ). Finally, only a few measures with a low respondent burden (i.e., completion time less than 10 to 15 minutes) are also reliable and sensitive (CAQ, CHSA, PAQLQ, and Peds-QL-Asthma Module).

The majority of asthma measures have at least one limitation in terms of reliability, validity, sensitivity, responsivity, or clinical utility. With the exception of the PAQLQ, all measures lack an established MID, leaving health care providers with little guidance on how to interpret changes in scores. Respondent burden is a limitation of several measures (AMA, TACQOL-Asthma, and LAQ). Thus, because of the time they take to complete, these instruments are less feasible for use in routine care. In addition, the AMA only provides a total score, which limits providers' ability to isolate problem areas. Further, few asthma measures are available for both children and caregivers; of those with both patient- and proxy-report, cross-informant agreement is rarely reported. Finally, additional self-report measures are needed for children younger than 5 years of age.

Recommendation

To date, the PAQLQ is the most widely used asthma instrument. Research on the PAQLQ indicates good reliability and validity, and it is the only disease-specific HRQOL measure for asthma that has an established MID. The PAQLQ is responsive to both pharmacologic and behavioral interventions, and it has been translated into more than 30 languages. The corresponding parent-proxy measure (Pediatric Asthma Caregiver's Quality of Life Questionnaire) and the computerized/Web-based administration options add to the utility of this instrument. A pictorial version for children 5 to 7 years of age is currently in development.

Cystic Fibrosis Measures

Five measures are available to assess HRQOL in children and adolescents with cystic fibrosis (Table 14-3). All of these instruments assess symptoms as well as other areas of functioning. Although all measures demonstrate good reliability, validity has only been established for the FLZM-CF, CFQoL, and CFQ-R. Responsiveness to pharmacologic and/or behavioral interventions has been established for most measures, as well as the ability to differentiate between levels of disease severity and between ill and well states. All five CF HRQOL instruments have been translated into other languages; however, the CFQ-R is the only measure with both parent and child forms.

The five available HRQOL measures for CF have specific weaknesses. The FLZM-CF only has one item per scale, limiting its ability to reflect more complex constructs (e.g., treatment adherence). Additionally, this measure has a 4-week recall window, which is longer than ideal and may increase error.[83] The CFRSD captures information that is relevant to pulmonary exacerbations rather than using a multidimensional framework. Additionally, an MID value has not been established for several measures, limiting the interpretability of results. The CFQ-R is the only measure that extends downward to children 6 years of age, while the CFQoL, FLZM-CF, and CFRSD measures do not extend below 12 years of age.

Recommendation

The CFQ-R is the most widely used and well-established instrument for CF and is recommended for both clinical and research purposes.[35] The CFQ-R covers the widest age range (6 years of age and older), and a pictorial version for preschoolers is currently being evaluated. Advantages of the CFQ-R include its availability in more than 34 languages, an established MID of 5 points for the Respiratory Symptom Scale, and computerized administration and scoring. Further, domains of the CFQ-R are found to correlate with health outcomes, including $FEV_1\%$ predicted and BMI percentile. Sensitivity to change has been established for the CFQ-R in several clinical trials.[84-85] In fact, the Respiratory Symptom Scale was used as a primary endpoint in the drug registration trial for AZLI.[11]

Vocal Cord Dysfunction Measures

To date, three HRQOL measures for vocal cord dysfunction have been developed for pediatric populations. All measures are completed by parents and offer the advantage of brevity and minimal respondent burden (Table 14-4). Additionally, these instruments demonstrate good test-retest reliability and discriminant and convergent validity. However, internal consistency on the pVHI has not been reported.

All of these measures are limited by their reliance on parents or caregivers as informants, and thus they do not capture the patient perspective. Additionally, none of the instruments has an established MID, and additional research on responsiveness is needed. Lastly, the PVOS consists of only four items, does not provide scores across different domains of functioning, and has lower reliability in parents of children older than 11 years of age.

Recommendation

Based on these findings, we recommend the PVR-QOL. The development of HRQOL instruments that can be completed by pediatric patients themselves is an important next step for vocal cord dysfunction research.

TABLE 14-2 HRQOL MEASURES FOR CHILDREN WITH ASTHMA

MEASURE	NUMBER OF ITEMS AND DOMAINS	AGE RANGE AND RESPONDENT	COMPLETION TIME	PSYCHOMETRICS: RELIABILITY	PSYCHOMETRICS: VALIDITY
About My Asthma (AMA)[57]	Number of items = 55 Domains: Total score only	6-12 years Child No parent version	15-20 minutes	α = .93 Test-retest = .57	Moderately correlates with the PAQLQ Responsive to a week-long asthma day camp
Adolescent Asthma Quality of Life Questionnaire (AAQOL)[58-59]	Number of items = 32 Domains (6): Symptoms, medication, physical activities, emotion, social interaction, and positive effects	12-17 years Child No parent version	5-7 minutes	α = .70 to .93 Test-retest = .76 to .90	High correlation with PAQLQ (r = .81) Weak to moderate correlation with patient-rated symptom severity, number of hospitalizations, severity of coughing, and severity of wheezing (r's = .25 to .65)
*Childhood Asthma Questionnaires (CAQ)[60-61]	CAQ-A—Number of items = 14 Domains (2): QOL and distress CAQ-B—Number of items = 22 Domains (4): Active QOL, passive QOL, severity and distress CAQ-C—Number of items = 31 Domains (5): Active QOL, passive QOL, severity, distress, and reactivity	4-7 years Child 8-11 years Child 12-16 years Child No parent version	10-15 minutes	α = .60 to .63 for CAQ A α = .57 to .84 for CAQ B α = .50 to .80 for CAQ C Test-retest = .59 to .63 (CAQ A); .73 to .75 (CAQ B); .73 to .84 (CAQ C) ICC = .59 to .63 (CAQ A); .72 to .75 (CAQ B); .68 to .84 (CAQ C)	Discriminates between asthmatic and nonasthmatic children Correlated with parent ratings of asthma severity
Children's Health Survey for Asthma (CHSA)[63]	Child Version—Number of items = 25 Domains (3): Physical health, child activities, and emotional health Parent Version— Number of items = 48 Domains (5): Physical health, activity (child), activity (family), emotional health (child), and emotional health (family)	7-16 years Child 5-12 years Parent	Child completion time: 7-13 minutes Parent completion time not reported	α = .74 to .81 (Child) Test-retest = .88 to .91 α = .81 to .92 (Parent) Test-retest = .60 to .85 No cross-informant reliability reported	Correlated with parent reports of their children's health status, and treatment burden as measured by the Asthma Symptom Day-14 (ASD-14) Parent version correlated with disease severity as measured by symptom activity (i.e, number of days wheezing, coughing, tightness of chest) and medication use (i.e., number of times child used inhaler, nebulizer, bronchodilator)
*DISABKIDS - Asthma Module[64-65]	Number of items = 37 Generic Domains (6): Medication, emotion, social inclusion, social exclusion, limitation, and treatment Number of items = 11 Asthma-Specific Domains (2): Impact (consists of limitations and symptoms), Worry	"Smileys" version for children ages 4-7 years, child 8-14 years, child	Not reported	α = .86 to .92 (generic) α = .83 to .84 (asthma module) Test-retest = .42 to .53	Correlated with symptoms (cough), frequency of doctor's visits, and use of inhaled medications Discriminates between levels of disease severity Linked to International Classification of Functioning, Health and Disability (ICF)
*†Pediatric Asthma Quality of Life Questionnaire (PAQLQ)[66-68]	Number of items = 23 Domains (3): Activity limitations, symptoms, and emotional function	7-17 years Child Pictorial version for ages 5-7 in development	10 minutes	ICC = .84 to .95 Cross informant r=0.61 No internal consistency reported	Discriminates between levels of disease severity Established MID (0.5 on a 7-point scale) Converges with issues from asthma focus groups conducted by independent investigators Responsive to pharmacologic and behavioral interventions Used in clinical trials

Chapter 14

Measure	Number of items and Domains	Age / Respondent	Time	Reliability	Validity / Responsiveness
*†Pediatric Asthma Caregiver's Quality of Life Questionnaire[69]	Number of items = 13; Domains (2): Activity limitations and emotional function	7-17 years; Parent	Not reported	ICC = .80 to .85; *No internal consistency or cross-informant reliability reported*	Discriminates between levels of disease severity; Established MID (0.5 on a 7-point scale); Responsive to pharmacologic intervention; Used in clinical trials
Asthma-Related Quality of Life Scale (ARQOLS)[16]	Number of items = 35; Domains (5): Restriction of social life, physical disturbances, limitations in physical activity, daily inconveniences in managing the disease, and emotional distress	6-13 years; Child; No parent version	Not reported	α = .81 to .96	Responsive to pharmacologic intervention
TACQOL-Asthma[70]	Number of items = 68; Domains (5): Complaints (spontaneous asthma symptoms), situations (that provoke symptoms), treatment (visits to doctors), medication (use of, and emotions (negative emotions)	8-16 years; Child; Parent	Not reported	α = .60 to .85 (child); α = .64 to .82 (parent); Parent-Child agreement (ICC) = 64 to .76; *No test-retest reliability reported*	Discriminates between levels of disease severity, except in the complaint domain; Responsive to a behavioral intervention to promote medication adherence; Correlates with the PAQLQ
PedsQL-Asthma Module[71]	Number of items = 23; Generic Domains (4): Physical functioning, emotional functioning, social functioning, school functioning; Number of items = 28; Asthma-Specific Domains (4): Asthma symptoms, treatment problems, worry, communication	5-18 years; Child; 2-18 years; Parent	Not reported	α = .74 to .90 (child); α = .77 to .91 (parent); α = .58 to .85 (child); α = .82 to .91 (parent); Parent-child agreement (ICC) = .29 to .87; *No test-retest reliability reported*	Discriminates between healthy children and children with asthma; Correlates with the PAQLQ; Responsive to an evidence-based asthma management intervention (N = 10)
Life Activities Questionnaire for Childhood Asthma (LAQ)[72]	Number of items = 71; Domains (7): physical, work, outdoor, emotions and emotional behavior, home care, eating and drinking, and miscellaneous	5-17 years; Child; No parent version	Not reported	α = 0.97; Test-retest: r = 0.76	Not reported
How Are You? (HAY)[73]	Number of items = 32; Generic Domains (4): physical activities, cognitive activities, social activities, and physical complaints; Number of items = 40; Asthma-specific Domains (4): asthma symptoms, emotions related to asthma, self-concept, and self-management	8-12 years; Child; No parent version	20 minutes	α = .71 to .83; α = .61 to .81; ICC = .11 to .83	Discriminates between healthy and asthmatic children in terms of physical and social activities; Correlates with the Child Attitude Toward Illness Scale; Responsive to illness severity over time
Integrated Therapeutics Group Child Asthma Short Form (ITG-CASF)[74-75]	Number of items = 8; Domains (3): daytime symptoms, nighttime symptoms, and functional limitations	2-17 years; Parent only	Not reported	α = .84 to .92; *No test-retest reliability reported*	Correlates with asthma severity (p = .002), dyspnea (p = .03), and ER visits; Correlates with the number of days of school missed or limited activities for the child (r = −0.45) and parent (r = −0.25); Responsive to illness severity over time

*Denotes measures translated in different languages.

†Denotes the recommended measure.

Adapted with permission from Quittner AL, Modi A, Cruz I. Systematic review of health-related quality of life measures for children with respiratory conditions. *Paediatr Respir Rev.* 2008;9:220-232.

TABLE 14-3 HRQOL MEASURES FOR CHILDREN WITH CYSTIC FIBROSIS

MEASURE	NUMBER OF ITEMS AND DOMAINS	AGE RANGE AND RESPONDENT	COMPLETION TIME	PSYCHOMETRICS: RELIABILITY	PSYCHOMETRICS: VALIDITY
*Cystic Fibrosis Quality of Life Questionnaire (CFQoL)[76]	Number of items = 52 Domains (9): Physical, social, treatment issues; chest symptoms; emotional responses; concerns for future, interpersonal relationships, body image, and career	14 years to adulthood No parent version	Not reported	α = .72 to .92 Test-retest: >0.80; .74 for treatment issues	Discriminates between levels of disease severity Sensitivity to change following IV antibiotics, as measured by FEV_1 and BMI Correlates with total SF-36 scores (r's = .64 to .74)
*†Cystic Fibrosis Questionnaire—Revised (CFQ-R)[10,77–78]	Child Version—Number of items = 35 Domains (8): Physical, emotional state, social, body image, eating, treatment burden, respiratory, and digestion Adolescent/Adult Version Number of items = 50 Domains (12): Physical, emotional state, social, body image, eating, treatment burden, respiratory, digestion, role, vitality, health perceptions, weight Parent Version—Number of items = 44 Domains (11): Physical, emotional state, body image, eating, treatment burden, respiratory, digestion, vitality, school, weight	6-13 years Child 14 to adulthood Adolescent 6-13 years Parent *Pictorial version for children 3-6 in development*	10-15 minutes	α = .34-.73 (child); .55 to .94 (adolescent); .58-.90 (parent) Test-retest = .45 to .90 (teen/adult) Parent-child agreement = .27-.57	Teen/adult version is correlated with SF-36 Child version correlated with PedsQL Discriminates between healthy children and children with CF Discriminates between levels of disease severity Correlated with FEV_1, BMI, height, and weight Established 4 point MID on Respiratory Scale Sensitivity to change following treatment with IV antibiotics Used in many Phase III clinical trials as a primary endpoint Primary endpoint for approval of a new antibiotic
*Questions on Life Satisfaction—Cystic Fibrosis (FLZM-CF)[79]	Number of items = 9 Domains (9): Breathing difficulties/coughing, abdominal pain/digestive trouble, eating, sleep, routine therapy, adherence to daily therapy, significance for others, understanding, and free from disadvantage	12-17 years Child 16 to adulthood Adolescent No parent version	5-11 minutes	α = .80 Test-retest = .69	Child version correlates with KIDSCREEN Discriminates between healthy children and children with CF Adolescent/Adult version correlates with FEV_1 and amount of time spent doing treatments Discriminates between mild, moderate, and severe disease severity Responsive to change after inpatient rehabilitation, and following pulmonary exacerbations
*DISABKIDS—Cystic Fibrosis Module[80]	Number items = 37 Generic domains (6): Medication, emotion, social inclusion, social exclusion, limitation, and treatment Number items = 10 CF-specific domains (2): Impact (consists of limitations and symptoms), treatment	"Smileys" version for children 4-7 years Child 8-16 years Child	Not reported	α = .80 to .85 *No test-retest reliability reported*	Distinguishes between clinician-rated illness severity
*CF Respiratory Symptom Diary (CFRSD)[81–82]	Number of items = 16 Domains (3): Respiratory symptoms, emotional impact, activity impact	12+ years Child No parent version	Not reported	α = .72 to .87 Test-retest = 71 to .91	Differentiates between ill and well states Responsiveness is currently being evaluated as part of several clinical trials

*Denotes measures translated in different languages
†Denotes the recommended measure.
Adapted with permission from Quittner AL, Modi A, Cruz I. Systematic review of health-related quality of life measures for children with respiratory conditions. *Paediatr Respir Rev.* 2008;9:220-232.

TABLE 14-4 HRQOL FOR CHILDREN WITH VOCAL CORD DYSFUNCTION

MEASURE	NUMBER OF ITEMS AND DOMAINS	AGE RANGE & RESPONDENT	COMPLETION TIME	PSYCHOMETRICS: RELIABILITY	PSYCHOMETRICS: VALIDITY
Pediatric Voice Outcome Survey (PVOS)[86–87]	Number of items = 4	2-18 years Parent only	Not reported	α = .69 to .86 by age Test-retest = 0.89	• Discriminates between patients with and without tracheotomies (p = .004) • Discriminates between patients before and after adenoidectomy • Does not discriminate between healthy children and those with paradoxical vocal fold dysfunction
*Pediatric Voice-Related Quality of Life (PVR-QOL)[88]	Number of items = 10 Domains (2): social-emotional, physical-functional	2-18 years Parent only	Not reported	α = .96 Test-retest = 0.80	• Correlates with the PVOS (r = .70) • Responsive to change in 9 patients with adenoidectomy (p < .001) • Distinguishes between healthy children and those with vocal fold paralysis, vocal nodules, or paradoxical vocal fold dysfunction
†Pediatric Voice Handicap Index (pVHI)[89]	Number of items = 23 Domains (3): functional, physical, emotional Total and visual analog scale	4-21 years Parent only	Not reported	Test-Retest = .77 to .95 *No internal consistency reported*	• Discriminates between healthy children and those pre- or post-laryngotracheal reconstruction • Discriminates between children with benign vocal cord pathologies and other airway conditions

*Denotes the recommended measure.
†Denotes measures translated in different languages.
Adapted with permission from Quittner AL, Modi A, Cruz I. Systematic review of health-related quality of life measures for children with respiratory conditions. *Paediatr Respir Rev.* 2008;9:220-232.

Sleep-Related Breathing Disorders

Two measures are available to assess HRQOL in children with sleep-related breathing disorders (Table 14-5). Both instruments rely on parent-proxy reports of sleep disturbances, physical symptoms, and emotional functioning. These instruments extend down to children as young as 6 months of age, and they demonstrate adequate psychometric properties. While both measures can detect postsurgical change, only the OSA-18 has an established MID.

Despite the strengths of these measures, limitations exist with respect to utility and informant type. The OSA-18 uses a 1-month recall period, which increases the potential for recall bias and error. Further, the OSD-6 utilizes only one item per scale, which limits it ability to assess more complex constructs. Finally, both measures rely solely on parent or caregiver report, highlighting the need to develop patient-report instruments.

Recommendation

The OSA-18 is recommended due to the established MID. However, more research on the internal consistency of this measure is warranted.

Conclusions and Future Directions

The shift in medicine toward a patient-centered model of care is consistent with the PRO guidance established by the FDA.[3] This guidance outlined the steps needed for PRO development and highlighted the importance of including the patient perspective in the evaluation of new pharmacologic interventions. HRQOL instruments are one of the most commonly used types of PROs, and they provide a more comprehensive assessment of functioning across several domains (i.e., symptoms; physical, emotional, and social functioning; treatment burden). This information is useful for both research and clinical purposes; HRQOL assessment can track natural disease progression, evaluate responsivity to a behavioral or pharmacologic intervention, and guide clinical decision making. Several well-established HRQOL instruments exist for asthma, CF, vocal cord dysfunction, and sleep-related breathing disorders.

There is a need to develop disease-specific HRQOL measures for other pediatric respiratory disorders, including bronchopulmonary dysplasia, interstitial lung disease, ventilator dependency, and primary ciliary dyskinesia (PCD). Previous research on HRQOL for these pediatric populations has utilized generic measures. However, for

TABLE 14-5 HRQOL MEASURES FOR CHILDREN WITH SLEEP-RELATED BREATHING DISORDERS

MEASURE	NUMBER OF ITEMS & DOMAINS	AGE RANGE & RESPONDENT	COMPLETION TIME	PSYCHOMETRICS: RELIABILITY	PSYCHOMETRICS: VALIDITY
Obstructive Sleep Disorders-6 Survey (OSD-6)[90]	Number of items = 6 Domains (6): physical suffering, sleep disturbance, speech and swallowing difficulties, emotional distress, activity limitation, and level of concern	6 months to 12 years Parent only	Not reported	α = .80 across items Test-retest = .69 to .86	Responsive to change after adenotonsillectomy Correlates moderately with physician estimates of child's QOL Correlates with a global sleep-related QOL rating
*Obstructive Sleep Apnea-18 (OSA-18)[91]	Number of items = 18 Domains (5): Sleep disturbance, physical symptoms, emotional distress, daytime functioning, and caregiver concerns	6 months to 12 years Parent only	Not reported	Item-total correlations = .38 to .86 Test-retest = > .70 *No internal consistency reported*	Discriminates between mild, moderate, and severe sleep apnea Correlates with the OSD-6 and with Brouilette score Correlates with number of hourly apneic episodes, number of hypopneic events, and adenoid size Responsive to change after surgery Established MID

*Denotes the recommended measure.
Adapted with permission from Quittner AL, Modi A, Cruz I. Systematic review of health-related quality of life measures for children with respiratory conditions. *Paediatr Respir Rev.* 2008;9;220-232.

a complex condition such as PCD, which affects multiple domains of functioning, it is critical to assess HRQOL with a measure that captures disease-specific symptoms. In fact, initial steps are underway to develop a HRQOL measure for PCD.[92]

In conclusion, HRQOL measurement provides unique information on patients' symptoms, level of functioning, and response to treatment. Inclusion of these instruments has been shown to facilitate patient-provider communication, detect problematic areas of functioning that extend beyond physiologic symptoms, and enhance shared decision making. With the advent of technology,

the use of these instruments in clinical practice is on the rise and likely to become part of standard care for pediatric patients with chronic respiratory conditions. The integration of HRQOL measurement in both research and clinical practice is a critical step in promoting patient-centered care.

References

The complete reference list is available online at www. expertconsult.com

15 CHILDREN DEPENDENT ON RESPIRATORY TECHNOLOGY

HOWARD B. PANITCH, MD

Children who require technology for chronic respiratory insufficiency or failure constitute a small but varied group. The U.S. Congress Office of Technology Assessment (OTA) defined a technology-dependent child as "one who needs both a medical device to compensate for the loss of a vital body function and substantial and ongoing nursing care to avert death or further disability."[1] This definition does not take into account the site of care (i.e., hospital, home, or skilled facility) or credentials of the caregiver (i.e., professional nurse or trained layperson). Further, the OTA identified four separate groups of children that would be considered technology dependent. Two of these groups included children who were dependent on mechanical ventilation for at least part of the day and children who were dependent on other device-based respiratory support (e.g., tracheostomy tubes, airway suctioning, and supplemental oxygen use). This chapter will confine the discussion to those children who require technology for the treatment of chronic respiratory failure, a condition for which mechanical ventilatory support is required for at least 4 hours per day for 1 month or longer.[2-3]

Epidemiology

The large-scale need for chronic respiratory support of children began with the polio epidemics of the 1930s, 1940s and 1950s. The development of subspecialties in neonatology and pediatric critical care in the 1960s resulted in advances in medical therapies that allowed children with previously fatal conditions to survive, albeit occasionally with chronic conditions such as respiratory failure.[4] A focus on pediatric chronic respiratory failure did not occur in the United States until the early 1980s. In 1981, President Ronald Reagan waived the eligibility rules for Supplemental Security Income to allow Katie Beckett, a ventilator-dependent child, to be cared for at home without losing Medicaid benefits, thus bringing the population of children with chronic respiratory failure into the national spotlight.[5] In 1982, the Surgeon General then convened a Workshop on Children with Handicaps and Their Families, where he noted that advances in medical interventions created a new type of disability: infants who were chronically dependent on ventilatory support as a result of other medical interventions, which he referred to as "a creature of our new technology."[6]

The causes for chronic dependency on mechanical ventilation or supplemental oxygen can be categorized as: (1) those that affect the respiratory pump (respiratory muscles, rib cage, ventral abdominal wall); (2) those that affect respiratory drive; (3) extrathoracic and central airway lesions; and (4) pulmonary parenchymal and vascular abnormalities (Table 15-1). Individual patients can have more than one cause for chronic ventilator dependency, including neuromuscular weakness and severe kyphoscoliosis, anoxic encephalopathy with abnormal respiratory drive, recurrent aspiration, and obstructive sleep apnea.

There is no national registry that tracks the population of ventilator-assisted individuals in the United States. Center-specific surveys of children cared for in acute pediatric hospitals in the 1980s demonstrated that bronchopulmonary dysplasia (BPD) and noncardiac congenital anomalies were the most common diagnoses of infants and toddlers who required prolonged mechanical ventilation,[7-9] whereas spinal cord injury and underlying neuromuscular diseases were more common among those cared for in rehabilitation facilities.[10] In Massachusetts, surveys of children who received chronic mechanical ventilatory support outside of acute care hospitals throughout the state showed that the chief cause of chronic respiratory failure (CRF) in the 1980s[11] and early 1990s[12] was sequelae of prematurity or congenital malformations, but over the next 15 years the major causes of CRF were neuromuscular disease and central nervous system injury or malformations.[13] In addition, the number of children who received such care outside a hospital nearly tripled between 1990 and 2005.[13] National surveys from Canada, Europe, and Japan similarly demonstrated that neuromuscular disease and central nervous system injuries were the most common disorders for which chronic ventilation was used in children.[14-19] These diagnoses now represent the most common indications for chronic mechanical ventilation, which likely reflects a philosophical change toward providing chronic respiratory support to patients with progressive neuromuscular disorders,[20-21] an increasing role of noninvasive ventilation for these patients,[22] and a reflection of the types of patients who most commonly require prolonged care in pediatric intensive care units.[23]

The prevalence of children requiring chronic mechanical ventilation in most populations is unknown, but the number has grown over the last two decades. In 1987, the OTA estimated that there were between 600 and 2000 ventilator-dependent children in the United States.[1] Ten years later, extrapolations of a survey from Minnesota estimated that there were 17,824 ventilator-assisted individuals in the United States of whom 5534 would be younger than 21 years of age.[22] Survey data showed that subjects younger than 20 years of age represented about one third of all ventilator-assisted individuals in the state, with those younger than 11 years of age being the largest group and those 11 to 20 years of age accounting for the greatest increase since the prior survey in 1992.

TABLE 15-1 CONDITIONS LEADING TO TECHNOLOGY DEPENDENCE

Respiratory Pump

Neuromuscular diseases
Chest wall deformity/kyphoscoliosis
Spinal cord injury
Prune belly syndrome

Respiratory Drive

Congenital central hypoventilation syndrome
Brain/brainstem injury
Central nervous system tumors
Metabolic disorders

Airway

Craniofacial malformations
Obstructive sleep apnea
Tracheomalacia
Bronchomalacia

Pulmonary Parenchymal and Vascular Problems

Chronic lung disease of infancy (bronchopulmonary dysplasia)
Lung hypoplasia
Recurrent aspiration syndromes
Cystic fibrosis
Congenital heart disease

This survey included only patients in whom a backup ventilator rate was used; thus, the number was likely an underestimate. In the 1990s, the prevalence of children requiring chronic mechanical ventilation was estimated to be 0.5/100,000 in the United Kingdom,[16] 0.68/100,000 in Japan,[18] and 1.2 to 1.5/100,000 in the United States.[9,24] In 2004, it was estimated that 4,100 children (6/100,000) younger than 16 years of age received mechanical ventilation via tracheostomy outside the acute care setting throughout the United States.[25] No data are currently available for children supported by noninvasive positive pressure ventilation.

Goals of Therapy

The objectives of technology-dependent support are largely independent of the cause of respiratory failure. They include reversing or ameliorating the cause of respiratory compromise, extending life, improving physiologic function, and reducing morbidity.[26] In infants and young children, respiratory failure can also be associated with slow growth and developmental delay, so chronic ventilatory support is also used to promote these activities. Occasionally, ventilatory support is augmented during periods of physical activity to promote the child's potential for rehabilitation, or it is increased if the child fails to maintain adequate growth velocity. Thus, the desire to reduce support must be balanced with a more global view of the child's needs when formulating the daily prescription for mechanical ventilation.

Psychosocial development and quality of life can be enhanced when chronic ventilatory support can be safely accomplished outside the intensive care unit.[27] The home setting has long been considered the best place for

technology-dependent children in terms of their psychological and somatic development,[7,28–29] but excellent medical, psychosocial, and developmental support, including weaning from mechanical ventilation when appropriate, can be safely accomplished in inpatient rehabilitation facilities (within or outside the acute care hospital).[30–33] The setting for postacute care will depend on the degree of medical stability of the patient, the willingness and ability of family caregivers to provide care in the home, and community resources. Although the number of ventilator-dependent children has increased over the years and home care of this population has become more common, it should never be assumed *de facto* that home care is the best setting for an individual child or family; this can only be concluded once a full assessment of the child, family, resources, home care setting, and available alternative settings has been made. Additionally, the best location might change throughout a child's course, for instance as the child's medical condition improves or worsens, or if caregiver availability changes.

Pathophysiology of Respiratory Failure

Respiratory failure can result from an imbalance between the output of the respiratory pump and the load against which it has to work, development of respiratory muscle fatigue, inadequate respiratory drive, pulmonary parenchymal disease, or pulmonary vascular disease.[34] The disparity between the abilities of the respiratory pump and its load refer to either inadequate pump output for the imposed load, as in the case of a child with respiratory muscle weakness, or an increased load for the output. This could be the result of a reduction in lung compliance, an increase in pulmonary resistance, or stiffening of the chest wall itself. In theory, "pump failure" results in hypercapnia, whereas parenchymal disease causes hypoxemia. In practice, however, the two often coexist, and hypoventilation from pump failure will also result in hypoxemia. An understanding of the causes of respiratory failure often provides a rationale for the type of assisted ventilation that will provide the best support for the individual. It is critical to recognize that while chronic mechanical ventilation will not alter the ultimate prognosis for chronic progressive disorders (e.g., Duchenne muscular dystrophy, spinal muscular atrophy, or cystic fibrosis), its use can still prolong survival, relieve dyspnea, and improve daytime function and quality of life for children with such disorders.

Inadequate Pump Output: Neuromuscular Disease, Spinal Cord Injury

There is a typical progression of respiratory morbidity in patients with neuromuscular disease (NMD).[35] Once weakness of the respiratory muscles is present, airway clearance becomes compromised, predisposing patients to recurrent episodes of lower respiratory tract infections and atelectasis. This results in a decrease in lung compliance and therefore an increase in the load against which the respiratory pump must work. Infants and young children with NMD are more likely to experience complications from mucus plugging because their airways are smaller and peripheral airways contribute a greater proportion of intrathoracic resistance in children younger than 5 years of age.[36] Early in childhood, the chest wall of children with NMD is abnormally compliant[37]; as a result, the effect of chest wall recoil on lung volume and airway caliber is less, and this contributes to intrathoracic airway narrowing.

There are also ventilatory consequences of this alteration of chest wall compliance. In the young child with neuromuscular weakness and a highly compliant chest wall, much of the work of the respiratory muscles can be wasted as chest wall retractions reduce the contribution of the thoracic compartment to ventilation. Contraction of intercostal muscles can help maintain tidal volume, but at the cost of increased respiratory energy expenditure; thus, adequate ventilation can be maintained, but growth failure might ensue. In very young children, the imbalance between the highly compliant chest wall and relatively stiff lungs can result in an acquired *pectus excavatum* deformity.[38-39] Acquired chest wall deformity such as this has led to the theoretical concern that when chronic low-volume breathing is present in infants, it can also impair lung growth and development[40] (although this has never been demonstrated). Nevertheless, noninvasive ventilation has been used to correct or to prevent the development of pectus excavatum in young children with NMD.[38-39]

Over time, the chest wall of subjects with neuromuscular weakness becomes stiffer than normal because of prolonged periods of low tidal volume breathing without deep sigh breaths. This leads to the development of ankylosis around costovertebral joints with stiffening of ligaments and tendons. When present, the progression of kyphoscoliosis will contribute to a mechanical disadvantage around the costovertebral joint, making the respiratory muscles less efficient. The sum of these imbalances results in a restrictive pattern of lung function, with reduced vital capacity and total lung capacity. If subjects have significant expiratory muscle weakness, however, the residual volume and functional residual capacity can be normal or even slightly elevated, because the rib cage cannot be reduced below its normal resting volume.

As weakness progresses, patients experience episodes of hypoventilation during sleep, especially during rapid eye movement (REM) sleep. Obstructive apnea can also occur because of weakness of bulbar musculature. Initially, patients will demonstrate hypercapnia during sleep, but they will be able to maintain normocapnia while awake. As the severity of sleep-disordered breathing increases (either because of prolonged periods of nocturnal hypoventilation, mechanical alterations of the respiratory system, or both), central drive becomes blunted and the patient does not respond in an appropriate way to the challenge of elevated $PaCO_2$. At this point, diurnal hypercapnia will occur, but the daytime hypercapnia can be corrected if nocturnal mechanical support of breathing is instituted.[41] Further progression of weakness, however, will result in ineffective ventilation during the day and diurnal hypercapnia, even when nocturnal ventilation has been instituted.[42]

Timing of the progression of respiratory failure varies with different NMDs. In the absence of ventilatory support, infants with spinal muscular atrophy who are unable to sit typically die by 2 years of age.[43] In contrast, boys with Duchenne muscular dystrophy do not exhibit respiratory compromise until their second decade of life. Respiratory muscle weakness in congenital myopathies is often static, but as children grow their conditions deteriorate because their muscles cannot compensate for the increase in body mass. Often, respiratory failure ensues during the pubertal growth spurt.

Diaphragm paralysis results from cervical injury above C-3, or from phrenic nerve injury, often in the setting of birth trauma, cardiac surgery, or other thoracic surgery. Infants can occasionally compensate for unilateral paralysis, but bilateral diaphragmatic paralysis requires ventilatory support. When unilateral diaphragmatic paralysis causes respiratory failure, plication of the affected diaphragm often improves ventilation sufficiently that mechanical support is not required. If the paralysis is the result of trauma, plication does not prohibit recovery of diaphragm function.

Abnormal Respiratory Pump: Early-onset Scoliosis, Asphyxiating Thoracic Dystrophy, and Severe Kyphosis

The respiratory pump itself can present a load too great to be overcome by the muscles of respiration. Distortion of the thoracic cage from early-onset scoliosis results in a restrictive pattern of lung function.[44-45] A reduction in chest wall compliance can occur when the ribs are congenitally fused, the intercostal muscles are replaced by fibroconnective tissue after years of disuse, or costovertebral joints become ankylosed from chronic low–tidal-volume breathing without sigh breaths. Alternatively, distortion of the thoracic cage can place the inspiratory muscles at sufficient mechanical disadvantage to compromise their force-generating ability. Then the thoracic compartment is noncompliant, and the majority of the volume change that occurs with ventilation is in the abdominal compartment.

Abnormal Respiratory Drive: Congenital Central Hypoventilation Syndrome, Chiari Malformation, Brainstem Lesions, Leigh Disease

Several rare disorders result in an abnormal response to hypercapnia and hypoxemia. Congenital central hypoventilation syndrome (CCHS) represents a failure of the autonomic control of breathing and is caused by a defect in the paired *homeobox 2B (PHOX2B)* gene, which produces a transcription factor that is essential for the migration of neural crest cells and development of the autonomic nervous system.[46-48] There is a range of ventilatory abnormalities in children with CCHS. Some children present in the neonatal period with chronic alveolar hypoventilation and require around-the-clock ventilatory support, while others may not present until adulthood.[48] Often, as infants grow older, they are able to breathe adequately without support while awake, but they require ventilatory assistance during sleep and with acute illnesses. Because patients with CCHS do not respond appropriately to hypoxemia or hypercarbia, their mechanical ventilation strategy requires a mandatory rate to assure adequate ventilation. Since the underlying lung parenchyma and chest wall are normal, the delivered tidal volume should be normal as well.

Prader Willi syndrome and rapid-onset obesity with hypothalamic dysfunction, hypoventilation, and autonomic dysregulation (ROHHAD) represent two other disorders associated with potentially severe hypoventilation.[46–47] The majority of children with Prader Willi syndrome have a deletion of the long arm of chromosome 15, while the genetic abnormality leading to ROHHAD is currently unknown. Both conditions are associated with hyperphagia and rapid-onset obesity, but children with ROHHAD also have problems with salt and water balance. The presence of obesity in both conditions can also cause obstructive sleep apnea and contribute to sleep-related hypoventilation.

Children with Chiari malformation demonstrate a blunted response to hypercapnia, suggesting a central chemoreceptor problem.[47] They may also, however, have both central and obstructive apnea during sleep. Thus, assuring adequate minute ventilation and providing necessary distending pressure to overcome upper airway obstruction are both important strategies in supporting these patients. If the Chiari malformation is accompanied by myelomeningocele and kyphoscoliosis, adjustment of the tidal volume will be necessary.

Parenchymal Lung or Intrathoracic Airway Disease: Bronchopulmonary Dysplasia, Cystic Fibrosis, Tracheomalacia, Bronchiectasis

The majority of children in this category of respiratory failure are those with chronic sequelae of neonatal lung disease. Approximately 1.5% of all newborns develop bronchopulmonary dysplasia (BPD) (chronic lung disease of infancy),[49] making it the most common cause of chronic obstructive lung disease among infants. It is associated with lung hypoplasia resulting from arrest of alveolar development, but there is also evidence of parenchymal scarring, air trapping, and distortion of lung architecture. The central airways can become deformed from cyclic positive pressure distension, leading to acquired tracheomalacia or bronchomalacia. These abnormalities lead to a decrease in lung compliance and conductance, and thus an increase in respiratory pump load. Severe air trapping can impair diaphragm contractility by altering its length-tension relationships. These all can result in an unfavorable balance between respiratory pump output and load, leading to chronic respiratory failure and the need for prolonged mechanical ventilation. The energetics of breathing may constitute as much as 25% of the infant's caloric needs. Thus, if weaning from mechanical ventilation is too aggressive, some infants with BPD can maintain adequate gas exchange, but only at the expense of growth and development. The need for supplemental oxygen will depend on the extent of parenchymal damage, hypoplasia, or ventilation/perfusion mismatch. Most infants with BPD who require chronic mechanical ventilation develop respiratory failure while in the neonatal intensive care unit and do not recover before they are otherwise considered ready for discharge. Occasionally, however, chronic respiratory failure ensues after discharge in the setting of an acute viral lower respiratory illness. Prolonged mechanical ventilation is appropriate in both settings, as lung function is expected to improve with growth and postnatal lung development.

In recent years, chronic mechanical ventilation of patients with cystic fibrosis (CF) has been performed, first as a bridge to lung transplant, and subsequently as a palliative measure. Like other patients whose respiratory pump becomes inadequate for the load, patients with CF and severe airway obstruction develop a rapid, shallow breathing pattern that is inefficient.[50,51] When challenged with an increased load or imposed hypercapnea, the mechanics of the respiratory system limit the patient's response.[50–52] As obstruction worsens, dynamic compliance of the lung falls as well, contributing to an increased respiratory load.[51] At the same time, downward displacement of the diaphragm from hyperinflation places it in a less favorable mechanical position, contributing to inefficiency of the respiratory pump.

General Considerations for Home Care

Often, the need for chronic mechanical ventilatory support is determined following an acute illness, when the child is unable to wean from mechanical ventilation. In other children, the requirement for chronic mechanical ventilation is recognized following an abnormal polysomnogram, or identification of other nonacute indicators (e.g., poor growth or chronic dyspnea). No matter the presentation, once chronic mechanical ventilation has been determined to be necessary for the support of a child, the eventual site of long-term care must be determined. This requires assessment not only of the medical stability and suitability of the child, but also of the family as potential medical caregivers. Other decisions regarding the approach to the child's care (e.g., the performance of a tracheostomy) require careful consideration as to how the choice of the child's site of care will be affected.

A child's medical stability must be evaluated within the context of the site of care. The required level of stability at the time of transfer from a pediatric intensive care unit (PICU) will differ between home and a care site within a hospital or a subacute care facility (Table 15-2).[26,30] In any setting, the child must have a stable airway (natural or tracheostomy), have blood gas values that are appropriate for the underlying diagnosis, and not have care demands that exceed the resources of the site of care. When a child goes home supported by mechanical ventilation for the first time, there should be no changes in the medical plan for at least 1 week before discharge to assure that the child is adequately supported on the proposed regimen.

When a technology-dependent child is being discharged to home, two adults must be willing and able to learn and assume all aspects of the child's daily care, including dosages and indications for all medications being used, feedings, airway clearance and respiratory assessment, ventilator assessment and troubleshooting, and equipment care. If the child will receive mechanical ventilation through a tracheostomy, the family caregivers must also learn how to suction the artificial airway and perform routine and emergency tracheostomy tube changes. In addition, there must be adequate financial support from third-party payers to provide the equipment and supplies necessary to care for the child at home. The residence in which the child will be cared for must have adequate space for the child, equipment, and visiting health care

TABLE 15-2 CRITERIA FOR MEDICAL STABILITY

HOME	GENERAL HOSPITAL WARD/ TRANSITIONAL CARE FACILITY
Clinical	
Positive trend on growth curve	No need for 1:1 nursing care
Stamina for periods of play	No invasive monitoring
No frequent fevers or infections	No need for intravenous vasopressors or vasodilators
Physiologic	
Stable airway	Mature tracheostomy ≥ 1 week postoperatively
$PaO_2 \geq 60$ Torr in $FiO_2 \leq 0.4$	$SpO_2 > 92\%$ in $FiO_2 \leq 0.40$
$PaCO_2 < 50$ Torr (parenchymal disease) or < 45 Torr (chest wall or neuromuscular disease)	Stable blood gases within normal range for the diagnosis
No need for frequent ventilator changes	Stable ventilator settings ≥ 1 week

Adapted from Make BJ, Hill NS, Goldberg AI, et al. Mechanical ventilation beyond the intensive care unit. Report of a consensus conference of the American College of Chest Physicians. *Chest.* 1998;113:289S-344S; Ambrosio IU, Woo MS, Jansen MT, et al. Safety of hospitalized ventilator-dependent children outside of the intensive care unit. *Pediatrics.* 1998;101:257-259.

providers. The home must have running water, heat, electricity, and a working telephone. Entrances must be accessible for patients confined to a wheelchair.

The discharge plan must also include the amount of skilled nursing care the family will require. All families of children who cannot correct an airway or ventilator problem or call for help should be offered skilled nursing care for at least a portion of the day to allow caregivers to sleep with reassurance that the child's welfare is not at risk. Funding for these services, which are the most expensive component of the home care of technology-dependent children,[2] should be guaranteed by third-party payers with periodic reassessments established to determine ongoing needs. While there are no uniform criteria for establishing the number of nursing hours provided, it should be determined by the medical needs of the child, the capabilities of the family, and other demands on family providers (e.g., work, other children in the home). To allow caregivers time off from continuous medical care and monitoring of the child, funded respite care should also be built into the discharge plan as it has been repeatedly identified as an essential component of the home care plan to help relieve stress and caregiver burnout.[53-58]

Treatment of Chronic Respiratory Failure

Noninvasive Ventilation (NIV)
Noninvasive ventilation refers to correction of alveolar hypoventilation or upper airway obstruction without the use of artificial airways (i.e., endotracheal or tracheostomy tubes). Noninvasive ventilation is usually used

at night, rather than continuously, but if a child has a progressive disorder or experiences an acute decompensation, NIV can be used 24 hours per day.[59] For patients with NMD or chest wall restriction who develop symptomatic hypercapnic respiratory failure, 4 hours or more of nocturnal NIV per day can cause a sustained decrease in daytime $PaCO_2$ and resolution of symptoms related to sleep-disordered breathing.[60] For instance, nocturnal NIV corrected diurnal hypercapnia and severe nocturnal hypoventilation and maintained normal daytime $PaCO_2$ for an extended period in a group of 23 young men with Duchenne muscular dystrophy.[61] In this series, nocturnal NIV was associated not only with improved survival (85% at 1 year, and 73% from 2 to 5 years), but also with sustained improvement in daytime gas exchange throughout the 5-year duration of the study.

The proposed mechanisms by which nocturnal NIV improves overall function in patients with restrictive disorders include resting of the respiratory muscles to reverse fatigue,[62] improving lung and chest wall mechanics by reversing areas of microatelectasis and increasing chest wall excursion,[60,63-66] and resetting central chemoreceptor sensitivity to CO_2.[60,63] These mechanisms are not necessarily mutually exclusive, but evidence that NIV improves lung or chest wall mechanics in a sustained way is lacking. Several series involving subjects with a variety of neuromuscular diseases failed to demonstrate an increase in vital capacity after the institution of NIV,[60,63-65] and the institution of NIV in young men with Duchenne muscular dystrophy before the onset of respiratory failure failed to slow the expected decline in vital capacity.[66] Furthermore, direct measurements of lung and chest wall compliance after 3 months of NIV did not change in a series of 20 patients with neuromuscular disease and restrictive defects.[60] By contrast, the investigators demonstrated enhanced responsiveness to CO_2 in these subjects after 3 months of NIV, suggesting a resetting of central chemoreceptors and enhancement of respiratory drive. Another study showed that nocturnal NIV can restore CO_2 responsiveness by an alternate method: reduction of respiratory muscle fatigue and improvement in respiratory muscle endurance.[42] Investigators calculated the tension time index of the respiratory muscles (a noninvasive measurement of the likelihood of muscle fatigue) in 50 subjects with Duchenne muscular dystrophy just after they ended a night of NIV support (8 AM) and again just before they resumed nocturnal NIV (8 PM). To assess respiratory muscle endurance, the authors also measured the time to fatigue (T_{lim}) after pressure threshold loading under the same conditions. There was a progressive increase in the tension time index and a decrease in T_{lim} that correlated with progression of symptoms. In the most affected subjects, however, the tension time index decreased and T_{lim} increased significantly following a night of NIV support. Thus, these data suggest that nocturnal NIV can unload weakened respiratory muscles, thereby improving their daytime capacity and reducing their fatigability.

While noninvasive ventilation is usually confined to those who require support for 16 hours per day or less, it has been used successfully in patients who require continuous support.[59,67] This can be achieved by either a nasal interface or a mouthpiece.[59,67–68] Contraindications include poor glottic function, inability to achieve adequate ventilation noninvasively, patient preference, and lack of caregiver expertise.[59] However, sometimes NIV has been used successfully in infants with spinal muscular atrophy and children with static encephalopathy who have impaired glottic function.[69]

Complications of positive pressure NIV are related either to the interface itself or misdirection of the applied pressure. Choices of nasal or oronasal interfaces for infants and small children are limited, so adaptation of adult interfaces is often necessary.[70] Poorly fitting interfaces lead to leaks that not only interfere with adequacy of ventilation, but can also cause eye irritation. In response, straps are often tightened to reduce the leak. This can cause facial erythema, or if the pressure is applied long enough, skin ulceration can occur.[71] Use of a custom-molded mask[71] or an alternate interface with different pressure points can reduce this complication, but attention to skin integrity is an integral component of care for the child receiving positive pressure NIV. Skin ulceration can preclude the ability to provide effective NIV and force a decision to advance to tracheostomy. Prolonged application of pressure by nasal interfaces on the growing face has been associated with midface flattening.[71–73] Although special devices have been created to correct this,[73] to avoid the problem one should consider the use of more than one interface with different pressure points, or a custom molded mask.[74]

High flows related to NIV can cause nasal congestion and mouth dryness[75]; humidifying the circuit can ameliorate these deleterious side effects. The positive pressure applied during NIV has been associated with ear and sinus pain in adults,[76] and higher positive pressures can cause aerophagia and gastric distension, which, in turn, can impair the effectiveness of NIV by creating abdominal competition for lung expansion.

Ventilation via Tracheostomy

Invasive ventilation via tracheostomy is typically used in infants and children with parenchymal lung or congenital heart disease. In addition, it is used in young children who require continuous mechanical ventilation, those with severe craniofacial malformations (or other causes of upper airway or central airway obstruction that cannot be corrected by NIV), and those with severe developmental delay.[3,8,25] Whenever possible, relatively small tracheostomy tubes are used to allow for a leak.[26,77] This facilitates speech and avoids damage to the tracheal wall. When the leak around the tracheostomy tube is large, however, effective mechanical ventilation can be compromised. This is especially true if the child is being ventilated in a volume-control mode, since the large leak will prevent adequate development of intrathoracic pressure to expand the chest because the ventilator breath escapes through the mouth and nose. The leak may be variable, so that even when mechanical ventilation is adequate during awake hours, significant hypoventilation can occur during sleep.[78] This is remedied either by changing to a pressure control mode of ventilation or by using a cuffed tracheostomy tube.

The presence of a tracheostomy increases the complexity of care for most patients requiring ventilatory assistance. Caregivers must be taught how to suction, clean, and change the tracheostomy tube and how to assess for displacement and obstruction.[77] The presence of a tracheostomy tube interferes with the child's speech and swallowing, increases the risk for infection and aspiration, and is associated with airway complications (e.g., infection at the stoma site, granuloma formation, tracheal stenosis, and traumatic tracheoinnominate or tracheoesophageal fistula formation).[79–81] While the presence of a tracheostomy alone can increase caregiver stress,[82] in select situations (e.g., the need for continuous ventilatory assistance and difficulty with secretion management in a young child) it can ease the care burden. Thus, the decision to advance from noninvasive to invasive ventilation must be individualized, considering the impact on both the child and the child's caregivers.

Options for Ventilatory Support
Body Ventilators

Initially, negative pressure body ventilators were used to augment the ventilatory efforts of patients with restrictive lung disease.[76] Devices such as the iron lung (tank ventilator), chest shell, poncho, and cuirass ventilators can all successfully reverse respiratory failure in children.[76,83–84] Negative pressure body ventilators, however, are cumbersome and can cause upper airway obstruction.[76,84–85] This may result from phasic collapse of the epiglottis or a lack of pre-inspiratory upper airway muscle activation before the ventilator supplies a negative pressure breath.[86–87] Negative pressure ventilators are difficult to get into and out of; thus they are not well suited for subjects who require frequent access for care. They are not portable, so the user cannot readily travel, or sleep at other people's homes. A negative pressure ventilator, however, can be an excellent alternative for the patient who cannot tolerate placement of a nasal device or the sensation of nasal positive pressure. Positive pressure body ventilators, like the pneumobelt, are used only to a limited degree in children. The pneumobelt must be used while the patient is in a seated position, so it is not suitable for treatment of nocturnal hypoventilation.

Positive Pressure Devices

The most common way for children to receive ventilatory assistance noninvasively is by positive pressure delivered via nasal, oronasal, or mouthpiece interface. Application of positive pressure can relieve upper airway obstruction as well as improve minute ventilation and unload inspiratory muscles. The source of positive pressure can be a portable volume or pressure preset ventilator, bi-level positive airway pressure (B_iPAP) device, or continuous positive airway pressure (CPAP) device. B_iPAP and CPAP devices use a blower to generate flow adequate to achieve the desired pressure set by the practitioner. Portable ventilators use pistons or turbines to generate the selected volume or pressure, and can do so at lower flow rates. Newer positive pressure ventilators also can provide continuous flow that allows for spontaneous breathing without imposing additional work and dead space. In general, B_iPAP units are smaller than portable ventilators.

They operate more quietly, compensate for leaks better, and are also less costly than portable ventilators.[88] On the other hand, B$_i$PAP devices cannot generate such high peak pressures and have higher rates of energy consumption than portable ventilators.[89] Unlike portable ventilators, most B$_i$PAP devices do not contain an internal battery. Because they use a single limb circuit for inspiration and exhalation, they also are more likely to promote rebreathing than systems with a double-limb circuit.

Some consider that CPAP is not a form of noninvasive ventilation, since the patient receives neither mandatory breaths nor assistance during spontaneous efforts. CPAP can, however, unload respiratory muscles and enhance minute ventilation by relieving upper airway obstruction, offsetting intrinsic PEEP, or improving lung compliance. B$_i$PAP devices provide pressure support ventilation, in which the patient's spontaneous effort is supported to a preset pressure. The supported breath is initiated by the patient, and the support is cycled off when inspiratory flow falls to a preset percent of peak flow. Many B$_i$PAP devices have, in addition to a spontaneous mode, timed or combined spontaneous/timed modes in which mandatory breaths can be delivered in the event the patient's drive or ability to trigger the machine is inadequate. The sensitivity of trigger and cycle variables differ according to manufacturers,[90-91] making some machines a poor choice for infants or patients who are very weak.[92] In such circumstances, the practitioner can set a mandatory rate higher than the child's spontaneous rate to overcome the mechanical shortcomings of the system.[69] When supplemental oxygen is required, the amount bled into the system can mask the patient's inspiratory efforts by contributing additional flow that must be overcome to trigger the device. The final FiO$_2$ delivered to the patient will vary depending not only on the flow rate of oxygen bled into the system, but also on where in the circuit the oxygen is introduced and the inspiratory pressure measured.[93] It is unusual to be able to deliver an FiO$_2$ above 0.5 to 0.7 noninvasively.[93-94]

Older portable ventilators, which are still in use, are able to provide only volume-preset breaths in which a desired tidal volume is set by the practitioner. Breaths can be delivered in synchronized intermittent mandatory ventilation (SIMV) mode, where the patient breathes spontaneously but unsupported through the ventilator circuit in between mandatory positive pressure breaths delivered according to a set rate, or in Assist/Control (A/C) mode. Here, the practitioner sets a rate at which mandatory breaths are delivered, but if the patient wishes to breathe above that rate, each effort results in a fully supported positive pressure breath. Such machines also require the use of an external PEEP valve if end-distending pressure is required for the patient. When large leaks are present in children with tracheostomies who use this type of ventilator, it is usually not possible to maintain the set PEEP.

Newer portable ventilators can provide either pressure preset or volume preset breaths, pressure support breaths, and continuous flow. Thus, they are more versatile, allowing for more modes of ventilatory support that can enhance ventilator-patient synchrony and hence patient comfort. They can be used to provide CPAP with or without pressure support, SIMV with or without pressure support, and A/C ventilation. Both trigger and cycle variables can be adjusted on most models. All have internal batteries, and marine batteries or newer lightweight lithium batteries allow for their use away from an electrical power source for several hours.

No single type of positive pressure device is ideal for all patients. Patient characteristics, as well as machine characteristics (e.g., trigger and cycle sensitivities and sensitivity to leaks) can influence the degree of patient-ventilator dys-synchrony and adequacy of ventilatory assistance.[90-92] Patients who breathe spontaneously will benefit from features such as continuous flow and pressure support. Patients with no spontaneous respiratory effort (e.g., children with cervical spinal cord injury) do not require such accessories, and their presence can occasionally be detrimental; in the setting of a large leak around the child's tracheostomy or interface, the leak will be interpreted by the ventilator as a patient-initiated breath and will result in unintended excessive ventilation or ventilator autocycling. If trigger or cycle sensitivities are not adequate, the child will make inspiratory efforts that are not supported or have to exhale while the device continues to provide a positive pressure breath.[95] In the best circumstances, the needs of the child are matched to the capabilities of the device, and interactions between device and child are assessed critically before the child is given the machine for long-term use.[92]

Ancillary Equipment

In addition to the actual ventilator, other equipment needs of children requiring chronic mechanical ventilation will vary depending on the interface being used (noninvasive versus tracheostomy), how many hours the child can tolerate being without ventilator support, and whether or not the child spends most waking hours in a wheelchair. In addition, how far the child lives from the medical center or durable medical equipment company, and how frequently power outages occur in the child's community are important considerations.

Children who use nasal or oronasal interfaces should have a second, different-style interface available to interchange with the primary one. In this way, different areas of the face are exposed to pressure from the mask, and discomfort or skin injury can be minimized or avoided. Small children, those who perspire excessively, and those who have difficulty controlling secretions should have backup headgear available for noninvasive interfaces. Fixation devices for noninvasive interfaces come in a variety of materials and, often because nasal interfaces are used that were designed for adults, straps must be altered or extra hook and loop (Velcro) straps added to fit the child's head and keep the interface in place. Whenever the mask or tubing touches the child's skin, adequate padding must be provided and frequent assessments performed to avoid skin injury. Children with tracheostomies should have a second tracheostomy tube available for emergencies and another tube one size smaller in case there is difficulty reinserting the tube during an unplanned tube change. To avoid skin breakdown under the ties, children who drool excessively may require extra tracheostomy tube holders to allow for frequent changes. Twill tape, Velcro, neoprene, and beaded-chain tracheostomy holders all are available and are chosen based on patient/family preference and the experiences of the health care team. Standards for tracheostomy care in children have been published that detail the equipment required for their use.[77]

Home mechanical ventilators are reliable pieces of equipment. In a survey of 150 ventilator users followed over 1 year, of whom 44 were 18 years of age or younger, defective equipment or ventilator failure occurred on average only once per 1.25 years of continuous ventilator use.[96] Of the 189 incidents of suspected ventilator failure, actual equipment malfunction or failure was responsible for the report in only 73 (39%). Two patients required re-hospitalization, and in both cases a change in the patient's condition that mimicked equipment failure, rather than a true ventilator malfunction, was the cause for re-hospitalization. Nevertheless, if a child cannot tolerate absence of ventilatory support for more than 4 hours of the day[26] or if the child lives more than 1 hour from the tertiary care center or home equipment company,[96] the child should have a second ventilator and complete circuit setup in the home in case of emergency. If the child spends most of the day in a wheelchair, two setups are usually made available: one setup is left on the chair for daytime use, and a second setup is kept at the bedside. To ensure proper functioning, mechanical ventilators and other equipment should undergo routine checks at least monthly and should receive preventive maintenance as needed.[26] These checks should include not only assessment of various ventilator functions (e.g., inspiratory and expiratory pressures, trigger sensitivity, oxygen delivery, alarms) but also of whether the actual settings match the patient's prescription.[97]

Most of the newer ventilators designed for home use have an internal battery that can be used during transfers or in the case of a brief power outage. Usually the internal battery life is only about 1 hour, however, and will vary with the amount of support required by the child.[98] External batteries are necessary when the child is expected to spend longer periods of time away from an electrical power source. These batteries can last up to 12 hours, again depending on the child's ventilator requirements.[98] Some systems also permit the ventilator to use power from the battery of an electric wheelchair to reduce the bulk of equipment that must be transported. Batteries enhance the child's portability and can be used in emergencies when electrical power is not available, but if the child lives in an area where electrical power outages are frequent, a backup generator may be required to keep the child safely at home during outages and to run other equipment like suction machines and monitors.

Infants and children who are supported by mechanical ventilation via tracheostomy require humidification of the ventilator circuit, since bypassing the natural upper airway results in delivery of cool, dry air to the central airways. This can result in ineffective secretion clearance and plugging of the artificial airway. Inspired gas should be humidified to 28 to 35 mg/L and should be heated to 29° to 35° C.[77,99] This can be achieved with heated humidifiers or heat-moisture exchangers. The effectiveness of heat moisture exchangers varies by manufacturer,[100] and

their efficiency decreases with increasing tidal volume, inspiratory flow, and minute ventilation.[99] Heat moisture exchangers are not as efficient as heated humidifiers in infants and small children, and should be confined to use during travel or waking hours, with a heated humidifier used during sleep. The addition of heating devices to the ventilator circuit can increase ventilatory demands; heated humidifiers increase ventilator circuit compliance, and heat moisture exchangers add dead space to the circuit. In both cases, the set tidal volume may have to be increased to accommodate these changes. Children who use noninvasive ventilation do not necessarily require humidification of the circuit. Patients who complain about nasal congestion or dryness, however, can benefit from addition of humidification to the circuit, and often patients are more comfortable when the delivered air is humidified.

Patients ventilated via tracheostomy, and those with neuromuscular or neurologic conditions using noninvasive ventilation require suction equipment. Both stationary and portable devices should be available to afford patients freedom to leave the home.[56] Portable suction machines are capable of developing pressures in excess of the 60 to 150 Torr recommended for airway suctioning.[101] All patients with tracheostomies and those who use noninvasive ventilation to treat alveolar hypoventilation require a manual ventilation system (e.g., self-inflating resuscitation bag) for use with suctioning or during emergencies. Patients with impaired cough can use a self-inflating bag to provide insufflation before manually assisted cough, or they can use specialized equipment (e.g., a mechanical insufflator) to aid with airway clearance.[56]

Home positive pressure mechanical ventilators have internal alarms, as do many newer B_iPAP machines. These include low-pressure or patient-disconnect alarms and power failure, low-battery, high-pressure, apnea, low–minute volume, and low–tidal volume alarms. These alarms provide early warning in the case of machine failure, ventilator disconnection, inadvertent decannulation, tracheostomy tube obstruction, or excessive leak of a noninvasive circuit. The low pressure alarm present on ventilators delivering positive pressure via tracheostomy is typically set 5 cm below the desired peak pressure to be delivered.[26] However, the low pressure alarm might not sound in the setting of an inadvertent decannulation when used with children who require small tracheostomy tubes (<4.5 mm inside diameter) because of the high resistance of the tube.[102] For this reason, additional monitoring with external devices is used for early detection of emergency situations.

The use of external monitors remains practice-driven, not data-driven. No author advocates recreating an ICU environment at home, but considerable differences of opinion exist regarding the roles of home cardiorespiratory impedance monitoring, pulse oximetry, and capnometry.* Monitoring practice also varies depending on the method of ventilatory assistance, between tracheostomy-delivered, noninvasive positive pressure, and negative pressure ventilation.[13] Impedance monitors are advocated generally by some[4,104] or for use in certain circumstances, such as when a child requires a tracheostomy tube smaller than 4.5 mm.[26]

---

*References 3, 4, 26, 56, 103, and 104.

Others feel that such monitoring is both redundant and unnecessary.[103] Importantly, the cardiorespiratory monitor will not alarm in the event of a tube obstruction, inadvertent decannulation, or ventilator disconnection until the child has become hypoxemic enough to experience bradycardia. Pulse oximetry monitoring is not universally advocated,[103–104] but when employed it can be used to fulfill several functions. It is used as a surveillance device, with continuous oximetry monitoring recommended when the child is asleep or unattended.[3] A decrease in death and severe hypoxic encephalopathy related to airway accidents has been attributed to its use in this fashion,[9] as oximetry will detect hypoxemia associated with ventilator failure, tube obstruction, or accidental disconnection sooner than these events can be discovered by cardiorespiratory monitoring. Pulse oximetry is also used to assist in weaning supplemental oxygen or ventilator support, and as an early warning of lower respiratory tract complications (such as bronchospasm or infection) that might require an increase in ventilatory support. Pulse oximetry monitoring is an integral component for patients with neuromuscular disease, where hypoxemia heralds the need for increased airway clearance, or delay in airway extubation to noninvasive ventilatory support after an acute illness.[69] Importantly, absence of nocturnal hypoxemia by pulse oximetry monitoring does not preclude significant episodes of hypercapnia in children who require nocturnal ventilation for treatment of alveolar hypoventilation.[105] Capnometry or capnography is not advocated by all,[103] but its intermittent use can help in assessing a child's ability to sustain adequate ventilation during weaning trials. Continuous capnography or capnometry is not indicated for home monitoring. Recently, a transcutaneous oximeter/capnometer was shown to be accurate and effective in assessing gas exchange in children with chronic respiratory failure using noninvasive ventilation at home.[105]

In general, the recommendation for external monitoring must be individualized. While such monitoring can be lifesaving, the monitors themselves can also increase caregiver stress and anxiety.[82] False alarms can disrupt parents' sleep, contributing to caregiver sleep deprivation.[54,106] No monitoring system can fully replace direct patient observation, and none of the external monitors should be considered as a surrogate for appropriate ventilator alarms.

Patient Follow-up

The course of children with chronic respiratory failure is either one of gradual improvement with ability to be liberated from mechanical ventilation, or a trajectory of worsening, depending largely on the natural history of the underlying disease. The frequency with which children need to be seen will vary according to where they are in their disease process and the comfort of the health care team and family with performing interventions at home. For instance, an adolescent with Type 2 spinal muscular atrophy (SMA) might require only semiannual visits once growth has stopped and progression of the underlying disease is slow. An infant with Type 1 SMA is likely to require visits every 2 to 3 months to reassess adequacy of ventilation and airway clearance.

Children with chronic respiratory failure can be weaned partially or completely from mechanical ventilation in postacute rehabilitation facilities[32–33] or in the home. In our practice, once a child has demonstrated tolerance for reduction in ventilator support during an office visit, the family is given guidelines for reduction in support and clinical indicators for tolerance of reduction of support. During weekly telephone interviews, changes in vital signs, weight gain, tolerance for physical activity, and overall mood are assessed, and if the child tolerates the reduction in support, orders are given for continued slow reduction of ventilator assistance. Often several days of reduction are required before intolerance becomes apparent, either through an alteration in mood, a reduction in activity, or a failure to continue to gain weight. Thus, reductions occur only weekly or at most twice weekly. A 20% increase in heart rate or respiratory rate from the resting condition or the failure to maintain adequate gas exchange as determined by oximetry and capnometry are indicators to curtail further weaning immediately. There is no single best way to liberate a child from mechanical ventilation. Some practitioners gradually reduce the level of pressure support or number of mandatory breaths delivered to the patient. Our practice usually is to begin weaning trials either to CPAP or completely off support for short periods once or twice a day, returning the child to the usual level of support for the duration of the day. The weaning trials are gradually lengthened as tolerated while the child is awake until the child is breathing independently for all waking hours. Further reduction of support then occurs during naps, and finally during sleeping hours overnight. The ability to liberate a child from daytime mechanical ventilation, even if nocturnal support is still required, minimizes the need for community health services and promotes school attendance.[107]

If a child undergoes tracheostomy placement to facilitate chronic mechanical ventilation and is weaned from ventilator support, decannulation of the trachea should be considered. There is no single best approach to tracheal decannulation. Most authors recommend bronchoscopy before attempted decannulation to assess for airway obstruction from granulation tissue, suprastomal collapse, tracheomalacia, enlarged tonsils or adenoids, and vocal cord paralysis.[108–110] Once airway patency is assured, the tube is often downsized and capped for a period of time,[109–111] whereas other authors simply remove the tube.[112] In all cases, however, the child is hospitalized for observation for 24 to 48 hours to be certain that airway compromise does not develop after tube removal. Polysomnography with the tube downsized and capped can be used as an adjunct when concern about patency of the airway during sleep affects the decision to decannulate the airway.[111] In each case, the approach to tracheal decannulation should be tailored to the individual's condition.[109]

Children with tracheostomies require routine tube changes. Recommendations, based on practice rather than evidence, range from daily to monthly with most experts suggesting a weekly timetable.[77] More frequent changes may be required in the setting of an acute infection when thick secretions can obstruct the tube. Bacterial colonization of the airway is almost ubiquitous in patients with tracheostomies,[113] but most experts do not advocate the routine use of oral or inhaled antimicrobials for prophylaxis against pneumonia.[114] While *Pseudomonas aeruginosa* and *Staphylococcus aureus* are the two most commonly isolated organisms from patients on long-term mechanical ventilation, anaerobes may also play an important role and should be considered when antimicrobial treatment is contemplated.[115] Routine bronchoscopic evaluation to assess for airway lesions or narrowing, and appropriate sizing of the tube, is recommended every 6 to 12 months or more frequently in a child experiencing rapid changes in growth or medical condition.[77] In the absence of bleeding or difficulty with tracheostomy tube changes, however, some otolaryngologists do not perform routine bronchoscopic evaluation.

Infants and toddlers with BPD experience exacerbations of respiratory failure most commonly as a result of acute wheezing illnesses and nonbacterial respiratory infections. During such episodes, ventilatory support may have to be increased to meet demands. The first intervention for respiratory distress in a child with a tracheostomy is to perform a tracheostomy tube change to be sure there is no partial obstruction of the tube causing the distress. Occasionally, antimicrobials are administered when tracheal secretions remain purulent, elevated neutrophils are identified on sputum Gram stain, and a predominant bacterial organism is recovered from the sputum culture.[114] Thereafter, if minor changes in ventilator support do not correct gas exchange abnormalities, or if the family or skilled caregivers are not comfortable with continuing care at home, the child should be hospitalized for care.

Patients with neuromuscular weakness may experience acute deterioration in respiratory function when impaired mucus clearance leads to atelectasis, or respiratory infections cause increased mucus production with airway obstruction. The first intervention is to increase airway clearance to resolve the obstruction or to keep pace with increased mucus production. Experts also recommend judicious use of antimicrobials for respiratory infections,[43] even when the illness begins as a viral infection, presumably because stasis of mucus predisposes to secondary bacterial infections. Patients supported by NIV may require longer (up to continuous) periods of ventilatory support during the acute illness, or an increase in applied positive pressure. Distending pressure (expiratory positive airway pressure, EPAP) is often increased to overcome atelectasis, while inspiratory positive airway pressure (IPAP) may have to be increased to offset increases in airways resistance or a decrease in lung compliance. If the child requires airway intubation for an acute illness, some experts advocate waiting until the child has weaned from supplemental oxygen before attempting extubation to noninvasive support.[69] Progression of the underlying neuromuscular disease can lead to inadequate support, so symptoms of sleep-related hypoventilation should be sought at each office encounter and reassessment of ventilatory requirements during sleep should occur at least annually.[116]

Outcomes

Weaning from Ventilator Support
The underlying cause of respiratory failure is the principal determinant of whether a child eventually will be liberated from ventilator support.* Several studies suggest

that children who receive chronic mechanical ventilation for parenchymal lung disease (e.g., bronchopulmonary dysplasia) or central airway lesions (e.g., tracheomalacia) are more likely to be able to wean from mechanical ventilation than those with neuromuscular weakness or multiple congenital anomalies.* This finding likely reflects the propensity for improvement in a child's lung mechanics or respiratory pump function over time in the former group, and deterioration in lung and respiratory pump function in the latter. One of these reviews, in which 20% of the 228 patient cohort carried a diagnosis of central hypoventilation syndrome, included transitioning from chronic mechanical ventilation to diaphragm pacing as a reflection of successful weaning.[118] Severity of underlying disease also may influence weaning outcome. Of 35 children requiring chronic mechanical ventilation via tracheostomy in association with congenital heart disease, only those patients with less severe underlying disease, as reflected by a Risk Adjustment for Congenital Heart Surgery (RACHS-1) score ≤ 3, were able to wean from mechanical ventilation.[119]

Survival
There is no question that chronic ventilatory support, even when confined to nocturnal use alone, improves survival among patients with neuromuscular and other restrictive chest wall diseases. In the absence of ventilatory support, mean duration of survival for patients with Duchenne muscular dystrophy and diurnal hypercapnia was 9.7 months.[121] In contrast, among 23 young men with Duchenne muscular dystrophy and diurnal hypercapnia who began NIV, survival was 85% at 1 year and 73% at 5 years.[61] Because of the increased longevity of patients with diseases such as Duchenne muscular dystrophy resulting from improved respiratory care and other technologies, new complications and medical issues are being described that will require greater recognition and surveillance.[122-123]

Among all children with chronic respiratory failure, the greatest predictor of long-term survival is prognosis of the underlying condition.[124] Teague abstracted from published reports the average 5-year cumulative survival of 265 pediatric patients and reported an approximately 85% survival in children treated with home mechanical ventilation between 1983 and 1998.[124] Of the 137 patients with neuromuscular diseases who were receiving home mechanical ventilation, the 5-year cumulative survival estimate was 75%. Once again, severity of the underlying disease has been suggested as a predictor of survival in some diseases; the cumulative 5-year survival of children with chronic respiratory failure associated with congenital heart disease was 68%, but it was 90% when considering only those with a RACHS-1 score of ≤ 3, and merely 12% for those with a score ≥ 4.[119]

Most studies suggest that the primary cause of death of ventilator-dependent children cared for outside the hospital relates to progression of the underlying disease.[8,120,124-125] A recent single-center review, however, noted that death among ventilator-dependent children was often unexpected and may have been related to

*References 3, 4, 32, 107, and 117–120.

*References 3, 32, 107, 117, 118, and 120.

co-morbidities as well.[118] While it is unlikely for ventilator malfunction to be the cause of death, one series in which 17 patients died over a 20-year period described three deaths resulting from unwitnessed ventilator disconnections and one from an overnight power failure of a negative pressure body ventilator, leading the author to speculate that at least three and perhaps as many as seven deaths could have been prevented if the patients had been monitored visually or electronically.[10]

The presence of a tracheostomy increases the risk of death as well as other negative outcomes. Edwards and colleagues calculated that tracheostomy-related deaths accounted for 8% of all reported deaths among published accounts.[118] In their cohort, tracheostomy-related deaths were responsible for 19% of all deaths, with complications that included obstruction of the tube, bleeding from tracheal granulomas, and misplacement of the tracheostomy tube into a false track. Downes and Pilmer compared the incidence of life-threatening tracheostomy-related accidents between ventilator-dependent children cared for in the home and those cared for in the hospital in the early 1980s.[9] Although low, they found the rate to be eight times greater among those cared for in the home (2.3/10,000 patient days) versus the pediatric ICU (0.3/10,000 patient days). The authors speculated that recent use of home pulse oximetry has helped to reduce the disparity. Tracheostomy-related deaths have also been reported after children have already been weaned from chronic mechanical ventilation. Of 30 deaths among 101 infants with chronic respiratory failure over an 18-year period, 10 occurred after ventilation had been discontinued.[8] Six of the deaths were considered airway-related accidents, and all but one occurred following hospital discharge.

Quality of Life

When surveyed, ventilator-dependent children generally view the use of the ventilator as something positive, because it helps them breathe more easily, giving them more energy and an overall sense of better health.[126–127] Mechanical ventilatory support is associated with a reduction in hospital admission frequency, improved sleep quality, and better daytime functioning in children with nocturnal hypoventilation from neuromuscular and chest wall disorders.[128–130] Subjects who have diurnal hypercapnia or who complain of dyspnea by the end of the day experience relief of dyspnea by using daytime mechanical ventilator support for as little as 2 hours in the afternoon.[42] When surveyed, the quality of life of patients with neuromuscular disease is independent of the need for mechanical ventilation.[131] Ventilator users have a generally positive outlook and are interested in making future plans.[130,132–134] Ventilator-dependent children attend school, including college and graduate school, and also vacation with their families.[130,133] They are generally happy with how they spend their time, although adolescents with chronic respiratory failure may be less satisfied with their daily activities than are younger children.[133] Children who are dependent on mechanical ventilation view their equipment as adaptive technology, in much the same way that a wheelchair helps with mobility.[126] Nevertheless, children who are ventilator users feel ostracized by people outside of immediate friends and family because of their need for breathing support,[53,126–127] and families express feelings of isolation because of the child's disability.[53]

In fact, there is disparity between the perceived good quality of life of ventilator-dependent children and that of their families. Home care of a ventilator-dependent child is stressful, and the degree of stress increases with the duration of care.[53,134–136] Parents focus more on the possibility of their child's death and dying than do the ventilator users themselves.[53,126] Additionally, home care of ventilator-dependent children adversely affects the health of caregivers, resulting in sleep disruption and inadequate amounts of sleep, feelings of depression and being overwhelmed, as well as limited time for the caregiver to pursue health-promoting activities.[54,135,137] Nevertheless, parents typically express a desire to have their child at home and satisfaction with their choice to do so.[53,55] Regardless of these stresses, parents and ventilator users themselves typically rate the child's quality of life higher than do health professionals,[21,138] and recognition of this by parents adds to their sense of frustration and isolation.[53,126]

■ SUMMARY

The number of children who require prolonged mechanical ventilatory support continues to increase as a result of improved care of critically ill neonates, infants, and children and changing practices regarding children with neuromuscular diseases. Whereas negative pressure body ventilators gave way to positive pressure ventilation via tracheostomy in the 1970s and 1980s, recent trends have been toward noninvasive positive pressure ventilation. Significant improvement in equipment, monitoring, and understanding of the pathophysiology of respiratory failure has led to a wider array of therapeutic options that benefit patient tolerance. Significant challenges remain, especially with regard to designing interfaces and equipment for very young patients, supporting patients and their families to avoid caregiver fatigue, and improving general societal access. This includes access to public transportation, housing choices (e.g., group homes for ventilator-assisted individuals), and employment opportunities. Older children who remain ventilator-dependent will require programs designed to transition their care to adult care providers.

Suggested Reading

Make BJ, Hill NS, Goldberg AI, et al. Mechanical ventilation beyond the intensive care unit. Report of a consensus conference of the American College of Chest Physicians. *Chest.* 1998;113:289S–344S.

Mehta S, Hill NS. Noninvasive ventilation. *Am J Respir Crit Care Med.* 2001;163:540–577.

Pilmer SL. Prolonged mechanical ventilation in children. *Pediatr Clin North Am.* 1994;41:473–512.

Sherman JM, Davis S, Albamonte-Petrick S, et al. Care of the child with a chronic tracheostomy. *Am J Respir Crit Care Med.* 2000;161:297–308.

Teague WG. Long-term mechanical ventilation in infants and children. In: Hill NS, ed. *Long-term mechanical ventilation.* vol. 152. New York: Marcel Dekker; 2001:177–213.

References

The complete reference list is available online at www.expertconsult.com

16 TRANSITION FROM PEDIATRIC TO ADULT CARE

Donald Payne, MD, FRACP, FRCPCH, and Andrew Kennedy, MD

Children and adolescents with chronic respiratory disease become adults with chronic respiratory disease. As a result of ongoing improvements in health care, this is now increasingly the norm rather than the exception. Professionals who look after children and adolescents with chronic illness therefore have a responsibility to consider how their patients' health care needs will continue to be met as they become adults. This chapter, a new addition to this textbook of respiratory disorders in children, discusses the background to transition from pediatric to adult health care and provides a practical approach to assist health professionals, administrators, patients, and families to plan and negotiate the process.

■ WHAT IS TRANSITION?

Transition, as defined by the Society for Adolescent Health and Medicine in the United States, is a "purposeful, planned process that addresses the medical, psychosocial and educational/vocational needs of adolescents and young adults with chronic physical and medical conditions as they move from child-centered to adult-oriented health care systems."[1] There is a wide range of chronic pediatric respiratory disorders that persist through adolescence into adulthood (Table 16-1). For some, such as cystic fibrosis, models of transition are already relatively well established, with the existence of recognized specialist adult centers and clear pathways to facilitate the move from pediatric to adult care.[2–5] For other rare (e.g., primary ciliary dyskinesia) or more heterogeneous conditions (e.g., bronchiectasis), transition models are less well established.[6,7] Finally, there is an increasingly large cohort of adolescents and young adults growing up with respiratory disorders (e.g., chronic lung disease associated with extreme prematurity, muscular dystrophy, or ventilator-dependent airway malacia) with which adult health professionals may have had little or no clinical experience and minimal training.[8–10] These young adults may have associated co-morbidities, (e.g., significant neurologic disease or cognitive impairment) that present an additional challenge to ensuring a successful transition.

■ WHY IS TRANSITION IMPORTANT?

Before outlining some of the practical steps involved in developing a transition plan, it is important to consider why the process needs to be addressed at all. Why should patients and families, who have developed a trusting and collaborative relationship with their health care providers over many years, have to leave this behind and develop a completely new set of relationships? There are a number of aspects to this question. These include acknowledging the process of adolescent development, the emerging health care needs and patterns of morbidity in adulthood, and the differences between pediatric and adult models of care.

Understanding Adolescent Development

For adolescents and young adults with a chronic respiratory disorder, the transition from pediatric to adult health care is just one of a number of transitions they will encounter. Adolescence refers to the developmental stage between childhood dependence and adult independence. During this time, individuals begin to establish their own identity and self-image and take on adult roles (Table 16-2).[11] Key tasks that adolescents and young adults usually complete include developing independence from parents or caregivers, forming relationships outside the family, and providing for themselves financially. Significant transitions during this period include leaving school and joining the workforce or enrolling in higher education, moving away from the parental home, and possibly becoming parents themselves. Health professionals who work with adolescents and young adults need to acknowledge and understand this process of adolescent development and recognize that the transition from pediatric to adult health care occurs within the wider context of a more general transition from childhood to adulthood.

Seen within this context of increasing independence and autonomy, transition to adult care thus sends a powerful message to young people with chronic illness that they have a future and that they are expected to participate in and contribute to society as adults.[12] Remaining within the pediatric health care system may give the impression that living life as an adult is unlikely to be achievable. With increasing age and maturity, many young people become increasingly uncomfortable being cared for in a child-centered setting. A danger of not addressing transition to adult care is that they may become lost to follow-up when they decide for themselves that they have outgrown their pediatrician.

It is also important to be aware that some young adults with chronic illness (e.g., those with muscular dystrophy or severe neurologic impairment) will never be able to attain the same degree of independence as that achieved by their healthy peers. However, this does not mean that these young adults should be looked after within a pediatric model of care indefinitely. There are many ways to acknowledge a young person's development into adulthood (seeing them on their own, discussing age-appropriate topics, providing them with opportunities

TABLE 16-1 PAEDIATRIC RESPIRATORY DISORDERS THAT MAY PERSIST INTO ADULTHOOD

- Cystic fibrosis
- Asthma
- Primary ciliary dyskinesia
- Other causes of bronchiectasis (e.g., immunodeficiency, postinfectious)
- Interstitial lung disease
- Chronic lung disease of prematurity
- Obliterative bronchiolitis
- Neuromuscular disorders (e.g., muscular dystrophy)
- Tracheomalacia/bronchomalacia
- Lung transplant recipients

TABLE 16-2 TASKS OF ADOLESCENCE

- Separate from parents
- Develop a coherent sense of self
- Come to terms with physical self
- Come to terms with sexual self
- Develop mature altruistic relationships
- Develop financial independence

to be involved in decision making), even if their physical independence is limited. These issues are discussed in more detail later in the chapter. For young adults who are physically dependent on others for providing aspects of their care, one obvious example of emerging adulthood can be seen when this assistance is no longer provided by parents, but by other adults (e.g., friends or partners).

Adult Health Care Needs and Patterns of Morbidity

Pediatricians are trained to deal with children and, increasingly, with adolescents.[13] However, few are trained to provide care for adults. In the same way as pediatricians recognize that it is inappropriate for adult-trained physicians to manage young children, it also becomes increasingly inappropriate for pediatricians to continue to care for their patients once they have completed the tasks of adolescence and are living their lives as adults. While pediatricians may feel relatively confident and competent managing certain disease-specific aspects of respiratory disorders such as asthma or bronchiectasis, more general areas of adult health care (e.g., sexual and reproductive health, cardiovascular problems, or liaison with employers) are likely to be less well managed. There are some clinics (e.g., for cystic fibrosis) in which the same team provides care for children, adolescents, and adults. However, in the interest of optimal health care, it is important that whatever model is employed, professionals who manage adults with chronic respiratory disease receive adequate training in general adult health issues.

Differences Between Pediatric and Adult Models of Care

Logistical and financial considerations also come into play when considering transition. Pediatric and adolescent medical departments are not designed or funded to provide care for adults. Budgets are limited, and staffing, equipment, and hospital systems are designed to provide high-quality and developmentally appropriate care for infants, children, and adolescents, rather than adults. At some point, a decision must therefore be made to transfer adolescents and young adults with chronic illness to a unit that can provide developmentally appropriate care for young adults.

What Is the Evidence Base for Transition?

Over time, a number of principles regarding the transition process have been developed, which have gained widespread consensus.[14–18] However, the evidence base for specific transition programs is small. A number of studies have highlighted problems associated with unsuccessful transition from pediatric to adult care, in different subspecialty areas. These include unexpected transplant rejection following transfer to adult care in young adults who had received renal transplants in childhood[19] and the deaths of young adults with congenital heart disease who were cared for by clinicians lacking specific training in the management of these conditions.[20] The absence of an appropriately trained adult team is a significant barrier to successful transition, as discussed later in the chapter. Less extreme consequences of unsuccessful transition to adult care include loss of young adult patients to follow-up, frequent missed appointments, and deterioration in disease control.[21] For young people with chronic respiratory disease, there is a very real possibility that lack of regular contact and follow-up with the medical team over a number of years can result in a major and potentially irreversible deterioration in lung function and quality of life.[22] Traditionally, the adult model expects patients to take responsibility for their own care. If they do not attend for regular outpatient review, they are less likely to be contacted and followed up than if they are being managed within a pediatric setting. A challenge for adult physicians is to recognize and understand that adolescents and young adults are still developing and that they may continue to need a greater degree of involvement by the health care team, at least for the first few years after transfer. Duguépéroux and colleagues have described outcomes for young adults with cystic fibrosis 1 year after transfer to an adult center and demonstrated that the clinical status of the patients transferred remained stable, with an increase in the mean number of outpatient attendances in the year after transfer to the adult center, compared to the year before.[3]

■ TRANSITION: A PRACTICAL APPROACH

Transition refers to the process of preparing adolescents and young adults for the move to the adult health care system and to an adult health team. It is widely acknowledged that this is a continuous process leading to the single event of transfer of care. The transition process needs to be planned in advance and begin early. While there are certain elements of transition that are disease-specific, there are many aspects that are generic to all chronic illness. Russell Viner, a leading advocate for

adolescent and young adult health in the UK, has summarized the approach to transition as follows[23]:
- Prepare young people and their families well in advance for moving from pediatric to adult services
- Ensure that they have the necessary skill set to survive and thrive there
- Prepare and nurture adult services to receive them
- Listen to young people's views

Preparing Young People for Transition

Preparing young people and their families for transition involves discussing the process with them early. Some suggest making transition a topic of discussion from the moment of diagnosis. In practice, this may prove difficult, given the amount of information that families have to take in at the time of diagnosis of a chronic illness. However, the prospect of transition to adult care is an issue that needs to be brought up in any discussion of long-term prognosis—a subject that usually arises in conversations at an early stage. For older children and adolescents, there is no "right" time to start increasing the focus on transition. However, the consensus is that the emphasis on transition should increase as children enter adolescence, often at the same time as they move from primary to secondary school. Transition is one aspect of the wider process of providing developmentally appropriate health care for adolescents. Health professionals can employ certain practical strategies to help promote healthy adolescent development and prepare adolescents for their subsequent move to adult care. These strategies include the following:
- Seeing adolescents on their own, separate from their parents, for part of the consultation
- Emphasizing the importance of confidentiality
- Discussing understanding of their illness and actively promoting self-management
- Addressing general adolescent health issues, in addition to those related to their specific condition

Seeing adolescents alone for part of the consultation is a visible way of demonstrating to them and their families that adolescence is a time of developing independence. It conveys a message to the whole family that it is appropriate for the adolescent to begin to take increasing responsibility for his or her own health.[24] A major advantage of seeing adolescents alone is that it increases the chance that they will talk. Asking questions about school, friends, and activities shows an interest in the adolescent as an individual, rather than his or her disease. This allows time for rapport to develop and provides an opportunity to see how the young person's illness fits in with the rest of his or her life—in particular, whether or not the adolescent sees his or her condition and its treatment as a priority.

Table 16-3 shows the HEADSS framework, used widely around the world, which is a helpful guide for clinicians to use when interviewing adolescents.[25] HEADSS begins with relatively unthreatening questions about home, school, and activities. These have the dual purpose of gathering information and allowing time to develop rapport. However, difficulties in these areas (e.g., prolonged school absence, no hobbies or interests)

TABLE 16-3 HEADSS

H Home
- Where do you live? Who lives with you?
- How do you get along with the people you live with?
- Who would you talk to if you had a problem?

E Education (or employment)
- Which school do you go to? Which year are you in?
- Which subjects do you enjoy? What are you good at?
- Who do you spend time with at school? What are the teachers like?

A Activities
- What do you enjoy doing outside of school?
- Are you in any clubs or sports teams?
- Who do you meet up with at weekends?

D Drugs
- Do any of your friends smoke cigarettes or drink alcohol? How about you?
- How much do you smoke/drink? Every day? On weekends?
- Have you ever tried marijuana or other drugs?

S Sexuality
- Do any of your friends have girlfriends/boyfriends? How about you?
- Have you ever had sex? Do you use condoms/the pill?

S Suicide
- How would you describe your mood? Do you ever get really down?
- Some people who feel really down often feel like hurting themselves or even killing themselves. Have you ever felt like that?
- Have you ever tried to hurt yourself?

From Goldenring JM, Cohen E. Getting into adolescent heads. *Contemp Pediatr.* 1988;July:75-90.

may be a reflection of poor disease control or other underlying problems, such as anxiety or depression. As discussed later in the chapter, mental health problems and health risk behaviors such as smoking, alcohol and other drug use are common in adolescents with chronic illness and always need to be considered.[26–29] It is essential that such a risk and protective health screen is used at the outset of adolescence and continually revisited and updated.

Establishing Confidentiality

When seeing adolescents on their own, it is essential to explain at the outset that the conversation will remain confidential and that, while you may have to consult with colleagues, information will not be discussed with parents, without the adolescent's permission. The limits of confidentiality must also be made explicit. The disclosure of any activity that puts the young person at serious risk of significant harm (such as suicidal thoughts or physical/sexual abuse) cannot remain confidential. Neither can the disclosure of activities that put others at risk. If adolescents are assured of some degree of confidentiality, they are more likely to speak frankly.[30] In practice, this increases the chances of being able to address issues that can have a major impact on disease control (e.g., treatment adherence, smoking, and anxiety), thus opening up the real possibility of providing effective health care.[31]

Actively Promoting Self-Management

Self-management of chronic disease is a major focus of adult programs. Pediatricians can assist in helping adolescents to develop self-management skills through the gradual process of increasing the focus on the adolescent, rather than their parents, during each consultation. As mentioned earlier in the chapter, this is helped by seeing adolescents on their own. Discussions should focus on the understanding of their illness, their priorities and goals, the reasons for and the effects of adhering to a specific treatment regimen, and ways to minimize the impact of the illness on their day-to-day life. Over time, other practical issues can be discussed. These include how to book or reschedule an appointment, obtaining prescriptions and knowledge of any fees payable, whom to contact in an emergency, and how to get to the adult clinic (e.g., public transport, parking). These are issues common to all chronic illnesses, and when addressed can help to reduce the anxiety around the eventual transfer of care to an adult center.[32] To assist in this process, many transition programs have developed checklists that patients and professionals can use to track each individual's progress through adolescence and identify issues that may need to be addressed at specific times. An example is shown in Table 16-4, and others are available on the transition websites listed in the Suggested Reading at the end of the chapter.[15,16]

TABLE 16-4   TRANSITION READINESS: SAMPLE CHECKLIST FOR A 15- TO 16-YEAR-OLD

Independence

Sees health professional alone for some of the consultation
Understands about confidentiality (and its limits)
Feels comfortable asking questions during the consultation

Awareness of transition and transfer

Understands that transfer to the adult center will occur within the next 2 to 3 years
Understands some of the differences between paediatric and adult health care
Knows which adult center he or she will be going to and where it is

Self-management

Understands his or her medical condition and can explain it to a friend
Understands his or her treatment regimen (what the treatments do, why they are important, and the side-effects)
Able to administer own medication/treatment
Able to discuss any difficulties with adherence to treatment
Knows whom to contact in an emergency
Beginning to know how to make appointments, obtain new prescriptions

General adolescent health

Able to discuss body image, healthy eating, exercise
Has discussed sexual health/fertility with his or her doctor
Has discussed alcohol, smoking, and other drug use—impact on their health
Able to discuss mood (anxiety, depression)
Able to identify support systems outside the family and how to access psychological support if required

Educational and vocational planning

Has discussed school, plans for the future
Able to discuss any difficulties at school (attendance, bullying, subject difficulties)

Addressing General Adolescent Health Issues

Health professionals who work with adolescents need to acknowledge and understand the process of adolescent development and be aware of both the impact of emerging adolescent behaviors on disease management, as well as the effect of a chronic respiratory disorder on normal adolescent development.[33,34] Regular appointments and hospital admissions, time off school, limitation of normal activities, and reduced ability to interact with peers can inhibit an adolescent's path toward independence. Parents may also find it difficult to let go. It is therefore important that health professionals monitor their patients' progress through adolescence and identify problems when they arise.

Certain features of adolescence, such as engaging in exploratory behaviors (e.g., smoking, drug use) and challenging authority (e.g., reluctance to adhere to a regular treatment regimen, nonattendance at appointments), may lead to poor disease control.[26] The available data suggest that adolescents with chronic illness are as likely, or more likely, to engage in health-risk behaviors as their healthy peers.[26–29,35] The effects of certain behaviors, such as smoking, on health outcomes are more pronounced in adolescents with chronic respiratory disease than in those without.[24,36] Adolescents with chronic illness are more likely to suffer from anxiety and depression, which may also have a considerable impact on health outcomes and on their ability to manage their illness.[37,38] Health professionals therefore need to develop confidence in discussing health-risk behaviors and mental health problems with their adolescent patients and be able to offer support along with access to more specialized services (e.g., clinical psychology or psychiatry) when appropriate. In support of this approach, a recent study in primary care involving adolescents 11 to 16 years of age demonstrated that adolescents had more positive perceptions of their primary care physician when sensitive issues such as drugs, sex and mental health were discussed.[39] The adolescents studied were also more likely to take an active role in their treatment if the consultation included the discussion of these types of sensitive topics.[39]

Providing this level of care for adolescent patients requires that systems be organized to facilitate the process, such as scheduling longer appointment times for young people. This has significant implications for the provision of appropriate resources. However, taking a long-term view, the argument for providing intensive input during adolescence and young adulthood is that this will lead to improved health outcomes and reduce the potential for unscheduled emergency visits and hospital admissions, which account for the majority of the health care costs associated with chronic illness.

Providing an environment where patients can be seen alone in suitable physical surroundings (i.e., not surrounded by younger children) is also important. Simple measures can be very effective, such as considering the color scheme of the clinic area, the furniture, and the reading material available (e.g., age-appropriate magazines, health promotional literature). The participation of young people in the design of clinical areas is extremely valuable and is likely to increase the chances of their remaining engaged in their own health care.[40]

Preparing Adult Services to Receive Young People with Chronic Respiratory Disorders

A successful transition requires there to be an adult service that is willing and able to receive young people with chronic illness and to provide high-quality care. For cystic fibrosis, the existence of specialist adult centers is well established, and the models of transition are those to which other subspecialties often look for guidance. Transition programs for asthma, a much commoner condition than cystic fibrosis, are less well established, probably because most young adults with persistent asthma do not require the same level of specialist, multidisciplinary input as young adults with cystic fibrosis.[41] However, for children and adolescents with severe or treatment-resistant asthma, transition and transfer to a specialist adult center will be required.[42]

For young adults with rarer conditions, the challenge for pediatric health professionals is to identify suitable colleagues in the adult system who have the skills and training to provide ongoing care. The absence of suitable providers is one of the reasons why some patients may remain under the care of the pediatric team indefinitely. In the longer-term, one of the many roles for pediatricians to play is that of advocates for the provision of suitable training programs for adult physicians. Good communication, collaboration and respect between pediatric and adult units are essential. Depending on the availability of services and personnel, different models of transition and eventual transfer may develop. One option is the establishment of a regular joint clinic for adolescents and young adults, involving both pediatric and adult teams, which may be based either at one center or the other, or rotate between the two. Another model is for patients to have one or two appointments at the adult center, while still being seen at the pediatric center prior to the eventual final transfer of care to the adult center. With this type of arrangement, it is important to make clear who should be the first port of call in an emergency. There is no evidence that any one model is superior to another, and, in practice, the model developed will depend on a variety of factors. These include the number of patients to be transitioned and the availability of appropriately trained staff, funding, and clinic space. More important than the precise model of transitional care employed is the need for all health professionals who work with adolescents and young adults to recognize and understand the process of adolescent development and to incorporate this into their day-to-day practice.

Listening to Young People's Views

It is vital to involve adolescents and young adults in the transition process.[23] This means ensuring that they not only participate actively in their own individual transition and transfer to adult care, but also that they are involved in the planning of the wider program of transition. The Royal College of Paediatrics and Child Health in the UK has recently published guidelines to promote the participation of children and young people in the planning of health services.[40] Transition programs are much more likely to be successful if they incorporate the views and ideas of the young people they are designed to support.

BARRIERS TO TRANSITION

In addition to the participation of adolescent and young adults in the process, successful transition requires health professionals to advocate continually for the needs of this group and for the provision of adequate services. As mentioned earlier in the chapter, a major barrier to successful transition is the absence of appropriately trained health professionals within the adult health care system.[20] Where adult services are lacking, pediatricians need to provide training for their adult colleagues, while adult health professionals need to acknowledge and embrace the need to provide a clinical service for the increasing number of young adults with chronic respiratory disorders who will be moving to adult care. This process also needs the support of the health service administrators and politicians who control the funding. Above all, it requires a shift in attitude and culture of all concerned in order to recognize and understand the importance of adolescent and young adult health.[43]

Where adult services exist, a lack of trust and respect between the pediatric and adult center can hamper transition. Parents may also feel concerned about the move, and their concerns therefore must be recognized and addressed early. Guidelines for transition recommend that a nominated individual is identified who is responsible for the overall transition process (a transition coordinator). This role may be performed by any member of the health care team. The coordinator should ensure that all aspects of the process have been considered and follow up on any difficulties encountered. One of the coordinator's roles should be to facilitate communication between the pediatric and adult centers and to provide a written summary of the young person's condition in advance of the transfer date. Financial considerations and health insurance coverage are also key issues.[41] With increasing age, the rules regarding eligibility for certain services and allowances may change. For example, financial support or equipment, which is provided during childhood, may not be available indefinitely. These issues therefore need to be anticipated well in advance.

SUMMARY

Transition from pediatric to adult care is one aspect of the wider provision of health services for adolescents and young adults. An understanding of the health issues affecting this group along with specific training in adolescent and young adult health is essential for all health professionals. The number of young adults with chronic respiratory disorders of childhood is only going to increase, as will the range of specific disorders that adult physicians will need to be competent to manage. For pediatric and adult respiratory physicians, the clinical landscape is changing. The challenge is there to be met.

Suggested Reading

Boyle MP, Farukhi Z, Nosky ML. Strategies for improving transition to adult cystic fibrosis care, based on patient and parent views. *Pediatr Pulmonol.* 2001;32:428–436.

Department of Health/Child Health and Maternity Services Branch. *Transition: getting it right for young people. Improving the transition of young people with long term conditions from children's to adult health services.* London: Department of Health; 2006.

Goldenring JM, Cohen E. Getting into adolescent heads. *Contemp Pediatr.* 1988;75–90 July.

New South Wales Health Department, Australia. *Transition Care - Helping young people move successfully from child to adult health services.* Available at www.health.nsw.gov.au/gmct/transition; Accessed 26.09.10.

Rosen DS, Blum RW, Britto M, et al. Transition to adult health care for adolescents and young adults with chronic conditions: position paper of the Society for Adolescent Medicine. *J Adolesc Health.* 2003;33:309–311.

Rosen DS. Transition to adult healthcare for adolescents and young adults with cancer. *Cancer.* 1993;71:3411–3414.

Royal Children's Hospital, Melbourne, Australia. *Transition to adult health services.* Available at www.rch.org.au/transition; Accessed 26.09.10.

Sawyer S, Drew S, Duncan R. Adolescents with chronic disease - the double whammy. *Aust Fam Physician.* 2007;36:622–627.

Tuchman LK, Schwartz LA, Sawicki GS, et al. Cystic fibrosis and transition to adult medical care. *Pediatrics.* 2010;125:566–573.

Viner RM. Transition of care from paediatric to adult services: one part of improved health services for adolescents. *Arch Dis Child.* 2008;93:160–163.

References

The complete reference list is available online at www.expertconsult.com

17 LONG-TERM CONSEQUENCES OF CHILDHOOD RESPIRATORY DISEASE

Manjith Narayanan, MD, DNB(Paediatrics), MRCPCH, PhD, and
Michael Silverman, MD

RELEVANCE OF LONG-TERM CONSEQUENCES

The after-effects of childhood respiratory diseases are increasingly encountered in adult life, not because of an increased incidence of childhood respiratory disease, but due to increased survival. For example, in the UK, the proportion of all patients with cystic fibrosis older than 16 years of age increased from 24.7% to 43.2% between 1985 and 2003.[1,2] Survival after extreme preterm birth, with attendant respiratory problems (e.g., chronic lung disease of prematurity) has increased three-fold between 1979 and 1997.[3]

At the same time, there is a growing recognition that many supposedly adult respiratory disorders have their roots in childhood. The recent update published by the Global Initiative for Chronic Obstructive Lung Disease[4] stresses that genetic factors, early life exposures (e.g., environmental tobacco smoke, ETS), and insults to lung growth and development are important risk factors for chronic obstructive pulmonary disease (COPD). Observations such as these have increased interest in the childhood origins of adult disorders and placed responsibility on pediatricians to raise awareness among those who deal with lung diseases in adults.

Lung growth (as determined by lung function tests) occurs up to late adolescence in females and early adulthood (about 21 years of life) in males.[5] Any insults occurring before this process is complete could affect the final size, structure, and function of the lung as individuals enter adulthood, potentially leading to earlier senescence. The adult lung is therefore likely to carry an imprint of childhood diseases and environmental exposures. The alveolar complement of the lung was thought to be complete by 3 years of age.[6] However, there is growing evidence for continued alveolarization throughout the period of lung development.[7] On the one hand, this presents an opportunity to correct deficits resulting from early life insults. Conversely, insults in late childhood and adolescence could affect alveolarization.

PATTERNS OF LONG-TERM OUTCOME

Childhood respiratory diseases can have various patterns of long-term outcome (Table 17-1), depending on the nature and timing of lung insults. The various patterns are discussed in the following paragraphs.

Fetal and Perinatal Disorders

One of the characteristics of fetal and perinatal disorders is the association between the gestational age at which the pathologic process starts and the long-term outcome.

In congenital diaphragmatic hernia (CDH), earlier herniation is related to greater degree of pulmonary hypoplasia and therefore worse outcome (Fig. 17-1).[8] A residual lung capacity of less than 50% predicted is associated with poorer prognosis. Typically most deaths occur in the first 30 days of life (31% in Bedoyan's series),[9] and mortality is low in postneonatal survivors (~1.5%). Long-term survivors have evidence of impaired lung function in late childhood[10] and adulthood,[11] apparently without physical limitation or reduced quality of life.[11] Similarly, chronic lung disease of prematurity (CLD) is more common and more severe in children born at an earlier gestation.[12,13] There is a trend toward improvement in lung function over time in long-term survivors.[14] However, the nature of CLD continues to change over time as even more immature infants survive.

In survivors of early developmental disorders, the outcome may be worsened by additional insults such as infections (severe RSV infections), environmental exposures (ETS), or co-existing anomalies (such as patent ductus arteriosus [PDA] in CLD survivors). Conversely, prognosis may be improved by prevention of these secondary insults (e.g., palivizumab to prevent RSV infections). The hallmark of developmental disorders is the trend for improvement in lung function between secondary insults.

Acute Respiratory Illnesses

Most acute insults that occur in healthy children resolve without long-term adverse outcomes. However, severe respiratory infections before 5 years of age are associated with a lower forced expiratory volume in 1 second (FEV_1) at 14 years of age and a greater decline in normalized lung function between 14 and 50 years of age.[15] Occasionally an acute insult can trigger long-term changes in airways (e.g., postpertussis bronchiectasis, postadenoviral obliterative bronchiolitis [OB]), thus leading to poorer outcome. While these long-term changes may sometimes be "idiosyncratic" or genetically mediated, there is evidence that they may be more common in socially disadvantaged or 'indigenous' populations.[16–18] Postadenoviral OB is also related to the severity of acute insult[18] and may follow the pattern shown in Figure 17-2.

Chronic Diseases in Childhood

There are two patterns of chronic respiratory diseases in childhood with distinct patterns of long-term outcome: the episodic pattern and the persistent pattern. These are discussed in the following paragraphs.

TABLE 17-1

PATTERNS OF LUNG DISEASE	EXAMPLES USED IN TEXT
Fetal and perinatal disorders	Congenital diaphragmatic hernia, chronic lung disease of prematurity
Acute respiratory illness	Respiratory tract infections, postadenoviral obliterative bronchiolitis
Chronic episodic disease	Asthma
Chronic persistent disease	Cystic fibrosis
Adult disease with origin in childhood	Chronic obstructive pulmonary disease

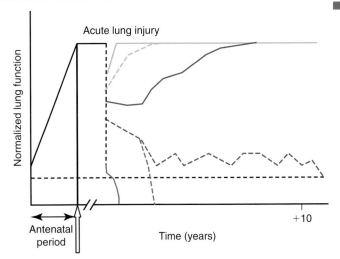

FIGURE 17-2. Schematic representing the factors influencing outcomes following acute insults in previously normal children. *X-axis* represents the timeline with *black arrow* showing time of birth. *Horizontal dotted line*, lung function incompatible with life; *vertical dotted line*, acute insult; *orange line*, severe acute injury incompatible with life; *green line*, mild insult resulting in recovery to normal function; *green dotted line and blue line*, insults of progressively greater severity taking longer to recover; *blue dotted line*, severe acute insults are more prone to develop complications which then assume the course of a chronic disease or may lead to death in more severe cases (*orange dotted line*).

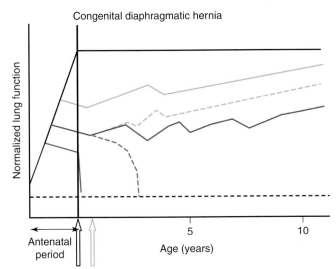

FIGURE 17-1. Schematic representing the factors influencing outcomes following congenital diaphragmatic hernia. *X-axis* represents the timeline with *black arrow* (and black vertical line) showing time of birth and *green arrow* showing timing of surgery. Horizontal solid black line represents lung function associated with normal lung development. *Horizontal dotted black line* represents lung function incompatible with life. *Orange line*, earlier herniation, lower overall lung function and poor outcome (death). *Green line*, later herniation with better outcome. *Blue line*, herniation occurs leaving sufficient lung function to sustain life following surgery showing a typical pattern of decreased lung function during secondary insults and improvement of lung function during intervals between insults. Outcome depends on frequency and severity of secondary insults (*green dotted line*, fewer secondary insults, and *orange dotted line*, severe secondary insult leading to death).

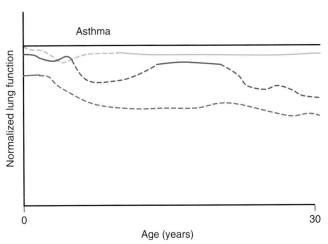

FIGURE 17-3. Schematic to illustrate long-term outcomes of childhood asthma. *Black line*, controls; *green line*, transient wheezy illness; *blue line*, relapsers; *orange line*, persistant disease. *Dotted lines* imply symptoms. (From Sears et al and Phelan et al.[20,21])

Episodic Pattern

Episodic exacerbations with interludes of relative normality are the classic pattern in many common pediatric lung diseases, notably asthma. Multiple phenotypes of asthma have been described, and some have been based on the long-term temporal pattern of the disease.[19] In a longitudinal cohort study conducted in New Zealand, Sears and colleagues[20] reported that about 36% of childhood asthma resolves, about 14% have persistent disease to adulthood, and about 13% have recurrence in later life after a disease-free adolescence (Fig. 17-3). Some phenotypes of asthma are associated with interval symptoms and slow decline in lung function akin to a persistent chronic disease.

Long-term outcome has been associated with the severity of disease in early life. For example, Stern and associates

reported that persistent wheezing in early life, along with low lung function at 6 years of age are associated with early adulthood asthma.[22] Many follow-up studies report a link between adult outcomes and severity of childhood asthma.[21] This may be because of a causal link (remodeling) but may also be simply due to lifelong predilection to asthma.

Persistent Pattern

Some chronic respiratory diseases of childhood follow a persistent pattern characterized by a slow decline of lung function with time. The course may be punctuated by superimposed insults (e.g., infections) that may cause intermittent rapid decline in lung function (acute on chronic pattern). Cystic fibrosis (CF), for example, may present as a severe, rapidly progressive life-limiting

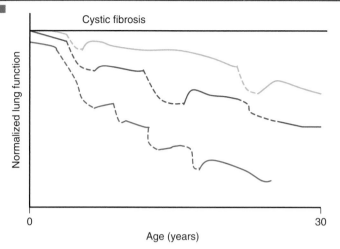

FIGURE 17-4. Schema showing outcomes in CF. *Black line,* controls; milder disease *(green)* is associated with less frequent exacerbations *(dotted lines)* and slower progression of lung disease in the interval period when compared with moderate disease *(blue)* and severe disease *(orange).* The outcomes are modified by genotype, colonising pathogen, institution of appropriate treatment regimen[23] and other general factors (see mechanisms). The overall trend in lung function is gradual decline except for some recovery following treatment of acute exacerbations.

disorder or as a mild disorder with near-normal life expectancy (Fig. 17-4). Outcome may be related to genotype. For example, ΔF508 homozygotes are significantly underrepresented in middle-age CF survivors.[23] Long-term outcome may be worsened by chronic infection with certain pathogens. CF is an example of modification of outcomes by therapeutic advances.[1]

Adult Diseases That Have Their Origin in Childhood

There is growing recognition that some diseases that manifest in adulthood have their origins in exposures and risk factors that occur in childhood (Fig. 17-5).

For example, it has been increasingly acknowledged that many childhood environmental and genetic risk factors have an important role in the origin of COPD. In the analysis of longitudinal data from the European Community Respiratory Health Survey (ECRHS) I and II,[26] it was shown that "childhood disadvantage factors" were at least as important as heavy smoking in the etiology of COPD. Detecting and modifying such risk factors will have an important role in the management of COPD in the future and will fall into the realm of pediatric pulmonology.[4]

■ MECHANISMS INVOLVED IN LONG-TERM CONSEQUENCES

The common patterns described above are useful as general descriptors of outcomes of the various classes of lung disease in children. Prediction rules are rarely accurate enough for individual children, even for a common condition such as asthma.

The various factors explored below influence the outcome of childhood respiratory illnesses in general. While the current body of evidence is mainly from epidemiologic associations, progress is being made in understanding the mechanisms that connect these risk factors to outcome. The current body of research already shows that many of these

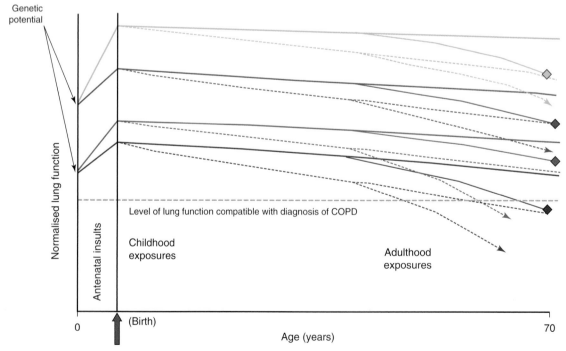

FIGURE 17-5. Tracking of lung function and childhood origin of COPD: An analysis of normalised lung function against age shows the additive influence of antenatal and childhood insults on lung function and how this predisposes to adult COPD. The slopes depend on degree of exposure and severity of each insult. Does not take into account instances where insults on the lung are time limited. *Grey dotted line,* lung function compatible with diagnosis of COPD; *black arrow,* birth. *Green,* normal genetic potential, no antenatal insults; *blue* normal genetic potential with antenatal insults (e.g., maternal smoking/IUGR); *red,* lower genetic potential, no antenatal insults; *brown,* lower genetic potential with antenatal insults. *Solid lines,* no postnatal insults to the lung; *dotted lines,* added childhood risk factors; *lines that end in arrowheads,* added adulthood risk factors.[22,24–28]

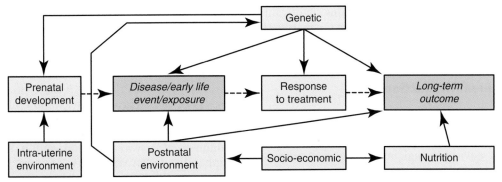

FIGURE 17-6. Complex interplay of factors that affect long term outcomes of disease. The response to treatment may be restorative (e.g., lung transplantation) or adverse (e.g., chemotherapy).

factors act in additive or multiplicative ways with each other and are therefore complex to interpret (Fig. 17-6).

Genetic Factors

These are probably the most important of the factors affecting outcome. They can determine the susceptibility to a disease, response to treatment, or impact of additional environmental exposures.

Susceptibility to Disease

Certain single nucleotide polymorphisms (SNPs) are associated with increased risk of asthma. These include tumor necrosis factor–α guanine to adenine substitution in nucleotide 308 (TNF-α 308 G > A)[29] and dipeptidyl peptidase 10 (DPP10 rs13392783 G > A).[30] Similarly, there are genetic contributions to susceptibility to BPD[31] and severe bronchiolitis.[32]

Pharmacogenetics

There is emerging evidence that patient responses to β-agonists, corticosteroids, and leukotriene receptor antagonists in children with asthma are dependent on genetic factors.[33]

Modifying Long-term Outcome

Certain polymorphisms in the *ADAM33* gene are not only associated with fetal lung development, but also with accelerated decline of lung function in asthmatics.[34] The latter is postulated to be due to the involvement of this gene in airway remodeling.

Tracking of Lung Function and the Fetal/Childhood Origin of COPD

Recent evidence indicates that in otherwise healthy children, adjusted lung function tends to track along centiles. In a longitudinal cohort study,[22] infants on the lowest quartile of lung function remained in the same quartile as adolescents and young adults. Data from the ECRHS study[26] suggests that adjusted adult lung function also tracks. These studies, taken together, imply that infants born with poor lung function will be at significantly higher risk of developing COPD in adulthood (Fig. 17-5). Genetic factors may be responsible for the link between "early life disadvantage," poor lung function in early life, poor lung function in adulthood, and COPD.[22,26,27] In the Genetic Research in Isolated Populations (GRIP) study,[35]

certain SNPs (TGFβ1-509 C > T, TGFβ1 Leu10Pro) were strongly associated with severity of COPD.

Environment

Environmental Tobacco Smoke

The best researched (and perhaps the most dangerous) environmental agent that affects childhood lung disease is passive exposure to ETS.

ETS increases susceptibility to disease. ETS has been a subject of a series of reviews by Strachan and Cook. It is known, among other effects, that it increases the incidence[36,37] and prevalence of wheeze and asthma;[38] increases the incidence of lower respiratory tract illness (LRTI) in children younger than 2 years of age;[39] and increases hospital admission rates for acute LRTI, bronchiolitis, and pneumonia.[40] It is known to decrease lung function in children.[41,42] ETS may act by inducing chronic inflammation in the airways or exacerbating hypersensitivity reactions to allergens.[37]

ETS modifies pre-existing disease. ETS worsens the outcome in almost all lung disease in children. For example, in asthma, reducing ETS exposures in children has been associated with a decreased number of episodes of poor asthma control.[43] In cystic fibrosis, ETS exposure is associated with significantly lower lung function tests (LFT) in cross-sectional studies and a significantly greater decrease in lung function in longitudinal studies.[44]

Air Pollution

There is evidence that air pollution may be one of the factors associated with induction of asthma.[37] Studies linking air pollution and asthma are complicated by the presence of many confounding factors. In a prospective study of schoolchildren in California,[45] air pollution was associated with significantly decreased growth in lung volumes, after adjustment for confounding factors. Air pollution can thus be a significant factor leading to poor outcome in childhood respiratory diseases.

Intrauterine Environment

Most airway and lung vascular development occurs in intrauterine life, and it is no surprise that antenatal events affect postnatal lung function. Evidence from cohort studies shows that intrauterine growth retardation (IUGR) is associated with poor lung function Z-scores in children

8 to 9 years of age.[46] This association remains significant after adjusting for confounding factors (e.g., maternal smoking and social status).

Gene-Environment Interactions

The close interplay of environmental exposures with genetic makeup is increasingly apparent. It can help explain the differences in outcome between children with similar levels of environmental insults. Some examples are explained in the following paragraphs.

Detoxification Genes

The role of the antioxidant glutathione S-transferase (GST) system of genes in wheeze has become clearer. Gilliland and colleagues[47] have shown that prenatal exposure to ETS is associated with postnatal asthma in *GSTM1*-null but not *GSTM1*-positive children. Kabesch and coworkers[48] have shown an interaction between *GST* genes and ETS exposure in asthma and wheezing illnesses in schoolchildren.

Epigenetics

Epigenetic alterations are heritable differences in gene expression that do not involve mutations of the DNA sequence.[49] There is evidence linking traffic-related air pollutants with epigenetic changes (gene methylation) and doctor-diagnosed asthma below 5 years of age.[50] It is postulated that fetal exposure to ETS can lead to epigenetic changes,[51] which then contribute to disease such as asthma later in life.[47]

"Modifier Genes" and Environmental Exposures

In cystic fibrosis, there is evidence that ETS causes greater adverse effect on lung function in the presence of certain mutations of modifier genes (e.g., *TGF β1-509 TT*).[44]

Social/Personal

Nutrition

Poor nutrition is associated with poor lung function. In a survey of 14,120 participants, higher serum levels of vitamin A, vitamin C, vitamin E, selenium, calcium, chloride, and iron were associated with better lung function (FEV_1) after adjusting for confounding variables.[52] The association between vitamin D level and COPD may have some of its origins in early life.[53]

Socioeconomic Factors

The role of socioeconomic factors in long-term outcome is well known but difficult to separate from other confounding factors. Jackson and colleagues[54] showed that children from lower socioeconomic status had lower LFTs as adults and greater fall of LFTs on longitudinal analysis. This effect remained after adjusting for the effect of exposure to ETS and the presence of asthma. Other factors that could lead to this relationship could be exposure to environmental pollutants, poor nutrition, and psychosocial factors such as stress and depression. This illustrates the problem of causal inference in epidemiology.

■ MEASURING AND PREDICTING LONG-TERM OUTCOME

Lung Function Tests

Serial Spirometry

Spirometry has been the tool of choice for monitoring the progress of most chronic diseases in children. However, it should be placed in appropriate context when predicting long-term outcomes because it is a test of large- and medium-sized airway function and is not sensitive to peripheral conductive airway or intra-acinar disease.[55] Spirometry alone is inappropriate as a measure of the function of the gas-exchanging zones of the lungs.

Tests of the Lung Periphery

New techniques have been developed in the past few years to monitor peripheral lung structure and function. Lung clearance index (LCI), an index of ventilation inhomogeneity measured by multibreath washout, has been shown to be a sensitive, robust, and repeatable technique to measure peripheral airway function.[56] Being effort-independent, it has the potential to be applied to toddlers.[57] LCI was more sensitive than traditional lung function tests in discriminating CF from normals in detecting *Pseudomonas* colonization in children with CF[57] and monitoring response to treatment in CF.[58] Similarly it is more sensitive than spirometry in detecting persistent airway dysfunction in children with well-controlled asthma.[59]

Imaging Techniques

High-Resolution Computed Tomography

High-resolution computed tomography (HRCT) has been used to monitor the extent of lung disease in CF. A multicenter trial[60] has concluded that HRCT is a sensitive, specific, and reproducible outcome measure in CF. While LCI reflects the function of the peripheral airways as a whole, HRCT provides structural localization. Therefore, these two techniques are complementary in assessment of lung disease. The main drawback of HRCT is the associated exposure to ionizing radiation.

Hyperpolarized Helium-3 Magnetic Resonance

Hyperpolarized Helium-3 magnetic resonance (HHe3MR) is a research tool that has the potential for future clinical applications. Apparent diffusion coefficient (ADC) measured by HHe3MR is a means of measuring the average size and size distribution of alveoli and acinar airspaces[61] without recourse to histology. Because it involves only a short breath-hold time (about 5 to 10 seconds), this technique can be applied to children as young as 5 years of age.[7,62] This technique has already found applications in BPD, CF, and COPD.[63,64] It is well-suited for tracking acinar structures on a longitudinal basis because of its high repeatability and lack of exposure to ionizing radiation.

Laboratory-Based Tests

Various microbiological and biochemical tests that predict outcomes in particular diseases (e.g., colonization with *Pseudomonas* spp. in CF) are discussed in other individual chapters.

Combined Approach

Prediction scores that combine various modalities and clinical assessment to predict outcomes are being developed. An example is the recently published pulmonary outcome prediction (POP) score for CF.[65]

Future Directions

It is only a matter of time before genetic testing for mutations described above become available to inform prognosis of various respiratory diseases. Given the polygenic cause of most chronic diseases (the importance of environmental exposures and underlying developmental processes), it seems unlikely that genetics alone will ever be a sufficient predictor of long-term prognosis. Current and future lifelong cohort-based studies will hopefully provide sufficient long-term data to lead to better prediction scores. Intervention studies to examine causal mechanisms may shed further light on long-term outcomes.[66]

▮▮▮ CAN LONG-TERM OUTCOMES BE MODIFIED?

Prevention

Avoidance of noxious environmental exposures may improve the long-term outcomes of certain lung diseases.[43] Better nutrition is known to decrease the incidence of chronic lung disease following prematurity.[67]

Therapy

New therapeutic advances have improved long-term outcomes in some cases. For example, therapies aimed at preventing respiratory infections have greatly improved the outcomes of cystic fibrosis.[1] Children with nonprogressive neuromuscular diseases have been helped by new noninvasive ventilation techniques. However, the long-term impact of many therapies (e.g., nitric oxide therapy, high-frequency oscillatory ventilation, and extracorporeal membrane oxygenation in CDH) remains a matter of debate, though they have been shown to be effective in managing the acute stage of illness.[68] Stege and colleagues[69] have pointed out the effects of case selection bias and the use of historical controls in skewing outcome trials of CDH. Sinha and associates[12,13,70] found in a systematic review that there were no studies of corticosteroids in asthma looking at long-term outcomes. However, it may be impractical and sometimes even unethical to conduct randomized studies on long-term outcomes when short-term effects are clearly beneficial.

Modification of Lung Growth

There is exciting evidence of the possibility of long-term alveolarization in humans.[7] Given this possibility, lung resection surgery in childhood takes on an entirely new dimension. Postpneumonectomy alveolarization has been described in mature mammals, and there is no reason why this should not happen in humans. There is evidence of normalization of alveolar structure in school-age survivors of extreme preterm birth.[63] It may only be a question of sustaining nutrition and preventing infection to allow the natural human growth process of alveoli to come to the rescue. Although the early promise of retinol/retinoic acid in this area has not been sustained, there is also the possibility of developing medications designed to augment this process.

References

The complete reference list is available online at www.expertconsult.com

18 DRUG ADMINISTRATION BY INHALATION IN CHILDREN

David E. Geller, MD, and Allan L. Coates, MDCM, B Eng (Elect)

Topical administration of drugs to the lower respiratory tract by inhalation is a mainstay of treatment for pulmonary disorders in children. Current treatment guidelines emphasize the importance of inhaled corticosteroids and bronchodilators for controlling asthma and of inhaled mucus-active agents and antibiotics for controlling lung disease in cystic fibrosis (CF).[1,2] Another emerging area is the use of aerosols for systemic delivery of small molecules, peptides, and proteins by utilizing the large surface area of the lung as a sponge to absorb drugs that would otherwise be degraded in the gut or inactivated by first-pass metabolism in the liver, or those that require injection.

For treatment of airways diseases such as asthma, the use of inhaled medications has distinct advantages over other routes of administration. First, the onset of action of inhaled drugs such as bronchodilators is much faster than with oral medications.[3] Second, the therapeutic index is much better in that smaller doses can be delivered topically to the site of action, while reducing systemic exposure and side effects (e.g., corticosteroids for treatment of airway inflammation). While the concept of drug inhalation may seem very simple, the challenges of successful delivery of drugs to the lungs are much greater than those for oral or systemic drug delivery. The respiratory tract has evolved to filter out foreign materials and exclude entry into the lower airways, with barriers that include the nose, the pharynx, and airway branch points. Cough, mucociliary clearance, and uptake by alveolar macrophages may limit the residence time of drugs in the airways. Therefore, aerosol formulations, devices, and breathing techniques must be able to bypass these defenses to deposit and facilitate retention of therapeutic agents in the lungs. The success of aerosol delivery depends upon several complex, interrelated variables. Since improper use of aerosol devices is associated with poorer clinical outcomes,[4] it is essential that caregivers be familiar with aerosol principles and the operation of aerosol delivery systems so they may advise and train their patients properly.

This chapter will help caregivers develop a greater understanding of the underlying principles and practical concerns of drug administration by aerosol, including factors that govern aerosol deposition and sources of variability. We will also discuss the most commonly used aerosol delivery systems: pressurized metered-dose inhalers (pMDIs), dry-powder inhalers (DPIs), and wet nebulizers. We will point out the advantages and disadvantages of each and provide information regarding the appropriate choice of devices. Finally, we will discuss a number of newer and very innovative drug formulations and aerosol devices being developed for future use that may solve many of the limitations of current systems.

■ AEROSOL PRINCIPLES

Aerosols are suspensions of liquid or solid particles in a carrier gas. Therapeutic aerosols are generated by several different means, including atomization by pneumatic, ultrasonic, hydraulic or electrostatic processes, dispersion in an evaporative propellant, or dispersion of a dry powder into air. The physical form of the generated aerosol may be solid particles, liquid droplets, solutions, or suspensions.

The therapeutic response to an inhaled drug depends on the quantity that bypasses the upper airway and deposits in the lungs, the regional deposition in the central and peripheral airways, and how well the drug distribution matches that of the receptor or target.[5] There are three main mechanisms of aerosol deposition: inertial impaction, sedimentation, and diffusion.[5,6] Inertial impaction occurs in the upper airway and in the first few generations of bronchi, where airflow is faster and more turbulent. The chances of impaction are proportional to the particle size and velocity (i.e., larger and faster particles have a greater chance of impacting on an airway surface). Impaction also occurs at bends and branch points in the airways, as the particle momentum may be too great to follow the air stream more distally. With successive generations, the cross-sectional area of the airways increases and the velocity of airflow decreases and becomes more laminar. In these peripheral airways, gravitational sedimentation is the predominant mechanism of deposition. Clearly, longer residence time favors settling of small particles in the peripheral airways, which can be accomplished with slower inhalation, larger inhaled volume, or increased breath-holding time. For particles much less than 1 μm, transportation by diffusion rather than bulk flow and deposition by electrostatic forces become important. Due to the large surface areas relative to mass, submicronic particles settle very slowly and may be exhaled before they contact the respiratory epithelium.

Numerous variables are involved to determine aerosol deposition, including particle size, breathing pattern, and method of inhalation, as well as the anatomic and functional status of the lungs (Table 18-1). Data that contribute to our knowledge about these variables come from mathematical models,[7] in vitro assessments,[8] deposition studies using gamma scintigraphy or positron emission tomography (PET),[9] pharmacokinetic (PK) studies,[9] and clinical trials. Each approach has its own advantages and drawbacks.

TABLE 18-1 DETERMINANTS OF AEROSOL DEPOSITION

AEROSOL FACTORS	PATIENT FACTORS
Particle size	Age
Particle velocity	Inspiratory flow rate
Hygroscopic properties	Breathing pattern (inspiratory volume, rate)
Drug viscosity and surface tension	Nasal versus mouth breathing
Suspension versus solution	Anatomy (upper and lower airways) Disease severity Physical and cognitive ability Adherence, contrivance

AEROSOL VARIABLES

Of the aerosol-related variables listed in Table 18-1, the single most important factor is the size of the particles. The range of particle sizes encountered by patients of respiratory physicians is large—from <0.1 μm for particles in tobacco smoke or smog to tens of microns for therapeutic nasal sprays. Most pharmaceutical aerosols are polydisperse (or heterodisperse), consisting of a range of particle sizes. The size distribution of an aerosol can be described in terms of the frequency with which either particle number, particle volume, or particle mass occurs as a function of diameter. The count median diameter (CMD), volume median diameter (VMD), and mass median diameter (MMD) are the particle diameters above and below which half the number of particles, half the volume of the aerosol, and half the mass of the aerosol distribution resides, respectively. VMD and MMD are identical if all the particles in an aerosol have the same density (as in a nebulized solution). CMD is not very meaningful for

therapeutic aerosols because it is the mass of the delivered drug that determines effect. The mass of a spherical particle is related to the cube of the radius, thus a particle with a 5-μm diameter carries the same mass as 1000 particles with 0.5-μm diameters.

Particles may have irregular shapes, making it difficult to describe their size, and they may have high or low densities. The aerodynamic behavior of particles can be described by the aerodynamic diameter, which is the size of a spherical particle of unit density (like water) that has the same settling velocity as the particle in question. Measurement of the mass median aerodynamic diameter (MMAD) helps to define the behavior of inhaled particles with different shapes and densities, and it has the advantage of being able to measure the particle size of aerosolized suspensions. The degree to which the aerosol is polydisperse is given by the geometric standard deviation (GSD, or σ_g), which is the ratio of the diameter at 84.3% of the mass of the aerosol to that at 50% of the distribution.[10] The larger the σ_g, the more the aerosol is polydisperse. Most medical aerosol devices produce particles with a variable size range that exhibit a Poisson distribution with a large number of small particles and a progressively smaller number of larger particles. By plotting the logarithm of the diameter against the probability distribution of volume (or mass), this distribution results in an approximation of a bell-shaped curve, which is referred to as *log normal*[11] (Fig. 18-1).

In general, particles smaller than 5 μm are best able to negotiate the curves of the posterior pharynx and beyond the vocal cords to deposit in the lower airways. While carrying much more drug, larger particles (>5 μm) may be too large to penetrate below the vocal cords in adults.[12,13] Particles <1 μm may not have enough time to settle and are more likely to be exhaled, though this may not be as true in patients with obstructed airways. Therefore, the proportion of drug mass contained in particles between 1 to 5 μm or <5 to 6 μm has historically been dubbed the *respirable fraction (RF)*. However, this term is very

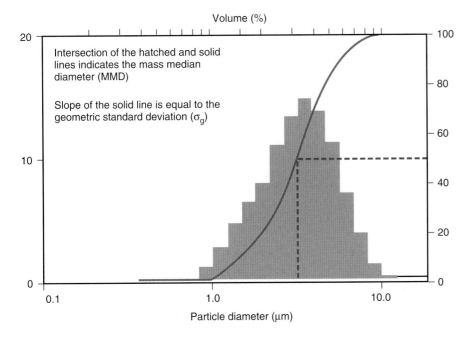

FIGURE 18-1. The particle size distribution of a medical aerosol generator that has been measured by laser diffraction. Each bar to the histogram represents a size band of particles (the height of the bar represents the percentage of the sample within that band). The scale on the left is used to read the histogram; the scale on the right is used to read the cumulative plot represented by the solid line going through the histogram. The particle size that corresponds to 50% on the cumulative curve is the MMD—in this case 3.3 μm. The slope of the line at the 50% point corresponds to the geometric standard deviation.

misleading because the *in vitro* assessment of RF overestimates the amount that deposits in the lungs. Unfortunately, no single particle-size fraction can accurately represent the complex relationships between drug formulation, delivery system characteristics, and how they interact with the human airways.[14] Therefore, to simplify nomenclature, the term *fine-particle fraction* (FPF) is used to describe the fraction of aerosol with the highest potential to deposit in the lower airways, and *fine-particle dose* (FPD) refers to the mass of drug contained in the FPF. The FPD definition varies somewhat between investigators, but it usually approximates the ranges described earlier in the chapter.

■ PARTICLE SIZE DISTRIBUTION MEASUREMENT

Since particle size is such an important parameter of aerosol delivery, it should not be surprising that many aerosol measurement techniques are used. Different techniques for particle sizing may give very different results from one another, making it difficult to compare and interpret study results or promotional materials. While an extensive review of the technology is beyond the scope of this chapter, detailed reviews cover virtually all aspects.[14–16]

Briefly, there are two principle methods of determining the size distribution of an aerosol. One is based upon the physical measurement of size, and the second is based upon the aerodynamic behavior of the particles. The first uses laser diffraction technology, based on the ability of small particles to diffract light at their edges, and is the method of choice for measuring the particle size distribution of droplets from solutions produced by nebulization. The main advantage of the laser diffraction technique is that it can measure particle size distributions very rapidly. However, this technique measures particle volumes (VMD) and does not measure the drug itself. For drugs such as albuterol and tobramycin, which are dissolved in solution, droplet volume accurately reflects drug distribution in the various-sized particles. However, for suspensions such as budesonide, many of the drug particles are 2 μm or larger, so that some droplets may be too small to carry any drug and laser diffraction particle sizing gives an erroneously small measurement.[17]

Cascade impaction techniques use the laws of aerodynamics to measure particle size distributions. The aerosol is drawn into a device that has several stages with jet arrays that diminish in size with each stage. There is a collection system at each stage: a plate as used in a cascade impactor,[18] or a pool of liquid as used in a liquid impinger.[19] Larger particles fail to remain suspended in the air stream and impact on the plate at an early stage, whereas smaller particles are able to pass through to one of the later stages. By assaying the amount of drug from each plate or liquid stage, it is possible to calculate the particle size distribution, since each plate or stage removes a specific size range of particles from the flow of aerosol. This technique is very labor-intensive compared to laser diffraction, but it allows direct measurement of the drug of interest, ignoring the particle size of any excipients in the formulation.

For those reasons, cascade impaction is used for measuring aerosol characteristics from pMDIs, DPIs, and nebulized suspensions. Impactors can allow heat transfer and evaporation to occur, giving an artificially smaller distribution.[20] However, if these factors are controlled for, inertial impaction techniques agree well with the laser light diffraction techniques.[20,21] Finally, it is imperative to remember that although it is very important, particle size is only one of the many variables that determine aerosol deposition in the airways, and it should not be used alone to judge the quality or efficiency of an aerosol delivery device.

■ PATIENT-RELATED VARIABLES

Aerosol deposition and distribution in the airways is also dependent on the patient variables listed in Table 18-1. There is a large variability in deposition between subjects due to these host factors; something that would not be tolerated in oral or intravenous formulations. For example, in pharmacokinetic studies of inhaled antibiotics in CF, the standard deviation often approaches the value of the mean for serum and sputum drug levels.[22]

Inspiratory flow rate is one of the most important of the patient variables. Larger and higher-velocity particles have the greatest inertia and the highest probability to impact in the upper airways. The more slowly one inhales, the more likely the particles will bypass the upper airway and deposit in the lung. To emphasize this point, it was recently demonstrated that by using a nebulized aerosol with MMAD of 9.5 μm, and breathing with a large tidal volume and very slow inspiratory rate (4.8 Lpm), almost twice the lung deposition was achieved than with an aerosol with MMAD 5.0 μm and regular tidal breathing.[23] By slowing inspiration enough, even these larger particles (not normally considered "respirable") could navigate beyond the upper airway. Thus, slow inhalation is recommended for both pMDIs and nebulizers to optimize deposition. For DPIs, a faster inhalation is required to de-aggregate the powder.

Age plays a large role in aerosol deposition, with younger patients having higher upper airway deposition and lower lung deposition.[24,25] Larger inhaled volume is associated with greater lung deposition, and lower respiratory rates increase lung deposition because the dwell time in the lungs is longer, allowing for sedimentation of particles to occur.[25–27] These factors favor lung deposition in adults versus young children, and healthier versus sicker patients. Breath-holding at the end of inspiration is useful when using a breath-actuated device or a pMDI, but not when using a continuously operating nebulizer (because aerosol is wasted during the breath-hold). Of course, very young children cannot perform a breath-hold, which may contribute to a lower deposited fraction than that observed in older children and adults.

Lower airway geometry and pathology govern the distribution of an aerosol.[28] For example, CF patients with worsening lung disease may have increased total lung deposition versus healthy subjects, but the aerosol deposits mostly in the central airways and at sites of obstruction.[25,26,29,30] As airway obstruction increases, there is less homogeneous distribution of aerosol, and poorly ventilated areas may receive no drug at all.[5,31] In patients with the most airway obstruction, this patchy aerosol distribution may reduce the therapeutic response to some aerosolized drugs.

Upper airway geometry is also important, as it is the body's first defense against foreign material entering the respiratory system. The nasal passages force inspired airborne particles to flow though a series of convoluted turns, and some particles come into contact with the mucosa (which is lined with ciliated columnar epithelial cells and a blanket of mucous) and become entrapped. This arrangement can be highly effective and may take out particulate matter as small as 1 μm.[11] Nasal breathing can filter half of an aerosol drug before it can reach the lower airway,[32] so converting a child from a mask to a mouthpiece is recommended as soon as they can understand how to use mouthpiece devices. Also, there is a negative correlation between whole lung deposition from an inhaler and its variability, suggesting that the interaction between aerosol plumes and variable upper airway geometries in different subjects is the major cause of the high variability in lung deposition.[33]

Treatment with aerosolized drugs may involve children from early infancy to college age, and with varying degrees of lung disease. While all of the aerosol principles apply, achieving successful aerosol delivery in infants and small children is the most challenging. They have small upper and lower airways, fast breathing rates, and lower inhaled volumes. Breathing patterns are variable, depending on sleep state and degree of health. Infants are nasal breathers, which may filter the aerosol, and many children become fussy or cry during aerosol administration, which dramatically decreases lung dose.[34] The deposited lung dose in infants is many-fold smaller than in older children and adults, but their lungs are also much smaller. Lung deposition tends to be proportionate to size, so adjusting the nominal dose of an aerosol drug for children is not always necessary. Finally, while there are no clinical data yet, there is support for the idea that a 5-μm particle size cutoff may be too large for infants and young children.[35] In vitro experiments with a model of a 9-month-old's airway, and scintigraphy studies in toddlers suggest that an upper cutoff of 2.5 to 3 μm is more appropriate for young children.[36,37]

Finally, all instructions to the patients are of no avail if the child is physically or developmentally unable to use a prescribed device, or if there is little adherence to recommended therapy. Adherence to asthma medications is poor[38]; prescribed medications are underused approximately 50% of the time. There is no evidence that adherence is improved by changing to a different inhaler device (be it small or unobtrusive), even though such devices are often marketed on the basis that they are more acceptable to a patient and therefore will be used more. With improvements in technology, it is likely that drug delivery devices will be available that can both monitor and prompt patient use. In the meantime, thorough education and re-education of patients and their caregivers is necessary regarding the purpose of the prescribed medication and how to use, clean, and maintain their delivery devices.

PRESSURIZED METERED-DOSE INHALERS

The pMDI has a pressurized chamber that holds a propellant and the drug, either in suspension or solution (Fig. 18-2). Previously the propellant was a chlorofluorocarbon (CFC) that was a liquid under pressure, but as soon as it was released to atmospheric pressure it "flashed" and became a gas. More recently, in keeping with the Montreal Protocol to reduce the harmful effects of fluorocarbons on the ozone layer, the propellant has been changed to hydrofluoroalkane (HFA). It cannot be assumed that CFC and the replacement, HFA inhalers, are equivalent in every situation. For example, the HFA beclomethasone dipropionate (BDP) pMDI was reformulated as a solution rather than the older CFC suspension, and it emits drugs in much smaller particles (MMAD approximately 1 μm) and in a gentler plume, which results in an increased lung dose and less upper airway deposition of the medication. Scintigraphy studies of this HFA BDP inhaler show an average lung dose of 50% of emitted dose,[39] and clinical studies show that compared to the older CFC formulation less than half the dose of the HFA formulation is necessary to achieve the same improvement in pulmonary function.[40]

For drugs that are not in solution, it is necessary to shake the device before use to disperse the propellant and suspended drugs evenly so that consistent amounts of drug will be emitted with activation. Additions of surface active material and manipulations of polarity further facilitate the dispersion of the suspension. The emitted aerosol from some HFA formulations is warmer and less dense than that from the CFC-containing metered-dose inhalers, and patients may experience a different feel and taste when taking their inhalers. They should be warned about this and reassured that it does not mean that the inhaler is not working properly.[41] A further advantage of the HFA metered-dose inhaler may be enhanced

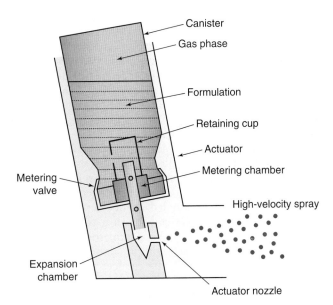

FIGURE 18-2. Schematic of a pMDI.

dose-to-dose reproducibility.[42] Unlike CFC inhalers, the dose released is unaffected by storage orientation or ambient temperature.[43]

In addition to a drug reservoir, there is a metering chamber of a fixed volume. The actual amount of drug contained in this chamber depends on the volume of the chamber and the concentration of drug within the propellant. While rigorously controlled at the time of manufacture, multiple activations without shaking can result in higher concentrations of drug if the device is held in the operating position and the drug settles, or in lower concentrations if the propellant is concentrated around the opening to the metering chamber at the time of refilling after activation.

The "flashing" process that occurs when the aerosol propellant mixture leaves the inhaler is never instantaneous, and until it has occurred completely, the droplets containing the drug have a greater size distribution than the drug particles alone. The velocity of the plume leaving the orifice is in the order of 25 to 30 m/sec, but it is rapidly slowed by the resistance of the air. If the device is activated when held between the lips during a vigorous inspiration, whether or not the particles in the plume will become small enough through loss of propellant and slow enough not to affect the posterior pharynx depends on the plume velocity and particle size and the distance traveled, which depends on the size of the patient.

Unlike early dry-powder preparations for which high levels of humidity became a problem, in a pMDI the drug is completely protected from the environment. However, "flashing" requires energy, specifically heat, and perhaps more important, the pressure inside the reservoir is very dependent on the ambient temperature. Hence, in cold climates the pMDI may be too cold to completely empty the metering chamber, and the droplets may not flash but may rain out in the mouth. The effect of temperature is less of a problem with newer HFA inhalers.

A pMDI alone, especially for inhaled steroids, is not recommended in children, as coordination between inhalation and actuation of the pMDI is rarely perfect, and upper airway deposition may result in topical side effects such as thrush or hoarseness. Since the development of the pMDI in the 1960s, it has been recognized that add-on devices are needed to improve drug delivery. Add-on devices include valveless spacers and valved holding chambers (VHCs). The word *spacer* refers to a device that increases the volume between the pMDI and the patient. This reduces the "ballistic" component by allowing complete flashing of the propellant and a reduction in particle speed, thus potentially reducing upper airway deposition. However, spacers have no valves and still require active coordination of the patient. Pressurized MDIs with VHCs are regarded as the most convenient system for the delivery of anti-asthma drugs to children younger than 5 years of age and delivery of inhaled corticosteroids to older children. They present the child with a relatively static cloud of aerosolised drug, thus reducing the need to coordinate actuation of the MDI with inhalation. The lack of a ballistic component markedly reduces the oropharyngeal deposition of drug, which in turn reduces the likelihood of local side effects. In the case of steroids with significant gastrointestinal absorption (e.g., BDP), use of

a VHC significantly reduces the amount of swallowed drug available for absorption, thus reducing potential systemic side effects. VHCs vary greatly in size, shape, valve position and design, and anti-static properties. These differences result in highly variable drug delivery among devices. Manufacturers make frequent modifications to their add-on devices (sometimes every 2 to 3 years), so by the time a paper comparing VHCs is published, it may no longer be relevant. Likewise, performance of VHCs with newer HFA inhalers cannot be inferred from studies of older CFC inhalers used with the same VHCs. As with nebulizers, the prescribed (nominal) dose may bear little resemblance to the amount of drug inhaled if different add-on devices are used to deliver the same drug. The addition of a facemask to VHCs has revolutionized the treatment of infants and young children with asthma. However, drug will only be delivered if the facemask fits the child's face and forms a complete seal without leaks. It has recently been shown that a facemask that was recommended for many years for use with an inhaled steroid may have delivered little of any drug to young children due to problems in obtaining a seal between the child's face and the mask.[44] Delivery by a mouthpiece is more efficient, and patients should use this in preference to a facemask when possible.

Both pMDIs and VHCs have advantages and disadvantages. pMDIs are relatively inexpensive, convenient to carry, and quick to use. However, they are very difficult to use correctly. For optimum drug delivery, the pMDI requires a high degree of coordination and psychomotor skill. The ideal closed-mouth technique is when the patient holds the mouthpiece between the lips and teeth, and begins inhalation slowly, almost simultaneously with actuation, followed by breath holding for about 10 seconds. The open-mouth technique uses the same sequence, but the patient fires the pMDI about 2 to 3 cm in front of a wide-open mouth, allowing some slowing of particle velocity and using the oropharynx as a small spacer. In practice, few adults and even fewer children can correctly use a pMDI, and even health care professionals have inadequate skills with pMDIs.[45] The variability of drug delivery to the lower respiratory tract between patients is extremely high. It is also surprisingly high within the same subject. Until recently, there was no reliable way that one could tell when the device was empty, but now most pMDIs have incorporated a dose counter.

Some manufacturers addressed the problem of coordination in pMDIs by developing breath-actuated pMDIs. These incorporate a mechanism that is activated during inhalation and fires the inhaler. This approach reduces the need for the patient or caregiver to coordinate pMDI actuation with inhalation.[46] However, patients may still stop inhaling when the pMDI is actuated due to the cold propellant effect.[47] Use of these devices for delivery of albuterol should be restricted to older children and adults. Evaluation of their efficacy in children younger than 5 years of age is limited.[48] A scintigraphy study showed excellent lung deposition using a breath-actuated pMDI of HFA-BDP.[49] Oropharyngeal deposition of steroids using these devices is still high and is minimized by the use of the conventional pMDI and VHC instead.

While MDIs are easy to carry and conceal for the self-conscious adolescent, VHCs are not. Side effects from systemic absorption of albuterol that deposited outside the lung are rare, so an add-on device is not essential for albuterol in a child with good technique. In contrast, it is sensible to reduce the deposition of steroids in the upper airway. One often-neglected issue is that the plastic used in some VHCs carries a high static electrical charge when new that will remove most of the medication. However, rinsing in mild detergent followed by a water rinse and air drying will remove most of the static electricity.[50] Failure to do this will mean that many days of multiple doses may be administered until the plastic has completely discharged. This often results in the diagnosis of refractory asthma that has resolved by the time the patient reaches the pediatric respiratory physician. In reality, all that has happened is that while waiting for the appointment, the static charge was reduced by coating the chamber with repeated doses so the subsequent doses were delivered effectively. The use of modern materials in VHCs (e.g., charge-dissipating plastics) removes much of the static charge, allowing a longer time between actuation and inhalation.[51] Pulmonary deposition in infants using a CFC pMDI correctly with a VHC results in a pulmonary delivery of about 2%,[52] and even the best of devices in adults achieve a delivery of less than 50% of the released dose, with large variability. However, as Tal and colleagues have argued,[52] on a mg per kilogram of body weight basis, 20% deposition from a pMDI and VHC in a 70-kilogram adult is very similar to 2% in a 7-kilogram infant. In children there are large variations, even when technique is good.[35] As mentioned earlier, nose breathing will remove more of the aerosol particles than mouth breathing, so as soon as a child is old enough to use a mouthpiece rather than a facemask, he or she should be switched. Interestingly, as add-on device design improves over time, so may the bioavailability of the inhaled drugs. One study comparing VHCs in young children showed that serum levels of fluticasone (which reflects the lung dose) averaged over 70% higher when using a nonstatic VHC versus a standard VHC of the same brand.[53] Since actual drug delivery varies so widely, it is prudent to adjust the dose of inhaled steroids to the minimum required to maintain disease control.

DRY-POWDER INHALERS

DPIs are widely used to deliver the same types of drugs as pMDIs (i.e., long-acting β2-agonists, anticholinergics, and anti-inflammatory drugs). However, DPIs are breath-actuated devices that do not require a coordinated press-and-breathe effort as with pMDIs. There are a variety of DPI device types, including capsule-based single-dose devices, multi-dose devices with a bulk-drug reservoir, and multi-dose devices with individual doses protected by foil. The common characteristic of both MDIs and DPIs is that a single activation results in a known ("metered") dose of drug to be released from the device. Unfortunately, there is a common misconception that precision in the amount of drug released from the DPI translates into a similar level of precision in the amount of drug delivered. This is far from the case. DPIs require the patient to generate the energy needed to both disperse and deliver the drug. For children with poor inspiratory efforts, delivery can be quite variable, although numerous clever features have been incorporated into many devices so that there is consistency after a certain minimal inspiratory flow has been achieved. As with any other aerosol, the size of the particle is fundamental to the eventual site of delivery. While there a number of ways to produce particles less than 5 μm including milling and spray drying, these particles tend to be bound together by electrostatic, Van der Waal and capillary forces. Hence, fine particles have poor flow characteristics and tend to be quite difficult to disperse. To address this problem, some formulations loosely bind the small drug particles to a larger excipient particle such as lactose. These particles, in the range of 30 to 60 μm, have much better flow characteristics. The preparation is then packaged in some form of metering device. The device is prepared for use by piercing the blister pack or capsule, or loading the outflow track, after which the patient inhales forcefully. The inspiratory air is forced to go through a system that generates high turbulence in order to separate the drug particles and the excipient. The small drug particles can then deposit below the vocal cords while the excipient impacts on the posterior pharynx. Flows required are generally in the 30 L/min range or higher. Most devices are designed so that flows in excess of the minimum do not give rise to variable output. However, flows less than the minimum can result in failure to separate drug particles from one another or the excipient from the drug and poor pulmonary deposition. Not only does the inspiratory energy have to be high enough to de-aggregate the powder, but the inspired volume has to be adequate to carry the particles deep into the lungs. Therefore DPIs are not recommended for children younger than 5 to 6 years of age.

There are many advantages of DPIs, including compactness and portability, rapid delivery time, and no need for hand-breath coordination. Multi-dose DPIs also have dose counters so the patient can recognize when the prescription needs to be refilled. Like pMDIs, most drugs delivered currently by DPI are in microgram quantities, though it is possible to develop formulations for DPIs that can be delivered in very high doses. Examples of this capability include inhaled mannitol powder for airway clearance[54] and inhaled colistin for CF airway infection.[55] Other novel formulations for high-dose delivery will be discussed later. DPIs also have some drawbacks. When used to deliver steroids, they still have the disadvantage of significant upper airway deposition of drug. They are effort dependent as previously stated, so there are limitations of age and disease severity to consider. Dry-powder formulations are sensitive to humidity, so exhaling into the device may cause clumping of particles. Perhaps the biggest challenge with current DPIs is that there are many types of inhalers, and learning how to use one type does not make use of a different type intuitive (Fig. 18-3).[56] To add to the confusion, there are no DPI formulations currently available for short-acting β2-agonists. Thus if a patient learns how to use a DPI for controller asthma therapy, he or she still needs to learn how to use a pMDI

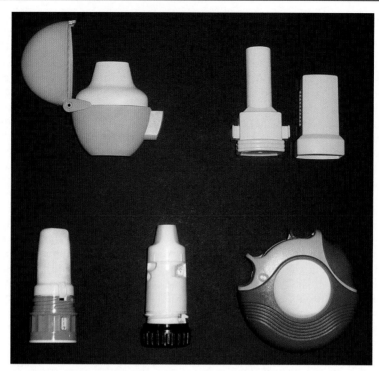

FIGURE 18-3. Types of dry-powder inhalers. Top row: single-dose inhaler HandiHaler and Aerolizer. Bottom row: multidose inhalers Twisthaler, Flexhaler, and Diskus.

or nebulizer for rescue medication. Learning different techniques for controller and rescue medications can be very confusing and can lead to what has been dubbed "device delirium."[57]

NEBULIZERS

Pressurized MDIs and DPIs tend to be somewhat complex and dependent upon the physical properties of the agents being aerosolized. The development of this type of drug device combination is both expensive and lengthy and, as a result, is largely restricted it to agents that are in widespread use (e.g., agents used in the treatment of asthma). For diseases with low prevalence (e.g., CF), no pharmaceutical companies were willing to invest the resources necessary to develop specific drug-device aerosol delivery systems until recent years. Consequently, two phenomena occurred historically. First, companies that developed novel aerosol treatments for CF utilized off-the-shelf inexpensive nebulizers as the least expensive path to regulatory approval (though it added significant time burden for patients). Second, because the theory and science of treating CF lung disease with topical aerosols advanced more quickly than delivery device technology, many physicians resorted to treating CF patients using commercially available nebulizers to aerosolize drugs that were not originally intended for aerosol delivery. At present, some drugs are approved with specific nebulizers, though clinicians may still substitute a different type of nebulizer for the approved device. Since there is a very large variability of particle size and output characteristics between nebulizers,[58] this practice may result in delivery of much higher lung doses (which risks increased toxicity with some drugs)

or much lower lung doses (which risks reduced efficacy). The decision by the individual prescribing physician to use an off-label drug or delivery device circumvents the quality-control mechanisms of the governmental drug regulating bodies (e.g., the Food and Drug Administration, FDA). Failure to match the delivery device to the agent being nebulized[59] and use of the aerosol route of administration for agents not intended for this purpose[60] can, and sometimes does, lead to problems. A recently published consensus document recommended that new devices and compounds be studied properly before using them in patients to avoid the potential problems that can otherwise occur.[61]

Another reason for choosing nebulization over pMDIs or DPIs has to do with the potency of the drug being aerosolized. For example, albuterol is potent in the microgram range, whereas tobramycin is only potent in the milligram range, so the volume of liquid that must be delivered to the lungs becomes a limiting factor for MDIs. While a DPI has been developed to deliver tobramycin,[62] the relatively large amount of drug needed for effect compared to most asthma medications delivered by DPIs does have its challenges. Some of the indications for nebulized drugs are listed in Table 18-2.

Nebulization can be accomplished by ultrasound, compressed-air jet, or vibrating-perforated-membrane technologies, or by a piston that forces liquid through tiny holes. This last system is discussed later in the chapter in the section entitled "Future Directions for Aerosol Delivery." The ultrasonic method uses a piezoelectric crystal that rapidly vibrates the nebulizing solution placed in a compartment directly above. The liquid vibrates to the extent that droplets become separated from the surface (Fig. 18-4). The cloud of droplets can be carried to the patient for inhalation by directing a flow of air across the surface of the solution. Depending on the

TABLE 18-2 THERAPEUTIC INDICATIONS FOR NEBULIZED THERAPY IN CHILDREN

Asthma
β2-agonists
Anticholinergics
Corticosteroids
Croup
Budesonide
Epinephrine
Cystic fibrosis
Antimicrobials
rhDNase
Hypertonic saline
Bronchiectasis
Antimicrobials
Pulmonary hypertension
Prostacyclin
Immunization
Measles vaccine

type of ultrasonic nebulizer, the particle size distribution may be quite appropriate for inhalation, and many of these nebulizers are capable of producing large amounts of aerosol per unit time. In general, ultrasonic nebulizers tend to have larger particle size distributions than jet nebulizers, but there is considerable overlap, which is very device dependent. However, there are some disadvantages of ultrasonic nebulization. Some (although not all) have a relatively large residual volume (V_r), which is the volume remaining in the device at the end of effective nebulization. This results in wasted drug. A second theoretical disadvantage is the heat generated by the ultrasonic process, which can denature any proteins in the agents being nebulized.[63] Another limitation of this method is that some drugs (e.g., budesonide) are available only as suspensions rather than solutions. Since the vibrations of the ultrasonic nebulizer are at the surface of the liquid, suspended particles below the surface can settle, thus reducing output of the drug significantly.[64] The viscosity of the agent being nebulized can affect output. Ultrasonic devices are not disposable and require vigilant cleaning and disinfection for infection-control purposes.

Somewhat analogous to ultrasonic nebulizers, but clearly an advance, are vibrating membrane devices. With vibrating mesh technology, aerosol is generated by extruding fluid though precision-drilled holes (Fig. 18-5). This requires much less energy, which means that they can be battery driven and are much quieter. Since there are no baffles and the particle size is determined by the size of the holes and the physical properties of the solution being nebulized (primarily surface tension and viscosity), the aerosol droplets are much more uniform than those produced by jet nebulizers. The "tradeoff" with regard to particle size is that although smaller particles may be desired, the smaller the precision holes, the slower the aerosol generation. When nebulizing solutions with viscosities close to water, the vibrating mesh devices have a much faster output. Because of the absence of a baffling system and surfaces to trap droplets, these devices have a very low V_r and can be highly efficient.[65] The Pari eFlow is a platform of devices that has been used in the development of several CF drugs, including the recently-approved aztreonam solution for

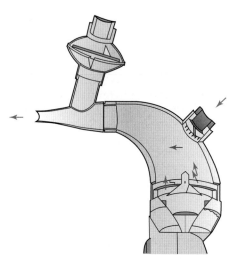

FIGURE 18-4. This ultrasonic nebulizer relies on the vibration of a piezo electric crystal to produce an aerosol. When the patient inhales, air is entrained through the device, capturing the aerosol that is generated for inhalation. The patient then breathes out through the filter at the top, which stops drug-laden air from contaminating the surroundings.

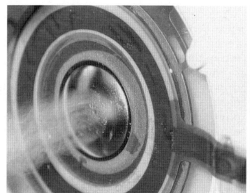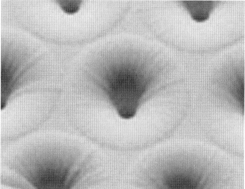

FIGURE 18-5. Examples of vibrating perforated-membrane technology. On the left, the aerosol generator from a Pari eFlow device shows the aerosol being generated from the "mesh," which is driven by the surrounding piezo element. On the right, a magnified view of a perforated membrane used in Aerogen nebulizers is shown.

inhalation (AZLI) that only takes 2 to 3 minutes to nebulize for CF patients with chronic *Pseudomonas* airway infections.[66] The product was designed as a drug-device combination, and this particular eFlow device (called Altera) is meant to be used only with AZLI. In fact, because increased efficiency could lead to overdosing of some drugs (e.g., albuterol or tobramycin), the Pari eFlow Rapid was designed as an open device for other CF drugs to speed drug delivery, but match the other performance characteristics of jet nebulizers that have been approved for use with these drugs. A number of vibrating membrane devices are available, each with similarities and differences. The similarity is the electronic circuit that senses both the membrane and the physical properties of drug being nebulized and adjusts the frequency of the membrane to the resonant frequency. Because of both efficiency and greater flow through the membrane compared to the output of a jet nebulizer, they can often shorten treatment time compared to other devices.[67] For diseases such as CF, where lack of adherence to medically recommended therapies is common, often due to time requirements of the therapy, devices that reduce total treatment time would, hopefully, promote better adherence to all aspects of CF treatment. However, there are some drawbacks. One is the initial high cost that makes these devices reusable rather than disposable. Thus, they require complicated cleaning and sterilization procedures for infection control. As long as the drug being nebulized is a solution with relatively low viscosity, good output rates are easily achieved, so nebulization times can be minimized. However, increasing viscosity may compromise performance of these devices, even more than with jet nebulizers. If the drug of choice is a suspension, the particles may be too large to pass through the membrane, resulting in clogging, low output, or both. Similar problems may occur with protein aqueous solutions, such as those that might be used for lung gene therapy. They also tend to be more expensive than traditional jet nebulizers, although the price difference lessens when the cost of the external compressor needed to drive jet nebulizers is considered.

While many options exist, jet nebulization is still widely used in both the home and hospital setting. Jet nebulizers range widely in cost and performance, but the less expensive ones are disposable so complicated cleaning procedures are less necessary. Jet nebulization is a comminution process where a high-velocity gas jet fragments a film of liquid into droplets of varying sizes (Fig. 18-6). Passing compressed air through an extremely small orifice generates the high-velocity jet. At the exit of this orifice are one or two capillary "feed" tubes that lead to the well of the reservoir containing the nebulizing solution. Forcing a jet of gas to travel at high velocity will result in a reduction of air pressure at the sides of this jet stream. As a result of this Bernoulli effect, liquid from the reservoir will be drawn up the capillary tube, spread out to the exit of the jet orifice, and be fragmented by the stream jet. Another method of shearing the liquid film into aerosol is employed by the Ventstream and Sidestream nebulizers (both by Medic-Aid Ltd., Pagham, UK). Rather than shearing the liquid film at a 90-degree angle, the shearing takes place

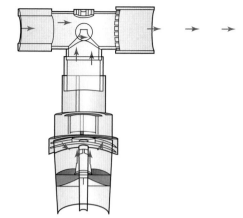

FIGURE 18-6. The inside of the Cirrus jet nebulizer is shown. Air under high pressure passes through a small hole as it expands, and the negative pressure generated sucks the drug solution or suspension up the feeding tube, where it is atomized. The atomized drug either impacts on the baffle, returns for re-nebulization, or leaves the nebulizer.

over the surface of the liquid film, resulting in a less violent process. In both these methods, the range of particle sizes is considerable, ranging from 0.1 to 30 μm. By forcing this air containing aerosol droplets through a series of baffles, the larger particles are removed by inertial impaction and will run back to the reservoir to be renebulized, the fate of 99% of the droplets generated.[68] With greater nebulizing flow, a larger number of small particles are generated by the jet and fewer large particles survive the baffling process, giving rise to a smaller particle size distribution. The goal is to have the majority of the remaining particles within the fine particle fraction (≤5 μm diameter). Particles that are small enough to escape inertial impaction may leave the nebulizer and deposit in the airway during inspiration, or are lost to the atmosphere during the expiratory phase. Particles can also "rain out" in the nebulizer. Since the internal volume of the nebulizer and gas flow determine the suspension time of a particle within the nebulizer, higher nebulizing flow will increase output and reduce rain out. In general, one can achieve higher nebulizing flows such as these by using tanks of compressed gas or piped-in medical gases, which result in increased rates of output and smaller particle size distributions than home-based compressor units.[69] The particle-size difference between aerosols generated by home compressors versus compressed-gas sources may have an effect on the intrapulmonary dose.

The process of jet nebulization is very violent and may destroy complex molecules, such as lipid-DNA complexes or proteoliposomes.[70] This places considerable physical demands on the equipment. Repetitive use of disposable devices in the laboratory can lead to degradation of particle size distribution when the device is driven by a 50-psi source of compressed air, although the clinical significance of this is questionable with the use of a compressor in the home environment.[71] However, the plastic in disposable devices may not stand up to proper cleaning, and failure to adequately clean the device leads to significant bacterial contamination.[71] On the other hand, reusable devices are built with material that will withstand the high flows and pressures over a prolonged period of time as well as repetitive cleaning.

In the standard unvented nebulizer (see Fig. 18-6), the only inlet to the nebulizer (once charged) is the driving flow, and the only outlet is the exit of this flow carrying the suspended droplets. This outlet is usually connected to a combination of a T-piece and a mouthpiece (or a facemask for children who are too small to use a mouthpiece). The aerosol output of this type of device is independent of any respiratory activity of the patient. The output will remain constant during inspiration when drug is inhaled into the patient's airway, and also during expiration when the aerosolized drug is lost to the atmosphere. The expiratory time usually exceeds the inspiratory time, often approaching 60% of the respiratory cycle for children with CF breathing through a nebulizer,[72] and the ratio of expiration to inspiration appears to increase with worsening airflow obstruction.[73] In other words, unvented nebulizers, almost by definition, are very inefficient simply due to the pattern of breathing. Low fill volumes (e.g., the 2-mL nebule containing budesonide), coupled with a V_r that is usually at least 0.5 mL and can be over 1 mL, further decrease the level of efficiency. The Sidestream nebulizer incorporates an adaptation to increase the rate of output by allowing air to be drawn into the device by the Venturi action of the flow from the compressor (Fig. 18-7). This greatly increases the rate of aerosol leaving the device, which can shorten treatment time but does nothing to reduce the waste of aerosol during expiration.

In order to increase efficiency, it is necessary to minimize losses during the expiratory phase. This can be accomplished in three ways. First the device can be engineered to increase its output during inspiration relative to expiration by utilizing inspiratory flow that is entrained into the device through a system of one-way valves. Second, the device can be "breath actuated" so that nebulization occurs only during inspiration, which can be detected electrically or mechanically. The third approach is to have a valved holding chamber between the aerosol generator and the mouthpiece that captures and stores aerosol generated during expiration, which is then inhaled during the first part of inspiration. All three systems have advantages and disadvantages.

The breath-enhanced nebulizer shown in Figure 18-8 has valves that direct inspiratory flow though the nebulizer and expiratory flow away from the nebulizer. This causes particles that would normally "rain out" when using a standard unvented nebulizer, to be swept into the airway because of the enhanced flow through the nebulizer during inspiration. During expiration, increased rain out occurs and the drug returns to the reservoir for re-nebulization. Such breath-enhanced nebulizers increase aerosol output during inspiration and become "quiescent" during expiration, which minimizes drug waste. Figure 18-9 shows the comparison of a standard unvented nebulizer to a "breath-enhanced" nebulizer—both widely used in the treatment of CF. The difference can be seen in the rate of output within the RF for both types of nebulizers. For an adult with CF, it is estimated that the breath-enhanced PARI LC Jet Plus nebulizer (PARI Pharma GmbH, Munich, Germany) would double the deposition of inhaled tobramycin compared to the unvented device.[74] Similar results have been shown *in vivo* by direct comparison of the breath-enhanced Ventstream nebulizer and the unvented Hudson 1730.[75]

The second approach is breath activation where aerosol is only generated during inspiration, thus reducing waste. The first example is the Halolite (Medic-Aid Ltd., Pagham, UK), which senses the patient's breathing pattern and delivers a pulse of aerosol at the start of inspiration based on the previous three breaths for a pre-programmed finite number of breaths. The Halolite and its successor "smart devices" (discussed later in the chapter) can deliver a precise dose of medication to the airway, an advantage for a

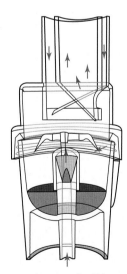

FIGURE 18-7. A cutaway drawing of a Sidestream nebulizer is shown. The Sidestream is similar to a conventional jet nebulizer, but it has a vent at the top of the device. As air under high pressure from the compressor passes through the small hole (known as the Venturi) within the device, it expands and rapidly creates a negative pressure. The open vent allows extra air to be drawn through the nebulizer as a result of this negative pressure. The extra air entrained through the nebulizer captures more aerosol drug from the device. This device does not necessarily deliver more drug, but it significantly shortens nebulization times.

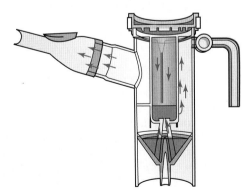

FIGURE 18-8. A drawing of a PARI LC Plus nebulizer is shown. The PARI LC differs from a conventional nebulizer in that a vent at the top of the nebulizer opens when the patient breathes in, thus allowing extra air to be entrained through the device. This extra air carries with it more aerosol than would normally have been deposited within the device and re-nebulized. Drug delivery is increased, as proportionally more drug is inhaled during inspiration than is lost during the expiratory phase when the valve at the top of the nebulizer closes.

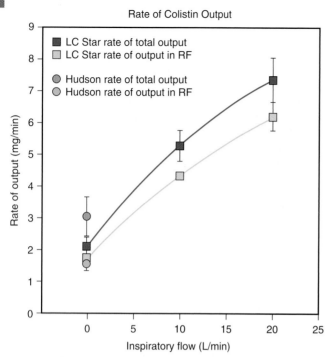

Rate of Colistin Output

FIGURE 18-9. The rate of output of colistin from an unvented (Hudson Updraft II) and a breath-enhanced (PARI LC Star) nebulizer in relation to entrained flow. The breath-enhanced nebulizer dramatically increases the rate of output (both total and that in the respirable fraction), whereas the inspiratory flow (entrained flow plus nebulizer driving flow) has no effect on the unvented nebulizer. (Modified from Katz SL, Ho SL, Coates AL. Nebulizer choice for treatment of cystic fibrosis patients with inhaled colistin. Chest. 2001;119:250-255.)

drug with a narrow therapeutic safety profile.[76] A simpler system, the AeroEclipse II (Trudell Medical International, London, Canada) is disposable breath-actuated nebulizer that generates aerosol only when the patient's inspiratory flow exceeds 15 L/min. This type of device[76] produces no aerosol during expiration, which virtually eliminates environmental contamination—a significant issue with aerosolized antimicrobials, especially in a hospital setting. The only drug wastage that occurs with breath-actuated devices is from that remaining in the device at the end of nebulization. However, both devices require that the patient breathe on a mouthpiece, and in the latter case small children may not have a sufficiently long portion of inspiration during which flow is greater than 15 L/min to activate nebulization. While both devices require an internal or external source of compressed air, the demands of the AeroEclipse II are roughly 6 to 8 L/min from a controlled 50 psi, which is significantly greater than that produced by a standard home compressor.

A third technique to increase efficiency employs an aerosol holding chamber with valves to minimize expiratory losses,[67,77] an example of which is the PARI eFlow. This device generates aerosol at a constant rate into a small chamber. During inspiration, a set of one-way valves open to allow entrained air to sweep the aerosol from the chamber into the patient. During exhalation, the valves close and an expiratory valve in the mouthpiece opens to direct expired air away from the chamber, thus allowing newly produced aerosol to be stored for the next inhalation. One way to customize the eFlow for various

purposes is to change the size of the aerosol chamber to alter how much aerosol can be captured in this way.

A number of other factors influence nebulizer efficiency. Various geometrical configurations of different nebulizers will result in different values for V_r.[59] The relative humidity of the driving gas flow is another factor. For example, most home compressors are considered a "wet" gas source because ambient water vapor is compressed to the saturation point. In contrast, tanks of compressed air and oxygen, or hospital gases from a wall outlet, are dry gas sources. When utilizing a wet source, there is less evaporative loss and less concentration of the drug in the V_r, therefore nebulized drug output is increased.[78] Historically, evaporative losses were not always considered when reporting nebulizer output,[79] though now it is recognized that failure to do so can lead to significant errors.[80] From the clinical perspective, if the nebulizer fill volume is 2 mL (e.g., a nebule of budesonide) and the V_r is 0.5 mL, driving the nebulizer from a dry gas source will result in almost half of the drug remaining behind in the nebulizer at the time of "dryness." Both increasing the fill volume and using a "wet" gas source would improve nebulizer efficiency, the former being the most important factor.

There are several types of nebulizers with highly variable levels of efficiency. Drug dosing that does not consider nebulizer/compressor efficiency can result in marked underdosing or very significant overdosing.[76,81] Hence, most drugs that are commonly administered by nebulization have a very wide therapeutic safety margin.

One of the principle advantages of using jet nebulizers is that little cooperation from the patient is required, especially where the nebulizer is connected to a mask that is secured to the face of a small child. However, Everard and colleagues[82] have shown with an *in vitro* model that moving the mask just 2 cm from the "face" reduces delivery of the nebulized drug by up to 85%. A mouthpiece should be used whenever possible. Another general recommendation involves the use of the appropriate fill volume. All devices have a Vr, which may be somewhat reduced by tapping the nebulizer walls during nebulization. The factors already mentioned ultimately determine the V_r of a particular nebulizer.

Jet nebulizers have evaporative losses of solvent during operation, resulting in a more concentrated drug in the V_r than at the beginning of nebulization. Hence, aerosol output can be increased for a given dose of drug by increasing the charge volume, although the cost will be a longer nebulization time. In principal, 4 mL is ideal for many devices[83] because drug output for volumes ≤3 mL are lower and device-dependent. That said, most nebulized drugs come in prepackaged ampules ranging from 2 to 5 mL. The clinical trials that led to approval of these drugs were conducted with the known inefficiencies of the devices, so changing the fill volume may change the risk-benefit ratio of a particular drug.

Finally, in this age of increasing concern about health care expenses, issues of cost-effectiveness must be taken into account. In hospital, the actual cost of treatment is a combination of the cost of the nebulizer, the cost of the medication being nebulized, and the labor costs of administration. At home, costs include those of the compressor. While labor may be less of an issue at home, inefficient nebulizers that require longer nebulization times may reduce adherence to recommended treatment (which has its own associated costs). For any agent other than the least expensive drugs, the cost of the drug and the efficiency of the nebulizer, rather than the cost of the device, determines the cost-effectiveness of drug delivery.

■ HOW TO CHOOSE A DELIVERY DEVICE

Each of the aerosol delivery systems has advantages and disadvantages. These are outlined in Table 18-3. There is a large body of literature that compares the efficacy of inhaled bronchodilators and corticosteroids delivered by different devices, with various claims of superiority or equivalence between devices. A comprehensive review of this literature examining a variety of clinical settings including the home, emergency department, hospital, and intensive care unit concluded that each of the aerosol devices can work equally well *in patients who can use these devices appropriately.*[84] Patients must be evaluated for their understanding and capability of using aerosol devices, and they must be taught proper techniques for use and maintenance of the devices. There are strong caregiver biases that favor the use of one device over another, which may serve the majority of patients well but fall short in others. For example, the pMDI is used exclusively for asthma drugs in many centers and countries, for both hospitalized and ambulatory patients. However, pMDI technique is the most difficult to teach and learn, leading to multiple errors that can affect efficacy.[4] Also, although in young children the pMDI coupled with a VHC and mask is very popular, repeated crying has been observed in as many as 38% of these children, which can significantly

TABLE 18-3 ADVANTAGES AND DISADVANTAGES OF COMMON AEROSOL DEVICES

DEVICE	ADVANTAGES	DISADVANTAGES
Jet nebulizer with compressor	• Easy technique (quiet tidal breathing) • May be used at any age • Can deliver large doses (e.g., antimicrobials) • Can use with any disease severity • Can deliver wide range of medication types • Some models are small and portable with DC or battery power • Can use with artificial airways, mechanical ventilation	• Some technique is required (need to inhale by mouth if using mouthpiece) • More expensive • Noisy (if compressor driven) • Longer treatment times • Requires power supply • Requires regular servicing, cleaning, and disinfection • Some drugs contain preservatives; osmolality and pH may vary • Large variability in drug output and aerosol characteristics between different brands (portable models generally are slower and have larger particle size)
Ultrasonic nebulizer	• Same general advantages as jet nebulizer • Faster aerosol output • May be handheld • Quiet operation • Portable and may be run by rechargeable batteries	• Poor delivery of suspensions (like corticosteroids) • In general, larger particle size than jet nebulizers • More expensive than jet nebulizers
Pressurized metered-dose inhaler	• Convenient, multidose • Compact, portable • Rapid delivery time • Dose counters more common	• Difficult technique; requires coordination of actuation and inhalation • High oropharyngeal deposition of drugs (topical side effects possible) • Limited number of drugs; only small doses possible • Not recommended for young children without add-on device • Nozzle may clog with some HFA inhalers
Breath-actuated metered-dose inhaler	• Helps overcome coordination difficulties • Popular with children older than 5 years of age who require bronchodilator therapy	• Does not eliminate throat deposition • Cannot use with add-on devices • Not recommended for children younger than 5 years of age
Pressurized metered-dose inhaler plus add-on device (spacer, holding chamber)	• Convenient • Allows patients of any age to use pMDI (including infants/young children) when used with facemask • Markedly reduces oropharyngeal deposition of drug • Use of antistatic spacers reduces variability of drug delivery • May be used to administer bronchodilators in emergency situations	• Still requires correct technique • Highly variable drug delivery between brands • Some devices affected by static on spacer walls, resulting in variable drug output • Holding chambers with inspiratory valves are recommended over spacer devices without a valve • Add-on devices require cleaning and replacement after several months of use
Dry-powder inhaler	• Convenient • Compact, portable • Rapid delivery time	• Effort-dependent particle size and drug output • Vulnerable to humidity • Limited to children older than 5 years of age • High oropharyngeal drug deposition • Multiple types (multi-dose, single dose, design differences) • Short-acting bronchodilators not available in DPI; need to provide a different device, which may confuse the patient

reduce the lung dose.[85] There is no "one size fits all" when it comes to aerosol devices.

The complex relationship between caregivers, suppliers, pharmacies, insurers, hospitals, and patients will influence the choice of aerosol device for a child.[57] The following questions will factor into the choice of device:

1. Which device can deliver the desired drug?
2. Is the device appropriate for the age, comprehension, and capability of the child?
3. Is the drug/device covered by the child's third-party payor?
4. Can the same device type be used for all prescribed inhaled drugs for the child?
5. Which device would be the most convenient, least expensive, most portable, and most time-saving?
6. For which devices can the care provider teach the proper technique?
7. Which device does the patient and/or parent prefer?

The American Association of Respiratory Care provides an invaluable guide with detailed instructions on how to use and care for aerosol-delivery devices.[56]

NEBULIZER USE FOR VENTILATED PATIENTS

Many patients receive inhaled therapy during mechanical ventilation. They range from tiny infants receiving inhaled surfactants to older children receiving medication for treatment of acute severe asthma. Unfortunately, the use of aerosolized medications for ventilated patients is largely supported by only anecdotal evidence. One of the biggest issues is optimizing the amount of drug delivered to the lung. Factors that affect drug deposition may be divided into those related to the ventilator, those related to the ventilator circuit, those affected by the choice of nebulizer or drug delivered, and finally those factors determined by the patient and his or her disease.[86-89]

Optimized deposition occurs during synchronized ventilation but is reduced if the patient inappropriately triggers ventilation or is fighting the ventilator. Increasing the patient's tidal volume will increase drug deposition from a nebulizer. While keeping the minute volume constant, an increase in respiratory rate will decrease the lung delivery of aerosol. This is because a greater proportion of the inspired air is used to move aerosol in the functional dead spaces of the circuit and the respiratory tract. Nebulized aerosol is only delivered to the patient during inspiration. Therefore, if the patient has a short inspiratory phase or a prolonged expiratory phase, aerosol delivery will be reduced. This may be due to either inappropriate settings of the ventilator or the patient's illness (e.g., a patient with airway obstruction, such as asthma, who has prolonged expiration). The inspiratory waveform will differ according to the mode of ventilation chosen.

Other factors that affect the deposition of aerosol include the endotracheal (ET) tube, heating and humidification of inspired gases, and gas density. The ET tube provides a significant obstruction to aerosol delivery if it is coated with secretions as these promote turbulent airflow. Ventilator gases are normally heated and humidified, but high humidity may cause a rapid increase in particle size. A small number of studies have demonstrated that using non-humidifying gases while delivering nebulized drugs can double aerosol

delivery to the lung. However, this is not generally recommended. Low-density gases are less likely to demonstrate turbulent flow, and several studies have shown that by using low-density gases (e.g., heliox), lung deposition of drug may be improved by up to 50%. The ventilator must be designed for use with heliox. If heliox is used to power the nebulizer, the effect on drug output must be determined.

Many different nebulizers are available for use with ventilated patients. Aerosols may be generated continuously throughout ventilation, or they may be timed to coincide with inspiration. Aerosol delivery may be given continuously or intermittently. Some nebulizers run off the ventilator driving gas flow and are synchronized so that the driving gas flows only during inspiration. However, the timing of the gas flow may be such that there is a delay between the start of the inspiration and aerosol production. The most efficient position of a nebulizer in a ventilatory circuit is in the inspiratory limb at least 30 cm from the endotracheal tube. In this position, the inspiratory tube appears to act as a reservoir for nebulized drug. A number of patient-related factors may also affect drug deposition. These include the severity of the disease (e.g., more central deposition of inhaled drugs with airway obstruction), the presence of hyperinflation, and ventilatory retractions. Drug delivery is enhanced if the patient and ventilator are working in synchrony and is reduced if the patient is "fighting" the ventilator.

In addition to conventional jet and ultrasonic nebulizers, two other devices have been proposed for use with ventilated patients. The first is a mesh-based system in which liquid is forced through a rapidly vibrating mesh and aerosol droplets are formed as the liquid extrudes through the pores in the mesh. No gas flow is needed, and these devices are small and highly efficient. A different approach is to inject liquid through a fine catheter that has been passed through the endotracheal tube, thereby bypassing the upper airway. Production of aerosol occurs at the end of the catheter. High delivery rates have been found with this system during *in vitro* experiments.

PMDIs may also be used with adaptors that attach directly to the endotracheal tube or elsewhere in the inspiratory ventilator circuit. Impaction on surrounding structures after actuation means that much drug is lost on the walls of the tubing and ET tube. Incorporating a spacer device into the circuit increases the drug delivery from the MDI considerably and, like the nebulizer, the spacer is best placed in the inspiratory limb approximately 30 cm from the ET tube.[90-93]

It is important that any devices used to deliver inhaled medicines are thoroughly tested and their efficacy understood both in the clinical setting for which they are intended, and with the drugs that will be used. Unfortunately, there is limited research on the delivery of aerosolized medications to children on ventilators.

FUTURE DIRECTIONS FOR AEROSOL DELIVERY

There have been many forces driving the technological development of novel techniques and aerosol delivery systems. The ban on chlorofluorocarbons has led to the development of alternate propellants, the redesign of pMDI components, and the development of non-propellant devices. The need to deliver expensive or complex therapeutic moieties (e.g., proteins, liposome-drug complexes, genes)—some with a narrow therapeutic index—led to the design of devices and formulations that reduce drug waste, speed delivery times, and improve targeting precision. The latter is very important for systemic delivery of inhaled drugs (e.g., insulin) that require the dose to be delivered to the lung periphery where the large surface area can absorb the drug more effectively. The novel aerosol devices described in the following paragraphs address one or more of the limitations of current systems.

The Respimat (Boehringer Ingelheim, Ingelheim, Germany) is a small, propellant-free, multidose device that employs a spring mechanism to push liquid through nozzles to generate a "slow mist" aerosol over 1 to 1.5 seconds (Fig. 18-10). It has the convenience of a pMDI but improves ease of use by slowing the particle cloud to allow for easier coordination of actuation/inhalation, and reduction in throat impaction. Lung deposition in adults averages 40% with this device.[94] The aerosol qualities are not dependent on propellants or inspiratory effort (unlike pMDIs and DPIs, respectively). The Respimat does not require a spacer, battery, or electrical power source. The drug is in solution form rather than suspension form, so shaking is not required; it still requires some coordination of actuation and inspiration that may preclude the use of the Respimat in very young children. The Respimat is available in some countries for asthma drugs. Another slow-mist device is the AERx Pulmonary Drug Delivery System (Aradigm, Hayward, California) in which a piston drives the drug through microscopic pores in blister packs while the patient inhales. One version has an electronic processor that monitors and guides the patient's inspiratory flow and breath-hold, releases drug only when inspiratory flow is optimal, conditions the temperature of the entrained air, and can monitor adherence. A less expensive mechanical version was also developed for formulations that do not require such precision of dosing. The AERx has been studied with a variety of drugs for pulmonary and systemic delivery, but it is not yet approved.

The AERx was one of the first so-called "smart devices" that operate in various ways to improve lung targeting and delivery efficiency. A trio of devices makes use of a technique called adaptive aerosol delivery (AAD, Philips Respironics). The HaloLite previously described was the first generation of these devices, and the ProDose is the second-generation device. Both devices use jet nebulizers and compressors, but they have electronics to monitor and adapt to the tidal breathing pattern, releasing aerosol only during the first portion of inhalation, with no wasted drug during exhalation. A microchip inserted in the ProDose includes information about the dose, frequency of administration, lot number, and expiration date. The ProDose is used in some European countries for delivery of colistin, and it is licensed for delivery of iloprost for the treatment of pulmonary hypertension. However, the HaloLite and ProDose have some of the same limitations as other jet nebulizers, including power source requirement, noise, high V_r, and long treatment duration. The I-neb is the third-generation AAD device that addresses some of these limitations. It incorporates vibrating perforated membrane technology, making it portable, battery-operated, and silent, with a low V_r to reduce drug waste (Fig. 18-11) The I-neb can operate in two modes. The tidal breathing mode is the same as the predicate devices that deliver drug during spontaneous tidal breathing to the inspiratory portion only. There is no control over how fast or deeply the patient breathes in this mode. However, by slowing down the inspiratory flow, there will be less upper airway impaction, higher lung deposition, and more even drug dispersion with far less variability of lung dose.[95] Taking this into account, the "targeted inhalation mode" was developed to improve the precision of dosing. A high-resistance mouthpiece restricts inspiratory flow to about 20 L/min, and the device uses a tactile indicator to coach the patient to inhale slowly and deeply, for as long as 9 seconds, depending on his or her capability. Aerosol is produced for all but the last 2 seconds of inspiration to allow the droplets to travel further in the lung to deposit. With this mode, over 70% of the emitted dose is deposited in the lungs, and treatment times can be reduced versus tidal breathing.[96,97] Also, the I-neb has an accessory

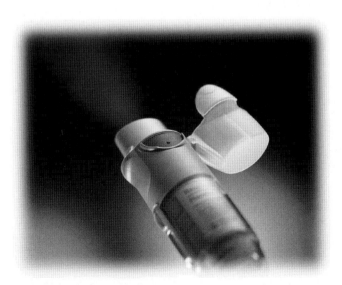

FIGURE 18-10. The firing of a Respimat slow-mist inhaler.

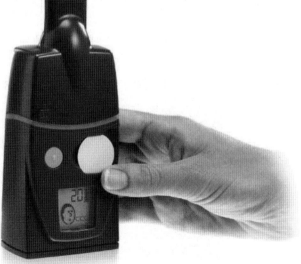

FIGURE 18-11. The portable I-neb device has an LCD screen and a memory disc.

device that monitors how and when the device is used so adherence patterns can be studied. The I-neb is replacing the ProDose for colistin and iloprost delivery (tidal breathing mode) and is being developed for use with many other formulations.

Another device called the Akita (Activaero, Gemunden, Germany) device allows individualized controlled inhalations in combination with either a jet nebulizer or an eFlow vibrating mesh (Fig. 18-12).[98] The Akita stores a patient's pulmonary function on a "smart card" that tells the device when to pulse the aerosol during inspiration, depending on the drug target (early inspiration for distal airway deposition or late inspiration for large-airway targeting). When the patient starts to inhale, the Akita supplies air from a compressor at a constant, slow flow of 12 to 15 L/min. By controlling the breathing pattern with devices such as the I-neb and Akita, aerosol deposition in the lung is greater, distribution is more uniform, variability is reduced, and treatment time is shorter. Currently, the high expense of these devices limits them to high-cost drugs, so the device costs are buried in the expense of a drug-device

combination. But the breath-control technique holds great promise for many drugs in development.

Finally, some technological advances have occurred with drug formulations, rather than delivery devices. For example, one of the difficulties with DPIs is the difficulty in de-aggregating the milled particles that have high cohesive forces. A different approach uses an emulsion-based spray-drying process that is designed to create porous particles with a sponge-like morphology (Fig. 18-13). Because of their low density, these light-porous particles behave aerodynamically similar to a very much smaller droplet of unit density. They also have fewer contact points than milled particles, leading to improved dispersion of the powder with less patient effort. These powders can be delivered with very simple inhaler devices, and this technology has been used to develop drugs for both pulmonary and systemic delivery, including small molecules, peptides, and proteins. Pulmosphere technology (Novartis Pharmaceuticals) allowed for a high payload of drug and was shown to significantly reduce the time burden for CF patients taking inhaled tobramycin.[62] This DPI formulation was recently approved in several countries. There are still lower age limits for new DPI formulations, and some patients may not tolerate a high payload powder formulation, but the lower time burden from shorter delivery times and no need for cleaning and disinfection is a tremendous advantage.

SUMMARY

Aerosol therapy in the treatment of respiratory diseases in children has had a long and increasingly successful history, especially in CF and asthma. However, safe and effective treatment depends on understanding the advantages and limitations of both the medications and the delivery devices. The use of the respiratory tract to deliver systemic pharmaceuticals for treatment of pain, diabetes, pulmonary hypertension, and other conditions is becoming a reality as delivery systems with high degrees of efficiency and reproducibility are becoming available.

References

The complete reference list is available online at www.expertconsult.com

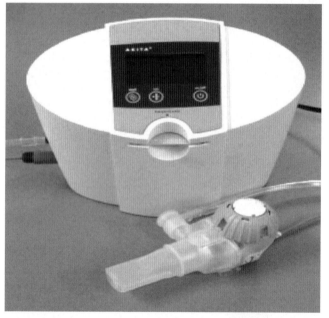

FIGURE 18-12. The Akita device with a vibrating perforated membrane nebulizer, which is used to maximize efficiency.

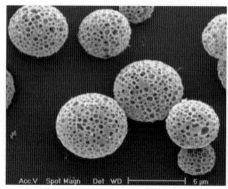
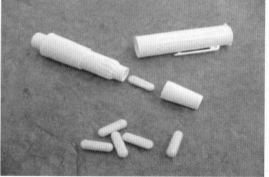

FIGURE 18-13. Light, porous particles from spray-dried emulsions (left) behave aerodynamically like small particles and can be delivered by simple capsule-based dry-powder inhalers.

19 PHYSICAL THERAPIES IN PEDIATRIC RESPIRATORY DISEASE

MICHELLE CHATWIN, BSc, PhD, RUTH WAKEMAN, BSc (HONS) PHYSIOTHERAPY, MSc, AND SARAH WRIGHT, GRAD DIP PHYS

Pediatric physical therapy (physiotherapy) spans a broad range of treatment—from advice to nonpharmacologic interventions for patients with a variety of respiratory conditions. Physiotherapists are an essential part of the multidisciplinary team. Physiotherapy can be administered from birth to old age in the community, outpatient, ward, or intensive care setting.

Prior to pediatric physiotherapy, one must obtain informed consent from caregivers and age-appropriate assent from the child. Treating children can be difficult and challenging, and these sessions are easier when children are cooperative and compliant. One can often attain a child's cooperation by using persuasion and distraction.

Physical therapy treatments should never be carried out routinely and should always be tailored to the individual after a detailed assessment.[1,2] The effect of interventions should be constantly re-evaluated. The timing of physiotherapy treatments can be important; for example, airway clearance should be timed before feeds or delayed for a sufficient time after feeds in order to avoid vomiting and aspiration. Likewise, physiotherapy should be timed around analgesia when clinically necessary.

GENERAL PRINCIPLES OF PHYSIOTHERAPY

Physiotherapy often focuses on treating or alleviating generic problems that are amenable to intervention rather than being disease-specific (Fig. 19-1). In some instances, however, interventions are selected based upon the underlying disease process (e.g., primary ciliary dyskinesia [PCD] versus cystic fibrosis [CF]), whereby the elements of the mucociliary escalator affected by the disease process may differ (predominantly ciliary dysfunction versus altered sputum rheology). The pediatric respiratory physiotherapist/therapist will perform a wide variety of roles. The professionals and their training vary internationally. In the United Kingdom, physiotherapists are able to treat patients without a referral from a medical doctor and are therefore independent practitioners.

The respiratory physiotherapist/therapist needs physiologic knowledge and practical skills to perform a competent respiratory assessment of the child. From this assessment, problems amenable to physiotherapy are identified and treatment strategies are recommended and implemented. Physiotherapists may also assess the response to inhaled pharmacologic agents (e.g., bronchodilator response and nebulized antimicrobial bronchoconstriction trials) (Chapter X), provide education in inhaler and nebulizer techniques, and advise on the optimal timing of inhaled medications with respect to sessions of respiratory physiotherapy. They can also assess the need for home oxygen therapy by performing exercise testing with oximetry.[3] Physiotherapists may also help to identify potential causes for respiratory problems (e.g., gastroesophageal reflux during airway clearance). This should then be re-evaluated by the medical team. If it is felt that pulmonary secretions are a result of aspiration secondary to uncoordinated swallowing, then a speech and language assessment is warranted (see Section IX, Aerodigestive Disease).

ROLE OF PHYSIOTHERAPY IN PEDIATRIC RESPIRATORY DISEASE

Physical therapies are essential in the removal of excess bronchopulmonary secretions (Table 19-1) and maintaining and improving exercise capacity. Physical therapy can support ventilation using continuous positive airway pressure (CPAP) or noninvasive ventilation (NIV). Physical therapy should include postural education where appropriate and it can be used to prevent, correct or improve postural problems, such as kyphosis in CF patients (Fig. 19-2). Postural education can also be helpful in musculoskeletal dysfunction, in children with contractures that inhibit function, or in children with pain limiting range of motion, mobility and ability to breathe normally. Poor posture leads to tightening of the respiratory muscles that can lead to chest wall deformity and may contribute to decline in pulmonary function. It is therefore essential that patients with chronic lung disease have a postural assessment and treatment of any musculoskeletal disorders identified.

Specifically in neuromuscular disease (NMD), physical therapy is essential to maintain ambulation or facilitate standing where possible, to improve lung function. Optimizing the maturing musculoskeletal and neuromuscular systems of a child with CF may play an important role in the long-term outcome of the child's mental and physical state.[4] It is essential that children with chronic lung disease should also be asked about urinary and fecal incontinence, in a private and empathetic setting. Reluctance to cough may be because of fear of incontinence. Physical therapies should be directed towards managing this problem.[5,6]

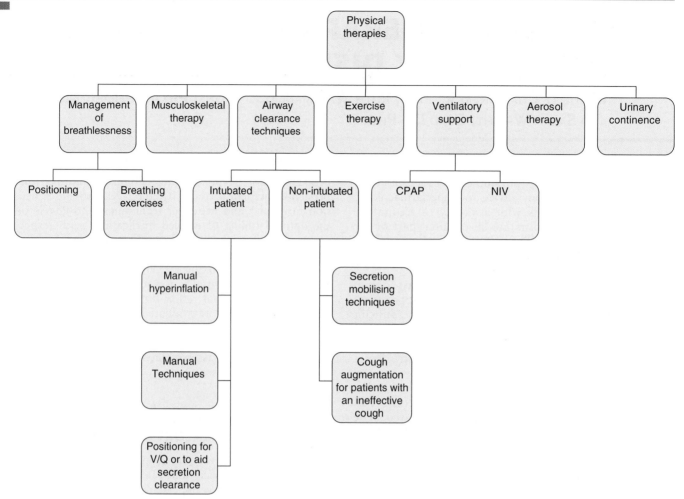

FIGURE 19-1. The physical therapies that can be offered to a child with respiratory disease are shown. *V/Q*, ventilation perfusion; *CPAP*, continuous positive airway pressure; *NIV*, noninvasive ventilation.

■ RESPIRATORY PHYSIOTHERAPY IN SPECIFIC CONDITIONS

Cystic Fibrosis and Non-Cystic Fibrosis Bronchiectasis (Including Primary Ciliary Dyskinesia)

Airway Clearance

Airway clearance treatment options will depend on the child's age and ability to participate in treatment. There are a wide variety of airway clearance techniques (ACTs) (Table 19-2). No single best technique has been identified.[2,7-12] The vast majority of research is focused on CF, and the therapist should not assume that the findings all apply to non-CF bronchiectasis.

The technique should be tailored to the individual, and choice is dependent on efficacy, simplicity of use, and cost.[1,2] A good starting point is with the technique that is simplest to use and that impinges least on the patient's life.[13] The term *airway clearance* describes a number of different treatment modalities that aim to enhance the clearance of bronchopulmonary secretions.[14] Through clinical reasoning, the therapist will decide the aim of treatment and the specific issue (or issues) to be addressed. Lannefors and colleagues clearly identified the following four stages of airway clearance, and they are the cornerstones to decision making.[15]

1. To get air behind mucus to open up the airways
2. To loosen/unstick the secretions from the small airways
3. To mobilize the secretions through the airways to the larger airways
4. To clear the secretions from the central airways

As discussed earlier in the chapter, the age and adherence of the individual and caregivers as well as the disease severity will impact the modalities introduced and in what combination. In the infant, manual techniques[16] and positioning[17] are commonly used, however the introduction of infant positive expiratory pressure (PEP)[18] and assisted autogenic drainage (AAD)[19] have provided alternative strategies. These highlight the focus on enhancing changes in air flow and ensuring the move from "passive" techniques to a more dynamic approach for toddlers. The use of movement is encouraged, as it is not only more effective but also realistic in this age group.

As the child gets older and can become an active participant in therapy, the emphasis will change. The therapist can incorporate techniques that augment volume and introduce the concept of a change in expiratory flow; in

TABLE 19-1 STRATEGIES USED FOR AIRWAY CLEARANCE AND TO ENHANCE VENTILATION AND GAS EXCHANGE

Positioning

Positioning can be used to optimize respiratory function. Supine positioning is the least beneficial (unless there is respiratory muscle weakness with diaphragmatic sparing), while prone positioning has been shown to improve respiratory function with a reduction in gastroesophageal reflux and in energy expenditure.[79] Ventilation in infants and small children is preferentially distributed to the uppermost regions. In acutely ill children with unilateral lung disease, care should be taken if positioning the child with the affected lung uppermost because this position may cause a rapid deterioration in respiratory status.

Precautions: Prone (unless during play) should only be used in the hospital environment where the child can be monitored.

Manual Hyperinflation

The aims of manual hyperinflation are to enhance mobilization of secretions by increasing expiratory flow, re-inflate atelectatic areas, and improve gas exchange. The technique involves disconnecting the patient from mechanical ventilation to provide temporary manual ventilation. Patients receive normal tidal volumes coupled with an increased tidal volume using a 500 mL infant bag (or a 1 L bag for older children). A manometer is applied to the circuit to monitor pressures. As a general guide, manual hyperinflation ventilation pressures should not exceed 10 cm H_2O above the ventilator pressure. Flow rates of gas should be adjusted according to the child: 4 L/min for infants, increasing to 8 L/min for children.

Contraindications and precautions: Hemodynamic instability, undrained pneumothorax, severe cystic or bullous lung disease, severe bronchospasm, High PEEP.

Intermittent Positive Pressure Breathing (IPPB)

IPPB has been shown to augment tidal volume by delivering positive pressure via a mouthpiece or mask. By increasing tidal volumes, this device utilizes collateral ventilation and gets air behind secretions to mobilize them. IPPB has been shown to help with clearance of secretions when simpler airway clearance techniques are not maximally effective (e.g., patients who are fatiguing and have chronic sputum retention, postoperative patients, or patients with neuromuscular disease who are unable to take a deep breath).

Precautions: Oxygen-sensitive patients, postoperative air leak, hemodynamic instability, pneumothorax, lung abscess, bronchial tumors, and severe bronchospasm.

Noninvasive Positive Pressure Ventilation (NIV) and Continuous Positive Airway Pressure (CPAP)

NIV and CPAP require the provision of positive pressure through the patient's upper airway using a full facemask, nasal mask, or lip seal device. The aims of CPAP are to improve oxygenation, decrease the work of breathing, and prevent upper airway collapse. The aims of NIV are to decrease breathlessness by providing ventilatory support and importantly to improve oxygenation and decrease arterial carbon dioxide levels. NIV and CPAP may be required postoperatively or for patients with neuromuscular weakness, upper airway obstruction, or chronic lung disease.

Precautions: Frank hemoptysis, pain, large bullae, vomiting (when full facemask is used), hemodynamic instability, and undrained pneumothorax.

Incentive Spirometry (IS)

Incentive spirometry is designed to mimic natural sighing or yawning by encouraging the patient to take long, slow, deep breaths. This is accomplished by using a device that provides patients with visual or other positive feedback when they inhale at a predetermined flow rate or volume and sustain the inflation for a minimum of 3 seconds. The aim of this maneuver is to open up atelectatic areas and improve lung volumes with visual feedback.

Precautions: Children with ventilatory failure.

Active Cycle of Breathing Techniques (ACBT)

ACBT has been shown to be effective to clear bronchial secretions and to improve lung function without causing hypoxemia. The technique consists of (1) breathing control (BC), which is a resting period of gentle relaxed breathing at the patient's own rate and depth, (2) thoracic expansion exercises (TEE), which are 3 to 5 deep breaths emphasizing inspiration, and (3) forced expiration technique (FET, or "huff"), which combines 1 to 2 forced expirations followed by a period of BC. The technique is flexible and can be performed in any position. It can be adapted for young children into blowing games. The patient carries out cycles of BC, TEE, BC, and FET. If the secretions are in the lower airways, the cycle will incorporate more cycles of TEE and BC.

Autogenic Drainage (AD)

AD aims to maximize air flow within the airways, improve ventilation, and clear secretions. AD utilizes gentle breathing at different lung volumes to loosen, mobilize, and clear bronchial secretions. The patient breathes in and holds his or her breath for 2 to 4 seconds (the hold facilitates equal filling of the lung segments). Expiration is performed keeping the upper airways open (as if sighing). The expiratory force is balanced so that the expiratory flow reaches the highest rate possible without causing airway compression. This cycle is repeated at different lung volumes, while collecting secretions from the peripheral airways and moving them toward the mouth. Patients need to have a good understanding of the technique, and their lungs to be able to move the secretions effectively.

(continued)

TABLE 19-1 STRATEGIES USED FOR AIRWAY CLEARANCE AND TO ENHANCE VENTILATION AND GAS EXCHANGE—Cont'd

Positive Expiratory Pressure (PEP)

PEP can be delivered via a mouthpiece or, more traditionally, via a mask. PEP has been hypothesized to have an effect on the peripheral airways and collateral channels of ventilation. In addition, the increase in lung volume may allow air to get behind the secretions and assist in mobilizing them. Usually PEP consists of a mask with a one-way valve to which expiratory resistance is added. A manometer is inserted into the circuit between the valve and resistance to monitor the pressure, which should be 10 to 20 cm H_2O during mid-expiration. The child usually sits with his or her elbows on a table and breathes through the mask for 6 to 10 breaths with a slightly active expiration.

Contraindications and Precautions: Hemodynamic instability, pneumothorax, severe bronchospasm.

Acapella

This device combines an oscillation of the air within the airways during expiration. It consists of a counterweighted plug and magnet to create air flow oscillations. The Acapella also produces positive expiratory pressure. It can be used in any position. The patient takes 6 to 8 breaths through the device followed by huffing.

Contraindications and Precautions: Hemodynamic instability, pneumothorax, severe bronchospasm.

Flutter

This device combines an oscillation of the air within the airways during expiration. It consists of a small plastic pipe with a high-density ball enclosed in a small cone. Breathing through the pipe and against the ball creates positive expiratory pressure and oscillation within the airways. The flutter device requires correct positioning in order to get maximum vibrations. The device can be used with the patient in the lying or sitting position and has been shown to decrease sputum viscosity. Usually patients will perform 4 to 8 deep breaths followed by a forced expiration.

Contraindications and Precautions: Hemodynamic instability, pneumothorax, severe bronchospasm.

High-Frequency Chest Wall Oscillation (HFCWO)

HFCWO provides compression of the chest wall at frequencies of 5 to 20 Hz. The compressive force is usually via an inflatable jacket that is adjusted to fit snugly over the thorax. The air pulse generator then delivers intermittent positive air flow into the jacket. As the jacket expands and compresses the chest wall, it produces a transient/oscillatory increase in air flow in the airways and vibrates secretions from the peripheral airways toward the mouth.

Contraindications and Precautions: Hemodynamic instability, pneumothorax, severe bronchospasm, rib fractures.

Intrapulmonary Percussive Ventilation (IPV)

IPV is a modified method of intermittent positive pressure breathing (IPPB). It superimposes high-frequency mini-bursts of air (50 to 550 cycles per minute) on the individual's intrinsic breathing pattern. This creates an internal vibration (percussion) within the lungs. Internal or external vibration of the chest is hypothesized to promote clearance of sputum from the peripheral bronchial tree. IPV may provide ventilatory support in patients with neuromuscular disease. IPV devices include: IMPULSATOR—F00012, IPV1C—F00001-C, IPV2C—F00002-C. (Percussionaire Corporation, USA; IMP II, Breas, Sweden).

Contraindications and Precautions: Hemodynamic instability, pneumothorax, severe bronchospasm, Lyell's syndrome.

Manual Techniques

Chest percussion (chest clapping) is carried out using a hand, fingers, or facemask and is generally well tolerated and widely used in small children and infants. Chest vibrations involve the application of a rapid extra thoracic force at the beginning of expiration, followed by oscillatory compressions until expiration is complete. The compression and oscillation applied to the chest are believed to aid secretion clearance via increasing peak expiratory flow to move secretions toward the large airways for clearance via suction or a cough. In infants, the closing volume is the lung volume at which closure of the small airways occurs. Therefore, one needs to be careful with techniques (assisted coughing and end-expiratory shaking and vibrations) in infants because there may be a worsening of atelectasis.

Precautions: Patients with osteoporosis/osteopenia and coagulopathies. Manual techniques may not be appropriate in premature infants.

Postural Drainage (PD)/Gravity-Assisted Positioning (GAP)

This is the use of gravity-assisted positioning to drain lung areas of secretions. The positions can include the head-down position, which has been debated to cause an increase in gastroesophageal reflux. In reality, this is only an issue if the gastroesophageal reflux is not treated. If specific areas of the lungs are affected, then the appropriate positioning should be used to facilitate airway clearance. Postural drainage can be particularly affective in patients with CF, bronchiectasis, and PCD.

Precautions for Head-Down Positioning: Raised intracranial pressure, preterm infants, and patients with abdominal distension.

TABLE 19-1 STRATEGIES USED FOR AIRWAY CLEARANCE AND TO ENHANCE VENTILATION AND GAS EXCHANGE—Cont'd

Manually Assisted Coughing (MAC)

The aim of the manually-assisted cough is to increase expiratory air flow by either compression of the chest wall or abdomen. Synchronous compression of the abdomen causes a sudden increase in abdominal pressure, which in turn causes the abdominal contents to push the diaphragm upward, thus increasing expiratory air flow. The increase in expiratory air flow assists in moving airway secretions toward the mouth. MAC is a simple, effective technique that can be used anywhere, and some patients are able to perform their own MAC. This technique is most effective when the child can cough to command (usually >2 years of age).

Precautions: Raised intracranial pressure, preterm infants, abdominal distension, and unstable spinal cord injury.

Maximum Insufflation Capacity (MIC)

The aim is to produce a MIC by breath stacking, intermittent positive-pressure breathing (IPPB), or glossopharyngeal breathing (GPB). MIC can be augmented by a noninvasive ventilator set in volume mode or a resuscitation bag and mask with or without a one-way valve, depending on the patients' ability to hold his or her breath. After the first assisted breath, the patient is instructed not to expire and to take a second assisted breath. This may repeated for a further 1 to 3 breaths to augment a greater inspiratory VC beyond that of the patients spontaneous VC. MIC has been shown to be an effective method of improving cough strength and improving secretion clearance.

Contraindications and Precautions: Hemodynamic instability, pneumothorax, severe bronchospasm.

Mechanical Insufflation/Exsufflation (MI-E)

All of these devices clear secretions by (gradually) applying positive pressure to the airway (insufflation) and then rapidly shifting to negative pressure. The rapid shift in pressure produces a high expiratory flow of 6 to 11 L/sec, simulating a natural cough. The device has been shown to improve peak cough flow in patients with spinal cord injury and neuromuscular disease. This technique is most effective when the child can cough to command (usually >2 years of age), but it also can be used in younger children.

Precautions: Raised intracranial pressure, preterm infants, abdominal distension, and pneumothorax.

Nasal Pharyngeal and Oral Suction

If the child is unable to clear secretions with the airway clearance techniques previously described, nasopharyngeal or oropharyngeal suctioning may be indicated. Nasopharyngeal suctioning is required in children until they are old enough to cough voluntarily and effectively. Nasopharyngeal suctioning uses an appropriate-size catheter, and it is an unpleasant experience. Prior to suctioning, the patient must be adequately oxygenated. Supplemental oxygen should be available during the procedure. If secretions have collected at the back of the throat, oral suction to the back of the mouth may be sufficient.

Precautions: Raised intracranial pressure, epistaxes, craniofacial abnormality, severe bronchospasm, and stridor.

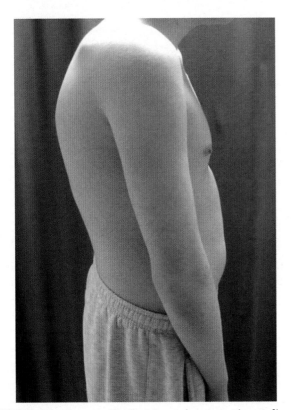

FIGURE 19-2. The onset of kyphosis in a male patient with cystic fibrosis.

many cases this is a forced expiration.[20] Forced expiration or "huffing" is integral to many techniques and utilizes the theory of the equal pressure point to move mucus to the larger airways.[21] It is also a valuable assessment tool for children as chest palpation during a "huff" can often be abnormal, with crackles being palpable, even when there are no abnormalities on auscultation. In young children, forced expiration will start as blowing games and then become a more formal component of ACT.

With increasing ability to participate, the active cycle of breathing techniques (ACBT),[17,22] can be taught and used in postural drainage (PD) positions (see Table 19-1). Physiotherapy may consist of modified PD targeting the area of lung affected or rotating through different areas to ensure that the lung fields are clear.[16] Other techniques such as autogenic drainage (AD) also can be considered.[23] In addition, many adjuncts are available, with PEP[24] or oscillatory PEP[25,26] commonly used to facilitate clearance and to help move toward independence, if appropriate. Devices include the Flutter device (Clement Clarke International Limited, Harlow, Essex, UK), the Acapella (Henleys Medical, Welwyn Garden City, Hertfordshire, UK), the PEP Mask (Astratech, Stonehouse, Gloucestershire, UK), the TheraPEP (Smiths Medical, Watford, UK), and the Pari PEP (Pari Medical, West Byfleet, Surrey, UK). Several of these devices can be used in combination with inhaled medications (e.g., hypertonic saline) or in conjunction with exercise.

TABLE 19-2 PHYSIOTHERAPY OPTIONS FOR DIFFERENT AGES

TECHNIQUES AND ACTIVITY OPTIONS	INFANTS	TODDLER TO PREP	PRIMARY SCHOOL AGE	TEENS	ADULTS	COMMENTS
Conventional Techniques						Conventional techniques (often re-introduced when the patient is unwell or in the hospital) are combined with other techniques to maximize clearance.
Positions (+/– modified)	+++	+++	+/++	+/++	+/++	
Chest percussion (patting)	+++	+++	+/++	+/++	+/++	
Chest vibration	+	++	+/++	+/++	+/++	
Activity and Exercise						Exercise must be modified according to interests, abilities, and health status. Many young people with CF can participate in high-level sports. Exercise can be combined with other ACTs.
"Physio play" (e.g., tickles,	+++	+++	+	×	×	
bouncing, sports, aerobic	×	×	+/++	+++	++	
fitness, gym, weights,	×	×	×	++/+	+++	
interval training, core	×	×	+/++	++/+++	+++	
stability exercise,	×	+	++	+++	+++	
stretches)	++	++	++	+++	+++	
Active family/lifestyle	+++	+++	+++	+++	+++	
Breathing Exercises						Breathing exercises are introduced at around 3 to 5 years of age, and they remain an active part of adult techniques.
Blowing games	×	++	++	×	×	
"Bubble" (underwater)	×	+	+	×	×	
PEP	×	++	+++	+++	+++	
Huffing, forced expiration	×	+	++	+++	+++	
Active Cycle of Breathing	+	×	×	+ /++	+++	
Autogenic drainage (AD)						
Positive Expiratory Pressure (PEP)						PEP and oscillating PEP are widely used with parent coaching by young people and independently by adults. Some also can be combined with inhalations.
PEP Mask	+	++	+/++	+/++	+/++	
PEP + Mouthpiece	×	+	+++	+++	+++	
Flutter	×	×	+	++	++	
Acapella	×	×	+	++	+++	
Quake	×	×	×	×	×	
High-Frequency Chest Wall Oscillation (HFCWO)	×	+	+	+	+	Needs individual evaluation. Best to combine with other techniques. Very costly.
Mechanical Insufflation/ Exsufflation (MI-E)	+	+	+	+	+	Needs individual evaluation. Best to combine with other techniques. Benefit in neuromuscular disease. Very costly.

Code: +++, very frequently used; ++, often used; +, may be used: depends on individual factors, risks versus benefits; ×, rarely or never used: not recommended.

High-frequency chest wall oscillation (HFCWO) with the Vest (Hill-Rom, St Paul, MN) or Smart Vest (Electromed, New Prague, MN)[27] is widely used across North America. Although evidence indicates that it may be less effective than other therapies,[27,28] it still can be considered for specific individuals. One other device that may be of benefit is intrapulmonary percussive ventilation (IPV) devices (IMPULSATOR-F00012, IPV1C-F00001-C, IPV2C-F00002-C, Percussionaire Corporation, USA; IMP II, Breas, Sweden). Previous studies have investigated sputum mobilization in cystic fibrosis patients by comparing the use of IPV to other modes of airway clearance (e.g., postural drainage and percussion, HFCWO, and the Flutter device).[29–31] These studies have shown IPV to be as effective as the other methods of airway clearance in sputum mobilization.

Regular review of ACT is advised to ensure continuing effectiveness and concordance with therapy; appropriate adjustments to treatment can be made as necessary.[32,33] It is important that the regimen is specific to each individual's changing needs, and as they get older their understanding for doing treatment and its goals must be clear. There is debate worldwide regarding the introduction of ACT prior to diagnosis of bronchiectasis. There is consensus in the symptomatic patient, where response to treatment is evident; however, there is less agreement in the asymptomatic patient.[14] Chest physiotherapy does not need to be routinely performed unless the underlying diagnosis affects the normal mechanisms of airway clearance. In CF, there is evidence that inflammation and infection are present early in life.[34] In addition, for CF or PCD, it would seem unethical to wait for airway damage to occur, as the child will never have normal mucociliary clearance.

Gastroesophageal Reflux

The relationship between ACT (particularly gravity-assisted positions) and gastroesophageal reflux (GER) remains unclear. Button and colleagues reported an increased incidence of GER with head-down tilt compared to modified positions in infants with CF.[35] However, this was not supported by Phillips and coworkers, who identified the sitting position as most likely to cause GER in children with respiratory symptoms. These conflicting findings identify a key problem within physiotherapy where there are so many variations in regimens, outcome measures, and overall management.[36] Physiotherapists must be aware of the possible risks with treatment and modify their therapies accordingly; thus one should not base the decision on whether gravity will induce reflux, but whether it is necessary to tip at all. Few therapists would tip a 4-week-old asymptomatic CF infant, but in a 1-year-old child with PCD that is at risk of developing acute large airway mucus impaction and lobar changes, postural drainage should form part of the treatment.

Ventilatory Support

As the disease progresses, devices that provide some inspiratory ventilatory support may be the treatment of choice. The use of NIV to reduce the work of breathing, facilitate inspiration, and correct respiratory failure is widely used in the adult setting. However a recent review of its use in CF children[37] demonstrated a need for more evidence and protocols to identify indications for use.

Inhalation Therapies

Effective treatment in this group of patients might need to be supported by inhaled therapies such as bronchodilators; mucolytic agents such as hypertonic saline and deoxyribonuclease (RhDNase); antimicrobials (Fig. 19-3); and, where indicated, oxygen therapy.[38,39]

Asthma

A crucial part of physical therapy management of asthma is education of the child and parents. It is important to ensure ongoing adherence to prescribed medication (see Chapter 47). Physiotherapy includes advice on exercise. In some children, breathing retraining using a reduced volume and/or frequency, with relaxation, can reduce symptoms and therefore improve quality of life. Several groups advocate specific techniques, but it is important to stress that these techniques are adjunctive to medication and are not replacement therapy. Routine airway clearance is rarely indicated in asthmatic patients. Airway clearance may be indicated in the mechanically ventilated asthmatic patient or following an acute exacerbation where mucus plugging is a factor (see Table 19-1). It is important to remain aware that airway clearance techniques may exacerbate bronchospasm.

Breathing Pattern Disorders

This is a particularly challenging area. It is important that the child undergo a full assessment prior to referral for physical therapies to rule out organic disorders (e.g., croup, asthma) and neurologic disorders (e.g., Rett syndrome). A careful history should be taken to investigate when symptoms are present. If the child is symptom-free

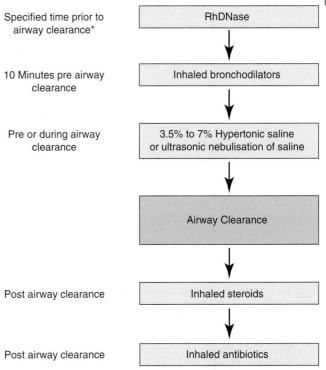

FIGURE 19-3. The timing of inhaled therapies around physiotherapy. The algorithm is individualized to the patient. Obviously, the patient will not necessarily take all of the inhaled therapies listed in Figure 19-1. *RhDNase*, Deoxyribonuclease.
* RhDNase should not be given immediately prior to airway clearance.

during sleep, this may help to refine the diagnosis. If the child is suffering from a psychogenic disorder or other abnormal breathing patterns (e.g., hyperventilation syndrome and sighing dyspnea), then physiologic input will be of benefit to identify triggers and provide advice on how to cope with them. Breathing re-education is essential in this group of children and adolescents. Breathing retraining incorporating reducing respiratory rate and/ or tidal volume should be offered as a first-line treatment for hyperventilation syndrome, with or without concurrent asthma. Identification of precipitating factors (e.g., sighing) and other triggers is important.

Chest Wall Disorders

Physical therapies in chest wall disease are aimed at maximizing lung function. This includes pulmonary rehabilitation,[40] manual musculoskeletal therapies for postural pain, and initiation of NIV in the hypercapnic patient.[41]

Neuromuscular Disease

The ability to clear bronchopulmonary secretions is essential to prevent sputum retention and associated complications, including lower respiratory tract infection. An effective cough is a vital mechanism to protect against respiratory tract infections, which are the commonest cause of hospital admission in patients with respiratory muscle weakness from neuromuscular disease (NMD).[42] An intact afferent and efferent pathway is required for an effective cough. Reduced airway sensation will fail to elicit a cough in response to a noxious stimulus. The efferent pathway may be weakened by diseases of the nerves (upper or lower motor neuron), neuromuscular junction, or muscles.

The act of coughing involves the following three main components[43]:

1. Deep inspiration up to 85% to 90% of total lung capacity
2. Glottic closure, which requires intact bulbar function so a rapid closure of the glottis occurs for approximately 0.2 seconds
3. Effective contraction of the expiratory muscles (abdominal and intercostal muscles) to generate intrapleural pressures of >190 cm H_2O.

If one or more of these three components are impaired, the cough will be less effective[44] and the individual may be unable to produce the transient flow spikes essential for an effective cough[45] (Fig. 19-4). Cough strength can be measured by peak cough flow (PCF). PCF is the result of an explosive decompression that generates a flow rate as high as 360 to 944 L/min^{-1} in children older than 12 years of age.[46] It is important not to quote adult PCF threshold values for children younger than 12 years of age.

Physical therapies involve measuring PCF. Poponick and coworkers[47] demonstrated that acute viral illness was associated with a reduction in vital capacity (VC) due to reduced inspiratory and expiratory respiratory muscle strength (by 10% to 15% of baseline values). This reduction in inspiratory and expiratory muscle strength will also cause a decline in PCF, possibly to the critical level of 160 L/min^{-1}, which has been reported in the adult literature.[48] Assisted cough techniques should be targeted to whichever component of the cough is reduced. For example, if there is only expiratory muscle weakness, then a manually assisted cough (MAC; an abdominal thrust or costal lateral compression after an adequate spontaneous inspiration or maximal insufflation) will improve PCF.[49,50] If there is inspiratory muscle weakness, then the inspiratory component can be supported

with a maximum insufflation capacity (MIC), which is a series of deep breaths to total lung capacity (TLC) via a facemask attached to a one-way valve and Ambu bag[51] (see Table 19-1). If there is both inspiratory and expiratory muscle weakness, then the inspiratory component can be supported with MIC and expiratory component with MAC.[49] If the cough is extremely impaired, the patient may require mechanical insufflation/exsufflation (MI-E) (Cough Assist, Philips Respironics, Andover, MA; NiPPY Clearway B&D Electromedical, Warwickshire, UK; or Pegaso, Dimla-Italia, Bologna, Italy).[52,53] This device clears secretions by (gradually) applying a positive pressure to the airway (insufflation), and then rapidly shifting to negative pressure (exsufflation). The rapid shift in pressure produces a high expiratory flow, simulating a natural cough (see Table 19-1).

In pediatric patients with NMD, MI-E has been provided as part of a protocol in patients with a PEmax of 20 cm H_2O or less.[54] MI-E has also been shown to expedite secretion removal[55] and prevent intubation.[56] A combination of NIV and MI-E in spinal muscular atrophy type I has been associated with increased life expectancy when compared to the untreated natural history in observational studies.[57-60]

NIV may also have a role in preventing chest wall deformity in NMD.[60,61] Physical therapies that consist of secretion-mobilizing techniques in NMD may need to provide ventilator support. Such options include IPV (see the section entitled "Cystic Fibrosis and Non-Cystic Fibrosis Bronchiectasis Including Primary Ciliary Dyskinesia" and Table 19-1), a modified ACBT (adjusting the patients NIV settings), or HFCWO on NIV (see Table 19-1). Patients who use NIV should not be taken off their ventilator for physiotherapy or transferred to continuous positive airway pressure (CPAP). Some patients with NMD are provided with NIV to decrease their work of breathing and augment tidal volumes to enhance ACT. The ACBT can be modified by using NIV to provide deep breaths that mobilize secretions with or without manual techniques, followed by an assisted cough technique.

Spinal Cord Injury

Physical therapies need to be appropriate to the level of the spinal cord injury. Cervical spinal cord injuries may require ventilator support in the form of NIV or, in higher spinal cord injuries, tracheostomy intermittent positive pressure ventilation (TIPPV). Patients may need to be taught MIC (see the section entitled "Neuromuscular Disease" and Table 19-1) to promote chest wall stretching,[62] along with lung growth and development. For injuries that included the thoracic spine, MAC should be taught[63] (see the section entitled "Neuromuscular Disease" and Table 19-1). Patients who are significantly weak are likely to benefit from MI-E. Abdominal binders may be required to minimize the effect of postural hypotension and aid in respiration.[64,65]

Preoperative Preparation for Surgery

It may be desirable to teach physical therapies to high-risk children prior to surgery, for example patients with co-existing respiratory conditions that may predispose

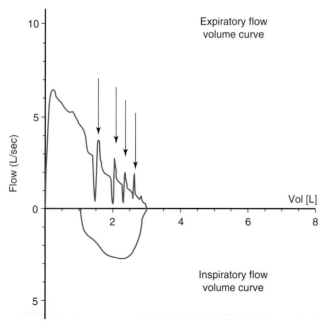

FIGURE 19-4. A series of cough spikes is superimposed on the maximal expiratory flow. Cough flow spikes are highlighted (arrows).

to postoperative respiratory atelectasis and infection, or patients with reduced mobility. This may help to reduce anxiety, and teaching breathing exercises may ensure that the child has a better understanding of the necessary techniques. The family will also understand the importance of early mobilization when applicable. For children undergoing abdominal and cardiothoracic surgery, supportive coughing techniques can be taught.

Postoperative Management

Postoperative physical therapies differ depending on the patient's status. Intubated and mechanically ventilated children require thorough assessment to identify any need for physiotherapy. Manual hyperinflation or other manual techniques may be indicated when areas of atelectasis or retained secretions are identified (see Table 19-1). Early mobilization is essential once the child is extubated. Breathing exercises such as ACBT may be appropriate (or blowing games in younger children) if secretion retention is an issue. Incentive spirometry can give visual feedback and encourage the child to take deeper breaths in an attempt to resolve atelectasis.[66] If there is a significant amount of atelectasis with a decline in oxygen saturation, CPAP may be warranted. Intermittent positive pressure breathing (IPPB) (Bird Mark 7, Viasys Health Care, Bilthoven, The Netherlands)[67] may be of benefit for older children with sputum retention.[68,69]

Exercise therapy is an essential part of postoperative care, and endurance training has a favorable influence on pulmonary function in patients after surgical correction of scoliosis.[70] A rehabilitation program should be included in the management of patients after spinal fusion combined with thoracoplasty.

Airway Structural Disorders

With the diagnosis of tracheomalacia and bronchomalacia via bronchoscopy increasing, physiotherapists are building evidence for the use of PEP. It is hypothesised in children with some structural abnormalities, that PEP can increase airway stabilisation and enhance cough expiratory flow.[70a] It is well known that children with airway malacia are prone to recurrent respiratory infections,[70b] and further research needs to be undertaken into the role of physiotherapy.

Interstitial Lung Disease

There is little published evidence on physiotherapy for interstitial lung disease. Studies in adult patients have shown an improvement with exercise training in patients with this disease.[71–73] Adult patients with more advanced disease may benefit from ambulatory oxygen therapy and breathlessness management. Physical therapies for this condition include positioning to ease breathlessness. Given the very different spectrum of interstitial lung diseases in children (see Section IX of this book), recommendations based on adults should only be adopted with extreme caution, and a detailed individualized assessment is essential.

▰ CONDITIONS NOT GENERALLY AMENABLE TO PHYSIOTHERAPY

Acute Laryngotracheobronchitis (Croup)

Physical therapies are usually contraindicated in the spontaneously ventilating child with croup. However, other techniques may be indicated if the child is intubated and mechanically ventilated, and secretions cannot be cleared by suction airway clearance alone.

Pertussis

Any physical therapies during the acute phase of pertussis can precipitate paroxysmal cough and its complications. If the child is mechanically ventilated, paralyzed, and sedated and there are issues with retained secretions, airway clearance techniques may be of benefit (see Table 19-1). In the child with persistent lobar collapse, and in whom the paroxysmal cough phase has ended, appropriate airway clearance techniques can be taught.

Inhaled Foreign Body

Physical therapy is not indicated to remove the foreign body. These children require bronchoscopic removal of the material, usually with a rigid bronchoscope. After bronchoscopic removal, postural drainage, manual techniques, and breathing exercises may be necessary to clear excess secretions that have accumulated in the obstructed airway behind the foreign body.

Pulmonary Edema

Airway clearance techniques are not indicated for pulmonary edema; however in some situations CPAP or NIV may be an appropriate strategy to help children with significant work of breathing while waiting for diuresis or other medical strategies to take effect.

Lobar Pneumonia and Empyema

There is little evidence to support chest physiotherapy to treat lobar pneumonia[74,75] or empyema.[76] The pathophysiology of both conditions indicates that physiotherapy will not be effective in the acute stages or even during resolution phase when secretions can appear in the airways; previously healthy children have the capability to clear these independently, with particular focus on mobilization. However, specific airway clearance techniques may be required in children with conditions that may alter muscle tone (e.g., cerebral palsy), mobility/muscle strength (e.g., neuromuscular conditions), or mucociliary clearance (e.g., bronchiectasis).

Bronchiolitis

Physical therapy is counterproductive during the acute stage of bronchiolitis. Mechanically ventilated infants will need careful assessment and may benefit from airway clearance techniques if there is secretion retention.

Chest physiotherapy has not been shown to reduce length of hospital stay, oxygen requirements, or severity clinical score,[77] and intervention should be based on specific focal signs or co-morbidities. In these cases, physiotherapy may need to be modified to reduce the impact on the infant's work of breathing and should be continually re-assessed.

In children with normal lung defense mechanisms and function, chest physiotherapy is very unlikely to be of benefit for acute respiratory disorders. However, lack of evidence does not mean that this should be extrapolated to all children. It is imperative that the therapist is able to assess the patient and liaise with the medical team regarding the necessity of intervention so that appropriate treatment is provided.[78]

◼ SUMMARY

Physical therapy is well established as part of the management of many respiratory conditions, in particular for children requiring mechanical ventilation and those with chronic disorders such as bronchiectasis or neuromuscular conditions. Over the past few decades the profession has evolved, and a wide variety of techniques and modalities are available with a growing evidence base. Fundamentally, the key to effective physiotherapy is identifying the physiologic issue, deciding whether physiotherapy strategies can assist, and identifying outcomes that can be measured. The latter must include both positive and negative effects so the therapist can assess the risk and take an informed approach to patient care.

Suggested Reading

Balfour-Lynn IM, Field DJ, Gringras P, et al. Paediatric Section of the Home Oxygen Guideline Development Group of the BTS Standards of Care Committee. BTS guidelines for home oxygen in children. *Thorax*. 2009;64(suppl 2):ii1–ii26.

Chatwin M, Bush A, Simonds AK. Outcome of goal-directed non-invasive ventilation and mechanical insufflation/exsufflation in spinal muscular atrophy type I. *Arch Dis Child*. 2011;96:426–432.

Cystic Fibrosis Foundation, Borowitz D, Parad RB, Sharp JK, et al. Cystic Fibrosis Foundation practice guidelines for the management of infants with cystic fibrosis transmembrane conductance regulator-related metabolic syndrome during the first two years of life and beyond. *J Pediatr*. 2009;155(6 suppl):S106–S116.

Niggemann B. How to diagnose psychogenic and functional breathing disorders in children and adolescents. *Pediatr Allergy Immunol*. 2010;21:895–899.

Prasad S, Main E, Dodd M, et al. Association of Chartered Physiotherapists. Finding consensus on the physiotherapy management of asymptomatic infants with cystic fibrosis. *Pediatr Pulmonol*. 2008;43: 236–244.

Pryor JA, Prasad SA, eds. Physiotherapy techniques. In *Physiotherapy for Respiratory and Cardiac Problems*. 4th ed. Vol 1. Edinburgh: Elsevier Limited; 2008:632.

Simonds AK. *Non-Invasive Respiratory Support: A Practical Handbook*. 3rd ed. Vol 1. London: Hodder Arnold; 2007:370.

References

The complete reference list is available online at www. expertconsult.com

20 MODERN MOLECULAR THERAPIES FOR RESPIRATORY DISEASE

GWYNETH DAVIES, MBCHB, ERIC W.F.W. ALTON, FMEDSCI, AND JANE C. DAVIES, MB, CHB, MRCP, MRCPCH, MD

This chapter describes the key novel therapeutic approaches that have reached the respiratory clinical and research arena in recent years. These include gene- and cell-based therapies, biologic therapies (including monoclonal antibodies), and small molecules. The emphasis is on the background and scientific rationale for these approaches. Where appropriate, examples of molecular therapies that are relevant to aspects of pediatric respiratory disease are given. However, the reader is asked to refer to relevant chapters for a more detailed description of emerging and current therapies for specific diseases.

Over recent years, a range of novel therapeutic targets and potential agents for treating respiratory diseases have been identified, thanks largely to an increased understanding of underlying mechanisms and pathophysiology of disease at the molecular level. In the scientific and regulatory community, distinction is often made between so-called "biological therapies" and small molecules. Universally accepted definitions remain elusive, however biological therapies are generally considered those that are derived from living sources (i.e., human, animal, bacterial, viral) and include antibodies, proteins, peptides, cytokines, receptors, vaccines, and gene- and cell-based therapies. Biological therapies differ in several key features from small-molecule agents. They tend to have a longer duration of action than small-molecule drugs. Also, they usually are at least several thousand kilodaltons (kDa) in size, and because they are too large to traverse gut barriers, administration is commonly parenteral. In contrast, the size of small-molecule agents (<1 kDa) generally permits enteral routes of administration.

Biological therapies are considered attractive because they have a greater potential selectiveness of targets over conventional small-molecule therapies. However, they also have a greater potential to induce an immunogenic response in the host than their small-molecule counterparts. Proteins can be recognized as foreign by the host, and an immunologic response will ensue. Importantly, antibodies can thus form in response, which may reduce or neutralize the therapeutic effectiveness of the agent, depending on the antigenic protein eliciting the reaction. Increasing the human (rather than bacterial or animal) protein components of such agents (e.g., by "humanizing" a monoclonal antibody; see later in the chapter) may reduce immunogenicity. Furthermore, a targeted approach with biological agents that have the capacity for profound effects on immunomodulation can have both desirable and undesirable consequences. Several high-profile cases have highlighted the importance of monitoring adverse events both in the acute and long-term (postmarketing approval) setting.

During recent years, the development of biological therapies has become big business (accounting for 17% of global pharmaceutical sales in 2009). However, historically, drug development and marketing has been concerned primarily with small-molecule drugs. Development of new small-molecule drugs continues to be important, and, in the field of respiratory medicine, there are several prime candidates in the pipeline. The processes involved in the identification, screening, and preclinical development of small-molecule drugs has evolved substantially over recent decades. This reflects both advances in molecular techniques and increased understanding of the underlying mechanisms of disease (and identification of potential novel drug targets).

Drug development typically starts with identification of a therapeutic target, which may be site-, cell- or receptor-specific. Candidate compounds are then investigated for their ability to modulate this target. These can be either selectively or randomly chosen; the latter clearly requires high-throughput screening techniques—automated assays that allow high numbers of potential compounds to be screened quickly. By either traditional or high-throughput methods, "lead" compounds that show potential are identified and taken forward for further preclinical assessment. Optimization to improve selectivity of the desired target, pharmacokinetics, and preclinical toxicology follows. The agents that are considered promising at the end of this process may proceed to clinical trials. It has been estimated that 1 in every 1 million compounds evaluated makes it through to the marketing stage. The potential number of drug targets has increased markedly in the post–human-genome era, so efforts have been made to rationalize the screening of any potential target.

GENE THERAPY

Gene therapy is based on the premise that exogenous DNA (which can be made to reach the inside of a host cell, most commonly the nucleus) can produce the protein of choice with the aim of ameliorating disease. This can be a protein, the function of which is missing in the disease (e.g., cystic fibrosis transmembrane conductance regulator [CFTR] or alpha-1-antitrypsin) or a therapeutic protein (e.g., an anti-inflammatory cytokine). Because cystic fibrosis (CF) is the only respiratory condition affecting the pediatric population for which gene therapy has been extensively researched, it will therefore be the focus of this section.

Only 1 year after the discovery of the *CFTR* gene, the first description of *in vitro CFTR* cDNA transfer was reported, which paved the way for early animal experiments.

Since then, over 20 clinical trials have been conducted worldwide. The majority of clinical approaches have utilized gene-transfer agents (GTAs, sometimes termed *vectors*) to carry the DNA into the cell; although naked DNA is capable of transfection, efficiency is extremely low. GTAs include (1) genetically-modified viruses (which can enter cells and express genes but do not possess reproductive capacity and therefore do not lead to infection and (2) synthetic agents (e.g., liposomes, lipoplexes, and nanoparticles).

The first trials used modified adenoviral vectors administered to either the nose or lower airway. Vector-induced inflammation was observed in some of these and was thought to relate both to dose and mode of delivery, with bronchoscopic instillation appearing more problematic than nebulization. Subsequent trials with reduced doses of virus administered via nebulizer have not encountered such significant side effects. Some studies have reported transgene expression based on mRNA and functional (bioelectrical, potential difference) changes. The key problem with viral vectors is the inability to administer them repeatedly, subsequent applications resulting in little or no gene expression.[1,2] The neutralizing antibody response, which together with cell-mediated immunity is responsible for this phenomenon, appears to depend on the route of administration (low with airway, variable with myocardium and skin, and high with the hepatic route) rather than the dose of vector.

Adeno-associated virus (AAV) has also been used as a GTA and was assessed in CF patients with the novel approach of using preexisting antrostomies into the maxillary sinus for ease of administration and assessment.[3] Ten patients received escalating doses in an unblinded fashion with no significant inflammatory response. Gene transfer was confirmed with measurable DNA up to 41 days after administration, but assessment of expression was difficult. Functional assessment with potential difference (PD) responses to isoprenaline and amiloride demonstrated some changes, although numbers were small. Subsequently, levels of the anti-inflammatory cytokine IL-10 were shown to have increased, despite other markers not changing.

AAV has been administered repeatedly to the lung in two trials conducted by the same group.[4,5] In the first of these, 37 patients received repeated doses via nebulizer; improvements in FEV1, IL-8, and IL-10 were reported, although molecular confirmation of expression was difficult once again. On the basis of these results, a larger trial was conducted on over 100 patients. Unfortunately, although there were no significant safety concerns, improvements in clinical efficacy outcomes were not observed in the second trial.

As an alternative, several nonviral or synthetic approaches have been reported; the majority of these trials have used lipid-based gene-transfer agents. To summarize, nasal administration has been relatively free of side effects. Efficacy has been variable, with some positive results both in molecular and functional assays. One trial has demonstrated that repeat administration is feasible, with no decrease in efficacy of subsequent doses. Our group conducted a placebo-controlled trial of liposome-mediated *CFTR* to the nose and lungs of CF patients.[6]

Administration was well-tolerated, although mild respiratory symptoms were seen in both groups. In addition, those in the treatment group reported mild influenza-like symptoms within the first 24 hours, which may relate to the presence of unmethylated CpG groups on the bacterially-derived DNA. Importantly, these symptoms were not reported after nasal administration, suggesting that for safety at least, the nasal epithelium may not be a good surrogate site for such trials. This was the first trial to assess functional (PD) change in the lower airway; the parameters of sodium absorption did not change (a common feature of all gene therapy trials), but there was a significant increase in chloride secretion in the active group to approximately 25% of non-CF values. Most recently, compacted DNA nanoparticles were administered to the nasal epithelium of 12 CF patients; some correction of chloride transport was observed on nasal PD, and the dose was well-tolerated.[7]

It remains unclear how the degree of molecular efficacy demonstrated might relate to *clinical* benefit. The UK CF Gene Therapy Consortium (www.cfgenetherapy.org.uk/) was formed several years ago from the three centers in the UK with CF clinical trials experience: Oxford University, Edinburgh University, and Imperial College London/ Royal Brompton Hospital. The purpose of the collaboration was to streamline efforts, rationalize resources, and hopefully thereby advance progress more rapidly. The clinical trials discussed earlier in the chapter had largely already been reported, from which proof of principle had been confirmed for both viral and nonviral gene-delivery methods. The primary aim of the Consortium is to develop gene therapy to produce *clinical* benefit in CF. We are currently focused on two waves of research: Wave 1 is a program to determine whether such clinical benefit is achievable with the best currently-available gene-transfer agent; Wave 2 explores a novel approach not yet ready for clinical use.

Gene therapy approaches are also being explored for alpha-1-antitrypsin deficiency, lung cancers, acute lung injury, and a variety of inflammatory lung diseases including lung fibrosis and asthma. Of these, the only disease of any major relevance to the pediatric population is perhaps asthma. Gene therapy approaches are at the preclinical stage and include interferon-gamma, IL-12, and glucocorticoid receptor gene transfer. The multifactorial nature of this disease has led some investigators to hypothesize that conventional gene therapy is unlikely to succeed and that other approaches such as antisense molecules (see later in the chapter) may be more applicable. The other consideration is whether a disease such as asthma merits such molecular approaches, given the treatments already available, and whether funds would be better spent promoting treatment adherence.

CELL-BASED THERAPIES

Over recent decades, cell-based therapies have captured the attention of the scientific community and wider public domain alike. Potential approaches include stem cells and regeneration, immunotherapy, and the use of cells as drug-delivery agents to a specific site of interest. Cell-based therapies may involve the harvesting, modification, and delivery of a patient's own cells (autologous) or the delivery of nonautologous cells (allograft). While perhaps benefiting from being widely rather than individually applicable, allografts may require the concurrent use of immunosuppressants because the patient's immune system might recognize the cells as foreign.

Stem cells are cells that have the potential to develop into all (pluripotent) or a limited range (multipotent) of cells in the body. They also have the capacity for self-renewal while retaining their original undifferentiated state. There is interest in the potential for stem cells to differentiate and populate specific cellular populations or tissues within the body. In respiratory medicine, there is interest in the potential for either endogenous or exogenous stem cells to regenerate and repair abnormal or damaged lung or airway tissue.

Stem cells can be isolated from human embryos (embryonic stem cells, ESC) and many individual tissues in the body. Strictly speaking, these "adult" stem cells are multipotent rather than pluripotent (as is the case for ESCs) (Fig. 20-1). They are also sometimes referred to as *somatic stem cells* or *progenitor cells*. Tissue-specific stem cells and progenitor cells are thought to play a role in regeneration and repair. They are able to self-renew and can give rise to differentiated cells. Whereas in some organs these cells have been well characterized, in the lung this is less clear. However, basal cells in the proximal airways, Clara cells more distally, and type II pneumocytes have been reported to possess progenitor characteristics.

In theory, delivery of stem cells to the airway could lead to the regeneration of local cellular populations and the restoration of normal physiologic function. The mode of delivery of any stem cell is important for likely efficacy. Systemic administration via the bloodstream creates the challenge of the cells correctly (and specifically) engrafting the tissue of interest. For these reasons and due to its relative accessibility, cell-based therapies have also focused on topical delivery to the lung and airway. Some studies suggest that airway or alveolar epithelium can engraft from administration of adult stem cells in animal models. In CF, cell-based therapies have been considered as a potential way of restoring healthy airway epithelium, although in mouse models, results to date have demonstrated very low levels of engraftment; a degree of damage to host tissue appears to be required, and alveolar regions seem to be easier to repopulate than the airways.[8-11]

ESCs have the ability to self-renew and can differentiate into a wide variety of different cell types, including lung progenitor cells. This has led to interest into whether such cells could "replace" those damaged as a result of acute lung injury. A recent study of bleomycin-induced lung injury in mice reported normal function of ESC-derived alveoli with improvements in arterial oxygenation and survival.[12] However, the potential for malignant transformation remains a serious concern with this approach.

Mesenchymal stem cells (MSCs) have also been investigated as potential modulators of airway inflammation. They are found predominantly in the bone marrow, albeit at low frequency, and give rise to cells of endodermal, ectodermal and mesodermal origin. Adult bone marrow–derived MSCs have been shown to differentiate into airway epithelium (bronchial and alveolar), vascular endothelium, and stromal cells. MSCs can migrate to sites of tissue injury and have also been shown to secrete cytokines involved in the inflammatory response. In a mouse acute lung injury model, improvement in mortality, inflammation, and injury were seen following systemic or intrapulmonary administration of MSCs.[13] Markers of inflammation can be altered without significant engraftment of cells, leading to a proposal that such cells are largely exerting "paracrine" effects. The other potential advantage of mesenchymal stem cells is that they do not seem to induce significant host immunologic responses. The encouraging results from mouse studies in terms of altering the inflammatory and immune response have led to their evaluation in man. At the time of this writing in 2010, Osiris Therapeutics (Osiris Therapeutics Inc, MD) are undertaking a placebo-controlled phase II trial of adult mesenchymal stem cells in adult patients with moderate to severe chronic obstructive pulmonary disease. Six-month interim results reported product safety but no significant difference in lung function between treatment and placebo groups.[14] No clinical trials of MSCs have been undertaken in children with respiratory disease.

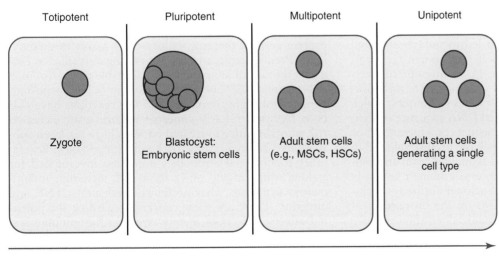

Totipotent	Pluripotent	Multipotent	Unipotent
Zygote	Blastocyst: Embryonic stem cells	Adult stem cells (e.g., MSCs, HSCs)	Adult stem cells generating a single cell type

Increasing differentiation →

FIGURE 20-1. Stem cells and differentiation capacity. *MSC,* Mesenchymal stem cell; *HSC,* haematopoetic stem cell.

In addition to CF and acute lung injury, other lung conditions relevant to childhood for which cell-based therapies are being explored include asthma and pulmonary vascular disease. *In vitro* and animal models have been used to mimic these conditions. There is interest in the use of mesenchymal stem cells in asthma because of the potential immunomodulatory actions. In pulmonary hypertension, endothelial progenitor cells have been administered in clinical trials involving both adult and pediatric participants. Approaches have included combining the technologies of gene- and cell-based therapies, for example by transducing autologous endothelial cells to express endothelial nitric oxide synthase (eNOS).

Cell-based therapies for respiratory diseases remain predominantly at the preclinical stage at present. Many unknowns remain, and transition to the clinic will depend on safety as well as efficacy profiles from preclinical models and clinical trials. Greater understanding of the control of cell proliferation will help determine whether such approaches carry any additional unfavorable risks (e.g., tumorigenesis), particularly if such therapies are administered in early life.

◼ MONOCLONAL ANTIBODIES

As therapeutic agents, monoclonal antibodies are designed to interact with a specific target to ameliorate disease or the downstream consequences thereof. Targets that have been exploited for therapeutics include cell surface receptors, cytokines, and immunoglobulins.

Monoclonal antibodies are those produced from a single clone of B lymphocytes. Antibodies have two distinct regions: the constant region (Fc domain) and the variable region (the fragment antigen-binding or Fab domain). The variable region contains one or more specific sites for recognition and binding of a particular antigen, termed *epitopes*. Monoclonal antibodies are identical with respect to their constant and variable regions, therefore each antibody interacts with the same epitope.

Monoclonal antibodies were first developed over 35 years ago by Köhler and Milstein, who fused immortal myeloma cells with mouse B lymphocytes derived from the spleen and created a "hybridoma."[15] The fused cells could be subsequently cultured *in vitro* and a single clone of specific antibody produced. The early administration of mouse-derived antibody in man led to unfavorable and often severe immune responses in the human recipient. Modifications have been made in an attempt to overcome this limitation. Clones of antibodies are now usually produced using recombinant DNA techniques, which involve the creation of the desired DNA sequence by artificially combining two or more sequences. Humanized or chimeric monoclonal antibodies have been developed in which the important amino acid sequences from an original mouse antibody are grafted onto a human antibody sequence. Designation of a monoclonal antibody as chimeric or humanized is dependent on the proportion of human sequences present (humanized antibodies have more). The higher the proportion of human protein, the lower is the likelihood of cross-species immunologic reactions. In chimeric antibodies the constant region of the antibody is human, whereas the variable region remains murine in origin. Examples (with FDA-approved indications in brackets) of chimeric antibodies used as therapeutic agents include infliximab (inflammatory bowel disease and rheumatoid arthritis) and rituximab (B cell non-Hodgkin's lymphoma). In humanized monoclonal antibodies, the variable region is composed of mouse and human components. Examples of humanized monoclonal antibodies include omalizumab (asthma) and palivizumab (RSV). Production of fully human monoclonal antibodies is technically challenging. At the time of this writing, there are no human monoclonal antibodies approved for respiratory disease; the two FDA-approved human monoclonal antibodies are for autoimmune disorders (adalimumab) and colorectal cancer (panitumumab).

Naming of monoclonal antibodies currently follows a system of stems and sub-stems described by the World Health Organization for International Nonproprietary Names (INN).[16] This enables identification of the background and origin of the monoclonal antibody. Monoclonal antibodies are recognized by the general stem "-mab." A sub-stem then provides information about the source of the product (Table 20-1). A further sub-stem placed prior to this identifies the disease or target class.

The target epitope for monoclonal antibodies may be early or late in terms of disease pathogenesis. For example, they may be produced to interact with a specific receptor to prevent viral entry to a host cell, or instead target an undesirable inflammatory mediator. To date, two monoclonal antibodies have been licensed for clinical use in respiratory diseases: omalizumab and palivizumab; however several others are undergoing current evaluation in clinical trials. Omalizumab is a recombinant humanized IgG1 monoclonal antibody that is produced by grafting sections of mouse IgG Fab regions onto human IgG antibodies. The final antibody contains less than 5% nonhuman residues. Binding of omalizumab to the constant region (cε3) of IgE prevents IgE acting on proinflammatory cells including mast cells and basophils.[17] Omalizumab was licensed by the FDA in 2003 as an add-on therapy for adults and children 12 years of age and older with moderate to severe asthma and a positive RAST or skin prick evidence of at least one perennial aeroallergen, and symptoms inadequately controlled with usual maintenance therapy with inhaled steroids. It is generally well tolerated, although, in common with any protein-derived therapy, it does carry a risk of anaphylaxis. Premarketing and postmarketing surveillance estimates the risk of anaphylaxis attributable to omalizumab to be around 0.2%, with early reactions (<2 hours postadministration) most common; but late reactions have also been reported.[18] Early concerns regarding an increased risk of malignancy in treated patients have not been substantiated following postmarketing surveillance. Several other monoclonal antibodies are being investigated for asthma with targets other than IgE, including inflammatory cytokines, glycoproteins, interleukins, TNF, and integrins. There are some concerns regarding the potential adverse effects of agents targeting the immune system with cytokines involved in the systemic inflammatory response, in particular with regards to severe infections (including tuberculosis) and malignancy. Whether these

TABLE 20-1 SUB-STEMS FOR NAMING MONOCLONAL ANTIBODIES

SUB-STEMS FOR SOURCE OF PRODUCT		SUB-STEMS FOR DISEASE OR TARGET CLASS	
ABBREVIATION	SOURCE	ABBREVIATION	SOURCE
u	Human	ba(c)	Bacterial
o	Mouse	ci(r)	Cardiovascular
a	Rat	fung	Fungal
e	Hamster	le(s)	Inflammatory lesions
i	Primate	li(m)	Immunomodulatory
xi	Chimeric	os	Bone
zu	Humanized	vi(r)	Viral

Naming of monoclonal antibodies according to sub-stems, as defined by the World Health Organization International Non-Proprietary Names (INN).[16] Examples are given for the origin and disease or target of the monoclonal antibody according to the INN abbreviation.

risks are also intrinsically linked to the underlying disease remain to be further understood.

At the time of this writing, palivizumab is the only FDA-approved monoclonal antibody for the prevention of an infectious disease. It is an RSV-neutralizing antibody, thought to act by inhibiting virus-to-cell and cell-to-cell fusion by preventing conformational changes in F protein.[19]

In an attempt to find an antibody with improved efficacy, other humanized monoclonal antibodies that bind to RSV F protein (e.g., motavizumab, which binds to the RSV F protein with a greater affinity) are being evaluated. Monoclonal antibodies are also being evaluated as potential therapies for interstitial lung diseases and pseudomonas infection in cystic fibrosis.

NON-ANTIBODY PROTEIN AND PEPTIDE-BASED THERAPIES

In addition to monoclonal antibodies, several protein- and peptide-based therapies for respiratory disease are in development. These include both novel and existing molecules identified through drug development programs to have specific molecular interactions in the disease pathway of interest. For example, specific receptors implicated in disease pathogenesis may be created using DNA recombinant technology. Altrakincept (Immunex Corporation, Seattle, WA) is a soluble recombinant extracellular portion of the IL-4 receptor. IL-4 has been recognized as a key target for novel therapeutic agents in asthma as it is a proinflammatory cytokine involved in the TH2 response. Soluble IL-4 receptors can bind to circulating IL-4, thus inactivating it. In initial small-scale clinical studies involving adult asthmatic patients with moderate disease severity, lung function and symptom scores were better preserved in the treatment group rather than the placebo group following discontinuation of inhaled steroid therapy.[20] However, no efficacy has been seen in larger studies.[21] There is no published literature for IL-4R administration in childhood.

Other protein- and peptide-based therapies for respiratory diseases have been developed through the use of molecular techniques to artificially create agents with pharmacologic similarities to existing nonhuman products (e.g., porcine surfactant). In the case of surfactant therapy, synthetic agents have been produced that do not contain any of the proteins found in natural surfactant. Rather they are based on synthetic phospholipids and chemically or genetically engineered peptide analogs of surfactant proteins B or C. At the time of this writing, they are still in the phase of clinical trial evaluation and have not been FDA-approved. In addition to traditional routes of administration via an endotracheal tube, products with an aerosol route of administration are under development.

OLIGONUCLEOTIDE THERAPIES

Oligonucleotides are short nucleic acid polymers, typically with 20 or fewer base pairs. The lung is considered a relatively attractive organ system for such therapies due to its accessibility via the topical route, rather than by systemic administration.

Antisense Oligonucleotides

Antisense oligonucleotides are short, single-stranded DNA molecules that interact with messenger RNA to prevent translation of a targeted gene. Their DNA sequence is complementary to the specific mRNA target; binding leads to degradation of the DNA sequences with failure of protein production. Respiratory areas for which antisense oligonucleotides are being explored include asthma, other inflammatory lung diseases, and viral lung infections. Targets include cytokines and their receptors, and transcription factors involved in the asthmatic inflammatory response. For example, $p38\alpha$ mitogen-activated protein kinase (MAPK) antisense oligonucleotide has been shown to attenuate airway inflammation in a mouse asthma model.[22] At the time of this writing, Altair Therapeutics is undertaking phase II trials of an antisense oligonucleotide therapy (AIR645) targeting the alpha subunit of the IL4 receptor (involved in activating the Janus kinase/signal transducers and activators of transcription [JAK/STAT] pathway and neutrophilic inflammation) in patients with asthma. To date, the only antisense therapy approved by the FDA is one directed at cytomegalovirus retinitis.

RNA Interference

RNA interference (RNAi) is the regulation of specific gene expression through the silencing of messenger RNAs. This process occurs in the body naturally, for example in cellular defense against viral infection. The potential actions of RNAi have lead to enthusiasm as a potential novel approach to treatment, and several avenues are being explored relevant to respiratory disease, including viral respiratory infections (respiratory syncytial virus, parainfluenza, and human metapneumovirus), asthma, and cystic fibrosis.

Small interfering RNAs (siRNAs) are short RNA sequences involved in the RNAi pathway. These are being evaluated in a number of diseases, in particular inflammatory disorders.

Although this is a very new technology, there has been extensive preclinical evaluation of the potential of siRNAs as therapeutic agents over recent years. While specific immunity for siRNAs is likely privileged, they can potentially activate innate immune responses; therefore, careful monitoring of any adverse events will be paramount. In addition to ensuring that the mechanism of action is highly specific, it is important to understand these responses when evaluating a potential role in the clinic. The respiratory system is considered a prime target for siRNA therapies due to the accessibility of the airway surface. However, despite the apparent ease of access, the major challenge to these therapies is of effective intracellular delivery. Preclinical work is ongoing to assess the best way of delivering siRNAs, including the use of viral and nonviral vectors to facilitate cellular entry.

Alnylam Pharmaceuticals began clinical trials of a siRNA targeting RSV infection in 2006. ALN-RSV01 (Alnylam Pharmaceuticals, Cambridge, MA) is an siRNA that is directed against the mRNA of the virus's nucleocapsid (N) protein, which aims to prevent viral replication. SiRNAs directed at RSV RNA polymerase protein have shown promise in mouse models, where replication of RSV was reduced following direct administration of siRNA in RSV-infected mice.[23] Phase II trials of this agent started in 2007, with volunteers given the siRNA or placebo as a nasal spray for 2 days before and until 3 days after experimental infection with RSV. Results included a 38% decrease in culture-defined RSV infections and a 95% increase in the number of uninfected subjects.[24] This is an encouraging proof-of-concept study, although future research is needed to demonstrate the role of this siRNA in environmentally acquired RSV infection, including potential influence on the acquisition of lower respiratory tract infection (which is responsible for the greatest morbidity). At the time of this writing, ALN-RSV01 is being evaluated in RSV-infected adult lung transplant patients.

The coming decade will determine whether siRNAs live up to the often very impressive results seen *in vitro* and translate into clinical therapeutics, or whether the key *in vivo* delivery difficulties will prevent this progress.

Toll-like receptors and CPGS

Toll-like receptors (TLRs) have been recognized as key players in the innate immune response. Targeting these receptors is therefore a potential immunomodulatory strategy relevant to respiratory disease. TLRs function as allergen or infective stimuli "detectors" and play an important role in immune defense. Ten human TLRs have been identified, with each playing a role in antimicrobial or antiviral response. TLR9 has received particular attention in respiratory disease, notably asthma. TLR9 is able to differentiate nonhuman from human DNA, according to the presence or absence of cytosine guanine dinucleotide (CpG) motifs. CpGs occur predominantly in nonhuman (e.g., bacterial) DNA. Interestingly, administration of CpG DNA motifs has been shown to modulate the Th1/Th2 response, with signaling via a TLR9 pathway.[25,26] CpGs administered concurrently with a known allergen can modify the resultant inflammatory response by increasing Th1 responses (and thus dampening Th2 responses). It is therefore perhaps not surprising that both CpG- and TLR-based therapies are seen as potential therapeutic strategies for diseases such as asthma. In addition to allergic inflammation, TLR agonists may improve immunity to infection or reduce inflammation in response to infectious stimuli. Whether or not agents acting via these pathways are effective tools in respiratory disease remains to be demonstrated.

▬ DINUCLEOTIDES

Although dinucleotides could be considered under the oligonucleotide section discussed earlier in the chapter, their mechanism of action is different, so they will be described separately. They are not aimed at interfering with protein translation (being composed of only two nucleic acids, they would be unlikely to be specific enough for a gene of interest; longer chains are required for this purpose). Rather, they are used as receptor agonists or antagonists. The $P2Y_2$ purinergic receptor agonist denufosol tetrasodium (Inspire Pharmaceuticals, Durham, NC) is a dinucleotide being evaluated as a potential novel therapy for CF. Activation of $P2Y_2$ induces chloride secretion via calcium-activated (non-CFTR) chloride channels, which potentially enhance airway hydration and improve mucociliary clearance. A recent placebo-controlled phase III trial of denufosol in 352 CF patients 5 years of age and older with baseline FEV1 ≥75% reported a small improvement in absolute FEV1 change after a 24-week treatment period. In comparison to the overall study population, subgroup analysis demonstrated a greater improvement in lung function in adolescent patients and those on minimal pharmacotherapy.[27,28] A further phase III trial is in progress.

▬ NONBIOLOGICAL SMALL-MOLECULE THERAPIES

CF is a good example of a disease where increased understanding of the genotypic and phenotypic mechanisms has facilitated the development of disease-modifying small-molecule therapies (Figure 20-2). Both traditional and high-throughput screening processes have been

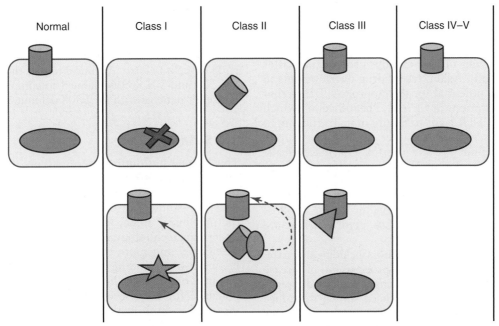

FIGURE 20-2. Schematic representation of mutation classes in cystic fibrosis and mechanism of action of novel CFTR therapies. Class I mutations with a premature stop codon prevent full-length CFTR from being produced. These mutations are being targeted with therapies that allow ribosomal read-through *(orange star)*. Class II mutations, in which CFTR is misfolded and does not traffic to the cell membrane, may be treated with "correctors," which increase the cell surface expression of CFTR *(orange oval)*. Class III mutations are associated with abnormal CFTR functioning in the cell membrane and may be treated with "potentiators," which restore channel function by increasing open probability *(orange triangle)*.

used to identify potential compounds that target defective or absent CFTR, and several of these are currently being evaluated in clinical trials. These compounds are referred to as CFTR "modulators" and include drugs that target defects in *CFTR* transcription, processing, and function (see Chapter 50). Understanding of the phenotypic manifestation of a particular disease-causing mutation in CF allows the use of assays in high-throughput screening that can identify any impact on CFTR function. Assays measuring anion conductance across cell membranes act as a "readout" for CFTR function. Novel agents have also been identified using assays detecting other outcomes. For example, the increased presence of CFTR protein in the cell membrane (as a "readout" of improved trafficking of CFTR to the apical surface) has identified the phosphodiesterase inhibitor sildenafil as a potential therapy for patients with F508 del mutations.

Targeting Post-Transcriptional Regulation

Stop codons are nucleotide triplets in mRNA that serve an important role in signaling the end of protein coding sequences. Premature stop codons are those that are present in mRNA prior to their normal position in the gene. This means that the message to create the protein of interest is incomplete; thus only incomplete (commonly referred to as *truncated*) protein is formed. Small molecules that allow the read-through of premature stop codons are being evaluated for diseases with this genetic basis (e.g., class I mutations in CF, where full-length CFTR protein is not produced).

The aminoglycoside gentamicin was initially shown to possess such capabilities, but concerns over the adverse safety profile of this group of agents (renal toxicity and sensorineural deafness) led to a search for other potential candidates. One such candidate is the oral small-molecule agent PTC124 (PTC Therapeutics, South Plainfield, NJ). This was identified by a high-throughput screening process involving over 800,000 compounds. PTC124 has been evaluated in both adults and children with at least 1 nonsense mutation in CFTR in early-phase clinical trials. Changes toward normal have been seen in nasal PD measurements (a bioelectrical test of CFTR function) in the majority of adults[29] and in around half of children.[30] An increased proportion of airway epithelial cells expressing CFTR detected by immunofluoresence was also seen.[30] These phase II trials involved CF patients from Israel (adults) and Europe (children). The results were in contrast to the lack of efficacy seen in a phase II trial of PTC124 in the United States.[31] The reasons for the discrepant trial outcomes remain unknown. Multicenter phase III trials designed to assess clinical benefit are currently in progress.

Nonsense mutations leading to premature stop codons have also been found in patients with primary ciliary dyskinesia (PCD). PCD is not a single gene disorder, but mutations in the *DNAH5* gene have been found in a high number of patients, particularly those with outer dynein arm defects,[32,33] and most are nonsense mutations. PTC124 is being investigated *in vitro* as a novel treatment for PCD. Like CF, current treatments for PCD are supportive, and therefore the theoretical advantages of this treatment approach could ultimately change management (targeting the cause rather than consequences of disease), albeit only in certain subgroups of patients.

Targeting Disease-Causing Protein Abnormalities

Small-molecule therapies also are being developed to target an underlying disease-causing protein (i.e., after protein translation). Again, recent drug developments in CF illustrate the potential for this approach. Drugs that target class II mutations in CF (e.g., Phe508Del) in which a misfolding of CFTR leads to failure of its trafficking to the apical cell membrane are referred to as *correctors*. The oral compound VX-809 (Vertex Pharmaceuticals/ Cystic Fibrosis Foundation Therapeutics, Inc.) has been identified as a potential agent.[34] Functional evidence of efficacy as assessed by sweat chloride has been demonstrated in adult CF patients homozygous for the F508del class II mutation, and early-phase clinical trials are ongoing.

Similarly, phosphodiesterase inhibitors including sildenafil, vardenafil, and tadalafil may also prove useful in disease caused by class II mutations. Using an inhaled preparation, these drugs have recently been shown to induce changes toward normality in nasal potential difference measurements in F508Del mice.[35] Their potential clinical efficacy has not yet been assessed in CF.

In CF patients with class III mutations (CFTR protein is expressed in the cell membrane but lacking function), novel small-molecule drugs that open CFTR, thereby restoring chloride ion secretion ("potentiators"), are also in the development pipeline. Candidates include VX-770 (Vertex Pharmaceuticals/Cystic Fibrosis Foundation Therapeutics, Inc.) and phosphodiesterase inhibitors such as sildenafil. VX-770 is being evaluated in patients with the most common Class III mutation, G551D; early-phase studies demonstrated evidence of functional improvement in CFTR with nasal PD and sweat chloride measurements.[36] Phase III studies involving both pediatric and adult patients are in progress.

There is also current interest in the potential synergistic effect of combining small-molecule drugs in CF. Along with a potential to work beyond the boundaries of a specific mutation class, this would greatly increase the potential number of CF patients that would benefit from any such therapies. There is evidence that combinations of potentiator and corrector compounds can restore function in F508 del cells *in vitro*. A clinical trial of the combination of VX-770 and VX 809 is planned to commence in the near future for patients with the F508 del mutation.

■ SUMMARY

This chapter has outlined several types of modern molecular therapies for respiratory disease. These therapies range from those being used as treatments (tested in large Phase III studies) through to those currently firmly in the preclinical arena. Although varied in approach and underlying technology, their aim is to target disease more specifically and more efficaciously than has been possible with long-standing conventional therapies. But with this new opportunity has come new risks in terms of the potential for adverse effects of therapy. Understanding these risks—both in the short-term and long-term—will prove key to the ultimate success in fundamentally changing our approach to treating lung disease in childhood.

Suggested Reading

Griesenbach U, Alton EW, UK Cystic Fibrosis Gene Therapy Consortium. Gene transfer to the lung: lessons learned from more than 2 decades of CF gene therapy. *Adv Drug Deliv Rev.* 2009;61:128–139.

Retsch-Bogart GZ. Update on new pulmonary therapies. *Curr Opin Pulm Med.* 2009;15:604–610 (This article is about cystic fibrosis therapies).

Séguin RM, Ferrari N. Emerging oligonucleotide therapies for asthma and chronic obstructive pulmonary disease. *Expert Opin Investig Drugs.* 2009;18:1505–1517.

Sueblinvong V, Weiss DJ. Stem cells and cell therapy approaches in lung biology and diseases. *Transl Res.* 2010;156:188–205.

References

The complete reference list is available online at www.expertconsult.com

III

Respiratory Disorders in the Newborn

21 CONGENITAL LUNG DISEASE

Robin Michael Abel, BSc, MBBS, PhD, FRCS (Eng Paeds),
Andrew Bush, MD, FRCP, FRCPCH, Lyn S. Chitty, PhD, MRCOG,
Jonny Harcourt, FRCS, and Andrew G. Nicholson, FRCPath, DM

The increased skill and widespread application of antenatal ultrasound has allowed precise early diagnosis of many congenital malformations but has brought new problems with it. Recent UK National Screening Committee guidelines recommend that all women be offered a detailed fetal anomaly scan at around 20 weeks gestation to confirm the gestational age and examine the fetal anatomy in detail. Many parents are now faced with having to decide what to do for a baby who is affected by one of many different abnormalities, some of which would have previously escaped detection. The natural history of many of these malformations is unknown, and so health professionals can have difficulty offering accurate information to parents faced with the unexpected diagnosis of an abnormality in their baby. The diagnosis of fetal lung lesions is one good example. Early reports published in the 1980s described a poor outcome for fetuses with lung masses detected in the second trimester. However, these studies were biased by a high incidence of intervention, including termination of pregnancy. With increasing use of antenatal ultrasound and the detection of many less obvious lesions, it has become clear that many abnormalities disappear or regress considerably by term if conservative management is followed. Indeed, as we will demonstrate in this chapter, the outcome for such fetuses is very good in general, and the dilemma now is whether to pursue conservative or surgical management in an asymptomatic infant. Further confusion arises as to how these malformations should be described. The nomenclature of congenital lung disease was never very clear. Terms such as *sequestrated segment, cystic adenomatoid malformation, hypoplastic lung,* and *malinosculation* (Latin: *mal*=abnormal; *in*=in; *osculum*=mouth; defined as "the establishment of [abnormal] communications between already existing blood vessels or other tubular structures that come into contact") were used to describe abnormalities that often overlap. Now, however, they are

used inconsistently before and after birth. For example, congenital cystic adenomatoid malformation (CCAM) is used by perinatologists to describe a lesion that may well disappear before birth; however, the term is used postnatally to describe an abnormality that may require lobectomy. CCAM may have a pulmonary arterial supply or be supplied like a sequestration from systemic arteries, and histologic features of these lesions may overlap. Furthermore, overlap lesions that contain features of two or even three pathologic entities are common.[1-3] New imaging modalities such as magnetic resonance imaging (MRI) now allow delineation of blood supply with increasing precision. New treatment options (e.g., fetal surgery and postnatal embolization of feeding vessels) have become available; however, the availability of a procedure is not necessarily the best indication for its performance. A complete reappraisal of the diagnosis, investigation, and management of congenital lung disease is thus timely.

CLINICAL APPROACH

To clarify the dialog among various professionals (i.e., obstetricians, perinatologists, pediatric surgeons, pathologists, pediatricians), it is suggested that the following principles be followed:[4]

1. What is actually seen should be described without indulgence in embryologic speculation, which later may be proved wrong. Clinical descriptions should not include assumptions of pathology, since the same clinical appearance (e.g., a multicystic mass) may have different pathologic etiologies. Indeed, specific antenatal diagnoses often have to be revised after postnatal excision of the lesion.[5]
2. The description should be in common language, discarding Latin.

3. The lung and associated organs should be approached in a systematic manner, because abnormalities are often multiple and associated lesions will be missed unless carefully sought.

4. Pathologic descriptions should describe what is actually seen (epithelial and mesenchymal elements), which may then be related to a diagnostic category (CCAM). However, even distinguished pathologists disagree over the classification of excised specimens, underscoring that clinicians seeing grayscale images are most unlikely to get it right.[7,8]

Describe What Is Actually Seen

The recommendation to describe what is actually seen should be followed by the clinician both before and after birth. In principle, antenatal ultrasound abnormalities should be described using terms such as *increased echogenicity with large, small, or multiple cysts* rather than as "CCAM," which is and remains a histologic diagnosis only. The presence or absence of abnormal feeding vessels may be defined using color or power Doppler. Other features such as mediastinal shift should also be described. In the postnatal period, a radiographic abnormality should be described as solid or cystic. If cystic, the cysts are either single or multiple, and the uniformity and thickness of the walls should be described. They may be filled with air, or partially or completely with fluid; moreover, their size should be recorded. Postnatally, an air-fluid level suggests that the abnormality is connected to the tracheobronchial tree, accounting for the gas in the cyst. If the lesion has been excised, the pathologist should describe the tissues found (e.g., epithelial, mesenchymal) and the contents of any cysts that may be present, thus giving a simple description of what is seen under the microscope. Only then is it relevant to make a pathologic diagnosis such as one of the various histologic types of CCAM (see subsequent sections). Any classification system that is to be robust cannot be based on embryologic speculation.

Use Common Language

Many terms are ambiguous and are best avoided. For example, *hypoplastic lung* could be taken as meaning a lung that is small but otherwise normal, or small because the underlying structure is abnormal; the term *congenital small lung (CSL)* avoids such ambiguity. The use of the term *emphysema* in *congenital lobar emphysema* is another source of confusion because it implies lung destruction, whereas in at least some variants (e.g., polyalveolar lobe) there may be too many, not too few alveoli. What is actually seen is a *congenital large hyperlucent lobe (CLHL)*, a term that should be used in clinical practice. Throughout this chapter, unwarranted established terms will be given in parentheses after the proposed new term; for the convenience of the reader, new terms will be spelled out in full, with the abbreviated form given in parentheses. A summary comparison of old and new nomenclature is provided in Table 21-1.

TABLE 21-1   NEW AND OLD TERMS USED TO DESCRIBE THE CLINICAL, BUT NOT PATHOLOGICAL, APPEARANCES OF CONGENITAL LUNG MALFORMATIONS

NEW NOMENCLATURE	OLD TERMS SUPERCEDED
Congenital large hyperlucent lobe (CLHL)	Congenital lobar emphysema Polyalveolar lobe
Congenital thoracic malformation (CTM)	Cystic adenomatoid malformation (Types 0 to 4 pathologically) Sequestration (intrapulmonary and extrapulmonary) Bronchogenic cyst Reduplication cyst Foregut cyst
Congenital small lung (CSL)	Pulmonary hypoplasia
Absent lung, absent trachea	Agenesis of lung, tracheal aplasia
Absent bronchus	Bronchial atresia

Use a Systematic Approach

The lung can be considered to be formed from six "trees": bronchial, arterial (systemic and pulmonary), venous (systemic and pulmonary), and lymphatic. There are no known abnormalities of bronchial venous drainage, so only five trees have to be considered in practice. There are three other areas wherein malformations may affect the respiratory system and thus should also be assessed. These are (1) the heart and great vessels, (2) the chest wall, including the respiratory neuromuscular apparatus, and (3) the abdomen. Finally, the possibility of multisystem disease (e.g., tuberous sclerosis) should be considered. Each patient suspected of having a congenital lung malformation should be systematically evaluated along these lines if important coexistent abnormalities are not to be missed. The importance of a systematic approach to treatment, with an appropriate evaluation of all trees and associated systems before embarking on treatment, cannot be overstated.

Keep Clinical and Pathologic Descriptions Separate

This is an extension of the principle of describing what is seen. Black-and-white images on a scan are unlikely to be pathognomonic of a single histologic entity. It is more logical to describe the clinical appearances and construct a pathologic differential diagnosis. Only after excision of the lesion can the pathologist make an appropriate diagnosis from examination of the excised specimen.

EPIDEMIOLOGY OF CONGENITAL MALFORMATIONS OF THE LUNG

There is a paucity of high-quality, population-based epidemiologic studies. The requirement for a high-quality study to be performed is for all women in a large population to have access to diagnostic quality, mid-trimester ultrasound scans that are properly interpreted by experienced radiologists. The European Surveillance of Congenital Anomalies (EUROCAT) is the largest network of population-based registers for the epidemiologic surveillance of congenital anomalies including congenital thoracic malformations (CTMs). Current data are collected from 43 European registries in 20 European countries[7] but still only capture less than 30% of Europe's birth population.[7] In 2008, EUROCAT reported 222 fetuses with CTMs giving an incidence of 4.44/10,000 (which included live births, fetal deaths, and terminations of pregnancy). Although it is the best currently available data, EUROCAT prevalence data must be treated with caution because it is a relatively limited sample.

AGE-RELATED PRESENTATIONS OF CONGENITAL LUNG DISEASE

A complete review of congenital lung disease might also include a few disorders that are acquired *in utero*, such as congenital pneumonias (discussed in Chapter 22), but this chapter is limited to the stricter definition of developmental disorders. There is an overlap with the developmental components of pediatric interstitial lung disease,[9] and these are described in detail in Chapter 55. We will first describe the age-related clinical presentations of congenital lung disease (Table 21-2), and then we will consider, tree by tree, the important abnormalities encountered.

Antenatal Presentation

Antenatal presentation is usually associated with an abnormality detected at the time of a routine fetal anomaly scan, as described in detail later in the chapter.

TABLE 21-2 PRESENTATION OF CONGENITAL LUNG DISEASE BY AGE

AGE	PRESENTING FEATURE
Antenatal	Intrathoracic mass Pleural effusion Fetal hydrops Oligohydraminios or polyhydramnios Other associated abnormalities discovered
Newborn	Respiratory distress Stridor Bubbly secretions in mouth, unable to swallow Failure to pass nasogastric tube Unable to establish an airway Cardiac failure Chance finding Cyanosis in a well baby Poor respiratory effort
Later childhood/ adulthood	Recurrent infection (including tuberculosis, aspergillus) Hemoptysis, hemothorax Bronchiectasis, bronchopleural fistula Steroid-resistant airway obstruction Cardiac failure Malignant transformation Cyanosis Coughing on drinking Chance finding of mass or hyperlucent area on chest radiograph Air embolism (rare)

However, abnormalities of amniotic fluid volume may also be associated with underlying pulmonary pathology. This may be secondary, as in bilateral CSL (pulmonary hypoplasia) associated with both early-onset oligohydramnios (e.g., caused by bilateral renal dysplasia/agenesis or first-trimester or early second-trimester rupture of the membranes) or polyhydramnios associated with conditions such as the Pena-Shokeir phenotype or antenatal onset of severe spinal muscular atrophy (wherein severe neuromuscular disease prevents normal respiratory movements and lung development). Another possibility is compression of the fetal esophagus by a mass, preventing normal swallowing of amniotic fluid. In other situations, there is a primary pulmonary anomaly (e.g., tracheoesophageal fistula [TEF] or laryngeal/tracheal agenesis) that causes the polyhydramnios. Other presentations include short limbs in those skeletal dysplasias associated with bilateral CSL secondary to small chests and short ribs (e.g., Jeune syndrome of asphyxiating thoracic dystrophy), or talipes and polyhydramnios in congenital myotonic dystrophy.

Presentation in the Newborn Period

Not all lesions are detected prenatally, although postnatal presentation is becoming less common with increasing use and improvements in technology and sonographic skills. Late detection may particularly be an issue in diaphragmatic hernias, some of which do not present with sonographic findings until after the time of the routine anomaly scan or indeed well after birth. Large airway obstruction as the primary problem is suggested by stridor, failure to pass an endotracheal tube (ETT), or successful passage of the ETT but inability to establish ventilation. This last condition may be due to a TEF as well as to large airway stenosis or complete obstruction. Respiratory distress in the absence of major airway disease may be due to disorders of the lung parenchyma. These include a large cystic or solid CTM, the presence of unilateral or bilateral small lungs, and congenital pleural effusion or lymphatic disorder. Vascular abnormalities may present at this time. One such group are aortopulmonary collaterals supplying either a CSL or a CTM. These act hemodynamically as systemic arteriovenous malformations and may cause high-output heart failure. Abnormalities of venous drainage, such as "scimitar" syndrome (hemianomalous pulmonary venous drainage to the inferior caval vein), may also present as heart failure or enter the differential diagnosis of pulmonary hypertension in the newborn period. Other vascular problems that may present at this time include alveolar-capillary dysplasia (discussed in Chapter 55) and pulmonary arteriovenous malformation (PAVM), which may present as cyanosis in a well infant (not with heart failure, unless there is an associated systemic, usually cerebral, arteriovenous malformation). Chest wall disease (e.g., diaphragmatic hernia and asphyxiating dystrophy) presents as respiratory distress with difficulty in establishing ventilation. By contrast, neuromuscular disease (e.g., severe spinal muscular atrophy or myotonic dystrophy with maternal inheritance) is characterized by inadequate or absent respiratory effort but with ease of establishing ventilation, unless there are associated unilateral or bilateral CSLs. This last group of conditions is covered in Chapter 15. The differential diagnosis of a cystic abnormality detected postnatally but not antenatally includes cysts secondary to infection[10] or pulmonary interstitial emphysema,[11] which may present in localized form, even in a term baby who has not been artificially ventilated.

Later Presentation of Congenital Lung Disease

Congenital lung disease may present later in childhood, or even in adult life. Respiratory distress as the sole presenting feature of congenital lung disease is rare after infancy. Many CTMs can present as an asymptomatic radiologic abnormality, including a focal solid or cystic mass, or hyperlucency. Unilateral CSL may also be a chance finding, and, if right-sided, may mimic mirror-image arrangement. A cystic CTM enters the differential diagnosis of recurrent pneumonia in the same location, with failure of radiologic clearing between bouts or atelectasis due to large airway compression. More rarely, a cystic CTM may present as a lung abscess, focal bronchiectasis, pneumothorax, air embolism,[12] hemoptysis, or hemothorax—or even with malignant transformation. However, it must be stressed that this last condition is very rare and is described in more detail later in the chapter. The occurrence of any of this formidable but rare list of complications is extremely unusual in the first 2 years of life. Other conditions presenting with hemoptysis are any abnormalities characterized by abnormal systemic arterial supply and PAVM. The latter condition also may present with progressive cyanosis in a well person, which may lead to polycythemia or with systemic abscess or embolism (including cerebral) due to bypass of the pulmonary vascular filter.

Another important presentation of congenital lung disease is as "steroid-resistant asthma." Large airway narrowing such as tracheomalacia, vascular ring, or pulmonary artery sling, or complete cartilage rings enter the differential diagnosis; important physiologic clues come from the inspiratory and/or expiratory amputation of the flow-volume curve, and the presence of a normal residual volume in the face of a greatly reduced FEV_1/FVC ratio (ratio of forced expiratory volume in one second to forced vital capacity).

Tracheoesophageal fistula and diaphragmatic hernia are considered the archetypal conditions presenting in the newborn period. However, both can present late. Tracheoesophageal fistula may present with recurrent bouts of coughing after drinking, or hemoptysis. Symptoms may have been present for more than 15 years.[13] Diaphragmatic hernia usually presents with gastrointestinal symptoms later on, although abrupt presentation with respiratory distress has been described.[14] Whether some of these late-presenting hernias are truly congenital has been disputed.

It can be seen from the foregoing that congenital lung disease is not necessarily rare and esoteric and important only up to the stage of early infancy, but that in many

clinical scenarios it is worth asking, "Could there be a congenital thoracic disease present?" when considering the differential diagnosis.

◼ ANTENATAL DIAGNOSIS AND TREATMENT

What Can We Diagnose and When?

Fetal lung abnormalities are increasingly detected prenatally as a result of advances in ultrasound imaging improving diagnosis and also because fetal anomaly scanning is now routinely offered to many women in the developed world. A fetal lung lesion is suspected either when a mass (cystic or solid) is identified in the thorax or because of mediastinal shift (Table 21-3). The opportunity to identify an intrathoracic anomaly in the antenatal period permits further investigations and occasionally offers the potential for intrauterine therapy. It also identifies fetuses that may benefit from delivery in a center that offers tertiary-level neonatal support and the option of early postnatal surgical intervention. Many of these lesions can be detected around 20 weeks gestation, but late presentation is well recognized for some, in particular diaphragmatic hernias and pleural effusions. Such lesions may not be detected until an incidental scan in the third trimester is undertaken, or indeed until sometime after birth when clinical signs appear. It must also be recognized that a sonographic diagnosis can only describe the macroscopic nature of the lesion, and a definitive diagnosis for many anomalies must await definitive radiologic or histologic diagnosis after birth. Many reported studies are seriously limited because they base conclusions solely on prenatal ultrasound or postnatal imaging, which is often limited to plain radiology. While advances in technology have improved antenatal diagnosis of lesions that may benefit from early postnatal intervention, many of the abnormalities detected appear to resolve spontaneously or are clinically silent. The pediatrician is frequently faced with a new dilemma—how to manage the well infant with a lesion that would not have been brought to medical attention were it not for antenatal imaging.

What is the natural history of some of these lesions? Do they require intervention, or are they benign variants? This section will present an overview of the antenatal

TABLE 21-3 DIFFERENTIAL DIAGNOSIS OF FETAL INTRATHORACIC LESIONS

SOLID LESIONS	CYSTIC LESIONS
Microcystic adenomatoid malformation	Macrocystic adenomatoid malformation
Pulmonary sequestration	Congenital diaphragmatic hernia
Right-sided diaphragmatic hernia	Bronchogenic cyst
Tracheal/laryngeal atresia	Mediastinal encephalocele
Rhabdomyoma	Pleural and pericardial effusions
Mediastinal teratoma	

diagnosis and management of the more common types of congenital intrathoracic abnormalities. Postnatal management of the abnormalities is discussed in subsequent sections.

In addition to fetal ultrasound, in recent years there has been an increasing use of fetal MRI to further define pathology detected with ultrasound. There are reports of its use for the delineation of fetal cystic masses,[15] but how much MRI adds to the ultrasound diagnosis remains to be demonstrated. It may be more sensitive to small lesions than ultrasound, but it is arguable whether detection of tiny abnormalities really matters. It has been shown to be superior to screening ultrasound for the diagnosis of congenital high-airway obstruction syndrome (CHAOS) when it changed the diagnosis in 70%, but in 9 of these 10 cases the MRI diagnosis was concordant with the referral center prenatal ultrasound findings.[16] However, it may be useful to accurately determine the level of airway obstruction in this condition.[17] MRI may also be of use to determine the location of feeding vessels in fetuses with pulmonary sequestration,[18] but further comparison with ultrasound-based methods is required before we can say whether it adds significantly to Doppler ultrasound methods. The role of MRI to determine lung volumes in fetuses with CDH or lung masses has been evaluated[19] and may ultimately prove superior to other ultrasound-based methods (see the paragraphs that follow).

Congenital Diaphragmatic Hernia

The etiology of congenital diaphragmatic hernia (CDH) is obscure, and a full review is beyond the scope of this chapter. Genetic studies have recently been reviewed.[20,21] More recent candidate genes include the *HLX* gene at chromosome 1q41-1q42,[22] dispatched 1 *(DISP1)*,[23] fibroblast growth factor (FGF) receptor-like 1 *(FGFRL1)*,[24,25] t-complex-associated-testis-expressed 3 *(TCTE3)*.[26] Interestingly, TCTE3 is also found in ciliary outer dynein arms. Animal

models suggest that nitrofen induced reduced cellular proliferation in the developing diaphragm may be important,[27] although it is possible that the primary abnormality is maldevelopment of the ipsilateral lung.[28]

The prenatal incidence of CDH is around 1 in 2000.[8] There is a wide variety of abnormalities associated with CDH, including aneuploidy (in particular trisomies 18 and 13), genetic syndromes, and structural abnormalities.[29] Many of these will result in a stillbirth or the pregnancy being terminated, so isolated CDH is much more common in neonates. Anomalies associated with CDH include neural tube defects (e.g., myelomeningocele), cardiac defects, and midline anomalies (e.g., cleft lip and cleft palate). Genetic syndromes such as Fryn's syndrome accounted for up to 10% of cases in some series.[29] The herniation of abdominal contents into the chest inhibits normal lung development, resulting in pulmonary hypoplasia,[30] which in isolated lesions is the main cause of death.

The diagnosis of a left-sided CDH is usually first suspected when mediastinal shift is observed and abdominal viscera are seen within the fetal thorax (Fig. 21-1). The most useful clue is usually the identification of a cystic structure (the stomach) in the chest together with the absence of an intra-abdominal stomach. The observation of peristalsis in the chest can also be a useful clue because loops of bowel may be difficult to distinguish from other cystic lesions. Paradoxical movements of the viscera in the chest with fetal breathing movements are also occasionally seen. Once alert to the possible diagnosis, the clinician doing a careful examination of the fetus in the coronal and parasagittal planes will be unable to identify the diaphragm. Right-sided CDH is more difficult to recognize because only the liver is herniated, and this is of similar echogenicity to liquid-filled lung tissue. Often the only clue is mediastinal shift, and this can be overlooked at the time of a routine anomaly scan unless the degree of shift is great. The diagnosis is sometimes made in the third trimester when a scan is performed because of

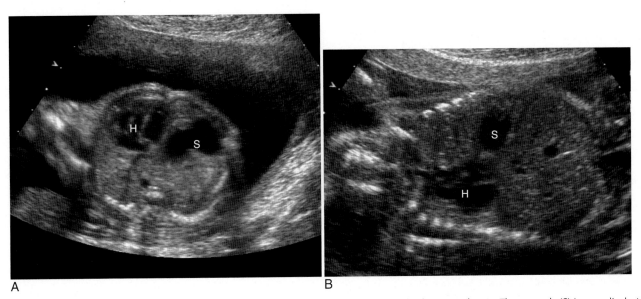

A   B

FIGURE 21-1. A, Transverse view through the thorax of a fetus at 20 weeks gestation with a diaphragmatic hernia. The stomach *(S)* is seen displacing the heart *(H)* to the right. **B,** In the longitudinal plane, no diaphragm can be seen and the stomach is in the chest.

polyhydramnios caused by increased intrathoracic pressure due to the presence of herniated abdominal contents in the chest. This prevents normal swallowing movements and results in late onset of increased amniotic fluid.

The overall prognosis for fetuses with CDH is poor, with the major causes of death being pulmonary hypoplasia or associated abnormalities. The time of diagnosis is related to outcome, with those diagnosed early faring the worst. Currently the best prognostic indicator of outcome, independent of gestation, is the lung-to-head-ratio (LHR), in which 2D-ultrasound is used to measure the size of the contralateral lung at the level of the four-chamber view of the heart. This value is compared to the value of that expected in a normal fetus (observed/expected LHR). Values of <0.25 indicate a low (<15%) chance of survival.[31] In a meta-analysis of 21 studies that fulfilled the entry criteria, 6 examined entirely unique heterogeneous parameters, and the remaining 15 examined LHRs and/or the presence of liver in the fetal thorax. Low LHR and the presence of the liver in the chest were poor prognostic features. The strongest association with lethal pulmonary hypoplasia was that of LHR >0.6 compared to <0.6, although more clinically relevant with the best positive predictive value for survival was that of LHR >1.0.[32] Another group suggested that a McGoon index (combined diameters of the pulmonary arteries indexed to the descending aorta,

cutoff value, 1.31) and particularly PAI (cutoff value, 90) were reliable methods for predicting mortality in CDH.[33] Other poor prognostic indicators include cardiac disproportion before 24 weeks gestation. Isolated left-sided hernias, an intra-abdominal stomach, and diagnosis after 24 weeks are favorable prognostic factors. In Europe, a combination of these variables is used in the evaluation of prognosis, but it is likely that MRI volumetry will shortly play a more significant role as it can measure total rather than unilateral lung size and demonstrate liver position.[19] Survival in cases with isolated left-sided CDH is now reported to be in excess of 60% (Table 21-4).[34]

Following the prenatal diagnosis of CDH, management should include a detailed search for other anomalies and fetal karyotyping. Expert fetal echocardiography is indicated because examination of the heart is complicated by distortion of intrathoracic contents. Consultation with a pediatric surgeon should be offered and, given the variable prognosis in terms of perinatal mortality as well as morbidity, termination of pregnancy is an option that should be discussed. Delivery of ongoing pregnancies should be planned in a center with neonatal intensive care and pediatric surgical facilities. In the event of fetal or perinatal death, a postmortem examination is to be recommended. This should include a genetic opinion to facilitate an accurate diagnosis of

TABLE 21-4 PROGNOSIS FOR ANTENATALLY DIAGNOSED CDH

AUTHORS	NUMBER	CHROMOSOME ABNORMALITY N %		% SURVIVAL OVERALL	% SURVIVAL AT < 24 WEEKS	% SURVIVAL AT > 24 WEEKS	% SURVIVAL IN ISOLATED CASES
Thorpe-Beeston et al., 1989[183]	36	11	31	25			60
Adzick et al., 1989[184]	38	6	16	24	0	38	38
Sharland et al., 1992[185]	55	2	4	27	26	40	28
Manni et al., 1994[186]	28	3	11	14	0	100	30
Bollman et al., 1995[187]	33	6	18	18			44
Dommergues et al., 1996[188]	135	14	10	19			30
Howe et al., 1996[189]	48	13	34	27	24	30	50
Geary et al., 1998[190]	34	5	15	18	31	33	38
Bahlmann et al., 1999[191]	19	1	7				
Betremieux et al., 2002[192]	31	4	13	38			60
Garne et al., 2002[193]	187	20	11	71			
Laudy et al., 2003[194]	261	0	0	50			
Dott et al., 2003[195]	249	18	7	19/54*			
Hendrick et al., 2004[196]	222	0	0	70			
Total	1376	103	13	32/35*	16	48	42

1 Only isolated left-sided CDH cases were included in study.
2 Only right-sided CDH cases were included in study.
* Overall survival has increased during the time period of the study from 19% (1968 to 1971) to 54% (1996 to 1999).
Where there is no figure for survival, data were not given in the publication.

any possible underlying syndrome, which may confer an increased risk of recurrence in future pregnancies. Open fetal surgery has been performed for CDH in order to occlude the airway; the continued secretion of lung liquid beyond the obstruction leads to expansion of the lung. The procedure is demanding and carries significant maternal risks as well as the possibility of precipitating preterm labor. A randomized controlled trial failed to show any benefit for open surgery for fetal airway occlusion.[35] In view of this, there has been a move to a less invasive approach that utilizes temporary FETO with a percutaneous approach under local anesthesia, and thereby minimizes risk to the mother.[36] A balloon is inserted into the trachea at 26 to 28 weeks aiming to stimulate lung growth. The occlusion is reversed at around 34 weeks either by removal of the balloon fetoscopically, ultrasound guided puncture of the balloon, or at the time of delivery using the EXIT (**EX** utero, **I**ntrapartum **T**reatment) procedure. In an animal study,[37] phasically inflating and deflating the intratracheal balloon led to better lung development than continuous airway occlusion. A large, pan-European study of 210 cases treated this way recently demonstrated an increase in survival in cases with severe left-sided CDH (as predicted using the LHR) from a predicted 24.1% to 49.1%, and in right-sided from 0% to 35.3%, despite a high incidence of early rupture of the membranes and around 30% delivering before 34 weeks gestation.[38] This trial only included cases with severe left-sided CDH and those with a right-sided lesion. A further trial is about to start, evaluating FETO (Fetoscopic EndoTracheal balloon Occlusion) in cases with less severe degrees of CDH.[36] Of note, tracheomegaly is described as a complication of fetal tracheal occlusion.[39]

CTM Subsequently Diagnosed Pathologically as CCAM

The etiology of CTMs (whether CCAM, sequestration, or others) is little known. Genetic studies have implicated Hoxb-5,[40] epidermal growth factor receptor,[41] brain type fatty acid binding protein-7,[42] fibroblast growth factor 7 and 9,[43] alpha-2 integrin, and E-cadherin.[44] CCAM is traditionally classified according to histologic and clinical findings; however, sonographic classification is best achieved by considering these malformations as either macrocystic (Fig. 21-2) or microcystic (Fig. 21-3).[45] The main differential diagnosis to consider with a macrocystic CCAM is diaphragmatic hernia. Differentiating features have been described earlier. However, in a series of 110 fetuses with a prenatal diagnosis of CCAM who were seen in the Fetal Medicine Unit at University College London Hospitals, 12 had other diagnoses, including 3 with a diaphragmatic hernia and 1 an eventration of the diaphragm (see Table 21-5).[46] In two of those with a diaphragmatic hernia, the correct diagnosis was made prenatally after serial scanning. In the other case of diaphragmatic hernia and that of the eventration, the correct diagnosis was made only on postnatal imaging.

Most CCAMs occur in isolation, although other abnormalities including bronchopulmonary sequestration and CDH have been reported to occur in association with CCAM, as have a broad range of extrapulmonary malformations including renal and cardiac anomalies.[29,47,48] Aneuploidy is not a recognized association.

In general, the prognosis for a fetus with a CCAM is good, with only a small number going on to develop hydrops, which is a poor prognostic sign (particularly if

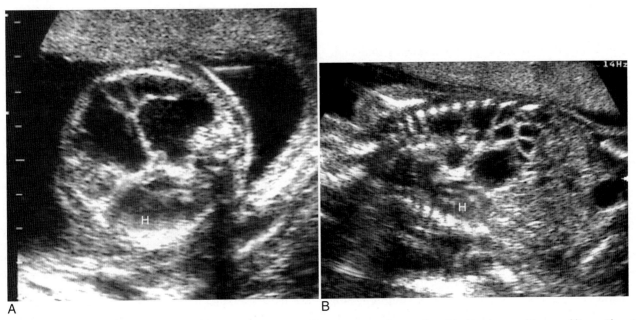

FIGURE 21-2. Axial (**A**) and longitudinal (**B**) views through the thorax of a fetus at 21 weeks gestation with skin edema and increased liquor. There is a large macrocystic congenital thoracic malformation. The heart *(H)* can be seen displaced to the left, and the whole chest appears to be full of abnormal lung tissue. In the longitudinal view, the diaphragm is displaced downward by the abnormally expanded lung tissue. The large cysts were aspirated and pleuroamniotic shunts were inserted to resolve the skin edema. The pregnancy continued to term; respiratory support was required at birth with surgery in the neonatal period. The child is now alive and well at school age.

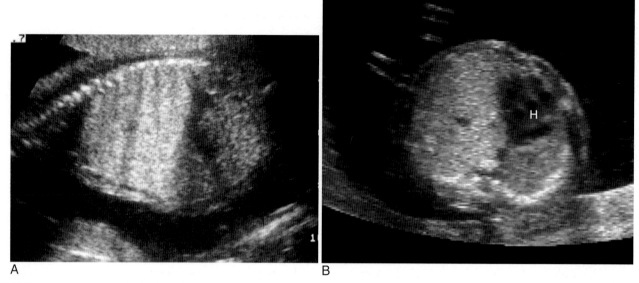

A   B

FIGURE 21-3. **A,** Parasagittal view through the chest of a fetus at 21 weeks gestation with a microcystic congenital thoracic malformation showing the echogenic wedge-shaped left lower lung behind the chest. In the axial view of the fetal chest (**B**), the abnormal lung can be seen causing marked mediastinal shift with the heart (H) lying in the right chest. The mediastinal shift resolved as pregnancy progressed, and the baby was well at birth. Postnatal imaging confirmed the presence of the lesion, and a conservative management policy was followed.

evident at the initial presentation in the second trimester). Traditionally, both polyhydramnios and mediastinal shift were considered poor prognostic indicators,[49] but more recent data suggest that these signs are less reliable than once thought. Accurate prediction of outcome for prenatally diagnosed lesions can be difficult following a single scan, because spontaneous *in utero* improvement is often observed (Table 21-5). Serial scans should be undertaken to detect those lesions that progress in size or display adverse prognostic features that may warrant consideration of intervention. In one series, pure hyperechogenicity versus mixed lesions, and later gestational age at birth, were associated with regression in size of the malformation.[50] Another group suggested that high mass thorax ratio, diaphragmatic eversion, and cystic predominance were adverse features.[51] It has been suggested that relating cyst size to head circumference may be a useful guide to prognosis.[52] However, before being too gloomy in prognosticating about large CTMs, it should be noted that even some large lesions may present late; a case report of a 33-year-old man presenting with a CTM occupying the whole of one hemithorax reminds us that even large CTMs are compatible with normal existence.[53]

There is very little agreement on definitions (even for something as basic as fetal hydrops) and only a limited evidence base with regard to the antenatal options for treatment, and there are no randomized controlled trials.[54] Most would agree that an expectant approach is best, reserving treatment for hydropic fetuses, or perhaps for the rare case with a rapidly expanding lesion in the last trimester. Even in large units, the performance of invasive interventions is unusual.[55] The least aggressive intervention is the administration of betamethasone to the mother.[56] It is said that up to 50% of fetuses may respond.[57] Whether repeated courses are

beneficial is not known,[57,58] and fetal death with this therapy has been reported.[59] When there are single or multiple large cysts (see Fig. 21-2) with associated hydrops or polyhydramnios, improvement has been reported with *in utero* decompression by thoracocentesis or the insertion of a shunt.[60] Intrauterine surgery to remove these lesions has also been reported.[36,60] Other surgical options that have been reported include fetal sclerotherapy in the second half of the pregnancy, which is the percutaneous injection of sclerosants such as Ethamolin (ethanolamine oleate) or Polidocanol (aethoxysklerol) under ultrasound guidance[61,62] and radiofrequency ablation, although fetal death has resulted from the latter approach.[51] It should also be noted that marked postnatal chest deformity has followed fetal shunt insertion.

The King's College Hospital group has reported on 67 fetuses with an antenatally diagnosed congenital lung malformation.[63] Of the 64 who were born alive, 42 underwent postnatal surgery. Surgery was performed in 45% of lesions showing late-gestation "resolution." Although there was some correlation between the antenatal appearances and the need for surgery, this was not usefully predictive for an individual, and the need for operation was judged on postnatal features rather than clinical need. In general, the approach to the postnatal management of neonates with prenatally diagnosed cystic lung lesions is very variable. Some feel that all lesions should be surgically removed, and others favor a more conservative approach (see Table 21-5). At University College London Hospitals, we have seen 110 fetuses with cystic lung lesions in the last 15 years, of whom 100 are alive, 20 having had surgery. This is a much lower proportion than in the King's series and demonstrates the varying approach to management (see Table 21-5). In all cases, early consultation with neonatal and pediatric surgical staff is helpful for parents.

TABLE 21-5 REPORTED OUTCOMES AND POSTNATAL MANAGEMENT IN RECENT SERIES OF CYSTIC LUNG LESIONS

	TOTAL	RESOLVED IN UTERO	ALIVE	OTHER DIAGNOSIS	TOP	IUD/ PND	POSTNATAL MANAGEMENT SURGERY EMERGENCY	ELECTIVE	CONSERVATIVE
*Kunisaki et al., 2007[197]	12	0	9	5	0	**3	4	5	0
Illanes et al., 2005[198]	48	22 (5)	39	5	3 (**1)	**6	0	23	6 (+5 ltfu)
Pumberger et al., 2003[199]	35	11 (6)	29	3	4	2	4	17	2
Laberge et al., 2001[200]	48	23 regressed	36	4	7	5	Not reported	Not reported	Not reported
De Santis et al., 2000[201]	17	3	14	0	2	2	4		6 (+ 2 ltfu)
Miller et al., 1996[202]	17	0	12	0	3	2	12		0
Sauvat et al., 2003[203]	29	4 (4)	29	0	0	0	3	14	12
Davenport et al., 2004[63]	67	8 (1)	64	7	1	4	42		12 (+10 ltfu)
Lacy et al., 1999[204]	23	9 (4)	19	5	4	1	5		13
Calvert et al., 2006[205]	19	0	19	0	5	2	3	13	3
UCLH	110	11 (9)	100	12	7	3	12	8	46 (+ 17 PND awaited and 4 ltfu)

*, All large lesions; **, all severe hydrops; +, reports antenatally diagnosed cases who were asymptomatic only. ( ), cases with no signs on postnatal imaging either; other diagnosis (e.g., CDH, tracheal atresia). From Bush A, Hogg J, Chitty LS. Cystic lung lesions—prenatal diagnosis and management. *Prenat Diagn.* 2008;28:604-611, with permission from Wiley Blackwell.

The issues of postnatal management are discussed in more detail later in the chapter. Where a lesion has persisted or increased in size and mediastinal shift persists in the third trimester, delivery in a center with neonatal intensive care and surgical facilities should be considered. In all cases, careful postnatal follow-up should be undertaken, with computed tomography (CT) being offered to all. It is well documented that lesions that have apparently involuted completely *in utero* are still present when examined by CT after birth.

CTM Subsequently Diagnosed Pathologically as Bronchopulmonary Sequestration

In the fetus, a sequestrated lobe of lung is most often identified as a mass of uncertain origin in the chest or subdiaphragmatic area. Rarely, bilateral communicating sequestrations may be seen.[64] Prenatally it is not possible to make a definitive diagnosis unless an independent blood supply is demonstrated using Doppler ultrasound, although it should be noted that a CCAM might also have an aortic blood supply. The use of the generic term *CTM* may thus be appropriate in this context. The sequestrated lobe usually appears as an echogenic mass in the chest (Fig. 21-4) or abdomen (Fig. 21-5). It can be associated with hydrops, mediastinal shift, and polyhydramnios (see Fig. 21-4). The prenatal management of fetuses with lesions suspected to be a sequestration is much as for those with a suspected CCAM; serial scanning should be undertaken, and the fetus should be delivered in a tertiary unit if there is significant mediastinal shift in the third trimester. Spontaneous improvement *in utero* has also been reported.

Upper Respiratory Tract Atresia

Laryngeal or tracheal atresia are rare malformations that may be isolated or found in association with other abnormalities or genetic syndromes, the most common of

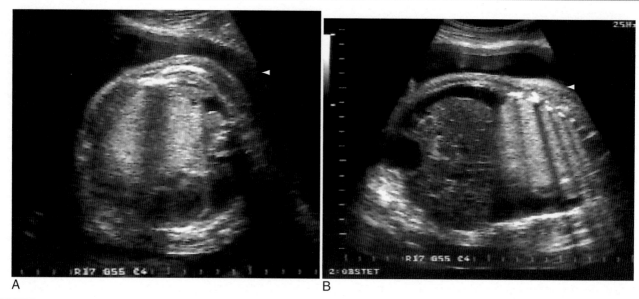

FIGURE 21-4. Axial (**A**) and longitudinal (**B**) views through the thorax of a fetus at 34 weeks gestation with hydrops and polyhydramnios. The large echogenic mass can be seen occupying most of the chest. There is a significant rim of ascitic fluid in the abdomen as well as pleural effusions in the chest. Preterm labor ensued after amniodrainage. Resuscitation failed, and a postmortem examination demonstrated a sequestrated lobe with associated pulmonary hypoplasia.

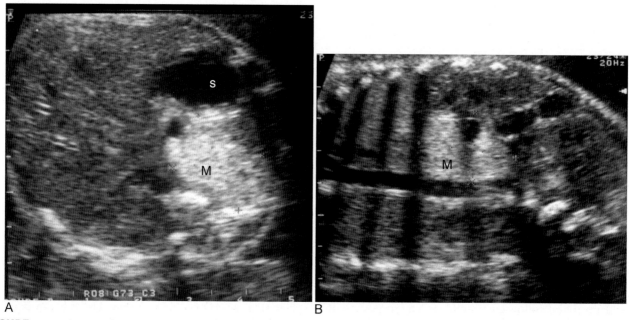

FIGURE 21-5. Axial (**A**) and longitudinal (**B**) view through the abdomen of a fetus at 22 weeks gestation. Note the echogenic mass *(M)* related to the diaphragm lying behind the stomach *(s)*. An ultrasound-guided needle biopsy after birth confirmed this to be a pulmonary sequestration. This subsequently resolved spontaneously in early childhood.

which is Fraser syndrome.[29] The diagnosis of laryngeal or tracheal obstruction should be suspected when enlarged, uniformly hyperechogenic lungs are seen on ultrasound (Fig. 21-6). Other sonographic features include cardiac and mediastinal compression, flattening or convexity of the diaphragms, hydrops, and polyhydramnios. A dilated, fluid-filled upper trachea can also be seen in tracheal atresia (Fig. 21-7). The differential diagnosis of laryngeal or tracheal atresia includes subglottic stenosis and bilateral microcystic CCAM. When associated with

Fraser syndrome, there may be renal anomalies, syndactyly of fingers and toes, and cryptophthalmos (membrane-covered eyes). The prognosis is invariably poor, and the option of termination of pregnancy should be discussed. Parents should also have the opportunity to discuss the prognosis with a pediatric surgeon, and, if the pregnancy is continued, delivery should be planned in a unit with neonatal intensive care and pediatric surgical facilities. *Ex utero* intrapartum treatment (EXIT procedure) has been reported (see later in the chapter).

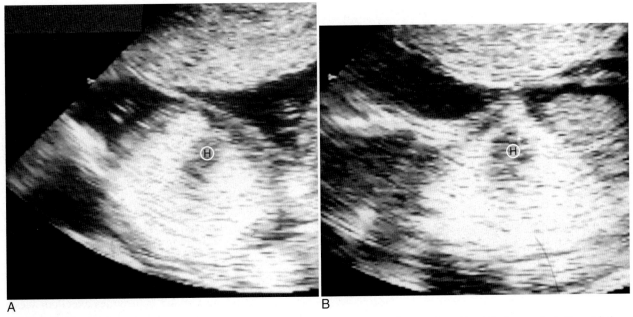

FIGURE 21-6. Axial (**A**) and longitudinal (**B**) views through the thorax of a fetus at 19 weeks gestation with tracheal agenesis. In the axial plane (**A**), the lungs are completely bright and can be seen compressing the heart (*H*). In the longitudinal plane (**B**), the diaphragms are displaced downward by the expanded lung tissue.

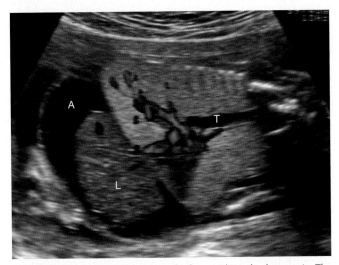

FIGURE 21-7. Longitudinal view of a fetus with tracheal agenesis. The heart can be seen highlighted by the color Doppler with the abnormally dilated trachea (*T*) seen as a fluid-filled structure in the mediastinum. The lungs bulge downward into the ascites (*A*) in the abdominal cavity in which the liver (*L*) can be seen.

▰ POSTNATAL FEATURES OF CONGENITAL LUNG DISEASE: AIRWAY AND LUNG PARENCHYMA

Congenital Abnormalities of the Upper Airway

This section will detail the variety of different congenital abnormalities that involve the upper airway and will deal with clinical problems involving the larynx and trachea. Though this section will not cover the complete spectrum of congenital disorders that can cause respiratory disorder in neonates, the pediatric otolaryngologist will be experienced in dealing with airway problems due to congenital abnormalities involving the whole airway from the anterior nares to the bronchi. The abnormalities may be intrinsic or extrinsic to the airway and be single or multiple. The spectrum of disorders is detailed in Tables 21-6 and 21-7.

These abnormalities may present with immediate respiratory distress at delivery but may equally be more subtle in their clinical symptoms and signs. Airway abnormalities should be considered in the presence of an abnormal cry, weak or husky voice, or recurrent crouplike episodes. Difficulties with feeding may also be a feature of airway

TABLE 21-6 CONGENITAL CONDITIONS ABOVE THE LARYNX AND TRACHEA THAT CAUSE NEONATAL AIRWAY OBSTRUCTION

Intrinsic

Nose	Atresia (absence) (e.g., arhinia)
	Choanal atresia (complete obstruction)
	Piriform aperture stenosis (narrowing)
	Severe craniofacial abnormalities (e.g., hemifacial microsomia [Goldenhar's syndrome] and the mid-facial syndromes [Apert's or Crouzon's syndrome])
	Tumors (e.g., teratoma, dermoid, glioma)
Oral cavity and oropharynx	Macroglossia (e.g., Pierre-Robin sequence)
	Retrognathia (e.g., Treacher-Collins syndrome)

Extrinsic

Viscerocranial and neck masses	Lymphatic malformations (e.g., cystic hygroma)
	Vascular malformations (e.g., arteriovenous malformation)
	Vascular tumors (e.g., capillary hemangiomas)
	Encephaloceles

TABLE 21-7 CONGENITAL ABNORMALITIES OF THE LARYNX AND TRACHEA

Larynx	Laryngeal atresia and webs
	Laryngeal cleft
	Laryngomalacia
	Vocal cord paralysis
	Saccular cysts and laryngoceles
	Subglottic hemangiomas
	Congenital subglottic stenosis
Trachea	Tracheomalacia
	Congenital tracheal stenosis
	(complete tracheal rings)

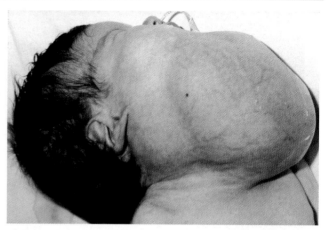

FIGURE 21-8. Severe neonatal upper airway obstruction due to cystic hygroma. (Reproduced courtesy of CM Bailey.)

abnormalities such as laryngomalacia or laryngeal cleft. In these situations, there may be recurrent episodes of aspiration with feeding (laryngeal cleft) or respiratory distress and gastroesophageal reflux (laryngomalacia)

Management of Neonatal Respiratory Distress

Severe Distress at Birth

Immediate examination in the delivery room may provide an obvious diagnosis by the pediatric staff, such as a major craniofacial abnormality. Severe airway problems such as congenital tracheal stenosis may, however, have no external physical signs.

It is not unusual for children to be intubated for safety before a more definitive diagnosis is made. If the obstruction seems to be nasal (e.g., in choanal atresia), it may be confirmed by the inability to pass a nasal catheter through either nostril. The airway can be stabilized by using an oral airway to allow oral respiration while definitive diagnosis and surgical treatment is planned. Conversely, with oral/oropharyngeal obstruction (e.g., in Pierre-Robin sequence), the airway may be improved by simply nursing the child prone. However, a nasopharyngeal airway (NPA) might be necessary if the obstruction is not easily relieved. This is a very reliable method and may avoid the necessity of a tracheostomy. As the child grows, the NPA may only be necessary during sleep.

If intubation is extremely difficult, it may be appropriate to consider immediate tracheostomy to avoid the risk of the endotracheal (ET) tube becoming dislodged and failure to re-intubate. This might be considered with a large cystic hygroma (Fig. 21-8). If the anatomy of the neck is very abnormal, it may be useful to pass a rigid bronchoscope to allow ventilation and act as a marker for the trachea within the distorted anatomy of the neck.

Assessment of the Nonintubated Neonate

A child who has chronic or episodic stridor may be examined with a flexible endoscope to assess the upper airway. This is a safe procedure provided that the following is available:
1. Small diameter endoscope (ideally 1.8 mm)
2. Access to pediatric resuscitation equipment and personnel, especially skilled pediatric anesthesiology
3. Stable neonate (minimal oxygen or air pressure support).

This is an excellent method for making a preliminary assessment of the airway. It provides excellent views of the posterior choanae, nasopharynx, oropharynx, and hypopharynx as well as the laryngeal inlet and vocal cords. However, the subglottis and upper trachea are not easily visualized, and a variety of laryngeal abnormalities (e.g., laryngeal cleft) may not be apparent. In many cases, it does avoid the need for more formal endoscopic examination of the upper airway and has shown itself to be a safe and reliable method in experienced hands.

In cases in which symptoms are significant and flexible endoscopy or imaging has not made a diagnosis, a microlaryngoscopy and bronchoscopy (MLB) is indicated. The preparation for the procedure includes a close discussion of the case with the pediatric anesthetist. It is ideal to have the child spontaneously breathing throughout the procedure and to avoid intubation, particularly if a subglottic stenosis is suspected, as this intervention may cause swelling within a compromised airway and lead to a sudden and severe obstruction. The larynx should be sprayed with a metered dose of local anesthetic and a nasopharyngeal airway introduced to support the breathing with both adequate oxygen support and positive pressure if the mouth is closed or the laryngoscope occluded. However, it should be noted that local anesthesia of the larynx may worsen the appearances of laryngomalacia.[65] The procedure should be done in a standardized fashion as follows:
1. *Global view of the larynx within the pharynx*—to view supraglottic lesions (e.g., cysts or laryngomalacia).
2. *Microlaryngoscopy*—using the microscope allows two-handed maneuvers. The larynx is probed to check for a laryngeal cleft and crico-arytenoid joint mobility. Glottic and subglottic lesions are usually self-evident.
3. *Rigid bronchoscopy*—tracheoscopy and bronchoscopy. Ventilation is supported through the sidearm of the bronchoscope, and the image is viewed on a screen (Fig. 21-9).
4. *Dynamic movements of the supraglottis and vocal cords*—with a 30-degree telescope while the child is waking up.

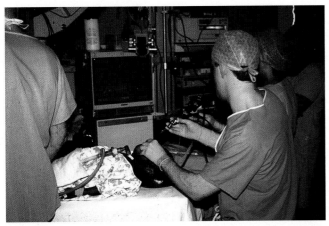

FIGURE 21-9. Rigid bronchoscopy in a tracheostomised patient (the tube will be removed after the upper trachea has been examined). The image is displayed on screen.

Assessment of the Intubated Neonate

Neonates whose respiratory distress is so severe that they need to be intubated represent a significant challenge for diagnosis. Optimally, a child should initially be managed for a trial of decannulation including the following:

1. Systemic corticosteroid treatment, if not contra-indicated
2. Regular tracheobronchial toilet prior to trial of extubation
3. Treatment of gastroesophageal reflux, if present
4. Extubation onto a nasopharyngeal prong with CPAP
5. Early adrenaline (epinephrine) nebulizer treatment if failing

If the extubation fails, the child may merit an MLB. This is a potentially dangerous procedure in a child with a severely compromised airway and should be considered in conjunction with all the pediatric medical staff involved as well as the family of the patient. The child's medical condition may need to be optimized in readiness for surgery. An early discussion with the pediatric anesthetic staff is important to plan details of the procedure. Consent for an emergency tracheostomy will need to be given by the patient's family.

If the initial intubation was judged to be difficult, then the ET tube should be left *in-situ* for as long as possible. The child should be self-ventilating and not paralyzed. With the child in a supine position, the oral cavity, nose (if necessary), and pharynx should be examined with rigid endoscopes (and possibly a microscope) or other endoscopes. It may be possible to pass a fine rigid endoscope alongside the ET tube and into the trachea to allow visualization of the lower airway without removing the tube. Alternatively, a rigid bronchoscope may be used once the tube has been removed. Another alternative is to pass a flexible endoscope through the ET tube that has been gently withdrawn into the larynx or pharynx, thus allowing the lower airway to be visualized.

An MLB can be combined with any procedure that will improve the chances of extubation (e.g., aryepiglottoplasty in the presence of severe laryngomalacia). The child should be sent back to the intensive care unit with the ET tube *in situ,* and the further trial of extubation should be attempted after a short period of recovery (depending on the surgical insult of the procedure).

Congenital Abnormalities of the Larynx

Laryngeal Webs and Atresia

The larynx develops from the endodermal lining of the cranial end of the laryngotracheal tube and from the surrounding mesenchyme derived from the fourth and sixth pairs of branchial arches. The epithelium proliferates rapidly, and this leads to an occlusion of the laryngeal lumen, which recannalizes by the tenth week of gestation. Failure to re-establish a complete lumen leads to either a laryngeal web or, in extreme cases, to complete atresia.

Laryngeal Atresia

Laryngeal atresia was traditionally said to be incompatible with life, but with the advent of prenatal diagnosis there is the possibility of planned immediate airway treatment. This type of anomaly and similar gross abnormalities (e.g., laryngeal cysts) have been given the label of *congenital high airway obstruction syndrome (CHAOS).*[66] It is characterized by ultrasound findings of large echogenic lungs, a dilated airway distal to the obstruction, an inverted diaphragm, and massive ascites. The early prenatal diagnosis provides two possible choices for airway intervention as follows:

1. *Fetal Intervention.* It has proved technically possible to introduce a tracheostomy while still *in utero,* though the operation may lead to fetal distress and delivery of the child.[67]
2. Ex utero *intrapartum treatment (EXIT).* The principle of this management is to allow the infant's oxygenation to be maintained by the uteroplacental circulation for as long as possible. This can be prolonged by anesthetic treatment to produce uterine relaxation, though this relaxation must be reversed just before the cord is clamped to prevent uterine atony and excessive maternal bleeding. The hysterotomy is ultrasound-controlled to prevent damage to the placenta. Limited exposure of the fetus also helps in maintaining the uterine volume and fetal temperature.[68]

EXIT survivors have shown a reasonably benign natural history with gradual recovery of diaphragmatic and pulmonary function. There are no large series reports of long-term surgical reconstruction in these patients.

Laryngeal Webs

The majority of these anomalies involve the anterior glottis (Fig. 21-10). There is a strong association with velocardiofacial syndrome (chromosome 22q11.2 deletion), and the genetic abnormality is found in the majority of patients with anterior glottic webs—even those with no overt clinical features of the complete syndrome.[69] They present with either aphonia or an abnormal cry or airway obstruction. The web may be a thin band between the vocal cords of variable extent but may often involve an abnormal cricoid ring with an associated anterior subglottic stenosis. If the web is thin, then division is simple

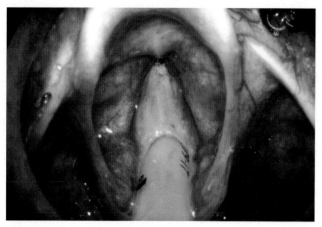

FIGURE 21-10. Congenital laryngeal web associated with anterior subglottic stenosis. (Reproduced courtesy of CM Bailey.)

with either a laser or surgical instruments; however, there is a high rate of re-stenosis. This may be prevented by the temporary placement of a keel (a flat plastic stent) between the divided vocal cords and held in place with a looped suture through the soft tissues of the anterior neck. This is subsequently removed when epithelial healing is complete and the risk of re-stenosis is small. There is considerable risk of granulation from a synthetic keel, and an alternative is using an autograft to stent and also line the vocal cords.[70]

If there is an associated anterior subglottic stenosis, conventional techniques of laryngotracheal reconstruction are appropriate and effective.[70] Posterior glottic webs are usually acquired from prolonged intubation but rarely may be congenital in origin. They are manifested as an interarytenoid web and usually present with airway obstruction. Tracheostomy is usually necessary for 3 to 5 years, as definitive corrective management has not been established.

Laryngeal Cleft
The lower respiratory tract forms from the *laryngotracheal diverticulum*, which extends from the primitive pharynx. It becomes separated from the foregut by longitudinal ridges called *tracheoesophageal folds*, which fuse to form a partition known as the *tracheoesophageal septum*, which divides the laryngotracheal tube and the esophagus. Failure of the septum leads to the formation of a laryngeal cleft.

Laryngeal clefts are associated with TEF and may be a missed diagnosis as an explanation for recurrent aspiration following surgical repair of a TEF. They may also be a part of the G syndrome, the spectrum of which may also include cleft lip and cleft palate, hypertelorism, and hypospadias.

Laryngeal clefts are variable in length and may be classified as follows:

Type 1   Inter-arytenoid
Type 2   Cricoid cleft—partial
Type 3   Complete cricoid cleft—extending into the
             cervical trachea
Type 4   Laryngo-tracheal cleft—extending into the
             thoracic trachea

Patients with laryngeal clefts usually present with recurrent aspiration and cyanotic episodes with feeding, though neonates with more extensive clefts may demonstrate respiratory distress. The diagnosis may be made from videofluroscopy, but endoscopic examination is the gold standard. Indeed, during all routine endoscopic examinations of the airway, a probe should be introduced between the arytenoids cartilages to screen for this defect.

Infants with laryngeal clefts should be assessed and aggressively treated for gastroesophageal reflux (including medical as well as surgical treatment such as Nissan's fundoplication), as this significantly improves the outcome of surgical intervention.

Management of Type 1 Clefts
Conservative management of inter-arytenoid clefts should be the initial choice, with swallowing therapy particularly aimed at thickening feeds to prevent aspiration. If this fails, endoscopic repair is advocated. Through a laryngoscope, the mucosa is cut from the inner margins of the cleft, which are then sutured together (Fig. 21-11).

Management of Type 2 and 3 Clefts
Some smaller type 2 clefts may be easily closed with an endoscopic technique, but for more extensive defects there are difficulties of access and instrumentation, particularly beyond the second tracheal ring.[71] Open procedures usually involve an anterior approach, as this avoids damage to the recurrent laryngeal nerves. A vertical laryngofissure is performed and the cleft is closed with either direct suturing or with interposition of a fascial graft. A tracheostomy may be necessary if prolonged postoperative ventilation is anticipated, but with shorter clefts 7 to 10 days of postoperative intubation may suffice to stent the surgical segment.[72]

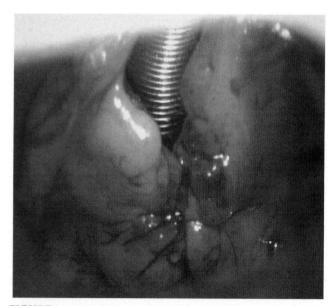

FIGURE 21-11. Endoscopic repair of laryngeal cleft type 1.

Management of Type 4 Clefts

To repair the thoracic segment, these patients require a thoracotomy, possibly via a posterolateral approach, and this may require the child to be maintained on extracorporeal circulation. This is combined with an anterior cervical approach to repair the upper cleft. If the tracheoesophageal folds are very basic, it may be necessary to close off the esophageal sphincters and to use the whole of the undivided foregut as the airway. Because treatment entails significant morbidity and mortality, the decision on whether or not to operate should be based upon the associated co-morbidity and fully informed parental choice.[73]

Laryngomalacia

Laryngomalacia is the most common congenital abnormality of the upper airway. Despite its relative frequency, the underlying pathologic mechanisms are poorly understood. The term *laryngomalacia* is a misnomer. There is no histologic evidence of an abnormality of the tissue of the supraglottic, and in particular the cartilage of the epiglottis is unremarkable. It is not an immature state of the supraglottis, as it is no more frequent among severely premature neonates as compared to full-term babies.

The larynxes of children with this condition show a variable spectrum of characteristic macroscopic abnormalities, which cause or are caused by a dynamic anomaly of the supraglottis. These include the following:

1. The aryepiglottic folds are short and very vertical, curling the epiglottis into an omega shape.
2. Prominent cuneiform and corniculate cartilages lie over the arytenoid cartilages, which prolapse into the airway.
3. A loose, redundant mucosal covering of the aryepiglottic fold prolapses into the airway.

It has been suggested that these facets of laryngomalacia are produced by an incoordination of the laryngeal muscles due to neuromuscular immaturity. This leads to a mistiming of laryngeal movements and tends to cause indrawing and lengthening of the supraglottic structures. However, laryngomalacia may just be a structural variation.

The principal symptom of laryngomalacia is inspiratory stridor with noisy respiration. The onset of the stridor is usually within the first week of life but characteristically is not with the first breath. There may be associated feeding problems, with the child becoming distressed and regurgitating from the efforts of inspiration. Feeds are often short, and, if severe, the child may fail to grow. The vast majority progress very well despite the stridor, and management consists of confirming the diagnosis with flexible endoscopy and reassurance for the parents. The symptoms tend to resolve in the second year of life, though may become louder as the child becomes more active, particularly at the stage of crawling. The laryngeal abnormality may persist into adulthood, and occasionally the condition will present as inspiratory stridor in teenagers undertaking extremes of exercise. However, exercise-induced vocal cord dysfunction is a more likely cause of such symptoms.[74,75]

Active Treatment

In a minority of patients (<10%), the child will fail to adequately gain weight. In this situation, the traditional treatment was tracheostomy. A surgical alternative is aryepiglottoplasty ("supraglottoplasty"), which involves surgical relief of the tight aryepiglottic folds and/or removal of the cuneiform/corniculate and/or redundant mucosal covering. This can be performed with micro-scissors, a laser, or a microdebrider.[76] There are serious potential complications of excessive removal of the supraglottic tissues. This includes supraglottic stenosis and aspiration. To avoid this, the surgery should be as limited as possible and, if necessary, unilateral, with the option to repeat if there is inadequate symptom improvement. The surgery is very successful in controlling severe airway obstruction, but less so if there is concomitant cerebral palsy. Feeding problems often improve but still may be significant in a minority of patients.[77]

Vocal Cord Paralysis

Congenital vocal cord paralysis (VCP) may be unilateral or bilateral. When only one side is affected, it is usually the peripheral nerve that is nonfunctioning, and it is a more common finding on the left than on the right. This is because of the longer course of the left recurrent laryngeal nerve, which loops around the ligamentum arteriosum in the thorax. VCP may be associated with cardiac or great vessel abnormalities or be due to birth trauma. Bilateral VCP is more likely to be associated with a lesion of the central nervous system such as hydrocephalus or the Arnold Chiari abnormality. Later presenting VCP may be due to underlying neuromuscular disease.[78,79]

Diagnosis of VCP may be made using a flexible endoscope, but an assessment of vocal cord movement should be part of a standardized endoscopic evaluation of the pediatric airway. At completion of the laryngoscopy and tracheoscopy/bronchoscopy, the vocal cords should be visualized with a 30° telescope, while the child's level of anesthesia is progressively lightened. It is only in the first stages of anesthesia that active abduction of the vocal cords is seen. Movements of the vocal cords in deeper stages of anesthesia are usually passive. During inspiration, the high velocity of air movement reduces lateral pressure at the glottis (as a result of Bernoulli's principle) and the elastic vocal cords passively adduct. During expiration, the opposite movement is seen. Activity of the vocal fold is typified as abduction during inspiration (to reduce the upper airways resistance) and the anesthetist should call out when the child is inspiring so that the active movements can be identified.

Unilateral VCP may be a delayed diagnosis as there will often be no associated airway obstruction. The voice will sound breathless and hoarse, but there may be remarkable good compensation, with good apposition by the mobile vocal cord to the paralyzed side, allowing reasonable phonation. It is mandatory to image the whole length of the left recurrent laryngeal nerve to screen for anomalies in the skull base, neck, and thorax. If compensation is inadequate, improved apposition with the contralateral vocal cord may be achieved by vocal cord bulking with injection of collagen, fat, or other materials, or by medialization of the whole cord by laryngeal framework surgery.

Bilateral VCP will produce immediate stridor at birth, which may be biphasic but is usually predominantly inspiratory. If the infant is intubated, this should be very easily done and relieves the stridor, which gives a clue to the diagnosis. Treatment with a tracheostomy, while awaiting spontaneous resolution of the VCP, is the traditional treatment. However not all children with bilateral VCP will need airway intervention. It may be possible to avoid a tracheostomy in nearly 50% of cases if the child is closely monitored and adequate home support is provided.[80] Treatment of the primary neurologic abnormality will obviously be of potential benefit.

The upper airways resistance associated with bilateral VCP can be reduced by excising part of the vocal cord or arytenoid cartilage on one side. The cord can also be lateralized with open surgery. This will obviously affect the potential for vocal quality but may allow decannulation for those who have a tracheostomy. There is no universal agreement about the age at which one should abandon hope of spontaneous recovery of vocal cord movement and consider surgical movement of the cord(s). There are reports of recovery occurring as late as 11 years of age, though many suggest that if there is no evidence of activity by 2 years of age, then it can be presumed that it is a permanent condition and that cord surgery should be considered to try and achieve reversal of the tracheostomy. There is a minor risk of aspiration after vocal cord resection, so the procedure should only be considered with caution in the presence of significant feeding problems.

Saccular Cysts and Laryngocoeles

The saccule is a blind ending structure that opens into the laryngeal ventricle, the lateral space between the true and false vocal cord. It runs in an anterior-superior direction and is usually of modest size in the normal larynx. It is lined by pseudostratified columnar epithelium and contains serous and mucous glands. A laryngocele is an abnormally enlarged laryngeal saccule and is air-filled. The condition is a rare congenital abnormality but may produce significant airway obstruction. It may be entirely within the confines of the larynx or extend into the neck via the thyrohyoid membrane. If the lesion is small in size, it may be excised using an endoscopic approach. Alternatively, an open operation may be necessary for larger lesions, with the possible need for a prior tracheostomy to ensure an adequate airway postoperatively.

Saccular cysts are mucous filled and are found in the false vocal cord or aryepiglottic fold (Fig. 21-12). They are presumed to arise from a part of the saccule that has become sealed off from its outlet into the ventricle. They may be massive and cause immediate and severe airway obstruction. Standard endoscopic therapy is aspiration and marsupialization with scissors or laser. There is a high rate of recurrence, and open resection may eventually become necessary.[81]

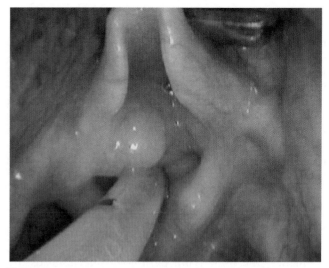

FIGURE 21-12. Congenital saccular cyst of aryepiglottic fold.

Subglottic Hemangioma

Subglottic (and tracheal) hemangiomas (Fig. 21-13) are benign vascular tumors that may be multiple in site in the head and neck and may be enormous in size. Their natural history is of a rapid growth phase for 12 to 18 months followed by a period of involution and final resolution. They are more common on the left side than the right. They are usually asymptomatic at birth but cause increasing airway obstruction from about 3 month of age. They are usually diagnosed during endoscopic examination of the upper airway, precipitated by the onset of airway symptoms. Diagnosis does not require formal biopsy as the presence of an asymmetric compressible bluish mass in the subglottic area is highly characteristic and biopsy will precipitate brisk bleeding, though this should be easily manageable with compression from an ET tube.

Management of this condition was traditionally controversial with a variety of surgical, chemotherapy and radiotherapy approaches including the following:
1. Systemic or intralesional corticosteroids
2. Laser excision
3. Open excision

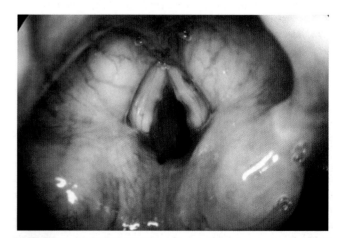

FIGURE 21-13. Subglottic hemangioma. (Reproduced courtesy of CM Bailey.)

4. Adjuvant treatment with alpha-interferon, cyclophosphamide, or vincristine
5. Radiotherapy—external beam or brachytherapy

There has been a recent chance discovery that propanolol produces a rapid regression of the disease, first noted in children who were being treated for cardiopulmonary conditions.[82] There have now been multiple reports of successful treatment of hemangiomas with propanolol, which has a well-documented safety and side-effect profile. A dose of 2 to 3 mg/kg/day divided into two to four doses per day is recommended, with initial monitoring of pulse, blood pressure, and blood glucose levels.[83] Tapering of treatment at 12 months, after a check MLB, may be appropriate depending on the size and extent of the original lesion.

Subglottic Stenosis

Differentiating between congenital and acquired subglottic stenosis may be difficult, particularly as any severe obstruction may lead to intubation, which is the single most common factor in acquired stenosis. Congenital stenosis is undoubtedly a separate entity and will often present in the first year of life with recurrent episodes of croup. The condition is typified by an abnormality of the cricoid cartilage, with prominent lateral shelves producing an elliptical subglottic space.

Diagnosis will be by endoscopic examination, and this should be combined with a careful inspection of the mobility of the vocal cords and cricoarytenoid joints. If the subglottic space only allows an ET tube two sizes smaller than that expected for a child of that age, then surgical treatment should be considered. Avoidance of a tracheostomy should be pursued. The condition can be managed with either of the following:

1. Laryngotracheal reconstruction (LTR). Rib cartilage is used to hold open a vertical slit in the cricoid and upper trachea, either in the anterior wall alone or as separate anterior and posterior grafts.
2. Cricotracheal resection (CTR). The stenotic segment is excised with direct anastomosis of the airway. This is technically difficult when the stenosis involves the vocal cords.

A single-stage procedure is ideal (though not possible in all cases). Postoperatively the child is intubated for 7 to 10 days prior to a trial of extubation. Airway reconstruction has been shown to have good outcomes, even in the presence of concomitant anomalies.[84]

Congenital Abnormalities of the Trachea

Tracheomalacia

Tracheomalacia is an abnormal collapse of the trachea due to localized or generalized weakness of the tracheal wall (Fig. 21-14). Microscopically specimens show an increase in the ratio of muscle to cartilage. It is subdivided into primary or secondary, though either form can be congenital. In primary tracheomalacia, there is an intrinsic abnormality of the tracheal wall, whereas in secondary cases there is extrinsic compression. In congenital

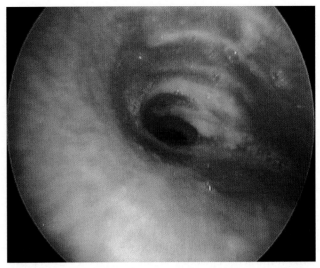

FIGURE 21-14. Tracheomalacia, acquired secondary to cardiac surgery. Note the retained mucopurulent secretions.

cases, this is usually in association with cardiovascular abnormalities including the following (discussed in more detail later in the chapter):

1. *Double aortic arch*—surrounds the trachea, producing a concentric compression
2. *Anomalous innominate artery*—compresses the right anterior trachea
3. *Pulmonary artery sling*—compresses the right main bronchus

Congenital tracheomalacia may be associated with bronchomalacia, particularly in more generalized cases. It may also be found with other tracheal abnormalities such as TEF or laryngeal cleft. Though they may coexist, there is no connection with laryngomalacia.

The clinical manifestations of the condition are very variable, and it is often a diagnosis that can only be reliably made by endoscopy. There is likely to be stridor, which is usually expiratory as the obstruction is predominantly intrathoracic. There are usually recurrent acute episodes of stridor and dyspnea, during which the child may become cyanosed and moribund ("dying spells"). This may be precipitated by severe crying, coughing, or even feeding. The symptoms are usually apparent in the immediate neonatal period but may deteriorate in the first and second year of life, in an almost stepwise manner.

Diagnosis is essentially by endoscopy. For the pediatric otolaryngologist, this is most often with rigid bronchoscopy. The pediatric airway is very elastic and may collapse during forceful inspiration and certainly during coughing fits. The membranous part of the trachea also tends to bulge forward, giving the impression of a narrow airway. During endoscopy, it is important that the child is adequately anesthetized to avoid coughing while there is still spontaneous respiration. There is no generally accepted definition of the degree of collapse that can be taken as abnormal, but it seems reasonable to suggest that more than 25% reduction of the lumen is a significant finding and that greater than 50% is likely to be symptomatic. As well as overdiagnosis, it is possible to miss the condition if the trachea is splinted by the bronchoscope or if there is excessive positive end-expiratory pressure applied by the anesthetist through the sidearm of the instrument. The procedure should involve a detailed laryngoscopy to screen for a laryngeal cleft and active vocal cord movements should be confirmed, particularly if there has been tracheal surgery for a TEF or cardiovascular surgery for a vascular anomaly.

The diagnosis may be made (and later confirmed and quantified by bronchoscopy) with multiple detector CT scans; however, the radiation dose is significant but can be reduced with variation of the expiratory phase of the investigation.[85]

Treatment

Though the condition may progress in the first couple of years of life, it is generally self-limiting and if mild requires no active treatment. The patient's family should, however, be taught cardiopulmonary resuscitation, particularly if the acute episodes are severe and they can be provided with a facemask and ventilation bag. There may be associated recurrent respiratory infections, and training in home chest physiotherapy may need to be provided. In more severe cases, active treatment might be considered, though many of the choices have severe potential complications and should only be utilized in the face of extreme circumstances:

1. *Surgery for Abnormal Vasculature.* This may relieve the compression though once the tracheal wall has become weakened from external pulsatile pressure, it may not immediately recover following removal of the anomalous vessel.
2. *Aortopexy.* A suture through the adventitial lining of the aortic arch and the periostium of the sternum is used to pull the arch forward. As the anterior tracheal wall is intimately connected to the aortic arch with fascial tissue, it is also towed forward, thus widening the tracheal lumen. There may be a failure of the suture, and there is a risk of damage to the aortic arch itself. This procedure can be performed via a thorascopic approach, which has the potential of reducing operative morbidity.[86]
3. *Tracheostomy.* This is very effective for short-segment tracheomalacia but is unsatisfactory when the distal trachea is involved. The tube tip has to pass through the segment to stent it; custom-made tubes can be manufactured to optimize the length. However with a distal segment, the tube tip may pass into the right main bronchus on neck flexion and may not adequately stent the tracheomalacic segment on neck extension.
4. *Nasal or tracheostomy continuous positive airway pressure (CPAP).* A pneumatic splint of the segment can be achieved with CPAP via a tight-fitting facemask, or tracheostomy if the former is not tolerated, particularly with collapse at the carina (and in association with bronchomalacia).
5. *Segmental resection.* This is suitable for short-segment collapse if the obstruction is severe. An end-to-end anastamosis is used to reconstitute the trachea.
6. *Internal Stents.* These are typically made from siliconized plastic or are designed as expandable metal tubes. Stents may be highly effective at maintaining the lumen of the trachea but can be difficult to introduce

down a bronchoscope and may be complicated by displacement, granulation tissue, and infection.
7. *Cartilage grafting.* Rib cartilage grafts can be used to stiffen the tracheal wall, but if near to half of the tracheal wall is replaced there can be slow or incomplete re-epithelialization.

Congenital Tracheal Stenosis (Complete Tracheal Rings)

In this very rare condition, there is a segment of the trachea, often distal, where the tracheal rings are truly complete. It is often found in combination with other regional abnormalities, particularly cardiac, including pulmonary artery sling. If the lumen of the trachea is small, this may not be compatible with life. Alternatively, the child may suffer immediate respiratory distress in the delivery room that is not relieved by intubation or even tracheostomy. Extracorporeal oxygenation may be necessary to allow time to consider a surgical remedy.

If the child is relatively stable, it may not be necessary to consider any form of tracheal surgery, and there is potential for airway growth with the child. It may, however, become necessary as the child grows if exercise tolerance is severely limited.

Surgical options include the following:
1. *Resection of the stenotic segment.* The innate elasticity of the pediatric trachea means that quite a long segment may be excised and the trachea reconstituted. It has been suggested that this is possible when up to eight rings are involved.
2. *Reconstruction of the stenotic segment.* There are many described procedures aimed at reconstructing the anterior wall of the stenotic segment after it has been opened in a vertical plane. These include pericardial patch tracheoplasty, slide tracheoplasty, homograft tracheal transplantation, free tracheal autograft (partially excised segment used to patch the remainder), and costal cartilage autograft.

The multiplicity of surgical techniques reflects the relatively poor outcome in severely symptomatic patients,[87] and careful discussion with the family is imperative to come to a balanced view of the potential outcome of surgery.[88]

Tissue-engineered tracheal transplantation represents an exciting avenue of future research and developing surgical techniques for this condition. Previous homograft operations have been complicated by inflammatory reactions in the airway. A decellularized human donor trachea, colonized by the recipient's epithelial cells and chondrogenic mesenchymal stem cells, is envisaged as an ideal tracheal graft, and this technique has already been used in an adult with end-stage airway disease.[89]

BRONCHIAL ABNORMALITIES

Congenital Bronchial Stenosis and Atresia

Congenital stricture of the bronchus occurs predominantly in a main-stem or middle lobe bronchus and can produce acute or chronic pulmonary infection. Inflammatory scarring of the congenitally stenosed bronchus provides an ideal environment for distal suppuration, atelectasis, and bronchiectasis. Atresia is usually asymptomatic and detected incidentally on radiography, but it may present with recurrent infection. The airway may be blocked by a simple membrane, or there may be a discontinuity. It often results in cystic degeneration of the lobe distal to the obstruction before birth because fetal lung liquid continues to be secreted and cannot drain into the amniotic cavity. The distal airspace is often cystic and filled with mucus, and it is typically in continuity with an area of distal hyperinflation. The mechanism of this hyperinflation is unclear, but it could involve either collateral ventilation through the pores of Kohn (although these are scanty in the newborn) or a ball-valve effect from intraluminal mucus, or both. Bronchial atresia may be very difficult to distinguish from a CTM until the lesion is excised. Infection and scarring may ensue, with symptomatic presentation. Failure to identify the congenital nature of the problem may lead to a misdiagnosis of mucus plugging. Unlike the situation with absent bronchus, there is no focal opacity in congenital large hyperlucent lobe (CLHL, congenital lobar emphysema). The continuity of the cyst with the distal airways and the hyperinflation of the distal lung distinguish absent bronchus from bronchogenic cyst (the nomenclature of which is discussed later in the chapter), but the two conditions are occasionally associated.

Abnormal Bronchial Origin and Bronchial Branching

Bronchi can arise from the gastrointestinal tract. Bronchial diverticula also possibly represent abnormal bronchial branching. The right upper lobe bronchus can arise from the trachea, particularly in association with the tetralogy of Fallot. An accessory cardiac lobe bronchus may arise from the intermediate bronchus. A tracheal origin of one or more of the right upper lobe bronchi ("pig bronchus") is usually of no clinical significance but may be a cause of recurrent right upper lobe collapse in an intubated patient if the ETT is low. The right lower lobe bronchus may also arise from the left bronchial tree, a "bridging bronchus." Lung segments may also cross over, with bronchial and arterial connections from the opposite side, usually from right to left. The crossover may simply be of vessels and bronchi, or include a tongue of parenchymal tissue, the "horseshoe" lung, where there is fusion of the lungs behind the heart.[90]

Disorders of Bronchial Laterality

Abnormal arrangements require consideration of what makes, for example, a right lung a right lung. It is not because it is in the right hemithorax. In clinical practice, the two most useful determinants of right lung morphology are the presence of three lobes, not two, and a very short main bronchus before the takeoff of the upper lobe bronchus. A third criterion is the presence of an eparterial bronchus (the branch of the right main bronchus given off about 2.5 cm from the bifurcation of the trachea, which supplies the superior lobe of the right lung). Mirror-image arrangement must be distinguished from the superficially similar congenitally small (hypoplastic) right lung with right-sided heart (dextroposition) by determining bronchial morphology. This is important because each has a different implication and requires different investigation. Mirror-image

arrangement may be a feature of primary ciliary dyskinesia (discussed in Chapter 71), whereas a CSL must have its vascular supply delineated (see later in the chapter).

The term *isomerism* is so entrenched that it is probably not feasible to replace it with, for example, *bilateral right lung,* which would be more logical. Nearly 80% of children with right isomerism (bilateral right lung) lack a spleen, leading to a risk of overwhelming pneumococcal sepsis. A similar proportion with left isomerism (bilateral left lung) have multiple small spleens. Ivemark syndrome consists of right isomerism (bilateral right lung), asplenia, a midline liver, malrotation of the gut, and a variety of cardiac abnormalities including a common ventricle, totally anomalous pulmonary venous drainage, and bilateral superior caval veins and right atria. Left isomerism (bilateral left lung) is associated with multiple small spleens (polysplenia), a midline liver, malrotation of the gut, partially anomalous pulmonary venous drainage, and cardiac septal defects. Although nonfamilial, Ivemark syndrome is confined to males, whereas the other isomerism syndromes can affect either sex. A syndrome of left bronchial isomerism, normal atrial arrangement, and severe tracheobronchomalacia has been described,[91] extending the spectrum of left isomerism (bilateral left lung). Recently, the spectrum of primary ciliary dyskinesia has been broadened to include isomerism sequences[92] (see Chapter 71). Occasionally, a CSL may be so abnormal that its morphology can only be described as *indeterminate.* The contralateral lung morphology is, however, usually obvious. Quite commonly, minor deviations from the normal bronchial branching pattern may be seen, which one study suggested may be associated with spontaneous pneumothorax.[93]

Other Disorders of the Bronchial Walls

Abnormalities in bronchial wall caliber may result in all or part of the bronchial tree being too large or too small. These may present with recurrent infections, steroid-unresponsive wheeze, or stridor. Congenital tracheobronchomegaly (Mounier-Kuhn syndrome) is characterized by tracheomalacia and bronchiectasis, with greatly dilated major airways. It usually presents in middle age, but childhood cases have been reported. There are saccular bulges between the cartilages. Bronchial clearance is impaired, resulting in recurrent respiratory infection. This syndrome, which may be inherited as an autosomally recessive trait, generally presents between 30 and 50 years of age and is more common in males. It is occasionally associated with Ehlers-Danlos syndrome, cutis laxa, or Kenny-Caffey syndrome (an extremely rare hereditary skeletal disorder characterized by thickening of the long bones, thin marrow cavities in the bones (medullary stenosis), and abnormalities affecting the head and eyes). True congenital bronchiectasis is much rarer than previously thought.

The bronchial lumen may be narrowed by complete cartilage rings (Fig. 21-15). There may be an associated pulmonary artery sling. A short segment of narrowing, situated relatively distally in the airway, may require no treatment. If ventilation is critically compromised,

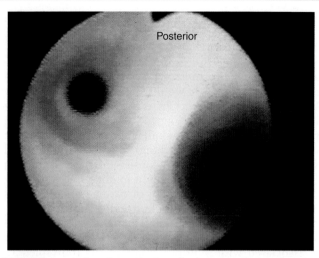

FIGURE 21-15. Bronchoscopic view of a single complete cartilage ring at the origin of the right main bronchus.

surgical excision or a Z-plasty may be indicated. Bronchoscopic balloon dilatation should probably be considered experimental. It is wise to ensure that the distal lung is normal before embarking on treatment; if the small airway is part of a generally maldeveloped segment, then enhancing ventilation may in fact only increase dead space ventilation.

Congenital bronchomalacia may be isolated, often with a good prognosis, at least in the short term, or it may be associated with other congenital abnormalities (including connective tissue disorders and Larsen and Fryn syndrome). Williams and Campbell described a syndrome of diffuse bronchomalacia that affects the second to the seventh generations of bronchi.[94] Its occurrence in siblings and the very early onset of symptoms suggests a congenital etiology. Bronchomalacia may also be secondary to other congenital abnormalities, such as vascular rings. A rare cause of congenital tracheobronchomalacia is the presence of esophageal remnants in the wall of the trachea, generally associated with esophageal atresia and TEF. Fixed bronchial narrowing may be due to defects in the wall (e.g., complete cartilage rings) or extrinsic compression by an abnormal vessel or cyst. In older children, this may be suspected from the appearances of the spirometric flow-volume loop (Fig. 21-16).

Pulmonary Agenesis, Aplasia (Absent Lung), and Hypoplasia (Small Lung)

Bilateral pulmonary agenesis is a rare malformation that may occur in anencephaly. Unilateral pulmonary agenesis is slightly more common, with absence of the carina and the trachea running directly into a single bronchus. Pathologically, the sole lung is larger than normal; this enlargement is true hypertrophy and not emphysema. Associated ipsilateral congenital abnormalities are common.[95] There may be an association with duplications of chromosome 2.[96] The mortality of right-sided agenesis is twice that of left-sided agenesis; this is probably a result of more severe mediastinal and cardiac displacement. Unilateral pulmonary aplasia, the most common variant, consists of a carina and main-stem bronchial stump with absence of the distal lung. In this situation, secretions can pool in the stump, become infected, and possibly spill over to infect the sole lung. Lobar agenesis and aplasia are rarer than complete absence of one lung and usually affect the right upper and middle lobes together. Pulmonary hypoplasia (CSLs) consists of incompletely developed lung parenchyma connected to bronchi that may also be underdeveloped depending on when the presumed causal insult took effect in embryogenesis. There are a large number of causes of CSLs (Tables 21-8 and 21-9). The alveoli are reduced in number or size (numbers are assessed by counting alveolar wall intercepts on a line from the terminal bronchiole to the interlobular septum). However, hypoplasia is perhaps best considered to be present in term babies when the lung–to–body weight ratio is less than 0.012. There is a high incidence (around 50%) of associated diaphragmatic, cardiac, gastrointestinal, genitourinary, and skeletal malformations, as well as frequent variations in the bronchopulmonary vasculature. Correction of any

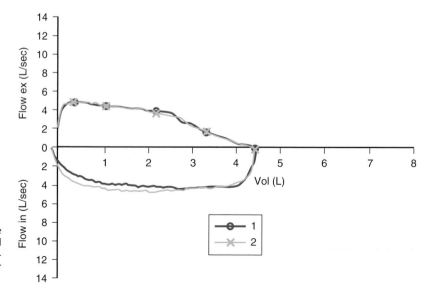

FIGURE 21-16. Typical appearance of the flow-volume curve in fixed upper airway obstruction. There is marked abrupt attenuation of inspiratory and expiratory flow, persisting until late near complete emptying, and then near complete filling of the lungs.

TABLE 21-8 CAUSES OF BILATERAL CONGENITAL SMALL LUNGS

SYSTEM FAULT	EXAMPLE
Lack of space	Abnormal thoracic, abdominal, or amniotic cavity contents (See Table 21-9)
Abnormal vascular supply	Pulmonary valve or artery stenosis Tetralogy of Fallot
Neuromuscular disease	CNS, anterior horn cell, peripheral nerve or muscle disease (particularly severe spinal muscular atrophy and myotonic dystrophy inherited from mother) reducing fetal breathing movements

TABLE 21-9 CONGENITAL SMALL LUNGS DUE TO EXTRAPULMONARY MECHANICAL FACTORS

Abnormal thoracic contents	Diaphragmatic hernia Pleural effusion Large congenital thoracic malformations
Thoracic compression from below	Abdominal tumors Ascites
Thoracic compression from the sides	Amniotic bands Oligohydramnios (any cause) Asphyxiating dystrophy/scoliosis or other chest wall deformity

underlying abnormality, if feasible (either postnatally or antenatally) may permit growth of alveoli. However, airway branching is complete by 16 weeks, so airways will not branch after a causal abnormality has been corrected, and because the airway pattern is abnormal, alveolar numbers are never likely to be normal.

Ectopia

Ectopia is the growth of normal tissue in an incorrect anatomic position. In relation to the lung, ectopia comprises either nonpulmonary tissues being present in the lung or lung tissue outside the thoracic cavity.[97,98] In relation to extrapulmonary tissues, ectopic glial tissue is well recognized within the lung, with nodules of glial tissue being implanted in anencephalics or due to embolization in relation to intrauterine trauma. Adrenocortical tissue, thyroid, liver, and skeletal muscle have also been described in the lung, and pancreatic tissue has been found in intralobar sequestrations. Ectopic lung tissue may be found in the neck, chest wall, and even in the abdomen, although some ectopias represent extralobar sequestrations. Alternative terms for this occurrence include congenital pneumatocele and congenital pulmonary hernia, although they are best regarded as true ectopias. Entire kidneys may also be intrathoracic in location.

CONGENITAL CYSTIC LESIONS

Numerous pathologic conditions present with cystic changes in the lung, with acquired lesions outnumbering those that are developmental in origin. In this section, we will discuss the pathology of developmental lesions. It is usually only after surgical excision that accurate pathologic diagnoses can be made.

Foregut (Bronchogenic) Cysts

Foregut cysts (clinically, cystic CTMs) can be defined as closed epithelium-lined sacs developing abnormally in the thorax from the primitive developing upper gut and respiratory tract. When these structures differentiate toward airway and contain cartilage in the wall, they are termed *bronchogenic cysts*, while those developing toward the gut are termed *enterogenous cysts*, although they are most likely of common origin from abnormal division of the embryonic foregut.[99] Bronchogenic cysts are the most common cysts in infancy, although many do not present until adulthood. About 50% are situated in the mediastinum close to the carina, and less frequently they are adjacent to the esophagus and alongside the tracheobronchial tree. More uncommonly, they are found within the lung parenchyma, and exceptionally in sites such as below the diaphragm, pericardium, presternal tissues, and skin. Foregut cysts are usually single, unilocular, and more common on the right. They may have a systemic blood supply. Symptoms often relate to compression of the airways or complications (e.g., hemorrhage or infection), which may be reflected in the macroscopic appearance when the wall is thickened by fibrous scarring or shows brown discoloration due to chronic bleeding (Fig. 21-17). Microscopic examination shows a cyst lined by respiratory-type epithelium, although there may be squamous metaplasia and even ulceration with a foreign body–type granulomatous reaction, depending on

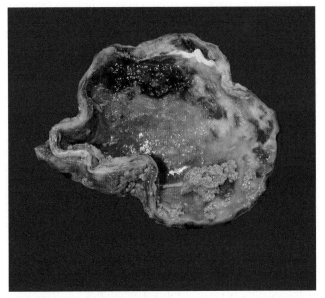

FIGURE 21-17. Mediastinal bronchogenic cyst. The inner surface of this unilocular cyst is partly haemorrhagic and partly covered by purulent debris, which is indicative of recurrent infection.

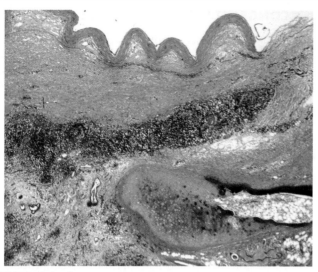

FIGURE 21-18. Mediastinal bronchogenic cyst. The lining of the cyst is mainly denuded, while the wall is chronically inflamed. Note the cartilage plate that indicates bronchogenic origin.

secondary phenomena. The wall is often fibrous and inflamed, and it may contain seromucous glands and cartilage plates (Fig. 21-18). In the absence of cartilage, such a cyst should be termed a *simple foregut cyst.*

Enterogenous cysts are subdivided into esophageal and gastroenteric (duplication) cysts, the former being more common. Esophageal cysts are intramural and do not involve the mucosa. They are lined by either squamous or respiratory-type epithelium. Gastroenteric cysts, in contrast, are typically unconnected to the esophagus but may be in close association with the vertebrae, often in the region of the sixth to the eighth. Symptoms are typically due to pressure, infection, or hemorrhage, and there may also be symptoms in association with the vertebral anomalies. In infants, they are a common cause of a posterior mediastinal mass and are typically paravertebral in location. They may extend across the diaphragm. The cysts are often saccular and are lined by gastric or intestinal mucosa with a muscle layer akin to the muscularis propria. Gastric mucosa may cause symptoms due to ulceration. Malignant transformation is exceptionally rare but is reported in gastroenteric cysts.

Congenital Cystic Adenomatoid Malformation (CCAM)

The term *CCAM* (clinically, cystic CTM) encompasses a spectrum of variably sized cysts with differing histology. The reported incidence is between 1 in 25,000 and 1 in 35,000, although, as with many conditions, the advent of antenatal ultrasound is causing us to revise upward our estimates of prevalence. The relationship between different types and with other malformations is contentious, and their etiology is obscure. Some view them as defects that relate to insults to the pulmonary airways during maturation—hence the proposed alternative term *congenital pulmonary airway malformation*, or here, the more generic *congenital thoracic malformation (CTM).* Pathologically, five types (types 0 to 4) have been proposed by Stocker, the speculation being that they represent malformations that relate to insults at different levels

of the airways. In this classification system, type 0 (a condition formerly described as *acinar dysplasia*) is described as bronchial; type 1 as bronchial/bronchiolar; type 2 as bronchiolar; type 3 as bronchiolar/alveolar duct; and type 4 as peripheral.[6] Although lesions are not obviously distributed along the bronchial pathway, there is a high incidence of associated abnormalities of the bronchial tree on detailed analysis, and furthermore, vascularity and cellular composition in CCAMs corresponds to that seen in airways during gestation. This histologic classification is useful because it permits identification of certain histologic patterns that rarely undergo malignant transformation in association with certain subtypes. However, this system has not been universally accepted, as discussed in the following paragraph, and many pathologists limit classification of CCAMs to types 1 and 2.[7]

Type 0 CCAM

Type 0 CCAM is also termed *acinar dysplasia.*, The condition is rare, incompatible with life, and typically associated with other abnormalities. The lungs are small and firm, and histology shows bronchial-type airways with cartilage, smooth muscle, and glands that are separated only by abundant mesenchymal tissue. This condition is discussed in more detail in Chapter 22.

Type 1 CCAM

Type 1 is the most common type of CCAM and has the best prognosis. This is because these malformations are usually localized and affect only part of one lobe. Most present in the perinatal period or *in utero,* but rare cases can present later. Cysts are usually multiloculated and range considerably in size, although type 1 CCAMs are larger than 2 cm in diameter by definition (Fig. 21-19). There is no relationship between age and cyst size. Microscopically there is a sharp boundary between the lesion and the adjacent normal lung, but there is no capsule. The cystic spaces are lined by pseudostratified ciliated columnar epithelium, and mucous cell hyperplasia is seen in 35% to 50% of cases (Fig. 21-20). Arbitrarily, hyperplasia is defined as mucous cell proliferation confined to the cyst, while extensions of this process into the alveolar parenchyma with lepidic growth pattern is classified as bronchioloalveolar carcinoma.[100] This latter complication is considerably rarer, and it has been argued that such proliferations are not neoplastic. However, occasional cases have metastasized, and molecular studies have shown chromosomal aberrations in the mucous cells similar to those seen in adenocarcinomas of nonsmokers. Therefore such proliferations should be regarded as mucinous adenocarcinomas, with a very good prognosis following complete resection.

Type 2 CCAM

Type 2 CCAM is the second most frequent type. These malformations generally cause respiratory distress in the first month of life and may be associated with renal agenesis, cardiovascular defects, diaphragmatic hernia, and syringomyelia, which often have an additional adverse effect on the prognosis. Occasional cases present later in childhood with infection. Macroscopically, the lesions are spongelike, comprising multiple small cysts.

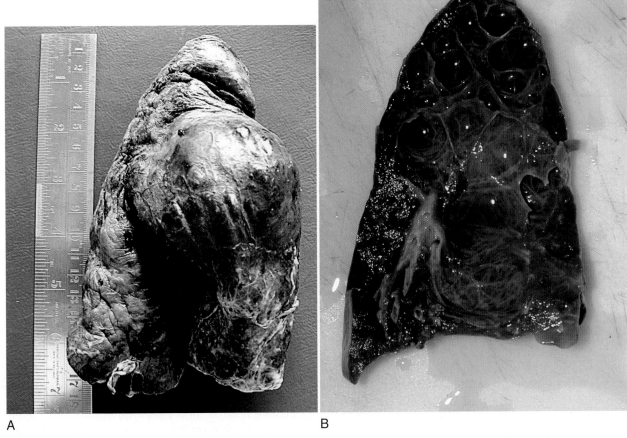

A   B

FIGURE 21-19. Type 1 CCAM. **A,** A cystic lesion bulges to fill most of the lower lobe. **B,** The cut surface shows a multiloculated cyst replacing most of the parenchyma.

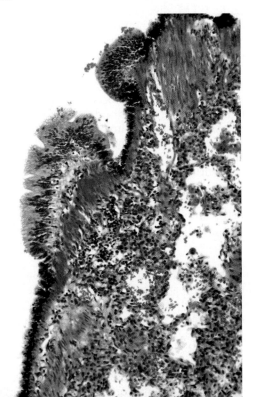

FIGURE 21-20. Type 1 CCAM. The cyst lining is mainly of respiratory type, although mucous cell hyperplasia is not infrequently seen.

Microscopically, the cystic airspaces relate to a relative overgrowth of dilated bronchiolar structures that are separated by alveolar tissue, which appears comparatively underdeveloped. Occasional examples contain striated muscle, although this has no clinical significance.

Type 3 CCAM

Type 3 CCAMs are uncommon and occur almost exclusively in male infants. They typically involve and expand a whole lobe, and the others are compressed. It may cause hypoplasia in the remaining pulmonary tissue. Macroscopically, lesions appear solid and not cystic. Microscopically, there is an excess of bronchiolar structures separated by airspaces that resemble late fetal lung. There is also a virtual absence of small, medium, and large pulmonary arteries within the lesion. Some regard this lesion as identical to pulmonary hyperplasia.[7]

Type 4 CCAM

Type 4 CCAMs are also very rare and comprise peripheral thin-walled cysts that are often multiloculated. The cystic spaces are typically lined by alveolar type I or type II cells, and the intervening stroma are thin and comprise loose mesenchymal tissue (Fig. 21-21). Their etiology is obscure, and there is likely a spectrum of disease between these lesions and type 1 pleuropulmonary blastomas. Certainly, if the stroma of a suspected type 4 CCAM is even focally hypercellular, classification and management as type 1

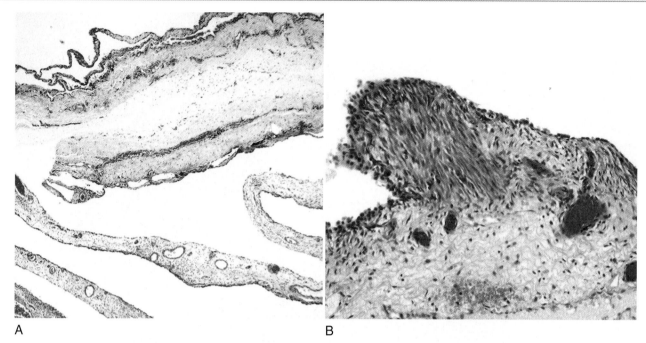

A   B

FIGURE 21-21. Type 4 CCAM. **A,** These cysts are lined typically by pneumocytes with loose and myxoid fibrous stroma composing the walls of variably sized thin-walled cysts. **B,** Care must be taken to ensure that no blastematous elements are present, which would indicate a diagnosis of pleuropulmonary blastoma.

pleuropulmonary blastoma is recommended, and it has been proposed that such lesions lacking a blastematous component are better classified as regressed pleuropulmonary blastomas rather than type 4 CCAM.[7,100,101]

Postnatal Treatment Decisions in Congenital Cystic Lung Disease

Decisions about the treatment of a CTM that is symptomatic are straightforward, either because of its size, compression of nearby structures, or because it has developed a complication such as infection. Once a previously asymptomatic cystic lesion has become infected, it is probably safe to assume that recurrent infections are inevitable, and the lesion should be excised (Fig. 21-22). If medical management has failed,

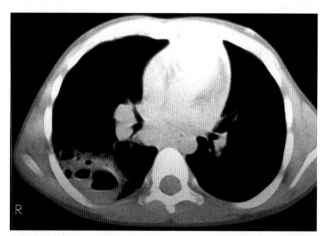

FIGURE 21-22. CT scan of a right sided, thin-walled, multicystic congenital thoracic malformation with air fluid levels. The CTM is the seat of recurrent infection.

then surgical removal is indicated, conserving as much normal lung as possible. If the lesion is discovered as a chance finding on a chest radiograph, it is likely to be excised to establish the diagnosis and exclude a malignancy.

No area is more controversial than that of the asymptomatic CTM discovered on antenatal ultrasound. A chest radiograph should be done postnatally in the asymptomatic child. However, this is only around 60% sensitive, so further imaging, usually HRCT, is advised to delineate the abnormality. The question about what to do next then arises. Even surgeons, who almost by definition are interventionists, cannot agree.[102] There are not enough natural history data to give sound advice to parents. Trivial lesions are usually left alone, but some resect even tiny malformations to try to reduce the risk of malignancy. However, there is no evidence that this policy works (see later in the chapter). Reasons for operation on an asymptomatic CTM also include prevention of nonmalignant complications, allowing optimal lung growth, and prevention of malignant transformation. Unfortunately, there are important evidence gaps in all three areas.

Prevention of (Nonmalignant) Complications
The main risk is probably infection. If the CTM is cystic, then it is likely (but unproven) that infection will occur sooner or later.[103] The best information is from a recent meta-analysis.[104] There were 41 series published between 1996 and 2008 describing 1070 patients, nearly 80% of whom had an antenatal diagnosis of CTM. 505 reached infancy without surgery of whom only 16 (2.3%) became symptomatic. Complications were significantly less likely after elective surgery. Furthermore, previous pneumonia is a risk factor for the need to convert video-assisted

thoracic surgery (VATS) to open thoracotomy.[105] The authors recommended surgery before 10 months of age, although the numbers who actually became symptomatic were too small to be dogmatic. Clearly surgery will prevent nonmalignant complications of CTM, but if all CTMs were operated on, many unnecessary operations would be performed.

A final consideration in this section is that removal of a CTM may reveal that it was not as "asymptomatic" as was thought preoperatively. A single paper suggested that histiocytic inflammation may be a feature of some CTMs,[106] although no data about symptoms were given, and there was no evidence of chronic infection. However, anecdotally the occasional infant who undergoes resection of an apparently asymptomatic malformation becomes much more alert and lively, and the family realizes that in fact he or she was not quite as well as was thought prior to resection of the CTM.

Optimizing Lung Growth

It seems likely that operative removal of a large mass would allow the residual lung to expand. However, evidence in support of this is scant. Indeed, CLHL may cause considerable mediastinal shift in asymptomatic infants, but as the child gets older the shift regresses, and there is no evidence of interference with lung growth or function. Indeed, CLHL may be a chance finding in a completely asymptomatic adult. Hence we do not believe that optimizing lung growth is a credible indication for removal of an asymptomatic CTM.

Preventing Malignant Transformation

This is a vexing and difficult issue. A few definite background statements can be made:

- Primary intrathoracic malignancy in childhood is very rare. For most but not all types of CTM, there is no evidence of an increased risk, and cytogenetic studies are reassuring.[107]
- There are isolated case reports and case series documenting the coexistence of a CTM and primary intrathoracic malignancy (reviewed in[108]).
- Even complete removal of a CTM does not prevent development of a malignancy.[109,110]

There is debate as to whether some CTMs may evolve into a pleuropulmonary blastoma (PPB), or whether in fact they represent a regressed PPB. Registry data suggest that those with bilateral CTMs; a family history of PPB, lung cysts, or renal anomalies; or a close relative with a childhood malignancy (especially Wilm's tumor or medulloblastoma) are at particular risk.[101,111,112] Recently, heterozygous germline mutations in DICER1 have been shown to be important in PPB.[113] Nonetheless, even after defining a high-risk group and removing the CTM, there is no established protocol for postoperative follow-up.

Conclusion

The uncertainties as to what is best to do must be shared honestly with the family. There is no right answer in the asymptomatic child, and this needs to be acknowledged. Whatever therapeutic decisions are made, follow-up to obtain natural history data is recommended.

Pulmonary Sequestration

Etiology of these lesions is not clear, and, specifically, genetic studies have tended to lump sequestrations and CCAMs together (probably logically). The classical definition of sequestration is pulmonary tissue that is isolated from normal functioning lung and is fed by systemic arteries. The intrapulmonary variant is contained within otherwise normal lung parenchyma. The less common extralobar sequestration is divorced from and accessory to the lung. Sequestrations may also connect to the esophagus or stomach, as well as contain pancreatic tissue; they also may show histologic features of adenomatoid malformations. These complicated lesions are perhaps best classified pathologically as complex *bronchopulmonary-foregut malformation*, if the simpler term CTM is not to be used.

Their etiology is far from understood, with various proposed theories. Some workers have suggested that intralobar sequestration is acquired when a focus of infection or scarring acquires its blood supply from a systemic collateral, basing this on the relative sparsity of other malformations associated with this type of sequestration and its rarity in perinatal autopsies. Those who believe sequestration to be congenital generally propose that accessory lung buds are fundamental to both forms of pulmonary sequestration and liken them to intestinal duplications, with subsequent acquisition of a blood supply from the nearest and most convenient source, which happens to be systemic.

Intralobar sequestrations are usually found in the posterior basal segment of the left lower lobe and extralobar sequestrations beneath the left lower lobe. About 15% of extralobar sequestrations are abdominal. The intralobar sequestration is encircled by visceral pleura and has no pleural separation from the rest of the lobe. The remainder of the affected lobe and lung is normal, unless secondary changes such as infection have supervened. More than half the cases of intralobar sequestration are diagnosed after adolescence, and symptoms in neonates and infants are uncommon. Extralobar sequestration is generally detected in infancy because of associated malformations, and it affects males four times more frequently than females. Though much rarer, intralobar sequestrations also may be associated with other malformations.

Both types of sequestration have certain similar pathologic characteristics as well as clear-cut differences. In both types, the pulmonary tissue is largely cystic and contains disorganized, airless alveoli, bronchi, cartilage, respiratory epithelium, and a systemic artery. It is often secondarily infected, bronchiectatic, or atelectatic, and may show histology of a CCAM, particularly type 2 CCAM in extralobar variants.[114,115] The aberrant arteries may arise from the thoracic or abdominal aorta and, in the latter instance, may pierce the diaphragm and run through the pulmonary ligament before reaching the sequestration. The elastic vessel walls may become atherosclerotic, and the lumen varies considerably in size. In intralobar sequestrations, the systemic arteries are likely to be large, and the veins drain into the pulmonary system; in extralobar variants, the systemic arteries are small and the venous drainage is likewise systemic through the azygos system. The pulmonary vessels may show features of hypertension, although this does not appear to be of clinical significance.[115]

Treatment of sequestration is conventionally by surgical excision. As with CTMs, the vascular supply should be carefully delineated by preoperative investigations (see later in the chapter), and embolization of aortopulmonary collaterals should be considered. There is a small series of definitive treatment by embolization, in some cases very early in life. The results are better for solid lesions; cystic components do not respond so well.[116]

Congenital Large Hyperlucent Lobe (Congenital Lobar Emphysema)

A rare condition, CLHL presents in 50% of cases in the neonatal period; otherwise it presents in early infancy. Some cases are caused by easily identifiable partial obstruction, such as mucosal flaps or twisting of the lobe on its pedicle. However, in many cases, a deficiency of bronchial cartilage is thought to be the cause, leading to inappropriate collapse of the airway and the trapping of air. Histologically, the majority of cases show normal radial alveolar counts but with no apparent maturation with age when compared to age-matched controls, suggesting a postpartum arrest of acinar development within affected lung tissue. A minority of cases, however, show true alveolar hyperplasia with increased radial alveolar counts; this sometimes is referred to as a *polyalveolar lobe*.[117] The condition affects the left upper (42%), right middle (35%), right upper (21%), and lower lobes (2%). The affected lobe cannot deflate, but overdistends and displaces adjacent lobes, and subsequently the mediastinal structures. The emphysematous lobe may herniate into the contralateral hemithorax, usually through the anterior mediastinum. The condition may be diagnosed antenatally (see earlier in the chapter), present as respiratory distress (often with consequent failure to thrive in infancy), or be a chance finding on a chest radiograph taken later in life.

Presentation in Infancy

Clinical features of infantile lobar emphysema are those suggestive of a tension pneumothorax: hyperresonance of the affected hemithorax associated with diminished breath sounds and deviation of mediastinal structures to the contralateral side. Usually, a chest radiograph will demonstrate a hyperlucent lobe with features of compression and collapse of adjacent lung and depression of the ipsilateral diaphragm (Fig. 21-23). The mediastinum is deviated, and the contralateral lung may be collapsed. Occasionally, initial chest radiographs may demonstrate an opaque lung field. This then clears and the affected lung becomes overinflated and hyperlucent on the radiograph. Ventilation-perfusion (V/Q) scanning may demonstrate delayed uptake and clearance of isotope and reduced blood flow in the affected lobe. This investigation is particularly useful if it is unclear whether the problem is a pathologically distended lobe on one side or a congenitally small contralateral lung, with secondary physiologic overexpansion. Bronchoscopy may reveal causes of intrinsic obstruction and permit the removal of a foreign body or inspissated secretions. An echocardiogram is valuable in evaluating the heart and great vessels, while a contrast CT scan is useful in evaluating the anatomy of the emphysematous lobe—its size and relations, and whether it has herniated into the contralateral hemithorax. It is useful in demonstrating the nature of adjacent lobes of the lung. This investigation is also useful in excluding contralateral pulmonary hypoplasia.

Differential Diagnosis

There are two broad groups of differential diagnoses. The first is any intrinsic or extrinsic cause of failure of airspace emptying. Intrinsic partial obstruction may result from

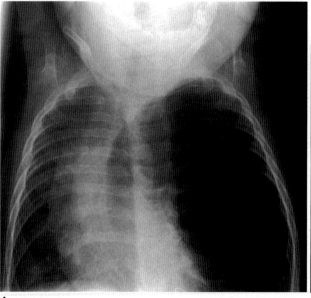

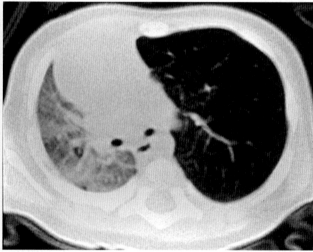

A   B

FIGURE 21-23. Chest radiograph and CT scan of a congenital large hyperlucent lobe in a patient with congenital lobar emphysema.

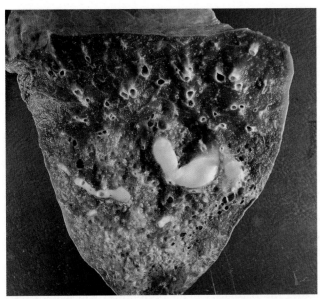

FIGURE 21-24. Bronchial atresia. The cut surface of the lung shows dilated airways plugged with mucus with surrounding microcystic changes. Dissection showed atresia at the origin of the apical segmental bronchus.

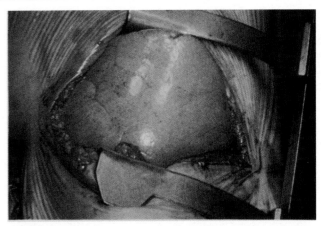

FIGURE 21-25. Surgery for congenital large hyperlucent lobe (congenital lobar emphysema). The hyperexpanded lobe protrudes out of the thoracotomy incision.

inspissated mucus or aspirated material. Endobronchial granulomas due to endotracheal suction may result in obstruction of the airway as well.[118] Intrinsic obstruction due to bronchial atresia of the affected lobe is well recognized (Fig. 21-24). The affected parenchyma is ventilated collaterally, through the pores of Kohn, from adjacent normal lung. Extrinsic compression of bronchi due to congenital heart disease or anomalies of the great vessels usually presents as emphysematous changes of more gradual onset, often after the neonatal period. Less common causes of extrinsic compression include bronchogenic cysts. The second big group is any cause of loss of lung volume on the contralateral side. Other causes include absent lung, and lobar or lung collapse due to bronchial obstruction. Mediastinal shift with an opaque large lung, an occasional early finding in congenital large hyperlucent lobe, should be distinguished from other causes of unilateral opacification and contralateral mediastinal shift in the neonate (e.g., chylothorax, CDH, or airless CTM).

Treatment
Children who do not suffer respiratory compromise can be managed conservatively. Their outcome is comparable to that of children managed by resection of an emphysematous lobe (Fig. 21-25); the distended emphysematous lobe does not compromise the growth and development of adjacent lung.[119] Lobectomy is indicated in the event of respiratory distress, which rarely, if ever, develops *de novo* beyond the newborn period. The actual surgical technique is as for any other lobectomy. Ventilation in this circumstance may be difficult. Low-pressure high-frequency oscillation has been advocated to prevent barotrauma to the affected lobe and further respiratory compromise to the adjacent lung.

ABNORMAL CONNECTIONS BETWEEN THE BRONCHIAL TREE AND OTHER STRUCTURES

Tracheoesophageal Fistula and Esophageal Atresia

Etiology
The environmental, chromosomal, and genetic abnormalities implicated in these conditions have recently been reviewed.[120–123] Recently deletions in the glutathione S-transferase gene have been implicated in isolated esophageal atresia.[124] Genetic factors implicated in esophageal atresia as part of a syndrome include CHD7 in familial CHARGE syndrome (Coloboma of the eye, Heart defects, Atresia of the nasal choanae, Retardation of growth and/or development, Genital and/or urinary abnormalities, and Ear abnormalities and deafness),[125] *FOXF1* and the 16q24.1 *FOX* transcription factor gene cluster,[126] polyalanine expansion in the *ZIC3* gene[127] (both VACTERL: Vertebra abnormalities, Anal Atresia, Cardiovascular anomalies, Tracheoesophageal fistula, Esophageal Atresia, Renal or Radial abnormalities, Limb defects), and a 5.9 Mb microdeletion in chromosome band 17q22-q23.2 associated with TEF and conductive hearing loss.[128]

Pathology
If there is incomplete mesodermal separation of the primitive foregut, then a fistula may develop between the esophagus and the trachea (Fig. 21-26). Most commonly, they are associated with esophageal atresia, with about 85% of such cases being associated with a fistula. Typically, the proximal part of the esophagus ends in a blind sac and the distal part takes origin from the lower part of the trachea. The upper blind pouch is large and substantial, and it usually ends about 8 cm from the superior alveolar ridge in the region of the azygos vein. Conversely, the lower esophageal segment is small and originates from the region of the distal posterior membranous trachea, carina, or right main-stem bronchus.

Instances of communication between the trachea and the esophagus with an otherwise normal esophagus occur in about 3% of TEFs (see Fig. 21-26). Although symptoms

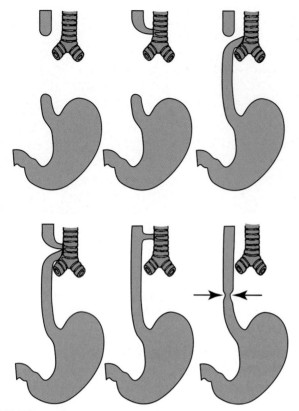

FIGURE 21-26. Types of tracheoesophageal fistulae.

from this congenital abnormality are fairly gross, the diagnosis is often delayed, with considerable respiratory morbidity due to aspiration and infection. The tracheoesophageal connection is almost always small, and the majority are found in the neck, from below the larynx to the thoracic inlet. Occasionally, a bronchus may communicate with the esophagus.

Associations

Tracheoesophageal fistula is more common in first and twin pregnancies of mothers of increasing age. About two thirds have an associated abnormality of some sort.[129] Of the live births, 20% have birth weight below the 5th percentile. More than 50% of infants with esophageal atresia have associated anomalies. These are most common in pure esophageal atresia without fistula and least common in H-type fistulas. Infants with this association have a high mortality rate. Almost 80% have cardiac anomalies, these being the principal cause of death. Esophageal disease is also part of CHARGE syndrome, which carries a high mortality. Chromosomal abnormalities are reported in 6% of cases, in trisomy 13, 18, and 21 in particular.[130] Other associations include Potter's syndrome (bilateral renal agenesis), Pierre Robin, polysplenia, and DiGeorge sequences. The incidence of cardiac anomalies has been reported to be between 30% and 50% in various series. There is also a significant incidence (47%) of tracheobronchial anomalies,[131] ranging from tracheomalacia, abnormal nonciliated epithelium, lung agenesis, and hypoplasia or ectopic bronchi, to glossoptosis and airway obstruction. Pharyngeal function and aspiration on deglutition is common. The incidence of vertebral and

skeletal anomalies, including sacral agenesis, hemivertebrae, and rib and radial anomalies is 20% to 50% overall. Cases with associated cleft lip[132] and duodenal atresia are higher risk.

Presentation

The incidence of esophageal atresia is 1 in 2500. Maternal polyhydramnios has been reported in 85% of cases with pure esophageal atresia and 32% of those associated with TEF. Diagnosis by antenatal ultrasound is unreliable, with up to 50% false-positives.[133] At birth, the baby is commonly frothing, choking, and suffering cyanotic episodes despite oral suction. If the condition is suspected, the initial examination should be carefully performed to identify any associated anomalies. The effect of birth weight and associated anomalies on survival is given in Tables 21-10 and 21-11. An attempt should be made to pass an orogastric tube. Acid fluid may be aspirated from the tube if gastric contents reflux into the upper pouch across the fistula. A plain radiograph will demonstrate the tube coiled in the upper pouch and may identify pulmonary abnormalities such as consolidation of the right upper lobe due to aspiration, plethoric lung fields due to cardiac anomalies, and vertebral and rib anomalies. The radiograph will reveal the presence or absence of gas

TABLE 21-10   WATERSON CLASSIFICATION OF OESOPHAGEAL ATRESIA, WITH SURVIVAL FIGURES

GROUP	CLASSIFICATION	SURVIVAL
A	Birthweight >2500 g, otherwise well	100%
B	Birthweight 2000 to 2500 g, otherwise well	85%
	Birthweight >2500 g, moderate anomalies	
	Noncardiac anomalies including patent ductus arteriosus	
	Ventricular septal defect and atrial septal defect	
C	Birthweight <2000 g, severe cardiac anomalies	65%

TABLE 21-11   SPITZ CLASSIFICATION OF OESOPHAGEAL ATRESIA, WITH SURVIVAL FIGURES

GROUP	CLASSIFICATION	SURVIVAL
I	Birthweight >1500 g without congenital heart disease	97%
II	Birthweight <1500 g or major congenital heart disease	59%
III	Birthweight <1500 g and major congenital heart disease	22%

in the stomach, indicating the presence or absence of a TEF. The intestinal gas pattern should be carefully examined on the abdominal radiograph to try to exclude distal intestinal atresia. An echocardiogram is useful to identify intracardiac structural anomalies and the possibility of a right-sided aortic arch.

Preoperative Care

The preoperative care for this condition should start from the moment it is suspected. Continuous suction of the oropharynx is important to reduce the risk of aspiration and protect the airway. A sump sucker such as a replogle tube is useful because it permits continuous suction and protects the esophageal mucosa from direct suction-related trauma.[133] Cyanotic episodes have been reported with the use of this form of suction of the upper pouch. This is thought to be due to the generation of excessive negative pressure causing ineffective inspiration. The infant should be nursed prone. If pulmonary consolidation is identified, then physiotherapy and postural drainage should be employed.

Surgery

A right thoractomy[134] by extrapleural approach with end-to-end single-layer anastomosis and division of fistula remains the most common technique for the majority of children presenting with esophageal atresia and TEF. Routinely, the infant is fed by a transanastomotic tube. The use of intercostal drains and postoperative contrast studies varies among institutions and cases.[135] A variety of approaches have been proposed for those cases of esophageal atresia with a large distal fistula presenting with respiratory compromise due to gastric distention: endotracheal intubation beyond the fistula orifice, Fogarty balloon occlusion of the fistula, and formation of gastrostomy. More recently, urgent thoracotomy and fistula ligation with primary or subsequent repair of the atresia has gained wider acceptance. Several preoperative and perioperative techniques have been proposed for cases wherein the distance between the proximal and distal segments is wide. The absolute length of the gap is not so relevant as its relation to the size and strength of the wall of the esophageal segments. Per pouch bougienage either preoperatively or perioperatively to shorten the gap has been widely described and more recently modified.[136] Perioperative techniques to facilitate primary anastomosis include the use of circular, transverse, or spiral myotomies of the upper pouch. More recently, alternative techniques have been proposed to repair long-gap esophageal atresia.[136] An alternative approach, described by Scharli,[137] is to mobilize the gastric cardia into the chest by thoracoabdominal approach, permitting division of the left gastric artery. Favorable long-term results of this approach have been reported.[138] The primary thoracoscopic repair of esophageal atresia and TEF is well described. The possible advantages of this approach are being assessed.[139-141] Failing these techniques, the only option may be esophageal replacement by colonic, ileocolic, or gastric interposition. Each technique is associated with vagotomy and requires a gastric drainage procedure. Proponents of each approach have described good results. More recently, gastric transposition has become a well-established substitute for esophageal replacement.[142] What is clear is that the advantages or otherwise of this plethora of surgical techniques will only be determined if careful follow-up studies are undertaken.

Postoperative Course

Even after completely successful surgery, tracheomalacia is common, and the well-known brassy "tracheoesophageal fistula cough" (TOF cough, as it is known in Europe) is a feature. Recurrent aspiration leading to bronchitis and bronchopneumonia is frequent. A missed diagnosis of laryngeal cleft should always be considered (see earlier in the chapter). Occasionally, tracheomalacia may be so severe as to be life-threatening, but generally the cough sounds more impressive than the consequences. Up to 17% of patients may require fundoplication for postoperative gastroesophageal reflux, and 25% have dysphagia at 2 years.[129] The early mortality associated with this condition is often related to the associated malformations. The long-term outcome is good.[143]

Other Abnormal Connections

Rare cases of direct communication between the bronchial tree and congenital cysts have been described. Congenital bronchobiliary fistula as part of upper gastrointestinal tract duplication is a source of bile in respiratory secretions. Rarely, a CTM may connect with the stomach and be associated with abdominal visceral malrotation.

CONGENITAL DISEASE OF THE PULMONARY ARTERIAL TREE

When surgery is contemplated for any CTM, it is important that any abnormal vasculature is identified in advance. Inadvertent severing of anomalous systemic arteries has led to fatal hemorrhage, whereas ligation of anomalous veins from adjacent nonsequestered lung has led to infarction of normal tissue. The pulmonary and systemic arterial trees must be considered separately. Systemic arterial abnormalities of the great vessels of the mediastinum can be separated into those of the bronchial circulation (normally 1% to 2% of the left ventricular output) and other pathologic collaterals. The pulmonary capillary bed may be bypassed, leading to direct arteriovenous communication, or absent, resulting in minimal pulmonary arteriovenous connections.

Disorders of Pulmonary Artery Arrangement

Pulmonary arterial and venous arrangement generally mirrors bronchial arrangement. Exceptions to this rule include congenital origin of the left pulmonary artery from the right (pulmonary artery sling) (Fig. 21-27). Presentation is as with any vascular ring (see earlier in the chapter). In this condition, the left pulmonary artery has to traverse the mediastinum from left to right, compressing the trachea as it does so. There may also be a crossover arterial segment, with the right upper lobe supplied by a branch from the left pulmonary artery, so

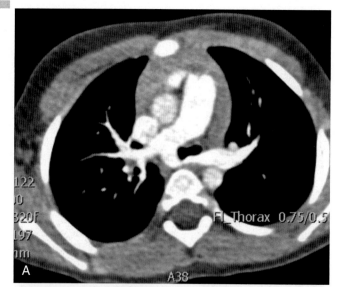

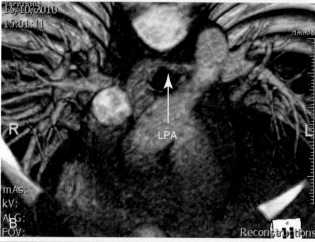

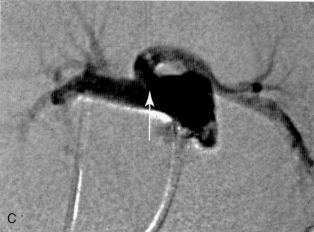

FIGURE 21-27. Pulmonary artery sling. **A,** CT scan with contrast showing the left pulmonary artery (*PA*) taking origin from the right PA, and running behind the carina and compressing it. **B,** Reconstruction showing the course of the left PA. **C,** Digital subtraction angiogram. The left PA takes origin from the right PA (*arrow*).

preoperative pulmonary angiography is essential. Surgical repair of a sling with a crossover may result in infarction of the right upper lobe if the abnormal vessel has not been discovered. Another association is complete cartilage rings (mentioned earlier), and the infant should be

evaluated for this anomaly, probably before undergoing surgery. Isolated crossover pulmonary artery branches in the absence of bronchial crossover are occasionally seen. They cross the mediastinum to supply lung segments, which often are abnormal in other ways.

Absent or Small Pulmonary Artery

Either lung may be affected by unilateral absence of a pulmonary artery, and the defect may be isolated or associated with other cardiovascular anomalies, typically tetralogy of Fallot with an absent left pulmonary artery and patent ductus arteriosus with an absent right pulmonary artery. There is an association with absent pulmonary valve syndrome. Symptoms may not arise until adult life, when they are generally due to pulmonary infection or hemorrhage. When there is only a short section absent, patients may be amenable to surgical correction, but usually the pulmonary vasculature is absent in much of the lung; histologic examination reveals hypertrophied bronchial arteries and often areas of dense fibrous scarring (Fig. 21-28). Normal pulmonary blood flow *in utero* and in the early postnatal period is needed for normal lung development. Before birth, less than 5% of the cardiac output reaches distal to the arterial duct, so it may seem surprising that interference with this small flow leads to underdevelopment of the alveolar bed and its vasculature; however, there is considerable experimental evidence and clinical observation to confirm that this is so. Congenitally small unilateral pulmonary artery usually is seen in association with an ipsilateral small lung. However, it is unclear whether the primary abnormality is related to blood flow or if both the small lung and the abnormal blood supply are due to an unknown primary event.

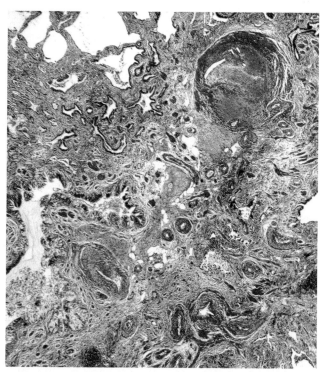

FIGURE 21-28. Absence of the pulmonary artery. The parenchyma lacks pulmonary arteries but shows very prominent bronchial arteries instead.

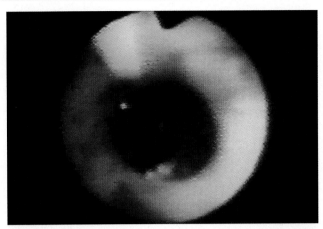

FIGURE 21-29. Iatrogenic complete infarction of the trachea, which is black and necrotic. The child had undergone a unifocalization procedure in which the bronchial arteries had been stripped from the airways and anastomosed to create a pulmonary trunk. The child is intubated (the blue line marks the endotracheal tube).

Pulmonary stenosis may affect lobar and segmental vessels as well as the main pulmonary arteries, and the narrowings may be multiple. Unilateral absence of a pulmonary artery leads to the lung on that side receiving only a systemic blood supply, either through anomalous systemic arteries or enlarged bronchial arteries. Individuals with isolated unilateral absence may lead a normal life, or symptoms may not arise until adult life; one third remain completely asymptomatic. Symptoms include pulmonary infection or bleeding from bronchopulmonary anastomoses. Ipsilateral lung tumor and pulmonary hypertension have been reported.[144] Clinically, the condition may be difficult to distinguish from embolic occlusion and obliterative bronchiolitis. The presence of other congenital defects would militate against these, and the absence of mosaic attenuation on CT scan would point away from obliterative bronchiolitis.

It is worth noting an iatrogenic complication related to an abnormal pulmonary blood supply in children with pulmonary valve atresia and supply of the lungs solely by systemic arterial blood. In the surgical procedure of unifocalization, the collateral circulation is used to create an artificial trunk supplying the whole of the lung, which can then be anastomosed to the right ventricle via a conduit. We have reported on children with severe postoperative bronchial ischemia (and even total infarction) as a result of excessively vigorous stripping of the bronchial circulation from the airways (Fig. 21-29).[145]

One or both pulmonary arteries may take origin from the aorta.[146] Bilateral origin from the aorta is part of the spectrum of common arterial trunk and usually will present to the pediatric or fetal cardiologist. Unilateral origin of a pulmonary artery from the aorta may be an isolated abnormality, sometimes presenting with persistent tachypnea.

CONGENITAL DISEASE OF THE SYSTEMIC ARTERIAL TREE

Two groups of abnormalities are relevant to the lung. The first includes those that produce a vascular ring. Although numerous variations from the normal aortic

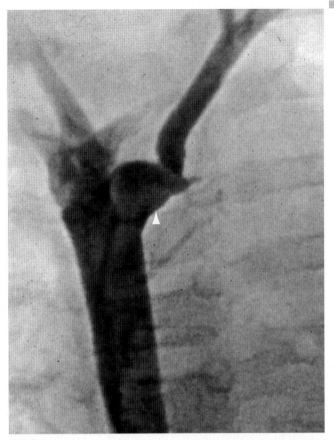

FIGURE 21-30. Digital subtraction angiogram showing a right-sided aortic arch with aberrant origin of the left subclavian artery from a diverticulum of Kommerell *(arrow)*. A left-sided ligamentum arteriosum completed the vascular ring.

arch development have been reported, only a few distinct patterns can produce extrinsic tracheal obstruction, and even these may be incidental findings without clinical correlation. The most likely types that compromise the trachea and esophagus, singly or together, are (1) right aortic arch with left ligamentum arteriosum or patent ductus arteriosus, (2) double aortic arch, (3) anomalous innominate or left carotid artery, (4) aberrant right subclavian artery, usually in association with a diverticulum of Kommerell (Fig. 21-30), and (5) pulmonary artery sling (see Fig. 21-27) (origin of left pulmonary artery from right pulmonary artery, sometimes with a crossover segment from the left artery supplying the right upper lobe). Right aortic arch and double aortic arch account for the largest number. The common denominator in these arch anomalies is compression and narrowing of the tracheoesophageal complex. Presentation is with stridor, or steroid-resistant asthma, and surgical treatment is recommended. If there is doubt about the extent of any compression, for example, in the case of right aortic arch and aberrant right subclavian artery, which may be a normal variant, then a preoperative bronchoscopy should be performed. The second group of systemic arterial abnormalities includes collateral vessels arising from the aorta and supplying all or part of one or both lungs, a CTM, or even supplying a part of what is an otherwise normal lung.[147] They are also found if the pulmonary artery is absent and may also be part of complex arteriovenous malformations. They may also be an isolated finding. These vessels may be hypertrophied bronchial arteries or abnormal nonbronchial arteries; there may be multiple collaterals.[148] This last group may be seen in association with direct pulmonary arteriovenous connections ("PAVMs"). Aneurysm of aortopulmonary collateral vessels has been described.

Dieulafoy's disease is most commonly found in the gastrointestinal tract, but a few cases have been reported in the lung. Patients generally present with massive hemoptysis and are found to have an isolated bronchial artery that is often dilated and tortuous, running within the subepithelial stroma.

CONGENITAL DISEASE OF THE PULMONARY VENOUS TREE

Abnormal Pulmonary Venous Drainage

Anomalous pulmonary veins result in blood from the lungs returning to the right side of the heart rather than entering the left atrium. The anomalous veins may join the inferior vena cava vein or hepatic, portal, or splenic veins below the diaphragm, or above the diaphragm they may drain into the superior vena cava vein or its tributaries, the coronary sinus, or the right atrium. Anomalous pulmonary venous drainage may be obstructed or unobstructed. The anomaly may be total or partial, unilateral or bilateral, and isolated or associated with other cardiopulmonary developmental defects. These include bronchial isomerism, mirror-image arrangement, asplenia, pulmonary stenosis, patent arterial duct, and a small interatrial communication. The type of isomerism gives a good indication as to whether the anomaly is total or partial, right-sided isomerism suggesting totally anomalous veins and left-sided isomerism suggesting a partial anomaly. Occasionally, the anomalous vein runs much of its course buried within the lung substance. Anomalous pulmonary venous connections are often narrow, and this may cause relatively mild pulmonary hypertension. Unilateral anomalous venous drainage may be part of complex lung malformations; it may also be seen in association with what appears to be a simple lung cyst. This underscores the need for accurate delineation of all abnormalities, even in straightforward-appearing cases. Minor abnormalities of venous connection (e.g., a segment draining directly into the azygos system) are not uncommon and usually not of practical significance.

Scimitar syndrome is a particular clinical problem characterized by a small right lung, resulting in the heart moving to the right (cardiac dextroposition) and an abnormal band shadow representing the abnormal venous drainage to the systemic veins (Fig. 21-31), fancifully compared to a scimitar (a sign that is in fact often absent). Infants with this condition presenting in heart failure have a worse prognosis, often because of associated abnormalities, among which may be malformations in the left side of the heart. Aortopulmonary collaterals should be sought and occluded. More invasive treatment options include re-implantation of the vein or pneumonectomy. Severe pulmonary hypertension

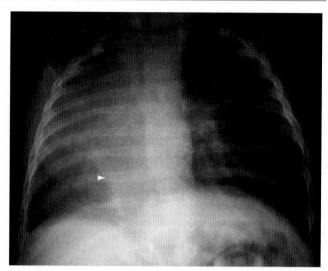

FIGURE 21-31. Scimitar syndrome (congenital small right lung, venous drainage to the inferior caval vein). The abnormal right-sided venous drainage is arrowed.

is an adverse prognostic feature. An association with horseshoe lung has been described; this usually causes early death, but occasional long-term survival has been reported.[149,150]

Congenital Absence of the Pulmonary Veins

Absence of the pulmonary veins or narrowing of their ostia into the left atrium results in pulmonary venous obstruction. It may also be associated with partial anomalous pulmonary venous drainage. The atresia may be unilateral (Fig. 21-32) or bilateral, but in either case severe hypertensive changes develop in both lungs. Congenital pulmonary vein atresia carries a very poor prognosis; few children with the condition survive longer than a year. Stenting the ostia via cardiac catheterization has been reported.

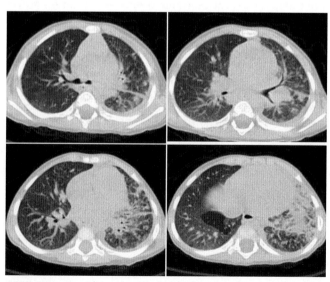

FIGURE 21-32. CT scan showing changes associated with absent left pulmonary veins. The left lung is engorged, with dilated lymphatics and a left-sided pleural effusion.

ABNORMALITIES OF THE CONNECTIONS BETWEEN THE PULMONARY ARTERIAL AND VENOUS TREES

Congenital Alveolar Capillary Dysplasia

Congenital alveolar capillary dysplasia represents a misalignment of lung vessels due to a failure of the capillaries to grow in appropriate number and location within the alveolar tissue of the lung (often associated with abnormally sited pulmonary veins within bronchovascular bundles). The disorder is an unusual cause of congenital pulmonary hypertension, persistent fetal circulation, and respiratory distress in the newborn. Congenital alveolar capillary dysplasia is discussed in detail in Chapter 55 and will not be considered further in this chapter.

Pulmonary Arteriovenous Malformations

Etiology

Many cases of pulmonary arteriovenous fistula are associated with hereditary hemorrhagic telangiectasia (HHT; Osler-Weber-Rendu disease). HHT is a genetic vascular disorder characterized by epistaxis, telangiectasia, and visceral manifestations including PAVMs. The two known disease types, HHT1 and HHT2, are caused by mutations in the endoglin *(ENG)* and ACVRL1 *(ALK-1)* genes, respectively.[151,152] A third locus has been described on chromosome 5[153]; the exact gene is not yet known. Recently, *SMAD4* mutations have been described in HHT with juvenile polyposis syndrome.[154]

Clinical features of PAVMs constitute an important group of abnormalities that potentially involve systemic and pulmonary arterial and venous trees (Fig. 21-33). They represent a direct intrapulmonary connection between pulmonary artery and vein without an intervening capillary bed. This cavernous arteriovenous aneurysm is an uncommon cause of symptoms in the pediatric age group and is often diagnosed in adults. Presentation is with cyanosis, hemoptysis, or neurologic complications (see later in the chapter). The chest radiograph may be normal, but usually well-defined single or multiple opacities are seen, with vessels connecting them to the hila, which are strongly suggestive of the diagnosis. Fistulas occur in the lower lobes in about 60% of cases; they are single in 60% and unilateral in 75%. Macroscopically, lesions can be peripheral or central and may simulate a saccular, cavernous hemangioma because of its aneurysmal swelling. The fistula is fed by at least one afferent artery, usually pulmonary and less often bronchial, and may be drained by several veins, almost always pulmonary. In 80%, there is a single feeding pulmonary artery and a single draining pulmonary vein. There are numerous communications between artery and vein in this tortuous, dilated, wormlike vessel mass. On microscopic examination, the arteriovenous fistula is lined with vascular endothelium.

Diagnosis

Diagnosis is confirmed by documenting an abnormal right-to-left shunt at the pulmonary vascular level, either by contrast echocardiography (the contrast being a peripheral injection of microbubbles,) a technetium Tc 99 m macroaggregate lung perfusion scan with shunt quantification by counting over the kidneys and brain, or (increasingly) CT angiography. The large connections may have both a systemic and a pulmonary arterial supply (see earlier in the chapter).

Treatment

When planning therapy, it is important to know if there is a systemic component, since this may cause high-output cardiac failure. Furthermore, whereas embolization of an abnormal pulmonary arteriovenous connection via the feeding pulmonary artery may be curative, more extensive procedures may be needed to deal with systemic arterial components. Embolization for PAVMs with a feeding artery ≥3 mm is the preferred treatment option,[155] even if they are extensive. Various devices, including the Amplatzer, have been used.[156–159] Although lung transplantation has been reported for this condition, the results are clearly inferior. Multiple procedures may be necessary. In one series, about 33% of patients obtained normal oxygen saturation and 15% an improved exercise tolerance; generally embolization, even of major multiple PAVMs is preferable to transplantation. Diffuse microscopic disease is more difficult to treat, but there is some evidence that embolization may reduce the prevalence of neurologic complications.

HHT is associated with AVMs in the brain and elsewhere. Pulmonary complications include PAVMs, pulmonary hypertension secondary to high-output cardiac failure with systemic AVMs, and primary pulmonary hypertension.[160] The extent to which screening for, in particular, cerebral AVMS is worthwhile is controversial.[161–162] This and other aspects of the multisystem management of the condition are beyond the scope of this chapter.

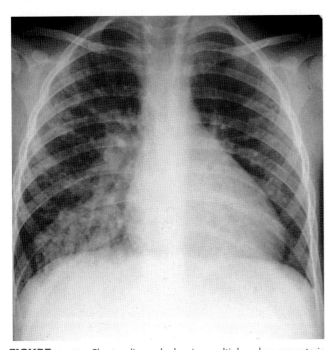

FIGURE 21-33. Chest radiograph showing multiple pulmonary arteriovenous fistulae, in particular in the right lower lobe.

Complications

Complications of PAVMs are related to the bypassing of the filtration function of the pulmonary circulation, and hyperviscosity due to polycythemia secondary to systemic arterial hypoxemia. Pulmonary hypertension does not develop because there is no alveolar hypoxemia. The patient may develop systemic, in particular cerebral, abscess or thrombosis. Particular care is needed during prolonged periods of immobility in the patient with hyperviscosity. If the child is treated before puberty, further embolizations may be needed for recurrence of PAVMs after the pubertal growth spurt.

■ CONGENITAL DISEASE OF THE LYMPHATIC TREE

This tree is the hardest to delineate, and in most malformations it will not be relevant. Lymphatic tree disorders usually require histologic confirmation. Lymphatic hypoplasia of varied distribution underlies the yellow nail syndrome in which lymphedema is accompanied by discoloration of the nails and pleural effusions. Though inherited, it may not be manifest until adult life. Klippel-Trenaunay syndrome, usually characterized by varicosities of systemic veins, cutaneous hemangiomas, and soft-tissue hypertrophy, is another congenital disorder in which pleuropulmonary abnormalities are described, including pulmonary lymphatic hyperplasia, pleural effusions, pulmonary thromboembolism, and pulmonary vein varicosities. Congenital chylothorax is described in Chapter 22.

Congenital pulmonary lymphangiectasia may be either secondary to obstruction to pulmonary lymphatic or venous drainage, or primary, the latter either limited to the lung or part of generalized lymphangiectasia. There is a high association of primary pulmonary lymphangiectasia with other congenital abnormalities, particularly asplenia and cardiac anomalies. It causes severe respiratory distress and has been generally thought to be fatal in the neonatal period, but milder cases with prolonged survival have been described, and indeed presentation may be delayed until adult life.[163,164] The lungs are heavy, with widened interlobular septa, and on the visceral pleural surface there is a pronounced reticular pattern of small cysts that accentuates the lobular architecture of the lungs. The cysts measure up to 5 mm in diameter and are situated in the interlobular septa and about the bronchovascular bundles. The cysts are elongated near the hila of the lungs. Microscopy confirms that the cysts are located in connective tissue under the pleura, in the interlobular septa, and about the bronchioles and arteries. Serial sections show that they are part of an intricate network of intercommunicating channels that vary greatly in width and are devoid of valves. The cysts are lined by an attenuated simple endothelium. The absence of multinucleate foreign body giant cell reaction distinguishes this condition from interstitial emphysema. The clinical history is also quite different; interstitial emphysema is usually (but not invariably) a complication of positive pressure ventilation in a very preterm infant.

■ OTHER RELEVANT ISSUES

Congenital Disorders of the Chest Wall

Disorders of the bony ribcage and scoliosis are described in Chapter 43. Here we will concentrate on diaphragmatic disorders. Disorders of fetal breathing movements are beyond the scope of this chapter, but these are essential for normal lung development. The abdomen is part of the chest wall, and any disorder that increases abdominal contents before birth (e.g., fetal ascites or a large tumor) will impede lung development and cause bilateral CSL.

Congenital Diaphragmatic Hernia

Pathologic Anatomy

Eighty percent of CDHs are left-sided, through the left pleuroperitoneal canal. Bilateral CDHs are rare. The defect is within the diaphragm itself; there is usually no associated membranous sac. The diaphragm itself may be well developed or significantly deficient, especially at its origin from the twelfth rib. Intestine, stomach, liver, and spleen may all herniate into the chest. A nonmuscular membranous sac is present in 10% to 15% of cases, signifying the early occurrence of this lesion before closure of the pleuroperitoneal canal. Associations of this condition are discussed in the "Antenatal Presentation" section under "Age-Related Presentations of Congenital Lung Disease" earlier in the chapter.

Postnatal Presentation

The diagnosis of CDH is usually made antenatally. From birth, infants may present with a variety of symptoms and signs. Typically, the abdomen is scaphoid (Fig. 21-34), the chest is funnel-shaped, and the trachea and mediastinum are deviated to the contralateral side. The infant may be entirely well or suffer from several problems ranging from choking episodes to apneas to acute respiratory failure. Rarely, late presentation may be associated with chronic gastrointestinal symptoms.[165] The diagnosis of CDH is confirmed by a plain radiograph of the chest and abdomen (Fig. 21-35) after the passage of a nasogastric tube. The plain film is a poor indication of the

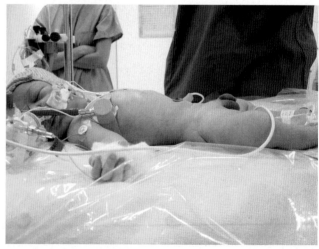

FIGURE 21-34. Scaphoid abdomen in congenital diaphragmatic hernia.

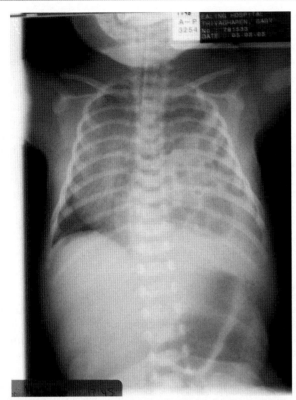

FIGURE 21-35. Plain radiograph demonstrating a left-sided congenital diaphragmatic hernia. There are obvious gas-filled loops of bowel in the chest.

degree of pulmonary hypoplasia.[166] If doubt persists, then an ultrasound scan of the chest demonstrating intrathoracic intestinal peristalsis is helpful. An echocardiogram should be performed to exclude intracardiac anomalies; fetal echocardiography should, however, have been part of the antenatal diagnostic workup. The postnatal differential diagnosis of CDH is similar to the prenatal one and includes extensive congenital cystic disease of the lung, Morgagni anterior diaphragmatic hernia, paraesophageal hiatus hernia, and eventration of the diaphragm.

Surgery
The management of CDH is no longer regarded as a surgical emergency. The initial management is to stabilize the infant and optimize respiratory function. Delayed surgical repair has become generally more accepted, with lower mortality rates than have been seen with immediate repair. The exact timing of surgery remains controversial. Many studies have reported varying periods of delay before surgery. One of the principal advantages of this strategy has been related to pulmonary artery pressures falling toward more normal values.[166] The operative repair may be by thoracotomy or by subcostal or transverse abdominal approaches. The advantage of an abdominal approach is that it permits identification and correction of an associated intestinal malrotation. The laparoscopic repair of CDH has been described.[167] The principle of repair is as with any other hernia: reduction of herniated viscera, identification and excision of any hernia sac, and repair of the defect. Usually, repair may be achieved primarily following adequate mobilization of the defect's margins. Occasionally, this is not possible because the size of the defect prevents primary suture repair. In these

circumstances, a prosthetic patch may be required. An autologous muscle flap is preferred by many surgeons.[168] Should anticoagulation therapy be required, if ECMO therapy is anticipated, then some surgeons would prefer to minimize any dissection to reduce the risk of postoperative bleeding secondary to anticoagulation for ECMO. In these circumstances, the mobilization of the defect margins is less and the use of prosthetic patches is greater. For the same reason, malrotation will not be corrected. An intercostal chest drain is placed in the ipsilateral hemithorax by some surgeons to drain any subsequent pneumothorax or chylothorax. The negative pressure associated with such a device has been reported to increase barotrauma to the hypoplastic lung.[169] Some surgeons will leave the drain *in situ*, only to have negative pressure applied in the event of an accumulation that requires drainage. A thoracoscopic approach to the repair of CDH has been described. Individual centers describe that the only relative contraindication to this approach is the use of ECMO.[170] Longer operation times and higher recurrent hernia rates have been described, leading the authors to advocate the routine use of larger, wider prosthetic patches rather than primary repair of CDH if a laparoscopic approach is used. These findings have been confirmed in the most recent and wide-ranging literature review of this surgical option,[171] leading the authors to advocate a registry and review of this technique for further assessment. The need for registries and long-term follow-up is a recurring theme in this field.

Chylothorax complicating repair of CDH is well recognized. It may be a persistent complication associated with significant morbidity. Octreotide has been advocated in the management of this complication.[172] A thoracoabdominal shunt might be considered in this and other causes of chylothorax.[173]

Outcome
Survival of neonates reportedly varies between 39% and 95% after repair of CDH. The large variation in mortality reflects the varying severity of the pulmonary hypoplasia and abnormal pulmonary vascularity, as well as variations in the period and technique of preoperative stabilization, perioperative and postoperative mechanical ventilation, and the use of ECMO. If ECMO has to be used, the outlook is not good. Only about one third of patients thus treated survive to a year of life, and substantial comorbidity (respiratory, gastrointestinal, neurodevelopmental) is common.[174] Stege and colleagues have demonstrated that the survival of this condition within one well-circumscribed geographic locus has remained unchanged over 11 years despite the advent of new therapies. The mortality increased with the presence of other malformations.[175] A variety of neurologic abnormalities (including motor and cognitive anomalies, gastroesophageal reflux and foregut dysmotility, and skeletal anomalies) have been reported in infants surviving management of this condition.[176] Significant respiratory and nutritional problems associated with gastroesophageal reflux can occur but often tend to improve with time. Respiratory findings reported in survivors include a range of abnormalities on imaging, from a complete normal examination to ipsilateral lucency on the chest radiograph. Lung function may be normal, or there may be obstructive or restrictive disease. V/Q scans are almost invariably abnormal. Bronchial hyperreactivity is also described, but the pattern

of challenge testing suggests distal airway dysfunction rather than airway inflammation. It is suggested that most of these functional abnormalities relate to the intensity of ventilation in the perioperative period, rather than the degree of pulmonary hypoplasia at birth. However, pulmonary hypoplasia is obviously a critical determinant of survival. The incidence of gastroesophageal reflux has been reported as higher in those diaphragmatic hernias that were repaired directly.[177] Postoperative failure to thrive due to gastroesophageal reflux and oral dysfunction is common. The overall outcome of the condition is known to be worse when it is found to occur within certain syndromes such as Fryn's.

Anterior Diaphragmatic Hernia

Anterior diaphragmatic hernias occur through the foramen of Morgagni (Fig. 21-36)—a potential space that transmits the internal mammary artery, lying between the sternal and costal attachments of the diaphragm. They are much rarer than Bochdalek's hernia and tend not to present in the neonatal period. If unilateral, they occur more often on the right side than on the left side and are almost always associated with a hernial sac. Often, these hernias are bilateral, and the hernial sacs may

communicate with each other or with the pericardium.[178] Anterior diaphragmatic hernias may occur as an isolated morphologic malformation, but they often are associated with cardiac anomalies and are the diaphragmatic defect associated with the pentalogy of Cantrell. The principles of repair are similar to those for Bochdalek's hernia. Since the diaphragmatic defect is smaller and more easily repaired, prosthetic patches or autologous grafts are far less frequently required than with Bochdalek's hernia. Abdominal and thoracic approaches have been described for open repair.[179] Laparoscopic repair is now well established. The long-term outcome following repair is excellent, principally determined by the nature of any associated anomalies. There may be mild air flow obstruction and bronchial hyperreactivity to methacholine, possibly related to distal airway dysfunction. Chest asymmetry and scoliosis are also not uncommon.

Diaphragmatic Eventration

Eventration of the diaphragm may be congenital or acquired (Fig. 21-37). The congenital lesion is far rarer than the acquired one, which is most often either an injury to the phrenic nerve acquired during difficult instrumental

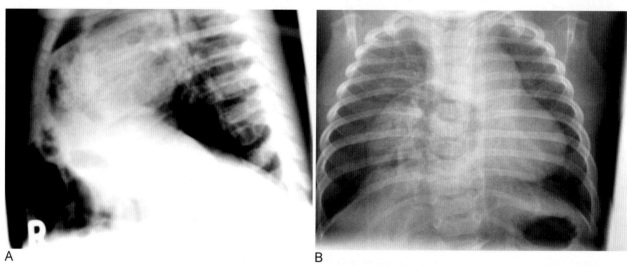

A   B

FIGURE 21-36. Lateral (**A**) and posteroanterior (**B**) chest radiograph showing a Morgagni hernia.

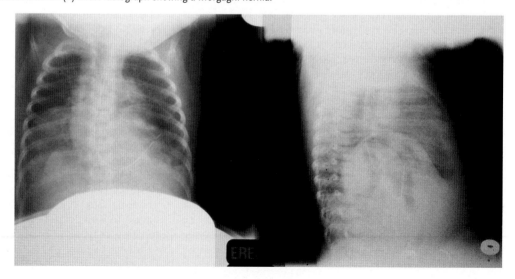

FIGURE 21-37. Bilateral eventrations of the diaphragm.

delivery, insertion of chest drain for pneumothorax, or cardiac surgery. Should the lesion result from difficult (often breech) delivery, then it may be associated with Erb's palsy. The congenital lesion results from an incomplete development of the muscular portion of the diaphragm or its innervation. This has been described in neonatal cases of fetal rubella and cytomegalovirus infection. The defect is more common on the left side than on the right side and usually presents as a moderate to complete thinning of the diaphragmatic muscle fibers. In extreme cases, it may be very difficult pathologically to differentiate the lesion from a CDH. Bilateral lesions are rare. Several associated anomalies have been described with the congenital form of diaphragmatic eventration: rib and cardiac anomalies, renal ectopia, and exomphalos. Presentation is usually as a chance finding on a chest radiograph taken for other purposes. The diagnosis is confirmed by ultrasound examination demonstrating paradoxical movement of the diaphragm. Usually no treatment is needed, and the radiologic appearance improves with time. Bilateral large eventrations may need repair, and the best approach is through the chest, followed by radial incision and plication of the diaphragm using a nonabsorbable suture.

CONGENITAL CARDIAC DISORDERS

Cardiac malformations may be coincidental to or a fundamental part of a pulmonary malformation. They are sufficiently common that echocardiography should be a routine part of the workup of most suspected congenital lung abnormalities. Coincidental malformations are seen with, for example, congenital large hyperlucent lobe. Around 10% have an atrial or ventricular septal defect. Lung abnormalities in which heart disease is fundamental include those with the pulmonary atresia spectrum (see earlier in the chapter). By definition, lung blood supply is abnormal. However, these cases usually present to pediatric cardiologists and are beyond the scope of this chapter. It should be noted that vascular compression of the airways in the setting of congenital heart disease is not uncommon and may be referred to the pediatric pulmonologist.

MULTISYSTEM CONGENITAL DISORDERS THAT AFFECT THE LUNG

Most congenital lung abnormalities are isolated, but a few are part of a more generalized disorder. Tuberous sclerosis may affect the lung as well as kidneys, heart, and brain. Complex abnormalities of lung development may be associated with chromosomal abnormalities. Micronodular type II pneumocyte hyperplasia is largely though not exclusively confined to patients with tuberous sclerosis, of which it is a particularly rare manifestation. It is a multifocal microscopic lesion that usually has no clinical significance, but in rare cases the lesions are of an appreciable size and so numerous that pulmonary function is compromised and the patient complains of breathlessness. The hyperplastic cells show no atypia and appear to be devoid of any malignant potential. Micronodular type II pneumocyte hyperplasia may be seen in otherwise normal lungs or in association with pulmonary lymphangioleiomyomatosis. Unlike lymphangioleiomyomatosis, it affects tuberous

sclerosis patients of either sex, and the hyperplastic type II cells fail to stain for HMB-45.

Rare metabolic diseases may affect the lung. These include Niemann-Pick, and lysinuric protein intolerance. They also enter the differential diagnosis of pediatric interstitial lung disease (see Chapter 55).

ROLE OF SPECIFIC INVESTIGATIONS

This section discusses possible investigations and their role, and it does not imply that all should be performed on every child. A selective approach is essential.

Chest Radiography

All infants in whom any suggestion of a lung malformation has been made antenatally will require a chest radiograph before discharge. In many it will be normal, but subsequent, more detailed imaging may reveal tiny malformations. Specific points in the chest radiograph in the context of congenital lung disease include the determination of bronchial arrangement and the side of the aortic arch (Fig. 21-38); a right-sided arch may be a normal variant of no concern but may give a clue to the presence of a vascular ring.[180] A normal chest radiograph does not exclude a significant CTM (see earlier in the chapter).

Ventilation:Perfusion Scanning

Although this technique gives useful functional information, in general its use in investigating congenital lung disease is declining as CT and MRI increasingly give

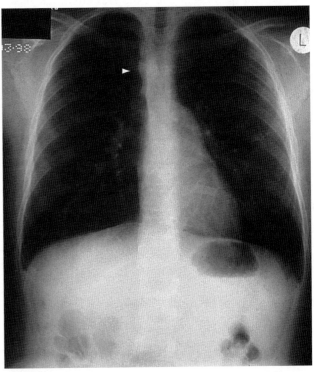

FIGURE 21-38. Right-sided aortic arch (arrow). Note the tracheal compression by the associated vascular ring.

better anatomic and functional images. Unilateral absent perfusion and ventilation is seen in complete absence of one lung. Unilateral absence of perfusion, which may be combined with secondary abnormalities in ventilation, is seen in unilateral absence of the pulmonary artery, unilateral origin of pulmonary artery from aorta, and unilateral absence of pulmonary veins. Bilateral absent or greatly reduced perfusion is seen in common arterial trunk (truncus arteriosus); the pattern of ventilation is normal. Focal defects are seen with large CTMs. Increased uptake of radiolabeled microspheres given by peripheral vein injection is seen in the brain and kidneys as a feature of PAVMs (as well as in congenital heart disease with right-to-left shunt) and has been used to quantitate shunt. Split lung function may be useful in determining whether operation on a unilateral bronchial or pulmonary artery stenosis is advisable. In cases of doubt, V/Q scanning can differentiate congenital large hyperlucent lobe from hyperinflation of a normal lobe secondary to contralateral CSL or lobar atelectasis; in this case, the lucent area is functional, whereas congenital lobar emphysema causes a filling defect.

Ultrasound Scanning (Including Echocardiography)

Cardiac abnormality is so important when considering congenital lung malformations that it is wise to include an echocardiogram as part of the investigation of many (if not most) infants with suspected congenital lung disease. Indeed, antenatal ultrasound will have already detected many cardiac abnormalities. Echocardiography detects relevant abnormalities of the systemic arteries in the mediastinum, such as double aortic arch and aberrant origin of subclavian artery. The pulmonary arteries and veins should be imaged and unilateral abnormal (hemianomalous) venous drainage excluded. Injection of saline into a peripheral vein allows detection of a right-to-left shunt; in such cases, bubbles appear in the left atrium. Pulmonary artery pressure may be estimated from the Bernoulli equation if there is physiologic tricuspid or pulmonary regurgitation. It may be possible to image abnormal collateral arteries arising from the abdominal aorta. Parenchymal ultrasound imaging is generally less helpful. Defects in the diaphragm may be identified and pleural disease confirmed. Ultrasound is useful in differentiating thymic abnormalities from mediastinal cysts.

Computed Tomography

Computed tomography gives the best images of parenchymal abnormalities and is currently probably the first investigation of choice in an adult with suspected CTM. A cystic CTM large enough to have the potential to be infected may be invisible on chest radiographs, so CT is recommended for all infants in whom an antenatal diagnosis of a lung malformation has been made, even if the chest radiograph after birth appears normal (see earlier in the chapter). Scanning after contrast injection, especially using modern reconstruction techniques, may delineate abnormal aortopulmonary collaterals, obviating the need for angiography (Fig. 21-39).

Magnetic Resonance Imaging

At present, MRI requires general anesthesia in small children, but the lack of radiation exposure and ability to reconstruct vascular anatomy make this an attractive technique. MRI is the best way of detecting extension of a neurogenic tumor into the spinal canal. It can also be used to image any airway compression and its cause.

Barium Swallow

A Barium swallow investigation may be used to diagnose a vascular ring (Fig. 21-40), but increasingly its use is superseded by CT or MRI angiography. If the appearances are those of an anomalous subclavian artery, which may be a variant of no consequence, airway compression may be confirmed with a bronchoscopy. A barium swallow cannot rule out an H-type TEF.

Esophageal Tube Injection

Abnormal connections between the esophagus and the trachea or a CTM are best delineated by a tube esophagram. The pressure injection of barium will reveal a connection that a simple barium swallow will miss. This investigation is only needed in selected cases, in which either the malformation is close to the bronchial tree, or severe infection (particularly anaerobic) is a feature.

Angiography

In complex cases, angiography may be necessary before surgery. However, the increasing use of CT and MRI to delineate vascular anatomy means that invasive investigation is now needed much less often. The operator must completely delineate the anatomy of the pulmonary and systemic trees, including establishing whether there are any arterial collaterals (see earlier in the chapter). It should be remembered that a CTM may be supplied from the coronary, internal mammary, intercostal, or subclavian arteries. At the same time, any embolization that might be indicated can be performed, including occlusion of PAVMs and systemic arterial collaterals (Fig. 21-41). This may be the only treatment required, or the occlusion of large aortopulmonary collaterals to a CTM may make subsequent surgery safer. It should be stated that the role of embolization in congenital disorders of the lung, other than pulmonary arteriovenous fistula, is controversial.

Bronchoscopy

The most clear-cut use of bronchoscopy is in the investigation of stridor (see earlier in the chapter). In all but typical cases of laryngomalacia, this investigation should be performed at an early stage. Multiple causes of stridor are not uncommon, and all of the accessible respiratory tract should be examined. Bronchoscopy should not be delayed by performing a series of nondiagnostic imaging studies. In

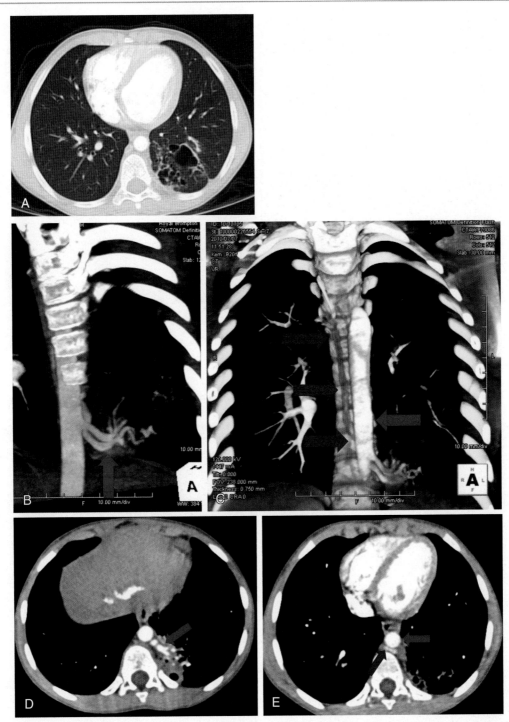

FIGURE 21-39. CT scan with contrast injection investigation of a left-sided congenital thoracic malformation. **A,** Note the large, multicystic CTM in the left lower lobe. **B,** The reconstruction shows that there are large aortopulmonary collaterals to the mass *(red arrow).* **C,** The venous drainage *(blue arrows)* passes behind the aorta *(red arrow)* and cranially to drain into the azygous system. **D,** The CTM is supplied by collaterals arising from the aorta below the diaphragm. **E,** Note the venous drainage *(blue arrow)* lying behind the aorta *(red arrow).*

other contexts, bronchoscopy is probably best combined with other procedures requiring a general anesthetic, such as angiography (see earlier in the chapter). Other than for the investigation of stridor, an anesthetic can rarely be justified solely for bronchoscopy in the context of congenital lung disease. Ideally, the procedure should be performed under general anesthesia via a facemask, so that the whole of the airway including the larynx can be inspected under

conditions of quiet respiration. First, bronchial arrangement can be verified. Second, abnormalities of the bronchial wall such as complete cartilage rings or compression by a vascular ring can be ascertained. Finally, the presence of blind-ending bronchial stumps can be determined; these may act as a reservoir for infection. Another role for bronchoscopy is the assessment of airway narrowing in the case of aberrant origin of the left subclavian artery.

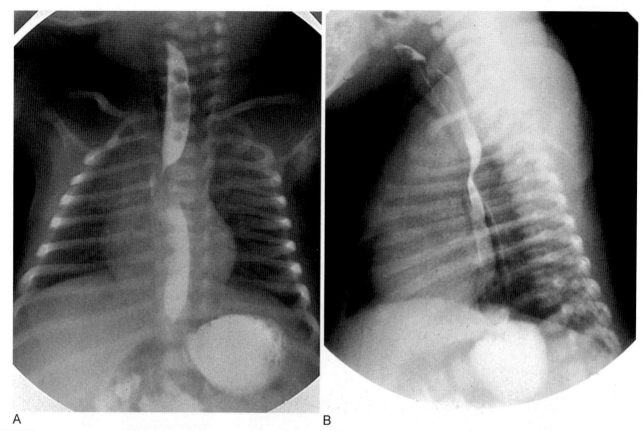

FIGURE 21-40. Barium swallow showing the indentation of a vascular ring (double aortic arch). **A,** Posteroanterior view. **B,** Lateral view.

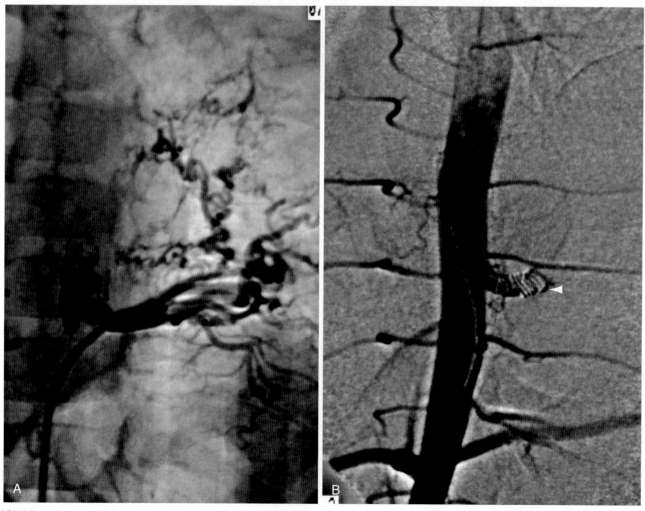

FIGURE 21-41. Digital subtraction angiogram before (**A**) and after (**B**) coil embolization of a large aortopulmonary collateral supplying a cystic congenital thoracic malformation in the left lower lobe. The arrow in **B** points to the site of the coil occlusion.

This may be a harmless normal variant or may cause significant airway narrowing if a left arterial ligament completes a vascular ring. In doubtful cases, bronchoscopic inspection of the airway is indicated. Finally, H-type fistula may be missed on esophageal tube injection and only detected by bronchoscopy.

Low-Contrast Volume Bronchography

Airway malacia can be visualized directly and further documented by performing a limited bronchogram with a soluble contrast medium.[181] Unlike the bronchograms carried out before the advent of CT scanning, the purpose is to delineate the major airways, not to achieve alveolar filling, and only very small volumes of water-soluble contrast are required.

SPECIFIC TREATMENT ISSUES

Details of the treatment of specific conditions can be found in the foregoing sections. For many abnormalities, surgery is the best and definitive treatment. For all but the smallest, sickest infants, lobectomy is a safe and well-tolerated procedure, with few if any significant sequelae. Segmentectomy may even be feasible in some cases, with preservation of normal lung tissue.[182] However, pneumonectomy carries a significant mortality in infancy. There is also considerable long-term morbidity, in particular scoliosis, which may worsen dramatically during the pubertal growth spurt. In general, asymptomatic congenital cystic disease merits surgery because it is likely that there will be a complicating infection of the cyst eventually, which may make the operation more difficult.

It should be remembered that children with complex malformations (e.g., unilateral CSL with abnormal vasculature) may be asymptomatic for long periods despite a formidable list of abnormalities. A conservative approach, perhaps occluding any aortopulmonary collaterals, may be adequate.

LONG-TERM FOLLOW-UP

There are several issues to be considered, including the effects of previous treatment (usually lung resection) and the needs of the child with a malformation that is being managed conservatively.

In general, lobectomy is well tolerated. The effects of lung resection have been reviewed[143]; issues include the total amount of resection and the age at operation (and thus the possibility of new lung tissue formation). Human and animal data are difficult to interpret, but in general it is extent, not age, of resection that is important. A related issue is whether a large malformation, such as a CLHL can so compress normal lung as to interfere with its growth. The evidence seems to be that this is not the case, and that even very large lobes can be left intact unless the infant is symptomatic.

SUMMARY

Congenital lung disease can present at any time from 20 weeks of gestation to old age and should at least be considered as part of the differential diagnosis in many clinical situations. The lesions may regress to virtually nothing, or require relatively straightforward surgery, or be among the most complex therapeutic challenges encountered. The chief need is for information about the long-term consequences of many of the lesions diagnosed antenatally, so that more precise counseling can be provided. Children with congenital lung disease should be enrolled in registries and followed in a systematic manner. Another need is for refinement of MRI scanning so that it can be performed without general anesthesia and give more precise information about parenchymal abnormalities, to obviate the need for radiation exposure.

Finally, when this chapter was updated, it was clear that underlying genetic abnormalities are being discovered for a number of congenital malformations. This is undoubtedly a fruitful area for further study and will require the formation of consortia of interested multidisciplinary teams and basic scientists to move the field forward.

Suggested Reading

Bush A. Prenatal presentation and postnatal management of congenital thoracic malformations. *Early Hum Dev.* 2009;85:679–684.

Bush A, Hogg J, Chitty LS. Cystic lung lesions—prenatal diagnosis and management. *Prenat Diagn.* 2008;28:604–611.

Deprest JA, Flake AW, Eduard Gratacos E, et al. The making of fetal surgery. *Prenat Diagn.* 2010;30:653–667.

Hsu CC, Kwan GN, Thompson SA, et al. Embolisation therapy for pulmonary arteriovenous malformations. *Cochrane Database Syst Rev.* 2010;(5): CD008017.

Knox EM, Kilby MD, Martin WL, et al. In-utero pulmonary drainage in the management of primary hydrothorax and congenital cystic lung lesion: a systematic review. *Ultrasound Obstet Gynecol.* 2006;28:726–734.

Knox E, Lissauer D, Khan K, et al. Prenatal detection of pulmonary hypoplasia in fetuses with congenital diaphragmatic hernia: a systematic review and meta-analysis of diagnostic studies. *J Matern Fetal Neonatal Med.* 2010;23:579–588.

Lansdale N, Alam S, Losty PD, et al. Neonatal endosurgical congenital diaphragmatic hernia repair: a systematic review and meta-analysis. *Ann Surg.* 2010;252:20–26.

Langston C. New concepts in the pathology of congenital lung malformations. *Semin Pediatr Surg.* 2003;12:17–37.

Stanton M, Njere I, Ade-Ajayi N, et al. Sytematic review and meta-analysis of the postnatal management of congenital cystic lung lesions. *J Pediatr Surg.* 2009;44:1027–1033.

Zach MS, Eber E. Adult outcome of congenital lower respiratory tract malformations. *Thorax.* 2001;56:65–72.

References

The complete reference list is available online at www.expertconsult.com

22 RESPIRATORY DISORDERS IN THE NEWBORN

Anne Greenough, MD (Cantab), MBBS, DCH, FRCP, FRCPCH, Vadivelam Murthy, MD, and Anthony D. Milner, MD, FRCP, DCH

Respiratory disorders are the most common cause of neonatal unit admission and a major cause of neonatal mortality and morbidity. This chapter describes the etiology, presentation, management, and outcome of neonatal respiratory disorders, as well as the initiation of respiration at birth and resuscitation. Relevant congenital anomalies are described in Chapter 21.

▬ RESPIRATORY DEPRESSION AT BIRTH

Initiation of Respiration at Birth

Fetal breathing activity is essential for normal lung growth. It can be detected as early as 14 weeks of gestation in the human. The amount of time the fetus spends breathing increases with advancing gestational age. Fetal breathing activity ceases during labor. At birth, one of the most important stimuli to initiate breathing is cooling. In addition, audiovisual, proprioceptive, and touch stimuli recruit central neurons and increase central arousal.[1] The central chemoreceptor areas are activated at birth, as indicated by the expression of immediate early genes, such as *c-fos;* skin cooling may be involved in this activation. Also, a switching on of genes encoding neurotransmitters involved in respiratory control occurs. Hypoxia mediated by central chemoreceptors is important to the onset of respiration, but peripheral chemoreceptor activity is not critical. Birth is also associated with the removal of respiratory inhibitory mechanisms, including prostaglandins and adenosine. Prostaglandin E_2 inhibits fetal breathing movements (FBM), and prostaglandin inhibitors (e.g., indomethacin) stimulate FBM. Plasma concentrations of PGE_2 decrease at birth, and it has been suggested that this may be important for the onset of respiration. PGE_1 and E_2 depress ventilation in the neonate. The median time for the onset of respiratory activity in the healthy full-term neonate has been demonstrated to be 10 seconds.[2] A high negative inspiratory pressure (>20 cmH$_2$O) was required to overcome the high flow resistance and inertia of liquid in the airways, as well as the surface tension at the air-liquid interface.[3] Expiration is also active for the first few breaths to aid the distribution of ventilation and further fluid clearance from the lungs. A functional residual capacity (FRC) is formed following the first breath in over 95% of infants. Following vaginal delivery, the FRC is usually fully formed by 2 hours, but compliance increases more slowly over the first 24 hours as lung liquid is gradually absorbed.

Respiratory Depression at Birth

Failure of adequate initiation of respiration at birth can occur because of birth depression (asphyxia), drugs that depress respiration, trauma to the central nervous system, anemia, sepsis, and congenital malformations. It is more common in prematurely born infants, and the requirement for active resuscitation is inversely related to gestational age at birth. In newborn animals, after acute postnatal asphyxia there is an early period of apnea, which is called *primary apnea.* Primary apnea can last up to 10 minutes, but usually after 1 or 2 minutes gasps occur with increasing frequency until the last gasp. The period of apnea that follows is called *secondary* or *terminal apnea.* During this time, the heart rate falls rapidly, but it may continue for at least 10 minutes after the last gasp. The blood pressure falls, paralleling the changes in heart rate, and a severe mixed academia and hyperkalemia develop. If the infant is in primary apnea, he or she can be provoked to breathe by peripheral stimuli (e.g., being rubbed with a warm towel), whereas in secondary apnea active resuscitation by positive pressure ventilation is required. The newborn can survive at least 20 minutes of complete oxygen deprivation as the neonatal brain can metabolize lactate and ketones. In addition, infants have large glycogen stores in their brain, liver, and myocardium, which can be metabolized anaerobically to produce energy. Growth-retarded infants, who have low glycogen stores, are less able to withstand oxygen deprivation. Birth depression can result in hypoxic ischemic encephalopathy, convulsions, and abnormal neurodevelopmental outcome. Affected infants may also suffer myocardial ischemia and heart failure, pulmonary hemorrhage, and acute tubular necrosis. Respiratory distress is worsened by asphyxia as pulmonary blood flow falls during asphyxia, but after the asphyxia has ceased there is a reactive hyperemia. This is associated with fluid transudation and edema; the protein-rich edema fluid inhibits surfactant function, and any persisting academia inhibits surfactant synthesis. At 1 and 5 minutes following birth, the infant's color, respiratory activity, heart rate, tone, and response to stimuli are assessed and the Apgar scores are calculated. A low Apgar score at 5 minutes is associated with the development of long-term neurologic problems.

Delivery Room Resuscitation

Approximately 10% of infants require some form of resuscitation, and approximately 2% require intubation and positive pressure ventilation. The International Liaison Committee on Resuscitation (ILCOR) and American Heart Association/American Academy of Pediatrics (AHA/AAP) have produced consensus statements on the procedures that should be followed if a newborn fails to breathe adequately; the following remarks reflect their recommendations.[4,5] Infants who fail to establish regular respiration by

1 minute but have a heart rate in excess of 80 bpm should be provided with facial oxygen. Routine oropharyngeal suction should not be undertaken as it will inhibit the onset of respiratory effort if applied too vigorously.[6] If the infant fails to show an immediate response but still has a heart rate in excess of 80/min, facemask resuscitation should commence using inflation pressures of 25 to 30 cm H_2O and inspiratory times of 2 to 3 seconds for 5 breaths to aid the formation of a functional residual capacity. This is most easily achieved using a round facemask and a T-piece in the inspiratory line, as bag-and-mask systems produce more variable inflation pressures and tend to deflate in less than 1 second. Resuscitation should then continue with inflation times of 0.5 to 1 seconds at approximately 30 inflations per minute. This is successful in the majority of term infants. Intubation and ventilation should be undertaken in infants in whom facemask ventilation fails to produce an improvement in oxygen saturation or respiratory efforts within 30 seconds or who have a heart rate that is either below 60 bpm at birth or falls despite basic resuscitation using the same ventilatory settings. Results from randomized trials have highlighted that the onset of spontaneous breathing and crying were significantly delayed in infants being resuscitated with 100% oxygen rather than air and that the use of air significantly reduces mortality and tends to reduce the incidence of severe hypoxic ischemic encephalopathy.[7] As a consequence, the current consensus is that resuscitation with air is at least as good as 100% oxygen for most asphyxiated term infants, but some infants may require supplementary oxygen.

External cardiac massage should be commenced in all infants whose heart rate is below 60 bpm and who fail to improve within 30 seconds of onset of adequate ventilatory support. Cardiac massage is best achieved by placing both hands around the chest so that the thumbs are over the lower part of the sternum and the fingertips close to the spine. The sternum is then depressed by one third of the diameter of the chest, approximately 2 cm. A ratio of three compressions to one inflation, with a rate of 120 "events" (that is 90 compressions and 30 inflations) per minute is recommended. Chest compressions can be discontinued once the heart rate exceeds 80 bpm. If the heart rate fails to improve on commencing external cardiac massage, adrenaline should be given. The preferred route is intravenously via the umbilical vein[5] (0.1 to 0.3 mL/kg of 1:10,000 strength) rather than injecting down the endotracheal tube. Administration of sodium bicarbonate (a dose of 1 to 2 mEq/kg of a 0.5 mEq/ml solution given over at least 2 minutes[8] should be restricted to those with prolonged arrest, as giving bicarbonate may reduce cerebral blood flow and may lead to intracranial hemorrhages in preterm infants because of the large osmotic load. Naloxone (0.1 mg/kg intravenous/intramuscular)[8] should only be given to infants who are receiving adequate ventilatory support and if the infant's respiratory depression has resulted from maternal opiate administration. Naloxone should not be given to the newborns of opiate-addicted mothers, as this will precipitate acute withdrawal symptoms. Group O Rh-negative blood (10 ml/kg body weight) should be given over 5 to 10 minutes if the infant is hypotensive due to blood loss. If there is no response to 30 minutes of full resuscitation, consideration

should be given to stopping resuscitative measures as the infant's prognosis is very poor. It is important, however, to consider any underlying conditions that may make the infant difficult to resuscitate (e.g., congenital diaphragmatic hernia, pneumothorax, or hypoplastic lungs).

Resuscitation of Preterm Infants

Preterm infants present a greater problem than term infants. On one hand, they often have insufficient surfactant in their lungs, which results in low compliance. This indicates that high inflation pressures should be used, yet there is evidence that the use of excess ventilatory tidal volumes (volutrauma) may increase the incidence of chronic lung disease.[9] Volutrauma may occur at resuscitation if rapid lung expansion is attempted; prematurely born lambs given six manual inflations of 35 to 40 mL/kg, compared with those not "bagged" at birth, had poorer lung function at 4 hours of age as indicated by lower inspiratory capacities,[10] and those exposed to high tidal volumes at resuscitation had a poorer response to surfactant therapy.[11] A compromise is to initially attempt to resuscitate preterm infants with inflation pressures of 18 to 20/5 cm H_2O, but to increase the peak pressures if there is no response.[12] There is limited information on whether initial inflation times in excess of 1 second are beneficial in preterm infants, although a single study found that an initial inflation pressure of 20 to 25 cm H_2O maintained for 20 seconds, followed by continuous positive airway pressure reduced the incidence of chronic lung disease.[13] Among prematurely born infants, use of air at resuscitation may fail to achieve target oxygen saturations in the first 3 minutes after birth.[14] Resuscitation, however, can be effective when initiated with 30% oxygen, which is then adjusted to the infant's needs.[15] There is little evidence that either adrenaline or external cardiac massage have a role in role in the resuscitation of infants born at less than 26 weeks of gestation. It is important to maintain normal body temperature during the stabilization of very premature infants; plastic bags or plastic wrapping in combination with overhead radiant heat is more effective than the conventional drying and wrapping approach.[16]

■ CONTROL OF BREATHING

A loose complex of respiratory neurons ("center") that lie within the ventrolateral region of the brainstem generate the respiratory cycle. The phasic transition from inspiration to expiration is modulated by input from the slowly adapting pulmonary stretch receptors and pontine neurons; suppression of either input prolongs inspiration (apneusis). The rhythm is transmitted to spinal motor neurons and cranial premotor neurons; the latter control the activity of airway muscles. Afferents from the forebrain, hypothalamus, central and peripheral chemoreceptors, muscles, joints, and pain receptors are integrated into the "center." Most areas contain multiple neuromodulators that are partly released from the same neurons, thus neuromodulation occurs at all level of integration.[17] The number of intersynaptic connections reaches a peak towards the end of fetal life. The excitatory neurotransmitter, glutamate, excites receptors involved in generating and transmitting respiratory rhythms to spinal and cranial respiratory neurons. Serotonin (5HT) neurons in the medulla oblongata compose a critical system in the modulation of autonomic and respiratory effector neurons[18]; serotonin's most consistent effect is to restore a normal breathing pattern in hypoxia or ischemia. Opioids (endorphins and exogenous drugs) decrease respiration by peripheral and central actions; the latter are due to suppression of recurrent excitation by glutaminergic inputs within the primary respiratory network. Both γ-aminobutyric acid (GABA) and glycine are essential for generating respiratory rhythm; they are released by late and postinspiratory neurons and turn off inspiratory neurons, thus facilitating the transition from inspiration to expiration. Deficiency of glycinergic inhibition in knockout mice results in a slower frequency of breathing.

Central and peripheral chemoreceptors modify respiratory activity in response to changes in blood gases. The central chemoreceptors are situated near the ventral surface of the medulla and respond to changes in carbon dioxide/pH and oxygen. The peripheral chemoreceptors are situated at the bifurcation of the common carotid arteries (carotid bodies) and above and below the aortic arch (aortic bodies). In the fetus, the arterial chemoreceptors are active but have reduced sensitivity. The peripheral chemoreceptors are not essential for the initiation of respiration and are virtually silenced when the arterial oxygen level rises at birth. Resetting of the carotid chemoreceptors to hypoxia occurs within 24 to 48 hours of birth[19]; this may result from changes in dopamine levels. The fetus responds to hypoxia with a suppression of ventilation; the hypoxic suppression of ventilation is mediated by the lateral part of the lower pons. In response to hypoxia, there is a redistribution of the circulation to favor the heart, brain, and adrenals; this minimizes oxygen consumption and conserves oxygen supplies for vital organs. Hyperoxia stimulates continuous fetal breathing. In the perinatal period, the newborn has a biphasic response to hypoxia—a transient increase in minute ventilation followed by a decrease to or below baseline levels. The initial increase in ventilation is probably due to activation of peripheral chemoreceptors, and the subsequent reduction in ventilation may result from a fall in carbon dioxide tensions following the initial hyperventilation or the suppressant effect of hypoxia, which occurs in the fetal state and persists into the neonatal period. Very immature infants respond to hypoxia in a similar fashion to fetuses that is with apnea. The biphasic response to hypoxia disappears at 12 to 14 days, and the adult pattern is then seen (i.e., stimulation of breathing without depression). Exposure to a hyperoxic gas causes a temporary suppression of breathing due to withdrawal of peripheral chemoreceptor drive. After a few minutes of hyperoxia, ventilation increases to above control levels probably because of hyperoxic cerebral vasoconstriction resulting in increased brain tissue carbon dioxide. Immaturity and prolonged exposure to supplementary oxygen reduce the response to hyperoxia. The fetus and newborn respond to increased carbon dioxide levels with an increase in breathing activity. The slope of ventilatory response to carbon dioxide is less in term infants during active than quiet sleep and in preterm infants, but it increases with postnatal growth.

Respiratory activity is also affected by stimulation of respiratory reflexes. Hering and Breuer described three respiratory reflexes; an inflation, an expiratory, and a deflation reflex. The Hering-Breuer inflation reflex is stimulated by lung inflation and results in cessation of respiratory activity. In the newborn, the reflex produces a pattern of rapid, shallow tidal breathing and operates within the tidal volume range. In older subjects, the reflex prevents excessive tidal volumes and can only be stimulated if the inflating volume is increased above a critical threshold.[20] The Hering-Breuer expiratory reflex is stimulated if inflation is prolonged; the active expiration seen in infants ventilated at slow rates and long inflation times, and which may result in pneumothoraces, may be a manifestation of this reflex.[21] In animal models, the Hering-Breuer deflation reflex is evidenced by a prolonged inspiration generated in response to deflating the lung rapidly or following an unusually vigorous expiratory effort that takes the lung below its end expiratory level.[22] In the newborn, this reflex may have a role in maintaining the functional residual capacity. Head's paradoxical reflex, also called the *inspiratory augmenting reflex* or *provoked augmented inspiration*, is the underlying mechanism of the first breath and sighing. A rapid inflation stimulates a stronger diaphragmatic contraction. The reflex improves compliance and reopens partially collapsed airways[23]; it has an important role in promoting lung expansion during resuscitation. Rapid chest wall distortion via the intercostal phrenic inhibitory reflex results in a shortening of inspiratory efforts. This reflex response is inhibited by an increase in FRC or applying continuous positive airway pressure (CPAP). The mechanism may be improved chest wall stability.[24] Inhalation of toxic gases such as nitrogen dioxide and sulfur dioxide causes a change in the frequency and depth of respiration via stimulation of subepithelial chemoreceptors in the trachea, bronchi, and bronchioles. The response is less in REM sleep and in the premature infant.[25] The presence of upper airway reflexes results in cold exposure stimulating breathing via trigeminal afferents in the facial skin, whereas irritant stimuli to the nasal mucosa cause inhibition of breathing. The laryngeal chemoreceptors defend the lower airway from inhalation. Maturation of the laryngeal chemoreflex is characterized by an increase in coughing and a decrease in swallowing and apnea.[26]

Periodic Breathing

Periodic breathing is characterized by regular cycles of breathing of 10 to18 seconds duration, which are interrupted by pauses of at least 3 seconds in duration. This pattern recurs for at least 2 minutes. Periodic breathing is a benign condition and not a precursor of significant apnea. The frequency of periodic breathing decreases with increasing postmenstrual age and administration of methylxanthines and increases with increases in altitude.

Apnea

Apnea is defined as cessation of breathing for at least 10 seconds; a duration of at least 20 seconds is frequently used to diagnose significant apneas, as normal infants do not have apneas of greater than 20 seconds. Apneas are classified as central, obstructive, or mixed. Central apnea is characterized by total cessation of inspiratory efforts without upper airway obstruction, whereas in obstructive apnea the upper airway is obstructed (so there is no airflow despite chest wall movements). Mixed apnea, a combination of central and obstructive apneas, accounts for 50% of all apneas; 40% are central, and 10% are obstructive. Bradycardia may occur within a few seconds of onset of apnea with accompanying changes in blood pressure and cerebral blood flow velocity. In infants without adequate cerebrovascular autoregulation, cerebral perfusion may decrease to very low levels during prolonged apnea and potentially exacerbate hypoxic-ischemic brain injury. The incidence of apnea of prematurity is inversely related to gestational age and usually resolves by about 37 to 40 weeks postmenstrual age. Other causes of apnea include infection, intracranial abnormality or hemorrhage, anemia, metabolic disorders (especially hypoglycemia and temperature instability), and gastroesophageal reflux (GER) (see later in the chapter). Certain pharmacologic agents can cause apnea, including barbiturates and sedatives.

Minor episodes of apnea respond to stimulation. Additional treatment is required if the apneas are frequent or severe or are associated with prolonged desaturation. Treatment with methylxanthines, theophylline, and caffeine reduces apnea in preterm infants. Caffeine is the preferred agent because once-a-day dosing is possible due to its longer half-life, and it has a higher therapeutic index than theophylline. Side effects of theophylline include hyperactivity, tachycardia, cardiac dysrhythmias, feeding intolerance, and seizures. Caffeine treatment in infants with or at risk for apnea of prematurity has also been shown to reduce BPD[27] and improve survival without neurodevelopmental delay.[28] Prophylactic caffeine reduces apnea/bradycardia and episodes of oxygen desaturation in preterm infants following postoperative anesthesia.[29] Doxapram, a respiratory stimulant, has been used to treat apnea but has many side effects, and any long-term effects need to be investigated. Inhalation of low-dose CO_2 may also reduce apneas, but again long-term effects have not been assessed.[30] Infants with troublesome apnea despite treatment with methylxanthines may benefit from CPAP. The frequency of apnea is decreased by increasing the functional residual capacity, stabilizing oxygenation, and/or by splinting the upper airway. CPAP is effective in infants whose episodes are precipitated or prolonged by pharyngeal obstruction. CPAP distends both the pharynx and laryngeal aperture and so prevents mixed and obstructive apneas, but it has no effect on central apnea. Infants with severe and refractory apnea may need to be intubated and supported by mechanical ventilation; minimal ventilator settings should be used to reduce the risk of volutrauma.

Gastroesophageal Reflux

GER should be suspected in neonates with recurrent respiratory problems, especially if there is right upper lobe collapse or consolidation on the chest radiograph. Although apnea may be the presenting symptom of GER in some premature infants, in most infants GER is unrelated to apnea.[31] In those with recurrent apneas, only approximately 10% were temporally related to GER,[32] and treatment with metoclopramide and ranitidine did not reduce bradycardic episodes in preterm infants with GER.[33] In asymptomatic preterm infants, there was no significant correlation between the amount of acid GER and the number of either obstructive or total apnea episodes.[34] The diagnosis may be suggested by the demonstration of significant levels of fat-laden macrophages or Pepsin in the tracheobronchial secretions, or more usually by radiological or pH or impedance probe demonstration of reflux. Apnea preceded by a fall in pH to less than 4, recorded by a probe placed in the esophagus, is diagnostic of reflux-stimulated apnea. Although pH monitoring is often considered the standard diagnostic test, its use is limited in preterm infants, as their gastric pH is >4 for 90% of the time. Impedance testing, which will detect non-acid reflux, is an alternative, but there is no evidence that non-acid reflux causes symptoms or reflux disease.[35] Before undertaking a Nissan's fundoplication, a contrast study should be undertaken to confirm reflux.

Episodes of troublesome apnea with complications (e.g., recurrent aspiration attributed to apnea) should be treated, but apneas in general should not be treated with anti-reflux medication.[35] The volume of feed given at any one time should be reduced, and the infant should be given frequent small-volume feeds or feeds continuously. If the symptoms persist, "thickeners" should be given or nasojejunal feeding instituted. In the presence of gastric acid, alginates precipitate forming a gel that floats on the surface of the gastric contents and provides a relative neutral barrier; Gaviscon (sodium alginate) can increase the sodium content of feed, which may be undesirable in very prematurely born infants.[36] Nursing the infant prone can reduce GER. Antacids should be given to infants who have esophagitis. Proton pump inhibitors (e.g., lansoprazole) have been administered to infants with GER but were not more effective than placebo in a randomized trial of infants 1 to 12 months of age.[37] Prokinetic agents have been used in infants with GER. Erythromycin binds to motilin receptors and stimulates gastric antral contractions and induces antral migrating motor complexes, which are important for gastric emptying. Treatment with erythomycin was associated with more positive effects in improving feeding intolerance when a higher dose (40-50 mg/kg/day) was used or the treated infants were 32 weeks gestational age or older.[38] Infants who have troublesome GER resistant to all the previously mentioned treatments may require a fundoplication, however this is rarely required.[38a]

◼ RESPIRATORY DISTRESS SYNDROME

Approximately 1% of infants develop respiratory distress syndrome (RDS). The risk of RDS is inversely proportional to gestational age. Babies with RDS have noncompliant lungs, which contain less surfactant than normal (see later in the chapter). Hyaline membranes line the terminal airways, hence the alternative name of *hyaline membrane disease.*

Pathophysiology

RDS is due to immaturity of the lung resulting in surfactant deficiency. Poor clearing of lung fluid, inadequate respiratory efforts, and underdeveloped chest wall and respiratory muscles compound the infants problems. Surfactant is produced in alveolar type II cells, which are cuboidal cells covering about 2% of the alveolar surface and account for 15% of the cell numbers. They differentiate from the columnar epithelium during the canalicular phase of development but are not prominent until about 24 weeks of gestation. Surfactant is a complex mixture of substances including phospholipids, neutral lipids, and proteins. Lipids are the major constituent of surfactant; the most important are phosphatidylcholine and phosphatidylglycerol, representing 70% to 80% and 5% to 10% of the lipids respectively. Approximately 60% of the phosphatidylcholine is saturated, and the primary saturated fatty acid is palmitic acid, hence it is called *disaturated palmityl phosphatidylcholine (DPPC)*. Phosphatidylinositol, phosphatidylserine, and phosphatidylethanolamine make up a further 10% of the lipids in surfactant. About 10% of the total lipids in surfactant are neutral lipids: cholesterol, triacylglycerols, and free fatty acid. Cholesterol alters the fluidity and organization of lipid-rich membranes. Sphingomyelin represents less than 2% of surfactant lipid.

Surfactant is synthesized in the endoplasmic reticulum; the phospholipid then moves via intracellular pathways to the lamellar bodies, which unravel to highly surface active tubular myelin. There is direct transition from the tubular myelin to the surface film, with absorption of a mixture of saturated and unsaturated phospholipids. The surface film is then refined by selectively squeezing out unsaturated phospholipids, generating small vesicular forms of surfactant, which have poor surfactant activity. They are mainly taken up by type II cells, although some are degraded by macrophages or lost from the airways. The loss of surfactant into the airways is proportional to the rate and depth of respiration and can be reduced by addition of continuous positive airway pressure. Surfactant lost in this way is swallowed or, in fetal life, moves into the amniotic fluid. Surfactant may be degraded locally in the alveoli and small airways, the breakdown products being absorbed and recycled by the alveolar cells. More than 90% of the phosphatidylcholine on the alveolar surface is reprocessed, the turnover time being approximately 10 hours. There is negative feedback regulation of surfactant production, which is mediated by surfactant protein A binding to type II cells. Surfactant secretion is controlled by stretch receptors and stimulated by alveolar distension. β-adrenergic receptors on alveolar type II cells, which increase in number toward the end of gestation, also control secretion.

The palmitic acid residues of DPPC are nonpolar and hydrophobic and orient toward the air, whereas the head group of phosphatidylcholine is polar and hydrophilic and associates with the liquid phase. DPPC is a symmetrical molecule, and the two straight hydrophobic fatty acid chains allow close packing of the monolayer. Compression of such a monolayer results in it being changed from a liquid to a condensed gel or solid state. As the radius decreases, the presence of an insoluble surface film means that the surface tension is reduced and the "solid" monolayer formed in expiration promotes stability of the alveoli and prevents atelectasis. The reduction in surface tension decreases the work of breathing and prevents transudation of fluid; in conditions of high surface tension, fluid is sucked into the alveolar spaces from the capillaries. DPPC is relatively rigid at body temperature and cannot move rapidly enough to maintain a surface monolayer during the respiratory cycle; hence a "spreading" agent such as phosphatidylglycerol (PG) is required. Initially, PI is the primary acidic phospholipid, but with increasing lung maturation PI is replaced by PG. In RDS, PG is absent and there are also low levels of phosphatidylcholine, which is relatively unsaturated. As a consequence, the resulting monolayer formed in expiration is unstable and does not reduce surface tension effectively; once the monolayer has been refined, there is so little DPPC available the alveoli are of small size. Thus, infants with RDS have a low functional residual capacity and noncompliant lungs and their work of breathing is increased. The alveolar hypoventilation results in ventilation perfusion imbalance and hypoxia. The increased alveolar surface tension secondary to the lack of surfactant promotes the flow of protein-rich fluid from the intravascular space to the interstitium and the alveolar spaces. This leak is increased as hypoxia damages the integrity of the alveolar capillary membrane. These plasma proteins inhibit surfactant function by adsorbing onto the alveolar surface. The infant's lungs then become stiffer and more atelectatic, and a vicious cycle occurs.

The four surfactant-associated proteins, SP-A, SP-B, SP-C, and SP-D compose 5% to 10% of surfactant by weight. SP-A is composed of 248 amino acids and belongs to the calcium-dependent collectin family of proteins. The human gene is located on chromosome 10; gene expression occurs exclusively in type II pneumocytes. The synthesis of SP-A increases after 28 weeks of gestation. The roles of SP-A include determining the structure of tubular myelin, the stability and rapidity of spreading and recycling of phospholipids. SP-A and SP-D are part of the innate host defense against infection. As collectins, they target carbohydrate structures on invading microorganisms, particularly bacteria, resulting in agglutination and enhanced clearance. SP-A binds endotoxin and a wide range of Gram-positive and Gram-negative organisms, thus promoting phagocytosis and killing of microorganisms by alveolar macrophages. It acts also as an opsonin for the phagocytosis of viruses, such as herpes simplex, influenza A, and respiratory syncytial virus. SP-A increases nitric oxide production by macrophages to promote pathogen killing. SP-A polymorphisms have been associated with severe respiratory syncytial virus infection and increased risk of bronchopulmonary dysplasia (BPD).[39] The *SP-B* gene is located on chromosome 2. The mRNA for SP-B is detectable in the epithelial cells of bronchi and bronchioles at 12 to 14 weeks of gestation and after 25 weeks in type II cells. SP-B is required for the formation of tubular myelin and increases the spreading of surfactant phospholipids onto an air-water interface. SP-B is important for surface activity; SP-C and SP-B together are more effective. SP-B can also protect the pulmonary surfactant film from inactivation by serum proteins.[40] The absence of SP-B is associated with markedly decreased phosphatidylglycerol and an additional aberrant SP-C peptide. DPPC synthesis is preserved in SP-B deficiency, but SP-C cannot be processed to its active peptide and no secretion of normal surfactant occurs. In SP-B knockout mice, lamellar bodies and tubular myelin structures are absent. SP-B deficiency is an autosomal recessive inherited disorder and causes lethal hypoxemic respiratory failure. The gene frequency of the 121ins2 frame shift mutation (which accounts for 60% to 70% of cases) is 1 per 1000 to 3000, and the estimated disease incidence is 1 in 1.5 million.[41] Partial deficiencies of SP-B with less severe clinical courses have now been reported.[42] SP-B polymorphisms may explain differences in the risk of RDS between African-American and Caucasian subjects and between males and females. The *SP-C* gene is located on chromosome 8. The mRNA for SP-C is present early in lung development at the distal tips of the branching airways, but subsequently occurs only in the type II cells. SP-C enhances surface adsorption and spreading of phospholipids and may play a role in enhancing the re-uptake of phospholipids. SP-C mutations have been associated with interstitial lung disease presenting in newborns and children.[43] SP-B and SP-C mutations are reviewed in more detail in Chapter 56. SP-D production begins in the bronchiolar and terminal epithelium from about 21 weeks of gestation. SP-D expression is widely distributed in epithelial cells in the body; in the lung SP-D expression occurs in the type II cells, Clara cells, and other airway cells and glands. Glucocorticoids increase SP-D expression. SP-D is involved in the immune function of the lung, binding to a variety of complex carbohydrates and glycolipids, and it may have a role in host defense functions in the lung by interacting with the surfaces of bacteria and other microorganisms. An SP-D polymorphism has been associated with a lower number of repetitive surfactant doses and a lower requirement for supplementary oxygen at day 28.[44]

Many factors influence lung maturation and surfactant production and hence whether an infant develops RDS. Both cortisol and thyroxine increase lung maturation. β-adrenergic drugs increase the amount of intracellular cAMP, thus increasing the production and secretion of surfactant. Insulin delays the maturation of alveolar type II cells, decreasing the proportion of saturated phosphatidylcholine and inhibiting SP-A and SP-B mRNA accumulation and SP-A gene expression in vitro.[45] In addition, infants of diabetic mothers have delayed appearance of phosphatidylglycerol. Pulmonary maturity may also be delayed in infants with severe hemolytic disease of the newborn; this may be because of increased levels of insulin due to beta-islet cell hypertrophy. Boys are much more likely to develop RDS than girls, with a male-to-female ratio of 1.7:1; boys are also more likely to die from the disease. Boys' lungs are approximately 1 week more immature than girls' lungs; they have delayed maturation of the L:S ratio and late appearance of phosphatidylglycerol due to inhibition of synthesis by fetal androgens. Androgens delay lung maturation through their action on lung fibroblasts.[46] African babies have a lower incidence of RDS compared to Caucasian babies—60% to 70% of that of Caucasian babies of the same gestational age; in one series, only 40% of African infants less than 32 weeks gestational age developed RDS compared to 75% of the Caucasian infants.[47] Allelic variation in the *surfactant protein A* gene has been reported between Caucasian-Americans and Nigerians. Asphyxia, hypoxia, hypotension, and hypothermia can impair surfactant synthesis and/or increase alveolar capillary leakiness. Exposure to cold results in impaired surfactant function; below 34° C, DPPC cannot spread to form an adequately functioning monolayer. Caesarean section carried out before labor increases the risk of both RDS and TTN. A review of nine studies in which the outcome by mode of delivery in at-term or near-term infants was assessed demonstrated that elective caesarian section was associated with an average two- to three-fold increased risk of respiratory morbidities.[48] Each week of gestational age after 35 weeks reduces the risk of respiratory symptoms, particularly if primary caesarian section is performed.[49] Pneumothorax has also been reported to be increased following caesarian section compared to vaginal delivery.[50] Increased intrauterine inflammation decreases the risk of RDS, hence there is a lower incidence of RDS following chorioamnionitis.[51] There is a genetic predisposition to RDS; families in which several relatively mature babies have developed RDS have been reported. Specific alleles of the *SP-A* and *SP-B* genes associate interactively to increase susceptibility to RDS (see earlier in the chapter).[41,52]

Clinical Presentation

In the absence of exposure to antenatal steroids or prophylactic surfactant, infants with RDS present within 4 hours of birth with tachypneic (respiratory rate > 60 breaths/min), intercostal and subcostal in-drawing, sternal retraction, and nasal flaring. Affected infants also have a grunt during expiration. The infant continues to contract the diaphragm in an attempt to delay any reduction in lung volume and simultaneously contracts the constrictor muscles of the larynx to close the upper airway; contraction of the abdominal muscles then results in an explosive exhalation of air, the grunt. The lungs are noncompliant and of small volume; in severe disease the FRC may be as low as 3 mL/kg, whereas the FRC is 25 to 30 mL/kg in recovering babies. In infants who do not receive exogenous surfactant over the first 24 to 36 hours after birth, the dyspnea worsens due to the disappearance of the small quantities of surfactant present in an infant with RDS and the inhibitory effect of plasma proteins on surfactant, which leak onto the alveolar surface in the early edematous stage of lung damage. At approximately 36 to 48 hours of age, endogenous surfactant synthesis commences and the infant's respiratory status improves: this is associated with a spontaneous diuresis. Recovery from RDS can be expected by 1 week of age, although respiratory support still may be required because of the development of complications. Nowadays this classical presentation is unusual, as exogenous surfactant is given; relatively mature infants so treated are frequently in room air by 48 hours of age.

Diagnosis and Differential Diagnosis

Diagnosis of RDS is made on clinical history (including premature birth) and chest radiograph appearance. The chest radiograph shows diffuse atelectasis that results in fine granular opacification in both lung fields and an air bronchogram where the air-filled bronchi stand out against the atelectatic lungs (Fig. 22-1). If the disease is severe, the lungs may be so opaque that it is impossible to distinguish between lung fields and the cardiac silhouette; this is called a *whiteout*. If the radiograph is taken during the first 4 hours, the retention of fetal lung fluid can make interpretation difficult. As the fluid clears, the chest radiograph appearance may show marked improvement. Antenatally, fetal lung maturity can be assessed by sampling amniotic fluid. This is because as the fluid secreted by the fetal lung moves out into the amniotic fluid, it carries surfactant. As the lung matures, the amount of DPPC (lecithin) in the amniotic fluid increases, but the amount of sphingomyelin remains unchanged throughout gestation; thus lung maturity can be assessed from the ratio of lecithin to sphingomyelin (L:S ratio). The lower the L:S ratio, the more likely that the infant will develop RDS: 21% of infants with a ratio of 1.5 to 2.0 are affected, compared to 80% with a ratio <1.5. An L:S ratio <2 predicts RDS with an accuracy of only 54%. An L:S ratio >2.0 usually is associated with lung maturity, and in 95% of cases it will predict the absence of RDS. A mature L:S ratio, however, can be associated with RDS in the infants of diabetic mothers or infants with rhesus disease; in these cases, the abnormality is phosphatidylglycerol deficiency. Further problems in interpreting the L:S ratio can occur when the specimen is contaminated with blood, meconium, or vaginal secretions. The L:S ratio also can be assessed in

fluid from the pharynx or stomach. Pulmonary maturity can be estimated by measuring the level of serum SP-A in cord blood using an enzyme-linked immunosorbent assay (ELISA) system, but the tests are expensive and time-consuming. However, tests of surfactant maturity are now rarely employed, as most clinicians give exogenous surfactant very soon after birth to all infants born below a certain gestational age. The exact cutoff will depend on local resource issues, but infants younger than 28 weeks gestational age usually receive prophylactic surfactant.

It is impossible to differentiate severe early-onset septicemia from RDS, and both conditions may co-exist. Therefore, all dyspneic newborns should have appropriate bacterial cultures taken, and antimicrobials should be administered from the earliest signs of respiratory illness because without treatment, early-onset septicemia can be fatal within hours. Penicillin and gentamicin act synergistically against group B streptococcus and are also effective against many organisms that cause early-onset septicemia and pneumonia. In babies with RDS who are stable or are improving, antimicrobials should be stopped when negative culture results are notified at 48 to 72 hours. Infants with RDS may have co-existent pulmonary hypertension, their oxygen requirement will be out of proportion to their chest radiograph appearance, and they frequently have a poor response to surfactant therapy. Respiratory distress that presents after 4 to 6 hours of age is usually due to pneumonia; the differential diagnosis includes air leak, heart failure secondary to congenital heart disease, or aspiration.

Management

The management of an infant who is at high risk of RDS begins in the labor suite. Practice differs, as some clinicians prefer to place very preterm babies immediately on nasal CPAP (nCPAP), some intubate infants to give them surfactant and then immediately extubate onto nCPAP (INSURE technique), and others prefer keeping the infant intubated until further assessment can take place on the neonatal intensive care unit (NICU) (see later in the chapter). On arrival in the NICU, the infant should be put in an incubator that has been prewarmed to 35° to 36° C or placed under a radiant heater and carefully examined, including measurement of the head circumference and weight. Appropriate monitoring should be implemented to measure blood pressure, and an umbilical arterial catheter (UAC) or peripheral arterial cannula should be inserted to facilitate PaO_2, $PaCO_2$ and pH measurements if the infant has more than mild RDS. A blood sample should be obtained to estimate the hemoglobin level, white blood cell count, and coagulation status, and for culture. A chest radiograph should be taken, preferably after inserting the UAC. Vitamin K and antimicrobials should be given (see earlier in the chapter) and surfactant should be administered if it has not been given in the labor ward. It is then important to handle the infant as little as possible, as this can result in hypoxia. As a consequence, chest physiotherapy and routine endotracheal suctioning are contraindicated in the first 24 to 48 hours. If the blood pressure monitoring reveals the infant to be hypotensive and this is due to anemia, the first transfusion (15 mL/kg)

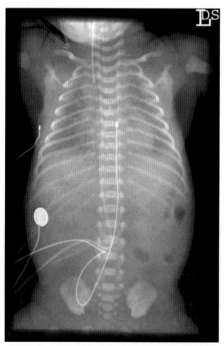

FIGURE 22-1. Chest radiograph of an infant with severe respiratory distress syndrome. Note the diffuse reticulogranular appearance with an air bronchogram.

usually should be given by infusion over 10 to 15 minutes; thereafter transfusions should be given more slowly at a rate guided by the condition of the neonate. Low blood pressure, however, has a poor correlation with poor perfusion in the first 48 hours after birth in sick preterm infants,[53] and infants who are apparently hypotensive on gestational age criteria but with good perfusion may have as good an outcome as normotensive patients.[54] Hence, it is important to treat only those "hypotensive" infants who are symptomatic. Blood loss after birth is usually iatrogenic, but a sudden drop in the hemoglobin level in an infant with RDS suggests the development of an intracerebral hemorrhage. Ventilated preterm neonates tolerate anemia poorly and should be transfused with blood from a CMV-negative donor, which is routine NICU practice; the blood should be irradiated to avoid the risk of graft-versus-host disease. Maintaining a higher rather than a lower hemoglobin threshold for transfusion resulted in more transfusions, but no significant difference in other outcomes in one trial.[55] Only if the infant has a clinically important patent ductus arteriosus (PDA) should he or she receive furosemide (1 mg/kg) during the transfusion. If the hypotensive neonate's hemoglobin is not low, saline should be given rather than albumin because the response to albumin is not better than that to saline, and albumin has more adverse effects.[56] If the neonate is severely hypoxic or acidemic, cardiac function may be impaired; this should be confirmed by echocardiography. In such circumstances, volume expansion will be poorly tolerated and inotropes are the preferred treatment for hypotension. Renal function is often impaired in RDS, and urine production may be less than 1 mL/kg/hour. Peripheral edema, however, is usually due to leaky capillaries. Infants with RDS should be given 40 to 60 mL/kg/24 hours of a 10% dextrose solution, and fluid intake should be subsequently guided by electrolyte levels and change in the infant's weight. High fluid intake in the first days after birth increases the risk of PDA.[57] The ill neonate will lose about 1% to 3% of body weight per day. A greater loss may indicate dehydration, whereas static or increased weight suggests that too much fluid has been given. Sodium and potassium usually do not need to be added to the fluid intake for the first 36 to 48 hours, but calcium may be required. A diuresis occurs around the time the infant's lung function improves; at this time, the fluid input should be increased to prevent dehydration. Since the protein and caloric reserves of the very low birth weight (VLBW) neonate are small, it is essential that some form of nutrition is given as soon as possible after birth. It is important to introduce enteral feeds as soon as possible, as the prolonged absence of enteral feeding compromises gut growth and development. Thus, enteral feeding should be started once bowel sounds are present in a ventilated neonate who is appropriately grown and has passed meconium. Neonates with severe respiratory illness, however, may have an ileus and delayed gastric emptying; as a consequence, enteral feeding is initially not feasible. Parenteral nutrition should be given until an adequate enteral intake has been achieved. There is no evidence to suggest that chest physiotherapy reduces respiratory morbidity in infants with RDS,[58] and it should be avoided because some infants will have pulmonary hypertension.

Surfactant given as a "rescue" therapy improves the outcome of babies with established RDS, resulting in a reduction in pneumothorax, mortality, and the combined outcome of mortality and BPD. Surfactant is, however, more efficacious given prophylactically or early rather than selectively or as rescue therapy.[59-61] Benefits are shown after a single dose of 100 mg/kg, but most studies demonstrate that better results are obtained with more than one dose. Many clinicians usually give two doses of a natural surfactant. Meta-analysis of the results of randomized trials highlighted that administration of natural (animal-derived) rather than synthetic surfactant was associated with a significant reduction in mortality and pneumothorax.[62] Synthetic surfactants are now available that contain proteins. One includes a polypeptide KL4 composed of lysine and leucine that mimics the effects of SPB. This surfactant appears to be resistant to the inhibitory effects of proteins on the alveolar surface as natural surfactants, but it has not been shown to improve 36-week PMA outcomes.[63] Not all babies (including those with a PDA, cardiogenic shock, pulmonary hypertension, or an air leak) respond to surfactant; failure to respond marks out a group of babies with a poorer prognosis. Transient hypoxemia and bradycardia may be present during surfactant administration. However, if care is taken with the surfactant instillation, there will be only transient perturbation in cerebral hemodynamics and either no effect or even a slight reduction in the incidence of cerebral hemorrhage. No increased risk of infection has been found, although instilling surfactant could theoretically swamp the alveolar macrophages. Massive pulmonary hemorrhage, however, has been noted following surfactant administration, and the occurrence has been doubled by the use of a synthetic surfactant. Follow-up studies have demonstrated that surfactant treatment is not associated with additional neurologic deficits or an increase in severe retinopathy of prematurity, but better long-term lung function.

Some infants have relatively mild RDS and require only warm humidified supplementary oxygen. Automated adjustment of the inspired oxygen concentration can improve maintenance of oxygenation within an intended range compared with routine and even dedicated care and for prematurely born infants on ventilators.[64] If their disease is more severe, continuous distending pressure is required to prevent atelectasis and improve oxygenation. CPAP can be delivered via endotracheal tube, facemask, a tube into one nostril, a pair of tubes into both nostrils, or a binasal tube. The devices can be connected via a T-piece circuit to a standard neonatal ventilator or a dedicated device; nowadays, a binasal system is most frequently employed. The method of administration of CPAP may influence its efficacy, but irrespective of the type of nasal device used, nasal trauma is common and is significantly related to the duration of nCPAP.[65] Increasing the level of CPAP increases lung volume and hence improves oxygenation, but it is possible to cause overdistension and carbon dioxide retention; infants may also suffer air leak. There are now reports of nCPAP use in the labor suite and to provide ongoing respiratory support, in preference to intubation and ventilation. Such a policy has been described as a gentler form of ventilation, as it has been reported to be associated with a lower incidence of BPD, but this has not been confirmed in the randomized trials performed to date.[66,67] Indeed in one trial[66] there was a three-fold increase in the pneumothorax in the CPAP arm. There is too little evidence to evaluate the efficacy of prophylactic CPAP commenced after birth regardless of respiratory status, but as there was a trend for some adverse outcomes, it cannot be recommended.[68] In other centers, immature infants are intubated in the labor suite to receive prophylactic surfactant (see later in the chapter) and then ongoing respiratory support is provided by mechanical ventilation; more mature infants (older than 28 weeks gestational age) are intubated and ventilated because of worsening respiratory distress and/or a major or recurrent troublesome apnea. Conventional mechanical ventilators deliver intermittent positive pressure inflations and positive end-expiratory pressure (PEEP). The ventilator inflations are delivered at a preset rate, which may be out of synchrony to the infant's respiratory efforts, which can lead to the development of air leak (see later in the chapter). In randomized trials, using ventilator rates of at least 60 bpm has been associated with a reduction in the incidence of pneumothorax[69]; the likely mechanism is that faster rates resulted in synchronization of the infant's respiratory efforts with the ventilator inflations. The only benefit of assist-control ventilation or synchronized intermittent mandatory ventilation (patient triggered modes), which also can synchronize the infant's respiratory efforts, however, was a shortened duration of weaning.[69] Volutrauma/barotrauma has been incriminated in the causation of BPD; as a consequence, forms of ventilatory support that deliver a constant tidal volume (volume-targeted ventilation) have been investigated. Meta-analysis of the randomized trials to date demonstrates that they do not reduce the incidence of BPD.[70] The airway pressure waveforms delivered by the different ventilator types varies[71]; which is the most efficacious has not been determined. The results of physiologic studies have demonstrated that the level of volume targeting can also influence short-term outcomes[72,73]; whether this translates into long-term benefits needs to be assessed. An alternative approach has been to use volumes much less than the tidal volume. During high-frequency jet ventilation (HFJV), high-velocity "bullets" of gas are fired at rates of 200 to 600 per minute, and this entrains gas down the endotracheal tube. High-frequency oscillatory ventilation (HFOV) usually is delivered at frequencies between 10 and 15 Hz. Randomized trials have yielded conflicting results regarding whether use of HFJV reduces BPD; HFJV, however, may be helpful in infants who have already suffered the consequences of barotrauma. Its use has been associated with more rapid resolution of PIE. Randomized trials comparing HFOV to conventional ventilation have also yielded conflicting results, but a meta-analysis of the results has demonstrated that prophylactic HFO (i.e., commencing within the first 12 hours after birth) is associated with a modest but significant reduction in BPD, with no excess of ICH or PVL.[74] In infants with severe RDS, transfer to HFOV can improve oxygenation if a high-volume strategy is used (i.e., the mean airway pressure is increased to optimize lung volume). There has been only one randomized trial comparing HFOV to conventional ventilation in prematurely born infants with severe respiratory failure; HFOV use was associated with a significant reduction in new pulmonary air leaks, but an increase in intracerebral hemorrhage.[75] Pulmonary hypertension should be suspected in infants with RDS, whose hypoxia is more severe than would be anticipated from their chest radiograph appearance. The management of affected infants is described in the "Pulmonary Hypertension of the Newborn" section.

Preventative Strategies

Antenatal steroids that cross the placenta (i.e., synthetic steroids such as dexamethasone or betamethasone) mature the fetal lung, inducing the enzymes for surfactant synthesis and the genes for the surfactant proteins, increase anti-oxidant activity, and reduce oxidative stress.[76] Randomized trials have demonstrated that administration of dexamethasone or betamethasone significantly reduces the incidences of RDS, neonatal death, cerebral hemorrhage, and necrotizing enterocolitis.[77] Benefit is maximal in infants delivered between 24 and 168 hours of maternal therapy being started; but benefit is seen in infants whose mothers have received less than 24 hours of treatment. Antenatal steroids do not increase the risk of infection in pregnancies complicated by premature rupture of the membranes (PROM); indeed they have a beneficial effect. Glucocorticoids should also be given in diabetic pregnancies and the insulin regime altered as necessary during the brief period of hyperglycemia resulting from the steroid treatment. Data from animal models have highlighted that repeated doses have beneficial effects on lung function but can have adverse effects on brain function and fetal growth[78]; randomized trials have highlighted similar effects in infants with reductions in weight and head circumference.[79] Guidelines for antenatal steroid use have been produced by the Royal College of Obstetricians and Gynecologists and the U.S. National Institutes of Health. Their recommendations include that antenatal treatment with corticosteroids should be considered for all women at risk of preterm labor between 24 and 36 weeks. Betamethasone (two doses 24 hours apart) rather than dexamethasone (four doses 12 hours apart) is preferred, as in an observational study betamethasone was associated with a lower occurrence of cystic periventricular leukomalacia[80] and in an uncontrolled study was associated with lower rates of RDS and BPD. Corticosteroids should be given unless immediate delivery is anticipated. In the absence of chorioamnionitis, antenatal corticosteroids are recommended in pregnancies complicated by preterm and prolonged rupture of the membranes and in other complicated pregnancies, unless there is evidence that corticosteroids will have an adverse effect on the mother. Thyroid hormones induce surfactant synthesis, but meta-analysis of the results of eleven trials demonstrated that antenatal administration of TRH (which, unlike T_4, T_3, or TSH does cross the placenta) did not reduce the risk of neonatal respiratory distress or BPD. Indeed, there were adverse effects, an increase in requirement for ventilation, and a greater likelihood of the treated infants having a low Apgar score at 5 minutes.[81] Antenatally administered TRH can also produce transient suppression of the pituitary thyroid axis and complications in the mother, including nausea, vomiting, and increased blood pressure. Other drugs, including aminophylline and ambroxol, have been used in animal experiments to mature the surfactant synthetic pathways. The effect of antenatal betamimetics on the human neonate appears to be small, although, in a randomized controlled trial, infants whose mothers had received an infusion of terbutaline prior to elective delivery had significantly better lung function.[82] Benefit from ambroxol has been reported, but this is not a consistent finding.

Prophylactic versus selective (i.e., when RDS is established) surfactant administration has been associated with significant reductions in neonatal mortality, BPD, and pneumothorax[61] and early versus late reductions in neonatal mortality and pneumothorax.[83] In one recent randomized study, prophylactic surfactant was not superior to nCPAP and early selective surfactant in decreasing the need for mechanical ventilation at 5 days.[84] Positive effects of both synthetic and natural surfactants have been reported. Meta-analysis of two randomized studies highlighted that the use of a synthetic protein-containing surfactant (i.e., Lucinactant, which contains a functional SP-B mimic, leucine, and lysine repeating units [KL4]) did not significantly improve 36-week PMA outcomes.[85]

Mortality and Morbidity

Overall the mortality from RDS is between 5% and 10%; the mortality rate is inversely proportional to gestational age. The acute complications of RDS include air leaks, patent ductus arteriosus, and pulmonary hemorrhage. These are discussed in the relevant sections below. Bronchopulmonary dysplasia, defined as oxygen dependency 28 days after birth, develops in more than 40% of infants born prior to 29 weeks of gestation.[86] This condition is described in detail in Chapter 23. Severely affected infants may require prolonged mechanical ventilation (see Chapter 15). In addition, infants with RDS may suffer an intracerebral hemorrhage or periventricular leukomalacia—both conditions increasing the risk of adverse neurodevelopmental outcome. The latter is particularly common in infants born prior to 26 weeks gestational age.[87]

◾ ACUTE RESPIRATORY DISTRESS SYNDROME

Acute respiratory distress syndrome (ARDS) can occur following asphyxia, shock, sepsis, or meconium aspiration syndrome. Asphyxia results in damage to the myocardium and the associated severe metabolic academia in depressed myocardial contractility, which leads to heart failure and pulmonary edema. Asphyxia also damages the pulmonary blood vessels, and ARDS will develop if the leak of protein-rich fluid onto the alveoli is large. ARDS presents with tachypnea (respiratory rate of at least 100/min) rather than with retraction or grunting in at-term infants within the first 1 or 2 hours after birth. The tachypnea results from stimulation by metabolic academia, damage to the central nervous system, and/or pulmonary edema. Infants with ARDS are severely hypoxemic. The chest radiograph demonstrates diffuse pulmonary infiltrates, and in severe cases a whiteout will be present. Surfactant administration can improve oxygenation in ARDS and is most effective if given early and in larger doses than used in RDS. A high PEEP level should be used in an attempt to restore the FRC to normal values and improve oxygenation. High-volume strategy HFOV can also improve oxygenation, particularly in patients who have had a positive response to PEEP elevation. Fluid intake should initially be restricted to 40 mL/kg/24 hours, and furosemide should be administered if heart failure is present. If the infant is anemic and there is co-existing myocardial asphyxial injury, a blood transfusion should be given slowly with a diuretic. However, if the anemia is severe, then a single-volume exchange transfusion using packed red blood cells should be undertaken. Broad-spectrum antimicrobials (usually penicillin plus an aminoglycoside) should be administered, but aminoglycoside levels must be carefully monitored because these infants are at risk of renal dysfunction. The mortality of ARDS is high, particularly in infants who develop secondary infection or do not respond to elevation of their PEEP level. Air leaks and infection are commonly seen in infants with ARDS.

◾ TRANSIENT TACHYPNOEA OF THE NEWBORN

Transient tachypnea of the newborn (TTN) occurs in 4 to 6 per 1000 at-term infants. An incidence of 10 per 1000 has been reported in premature infants,[88] but coexisting problems (e.g., RDS) may mask the presentation. TTN is due to delayed fetal lung fluid clearance[89]; neonates with TTN have an immaturity of the lung epithelial transport[90] (see later in the chapter). In fetal life, the lung is filled with liquid; fetal lung fluid is produced initially at a rate of 2 mL/kg/hour, increasing to 5 mL/kg/hour at term. It contributes one third to one half to the daily turnover of amniotic fluid. Compared to either amniotic fluid or plasma, lung liquid has a high chloride concentration, but a low bicarbonate and protein concentration. The secondary active transport of chloride ions from the interstitial space into the lung is the main force for lung liquid secretion, sodium ions, and water following passively down electrical and osmotic gradients. The presence of lung liquid is essential for normal lung development; chronic drainage results in pulmonary hypoplasia. The volume of fetal lung liquid is regulated by the resistance to lung liquid efflux through the upper airway; a pressure in the lumen of the lung is generated that is approximately 1 cm of water greater than that in the amniotic cavity. During labor and delivery, the concentration of epinephrine increases, the chloride pump responsible for lung liquid secretion is inhibited, and lung liquid secretion ceases. In addition, lung liquid resorption commences as the raised epinephrine levels stimulate sodium channels on the apical surface of the pulmonary epithelium, via which fetal lung liquid absorption occurs. Thyroid hormone and cortisol are necessary for maturation of the response of the fetal lung to epinephrine; steroids are highly effective in enhancing the expression of highly selective sodium channels in the lung epithelial cells.[91] Exposure to postnatal oxygen tension increases sodium transport across the pulmonary epithelium. Although some liquid is squeezed out under high vaginal pressure during the second stage of labor, the majority is absorbed into the pulmonary lymphatics and capillaries. Air entry into the lung displaces liquid from the terminal respiratory units into the perivascular space, the hydraulic pressure in the pulmonary circulation is reduced, and blood flow is increased. As a consequence, the effective vascular surface area for fluid exchange is increased, facilitating water absorption into the pulmonary vascular bed. The replacement of lung liquid by air is largely accomplished within a few minutes of birth.

TTN is more common in infants who are born by caesarean section without labor[92] because lung fluid clearance will not have occurred. Respiratory distress is more likely to occur if a caesarean section without labor is performed at 37 rather than 38 weeks of gestation.[92] Surfactant deficiency may be important in the pathogenesis of TTN. Other risk factors for TTN include male sex and a family history of asthma. Infants of asthmatic mothers may have a genetic predisposition to β-adrenergic hyporesponsiveness. Resorption of fetal lung fluid is a catecholamine-dependent process and β1 and β2 adrenoreceptor polymorphisms (known to alter catecholamines) are operative in TTN.[93]

Infants with TTN are tachypneic with respiratory rates up to 100 to 120 breaths/minute. However, they rarely grunt because their lungs are not atelectatic. The chest may be barrel-shaped as a result of hyperinflation. The chest radiograph shows hyperinflation, prominent perihilar vascular markings due to engorgement of the periarterial lymphatics (Fig. 22-2), edema of the interlobar septae, and fluid in the fissures. Cerebral irritation from subarachnoid blood or perinatal hypoxic ischemia should be considered in the differential diagnosis of a tachypneic infant, but such infants have a respiratory alkalemia. The chest radiograph appearance of TTN may be mimicked by heart failure.

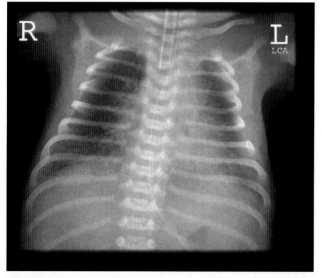

FIGURE 22-2. In transient tachypnea of the newborn, severe changes with widespread consolidation are indistinguishable radiologically from infection. Rapid clearance of the abnormalities within 24 hours confirmed the diagnosis.

Management includes supplementary oxygen; very unusually infants with TTN have been reported to require very high concentrations of oxygen or even mechanical ventilation. Intravenous antimicrobials should be administered until infection has been excluded and nasogastric tube feeds should be withheld until the respiratory rate settles. Diuretics appear to be of no benefit, but they have only been adequately investigated in one randomized trial.[94] By definition TTN is self-limiting, and affected infants have usually made a complete recovery within a few days of birth. Complications are rare, though air leaks may occur, particularly if the infant has required CPAP or IPPV. There is debate as to whether infants who had TTN are more likely to wheeze at follow-up.

PNEUMONIA

Early-Onset Pneumonia

Early-onset pneumonia is generally diagnosed if clinical presentation is in the first 48 hours after birth.[95] It is acquired transplacentally or during labor or delivery; ascending infection is particularly likely if there is prolonged rupture of the membranes. Transplacentally acquired organisms, which can cause pneumonia, include *Listeria monocytogenes, Mycobacterium tuberculosis, Treponema pallidum,* rubella virus, cytomegalovirus (CMV), herpes simplex virus (HSV), adenovirus, and influenza type A virus. Sixty to 70% of cases caused by ascending infection are due to *Streptococcus agalactiae* (group B streptococcus, GBS). There are seven identifiable subtypes of GBS based on capsular polysaccharide antigens; most neonatal infections are caused by types I, II, and III. The incidence of early-onset GBS sepsis is 1.8 per 1000 live births in the United States and 0.3 to 1 per 1000 in the United Kingdom. *Escherichia coli (E. coli)* is the second most common cause of early neonatal sepsis. Approximately 40% of *E. coli* strains that cause early-onset sepsis possess the capsule type K1, which confers antiphagocytic properties and resistance to complement mediated killing. Pregnancy is associated with an increased carriage of K1 strains, which are then vertically transmitted. Other organisms that cause ascending infection include *Haemophilus influenzae, Streptococcus pneumoniae, Listeria monocytogenes, Klebsiella pneumoniae,* Candida albicans, adenovirus, CMV, HSV, and echovirus.

Risk factors for early-onset pneumonia include prolonged rupture of the membranes, premature labor, and organisms present in the vagina. Other risk factors for GBS infection include chorioamnionitis, prolonged labor, and frequent pelvic examinations in labor. Vaginal and rectal carriage rates of GBS are reported to be between 7% and 23%. Infants at highest risk of GBS infection are those whose mothers, although having GBS in their vagina, have little or no circulating anti-GBS immunoglobulin. Approximately 1% of infants born vaginally to mothers who carry GBS at the time of birth become infected. The most important reservoir for transmission of *Listeria monocytogenes* to humans is food (especially dairy products) contaminated by infected farm animals. Women infected with HIV are considerably more susceptible to *L. monocytogenes* than the general population. Herpes simplex virus is usually transmitted during delivery through an infected maternal genital tract.

Clinical Presentation and Diagnosis

Infants with transplacentally acquired infection present at birth and those infected with organisms acquired from the birth canal present within the first 48 hours after birth. The infant typically suffers progressive respiratory distress and has signs of systemic sepsis, which develop within a few hours of birth. Infants who are frankly septicemic with poor peripheral perfusion, cyanosis, and inadequate respiration have a poor prognosis. Most cases of GBS pneumonia present within the first 4 to 6 hours. If the infant does not receive prompt treatment, the condition rapidly deteriorates; the infant will require intubation and ventilation for apnea and will develop pulmonary hypertension. Infants with congenitally acquired Listeria infection are often extremely ill at birth with severe pneumonia and hepatomegaly. Diarrhea and an erythematous skin rash may occur. Characteristically, affected infants have small pinkish-grey cutaneous granulomas; these granulomas are widespread in lung, liver, and nervous system. More typically, infants with early-onset pneumonia have respiratory distress with nonspecific signs (e.g., poor feeding and irritability); they may be febrile or hypothermic.[95] Neonates with HSV infection can present with local or disseminated disease, pneumonitis, hepatitis, and/or DIC with or without encephalitis or skin disease.[95]

The chest radiograph appearance is varied; there can be lobar (Fig. 22-3) or segmental consolidation, atelectasis, or diffuse haziness or opacification (Fig. 22-4). In addition, pleural effusions may occur, particularly if the pneumonia is the result of bacterial or fungal infection. Rarely, there is abscess or pneumatocele formation. These complications are most likely to occur with staphylococcal or coliform pneumonia. GBS is easy to

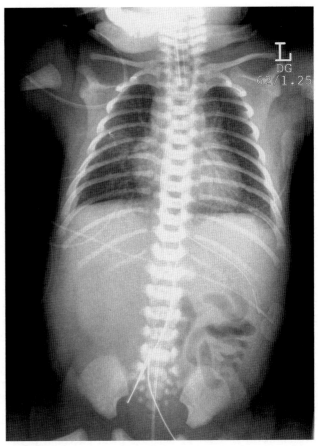

FIGURE 22-4. Group B *streptococcus* pneumonia mimicking respiratory distress syndrome. The focal consolidation in the posterior segment of the right upper lobe is more suggestive of GBS pneumonia.

culture and will usually grow from surface swabs and the gastric aspirate. *Listeria* can be isolated from the first meconium passed. In addition to appropriate cultures from the infant, histologic evaluation and culture of the placenta should be undertaken and serological testing of the mother and infant for syphilis or viral agents should be considered. If infection due to herpes is likely, viral cultures from the maternal lesions and the infant should be obtained. Case fatalities for pneumonia are higher for low birth weight (LBW) infants and for those with early-onset rather than late-onset pneumonia.[95]

Treatment

All infants with respiratory distress should receive antimicrobial treatment (see earlier in the chapter). Initial treatment for early-onset pneumonia should be a combination of ampicillin or benzylpenicillin, and an aminoglycoside. Modification to that regime may be necessary once the culture results are known or there is good reason to suspect a particular organism; for example, *H. influenzae* with ampicillin resistance are emerging, and cefotaxime should be added if *H. influenzae* sepsis is suspected. Cefotaxime and ceftriaxone are used for *E. coli* sepsis, but for infection with *Listeria* the most effective antimicrobial therapy is ampicillin

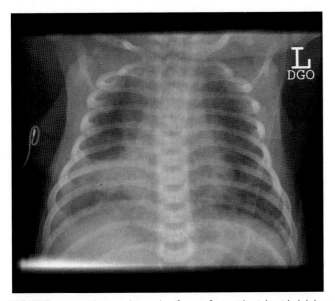

FIGURE 22-3. Chest radiograph of an infant with right-sided lobar pneumonia.

plus gentamicin; *Listeria* are resistant to all third-generation cephalosporins. Antimicrobial therapy should continue for at least 10 days, but for 3 weeks if the pneumonia is due to *Staphylococcus aureus.* Long-term intravenous therapy should be given if there is abscess formation. Empyemas should be drained, and intravenous antimicrobials should be administered for at least 2 weeks. It is important to prevent vertical transmission of GBS by giving intrapartum antimicrobial prophylaxis (penicillin or ampicillin) to women who have been identified by screening in pregnancy to carry GBS and/or have risk factors. Risk factors include a previous infant with GBS disease, GBS in the maternal urine during pregnancy, preterm labor, ruptured membranes for more than 18 hours prior to delivery, and intrapartum fever. High-dose acyclovir (20 mg/kg/q8hr for 14 to 21 days) can halve the mortality rate in HSV.[95]

Late-Onset Pneumonia

The majority of cases of late-onset pneumonia on a NICU occur in ventilated prematurely born infants. The most common responsible bacteria are coagulase-negative *Staphylococci,* coagulase-positive *Staphylococci* (including *S. aureus*), and Gram-negative bacilli (including *Klebsiella, E. coli,* and *Pseudomonas*). Infants may acquire tuberculosis by transplacental spread, aspiration, or ingestion of infected amniotic fluid or by airborne inoculation from close contacts.[95] The clinical presentation is nonspecific.[96] Atypical bacterial pathogens (e.g., *Chlamydia trachomatis*) are well-recognized causes of late-onset pneumonia. The risk of pneumonia developing in a neonate with maternal colonization is 7%.[95] Viruses can also cause late-onset pneumonia; these include RSV, influenza virus, parainfluenza virus, adenovirus, and rhinovirus. Viral pneumonia usually occurs when there are high levels of infection in the community, resulting in nosocomial infection. Fungal infections are a significant problem if infants have had prolonged exposure to antimicrobials, particularly third-generation cephalosporins; pneumonia occurs as a result of blood-borne spread. Small for dates VLBW infants are at increased risk of nosocomial pneumonia.[97] Lateral rather than supine positioning of ventilated infants may make them less likely to contract bacterial colonization.[98] Active surveillance and strict adherence to hand hygiene has been reported to be effective in controlling NICU-acquired infections by *P. aeruginosa.*[99] Cytomegalovirus pneumonia may follow from feeding with thawed frozen breast milk from HCMV-Ig-positive mothers.[100]

The development of pneumonia in a ventilated infant will present as an increasing requirement for ventilatory support. Initial treatment should be a third-generation cephalosporin and vancomycin, as the most likely infecting organism will be a coagulase-negative staphylococci. The choice of antimicrobials should be modified according to local knowledge and, if necessary, according to culture results. If the infant is already on antimicrobials, the regime should usually be changed and the spectrum of cover broadened. Two weeks of oral erythromycin is recommended for chlamydial pneumonia.[97]

Aspiration Pneumonia

This occurs in infants with GER or with sucking or swallowing incoordination. Aspiration can result in physical obstruction because inhaled curd is particulate. The resultant airway obstruction can lead to lung collapse (Fig. 22-5) and/or consolidation and can predispose to infection. Chemical irritation occurs with the aspiration of acidic gastric contents. The infant may initially be asymptomatic if the aspiration is due to GER. However, if there is massive regurgitation the infant may be found cyanosed and apneic or gasping, and crepitations and rhonchi on auscultation will be heard. A new area of consolidation on the chest radiograph, particularly in the right upper lobe, is suggestive of aspiration (Fig. 22-6).

Following the episode of aspiration, the airway should be cleared and the infant may require supplementary oxygen or even ventilatory support. Broad-spectrum antimicrobial

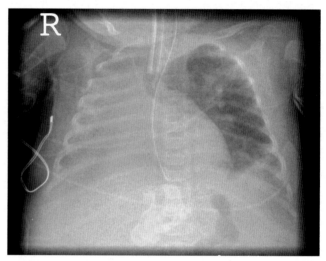

FIGURE 22-5. Aspiration with right lung collapse and herniation of the left lung across the mediastinum.

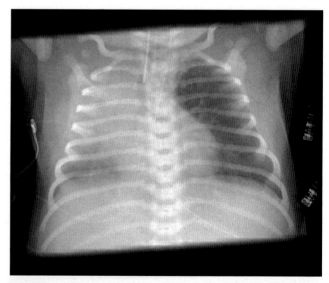

FIGURE 22-6. Aspiration with predominantly right upper lobe changes in an infant with sucking and swallowing incoordination following severe birth depression.

cover should be given, usually flucloxacillin and an aminoglycoside, for at least 5 days. If the infant has an area of consolidation, regular physiotherapy should be undertaken and the infant should be positioned to optimize drainage from the affected lobe.

INTERSTITIAL LUNG DISEASE

Interstitial lung disease is a consideration in the differential of a newborn with severe respiratory distress or in preterm infants with out-of-proportion clinical findings. These conditions may include surfactant dysfunction mutations in *SP-B*, *SP-C*, *ABCA3*, and *NKX2.1* genes; alveolar capillary dysplasia with misalignment of pulmonary veins; or pulmonary interstitial glycogenosis (PIG). Though these diseases individually are an uncommon cause of respiratory distress in neonates, collectively they may be more common and require consideration. Interstitial lung disease is covered in detail in Chapters 55 and 56.

MECONIUM ASPIRATION SYNDROME

Meconium staining of the amniotic fluid occurs in 8% to 20% of pregnancies; 5% of babies born through meconium-stained amniotic fluid will develop meconium aspiration syndrome (MAS). Prolonged severe fetal hypoxia can stimulate fetal breathing with inhalation of amniotic fluid that contains meconium, or the inhalation can occur perinatally if the airway contains meconium-stained amniotic fluid. Meconium aspiration is a disease of term or postterm babies; the prevalence is 10% or more after 38 weeks gestational age but 22% in babies of 42 weeks gestational age. Meconium staining of the liquid occurs in less than 5% of preterm pregnancies, and if it does occur suggests infection. Passage of meconium relates to motilin levels. Motilin is produced mainly by the jejunum and stimulates peristalsis. Levels are very low in preterm infants and nonasphyxiated term infants, but are raised in asphyxiated term babies who pass meconium intrapartum.

Meconium is sticky and composed of inspissated fetal intestinal secretions. When inhaled it creates a ball-valve mechanism in the airways; air can be sucked in, but it cannot be exhaled. The result is gas trapping and lung overdistension, which predisposes to air leaks. Meconium is also an irritant, and inflammatory cells and mediators are released in response to its presence in the airways. An inflammatory pneumonitis with alveolar collapse develops. The pulmonary artery pressure is increased, as the inflammatory response results in release of vasoactive substances that cause vasoconstriction. Although meconium is initially sterile, its presence in the airway predisposes to pulmonary infection because of its organic nature, particularly with *E. coli*. In addition, as meconium may inhibit phagocytosis and the neutrophil oxidative burst, bacteria can grow in meconium-stained amniotic fluid. Meconium (particularly, the chloroform-soluble phase: free fatty acids, triglycerides, and cholesterol) inhibits surfactant function and production in a concentration-dependent manner.

Clinical Presentation

Infants with MAS are tachypneic, their respiratory rate may exceed 120 breaths/minute, and they have intercostal and subcostal retractions and use their accessory respiratory muscles. They are frequently hypoxic due to ventilation-perfusion mismatch and pulmonary hypertension. However, carbon dioxide levels are not usually elevated unless the disease is severe. The meconium in the airways causes widespread crackles, and affected infants have an overdistended chest because of air trapping. In mild cases recovery may occur within 24 hours, but those who require ventilation are frequently still symptomatic at 2 weeks of age and may remain oxygen dependent beyond the neonatal period. Early chest radiographs demonstrate widespread patchy infiltration (Fig. 22-7) and overexpansion; small pleural effusions occur in approximately 20% of patients. In severe cases, by 72 hours of age the appearance is often changed to that of diffuse and homogeneous opacification of both lung fields, because of pneumonitis and interstitial edema. The changes gradually resolve over the next week, but in severe cases the chest radiograph appearance may merge into the pattern seen in BPD. Air leaks, in particular pneumothorax and pneumomediastinum, are very common, occurring in approximately 20% of infants. If there has been severe intrapartum asphyxia, there may be ECG changes suggesting subendocardial ischemia, and the echocardiogram will show reduced cardiac contractility. In those with pulmonary hypertension, echocardiography will demonstrate right-to-left shunting at ductal and atrial levels.

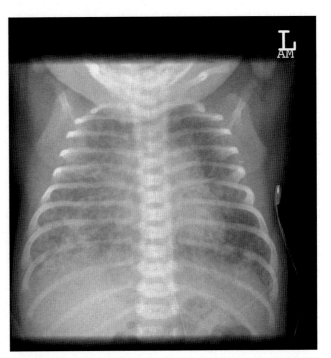

FIGURE 22-7. Chest radiograph of an infant with meconium aspiration syndrome with diffuse patchy infiltration bilaterally.

Management

In the initial stages of the illness, sufficient supplementary oxygen should be given to maintain the oxygen saturation levels at 95% and the arterial oxygen level greater than 10 kPa. Warmed, humidified oxygen should be delivered into a headbox, even if the infant requires up to an oxygen concentration of 80%, providing there is no respiratory acidosis. CPAP may improve oxygenation but will increase the risk of pneumothorax, thus it is not recommended in MAS. Intubation and ventilation are indicated if $PaCO_2$ rises above 8 kPa (60 mm Hg), particularly if the infant is hypoxic. However, if the infant has hypoxic ischemic encephalopathy (HIE), more rigid control of blood gases is required. Babies with MAS can be very difficult to ventilate; theoretically, a long expiratory time and low a level of PEEP should be used, but elevation of PEEP may be necessary to improve oxygenation, although this maneuver will increase the risk of pneumothorax. A neuromuscular blocking agent should be administered because infants with MAS often "fight the ventilator," hence increasing their risk of an air leak (see later in the chapter). In infants with severe disease and pulmonary hypertension, HFOV, particularly if used with nitric oxide (NO), and NO used in conjunction with conventional ventilation can improve oxygenation and reduce the need for extracorporeal membrane oxygenation (ECMO). If the oxygenation index is >40, results of a randomized trial demonstrated that ECMO improved survival.[103] Overall, more than 90% of babies with MAS who are managed with ECMO survive. Meta-analysis of the results of the four randomized trials demonstrated that surfactant administration does not influence mortality, but in two trials it was associated with significant reduction in the risk of requiring ECMO (number required to treat = 6), but no other statistically significant reductions in other outcomes.[104] Administering the surfactant by dilute surfactant lavage rather than bolus may be more effective in improving gas exchange.[105] Broad-spectrum antimicrobials (penicillin and gentamicin) should be given.

Preventive Strategies

Avoidance of postterm delivery is the most important factor in reducing MAS. In uncontrolled studies, meticulous clearing of the airway at delivery has been reported to reduce the incidence of MAS. However, in a meta-analysis of the results of four randomized trials, no significant benefit of routine endotracheal intubation and suctioning at birth over routine resuscitation (including oropharyngeal suction of vigorous term meconium-stained babies) was demonstrated[106]; however, MAS, HIE, and mortality rates in that systematic review were low. Nevertheless, on the evidence to date, intubation and suctioning should be restricted to newborns who are depressed (i.e., they have a heart rate less than 100 bpm, poor respiratory effort, and poor tone). Direct endotracheal suctioning is only indicated if meconium is seen below the cords. Compression of the neonatal thorax is not recommended because it is unlikely to prevent gasping, and compression of the thorax can stimulate respiratory efforts. Whether instillation of water or saline into the lower respiratory tract is useful

is controversial; an increase in wet lung has been noted following this procedure. If the infant requires mechanical ventilation, then tracheal suction with saline lavage can result in an improvement in airway resistance. Aspiration of the stomach may prevent subsequent inhalation following vomiting or reflux of previously swallowed meconium. Routine gastric lavage prior to feeding in one study, however, did not decrease the incidence of MAS in babies born through meconium-stained fluid. There is an inverse relationship between amniotic fluid volume and fetal heart rate decelerations, possibly due to either cord or head compression. Amnioinfusion to maintain amniotic fluid volume during labor is undertaken to try and stop such compression and hence reduce the likelihood of MAS. Results of a meta-analysis suggested that amnioinfusion, particularly in settings of limited perinatal surveillance, improved perinatal outcome with significant reductions in MAS, HIE, and NICU admission.[107] There are, however, adverse outcomes of amnioinfusion, including increased incidences of cord prolapse, infection, and requirement for instrumental delivery. Suppression of fetal breathing movements by maternal narcotic administration, although successful in a baboon model, did not reduce the incidence of MAS in two clinical series.

Mortality and Morbidity

Mortality rates are between 4% and 12%; the majority of deaths are from respiratory failure, pulmonary hypertension, or air leaks. Fifty percent of babies who require mechanical ventilation because of MAS suffer an air leak. BPD is a rare complication of MAS. Neurologic sequelae occur in infants with coexisting HIE. MAS is associated with long-term respiratory morbidity; lung function abnormalities, including increased bronchial hyperreactivity, have been reported, and up to 40% of those who have had severe MAS may go on to develop asthma at school age.

▬ PERSISTENT PULMONARY HYPERTENSION OF THE NEWBORN

Infants with persistent pulmonary hypertension of the newborn (PPHN) have right-to-left shunts at the level of the ductus arteriosus and the foramen ovale. PPHN has been called *persistent fetal circulation,* but this is inaccurate as the high-flow, low-resistance circuit through the placenta present in the fetal circulation is missing.

Changes in the Circulation at Birth

In the fetus, the pulmonary vascular resistance is high, but within the systemic circulation there is a low-resistance component, the placenta. There is shunting across the patent ductus arteriosus, and only approximately 10% of the right ventricular output enters the pulmonary circulation. At birth, removal of the placenta from the circulation reduces venous return through the inferior vena cava to the right atrium. This results in lowering of the right atrial pressure at a time when the left atrial pressure is increased because of the increased pulmonary venous return, hence the foramen ovale closes. The flow through the ductus venosus is diminished, and passive closure of the ductus venosus occurs within 3 to 7 days after birth. Pulmonary vascular resistance (PVR) falls rapidly in the first minutes after birth, and then more gradually over the next days. The fall in PVR is associated with a structural reorganization and thinning of the vessel walls. It is a consequence of lung aeration, which results in opening up the pulmonary capillary bed, an acute lowering of PVR, and an increase in pulmonary blood flow. This is due both to a mechanical effect and oxygenated blood passing through the pulmonary circulation. Inflation of the lungs stimulates pulmonary stretch receptors, which leads to reflex vasodilation of the pulmonary vascular bed. Mechanical expansion creates surface forces at the gas-liquid interface within the alveoli, which physically expand small blood vessels and decrease perivascular pressure. The majority of the changes in cardiopulmonary hemodynamics occur by 8 hours, although some degree of right-to-left ductal shunting may be found up to 12 hours after birth. In most infants, the ductus arteriosus closes by 24 hours of age, but there is a significant delay in ductal closure in infants with pulmonary hypertension. PVR is high in the fetus because of the low oxygen tension and low prostaglandin (PGI_2) and nitric oxide (NO) levels and the presence of vasoconstrictor substances, such as endothelin-1 (ET-1). PGI_2 production and release is increased by pulmonary tissue stretch. PGI_2 participates in the reduction of pulmonary vascular resistance accompanying ventilation, but it is not essential for maintaining low pulmonary vascular resistance once it is established. The vasodilator effects of exogenous PGI_2 are blocked by NO synthase inhibitors, which suggests that NO modulates PGI_2 activity. NO is produced by the vascular endothelial cells; NO synthase acts on L-+arginine to form citrulline and NO. NO then diffuses into the smooth muscle cells stimulating guanylate cyclase and increasing guanosine monophosphate production, which results in smooth muscle relaxation. Increased fetal oxygen tensions augment endogenous NO release, and pharmacologic NO blockade attenuates the rise in pulmonary blood flow after birth. Decreased production of endogenous vasoconstrictors (e.g., thromboxane and ET-1) may also participate in the decrease in PVR at birth. In neonates with hypoxia and severe pulmonary hypertension, ET-I levels are raised. In pulmonary hypertension that accompanies sepsis due to group B streptococci or other organisms, thromboxane A_2 may cause initial severe arterial spasm followed by increased vascular permeability and an increased lung fluid content. The increased capillary permeability in sepsis-induced pulmonary hypertension appears to be due also to the action of bacterial endotoxins sequestering white cells in the lungs, where they release vasoactive agents such as tumor necrosis factor. Raised levels of other vasoconstrictors (e.g., the leukotrienes LTC4 and LTD4) have been found in some neonates with pulmonary hypertension; the levels fell with successful therapy.

Pathophysiology

Pulmonary hypertension in the neonate may be primary or secondary to conditions including severe intrapartum asphyxia, infection, pulmonary hypoplasia, drug therapy (e.g., the use of PGSI before delivery), alveolar capillary dysplasia, congenital heart disease, or overventilation. The neonatal pulmonary vasculature is extremely sensitive to changes in pH, PaO_2, and $PaCO_2$; perinatal or postnatal hypoxemia and metabolic or respiratory academia can cause marked pulmonary arterial spasm and pulmonary hypertension. A rise in the hematocrit can cause pulmonary hypertension, but polycythemia is not a consistent feature of neonates with pulmonary hypertension. Pulmonary hypertension in the neonate is often characterized by varying degrees of vascular remodeling and decreased arteriolar number. The pulmonary hypertension, which occurs in infants with congenital diaphragmatic hernia or in other conditions associated with pulmonary hypoplasia, is due to a reduction in the number of intralobar arteries and increased muscularity of the arteries. Following chronic hypoxia *in utero*, excessive muscularization of the pulmonary arterioles is found and muscle extends into the normally muscle free intra-acinar arteries; such changes are seen in extremely small for dates infants. In other infants, there is a normal arteriolar number and muscularization, but the normal decrease in pulmonary vascular resistance after birth fails to occur. Persistent pulmonary hypertension may also be due to alveolar capillary dysplasia with congenital misalignment of the pulmonary veins. This condition is usually sporadic, but rarely family occurrence has been reported (See Chapter 55).

Clinical Presentation

Infants with primary pulmonary hypertension of the newborn (PPHN) usually present within 12 hours of birth; affected infants are cyanosed but have only mild respiratory distress, and grunting is rare. The second heart sound is loud because of the rise in pulmonary arterial pressure. There may be a soft systolic murmur due to tricuspid or occasionally mitral incompetence. In neonates who are critically ill because of group B streptococcal infection, severe asphyxia, or congenital diaphragmatic hernia, pulmonary hypertension appears within 6 hours of birth; these infants also have the clinical features of their underlying condition.

Diagnosis and Differential Diagnosis

Pulmonary hypertension is diagnosed in an infant with severe hypoxemia when the hypoxemia is disproportionately severe for the radiologic abnormalities (Fig. 22-8), there is evidence of a right-to-left ductal shunt with a lower level of oxygenation in the distal aortic blood (obtained from an umbilical artery catheter) compared to the preductal blood (obtained from the right radial artery), and the echocardiograph demonstrates a structurally normal heart. Echocardiography is important, not only to establish the diagnosis, but also to exclude cyanotic congenital heart disease. In primary pulmonary hypertension, chest radiograph changes are often minimal; in secondary pulmonary hypertension, the chest radiograph appearance will be that of the underlying lung disease, but the appearance will be less severe than anticipated for the severity of the hypoxemia. The most important differential diagnosis

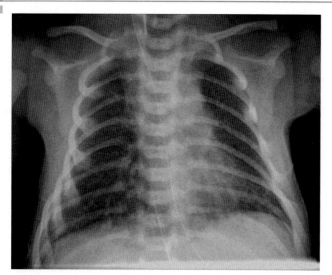

FIGURE 22-8. Chest radiograph of an infant with severe PPHN who had severe hypoxia despite relatively mild radiologic abnormalities.

is cyanotic congenital heart disease, but when this presents in the first 12 hours it is usually with heart failure, distinctive murmurs, and obvious changes on the chest radiograph and electrocardiogram. The response to ventilation with 100% oxygen can help to distinguish the two conditions; in some infants with pulmonary hypertension, the arterial oxygen level will increase to above 13 kPa (100 mm Hg), whereas in cyanotic congenital heart disease it will not rise above 5 to 6 kPa (37.5 to 45 mm Hg). Not all neonates with pulmonary hypertension, especially those with sepsis or a congenital diaphragmatic hernia, however, have a large improvement in oxygenation in response to 100% oxygen. Alveolar capillary dysplasia should be suspected in infants with pulmonary hypertension that is unresponsive to maximal cardiorespiratory support and who cannot be weaned from ECMO; in such cases, a lung biopsy can establish the diagnosis.

Treatment

Minimal handling is important because it is easy to precipitate severe hypoxemia in infants with pulmonary hypertension. As a consequence, endotracheal tube suctioning should only be performed when essential to maintain endotracheal tube patency and chest physiotherapy is contraindicated. Monitoring must be continuous. The size of the right-to-left shunt is in part dependent on the systemic blood pressure, thus aggressive therapy should be used to achieve an appropriate systemic blood pressure. The hemoglobin level should be kept >13 g/dL (PCV 40%) to maximize oxygen transport to the tissues, but if polycythemia (central packed cell volume greater than 70%) is present, a dilutional exchange transfusion should be undertaken. Broad-spectrum antimicrobial cover should be given. Infants should be ventilated if their PaO_2 is <5 to 6 kPa (37 to 45 mm Hg) in 70% oxygen. If mechanical ventilation is needed, the level of inspired oxygen should be sufficient to achieve a PaO_2 of at least 8 to 9 kPa (56 to 63 mm Hg); the pH should be kept above 7.25, and the $PaCO_2$ should be kept in the range of 4.8

to 5.5 kPa (35 to 40 mm Hg). Hyperventilation to reduce the $PaCO_2$ to 2.5 to 3.5 kPa is no longer recommended because it may result in a reduction in cerebral blood flow. Although no long-term adverse sequelae have been described in babies born at term, hypocapnia in preterm babies has been linked to the development of periventricular leukomalacia. Hyperventilation can also cause barotrauma, resulting in air leaks and BPD. High inflating pressures and PEEP levels can result in lung overdistension and worsen pulmonary vascular resistance. Alkalosis can promote pulmonary vasodilation, but such a strategy should not be maintained for a prolonged period, as persisting alkalemia increases the hypoxic reactivity of the pulmonary vasculature, thus tending to perpetuate the pathophysiology of pulmonary hypertension. Neuromuscular blocking agents should be administered to full-term babies to prevent them fighting the ventilator. Anecdotally, high-frequency oscillatory and jet ventilation have been used with improvements in oxygenation. ECMO is an effective rescue therapy for infants with pulmonary hypertension.

A variety of vasodilator drugs have been used to treat infants with pulmonary hypertension. Between 25% and 50% of affected babies respond to tolazoline hydrochloride, but this is not a specific vasodilator and hypotension is a common side effect. Other side effects include renal failure and gastrointestinal hemorrhage. Prostacyclin (PGI2) is an effective pulmonary vasodilator, but it is nonselective and has side effects. Tolazoline and PGI2 have been given via inhalation to avoid side effects associated with systemic administration, but there is no long-term experience of this mode of delivery at the time of this writing. Magnesium sulfate administration improves oxygenation, but it is less effective than inhaled nitric oxide (iNO) and has more side effects. Magnesium levels must be carefully monitored, as hypermagnesemia can cause sedation, muscle relaxation, hyporeflexia, hypotension, and calcium and potassium disturbances. Phospodiesterases (PDE) catalyze the hydrolytic cleavage of the 3' phosphodiesterase bond of the cyclic nucleotides (cGMP and AMP), which play a central role in pulmonary vascular smooth muscle relaxation. PDE inhibitors used to treat neonates with pulmonary hypertension include dipyridamole (a nonspecific PDE5 inhibitor), milrinone (a PDE3 inhibitor), and sildenafil (a PDE5 inhibitor). Milrinone administration has been associated with improvement in oxygenation in neonates unresponsive to iNO, but some infants developed severe ICH.[108] Sildenafil has been shown to selectively reduce pulmonary vascular resistance in both animal models and humans.[109] Rapid infusion of a loading dose of sildenafil may cause hypotension, a dosing regimen with loading at 0.4 mg/kg delivered over 3 hours and maintenance of 1.6 mg/kg/day was well tolerated in neonates with severe pulmonary hypertension.[110] Sildenafil has been used to support infants as they are being weaned off of iNO.[111] Other agents are calcium channel antagonists such as Diltiazem[112] and endothelin receptor antagonists such as Bosentan.[113] Successful use, however, has only been described in a few case reports, though use in centers with experience in pulmonary hypertension may be more common.

As mentioned earlier in the chapter, NO is a vasodilator substance that relaxes vascular smooth muscle. When NO is inhaled, it diffuses across the capillary membrane and activates guanylate cyclase in the pulmonary arteriolar smooth muscle. The resulting increase in cGMP causes smooth muscle relaxation. NO then binds rapidly to hemoglobin, and once bound is inactivated and therefore produces no systemic effects. Levels of up to 80 ppm have been used, but in term infants 5 ppm appears as effective as higher doses.[114,115] However, lower doses (2 ppm) are not effective and may diminish the clinical response to higher doses and have adverse sequelae.[116] It has been recommended to start at 20 ppm in term newborns with PPHN; increasing to 40 ppm usually does not improve oxygenation in infants who have failed to respond to 20 ppm.[117] Administration of NO to infants with pulmonary hypertension improves oxygenation, but not all babies respond. A poor response, which occurs in infants with severe parenchymal disease, systemic hypotension, myocardial dysfunction, pulmonary vein stenosis, or structural pulmonary abnormalities such as pulmonary hypoplasia or dysplasia, is predictive of a poor outcome. It is important to wean inhaled NO as soon as oxygenation has improved and the infant is stabilized, otherwise tolerance may occur. Unfortunately, NO has side effects; it reacts rapidly with oxygen to form nitrogen dioxide, which is toxic to the lung. The nitrosylhaemoglobin produced by NO binding to hemoglobin is rapidly converted to methemoglobin, which is then reduced by methemoglobin reductase in erythrocytes. Immature infants and those of certain ethnic groups (including those of Turkish and American Indian origin) have low levels of methemoglobin reductase. These problems are more likely if high concentrations of NO are used for prolonged periods in high inspired oxygen concentrations. NO administration has been associated with an increased bleeding time. Other potential side effects include surfactant dysfunction and mutagenicity.

In term babies, meta-analysis of the results of randomized trials demonstrated that use of inhaled NO was associated with an improvement in oxygenation and a reduction in the combined outcome of death or need for ECMO; the effect was due to a reduction in the need for ECMO.[118] The combined intervention of inhaled NO and HFOV may be more successful than the use of inhaled NO or HFOV alone in rescuing infants at or near term with severe respiratory failure,[119] reflecting that the efficacy of inhaled NO is improved if combined with a strategy to improve lung volume. No excess of adverse neurodevelopmental outcomes has been demonstrated in babies exposed to iNO in randomized trials.[120–122] No significant long-term benefits of iNO have been demonstrated in babies with CDH, and they have a higher incidence of sensorineural hearing loss.[123] Meta-analysis of eleven randomized trials demonstrated that the effect of iNO in preterm babies depended on the timing of administration and the population.[124] Early rescue treatment based on oxygenation criteria did not affect mortality or BPD rates, and there was a trend toward an increase in ICH. Early routine use for intubated infants, however, was associated with a just significant reduction in the combined outcome of death or BPD and a reduction in the incidences of severe ICH and PVL. In a subsequent large trial in which preterm infants were randomized to early, prolonged, low-dose iNO therapy, no significant differences were demonstrated in any important outcomes.[125] Use of iNO after 3 days based on an elevated risk of BPD showed no effect on BPD.[125]

Mortality and Morbidity

The mortality varies according to the underlying condition. The mortality rates are between 10% and 20% in infants who require ECMO because of primary pulmonary hypertension or pulmonary hypertension complicating RDS or MAS. In babies with group B streptococcal sepsis, the mortality rate ranges from 10% to 50%, with most babies dying from irreversible hypoxia or myocardial failure. Alveolar capillary dysplasia is a uniformly fatal condition. BPD occurs in infants who have required a high level of prolonged respiratory support, and neurologic damage may be sustained in infants who have suffered severe hypoxia.

▆ SECONDARY PULMONARY HYPOPLASIA

Secondary pulmonary hypoplasia can result *in utero* from reductions in intrathoracic space, fetal breathing movements (FBM), or amniotic fluid volume. Reduction in intrathoracic space occurs with small chest syndromes (particularly asphyxiating thoracic dystrophy or Jeune syndrome), cystic adenomatoid malformation or sequestration of the lung, congenital diaphragmatic hernia (CDH), and pleural effusions. Infants with anterior abdominal wall defects (AWDs) can have abnormal lung growth as, *in utero*, they have a reduction in viscera in the upper part of the abdominal cavity and hence an inadequate framework for chest wall and diaphragmatic[126] development. Intrathoracic compression by pleural effusions may explain the association of hydropic fetuses due to rhesus isoimmunization and pulmonary hypoplasia, but an immune mechanism may also operate. Cessation or reduction of FBM is responsible for the abnormal lung growth in certain neurologic or neuromuscular diseases presenting *in utero* (e.g., Werdnig-Hoffman disease and myotonic dystrophy inherited from the mother). There is, however, considerable debate regarding the relevance of absent FBM in other conditions associated with abnormal lung growth (e.g., oligohydramnios resulting from PROM). Experimental production of oligohydramnios, by chronic drainage of amniotic fluid or urinary tract obstruction, is associated with the development of pulmonary hypoplasia. Reduction in the production of amniotic fluid can occur with fetal renal abnormalities (e.g., Potter's syndrome or uteroplacental insufficiency). Pulmonary hypoplasia can occur in fetuses with bladder outlet obstruction, but also in those with renal dysplasia/hypoplasia or multicystic kidneys; possible mechanisms include reduced renal proline production and thoracic compression, as well as reduced amniotic fluid volume.[127] Loss of amniotic fluid following PROM or amniocentesis has also been associated with pulmonary hypoplasia or at least lung function abnormalities suggestive of abnormal lung growth.[128,129] The timing of onset of the oligohydramnios in pregnancies complicated by PROM is critical; pulmonary hypoplasia only occurs if the onset of membrane rupture is prior to 26 weeks of gestation. Review of 28 studies demonstrated that the gestational age at PROM rather than the latency period or degree of oligohydramnios was the better predictor of pulmonary hypoplasia; onset at 20 weeks had 70% sensitivity and 73% specificity.[130] Congenital sepsis also predicted perinatal mortality following PROM.[131] Abnormal lung development, however, is not an invariable consequence of early-onset oligohydramnios; in one cohort, 23% of patients who had membrane rupture prior to 20 weeks of gestation had no clinical signs suggestive of pulmonary hypoplasia.[132] Pulmonary hypoplasia has also been described in infants with trisomy 18 or 21.

Clinical signs are similar to those seen with primary pulmonary hypoplasia. Some with mild pulmonary hypoplasia are apparently asymptomatic but on inspection are tachypneic. Others suffer severe respiratory distress from birth and require ventilatory support. Infants with pulmonary hypoplasia have small-volume noncompliant lungs, and their chest wall is disproportionately small with respect to the abdomen. In addition, infants with secondary pulmonary hypoplasia may have associated congenital anomalies (e.g., diaphragmatic hernia/eventration, anterior AWD, dislocated hip, and/or talipes). They may also have the features of neuromuscular diseases such as Werdnig Hoffman disease or congenital dystrophia myotonica inherited from the mother. "Dry lung syndrome" has been described following oligohydramnios due to PROM and is likely to be due to functional compression. Affected infants are difficult to resuscitate requiring high peak inflating pressures; the requirement for high pressures may continue for 48 hours, but then the infants make a spontaneous recovery, indicating they have no structural abnormality.[133]

On antenatal ultrasound examination, oligohydramnios and abnormalities commonly associated with pulmonary hypoplasia (e.g., pleural effusion and CDH) can be identified. A variety of techniques to diagnose pulmonary hypoplasia antenatally have been investigated, including the development of reference ranges of fetal chest growth related to gestational age, relating the thoracic to the abdominal circumference, and calculating the thoracic-to-heart ratio or the thoracic-to-head ratio. In addition, fetal lung volume can be assessed by echoplanar magnetic resonance imaging or 3-D ultrasound. Postnatally on the chest radiograph, the ribs may appear crowded with a low thoracic-to-abdominal ratio (Fig. 22-9) and a classically bell-shaped chest (Fig. 22-10), however the lung fields are clear unless there is coexisting RDS. Pneumothorax or other forms of air leak are frequently present. The chest radiograph may also demonstrate features of the infant's underlying condition (Figs. 22-11 and 22-12). Pathologically, pulmonary hypoplasia is diagnosed if the lung weight to body weight ratio is <0.015 in infants born before 28 weeks of gestation and <0.012 in infants born after 28 weeks of gestation; in addition, there is a radial alveolar count of less than 4%.

Antenatally diagnosed pleural effusions can be chronically drained by thoracoamniotic shunts, which will facilitate ease of resuscitation.[134] *In utero* surgery has

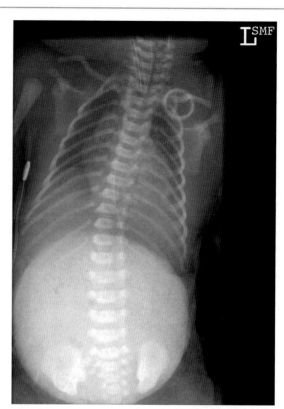

FIGURE 22-9. Pulmonary hypoplasia in association with an abdominal wall defect. The radio-opaque area is the silo containing the gastroschisis.

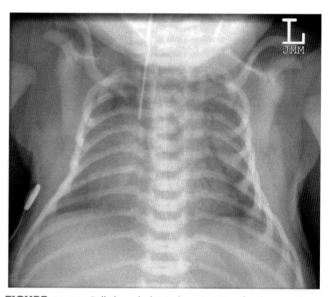

FIGURE 22-10. Bell-shaped chest characteristic of pulmonary hypoplasia. This infant had bilateral renal agenesis. The trachea appears deviated to the right because of some secondary right-sided collapse.

been undertaken for infants with CDH, but this has been problematic. As a consequence, the efficacy of reversible tracheal "obstruction" is being investigated in cases predicted to be at high risk of fatal pulmonary hypoplasia.[135] The rationale for this approach follows from the observation that obstruction of the upper respiratory tract, as occurs in laryngeal atresia, results in larger than normal lungs. For fetuses with renal malformations,

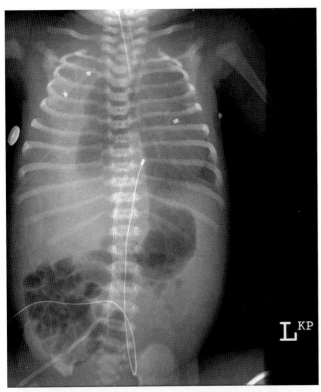

FIGURE 22-11. Chest radiograph of an infant with right-sided pleural effusion. The two radio-opaque dots on each side of the chest represent the ends of the thoracoamniotic shunts; the shunt on the right side is lying entirely within the chest, resulting in a large effusion accumulating and pushing the mediastinum across to the left. There are UAC and UVC catheters in place.

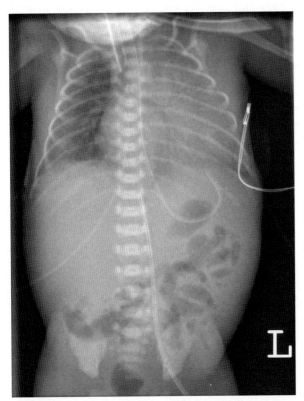

FIGURE 22-12. Pulmonary hypoplasia in an infant with trisomy; the infant has the characteristic gracile ribs and also has a large heart due to critical pulmonary stenosis.

antenatal therapy is directed at relieving urinary obstruction, but vesicoamniotic shunting has a high morbidity and whether it improves pulmonary outcome requires quantitative evaluation.[12] If an infant with pulmonary hypoplasia requires ventilatory support, the minimum pressures compatible with acceptable gases should be used, as these infants are at high risk of air leaks. Low-pressure, fast-rate ventilation or HFOV[136] can be helpful in some infants, but ECMO is usually contraindicated as the infants do not have a reversible condition. Pulmonary vasodilators can be useful if there is coexisting pulmonary hypertension; in a small series, administration of iNO was associated with improvement in oxygenation in infants with pulmonary hypertension associated with suspected pulmonary hypoplasia following oligohydramnios and PPROM.[137] Home oxygen therapy allows early discharge, but parents need to be counseled that supplementary oxygen may be required for many months. Every attempt should be made to reduce further compromise to the lungs; full immunization is essential, and RSV prophylaxis should be considered.

Infants with Potter's syndrome (large, low-set ears, prominent epicanthic folds, and a flattened nose, and postural limb defects) die in the neonatal period. There is also 100% mortality rate in infants with oligohydramnios syndrome (pulmonary hypoplasia, abnormal faces, and limb abnormalities) due to PROM. In less severely affected infants, the perinatal mortality rate has been reported to be approximately 50% if membrane rupture occurs between 15 and 28 weeks.[138] In one series,[139] survival rate to hospital discharge among liveborn infants from pregnancies complicated by membrane rupture prior to 24 weeks of gestation with PPROM of >14 days in duration was 70%. Infants with pulmonary hypoplasia who remain on high-pressure ventilation and high inspired oxygen concentrations at the end of the first week are in an extremely bad prognostic group. It is our experience that such infants rarely go home, and if they do, they go with home oxygen therapy and they die in the first 2 years following infection. Infants born following oligohydramnios can suffer limb abnormalities due to the compression[140]; the reported incidence varies from 27% to 80%; they also suffer from long-term respiratory problems, including BPD and recurrent episodes of wheezing and coughing.[141] In addition, neurologic or developmental deficits are more common, being reported in 28% of infants born after preterm rupture of the membranes prior to 26 weeks of gestation.[142]

AIR LEAKS

Pneumothorax

Spontaneous pneumothoraces occur immediately after birth due to the high transpulmonary pressure swings generated by the first spontaneous breaths. Chest radiographs obtained on consecutive newborns demonstrated that 1% of newborns had an air leak, but only 10% of the affected infants were symptomatic. Pneumothoraces more usually occur as a complication of respiratory disease or a congenital malformation, particularly if there is uneven ventilation, alveolar overdistension, and air trapping, and the infant is receiving ventilatory support. Approximately 5% to 10% of ventilated babies develop an air leak; they are particularly likely to occur in babies who fight the ventilator and actively exhale during ventilator inflation (active expiration). Rarely, pneumothoraces occur as a result of a direct injury to the lung, for example by perforation from suction catheters or introducers passed through the endotracheal tube or by central venous catheter placement.

Small pneumothoraces may be asymptomatic and diagnosed on a chest radiograph taken for other reasons. If an infant suffers a large pneumothorax, he or she frequently deteriorates dramatically with marked respiratory distress, pallor, shock, and deterioration in oxygenation. A tension pneumothorax results in a shift of the mediastinum and abdominal distension due to displacement of the diaphragm. Pneumothorax causes and aggravates hemorrhage into the germinal layer and cerebral ventricles of preterm infants. A chest radiograph should be obtained if a pneumothorax is suspected, unless the infant's clinical condition makes emergency drainage mandatory. A large pneumothorax is associated with absent lung markings and a collapsed lung on the ipsilateral side. If the pneumothorax is under tension, there will also be eversion of the diaphragm, bulging intercostal spaces, and mediastinal shift (Fig. 22-13). A small pneumothorax, however, may only be recognized by a difference in radiolucency between the two lung fields (Fig. 22-14). Unusually the appearance of either lobar emphysema or cystic adenomatoid malformation of the lung may resemble a pneumothorax. In a preterm infant with a thin chest wall, transillumination with an intense beam from a fiberoptic light will demonstrate an abnormal air collection by an increased transmission of light, but PIE can give a similar appearance.

Asymptomatic pneumothoraces do not require treatment, but the infant should be carefully observed. Nursing an infant with a pneumothorax in an inspired oxygen concentration of 100% favors resorption of the extraalveolar gas, but this strategy should not be used in infants at risk of retinopathy of prematurity. If the

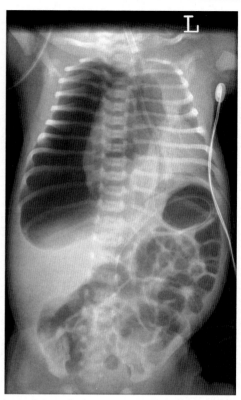

FIGURE 22-13. Tension right pneumothorax with eversion of the diaphragm.

infant is symptomatic or has a tension pneumothorax, the pneumothorax must be drained. If the infant is in extremis and there is no time for insertion of a chest drain, emergency aspiration should be undertaken with an 18-gauge butterfly needle, which is attached to a three-way tap held underwater in a small sterile container. The needle is inserted through the skin in the second intercostal space anteriorly, and then the skin and needle are moved sideways before advancing the needle through the underlying muscle; this reduces the likelihood of leaving an open needle track for entry of air

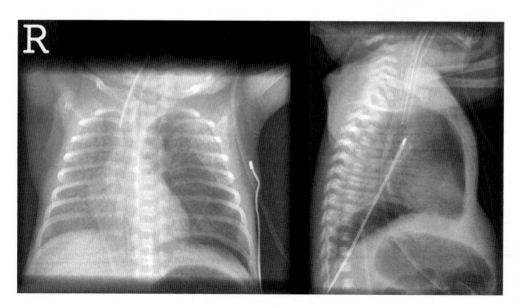

FIGURE 22-14. Left-sided pneumothorax, demonstrated by a discrepancy in the translucency of the two lung fields and a small rim of basal free air. The lateral chest radiograph demonstrates the free air.

once the needle has been removed. Following emergency drainage, a chest tube (French gauge 10 to 14) should be inserted under local anesthesia through either the second intercostal space just lateral to the midclavicular line or the sixth space in the midaxillary line. The tip of the chest tube should be placed retrosternally to achieve the most effective drainage; whether the drain has been positioned correctly should be checked on a lateral chest radiograph (Fig. 22-15). Complications of malpositioned tubes include traumatization of the thoracic duct resulting in a chylothorax, cardiac tamponade due to a hemorrhagic pericardial effusion, and phrenic nerve injury. Once inserted, the tube should be connected to an underwater seal drain with suction of 5 to 10 cm H_2O. Heimlich valves are useful during transport, but they can become blocked so should not be used for long-term drainage. The chest drain can be removed 24 hours after there is no further bubbling of air into the water seal.

To prevent air leaks, it is important to stop infants breathing out of phase with the ventilator (active expiration or asynchrony). This can be achieved by administration of a neuromuscular blocking agent, but as this has side effects, including fluid retention, many clinicians prefer to administer analgesics and/or sedatives to try and suppress respiratory activity. Although they have benefits, administration of analgesics and/or sedatives (e.g., fentanyl, morphine, diamorphine, midazolam, or chloral hydrate), however, have not been demonstrated in randomized trials to reduce the pneumothorax rate, and they also have side effects. An alternative strategy to prevent pneumothoraces is to use a form of ventilatory support, which encourages the infant to breathe synchronously with the ventilator (i.e., inspiration and inflation are coinciding). Use of a faster rate (60/min) rather than a slower rate (30 to 40/min) during conventional ventilation has been associated with a reduced risk of pneumothorax development (relative risk 0.69, CI 0.51, 0.93),[69] but randomized trials have failed to demonstrate that either patient-triggered ventilation or high-frequency oscillation are efficacious in that respect. Surfactant administration is associated with a lower risk of pneumothorax development (see earlier in the chapter).

Pulmonary Interstitial Emphysema

The incidence of pulmonary interstitial emphysema (PIE) is inversely related to birth weight. It has rarely been described in spontaneously breathing infants and occurs mainly in neonates with RDS supported by positive-pressure ventilation and exposed to high-peak inspiratory pressures and/or malpositioned endotracheal tubes. PIE commonly involves both lungs, but it may be lobar in distribution. It frequently occurs with either a pneumothorax or pneumomediastinum. In surfactant-deficient infants, rupture of the small airways can occur distal to termination of the fascial sheath. Gas then dissects into the interstitium and becomes trapped within the perivascular sheaths of the lung, resulting in PIE. The trapped gas reduces pulmonary perfusion by compressing the vessels and interfering with ventilation. As a result, affected infants are profoundly hypoxemic and hypercarbic. PIE is usually diagnosed when a chest radiograph is obtained on a severely ill neonate. The chest radiograph demonstrates hyperinflation and a characteristic cystic appearance, which may be diffuse, multiple, or small nonconfluent cystic radiolucencies (Fig. 22-16). Severe mediastinal compression can result from the PIE (Fig. 22-17). At a later stage, large bullae may appear. The appearance may be confused with lobar emphysema or with cystic adenomatoid malformation of the lung, especially if localized.

If the PIE is localized, the infant should be nursed in the lateral decubitus position with the affected lung dependent and hence underventilated, this promotes partial or complete atelectasis. Selective bronchial intubation to bypass the affected lung for 24 to 48 hours may also be associated with resolution of the PIE; selective intubation of the left main bronchus can be difficult, and adequate blood gases cannot be maintained in some infants if only one lung is ventilated. Despite such maneuvers, if the PIE persists and compresses adjacent normal lung parenchyma, resection of the affected area may be necessary to alleviate respiratory distress. If the infant has widespread PIE, the PEEP and peak-inflating pressures should be reduced to the minimum compatible with acceptable gases and the infant should be paralyzed to try and avoid extension of the air leak. Transfer to high-frequency jet, flow interruption or oscillatory ventilation or continuous negative pressure with intermittent mandatory ventilation have all been anecdotally described as improving gas exchange in infants with PIE

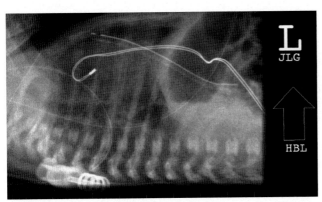

FIGURE 22-15. Lateral chest radiograph demonstrating appropriate retrosternal placement of the chest drainage tube.

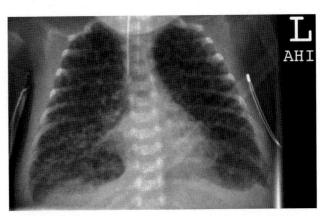

FIGURE 22-16. Severe bilateral pulmonary interstitial emphysema.

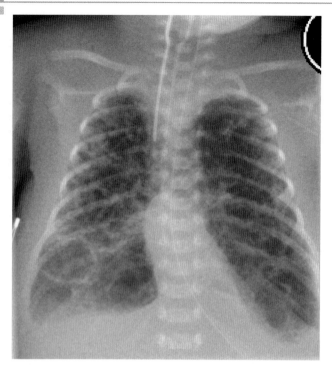

FIGURE 22-17. Severe mediastinal compression. Note the large cystic bullae at the lower bases.

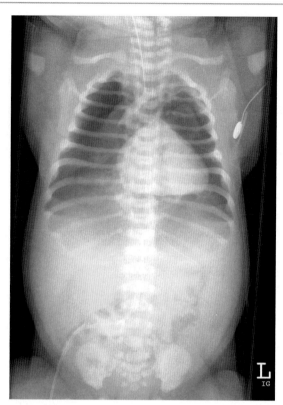

FIGURE 22-18. Bilateral pneumothoraces with elevation of the thymic shadow, indicating air in the mediastinum and air inferior to the diaphragmatic surface of the heart.

and respiratory failure that is poorly responsive to conventional ventilation. If such strategies fail and the infant is in extremis, linear pleurotomies, scarifing the lung through the chest wall to create an artificial pneumothorax, may help to decompress the PIE. Pneumatoceles can develop as a complication of PIE, pneumothorax, or pneumomediastinum; in one case series,[143] the majority responded to a decrease in MAP or extubation. Rarely infants develop persistent PIE. There is a poor prognosis if this affects multiple lobes; in those with progressive localized disease, early surgical resection should be considered.[144] The mortality from diffuse PIE has been reported to be high, but the studies generally predated the routine use of antenatal steroids and postnatal surfactant. The incidence of BPD is increased following diffuse PIE.

Pneumomediastinum

Pneumomediastinum occurs in approximately 2.5 per 1000 live births. An isolated pneumomediastinum rarely causes severe symptoms. Pneumomediastinum, however, usually coexists with multiple air leaks in severely ill ventilated babies. On the chest radiograph, a pneumomediastinum appears as a halo of air adjacent to the borders of the heart, and on lateral view there is marked retrosternal hyperlucency. The mediastinal gas may elevate the thymus away from the pericardium, resulting in a crescentic configuration resembling a spinnaker sail (Fig. 22-18). An isolated pneumomediastinum usually requires no treatment. In term infants, use of a high inspired oxygen concentration is associated with resorption of the extraalveolar air. Drainage of a pneumomediastinum is difficult because the gas is collected in multiple independent lobules, and multiple needling and tube drainage may be required.

Pneumopericardium

A pneumopericardium is usually accompanied by other air leaks (e.g., a pneumomediastinum, widespread PIE, or tension pneumothorax), which suggests that the gas enters the pericardium through a defect in the pericardial sac, probably at the pericardial reflection near the ostia of the pulmonary veins. The majority of cases occur in ventilated prematurely born babies. A pneumopericardium causes cardiac tamponade with sudden hypotension, bradycardia, and cyanosis. The chest radiograph demonstrates gas completely surrounding the heart, outlining the base of the great vessels, and contained within the pericardium. Gas can be seen inferior to the diaphragmatic surface of the heart, differentiating this abnormality from a pneumomediastinum, in which the mediastinal gas is limited inferiorly by the attachment of the mediastinal pleura to the central tendon of the diaphragm (see Fig. 22-18). All symptomatic pneumopericardia should be drained immediately by direct pericardial tap via the subxyphoid route. The blood pressure should be monitored continuously, and the tap repeated if bradycardia or hypotension recur. Catheter drainage may be necessary if the pericardial air re-accumulates. The mortality of symptomatic pneumopericardia is between 80% and 90%, and many survivors have neurologic sequelae.

Pneumoperitoneum

A pneumoperitoneum may result from perforation of the gut or by gas dissecting from the chest through the diaphragmatic foramina into the peritoneum. The latter scenario is particularly likely in ventilated babies who have a pneumothorax and a pneumomediastinum. If the pneumoperitoneum is large, the diagnosis can be made from the anteroposterior radiograph (Figure 22-19), but it is better shown in a horizontal-beam lateral, (Figs. 22-20 and 22-21); a right lateral radiograph may be required to demonstrate smaller leaks (Fig. 22-22). Treatment is only necessary if the abdomen is under sufficient tension to cause respiratory embarrassment; then the pneumoperitoneum should be drained either by needle aspiration or by inserting a drainage tube.

Systemic Air Embolism

The majority of infants who suffer a systemic air embolism have other air leaks. Affected infants deteriorate suddenly, with pallor, cyanosis, hypotension, and bizarre irregularities on their echocardiogram. On the chest radiograph, gas can be seen in the systemic and pulmonary arteries and veins. Early withdrawal of air from the umbilical artery catheter may be of benefit, particularly if the leak is small or has been introduced through an intravascular line, but the condition is usually fatal.

PATENT DUCTUS ARTERIOSUS

During fetal life, blood is shunted from the right heart via the pulmonary artery through the ductus arteriosus to the aorta, and the lungs are "bypassed." At birth, the ductus arteriosus begins to constrict with the onset of breathing. In the majority of infants, the ductus arteriosus has

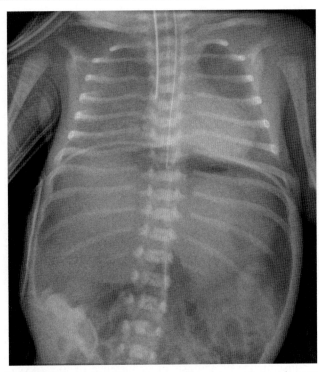

FIGURE 22-20. Pneumoperitoneum. This anteroposterior abnormal radiograph shows a large collection of free air.

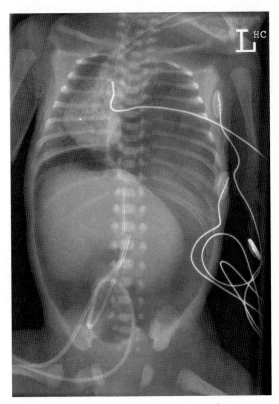

FIGURE 22-19. Large pneumoperitoneum. The mediastinum is pushed to the right by free air in the left chest. UAC and UVC catheters are in place.

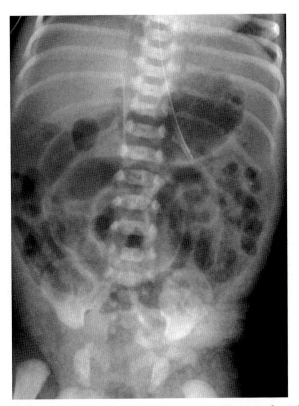

FIGURE 22-21. Pneumoperitoneum. The horizontal beam confirms the large amount of free air.

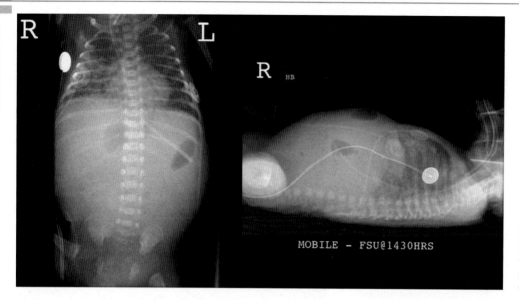

FIGURE 22-22. This anterior-posterior abdominal radiograph shows a small pocket of nonanatomic air. The horizontal beam demonstrates a free collection, confirming the diagnosis of a pneumoperitoneum.

closed by 24 hours of age, and in 90% will have closed by 60 hours of age. Ductal closure is delayed in infants with pulmonary hypertension and respiratory failure as a consequence of acidosis or persistence of low oxygen tensions; in such circumstances, prostaglandin E_2 levels remain high. The incidence of PDA is inversely related to gestational age. The incidence of PDA in term infants has been estimated to be 57 per 100,000 live births, whereas 55% of ELBW infants will have a symptomatic PDA.

Clinical Presentation and Diagnosis

A hemodynamically significant PDA presents either as a failure of improvement in an infant with RDS or an acute deterioration that necessitates an increase in respiratory support. Some infants will present when they are extubated from the ventilator. The increased pulmonary blood flow is associated with a decrease in pulmonary compliance. The infant is unable to maintain small airway patency without PEEP and hence collapses on extubation. Infants with a hemodynamically significant PDA have tachycardia, bounding pulses, an active precordium, and sometimes a murmur, although the latter might be absent. The typical ductal murmur is systolic (in about 75% of cases), but it can be continuous and is best heard at the upper-left sternal edge. As the pulmonary vascular resistance falls, the left-to-right shunt through the ductus increases and the peripheral pulses become bounding. This reflects the widened pulse pressure due to blood being shunted from the high-pressure systemic circulation into the lower pressure pulmonary circulation. The left-to-right shunt means higher blood flow in the lungs, resulting in the infant being tachypneic, and crackles heard at the lung bases. The chest radiograph (Fig. 22-23) demonstrates cardiomegaly, pulmonary plethora, and a wide angle between the left and right main bronchi due to left atrial dilation. The diagnosis can be confirmed by echocardiography; echocardiographic signs of a ductal shunt precede the development of overt clinical signs by on average 3 days. Typical echocardiographic findings of a moderate to large left-to-right ductal shunt are bowing of the interatrial septum to the right

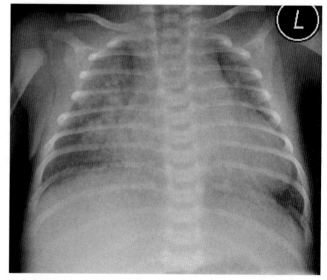

FIGURE 22-23. Chest radiograph of an infant with symptomatic patent ductus arteriosus. Note the large heart and increased pulmonary vascular markings.

with enlargement of the left atrium and ventricle and left atrium enlargement with a left atrial: aortic root (LA:Ao) ratio >1.4:1.[145] Color Doppler examination reveals a continuous flare in the main pulmonary artery from the arterial duct. The size of the shunt can be determined from the ductal size on color Doppler examination, the LA:Ao ratio, and whether the diastolic flow in the descending aorta is reversed during diastole. If the shunt is large, flow reversal will be throughout diastole. Echocardiographic examination is also important to exclude other congenital heart abnormalities.

Management

Some PDAs will close spontaneously. This is less likely in infants born between 23 and 25 weeks of gestation; such infants are also more likely to be refractory to treatment.[146] Initial management of an infant with a PDA usually includes fluid restriction, although there have been no randomized trials demonstrating that fluid restriction in infants with a hemodynamically significant PDA promotes ductal closure. Diuretics are frequently given, but theoretically furosemide might promote ductal patency via its effect on renal prostaglandin synthesis; administration of furosemide before each dose of indomethacin is not recommended because it can result in significant increases in serum creatinine and hyponatremia and no increase in urine output.[147] Early randomized trials demonstrated that fluid restriction reduced the likelihood of a PDA. These results, however, have not been confirmed in a study that has included infants routinely exposed to antenatal corticosteroids and postnatal surfactant.[148] If there is no improvement following fluid restriction for at least 24 hours (providing there are no contraindications, such as poor renal function or a low platelet count), treatment with indomethacin or ibuprofen should be considered. Indomethacin is a nonselective cyclooxygenase inhibitor, reducing the synthesis of prostaglandin E. Ductal closure is achieved with indomethacin treatment in 48 hours in approximately 70% of infants. Indomethacin can be given as three doses 12 hours apart or for 6 or 7 days at 24-hourly intervals; results from randomized trials have highlighted that the prolonged course did not result in a statistically significant difference in PDA closure, retreatment, reopening, or ligation rates, but an increased risk of NEC.[149] Increasing indomethacin concentrations above the levels achieved with a conventional dosing regime is not recommended because it does not significantly increase PDA closure and increases the rates of moderate/severe ROP and renal compromise.[150] Indomethacin treatment has a number of side effects, including gastric or bowel perforation and reduction in renal function. Administration by infusion rather than bolus is associated with less alteration in cerebral, renal, and mesenteric circulation, but the clinical meaning of such an effect remains uncertain.[151] There are two isoforms of the cyclooxygenase: COX-1 and COX-2. The former is primarily involved in basal physiologic processes in the kidney. Like indomethacin, ibuprofen also inhibits both isoforms of the cyclooxygenase inhibitor, but it appears to have less impact on urine output.[152,153] Indomethacin is more potent against COX-1. Ibuprofen is similarly effective to indomethacin with regard to PDA closure,[154] but the rate of NEC was reduced for ibuprofen.[153] In a large randomized study, prophylactic indomethacin in infants with a PDA did not reduce the incidence of BPD and was associated with a higher incidence of BPD in infants without PDA.[154] Given the side effects of indomethacin, prophylactic treatment cannot be recommended. Meta-analysis[155] of the results of trials of prophylactic treatment with ibuprofen demonstrated that it reduces the incidence of PDA, the need for rescue therapy, and surgical closure, but it does not improve any other short-term outcomes. Prophylactic ibuprofen given to infants with nonsymptomatic PDAs in the first 72 hours after birth was associated with a trend toward decreased PVL, but it had no significant effect on any other outcome.[156] Meta-analysis of the results of randomized trials demonstrated that ibuprofen is as effective as indomethacin in closing a PDA and reduces the risk of NEC and transient renal insufficiency;

as a consequence it was concluded that ibuprofen was the preferred treatment.[53] Surgical closure is reserved for infants in whom there is a contraindication to indomethacin administration or when treatment has been ineffective. The risk of treatment failure is increased by sepsis and more common in very immature infants.[157] Despite surgical closure, infants may still go on to develop BPD.[158] Treatment failure has been associated with a significantly increased risk of BPD.[157] Infants who undergo surgical closure compared to those who respond to indomethacin are smaller and more premature and more likely to develop BPD.[159] Prophylactic ligation (ligation in the first 24 hours regardless of whether the PDA was symptomatic) is not recommended as it was associated with an increased incidence of BPD in a randomized trial.[160] Surgery can be performed safely on the NICU, and this has the advantage of avoiding the risks inherent in patient transfer.[161]

Mortality and Morbidity

BPD is significantly increased in infants who have had a PDA, particularly if they have also suffered a nosocomial infection. If the PDA is large, there is a diastolic steal, thus retrograde diastolic flow develops in the cerebral circulation and the descending aorta, renal blood vessels, and mesenteric blood vessels. Due to compromised gut (diastolic) blood flow, the incidence of necrotizing enterocolitis is increased in infants who have had a PDA.

▰ PULMONARY EDEMA

Pulmonary edema occurs when there is leakage of fluid from pulmonary capillaries into the interstitium and alveoli. This can occur when the pulmonary capillary pressure is greater than the plasma oncotic pressure or there is disruption of the barriers between the vascular space and the lung interstitium. Increased lung microvascular pressure occurs most commonly if there is a large left-to-right shunt from a PDA, but it can occur in infants with cardiac disease (e.g., in severe forms of total anomalous pulmonary venous drainage). In addition, cardiac arrhythmias, particularly tachyarrhythmias, can result in an acute onset of heart failure and pulmonary edema. Myocardial dysfunction or an overrapid infusion will exacerbate these problems. Altered capillary permeability occurs in ARDS or following any hypoxic insult. Fluid accumulates if the lymphatic system is overloaded, and thus pulmonary edema also occurs if there are abnormalities of the pulmonary lymphatic drainage. Initially, any excess fluid builds up in the interstitium; however as the fluid accumulates it disrupts the alveolar membrane, and fluid fills the alveoli.

The infant with pulmonary edema is tachycardic, pale, and sweaty and has poor volume peripheral pulses with reduced cardiac output. The chest radiograph demonstrates perihilar shadowing obscuring the vascular structures (Fig. 22-24) and linear septal shadows (Kerley B lines) in the lower part of the lungs; in the most severe cases, fluid may be visible in the horizontal and oblique fissures, cardiomegaly, and pericardial effusions. Cardiac causes of pulmonary edema can be diagnosed from the echocardiogram or electrocardiogram.

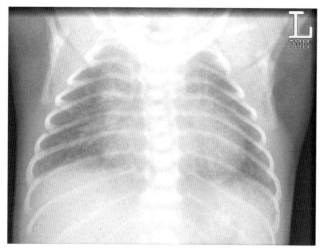

FIGURE 22-24. Pulmonary edema due to a large ventricular septal defect. Note also the gracile ribs of an infant with trisomy 13.

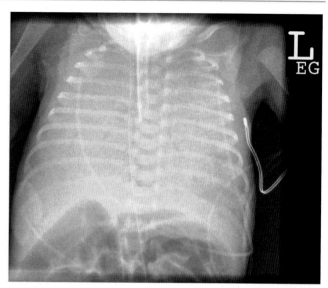

FIGURE 22-25. Chest radiograph of an infant with patent ductus arteriosus who suffered a massive pulmonary hemorrhage. The endotracheal tube tip is too low, as it abuts the carina.

Fluid input should be restricted and fluid overload avoided. Diuretic treatment is given to reduce the circulating volume and the clinical manifestations of pulmonary edema, but it may critically lower the cardiac output. Positive pressure ventilation may be needed to acutely stabilize the patient, and oxygenation can be improved by increasing the PEEP in infants who are already ventilated. Treatment of any underlying structural or functional cause is essential.

PULMONARY HAEMORRHAGE

Pulmonary hemorrhage occurs most commonly in VLBW babies who have heart failure secondary to a large pulmonary blood flow due to a PDA. Prophylactic indomethacin reduces the rate of early serious pulmonary hemorrhage, mainly through its action on the PDA, but it is less effective in preventing serious pulmonary hemorrhages that occur after the first week after birth.[162] Surfactant administration may increase the risk of pulmonary hemorrhage, particularly if a synthetic rather than natural surfactant is used.[163] Pulmonary hemorrhage also occurs following severe birth depression and in infants with hydrops due to Rhesus hemolytic disease, left heart failure, congenital heart disease, sepsis, fluid overload, and clotting abnormalities. Growth-retarded infants are more likely to suffer a pulmonary hemorrhage. Pulmonary hemorrhage is a severe form of lung edema with leakage of red cells and is better named *hemorrhagic pulmonary edema*. In most cases, the amount of blood lost is small because the hematocrit of the lung effluent is less than 10%.

Infants who suffer a massive pulmonary hemorrhage deteriorate suddenly with copious bloody secretions appearing from the airway. The infant is hypotensive because of blood and fluid loss and heart failure, and usually is limp and unresponsive. If the hemorrhage is secondary to heart failure, the infant may have tachycardia, the murmur of a PDA, hepatosplenomegaly, and a triple rhythm. Affected infants are dyspneic and cyanotic with widespread crackles and reduced air entry into their lungs. The chest radiograph usually demonstrates a whiteout with only an air bronchogram visible

(Fig. 22-25). A lobar pattern of consolidation may be found if the hemorrhage occurs in only part of the lung.

All infants with a massive pulmonary hemorrhage should be intubated and ventilated. Peak inflating pressures above 30 cm H_2O may be necessary to achieve acceptable blood gases. A high PEEP level should be used to help to redistribute fluid back into the interstitial space and to improve oxygenation. Neuromuscular blockade and sedation should be used until the hemorrhage is controlled. Although surfactant administration has been incriminated in increasing the risk of a pulmonary hemorrhage, once a hemorrhage has occurred a single dose of surfactant may improve oxygenation.[164] Frequent suctioning is initially required to prevent the copious bloody secretions from blocking the endotracheal tube. Physiotherapy, however, is not of proven value. Infection may cause a pulmonary hemorrhage, thus broad-spectrum antimicrobials should be administered, ensuring coverage against infection by *Staphylococcus* and *Pseudomonas*. Blood transfusions may be required, and it is important to support the blood pressure. Fluid input should be restricted, particularly if there is a coexisting patent ductus, and diuretics should be given if there is evidence of fluid overload.

The risks for death or for survival with neurosensory impairment are doubled in ELBW infants who have had a serious pulmonary hemorrhage.[162] Affected babies frequently require high-pressure ventilation, thus air leaks and BPD are common sequelae.

UPPER AIRWAY OBSTRUCTION

The presentation of upper airway obstruction depends on the site (see later in the chapter) and the magnitude of the obstruction. Tachypnea may be the only manifestation of a partial obstruction, whereas those with a complete obstruction will present with severe respiratory failure, which will be fatal if not promptly relieved.[165] This subject is discussed in more detail in Chapters 21 and 69.

Nasal Obstruction

Infants are obligate nasal breathers, thus any anatomic or functional obstruction will result in respiratory distress. Choanal atresia is the most common cause of true nasal obstruction, but it occurs in only 1 in 10,000 live births. It can be unilateral or bilateral, isolated or associated with other congenital abnormalities, such as in CHARGE syndrome (coloboma of the iris and retina, heart disease, atresia choanae, retarded growth, genital hypoplasia, ear defects). Infants with unilateral Choanal atresia may be asymptomatic until the nonaffected nares become blocked, for example with secretions. Infants with bilateral Choanal atresia classically appear normal when crying and mouth breathing, but respiratory difficulty appears as soon as they try to breathe through their nose. Less common causes of nasal obstruction include midnasal stenosis and choanal stenosis. Choanal atresia or stenosis can be diagnosed on a CT scan, but magnetic resonance imaging should also be employed to determine whether there are intracranial connections in suspected encephalocele, meningocele, and nasal glioma. Nasal causes of obstruction are relieved by an oral airway. Surgical intervention for choanal atresia includes opening the bony membrane, which is blocking the airway and insertion of tubes to maintain the airway; these are sutured in place for at least 4 weeks.

Pharyngeal Obstruction

Pharyngeal obstruction can occur if there is macroglossia or micrognathia. Craniofacial syndromes associated with oropharyngeal obstruction include Pierre Robin, hemifacial microsomia, and Crouzon's syndrome. If the tongue is too large or there is inadequate space for the tongue, it is displaced posteriorly into the hypopharynx, causing obstruction, particularly if the infant is nursed in a supine position. As a consequence, affected infants should be nursed prone.

Laryngeal Obstruction

Laryngeal obstruction can result from laryngeal polyps or cysts and dynamic causes, such as vocal cord palsy and severe laryngomalacia. Birth injury is responsible for 20% of vocal cord palsy; traction on the infant's neck during the delivery can result in damage to the recurrent laryngeal nerve; it can also occur following cardiac surgery such as duct ligation. Stridor occurring immediately after delivery should always raise the suspicion of a vocal cord palsy, but it may also be due to a laryngeal web, cyst, or stenosis. Bilateral vocal cord palsy can occur in infants with severe neurologic abnormalities. Affected infants have pharyngeal incoordination, and aspiration is common. Laryngomalacia presents during the first few days after birth. Laryngomalacia is most commonly due to prolapse of the aryepiglottic folds, which collapse on inspiration due to the negative airway pressure; the stridor, therefore, is worse on crying and feeding, but it tends to be better when the infant is at rest. Management is usually supportive, as the condition resolves over 12 to 24 months. Subglottic stenosis can be congenital, resulting from a malformation of the cricoid cartilage, but it is more commonly acquired secondary to intubation. Infants with acquired subglottic stenosis present with respiratory distress due to upper airway obstruction after extubation, and this condition should be suspected if there are intubation difficulties, particularly difficulty in siting an appropriate-sized endotracheal tube. Hoarseness suggests a laryngeal lesion, such as a laryngeal web or vocal cord palsy. Laryngeal obstruction is relieved by intubation, but not by an oral airway.

Lesions within the laryngotracheobronchial tree (e.g., stenosis) are sometimes visible on a chest radiograph or a highly penetrated filtered (Cincinnati) view. MRI is the investigation of choice for extrinsic lesions, particularly if vascular compression is suspected. Laryngoscopy can be used to diagnose dynamic conditions, but rigid laryngotracheobronchoscopy is the investigation of choice for all complex airway lesions.

Vocal cord palsy resulting from a birth injury or following an operative procedure is usually due to edema and inflammation and usually resolves with time. Spontaneous resolution is not the case if bilateral cord palsy is associated with a neurologic condition; as a consequence, affected infants may require a tracheostomy to protect the airway and a gastrostomy feeding tube for pharyngeal incoordination. The occurrence of acquired subglottic stenosis can be minimized by using appropriately sized endotracheal tubes with a leak around the tube. If there is no leak, airway edema should be suspected and pre-extubation corticosteroids and adrenaline nebulizers should be given. Nevertheless, some neonates require re-intubation because of stridor and airway compromise, and such infants should remain intubated for a period of "laryngeal rest." If extubation still fails after such a period, an endoscopic examination should be performed to determine the diagnosis. Surgical intervention for subglottic stenosis consists of a cricoid split or laryngeal reconstruction using rib cartilage; tracheostomy may be required (see Chapter 69 for a further discussion).

Suggested Reading

Barrington KJ, Finer NN. Inhaled nitric oxide for preterm infants: a systematic review. *Pediatrics.* 2007;120:1088–1099.

Been JV, Zimmermann LJI. Histological chorioamnionitis and respiratory outcome in preterm infants. *Arch Dis Child Fetal Neonatal Ed.* 2009;94:F218–F225.

Crowther CA, Alfirevic Z, Han S, et al. Thyrotropin-releasing hormone added to corticosteroids for women at risk of preterm birth for preventing neonatal respiratory disease. *Cochrane Database Syst Rev.* 2010;(1): CD000019.

Greenough A, Dimitriou G, Prendergast M, et al. Synchronised mechanical ventilation for respiratory support in newborn infants. *Cochrane Database Syst Rev.* 2008;(1): CD000446.

Henderson-Smart DJ, De Paoli AG, Clark RH, et al. High frequency oscillatory ventilation versus conventional ventilation for infants with severe pulmonary dysfunction at or near term. *Cochrane Database Syst Rev.* 2009;(3): CD002974.

Ng E, Shah V. Erythromycin for feeding intolerance in preterm infants. *Cochrane Database Syst Rev.* 2000;(2): CD001815.

Schmidt B, Roberts RS, Davis P, et al. Caffeine therapy for apnea of prematurity. *N Engl J Med.* 2006;354:2112–2121.

Stevens TP, Blenno M, Myers EH, et al. Early surfactant administration with brief ventilation versus selective surfactant and continued mechanical ventilation for preterm infants with or at risk for respiratory distress syndrome. *Cochrane Database Syst Rev.* 2008;(3): CD.

The International Liaison Committee on Resuscitation (ILCOR) consensus on neonatal resuscitation. *Pediatrics.* 2006;117:e978–e988.

References

The complete reference list is available online at www.expertconsult.com

23 BRONCHOPULMONARY DYSPLASIA

STEVEN H. ABMAN, MD

Improved survival of very immature infants has contributed to an increase in the number of infants who develop bronchopulmonary dysplasia (BPD). BPD is a chronic lung disease that occurs in roughly 10,000 to 15,000 infants per year in the United States alone. This has important health resource utilization implications, as follow-up studies have demonstrated that BPD infants require frequent re-admission to the hospital in the first 2 years after birth for respiratory infections, asthma, and related problems, and they have persistent lung function abnormalities as adolescents and young adults. BPD most commonly occurs in prematurely born infants who have required mechanical ventilation and oxygen therapy for acute respiratory distress,[1-4] but it also can occur in immature infants who have had minimal initial lung disease.[5-8] Although BPD is most commonly associated with premature birth, it can occur in term or near-term infants due to severe acute lung injury, as reflected by the need for high mechanical ventilator support or extracorporeal membrane oxygenation (ECMO) therapy.

Over the past 40 years, the introduction of prenatal steroid use, surfactant therapy, new ventilator strategies, aggressive management of patent ductus arteriosus (PDA), improved nutrition, and other treatments have resulted in dramatic changes in the clinical course and outcomes of premature newborns with RDS. Whereas the overall incidence of BPD has not declined over the past decade,[8] its severity has been clearly modulated by changes in clinical practice. There is now growing recognition that infants with chronic lung disease after premature birth have a different clinical course and pathology than had been traditionally observed in infants who were dying with BPD during the pre-surfactant era (Fig. 23-1).[6-12] The classic progressive stages with prominent fibro-proliferation that first characterized BPD are often absent, and the disease has changed to being predominantly defined by a disruption of distal lung growth; this has been termed "the new BPD."[5] In contrast to classic BPD, the new BPD develops in preterm newborns who may have required minimal or even no ventilatory support and relatively low inspired oxygen concentrations during the early postnatal days[6,7] (Fig. 23-2). At autopsy, the lung histology of infants who die with the new BPD displays more uniform and milder regions of injury, but impaired alveolar and vascular growth remain prominent (Table 23-1). The implications of how these changes in BPD alter long-term pulmonary outcomes remain unknown. The new BPD is likely the result of disrupted antenatal and postnatal lung growth that leads to persistent abnormalities of lung architecture. It is unclear whether such infants subsequently experience sufficient catch-up lung growth to achieve and sustain improved lung function over time. To date, no safe and effective preventative therapy for BPD has been identified, but there are promising new therapies directed either at reducing lung injury or improving lung growth.

Overall, BPD may perhaps be best considered as a "syndrome" rather than a single disease because etiologies, clinical course, and respiratory outcomes are diverse and modulated by therapeutic interventions. The changing nature of BPD suggests that a standard binomial definition will not adequately predict long-term pulmonary outcomes. Importantly, there is growing recognition that prematurity itself, even in the absence of BPD, and even in late preterm infants, is associated with significant late respiratory morbidity.[13,14] Importantly, there is a growing appreciation that interventions designed to prevent BPD should focus on late pulmonary and neurodevelopmental outcomes that have the most impact on the health and welfare of prematurely born children and their families, rather than short-term outcomes (e.g., supplemental oxygen requirement at 36 weeks corrected age). Such a change in thinking about BPD requires the development of multidisciplinary teams of health care professionals and clinician-scientists; an appreciation of the magnitude, nature and chronic manifestations of prematurity and BPD; and novel programs that provide continuity of long-term care. This chapter reviews the epidemiology, pathogenesis, pathophysiology, and long-term outcomes of infants with BPD.

DEFINITION

Despite extensive studies of premature infants with chronic lung disease, the definition of BPD remains problematic. BPD is usually defined by the presence of chronic respiratory signs, a persistent oxygen requirement, and an abnormal chest radiograph at 1 month of age or at 36 weeks postconceptional age. Unfortunately, this definition lacks specificity and fails to account for important clinical distinctions related to the extremes of prematurity and wide variability in criteria for the use of prolonged oxygen therapy. The need for supplemental oxygen at 1 month of age in infants born at 24 or 25 weeks gestation may represent lung immaturity and not the results of "lung injury," and such infants may or may not develop chronic respiratory disease. A National Institutes of Health–sponsored conference led to the suggestion of a new definition of BPD that incorporates many elements of previous definitions but attempts to categorize BPD severity according to the level of respiratory support required near to term[15] (Table 23-2). The potential advantage of this approach is that BPD is defined as a spectrum of disease with early markers that may be predictive of long-term pulmonary morbidity. Preliminary studies suggest that this grading of BPD severity is associated with the degree of abnormal lung function during infancy.[16] Another approach to determine the severity of BPD is to assess chest radiographs, but for many infants with chronic oxygen dependency, the chest x-ray only demonstrates small volumes

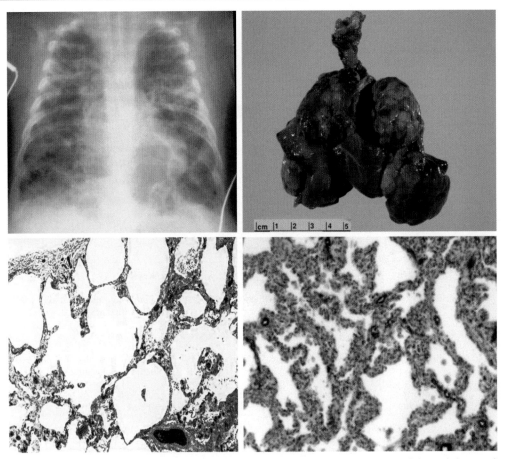

FIGURE 23-1. Radiographic, anatomic, and histologic features of severe bronchopulmonary dysplasia. Upper-left panel shows a chest radiograph with hyperinflation, diffuse but patchy parenchymal infiltrate, and cor pulmonale. Upper-right panel shows gross appearance of severe fibroproliferative bronchopulmonary dysplasia. Note the cobblestone pattern with pseudofissures. Lower-left panel shows marked alveolar simplification in an older child who died from a nonrespiratory cause. Lower-right panel shows immunostaining for factor VIII to highlight a dysmorphic and simplified vascular bed.

"Classic BPD"   "New BPD"

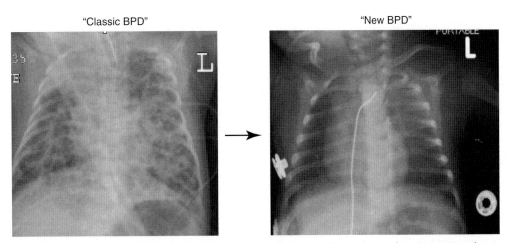

FIGURE 23-2. Chest radiographs illustrating the transition from severe bronchopulmonary dysplasia (Northway Stage IV) in the presurfactant era (classic BPD) compared with a typical x-ray pattern from the new BPD.

with hazy lung fields (Fig. 23-2). Various scoring systems have been developed and may predict chronic oxygen dependency and troublesome respiratory symptoms at follow-up.[17,18]

An additional problem in defining BPD is the wide center-to-center variability in diagnosing the need for supplemental oxygen. A survey from the Vermont Oxford Network revealed striking variations in thresholds for instituting supplementary oxygen based on pulse oximetry, ranging from <84% to <96%, with only 41% of the respondents using the same criteria (<90%).[19] This alone has a marked impact on the reported incidence of BPD. For a given study population, the incidence of BPD decreased from 37% to 24% if the need for supplemental oxygen

TABLE 23-1 CHANGING PATHOLOGIC FEATURES OF BPD

PRE-SURFACTANT ERA ("OLD BPD")	POST-SURFACTANT ERA ("NEW BPD")
Alternating atelectasis with hyperinflation	Less regional heterogeneity
Severe airway epithelial lesions (e.g., hyperplasia, squamous metaplasia)	Rare airway epithelial lesions
Marked airway smooth muscle hyperplasia	Mild airway smooth muscle thickening
Extensive, diffuse fibroproliferation	Rare fibroproliferative changes
Hypertensive remodeling of pulmonary arteries	Fewer arteries but "dysmorphic"
Decreased alveolarization and surface area	Fewer, larger, and simplified alveoli

TABLE 23-2 NIH CONSENSUS CONFERENCE: DIAGNOSTIC CRITERIA FOR ESTABLISHING BPD

	GESTATIONAL AGE	
	<32 Weeks	**>32 Weeks**
Time point of Assessment	36 weeks PMA or discharge to home, whichever comes first	>28 d but <56 d postnatal age or discharge to home, whichever comes first
	Treatment with oxygen >21% for at least 28 d	
Mild BPD	Breathing room air at 36 wk discharge, whichever comes first	Breathing room air by 56 d postnatal or discharge, whichever comes first
Moderate BPD	Need for <30% O_2 at 36 wks PMA or discharge, whichever comes first	Need for <30% O_2 to 56 d postnatal or discharge, whichever comes first
Severe BPD	Need for >30% O_2 +/– PPV or CPAP at 36 wks PMA or discharge, whichever comes first	Need for >30% O_2 +/– PPV or CPAP at 56 d postnatal age or discharge, whichever comes first

PMA, Postmenstrual age; *PPV,* positive pressure ventilation; *NCPAP,* nasal continuous positive airway pressure.

was defined by accepting oxygen saturations above 92% or 88% while breathing room air, respectively.[20] Use of an oxygen reduction test may better help to diagnose ongoing supplemental oxygen requirements[20,21] (Table 23-2). Further work is needed to identify early physiologic, structural, and genetic or biochemical markers of BPD (which are predictive of critical long-term endpoints) such as the presence of late respiratory disease evidenced by recurrent hospitalizations, reactive airways disease, the need for prolonged oxygen, the need for respiratory medications, or exercise intolerance during childhood.

EPIDEMIOLOGY

Pulmonary immaturity is the primary risk factor for BPD due to incomplete structural and biochemical development, including inadequate surfactant, antioxidant, and anti-protease activities.[22] As described earlier in the chapter, the epidemiology of BPD has changed dramatically over the past 40 years. In the early 1960s, oxygen and mechanical ventilation were selectively used for premature infants with acute respiratory failure due to apnea and hyaline membrane disease. As these therapies were applied more widely, there was a growing recognition of premature infants who survived but developed chronic pulmonary disease with hypoxemia and chest radiographic abnormalities. In 1964, Shepard and colleagues reported that 50% of premature neonates who received oxygen and mechanical ventilation developed chronic

lung disease.[23] In 1967, Northway and co-workers provided a comprehensive characterization of the clinical, radiologic, and pathologic features of chronic lung disease in infants who had received high concentrations of oxygen and mechanical ventilation from birth.[1] On average, these premature infants were born at 34 weeks' gestation and weighed 2200 grams, yet their mortality was 67%, and the surviving infants had persistent respiratory distress and abnormal chest radiographs beyond the first 4 weeks after birth. In the latter study, the term *bronchopulmonary dysplasia* was first applied, referring to the striking disruption of airway structure. This seminal study identified the interactive roles of three key pathogenic factors: lung immaturity, acute lung injury, and inadequate repair of the initial lung injury. This basic concept still provides an important paradigm for our current understanding of BPD.

Currently, most infants who develop BPD are born with extreme prematurity, and 75% of cases have birth weights <1000 grams.[6-8] The risk of BPD increases with decreasing birth weight; the incidence has been reported to be as high as 85% in neonates between 500 and 699 grams, but only 5% in infants with birth weights over 1500 grams. Implications regarding the impact of extreme premature birth on lung growth and structure are best appreciated in the context of the stages of lung development (Fig. 23-3). The fetal lung at 24 weeks' gestation is generally at the late canalicular or early saccular stage of growth, which is characterized by immature airway

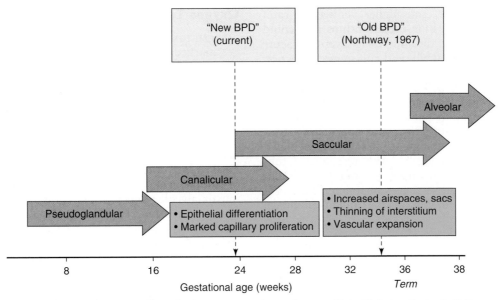

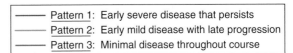

FIGURE 23-3. Relationship between the stages of lung development, gestation, and average birth of infants with classic BPD versus the more extreme premature newborn that typifies the new BPD.

structure, undifferentiated epithelial cells, a paucity of capillaries, and reduced surface area. Thus, premature birth and injury at this early stage of development has profound implications for the risk of BPD, which provides additional challenges in addition to those of premature birth at later stages of lung development.

Although the overall incidence of BPD is reported at about 20% of ventilated newborns, marked variability exists between centers.[24] This variability likely reflects regional differences in the clinical definitions of BPD, the number of inborn versus outborn infants, the proportion of newborns with extreme prematurity, and specific patient management. In the most immature infants, even minimal exposure to oxygen and mechanical ventilation may be sufficient to contribute to BPD. A recent report demonstrated that about two thirds of infants who develop BPD have only mild respiratory distress at birth[8] (Fig. 23-4). Others have observed the recognition of this change in patterns of respiratory diseases[6,7,25] and have emphasized the importance of enhancing our understanding of the mechanisms of progressive respiratory deterioration and the lack of clinical improvement during the first week of life.

Epidemiologic studies of BPD have identified many factors that modify BPD risk. Endogenous factors linked with BPD include gestational immaturity, lower birth weight, male sex, white or nonblack race, family history of asthma, and being small for gestational age.[26–35] Additional perinatal risk factors for BPD include: absence of maternal glucocorticoid treatment, lower Apgar scores, perinatal asphyxia, and respiratory distress syndrome. Recent studies have strongly implicated prenatal factors, including maternal smoking, pre-eclampsia, chorioamnionitis, and intrauterine growth restriction as key factors in the risk for BPD after preterm birth.[36–40] However, the interactions of prenatal and postnatal factors, such exposure to hyperoxia in growth-restricted infants or after endotoxin, may be critical factors as well.

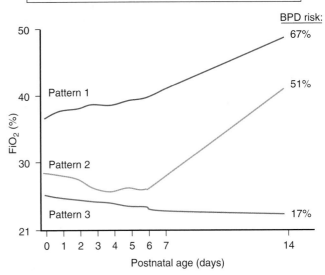

FIGURE 23-4. Changing patterns of respiratory disease with risk for bronchopulmonary dysplasia. (Modified from Laughon M, Alfred EN, Bose C, et al. Patterns of respiratory distress during the first 2 postnatal weeks in extremely premature infants. *Pediatrics.* 2010;123:1124-1131.)

Early respiratory support and related findings are also associated with BPD risk. Such markers include a greater severity of initial pulmonary disease, pneumothorax, pulmonary interstitial emphysema, and severe atelectasis.[31,41] BPD risk also has been linked with other early neonatal influences, including patent ductus arteriosus,[7,25] pulmonary edema,[42] higher weight-adjusted fluid intake, earlier use of parenteral lipid, light-exposed parenteral nutrition, and duration of oxygen therapy. Among at-risk infants, the duration and approach to mechanical ventilation (including the use of high inspired oxygen, high peak inspiratory pressure, lower positive end expiratory pressure, and higher ventilation rate) are also associated with BPD—relationships that could be causal or simply reflect the underlying severity of acute respiratory disease.[43] Kraybill, and colleagues' detection of increased BPD risk associated with hypocarbia (indicated by highest PCO_2 <40 at 48 or 96 hours) suggests that aggressive ventilation can contribute to lung injury and BPD.[31] Colonization or infection with *Ureaplasma urealyticum* and postnatal sepsis also appear to predispose to BPD.[44,45] Epidemiologic studies of BPD yielded a number of predictive models.[46,47] Although none is routinely applied currently in caring for infants at risk of BPD, such models might serve as valuable tools for providing risk adjustment for clinical trials and other clinical research studies.

PATHOGENESIS

Preterm infants are especially susceptible to injury caused by mechanical forces, oxidative stress, and inflammation due to the extreme structural and biochemical immaturity of the preterm lung. As Northway first observed, BPD has diverse, multifactorial etiologies, including hyperoxia, ventilator-induced lung injury, inflammation, and infection[1] (Fig. 23-5). Animal studies suggest that lung injury due to each of these adverse stimuli is at least partly mediated through increased oxidative stress that further augments inflammation, promotes lung injury, and impairs growth factor–signaling pathways. Over the past decades, there has been growing recognition that prenatal factors including chorioamnionitis, placental dysfunction, pre-eclampsia, intrauterine growth restriction, and genetic factors are especially important in the development of new BPD.[37–40] How these epidemiologic observations are mechanistically linked with premature birth and poor respiratory outcomes are currently under intense laboratory and clinical investigation.

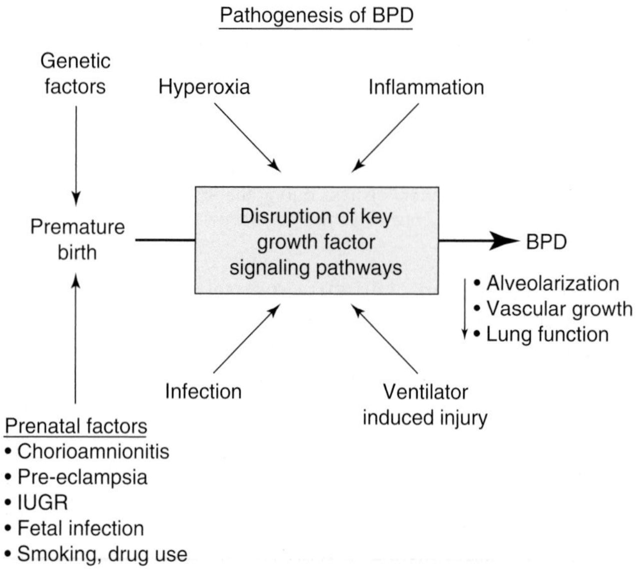

FIGURE 23-5. Pathogenesis of bronchopulmonary dysplasia: multifactorial mechanisms.

Oxygen Toxicity

Oxygen toxicity due to high levels of supplemental oxygen markedly increases the production of reactive oxygen species (ROS), which overwhelm host antioxidant defense mechanisms in the immature lung, and thus cause adverse molecular, biochemical, histologic, and anatomic effects.[1,48,49] Prematurely born infants are especially vulnerable to oxidative stress because their lungs are relatively deficient in antioxidant enzyme systems (e.g., superoxide dismutase, catalase, and others) at birth.[22] Early animal studies clearly demonstrated that high levels of supplemental oxygen promote lung inflammation, impair alveolar and vascular growth, and increase lung fibroproliferation. Experimentally, even relatively mild levels of hyperoxia may be sufficient to induce oxidative stress and impair growth of the immature lung.

A promising method for preventing the development of BPD appears to be prophylactic supplementation of human recombinant antioxidant enzymes.[50] In a multicenter randomized controlled trial, intratracheal treatment of premature infants at birth with recombinant human CuZnSOD (rhSOD) was associated with fewer episodes of respiratory illness (i.e., wheezing, asthma, pulmonary infections) and less need for treatment with bronchodilators or corticosteroids at 1 year corrected age.[51] This suggests that rhSOD may prevent long-term pulmonary injury from ROS in high-risk premature infants.

Ventilator-Induced Lung Injury (VILI)

Mechanical ventilation can induce injury through "volutrauma," in which phasic stretch or overdistention of the lung can induce lung inflammation, permeability edema, and subsequent structural changes that mimic human BPD—even in the absence of high levels of supplemental oxygen.[52,53] Aggressive mechanical ventilation with hypocarbia has been associated with the development of BPD, as reports have shown an inverse relationship between low $PaCO_2$ levels and BPD development.[31] High tidal volumes should be avoided during mechanical ventilation and even during resuscitation in the delivery room.[53] In an experimental study demonstrating a relationship between the size of manual inflations and lung damage in lambs, adverse effects were demonstrated even with inflations of 8 mL/kg.[54–57] Although small tidal volumes may reduce the risk for VILI in preterm infants, failure to recruit and maintain adequate functional residual capacity (FRC), even with low tidal volumes, is injurious in experimental models.[56] Despite some data suggesting that alternate strategies such as nasal continuous positive airway pressure (nCPAP) and high-frequency ventilation may reduce the risk for BPD, a striking center-to-center variability remains, and meta-analysis has not shown uniform benefits.[53]

Inflammation

Experimental and clinical studies have shown that inflammation clearly plays a central role in the pathobiology of BPD.[58] Oxygen toxicity, volutrauma, and infection can induce early and sustained inflammatory responses that promote the recruitment and activation of neutrophils, which persists in infants who develop BPD.[59,60] Levels of multiple pro-inflammatory cytokines (e.g., interleukins (IL) IL-1beta, IL-6, and soluble ICAM-1) and growth factors (e.g., transforming growth factor-β (TGR-β), vascular endothelial growth factor, and others) are present and altered in lung lavage and blood samples from premature infants who subsequently develop BPD versus controls.[61,62] IL-1beta induces the release of inflammatory mediators, activating inflammatory cells and up-regulating adhesion molecules on endothelial cells. ICAM-1 is a glycoprotein that promotes cell-to-cell contact. Direct contact between activated cells leads to further production of pro-inflammatory cytokines and other mediators. Each, such as IL-8, which induces neutrophil chemotaxis, inhibits surfactant synthesis, and stimulates elastase release.[60,63] The levels of collagenase and phospholipase A2 are also increased, and oxidative modification results in inactivation of alpha-1-antiprotease, which further tips the protease-antiprotease imbalance to favor injury. Lung inflammation is associated with loss of endothelial basement membrane and interstitial sulphated glycosaminoglycans,[65] which are important in inhibiting fibrosis. TNF-alpha activity increases late, with peak levels between 14 and 28 days.[66] TNF-alpha and IL-6 induce fibroblast and collagen production.[58,67,68] Increased TGF-β and impaired VEGF signaling have been strongly linked with the risk for BPD.[69–72] Leukotrienes are present in high levels in the lungs of infants developing BPD and remain elevated even at 6 months of age.[73,74]

Evidence that a systemic inflammatory response contributes to the pathogenesis of BPD led investigators to explore the contributions of antenatal, perinatal, and postnatal inflammation to lung injury.[75] Observational studies have suggested an association between amniotic fluid markers and placental and umbilical cord pathology of chorioamnionitis with BPD.[76–78] The combined effects of antenatal infection or inflammation and clinical factors might contribute to the occurrence of BPD via a number of mechanisms: direct injury of pulmonary parenchyma, disruption of the developmental milieu, impaired angiogenesis,[70–72,79,80] or activation (priming) of immune cells in the lung, thus provoking an exaggerated inflammatory injury in response to a variety of prenatal, perinatal, and postnatal insults.[75] BPD may be increased in infants whose mothers had chorioamnionitis.[76] This is because intraamniotic endotoxin exposure can disrupt alveolar and vascular development and thus lead to a decreased alveolar number and pulmonary hypertension (PH).[81] In a case-control study of 386 infants born at or below 1500 grams (after adjusting for other BPD risk factors), chorioamnionitis alone appeared to be associated with reduced risk of BPD; however, chorioamnionitis followed by 7 days of mechanical ventilation or postnatal sepsis had a synergistic effect that substantially increased the risk of BPD.[82] These data suggest that chorioamnionitis might make the lung more susceptible to postnatal injury from a "second hit" of hyperoxia or ventilator-induced injury. Alternatively, these findings also suggest variable effects of chorioamnionitis on lung maturation versus arrested development, in which greater prenatal injury is reflected by an increased need for more ventilator and oxygen support.[81]

Although controversial, several studies note a significant association between PDA and BPD, and that this effect is potentiated by infection.[83] Fluid overload resulting in worsening lung function may explain the association of PDA and BPD.

Genetic Susceptibility

The risk for developing BPD is now recognized as being markedly influenced by complex interactions between genetic and environmental risk factors.[84,85] Variability in the incidence and severity of BPD among premature infants with similar environmental risk factors suggests that genetic susceptibility plays a critical role in the pathogenesis of BPD. Parker and colleagues first reported that genetic factors increase the risk for BPD in preterm twin pairs independent of birth weight, gestational age, gender, RDS severity, PDA, infection, antenatal steroids, and other factors.[86] A subsequent study of 450 sets of preterm twins found that after controlling for the effects of covariates, genetic factors accounted for 53% (p = 0.004; 95% CI: 16% to 89%) of the variance in liability for BPD. A significant increase in concordance rates of BPD in monozygotic versus dizygotic twins further suggests a strong role for genetic susceptibility in the development of BPD. In fact, these findings suggest at least as strong a role for genetic factors in BPD as observed in such complex diseases in adults as systemic hypertension (30%), cancer (42%), and psychiatric disorders (>60%).[87–89] Lavoie and colleagues found that genetic effects accounted for about 80% of the observed variance in BPD susceptibility.[90] Numerous genes are required for normal lung growth and development, and they are likely to contain sequence variations that modulate the risk for BPD. Published studies have identified several potential candidate genes, especially regarding surfactant proteins and cytokines.[91–96] However, many studies report small sample sizes, and the findings from most of the studies have not been replicated in subsequent cohorts. The current challenge is to specifically identify the candidate genes that contribute to the development of BPD and their interaction with the specific environmental stimuli that adversely affect lung injury, repair, and structure after preterm birth.

▅ PATHOPHYSIOLOGY

Respiratory Function

Multiple abnormalities of lung structure and function contribute to late respiratory disease in BPD (Fig. 23-6). Chronic respiratory signs in children with BPD include tachypnea with shallow breathing, retractions, and paradoxical breathing pattern; coarse rhonchi, crackles, and wheezes are typically heard on auscultation. The increased respiratory rate and shallow breathing increase dead space ventilation. Nonuniform damage to the airways and distal lungs results in variable time constants for different areas of the lungs. Inspired gas may be distributed to relatively poorly perfused

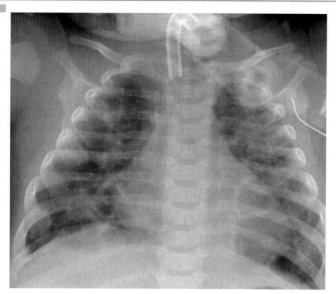

FIGURE 23-6. Chest radiograph of BPD infant with tracheostomy and chronic ventilation.

lung, thereby worsening ventilation-perfusion matching. Decreased lung compliance appears to correlate strongly with morphologic and radiographic changes in the lung. Dynamic lung compliance is markedly reduced in infants with established BPD, even in those who no longer require oxygen therapy.[97] The reduction in compliance is due to small airway narrowing, interstitial fibrosis, edema, and atelectasis. Increased airway resistance can be demonstrated even during the first week after birth in preterm neonates at risk for BPD.[98] Infants with BPD at 28 days of age have an increased total respiratory and expiratory resistance with severe flow limitation, especially at low lung volumes.[99] The presence of tracheomalacia may also result in air flow limitation, which is worsened by bronchodilator therapy.[100] In the early stages of BPD, the functional lung volume is often reduced due to atelectasis, but during later stages there is gas trapping with hyperinflation. The use of pulmonary function testing to follow the progression of BPD and the response to therapeutic interventions has increased but is still not commonly applied in the clinical setting.

Established BPD is primarily characterized by reduced surface area and heterogeneous lung units in which regional variations in airway resistance and tissue compliance lead to highly variable time constants throughout the lung. As a result, mechanical ventilation of severe BPD, especially beyond the first few months of life, requires strikingly different ventilator strategies than commonly used earlier in the disease course. Such strategies generally favor longer inspiratory times, larger tidal volumes, higher PEEP, and lower rates to allow more effective gas exchange and respiratory function.[101] Although the new BPD has been characterized as an arrest of distal lung and vascular growth, most of these observations were based on lung histology, and evidence that provided direct physiologic data to support this finding was lacking. Recent work by Tepper and colleagues has demonstrated the

important finding of reduced lung surface area in infants with BPD by utilizing novel methods of assessing diffusion capacity.[102]

Pulmonary Circulation

Acute lung injury also impairs growth, structure, and function of the developing pulmonary circulation after premature birth.[103,104] Endothelial cells are particularly susceptible to oxidant injury due to hyperoxia or inflammation. The media of small pulmonary arteries may also undergo striking changes, including smooth muscle cell proliferation, precocious maturation of immature pericytes into mature smooth muscle cells, and incorporation of fibroblasts into the vessel wall and surrounding adventitia.[105] Structural changes in the lung vasculature contribute to high pulmonary vascular resistance (PVR) due to narrowing of the vessel diameter and decreased vascular compliance. Decreased angiogenesis may limit vascular surface area, causing further elevations of PVR, especially in response to high cardiac output with exercise or stress. The pulmonary circulation in BPD patients is further characterized by abnormal vasoreactivity, which also increases PVR[106,107] (Fig. 23-7). Abnormal pulmonary vasoreactivity is evidenced by a marked vasoconstrictor response to acute hypoxia.[107,108] Cardiac catheterization studies have shown that even mild hypoxia causes marked elevations in pulmonary arterial pressure, even in infants with modest basal levels of PH. Maintaining oxygen saturation levels above 92% to 94% effectively lowers pulmonary arterial pressure.[107] Strategies to lower pulmonary arterial pressure or limit lung injury to the pulmonary vasculature may limit the subsequent development of PH in BPD.

Early injury to the lung circulation leads to the rapid development of PH, which contributes significantly to the morbidity and mortality of severe BPD. Even in early reports of BPD, PH and cor pulmonale were recognized as being associated with high mortality.[109,110] Persistent echocardiographic evidence of PH beyond the first few months has been associated with up to 40% mortality in infants with BPD.[110] High mortality rates have been reported in infants with BPD and severe PH, especially in those who require prolonged ventilator support[111] (Fig. 23-8). Although PH is a marker of more advanced BPD, elevated PVR also causes poor right ventricular function, impaired cardiac output, limited oxygen delivery, increased pulmonary edema, and perhaps a higher risk for sudden death.

In addition to the adverse effects of PH on the clinical course of infants with BPD, the lung circulation is further characterized by persistence of abnormal or "dysmorphic" growth of the pulmonary circulation, including a relative paucity of small pulmonary arteries with an altered pattern of distribution within the interstitium of the distal lung.[112–114] In infants with severe BPD, decreased vascular growth occurs in conjunction with marked reductions in alveolar formation, suggesting that the new BPD is primarily characterized by growth arrest of the developing lung. This reduction

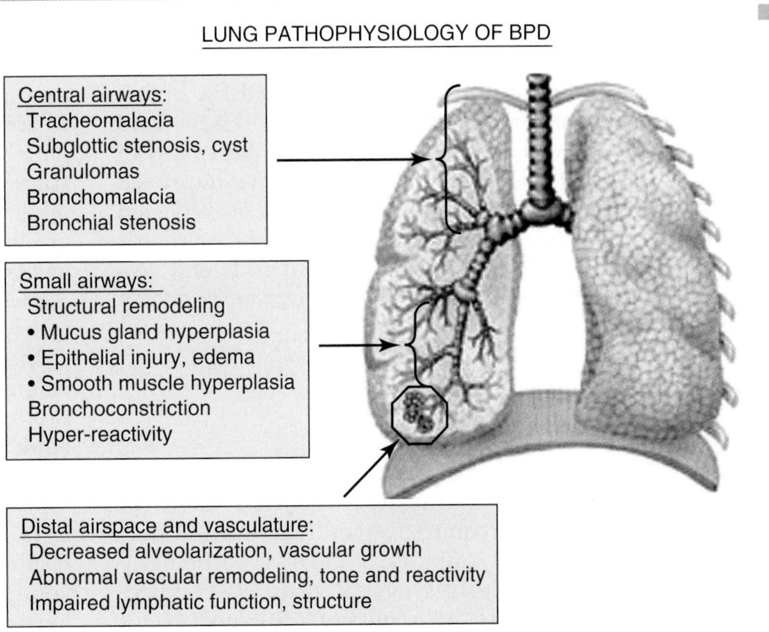

LUNG PATHOPHYSIOLOGY OF BPD

Central airways:
Tracheomalacia
Subglottic stenosis, cyst
Granulomas
Bronchomalacia
Bronchial stenosis

Small airways:
Structural remodeling
• Mucus gland hyperplasia
• Epithelial injury, edema
• Smooth muscle hyperplasia
Bronchoconstriction
Hyper-reactivity

Distal airspace and vasculature:
Decreased alveolarization, vascular growth
Abnormal vascular remodeling, tone and reactivity
Impaired lymphatic function, structure

FIGURE 23-7. Lung pathophysiology of bronchopulmonary dysplasia.

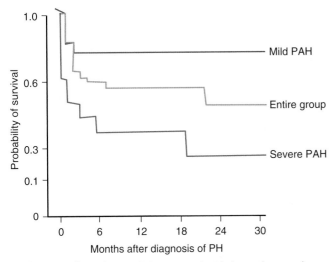

FIGURE 23-8. High mortality associated with late pulmonary hypertension in bronchopulmonary dysplasia. (Modified from Khemani E, McElhinney DB, Rhein L, et al. Pulmonary artery hypertension in formerly premature infants with bronchopulmonary dysplasia: clinical features and outcomes in the surfactant era. *Pediatrics.* 2007;120:1260-1269.)

Clinical studies have shown that the metabolic function of the pulmonary circulation is also impaired, as reflected by the impaired clearance of circulating norepinephrine (NE) across the lung.[115] Normally, 20% to 40% of circulating NE is cleared during a single passage through the lung, but infants with severe BPD have a net production of NE across the pulmonary circulation. It is unknown whether impaired metabolic function of the lung contributes to the pathophysiology of BPD or is simply a marker of severe pulmonary vascular disease. It has been speculated that high catecholamine levels may lead to left ventricular hypertrophy or systemic hypertension—known complications of BPD.

Cardiovascular Abnormalities

In addition to pulmonary vascular disease and right ventricular hypertrophy, other cardiovascular abnormalities associated with BPD include left ventricular hypertrophy (LVH), systemic hypertension, and the development of prominent systemic-to-pulmonary collateral vessels. Infants with severe BPD can develop LVH in the absence of right ventricular hypertrophy. Systemic hypertension in BPD may be mild, transient, or striking and usually responds to medication.[116,117] The etiology remains obscure, but further evaluation of some affected infants reveals significant renal vascular or urinary tract disease. Interestingly, perinatal hyperoxia leads to late cardiovascular abnormalities in infant rats, suggesting that oxidative stress and related mechanisms cause chronic changes in the systemic circulation as well as the pulmonary vasculature.[118] A recent report showed that left ventricular diastolic dysfunction can contribute to lung edema, diuretic dependency, and PH in some infants with BPD.[119]

Prominent bronchial or other systemic-to-pulmonary collateral vessels were noted in early morphometric studies of infants with BPD and can be readily identified in many infants during cardiac catheterization. Although

of alveolar-capillary surface area impairs gas exchange, thereby increasing the need for prolonged supplemental oxygen and ventilator therapy; this causes marked hypoxemia with acute respiratory infections and late exercise intolerance and further increases the risk for developing severe PH. Experimental studies have further shown that early injury to the developing lung can impair angiogenesis, which contributes to decreased alveolarization and simplification of distal lung airspace (the "vascular hypothesis").[79] Thus, abnormalities of the lung circulation in BPD are not only related to the presence or absence of PH, but more broadly, *pulmonary vascular disease* after premature birth as manifested by decreased vascular growth and structure also contributes to the pathogenesis and abnormal cardiopulmonary physiology of BPD.

these collateral vessels are generally small, large collaterals may contribute to significant shunting of blood flow to the lung, resulting in edema and the need for higher levels of supplemental oxygen. Collateral vessels have been associated with high mortality in some patients with both severe BPD and PH. Some infants have improved after embolization of large collateral vessels, as reflected by a reduced need for supplemental oxygen, ventilator support, or diuretics. The contribution of collateral vessels to the pathophysiology of BPD, however, is poorly understood.

LONG-TERM OUTCOME

Most follow-up data have been obtained from patients from the pre-surfactant era. Approximately 50% of infants with BPD will require hospital re-admission during early childhood for respiratory distress, particularly if they develop respiratory syncytial virus (RSV) infection.[120] Importantly, late re-admissions are not exclusively a problem of preterm infants with BPD; increased re-hospitalizations, including the need for intensive care, are also observed in late preterm infants without BPD.[121] This high rate of hospitalization generally declines during the second and third year of life,[122] but lung function studies often show limited reserve even in patients with minimal overt respiratory signs.[123,124] This observation likely explains the severity of presentation in some infants with BPD after acquiring RSV or other infections. Chest x-ray findings during follow-up are generally nonspecific, typically including hyperinflation with peribronchial cuffing and scattered interstitial infiltrates consistent with fibrosis, edema, or atelectasis. These findings tend to clear with age and are very insensitive markers of changes in lung function. In older infants with BPD, CT scans give more detailed information, but the clinical utility of serial CT scans during follow-up is uncertain. In selected patients, however, CT scans may help to identify localized area of disease (e.g., large cysts) that may require surgical resection.

Infants with severe BPD often develop chronic obstructive pulmonary disease (COPD), but impaired flows may reflect disproportionate or abnormal growth patterns between airways and the distal lung. In the majority of BPD infants, lung growth and remodeling during infancy results in progressive improvement of gas exchange, lung function, and level of oxygen therapy; few BPD patients remain oxygen dependent beyond 2 years of age. Lung function is usually in the low-normal range by 2 to 3 years of age, but air flow abnormalities may remain. Infants with BPD have reduced absolute and size-corrected flow rates in comparison with age- and size-matched control patients, suggesting poor airway growth with age. Filipone and colleagues have reported a strong correlation between V_{max} FRC at 2 years of age with FEV_1 at school age, suggesting persistent air flow limitation in selected patients with BPD.[125]

Although pulmonary function in most survivors with BPD improves over time and permits normal activity, abnormalities detected by pulmonary function testing often persist through adolescence, including increased

airway resistance and reactivity.[126] Additionally, abnormal distal lung structure with alveolar simplification and decreased tethering of small airways may also contribute to reduced flow and apparent airways disease in infants with BPD.[101] Unfortunately, comprehensive longitudinal studies of the pulmonary course and lung function of adult patients with a previous history of premature birth are lacking. Northway[127] reported persistent evidence of gas trapping and airway reactivity in young adults and adolescents with BPD, but these patients were treated nearly 3 decades ago.

More studies are needed to determine the long-term respiratory course of premature neonates, with or without severe BPD, and their relative contribution to the growing adult population with COPD. The lung function abnormalities seen in BPD patients translate into late respiratory symptoms and hospitalizations. Follow-up studies have shown an increased incidence of wheezing and other respiratory symptoms continuing into adolescence and young adulthood.[125,128] It is important to determine the long-term outcome of children who are diagnosed with the new BPD. Although infant pulmonary function studies at 1 year of age would suggest less air flow limitation than those with "old BPD,"[129,130] new BPD infants have impaired antenatal lung growth, and altered lung function may persist due to slow or failed lung growth.

PREVENTION

As described earlier in the chapter, diverse mechanisms contribute to the pathogenesis of BPD, which perhaps makes it less surprising that there is no single therapy or prevention strategy except for the prevention of premature birth. The use of antenatal steroids in mothers at high risk of delivering a premature infant reduced the incidence of neonatal death and RDS by 50%[131] but failed to decrease the incidence of BPD—even in combination with postnatal surfactant. Similarly, thyrotrophin-releasing hormone therapy did not reduce BPD in randomized trials.[132] Exogenous surfactant therapy reduces the combined outcome of death and BPD, but not BPD alone. Arguably, this may be due to the increased survival of very immature infants at high risk of BPD.

The association of volutrauma with the development of BPD has led to the use of strategies, such as permissive hypercapnia, to minimize lung injury.[133] Various ventilator devices and strategies have been assessed regarding their ability to reduce BPD. Meta-analysis of randomized trials has demonstrated that patient triggered ventilation does not reduce BPD but, if started in the recovery phase of RDS, significantly shortens weaning from mechanical ventilation.[134] The results of randomized trials of high-frequency oscillatory ventilation (HFOV) or high-frequency jet ventilation (HFJV) have been inconsistent. Two large studies that incorporated prenatal steroid and surfactant replacement therapy yielded different results. In one study (which restricted entry to very low birth weight infants with moderate to severe hypoxemic respiratory failure following surfactant administration), there was a significant benefit from HFOV of higher survival without BPD.[135] No substantial benefit or adverse effects of HFOV were found in the other study, however, which randomized premature infants (younger than 29 weeks) within 1 hour of birth regardless of the degree of lung disease.[136] An explanation for those conflicting results may be that in the current era that includes the use of modified conventional ventilation strategies, pulmonary benefit from HFOV may only be demonstrable in infants with moderate to severe disease. Clearly, the strategy applied for either conventional or HFOV are more important than the device itself. HFOV is frequently used as "rescue" therapy in premature newborns with severe respiratory failure despite treatment with exogenous surfactant. Whether such an approach reduces BPD or improves long-term outcomes requires appropriate testing.

Although no optimal ventilation mode has emerged, it is clear from physiologic studies that tidal volumes and inspired oxygen concentrations should be reduced as low as possible to avoid hypocarbia, volutrauma, and oxygen toxicity, and lung recruitment strategies should be employed. An alternative approach to reduce BPD has been to avoid intubation and mechanical ventilation by using early nCPAP. A study comparing the outcomes of premature infants weighing 500 to 1500 g at birth who were treated in either Boston or New York reported that the incidence of BPD was significantly higher in Boston (22%) compared to New York (4%), even after adjusting for baseline risk factors such as severity of prematurity.[137] Many centers now minimize their use of mechanical ventilation, preferring nCPAP with or without exogenous surfactant and report low incidences of BPD in high-risk infants. A recent multicenter trial demonstrated no difference in BPD or death between infants randomized to early nCPAP or early surfactant.[138] However, early nCPAP reduced the need for subsequent intubation and was associated with a reduced rate of steroid prescription and shorter duration of ventilation.

Although fluid restriction in the first week after birth does not reduce BPD,[139] it is important to avoid fluid overload, administration of colloid, and sodium supplementation. Aggressive treatment of symptomatic PDA may reduce the severity of BPD, but this remains controversial. Appropriate nutritional support is critical in helping to promote normal lung growth, maturation, and repair. Rapid weight gain and crossing of centiles, however, may be undesirable, particularly in small for gestational age infants.[140] Meta-analysis of seven randomized trials has demonstrated that systemic supplementation with vitamin A in sufficient quantities to establish normal serum retinol concentrations reduces oxygen dependence at 36 weeks postmenstrual age (PMA).[141] However, follow-up studies showed no improvement in long-term respiratory outcomes in vitamin A–treated infants.

Corticosteroid therapy, primarily directed at reducing lung inflammation, is one of the most controversial areas of BPD care. Acute treatment with steroids improves lung mechanics and gas exchange and reduces inflammatory cells and mediators in tracheal samples of patients with BPD.[142,143] Meta-analysis of randomized trials suggest that corticosteroids reduce chronic oxygen dependency at 28 days and 36 weeks PMA if administered systemically in the first 96 hours.[143,144] However, there are significant concerns regarding increased mortality and adverse effects on head growth, neurodevelopmental outcomes, and lung structure.[145,146] Additionally, a high incidence of gastrointestinal perforation was reported in one study.[147] Other side effects include systemic hypertension, hyperglycemia, cardiac hypertrophy, poor somatic growth, sepsis, intestinal bleeding, and myocardial hypertrophy. Currently, the routine use of early, high-dose steroids in premature newborns is strongly discouraged, as reflected in editorial statements from the American Academy of Pediatrics.[148] The adverse findings, however, are generally based on data from older studies that have used high doses of dexamethasone for prolonged periods of time, and many questions persist regarding the risk-benefit relationship with the use of other steroids for shorter study periods. As a result, some centers advocate the use of steroids at lower doses and shorter durations (5 to 7 days) in ventilator-dependent infants with severe, persistent lung disease.

To avoid the adverse effects associated with systemic administration, steroids have also been given by inhalation, but no significant benefits have been observed using this route.[149] The major effect of inhaled betamethasone in a multicenter randomized trial was to decrease the perceived need for the use of systemic steroids.[150] Fluticasone proprionate is a more potent steroid, but when given by inhalation was associated only with a lower chest radiograph score and unfortunately a higher systolic blood pressure.[151] The early use of low doses of hydrocortisone may reduce BPD, but adverse effects such as gastrointestinal perforation have been reported.

In addition to corticosteroids, several pharmacologic approaches or supplements have been explored in order to reduce the risk for BPD. One of the most intriguing findings arose from a large-scale clinical trial that was initially developed to examine the effects of early and prolonged use of caffeine on late neurocognitive outcomes. Analysis of other endpoints related to this study suggested that caffeine may reduce the risk of BPD by nearly 50%.[152] This effect is more striking than the benefit previously observed with vitamin A treatment.[141] Although mechanisms through which caffeine reduced BPD risk are uncertain, treated infants had a decreased need for surgical PDA closure and earlier discontinuation of respiratory support.

In clinical studies, inhaled nitric oxide (iNO) therapy acutely lowered pulmonary vascular resistance (PVR) and improved oxygenation in patients with PH in various settings, including premature infants with severe RDS and established BPD.[153-155] Experimental data have demonstrated that iNO therapy may be lung protective in several animal models of experimental BPD and, importantly, may be associated with increased alveolar and vascular growth.[156,157] The potential role of iNO in the prevention of BPD has received considerable attention over the past decade, but its routine use for this purpose remains controversial.

The results of randomized trials for the prevention of BPD have yielded conflicting results. In an early multicenter trial of low-dose iNO therapy (5 ppm) in severely ill premature newborns with RDS who had marked hypoxemia despite surfactant therapy (i.e., a/A O_2 ratio ≤0.10) and an estimated mortality of 53%, iNO acutely improved PaO_2. Although improvement in survival was not demonstrated partly due to the small size of this study, the duration of mechanical ventilation was reduced and the frequency or severity of intracranial hemorrhage was not increased.[153] In a single center study, Schreiber and colleagues reported that iNO reduced the combined endpoint of mortality and BPD in premature infants who required mechanical ventilation and also reduced the incidence of severe intracranial hemorrhage and periventricular leukomalacia.[158] A large multicenter trial, however, did not demonstrate similar benefit in a population of premature newborns with moderate respiratory failure, but showed a 50% reduction in BPD and death in preterm infants who weighed more than 1000 g at birth.[159] Another large multicenter study suggested that prolonged iNO therapy at higher doses reduces BPD when started before the second week of life and improves some respiratory outcomes during infancy.[160] However, a third large-scale study showed no effects when administered to preterm infants with minimal respiratory disease.[161] Overall, these findings suggest that iNO therapy may lower the risk for BPD in some preterm infants. However, due to the differences between studies (including gestational age, onset and duration of therapy, dose, and related questions), recommendations for its routine use for the prevention of BPD was not supported at a recent NICHD-sponsored Consensus Conference.[162]

TREATMENT

A general evaluation and treatment for infants with significant BPD is described in the following paragraphs. Supplemental oxygen remains a mainstay of therapy for infants with BPD, yet the most appropriate target for oxygen saturation levels remains controversial. Growing concerns regarding the adverse effects of even moderate levels of oxygen therapy have led many neonatologists to accept oxygen saturations below 85% to 90% early after birth of preterm newborns.[163] Studies have shown that levels of ≤92% compared to ≥95% are associated with a shorter duration of supplemental oxygen requirement[164] and perhaps fewer respiratory exacerbations.[165] Results from a large multicenter trial found that targeting oxygen saturations between 85% and 89% was associated with higher mortality but less retinopathy of prematurity and no difference in BPD diagnosis in comparison with infants treated with oxygen saturations targeted between 91% and 95%. Currently, most pulmonologists recommend maintaining infants with established BPD at oxygen saturations of 92%, with slightly higher levels for BPD infants with growth failure, recurrent respiratory exacerbations, or PH. Concerns persist that targeting higher levels (>95%) may be associated with ongoing lung injury due to oxidative stress. Prolonged monitoring of oxygenation while awake, asleep, and during feeds is important to ensure the avoidance of hypoxia while adjusting oxygen therapy.

In most NICUs, nCPAP or high-flow nasal cannulas are used to maintain adequate oxygenation and ventilation while avoiding the need for prolonged ventilation or re-intubation. Whereas several studies have examined the role of early nCPAP in lieu of endotracheal intubation during the first week after birth, there are no studies regarding benefits of the prolonged use of nCPAP in established BPD with chronic respiratory failure. In some infants with BPD, signs of severe respiratory distress persist despite nCPAP or high-flow nasal cannula therapy, including marked dyspnea, head-bobbing, retractions, tachypnea, intermittent cyanosis, and CO_2 retention. If subsequent attempts at weaning are not successful, these infants may benefit from re-intubation and the consideration of tracheostomy for chronic ventilator support. The timing and patient selection for tracheostomy and the commitment to more prolonged ventilator support is highly variable between centers. Tracheostomy and chronic ventilator support may provide a stable airway to allow for more effective ventilation and less respiratory distress, with enhanced cardiopulmonary function as reflected by lower oxygen requirements and less PH. Greater respiratory stability often improves tolerance of respiratory treatments, physical therapies, and handling by staff and family members, thereby improving maternal-infant interaction and neurodevelopmental outcome. Detailed care of ventilator-dependent BPD infants is beyond the scope of this chapter, but successful management requires well-organized, multidisciplinary teams to address the complexity of issues.

Drug Therapies

Multiple pharmacologic therapies have been used in the management of BPD, including diuretics, bronchodilators, and steroids. Despite observations that suggest acute improvement with many of these interventions, data are limited regarding the long-term safety and efficacy of many drugs used in infants with BPD.

Diuretics

Diuretics improve pulmonary compliance and airway resistance by reducing lung edema. Two Cochrane Systematic Reviews assessed the effects of loop diuretics (furosemide) and those acting on the distal renal tubule (thiazides and spironolactone) for preventing or treating BPD in preterm infants.[166,167] Chronic furosemide therapy can improve oxygenation and lung compliance in infants with BPD.[166] A small study suggested that furosemide (1 mg/kg 12-hourly intravenously or 2 mg/kg 12-hourly orally) can improve weaning from the ventilator when compared with a placebo.[168] Aerosolized furosemide can acutely improve lung mechanics, but data are lacking regarding its chronic use.[169] Thiazides and spironolactone can improve lung function, but this finding has not been consistent.[167-171] The use of alternate-day furosemide may sustain improvements in lung function while minimizing risks for electrolyte imbalance and nephrocalcinosis.[171] While diuretics generally cause short-term improvements in lung compliance, there is little evidence of sustained reduction in ventilator support, length of hospital stay, or other long-term outcomes.

Bronchodilators

Infants with BPD have airway smooth muscle hypertrophy and often have signs of bronchial hyperreactivity that acutely improve with bronchodilator therapy; but response rates are variable.[172-174] Data showing long-term benefit of bronchodilators, (including β-agonists and anticholinergic agents) for the prevention or treatment of BPD are lacking.[174] In addition to their roles in apnea, aminophylline and caffeine can reduce airway resistance in infants with BPD and may have an additive effect with diuretics. Methylxanthines can improve weaning of infants from mechanical ventilation,[175] but side effects such as jitteriness, seizures, and gastroesophageal reflux are recognized. As described above, caffeine use has been shown to reduce BPD, PDA, and cerebral palsy.

Steroids

Steroids are generally used to reduce lung inflammation in BPD. Systematic reviews of RCTs examining the potential benefits and risks of systemic glucocorticoids are based on postnatal timing of treatment: early (7 to 14 days) and late (>3 weeks) treatment.[176-178] With early glucocorticoid therapy, there is a reduction in neonatal mortality and a trend toward reduction in mortality before discharge. Treatment for 7 to 14 days led to earlier extubation and decreased the diagnosis of BPD at 36 weeks. However, side effects included systemic hypertension and cardiac hypertrophy. Late systemic glucocorticoids also enhanced weaning from mechanical ventilation but did not reduce mortality. Overall, glucocorticoid treatment improves lung mechanics and gas exchange, facilitating earlier extubation. Although commonly used in infants with asthma, inhaled steroids have not consistently showed improvement in lung function in BPD. However, one study showed that inhaled steroids can improve the rate of successful extubation and reduce the need for systemic steroids.[179-181] As discussed earlier regarding BPD prevention, the side effects of poor head growth and neurocognitive outcomes with early and prolonged high-dose strategies are unacceptable risks for preterm infants at risk for BPD. However, steroid bursts (high doses for 3 to 5 days) may be helpful in the management of BPD infants with acute deterioration of lung function.

Antiviral Immunization

Infants with BPD are at increased risk of recurrent respiratory tract infections, especially those due to respiratory syncytial virus (RSV). Treatment with RSV immunoglobulin or RSV monoclonal antibodies is effective in preventing hospital re-admissions. A large multicenter study of palivizumab, a humanized monoclonal antibody against RSV, found that monthly injections of 15 mg/kg for 5 months reduced hospitalization rates for RSV infection by 5% in infants with BPD.[182] The American Academy of Pediatrics recommendations include the use of palivizumab or RSV-IVIG prophylaxis for infants and children <2 years of age with BPD who required oxygen therapy for their lung disease prior to RSV season. Older infants with more severe BPD may benefit from prophylaxis for two RSV seasons.[183]

Pulmonary Hypertension

The initial clinical strategy for the management of PH in infants with BPD begins with treating the underlying lung disease. This includes extensive evaluation for chronic reflux and aspiration, structural airway abnormalities (e.g., tonsillar and adenoidal hypertrophy, vocal cord paralysis, subglottic stenosis, and tracheomalacia), assessments of bronchial reactivity, improving lung edema and airway function, and other pulmonary considerations. Periods of acute hypoxia, whether intermittent or prolonged, can often contribute to late PH in BPD. A sleep study may be necessary to determine the presence of noteworthy episodes of hypoxia and whether hypoxemia has predominantly obstructive, central, or mixed causes. Additional studies that may be required include flexible bronchoscopy for the diagnosis of anatomic and dynamic airway lesions (e.g., tracheomalacia) that may contribute to hypoxemia and poor clinical responses to oxygen therapy. Upper gastrointestinal series, pH or impedance probe, and swallow studies may be indicated to evaluate for gastroesophageal reflux and aspiration that can contribute to ongoing lung injury. If findings are positive, or even if clinical suspicion remains high in the face of negative findings and in the setting of lung disease that fails to improve, consideration should be given to gastrostomy tube placement and fundoplication. For patients with BPD and severe PH who fail to maintain near normal ventilation or require high levels of FiO_2 despite conservative treatment, consideration should be given to chronic mechanical ventilatory support.

Despite the growing use of pulmonary vasodilator therapy for the treatment of PH in BPD, data demonstrating efficacy are extremely limited, and the use of these agents should only follow thorough diagnostic evaluations and aggressive management of the underlying lung disease. We strongly encourage cardiac catheterization prior to the initiation of chronic therapy. Current therapies used for PH therapy in infants with BPD generally include inhaled NO, sildenafil, endothelin-receptor antagonists (ETRAs), and calcium channel blockers. Calcium channel blockers (e.g., nifedipine) benefit some patients with PH, and short-term effects of these blockers in infants with BPD have been reported.[184] In comparison with an acute study of iNO reactivity in infants with BPD, the acute response to calcium channel blockers was poor, and some infants developed systemic hypotension.[155] In general, we generally use sildenafil or bosentan (an ETRA) for chronic therapy of PH in infants with BPD. Sildenafil, a highly selective type 5 phosphodiesterase (PDE-5) inhibitor, augments cyclic GMP content in vascular smooth muscle, and it has been shown to benefit adults with PH as monotherapy and in combination with standard treatment regimens.[185] In a study of 25 infants with chronic lung disease and PH (18 with BPD), prolonged sildenafil therapy as part of an aggressive program to treat PH was associated with improvement in PH by echocardiogram in most (88%) patients without significant rates of adverse events.[186] Although the time to improvement was variable, many patients were able to wean off mechanical ventilator support and other PH therapies, especially iNO, during the course of sildenafil treatment without worsening of PH. The recommended starting dose for sildenafil is 0.5 mg/kg/dose every 8 hours. If there is no evidence of systemic hypotension, this dose can be gradually increased over 2 weeks to achieve the desired pulmonary hemodynamic effect or a maximum of 2 mg/kg/dose every 6 to 8 hours. Data are largely lacking on other agents (e.g. ETRAs and prostacyclin analogs) in BPD infants who fail to respond to other approaches.

SUMMARY

Nearly 40 years after its original description, BPD has changed. However, it remains a significant complication of premature birth and is a persistent challenge for the future. BPD has evolved from the classical stages described initially to a disease characterized largely by inhibition of lung development. Future strategies that improve long-term outcomes will depend on successful integration of basic research on the fundamental mechanisms of lung development and response to injury, with studies that test novel interventions to lower the occurrence and severity of the cardiopulmonary sequelae of BPD.

Suggested Reading

Abman SH. Pulmonary hypertension in chronic lung disease of infancy. Pathogenesis, pathophysiology and treatment. In: Bland RD, Coalson JJ, eds. *Chronic Lung Disease in Early Infancy.* New York: Marcel Dekker; 2000:619–668.

Askie LM, Henderson-Smart DJ, Irwig L, et al. Oxygen saturation targets and outcomes in extremely preterm infants. *N Engl J Med.* 2003;349:959–967.

Balinotti JE, Chakr VC, Tiller C, et al. Growth of lung parenchyma in infants and toddlers with chronic lung disease of infancy. *Am J Respir Crit Care Med.* 2010;181:1093–1097.

Ballard RA, Truog WE, Cnaan A, et al. Inhaled nitric oxide in preterm infants undergoing mechanical ventilation. *N Engl J Med.* 2006;355:343–353.

Bland RD, Coalson JJ. *Chronic Lung Disease in Early Infancy.* New York: Marcel Dekker; 2000.

Bose C, van Marter LJ, Laughon M, et al. Fetal growth restriction and chronic lung disease among infants born before the 28th week of gestation. *Pediatrics.* 2009;124:e450–e458.

Castile RG, Nelin LD. Lung function, structure and the physiologic basis for mechanical ventilation of infants with established BPD. In: Abman SH, ed. *Bronchopulmonary Dysplasia.* New York: Informa Healthcare; 2010:328–346.

Hansen AR, Barnes CM, Folkman J, et al. Maternal preeclampsia predicts the development of BPD. *J Pediatr.* 2010;156:532–536.

Kallapur S, Jobe AJ, Kramer BW. Prenatal inflammation and immune responses of the preterm lung. In: Abman SH, ed. *Bronchopulmonary Dysplasia.* New York: Informa Healthcare; 2010:118–132.

Kinsella JP, Cutter GR, Walsh WF, et al. Early inhaled nitric oxide therapy in premature newborns with respiratory failure. *N Engl J Med.* 2006;355:354–364.

Laughon M, Alfred EN, Bose C, et al. Patterns of respiratory distress during the first 2 postnatal weeks in extremely premature infants. *Pediatrics.* 2010;123:1124–1131.

Lavoie PM, Pham C, Jang KL. Heritability of bronchopulmonary dysplasia, defined according to the Consensus Statement of the National Institutes of Health. *Pediatrics.* 2008;122:479–485.

Lee HJ, Kim EK, Kim HS, et al. Chorioamnionitis, respiratory distress syndrome and BPD in extremely low birth weight infants. *J Perinatol.* 2010;1–5.

Mercier JC, Hummler H, Durrmeyer X, et al. Inhaled nitric oxide for prevention of bronchopulmonary dysplasia in premature babies (EUNO): a randomized controlled trial. *Lancet.* 2010;376:346–354.

Northway Jr WH, Rosan RC, Porter DY. Pulmonary disease following respiratory therapy of hyaline membrane disease. *N Engl J Med.* 1967;276:357–368.

Schreiber MD, Gin-Mestan K, Marks JD, et al. Inhaled nitric oxide in premature infants with respiratory distress. *N Engl J Med.* 2003;349:2099–2107.

Vento M, Saugstad OD. Role of management in the delivery room and beyond in the evolution of bronchopulmonary dysplasia. In: Abman SH, ed. *Bronchopulmonary Dysplasia.* New York: Informa Healthcare; 2010:292–313.

Viscardi RM, Muhumuza CK, Rodriguez A, et al. Inflammatory markers in intrauterine and fetal blood and cerebrospinal fluid compartments are associated with adverse pulmonary and neurologic outcomes in preterm infants. *Pediatr Res.* 2004;55:1009–1017.

Watterberg KL, Demers LM, Scott SM, et al. Chorioamnionitis and early lung inflammation in infants in whom bronchopulmonary dysplasia develops. *Pediatrics.* 1996;97:210–215.

References

The complete reference list is available online at www.expertconsult.com

IV

Infections of the Respiratory Tract

24 MICROBIOLOGIC DIAGNOSIS OF RESPIRATORY ILLNESS: PRACTICAL APPLICATIONS

Chrysanthi L. Skevaki, MD, PhD, Nikolaos G. Papadopoulos, MD, PhD, Athanassios Tsakris, MD, PhD, FRCPath, and Sebastian L. Johnston, MBBS, PhD, FRCP, FSB

Respiratory tract infections (RTIs) constitute a major health problem, with significant cost and mortality rates worldwide. Laboratory methods for the identification of infectious agents that cause respiratory illness are aimed at (1) direct detection by microscopic or antigenic techniques, (2) isolation by means of culture and antibiotic susceptibility testing if needed, (3) serologic evidence of infection in the patient (antibody detection), and (4) molecular genetic detection.

Clinicians should be able to suggest the suspected etiologic agent to facilitate the most cost-effective diagnostic approach and prevent infections from occurring among laboratory staff. Moreover, information should be provided about patient's basic demographic data, clinical condition and history of present illness, antibiotic treatment, immune status, and recent travel or potential exposure. In general, the necessary prerequisites for a successful diagnosis are the collection of an appropriate respiratory and blood sample, prompt transportation in a suitable medium, and laboratory processing within an acceptable time interval.

LABORATORY DIAGNOSIS OF RESPIRATORY VIRAL INFECTIONS

Acute viral respiratory illnesses are the most common reason for hospitalization of children in the United States.[1] Respiratory virus diagnosis may be important for a number of reasons including epidemiologic studies; avoidance of hospitalization; reduction in hospital stay and diagnostic workup; decrease in rates of unnecessary antibiotic administration; timely antiviral treatment; and decisions on isolation of infected children to prevent hospital-acquired infections.

Brief Overview of Viruses Involved in Respiratory Illness

The most prevalent are rhinoviruses (RVs) or "common cold" viruses that belong to the picornavirus (small RNA) family, which also includes the enteroviruses (e.g., poliovirus, echovirus, and Coxsackie virus) as well as cardiovirus and aphthovirus. Over 100 RV serotypes have been identified; these are divided into major (90% of serotypes) and minor groups that use as their cellular receptor the intercellular adhesion molecule-1 (ICAM-1) and the low-density lipoprotein (LDL) receptor, respectively. RV-induced colds are closely related to social contact, and peaks are usually seen when children return to school after a vacation period. They usually cause mild disease, but one of the most prominent roles of RV is the triggering of asthma exacerbations.[2] Replication is more active in the nose compared to the mouth and pharynx. RVs, however, may also replicate in the lower airway, as demonstrated with the use of molecular biology-based detection techniques.[3] Although the severity of upper respiratory tract (URT) symptoms after RV infection does not differ between patients with asthma and normal subjects, both the duration and the severity of lower respiratory tract (LRT) symptoms are more pronounced in patients with asthma.[4] LRT epithelial cells of asthmatics demonstrate a deficient innate immune response to RV infection, resulting in diminished apoptosis and accentuated late cytotoxicity.[5,6] Furthermore, RV-infected LRT epithelium is a rich source of inflammatory mediators and growth factors that may trigger or propagate airway inflammation and remodeling.[7]

Respiratory syncytial virus (RSV) belongs to the *Pneumovirinae* subfamily and is a medium-sized (100 to 300 nm) RNA virus. Variations in the attachment glycoprotein of the viral envelope give rise to the two antigenically distinct strains of RSV, namely A and B. The majority of studies report that A strains are more common and produce more severe disease. RSV enters the body through the eye or nose and, to a lesser extent, through the mouth. The virus subsequently spreads along the airway mucosa, mostly by cell-to-cell transfer along intracytoplasmic bridges, and also through aspiration from the upper to the lower airway. RSV follows a well-characterized epidemiologic pattern, with yearly outbreaks occurring between October and May in temperate climates. In infants, maternal antibodies reach nondetectable levels at 6 months of age. At least half of the infant population becomes infected during their first RSV epidemic, and almost all children have been infected by 2 years of age. During the first infection, IgM is detected after the first week and IgG during the second week. RSV infection does not confer immunity, and re-infection is common throughout life. All immunoglobulin classes appear, and after three episodes, titers approximate those of adults.[8] Although infection usually leads to mild respiratory illness, which is indistinguishable from other viral infections of the RT, some infants have more severe disease. Bronchiolitis is the characteristic clinical manifestation of such infection. There is evidence that hospitalizations for bronchiolitis—now the most common reason for admission among neonates (>125,000 per year in the United States)—have considerably increased during recent decades and that hospitalized children have an increased probability of wheezing later in life (with immune status of the host probably playing an important role in the process).

Three types of influenza virus (IFV) have been identified; they are designated A, B, and C, and they belong to the orthomyxovirus family of viruses. They are negative-stranded segmented RNA viruses. The two IFV envelope glycoproteins hemagglutinin (H) and neuraminidase (N) determine both viral entry into target cells (by binding to sialic acids and fusing with cellular membrane elements) and the release of the virus. Infection with IFV occurs via respiratory droplets, and infected cells become round and swollen with pyknotic nuclei. The progressive changes in epithelial cells suggest that infection starts in the trachea and then ascends or descends. The epidemiology is characterized by yearly epidemics lasting for 6 to 8 weeks during late winter; each year, there is usually only one dominant type or subtype. Illnesses initially appear in children, among whom the incidence of infection is higher, virus shedding is prolonged, and transmission to the community is greater. Later in the epidemic, more adults are affected. Viruses are present in the community before and after the epidemic, causing illness at a low frequency. Antigenic variation readily occurs in H and N primary structures, giving rise to new subtypes (*antigenic shift*) and to intra-subtype changes (*antigenic drift*). Antibodies against H

appear 2 weeks after infection and are protective for the specific subtype that caused the disease. Type A IFV has been associated with pandemics that have occurred every 10 to 40 years. Swine flu (a new subtype of IFV A H1N1) was the agent responsible for the 2009 pandemic, with higher pediatric mortality and higher rates of hospitalizations in children and young adults than in previous seasons, while asthma appeared to be a significant risk factor for developing severe disease.

Human parainfluenza viruses (PIVs) include four RNA viruses, numbered 1 to 4, and belong to the *Paramyxoviridae* subfamily, together with mumps and measles. Each PIV has distinct epidemiologic and clinical characteristics, as well as different age distribution patterns. PIV 1 and PIV 2, members of the *Respirovirus* genus, are generally associated with laryngotracheobronchitis (croup), URT illness, and pharyngitis, whereas PIV 3, a member of the *Rubulavirus* genus, is also a major cause of infant bronchiolitis and is associated with the development of pneumonia in susceptible subjects. PIV 4 is rare and less well studied. PIV 1 occurs in biennial epidemics during autumn, coinciding with croup outbreaks; its peak incidence occurs in children 2 to 3 years of age. PIV 2 epidemics are less predictable; however, they more or less follow the biennial pattern of PIV 1, affecting mostly children younger than 5 years of age. PIV 3 is more frequent and infects infants <6 months of age in yearly epidemics during spring and summer. Infection is mediated by interaction of the viral H and N glycoproteins with cellular sialic acid receptors. Protective antibodies against H and N appear early (1 to 2 weeks after infection) and persist for several years. Several infections are needed, however, for full protection. For transmission, aerosol spread is considered important, although deposition on surfaces and subsequent self-inoculation may also occur. Virus replication can occur throughout the tracheobronchial tree, causing local inflammation; however, only mild and rapidly repaired focal tissue destruction is observed *in vivo*. In immunocompromised hosts, fatal giant cell pneumonia may develop. Central to the pathogenesis of PIV infection is the ability of these viruses to escape interferon-mediated immune responses.[9]

In contrast to the rest of the respiratory viruses, adenoviruses (AdVs) are deoxyribonucleic acid (DNA) viruses. This large family of viruses includes 6 subgenera and more than 50 serotypes. Their overall size is 70 to 90 nm; the virion is naked and contains 36 to 38 kb double-stranded DNA, encoding >50 polypeptides from both strands. Some of these proteins allow efficient endosomal lysis and escape, leading to genome entrance into the host cell nucleus. The propensity of AdVs to shut off the expression of host messenger RNA and induce excess synthesis of adenoviral proteins leads to an accumulation of such proteins as intranuclear bodies, which are incompatible with normal cell function. In upper airway epithelial cells, ciliary and microtubular abnormalities lead to defective mucociliary clearance. An important feature of AdV is its ability to persist in the host for a long time, through low-grade replication, or for even longer periods, with production of adenoviral proteins without replication of a complete virus. AdVs may cause pneumonia, bronchiolitis, or conjunctivitis, while infection after solid organ or bone marrow transplantation can induce severe myelosuppression. The duration of virus isolation is 3 to 6 weeks from the pharynx or stool of children with RTI and 2 to 12 months in immunosuppressed patients. Antibodies that bind to complement appear 1 week after infection, remain for 1 year, and recognize the hexone antigen, which is common for all AdVs. Neutralizing antibodies develop against the specific serotype that caused the infection, and the titer remains stable for over a decade.

Human coronaviruses (HCVs) are RNA viruses that were isolated during the mid-1960s. The majority of HCVs studied to date are related to one of two reference strains, designated OC43 and 229E, which differ extensively. NL63, which was isolated from an infant with bronchiolitis and conjunctivitis, is a new group I HCV that shares 65% sequence identity with 229E.[10] Human aminopeptidase N, which is present on lung, intestinal, and renal epithelial cells, has been identified as a receptor for HCV 229E. OC43 binds to major histocompatibility complex class I molecules. Viral replication has been demonstrated in the nasal mucosa, inducing inflammation, ciliary damage, and epithelial cell shedding, although its *in vivo* cytopathic effect (CPE) is not pronounced. Volunteers can be successfully infected by intranasal inoculation, although replication in the lower airway has not been confirmed. HCV causes approximately 15% of common colds, which are usually mild. In general, HCVs may cause milder LRT symptoms than other viruses, with some exceptions of more severe LRT involvement in young children and the elderly.

The Eastern Asia–based SARS epidemic has been attributed to a new HCV with limited homology to the other known HCVs.[11] Sequencing of the Tor2 isolate showed a number of distinctive features of its genome (e.g., several small, open reading frames between its genes) that are of potential biologic significance.[12] The virus causes diffuse alveolar damage, with interstitial infiltrates. After 3 to 7 days of fever, a nonproductive cough may progress to dyspnea and hypoxemia in 15% of patients. The associated mortality rate is 3% to 6% (or as high as 43% to 55% when considering patients older than 60 years of age), but it is much lower in children.[13] The appearance of IgM and IgG antibodies takes place at the same time, with the former remaining for 11 weeks and the latter for months and possibly for years.

Finally, a new respiratory RNA virus, human metapneumovirus (MPV) of the *Metapneumovirus* genus, was isolated in 2001 from the nasopharyngeal aspirates of young children in the Netherlands.[14] MPV was later shown to be responsible for a significant proportion of RTI in children worldwide. This new virus proved to have paramyxovirus-like pleomorphic particles on electron microscopy (EM), while there are two potential genetic clusters. The clinical symptoms of the children from whom the virus was initially isolated ranged from URT disease to severe bronchiolitis and pneumonia.[14] Subsequent studies, conducted in different locations and using mixed patient populations with various respiratory symptoms, established the association of this virus with acute respiratory illness in both the URT and LRT, and in all age groups.[15]

Treatment of Clinical Samples

Samples that are intended for polymerase chain reaction (PCR) should be maintained at −70° C in order to minimize degradation of nucleic acids. For the same purpose, tubes, solutions, and buffers that are used for the collection, transport, and processing of samples should be ribonuclease free.

Blood Specimen

Infrequently, blood may be collected for PCR on serum or cells (usually on white blood cells), antigen detection, or serology. PCR on white blood cells requires that whole blood be sent at room temperature in tubes that contain ethylenediaminetetraacetic acid (EDTA) or citrate (heparin may inhibit the polymerase during subsequent PCR) and that cells be extracted within 24 hours of collection. Antigen assays may also be performed on the Buffy coat; however, clotted whole blood is needed for PCR on serum. For serology, an acute sample of clotted blood is collected as early as possible during the course of the disease, and a convalescent sample is sent 2 to 3 weeks later. Ideally, at least 2 mL of blood is obtained, although in infants less will often suffice. The sample should arrive in the laboratory within 1 day and should not be frozen, as this will provoke hemolysis. In the laboratory, serum is separated from the clot and stored at −20° C for future processing.

Upper Respiratory Tract Specimen

Samples collected during the first days of symptoms (when viral shedding is maximal) lead to higher recovery rates. URT samples include material from the rhinopharynx and oropharynx, with the former providing a lower rate of contamination by lower respiratory components. Throat swabs should be collected vigorously to ensure that mucus and cellular material is obtained from the pharynx, while in older children throat gargles can be obtained. Nasal wash is shown to produce the highest viral detection rate and relatively low patient discomfort compared to swabs, aspirates, and brushings.[16] Specimens should be placed in viral transport medium (VTM) in the presence of antibiotics to inhibit bacterial growth. Usually this is contained in a small sterile bottle, and, after immersion, the wooden shaft of the swab is broken level with the neck of the container, the cap is replaced, and the fluid is gently agitated. VTM prevents drying and maintains viral viability during transport and contains either Eagle's minimum essential medium or Hank's balanced salt solution, along with fetal bovine serum or bovine serum albumin (BSA). When the time interval between collection and delivery is less than 2 hours, specimens should be transferred to the laboratory at room temperature; when the time interval is 2 to 24 hours, they should be transferred on ice. When the time interval is more than 24 hours, specimens should be surrounded by solid CO_2 and packed in an insulated container. Specimens suspected of containing RSV should not be frozen; they must be transferred to the laboratory as soon as possible. They can also be used to prepare slides for immunofluorescent detection, either by rolling the swab directly on the slide or after recovery of cells by centrifugation.

Lower Respiratory Tract Specimens

Specimens from the LRT are usually obtained in the setting of an immunocompromised child (early in the course of a pulmonary infection) or in the immunocompetent child with severe atypical pneumonia. Although induced sputum is often contaminated by oropharyngeal components that hinder viral recovery, it is an easily obtainable sample, at least in older children, in whom the success rate is >70%. Therefore, it is often used after either filtration through 200-nm membrane filters or dilution, usually in the presence of a reducing agent such as 0.1% dithiothreitol (DTT) to reduce the viscosity. Transtracheal and bronchial aspirates, and bronchial biopsy specimens are all considered better sources than sputum for both culture (in VTM at 4° C) and direct immunodetection of viruses in pelleted cells (a few drops in a container without VTM). Similarly, after mild centrifugation (10 minutes, $500 \times g$), both the supernatant and the pellet of bronchoalveolar lavage (BAL) are good sources for isolation and immunofluorescent detection of respiratory viruses.

Pulmonary biopsies are suitable for EM; BAL and nasopharyngeal aspirate (NPA) samples that are intended for EM should not be diluted with VTM because it contains salts and proteins that obscure the field and dilute viral particles.

Diagnostic Techniques

A variety of methodologies have been developed for the diagnosis of respiratory virus infections, each with different characteristics (Table 24-1).

Virus Cultures

Culture of a virus from a clinical specimen confirms the presence of viable virus.

Cell Culture

For each respiratory virus, there are a number of cell lines that allow its replication *in vitro* (Table 24-2). Susceptible cell cultures may undergo degenerative processes on exposure to respiratory viruses. The speed at which these appear is usually characteristic for a particular virus

(e.g., 2 to 5 days for RSV). The most common CPE patterns include syncytia formation (fusion of many cells in multinucleated structures), vacuolation (generation of large, bubblelike regions in the cytoplasm), and granular degeneration. Rounding and detachment are also common features (Fig. 24-1).

The dose that causes CPE in 50% of inoculated cells ($TCID_{50}$) is used to express the content of a given viral preparation (titer). Alternatively, when the cell monolayer is permitted to grow covered by a solid (agar) medium, the foci of virus-infected cells form plaques that may be stained by specific dyes (e.g., neutral red) in a manner different from uninfected cells, and these can be readily identified and counted.

Viruses that possess H (e.g., IFV and PIV) may be able to adhere to erythrocytes of the host in which they replicate. When a suspension of erythrocytes derived from a suitable species is added to the infected cell culture, they adhere in clumps after a certain period.

Rotation enhances the yield of a cultured virus, while liposomal and other agents added in the media, as well as centrifugation protocols, may increase the detection rate. In addition, a virus can be isolated by culturing cells from a biopsy sample. However, co-culture with helper cells often leads to higher recovery rates because this technique overcomes the viral inhibitory activity of certain tissue homogenates.

Cell culture can be used in two additional ways for the identification of respiratory viruses. First, sera from patients can be assessed for the ability to inhibit the CPE, plaque formation, or hemadsorption activity normally triggered by a stock viral solution of known infectivity. Conversely, virus strains isolated from patients can be exposed to specific immune sera known to prevent such activities, and the final result can be assessed on the cell culture.

In many cases, cell culture remains the gold standard, often achieving the highest sensitivity scores and providing an isolate for epidemiologic and typing purposes or antiviral susceptibility assays. However, it is a rather time-consuming process that demands several days to weeks and many skilled personnel before results

TABLE 24-1 COMPARISON OF RESPIRATORY VIRUS DIAGNOSTIC TECHNIQUES

METHOD CHARACTERISTICS	CULTURE	IMMUNOFLUORESCENCE (IFA, DFA)	ENZYME-LINKED IMMUNOSORBENT ASSAY (ELISA)	USE OF PROBES WITHOUT TARGET AMPLIFICATION	POLYMERASE CHAIN REACTION (PCR)
Speed	+	+++	+++	++	++/+++
Sensitivity	+++	++	++	++	++++
Specificity	+++	++	++	+++	++++
Quantitative measurement	++	++	++	+	+++
Ease of use	+	+	+++	+	++/+++
Cost	++	+	+	++	+++

Modified from Myint S. Recent advances in the rapid diagnosis of respiratory tract infection. *Br Med Bull*. 2002;61:97-114.

TABLE 24-2 CELL LINES COMMONLY USED FOR IDENTIFICATION OF RESPIRATORY VIRUSES

CELL LINE	ORIGIN	TYPE	VIRUS
A549	Human alveolar adenocarcinoma	Continuous	AdV, RSV
HeLa	Human cervical carcinoma	Continuous	AdV, RSV, RV
Hep-2	HeLa contaminant	Continuous	AdV, RSV
HEK	Human embryonic kidney	Primary	AdV
LLC-MK2	Monkey kidney	Continuous	IFV, PIV, HCV-NL63
MDCK	Canine kidney	Continuous	IFV
MRC-5	Human fibroblasts	Cell strain	AdV, HCV
MRC-c/C16	Human fetal lung fibroblasts	Continuous	HCV
Mv1Lu	Mink lung	Continuous	IFV
PMK	Monkey kidney	Primary	IFV, PIV
tMK	Monkey kidney	Continuous	MPV
Vero E6	Monkey kidney	Continuous	SARS-CoV
WI-38	Human lung fibroblasts	Cell strain	RV, HCV

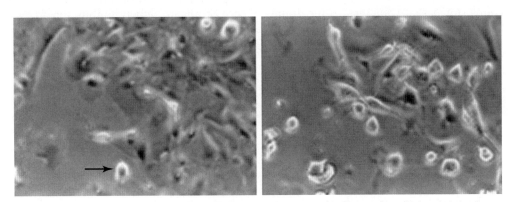

FIGURE 24-1. Cytopathic effect caused by human rhinoviruses *in vitro*. **A,** Primary cultures of human bronchial epithelial cells were infected by RV7 at a multiplicity of infection of 10, and characteristic shrinkage and rounding can be seen in some cells *(arrow)* 24 to 48 hours later, whereas the rest of the monolayer remains intact. **B,** At later time points, fully developed cytopathic effect gradually leads to cellular detachment, cell debris, and separation of the cell layer.

can be obtained. More rapid protocols that use a combination of cell culture with another detection method (e.g., immunofluorescence [IF]-, EM-, or PCR-based methods) have recently been developed. With these techniques, the sample is inoculated onto the culture, and the presence of replicating virus is verified after 24 to 48 hours by the second method.

In an interesting advance, IFV-susceptible, mink lung–derived Mv1Lu cells and the human adenocarcinoma A549 cell line were co-cultured in shell vials to detect respiratory viruses. The R-mix monolayers that can be used directly from cryopreserved vials are inoculated on coverslips with the clinical sample, and 24 hours later the coverslips are removed and stained with a mixture of antisera against many respiratory viruses. If a positive signal is present, cells from a parallel coverslip can be dispersed onto a suitable chamber containing multiple coverslips that can

be examined separately for the presence of individual respiratory viruses using monoclonal antibodies. Using this method, definitive results can be obtained within 2 days.[17] However, in conventional single-cell–culture CPE observation, the respective result takes approximately 10 days. Although of similar sensitivity to conventional cell culture and direct IF with respect to most respiratory viruses (IFV, PIV, and RSV), this method is less sensitive in detecting AdV.[18]

Eggs
Fertile eggs are used for the culture of respiratory viruses (e.g., IFV) after being chilled to prevent the release of red blood cells and subsequent virus loss due to cell adsorption. Inoculation into the amniotic cavity is used mainly for the isolation of such viruses from clinical samples. Harvesting is usually conducted 48 to 72 hours after inoculation.

Animals

Inoculation of a susceptible animal is a common practice for the detection of many viruses. In the SARS epidemics, for instance, one of the first tests to identify the virus was intracranial and intraperitoneal injection of clinical samples into suckling mice, with observation of the mice for 14 days for pathologic findings.[11] Other examples include AdV serotype 5, which when given intravenously to adult mice, kills them within 3 to 4 days, whereas other AdVs, when administered subcutaneously to newborn hamsters, cause their death within 4 to 12 days.

Detection of Whole Viruses by Electron Microscopy

This is the only method that allows direct inspection of viruses, detects pathogens that are difficult to cultivate, and is applied during epidemics of unknown etiology. Preparation of samples and negative staining techniques are fast, easy, and inexpensive processes. On the other hand, the sensitivity limit is approximately 10^6 viral particles/mL, which renders detection difficult after the first days of infection. Also, EM requires expensive equipment and skilled personnel and cannot differentiate between infectious and noninfectious organisms.

Fluid Samples

In a typical protocol, a 300- or 400-mesh grid is placed on a drop of sample for 5 to 15 minutes. After draining with filter paper, the grid can be stained. Fluid samples should be placed on support films, made either from Collodion films (2% solution in isoamyl acetate) or from the mechanically stronger 0.3% to 0.5% polyvinyl formal in ethylene dichloride (Formvar solution). The films are cast on a glass slide by experienced personnel, and grids are made by pressing the grid onto the film slide in the presence of water. A silver-gray rather than charcoal-gray or gold color coincides with optimal film thickness, and additional carbon coating under vacuum facilitates spreading of the sample, which improves the results. Glow discharging under the vacuum or treatment of the grids with a suitable agent (e.g., poly-L-lysine, Alcian blue, Cytochrome C, or BSA) is commonly used to overcome spreading problems.

Concentration of particles contained in BAL and NPA samples is recommended. This can be achieved with ultracentrifugation, ultrafiltration, or agar diffusion. With agar diffusion, a drop of suspension is placed on top of 2% agar, in which liquid and salts diffuse, leaving a film-coated grid containing the virus that can be drained on filter paper and stained for EM. The pseudoreplica technique is a variation whereby the drop is allowed to diffuse into the agar and then is irradiated and covered by Formvar film. Then the Formvar membrane is carefully removed and allowed to float onto a water surface. Grids are then applied on the replica membrane and picked up with the aid of filter paper.

Antibodies are also used for the concentration of viruses in suspension (clumping). For aggregation, the samples can be incubated with the antiserum, centrifuged, and placed onto grids with the pseudoreplica technique; alternatively, antiserum is mixed with agar, and a grid is placed onto the gel. Virus suspension is then added and allowed to absorb, followed by removal and staining

of the grid. In solid-phase immunoelectron microscopy, the film is coated with antibodies before incubation with virus suspension.

Immunoprecipitation techniques are particularly helpful when picornaviruses need to be detected. These viruses are so small that they sometimes appear similar to lipid droplets. Some viruses tend to clump in the absence of antiserum, reducing the specificity of this procedure. Viruses in suspension or on grids can be incubated with primary antiserum, allowed to aggregate, and after the antibody has been washed away, the preparation can be treated with a colloidal gold-labeled secondary antibody. Gold labeling has been used specifically to detect immune complexes in serum, as well as subviral particles. In a somewhat different approach, viruses are exposed to excess antibodies, resulting in extensive coating rather than aggregation of the viruses. This method allows specific identification and serotyping of viruses and can serve to assess the reactivity of convalescent serum against known viruses.

Finally, short-term culture of virus in vitro with harvesting before the appearance of the CPE is a good alternative for the enrichment of a sample. AdVs and paramyxoviruses can be detected in supernatants before a massive CPE occurs. On the other hand, AdV is membrane-associated and may be lost on removal of the debris with centrifugation.

An additional problem with NPA specimens is the presence of mucus, which inhibits spreading of the samples. These specimens can be treated with an equal volume of a DTT-containing buffer to break down the mucus.

Biopsy Specimens

Specimens should be placed in 2% to 5% glutaraldehyde in cacodylate or phosphate buffer and stored at $-20°$ C to maintain the tissue architecture and specifically localize the virus. Osmium fixation (1% to 2% OsO_4 in a 4-[2-hydroxyethyl]-1-piperazineethanesulfonic acid [HEPES] or a piperazine diethanesulfonic acid [PIPES]–based buffer) is also used. *En bloc* staining can then be conducted with uranyl acetate in veronal buffer. Otherwise, dehydration and embedding in resins should follow the fixation step. Although it is not optimal, formalin-fixed material and paraffin-embedded sections can also be used for EM after suitable treatment. Because the sample area used is limited, it is wise first to stain sections with suitable stains (e.g., toluidine blue) to select areas of particular interest (e.g., with a CPE) and then trim the sections further for thin sectioning. Viruses can also be seen by extracting solid tissue with a suitable buffer after homogenization or repeated freezing and thawing, and further treatment as a liquid sample. Thin sectioning is also the method of choice for identification of virus in cell culture. If the virus has triggered cell lysis, it can be detected in cell supernatant or medium (after ultracentrifugation is performed to remove the debris), followed by negative staining of the pellet. Cells can also be embedded in agar and further treated as tissue blocks.

Electron Microscopic Appearance of Respiratory Viruses

Table 24-3 summarizes the main morphologic characteristics of respiratory viruses. Picornaviruses and AdVs are naked virions of icosahedral symmetry and a round appearance on EM. AdVs have the higher size ranges

TABLE 24-3 MAIN MORPHOLOGIC CHARACTERISTICS OF RESPIRATORY VIRUSES

VIRUS	ENVELOPE	CAPSID SYMMETRY	GENOME	VIRION SIZE (NM)	PROJECTIONS (NM)	NUCLEOCAPSID SIZE (NM)
AdV	No	I	ds DNA	70–90		
RV	No	I	+ sRNA	24–30		
HCV	Yes	C	+ sRNA	80–150	20	10–20
SARS-CoV	Yes	C	+ sRNA	80–140	20–40	
IFV	Yes	H	– sRNA	80–120		9–15
PIV	Yes	H	– sRNA	150–250		12–18
MPV	Yes	H	– sRNA	150–600	13–17	
RSV	Yes	H	– sRNA	100–300	12	6–7

C, Complex; H, helical; I, icosahedral; +/– sRNA, negative or positive sense single-stranded RNA.

among naked virions, while picornaviruses are very small and are often confused with some tailless bacteriophage species. Immunoprecipitation techniques can be used in such cases. In addition, AdVs can degenerate, and individual capsomers may appear separately, forming hexagonal lattices. Enveloped respiratory viruses (e.g., IFV, PIV, and HCV) have a soft membrane that can become deformed during drying for negative staining. Thus, the particles may appear pleomorphic, and may vary in size. The enveloped respiratory viruses are spiked, rather than smooth. HCVs have long (20-nm) spikes on the surface, whereas paramyxoviruses and orthomyxoviruses contain projections that appear as a fringe on the outer side. However, even these forms can sometimes be confused with mitochondria or inverted bacterial membrane debris. Discrimination between orthomyxovirus and paramyxovirus families is often challenging.

The cellular location of viruses in thin sections of solid tissues also provides important evidence of their properties (e.g., DNA viruses replicate in the nucleus, whereas RNA viruses replicate in the cytoplasm). Naked viruses, such as AdVs, cause cell lysis and can be seen as round shells with a core of different density surrounded by dead cells. If the cytopathology is advanced, AdVs may be seen in both the nucleus and the cytoplasm. Picornaviruses cause swelling of the endoplasmic reticulum, and the ribosomes may appear as large beads on a string. Enveloped viruses acquire their membranes by budding through the nuclear envelope, through the plasma membrane, or into vesicles within the cells. There are some difficulties in discriminating virions from normal cell organelles (e.g., lysosomes and Golgi complexes); however viruses with spikes appear to have a thicker membrane than the cellular compartments. Nucleocapsids, which contain nucleic acids and viral proteins, are present in enveloped viruses and can be spherical, helical, or complex. PIVs, for instance, have helical filamentous nucleocapsids. AdVs can be discriminated from the otherwise similar but larger herpesviruses by the smaller size of their nucleocapsid.

Transmission electron microscopy (TEM) is a method of reference for the identification of many viruses. TEM allows detection of even one virus particle. However, it needs specialized and expensive instrumentation and skilled technicians. Moreover, it is unable to discriminate among viruses of the same family or among particular subtypes.

Other Whole-Virus Detection Methods
Fluorescent dyes can be used to stain a purified virus preparation and allow enumeration of virus in a solution consistent with data obtained by TEM. OliGreen (a dye that specifically binds to nucleotides) has been successfully used for the enumeration of AdV 5, RSV, and IFV A, and the method can be performed within 1 hour.[19] To that end, density-gradient–purified virus preparations are incubated with the dye and subjected to analysis in a modified-flow cytometer. This method also provides information about the virus genome size.

Antigen Detection
Antigen-based detection methods presuppose the knowledge or suspicion that a particular virus is present in the sample and preclude the discovery of unknown viruses. However, they are rapid, accurate, easy to perform, and do not depend on virus viability. Table 24-4 compares

TABLE 24-4 RAPID DIAGNOSTIC METHODS FOR RSV BASED ON ANTIGEN DETECTION COMPARED TO CELL CULTURE TECHNIQUES

METHOD	SENSITIVITY (%)	SPECIFICITY (%)
IFA/DFA	93-98	92-97
EIA	59-97	75-100
DIA	93	91
OIA	88-95	97-100

IFA/DFA, Indirect immunofluorescence/direct immunofluorescence; EIA, enzyme immunoassay; DIA, direct enzyme immunoassay; OIA, optical immunoassay.
Modified from Henrickson KJ, Hall CB. Diagnostic assays for respiratory syncytial virus disease. Pediatr Infect Dis J. 2007;26:S6-S40.

the sensitivity and specificity of these methods with cell culture detection of RSV. These features are of major importance for the surveillance and control of epidemic diseases (e.g., IFV infection) but are usually not recommended among the immunosuppressed, the elderly, and at times when prevalence is low in a community. Thus, the American Academy of Pediatrics does not recommend the routine use of antigen-detection assays for the diagnosis of RSV infection because it is thought that it does not influence the management of the patient who has been clinically diagnosed with bronchiolitis.[20] Viral antigens can be revealed based on the ability of the antigen to interact with an antibody or to elicit a specific immune response. In addition, specific functional assays (e.g., hemagglutination tests that assess the presence of particular proteins that are found in the envelope of orthomyxoviruses and paramyxoviruses) can be conducted to reveal the respective virus. These are described in the section on "Serologic Methods" later in the chapter.

Immunoassays

Immunoassays are laboratory tests based on the use of antibodies and are routinely used in the diagnosis of infectious diseases.

Immunofluorescence Immunofluorescence (IF) is based on the chemical conjugation of a fluorochrome with an antibody, without compromising either the ability of the fluorochrome to fluoresce or the specificity of the antibody. Fluorescein isothiocyanate and tetramethyl rhodamine isothiocyanate are the most widely used fluorochromes; the former fluoresces yellowish-green, whereas the latter appears reddish-orange. Fluorescein isothiocyanate seems to be more suitable for clinical samples because the background is more often red than green. In addition, red-fluorescing dyes (e.g., Congo red) can be used to stain all cellular components red and provide a contrast to the green fluorescence of fluorescein isothiocyanate. A fluorescence microscope is required for the detection of light emitted by excited fluorochrome, and the interpretation of results is partially subjective, depending on the experience of the examiner. In modern fluorescence microscopes with epi-illumination systems, light of selected wavelengths is deflected through the objective to the top surface of the sample. The resulting emitted light is directed to the observer through the objective, a dichroic mirror, a barrier filter, and the oculars. Each fluorochrome has specific fluorescence characteristics. For instance, fluorescein isothiocyanate absorption is at 495 nm, and emission is at 525 nm. With the available interference filters in fluorescence microscopes, 85% of transmitted light is between 400 and 500 nm (i.e., the visible part of the spectrum).

Practically, the sample should be fixed onto a slide first. Thereafter, it is incubated, either with a specific antibody conjugated with a fluorochrome (direct immunofluorescence assay [DIF]) or with a primary specific antibody and thereafter with a secondary antibody raised against the primary one that has been conjugated with the fluorochrome (indirect immunofluorescence assay [IIF]). The first method is less sensitive, but it avoids nonspecific staining of negative samples, as is often seen with the indirect method. However, the generation of primary conjugates

for many viruses is laborious and costly, whereas secondary conjugates may be common for several antigens. Incubation times are short for both procedures (30 to 45 minutes, 37° C), making IF a good method for rapid virus detection.

Viral samples can also be detected by IF with spin cultures, whereby suitable cell monolayers are grown on coverslips within flat-bottom vials. The sample is then applied on top of the coverslip, and the vial is centrifuged (650 to 900 × g, 30 to 60 minutes). This technique facilitates virus entry into the target cells, and usually the coverslip is removed, fixed, and stained for IF, 18 to 24 hours later.

DIF and IIF have been used for the development of a number of rapid tests for the detection of respiratory viruses. These can be accomplished within a few minutes, and they have become very popular due to their rapidity and ease of performance. Usually, a spot or slide containing the sample is prepared for every virus being tested, cytospun, and incubated with the monoclonal antibody. In a recent advance, a single spot can be used for the simultaneous detection of seven respiratory viruses (RSV, IFV A and B, AdV, and PIV 1 to 3).[21] A rhodamine label is used with the RSV antibody system, whereas fluorescein is used in all other cases. Thus, the development of a reddish-gold color in the spot suggests the presence of RSV particles in the sample, whereas a green color (fluorescein) is followed by a second reaction in another spot to determine which of the other viruses is present. The sensitivity of this method was greatly enhanced by centrifugation and was superior to that of enzyme immunoassay (EIA)–based protocols, but was inferior to that of cell culture.[22] Another IIF method proved more efficient than cell culture in detecting respiratory viruses in nasopharyngeal swabs.[23]

Radioimmunoassay There are two types of radioimmunoassay (RIA). In competitive RIA methods, a known quantity of radioactivity-labeled antigen competes with unlabeled antigen that is added (test sample). The inhibition of binding of labeled antigen depends on the concentration of unlabeled antigen in the clinical sample. The labeled antigen that is finally bound to antibody is measured and referred to as *bound antigen*, whereas the unconjugated labeled antigen is referred to as *free antigen*. To circumvent problems arising from the separation of bound antigen from free antigen in solid-phase RIA, the immunoreactant that is used first (antibody or antigen) is immobilized on a solid support. After each step, unwanted reactants can be removed readily by washing. In contrast to the laborious and expensive generation of labeled viral antigens, noncompetitive RIA methods use labeled antibodies. The former are more stable, with more predictable structures and biochemical properties. Noncompetitive RIAs are, therefore, more popular in diagnostic virology. In a technique known as *sandwich RIA,* unlabeled viral antibodies adsorbed to a solid-phase support are allowed to capture viral antigens present in the clinical sample. Then a radiolabeled antibody (indicator antibody) is allowed to bind to the captured viral antigens. This procedure can be either direct or indirect. In the latter case, a primary unlabeled indicator antibody is used initially, followed by incubation with a secondary radiolabeled antibody. In all of these procedures, free antibody is removed after the final incubation, and bound iodine-125-labeled antibody is measured.

Nasal aspirates are a suitable source for assessing the presence of respiratory viruses (e.g., RSV) with RIA. For the direct detection of viruses in tissue or cell culture,[125] I-labeled viral antibody is incubated with the cell mono-layers or tissue sections, and unbound labeled antibody is removed. The bound radioactivity is then measured. The radioactivity bound to the infected tissue or culture is then compared with the radioactivity bound to unin-fected control samples. Ratios exceeding 2:1 are considered positive. In the indirect version of this technique, the sample is first incubated with unlabeled antibody, followed by [125] I-labeled secondary antibody.

Enzyme Immunoassays As indicated by their name, EIAs are based on the conjugation of suitable enzymes (e.g., horseradish peroxidase, alkaline phosphatase [ALP]) to antibodies and their subsequent use for the qualitative and quantitative detection of antigens. Enzyme-labeled anti-bodies are reacted with substrates that generate soluble color products and are used to detect viral antigens (directly or indirectly) in tissues or cell cultures in cytoimmunoen-zymatic staining. Colored substrates can be observed with the naked eye, with light microscopy, with EM (in the case of electron-dense products), or they can be evaluated with a spectrophotometer. As in the IF methods described ear-lier in the chapter, infected and control cell monolayers and tissue sections on slides are fixed and incubated directly with enzyme-coupled antibody (or with an uncoupled pri-mary and an enzyme-coupled secondary antibody, in the indirect approach). Unbound enzyme conjugate is removed by washing, and the slides are incubated with enzyme sub-strates. After development of the colored product, the slides are rinsed, counterstained, and mounted in mount-ing medium to be observed under a light microscope.

A modification of the indirect approach includes an additional step whereby an antibody raised against the enzyme is incubated with the sample. Because this anti-body is also conjugated with enzyme, its sensitivity is greatly enhanced. Both peroxidase- antiperoxidase and ALP–anti-ALP are being used, and the final reaction products can be either soluble color complexes or insol-uble substrates that can be observed with the naked eye, observed with a light microscope, or measured with a spectrophotometer.

Avidin-biotin is another system that is widely used to increase sensitivity in such approaches. The bind-ing reaction between these two molecules is strong, and it occurs independently of the immune reactions in the assay. In a typical avidin-biotin complex protocol, biotin-conjugated primary antibodies are incubated with the samples, and after the unbound antibodies have been washed out, enzyme-conjugated avidin or streptavidin is added. The complex formed is monitored, with the final addition of substrate and mounting of the slide. In the indirect approach, an unlabeled primary antibody is first incubated with the sample, followed by secondary incubation with biotinylated antibody and the biotin-avi-din enzyme complex incubation.

Heterogenous EIA assays, in which unbound enzyme-labeled antibody is removed and incubation is relatively

long, are used for quantitation of viral antigens. Like viral RIA assays, quantitative EIAs use unlabeled antiviral antibody bound to a solid phase (e.g., microtiter plates, cuvettes). Unbound antibody is removed after adsorption, and nonspecific binding sites are blocked by blocking agents, such as BSA. After samples are added, unbound material is removed and enzyme-conjugated antibody is added. This antibody binds to antigen captured by solid-phase bound antibody. After removal of unbound mate-rial, enzyme substrate is added and the formation of the reaction product is measured. This measurement reflects the amount of enzyme bound to antigen that is retained in the solid phase. Control samples are always included to define the background levels of each modification. IFV, AdV, and RSV can be measured by these methods.

The cassette EIA method is based on the fact that large amounts of antibody can be bound to nitrocellu-lose, nylon, and other membranes. Such a membrane is attached to a plastic well, and the entire system is attached to a cassette containing a material that can absorb all waste fluid generated during the assay. The antibody and the controls can be dotted or slotted onto the membrane in separate wells. The method offers the advantages of increased sensitivity, reduced time required for its comple-tion, and detection of many different respiratory viruses from many samples. Based on the same principle, numer-ous variations are used, with different sensitivity scores. The solid phase, for instance, can be substituted by beads coated with antibody. After incubation with the sample, the beads can be transferred to the membranes and the assay can go on as a standard EIA. Alternatively, a clas-sic dot-blot apparatus can be used to place an antibody in dots on the membrane. The additional binding sites on the membrane are then blocked. Samples and controls can then be added as serial dilutions for quantitation, and waste fluids are collected from the associated vacuum sys-tem. However, although these systems are able to discrim-inate between serotypes of the same species (e.g., IFV A versus IFV B), they may not be as sensitive as cell culture or DIF in detecting virus.

Fluoroimmunoassay In time-resolved fluoroimmunoas-say (FIA), the unusually long fluorescence decay time of the lanthanide element Europium (Eu^{+3}) is used to discriminate the fluorescence decay characteristics of Europium-conjugated antibodies (Europium is first che-lated with ethylenediaminetetraacetic acid [EDTA]) from the fluorescence decay of clinical samples. In a represen-tative protocol, a microtiter plate or strip is coated with antibody and the remaining binding sites of the plates are blocked. The clinical sample is then added simultane-ously with the Europium-conjugated antibody, and after incubation, the unbound material is washed out. AdV, RSV, IFV, and PIV have been detected with time-resolved FIA, although sometimes with limited sensitivity.

Optical Immunoassay An advance in the field of anti-gen detection is optical immunoassay (OIA) technology. This allows direct visual detection of a macromolecule that is bound onto a molecular thin film. Binding causes an increase in the thickness of the optical surface (sili-con wafer film) that will alter the reflected light path and will be perceived as a color change that is observable with the naked eye. Practically, viral-specific antibodies are immobilized on the surface and allowed to capture extracted viral antigens that are placed directly onto the surface and incubated at room temperature for a short period. After addition of a suitable substrate, a positive result appears as a color spot, whereas in the absence of antigens in the sample, the background color remains unchanged. Commercially available tests for IFV and RSV can take as little as 15 minutes to be completed and do not require sophisticated laboratory equipment, although reported sensitivity varies.

Agglutination Assays

In the latex agglutination assay, antibody-coated nanoparticles from polystyrene, polyacrylamide, and other latexes; agarose beads; or colloidal gold agglutinate in the presence of viral antigens. In a typical protocol for respiratory viruses, a clarified and diluted NPA sample is mixed with antibody-coated latex particles on a microscope slide. The method is simple, and an agglutination reaction can be observed usually after 10 to 15 minutes, but the overall sensitivity and specificity are low.

Serologic Methods

As indicated by the name, serologic methods attempt to detect viruses in the host by assessing the presence of specific antibodies in blood samples, but sputum and urine also may be used. Serology is a rather sensitive, specific, and relatively cheap diagnostic technique that is also used to confirm the results of other methods. There are five classes of human immunoglobulins: IgG, IgM, IgA, IgE, and IgD. IgM antibodies represent approximately one tenth of serum immunoglobulins, while secretory IgA constitutes the first line of defense against mucosal viral infections. The four IgG subclasses (IgG1 to IgG4) have a longer half-life than the others (22 days) and are associated with long-term protection by triggering complement fixation (CFix) and improving the specificity of the immune response by binding to the surface of cytotoxic effector cells. Most viruses induce mainly IgG1 and IgG3 responses.

There are many potential antigens in each virus that may be presented at different time points in the course of infection. The primary antibody response to a virus is typically characterized by early onset of IgM production (peaking at 2 weeks) that declines later, followed by IgG production (reaching a plateau 2 weeks later) that may persist for years. When the antigen is localized in the mucosa, the immune response, driven by B cells of the interstitial lymphoid follicles (e.g., tonsils, Peyer's patches) also produces high quantities of IgA. Re-infection may result in overproduction of IgG by memory B cells, which may remain throughout life, together with a low or undetectable production of IgM. Infants younger than 6 months of age, however, mount a relatively poor IgG response, thus viral detection by isolation is the best way to diagnose a viral infection.

Diagnosis of the pathogen responsible for a recent infection may be achieved through detection of specific IgM in serum, 1 week after symptoms begin. Although useful clinically, this approach faces a number of problems upon evaluation of results. In some cases, patients remain seronegative during acute infection (e.g., 10% to 30% of patients with acute RSV infection, or 20% to 50%

of those with acute AdV infection). In other cases, IgM persists at high levels (even during convalescence), thus not representing recent infection. The presence of specific IgG is a cause of false-positive results when rheumatoid factor (RF) is also present in the serum, but also of false-negative results because of its competition with IgM. Such problems are minimized with the removal of IgG or RF pre-analytically, although the ideal way is the use of the μ-capture IgM technique.

Therefore, in most cases, blood samples should be collected at least twice during the course of an illness within a 2- to 3-week interval: in the acute phase (as soon as possible after the onset of disease and no later than 1 week) and during convalescence (at least 2 weeks after onset). Comparison of the antibody pattern in these two states allows safe demonstration of diagnostically significant active virus, and seroconversion is defined as a 4-fold increase in antibody titer. The long delay before a definite diagnosis is made limits its use in urgent decision making. However, in many cases rapid methods of antigen detection are inefficient (e.g., RSV detection in adults), and serologic testing is considered a reference method (e.g., Epstein-Barr virus [EBV] pharyngitis infection). Moreover, it is a fast automated method that remains the method of choice for archival material; it is as sensitive as PCR in detecting influenza infections.[24] It is also used to check on the effectiveness of vaccination and in confirming causation of illness (e.g., with AdVs and Enteroviruses that colonize the URT for a long time). On the other hand, serology is not indicated for immunosuppressed individuals, neonates, or infants because of their impaired immune responses.

Another major issue in antibody measurement is the type of antibodies targeted by the test. Thus, antibodies detected by EIAs may be different from those that confer neutralization activity. Neutralizing antibodies are raised against epitopes usually found on the surface of the virus, and upon binding to the virus, render it noninfectious by blocking its attachment to receptors or preventing uncoating of the virus. Neutralizing antibodies persist after viral infection; their measurement aims to determine vaccine efficacy and is used in epidemiologic studies rather than for the diagnosis of primary infection. In tests assessing neutralizing antibody, the serum sample is usually incubated with a viral preparation of known titer, and its ability to inhibit $TCID_{50}$ during CPE development in cell culture is assessed. Alternatively, the reduction in the ability of the viral preparation to form plaques can be measured. In the case of IFV for example, a titer 1:8 denotes protective immunity. Such tests are the method of choice for viral infections and can be performed in specialized laboratories.

There are three main ways to detect respiratory virus in the host serologically. Immunoassays (conducted in a manner similar to that described earlier for the detection of viral antigens) directly measure antibody-virus interaction through the use of labeled reagents. CFix and passive agglutination assays are based on the ability of virus-antibody interactions to interfere with the functions discussed earlier, but do not allow differentiation between antibody classes. Finally, assays such as hemagglutination inhibition allow the measurement of particular antibodies that specifically interact with viral surface proteins.

Possible cross-reactivity between viruses belonging to the same family and retrospective diagnosis are the main disadvantages of these methods, which do not necessarily produce comparable results because they detect antibodies of different types and specificity.

Immunoassays

As in the antigen detection immunoassays described earlier in the chapter, reporter molecules conjugated with antibodies (or antigens) allow the assessment of virus-antibody interactions. The reporter molecules may fluoresce (IF), have enzymatic activity for color-developing substrates (EIA), or have radioactivity (RIA).

Immunofluorescence In IF assays, purified hyperimmune animal sera or monoclonal antibodies are labeled with a fluorescent dye (e.g., fluorescein isothiocyanate). In a typical protocol, a serum sample is incubated with virus-infected cells that are fixed on a slide. After unbound material is washed out, the slide can be dried, mounted, and observed under a fluorescence microscope. Streptavidin-biotin and similar systems that are currently used provide greater flexibility and sensitivity in antibody detection. Background fluorescence is a common obstacle in IF procedures. In solid-phase FIA, the viral antigen is immobilized on an opaque solid-phase surface rather than a slide, and use of a fluorometer allows quantitation and automation. However, FIA instrumentation cannot discriminate between background and positive fluorescence.

IF is the method of choice for the diagnosis of EBV infection, where a single serum sample in the acute phase of pharyngitis is sufficient for the diagnosis of 90% to 95% of infectious mononucleosis cases with detection of capsid (VCA-M, VCA-G) and nuclear (EBNA-G) viral antibodies. IFA is easy to perform and inexpensive but can be time-consuming and requires an expensive fluorescence microscope and interpretation by skilled personnel. Only rare cases with ambiguous results require additional testing with Western blot or avidity tests (Table 24-5).

Enzyme Immunoassays EIAs are used to detect and quantitate antibody raised against viral antigens. Antigens are obtained from various sources, such as lysates from virus-infected cells. To that end, cells are washed, re-suspended in serum-free medium, and subjected to repeated freeze-thaw cycles. Virus is then clarified with ultracentrifugation, providing a rich source of antigens. Synthetic

peptides also may be used for antigen preparation. For IFV, this method is more sensitive than CFix, may discriminate between antibody classes, and may use antigens specific for virus serotypes or subtypes, but it needs standardization. Seroconversion for RSV, which may be delayed for 4 to 6 weeks, has been detected in 50% of infants younger than 6 months of age.

For indirect EIA, the antigen is bound to a solid-phase surface, and after incubation with the serum sample, bound antibodies are detected with an anti-human antibody enzyme conjugate. The more abundant IgG antibodies compete for antigens with the other classes and, thus, should be removed before IgM measurement. Nonspecific binding is common in this method, and impurities present in the antigen preparation may cause false-positive results. Pre-incubating the sera with uninfected cells may reduce this problem.

To increase the specificity of this method, inhibition (or competitive) EIAs have been used. In this case, serum antibodies are detected by their ability to block the binding of a known antibody conjugate to the antigen. The detector antibody can be added simultaneously or after the antigen and the serum sample. In this case, false-negative results can be caused by serum antibodies that do not compete with the conjugated antibody, but inhibit the ability of the antibody that is being tested to do so.

In the capture EIA method, anti-human immunoglobulin class-specific antibodies are first bound on a solid-phase (capture-phase) surface. After incubation with the serum sample, viral antibodies are bound on the capture phase, together with viral-unrelated antibodies. Viral antigens are added last and subsequently detected with an antigen-specific antibody conjugate. Because of the selective class-specific adsorption in the first step, this method avoids the problems caused by competition between antibody classes, particularly improving IgM detection. On the other hand, low-level IgG detection may be less sensitive due to the presence of large quantities of total IgG antibodies in serum.

Other Immunoassays When it is necessary to detect low levels of virus-specific antibodies in serum, standard immunoblot techniques (Western blot) can be used. Briefly, the protein content of semipurified virus propagated in cell culture is applied onto a nondenaturing polyacrylamide gel, and after electrophoretic separation, protein bands are transferred to a nitrocellulose or nylon membrane that can be cut into narrow strips and stored in the freezer. Serum samples can be diluted in buffer containing a protein that blocks free binding sites to reduce nonspecific binding, and then incubated with the membrane. After a washing step, bound antibodies are measured with the use of a radioactive or enzyme-labeled conjugate bound to a suitable secondary antibody. In dot immunobinding assays, viral antigens are bound in a dotted membrane. The membrane is then treated so that the potential protein-binding sites remaining in the membrane are blocked. The dots are then covered with small (e.g., 3-mm) strips saturated with the test serum. After a washing step, anti-human IgG conjugated with the appropriate enzyme is added, followed by incubation with the appropriate chromogen substrate. The intensity of the color spots is compared with that produced by the control sera to reveal

TABLE 24-5 ANTIBODIES FOR THE DIAGNOSIS OF INFECTIOUS MONONUCLEOSIS

EVALUATION	ANTIBODY AGAINST EBV ANTIGENS		
	VCA-M	VCA-G	EBNA-G
Seronegative	−	−	−
Present infection	+++	++	−
Recent infection	+	++	−
Past infection	−	+	+

−, Absence of antibodies; +, presence of antibodies; ++ or +++, presence of antibodies in high or very high titer.

specific antiviral antibodies. Dot immunobinding assays serve as qualitative rather than quantitative assays and are also subject to problems with nonspecific binding.

In radioimmunoprecipitation assays, antigen-antibody complexes formed after incubation of the serum being tested with viral antigens are cross-linked and immunoprecipitated with protein A or anti-human IgG antibody. The quantity of radioactivity bound in the precipitate can be measured and is proportional to the concentration of specific antibodies in the serum.

Avidity assays measure the relative degree of dissociation between specific antiviral antibodies and their respective antigens. During maturation of the immune response, the avidity (strength of the combined interaction of an antiserum with a pattern of antigens) of IgG antibodies remains high, whereas their concentration declines. Thus, sera from recent infection are characterized by high-avidity antibodies, and sera from re-infection have low-avidity antibodies. Practically, serum is incubated first with antigen bound to a solid-phase surface. The complex is then allowed to dissociate in the presence or absence of urea, and the relative degree of antibody dissociation (ratio of absorbance in the presence of urea to absorbance in the absence of urea) is measured by standard EIA methods.

Finally, three types of methods have been used to specifically measure IgM antibodies. First, in IgG absorption methods, an IgG absorbent (e.g., staphylococcal protein A, streptococcal protein G) is incubated with the serum, and after a centrifugation step, IgM antibodies can be measured in the supernatant. These absorbents are believed to be superior to anti-human IgG antibodies for this method, because the latter may also remove some types of IgM. However, staphylococcal protein cannot bind IgG3, and this could interfere with the accuracy of the method because viral antibodies may be significantly represented in this subclass. Streptococcal protein G, on the other hand, binds all IgG subclasses, but not IgM; accordingly, combinations of streptococci and protein A have been used to remove all IgG and IgA from serum samples before IgM measurement. IgA can interfere with IgM measurement, resulting in false-negative findings by competing with IgM for antigenic sites. Second, in one of the early IgM separation methods, rate zonal centrifugation allowed purification of the IgM subclass based on its higher sedimentation coefficient compared with that of the other antibody classes. Gel filtration takes advantage of the higher molecular weight of IgM compared with the other classes (900 versus 150 to 400 kd). However, serum lipoproteins and nonspecific cell agglutinins may be fractionated, together with IgM, and could interfere with the assay. Ion-exchange chromatography, based on the differential binding of IgM and IgG classes to anion-exchange resins, has been used, but the IgM yield is relatively low, whereas IgG and IgA may still be present in the IgM fraction after elution from the column. Third, in the popular IgM immunoassays, anti-human IgM-specific antibodies are employed. IIF and EIA are the methods typically used for IgM detection. Capture IgM assays show reduced nonspecific binding; in this method, solid-phase, fixed anti-human IgM antibodies separate IgM after incubation with the serum sample. The potential presence of

antiviral elements is further detected using labeled viral antigen or unlabeled antigen, followed by a labeled antigen-specific antibody. Detection of anti-PIV IgM has been also reported with the use of hemadsorption.

Complement Fixation

CFix systems take advantage of the fact that complement proteins bind, or "fix," to antigen-antibody complexes during the host immune response to a foreign antigen. If this antigen is cell-localized, then the deposition of complement elements will cause cell lysis. CFix to IgM is stronger (>1000 times/antibody molecule) than that to IgG. CFix antibodies can be raised against some or all viral proteins. Their titers increase slowly during primary infection, reaching lower levels than antibody titers detected by the other methods. In addition, they decline gradually, making this method less sensitive than others for the detection of viral infection. An additional problem is the interference of some serum elements (e.g., heparin, IgG aggregates) with complement formation. In a typical CFix assay, the serum sample is incubated with a particular antigen in the presence of a known amount of guinea pig complement. If a specific antibody is present in the serum, the complement will be bound and depleted from the solution. Subsequently, sheep erythrocytes coated with hemolysin (anti-sheep erythrocyte antibody) are added, and their lysis is proportional to the availability of complement proteins that did not react with the specific antibody during the first step. CFix may measure antibodies against IFV nucleoprotein (NP), which is common across strains of the same serotype and can discriminate between serotypes A and B, but not among subtypes. The antibodies tested are not protective and disappear in weeks or months. CFix can be used for the diagnosis of recent infection by testing for seroconversion, and, due to the fact that NP is stable, there is no need to prepare a new antigen every time a new IFV subtype emerges. The method is standardized but tends to become replaced by enzyme-linked immunosorbent assay (ELISA). CFix for RSV infection in infants younger than 3 months of age is not reliable.

In immune adherence agglutination assay, a rapid and more sensitive variation, *aggregation*, rather than lysis, of erythrocytes occurs and is measured. In this detection method, complement that is bound to antigen-antibody complexes is allowed to bind to C′3b receptors in human primate erythrocytes. Thus, agglutination of the erythrocytes reveals specific antibodies in the sample.

A simple technique used earlier for the detection of hemagglutinating activity–containing viruses (e.g., IFV and PIV) is the hemolysis-in-gel test. Erythrocytes from sheep or chicken were first sensitized by coupling to a viral antigen in a chromium chloride solution. After a washing step, the erythrocytes were suspended in an agarose gel–containing guinea pig complement. The serum sample was then loaded onto a well in the gel and allowed to diffuse. The presence of antibodies against the virus would lead to the formation of a zone of hemolysis around the well.

Anticomplement antifluorescence is a modified IF assay for the detection of CFix antibodies. In this assay, complement is added during or after exposure of virus-infected cells to the serum being tested. Any complement that is bound can then be detected with anti-C′3 antibody. Because nonspecifically bound IgG cannot trigger CFix, anticomplement antifluorescence assays do not have the common background problems associated with conventional IF.

Agglutination Assays

H or H-N proteins expressed in the envelopes of viruses such as IFV and PIV are able to bind to specific erythrocyte surface receptors and cause their agglutination. Practically, erythrocyte cross-linking leads to observable cell clumping. Hemagglutination inhibition tests measure the presence of specific antibodies in the sera that inhibit virus-mediated agglutination of erythrocytes. This is a sensitive assay that is affected, however, by both nonspecific H and agglutinin inhibitors present in the serum. Nevertheless, it is a particularly reliable method in IFV surveillance protocols, in which case titers ≥1:40 are considered protective, while 1:10 to 1:20 levels are less protective.[25,26]

Fusion proteins present in the envelope of viruses such as PIV and RSV allow their entry into cells by triggering fusion of the viral surface with the cell surface membrane. In the case of erythrocytes, fusion may lead to hemolysis. Hemolysis inhibition assays take advantage of these properties to measure the presence of antibodies in a serum sample that bind and block viral antigens and inhibit hemolysis. In this way, the hemolysis inhibition assay detects both anti-H and antifusion antibodies in the serum. In a typical protocol, serum dilutions are mixed and incubated with purified virus. A 10% suspension of suitable erythrocytes is then added. After some hours of incubation, the erythrocytes are removed by centrifugation and the optical density of the "cleared" supernatant is read with a spectrophotometer. A classic endpoint titer can then be calculated by defining the highest serum dilution that causes 50% inhibition of hemolysis.

In passive agglutination assays, sera are incubated with viral antigens attached to erythrocytes or to materials such as latex or bentonite. The particles or cells agglutinate in the presence of a specific antibody, forming precipitates in the bottom of the tubes. In the passive hemagglutination method, aggregates of erythrocytes develop due to "antibody bridges" formed between antigen-coated erythrocytes. These can be visible, even with the naked eye, and may detect low levels of antibodies.

Detection of Viral Nucleic Acids

A constellation of methods that gained increasing attention during recent years due to their increased sensitivity, specificity, reliability, and accuracy are genetic material-based methods, with PCR in the leading position. The common element in these methods is the isolation and partial purification of viral RNA or DNA and its subsequent detection and analysis in suitable molecular biology systems. Of course, the clinical significance of viral nucleic acid in a specimen needs to be determined because its presence does not always confirm that it is causing disease or that it is in an infectious state.

Hybridization

Hybridization-based protocols require the presence of single-stranded RNA or DNA. In this approach, a suitable oligonucleotide probe sharing a certain degree of homology that allows base pair matching with the single-stranded viral nucleic acid is allowed to anneal under stringent reaction conditions (hybridization). Whereas single-stranded RNA viruses provide ready-made yet labile genetic material, the double-stranded DNA content of AdV must first be denatured or dissociated by chemical (e.g., sodium hydroxide) or physical (heat) means. The resulting single-stranded DNA would return to its double-stranded configuration on removal of the dissociation agent. The probe can be labeled directly with enzymes or other reporter molecules. Alternatively, linker moieties (e.g., biotin or digoxigenin; the latter is more sensitive for in situ hybridization [ISH]) can be attached to probes and serve as bridges for the attachment of reporter molecules. In a typical protocol, the viral nucleic acid is isolated, purified, denatured, and bound to a nitrocellulose or nylon membrane. The denatured and labeled probe is incubated under carefully defined conditions with the viral nucleic acid, and unbound material is thoroughly washed out. A reporter molecule is then added (e.g., ALP-labeled streptavidin), and after a second incubation period the unbound reporter is washed out, and the final chromogen or other suitable substrate is added to give rise to a measurable signal.

Several hybridization-based techniques are used for viral nucleic acid detection (e.g., the molecular biology dot-blot and Southern blot protocols, liquid hybridization, and ISH). As suggested by its name, liquid hybridization allows the detection of nucleic acid that is free in solution rather than attached to a solid-phase surface. Microtiter plates and strips can be used in this method, increasing ease of handling. ISH allows the detection of virus in various sources, including cells and tissues grown or fixed on slides, respectively. ISH-based detection of RV in a human bronchial biopsy is shown in Figure 24-2. The method is very sensitive in RNA virus detection, with a limit of 30 to 100 viral genome copies per cell, and it sometimes may be even superior to PCR (with which it can be used in combination to increase overall sensitivity).

Polymerase Chain Reaction

PCR methods allow specific amplification of defined DNA sequences to a level at which they subsequently can be detected and can be applied to any virus for which part of the genome sequence is known. The majority of respiratory viruses are RNA viruses; therefore, an additional step of reverse transcription (RT) is required before their PCR detection in clinical samples. First, total RNA is extracted by standard molecular biologic techniques from samples that have been kept at −70° C in an appropriate virus transport medium. Alternatively, some samples may be placed directly into a denaturing solution to inactivate ribonuclease enzyme activity, and then stored or transported at room temperature. Extracted RNA is then reverse transcribed into complementary DNA (cDNA; e.g., with heat-stable reverse transcriptase isolated from a retrovirus, such as murine MoMuLV) and further amplified by PCR using virus-specific oligonucleotides (primers)

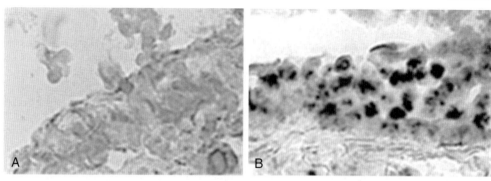

FIGURE 24-2. Detection of rhinovirus ribonucleic acid with *in situ* hybridization in a bronchial biopsy specimen obtained from a volunteer, **(A)** at baseline and **(B)** after experimental inoculation with rhinovirus. No signal could be observed in the baseline biopsy specimen, whereas an intense signal located at the bronchial epithelium *(black spots)* is present 3 days after nasal inoculation with the virus.

that have been designed with the aid of computer software. These primers are usually planned to amplify sequences that are 100 to 1000 base pairs long (amplicons) and can be designed so that they discriminate between different serotypes of the same virus. Nucleotide diversity that is frequently observed among different strains of a given virus species should also be taken into account, and areas of high homology should be selected for serotype-specific primer pairs design. Continuous cycles of denaturation, renaturation, and extension result in an exponential accumulation of the target DNA. The reaction is limited by the availability of substrate (nucleotides) and the possible competition between the target genome and other amplicons for the reaction's reagents. The amplicons then can be electrophoresed in a 1% to 2.5% agarose gel and visualized as DNA bands under an ultraviolet transilluminator following ethidium bromide or another DNA dye staining. This is readily accomplished within 1 working day, a fact that is of particular clinical importance.

To further improve the specificity and sensitivity of the test, the amplicons can be hybridized with labeled nucleic acid probes directed against regions of the amplicon. Alternatively, RT-PCR can be combined with EIA techniques that consist of hybridization of the amplicon with biotinylated RNA probes directed against the internal sequences of the amplicon. Time-resolved fluorometry has also been combined with PCR for the detection of picornaviruses. Moreover, in the "nested" PCR, PCR amplicons can be used as a source for a second round of PCR. In this approach, a second set of primers is designed against sequences that were localized internally in the sequences that were amplified in the first round. The method can be so sensitive as to detect a few particles of respiratory virus.[27] Nested-type PCR may not only increase sensitivity, but it also may discriminate between serotypes within viral species that are of similar size and thus are difficult to separate with gel from the first round of PCR. Discrimination within or between species can be also accomplished by digesting the amplicons with restriction endonucleases. Human RVs, for instance, can be discriminated from enteroviruses, which lack a BglI recognition site in their respective amplified sequence, based on the fact that their product remains undigested, retaining its original size after digestion with BglI restriction endonuclease[28] (Fig. 24-3).

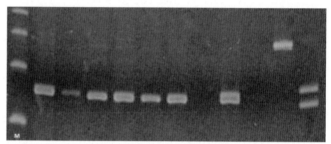

FIGURE 24-3. Detection of rhinovirus genetic material by reverse transcriptase polymerase chain reaction and its differentiation from enteroviruses. Picornavirus amplicons generated by the OL26-OL27 primer pair were digested with BglI. Rhinovirus *(lanes 1 to 6)* is detected as a single band with approximately 190 base pairs (bp) consisting of two almost identical bands. This easily allows differentiation from a poliovirus isolate *(lane 10)*, whose amplicon remains undigested (~380 bp) and from a coxsackie virus *(lane 11)*, which produces a duplet (~175 and 200 bp, respectively). *M,* DNA size marker.

In multiplex PCR, a mix of primer pairs is used, allowing simultaneous amplification and detection of several serotypes or viruses. Each primer pair demands different conditions for optimal target amplification, and therefore increased attention is needed upon development of this technique. For instance, Hexaplex (Prodesse, Waukesha, Wisconsin) allows prompt detection with high sensitivity and specificity of H1N1, H3N2, IFV A, IFV B, both RSV subtypes, and three of the four human PIVs in children.[29] The detection limits of multiplex RT-PCR protocols allow the identification of as few as 100 to 140 copies of viral particles/mL, or one $TCID_{50}$. This method can be at least as sensitive as combined tissue culture and IF methods. Combination with hybridization may further improve detection scores. In a combination of multiplex RT-PCR and enzyme hybridization assay, the amplicons of seven respiratory viruses (RSV A, RSV B, IFV A, IFV B, PIV 1, PIV 2, and PIV 3) were purified and hybridized with peroxidase-labeled probes into avidin-coated, 96-well microplates. The signal emitted after incubation of the complex with the substrate allowed the detection of almost twice as many positive clinical samples compared with conventional culture and IIF methods.[30] A multiplex PCR enzyme-linked immunosorbent assay that can detect seven respiratory viruses, in addition to the common respiratory pathogens *Mycoplasma pneumoniae* and *Chlamydia pneumoniae*, was less efficient in revealing

RSV and PIV 1, although it proved to be more sensitive than cell culture in detecting PIV 3, AdV, and IFV. Recent developments in this method include semi-quantitation of results with the use of specialized equipment and primers specific for additional viral and bacterial species (e.g., Reovirus, *Bordetella pertussis*), allowing for the detection of as many as 19 different microorganisms in a clinical sample.[31] Finally, multiplex PCR assays have been designed to discriminate between multiple subtypes within one species, as is the case with AdVs and picornaviruses.[32,33] In another approach, degenerate primers have been used to discriminate between AdV serotypes.[34]

Amplicons can also be subjected to sequence analysis to identify potential point mutations or deletions or specific serotypes. Cloning of PCR fragments that are generated with a series of partially overlapping or degenerate primers into bacterial plasmids allows sequencing of the entire viral genome, a laborious activity that is not necessary for usual clinical practice, but is indispensable when a previously unknown viral species is characterized (e.g. MPV) or when a high-risk epidemic from an initially unknown viral strain or mutation must be confronted efficiently and quickly (e.g. SARS). Heteroduplex formation between the amplicons may result in differential mobility of the product when run in a gel, and can be used for subtyping viral genomes. By combining, for instance, RT-PCR and heteroduplex formation, variant strains of IFV can be differentiated.[35]

In situ PCR allows the detection of viral genetic material and, furthermore, its localization at the cellular and tissue levels, providing information that is of particular importance for clinical pathology. Thus, paraffin-embedded fixed cells or tissue sections are treated with xylene and then digested with protease and DNAse solutions. The PCR mixture containing Taq polymerase is placed on top of it, and the entire slide is placed on an aluminum foil boat, transferred onto a conventional or modified PCR apparatus, and subjected to PCR amplification. If the one of the four deoxynucleoside 5'-triphosphates (dNTPs) that is present in the PCR mixture and is providing the nucleotide source is reduced and replaced by a modified nucleotide (e.g., biotinylated or digoxigenin-coupled deoxyuridine 5-triphosphate), then the emerging amplicons can be detected by incubation with an enzyme-labeled probe (e.g., ALP, anti-digoxigenin). Alternatively, in the absence of modified nucleotides, the amplified DNA can be detected by conventional ISH, conducted as described earlier in the chapter. Alternatively, the PCR mixture can be transferred to a test tube and run in an agarose gel or subjected to Southern analysis to identify the viral genomic fragments.

Real-Time Polymerase Chain Reaction

Recent advances in PCR technology allowed the development of real-time PCR, which is costly and requires appropriate instrumentation. On the other hand, real-time PCR can be more sensitive and time-efficient than conventional PCR, cell culture, and IF in detecting respiratory viruses in clinical samples.[36,37] Further, it is quantitative, allowing for assessment of the exact number of viral copies in a clinical sample. The final detection step employs either a fluorescent dye able to bind to double-stranded DNA (e.g., SYBR Green I) or a more specific hybridization probe (e.g., TaqMan, Molecular Beacons, Light Cycler probes) to monitor the presence and quantity of amplicons. For quantitative analysis as well as determination of the detection limits, serial dilutions of plasmid DNA containing a known amount of viral genome (virus genome equivalent) per microliter can be used as a standard reference solution.

In fluorescent dye SYBR Green protocols, the dye is incorporated into the amplicons in each cycle and assessment of fluorescing DNA is collected during each extension phase. However, such dyes bind to DNA, independent of the specific sequence, and thus can also detect undesired, nonspecifically amplified DNA. Thus, the specificity of the method is tested by the melting curves at which the final amplicon is briefly heated to denature (e.g., 95° C), allowed to re-associate at a lower temperature (e.g., 65° C, 15 sec), and finally re-denatured to 95° C by gradually increasing the temperature at a defined rate (e.g., 0.1° C/sec). The continuously measured fluorescence data recorded during this last stage are plotted against the temperature and allow calculation of the melting peak that characterizes a given amplicon under the conditions used. When the melting peak of a particular product coincides with the standard, it is considered specific. Highly sensitive one- and two-step, real-time PCR assays for the qualitative and quantitative detection of most respiratory viruses have been reported.[38,39]

In hybridization-based protocols, a specific probe sharing consensus homology with the sequenced strains of a viral species is labeled with a reporter fluorogenic dye (e.g., 6-carboxyfluoroscein) at the 5' end and a quencher dye (e.g., carboxytetramethylrhodamine) at the 3' end. The probe is present in the conventional PCR master mix (containing buffer, Mg^{+2} salts, dNTPs, water, and the primers) during PCR, and the real-time apparatus records the fluorescence emerging during time. The reporter dye fluorescence (e.g., 6-carboxyfluoroscein) is considered positive and, compared with the fluorescence emitted by a reference dye, present in the PCR master mix to normalize for non-PCR–related fluorescence fluctuations among samples. A threshold is usually set, above which a signal is considered positive.

Recent approaches to the detection of respiratory viruses include the development of multiplex real-time PCR protocols. A SYBR Green–based reaction, for instance, allowed simultaneous detection of IFV A, IFV B, and RSV, with specificity comparable to that achieved with commercially available rapid antigenic tests and considerably higher sensitivity scores.[40] Discrimination between the particular species was based on the specific melting temperature curves elicited by the amplicons. Limitations in the number of viruses and viral serotypes are inherent in the real-time approach, especially in the protocols using a labeled probe, because most platforms do not allow the simultaneous use of more than two fluorochromes. Using a more advanced apparatus that can detect up to four fluorochromes, Templeton and colleagues[41] succeeded in detecting both IFV serotypes, RSV, and all four PIV subtypes in a two-tube reaction. In their approach, the specific probes were labeled with different fluorochromes (i.e., 6-carboxyfluoroscein, Texas red, hexachlorofluoroscein, and cyanin 5); the overall reaction could be accomplished within 6 hours and proved to be more sensitive than cell culture, with detection limits ranging from 0.1 to 0.0001 $TCID_{50}$ of viral stocks of known titer, depending on the virus. Molecular methods allowing for simultaneous detection of 7 to 26 different viruses at the same time have been attempted.[21]

Other Methods

Advances in molecular biology continuously offer additional PCR- and hybridization-based methods. In a study, as few as 100 RNA copies of PIV (or one $TCID_{50}$) could be detected by probe hybridization and electrochemiluminescence or by using molecular beacons.[42] The first step in this approach, nucleic acid sequence–based amplification, was used. This technique employs avian myeloblastosis virus reverse transcriptase, together with ribonuclease H and T7 RNA polymerase, under isothermal conditions, and is able to directly amplify RNA. The use of nucleic acid sequences to amplify RNA with primers directed against the 5′ noncoding region of RV serotypes allows discrimination between RV subgroups.[43]

Complementary DNA-amplified restriction fragment length polymorphism (RFLP) allows the identification of previously unknown viral sequences. In this method, double-stranded cDNA is synthesized from viral RNA and digested with frequently cutting restriction endonucleases. Double-stranded adaptors are then ligated to the ends of the emerging restriction fragments and provide primer sites during PCR amplification. A second selective fragment amplification step is conducted by adding one or more bases to the PCR primers. If the complementary bases are present in the viral sequence, then successful amplification will occur. A modification of this method was successfully employed in the discovery of the NL63 HCV.[10]

Wang and colleagues used the powerful microarray technology to detect approximately 140 distinct viral genomes simultaneously, including most respiratory viruses.[44] To that end, 1600 oligonucleotides with a relatively greater length than those commonly used in array technology (70 versus 20 to 25 bases) were selected after a genome-wide BLAST analysis (Basic Local Alignment Search Tool, a method for rapid searching of nucleotide and protein databases) and ranked according to shared homology to regions of the viral genomes. Using an inkjet oligonucleotide synthesizer, these oligonucleotides are synthesized *in situ* and placed onto directed locations of a glass wafer.[45] The glass surfaces can then be hybridized, under strict conditions, with cDNA, PCR amplicons, RNA, or another form of genetic material derived from viral stocks, virally infected cells in cultures, or clinical samples. Human and cellular transcripts are also included to normalize against nonspecific hybridization. This material is labeled with cyanin 5 or cyanin 3, which provides red or green coloring, respectively, to allow color visualization of microarray data that are obtained after the arrays are scanned with confocal laser scanners and analyzed with suitable instrumentation and software. This method allows the detection of paramyxoviruses, orthomyxoviruses, AdVs, and picornaviruses from clinical samples. It can also detect and discriminate among all 102 RV serotypes, based on the

hybridization pattern obtained from each serotype. After human volunteers were experimentally infected with RV, the array could detect as few as 100 infectious RV particles in NPA samples.[44] Analysis of a small number of samples from naturally acquired colds showed different RV serotypes and PIV 1, which also has been confirmed by conventional RT-PCR. Although it is extremely promising, this technique needs further evaluation, including cost-effectiveness, before being applied in clinical practice.

Practical Considerations in the Use of Nucleic Acid–Based Techniques

The identification of a particular virus can be further, and without doubt, confirmed by restriction analysis or sequencing of the product and subsequent comparison with published genome databases. In addition, PCR-based methods have proved to be very sensitive, usually exceeding the sensitivity scores of cell culture techniques. However, false-positive or false-negative findings can be a problem, if certain practical measures in the handling of viral genetic material are not meticulously followed. First, preservation of the sample is of particular importance for the integrity of the viral genomic material. RNA, the genomic material of most respiratory viruses, is particularly vulnerable to degradation by RNAses that are present in all biologic samples and fluids. RNAse-free vials, solutions, and buffers should be used by specialized personnel in designated areas of the laboratory. In addition, if it takes too long for an NPA sample to be transported from the clinic to the laboratory, or if the sample remains on ice for too many hours instead of being placed in the freezer immediately, the sensitivity of the method can be unexpectedly low. Further, biologic fluids often contain substances that can inhibit PCR amplification (e.g., mucus). In this case, dilution of the sample or treatment with a suitable agent such as dimethyl sulfoxide may facilitate detection of the virus. The use of clinical samples spiked with stock virus or the inclusion of synthetic heterologous competitor RNA in the reaction may facilitate normalization of PCR outcomes.

On the other hand, PCR-based techniques are also subject to problems with contamination, especially if large numbers of samples are handled simultaneously. In the case of a nested PCR protocol, the first and second rounds of PCR should be conducted in separate areas, with separate sets of pipettes, and of course, with different plasticware, and several negative controls should be included for monitoring of contamination. If contamination occurs, replacement of the pipettes is required, as well as a review of laboratory and handling practices.

Techniques to Diagnose Respiratory Viruses in Clinical Practice

Threatening influenza pandemics and mortal epidemics of previously unknown respiratory viruses (e.g., SARS-CoV) require the use of rapid and reliable detection methods in clinical practice. Moreover, large epidemiologic studies are required to better define the involvement of these viruses in noninfectious diseases (e.g., asthma). These studies will help in drug development and the implementation of intervention strategies, even during an outbreak. Drugs are being developed that specifically block infection by individual viruses (e.g., anti-influenza neuraminidase inhibitors), but they are useless if the patient has been infected by another virus.

It is not possible to determine the optimal method for virus detection because many factors vary, depending on the particular conditions and the scope of the analysis (cost-effectiveness, time required, sensitivity, availability of skilled personnel, and laboratory equipment). A combination of methods, rather than a single one, is best used in particular cases because most protocols are not ideal or do not provide enough information. EM is still recognized as an indispensable method.[46] Although cell culture remains the gold standard, it is time-consuming and is being replaced by antigen-detection methods and molecular biological techniques. Their commercial availability, ease of performance, and rapidity have made antigen-based methods increasingly popular, especially in small units that lack advanced facilities. They can be accomplished within 15 minutes to a few hours. However, they can be inferior to cell culture in terms of sensitivity and are of limited value for the detection of some respiratory viruses. On the other hand, PCR has been widely used as a research tool during the last decade, and its clinical use is steadily increasing. PCR cannot, however, replace the use of cell culture in worldwide influenza surveillance, an aspect of classic virology that is vital for informing vaccine manufacture.[47]

Developing Techniques and Future Directions

Rapidity, high sensitivity and specificity, ease of use, and cost-effectiveness are the major requirements imposed on the respiratory viral detection field. In particular, the need for rapid diagnostics is likely to increase as more specific antiviral therapies enter the market. Although PCR-based analysis was the major breakthrough in recent years, none of the existing methods can be considered ideal, and usually a combination of techniques is used for more accurate results, increasing the costs, time, and skills required for analysis. Thus, combination of hybridization with electroluminescence or the use of molecular bonds is capable of detecting just a few PIV particles.[42] Other techniques, such as real-time loop-mediated amplification (LAMP),[48] nucleic acid sequence-based amplification (NASBA),[49] and asymmetrical multiplex PCR in combination with microarray hybridization[50] have shown similar sensitivity with conventional real-time PCR with regard to respiratory virus diagnosis. Additionally, the use of restrictive enzymes on a double cDNA helix that has been transcribed from viral RNA (cDNA-amplified RFLP), as well as 3' degenerate primers in a randomized PCR allow the amplification of genetic material of any virus in a clinical sample from patients with respiratory illness of unknown etiology.

Simultaneous and reliable detection of as many viruses as possible, in the shortest time possible, and ideally in a single test, is the goal of any novel and future technique. Although it is specific, sensitive, and reliable, multiplex real-time PCR can still detect a restricted number of viruses simultaneously. Nowadays, microarray technology is one of the most sensitive and high-throughput choices for concurrent diagnosis of many different viral strains (>100) or specific virus serotypes.[51] This technique

also can be combined with assays revealing expression patterns of target genes in the host, thus providing an overall picture, not only of viral presence, but also of host response.

Another combination that has also been used for detection of the SARS genome[52] is the use of molecular bonds connected to microspheres, which can detect multiple nucleic acids in solution, followed by conventional flow cytometry. Finally, some techniques such as surface plasmon resonance, quartz crystal microbalance and chromatometric functional polymers that do not use labeling may be used for direct detection of respiratory viruses.[53]

LABORATORY DIAGNOSIS OF RESPIRATORY BACTERIAL INFECTIONS

Bacteria rarely exist in mono-cultures, and species-species interactions can deeply affect the behavior of individual species. Moreover, bacterial load, virulence and pathogenicity, and the host's ability to mount an effective immune response all influence transition from mere contamination to colonization and infection.

Specimens for bacteriologic culture should be collected as soon as possible after the onset of disease and before the initiation of antimicrobial therapy. Optimal transport times depend on the volume of the sample, with small volumes of fluid (<1 mL) or tissue (<1 cm³) having to be submitted within 15 to 30 minutes to avoid evaporation, drying, and exposure to ambient conditions. Larger volumes in holding medium can be stored up to 24 hours; specimens should not be stored for longer than 24 hours under any circumstance. Some bacteria are particularly sensitive and should therefore be held at room temperature and immediately processed. Such bacteria include *N. gonorrhoeae, N. meningitidis, H. influenzae, S. pneumoniae,* and anaerobes. Delays of up to 6 hours result in minimal loss of colony-forming units (CFU) when transport media are used, but longer delays (even with the use of transport medium) result in significant losses of organisms. For delays beyond 6 hours, refrigeration improves recovery, except for the aforementioned organisms.

Upper Respiratory Tract Infections

Upper Respiratory Tract Specimens

Fresh pus, fluid, or tissue from the nose or nasopharynx (swab, wash, or aspirate), the sinuses (wash, aspirate, biopsy, scraping, or debridement), the gums and oral cavity (swab), as well as a pharyngeal swab from the tonsils and/or the posterior pharynx are the main URT biological specimens. Tympanocentesis is usually reserved for complicated, recurrent or chronic persistent otitis media. When the eardrum is intact, an aspiration is performed after cleaning the ear canal with soap solution, while a flexible shaft swab via an auditory speculum is used for collection of fluid (for aerobic culture only) when the eardrum is ruptured. Oral specimens should be collected with vigorous swabbing of the lesion, avoiding any areas of normal tissue following removal of oral secretions and debris from the surface of the lesion. Throat swabbing should be vigorous (with sampling of the posterior pharynx, tonsils, and inflamed areas while avoiding contact with the tongue and oral cavity) and should be transferred promptly to the lab in modified Stuart's or Amies medium with or without active carbon. For the diagnosis of group A streptococcal pharyngitis, which involves the performance of a rapid antigen detection assay and culture, two pharyngeal swabs should be collected (one swab/assay). Throat swab cultures in patients with epiglottitis should be collected by a physician only in a setting where emergency intubation can be immediately performed to secure a patent airway. Swabs for *N. gonorrhoeae* should be placed in charcoal-containing transport medium and plated immediately after collection. Nasal swabs for identification of *S. aureus* carriers should be premoistened with sterile saline, inserted 1 to 2 cm into the nares, rotated against the mucosa and transported in Stuart's or Amies medium. Nasopharyngeal aspirates (NPA), typically 0.5 mL, are collected over a 10-second procedure that involves introduction of a thin elastic catheter through the nasal cavity to a 5- to 7-cm depth or proportional to the distance between the nose and the ear. If the material does not pass into the container, the catheter may be washed off with saline or cut in order to obtain the specimen. The collection of nasopharyngeal wash is performed with installation of 1 to 2 mL of saline inside the nasal cavity of patients who have tilted their head backward (approximately 70%). Patients then lean forward, and the wash is collected in a sterile container or Petri dish. Nasopharyngeal swabs are collected with the help of flexible sterile swabs, which are passed through the nostrils until resistance is felt, and they are slowly rotated for 5 seconds to allow for mucus absorption. If possible, direct medium inoculation should be performed at bedside.

The material of the swab is important for the survival of certain microorganisms; cultures for *B. pertussis* are obtained by aspiration through a suction catheter or a Dacron or flexible wire calcium alginate swab of the nasopharynx. Samples intended for PCR for *B. pertussis* should not be collected with calcium alginate swabs, which is an inhibitor for the reaction, but with Dacron or rayon swabs. Cotton swabs contain fatty acids, which may be toxic for *B. pertussis*. For delays up to 24 hours, Amies medium with charcoal can be used, but Regan-Lowe medium is preferred for transportation times longer than 24 hours. Dacron swabs are also advocated for isolation of *C. pneumoniae*. Swabs without a buffer-type non-nutritive blood/charcoal transport medium (Stuart's or Amies) should not be used when transport is delayed more than a few hours because the specimen dries out and a lower microbial viability has been observed. This is of particular significance when clinically significant bacteria are present in low numbers or fastidious organisms such as anaerobes are involved.

Microscopic Examination

Microscopy following Gram staining is useful for the examination of paranasal sinus material, (normally sterile), pharyngeal smear, or material from the oral cavity for the detection of polymorphonuclear neutrophils (PMNs)

and some microbes (e.g., corynebacteria [diphtheria], spirochetes [Vincent angina] or *Candida* spp.) and nasopharyngeal smear for *C. diphtheriae* and *B. pertussis*.

Gram staining is not useful for the diagnosis of streptococcal pharyngotonsillitis or the detection of *N. meningitides* carriage because these cannot be discriminated over the nonpathogenic normal flora of the URT. Occasionally, other stains also may be used such as Loeffler's Methylene blue for *C. diphtheriae* (appear as pleomorphic, beaded rods with swollen/club-shaped ends and reddish purple metachromatic granules) and DIF for *Bordetella*.

Culture

Normally, the initial part of the nasopharynx is colonized mainly by *Staphylococcus* spp.; the middle part is colonized by nonpathogenic aerobic and anaerobic microorganisms as well as potentially pathogenic bacteria such as *S. pneumoniae, H. influenzae,* and *M. catarrhalis;* and the posterior part is colonized by flora similar to that of the oropharynx, in which α- and β-hemolytic *Streptococci* and anaerobes dominate. Bacterial pathogens implicated in URTI are: β-hemolytic group A *Streptococcus, S. pneumoniae, S. aureus, H. influenzae, M. catarrhalis, N. meningitidis, B. pertussis, C. diphtheriae, Klebsiella* spp. and other *Enterobacteriacae, Bacteroides* spp., *Fusobacterium* spp., *Borrelia* spp., *Arcanobacterium haemolyticum,* and other anaerobes.

To isolate distinct colonies, samples are inoculated on small areas of agar plates and then linearly on three consecutive areas using sterile loops. Pharyngeal smears are routinely cultured for *Streptococcus* group A on 5% sheep blood agar (SBA) or group A *Streptococcus* selective blood agar at 35° C for 48 hours in an environment of reduced oxygen achieved by anaerobic incubation or in air with multiple "stabs" through the agar surface. Low oxygen concentration allows the recovery of group C and G streptococci. The selective agar is easier to visualize because it inhibits accompanying flora but delays the appearance of colonies. Plates are checked for β-hemolytic colonies, and verification of the presence of *Streptococcus* group A versus group C and G is done based on the fact that the former microorganisms are catalase-negative and pyrolidonyl aminopeptidase–positive as well as with the help of bacitracin disks in the initial agar and antigen detection. A number of other pathogens may cause pharyngotonsillitis or may colonize the URT without causing disease, and their isolation may be important in patients with CF; organ transplantation; or ear, nose, and throat (ENT) disorders. Such bacteria include *C. diphteriae* (Loeffler's serum medium or potassium tellurite blood agar incubated at 5% CO_2, 48 hours, 35° C), *Arcanobacterium haemolyticum* (same culture media as for *S. pyogenes* but up to 72 hours incubation), *N. gonorrhoeae* (prompt inoculation on modified Thayer-Martin agar and incubation at 5% CO_2, 35° C, 72 hours), epiglottitis pathogens, which are mainly *H. influenzae* B and less frequently *S. pneumoniae,* and *S. pyogenes* (chocolate blood agar [CBA] with incubation at 5% CO_2, 35° C, 72 hours).

Nasopharyngeal specimens are useful for the diagnosis of infection by pertussis, diphtheria, and *Chlamydia* spp.; detection of the *N. meningitides, S. aureus,* and *S. pyogenes* carriage; and epidemiologic surveillance of *S. pneumoniae* antibiotic susceptibility among children. Such samples are usually inoculated on SBA (aerobically at 37° C, 48 hours) or CBA (5% CO_2, 37° C). Samples suspected for *B. pertussis* and *B. parapertussis* should be inoculated on Regan-Lowe charcoal agar with 10% horse blood and cephalexin and incubated aerobically under moist conditions (35° C, 5 to 7 days). Optimal recovery requires the use of the aforementioned medium with and without cephalexin because some strains do not grow in the presence of cephalexin. possible *N. meningitides* containing specimens should be transferred in Stuart's or Amies medium or directly inoculated on SBA, CBA, or, if interference with normal flora is expected, modified Thayer-Martin or other selective medium for incubation under 5% CO_2 at 35° C for 72 hours in a humidified atmosphere. For culturing *C. pneumoniae,* a nasopharyngeal swab is transferred in antibiotic-containing medium to permissive cell culture systems.

Selective media such as Canada colistin-nalidixic acid (CNA), or a selective and differential medium such as BBL CHROMagar *S. aureus* (BD Diagnostics, Sparks, MD), BBL CHROMagar MRSA (BD Diagnostics, Sparks, MD) or mannitol salt agar is helpful in differentiating *S. aureus* or MRSA (methicillin-resistant *S. aureus*) from other flora and is useful when interpreting large numbers of specimens.[54] Specimens from the inner ear may be inoculated on SBA and CBA and under anaerobic conditions on Brucella blood agar (BBA). Specimens from the paranasal sinuses, gums, or the oral mucosa can be inoculated on other media as well, depending on the occasion (e.g., MacConkey's for Gram negatives, Fildies for *H. influenzae,* media for anaerobes, *Capnocytophaga* spp.).

Following the isolation of the pathogen, serologic typing (e.g., *Streptococcus* group A, *H. influenzae* group B, *N. meningitidis* groups A, B, C) as well as antibiotic susceptibility testing are usually performed.

Lower Respiratory Tract Infections (LRTI)

Lower respiratory tract infections (LRTIs) are the third most important cause of mortality globally and are responsible for more than 4 million deaths annually.[55]

Blood Specimens and Culture

There are >100 pathogens that may infect the lower respiratory tract (LRT) and produce secondary bacteremia. Additionally, invasive techniques cannot be routinely used, and sputum samples cannot be easily obtained from young children. The detection of living microorganisms in the blood of an ill child is of great diagnostic and prognostic significance, and blood culture should be considered when there is fever (≥38° C), hypothermia (≤36° C), leukocytosis, or fever and neutropenia (<1000 PMN/mL). Semi-automated blood culture systems are present in nearly every clinical laboratory. Two or three separate blood cultures per 24 hours (ideally before initiation of treatment) should be collected under aseptic

conditions and directly into culture bottles from every child hospitalized with pneumonia. Avoidance of transport tubes allows bacteria to begin growing immediately, decreases the amount of anticoagulant to which bacteria are exposed (anticoagulant may be inhibitory for some bacteria), and decreases the risk of needlestick accidents among health care personnel. Skin should always be disinfected with povidone iodine (must be allowed to completely dry), 70% isopropyl alcohol, or iodine prior to venipuncture to minimize contamination with skin microorganisms. Obtaining blood for culture from intravascular catheters in the absence of peripheral blood culture should be discouraged because of the frequent isolation of coagulase-negative *Staphylococci* and other skin flora. However, if there is no other option, the line must be adequately disinfected and flushed of all inhibitory substances before the specimen is obtained. The amount of fluid flushed from the line is based on the weight and size of the child.[56] For infants, minimal discard volumes are in the range of 0.3 to 1.0 mL.[57] Media-containing resins are often used to adsorb antibiotics or inhibitory substances that may be present in a patient's blood and thus improve microbial detection. In infants and young children, 1 to 5 mL/culture and in older children 10 mL/culture provide optimal recovery for the diagnosis of sepsis.[58] In general, the total blood volume withdrawn for two bacterial cultures should not exceed 1% of the patient's total blood volume. Larger volumes of blood are necessary to maximize yield since 10% to 20% of pediatric patients may have low-grade bloodstream infections. Blood culture bottles that contain approximately 20 mL of broth and that accommodate an inoculation volume of up to 4 mL are available, thus allowing for a close approximation of the recommended blood-to-broth ratio necessary to diminish the effect of growth inhibitors. For the majority of patients, culture of the entire volume in a single (or additional) aerobic bottle is the most effective approach because anaerobic infections are rare among children. Patients at increased risk for anaerobic sepsis include immunocompromised children and those with infections located at areas outside the respiratory tract. Blood and tissue specimens for the diagnosis of Q fever *(C. burnetii)* should be frozen at −70° C until shipped, while clinical samples suspected of *Francisella tularensis* infection should be rapidly transported to the laboratory or frozen and shipped on dry ice. Prolonged incubation beyond 5 days is not necessary for automated instruments, although blind subculture may be needed if the patient is receiving antimicrobials at the time of blood collection.[59,60]

Positive blood culture bottles are initially evaluated by Gram staining of a smear, and subculturing on suitable media should commence, depending on the organism seen. Blood cultures are polymicrobial in 5% to 10% of cases. Therefore additional inoculation on a CNA or other medium inhibitory for Gram-negative organisms is recommended for smears indicative of Gram-negative bacilli, and on MacConkey's or related selective agar for smears showing Gram-positive organisms. Inoculation on media for anaerobes is advocated when the smear is suggestive of such microbes or when the organism is recovered from the anaerobic culture bottle only.

Blood isolates should be evaluated in relation to the clinical findings of a patient. Growth of common pathogens such as *S. pneumoniae*, *H. influenzae*, *S. aureus*, β-haemolytic *Streptococcus* group A or B, and *K. pneumoniae* demonstrates the etiologic microorganism. In specific groups of children, such as immunocompromised or hospitalized patients in intensive care units (ICUs), other uncommon pathogens may develop such as *Candida* spp., *Cryptococcus neoformans*, and others. Some bacteria (e.g., *Legionella* spp., mycobacteria, some *N. meningitidis* strains, and *N. gonorrhoeae*) cannot grow on routine media, and detection takes place by other methods such as lysis centrifugation. Growth of *Staphylococcus epidermidis* (coagulase-negative), corynebacteria, *Bacillus* spp. and propionibacteria is usually associated with contamination of the sample. In general, single cultures that are positive for any of these bacteria represent contamination, whereas multiple separate positive cultures are more likely to indicate a clinically significant bacteremia, which may result in sepsis, septic shock, or severe sepsis.

Blood cultures are positive in only <10% of pediatric RTIs due to either the characteristics of the pathogen, the fact that a microbe may not be causing bacteremia or it may be causing limited or intermittent bacteremia, insufficient sample collection, autolysis of a microbe during culture, prior antibiotic intake, or other factors.

Urine Specimens

Urinary samples may be used for the detection of antigens from pneumococcus, *H. influenzae*, and *Legionella*.

Lower Respiratory Tract Specimens

Candidate samples for processing include the non-invasive sputum and tracheobronchial aspirates (TBA through catheter), as well as the invasive transtracheal (percutaneous) aspirates, bronchial wash, bronchoalveolar lavage (BAL), protected bronchial brush (PBB), pulmonary aspirate, pulmonary tissue specimens (collected either via fine-needle transthoracic aspiration or open or thoracoscopic biopsies), and pleural fluid (via thoracocentesis). See Table 24-6 for sensitivity and specificity of these methods. Among these, percutaneous pulmonary and transtracheal aspirates and PBB specimens are the only samples, acceptable for culturing under anaerobic conditions. BAL is collected after washing of the lower airways with normal saline, which is aspirated at low pressure (<100 Torr) in order to avoid collapse and damage of the bronchial wall (a hemorrhagic specimen has a lower diagnostic value). For children <20 kg, the volume of the administered normal saline is 3 mL/kg divided into 3 equal parts, and the collected specimen is considered adequate when >40% of the instilled volume is returned back (the patient's age is usually inversely proportional to the percentage of aspirated fluid).[61] Indications for BAL include hospital-acquired pneumonia (ventilator-associated pneumonia [VAP], aspiration pneumonia); complicated community acquired pneumonia (CAP); CF; severe viral respiratory tract infections; mycobacterial, fungal, and parasitic infections; as well as pneumonia among immunosuppressed individuals. The PBB technique is applied since 1979 for collection of specimens mainly in the

TABLE 24-6 COMPARISON OF SPECIMEN COLLECTION TECHNIQUES INTENDED FOR CULTURE FROM THE LOWER RESPIRATORY TRACT

NON-BRONCHOSCOPIC TECHNIQUES	SENSITIVITY (%)	SPECIFICITY (%)
Collection of endotracheal secretions	38-100	14-100
Blind specimen collection (BBS)	74-97	74-100
Mini-BAL	63-100	66-96
Blind specimen collection with protected bronchial brush (BPBB)	58-86	71-100
Bronchoscopic Techniques		
Bronchoalveolar lavage (BAL)	42-93, 73*	45-100, 82*
Protected bronchial brush (PBB)	33-100, 67*	50-100, 95*

*Median value.
Modified from Baselski VS, Wunderink RG. Bronchoscopic diagnosis of pneumonia. *Clin Microbiol Rev.* 1994;7:533-558.

context of complicated bacterial CAP with introduction of a double telescopic catheter via a bronchoscope. On the other hand, saliva, oropharyngeal secretions, sinus drainage from the nasopharynx, swab samples, and 24-hour sputum collections are considered unsuitable for identification of organisms from the LRT.

At least 1 mL of any aforementioned LRT secretion should be transported in a sterile container, while tissue should be placed in an anaerobic transport system or a sterile screw-cap container with several drops of sterile saline to keep small pieces of tissue moist. Lavage specimens are collected in the trap, which is adjusted to the bronchoscope, while the PBB specimen is the brush itself that is cut and placed in a sterile container with 1 mL of sterile normal saline or Brain-Heart Infusion broth. A sucrose-phosphate-glutamate transport medium containing BSA is often used to transport *Rickettsiae*, *Mycoplasmas*, and *Chlamydiae*.[62] Occasionally, quantitative cultures of BAL or PBB specimens may help in distinguishing upper-tract contamination from lower-tract disease. If >10 mL of BAL is collected, the sample should be centrifuged prior to plating.

With the exception of CF patients, obtaining adequate sputum specimens in children may prove problematic, and the help of a physiotherapist is highly advisable. The latter aid in provocation of induced cough (e.g., with slight pressure over the cricothyreoid cartilage), mobilization of secretions (e.g., with vibration and percussion manipulations, huffing games), and bronchial drainage.[63] Preferably the first morning sputum before breakfast or alternatively sputum induced by the inhalation of aerosolized 0.9% to 7% sterile saline should be expectorated in a sterile container following appropriate oral hygiene with sterile water or normal saline and a toothbrush (without toothpaste for 5 to 10 minutes) to remove the normal oral flora. Tap water should be avoided because it may contain atypical mycobacteria or *Legionella* spp. and may obscure culture results. Occasionally, a Dacron or rayon swab is placed at the posterior pharynx of CF patients younger than 10 years of age for the induction of cough and collection of an LRT specimen (gagged or cough specimen), which is shown to have a high positive predictive value.[64] Alternatively, one can ask the patient to cough twice over a plate (or more than one plate possibly with different nutritive media), which is a more sensitive method compared to cough specimens.[65] In general, LRT specimens should be transferred to the laboratory within 2 hours at room temperature or stored for up to 24 hours at 2° to 8° C, with the exception of induced sputum that should be constantly kept at room temperature (up to 24 hours) since its collection. Sputum of CF patients may be preserved at 4° C for 24 hours without affecting the isolation of pathogens, which are of interest in this disorder.

Macroscopic and Microscopic Examination of an LRT Specimen

The appearance, color, consistency (e.g., purulent, mucoid, serous, bloody), quantity, smell, and presence of visible formations (e.g., Curschmann's spirals, *Actinomyces* granules) in LRT specimens should all be considered. The sample should be first vortexed and, if applicable, inoculated for a qualitative culture and then processed with equal volume of 0.5% to 2% N-acetyl-L-cysteine (Mucomyst) or DTT (Sputasol) solution if mucoid. Cell counts are determined with flow cytometry, and cytocentrifugation (600 to 800 rpm, 20 minutes) follows. Gram (or other) staining of the sediment and microscopic examination is necessary for evaluating the suitability of a sample. A number of >10 squamous epithelial cells (SECs)/100× objective microscopic field shows that the sputum sample contains saliva and is unsuitable. For endotracheal aspirates, specimens are acceptable when there are <10 SECs/average 100× field and bacteria detected in at least 1 of 20 such fields. In BAL, alveolar macrophages prevail (>90%), while the presence of >1% SECs indicates contamination with URT flora and renders the sample unacceptable. Unsuitable samples should be discarded, and the treating physician should be informed, except from the case of immunosuppressed patients, where samples are kept. Also, LRT specimens for the detection of *M. pneumoniae*, *Legionella* spp., dimorphic fungi, and *M. tuberculosis* should not be screened for adequacy and should be processed directly.

Specimens are also examined for inflammatory cells and the presence and characteristics of microbes such as how they Gram stain (positive versus negative); their shape (e.g., cocci versus diplococci, hyphae, blast cells), layout, and number; their intracellular or extracellular position; the prevalence of a single microbe population, and so on. Direct examination of the specimen with Gram staining along with compatible symptomatology is sensitive in only 10% of cases but has a specificity of 70% to 80%, which often allows for timely diagnosis and treatment of an LRTI since it is an easy, cheap, and fast method that provides information within 1 hour. Gram staining following processing with sterile normal saline in order to remove URT flora (washed sputum) demonstrates a sensitivity of 86%, 81%, and 91% and a specificity of 95%, 97%, and 98% for *H. influenzae*, *S. pneumoniae*, and *M. catarrhalis*, respectively.[66] Bacteria in Gram-stained smears should be reported if they are potential pathogens and should be reported as normal respiratory flora if they are insufficient in quantity or not representative of potential pathogens. Stained smears of patients with aspiration pneumonia are characterized by many PMNs and mixed intracellular respiratory flora, (commonly *Streptococci* and anaerobes) and should be discriminated from contaminating respiratory flora. The presence of intracellular microbes in alveolar macrophages of BAL has high sensitivity and specificity for the diagnosis of VAP. Depending on the suspected pathogen, other stains are modified (Kinyoun) acid fast stain *(Nocardia)*, Ziehl-Neelsen (mycobacteria), Giemsa, Gomori's Methenamine silver, Toluidine blue, and Calcofluor white (fungi and *Pneumocystis*). The absence of findings despite related clinical suspicion increases the probability of an atypical pneumonia due to mycoplasmas, mycobacteria, *Legionella* spp., parasites, and so on. Moreover, an endotracheal tube may add inflammatory cells to a tracheal aspirate, even in the absence of infection.

Culture of Lower Respiratory Tract Specimen

LRT bacterial pathogens include *S. pneumoniae*, *H. influenzae*, *M. catarrhalis*, *K. pneumoniae*, Enterobacteriacae, *P. aeruginosa*, *S. aureus*, *Legionella* spp., *Mycobacterium* spp., *Fusobacterium nucleatum*, *Chlamydia* spp., *M. pneumoniae*, *S. pyogenes*, *P. multocida*, *Bordetella* spp., *Pseudomonas* spp., *Nocardia* spp., *Prevotella melaninogenicus*, and various oropharyngeal flora anaerobes. *S. aureus* is found in the BAL fluid in 30% of CF children with an average age of 3 months.[67] The small-colony variant (SCV) phenotype of *S. aureus* is also common among these patients,[68] and the prevalence of MRSA is steadily increasing.[69] Non-encapsulate and non–type B capsulate *H. influenzae* are more common in children with CF than in older patients. *P. aeruginosa* is the most common pathogen cultured from CF sputum and may be seen early in infancy and often cultured intermittently thereafter. Eventually chronic infection develops, and this leads to a faster decline in lung function. Other bacteria, such as *Burkholderia cepacia complex*, *Burkholderia pseudomallei*, *Stenotrophomonas maltophila*, *Achromobacter xylosoxidans*, *Pandoraea apista*, and non-tuberculous mycobacteria are also commonly isolated from this patient population.

Positive cultures from blood or pleural fluid are obtained in only about 10% of pneumonias, while sputum cultures offer clinically useful information in 10% to 15% of cases only. Approximately 30% of patients with purulent sputum do not have clinically evident pneumonia, and only 60% of patients with pneumonia produce purulent sputum. Moreover, 10% of patients with nonpurulent sputum suffer from pneumonia and 40% to 50% of the samples are unsuitable for culture, even from patients with indicative symptomatology.

Qualitative (or Semiquantitative) Culture

Common Microbes: Sputum samples are initially centrifuged (1500 to 1800 × g, 15 to 20 minutes) and subsequently

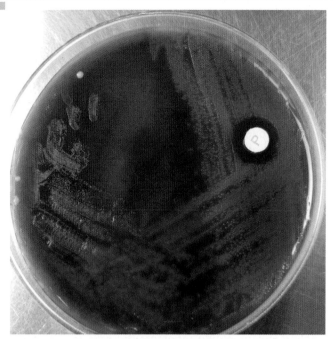

FIGURE 24-4. Culture of *Streptococcus pneumoniae* on blood Agar with an inhibition zone around the optochin disk *(P)*.

inoculated on SBA (35°C, 5% CO$_2$, 48 to 72 hours), CBA with 20,000 IU/L or 10 IU disk of bacitracin (35° C, 5% to 10% CO$_2$, 24 to 48 hours), and MacConkey's agar (35° C, aerobically, 24 to 48 hours) (Fig. 24-4). As with URT specimens, inoculation should be performed on a small part of the agar plate (~¼), and a sterile loop should be used to dilute the sample satisfactorily and obtain isolated colonies.

The same procedure is applied for bronchoalveolar brushings and washings, TBA, and BAL with additional inoculation on anaerobic CNA for the two latter. In the case of BAL fluid, it can also be cultured under anaerobic conditions on BBA, laked blood with kanamycin and vancomycin (LKV), and CNA. Table 24-7 features criteria for interpretation of LRT specimen cultures.

Uncommon Microbes: Special transport and culture media are used for some microbes such as *Hemophilus* spp. (Fildies medium at 35° C, 10% CO$_2$, 24 to 48 hours), *Legionella* spp. (buffered charcoal yeast extract with and without antimicrobial agents such as vancomycin, polymyxin B, and anisomycin; aerobically at 35° C, humidity, 5 to 10 days), *Chlamydia* spp. (prompt transport in antibiotic, e.g., gentamycin and nystatin containing media for 24 to 48 hours at 4° C, or for longer periods at –70° C, and inoculation in shell vials using McCoy cells for *C. trachomatis* and *C. psittaci*, and Hep-2 cells for *C. pneumoniae*), Burkholderia (Pseudomonas) cepacia in CF patients (*P. cepacia* selective agar and oxidative-fermentative-polymyxin B-bacitracin-lactose [OFPBL] agar), Mycoplasma pneumoniae (albumin and penicillin containing transport medium for up to 24 to 48 hours at 4° C, or for longer periods at –70° C and inoculation on Mycoplasma-Glucose agar, Methylene Blue-Glucose biphasic agar, or SP-4 agar for up to 3 weeks), SCV *S. aureus* (Mannitol Salt Agar) and *Nocardia* spp. (incubation up to 3 weeks at 35° C using the selective BCYE agar, while samples without significant cross-contamination may be inoculated on SBA, CBA, and Sabouraud with added bovine heart extract, Lowenstein-Jensen, and so on) (Fig. 24-5). For *Legionella* spp., the specimen is initially diluted 10-fold in a bacteriologic broth (e.g., tryptic soy or sterile water) to dilute inhibitory substances, and because this organism grows slowly, heavily contaminated samples should be subsequently disinfected from other bacteria by 1:10 dilution in KCl-HCl pH = 2.2, irrigation, and incubation for 4 minutes only at room temperature. In CF patients, it is now necessary to cultivate sputum for Nontuberculous *Mycobacteria* spp. (NTM), which is performed by treatment with 0.25% N-acetyl-L-cysteine-1% sodium hydroxide-5% oxalic acid for removal of *P. aeruginosa* and inoculation on Lowenstein-Jensen medium or automated liquid systems. Molecular techniques such as Accuprobe are used for typing.[70] If the sample is suitable for anaerobic culture, one can use the BBA, LKV agar (Laked blood

TABLE 24-7 INTERPRETATION OF BACTERIAL LOWER RESPIRATORY CULTURE RESULTS

SPECIMEN	PROBABLY SIGNIFICANT	PROBABLY INSIGNIFICANT	ADDITIONAL INFORMATION SUPPORTING SIGNIFICANCE
Spontaneous or induced sputum	Predominant organism present in Gram stain and culture Abundant PMNs	Organism not present in Gram stain and only 1 to 2+ growth in culture No abundant PMNs	Intracellular location of organism
Endotracheal tube aspirate	Predominant organism present in Gram stain and culture Abundant PMNs	Organism only 1 to 2+ growth in culture No abundant PMNs	Organism in >10^6 CFU/mL Intracellular location of organism
Bronchoalveolar lavage fluid	Predominant organism seen in every 100× field of Gram stain Quantitative culture detects >10^5 CFU of organism/mL	Organism not present in Gram stain Quantitative culture detects <10^4 CFU of organism/mL	Intracellular location of organism

PMN, Polymorphonuclear neutrophil.
Modified from Thomson RJ. Use of microbiology laboratory tests in the diagnosis of infectious diseases. In: Tan J, ed: *Expert Guide to Infectious Diseases.* Philadelphia: American College of Physicians, 2002, pp 1-41.

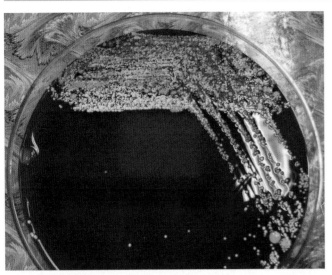

FIGURE 24-5. Sputum culture on sheep blood Agar with chalk-white colonies of *Nocardia* spp.

with canamycin and vancomycin), BBE (Bacteroides bile esculin) agar, and CNA.

Quantitative Culture Such cultures are necessary for the diagnosis of VAP, aspiration pneumonia, pneumonia in immunosuppressed individuals or CF patients, and tuberculosis. The most common microbial pathogens among ICU patients are: *S. aureus*, *P. aeruginosa*, *Enterobacter* spp., and multiresistant *Acinetobacter baumanii*. VAP is polymicrobial in 20% to 40% of cases, while the role of anaerobes has not been yet determined.[71] Aspiration pneumonia is usually attributed to oral flora anaerobes (e.g., *Bacteroides*, *Prevotella*, *Porphyromonas*, *Fusobacterium*, and anaerobic cocci), either alone or together with aerobes. Middle-lobe syndrome is usually due to *H. influenzae*, *S. pneumoniae*, and *S. aureus*.

Protected Bronchial Brush (PBB) Specimen A bronchial brush, which contains approximately 1 to 10 μL of secretions, should be placed in 1 mL of normal saline or common broth, transferred promptly to the lab, and homogenized with Vortex for 30 seconds. A smear is prepared by cytocentrifugation for Gram staining, and 10 and 100 μL samples are cultured in the appropriate culture media in aerobic and anaerobic conditions. A single colony in the agar plate corresponds to 10 CFU/mL of the initial sample, and this should be multiplied by the dilution factor of the sample in order to estimate the colonies/mL. Identification of ≥10³ CFU/mL (corresponding to 10⁶ CFU of original specimen/mL) is associated with active infection,[72,73] while lower counts represent possible cross-contamination.

Bal Five to 10 mL samples are used without prior centrifugation after 30 to 60 seconds vortexing, while 10 to 100 mL BAL is considered to contain 1 mL of bronchopulmonary secretions.[72,73] Culture is made by means of both calibrated loops and 100-fold successive dilutions.[74] Ten μL and 1 μl BAL are inoculated on agar media, and the respective 1:100 and 1:1000 dilution is noted. The agar plates are incubated at 35°C, aerobically for 4 to 7 days. Recovery of <10⁴ bacteria/mL is most likely to represent contamination, while >10⁵ bacteria/mL is indicative of active infection. Detection of 10⁴ to 10⁵ bacteria/mL

constitutes a "gray zone." The presence of intracellular bacteria in >5% to 7% of the total number of cells is associated with VAP.

Detection of Elastin Fibers in LRT Specimen

Elastin fibers in bronchoscopy samples derive from destruction of the parenchyma, which is associated with necrotic pneumonia from aerobic Gram-negative bacteria, Enterobacteriaceae (*Klebsiella* spp., *Enterobacter* spp.). Detection is simple with the use of KOH solution and is increased among patients with VAP or ARDS compared to normal subjects.[72,73] Elastin fibers may also be visualized microscopically in stained smears using a 10× objective.

Antigen Detection

Such assays allow prompt diagnosis of the underlying pathogen using any respiratory, blood, or urine specimen by means of DIF (e.g., diagnosis of pertussis), EIA with polyclonal or monoclonal antibodies causing Latex particle agglutination, OIA, and plaque or strip immunochromatography (e.g., diagnosis of group A *Streptococcus*, *S. pneumoniae*, *M. pneumoniae*, *C. pneumoniae*, *Legionella*). The reported sensitivity for EIA and OIA for the detection of group A *Streptococcus* is 60% to 95% but can be as low as 31%.[75] The Wellcogen-Latex urine test, which is applied on heated noncondensed urine, has been shown to have high sensitivity and specificity for the detection of *H. influenzae* type B among chidren,[76] while good results have also been obtained with the Directigen and Bactigen reagents for Latex among adults.[77] Membrane immunochromatography for the detection of *Legionella* antigen in urine provides a result within 15 minutes but covers serogroup 1 only. Urine detection of the polysacharitic antigen C, which is present in all pneumococcal serotypes, is performed with the use of the Binax NOW immunochromatography method (Binax, Portland, ME), with high sensitivity among children with documented invasive pneumococcal infection (bacteremia and segmental pneumonia).[78] However, the capability of this method to discriminate between patients with true pneumococcal disease and children with rhinopharyngeal carriage is questionable.[79-81]

Serology

This method is of particular importance for the diagnosis of pathogens responsible for atypical pneumonias. Immune response for *M. pneumoniae* is against glycolipids and proteins of the microbe. IgM may persist for months or years, while there is a variety of nonspecific antibodies that help in diagnosis.[82] CFix by incubation of the patient's serum with *M. pneumoniae* antigen and a defined quantity of guinea pig complement is used for the detection of anti-glycolipid antibodies, which gradually decrease after 1 month and remain low for 3 to 4 years.[83] A four-fold rise in titer or a titer ≥1:32 in convalescent serum sets the diagnosis. The sensitivity is 80% to 95% for the first criterion and 60% for the second. There are cross-reactions in 10% of patients with bacterial meningitis or pancreatitis.[83,84] CFix is mainly used for measurement of IgM and detection of recent infection among children,[82] and although inexpensive, this method can be technically demanding and time-consuming and is thus gradually replaced by ELISA, which is nowadays the method of choice. ELISA for IgM detection may diagnose infection using only one sample, if this is collected after the tenth day of illness. The method has a >99% sensitivity and 98% specificity when compared to samples positive with CFix. Only μ-capture IgM-ELISA is absolutely specific, while the specificity of other ELISA kits ranges between 25% and 90%.[85] Sensitivity is lower with IgG-ELISA.[86] Commercially available reagents with rapid membrane ELISA are easy to perform and give results in less than 15 minutes. ImmunoCard (Meridian) measures IgM antibodies and is reliable in children. Remel EIA detects total antibodies in sera with a CFix titer ≥1:64. They do not require specialized equipment, and they have a positive and negative predictive value of >90%.[83] Qualitative agglutination assays in card form and quantitative agglutination as microtiter plates are simple, and a titer ≥1:160 or four-fold increase is indicative of recent infection.[82] Cryoagglutinins are nonspecific IgM antibodies, appear 1 week after infection, and remain for 3 to 5 months. A titer of ≥1:32 is sufficient for a diagnosis, while higher titers are associated with more severe disease. They are detected in 50% to 60% of pneumonia cases, and cross-reactions with other bacterial and viral infections are observed.[83] A combination of μ-capture IgM-ELISA and PCR provides a >90% success rate during the acute phase of illness.

The surface antigens of *Chlamydia* and *Chlamydophila* lipopolysaccharide (LPS) produce a strong immune response. CFix detects anti-LPS antibodies, which are specific for the genus and common for all *Chlamydia*, and microfluorescence (MIF) uses an antigen from the elementary bodies, specific for the species.[87] The Centers for Disease Control and Prevention (CDC) considers *C. psittaci* infection confirmed when there is a compatible clinical presentation and one of the following laboratory findings: IgM titer ≥1:16 (MIF), positive culture, or a four-fold increase in titer with CFix or MIF (at least 1:32) in samples that are separated by a 2-week time interval. A titer of ≥1:32 in a serum sample with compatible clinical presentation is a possible case.[88] In the absence of a history of bird exposure, a positive result may be due to *C. pneumoniae* infection because of cross-reaction (common LPS).

MIF is the method of choice for the diagnosis of *C. trachomatis* pneumonia in infants, and only the titer of IgM ≥1:32 supports the diagnosis in neonates with compatible symptomatology. IgM (MIF) is present in virtually all neonates with pneumonia and about 30% of those with conjunctivitis due to the same pathogen. IgG does not help because maternal IgG titer is still high when the diagnosis of *C. trachomatis* is under investigation.

During the first infection with *C. pneumoniae*, IgM antibodies appear in 2 to 3 weeks from the beginning of disease, and IgG antibodies appear during the sixth to eighth week. During re-infection, IgM is absent or in low titers, and IgG appears in 1 to 2 weeks.[89] MIF is the most sensitive and only acceptable method for diagnosis but is cumbersome, and there are limited standardized and reliable reagents on the market. Therefore, with regard to the use of MIF for the diagnosis of *C. pneumoniae*, the CDC set a number of criteria and requirements for antigen

TABLE 24-8 RECOMMENDATIONS FOR THE USE OF MICROFLUORESCENCE FOR THE DIAGNOSIS OF *C. PNEUMONIAE* INFECTION

ANTIGEN	PURIFIED ELEMENTARY BODIES
Sample	Couple of serum samples with 4 to 8 weeks in between
Test course	Initial dilution 1:8 or 1:16 and 2-fold dilutions Removal of IgG with anti-IgG before testing for IgM
Results	Reading with ocular 10× and objective 40×
Evaluation	Acute infection: IgM ≥1:16 or 4-fold rise in IgG Possible acute infection: IgG ≥1:512 Hypothetical past infection: IgG ≥1:16
Quality assurance	Positive and negative control in every test Testing of positive control titer for consistency Maintenance of sera and reagents as indicated

Modified from Dowell SF, Peeling RW, Boman J, et al. Standardizing Chlamydia pneumoniae assays: recommendations from the Centers for Disease Control and Prevention (USA) and the Laboratory Centre for Disease Control (Canada). *Clin Infect Dis.* 2001;33:492-50.

preparation, suitability of sample, evaluation of results, and so on, that should be strictly followed (Table 24-8).

Upon a *Legionella pneumophila* infection, approximately 75% of patients seroconvert within weeks or months, and it is often necessary to examine several convalescent samples. IgM may remain for longer than 1 year and is thus a poor indicator of acute infection. IF is the reference method with 75% to 80% sensitivity and >99% specificity when the *L. pneumophila* serotype 1 antigen is used,[90] but the specificity is lower when the polyvalent antigen is used. For the diagnosis, seroconversion with a titer ≥1:128 is needed, while a titer of ≥1:256 is an indication of infection only during epidemics. ELISA may serve as a screening test, and its results need to be confirmed with IF. Agglutination assays permit the examination of multiple sera at the same time, have a high sensitivity and specificity, and are positive in 40% of cases during the first week of infection.

IF is the method of choice for *Coxiella burnetii* infection, and it has a high sensitivity and specificity without cross-reactions. About 90% of patients have detectable antibodies during the third week of infection that are gradually decreased within 12 months. IgM is no longer detected beyond 6 months. *C. burnetii* exists in two antigenic phases called phase I and phase II. Apart from a 4-fold increase, a titer of IgG ≥1:200 and/or IgM ≥1:50 against phase II is a strong indication of recent infection. There is a commercially available ELISA kit for the detection of phase II IgM, but the method is not standardized. Alternatively, agglutination assays and CFix have been attempted, but they lack in specificity.[91] Antibodies to phase I antigens of *C. burnetii* generally require a longer time to appear and indicate continued exposure to the bacteria (chronic Q fever).

Serology for *B. pertussis* has a sensitivity that ranges between 60% and 95%.[92] Reference laboratories use neutralization assays for the diagnosis of *B. pertussis,* while ELISA is the method of choice in clinical laboratories. IgM and IgA responses to toxin (PT) are a marker of infection, and 90% of patients have detectable IgG antibodies during the third to fourth week since the beginning of symptoms. Immune response depends on the age but also on prior exposure to the bacterium or to the antigen in the context of vaccination. This renders assessment difficult among vaccinated children. The acute phase sample is usually lost due to the delay in initiation of symptomatology. Comparison of antibody levels between mothers and children helps in the diagnosis of neonatal pertussis.

Antibodies G, A, and M against *F. tularensis* appear simultaneously during the first week after infection and remain for over 10 years, hence the presence of IgM does not prove recent infection. Agglutination assays are the method of choice, and a titer ≥1:160 is considered positive when there is compatible clinical presentation and no history of previous exposure or vaccination.

Detection of bacterial nucleic acid

The use of unsuitable culture media, transport media, and conditions as well as delays in transport may reduce the viability of a pathogen but may leave its nucleic acid still detectable. Also, nucleic acid persists in specimens after initiation of treatment[93,94] and may be detected in smaller and noninvasive specimens. On the other hand, due to the need for isolation of the organism for antibiotic susceptibility testing, cultures have been replaced by molecular methods only in cases in which the pathogens are of predictable susceptibility or the genetics of resistance are well defined, as with MRSA. Contribution of extracellular DNA and DNA that is derived from dead bacteria can be minimized by addition of propidium monoazide (PMA) to clinical samples before nucleic acid extraction. PMA enters cells whose structural integrity has been compromised, and intercalates with DNA, with which it cross-links upon exposure to a bright light source rendering it unsuitable to act as a PCR template. PMA treatment of samples generates bacterial community profiles that derive from DNA contained only intracellularly.

Species-specific PCR assays have been developed for numerous bacterial pathogens (e.g., *L. pneumophila, C. trachomatis, N. gonorrhoeae,* and *Mycobacterium* spp.) with greater accuracy and sensitivity of identification compared to conventional culture-based diagnostics. However, this approach requires a prediction to be made as to which is the most likely pathogen, as in the case of selective culture media. The nucleic acid–based assay for the detection *S. pyogenes* has a sensitivity of >90%, and by many it is considered sensitive and specific enough to obviate confirmatory culture.[95,96] PCR for the detection of *S. aureus* in nasal swabs is as sensitive as culture but provides faster results.[97] Detection of *B. pertussis* with PCR in a rhinopharyngeal sample is significantly more sensitive and specific compared to culture or IF and is the new gold standard of diagnosis.[98,99] In the cases of vaccinated patients, recent contact with an infected individual, sample collection during the paroxysmal stage of the illness, or after administration of antimicrobials, culture is often negative while PCR is positive.[98] Moreover, the sensitivity of this method for the identification of *Bordetella* spp. is higher among neonates and infants.[98,99] PCR for the detection of *M. pneumoniae* on a rhinopharyngeal aspirate or swab, or a throat swab, is the most sensitive and specific method.[100,101] Similarly, *C. pneumoniae* PCR is highly sensitive and specific, although a positive result may indicate carriage only.[100]

PCR using blood specimens (whole blood, plasma, or Buffy coat) is mainly applied for the detection of *S. pneumoniae, H. influenzae,* and meningococcus, and the sensitivity and specificity of the method depends on the specimen. Reliability of blood PCR may be affected by prior antibiotic administration, colonization of the rhinopharynx, insufficient removal of hemoglobin (extended presence of porphyrin complexes interfere with the action of DNA polymerase), and small number of infected cells.[102,103]

The more recent advent of real-time PCR allows prompt and accurate determination of bacterial load with even greater sensitivity.[104] Multiplex PCR systems that allow simultaneous detection of six respiratory bacterial species have also been developed.[105]

The most important phylogenetically informative region of bacteria is the 16 S rRNA gene, which contains both highly conserved and highly variable regions; and sequence analysis of this gene allows bacterial identification at the genus or species level. It can be performed either on strains of already isolated bacteria or directly on clinical samples, and it has been used for identification of previously unrecognized species.[106] The procedure involves nucleic acid extraction, amplification of the target sequence by PCR, sequence determination, and a computer software–aided search of a relevant sequence database. Disadvantages include the high cost of automated nucleic acid sequencers, lack of appropriate analysis software, and limited databases.

More effective means of resolving mixed bacterial PCR products generated from multispecies templates include MS-based approaches, which generate species identities depending on base composition signatures of the sequences amplified,[107] and ultra-high throughput sequencing,[108] which offers highly detailed bacterial community composition data.

References

The complete reference list is available online at www.expertconsult.com

25 ACUTE INFECTIONS THAT PRODUCE UPPER AIRWAY OBSTRUCTION

Ian M. Balfour-Lynn, BSc, MD, MBBS, FRCP, FRCPCH, FRCS (Ed), DHMSA, and Jane C. Davies, MB, ChB, MRCP, MRCPCH, MD

Upper airway obstruction due to acute infection is not uncommon in children, and many parents have experienced an anxious night with a "croupy" child. Although infants and young children are most commonly affected because they have relatively narrow upper airways, older children and adults can also have significant symptoms. Fortunately, these are mostly due to self-limiting viral laryngotracheobronchitis (LTB), but there is also a group of bacterial infections (e.g., epiglottitis, bacterial tracheitis, diphtheria, retropharyngeal abscess, and peritonsillar abscess) that can occasionally cause significant obstruction. It is the job of the emergency physician, pediatrician, pediatric pulmonologist, or otorhinolaryngologist to diagnose more serious infections promptly so that treatment can be instituted early and disastrous obstruction avoided. It is also important to recognize when a simple viral LTB is causing significant problems so that appropriate treatment can be given immediately. This chapter is clinically orientated and outlines the principal infective causes of upper airway obstruction, with an emphasis on diagnosis and treatment. Confusion exists regarding the nomenclature for these disorders, with some using the term *croup* to refer to any inflammatory disorder of the upper airway, whereas others restrict its use to subglottic disease (i.e., LTB, which is usually of viral origin). Therefore, for the sake of clarity term *croup* will be largely avoided in this chapter.

The consequence of these upper airway infections is usually stridor, which is a clinical sign and should not be considered a definitive diagnosis. This chapter briefly outlines the principles behind what causes stridor, which should clarify why this condition mostly affects infants and young children. The appendix in Holinger and colleagues' *Pediatric Laryngology and Bronchoesophagology* discusses the physics of air flow and fluid dynamics.[1] The laws of fluid dynamics are based on flow through fixed tubes and may not always apply to dynamic airways *in vivo*. Normally, air flow through the upper airways is laminar, and the moving column of air produces slight negative pressure on the airway walls.[2] Inflammation resulting from infection causes a degree of airway narrowing, which increases the flow rate through the narrowed segment (the Venturi effect). This, in turn, causes a reduction in the pressure exerted on the airway wall. This is the Bernoulli principle. In other words, negative intraluminal pressure increases. This enhances the tendency of the airway to collapse inward, further narrowing the airway and causing turbulent air flow. The respiratory phase (inspiration or expiration) has a differential effect on air flow, depending on whether the obstruction is intrathoracic or extrathoracic (Fig. 25-1).

Stridor is the sound made by rapid, turbulent flow of air through a narrowed segment of a large airway. It is most often loud, with medium or low pitch, and inspiratory. It usually originates from the larynx, upper trachea, or hypopharynx.[3] Progression of the disease process may make stridor softer, higher-pitched, and biphasic (inspiratory and expiratory). With the onset of complete obstruction, stridor may become barely audible as minimal air moves through the critically narrowed airway.[4]

The laryngeal anatomy of children makes them particularly susceptible to narrowing of the upper airways. The larynx of a neonate is situated high in the neck, and the epiglottis is narrow, omega-shaped (ω), and vertically positioned. The narrowest segment of the pediatric airway is the subglottic region (in adults, it is at the glottic level), which is encircled by the rigid cricoid cartilage ring. There is nonfibrous, loosely attached mucosa in this region that is easily obstructed in the presence of subglottic edema. Additionally, the cartilaginous support of the infant airway is soft and compliant, easily allowing dynamic collapse of the airways during inspiration. Young children have proportionally large heads and relatively lax neck support; this combination increases the likelihood of airway obstruction when supine.[5] Also, their tongues are relatively large for the size of the oropharynx. Simple mathematics shows why a small amount of edema has such a profound effect on the cross-sectional area and, hence, air flow. The diameter of the subglottis in a normal newborn is approximately 5 mm, and 0.5-mm edema in this region reduces the cross-sectional area to 64% of normal (area = $\pi \infty$ radius^2). Air flow is directly proportional to the airway radius to the fourth power (Poiseuille's law), so a small reduction in caliber has a major effect on flow rate. The same 5-mm airway with 0.5 mm edema will have a flow rate of only 41% of baseline, assuming that pressure remains unchanged—a situation that is not necessarily the case if the Bernoulli principle is in play. Because the caliber of the airway is almost inevitably reduced further in accord with the Bernoulli principle, and Poiseuille flow is not established, the flow rate is much further reduced and the work of breathing is greatly increased to maintain ventilation.

▰ VIRAL LARYNGOTRACHEOBRONCHITIS

Etiology

The most common etiologic agents are the parainfluenza viruses (PIVs), of which PIV 1 is found most frequently and leads to epidemics. PIV 2 may account for

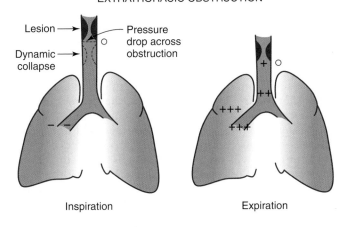

EXTRATHORACIC OBSTRUCTION

Lesion → Pressure drop across obstruction

Dynamic collapse

Inspiration   Expiration

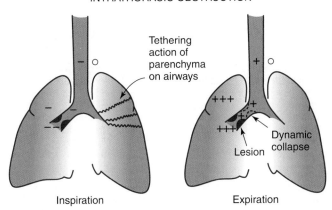

INTRATHORACIC OBSTRUCTION

Tethering action of parenchyma on airways

Dynamic collapse

Lesion

Inspiration   Expiration

FIGURE 25-1. The effect of the respiratory phase on extrathoracic and intrathoracic obstruction is shown. During inspiration, negative intratracheal pressure (relative to atmospheric pressure) leads to dynamic collapse of the extrathoracic airway, thus worsening the effects of an extrathoracic obstructive lesion. In contrast, intrathoracic obstruction improves during inspiration because the elastic recoil of the lung parenchyma opens the intrathoracic airways. During expiration, intratracheal pressure is positive relative to atmospheric pressure, opening the extrathoracic trachea and lessening the obstructive effect of lesions. In contrast, intrathoracic obstruction worsens because of lower pressure in the airways relative to the surrounding parenchyma, collapsing the airways. (From Loughlin GM, Taussig LM. Upper airway obstruction. *Semin Respir Med.* 1979;1:131-146.)

many sporadic cases, and PIV 3 is a less common cause of viral LTB, usually targeting the epithelium of the smaller airways and leading to bronchiolitic illness. The PIVs belong to the *Paramyxoviridae* family, along with respiratory syncytial virus, measles, mumps, and the recently identified human metapneumovirus.[6] Together the PIVs account for more than 75% of viral LTB cases, although other respiratory viruses (e.g., respiratory syncytial virus, rhinovirus, influenza virus, adenovirus, coronavirus, and enteroviruses) can produce a similar clinical syndrome. Herpesviruses tend to cause a more severe and protracted form of the disease. LTB can also occur with some systemic infections, such as measles, and less commonly, Mycoplasma. In general, however, it is not usually possible to identify the cause of infection from the child's symptoms because severity does not correlate with any particular etiologic agent.

Epidemiology

Viral LTB is the most common cause of infective upper airway obstruction in the pediatric age group. Affected children are usually of preschool age, with a peak incidence between 18 and 24 months of age.[7] Reported incidence rates vary from 1.5% to 6%, but less than 5% of these require hospital admission, and only 1% to 2% of those admitted require endotracheal intubation and intensive care.[8] This proportion has fallen dramatically since the use of corticosteroids has become routine. There is a male preponderance in children younger than 6 years of age (1.4:1), although both sexes appear to be affected equally at an older age. Cases may occur in epidemics, with those caused by PIV 1 particularly presenting in fall and winter months and infection with other organisms (including PIV 2) occurring more commonly as isolated infections. Infection is via droplet spread or direct inoculation from the hands. Viruses can survive for long periods on dry surfaces, such as clothes and toys, emphasizing the importance of infection-control practices.

Pathophysiology

Infection affects the larynx, trachea, and bronchi, although swelling and inflammation in the subglottic area leads to the characteristic clinical features of viral LTB. In addition to relative differences in airway size (discussed earlier in the chapter), it is suggested that poor cell-mediated immunity in younger age groups also accounts for differences observed between adults and children.[9] The epithelium of the subglottis possesses abundant mucous glands, secretions from which can further narrow the airway lumen in response to infection. The PIVs are trophic for the respiratory epithelium, binding in particular to ciliated cells via an interaction between the viral hemagglutinin-neuraminidase protein and its receptor, sialic acid. Other viral proteins (the F protein in particular) are important in membrane fusion and the passage of viral particles between cells. Many strains of PIV are cytopathic, with infection leading to the formation of giant cells and cell death. As with many infective processes, the ensuing inflammatory response is involved in the evolution of symptoms. Both polymorphonuclear and monocytic leukocytes infiltrate the sub-epithelium, which leads to vascular congestion and airway wall edema. In addition, the symptoms of viral LTB are believed to be caused by the release of spasmogenic mediators, leading to decreased airway diameter. This may result from a type I hypersensitivity response to PIV, and some authors have postulated a role for anti-PIV-specific immunoglobulin E (IgE) in the development of airway narrowing.[10] These factors may play a relatively greater role in patients with recurrent (spasmodic) croup, and these patients may have hyperreactivity of the extrathoracic and intrathoracic airways.[11] The etiology of recurrent, spasmodic croup remains unclear, with authors expressing differing views on whether it is usually virus-related[12] or is a separate disease entity; suggested triggers include gastroesophageal reflux and anatomical abnormalities in addition to an allergic predisposition.[13]

Clinical Presentation and Diagnosis

Mild

Most children are affected mildly by viruses that cause LTB.[7] The exact incidence remains unknown because many of them do not receive medical attention, but are managed by parents at home. Children have a barking cough and a hoarse cry or voice; these symptoms are worse in the evening and at night. They may also have inspiratory stridor on exertion, but stridor at rest is usually absent, as are other signs of respiratory distress. There is most commonly a coryzal prodrome accompanied by a low-grade fever, but children are not particularly unwell or toxic. They remain interested in their surroundings, are playful, and still eat and drink.

Moderate

Features of moderate viral LTB include those discussed earlier, but with inspiratory stridor present at rest, as well as a degree of respiratory distress manifest by chest wall recession, tachypnea, and the use of accessory muscles of respiration. There is usually accompanying tachycardia, but children remain interactive and are able to take at least liquids orally.

Severe

Progression from moderate to severe infection can occur rapidly and may be precipitated by the distress caused by clinical examination. Worrisome signs include those of increasing respiratory distress, with the child appearing anxious or preoccupied and tired. Drooling may occur, and the child will often refuse liquids or be unable to coordinate swallowing and breathing. However, the child with viral LTB will not appear toxic, with high fever and flushed face, as do those with the classic signs of bacterial epiglottitis (Table 25-1). Another difference is in the nature of the cough; a harsh, barking cough is not commonly associated with epiglottitis (in which there is often a muffled cough and cry). Restlessness and agitation are

TABLE 25-1 DIFFERENTIATION OF PRINCIPAL INFECTIVE CAUSES OF UPPER AIRWAY OBSTRUCTION

	VIRAL LARYNGOTRACHEO-BRONCHITIS	EPIGLOTTITIS	BACTERIAL TRACHEITIS	DIPHTHERIA	RETROPHARYNGEAL ABSCESS
Principal Organisms	Parainfluenza 1–3 Adenovirus Respiratory syncytial virus	*Haemophilus influenzae* *Streptococcus*	*Staphylococcus aureus* *Moraxella catarrhalis* *H. influenzae*	Corynebacterium diphtheria	Mixed flora, including *S. aureus*, *Streptococcus*, *H. influenzae*, anaerobes
Age Range	6 mo–4 yr (peak, 1–2 yr)	2–7 yr	6 mo–8 yr	All ages	<6 yr
Incidence	Common	Rare	Rare	Rare if vaccinated	Uncommon
Onset	Insidious Usually follows upper respiratory tract infection	Rapid	Slow, with sudden deterioration	Insidious	Gradual
Site	Below the vocal cords	Supraglottis	Trachea	Tonsils, pharynx, larynx, nose, skin	Retropharyngeal space
Clinical Manifestations	Low-grade fever Nontoxic Barking (seal-like) cough Stridor Hoarseness Restlessness	High fever Severe sore throat Minimal nonbarking cough Toxic Stridor Drooling Dysphagia Muffled voice position	High fever Toxic Brassy cough Stridor Hoarse voice Neck pain Choking	Fever Toxic Stridor Sore throat Fetor oris Cervical lymphadenopathy Bull neck	Fever Sore throat Neck pain and stiffness (especially on extension) Dysphagia Stridor (less common) Drooling Retropharyngeal bulge
Endoscopic Findings	Deep red mucosa Subglottic edema	Cherry-red or pale and edematous epiglottis Edematous aryepiglottic folds	Deep red mucosa Ulcerations Copious, thick tracheal secretions Subglottic edema, with normal epiglottis and arytenoids	Gray, adherent membrane on the pharynx	N/A
Intubation	Occasional	Usual	Usual	Occasional	Unusual
Therapy	Corticosteroids Nebulized epinephrine	Intubation (1–3 days) IV antibiotics	Intubation (3–7 days) IV antibiotics Tracheal suction	Diphtheria antitoxin IV antibiotics Immunization during convalescence	IV antibiotics ± surgery

late signs of airway obstruction of any cause, as is cyanosis, pallor, or decreased level of consciousness. Pulse oximetry should be performed, but limitations must be recognized. Oxygen saturation may be well preserved until the late stages of severe viral LTB, and it can lead to significant underestimation of respiratory compromise in a patient who is receiving supplementary oxygen. Conversely, desaturation may be seen in children with relatively mild airway obstruction (presumably reflecting lower airway involvement and ventilation-perfusion mismatch).[14] Pulsus paradoxus is present in this group with severe disease, but in clinical practice, it is difficult to assess, and attempts to do so could worsen symptoms by causing distress.

Recurrent or Spasmodic Croup

Symptoms are similar to those of the more typical forms of viral LTB, but children are often older, do not have the same coryzal prodrome, and may be afebrile during the episode. There may be links with atopy, often with a positive family history. Attacks often occur suddenly, at night, and may resolve equally quickly. Treatment must be guided by the degree of severity, and is similar to that for viral LTB. Some practitioners prescribe oral or inhaled corticosteroids (via a spacer device) to be kept at home and administered by the parents in case of an episode, although there is a paucity of evidence for or against this practice.

Non-Infective Causes of Acute Airway Obstruction

There are a number of non-infective causes of upper airway obstruction, and these must be considered in the differential diagnosis of infective causes (Box 25-1). Foreign body inhalation is the most common non-infective cause in children. Symptoms may partly mimic those of viral LTB and will depend on the location of the foreign body, the degree of resultant airway obstruction, and (to a lesser extent) the nature of the foreign body. Onset of symptoms may be either acute or insidious; a large foreign body may cause severe obstruction, whereas a smaller one may simply lead to laryngeal and tracheal irritation and airway edema. In cases of severe airway obstruction, the voice may be lost and

breath sounds quiet. This condition is an emergency and requires immediate visualization of the larynx and trachea and removal of the foreign body by a physician or surgeon experienced in this procedure. Occasionally, an unrecognized inhaled foreign body leads to chronic stridor. Acute upper airway obstruction may also result from the ingestion of caustic substances, with resulting pharyngeal burns, edema, and inflammation of the epiglottis, aryepiglottic folds, larynx, and trachea. This diagnosis is usually clear from the history. Rarely, angioneurotic edema may cause acute laryngeal swelling and airway obstruction. Patients appear nontoxic and may exhibit other signs of allergic disease, such as urticaria and abdominal pain. In hereditary angioneurotic edema due to C1 esterase deficiency, the family history may be positive, although the first presentation is more common in adults than in children.

There are numerous causes of chronic airway obstruction that are discussed elsewhere in this book. Confusion may arise when an upper respiratory tract infection unmasks a previously asymptomatic congenital abnormality. For example, mild subglottic stenosis may cause symptoms only with the additional burden of airway edema due to a simple viral upper respiratory infection. It is important to ensure that there is no history of intubation (which may have been brief, as in resuscitation of a newborn in the maternity unit) or of any coexisting signs (e.g., a cutaneous hemangioma) that may increase the index of suspicion for a congenital airway abnormality.

Who Should Be Evaluated?

Most children with viral LTB were previously well, have short, self-limiting symptoms, and make a full recovery. The lack of complete immunity and the variety of agents that can cause viral LTB mean that more than one episode is not uncommon, particularly in separate seasons. However, some children have symptoms that should lead to further clinical evaluation. These include multiple episodes, particularly if they are severe or frequent, symptoms that are particularly slow to resolve, and symptoms that occur between or in the absence of obvious infections. Evaluation of patients in this group is aimed at identifying an underlying airway abnormality that would predispose the child to more severe airway narrowing with viral infections, or that could cause problems independently of such infection. Investigation is usually centered on airway endoscopy. This must be performed in a unit and by an operator who is experienced in the technique because there is a risk in many of these conditions of exacerbating the airway obstruction. Spontaneous breathing is necessary to identify vocal cord problems or airway malacia, and anesthetic techniques must be carefully considered. If an inhaled foreign body is considered likely, rigid bronchoscopy is the study of choice. Additional studies that might be considered once the acute episode has resolved include plain lateral neck and chest radiographs, computed tomography or magnetic resonance imaging scan, contrast assessment of the upper airway (e.g., videofluoroscopy, barium swallow), and a

---

BOX 25-1 INFECTIOUS AND NONINFECTIOUS CAUSES OF ACUTE UPPER AIRWAY OBSTRUCTION

Infectious
Viral laryngotracheobronchitis
Epiglottitis
Bacterial tracheitis
Diphtheria
Retropharyngeal abscess
Peritonsillar abscess
Infectious mononucleosis

Noninfectious
Foreign body
Trauma
Caustic burns
Spasmodic croup
Angioneurotic edema

pH study. Polysomnography may help to determine the severity of chronic symptoms. Rarer causes of recurrent stridor (e.g., hypocalcaemia or angioneurotic edema) are diagnosed by blood testing.

Management of Viral Laryngotracheobronchitis

Management of viral LTB must be based on clinical assessment of severity. Such assessment should be based on the clinical features described earlier; there is no role for radiography in the assessment of acute airway obstruction. In skilled hands, plain lateral neck radiographs may demonstrate sites of obstruction, but this rarely influences management; it also wastes time and can be dangerous. The neck extension that is required could precipitate sudden worsening of airway obstruction, which can be fatal in severe cases. Several scoring systems have been devised,[15] and the most commonly applied system (the 17-point Westley scale, which assesses degree of stridor, chest retractions, air entry, cyanosis, and level of consciousness) has been well validated. However, these are mainly used in the context of clinical trials and are not a substitute for experienced clinical assessment.

Supportive Care

Children with mild croup can be managed at home. They should be treated with plenty of fluids and antipyretics as required. Because the vast majority of cases are of viral etiology, there is no role for the routine use of antibiotics in the absence of other features suggestive of bacterial infection. Parents should be warned that symptoms are usually worse at night.

Humidification

Both at home and in the hospital setting, humidified air (either steam or cool mist) has been used for more than a century to produce symptomatic relief from croup. Despite this, there is very little supportive published evidence; most early studies, some of which may have been underpowered, generally suggested no benefit.[16-18] A larger study of 140 moderately affected children showed no differences in signs or requirement for additional treatments with optimally delivered 100% humidity,[19] and the most recent Cochrane Systematic Review has also concluded there is no evidence of benefit.[20] Case reports have described severe burns caused by spilling of boiling water and facial scalds from the use of steam, so this type of treatment is not without the potential for harm.[21]

Corticosteroids

The use of corticosteroids has received much attention for more than a decade, and their therapeutic role is well established. Their mechanism of action, however, remains unclear, although is believed to relate to rapid-onset anti-inflammatory properties. The cumulative evidence strongly supports their use in children with moderate to severe symptoms, although there are still outstanding questions, including the optimal route of administration, the most appropriate dosing regimen, and the best oral agent.

The role of corticosteroids in the management of croup in children has been the subject of several Cochrane reviews, with the most recent update in November 2004.[22] In this review, the authors identified 31 studies that fulfilled their criteria for inclusion, namely, randomized controlled trials in children measuring the effectiveness of corticosteroids (any route of administration) against either a placebo or another treatment. A total of 3736 children were included, the majority from placebo-controlled trials. Outcome measures included the croup score (most commonly the Westley scale), the requirement for admission or return visit, the length of stay, and the requirement for additional therapeutic interventions. Overall, treatment led to an improvement in the croup score at 6 and 12 hours, but the improvement was no longer apparent at 24 hours. The length of time spent in either the emergency department or the hospital was also significantly decreased, as was the requirement for nebulized epinephrine. Importantly, and in contrast to the previous version of the Cochrane review, the authors concluded with funnel plots and other statistical methods that these results were not influenced by publication bias.[22] Since this publication, one further large randomized controlled trial (n = 720) studied mild croup (Westley score ≤ 2), and showed benefit of a single dose of dexamethasone, 0.6 mg/kg, in terms of return to medical care, resolution of symptoms, decreased loss of sleep by the child, and reduced parental stress.[23] In conclusion, the case for corticosteroids is now clear. In severe disease, rates of intubation are significantly decreased and the duration of intubation is reduced, and in moderate disease admission, the need for additional treatment and return visits are reduced.[8] More recent studies have focused attention on the optimal formulation, dose, and treatment regimen.

Optimal Route of Administration, Formulation, and Dosing Regimen

Studies included in the Cochrane review (discussed earlier in the chapter) and conducted since then have used the intramuscular, oral, or nebulized route to administer different corticosteroid preparations. This area has been recently well reviewed.[8] From the studies that have attempted to address the route of administration, nebulized, oral, and intramuscular routes appear, in general, to be roughly equivalent. Nebulization could potentially increase distress of the child and worsen upper airway obstruction, although it may be preferable in a child who is vomiting or having difficulty swallowing.

Similarly, studies using oral agents have used either dexamethasone or prednisolone, and both in varying doses. Many primary care physicians who visit homes do not routinely carry dexamethasone but do carry oral prednisolone. There is no strong evidence in support of one preparation over the other, although one recent study favored dexamethosone, which led to a reduced frequency of re-presentation.[24] In contrast, a recent Australian trial compared 1 mg/kg prednisolone with two doses of dexamethasone (0.15 and 0.6 mg/kg) and found no difference in croup score, requirement for further treatment, or re-presentation.[25] With regard to dexamethasone, 0.6 mg/kg has been the dose most widely used, but several recent studies have demonstrated that this dose may be higher than required and that 0.15 mg/kg is just as effective.[25-28] A practical approach might be to use dexamethasone, if available, at a dose of 0.15 mg/kg. If this preparation were not available at a home visit, prednisolone (at an equivalent dose of 1 mg/kg) could provide a useful substitute.

Nebulized epinephrine (adrenaline): Most clinical trials have used the racemic form of this drug,[29] although there is now evidence that the L-isomer used alone (which is the only available formulation in some units) may be equally effective.[30] The mechanisms of action are believed to be a combination of rapid reduction in airway wall edema and bronchodilation. It has a rapid onset of action (within 30 minutes), and the effect lasts for 2 to 3 hours. The recommended dose is 0.4 to 0.5 mL/kg (to a maximum of 5 mL) of the 1:1000 preparation that is put undiluted into the nebulizer pot. According to these studies, nebulized epinephrine has been shown to improve the croup score and reduce the likelihood of hospital admission, but it is less clear whether, when given with corticosteroids, it reduces the need for intubation. It should be used in any child who has severe signs and symptoms, and it should be considered for those with moderate signs and symptoms, depending on the signs of respiratory distress and possible response to corticosteroid administration. It can be administered in the home setting while awaiting an ambulance, but, clearly, any child requiring this treatment at home must be transferred promptly to the hospital for monitoring. Multiple doses may be administered, although the requirement for this must lead to consideration of the need for intensive care management. Although rebound worsening of symptoms after administration of nebulized epinephrine is often alluded to, in practice, this phenomenon does not appear to be a real risk. Traditionally, children treated with epinephrine have been admitted to the hospital, but recent studies have confirmed that discharge home is safe after 3 to 4 hours of observation if the child has made significant improvement.[31]

Other treatments for severe cases: Oxygen should be administered to any child with severe airway obstruction, even in the absence of severe hypoxia, because it will aid respiratory muscle function. As mentioned earlier, a child with severe respiratory distress and obstruction may have relatively normal pulse oximetry readings when breathing oxygen, which can be dangerous if misinterpreted by staff who are unaware of this limitation. Heliox (70% to 80% helium with 20% to 30% oxygen) has been used in both upper airway obstruction[32] and severe asthma, and it is the focus of a recent Cochrane review.[33] Only two small randomized controlled trials were identified, totaling 44 patients with severe croup. Heliox was compared with either 30% humidified oxygen or with 100% oxygen plus epinephrine. There was no additional benefit of Heliox, although further well-designed controlled trials were recommended. Some children with severe croup either do not respond to the usual therapies or are too severely compromised at presentation to permit their use. These children require urgent endotracheal intubation and mechanical ventilation to avoid potentially catastrophic complete airway obstruction and the serious sequelae of hypoxia and hypercapnia (e.g., hypoxic ischemic enceph-

alopathy). Intubation should be performed by the most experienced person available, and it should be attempted with an uncuffed endotracheal tube one size smaller than the usual size for the child.[34] Facilities for immediate tracheostomy must be available at the time of intubation. Children may have coexisting lower airway and parenchymal involvement that impairs gas exchange and may lead to slower than expected clinical improvement after intubation. Rarely, pulmonary edema may develop after relief of airway obstruction, particularly if the disease course has been prolonged. Most children without severe parenchymal involvement require respiratory support for 3 to 5 days.[34] This is one context in which multiple rather than single doses of corticosteroids are often administered. The timing of extubation will depend on the development of an air leak, indicating resolution of airway narrowing.[34] Re-intubation rates of approximately 10% have been reported.[35]

EPIGLOTTITIS

Etiology

Historically, *H. influenzae* type B (HiB) was responsible for almost all (approximately 99%) cases of epiglottitis in otherwise healthy children. Since the introduction of HiB immunization, other organisms have been implicated, including groups A, B, C, and G β-hemolytic streptococcus. Other responsible organisms include *Haemophilus parainfluenzae*, *Staphylococcus aureus*, *Moraxella catarrhalis*, *Pneumococcus*, *Klebsiella*, *Pseudomonas*, Candida, and viruses (e.g., herpes simplex, varicella, PIV, influenza).[2,36]

Epidemiology

H. influenzae type B vaccines were first licensed in the United States in 1988, with widespread immunization programs in place by the early 1990s. Since then, reported cases of invasive HiB disease (including epiglottitis) in children younger than 5 years of age have declined by 99%.[37] The same pattern has been repeated in Europe, with significant reductions in the United Kingdom.[38,39] Immunization was introduced in the United Kingdom in 1992, and, with immunization coverage exceeding 90%, the decline in incidence was more than 95%.[39] In 1998, the incidence in those younger than 5 years of age was 0.6 per 100,000, compared with 31 to 36 per 100,000 in England and Wales before the introduction of the vaccine.[39] However in 2003 there was a resurgence of Hib infections in the United Kingdom, which led to the launch of a booster program. Ethnicity plays a part in vaccine efficacy. Data from 1996 to 1997 in the United States show that the average annual incidence of HiB invasive disease per 100,000 children younger than 5 years of age was 0.5 among non-Hispanic whites, 0.6 among Asians and Pacific Islanders, 0.7 among non-Hispanic blacks, 0.7 among Hispanic Americans, and 12.4 among Native Americans and Alaskan natives.[37] Nevertheless, cases of epiglottitis due to HiB continue to be reported,[40] as do cases due to other organisms.[36]

Cases of invasive HiB occur principally in non-immunized children, but also rarely in some true vaccine failures. Clinical risk factors for vaccine failure include prematurity, Down syndrome, malignancy, developmental delay, and congenital or acquired immunodeficiency, principally reduced immunoglobulin concentrations (IgG$_2$ subclass, IgA, IgM) and neutropenia.[41] However, these factors explain fewer than 50% of cases of vaccine failures.[41] An HiB IgG antibody titer of ≥0.15 µg/mL confers protection from disease, but, given the natural waning in antibody levels, it is estimated that a titer of ≥1.0 µg/mL should provide long-term protection.[40] However, there may sometimes be qualitative functional problems with antibody responses that are not yet fully elucidated.

Epiglottitis tends to occur in children 2 to 7 years of age, but cases have been reported in those younger than 1 year of age.[2] Since the introduction of HiB vaccine, the peak age distribution has increased slightly.[42] A recent review of a national U.S. dataset from 1998 to 2006 has shown that the mean age of a patient admitted with epiglottitis is 45 years and the national mortality rate is 0.89%; there is a decrease in admissions for those under 18 years of age (with greatest risk at <1 year) and an increase in the 46- to 64-year-old group.[43] Most cases occur in the fall and winter.

Pathophysiology

Although HiB has a low point-prevalence of nasopharyngeal carriage (1% to 5%), most young children become colonized with HiB in the first 2 to 5 years.[44] The relationship between asymptomatic carriage, immunity, and the development of invasive disease is not clearly understood. Viral co-infection may have a role in the transition from colonization to invasion.[45] Colonies of HiB organisms reside in the nasal mucosal epithelium and submucosa. Invasive disease occurs when organisms disseminate from the mucosa of the upper respiratory tract via the bloodstream; bacteremia increases over a period of hours, and metastatic seeding can occur.[44] Thus, although situated in close proximity to the nose, the supraglottic area is likely to be affected via the bloodstream; direct spread along mucosal surfaces may also play a part. This may account for the relatively high yield of positive blood cultures in epiglottitis and the relatively low incidence of epiglottitis among carriers of HiB.

Epiglottitis is more correctly called *supraglottitis*. It is a bacterial cellulitis of the supraglottic structures, particularly the lingual surface of the epiglottis and the aryepiglottic folds.[2] Destruction of the infected epithelial tissue results in mucosal ulcerations, which may appear on the epiglottis, larynx, and trachea. The submucosal glands are involved as well, with the formation of abscesses. Infection of the epiglottis itself causes a local inflammatory response that results in a cherry-red edematous epiglottis when caused by HiB (Fig. 25-2), although it tends to be pale and edematous and accompanied by edematous aryepiglottic folds when caused by *Streptococcus*.[36,37] As supraglottic edema worsens, the epiglottis is displaced posteriorly, and it may obstruct the airway.

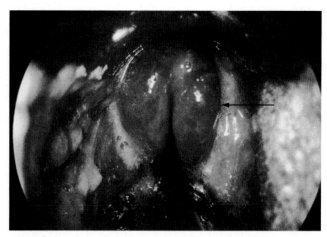

FIGURE 25-2. Swollen epiglottis *(arrow)* caused by acute epiglottitis in an intubated child. (From Benjamin B, Bingham B, Hawke M, et al. *A Colour Atlas of Otorhinolaryngology.* London: Taylor & Francis, 1995, p 292, with permission.)

Clinical Presentation and Diagnosis

Classic epiglottitis caused by HiB is a fulminant disease in an otherwise healthy child, who can be near death in a few hours. It is a medical emergency that can be alarming for the medical staff and devastating for the family. Epiglottitis clearly has not been eliminated, but due to its rarity there are concerns about a potential lack of familiarity with its management among emergency physicians, pediatricians, anesthesiologists, and otolaryngologists.[46] Up to 20% of infants with epiglottitis are misdiagnosed initially, usually with viral LTB.[4] Typically, there is a short history of fever, severe throat pain, stridor, and respiratory distress, but the symptoms progress rapidly. Children become toxic and tend to sit anxiously in the classic tripod position (sitting upright, with the chin up, mouth open, bracing themselves on their hands) as air hunger develops (Fig. 25-3). They often drool because they cannot swallow their secretions, and the voice is muffled due to pain and soft tissue swelling. Stridor may progress, and when marked, signals almost complete obstruction of the airways. Complete, fatal airway obstruction may occur suddenly and without warning. The most serious complication of this disease process (and any infective upper airway obstruction) is hypoxic ischemic encephalopathy resulting from respiratory arrest. This tragic complication is almost always preventable with clinical suspicion, prompt diagnosis, and correct management. However, a recent 13-year case series demonstrated that cardiac arrest occurred in 3 of 40 cases (7.5%), although there were no long-term sequelae.[40] Secondary sites of HiB infection may be present in approximately half of cases, and include meningitis, otitis media, pneumonia, and cellulitis; therefore, repeated physical examination during the admission is critical.[2] The pneumonia may contribute to poor gas exchange.

Generally, distinction from standard viral LTB is based on the older age of the child, the lack of history of upper respiratory tract infection, the speed of progression, the degree of toxicity, the extent of drooling, the use of the tripod position, and minimal cough (see Table 25-1).

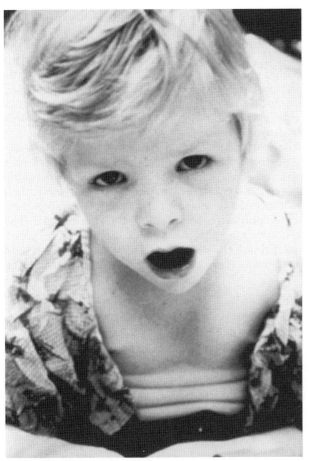

FIGURE 25-3. Characteristic posture in a patient with epiglottitis. The child is leaning forward and drooling, with a hyperextended neck. (Courtesy of Dr. Robert Berg.)

However, it is important to remember that most of these symptoms can be present in acute severe upper airway obstruction from other causes.

The presentation and clinical course of epiglottitis caused by various types of β-hemolytic streptococcal pathogens are similar to each other, but they differ from those associated with HiB.[36] The onset of disease is more gradual, but the resolution of tissue damage and the time to recovery are longer, with a mean intubation time of 6 days.[36,47]

Management

The first priority and key response to the diagnosis must be to secure the airway in a controlled environment. Physical examination (especially of the throat) and cannulation or venipuncture should be deferred because emotional upset and crying may precipitate complete airway obstruction. When epiglottitis is suspected clinically, the child (and parents) should be approached in a calm and reassuring manner. Oxygen should be given, even if the mask is held at a distance from the child's face. The child should be taken to the operating room, anesthetic room, or pediatric intensive care unit, and held by a parent. The child should be accompanied by a senior medical team that is skilled in airway management and carrying a laryngoscope, an endotracheal tube, and a percutaneous tracheostomy tray. If complete airway obstruction develops suddenly, performance of a Heimlich maneuver may relieve the obstruction temporarily; alternatively, forward traction may be applied to the mandible.

Inhalational induction of anesthesia is preferred. Laryngoscopy should then be performed and the diagnosis confirmed, based on the appearance of the epiglottic region, as described earlier in the chapter (erythema and edema of the supraglottis). Endotracheal intubation is then achieved using an orotracheal tube, which is later changed to a nasotracheal tube because this is less likely to be displaced. Although tracheostomy is rarely necessary, a surgical team should be prepared to perform this immediately if intubation is unsuccessful. Once the airway is secured, the emergency is over, and the remaining studies can be performed. Intravenous cannulation and blood sampling can be done. The white cell count is increased, and blood culture findings are often positive (70% in one series).[40] Airway secretions and swabs from the epiglottic region should be sent for bacterial culture and viral detection. Urinary antigen testing may be useful for those already receiving antibiotics.[45]

Some authors have advocated the use of a lateral neck radiograph if the child is stable before intubation, claiming it to be the "single most useful study."[2,5] We strongly disagree, and this is not our recommendation because it can precipitate respiratory arrest as a result of complete obstruction. We take the same view as Goodman and McHugh, who state that "plain radiographs have no role to play in the assessment of the critically ill child with acute stridor."[48]

Intravenous antibiotics are started and must cover HiB and *Streptococcus;* the response is usually rapid.[2] A third-generation cephalosporin (e.g., ceftriaxone or cefotaxime) is usually given and may be changed once antibiotic sensitivities are available. Antibiotics have traditionally been given for 7 to 10 days; however, a randomized controlled trial showed that a two-dose course of ceftriaxone was as efficacious as 5 days of chloramphenicol.[45] Contacts of patients with HiB should be given appropriate prophylaxis, usually rifampicin. There is some empiric evidence that corticosteroids may improve the course of epiglottitis, but racemic epinephrine has not been shown to be of benefit. The duration of intubation for epiglottitis due to HiB averages 1 to 3 days,[5,40] but it is longer when caused by *Streptococcus;*[3] as always, there is great individual variation. A decision to extubate may be made when an air leak develops around the endotracheal tube, but repeat endoscopy may be useful to aid this decision. Again, facilities for emergency tracheostomy must be available. Some give dexamethasone before extubation to reduce postextubation stridor.[4]

▄ BACTERIAL TRACHEITIS

Bacterial tracheitis has also been known as bacterial, or membranous LTB; nondiphtheritic laryngitis with marked exudate; and pseudomembranous croup.

Etiology

The most common pathogen is *S. aureus,* although other organisms implicated include HiB, α-hemolytic *Streptococcus, Pneumococcus,* and *M. catarrhalis.*[5] Occasionally, Gram-negative enteric organisms and *Pseudomonas aeruginosa* are isolated (the latter is associated with a more severe clinical course).[49] In a recent case series, *M. catarrhalis* (27%) was more common than S. aureus (22%), although this represents data from a single center over the course of 14 months.[50] One series of 94 cases over 10 years found that *M. catarrhalis* was associated with a greater rate of intubation: 83% versus 49% with other organisms, although they were a younger group.[51] In addition, PIV and influenza viruses are commonly isolated from tracheal secretions; measles and enteroviruses have also been detected. Although it may be a primary bacterial infection, bacterial tracheitis is considered secondary to primary viral LTB. Presumably, viral injury to the tracheal mucosa and impairment of local immunity predisposes to bacterial superinfection.

Epidemiology

Bacterial tracheitis is a rare disease, with the most recent large case series (from 1998) describing only 46 cases.[50] The peak incidence is during fall and winter, and it predominantly affects children 6 months to 8 years of age (mean 5 years of age). Most affected children were previously well, but it has been reported as a complication of elective tonsillectomy and adenoidectomy.[52] A large case series of life-threatening upper airway infections from Vermont in the United States between 1997 and 2006 showed that bacterial tracheitis has now superseded viral croup and epiglottitis, and was three times more likely as a cause of respiratory failure than the other two diagnoses combined.[53]

Pathophysiology

Bacterial tracheitis is characterized by marked subglottic edema, with ulceration; erythema; pseudomembranous formation on the tracheal surface; and thick, mucopurulent tracheal secretions. The thick exudate and sloughed mucosa frequently obstruct the lumen of the trachea and the main-stem bronchi.[2] The epiglottis and arytenoids are usually normal in appearance, although epiglottitis and bacterial tracheitis may coexist. Tracheal stenosis can be a complication, especially after prolonged intubation.[49]

Clinical Presentation and Diagnosis

The clinical picture is initially similar to that of viral LTB, with mild fever, cough, and stridor for several days. However, the patient's condition deteriorates rapidly, with a high fever and often a toxic appearance, with respiratory distress and airway obstruction. Other symptoms include choking episodes, orthopnea, dysphagia, and neck pain.[50] The clinical picture differs from that of epiglottitis in that its onset tends to be more insidious. Patients have a substantial brassy cough, are more able to lie flat, and tend not to drool

(see Table 25-1).[5] Children are more ill than with simple viral LTB and do not respond to expected therapies (e.g., corticosteroids or nebulized epinephrine). There may be other co-infections, particularly pneumonia. Other reported complications include cardiopulmonary arrest, with subsequent hypoxic encephalopathy and seizures, pneumothorax, subglottic stenosis, septicemia, toxic shock syndrome, pulmonary edema, and adult respiratory distress syndrome.[54]

The white blood cell count shows polymorphonuclear leukocytosis, often with a left shift. A lateral neck radiograph may show a hazy tracheal air column, with multiple luminal soft tissue irregularities due to pseudomembrane detachment from the soft tissue, but radiographs should be taken only after the patient is stabilized and safe. There are, however, no clinical or radiographic features capable of confirming the diagnosis.[2] This must be confirmed by upper airway endoscopy and a positive bacterial culture.

Management

Diagnostic endoscopy, which should be done under general anesthesia, is also therapeutic because it enables removal of secretions and sloughed tissue from the airway lumen. Rigid endoscopy may be necessary, and sometimes the procedure must be repeated. Many patients (especially younger ones) require endotracheal intubation and mechanical ventilation to overcome airway obstruction (reports of 50% to 100% intubation rates),[55] usually for 3 to 7 days. Frequent tracheal suction is necessary. In a recent series, 57% of patients required intubation, which is lower than the rate previously reported.[50] The decision to extubate is based on clinical improvement, with reduction of fever, decreased airway secretions, and development of an air leak around the endotracheal tube. Corticosteroids may be given before extubation. Tracheostomy is required less often than in the past. Initially, intravenous broad-spectrum antibiotics are given, and these can be refined once cultures and antibiotic sensitivities are known, usually for 10 to 14 days. Mortality is now uncommon.

◼ DIPHTHERIA

Etiology

Diphtheria is caused by toxigenic strains of the bacterium *Corynebacterium diphtheriae* and, less frequently, *C. ulcerans.* The organism may be isolated on bacterial culture of nasal and pharyngeal swabs, and serologic studies may detect antibodies to diphtheria toxin. Polymerase chain reaction can confirm *C. diphtheriae tox* genes.[56]

Epidemiology

Diphtheritic laryngitis was once the most common infectious cause of acute upper airway obstruction in children. Although it became uncommon due to widespread immunization programs started in the 1940s, it remains a serious disease in parts of the world. Large outbreaks occurred in the 1990s throughout Russia and the independent countries of the former Soviet Union (nearly 50,000 cases were reported). In 2005, 36 countries reported almost 13,000 cases to the World Health Organization, and 80% were from India.[57] The last childhood deaths reported in the UK were 1 in 1994 and 1 in 2008.[58] Most life-threatening cases occurred in unvaccinated or inadequately immunized persons, and it is important for children traveling to these countries, particularly for extended periods, to be vaccinated. A list of endemic countries is available on the Centers for Disease Control website *(wwwnc.cdc.gov/travel/ yellowbook/2012/chapter-3-infectious-diseases-related- to-travel/diphtheria.htm)*. Adults are particularly at risk because protective levels of diphtheria antibodies decrease progressively with time from immunization, so re-immunization is recommended before travel. The Third National Health and Nutrition Examination Survey of U.S. residents (1988 to 1994) indicated that fully protective levels (≥0.1 IU/mL) were found in 91% of children 6 to 11 years of age, but only in 30% of adults 60 to 69 years of age.[59]

Pathophysiology

Diphtheria is an acute disease, primarily involving the tonsils, pharynx, larynx, nose, skin, and, occasionally, other mucous membranes. In the milder, catarrhal form, there is no membrane formation, but in the more severe, membranous form, there is a characteristic lesion of one or more patches of an adherent grayish-white membrane, surrounded by inflammation. The toxin causes local tissue destruction at the site of membrane formation, which promotes multiplication and transmission of the bacteria.[60]

Clinical Presentation and Diagnosis

The incubation period is 1 to 6 days. Classic respiratory diphtheria is characterized by an insidious onset, and patients typically present with a 3- to 4-day history of upper respiratory infection. They have a fever, membranous pharyngitis with a sore throat, characteristic fetor oris, cervical lymphadenopathy, and sometimes edema of the surrounding soft tissues (bull-neck appearance). They may have a serosanguinous nasal discharge. Although not always present, the membrane is typically gray, thick, fibrinous, and firmly adherent, so it may bleed on attempted removal (Fig. 25-4). Laryngeal diphtheria most commonly occurs as an extension of pharyngeal involvement in children, leading to increasing hoarseness and stridor. The patient appears toxic, with symptoms of LTB, and signs of severe airway obstruction may develop quickly if the pharyngeal membrane dislodges and obstructs the airway. Complications include secondary pneumonia and toxin-mediated disease including myocarditis or cardiomyopathy, neuritis or paralysis, and adrenal failure with hypotension.[58] Cardiomyopathy can be predicted from a combination of a pseudomembrane score >2 (range is up to 4) and a bull-neck appearance.[61] Case fatality rates vary and can reach 20%, but the mor-

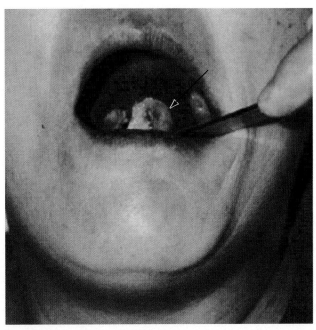

FIGURE 25-4. Diphtheritic membrane *(arrow)* extending from the uvula to the pharyngeal wall in an adult. (From Kadirova R, Kartoglu HÜ, Strebel PM. Clinical characteristics and management of 676 hospitalized diphtheria cases. Kyrgyz Republic 1995. *J Infect Dis.* 2000;181(Suppl 1):S110-S115. Photograph by P. Strebel.)

tality rate was only 3% in a series of 676 patients (30% younger than 15 years of age) reported from the 1995 Kyrgyz Republic outbreak.[62] Deaths are usually a result of airway obstruction, myocarditis/cardiomyopathy, or sepsis (disseminated intravascular coagulation and renal failure).

Management

Because diphtheria is now rare, a high index of suspicion is important to make the diagnosis and institute prompt treatment. Patients should be strictly isolated. Diphtheria antitoxin, which is a hyperimmune equine antiserum (available from the Centers for Disease Control and Prevention), should be administered without waiting for laboratory confirmation because it neutralizes circulating toxin, but not toxin bound to tissues. Antibiotics are not a substitute for antitoxin, but they are given to eradicate the organism, stop toxin production, and reduce the likelihood of transmission.[60] Intravenous penicillin or erythromycin is used, and once the child can swallow comfortably, treatment can be given orally, for a total of 14 days.[60] Mechanical ventilation and tracheostomy may be required. Intravenous dexamethasone has been given to children with laryngeal diphtheria and airway obstruction, and a small case series suggested that it was beneficial.[63] Because the disease may not confer immunity, patients should be given a diphtheria toxoid-containing vaccine during convalescence. Antibiotic prophylaxis (penicillin or erythromycin) is recommended for close contacts after nasal and pharyngeal specimens are taken, and immunization should be given to those who have not been vaccinated in the preceding 5 years.[60]

RETROPHARYNGEAL ABSCESS

Etiology

Retropharyngeal abscesses generally result from lymphatic spread of infection, although direct spread from adjacent areas, penetrating pharyngeal trauma (e.g., a fall with a pencil in the mouth), or foreign bodies can also play a role.[5] It has also been reported as a complication of adenoidectomy and adenotonsillectomy.[64,65] Infection is usually due to mixed flora, including *S. aureus* (methicillin-sensitive and resistant), various streptococcal species, HiB, and anaerobes.[66]

Epidemiology

The majority of cases occur in children younger than 6 years of age, probably due to the fact that retropharyngeal lymph nodes are so abundant at this age (they tend to atrophy later in life). Analysis of the U.S.-based Kid's Inpatient Database (KID) for 2003 covering 36 states revealed 1321 admissions with a mean age of 5.1 years, and 63% were boys; there were no deaths reported.[67] Another large series reported a median age of 3 years, with 75% of those affected younger than 5 years of age and 16% younger than 1 year of age.[66] In a large series from 1995 to 2006, there was a linear increase in incidence through the period.[68]

Pathophysiology

The retropharyngeal space (between the posterior pharyngeal wall and the prevertebral layer of deep cervical fascia) contains loose connective tissue and lymph nodes that drain the nasopharynx, paranasal sinuses, middle ear, teeth, and adjacent bones. The space extends from the base of the skull down to vertebra C7 or T1. Acute bacterial infection in this region may start as retropharyngeal cellulitis with localized thickening of the tissues, which can progress to purulent inflammation of the tissues and retropharyngeal adenitis. However, when this process is caused by lymphatic spread, it starts as adenitis. If liquefaction of one of the nodes occurs, an abscess can form and is usually contained within the inflammatory rind of the infected node.

Clinical Presentation and Diagnosis

Presentation is often nonspecific, and there may be overlap with the presentation of croup, epiglottitis, tracheitis, and peritonsillar abscess (see Table 25-1).[5] Children with acute epiglottitis tend to appear more toxic and progress to respiratory distress more rapidly.[69] Excluding causes secondary to foreign bodies or trauma, patients usually have a history of viral upper respiratory infection that lasts several days and then worsens. Children then have high fever, sore throat, dysphagia, poor feeding, neck pain, and stiffness. Limitation of neck extension and torticollis are more common than limited neck flexion.[66] Although the occurrence of neck signs with fever may

suggest meningitis, children tend not to be as toxic as those with meningitis. Further deterioration may lead to extrathoracic airway compromise, with drooling, stridor, and respiratory distress. The classical picture of stridor and airway obstruction seems to be less common now, and in a series of cases reported by pediatricians from 1993 to 1998, only 3% of 64 children in Salt Lake City had stridor or wheezing.[66] However in a series of cases from 2002 to 2007 from the same center, but published by the otolaryngologists, 14/130 (11%) presented with airways obstruction, and 50% required intubation, with an average age of 1.4 years.[70] Older series have reported a higher incidence of stridor. Reported rates include 71% in patients younger than 1 year of age, 43% in patients older than 1 year of age, and no stridor in those older than 3 years of age in a series of 31 children in Sydney, Australia[71]; a rate of 56% in 17 patients in Denver[72]; and a rate of 23% in 65 children in Los Angeles.[73] It is possible that the spectrum of disease is changing, but it is more likely that the diagnosis is being made earlier, before the airways are compromised.[66] Sometimes a retropharyngeal mass is visible in the mouth, seen as an asymmetrical bulge of the posterior pharyngeal wall (Fig. 25-5), or a neck mass (marked lymphadenopathy or parapharyngeal abscess) is visible and palpable. Complications include rupture of the abscess with aspiration, asphyxiation or pneumonia, extension to a mediastinal abscess, Lemierre's syndrome, and vascular complications (e.g., thrombophlebitis of the internal jugular vein and erosion through the carotid artery sheath).[64,69]

Once the child is stable and safe, a lateral neck radiograph with the neck in full extension may confirm the diagnosis. Widened prevertebral soft-tissue and air-fluid levels in the retropharyngeal space are all indicators.[5] The radiograph must be taken in the correct position (true lateral orientation, with the neck in extension, and, if possible, during full inspiration) to ensure that the

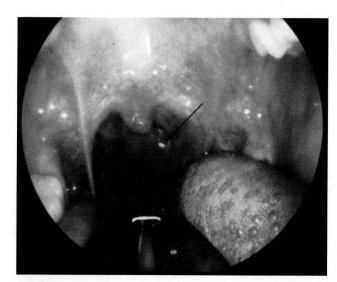

FIGURE 25-5. Retropharyngeal abscess behind and to the left of the uvula *(arrow)* is shown. The tongue is pressed down and to the left with a tongue depressor. (Photograph courtesy of the Otolaryngology Teaching Set, Department of Ear, Nose & Throat, Great Ormond Street Hospital for Children NHS Trust, London.)

retropharyngeal space is not falsely thickened.[66] A contrast-enhanced computed tomography scan is useful because it differentiates a fully developed abscess from cellulitis and delineates the full extent of the abscess. Blood cultures findings are usually negative, but the white blood cell count will be increased.

Management

Traditionally, management involves surgical drainage of the abscess (plus antibiotics). However, more cases are being managed by intravenous antibiotics alone, although surgery must be considered early if there is a compromised airway. In one older series, 25% of patients required no surgery,[72] but in the Salt Lake City series that covered 1993 to 1998, 58% of 64 patients had antibiotics alone, with no treatment failures.[66] Data from KID 2003 (discussed earlier in the chapter) showed that 57% of cases admitted did not require surgical drainage.[67] Many children start treatment with antibiotics before the diagnosis is made, and certainly retropharyngeal cellulitis can be treated with antibiotics alone. When necessary, surgical drainage is performed through the intraoral route. Care must be taken to avoid aspiration of the infected material. Occasionally, if there is extension lateral to the great vessels, external drainage through the neck is necessary. Mortality is rare now, with no deaths in recent reports.

■ PERITONSILLAR ABSCESS (QUINSY)

Etiology

A peritonsillar abscess is usually a complication of acute tonsillitis, but it may follow pharyngitis or a previous peritonsillar abscess. The infection usually involves mixed bacterial flora, with *Streptococcus pyogenes* the predominant organism. In a small series of children younger than 5 years of age, *Streptococcus viridans* was the most common organism detected.[74] In a large series of 457 children and adults in Israel, while *Streptococcus pyogenes* was the most common organism isolated, there was a sharp rise in anerobes cultured, particularly *Prevotella* and *Peptostreptococcus*.[75]

Epidemiology

Peritonsillar abscess is the most common deep-space head and neck infection in both adults and children. However, it is more common in young adults than in children. It tends to affect older children, and in one large, 10-year series, the mean age was 12 years of age, with two thirds of those affected older than 10 years of age.[76] In this series, 62% of cases occurred on the left side versus 38% on the right (with no obvious explanation).[76] There is no seasonal predilection. The reduction of antibiotic prescribing to children by general practitioners in the United Kingdom from 1993-2003 has not been accompanied by an increase in hospital admissions for peritonsillar abscess.[77]

Pathophysiology

Peritonsillar abscess is believed to arise from the spread of infection from the tonsil or the mucous glands of Weber, located in the superior tonsillar pole.[76] There is a spectrum of peritonsillar cellulitis that may then result in a collection of pus located between the tonsillar capsule (pharyngobasilar fascia), the superior constrictor, and the palatopharyngeus muscle.[76] There is a risk of spread through the muscle into the parapharyngeal space or other deep neck spaces. The abscess pushes the adjacent tonsil downward and medially, and the uvula may be so edematous as to resemble a white grape.

Clinical Presentation and Diagnosis

The child, who is already affected by acute tonsillitis, becomes more ill with a high fever and has a severe sore throat or neck pain, as well as marked dysphagia with referred earache. Absent or decreased oral intake can lead to dehydration, particularly in younger children.

Cervical lymphadenopathy is almost always present. The uvula is edematous and deviated to one side, and there is fetor oris. A striking feature may be trismus, with limited mouth opening. Examination may be difficult in a young, uncooperative child who refuses to open the mouth. The white blood cell count will be elevated.

The relevance of this condition to pediatric pulmonologists is that acute enlargement of the tonsils can cause airway compromise, and a ruptured abscess can lead to aspiration of infected material and subsequent pneumonia. In one large series of 169 children under 18 years of age, 8% presented with airway compromise.[78]

Management

Children may need intravenous fluids. Antibiotics are necessary, and intravenous penicillin is as effective as broad-spectrum antibiotics, although additional anaerobic coverage should be considered.[79] Analgesia is important. Corticosteroids are not uncommonly used but are of no obvious benefit (or harm).[78] Treatment often involves needle aspiration or incision and drainage; a meta-analysis of 10 studies with 496 patients revealed an average 94% success rate with simple needle aspiration.[80] Nevertheless, an initial period of medical treatment is appropriate in the absence of airway compromise and systemic toxicity, especially in younger children.[81] There is some debate among otolaryngologists about the role and timing of tonsillectomy, and peritonsillar abscess is no longer considered an absolute indication for tonsillectomy, although a history of recurrent tonsillitis prior to developing the peritonsillar abscess leads to a higher recurrence rate.[82]

■ INFECTIOUS MONONUCLEOSIS

Infectious mononucleosis is caused by Ebstein-Barr virus (EBV) and is common in adolescents and young adults. The clinical syndrome is characterized by fever, fatigue, malaise, lymphadenopathy, and sore throat. Diagnosis is confirmed by positive EBV serology, and positive heterophile antibodies (Monospot), although the latter are only positive in 50% of children and 90% of adults. The illness is usually self-limiting, but malaise and exhaustion can persist.

Some degree of airway obstruction is not uncommon (reported in 25% to 60% cases[58]), but significant airway compromise is rare, occurring in an estimated 1% to 3.5% cases.[83] Nevertheless, given the high frequency of EBV infection, this small proportion still represents many patients. Acute upper airway obstruction may occur, but the cardinal signs of acute obstruction (stridor and respiratory distress with recession and tachypnea) can be absent until late in the process.[84] Obstruction arises from a combination of inflammation and hypertrophy of the palatal and nasopharyngeal tonsils, edema of the pharynx and epiglottis, and pseudomembrane formation in the large airways.[85] Peritonsillar abscess formation is a rare complication that can further compromise the airway, and it is now believed that this is not significantly associated with the use of corticosteroids, which contradicts earlier reports.[86]

Management is with systemic corticosteroids (in the presence of obstruction) and supportive care, which may include ventilation. A tracheostomy is sometimes necessary. If corticosteroids do not help, the role of acute tonsillectomy has been advocated,[87] but it is controversial due to the high risk of perioperative bleeding.[85]

Suggested Reading

Bjornson CL, Johnson DW. Croup. *Lancet.* 2008;371:329–339.
Jenkins IA, Saunders M. Infections of the airway. *Pediatr Anesthesia.* 2009;19(suppl 1):118–130.
Johnson D. Croup. *Clin Evid.* 2004;(12):401–426.
Loftis L. Acute infectious upper airway obstructions in children. *Semin Pediatr Infect Dis.* 2006;17:5–10.

References

The complete reference list is available online at www.expertconsult.com

26 BRONCHITIS

Anne B. Chang, MBBS, FRACP, MPHTM, PhD

Bronchitis is a component of almost all (if not all) airway diseases. In the literal translation of the word, *bronchitis* refers to inflammation of the bronchus or bronchi. However, bronchitis has different major overlapping constructs based on duration (e.g., acute, subacute, chronic), inflammation type (e.g., neutrophilic, eosinophilic, lymphocytic, neurogenic), phenotype, and clinical syndromes (e.g., acute bronchitis, larygnotracheobronchitis, protracted bacterial bronchitis, aspiration bronchitis) (Fig. 26-1). A diagnostic entity may have varying types of airway inflammation (Table 26-1). For example, acute viral bronchitis is associated with both lymphocytic and neutrophilic inflammation. Although the type of airway inflammation does not distinguish etiology of the bronchitis in children, it provides supportive diagnosis. Cough is the dominant symptom when bronchitis is present, other than when bronchitis is very mild.

General Annotations on Cough

In countries where data are available, cough is the most common symptom that results in new medical consultations.[1,2] In the United States, 29.5 million doctor visits per year are for cough.[3] In Australia, acute bronchitis/bronchiolitis is consistently the most common new problem encountered by general practitioners, ranging from an annual rate of 2.2 to 3.2 per 100 encounters (1999 to 2009 data).[2] The burden of cough is also reflected in the billions of dollars spent annually on over-the-counter (OTC) cough medications, as well as the number of consultations (per child) sought for cough. In an Australian pediatric study, the number of medical consultations for coughing illness in the last 12 months was high: >80% of children had ≥5 doctor visits, and 53% had >10 visits.[4]

Evaluating Cough

Children with cough require a systematic evaluation and approach. A complete review of cough is beyond the scope of this chapter, and readers are referred elsewhere for an evidenced-based approach[5] and guidelines.[6–8] The overall evaluation entails defining the etiology (which includes assessing if further tests and or treatment are required); the exacerbation factors (e.g., exposure to environmental tobacco smoke [ETS]), and the expectations and effect on the child and family. Treatment should be etiology-based. When a clear etiology cannot be identified and medications are trialed, reassessment of the child is recommended in 2 to 3 weeks (the "time to response" for most medications).[6,7] Also, clinicians should be cognizant of the "time-period effect" and "placebo effect." The placebo effect is as high as 80% in cough studies.[9] The time-period effect[10] refers to the spontaneous resolution of cough with time. It has been described that parents who wanted medicine at the initial visit reported more improvement at follow-up, regardless of whether the child received drug, placebo, or no treatment.[11] Therefore, one must predetermine the time factor and *a-priori* definition of what constitutes an improvement in cough because the studies that do not predefine these issues have limited validity.

Defining Etiology

The most likely etiology depends on the setting; selection criteria of children studied; follow-up rate; and depth of clinical history, physical examination, and investigations performed. In defining the etiology, it is helpful to define cough types in accordance to different constructs. Pediatric cough can be classified in several constructs based on (1) timeframe (acute, chronic), (2) likelihood of an identifiable underlying primary etiology (e.g., specific and nonspecific cough), and (3) characteristic (wet versus dry). For clinical practicality, timeframe is commonly used, divided into acute (<2 weeks), subacute (2 to 4 weeks) and chronic (>4 weeks) cough. No studies have clearly defined when cough should be defined as chronic (variably defined from >4 to 8 weeks).[6–8] Cough related to an upper acute respiratory infection (ARI) resolves within 10 days in 50% of children and by 25 days in 90%;[12] Arguably, childhood chronic cough should be defined as persistent daily cough of >4 weeks. This duration includes a "safety factor" in the recognition that foreign body airway aspiration is not uncommon in children, and thus a systematic approach is required in those with chronic cough because they are likely to have a complicated ARI or other etiology.

Exacerbation Factors

When reviewing any child with cough irrespective of etiology, exacerbation factors including exposure to environmental pollutants (e.g., ETS) should be explored. However, outside of epidemiologic studies, chronic cough should not be simply ascribed to ETS exposure. Cohort studies on children with chronic cough have shown that cough resolution was still achieved in children exposed to ETS,[13,14] including a cohort with high exposure rates (56%).[13] This suggests that, while ETS is undoubtedly associated with increased coughing illnesses and is an important contributing factor, ETS alone is not the sole etiology. Other exacerbation factors include exposure to other pollutants[15] and secondary gain from having a cough (e.g., attention from parents, missing school).

Expectations and Effects

Parents of children with chronic cough do not have symptoms of anxiety or depression but are stressed.[4] This is in contrast to adults with chronic cough, which is

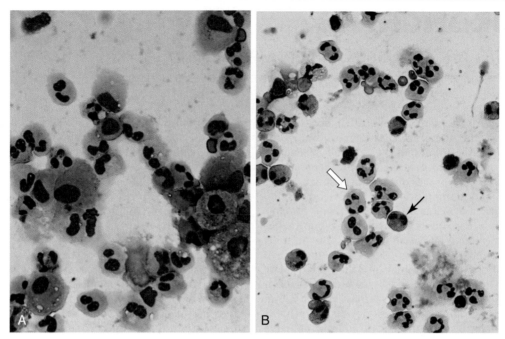

FIGURE 26-1. Micrographs of BAL cytospins showing different types of inflammation. **A,** Neutrophilic inflammation in BAL of a child with protracted bacterial bronchitis. **B,** BAL showing eosinophilic *(black arrow)* and neutrophilic *(clear arrow)* inflammation in a child with bronchiectasis and strongyloides infection.

TABLE 26-1 DOMINANT TYPE OF AIRWAY CELLULARITY IN COMMON CHILDHOOD DISEASES WITH BRONCHITIS

INFLAMMATION TYPE	EXAMPLES OF DISEASE	OTHER KEY AIRWAY MAKERS
Neutrophilic	Acute viral infection[69] Bronchiectasis[70,71] Cystic fibrosis[72] Protracted bacterial bronchitis[44] Chronic lung disease of prematurity[73] Severe bronchiolitis[74] Aspiration lung disease	Soluble intercellular adhesion molecule-1 Elevated IL-8, neutrophil elastase, TNF-α Elevated IL-8, neutrophil elastase, proteases Elevated IL-8, MMP-9 Proinflammatory cytokines and chemokines Myeloperoxidase, CD11b
Eosinophilic	Atopic asthma[75] Helminth infections (e.g., toxocara and strongyloides)*[71] Allergic bronchopulmonary aspergillosis*[76]	Elevated nitric oxide in steroid naïve Neutrophilic inflammation may also be present with elevated IL-8 and MMP-9[76]
Lymphocytic	Acute viral infection[69] Bronchiolitis obliterans[77] Autoimmune disease*[78]	Soluble intercellular adhesion molecule-1
Neurogenic	Post-RSV infection[79] Cough with gastroesophageal reflux[80]	substance P, nerve growth factor

*Data from nonpediatric studies.
IL, Interleukin; *MMP,* matrix metalloproteinase.

associated with the presence of depression and anxiety.[16] Thus clinicians need to be cognizant of the stress parents have when dealing with children with chronic cough and discuss expectations and fears. The reasons for parental fears and concerns include etiology of the cough, risk of choking, and the possibility of long-term respiratory damage.[4,17,]

Clinical Phenotypes or Syndromes of Childhood Bronchitis

While bronchitis is present in airway diseases, several clinical phenotypes of childhood bronchitis are characteristic and discussed in the following paragraphs. Other conditions associated with bronchitis (e.g., aspiration, asthma, bronchitis associated with other pathogens such as tuberculosis, and laryngotracheobronchitis) are discussed in other chapters. The precise mechanisms underpinning acute bronchitis will vary depending on the insulting agent (i.e., the properties of the infectious agent) and the host's characteristics (e.g., pre-existing conditions) and response (e.g., the host's innate and adaptive immunity, and genetic predisposition to intensity of inflammation).

Acute Bronchitis

Acute bronchitis has a dedicated code in the International Classification of Disease (ICD). It is a nonprecise term and often overlaps with other conditions of the respiratory tract. The most common cause of acute cough, acute bronchitis is caused by viral ARIs.[18] Fifty-six percent of children with ARI are still unwell 4 days after initial consultation. The percentage decreases to 26% on the 7th day and to 6% by the 14th day.[19] However, cough was not specifically reported in the study.[19] A systematic review on the natural history of acute cough in children 0 to 4 years of age in primary care reported that the majority of children improve with time, but 5% to 10% progress to develop protracted bronchitis or pneumonia.[20] A prospective community-based study in 600 families in Melbourne, Australia,[21] found that most acute bronchitis episodes last 2 to 5 days. Leder and colleagues[21] also described that children younger than 2 years of age were more likely to have at least one respiratory infection, a higher number of episodes per person, and the longest episode duration (6.8 days).[21] The frequency of ARIs was age-dependent, with a reduction in incidence with increasing age. Yearly rate per person was 3.8 in children 0 to 1 years of age; 3.3 in children 2 to 3 years of age; 2.8 in children 4 to 5 years of age; 2.2 in children 6 to 10 years of age; and 2 in children 11 to 20 years of age.[21] Bearing in mind the different definitions and sampling frames, studies from developing countries show higher rates of ARIs (3.7 to 14.9 per child per year).[21]

Etiology of Acute Bronchitis

Any pathogen that infects the respiratory tract can cause bronchitis. These include viruses, bacteria, mycoplasma, chlamydia, fungi, and helminths. However, only viruses, bacteria, mycoplasma, and chlamydia are considered in the clinical phenotype of acute bronchitis. Respiratory viruses are the most common etiology.[22,18] Importantly, 17% to 33% of infections involve co-infections with (single or multiple) viruses or bacteria.[23,24] In developed countries, both viral and bacterial infections are likely to be self-limited. Common respiratory viruses in children are human rhinovirus (HRV), coronaviruses, respiratory syncytial virus (RSV) (A and B), parainfluenza (1 to 3), influenza, adenovirus, and human metapneumovirus (hMPV).[18] In birth cohort studies,[22] the most common respiratory pathogens were found to be HRV, followed by RSV and coronavirus. More and more new respiratory viruses are being identified, and recent additions include subtypes of HRV, human enteroviruses (HEVs), and human parechoviruses (HPeVs).[25] Although some viruses are more commonly associated with certain syndromes

(e.g., RSV causes bronchiolitis and parainfluenza causes croup), any of these respiratory pathogens can cause acute bronchitis. With modern molecular techniques, co-infections are also found[25] in both symptomatic and asymptomatic children.[18,26] In a study on children with asthma exacerbations, viral co-detections occurred in 25.6% of children.[27] While co-infections were associated with lower asthma quality of life scores upon presentation than were single viral detections, the recovery phase (including symptoms of acute bronchitis) was not influenced by the presence or absence of virus.[25] There is no consensus in the literature about the relationship between clinical severity and co-detection of viruses. Persistence of symptoms is most likely to indicate a bacterial infection, either as a consequence of altered immunity from the initial viral insult[28] or a primary infection.[29]

Management of Acute Bronchitis

Viral ARIs are the most common cause of acute cough in children, and most affected children do not visit doctors. However when they do, children need to be assessed adequately for other respiratory etiologies (e.g., inhalation of a foreign body) and other infections (e.g., pneumonia and bronchiolitis). Complications develop in 8% to 12% of children with upper ARIs.[12] Fever alone, or fever with chest signs was found to be good predictors for complications in children with cough. However, the discriminatory ability is weak[30] and, to date, there is insufficient data to predict who will develop complications of acute bronchitis. Acute cough may also be the presenting symptom of an underlying disorder, and the presence of specific pointers (Table 26-2) should alert practitioners to the possibility of an underlying problem (e.g., a congenital/developmental respiratory or immunologic disorder). Differentiating uncomplicated ARIs from pneumonia has been relatively widely studied in developing countries where chest wall retractions and respiratory rate are good predictors of pneumonia.[31] Use of chest radiographs does not improve outcome in ambulatory children with acute lower respiratory infection.[32]

TABLE 26-2 POINTERS TO THE PRESENCE OF SPECIFIC COUGH*

Auscultatory findings such as crackles and wheezes
Cardiac abnormalities
Chest pain
Chest wall abnormality
Digital clubbing
Daily moist or productive cough
Dyspnea
Dysphagia
Exertional dyspnea
Hemoptysis
Immune deficiency (primary or secondary)
Neurodevelopmental abnormality
Recurrent pneumonia
Respiratory noises (stridor, wheeze)
Systemic symptoms (fever, weight loss, failure to thrive)

*Cough related to an underlying lung disease

Interventions

The American Academy of Family Physician's guidelines discourage the use of antimicrobials except when rhinosinusitis and cough is present and has not improved after 10 days.[33] Meta-analysis on antimicrobials for acute bronchitis (recent onset of productive cough without chronic obstructive pulmonary disease, sinusitis, or pneumonia) in children showed that patients receiving antibiotics were less likely to have a cough 7 to 14 days after initiation of treatment and less likely to show no improvement on the clinician's global assessment They were more likely to have shorter duration of cough, and feel ill.[30] However the benefits were small and translate into a reduction of symptoms for only a fraction of a day.[30] Thus the NICE recommends a "no antibiotic prescribing strategy or a delayed antibiotic prescribing strategy," unless the patient is systemically very unwell, has symptoms and signs that suggest serious illness or complications, or has high risk of serious complications because of pre-existing comorbidity (e.g., heart, lung, renal, liver, or neuromuscular disease; immunosuppression; cystic fibrosis; and young children who were born prematurely).[30] Other logical inclusions in this list are children with airway lesions with impaired airway clearance (tracheobronchomalacia), suppurative lung disease, and recurrent protracted bronchitis.

Parents' and caregivers' concerns and expectations should be determined and addressed, and advice about the usual natural history of the illness (up to 3 weeks for acute bronchitis) should be given.[30] OTC medications for cough confer no benefit in the symptomatic control of cough in children.[34,35] Moreover "OTC medications can be associated with significant morbidity and even mortality in both acute overdoses and when administered in correct doses for long periods of time."[36] The use of steam inhalation, vitamin C, zinc, echinacea, or lozenges for upper ARIs confer little benefit or have not been specifically examined for the symptomatic relief of cough.[37] A single RCT reported that treatment with nimesulide was associated with clinically significant improvement in cough and other signs and symptoms (rhinorrhea, nasal obstruction, pharyngeal redness, swelling of lymph nodes and cough), but this drug is not licensed in North America, the United Kingdom, Australia, or New Zealand because of safety concerns.[38] There is also no data of sufficient quality on the efficacy of Chinese herbs for acute bronchitis.[39] In ambulatory children with acute cough (1 to 10 days) with no history of asthma and a normal chest examination, oral albuterol was not effective in reducing cough frequency or duration in children.[40] In addition, β_2-agonists are not efficacious in reducing cough in children with acute bronchitis who do not have airflow obstruction.[41]

Protracted Bacterial Bronchitis

Acute bronchitis can progress to protracted bacterial bronchitis (PBB). PBB, a type of chronic airway inflammation in children, is a recently recognized clinical entity.[14] It was previously called various names including *chronic bronchitis*. Bronchitis related to suppurative lung disease is discussed in Chapter 30. The term *chronic bronchitis* should no longer be used as a diagnosis in children, as the etiologic underlying cause of any bronchitis that is chronic should be defined and appropriately treated.

Symptoms of PBB have long been recognized by pediatric pulmonologists (but have only been adequately characterized recently.[14,42–44] The original description of PBB required three criteria; (1) a history of chronic wet cough, (2) positive BAL culture ($\geq 10^5$ colony-forming units [CFU]/mL) (Fig. 26-2), and (3) response to antimicrobial treatment with cough resolution within 2 weeks.[14] PBB sometimes truncated to *protracted bronchitis (PB)* is clinically defined as (1) the presence of isolated chronic (>4 weeks) wet/moist cough, (2) resolution of cough with antimicrobial treatment, and (3) absence of pointers suggestive of an alternative specific cause of cough.[6,45] The criterion of demonstration of endobronchial airway infection by culturing respiratory pathogens from BAL is not feasible in the routine clinical setting.

PBB is differentiated from acute bronchitis by cough of shorter duration (≤ 2 weeks in acute bronchitis). Children with PBB are typically young (younger than 5 years of age) and do not have any other systemic symptoms such as clinical sinusitis or ear disease. Some parents may report a "wheeze." Tracheomalacia or bronchomalacia may coexist. On clinical assessment however, they usually do not have wheeze but a "ruttle or rattle" reflective of airway secretions.[42] Many of these children have been misdiagnosed as having asthma.[14,42] Their chest x-rays usually show peribronchial thickening or may be reported as "normal."[42,46] Like children with chronic cough, children with PBB have significant morbidity; parents typically have seen multiple medical practitioners for their child's chronic cough in the

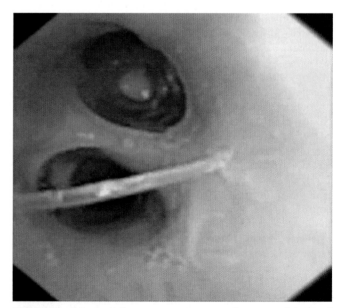

FIGURE 26-2. Bronchoscopic appearances of protracted bacterial bronchitis. A strand of mucus is present, just proximal to the left lower lobe bronchus, and there are prominent secretions in the lingula bronchus. The BAL cultured *H. influenzae* and *S. pneumoniae*, both at a density of $\geq 10^5$ CFU/mL. Polymerase chain reaction tests were negative for respiratory viruses (influenzas A and B, RSV, parainfluenzas 1 and 2, adenovirus, and human metapneumovirus), Mycoplasma, and Chlamydia.

last 12 months.[45] In PBB the child's cough resolves only after a prolonged course of appropriate antibiotics (12 to 14 days).

Pathogenesis of Protracted Bacterial Bronchitis

PBB is associated with bacterial infection in the airways,[42,14] and it is widely accepted that persistent bacterial infection is harmful.[47] The organisms most commonly identified in the airways (sputum or BAL) of children with PBB are common respiratory bacteria such as nontypeable *H. influenzae*, *S. pneumoniae*, and *M. catarrhalis*.[42,14] Transient viral ARIs in early childhood commonly precede PBB as the most common initiating event. However, colonization may be secondary to conditions that impair cough such as neuromuscular disease, mucus plugging in asthmatics, airway lesions that impede efficient airway clearance (e.g., tracheobronchomalacia), or mucosal damage secondary to aspiration. Tracheobronchomalacia is a common finding in children with PBB,[14] which may be a primary phenomenon (airway malacia predisposes to PBB through reduced efficiency in airway clearance) or a secondary phenomenon (malacia occurs as a consequence of intense airway inflammation).[48] Persistent airway colonization and neutrophilic inflammation may evolve to chronic mucus hypersecretion and further airway inflammation. In some cases, cumulative airway injury from recurrent or persistent bacterial infection can lead to bronchiectasis.[45] Repeated microbial exposure, especially during childhood, likely shapes later immune system responses.[49]

PBB is also likely to be heterogeneous, with neutrophilic airway inflammation developing by a variety of mechanisms. It is likely that an innate immune dysfunction or immature adaptive immune response is present, at least in a subgroup of these children. In 150 children without lung disease undergoing gastroscopy, a group of children with bacterial colonization, airway neutrophilia, and protracted cough was identified.[50] Bacterial colonization of the lower airways in these children was associated with reduced expression of both the toll-like receptor (TLR) -4 and the preprotachykinin gene, *TAC1*, that encodes substance P,[51] which also has a defensin-like function.[52] These data suggest that a dysfunction of innate immunity plays a role in PBB (at least in a subgroup of children), but the nature and duration of such immune dysfunction has been not defined.

Outcomes of Children with Protracted Bacterial Bronchitis

Long-term cohort data are currently not available. However, some children with PBB have recurrent episodes or a relapse of PBB weeks after initial treatment. These children should be investigated along the lines for a child with chronic suppurative lung disease (CSLD) (Chapter 30). It is also likely that recurrent PBB is a risk factor for chronic suppurative lung disease and bronchiectasis. Indeed it is highly likely that PBB, CSLD, and bronchiectasis represent part of a spectrum.[45] The likely link between PBB and bronchiectasis is based theoretically on a vicious circle hypothesis[53] and, experimentally, on old natural history data.[54,55]

Plastic Bronchitis

Plastic bronchitis is rare (and becoming more rare in the current era) and is characterized by the formation of bronchial casts that cause obstruction of the airways (Fig. 26-3). Bronchial casts have been divided into two types. Type I casts are inflammatory, consist mainly of fibrin with cellular infiltrates, and occur in inflammatory diseases of the lung. Type II, or acellular casts, consist mainly of mucin with a few cells and usually occur following surgery for congenital cardiac defects.[56] However analysis of casts may not fit neatly into either category.[57] Many etiologic factors have been associated with plastic bronchitis; these include cardiac defects (particularly after Fontan's procedure),[58] sickle cell disease (acute chest syndrome),[59] asthma, aspergillosis, pneumonia, cystic fibrosis,[60] pulmonary lymphatic disorders,[57] and neoplastic infiltrates.[61] The pathogenesis of cast formation is unknown but probably involves abnormal mucin accumulation, with reduced airway clearance and dehydration, in a genetically predisposed person.[57]

Children with plastic bronchitis usually present with cough and respiratory distress (with or without wheezing). Chest pain may also be present, and chest radiograph usually reveals atelectasis. Life-threatening events were higher in patients with cardiac defects (41%) than in those with asthma (0%, p = 0.02).[56] Diagnosis is made by bronchoscopy, which is also therapeutic (see Fig. 26-3). There are some case reports on the use of rhDNase.[59] Others have reported the use of inhaled corticosteroids, tissue plasminogen activator, macrolides, and inhaled heparin.[57] An alternative is direct instillation of dilute bicarbonate solution by fiberoptic bronchoscopy (used by

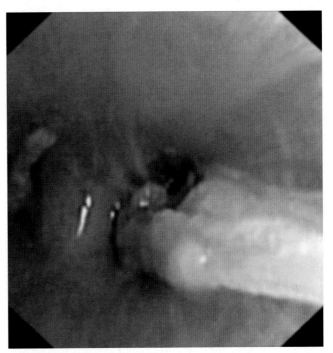

FIGURE 26-3. Bronchoscopic appearances of plastic bronchitis related to allergic bronchopulmonary aspergillosis and cystic fibrosis. The child presented with chronic cough and chest pain (no respiratory distress). The chest radiograph showed persistent changes in the lingula. The cast was removed bronchoscopically with resolution on the chest radiograph.

the author with resolution; unpublished data). It remains unclear which is the best treatment strategy. Reported mortality from plastic bronchitis is 16% and increases to 29% in patients with cardiac defects.[56]

Other Causes of and Contributors to Bronchitis

A complete review on the effects of pollutants and other possible causes of bronchitis (e.g., silent aspiration)[62] or associations (e.g., allergic rhinitis, gastroesophageal reflux) are described in other chapters. The most clinically important air pollutant in childhood bronchitis is tobacco smoke (*in-utero* and *ex-utero*). This has been extensively reviewed[63] and always requires addressing by counseling[64] and other modalities. Systematic reviews have described the link between cough and air pollution (indoors and outdoors).[15,65] It is increasingly appreciated in human and animal studies that environmental pollutants may have additive effects[66] and may influence the respiratory apparatus directly and indirectly through the immune system[67] and neural[68] pathways. However, irrespective of exposure, cough should not be simply ascribed to pollutants (see the "Exacerbation Factors" section) in clinical settings.

References

The complete reference list is available online at www.expertconsult.com

27 BRONCHIOLITIS

SAMINA ALI, MDCM, FRCP(C), FAAP, AMY C. PLINT, MD, MSC, AND TERRY PAUL KLASSEN, MD, MSC, FRCPC

Acute viral bronchiolitis is a clinically diagnosed condition characterized by a wheezing illness associated with an upper respiratory tract infection (URTI). It typically presents with coryza and low-grade fever that progresses to cough; tachypnea; hyperinflation; intercostal chest wall retractions; grunting; nasal flaring; and diffuse crackles, wheezes, or both.[1] Most definitions of bronchiolitis limit the affected age group to younger than 2 years of age, with some limiting it even further, to 12 months of age. Bronchiolitis is characterized by acute inflammation, edema, necrosis of small airway epithelial cells, increased mucus production, and bronchospasm.[2] Worldwide, it is one of the most common respiratory tract infections of infants.

INCIDENCE

Respiratory syncytial virus (RSV) is the most common etiology for bronchiolitis, with the highest incidence of infections in North America from December to April of each year.[3] In warmer climates, the first presentations of RSV tend to occur earlier, during the fall or summer months.[4]

In North America, bronchiolitis is the leading cause of hospitalization for infants younger than 1 year of age.[5,6] An estimated 75,000 to 125,000 American infants are hospitalized each year with this illness, representing approximately 2% to 3% of all children affected with bronchiolitis.[7,8] In both Canada and the United States, admissions for this illness have increased 1.4- to 2.4-fold over the last decade, and it has been associated with increasing morbidity and cost.[7,9] It is estimated that annual health costs associated with bronchiolitis reach $1 billion in the United States.[8]

CLINICAL PRESENTATION

Bronchiolitis is virally induced bronchiolar inflammation. As such, its clinical manifestations closely resemble those of an older child with asthma. There has been much debate about a definition for bronchiolitis as it is a clinical diagnosis and, as such, relies upon clinician judgment of presenting signs and symptoms. The American Academy of Pediatrics Clinical Practice Guideline defines bronchiolitis as "a constellation of clinical symptoms and signs including a viral upper respiratory prodrome followed by increased respiratory effort and wheezing in children less than two years of age."[2] Infants with bronchiolitis often have abnormal vital signs. For children with bronchiolitis, respiratory rate is often higher than 50 to 60 breaths per minute, and often heart rate is increased as well. Elevated body temperature may or may not be present; when present, fever may reach as high as 41° C. Oxygen saturation measurements by pulse oximeter are commonly used to assess children with bronchiolitis.

Although ubiquitous in most health care settings, pulse oximeters are not without their limitations; they can misread the oxygen saturation due to normal monitor variations (+/–2%), motion artifact, or poor placement.[10] Clinicians must take care to confirm a hypoxemic reading on a pulse oximeter, prior to initiating oxygen therapy. While there is no one clinical sign or symptom that accurately diagnoses hypoxemia, studies suggest that cyanosis, grunting, difficulty feeding, and level of mental alertness are predictive.[11] Manifestations of URTI, including mild conjunctivitis, otitis media, and pharyngitis, are present in many of the patients.

The clinical presentation of bronchiolitis can be quite variable, both over time and between patients. A child's manifestations may range from mild signs of respiratory distress with transient events such as mucous plugging, all the way to apnea and respiratory failure. Excessive nasal secretions may lead to upper airway obstruction, with both inspiratory and expiratory noise on auscultation. Increased work of breathing is manifested as nasal flaring, intercostal retractions, subcostal retractions, and use of accessory muscles. Upon auscultation, diffuse bilateral wheezes and crackles are often present; the expiratory phase of respiration also can be prolonged. Due to hyperinflation of the lungs secondary to air trapping, it is not uncommon to find the liver and spleen to be palpable in the abdominal exam of an infant with bronchiolitis.

As with any illness of early childhood, it is key to assess the hydration and feeding status of a child with bronchiolitis. This can be done through inquiry regarding total volume of fluid intake, number of wet diapers, presence of tears, and the child's activity level. If care is not taken to address fluid intake early in the child's course of illness, increased work of breathing combined with decreased intake can rapidly lead to dehydration.

Certain underlying conditions can predispose a child to a more turbulent course of illness with bronchiolitis. When inquiring about a child's medical history, care should be taken to inquire about prematurity, chronic lung disease, cardiac disease, immunodeficiency, and neuromuscular disorders.[12]

The utility of radiographs in the diagnosis of bronchiolitis is limited. When available, the radiographic findings tend to be nonspecific and include hyperinflation and patchy atelectasis. Occasionally, peribronchial infiltrates, consolidation, pleural fluid, or pneumonia may be seen.

ETIOLOGIC AGENTS

Respiratory syncytial virus (RSV) is the predominant etiologic agent for acute viral bronchiolitis, and 50% to 80% of cases are attributed to this virus.[13] Ninety percent of children will have been infected with RSV by

2 years of age.[14] Unfortunately, RSV infection does not result in long-term immunity, and re-infections are commonly experienced throughout childhood and into the adult years.

Recently, there has been a notable increase in the number of other viruses recognized as etiologic agents for bronchiolitis. This is due, in great part, to the availability of highly sensitive, molecular amplification-based diagnostic testing. These other viruses include rhinovirus, adenovirus, coronavirus, enterovirus, parainfluenza virus type 3, influenza, and the recently identified human metapneumovirus (HMPV).[12] HMPV is a new paramyxovirus that was first isolated in 2001 from young children with respiratory tract disease.[15] It is now thought to be responsible for up to 19% of cases of bronchiolitis and is considered the second most common cause of bronchiolitis, after RSV.[16] As with most respiratory viruses, there is seasonal variation in occurrence. Peak occurrence is in the late winter/early spring in North America and Europe, which is slightly after RSV's peak activity.[17]

PATHOLOGY

Acute viral bronchiolitis is characterized by extensive inflammation of the airways, increased mucus production, airway cell necrosis, and some bronchoconstriction.[18] RSV, the most common infecting virus in bronchiolitis, binds to toll-like receptor-4 (TLR-4) on epithelial cells, fuses its membrane with the cell membrane, and causes both direct cellular and ciliary damage and an indirect inflammatory effect on the respiratory tract.[19] The infecting virus (usually RSV) then replicates, causing epithelial cell necrosis and ciliary destruction.[16] This cell destruction triggers an inflammatory response, and infiltration of the submucosa with both neutrophils and lymphocytes (Fig. 27-1). Thick mucus plugs are created by increased mucus secretion from goblet cells combining with desquamated epithelial cells. These mucus plugs result in bronchiolar obstruction, leading to air-trapping and

varying degrees of lobular collapse. These mechanisms cause ventilation-perfusion mismatch, and ultimately hypoxemia.[20]

The immunopathogenesis of RSV bronchiolitis is still poorly understood. There is seemingly contradictory evidence regarding the role of T cells in the development of RSV bronchiolitis. Some studies show that specific T cells are required for pathology and actually enhance the severity of disease.[21,22] In contrast, recent studies have demonstrated that CD8+ T cells can protect against RSV-induced disease.[23,24] There is little doubt that T cells have an important role in RSV bronchiolitis. This is witnessed by the RSV vaccine trial in the 1960s in which the inactivated viral vaccine did not protect immunized children from natural infections.[25] In fact, it paradoxically led to more severe cases and two deaths in those who were immunized. Considering this historical issue and newer emerging evidence, it is likely that there are coexisting protective and disease-promoting adaptive immune mechanisms at play.[26] Future research should clarify this apparent conundrum.

DIAGNOSIS

The diagnosis of bronchiolitis is essentially based upon clinical presentation. The constellation of presenting signs and symptoms combined with the patient's age and the presence of a bronchiolitis-related virus in the community (usually RSV) make the diagnosis likely.

Laboratory testing of nasopharyngeal aspirates for bronchiolitis-related viruses can support patient diagnosis, aid with syndromic surveillance, and help inpatient bed assignment (see Chapter 24). For most cases of bronchiolitis, a clinical diagnosis is adequate, and viral testing adds little to routine management.[2] A blood gas (capillary, venous, or arterial) can aid with assessment of gas exchange and acidosis in a child with moderate to severe respiratory distress. If a child has poor oral intake and signs of dehydration, one can assess electrolyte

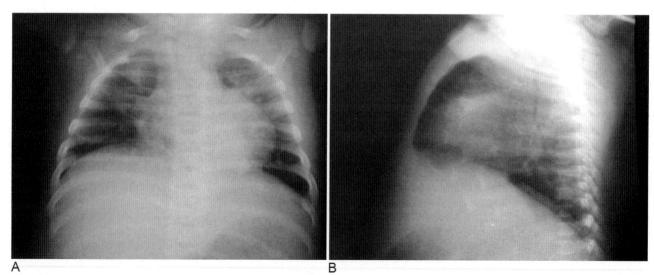

A   B

FIGURE 27-1. Histologic section of a bronchiole from an infant who died from acute severe RSV bronchiolitis. Peribronchiolar lymphoid infiltration and plugging of the lumen with exudate and cellular debris is shown. The surrounding alveoli are essentially spared. (Courtesy of Dr. W. Aherne.)

abnormalities and extent of dehydration can by measuring the plasma BUN, creatine, and electrolytes. If performed, the white blood cell count can range from low to normal to high, with counts as low as 5000 cells/mm³ or as high as 24,000 cells/mm³.[27] However, there are no laboratory tests that are specific to bronchiolitis, and as such, no single laboratory test can confirm or rule out the diagnosis of acute viral bronchiolitis.

Radiologic testing, mainly in the form of chest radiography, is commonly performed in children with suspected bronchiolitis. It is estimated that up to 60% of children presenting to the emergency department or admitted to an inpatient ward receive a chest radiograph.[28–30] Despite its high frequency of use, there is little evidence to support the effectiveness of this practice. In a large survey of 30 children's hospitals in the Unites States, performing chest radiographs for infants with bronchiolitis was associated with increased likelihood to prescribe antimicrobials and increased length of stay. This is likely due to the fact that bronchiolitis-related atelectasis is difficult to distinguish from consolidation on a radiograph.[1] A study of the utility of chest radiographs in acute bronchiolitis included 265 children who underwent radiography after a clinical diagnosis of bronchiolitis.[31] Ninety-three percent of the patients had "simple bronchiolitis" evident on imaging. The authors also concluded that risk of airspace disease was particularly low in children with hemoglobin oxygen saturations greater than 92% with mild-moderate distress.[31] If performed, a typical radiograph for a child with bronchiolitis will demonstrate hyperinflation, flattening of the diaphragms, peribronchial infiltrates, airway wall thickening, and (occasionally) patchy atelectasis (Fig. 27-2).[32] Currently, there is no evidence to support the routine use of radiographs in a child with typical bronchiolitis; further, there is no benefit evident, even if the child is to be admitted.

When considering the clinical diagnosis of bronchiolitis, it is important to also consider reasonable differential diagnoses. Other causes of respiratory distress to consider include upper airway obstruction (e.g., adenoidal hypertrophy,

retropharyngeal abscess), laryngeal obstruction (e.g., croup, foreign body), asthma, pneumonia, and metabolic disorders that mimick respiratory disease (e.g., salicylate poisoning, diabetic ketoacidosis, inborn errors of metabolism). Congestive heart failure (e.g., pre-existing congenital heart conditions, new-onset viral myocarditis) and parenchymal lung disease (e.g., exacerbation of cystic fibrosis, congenital lung disease) may also present in a fashion that is similar to bronchiolitis, or may be exacerbated by bronchiolitis.

■ MANAGEMENT PRINCIPLES

There have been two recent comprehensive evidence-based guidelines for the diagnosis, management, and prevention of bronchiolitis. It is reassuring to note that both the American Academy of Pediatrics (AAP) and the Scottish Intercollegiate Guideline Network (SIGN) performed comprehensive reviews of the literature that led to the same conclusions.[2,33] The cornerstone of bronchiolitis treatment remains supportive care. Most infants with mild bronchiolitis require no specific treatment and can be successfully treated at home. Infants with moderate to severe respiratory distress are often hospitalized; this is approximately 1% to 3% of all children with bronchiolitis. There is great variability in the clinical approach to treatment of bronchiolitis.[30,34–36] Despite four decades of research, there is much confusion and controversy regarding the treatment of this common life-threatening condition.[37] The following sections will attempt to summarize the currently available medical literature in order to support evidence-based decision making.

Fluid and Hydration Therapy

As previously stated, monitoring of fluid intake and hydration status is key in the assessment of an infant with bronchiolitis. If an infant can breastfeed, this should be highly encouraged, as it contributes to hydration and confers immunologic advantages. Breast milk has been shown to have neutralizing activity against RSV,[38] containing RSV immunoglobulins A and G as well as interferon-α.[39] It is estimated that approximately 30% of children admitted with bronchiolitis require fluid replacement therapy.[40] However, there is a lack of agreement on which method of fluid replacement should be used. Nasogastric feedings may be considered for a child who has decreased oral intake, with mild to moderate respiratory distress. When the respiratory rate exceeds 60 to 70 breaths per minute, there can be an increased risk of food aspiration into the lungs.[41] At this point, intravenous fluids should be considered for maintaining hydration. The evidence to determine the optimal route for fluid replacement in infants with bronchiolitis is currently inadequate. A large randomized multicenter trial is planned by an Australian pediatric emergency research collaborative, which may provide a definitive answer.[42]

Supplemental Oxygen

In the clinical setting, measurement of reduced oxygen saturations and the resultant use of supplemental oxygen is one of the major determinants of both hospital

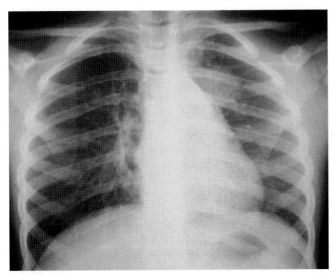

FIGURE 27-2. Chest radiograph of an infant with acute bronchiolitis. (Courtesy of Dr. ME Wohl.)

admission and length of stay.[43,44] Interestingly, there are no studies that examine the effect of oxygen on clinical recovery from bronchiolitis. A recent Cochrane Collaboration review of oxygen therapy for lower respiratory tract infections in children did not identify a single trial comparing oxygen therapy versus no oxygen supplementation.[11] To date, there is no clear direction as to what constitutes a safe admission or discharge hemoglobin oxygen saturation level.[45] The AAP recommends supplemental oxygen if the hemoglobin oxygen saturation is persistently below 90%.[2] Their suggested point of discontinuation of oxygen therapy is when the child's oxygen saturation can be maintained at or above 90% with room air *and* the child is feeding well, with minimal respiratory distress. Premature or low birth weight infants, as well as those with chronic lung disease or congenital heart disease may require further consideration when administering or discontinuing oxygen, as these children are likely to have lower tolerance for hypoxemia and a higher likelihood of severe disease.

Nasal Suctioning

Children with bronchiolitis often suffer from copious, thick nasal secretions. Their young age precludes effective self-clearing of the nasal passages, so nasal suctioning is commonly used both at home and in the hospital setting.[46] While it makes intuitive sense to continue with this practice, to our knowledge there is not a single trial that assesses the effectiveness of nasal suctioning for bronchiolitis.

Chest Physiotherapy

It might be thought that chest physiotherapy would improve the clearance of secretions associated with bronchiolitis and decrease ventilatory effort. However, a recent Cochrane review of three clinical trials of percussion and vibration (techniques used for chest physiotherapy in infants) versus no intervention does not support its routine use. This review concluded that for nonventilated infants with bronchiolitis, chest physiotherapy did not reduce the length of hospital stay or oxygen requirements or improve clinical severity scores.[47]

Albuterol/Salbutamol

Bronchodilators are commonly used in the management of bronchiolitis in North America. However, the evidence to support this practice is not very strong, and the practice remains controversial. A Cochrane review of 22 trials comparing bronchodilator (other than epinephrine) use with placebo for bronchiolitis included data from 1428 infants. Studies of both oral and inhalational short-acting β-2 agonists were included. There was a statistically significant but clinically modest improvement in the overall average clinical score of patients treated with bronchodilators.[48] Of note, there was no improvement in oxygenation. It appeared that bronchodilators have a greater effect in the outpatient setting rather than in the hospital

setting. However, patients receiving bronchodilators showed no improvement in hospitalization rates or duration of hospitalization. The authors of this review noted that the effectiveness of bronchodilators for bronchiolitis may have been overestimated, as many of the reviewed studies included patients with recurrent wheezing, a group thought to be clinically different from those with acute bronchiolitis. Overall, it would appear that short-acting β-2 agonists provide, at best, modest transient relief with no clear benefit to hospitalization rates or duration of hospitalization. As such, the AAP has recommended that bronchodilators should not be routinely used in the management of bronchiolitis. They do concede that a carefully monitored trial of an inhaled short-acting β-2 agonist can be considered, and its use can be continued if a beneficial clinical response is documented.[2]

Nebulized Epinephrine

Another commonly used bronchodilator for the treatment of bronchiolitis is nebulized epinephrine, or adrenaline. Just as with short-acting β-2 agonists, the AAP has recommended that nebulized epinephrine should not be routinely used in the management of bronchiolitis.[2] A Cochrane review of nebulized epinephrine for bronchiolitis reviewed 14 trials and included both inpatients and outpatients. For inpatient trials ($n = 5$), clinical score was improved in the epinephrine group, but oxygen saturation and admission rates did not differ.[49] Outpatient studies ($n = 3$) demonstrated short-term improvement in clinical scores, oxygenation, respiratory rate, and overall improvement of the patient. Of seven trials comparing epinephrine to salbutamol in both the inpatient and outpatient setting, it appeared that epinephrine might be the preferred drug for outpatients.[49] However, there was insufficient evidence to recommend epinephrine use in the inpatient setting. A carefully monitored trial of epinephrine can be performed for an individual patient, and its use should be continued only if a documented positive clinical response is noted. If the decision is made to test an inhaled bronchodilator, the current state of the evidence would seem to support a trial with epinephrine, first, as it appears to have a slightly greater effect than β-2 agonists. However, given the fact that epinephrine is not available for use in the home setting, the AAP suggests that a β-2 agonist trial might be appropriate in the clinic or nonhospital setting.[2]

Corticosteroids

Corticosteroids can be administered via inhalation or systemically (via oral, intramuscular, or intravenous route). Up to 60% of infants admitted to the hospital receive corticosteroid therapy.[50,51] As with many therapies for bronchiolitis, the use of corticosteroids is controversial.

Systemic corticosteroid use in bronchiolitis is a long and hotly debated topic. A recently completed Cochrane review conducted in 2010 included 17 trials with a total of 2596 infants.[52] Overall, the use of systemic corticosteroids did not demonstrate a benefit. The review concluded that glucocorticoids did not significantly reduce outpatient visits or length of stay for inpatients. Interestingly, a recent large multicenter, randomized 4-armed trial (*n* = 800 infants) examined the emergency department use of both oral corticosteroids and nebulized epinephrine in preventing hospital admission.[53] This study demonstrated a possible synergistic effect when combining the two medications in the treatment of bronchiolitis as demonstrated by reduced hospital admissions, as well as shortening both the time to discharge and the duration of some clinical symptoms. Bronchodilator and glucocorticoid synergy is a phenomenon that is well documented with β agonist/steroid use in asthma,[54–56] and it has also recently been seen in other smaller bronchiolitis studies.[57,58] In considering the synergy of epinephrine and oral glucocorticoids, this study should be considered exploratory, as the results were unexpected. Further studies will be required to confirm the finding.

The role of inhaled glucocorticoid use in infants with bronchiolitis has been examined in a systematic review to determine if there was any effect on the prevention of post-bronchiolitis wheezing. Five studies, including 374 infants, were included in the analyses and failed to demonstrate any effect on such wheezing, hospital re-admission rates, or use of bronchodilators.[59] The authors noted that the strength of their recommendations was negatively affected by the small number of participants and the clinical diversity of the studies. Of the two known studies that investigated the role of inhaled glucocorticoids for the treatment of the acute symptoms of the disease, neither has demonstrated any benefit.[60,61] Currently, there is no evidence to support the use of inhaled corticosteroids for acute or long-term benefit in bronchiolitis.

Mucolytics

Since it is known that mucous plugging plays a significant role in the small airway obstruction of bronchiolitis, it would seem reasonable that interventions that might thin airway secretions could improve clinical outcomes. Inhaled hypertonic saline and deoxyribonuclease (DNase) are two such interventions that have been successfully used in cystic fibrosis and are now being considered for bronchiolitis therapy.

While the exact mechanism of action remains unclear, nebulized hypertonic saline is thought to improve mucociliary clearance by causing osmotic movement of water into the airway. A recent Cochrane review of the effects of hypertonic saline reviewed four trials, with a total of 254 infants (189 inpatients and 65 outpatients). Three trials used 3% hypertonic saline combined with either nebulized epinephrine (two studies) or terbutaline (1 study); the remaining trial used nebulized hypertonic saline alone. Overall, patients treated with nebulized 3% hypertonic saline had a significantly shorter mean length of hospital stay (of almost 1 full day) and improved clinical severity scores compared to those who received nebulized normal saline.[62] They also demonstrated no adverse effects with its use. A recent emergency department–based randomized trial of hypertonic saline for bronchiolitis (which is not included in this review) would suggest that the effects of hypertonic saline are not seen immediately, as this trial demonstrated no effect on clinical severity in the first 2 hours posttreatment.[63] While the safety and efficacy evidence for the use of hypertonic saline is compelling, the trials in the review were small and few. Given the lack of adverse events and the possibility of improved outcomes, it seems reasonable to suggest the use of hypertonic saline in acute bronchiolitis. If one plans to use hypertonic saline, the current best recommendation would be to begin its use early, with the expectation that its beneficial effects would not be seen immediately post-use. DNase enhances mobilization of mucus by liquefying mucous plugs, which contain large amounts of lysed inflammatory cell DNA, in the airways.[8] There have been two trials of DNase for bronchiolitis reported in the current literature. To date, DNase has not been found to have any effect on length of stay, clinical severity scores, or duration of oxygen therapy.[64,65]

Leukotriene Modifiers

Leukotrienes are thought to contribute to the airway inflammatory response in bronchiolitis, thus the role of leukotriene modifiers has been explored for this illness. One small trial (*n* = 53) of daily oral montelukast (versus placebo) failed to demonstrate any difference in length of stay, clinical severity scores, or cytokine levels.[66] In a very large trial of 979 infants, RSV-positive infants were randomized to receive either oral montelukast or placebo.[67] In this study, montelukast did not improve the respiratory symptoms of post-RSV bronchiolitis in children. Currently, there is insufficient evidence to recommend leukotriene modifier use for bronchiolitis.

Heliox Inhalational Therapy

Heliox, a mixture of oxygen and helium, has been used for the treatment of acute asthma exacerbations since 1935.[68] A limited number of studies of heliox use in bronchiolitis have emerged over the last two decades. The mechanism of action for heliox inhalational therapy is not clearly understood. It is proposed that the decreased work of breathing and wheezing that occurs during heliox use might be due to increased flow rate or less turbulent flow, ultimately resulting in better ventilation of distal alveoli.[69] Heliox therapy has been traditionally reserved for the sickest patients. A recent Cochrane review of heliox therapy in bronchiolitis identified four intensive care unit (ICU) trials with a modest total number of patients (*n* = 84). While the patients benefited from a significantly lower mean clinical score in the first hour post–heliox therapy (versus air or oxygen therapy), there was no clinically significant reduction in rate of intubation, need for mechanical ventilation, or length of stay in the ICU.[70] At present, there is not enough evidence to routinely recommend the use of heliox therapy for severely ill children with bronchiolitis, and there is no evidence for its use in mild to moderately ill infants.

Antivirals

Ribavirin is an inhaled broad-spectrum antiviral agent that is sometimes, albeit controversially, used in the treatment of severely ill or high-risk infants with bronchiolitis.

It is the only antiviral agent licensed for use with RSV bronchiolitis, and it has been shown to provide limited clinical benefit.[16] A Cochrane review of twelve ribavirin trials for infants with RSV lower respiratory tract infections determined that its use may decrease the number of days of hospitalization and mechanical ventilation.[71] However, ribavirin did not reduce respiratory deterioration or mortality. Routine use of ribavirin is not recommended for children with bronchiolitis, as studies are limited, the drug is difficult to administer, and it is potentially toxic.

Antimicrobials

Despite bronchiolitis being recognized as a viral illness, antimicrobials are commonly prescribed. Reasons cited for antimicrobial use include high fever, young age, and concerns of bacterial superinfection.[72,73] A Cochrane review of the use of antimicrobials in bronchiolitis identified only one trial of ampicillin versus placebo, which demonstrated no difference in duration of illness or deaths between the two groups.[74] A recent moderate-sized study ($n = 295$) of antimicrobial use in infants with bronchiolitis demonstrated that there was no clinical advantage to using antimicrobials in the care of such children. The authors concluded that supportive measures without antimicrobials remained the standard of care in the hospital setting.[75] Given the results of this study and the low rates of serious bacterial co-infections in children with bronchiolitis, the routine use of antimicrobials cannot be recommended.

There has been some recent exploration of the effect of macrolide antimicrobials in lower respiratory tract disease. Macrolide therapy is thought to exert its effect through three potential mechanisms: antimicrobial (through direct bacterial killing action and indirect bacterial modulation), anti-gastroesophageal reflux (via its pro-motility effects), and anti-inflammatory (by altering the release and action of pro-inflammatory cytokines).[76] Currently, studies exist for the use of macrolides in bronchiolitis obliterans, cystic fibrosis, and bronchiectasis.[76] A recent small study ($n = 21$) of clarithromycin use in acute bronchiolitis suggests that this macrolide had a statistically significant effect on length of stay, use of β-2 agonists, and plasma levels of inflammatory markers.[77] While there is currently no role for the routine use of macrolide therapy in acute viral bronchiolitis, its role remains to be clarified by future research.

Ventilatory Support

When supportive care fails to lead to improvement in the clinical status of a child with moderate to severe respiratory distress, and respiratory exhaustion or failure is imminent, assisted ventilation is the next step. Endotracheal intubation and mechanical ventilation is the time-honored intervention. However, mechanical ventilation is not without risks and complications. As such, clinicians and researchers have considered nasal continuous positive airway pressure (nCPAP) as a less invasive alternative to ventilation. The proposed mechanisms of action for nCPAP in bronchiolitis include a pneumatic splinting effect, which then expands the airway diameter; improved air flow during exhalation; and a decrease in work of breathing.[78] Evidence is quite limited for the use of CPAP with only one trial identified.[79] A recent review of the topic found that there is no evidence that the use of nCPAP in bronchiolitis leads to lower rates of mechanical ventilation.[80] It is possible, however, that early use of nCPAP for moderate to severe bronchiolitis may lead to some modest improvements in cardiorespiratory parameters.[81]

Clinical Pathways

In reviewing the evidence for the treatment of bronchiolitis, it quickly becomes clear that there are many modalities of treatment available and many possible approaches to therapy. The near-exponential increase in evidence, opinions, and advice regarding the treatment of bronchiolitis, coupled with the demands of everyday clinical practice make it very challenging for the average health care professional to keep abreast of the latest approach. Clinical pathways aim to link evidence to practice in a condition-specific manner, thereby optimizing patient outcomes and clinical efficacy.[82] Studies specific to bronchiolitis show that implementation of evidence-based guidelines results in a decrease in the use of unnecessary nasopharyngeal virus testing (52%),[83,84] chest radiographs (14%),[83,84] and bronchodilators (10% to 17%).[83-85] In the reported studies, rate of admission decreased 30%, mean length of stay decreased 17%, and mean costs of respiratory care services decreased 72% to 77%.[83,84]

While clinical guidelines provide generic recommendations, clinical pathways outline the *specific* steps and timeframes in which to realize these said recommendations. A recent elaborate Cochrane review of 27 studies involving 11,398 patients suggests that the use of clinical pathways in general is associated with reduced in-hospital complications and improved documentation, without negatively impacting length of stay or hospital-based costs.[82]

Admission Criteria

There are no clear criteria for determining when to hospitalize children with bronchiolitis. Hospitalization can be considered for infants who have a respiratory rate greater than 60 to 70 breaths per minute or a hemoglobin oxygen saturation less than 90%; those with a history of apnea; and those who are lethargic or dehydrated. Factors that may influence disposition determination include prematurity, very young age, pre-existing cardiopulmonary disease, immunodeficiency, or neuromuscular disorder. An infant's social situation and caregiver exhaustion also play a role in decision making. A recently published abstract has identified that gestational age, heart rate, respiratory rate, respiratory distress assessment instrument score, and oxygen saturation on room air were significantly associated with the development of severe bronchiolitis in a cohort of Canadian infants with bronchiolitis.[86] The utility of such variables for predicting need for admission have yet to be determined.

PREVENTION

Frequent, thorough, and consistent hand hygiene has been shown to reduce the nosocomial spread of RSV.[87] This is a key infection-control principle both in the health care setting and in the home. RSV and other viruses can be spread through secretions, hand contact, and fomites. Viruses, including RSV, have been found on secretion-contaminated beds, toys, crib rails, and tabletops; such organisms can remain viable for many hours.[88,89] The Centers for Disease Control and Prevention has published detailed evidence-based recommendations regarding hand hygiene and antisepsis in the health care setting.[90] Of note, they recommend that hands should be decontaminated prior to and after direct contact with a patient, after contact with inanimate objects in the direct vicinity of a patient, and after removing gloves. Hand hygiene with antimicrobial soap is recommended for visibly dirty hands; otherwise, an alcohol-based rub is preferred.[91]

Currently, no vaccine exists for the prevention of RSV infection, which is the predominant etiologic agent for bronchiolitis. The development of a successful vaccine has been challenging, as immunity to multiple strains of the virus would be required. One would expect that a series of boosters would be necessary for the vaccine to be effective, as natural infection with the virus does not confer long-term immunity.[16]

Passive immunization to RSV has been accomplished through the development of two different products. Their use is currently recommended for infants who are considered at high risk for developing severe RSV bronchiolitis. The American Academy of Pediatrics' Subcommittee of Management and Treatment of Bronchiolitis has outlined groups of infants whom they consider to be high risk for severe RSV and its complications, and for whom they recommend Palivizumab (Table 27-1).[2]

RSV immune globulin (RSV-IG) was the first form of immunoprophylaxis to become available. It was an expensive therapy that required administration of a large volume (15 mL/kg) of fluid over a long period of time (2 to 4 hours). In a moderate sized (n = 249 subjects) randomized, blinded, multicenter trial of RSV-IG, there was an increased incidence of adverse events in the subgroup of infants with congenital heart disease, thus RSV-IG is not recommended for this group.[92]

Palivizumab is a humanized monoclonal antibody, and it has become the passive immunization agent of choice. It is administered as a monthly intramuscular injection over the 5 peak months of RSV season. In a large (n = 1502 subjects) randomized, double-blind, multicenter trial, palivizumab was associated with a 55% reduction in RSV-related hospitalizations, fewer overall days in the hospital, and a lower rate of ICU admissions.[93] These findings were further confirmed through similar results for a study of children with significant congenital heart disease.[94] Ease of administration and lack of interference with routine immunizations are the main considerations in choosing palivizumab over RSV-IG. Unfortunately, palivizumab is quite expensive, and it is estimated to cost $5000 to $6000 per season. Most of the economic analyses of RSV immunoprophylaxis have failed to demonstrate any overall savings in health care expenditure because of the large financial costs of immunizing all at-risk infants.[95–97] While the main advantage of palivizumab is related to its decrease in RSV-related *hospitalizations*, to date none of the five clinical randomized controlled trials have demonstrated a significant decrease in the rate of *mortality* attributable to receiving RSV immune prophylaxis.

DISEASE COURSE AND COMPLICATIONS

The majority of infants infected with RSV and other bronchiolitis-causing viruses develop a mild URTI during the first few days of illness. While some will only have URTI manifestations, up to 40% will then progress to

TABLE 27-1 RECOMMENDED HIGH-RISK GROUPS FOR RSV IMMUNOPROPHYLAXIS WITH PALIVIZUMAB

Risk Factor	Details of Risk Factor	IMMUNOPROPHYLAXIS	
		First RSV Season	Second RSV Season
Chronic lung disease (CLD)	Required medical therapy for CLD within 6 months before onset of RSV season	Y	
	More severe CLD requiring ongoing medical therapy	Y	Y*
History of prematurity	32-35 weeks gestation with 2 or more risk factors† (most benefit in first 6 months of life)	Y	
	Younger than 32 weeks gestation, with or without CLD	Y	
	29-32 weeks gestation (most benefit in first 6 months of life)	Y	
Congenital heart disease	Younger than 28 weeks gestation (most benefit in first 12 months of life)	Y	
Congenital heart disease	Cyanotic heart disease	Y	
	Taking medications for congestive heart failure	Y	
	Infants with moderate to severe pulmonary hypertension	Y	

From American Academy of Pediatrics Subcommittee on Diagnosis and Management of Bronchiolitis. Diagnosis and management of bronchiolitis. *Pediatrics.* 2006;118:1774-1793.
*Please note that data are limited for the use of immunoprophylaxis in the second year of life.
†Risk factors include child care attendance, school-aged siblings, exposure to environmental air pollutants, congenital abnormalities of the airway, and severe neuromuscular disease.

lower respiratory tract involvement (or bronchiolitis), with wheezing, crackles, and varying degrees of respiratory distress.[98] The mean duration of illness is 15 days, and the majority of these infections resolve uneventfully within 3 to 4 weeks.[30,99] Of note, up to 25% of infants with bronchiolitis remained symptomatic after 21 days of illness, in a recent prospective cohort study highlighting the prolonged disease course of this acute illness.[99]

Epidemiologic studies indicate that, while there is a very high degree of morbidity with bronchiolitis, there is low mortality. Over the last decades, it appears that mortality has remained stable for bronchiolitis. Of all children who are hospitalized with bronchiolitis, mortality rate estimates around 1%,[16,100,101] but rates are as high as 3.5% for children with underlying cardiac or chronic lung conditions.[102] Overall, rates of hospitalization have increased up to 2.4-fold.[7,9]

With bronchiolitis, apnea, or risk of apnea, is a cause for concern for caregivers and health care professionals alike and can often lead to hospitalization. Rates of apnea with RSV bronchiolitis range from 1.2% to 23.8%.[103,104] In a recent systematic review, it would appear that the rates of apnea in previously healthy term infants is less than 1%, while infants with risk factors (e.g., prematurity and congenital heart disease) carry a greater risk of occurrence.[105] Occurrence of prolonged or recurrent apnea is a consideration with regard to intubation of a patient; the risk of requiring intubation for hospitalized children with bronchiolitis is estimated at approximately 5%.[100]

Some studies have identified that up to 50% to 60% of children with bronchiolitis may have concomitant acute otitis media.[106,107] Unfortunately, there is no clinical feature that can reliably distinguish viral from bacterial ear infections. While tympanocentesis can reliably accomplish this differentiation, it is considered impractical for the average clinician to engage in this practice. When identified, acute otitis media is best treated as per the well-recognized AAP/American Academy of Family Physicians' guidelines.[108]

Serious bacterial infections, including bacteremia, urinary tract infection, and meningitis are a concern when evaluating febrile infants, including those with bronchiolitis. A number of studies have shown that febrile infants diagnosed with RSV infections are at significantly lower risk of serious bacterial infection when compared to children without RSV infection.[1,109–111] If a child has a bacterial infection, it is likely to be a urinary tract infection.[109] Very young febrile infants (younger than 3 months of age) with bronchiolitis require careful assessment for the source of their fever. For any febrile infant younger than 4 to 6 weeks of age, most clinicians would perform a full septic workup (including blood culture, blood count, catheter urine sample, chest radiograph, and lumbar puncture), and many would consider at least a partial if not full septic workup for infants between 6 weeks and 3 months of age.[112]

There have been reports of children with inappropriate secretion of antidiuretic hormone associated with bronchiolitis.[113,114] This should be kept in mind, and monitoring of fluid status and measurement of serum sodium levels should be performed, when appropriate, for infants receiving intravenous fluids.

A variety of cardiac manifestations of RSV have been noted, including myocarditis, arrhythmias, and complete heart block.[115–118] Sepsis-like syndrome, in the absence of a secondary bacterial infection, has also been known to occur in children with RSV infection.[104,119] Other extrapulmonary manifestations of severe RSV infection include focal and generalized seizures, focal neurologic findings, and hepatitis.[120]

■ LONG-TERM SEQUELAE

While hospitalization is a major notable outcome of severe bronchiolitis, it is not the only outcome. There are also longer-term complications including bronchiolitis obliterans, allergic sensitization, and the development of wheezing or (arguably) asthma later in life. Studies that attempt to link bronchiolitis in infancy with allergic sensitization and atopic illness have yet to produce clear answers. While some studies have demonstrated an association between the two entities,[121] others have not.[122,123]

■ BRONCHIOLITIS OBLITERANS

Bronchiolitis obliterans is a rare fibrosing form of chronic obstructive lung disease that follows a severe insult to the lower respiratory tract (see Chapter 59). It was first described by Lange in 1901.[124] Bronchiolitis obliterans results in partial or complete obliteration of the small airways (Fig. 27-3).[125] The exact incidence of childhood bronchiolitis obliterans is not known. The etiology of adult forms of bronchiolitis obliterans includes inhalational injuries, hypersensitivity pneumonitis, post-transplant, and autoimmune disorders.[126] In contrast, childhood bronchiolitis obliterans is most often seen after a severe lower respiratory tract infection. The most common associated viral etiology is adenovirus, especially serotypes 1, 3, 7 and 21,[127,128] however it has been suggested that RSV may cause it as well.[1] Table 27-2 outlines the varied possible etiologies for pediatric bronchiolitis obliterans.

The chain of events leading to bronchiolitis obliterans likely begins with an injury to the epithelial cells of the airways, causing transient derangements in cell function and necrosis. Local necrosis leads to intraluminal accumulation of fibrinopurulent exudate, inducing an overgrowth of the exposed myofibroblasts of the denuded submucosa.[124] The myofibroblast hyperproliferation leads to collagen and acid mucopolysaccharide deposition, with resultant narrowing of the bronchioles. Occasionally, a large intraluminal polyp known as a *Masson body* may develop secondary to histiocyte and capillary proliferation.

The clinical presentation of bronchiolitis obliterans may mimic acute viral bronchiolitis, but often without fever and rhinorrhea. Older patients may complain of dyspnea, cough, or decreased exercise tolerance. Physical findings are quite nonspecific, but expiratory wheezes or crackles may be heard on occasion. In the postinfectious setting, the infant may appear to partially recover from the acute illness, only to have persistent respiratory symptoms. Typically, the respiratory findings persist for more than 60 days.[129] Chest radiographs demonstrate dramatic hyperinflation and bilateral increase in interstitial markings. Bronchiolitis obliterans is most accurately diagnosed by microscopic examination of adequate biopsy material. Transthoracic

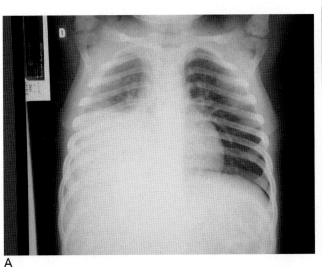
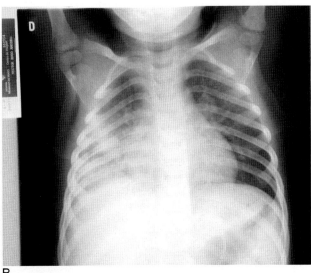

FIGURE 27-3. Histologic representation of bronchiolitis obliterans in an 18-month-old child who had severe adenovirus bronchiolitis one year before. The obliterated lumen of the bronchiole is filled with vascularized connective tissue. (From Wohl ME, Chernick V. State of the art: bronchiolitis. *Am Rev Respir Dis.* 1978;118:759.)

biopsy with two tissue site sampling is currently recommended for definitive diagnosis.[124] Because of the invasive nature of this type of diagnostic testing, criteria were created in the 1990s to reflect *bronchiolitis oblit-*

TABLE 27-2 POSSIBLE ETIOLOGIES FOR PEDIATRIC BRONCHIOLITIS OBLITERANS

Post-infectious	Adenovirus types 3, 7, and 21 Influenza Parainfluenza Measles Respiratory syncytial virus (RSV) Varicella Mycoplasma pneumoniae
Post-transplant	Chronic rejection of lung or heart/lung transplantation Graft-versus-host disease associated with bone marrow transplantation
Connective tissue disease	Rheumatoid arthritis Sjögren's syndrome Systemic lupus erythematosus
Toxic fume inhalation	NO_2 NH_3
Chronic hypersensitivity pneumonitis	Avian antigens Mold
Aspiration	Stomach contents: gastroesophageal reflux Foreign bodies
Drugs	Penicillamine Cocaine
Stevens-Johnson syndrome	Idiopathic Drug-induced Infection-related

From Moonnumakal SP, Fan LL. Bronchiolitis obliterans in children. *Curr Opin Pediatr.* 2008;20:272-278.

erans syndrome, and they take into account pulmonary function testing as a surrogate for graft dysfunction in lung transplant recipients.[130] High-resolution CT has become an important test in the diagnosis of bronchiolitis obliterans, with mosaic perfusion, vascular attenuation, and central bronchiectasis as key features.[131]

The morbidity and mortality for bronchiolitis obliterans remains uncertain. Post-adenovirus bronchiolitis obliterans seems to have low mortality, but high chronicity.[132,133] On occasion, gradual resorption of the fibrovascular connective tissue occurs, with a restoration of normal airway caliber and epithelium. The treatment for bronchiolitis obliterans in children is often difficult and unsuccessful. Azithromycin, a macrolide antimicrobial, appears to have been effective in the treatment of bronchiolitis obliterans, presumably acting via its postulated anti-inflammatory effects. Corticosteroids have not been shown to improve outcome, and experimental therapies include immunomodulators, monoclonal antibodies directed at the interleukin-2 receptor, and aerosolized cyclosporine.[124] The ultimate option for children with severe bronchiolitis obliterans is lung transplantation.

Up to one third of children with postinfectious bronchiolitis obliterans will develop Swyer-James syndrome[131] (or Macleod syndrome when diagnosed in adulthood). It is a long-term complication of postinfectious constrictive bronchiolitis of childhood. It also is associated with adenovirus pneumonia or bronchiolitis.[134] This syndrome describes the development of a unilateral hyperlucent lung with decreased vascularity and increased air trapping evident on plain radiographs. It develops due to postinfectious fibrotic healing of the immature lung, which leads to a decrease in the number of alveoli and pulmonary vessels. Imaging of Swyer-James syndrome demonstrates diffuse, asymmetric, patchy lobar or lobular air trapping that is almost often bilateral (Fig. 27-4).[135] Before the routine use of CT scan, it was believed that this syndrome was a unilateral phenomenon; this has since been disproved.[136]

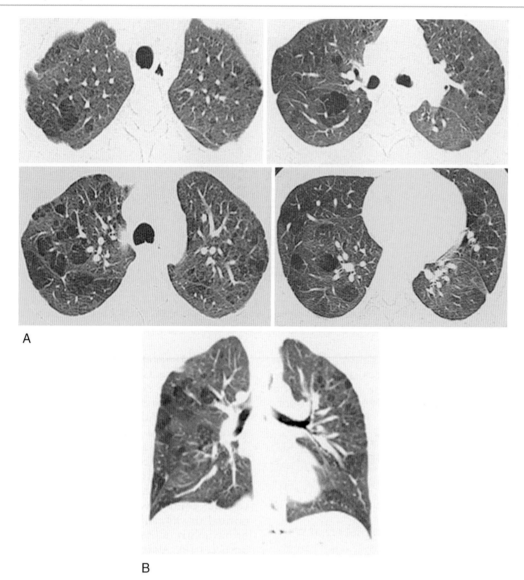

A

B

FIGURE 27-4. (A) High-resolution CT of the chest demonstrates asymmetric lobular air trapping with diminished vascularity shown in the lungs bilaterally from Swyer-James-Macleod syndrome. (B) Distribution of abnormality is better appreciated on the coronal reformatted image. (From Pipavath SN, Stern EJ. Imaging of small airway disease (SAD). *Radiol Clin North Am.* 2009;47:313.)

RELATIONSHIP TO ASTHMA

A relation between bronchiolitis in infancy and subsequent wheezing has been repeatedly demonstrated in the medical literature.[26] There is even some evidence to suggest that early RSV infection may affect pulmonary function in adulthood.[137,138] This association has led to much speculation and research into the mechanism behind this finding. The association may be causal (and RSV bronchiolitis actually leads to long-term changes in the lungs), or RSV infection simply may serve as a marker for a genetic or physiologic/ anatomic predisposition to future wheezing.[1] At present, it is clear that there is an association between infant bronchiolitis and subsequent development of asthma; however the exact nature of this relationship remains to be determined.

Suggested Reading

American Academy of Pediatrics Subcommittee on Diagnosis and Management of Bronchiolitis. Diagnosis and management of bronchiolitis. *Pediatrics.* 2006;118:1774–1793.

Hall CB, Weinberg GA, Iwane MK, et al. The burden of respiratory syncytial virus infection in young children. *N Engl J Med.* 2009;360:588–598.

Petruzella FD, Gorelick MH. Duration of illness in infants with bronchiolitis evaluated in the emergency department. *Pediatrics.* 2010;126:285–290.

Plint AC, Johnson DW, Patel H, et al. Epinephrine and dexamethasone in children with bronchiolitis. *N Engl J Med.* 2009;360:2079–2089.

Smyth RL, Openshaw PJ. Bronchiolitis. *Lancet.* 2006;368:312–322.

Zorc JJ, Hall CB. Bronchiolitis: Recent evidence on diagnosis and management. *Pediatrics.* 2010;125:342–349.

References

The complete reference list is available online at www. expertconsult.com

28 VIRAL PNEUMONIA

James E. Crowe, Jr., MD

Viral pneumonia is one of the most common maladies affecting infants and children throughout the world. Acute respiratory infection continues to be a leading cause of mortality in young children.[1] Of the estimated 8.795 million worldwide deaths in children younger than 5 years of age in 2008, infectious diseases caused 68% (5.970 million), with pneumonia causing the largest percentage (18%; 1.575 million; uncertainty range 1.046 million to 1.874 million).[1] About 40% of these cases are caused by viral infections. Pneumonia, a respiratory disease characterized by inflammation of the lung parenchyma, is usually caused by viruses, bacteria, or irritants. The term *pneumonia* refers to infection of the lung parenchyma and excludes the tissues of the airway such as the bronchi. However, it is thought that acute viral lower respiratory tract infections (LRTIs) in children affect all of the epithelial cells lining the airway, from the nasopharynx to the alveolar bed. Therefore, viral pneumonia is often a component of a more generalized respiratory tract infection syndrome.

INCIDENCE

It is well established that children younger than 5 years of age, especially infants, have a high burden of disease and hospitalization from respiratory syncytial virus (RSV), metapneumovirus influenza virus (MPV), and parainfluenza viruses (PIVs). However, studies conducted during the last several decades have struggled to define precise quantitative models for the incidence of these diseases. Most large studies were conducted in hospitals and thus lacked a known denominator of subjects at risk. These studies also varied by differences in geographic location of the study, type of hospital, age of the patients, season, criteria for admission, severity of disease, and number and type of diagnostic tests performed. The relatively new use of molecular diagnostic tests has increased our ability to diagnose virus infection, but comparison of data from these studies with data from cell culture–based studies is problematic.

Prospective, active population-based surveillance is needed to define incidence. The U.S. Centers for Disease Control and Prevention sponsored studies in young children who were hospitalized for acute respiratory illness from October 1, 2000, to September 30, 2001, in Monroe County, New York (Rochester area), and Davidson County, Tennessee (Nashville area).[2] Eligible children younger than 5 years of age were those who resided in surveillance counties and were hospitalized for febrile or acute respiratory illness. Viral culture and polymerase chain reaction identification of viruses from nasal and throat samples were obtained from all surveillance children, providing population-based rates of hospitalization for RSV, influenza virus, and PIV, as well as demographic, clinical, and risk factor assessment for each virus. Of the 592 enrolled children, RSV was identified in 20%, influenza in 3%, PIV in 7%, other respiratory viruses in 36%, and no detectable virus in 39%. Population-based rates of acute respiratory illness hospitalizations in children younger than 5 years of age were 18 per 1000. Virus-positive hospitalization rates per 1000 children were 3.5 for RSV, 1.2 for PIV, and 0.6 for influenza virus. Younger age (particularly younger than 1 year of age), African-American and Hispanic race/ethnicity, male gender, and presence of chronic underlying illness were associated with higher hospitalization rates.

ETIOLOGIC AGENTS

The etiologic agents that cause viral pneumonia are well defined. The cause of viral pneumonia varies depending on the age of the child, the setting in which the virus was acquired, the season, and the presence of medical or environmental risk factors. Although a very long list of viruses has been reported to cause pneumonia, the astute clinician can narrow the cause to a short list of potential agents using a careful medical history and physical examination. Common causes of viral pneumonia are shown in Box 28-1.

NEONATAL PNEUMONIA

Perinatal/Transplacental Acquisition

Bacteria, viruses, and noninfectious conditions (e.g., meconium aspiration) can cause pneumonitis at the time of birth. Viruses are infrequently the cause of this presentation, and pneumonia often is only part of a more generalized presentation of a systemic disease. Rubella and cytomegalovirus (CMV) infection associated with systemic disease in the mother can be associated with severe congenital or neonatal disease that probably is acquired by the transplacental route, presumably through the hematogenous spread of virus. Pneumonia manifests with signs of respiratory distress (e.g., retractions, grunting, tachypnea, and cyanosis) that sometimes requires immediate resuscitation and mechanical ventilation because of depressed respiration. Neonatal viral pneumonia can present with more nonspecific systemic signs of illness, such as apnea, bradycardia, poor peripheral perfusion, or temperature instability. These signs also are found frequently in bacterial pneumonia in the neonatal period. Usually, infants with congenital CMV or rubella pneumonia exhibit additional signs of congenital infection, such as petechiae, hepatosplenomegaly, and low birth weight. CMV infection is detected by testing the infant's urine in shell vial or conventional cell culture.

BOX 28-1 ETIOLOGIC AGENTS OF ACUTE ACQUIRED VIRAL PNEUMONIA IN CHILDREN, BY AGE

Perinatal
CMV
HSV types 1 and 2
Enteroviruses
Rubella

3 Weeks to 3 Months
RSV subgroups A and B
hMPV subgroups A and B
PIV type 3

4 Months to 4 Years
RSV subgroups A and B
hMPV subgroups A and B
PIV types 1, 2, and 3
Influenza A and B
Rhinoviruses
Adenoviruses

Older Children and Adults
Influenza A and B
Military recruits: Adenovirus types 4 and 7

Viruses That Are Less Common or That Cause Pneumonia in Certain Settings
Adenovirus types 1, 2, 3, and 5
Enterovirus spp.: echovirus, coxsackievirus
Coronaviruses, SARS-coronavirus
Epstein-Barr, CMV, human herpesvirus 6 (in the immunocompromised)
Varicella-zoster
Developing world: measles, mumps
Endemic areas: Hantavirus

TRANSMISSION FROM THE BIRTH CANAL

Herpes simplex virus (HSV) type I or II infection of the mother's cervix can lead to exposure of the infant during labor or birth by the mucosal route, including aspiration. HSV is capable of infecting the infant via an ascending route from the vagina; the risk of transmission from an infected mother is increased after prolonged rupture of the membranes during labor. The infection may be acquired without prolonged rupture of the membranes during the passage through the birth canal. Transmission is more efficient if the mother is suffering a primary infection, as opposed to a re-activation. The presence of visible herpetic lesions is not needed for transmission to the infant. Herpes simplex virus infection commonly presents in the second week of life. The medical history from the families of infants with pneumonia at this age should consider risk factors, and the physical examination should seek other manifestations of herpetic infection. The cytopathic effects of HSV have been observed in the lungs of infants with pneumonia caused by herpes infection. Systemic HSV infection should be treated with a prolonged course of intravenous acyclovir. Enteroviruses commonly cause symptomatic or asymptomatic infections of the gastrointestinal tract during the summer and fall months. Infected mothers can transmit an enterovirus infection to the infant during birth, and these infections can cause severe systemic disease including pneumonia. When viral infection is acquired from contaminated amniotic fluid or in the birth canal, the infant may not be affected clinically in the first hours or days after birth.

TRANSMISSION IN THE NURSERY

Nosocomial transmission of viruses in the early postpartum period occurs, with surprising efficiency in some cases. The most common cause of nosocomial pneumonia is RSV, which occasionally causes nursery outbreaks.[3] Such outbreaks can be especially devastating in a neonatal intensive care unit if premature infants who require mechanical ventilation become infected. In this setting, infection is usually transmitted by fomites or directly from infected personnel via nasopharyngeal secretions.

INFECTION IN THE FIRST WEEKS OF LIFE

The most common causes of pneumonia in the developed world in the first weeks of life are RNA respiratory viruses, especially RSV. RSV causes yearly winter epidemics in the community that result in the hospitalization of between 0.5% and 4% of infants, depending on the population. During the winter months, RSV is often the major cause of hospitalization of infants, and entire infant wards in many children's hospitals have been dedicated for cohorting of infants during the annual epidemics. Nosocomial spread of virus during the epidemics is common, but it can be minimized by strict attention to contact isolation and hand hygiene.

VIRAL PNEUMONIA DURING EARLY CHILDHOOD

A large panel of respiratory viruses is capable of causing pneumonia during childhood. RSV; human metapneumovirus (hMPV); PIV types 1, 2, and 3; influenza virus types A and B; and adenoviruses make up the majority of cases. RSV is still the most frequent cause of severe respiratory infections in infants after the first weeks of life and in young children, and it is responsible for 75,000 to 125,000 hospitalizations each year in the United States.[4,5] The role of rhinoviruses in causing LRTI such as pneumonia is under much discussion. Rhinovirus infection in children is so common that evidence for rhinovirus infection can be found frequently in children without symptoms of disease. Therefore, attributing causality to rhinovirus in cases of pneumonia is more difficult than with other viruses. Nevertheless, rhinovirus is present significantly more often in cases of childhood pneumonia, and some experts believe that rhinovirus is the most common etiology of all types of LRTI in children. Human rhinoviruses, members of the family *Picornaviridae*, were first isolated in the 1950s, and now there have been over 100 serotypes identified based on nucleotide sequence homologies. Human rhinoviruses were divided into two major genetic groups in the past: designated HRV-A and HRV-B. More recently, a new rhinovirus group, HRV-C, has been found in some patients with LRTI. PIVs, commonly associated with laryngotracheitis (croup syndrome), also cause pneumonia but in less discrete epidemics than those caused by RSV. PIV infections are common in the fall months but can occur at any time of the year. Influenza A and B viruses cause sharp winter epidemics.

In the developing world, measles virus is still a major cause of pneumonia, especially in the setting of malnutrition or vitamin A deficiency, and mumps virus can cause LRTI. Influenza virus type C and PIV type 4 cause upper respiratory tract disease, but their ability to cause lower respiratory tract disease is less clear. Severe acute respiratory syndrome (SARS) was caused by SARS-coronavirus, which was first recognized in Hong Kong during a 2003 epidemic, and this disease affected children.[6] Morbidity was high following SARS, with approximately one fourth of patients requiring intensive care and/or mechanical ventilation support. SARS morbidity and mortality are milder in children than they are in adults, and pneumonia was only one of the disease manifestations of what appears to be a systemic illness. Other more conventional human coronaviruses also cause some cases of pneumonia (e.g., the long-recognized OC43 and 229E strains or the more recently identified coronavirus NL63 and HKU1 strains).[7] Varicella-zoster virus can cause pneumonia during primary infection, especially in older subjects. Other viruses cause pneumonia less commonly (e.g., Epstein-Barr virus, CMV, and human herpesvirus).[6] The immuno-compromised are a special population at elevated risk for these infections, especially for CMV. Human bocavirus is a parvovirus that has been found in many respiratory secretions, but often in the same frequency in cases as in controls. Therefore, it is not clear that this agent is a significant cause of human disease.

The major features of the epidemiology of respiratory virus pneumonia caused by common agents was determined in the United States in detail mostly during the 1960s through the 1980s in a series of seminal longitudinal studies, such as the D.C. Children's Hospital studies,[8–11] Chapel Hill Pediatrics surveillance study,[12] the Vanderbilt Vaccine clinic surveillance studies,[13,14] the Tecumseh study of respiratory illness (Tecumseh, Michigan), and the Tucson Children's Respiratory Study. The principal viruses identified in association with pneumonia in otherwise healthy infants and children were RSV, PIV, and influenza viruses. These studies used cell culture–based or serologic detection for the most part, and it is fair to say that most of these studies did not have optimal culture systems for rhinoviruses or coronaviruses. More recently, very large studies using database methods, such as the U.S. National Hospital Discharge Survey data system[15,16] or the Tennessee Medicaid Database[17] (approximately 1% of U.S. children) have confirmed the earlier findings with larger numbers and added detail about the risk factors for severe disease. In the last several years, new data have emerged on the role of a newly identified paramyxovirus, hMPV,[18] which was shown to be one of the most common causes associated with LRTI in children.[19] Before 2001, studies could not address the epidemiology of this virus because it had not been discovered.

RISK FACTORS FOR PNEUMONIA

Most children are infected with the common respiratory viruses during the first years of life, but a minority suffers from lower respiratory tract disease or pneumonia to such an extent that it brings them to medical care. Studies have identified a number of risk factors for severe disease, especially young age, prematurity, preexisting lung disease (especially bronchopulmonary dysplasia), congenital heart disease, environmental exposure (smoking or wood fire heating), daycare, large number of siblings, low socioeconomic status, or birth near the start of the RSV season.[17] Exposures to infected children in the home or nosocomial exposure are pertinent historical risk factors.

PATHOGENESIS

Viral pneumonia is an infection of the cells surrounding the alveolar space. Alveolar walls thicken, and the alveolar space becomes occluded with exudates, sloughed cells, and activated macrophages. The clinical disease is distinguished by poor air exchange, first noted by poor oxygenation (detected by pulse oximetry or blood gas measurement) followed by CO_2 retention. The physiology of the disease reflects an inflammatory process that interferes with gas exchange, resulting in elevation of the alveolar-arterial Po_2 difference. Many cases of viral pneumonia in young children are also accompanied by inflammation of the bronchioles, and air trapping contributes to the poor level of gas exchange. Children compensate for respiratory compromise better than do adults, generally by increasing the respiratory rate. Children show a remarkable resilience when faced with respiratory compromise, even though their airways exhibit a much higher intrinsic level of resistance. Unrelieved tachypnea, however, can lead to exhaustion and respiratory failure. The histopathologic mechanisms underlying acute viral pulmonary disease in otherwise healthy children are not completely understood because lung tissue is rarely obtained for histology before mechanical ventilation or other medical interventions in previously healthy patients.

LIFE CYCLE OF THE VIRUSES *IN VIVO*

Despite significant advances in our understanding of the basic virology and molecular biology of these respiratory viruses based on *in vitro* studies, relatively little is known about the life cycle and spread of these viruses to the lung parenchyma *in vivo*. It is thought that the initial infection occurs in the nasopharynx after inoculation with contaminated respiratory secretions (fomite transmission) or exposure to large-particle aerosols containing virus. The viruses that cause pneumonia all have surface fusion proteins that mediate both virus-cell fusion and cell-cell fusion in monolayer cell culture. The viruses cause cytopathic effects following infection by inducing necrosis or apoptosis of infected cells. The viral fusion peptides of these viruses cause multinucleated cell (syncytium) formation in cell monolayer cultures. It is presumed that they cause syncytia formation *in vivo*, but the direct evidence for this is scarce. In fact, viruses that cause syncytium in nonpolarized cultured cells (i.e., cells that do not form tight junctions and segregate apical and basolateral cell membrane regions) often do not cause syncytia in polarized cell lines or primary cells in culture. Most of these viruses appear to infect both ciliated and nonciliated cells in culture. Impaired mucociliary clearance caused by infection of ciliated cells probably contributes to progression to pneumonia. Whether these viruses infect type I or II pneumocytes more efficiently is not known. Some of the respiratory viruses cause an abortive round of infection in cultured macrophages or dendritic cells. Infection of these antigen-presenting cell types may contribute to inflammatory disease of the lung.

The mechanism for spread of infection to the lower respiratory tract within days of inoculation is unknown. Virus probably spreads by microaspiration of infected secretions or by cell-to-cell spread. The rapid time course of spread *in vivo* suggests that aspiration of infected secretions results in direct inoculation of the lower respiratory tract. Autopsy of fatal RSV cases has demonstrated the presence of relatively little virus antigen, and pathologic changes in fatal cases can be patchy in distribution. Bronchoalveolar lavage and tissue specimens from hematopoietic stem cell transplant patients or autopsies evaluated by direct immunofluorescence or immunoperoxidase stains revealed epithelial cells and macrophages that stain positive for RSV proteins, and electron microscopy revealed occasional epithelial cells with cytoplasmic inclusions composed of filamentous virions. There are limited autopsy data from PIV-infected or influenza-infected humans. In summary, the population(s) of cells that are the primary target of respiratory virus infections in humans are probably epithelial in origin but have not been fully defined in normal hosts.

VIRUS RECEPTORS ON HOST CELLS

The hemagglutinin protein of influenza virus mediates virus attachment to a ciliated cell glycoconjugate terminating in sialic acid and causes fusion with an intracellular endosomal membrane at low pH. The PIV hemagglutinin-neuraminidase glycoprotein mediates attachment to sialic acid–containing host cell receptors. The RSV surface protein that mediates attachment is the RSV G (glycosylated) glycoprotein. Its cellular receptor is not fully understood, but this glycosylated protein binds to heparan sulfates and to the CX3CR1 protein (the specific receptor for the CX3C chemokine fractalkine) through a CX3C motif in the viral protein.[20] The viability of mutant RSV strains lacking the viral G protein indicates that this attachment protein is not strictly required for replication in cell culture or in rodents. The RSV F protein binds to toll-like receptor 4[21] and to heparan sulfates and interacts with the cellular protein RhoA[22] nucleolin[22a] but whether any of these serves as a principal protein receptor is not clear. An association between common toll-like receptor 4 genetic polymorphisms and severity of RSV disease has been reported.

INFLAMMATION

The magnitude and character of the inflammatory response in the airway appear to be highly regulated by epithelial cell–derived cytokines and chemokines that attract and activate specific subsets of leukocytes associated with airway inflammation. Cytokine secretion appears to be highly regulated by nuclear factor κB (NF-κB) transcription factors, which are dimers of structurally related proteins retained in the cytoplasm by association with the inhibitory κB proteins. Upon various cellular stimulations usually related to stress or pathogens, the inhibitors are degraded and the nuclear factors κB translocate to the nucleus, where they bind to κB DNA elements to induce transcription of a large number of genes, especially those associated with immune responses. Nuclear factor interleukin 6 (NF-IL-6) regulates expression of cytokine and adhesion molecule genes without increased transcription. RSV infection induces increased expression of several cytokines, including IL-6 and IL-8, which are transcriptionally regulated by NF-κB and NF-IL-6. These cytokine-regulated pathways appear to contribute to airway inflammation during pneumonia.

Immune cells also probably play a major role in the pathogenesis of disease. Infected epithelial cells appear to initiate a cascade of events that represent components of the innate immune response. When infected epithelial cells secrete IL-6 and IL-8 and other soluble factors, they recruit and initiate activation of immune effectors. The chemokine RANTES (regulated upon activation, normal T cell expressed and secreted) is a chemoattractant for eosinophils, monocytes, T cells, and basophils that is secreted in response to infection with viruses such as RSV. Eventually, adaptive immune effectors such as CD8+ T cells attack the virus-infected cells to eliminate the infection. This immune cytolysis is important to disease resolution but comes at the price of inducing some level of immunopathology. The cell surface factors that facilitate homing of lymphocytes to lung tissue are under investigation.

CLINICAL DISEASE

The clinical presentation of viral pneumonia includes increased respiratory rate and supracostal, intercostal, or subcostal retractions. Infants show nasal flaring, grunting, and marked retractions during severe disease. Vital signs reveal fever in about half of cases at presentation; fever higher than 103° F is much less common than in bacterial pneumonia but can occur. Systemic toxicity is less common than with bacterial infection because respiratory viruses (other than measles virus) rarely cause viremia. In fact, most respiratory viruses appear to be limited to the most superficial cells at the lumenal surface of the airway. Of the conventional respiratory viruses, influenza virus is the one that most frequently causes high fever and toxic appearance. Respiratory failure, heralded by a change in alertness due to hypoxia and CO_2 retention or decreased respiratory effort due to exhaustion, requires immediate action. Physical examination reveals crackles on auscultation, generally more prominent on inspiration. RSV disease in infants is commonly a mixed presentation of bronchiolitis and pneumonia, in which case expiratory wheezing is present in addition to inspiratory crackles. The viruses that cause pneumonia also cause upper respiratory tract infection. Therefore, concomitant coryza is common, complicated in about one third of cases with otitis media. Nasal obstruction caused by purulent nasal secretions contributes to the respiratory distress, especially in infants. Mild to moderate dehydration is common as a result of increased respiratory and other insensible losses, and poor oral fluid intake.

CLINICAL DIAGNOSIS OF PNEUMONIA

The terms *pneumonia* and *lower respiratory tract illness* have clinical, anatomic, and histologic definitions. *Lower respiratory tract illness* is defined clinically as the presence of crackles, rhonchi, or wheezes on physical examination or as infiltrates on a chest radiograph. Anatomically it is usually considered disease below the vocal cords. Pneumonia is an inflammation caused by infection of the lung parenchyma, comprising alveoli and interstitial tissue with possible extension to the bronchioles. Viral pneumonia during childhood is often one component of a lower respiratory illness that also affects the small and large conducting airways. For example, the most common presentation of severe RSV infection of infants is bronchiolitis and pneumonia.

RADIOGRAPHIC FINDINGS

Chest radiographs using the posteroanterior view are the principal diagnostic radiologic test for pneumonias. Children who have an effusion or an empyema identified on chest radiograph may need a computed tomography scan to define further the scope of the problem, but these complications are rare in viral pneumonia. Radiologic findings on chest radiographs of viral pneumonia are similar to those of bronchiolitis and reactive airways disease. The usual findings on chest radiographs are hyperaeration, prominent lung markings caused by bronchial wall thickening, and focal areas of atelectasis (Fig. 28-1). The hili may be somewhat prominent, but major hilar adenopathy is uncommon. The findings are commonly

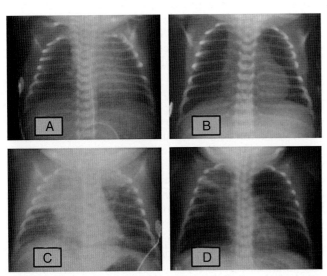

FIGURE 28-1. Chest radiographs from a premature infant who suffered RSV pneumonia early in life. **A,** This infant presented with neonatal respiratory distress syndrome (RDS) requiring mechanical ventilation; the radiograph shows a ground-glass appearance and lung volume loss from RDS on the day of birth. **B,** By 1 week of life, mechanical ventilation is discontinued and the lung fields normalize. **C,** At 6 weeks of life, the infant presented with an RSV-positive test and respiratory distress requiring mechanical ventilation; the radiograph shows diffuse interstitial infiltrates and atelectasis or pneumonia of the right upper lobe. **D,** By 7 weeks of life, the infant remained on a mechanical ventilator, but infiltrates and atelectasis were improving. (Radiographs courtesy of James Crowe, MD, Texas Children's Hospital.)

thought to differ from the typical case of bacterial pneumonia, which usually has been thought to present as lobar consolidation. It is true that most children with focal alveolar pneumonia have laboratory evidence of a bacterial infection, especially those with lobar infiltrates. However, half of the children with solely interstitial infiltrates on chest radiograph had evidence of bacterial infection in some studies.[23] Therefore, radiologic presentation of interstitial infiltrates alone does not distinguish between bacterial and viral pneumonia. One also cannot differentiate viral pneumonia from bronchiolitis or reactive airways disease on the basis of radiologic findings alone. Differentiation is based on non-radiologic factors such as the age of the patient and the clinical history. The chest radiograph in newborns with viral pneumonia usually shows bilateral diffuse densities or may have a granular appearance, similar to that found in hyaline membrane disease. When infection is congenital, radiographic changes may be present at birth, whereas the radiographs of infants infected during birth may be normal initially but can progress rapidly during the first days of life.

DIFFERENTIAL DIAGNOSIS

The differential diagnosis for nonviral causes of pneumonia varies by age. In newborns, group B streptococcus infection and hyaline membrane disease are the most common considerations. In infants, atypical organisms (e.g., *Chlamydia trachomatis* and *Ureaplasma urealyticum*) must be considered, as well as *Pneumocystis carinii* in children with immunodeficiencies or *in utero* exposure to human immunodeficiency virus. Common bacterial causes of pneumonia are *Bordetella pertussis*, *Streptococcus pneumoniae*, *Haemophilus influenzae* (mostly nontypable species in the era of universal immunization against type B), and *Mycobacterium* infections (including tuberculosis). In young children, *Mycoplasma pneumoniae*, *S. pneumoniae*, and *Mycobacterium* infections are important. In older children and adolescents, the atypical organisms *M. pneumoniae*, *C. trachomatis*, and *Chlamydia pneumoniae* remain important, and the bacteria *S. pneumoniae*, *B. pertussis*, and *Mycobacterium* species are considerations. *Histoplasma capsulatum* infection is relatively common in certain areas of the United States and causes an atypical pneumonia. *Cryptococcus neoformans* infection is also a consideration in immunocompromised patients.

Many published studies have addressed the differentiation of bacterial from viral pneumonia using clinical, radiologic, and routine hematologic tests, but these methods have not been found to be sufficiently reliable in differential diagnosis.[23–33]

Chest radiographic findings, total white blood cell count, erythrocyte sedimentation rate, and serum C-reactive protein have been used widely in children with community-acquired pneumonia of varying etiology to discriminate between bacterial and viral causes, but the specificities of these are not sufficient to determine the diagnosis in clinical practice. Lymphocytic predominance is usually present in the peripheral white blood cells during viral pneumonias, although this feature is also usually present in pertussis and atypical bacterial infections. Bacterial pneumonia requiring hospitalization on average causes higher fever than viral pneumonia, and it is more often associated with a fever higher than 103° F than is viral pneumonia. A lobar, segmental, or rounded well-defined pneumonia affecting a single lobe is more likely to be bacterial in etiology, as are cases associated with large pleural effusions, abscess, bullae, or pneumatoceles. A bedside cold agglutinins test may be positive in the case of viral pneumonia or mycoplasmal infection, thus it is not a particularly helpful test in distinguishing etiology.

LABORATORY DIAGNOSIS OF VIRAL ETIOLOGY

The specific cause of viral pneumonia can be identified by several methods with varying levels of stringency. Culture of virus in cell monolayer cultures is considered the gold standard. Viruses are identified by characteristic cytopathic effect and are confirmed by immunodetection using virus-specific antibodies and fluorescence detection. Culture techniques require a high level of expertise and generally are best performed on fresh specimens (e.g., secretions obtained by nasopharyngeal aspiration or nasopharyngeal swab). Rapid diagnostic tests for RSV and influenzas A and B based on the immunodetection of viral proteins in nasopharyngeal secretions are widely used, but their positive predictive value is more appropriate for use during epidemics, when the prevalence of positive tests is expected to be high. Antigen detection tests are not sensitive enough to determine that a hospitalized patient is no longer shedding infectious virus; therefore, negative tests should not be used to justify termination of contact precautions in a patient with viral pneumonia. Increasingly, clinical detection of viruses is being performed by molecular genetic techniques, such as reverse transcriptase–polymerase chain reaction followed by hybridization or sequence analysis. This technique identifies the presence of viral nucleic acid. Polymerase chain reaction tests tend to be more sensitive than cell culture during the period of viral clearance (1 to 3 weeks after infection). It is not clear how long viral RNAs are present following active infections, but evidence to date shows that they may persist for weeks or months, even when virus can no longer be cultured. Therefore, a positive polymerase chain reaction–based test must be used with caution because in some cases a positive test obtained during an acute pneumonia is actually related to a recent infection. Serology is helpful to diagnose or confirm infection, particularly in the clinical research setting. A four-fold increase in serum antibodies against a virus between the pre-infection period and after infection suggests a specific diagnosis, particularly when testing the binding to targets of functional antibodies. In practice, the use of serologic tests to diagnose the cause of pneumonia is difficult because the increase in antibodies in young children may not achieve a significant level until 6 to 8 weeks or more have passed.

CO-INFECTIONS

Single agents cause most cases of viral pneumonia, but co-infection does occur. Most careful studies in children have found evidence for the presence of two viruses in about 5% to 10% of cases of viral LRTI. There is little direct evidence in immunocompetent individuals that co-infection is characterized by a more severe clinical course than infection with a single agent. Bacterial superinfection does occur, but overt bacterial lung disease during viral pneumonia is unusual. Bacterial complication of viral pneumonia is suggested by an abrupt change in symptoms over several hours with appearance of generalized toxicity, and possibly with new radiographic findings of parenchymal consolidation or pleural effusions. Marked and changed leukocytosis (e.g., >20,000 cells/mm³ peripheral white blood cells) is suggestive of a bacterial process, but it is not particularly sensitive or specific. S. pneumoniae, H. influenzae, and Staphylococcus aureus are the most common bacteria involved in the complication of viral pneumonia, and influenza virus pneumonia is the most common viral pneumonia that is complicated by bacterial infection. Vaccine studies with a pneumococcal vaccine in a large population of children showed that a 9-valent bacterial polysaccharide vaccine prevented about one third of viral pneumonia cases, suggesting frequent interactions of bacteria and viruses that are not apparent by current methods of clinical evaluation.[34]

THERAPY

Most infants and children with mild viral pneumonia can be treated symptomatically as outpatients. Oxygen is required if there is grunting, flaring, severe tachypnea, and retractions, or if pulse oximetry indicates oxygen saturation below 90% to 92%, or arterial blood gas measurement indicates depressed Po_2 (<60 to 70 mm Hg). Retention of CO_2 is particularly concerning, especially in the face of tachypnea. Severe respiratory distress, hypoxia, and dehydration are among the indications for hospitalization. Care in the hospital is principally supportive, such as the delivery of supplemental oxygen and intravenous fluids, and the use of mechanical ventilation in the case of respiratory failure. The youngest infants with RSV pneumonia may require monitoring for the risk of apnea, although apnea usually presents near the beginning of the illness. Chest physiotherapy and mucolytics have unproven efficacy in viral pneumonia. If a specific viral diagnosis is made early in the course of illness, there are some antiviral medications available. Licensed drugs for influenza infection include the M2 ion-channel inhibitors amantidine and rimantidine, and the neuraminidase inhibitors oseltamivir and zanamivir. Many influenza viruses are resistant to the ion channel inhibitors, however. These antiviral compounds work best when therapy is initiated in the first days of infection and are particularly relevant for those with immunosuppression or preexisting cardiopulmonary disease. Ribavirin delivered as an aerosol is licensed for treatment of severe RSV infection, but recent studies have questioned its value. Most centers do not routinely treat otherwise healthy infants with RSV pneumonia with ribavirin. RSV intravenous immune globulin and palivizumab (an intramuscular injectable humanized monoclonal antibody directed against the RSV fusion protein) are available for prophylaxis against RSV disease and are indicated for children with chronic cardiopulmonary disease and other serious risk factors. Clinical trials of therapy of acute disease using these antibody preparations, however, have not shown this treatment to be effective during hospitalization. Antibiotic therapy does not improve the outcome in viral pneumonia and has not been shown to alter the risk of bacterial complication of viral pneumonia as a superinfection. Indiscriminate use of antibiotics in the setting of viral infection causes the selection of antibiotic-resistant bacteria. If secondary infection does occur, usually in hospitalized patients in intensive care units, the selected infecting bacterium may not be susceptible to conventional antibiotics. Therefore, specific diagnosis of the etiology of severe pneumonia suspected to be of viral etiology is warranted to minimize inappropriate antibiotic exposure, even when an antiviral therapeutic option is not anticipated.

COMPLICATIONS

Many of the common sequelae of bacterial pneumonia (e.g., persistent effusions, empyemas, abscess formation, and pneumatoceles) are distinctly uncommon following viral pneumonia. Therefore, the prognosis for most forms of viral pneumonia caused by conventional respiratory viruses is excellent. Most otherwise healthy children with uncomplicated pneumonia recover without sequelae. Complications during influenza pneumonia in children range from acute otitis media, sinusitis, and bacterial tracheitis to rare episodes of encephalitis, myositis, myocarditis, febrile seizures, encephalopathy, or Reyes syndrome. RSV disease is commonly complicated by otitis media. Immunocompromised children, those with underlying cardiopulmonary disease, and neonates are at the highest risk for severe sequelae. Pulmonary hypertension can complicate the course of neonatal pneumonia, and concomitant pulmonary hemorrhage due to vascular damage may follow. Pulmonary interstitial emphysema and other types of gas leaks can occur, especially during mechanical ventilation. Mortality is high in neonatal viral pneumonia, especially in premature infants in whom the disease may resemble severe hyaline membrane disease. Infants with severe viral pneumonia early in life who require mechanical ventilation or treatment with high concentrations of supplemental oxygen are at increased risk of chronic lung disease. Some cases of viral pneumonia, especially those due to rapid-onset severe adenovirus infection, can lead to bronchiolitis obliterans and hyperlucent lung syndrome. The prognosis for pneumonia due to more uncommon causes of viral pneumonia (e.g., varicella-zoster virus, SARS-coronavirus, and measles virus) can be guarded.

PROTECTIVE IMMUNITY

Serum-neutralizing antibodies appear to be most protective of the lower respiratory tract against severe disease caused by viruses. Probably this is a result of the close association of the intravascular space with the alveolus. The gradient of antibody transfer to the nasopharynx is quite steep in that there are about 300-fold higher levels of immunoglobulin G (IgG) antibodies in the serum than in the nasopharynx, but levels of IgG in the alveolus and serum can be quite similar.

High levels of IgG in the alveolus are probably caused by transudation. In higher areas of the airway, IgG antibodies may be transported to the lumen by the neonatal Fc receptor. Secretory IgA is uniquely suited for antiviral activity at the respiratory mucosal surface. Mucosal antibody secretion occurs locally, and polymeric IgA is taken up specifically by the polyimmunoglobulin receptor at the base of polarized epithelial cells, transcytosed in the apical direction, and secreted onto the mucosa. Antibodies may contribute to the resolution of acute primary infection of the lung. IgA and IgG RSV antibodies are present in the nasal secretions of infants early in infection, and the decrease in virus shedding in infants infected with RSV has been associated temporally with the detection of RSV-specific IgA in nasal washes. Laboratory studies and clinical trials provide strong evidence for the dominant role of antibodies in protection against re-infection. Maternal antibodies do not cross the placenta efficiently before 32 weeks gestation; therefore, premature infants are lacking the serum antibody protection against viral pneumonia that is conferred to term infants.

Cell-mediated immunity probably plays a primary role in the clearance of established respiratory virus pneumonia in humans. The best evidence to support this concept is that patients with defects in cellular immunity (e.g., recipients of hematopoietic stem cell transplantation or patients with cancer undergoing immunosuppressive chemotherapy) suffer more prolonged virus shedding or more frequent and more severe illnesses with RSV, MPV, influenza virus, or PIV type 3. The role in humans of cell-mediated immune effectors in protection against disease on re-infection or during virus challenge following immunization is less clear, however. Macrophages are abundant in the alveolar spaces of the lung. *In vitro* and *in vivo* data suggest that the resident pulmonary alveolar macrophage population actively suppresses the antigen-presenting function of lung dendritic cells (DCs) *in situ*. Low numbers of DCs and high numbers of macrophages have been noted in the human alveolar compartment, suggesting that the alveolar compartment may be less efficient for mounting an immune response. Human alveolar macrophages recovered during RSV infection can yield small amounts of RSV, but replication of RSV in alveolar macrophages is restricted. Inoculation of human alveolar macrophages with live or inactivated RSV induces increased secretion of cytokines, such as tumor necrosis factor, IL-6, IL-8, and IL-10.

Dendritic cells are distributed widely in the lung, where they are distinguished by their morphology and class II major histocompatibility complex antigen expression. DCs serve as potent pulmonary antigen-presenting cells. However, relatively little is currently known about how these cells respond to specific respiratory viruses at the mucosa. Recruitment of a wave of DCs into the respiratory tract mucosa appears to be a feature of the acute cellular response to local challenge with viral protein antigens or virus infection. Differentiation of DCs in the lung, homing of particular types of DCs to the lung, and crosstalk between adaptive immune cells and DCs in the lung are all areas of current research.

PREVENTION

The viruses that commonly cause viral pneumonia are ubiquitous, and every child becomes infected in the first years of life with most of the common respiratory viruses. It is not feasible to avoid or prevent exposure or infection completely; therefore, the practical goal is to avoid infection at a time of high risk and to prevent severe disease or complications during infection. Thorough hand hygiene, the use of contact isolation, and patient or provider cohorting are critical to the prevention of the nosocomial spread of infection to high-risk individuals in the hospital. Vaccination of at-risk individuals with licensed vaccines for seasonal influenza virus is wise. Influenza antivirals can be used effectively as a prophylactic treatment in some for the prevention of symptomatic influenza disease during an epidemic or immediately following exposure. Prophylactic treatments with an RSV monoclonal antibody (palivizumab, IM) can be used in infants at high risk of RSV disease, and these treatments prevent half or more of RSV hospitalizations during treatment. The combination of risk factors that best predicts susceptibility to hospitalization due to RSV is not entirely clear, but includes extreme prematurity, bronchopulmonary disease, and oxygen dependence. More subtle influences are important, but they affect risk incrementally. The use of the live attenuated measles-mumps-rubella vaccine is effective against measles and mumps disease, and varicella vaccine prevents severe disease caused by that virus. An adenovirus vaccine has been used effectively, but only in the military to prevent epidemic disease in adults who live in close quarters.

EXPERIMENTAL VACCINES

Candidate vaccines have been developed and tested for prevention of viral pneumonia caused by RSV; PIV types 1, 2, and 3; and hMPV. Both subunit and live attenuated RSV vaccines have been tested in phase I or II trials, and the live attenuated vaccines appear promising. The challenge for investigators is to identify or generate attenuated viruses that are sufficiently immunogenic to induce a protective response in newborns without causing any signs or symptoms of respiratory disease. Cold-passaged or bovine strain PIV type 3 vaccines have been tested extensively in humans, and they appear promising. To date, HMPV vaccine candidates have been generated, but they have not been tested in clinical trials.

References

The complete reference list is available online at www.expertconsult.com

29 COMMUNITY-ACQUIRED BACTERIAL PNEUMONIA

Paulo J.C. Marostica, MD, and Renato T. Stein, MD, MPH, PhD

Community-acquired pneumonia (CAP) is one of the most important health problems affecting children worldwide and is the leading single cause of mortality in children younger than 5 years of age. Its greatest impact is observed in developing countries, with more than 70% of the cases diagnosed in sub-Saharan Africa and Southeast Asia.[1] There are 4 to 5 million annual deaths reported in children younger than 5 years of age, again with the majority of these occurring in low-income populations.[2]

The proportion of pneumonia cases obtained from efficacy estimates of vaccine trials were used to demonstrate the burden of pneumonia caused by S. pneumoniae and Haemophilus influenza type b (Hib).[3,4] Over 13 million new cases of pneumococcal pneumonia were estimated with this strategy, with a global incidence of 2228 cases per 100,000 children younger than 5 years of age ranging from 462/100,000 cases in Europe to 3397/100,000 cases in Africa. The case fatality rate ranged from 2% in Western Pacific to 11% in Africa. Hib caused about 8 million cases of serious disease and 371,000 child deaths in 2000. The estimated global incidence of Hib pneumonia in the absence of vaccination was 1304 per 100,000 children younger than 5 years of age.

Pneumonia can be broadly defined as inflammation of lung tissue caused by an infectious agent that stimulates a response resulting in damage to lung tissue. Resolution of damage may be complete or only partial. Different definitions for pneumonia are found in the medical literature, varying from the detection of pulmonary pathogens in lung specimens to the presence of pulmonary infiltrates on chest radiographs, or clinical-based criteria such as tachypnea or retractions. For practical reasons, most experts define *pneumonia* as an association of clinical findings and radiographic evidence of infiltrates.[2,5] In less affluent countries, the preferred term is sometimes acute *lower respiratory tract infection (LRTI)*, possibly because of the difficulties in obtaining a chest radiograph. Not surprisingly, other common pediatric respiratory diseases may overlap this definition, especially viral bronchiolitis.

This chapter discusses bacterial pneumonias acquired in the community environment in children beyond the neonatal period. Pneumonias caused by viruses and other microorganisms are considered elsewhere in this book. Although in many real-life situations viruses may coexist with typical and atypical bacteria in the same child as causal agents for CAP, these nonbacterial agents are mentioned in this chapter only for the sake of comparison with bacterial disease in the diagnosis and treatment of CAP. The upper airways are commensally colonized by a variety of pathogens, differently from the lower respiratory tract, which is considered to be sterile. Bacterial infections are frequently preceded by viral (especially respiratory syncytial virus, or rhinovirus) or *Mycoplasma pneumoniae* infections. Impairment of the cough reflex, interruption of mucociliary clearance because of virus-induced changes in ciliary structure and function, and virus-induced enhancement of bacterial adherence are some of the mechanisms believed to be contributory in this chain of events eventually leading to CAP.

EPIDEMIOLOGY

The estimated median incidence of pneumonia in 2000 in children younger than 5 years of age in developing countries was 0.28 episodes per child-year, corresponding to 151.8 million new cases (8.7% of which are severe enough to require hospitalization). The estimated figures for developed countries are 4.08 million new cases, representing an incidence of 0.05 episodes per child-year. Variables such as nutritional status, age, crowding, and the presence of an underlying condition (in particular measles, especially in some African countries) influence morbidity and mortality rates caused by CAP.[2,6-9]

Air pollution is also a risk factor for childhood pneumonia, and this is especially important in many South Asian countries affected by heavy automotive traffic. A recent meta-analysis by Dherani and colleagues, despite finding an important heterogeneity among the reviewed studies, found an overall odds ratio of 1.79 for pneumonia in children exposed to unprocessed solid fuel use.[2,10]

Children attending daycare centers are also at an increased risk of acquiring pneumococcal infections, but these figures may change in the near future when general pneumococcal vaccination strategies are implemented in poor countries. Recent studies on the prevalence of capsulated Hib infections show a significant decline after efficient population-level immunization strategies, thus suggesting that this pathogen (which would have been responsible formerly for almost 20% of all CAPs) is less likely to cause CAP in vaccinated children.[11]

Respiratory syncytial virus (RSV) and influenza virus infections usually occur in late fall and winter months, and these pathogens may predispose infants and young children to bacterial CAP, especially if there are other risk factors present. In a cohort of children from rural Kenya followed from birth through three RSV epidemics, risk factors for LRIs associated with RSV were severe stunting, crowding, and number of children younger than 6 years of age living in the home.[12]

Although accurate data on pneumonia mortality are lacking for most developing countries, environmental changes, promotion of exclusive breastfeeding, immunization against *Pneumococcus* and *Haemophilus* B, and specific pneumonia case management would expect to reduce child mortality by 17%.[13]

INFLUENCE OF AGE IN ETIOLOGY

There are significant age-related differences in the etiology of CAP during childhood (Table 29-1). From birth to 20 days of life, most pneumonias are caused by group B streptococci or Gram-negative enteric bacteria. Viruses are the most frequent pathogens of CAP, especially in young children. *Chlamydia pneumoniae* and *M. pneumoniae* infections occur more often in school-age children and during adolescence, although there are many reports of these agents causing CAP in younger children as well.[14–16]

Infants in the first 3 months of life may present with cough, and respiratory distress associated with low-grade or no fever. This clinical picture may be caused by Chlamydia trachomatis, a variety of respiratory viruses, Bordetella pertussis, or possibly Ureaplasma urealyticum (the role of this agent is less clear). Staphylococcus aureus used to be a much more prevalent pneumonia pathogen in the first year of life, but its role has diminished in recent years. In children younger than 5 years of age, viruses are more frequently associated with a diagnosis of CAP than bacteria. The most commonly found bacteria are pneumococcus and atypical agents (*M. pneumoniae* and *C. pneumonia*).[17]

Frequency rates for *S. pneumoniae*, the most prevalent bacteria causing CAP, are less affected by age. *S. pneumoniae* is a common pathogen throughout both infancy and childhood, with the possible exception of the early postnatal period. *S. pneumoniae* infections are less influenced by immunization because many different serotypes, not all covered by vaccines, can cause disease. It is worth mentioning that pneumoccus immunization is standard practice in most affluent countries, but not in many developing countries.

Nontypable *H. influenzae* is less frequently associated with pneumonia than is *S. pneumoniae* in immunocompetent children, being occasionally found in case series from developing countries.[7–11,18,19]

CLINICAL FEATURES

Children with pneumonia do not necessarily present with an acute illness, and some may have no specific respiratory signs or symptoms.[20] Children with pneumonia may have clinical findings such as fever, chills, abdominal and/or chest pains, and productive cough, all of which suggest but do not prove typical bacterial pneumonia. On the other hand, a more gradual clinical onset associated with headache, malaise, nonproductive cough, and low-grade fever/no fever is more commonly associated with infection by atypical pathogens such as *M. pneumonia*.[19]

Wheezing is most frequently associated with viral, *Mycoplasma*, or *Chlamydia* infections, and it makes a bacterial cause unlikely in this setting. In the case series of pneumonias from Wubbel and colleagues, pneumococcal infection was the most frequent diagnosis among patients with a history of wheezing when this was not detected as a current clinical finding. On the other hand, viruses were the most frequent pathogens among those patients who wheezed.[9]

Tachypnea is a useful sign for the diagnosis of childhood pneumonia and is more specific and reproducible than auscultatory signs. Usually, the cutoff points are a respiratory rate of 60 breaths per minute in infants younger than 2 months of age, 50 breaths per minute for infants from 2 to 12 months of age, and 40 breaths per minute for children 1 to 5 years of age. Tachypnea is usually more sensitive and specific than crackles on auscultation, after a diagnosis of bronchiolitis or asthma has been excluded. The positive predictive value of this finding is high; this is why it is used to diagnose CAP in developing countries, where bacterial pneumonias are highly prevalent. By contrast, in affluent countries most children who present acutely with an increased respiratory rate have either bronchiolitis or asthma associated with a viral infection.[20–22]

Children can have pneumonia and fever without overt manifestations of respiratory disease. In a recent Canadian series of 570 pediatric patients with signs and symptoms suggestive of LRTI, fever was the most sensitive sign, while grunting and retractions were the most specific signs associated with alveolar infiltrates found on chest radiograph.[23] A retrospective study from the United States showed that 5.3% of children with fever and no signs of LRTI, respiratory distress, or hypoxia may have a confirmed diagnosis of pneumonia. The presence of cough as well as a longer duration of fever and cough was more likely associated

---

TABLE 29-1 MOST COMMON AGENTS CAUSING COMMUNITY-ACQUIRED PNEUMONIA, ACCORDING TO AGE GROUP

| | AGE | | | |
Newborns	1 to 3 Months	1 to 12 Months	1 to 5 Years	Older Than 5 Years
Group B Streptococcus	*Chlamydia trachomatis*	Viruses	Viruses	*S. pneumoniae*
Enteric gram-negative	*Ureaplasma urealyticum*	*Streptococcus pneumoniae*	*S. pneumoniae*	*M. pneumoniae*
	Viruses	*Haemophilus influenzae*	*M. pneumoniae*	*C. pneumoniae*
	Bordetella pertussis	*Staphylococcus aureus*	*C. pneumoniae*	
		Moraxella catarrhalis		

with occult pneumonia. When cough was absent, only 0.28% of the children had pneumonia.[24]

DIAGNOSIS

The diagnosis of pneumonia should be suspected in every child with fever, cough, tachypnea, respiratory distress, and crackles on chest auscultation. The presence of tachypnea is used by the World Health Organization in the diagnosis of pneumonia. The best way to assess respiratory rate is over a 60-second period with the child alert and calm. Other respiratory signs (e.g., retractions) also indicate pneumonia, but no sign by itself can be used to diagnose or to rule out pneumonia. There is better interobserver agreement over clinical signs than for auscultation of the chest, especially when examining infants where a high index of suspicion is paramount.[7]

The differential diagnosis includes viral bronchiolitis, asthma, cardiogenic causes of tachypnea, interstitial lung diseases, and chemical pneumonitis, especially secondary to aspiration syndromes. Infants and small children presenting with fever and respiratory signs are frequently sent for a chest radiograph and often receive antimicrobial treatment for a presumptive diagnosis of bacterial pneumonia. Neither white blood cell counts nor radiology can differentiate reliably between viral and bacterial etiologies, which may indeed coexist. Radiologic signs of bilateral interstitial lung infiltrates or atelectasis, signs of bronchitis (true wheeze on auscultation), and generalized hyperinflation, though not definitive markers, are very likely to identify viral pneumonias correctly (Fig. 29-1).

Tuberculosis should always be considered as a possible diagnosis, especially among children living in, or in families that have recently moved from, endemic areas. Nonresolving pneumonia with persistence or recurrence of radiologic findings should alert the physician to noninfectious primary causes or infection with bacterial agents such as *Mycobacterium tuberculosis*. Another important differential diagnosis is that of round pneumonias since

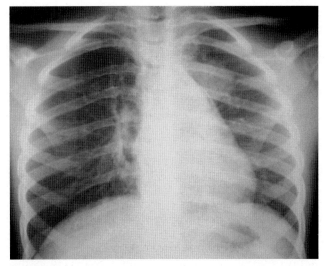

FIGURE 29-2. Round pneumonia. Opacity in the left upper segment, partially concealed by the mediastinal shadow.

secondarily infected congenital malformations or thoracic masses may have similar radiologic presentation (Fig. 29-2).

LABORATORY TESTS

Higher white blood cell counts and concentrations of C-reactive protein are seen in children with bacterial pneumonias, but there is great overlap with viral pneumonia, meaning that these findings are of little help clinically in the individual child.[17]

ETIOLOGIC DIAGNOSIS

Only a small proportion of CAPs will have a definite pathogen identified. Various approaches have been used to try to resolve this issue. Diagnostic methods for etiologic identification can be divided in microbiologic,

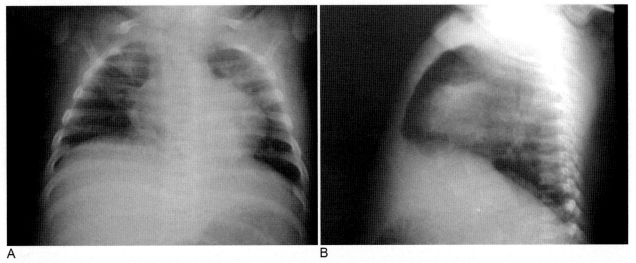

A   B

FIGURE 29-1. Viral pneumonia in a 6-month-old infant with respiratory syncytial virus–positive nasopharyngeal aspirate. **A,** Anteroposterior radiograph with bilateral interstitial infiltrates and patchy atelectasis. **B,** Lateral radiograph with hyperinflated lungs; increased anteroposterior volume, flattening of the diaphragm, and mediastinal air cushion.

immunologic, and DNA detection. The gold standard for etiologic diagnosis in CAP is either obtaining a lung puncture specimen or performing a bronchoalveolar lavage, but these are invasive methods and are unacceptable for routine clinical purposes (although BAL is helpful in non-responding patients and nosocomial or life-threatening infections). Although blood cultures may be considered a choice in some centers, the majority of children with CAP are appropriately managed without physicians using any laboratory tests.

Sputum examination is a possible alternative for respiratory secretion sampling. It is practical for adolescent and school-age children, but it should be interpreted with caution because upper airway commensals, which can be pathogenic to lower airways, usually contaminate the specimens. Furthermore, a child with lobar consolidation is unlikely to produce sputum in the acute phase of presentation. Zar and colleagues recovered pathogenic agents (*M. tuberculosis* in 9% and *Pneumocystis carinii* in 5.7%) from induced sputum samples (after 5% saline inhalation) in infants and young children with pneumonia from an area of high human immunodeficiency virus prevalence, suggesting a causative relation between these agents and pulmonary manifestations.[25] These authors also recovered the more usual CAP bacteria (*S. pneumoniae, S. aureus, H. influenzae,* and *Moraxella catarrhali*), but they could not establish with certainty that the lower respiratory tract was the source in these cases (since these bacteria are commensals in the upper respiratory tract). Bacterial cultures of the throat or nasopharynx do not correlate well with lung parenchyma cultures and are more likely to confound than to help, with the known exception of cystic fibrosis patients.[7,18,26]

Pleural fluid cultures may grow potential pathogens, but the usual practice of empiric antibiotic use in the early phases of the disease decreases the sensitivity of this method. However, pleural fluid should be aspirated for culture whenever technically feasible, unless the effusion is too small or there is fast clinical recovery.

Serologic Tests

Detection of bacterial antigens in urine or plasma has been used, but the results are conflicting, and sensitivity and specificity are both low. In August 1999, the U.S. Food and Drug Administration approved a rapid immunochromatographic test for pneumococcal antigen detection. The sensitivity and specificity are, respectively, 86% and 94% in urine for adult patients.[18] In children, a positive test may be associated with clinical infection but may also be secondary to nasal carriage. One possible advantage of antigen detection methods is that they do not depend on bacterial viability. Serology is useful for some agents such as *M. pneumoniae, C. pneumoniae,* and *S. pneumoniae,* but paired acute and convalescent titers are needed, resulting in the diagnosis being retrospective in most cases. In children younger than 6 months of age, there is only a weak immunologic response to capsular bacterial antigens, making this test less useful.[9,27]

Polymerase Chain Reaction

Polymerase chain reaction (PCR) has been used more recently as a diagnostic tool in respiratory infections. It may be applied to specimens from respiratory secretions, lung aspirate samples, or blood. Respiratory viruses, *M. pneumoniae, C. pneumoniae,* and other bacteria can be diagnosed by PCR. It is a good diagnostic tool in research and can be used by clinicians in special situations, but it does not differentiate carrier state from disease. It is possible that quantitative PCR may solve these problems if cutoff levels can be adequately defined. More details of these and other tests for viral detection can be found in other chapters.

▌ RADIOLOGIC FINDINGS

In general, chest radiographs are standard practice in hospitalized children for whom a diagnosis of pneumonia is being considered. The sensitivity of the test to diagnose pneumonia is approximately 75%. In the early stages, bacterial pneumonia not uncommonly presents with normal chest radiographs. There is also significant variation in interpretation of these radiographs in children. Specificity ranges from 42% to 100% in different studies because of varying definitions of pneumonia.[20]

A large proportion of children younger than 5 years of age with fever and leukocytosis, and without a definite source of infection may have radiographic abnormalities consistent with pneumonia. In a study by Bachur and colleagues, 26% of the patients younger than 5 years of age who presented to the emergency department with fever, leukocytosis greater than 20,000 cells/mm^3, and no clinical findings suggestive of pneumonia actually had a confirmed diagnosis of pneumonia on radiograph.[28] Therefore, a plain chest radiograph is part of the investigation of nonspecific clinical signs of infection in this age group.

Because chest radiographs do not change the outcome of LRTIs, guidelines do not recommend this examination for children older than 2 months of age who are cared for in an outpatient setting,[21,23,29] Even though not specific, the degree of respiratory compromise and the child's general appearance should be included in the decision-making process.

Although alveolar pneumonia is usually more frequently observed in infections by typical bacteria, compared with interstitial pneumonia (which occurs more frequently in viral pneumonias and after *Mycoplasma* or *Chlamydia* infections), it is usually impossible to make an etiologic diagnosis solely on the basis of chest radiographs.[7,19,20,27]

Another important issue is that no follow-up radiographs are needed to evaluate a CAP with good clinical response except for cases of round pneumonias, lobar collapse, or clinical deterioration.[21]

▌ STREPTOCOCCUS PNEUMONIAE

Streptococcus pneumoniae is the bacterial pathogen that most frequently causes pneumonia in children (Fig. 29-3). It is responsible for more than one half of the cases requiring hospital admissions.[20] In developing countries, it is estimated that 1 million children younger than 5 years of age die yearly

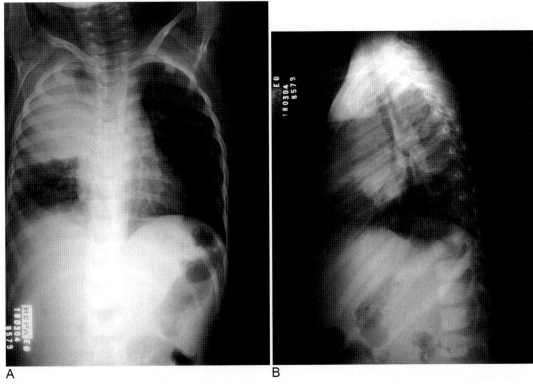

FIGURE 29-3. Pneumococcal pneumonia. Positive blood cultures for *Streptococcus pneumoniae*. Dense consolidation of upper and middle right lobes with air bronchogram. **A,** Anteroposterior view. **B,** Lateral view.

from bacterial pneumonias, and most of these are preventable with antimicrobial therapy.

Various pneumococcus serotypes have been implicated, with distinct prevalence rates in different parts of the world.[20,30] Prevalence of penicillin resistance also varies widely throughout different countries and continents. It can be very low or higher than 50%, as reported in case series from Africa and Asia.[31,32] One point that deserves attention is that the degree of penicillin resistance does not appear to cause adverse outcomes for pneumococcal CAP because high parenteral penicillin serum concentrations are achieved with usual dosage regimens (much higher than observed levels of resistance for these bacteria).

Antibiotic resistance is usually associated with changes in the penicillin-binding sites of the transpeptidases of the bacteria. It may be associated with cross-resistance to other beta-lactams and carbapenems. In 1997, in the United States alone, 92% of resistant pneumococcus strains were from serogroups 23, 6, 9, 19, and 14, which are covered by the current available conjugated vaccines. Resistance to macrolides (which has increased lately) is associated with the alteration of the 50S ribosomal binding site, preventing the drug from inhibiting protein synthesis or the presence of efflux pumps to macrolides. Macrolide resistance is more likely to occur with the widespread use of this class of antibiotics in the community.

OTHER BACTERIAL PATHOGENS

Haemophilus Influenzae Type B

This fastidious Gram-negative coccobacillus was once a more frequent cause of CAP, before the widespread use of appropriate *H. influenzae* type b immunization. It is

still an important cause of CAP in countries where these vaccines are not yet universally available. It is more frequently observed in children younger than 5 years of age. The most common mode of transmission is direct contact with respiratory secretions. The radiologic findings vary from linear infiltrates and hyperinflation to bronchopneumonia. Pleural effusion is a common feature.

Group A Streptococcus and *Streptococcus Pyogenes*

This is an infrequent cause of CAP nowadays. Pneumonia is not the leading presentation of group A streptococcal infections, with bacteremia and scarlet fever being common, and most significantly among small children. Measles, varicella, and influenza are also associated with co-infections from group A streptococcus since they seem to transiently affect host defenses and open room for commensal bacteria.

Staphylococcus Aureus

Staphylococcus aureus is secondary to inhalation of the infecting agent. In rare cases, it can be the result of bacteremic spread, usually in situations in which a predisposing factor is present (e.g., a catheter or IV drug use).

S. aureus pneumonia tends to present as an acute and severe illness, especially because many antibiotics commonly used to treat CAPs do not provide appropriate coverage for this agent. Radiologic findings include bronchopneumonia with alveolar infiltrates, which is more commonly unilateral. The infiltrates may coalesce and evolve to large areas of consolidation and cavitation. Destruction of bronchial walls may lead to air trapping and pneumatocele formation in at least 50% of cases. Pleural effusion and empyema are found in as many as 90% of cases. Pneumothorax and pyopneumothorax are common complications. In the case of hematogenic spread of *S. aureus*, the radiologic picture is one of multiple bilateral pulmonary infiltrates that may cavitate. An increase in white blood cell count is usual but is not sufficiently sensitive or specific to suggest the etiologic diagnosis. Although the appearance of staphylococcal pneumatoceles may be dramatic, usually once the infection is under control, the pneumatoceles resolve completely in the next few months.

Community-Associated Methicillin-Resistant *Staphylococcus Aureus*

In recent years, community-associated Methicillin-resistant *S. aureus* (CA-MRSA) has been increasingly recognized in otherwise healthy adults and children. CA-MRSA usually affects younger patients compared to what is observed in hospital-acquired MRSA, and it is often susceptible to clindamycin , trimethropim-sulfametoxazole, fluroquinolones, and tetracyclines. Many strains of CA-MRSA carry the gene for Panton-Valentine leukocidin, an exotoxin that is lethal to leukocytes, thus causing tissue necrosis, a high frequency of skin lesions, necrotizing pneumonia, and necrotizing fasciitis.[33]

■ GENERAL MANAGEMENT

Infants and children with mild and moderate LRTIs can be safely cared for at home. In this situation, the child usually should be re-examined within 48 hours after beginning treatment. According to the British Thoracic Society guidelines, an Sao$_2$ of 92% or less, cyanosis, respiratory rate greater than 70 breaths per minute, difficulty breathing, intermittent apnea, grunting, inability to feed, and a family incapable of providing appropriate observation or supervision are all indicators for hospital admission among infants.[21] In the case of older children, these indicators are a Sao$_2$ of 92% or less, cyanosis, respiratory rate greater than 50 breaths per minute, difficulty breathing, grunting, signs of dehydration, or a family incapable of providing appropriate observation or supervision. A Canadian board of experts includes also age younger than 6 months as lowering the threshold for admission.[7]

General management for hospitalized children include oxygen to keep saturation above 92%, antipyretics, and IV fluids if hydration is affected by severe respiratory distress or fatigue. Fluid intake should be carefully monitored because pneumonia can be complicated by hyponatremia secondary to the syndrome of inappropriate antidiuretic hormone secretion. The benefit of nasogastric tube feeding should be weighed against its potential for respiratory compromise due to obstruction of a nostril, or by worsening gastroesophageal reflux by interference with lower esophageal sphincter function.

There is no evidence-based data of a positive impact of chest physiotherapy in the management of CAP, and thus it is not currently indicated. Some studies have even shown increase in fever duration with the use of this practice.[21,34]

■ TREATMENT WITH ANTIMICROBIALS

Since viruses are the sole cause of many cases of pneumonia in childhood, it is appropriate not to treat every child with antibiotics. However, therapeutic decisions can be difficult because most tests do not adequately differentiate viral from bacterial infection in an individual child. An additional issue is the fact that some patients harbor mixed viral and bacterial agents.[9,18]

The problem of bacterial resistance to antibiotics has increased steadily in the last few years, and it is certainly preferable to restrict antibiotics as much as possible and to use narrow-spectrum agents whenever appropriate. It is believed that less antibiotic pressure limits the emergence of bacterial resistance.[18,26] Prior antibiotic therapy, day-care attendance, travel, exposure to infections, and coexisting morbidities are risk factors for resistance.[26] It is also important to keep in mind that, in an era of vaccines against *H. influenzae* type b and *S. pneumoniae*, previously effective antibiotic regimens may have to be re-evaluated.

Although no recent studies have addressed the issue, it is common sense to use them whenever bacterial pneumonia is the most probable diagnosis. This diagnosis is especially probable when CAP develops after several days of nonspecific respiratory illness.[18] Since a definitive etiologic diagnosis is more the exception than the rule, usually antibiotics are started on an empirical basis. Regional prevalences of CAP-causing agents should definitely be taken into account.

Few studies compare, in a well-designed fashion, different classes of antimicrobials for the treatment of childhood pneumonia. Since most children from affluent communities do well with very conservative treatment approaches, randomized controlled studies would have to involve large numbers of patients to be able to detect significant differences between treatments. Most of the existing recommendations are based on expert opinions.

Some studies have recently reviewed the issue of treatment duration. A multicenter study from Pakistan, which enrolled 2188 children between the ages of 2 and 59 months, showed equivalence of a 3-day or 5-day course of amoxicillin in the treatment of nonsevere pneumonia, diagnosed according to the World Health Organization's criteria. Of note were a low prevalence of positive radiographic findings (14%) and a relatively high rate (20%) of treatment failure.[35] Since most of the recommendations on antibiotic choice are a result of expert opinion, either alone or in consensus, the following recommendations are also based on the authors' view, based as much as possible on existing evidence.

Choice of Antibiotics

The choice of antibiotics is usually based on clinical features, prevalence data for different organisms in different age groups, and regional variations in pathogens. Though not a common feature, pneumococcus resistance rates of a specific locale should play importantly in the decision-making process.

When a causative agent is known, narrow-spectrum antibiotics are preferred. Table 29-2 shows appropriate

TABLE 29-2 CHOICE OF ANTIBIOTIC TREATMENT FOR COMMUNITY-ACQUIRED PNEUMONIA WHEN TYPICAL BACTERIA ARE IDENTIFIED

PATHOGEN	FIRST CHOICE	OTHER
Streptococcus pneumoniae, penicillin susceptible or intermediate	Penicillin, ampicillin, or high-dose amoxicillin	Cefuroxime, ceftriaxone, azithromycin
S. pneumoniae, penicillin resistant (MIC >2 mg/mL)	Second- or third-generation cephalosporins for sensitive strains; vancomycin	
Staphylococcus aureus	Methicillin/oxacillin	Vancomycin or teicoplanin (for MRSA)
Haemophilus influenzae	Amoxicillin	Amoxicillin/clavulanate, cefuroxime, ceftriaxone, other second- and third-generation cephalosporins
Moraxella catarrhalis	Amoxicillin/clavulanate	Cefuroxime

MIC, Minimum inhibitory concentration; *MRSA*, methicillin-resistant *S. aureus*.

antibiotic choices, based on bacteriologic tests and MICs. As discussed earlier in the chapter, penicillins (either IM, IV, or orally) can be used for most pneumococcal pneumonias, unless highly resistant strains are identified. As mentioned previously, in real-life situations, causative agents are rarely identified. In these cases, a model associating age and clinical presentation is probably the best guide.

Hospitalized patients with CAP caused by intermediate susceptible strains (0.1 to 1.0 mg/mL) respond well to adequate doses of beta-lactam antibiotics (e.g., 100,000–300,000 U/kg/day of penicillin). A possible exception warranting precaution would be the cases with very high resistance levels (MIC ≥2 mg/mL). Additional studies are required to determine at what level of penicillin resistance there should be a change in therapeutic strategy. One of the reasons for the better response in pneumonia may be the increased blood perfusion in alveoli as compared with those organs.[36,37] High doses of penicillin, ampicillin, and amoxicillin have been recommended whenever intermediate susceptible pneumococcus strains are considered. Some experts suggest an option with third-generation cephalosporins (e.g., ceftriaxone or cefotaxime) because these beta-lactams have greater affinity to pneumococcus. Data on clinical outcomes supporting these choices are scarce.

Neonates with CAP can be treated with a combination such as the use of IV ampicillin and gentamicin. Methicillin/oxacillin may be needed if the clinical picture is suggestive of *S. aureus* infection. For symptomatic children between 3 weeks and 3 months of age with interstitial infiltrates visible on chest radiograph, a macrolide should be used to cover for agents such as *C. trachomatis, B. pertussis,* and *U. urealyticum.* Children between 4 months and 5 years of age with CAP are most likely infected by pneumococcus, and amoxicillin, penicillin, or ampicillin are the drugs of choice (see Tables 29-1 and 29-2). Some experts suggest macrolides (e.g., azithromycin, clarithromycin, or roxithromycin) as optional choices because they cover both typical and atypical bacteria. Lately, pneumococci have become increasingly macrolide resistant, so it is our suggestion to leave macrolides as a second-line

treatment for situations in which atypical infections are either probable or confirmed by laboratory tests.

Infants and young children with CAP can receive ampicillin, amoxicillin, penicillin, or even a third-generation cephalosporin orally, unless this is prevented by vomiting, or when the patient is so sick that hospitalization and parenteral antibiotics are needed. In a review by the Cochrane Library, three controlled trials comparing oral with parenteral antibiotics in severe pneumonia according to the WHO criteria were evaluated. No differences in outcomes between oral and parenteral antibiotics were found. Since children with serious signs and symptoms (e.g., inability to drink, cyanosis, and convulsions) were not included, no definitive conclusions can be drawn from the review for this specific group of patients.[38] In regions of the world where *H. influenzae* type b immunization is not available, clinicians should consider amoxicillin/clavulanate, cefprozil, cefdinir, cefpodoxime proxetil, cefuroxime, or ceftriaxone as drugs of choice. The addition of a beta-lactamase inhibitor does not confer additional coverage for pneumococcus because this is not its resistance-associated mechanism.

Whenever there is a positive culture or a clinical picture suggestive of *S. aureus*, antibiotic coverage against this pathogen should be added (e.g., methicillin, oxacillin, clindamycin, or vancomycin in case of MRSA strains). CA-MRSA should be considered in cases of necrotizing pneumonia. Atypical bacteria are not common agents in infancy and early childhood and should be considered only for unresponsive cases. Vancomycin or teicoplanin should be reserved for severely ill patients, when coverage for high-resistant pneumococcus is desired, because overuse may lead to increased resistance from other pathogens. If the clinical and radiologic findings suggest the possibility of an atypical agent, then a macrolide is the first choice, and a beta-lactam will be added in cases of poor response.

As the scenario of CAP has changed in the last years mainly due the emergence of new or resistant pathogens, the WHO recently established a panel of experts to evaluate the available literature and to create evidence-based guidelines for the management of nonsevere pneumonia. In these guidelines, amoxicillin 50-mg/kg/day for 3 days in low HIV prevalence areas and 5 days in high prevalence areas was the preferred first-line drug, with co-trimoxazole as an acceptable option. Comparisons between different drug dosages of amoxicillin at either 45 or 90 mg/kg/day did not show significant changes in outcomes. When amoxicillin fails to improve pneumonia, high-dose amoxicillin (80–90 mg/kg per day) with clavulanic acid in order to cover *S. pneumoniae* and *H. influenza* is likely a reasonable choice. Cefuroxime and cefixime are reasonable options and could be taken into account whenever cost is not a main issue. For children over the age of 3, a macrolide or azalide (e.g., 50 mg/kg erythromycin in four divided doses for 7 days) may be added to the existing regimen during 5 to 7 days. The role of azithromycin, clarithromycin, and erythromycin is limited to extending the antimicrobial spectrum to atypical organisms, because these agents are relatively inactive against *H. influenzae*, and there is increasing resistance among *S. pneumoniae*. Thus, such choices should be tailored to treat organisms that fail first-line therapy.[39]

Pneumonia in HIV-positive children is usually more severe, but patients under co-trimoxazole prophylaxis against *Pneumocystis jirovecii* with nonsevere pneumonia can be treated with amoxicillin.

Table 29-3 and Box 29-1 summarize the aforementioned recommendations, including suggested drug regimens.

■ SLOWLY RESOLVING PNEUMONIAS

This term refers to persistence of either clinical or radiologic findings of pneumonia beyond the normal time course during which one would expect the infection to resolve. One such situation is when patients fail to respond to conventional treatment, and another is when clinical symptoms or radiologic signs persist, even in the presence of clinical improvement. It is generally accepted that between 48 and 96 hours after empiric "adequate" antimicrobial treatment, patients with CAP should show significant clinical improvement. During this period, it is not recommended that antimicrobials be changed unless there is clear evidence that other microorganisms not covered by the initial empiric choice of therapy are involved (e.g., *S. aureus* with developing pleural effusion or the presence

---

BOX 29-1 SUGGESTED ANTIBIOTIC DOSAGES FOR THE TREATMENT OF COMMUNITY-ACQUIRED PNEUMONIA

Penicillin 100,000 U/kg/day, q4h or q6h (if resistant strains are to be covered, up to 400,000 U/kg/day, for 7-10 days)
Ampicillin 50 mg/kg/day, q6h, for 7-10 days (PO) and 100-200 mg/kg/day q6h for 7-10 days (IV)
Amoxicillin 50 mg/kg/day, q8h or q12h, for 7-10 days (if resistant strains are to be covered, dose can be increased up to 100 mg/kg/day)
Amoxicillin/clavulanate 40 mg/kg/day of amoxicillin for 7-10 days
Oxacillin/nafcillin 150 mg/kg/day, q6h, maximum 12 g/day, for 14-21 days
Cefuroxime Oral 30 mg/kg/day, q12h, for 5-7 days
  IV 150 mg/kg/day, q8h, for 7-10 days
Ceftriaxone 50-75 mg/kg/day, qd, for 7-10 days
Cefotaxime 200 mg/kg/day, q8h, for 7-10 days
Cefprozil 15-30 mg/kg/day, q12h, maximum 1 g/day, for 7-10 days
Cefdinir 14 mg/kg/day, q12h, for 7-10 days
Cefpodoxime proxetil 10 mg/kg/day, q12h, maximum 400 mg/day, for 7-10 days
Azithromycin Oral 10 mg/kg/day, qd, for 3-5 days
Clarithromycin 15 mg/kg/day, q12h, maximum 1 g/day, for 5-7 days
Erythromycin 40 mg/kg/day, q6h, for 5-7 days
Vancomycin 40-60 mg/kg/day, q6h, for 7-10 days (14-21 days for *S. aureus*)
Gentamicin 7.5 mg/kg/day, q8h, for 7-10 days

---

of pneumatoceles, when initial therapy was with amoxicillin). Empyema or underlying lung abscess should be considered whenever there is persistence of fever with or without pleuritic pain (basal segment pneumonias may mimic acute abdominal pain). These situations often require additional management, rather than a change in antibiotic regimen (Fig. 29-4). These situations are discussed elsewhere.

Factors such as inappropriate choice of drugs, unexpectedly resistant microorganisms, inadequate dosage, or poor compliance if oral therapy has been chosen can result in slowly resolving CAP and should always be considered. Pneumonias that are either slow to resolve or unresponsive may be secondary to antibiotic failure. This may be the case with highly resistant strains of pneumococcus. In other instances, inappropriate choice of antibiotics may be an issue, as when there is inadequate coverage for atypical organisms. In endemic areas, tuberculosis should always be considered because its radiologic appearance may mimic usual bacterial pneumonia.

TABLE 29-3 CHOICE OF ANTIBIOTIC TREATMENT FOR COMMUNITY-ACQUIRED PNEUMONIA ACCORDING TO AGE AND CLINICAL PICTURE

AGE/CLINICAL PICTURE	INPATIENT	OUTPATIENT
Newborn	Ampicillin + gentamicin	—
3 weeks to 3 months, interstitial infiltrate, not toxic	Macrolides	Macrolides
4 months to 4 years	Penicillin or ampicillin; add macrolide if not responding	Amoxicillin
5 years and older: Alveolar infiltrate, pleural effusion, toxic appearance	Penicillin or ampicillin; add macrolide if not responding	—
5 years and older: Interstitial infiltrate	Macrolides; consider adding a beta-lactam if not responding	Macrolide
Necrotizing pneumonia	Oxacillin/nafcillin; Vancomycin. Consider adding third-generation cephalosporin	

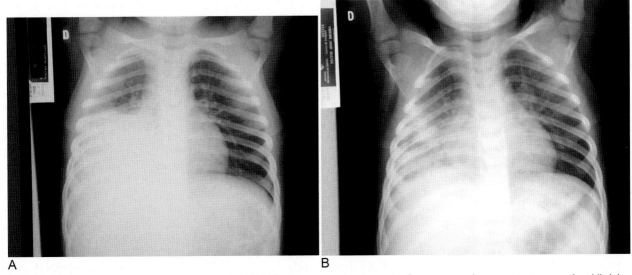

FIGURE 29-4. Slowly resolving pneumonia. **A,** A 3-year-old child with presumptive diagnosis of pneumococcal pneumonia. Lower and middle lobe consolidation is shown; treatment started with IV benzyl penicillin. This evolved into a pleural effusion, which later necessitated a thoracotomy. **B,** The same child, radiographed 3 weeks after first diagnosis; good clinical condition on discharge. Aeration of previously consolidated areas.

Inadequate host defenses or other coexisting diseases (e.g., ciliary dyskinesia, cystic fibrosis, and noninfectious causes) may also be associated with slowly responding or nonresponsive pneumonias. A number of differential diagnostic tests for such possible comorbidity should be considered, including bronchoscopy with bronchoalveolar lavage, chest computed tomography scan, and lung biopsies. Blood, pleural, and sputum cultures, as well as PCR should be considered for the diagnosis of possible atypical microorganisms.

Other conditions such as persistent alveolar collapse and/or atelectasis may be secondary to obstruction of the bronchial lumen, from either foreign body aspiration or lymph node enlargement. Congenital malformations such as pulmonary sequestration, bronchogenic cysts, or other mediastinal masses may also be causes for delayed radiologic improvement, especially if the appearance resembles round pneumonias. It is important to ensure adequate follow-up of all children with CAP who do not run a typical course with full resolution of their symptoms and signs.

NECROTIZING PNEUMONIA

Necrotizing pneumonia is characterized by necrosis and liquefaction of consolidated lung tissue, which may be complicated by solitary, multiple, or multiloculated radiolucent foci, bronchopleural fistulas, and intrapulmonary abscesses. Necrotizing pneumonia has been lately diagnosed more often as a complication of pediatric community-acquired pneumonia.[40] The majority of cases are confined to a single lobe, but some reports speak of multilobar involvement. Pneumatoceles are commonly associated, and they develop as a consequence of localized bronchiolar and alveolar necrosis, which allow one-way passage of air into the peripheral airways and alveoli.[41] Hemoptysis, high fever, leucopenia, hypoalbuminemia, and empyema are also frequent findings.[42]

Necrotizing pneumonia is usually secondary to pneumococcus (associated with nonvaccine serotypes), *Staphylococcus aureus,* or, less commonly, *Pseudomonas aeruginosa* infections. CA-MRSA is often associated with this clinical presentation, since this bacterium produces Panton-Valentine leukocidin, an exotoxin that causes tissue necrosis. In Europe, methicillin-sensitive *Staphylococcus aureus* (MSSA), producing the same exotoxin, was also implicated in the occurrence of necrotizing pneumonia.[43]

IMPACT OF VACCINES ON PNEUMONIA INCIDENCE

The two leading pathogens causing bacterial pneumonia in children 1 month to 5 years of age from developing countries are *Streptococcus pneumoniae* and *Haemophilus influenza* type b. Other preventable causes of pneumonia are pertussis and measles. Although vaccines against these agents have been available for several decades, many children still die from pneumonia caused directly by or as a complication of such pathogens, especially in developing countries. In 1980, before the widespread use of measles immunization in developing countries, there were more than 2.5 million deaths related to measles, and two decades later these figures were down to two thirds of this total. A number of studies evaluated the impact of Hib immunization in the prevention of childhood pneumonia, showing reductions of up to 44% in radiology-confirmed cases and up to 100% of bacteremic cases.

Five different randomized clinical trials were designed to evaluate the impact of pneumococcus conjugated vaccine (PCV) on pneumonia prevalence among children in different parts of the world, with seven-, nine-, or eleven-valent vaccines. These studies detected significant reductions (20% to 37%) of radiology-confirmed pneumonia, showing the importance of these pneumococcal serotypes as causes of pneumonia. In the United States, 3 years after

PCV introduction, a 39% reduction in pneumonia hospitalizations among children younger than 2 years of age was detected.[44]

PLEURAL EFFUSION AND EMPYEMA

Pleural effusion occurs when an inflammatory response to pneumonia causes an increase in permeability of the pleura with accumulation of fluid into the pleural space. It develops as a consequence of increased capillary permeability associated with parenchymal lung injury, favoring migration of inflammatory cells (neutrophils, lymphocytes, and eosinophils) into the pleural space. The process is mediated by a number of cytokines, such as interleukin (IL)-1, IL-6, IL-8, tumour necrosis factor (TNF)-alpha, and platelet activating factor, released by mesothelial cells lining the pleural space.

When germs enter the pleural space, pus appears, characterizing empyema.[45,46] Empyema occurs in about 1 in 150 children hospitalized with pneumonia.[47] Empyema may also be secondary to bronchiectasis and lung abscess. Rarely, empyema follows esophageal perforation, but this topic is out of the scope of this chapter.[48,49] There are three stages of parapneumonic pleural effusions and empyema. The exudative stage (stage I) usually last 3 to 5 days and consists of simple and sterile effusion. The fibrinopurulent stage (stage II) ensues 7 to 10 days after the first signs of the acute disease, with an increase in white blood cells and infection turning eventually into pus; there is deposition of fibrin on visceral and parietal pleura. Fibrinous and cellular debris may cause lymphatic channels blockage resulting in further fluid accumulation. Fluid may become loculated and, as a consequence, pus appears.[46] In the organizing stage, which takes place in 2 to 3 weeks' time, there is fibroblast infiltration of the pleural cavity, and the thin intrapleural membranes become thick and nonelastic, leading to tapping of the adjacent lung.

In a retrospective study from 8 different hospitals in Canada, Langley and colleagues described the main characteristics of hospitalized children due to empyema. Seventy-eight percent of the children were previously healthy and 57% were younger than 5 years of age, with the average age being 6 years; most cases occurred during winter.[50] In a series from the UK, parapneumonic pleural effusion and empyema, usually unilateral, was more common in boys than in girls, especially in infants and young children, and was more frequent during winter and spring.[49]

Streptococcus species, *Staphylococcus aureus, Haemophilus influenzae, Mycobacterium* species, *Pseudomonas aeruginosa,* anaerobes, *Mycoplasma pneumoniae,* and fungi are the most common pathogens that can cause empyema. Pneumococcus is the main agent associated with empyema. Recent data showing the increasing prevalence of community associated Methicillin-resistant *S. aureus* may change this scenario, and physicians may have to consider it as possible causative agent.[46-50] Anaerobic bacteria may be involved in aspiration pneumonia, especially in children with some degree of a neurodevelopment delay. Virus, *Mycoplasma pneumoniae,* and *Legionella pneumophila* may cause pleural effusions, but seldom cause empyema. Recently PCR techniques have increased the etiologic diagnosis of empyema (over 70% positive diagnoses against 8% to 76% for culture).[45]

Clinical Course

Either the child presents with typical, but usually more severe, signs of pneumonia or, what seems to be more frequently the case, after a few days of usual pneumonia symptoms, children become clinically worse, with persistent fever, and many times, respiratory distress. It is not uncommon that pleuritic pain is present. In cases where infection is located in the lower lobes, abdominal pain is quite often present. On physical examination, there will be reduced air entry and dull percussion over the affected area.[45] Unlike adults, where mortality rates around 40% are expected, the typical clinical outcome of children is one of full recovery.[49] Bronchopleural fistula, lung abscess, and perforation through the chest wall (empyema necessitatis) are uncommon complications in children.[48,49]

Diagnosis

Blood culture is recommended in order to identify the causative organism. Yet, positive blood cultures in patients with empyema vary from 10% to 22% in most series. Acute phase reactants are not helpful in detecting parapneumonic effusions or differentiating them from empyema. Other biochemical tests from the pleural fluid are usually inadequate to identify the causal agent or to differentiate empyema from an uncomplicated parapneumonic effusion.[45,49]

Chest radiographs should always be obtained when there are signs indicating an inadequate clinical course. Obliteration of the costophrenic angle and a rim of fluid may be seen ascending the lateral chest wall (meniscus sign) on posterior-anterior or anterior-posterior radiographs. If the film is taken when a child is supine, the appearance can be of a homogeneous increase in opacity over the whole lung field. A completely whiteout hemithorax may be seen in a big pleural effusion. Another radiographic finding of empyema is that of scoliosis, concave to the side of the collection, reflecting that the child may be choosing a protective position in order to avoid pain.

Loculation, defined as fluid not freely moving due to pleural fibrinous adhesions, can be diagnosed by evaluating the chest dynamically (i.e., in different positions) by means of plain radiographic films or by ultrasound. Statically, loculation can probably be inferred when a collection adopts a lenticular shape with internal convexity, while a freely moving collection should form an internally concave meniscus paralleling the chest wall.[46] Although chest radiographs are helpful in diagnosing pleural effusions, they are not useful for clinical follow-up because full radiologic recovery may be slow, and findings may be clinically not significant. Chest radiographs will become normalized in two-thirds of the children after 3 months after the acute event; 90% should have normal radiographs by 6 months, and all should have it clear by 18 months.[51,52]

Ultrasound (US) is very useful to differentiate between solid and liquid content in the chest and to mark the best spot for tube insertion in the case of empyema. It is particularly valuable in the case of a whiteout lung, where atelectasis, consolidation, and effusion should be differentiated. Either US or CT scans are advocated to identify fibrin deposition, but fibrinous septations are better visualized using US. US can estimate the size of the effusion, differentiate free from loculated pleural fluid, and determine the echogenicity of the fluid. It can be used to guide chest drain insertion or thoracocentesis with the radiologist or radiographer marking the optimum site for drainage on the skin. In most cases plain radiographs or US can distinguish abscess from a septated pleural effusion, although sometimes a CT is needed. US is considered essential in the management of children with parapneumonic effusions. The panel of experts from the British Thoracic Society recommends the referral of the patient if the attending site does not have such facilities.[49]

CT scans should not be used routinely unless another diagnosis is suspected (e.g., a tumor or abscess) because of radiation concerns in a growing child and because less invasive techniques usually suffice for diagnosis and management. CT allows examination of the entire thorax without being limited by the presence of air or bone compared with US. CT scans do not differentiate simple parapneumonic effusion from empyema. CTs usually do not visualize fibrin strands or loculations because they are too thin; they are usually best seen with US scans. CT scans can be helpful in complicated cases in order to identify parenchymal disease such as an intrapulmonary abscess. An irregular thick wall and a location in acute angle with the chest wall indicates an abscess, while visualization of pleural separation and compression of the adjacent lung both favor empyema. The idea here is that there is no role for CT scanning in children with empyema because it does not change management especially if a significant radiation dose will be required.[53] When a surgical approach is needed, a CT scan can be performed preoperatively in order to give the surgeon a greater anatomic delineation and better definition of the underlying lung parenchyma, in order to avoid misplacement of the instruments and/or a bronchopleural fistula.[46]

Pleural fluid should always be sent for Gram staining, microbiological testing, and, wherever possible, for PCR diagnosis. It is wise to also order culture for *Mycobacteria*. Cell counts should be evaluated, and when lymphocytosis is detected, tuberculosis or malignancies are more likely. In parapneumonic effusions, one should expect a predominance of neutrophils. Low glucose, low pH, and high LDH in adults have long been used to predict empyema development, but in children their role to guide management remains undetermined. Although it is probable that biochemical characteristics from parapneumonic effusions in children are no different from those in adults, such tests do not seem to change management or outcomes. Also, data from adult studies cannot be directly applied to children because empyema behaves differently in these two age groups. While sequelae occur in many adults, full recovery is the rule in children, although a temporary restrictive pattern can be seen in pulmonary function tests soon after hospital discharge.

Treatment

All children with parapneumonic effusion and empyema should be admitted to the hospital. General care of parapneumonic effusions includes supplemental oxygen and IV fluids when necessary, antipyretics, and IV antimicrobials. Children who need drainage of the effusion should be preferably managed at a tertiary center under the supervision of a specialist.

Different outcomes have been used to compare the efficacy of different treatment strategies, (e.g., length of hospitalization, radiologic resolution, or pulmonary function tests) because mortality rates are very low. Smaller effusions of less than 10 mm of thickness can usually be managed with antibiotics alone, and these should especially cover *S. pneumoniae*; *S. aureus* should be considered when pneumatoceles are present and the child is toxemic.

Although not based on specific randomized trials, a panel of experts from the British Thoracic Society recommends cefuroxime, co-amoxiclav, penicillin and flucloxacillin, amoxicillin and flucloxacillin, or clindamycin when effusion follows community-acquired pneumonia. Broader coverage should be initiated in cases of hospital-acquired pneumonia and following surgery, trauma, or aspiration. When a positive culture is available, choice of antimicrobials should be in accordance with sensitivity testing. The same panel recommends continuation of antibiotics for 1 to 4 weeks after discharge or even longer when there is residual disease.[49]

Antibiotics alone should not be the main strategy for managing enlarging effusions, or those that are big enough to cause respiratory distress Therapeutic options besides antibiotics are thoracocentesis, chest drain insertion with or without instillation of fibrinolytic agents, and surgical techniques such as VATS, mini-thoracotomy, and standard thoracotomy with decortication. Few studies compared repeated thoracocentesis versus catheter drainage. For the scarce data available and expert opinions it seem that the outcomes were similar with either approach, with the important advantage of the latter apparently causing less trauma to the child.[47] In prospective uncontrolled studies, where chest drain alone (i.e., without further surgical intervention) was used, the length of hospital stay varied between 14 and 24 days, and all children fully recovered.[47] Before tube insertion, clotting studies and platelet counts are only necessary in patients with known risk factors for bleeding. The chest drain should be inserted in the best site following US examination. It is important that the radiologist report the position of the patient during US so that it will be the same at the time of drain insertion. General anesthesia is the best choice for sedation, but local anesthesia should be used for pain control; a paravertebral block with bupivicaine or similar can be used to provide postoperative pain relief.

A chest radiograph should be obtained after the procedure to check tube position and to ensure there is no pneumothorax. The drain should be adequately protected so that it will not fall. The chest tube should be connected to a unidirectional flow drainage system, most frequently an underwater sealed bottle that must be kept below the level of the patient's chest. The drain is positioned 1 to 2 cm below the water level. Bubbling into the water bottle represents air in the pleural space (pyopneumothorax), and continuous bubbling is usually related to a bronchopleural fistula. Putting the drain under suction via the underwater seal may be an attempt to increase drainage, although this approach has not been adequately tested. It is suggested that the drain should be clamped for 1 hour once 10 ml/kg body weight is initially removed, to avoid the rare occurrence of re-expansion pulmonary edema. A chest drain should be removed when the child is well, being unnecessary to wait for complete drainage halt.[49]

Although drainage with tube thoracotomy and antibiotics may be all that is needed for the exudative stage, the presence of loculations and fibrinous adhesions may limit the success of this therapy.[54] The objectives of treatment of stage 2 empyema (fibrinopurulent) are treatment of infection, fluid removal, and debridement of the fibrinous layer of the pleura to allow the lung to expand.[48] In these situations, fibrinolytic drugs are used in order to lyse the fibrinous strands in loculated empyemas, thereby clearing lymphatic pores, which restore pleural fluid circulation. Different fibrinolytics (e.g., streptokinase, urokinase, and alteplase) have been studied in randomized clinical trials comparing to saline or to video-assisted thoracoscopic surgery (VATS), and the results were variable. The success rate of fibrinolytics is 80% to 90% in case series, with pain being the major side effect. Other possible side effects are fever and, less commonly, bleeding and allergic reactions.[47–49] Different dosing regimens of fibrinolytics have been used. In a study from the UK, urokinase 40,000 units in 40 mL of 0.9% saline was administered in the tubes, twice daily for 3 days to children 1 year of age or older, while 10,000 units in 10 mL normal saline was used in infants. A 4-hour dwell time was used. If the response is incomplete after 6 doses, additional urokinase doses can be given if necessary. In another pediatric study, urokinase 25,000 to 100,000 units (mean 3100 units/kg/day) was used once daily with a 1 hour dwell time. Alteplase was used in a dose of 0.1 mg/kg once daily with a 1-hour dwell time. These regimens were considered effective and safe by the British Thoracic Society panel of experts.[51,55]

A systematic review of the only three randomized clinical trials comparing VATS and fibrinolysis did not show significant differences between both treatments. There was no evidence of a clinically significant difference in length of stay between VATS and chest drain with fibrinolytics, except in one of the trials; insertion of a chest drain used with fibrinolytics was associated with lower hospital costs.[56–58] It should be emphasized that children virtually always recover, irrespective of the treatment they receive,[45,47,48,50] which means that length of stay may be shortened with operative procedures but that long-term outcome is not affected.

LUNG ABSCESS

Another possible complication of pneumonia is lung abscess. A pulmonary abscess is a thick-walled cavity that contains purulent material. The pathogenesis of lung abscess begins with inflammation of the parenchyma progressing to necrosis, cavitation, and abscess formation. The abscess may be secondary to predisposing conditions (e.g., pulmonary aspiration), especially in children neurodevelopmental delays, congenital malformations, immunodeficiency, or endocarditis. In the case of pulmonary aspiration, it is believed that it is associated with either large or frequently aspirated small volumes. Usually, the most dependent segments of the lung, especially the upper lobes and the apical segments of the lower lobes are affected. Primary abscesses are associated with a primary pulmonary infection, especially due to Gram-positive cocci (*S. pneumoniae, S. aureus, S. pyogenes*), or *Pseudomonas aeruginosa* and *Klebsiella*. *Streptococcus pneumoniae*, *Staphylococcus aureus*, *Pseudomonas aeruginosa*, anaerobic bacteria, and fungus cause secondary abscesses.

Clinical presentation of lung abscesses is similar to that of community-acquired pneumonias. Fever and cough are present in most patients. Other common signs are dyspnea, chest pain, anorexia, nausea, vomiting, malaise, and lethargy. One difference from CAP is that evolution may be indolent. A typical patient may show tachypnea, dull percussion, locally reduced air entry, and/or localized crepitations. The diagnosis is usually suspected or confirmed by a plain chest radiograph. A cavity with thick walls and air-fluid level is the characteristic finding, although the initial presentation may not be significantly different from a simple consolidation. Ultrasound is very useful in defining a diagnosis of lung abscess. It can help differentiate an abscess from a loculated empyema. Contrast-enhanced CT scan is thus usually considered to be the investigation of choice, showing a cavity with thick walls and central mobile fluid. It helps to differentiate abscess from empyema, necrotizing pneumonia, sequestration, pneumatocele, or underlying congenital abnormalities such as a bronchogenic cyst. It is the usual preferred test to guide an invasive drainage procedure.

The mainstay of treatment is the use of a parenteral antibiotic, usually recommended for 2 to 3 weeks, followed by 4 to 8 weeks of oral antibiotics. Penicillin with or without clindamycin, or metronidazole are the usual choices to cover the most prevalent pathogens. In most cases, this will be the only treatment, but interventional radiology-driven drainage or surgery can be considered. The routine use of CT-guided aspiration for abscesses and the more recent use of CT-guided pigtail drainage catheters at the time of presentation has been associated with a decrease in the length of hospital stay, but this needs to be confirmed by additional studies.[59]

Surgery is usually used as an intervention for failed medical therapy. In secondary abscess, the outcomes are more closely related to the predisposing factors. In the case of a primary abscess, the prognosis is usually good, no matter the choice of treatment. Complications of lung abscess are empyema, pyothorax, pneumothorax and, occasionally, bronchopleural fistula.[59,60]

References

The complete reference list is available online at www.expertconsult.com

30 BRONCHIECTASIS AND CHRONIC SUPPURATIVE LUNG DISEASE

Anne B. Chang, MBBS, FRACP, MPHTM, PhD, and Gregory J. Redding, MD

Today the most important cause of clinically significant bronchiectasis in affluent countries is cystic fibrosis (CF). However, worldwide there are more people with non-CF-related bronchiectasis than with CF-related bronchiectasis, and although regarded in affluent countries as an "orphan disease," bronchiectasis remains a major contributor to chronic respiratory morbidity in both affluent[1-3] and less affluent countries.[4,5] This chapter addresses bronchiectasis and chronic suppurative lung disease (CSLD) unrelated to CF. Other underlying pulmonary host defense deficiencies such as ciliary dyskinesia syndromes and immunodeficiencies are covered elsewhere in this textbook.

■ DEFINITIONS

Bronchiectasis and Chronic Suppurative Lung Disease (CSLD)

Bronchiectasis is a pathologic state of the conducting airways manifested by radiographic evidence of bronchial dilation and clinically by chronic productive or wet cough. Bronchiectasis can occur locally, producing recurrent cough and infectious exacerbations, or it can develop diffusely, resulting in generalized airway obstruction and destruction with eventual respiratory failure. The diagnostic criteria for bronchiectasis are based on radiographic features of chest high-resolution computerized tomography (c-HRCT). Bronchiectasis (radiologic diagnosis) also may occur in patients with interstitial lung diseases where traction on the airways causes secondary bronchial dilation. Traction bronchiectasis in the absence of recurrent or chronic wet cough is not considered further here because in recent years, the sensitivity of radiographic criteria derived from adults with bronchiectasis has been questioned when applied to children.[6,7]

CSLD describes a clinical syndrome where symptoms of chronic endobronchial suppuration exist with or without c-HRCT evidence of bronchiectasis. The presenting symptoms are identical to bronchiectasis, including a prolonged moist or productive cough responsive to antibiotics, hemoptysis, exertional dyspnea, increased airway reactivity, growth failure, and recurrent chest infections. However, the absence of physical signs and symptoms other than wet cough does not reliably exclude either bronchiectasis or CSLD. Lung abscess and empyema (previously included as CSLD) have distinct radiologic characteristics and are not discussed here. Whether bronchiectasis and CSLD are different clinical entities or simply reflect a spectrum of airway disease remains undetermined.[6] Both are chronic suppurative diseases of the airways and both respond to similar treatment regimens.[5,8,9]

The reliance of radiographic features to distinguish between bronchiectasis and CSLD is in question for several reasons:

1. It is unknown when radiologic changes consistent with bronchiectasis occur in the context of a patient with symptoms of CSLD/bronchiectasis. Adult-based studies have shown that bronchography (the old gold standard for diagnosis of bronchiectasis) is superior to c-HRCT scans in mild disease.[10,11] Recent studies have shown that contiguous 1-mm slices of c-HRCT images identify more bronchiectasis than conventional techniques (1-mm slice every 10 mm).[12,13] Hill and colleagues reported that the contiguous 1-mm slices protocol demonstrated 40 extra lobes with bronchiectasis not identified on conventional HRCT in 53 adults.[12] False-negative results are more likely to occur when the disease is mild and localized.[10] It is likely that in some children with symptoms of bronchiectasis, current c-HRCT protocols have insufficient sensitivity to detect early signs of this disorder.

2. A significant number of children have clinical characteristics of bronchiectasis, but their c-HRCT scans do not meet the criteria for radiologic bronchiectasis. Chest HRCT findings of bronchiectasis were derived from adult studies,[14] but scans in adults are not necessarily equivalent to those in children. Airway and morphologic changes in the lung occur with maturation and aging.[15,16] One of the key c-HRCT signs of bronchiectasis is an increased bronchoarterial ratio (defined as the diameter of the bronchial lumen divided by the diameter of its accompanying artery) of greater than 1 to 1.5. This ratio is influenced by age,[17] and a lower bronchoarterial ratio should be used in children to diagnose bronchiectasis. In young children (<5 years of age) the normal bronchoarterial ratio is around 0.5[18] and in older children (<18 years of age), the upper limit is less than 0.8.[7]

3. To fulfill the criteria of "irreversible dilatation," at least two c-HRCT scans are required. Performing more than one c-HRCT scan purely for diagnostic reasons may be impractical and poses safety concerns about cancer risks from radiation in children, adolescents, and young adults.[19]

4. The timing of c-HRCT scans to diagnose bronchiectasis is important. Chest HRCT scans performed in different clinical states, such as during an acute pulmonary exacerbation, immediately following treatment, or when clinically stable, may yield different results. C-HRCT scans are ideally performed in a "nonacute state," but this state may differ from a posttreatment state. The Liverpool group described bronchial dilatation resolving completely in 6 of 21 children with radiologically defined bronchiectasis when c-HRCT scans were repeated immediately following intensive medical therapy.[14]

Thus, we recommend that c-HRCT scans are best performed in a nonacute state, and bronchiectasis is best diagnosed if symptoms of CSLD are present, even if the c-HRCT does not fulfill current adult criteria of radiologic bronchiectasis.

EPIDEMIOLOGY AND PREVALENCE

Prevalence Across Time and Countries

In most affluent countries, the prevalence of childhood bronchiectasis has substantially declined since the 1940s. Field reported on 160 children with bronchiectasis over a 20-year period from the 1940s to the 1960s, noting a decline in the incidence from 48 cases per 10,000 people to 10 cases per 10,000 people.[20] By 1994, Nikolaizik and Warner found that only 1% of 4000 children referred to a respiratory specialty service had bronchiectasis.[21] The reduced incidence over time has been ascribed to reduced crowding, improved immunization programs, better hygiene and nutrition, and early access to medical care. However, bronchiectasis is now increasingly recognized worldwide as an important contributor to chronic respiratory morbidity in less affluent countries[22–24] and both indigenous[25] and nonindigenous populations in affluent countries.[1,26,27] Indeed, bronchiectasis is not rare in affluent countries[2,28,29] but is more common among disadvantaged groups such as the Alaskan Yupik children in the United States,[30] Aboriginal children in Australia,[31] and Maori and Pacific Islanders in New Zealand.[32] Among these populations, the prevalence of childhood bronchiectasis is 147 to 200 cases per 10,000 children.[30,31] Among Alaskan native people, the prevalence of bronchiectasis has not decreased over time despite dramatic reductions in tuberculosis and the development of modern immunization programs.[30] These estimates far exceed the prevalence of CF in mainstream communities in Australia and the United States (Australian CF prevalence is 3.5 cases per 10,000 people).[33] In the United States, the estimated prevalence rates based on a retrospective cohort study ranged from 4.2 cases per 100,000 people who were 18 to 34 years of age to 271.8 per 100,000 among those older than 75 years of age.[28] However, its prevalence is likely an underestimate because many cases in children and adults are misdiagnosed as "difficult asthma"[34,35] or chronic obstructive pulmonary disease (COPD). A proportion of adults with COPD (29% of 110) have underlying bronchiectasis.[36] Importantly, the majority of bronchiectasis in adulthood has its roots in childhood.[29,37,38] Recent studies of newly diagnosed adults with bronchiectasis have found that 80% of patients had chronic respiratory symptoms from childhood.[39]

Hospitalization rates for non-CF-related bronchiectasis in the United States also have increased in the last two decades; from 1993 to 2006 the age-adjusted rate increased significantly with an average annual increase of 2.4% among men and 3.0% among women.[40] The only available national incidence data are from New Zealand with a rate of 3.7 cases per 100,000,[26] almost twice that of CF. Those with bronchiectasis in the United States averaged 2.0 (95% confidence interval [CI] 1.7 to 2.3) additional days in hospital, 6.1 (95% CI 6.0 to 6.1) additional

outpatient encounters, and 27.2 (95% CI 25.0 to 29.1) more days of antibiotic therapy than those without the disorder.[28] The average total annual medical care expenditures were US$5681 ($4862 to $6593) higher for bronchiectasis patients than age, gender-matched controls with other chronic diseases such as diabetes, COPD, and congestive heart failure.[28]

Etiologic Risk Factors

Bronchiectasis is the end result of a variety of airway insults and predisposing conditions that ultimately injure the airways and lead to recurrent or persistent airway infection and destruction. Examples of these conditions are listed in Table 30-1. Bronchiectasis develops in some individuals when structural airway abnormalities, such as bronchomalacia, endobronchial tuberculosis, central airway compression, or retained aspirated foreign bodies impair mucous and bacterial clearance. Similarly, *persistent* airway injury and narrowing associated with bronchiolitis obliterans (due to viral injury or following lung transplantation) can lead to bronchiectasis. *Recurrent* airway injury, such as occurs with aspiration syndromes, also can result in bronchiectasis. Pediatric cohorts published during the last 20 years that describe the frequencies of these associated conditions are summarized in Table 30-2.

Another predisposing factor to bronchiectasis is the presence of inhaled irritants, including indoor and outdoor pollutants that stimulate mucous production in the presence of impaired airway clearance. Impaired upper airway defenses also may predispose to bronchiectasis, based on the common association between rhinosinusitis and bronchitis/bronchiectasis. Indeed, the sinuses and eustachian tubes have been considered a "sanctuary site" by some for bacterial pathogens and cytokines that may predispose to recurrent lower airway infection. Finally, there are variations in host inflammatory responses (e.g., cytokine and metalloproteinase levels) and counterbalancing anti-inflammatory mechanisms (e.g., antioxidants and anti-proteases), which may explain why some children develop bronchiectasis while others do not despite similar exposures and living conditions.

Previous Acute Lower Respiratory Infections (ALRIs)

It is well documented that ALRIs in children can lead to later respiratory morbidity and lung function abnormalities.[41,42] Epidemiologic studies have linked acute ALRIs from adenovirus and other infections with chronic bronchitis and productive cough later in childhood.[43–45] Recent large epidemiologic studies also have shown that those with ALRIs in early childhood are at risk of lower lung function in adulthood.[46–48]

There is little doubt that single severe ALRIs and multiple ALRIs in early childhood can lead to CSLD and bronchiectasis. In non-CF cohort studies, the majority of children with bronchiectasis have had previous pneumonic events with lobar or diffuse alveolar infiltrates.[30,49]

TABLE 30-1 CAUSES OF BRONCHIECTASIS

PRIMARY PATHOPHYSIOLOGY	DISEASES	MAJOR ASSOCIATIONS
Impaired immune function	Severe combined immunodeficiency Common variable immunodeficiency	Gastrointestinal bacterial infections
	Natural killer cell deficiency	EBV infection
	Bare lymphocyte syndrome	
	X-linked lymphoproliferative disease	
	Ectodermal dysplasia	Abnormalities of teeth, hair, eccrine sweat glands
	Ataxia-telangiectasia	Cerebellar ataxia, telangiectases
	Bloom syndrome	Telangiectatic, altered pigmented skin
	DNA ligase I defect	Sun sensitivity
	T-cell deficiency	Thymus aplasia
	HIV	
	Cartilage-hair hypoplasia	Short-limb dwarfism
Ciliary dyskinesia	Primary	Sinusitis
	Functional	
Abnormal mucous	Cystic fibrosis	Pancreatic insufficiency
Clinical syndromes	Young's syndrome	Azoospermia
	Yellow nail lymphedema syndrome	Nail discoloration
	Marfan syndrome	Phenotypic appearance
	Usher syndrome	Retinitis pigmentosa
Congenital tracheobronchomegaly	Mounier-Kuhn syndrome, Williams-Campbell syndrome	
	Ehlers-Danlos syndrome	Phenotype appearance
Aspiration syndromes	Recurrent small volume aspiration	Neurodevelopmental problems
	Primary aspiration	
	Tracheoesophageal fistula	
	Gastroesophageal reflux disease	
Obstructive bronchiectasis	Foreign body, tumors, lymph nodes	
Other pulmonary disease associations	Interstitial lung disease	Systemic disease, dyspnea
	Bronchiolitis obliterans	Past severe ALRI
	Allergic bronchopulmonary aspergillosis	Wheeze
	Bronchopulmonary dysplasia	Extreme prematurity
	Tracheobronchomalacia	Brassy cough
Others	Alpha-1 trypsin or protease inhibitor deficiency	Liver disease
	Posttransplant	
	Autoimmune diseases	
	Posttoxic fumes	
	Eosinophilic lung disease	

ALRI, Acute lower respiratory infection; *DNA,* deoxyribonucleic acid; *EBV,* Epstein-Barr virus; *HIV,* human immunodeficiency virus.

In a case-control study of childhood pneumonia and radiographically proven bronchiectasis, a strong association between pneumonia requiring hospitalization and bronchiectasis was found.[49] Children who had been previously hospitalized due to pneumonia were 15 times more likely to develop bronchiectasis. A dose effect also was shown; recurrent (>1) hospitalization for pneumonia and more severe pneumonia (episodes with longer hospital stays or oxygen requirement) increased the risk of bronchiectasis later in childhood.[49] Bronchiectasis was 3 times more likely in children with 4 to 5 episodes of pneumonia, and 21 times more likely if they had 6 or more occurrences of pneumonia. The overall number of pneumonias rather than the site of pneumonia was associated with bronchiectasis.[49] In an Alaskan cohort, there was no association between the lobe affected by the first ALRI and the eventually bronchiectatic lobe, but there was an association between the lobe most severely affected by ALRI and the lobes later affected by bronchiectasis.[30] Specific infectious etiologies were not described in these studies. An Italian study described recurrent ALRIs following pertussis or measles infection in 6 of the 23 children with bronchiectasis.[50]

TABLE 30-2 SELECTED STUDIES ON ETIOLOGIES OF CHILDHOOD BRONCHIECTASIS PUBLISHED IN LAST 20 YEARS

STUDY	NIKOLAIZIK ET AL[21]	EDWARDS ET AL[32]	SINGLETON ET AL[30]	KARAKOC ET AL[22]	CHANG ET AL[31]	KAPUR ET AL[169]	SANTAMARIA ET AL[2]
SETTING N (%)	CITY, ENGLAND N=41	CITY, NEW ZEALAND N=60	REMOTE, INDIGENOUS, ALASKA N=46	CITY, TURKEY N=23	REMOTE, INDIGENOUS, AUSTRALIA N=65	CITY, AUSTRALIA N=30	CITY, ITALY N=105
Postinfectious (severe pneumonia)	12 (29)	15 (15)	42 (92)	4 (17)	58 (90)	5 (16.6)	7 (6.7)
Tuberculosis	0	0	2 (4)	4 (17)	1 (1)	0	0
Inherited immune deficiency	8 (20)	7 (12)	0	4 (17)	2 (3)	7 (23)	11 (10.5)
Primary ciliary dyskinesia	7 (17)	0	0	3 (13)	0	1 (3)	25 (23.8)
Congenital malformations	6 (15)	1 (1)	0	0	1 (1)	3 (10)	0
Secondary immune defects	3 (7)	0	0	0	0	0	0
Aspiration of exogenous toxicants	2 (5)	1 (2)	1 (2)	0	0	0	0
Aspiration or GERD	0	6 (10)	1 (2)	0	3 (5)	1 (3)	4 (3.8)
Unknown	2 (5)	30 (50)	0	0	0	10 (33)	58 (55.2)
CF-like or CF	1 (2)	0	0	4 (17)	0	0	0
Interstitial lung disease	0	0	0	0	0	1 (3)	0
"Asthma"	0	0	0	4 (18)	0	0	0

CF, Cystic fibrosis; GERD, gastroesophageal reflux disease.

Some authors have suggested that bronchiolitis is an important precursor of bronchiectasis. However, in the Alaskan 5-year case-control follow-up of children hospitalized in infancy with severe respiratory syncytial virus (RSV) infections (hospitalization was required), they were not more likely to develop bronchiectasis.[51] In addition, hospitalizations for bronchiolitis among Indigenous Australian infants were not a risk factor for bronchiectasis.[31,49] Although measles, tuberculosis, pertussis, and severe viral pneumonia do not frequently cause bronchiectasis, these remain common ALRIs in less affluent countries; therefore, these infections are still considered important antecedents to childhood bronchiectasis.[23]

Upper Airway Infection and Aspiration

Mechanisms by which upper respiratory tract infections predispose to lower airway inflammation and injury are reviewed elsewhere.[52,53] Bacterial pathogens colonizing the nose and mouth are shed into saliva and contaminate the lower airways. Proinflammatory cytokines from the oropharynx also may be aspirated and augment neutrophilic inflammatory responses in the lower airways. Hydrolytic enzymes in infected upper airway secretions impair protective secretory molecules such as mucins in the lower airways and thereby predispose the lower airways to infection. In vitro studies have shown that some bacteria produce factors that cause ciliary slowing, dyskinesia, and stasis, setting the stage for chronic bacterial colonization of the lower airways.[54] Whether or not the concentration or persistence of these pathogens in upper airways represents a significant risk factor for development or progression of bronchiectasis is unknown. In indigenous Australian children with bronchiectasis, a study relating nasopharyngeal to bronchoalveolar lavage (BAL) bacteria found a high density and diversity of respiratory bacteria, along with strain concordance between upper and lower airways.[55] The study suggests a possible pathogenic role of recurrent aspiration of nasopharyngeal secretions.[55]

Bronchiectasis and other forms of suppurative lung disease have been described among individuals with neurologic and neuromuscular conditions that reduce the frequency and effectiveness of cough and also increase the risk of aspirating oropharyngeal contents. Brook reported on 10 children with such conditions who developed anaerobic pulmonary infections; six were notable for "poor oral hygiene."[56] Similar data have been reported in adults with COPD, where periodontal disease was associated with more severe airway obstruction.[57]

Public Health Issues

In 1949, Field wrote "Irreversible bronchiectasis is not commonly seen in the better social and economic classes. Good nutrition and home conditions probably give the child a better chance of more complete recovery from lung damaging disease."[58] Poor public health conditions, including malnutrition, crowding, lack of running water, and environmental pollution, increase the risk of ALRIs and bronchitis[59–62] and predispose children to recurrent infection and persistent airway mucous production in developing countries. In affluent countries, those communities with

higher prevalence of bronchiectasis also are those where poverty and low standards of housing are common.[30,31] In a qualitative study, community members and health care providers believed that potential contributing factors to acute and chronic lung diseases were smoke, dust, feeding practices, socioeconomic conditions, and mold.[63]

Macro malnutrition and selected micro malnutrition increase infection risks as each creates an immune deficiency state that leads to the malnutrition-infection-malnutrition cycle.[64] However, data on malnutrition specifically preceding bronchiectasis are limited and inconsistent. In Central Australia, children with bronchiectasis are three times more likely to have had malnutrition in early childhood before the diagnosis of bronchiectasis.[49] Seventeen percent of children had weight Z scores below the 2 standard deviations of World Health Organization (WHO) determined criteria.[31] In contrast malnutrition is uncommon in Alaskan children with CSLD.[30] One explanation for this difference may be the increased frequency of breastfeeding in Alaska, which approaches 80% among native Alaskan mothers.[65] Breastfeeding is a known protective factor against the development of bronchiectasis.[49] In addition, the role of depletion of micronutrients such as zinc and vitamin A may increase the risk of ALRIs, thus setting the stage for recurrent airway insults and subsequent long-term injury.[66] In Chile, increased arsenic exposure has been associated with a variety of chronic disorders including bronchiectasis.[67]

Bronchiectasis may itself predispose to malnutrition as a result of chronic pulmonary infection, diminished appetite, and reduced caloric intake. This scenario is best described in patients with CF.[68] The caloric needs and daily oxygen consumption of children with non-CF-related bronchiectasis have not been reported. One series described that children with bronchiectasis and low (<80%) baseline forced expiratory volume expired in 1 second (FEV$_1$)% predicted values and those with immunodeficiency had significantly lower body mass index at diagnosis, and they significantly improved after appropriate therapy was instituted.[5]

The effects of environmental tobacco smoke (ETS) on children's respiratory system are well known from both in utero and ex utero exposure and include reduced airway caliber and increased lower respiratory tract infections and middle ear disease. Reviews of ETS and its effects on the developing lung and accelerated lung decline are available elsewhere.[62] Exposure to indoor biomass combustion increases coughing illness associated with acute respiratory infections with an exposure-response effect.[69] Exposure to other indoor ambient pollutants (nitrogen dioxide, gas cooking) and traffic is also associated with increased cough in children in both cross-sectional and longitudinal studies.[70–72] There is no direct evidence of pollutants causing bronchiectasis, and the pathogenic role is likely to be indirect through an increased frequency of ALRIs and increased airway mucous production.

Genetics

The interplay between genotype and environment is increasingly recognized as the key in phenotypic expression of respiratory diseases.[73] An increased frequency of CFTR genotypes associated with cystic fibrosis, presenting as heterozygotes, has been described in several case series among adults with diffuse bronchiectasis.[74] While heterozygotes for alpha-1 antitrypsin also have been described more frequently in those individuals with diffuse bronchiectasis, a causal relationship remains controversial.[75] Published guidelines suggest optional screening for alpha-1 antitrypsin deficiency for patients with idiopathic diffuse bronchiectasis.[76] A Turkish study (where consanguinity of parents is common) described Transporter associated with Antigen Presentation (TAP) gene polymorphisms in their cohort of children with bronchiectasis.[77] It is interesting to note the high rate of consanguinity in several series of children with bronchiectasis from different countries.[24,78]

Aside from variations in specific gene frequencies, overexpression of innate pulmonary immune mechanisms, such as pro-inflammatory cytokine and adhesion molecule production and receptor expression, may contribute to the development of bronchiectasis in certain children. An increased or exaggerated neutrophilic response in Australian indigenous children as a group has been described.[79] Similarly, metalloproteinases (e.g., MMP-2 and -9) have been isolated from the sputum and BAL of bronchiectatic subjects, suggesting a role in airway destruction by gelatinases and collagenases.[80,81] Whether pro-inflammatory cytokine and collagenase overexpression are associated with early onset disease or particularly progressive disease in childhood remains unknown.

PATHOLOGY AND PATHOPHYSIOLOGY

The histopathology of bronchiectasis was first described by Laënnec[82] in 1819. It includes alterations in subsegmental bronchial structure accompanied by neutrophilic inflammation, intraluminal secretion accumulation, and obliteration of distal airways. There are accompanying changes of peribronchial inflammation and fibrosis, distal lung collapse, bronchial and pulmonary vascular changes, and pleural adhesions. The macroscopic and microscopic features of bronchiectasis change as the disease progresses. Classical papers on bronchiectasis divided morphologic types of bronchiectasis into tubular or cylindrical, early fusiform, late fusiform, fusosaccular, and saccular types as different stages in the progression of disease.[37] The most commonly used classification is that of Reid's subtypes: cylindrical, varicose, and cystic,[83] which were based on bronchographic findings. The latter findings are illustrated in Figure 30-1. More recent HRCT scoring systems describe cylindrical and saccular changes as markers of disease severity.[84] Saccular and cystic changes tend to reflect clinically more advanced, severe, and irreversible disease, but there are no published data on whether these changes reflect ongoing disease activity and progression.[84]

Macroscopically, the airways are tortuous and dilated, at times extending to the pleural surface. Early histologic changes include bronchial wall thickening, edema, presence of inflammatory cells, development of lymphoid nodules and follicles, and mucous gland hyperplasia. Intraluminal secretions are purulent or mucopurulent.

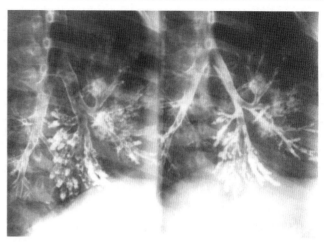

FIGURE 30-1. Varicose and cystic changes characteristic of severe bronchiectasis by bronchogram.

Microscopic changes include loss of ciliated epithelial cells and epithelial ulcerations. With time, chronic inflammation leads to squamous cell metaplasia and fibrotic obliteration of distal conducting airways and peribronchial tissue. As bronchiectasis becomes more severe, the airway walls become thin and saccular with destruction of the airway's muscular, elastic, and cartilaginous elements.[83,85] The saccular airway walls are composed of fibrous and granulation tissue with only remnants of normal tissue. In advanced disease, mucus-filled saccular airway changes can be severe enough to appear as cystic microabscesses.

Vascular changes accompany bronchial structural changes in bronchiectasis. Large bronchopulmonary anastomoses can develop, and total bronchial arterial blood flow is increased. Extensive precapillary anastomoses between the two arterial systems can serve as a shunt between the pulmonary and systemic systems, increasing cardiac work.[85] Bronchopulmonary vascular anastomoses most often occur near distal subsegmental bronchi that have undergone saccular changes. Abnormal bronchopulmonary anastomoses and enlargement of aberrant bronchial arteries are thought to be associated with the metabolic demands of hypertrophied muscle, lymphoid tissue, and peribronchial granulation tissue during the course of the organizing pneumonitis that precedes the development of bronchiectasis.[86] Additional vascular remodeling of the pulmonary arteries and aterioles occurs in association with chronic airway obstruction and alveolar hypoxia, predisposing patients to pulmonary hypertension and cor pulmonale in severe cases.

The initial trigger for the bronchiectasis process is unknown. Animal models of bronchiectasis suggest that inadequate mucous clearance and persistent infection are necessary prerequisites.[87] Mucous clearance in bronchiectasis is reduced by a combination of factors including airflow limitation[88,89]; abnormal quantity and quality of mucus produced[90]; and factors produced by bacteria that cause ciliary slowing, dyskinesia, and mucous stasis.[54] Mucociliary clearance of the debris is enhanced by cough, exercise, and hyperventilation[89,91,92] and is decreased in situations where airway caliber is diminished.[88,89] Decreased mucociliary clearance in turn leads to increased bacterial colonization and infection, setting up a vicious cycle.

Importantly, reduced mucociliary clearance is localized to the affected regions when bronchiectasis is produced by local injury rather than underlying deficiencies in pulmonary host defenses.[93] The role of bacteria in the pathogenesis of chronic lung infection has been reviewed by Stockley.[94]

Sputum markers of neutrophilic airway inflammation are found in adults with bronchiectasis, especially in those with chronic expectoration of mucopurulent sputum.[95] Although sputum production is excessive, sputum from Alaskan native children with stable idiopathic bronchiectasis is less viscous (by one third) less elastic (by one fifth), less adhesive (by half), and more transportable (by 50%) compared with sputum from children with CF.[96] Increased percentages of neutrophils, neutrophil elastase, myeloperoxidase, mellatoproteinases, tumor necrosis factor (TNF)-alpha, IL-8, and IL-6 have been described in lower airway secretions.[95,97,98] These generally reflect neutrophilic inflammation and are not specific to bronchiectasis. The intensity of the inflammation was worse in adults with more than 10^4 colony forming units of bacteria/gram of sputum.[95] However, even noncolonized subjects with bronchiectasis had a more intense bronchial inflammatory reaction than did control subjects.[95] Although antibiotics have been shown to reduce airway inflammation in some studies over a period of weeks,[99] other studies using antibiotics showed no effect on the sputum markers of inflammation despite clinical improvement.[100,101] An upsurge in systemic inflammatory response also has been reported.[102] However, there is a poor correlation between systemic and bronchial inflammatory mediators, suggesting that the inflammatory process is mostly compartmentalized to the airways.[100] Eosinophilic airway inflammation has been described in children[103] and adults with bronchiectasis.[98] There is, however, a paucity of data on BAL or sputum markers in children.

Exaggerated or persistent pulmonary inflammation present in bronchiectasis leads to increased lung destruction by many mechanisms.[98] The balance between proteases and anti-proteases are increasingly recognized in the protection of airways against hostile agents and destruction of lung tissue. Collagenase activity present in the BAL of adults with moderately severe bronchiectasis originates from neutrophils and bacteria. These collagenolytic proteases are likely contributors to increasing tissue destruction.[104] BAL from adults with bronchiectasis contains metalloproteinases (MMP-2, MMP-8, and MMP-9)[105] and collagenolytic proteinases of bacterial origin.[104] MMP-9 (but not tissue inhibitors of MMP-1) measured in exhaled breath condensate of children with non-CF-related bronchiectasis (42.8 ± 18.1 ng/mL) were similar to those with CF (48.9 ± 26.8) and significantly higher than controls (30 ± 3.7).[106] Endobronchial biopsies in adults with bronchiectasis demonstrated an overexpression of neutrophil matrix metalloproteinases.[105] Using sputum from adults with bronchiectasis, Shum and colleagues showed that serine proteases derived from neutrophils were responsible for degradation of proteoglycans in a model matrix and that the protease secretion was stimulated by TNF-alpha in the presence of cofactors isolated from bronchial secretions of patients with bronchiectasis.[107]

Additional pathogenic processes that contribute to persistence of airway inflammation and obstruction are associated with bronchiectasis. For example, resolution of inflammation is normally associated with the orderly removal of apoptotic inflammatory cells. and impaired removal of apoptotic inflammatory cells has been described in adults with bronchiectasis.[108] Increased airway permeability also has been described with bronchiectasis when purulent sputum and significant colonization of the respiratory tract by bacterial pathogens are present.[109] Upregulation of circulating adhesion molecules (E-selectin, intercellular adhesion molecule [ICAM]-1, and vascular adhesion molecule [V-CAM]-1) also have been suggested as playing a role in the pathogenesis of bronchiectasis.[105]

Expression of innate immune receptors (receptors TLR2, TLR4, and CD14) is increased in sputa of adults with bronchiectasis and neutrophilic asthma, accompanied by pro-inflammatory cytokines such as IL-8.[110] These findings are similar to that in children with protracted bacterial bronchitis,[111] a likely forerunner of bronchiectasis, if left untreated.[6] It is possible that some people with neutrophilic asthma have unrecognized CSLD or bronchiectasis. Indeed many of children with protracted bacterial bronchitis were previously misdiagnosed with asthma[35,112] that in some settings would have been classified as "difficult or severe asthma." In a recent study, 40% of newly referred adults with "difficult asthma" had bronchiectasis when adequately investigated.[34]

Natural History

Given the heterogeneity of etiologic factors and host responses, regional severity, and distribution of bronchiectasis, it is not surprising that the natural history is varied, ranging from mild respiratory morbidity to death from airway obstruction, pulmonary infection, and respiratory failure with hypercapnia. There are cases where bronchiectasis resolves radiographically with treament.[14] However, these children remain at risk of developing bronchiectasis and should be monitored regularly for reemergence of symptoms and obstructive lung disease. More often, bronchiectasis persists on HRCT but becomes less severe clinically, with fewer infectious exacerbations and less cough evident later in childhood. In a series of 46 children with HRCT-documented bronchiectasis, a third improved, a third remained symptomatic but stable, and a third worsened while receiving medical therapy.[30] Both Field and Landau and colleagues reported reductions in exacerbations during the second and third decade of life despite persistence of bronchiectasis radiographically.[113,114] What happens in the following decades is inferred from case series of adults with bronchiectasis, many of whom had onset of respiratory problems, if not bronchiectasis, in childhood. However, these series do not depict the era of minimal symptoms that occur at adolescence and anecdotally reappear at 35 to 40 years of age.

There are three published studies on longitudinal FEV_1 changes in children with non-CF-related bronchiectasis studied over variable intervals with varying results.[8,5,115] A British study (59 children over 2 years of age and

31 children over 4 years of age) found that lung function improves with intensive treatment but does not necessarily normalize.[8] Likewise an Australian study (52 children over 3 years of age and 25 children over 5 years of age)[8] found that lung function and anthropometric parameters remain stable over a 3- to 5-year follow-up period once appropriate therapy is instituted. Those with low function at diagnosis (FEV_1 % predicted < 80%) improved with time.[8] In contrast, a New Zealand (NZ) study of 44 children over 4.5 years of age found that FEV_1 declined at 1.9% per annum.[115] The explanations for this contrast are speculative but likely include the differences in age group (NZ[115] had an older group), differences in the children's ethnicity, and differences in health care. Also, the NZ cohort included cases of more extensive radiologic disease, with 89% having bilateral disease and a median of 4 having diseased lobes (95% multilobular). The Australian (Brisbane) study found that the only significant predictor of FEV_1 decline (in children over 3 years of age) was frequency of exacerbations requiring hospitalization.[5] The other two cohorts[8,26] did not examine for determinants of lung function decline.

Current data also suggest that delayed diagnosis is associated with poorer outcomes.[5,116,117] A large study of adults newly diagnosed with bronchiectasis showed that the decline in FEV_1 correlates (p < 0.0001) with the duration of chronic wet cough,[29] which is the most common symptom of bronchiectasis.[25] For each additional year of cough, FEV_1 % predicted declined by 0.51% in nonsmokers.[29] In the Brisbane longitudinal study, children diagnosed earlier (and hence managed appropriately earlier) were significantly younger and had better spirometric and growth parameters.[5] FEV_1% predicted decreased by 1.64% points for each year increase in age at diagnosis, but this was statistically nonsignificant (p = 0.19).

When bronchiectasis worsens, it may become increasingly saccular in appearance within a local lung region (Fig. 30-2). Alternatively, bronchiectasis can extend to additional airways, either because of endobronchial spread of infection or evolution of disease at multiple airway sites. The frequency with which bronchiectasis extends to new lung regions varies with different series, from 2% to 35%.[118,119] Local progression of disease rather than extension to new areas is probably more common.

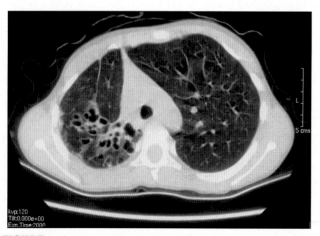

FIGURE 30-2. CT scan findings of saccular bronchiectasis in the right upper lobe of a 9-year-old boy.

The most severe cases of bronchiectasis have diffuse airway involvement and are accompanied by airflow limitation, with or without concomitant airway hyperreactivity. The diagnosis of asthma in the context of an underlying lung disease may be difficult. Wheeze and asthma symptoms are common in people with CSLD/bronchiectasis[120] although reported prevalence varies from 11% to 46%.[2,120] While some studies describe asthma as a cause of bronchiectasis, it is more likely that wheezing illness is a secondary or co-existent condition, or that asthma was initially misdiagnosed.[6,35] Asthmalike symptoms in adults with bronchiectasis may be associated with an accelerated decline in lung function.[121] King reported that increased use of bronchodilators led to a trend of a greater FEV_1 decline over time in adults.[27] The NZ cohort found that although the presence of asthma was associated with lower FEV_1 at diagnosis, asthmatics had a slower decline over the 5-year follow-up.[115]

Unfavorable prognostic factors for patients with bronchiectasis include presence of asthma, bilateral lung involvement,[114,122] and saccular bronchiectasis.[122] The advent of better antibiotics, inhaled antibiotics, long-term oxygen therapy, and improved nutrition have improved prognosis. The use of long-term oxygen therapy has reduced the progression of pulmonary vascular disease among children with cystic fibrosis. Cor pulmonale and right heart failure are now uncommon complications of advanced bronchiectasis.[123] In one pediatric study, echocardiography in 50 children with bronchiectasis found only one child with pulmonary hypertension.[31] In addition, chronic lung infection and inflammation are independent risk factors for developing cardiovascular disease in adults.[124,125] Among indigenous Australian groups, premature deaths in early adulthood (30 to 40 years of age) are unfortunately still common.[126] In a hospital-based cohort of 61 adults (mean age of 42 ± SD 15 years) in Central Australia (11.5% died within 12 months).[126] The mortality rate is somewhat related to setting; mortality rates in adults with bronchiectasis vary widely from a survival rate of 58% at 4 years (Turkey), a 75% survival rate at 8 to 9 years (Finland), to an 81% survival rate at 14 years (Scotland).[127] Pediatric-specific data are not available, but data from less affluent countries suggest that bronchiectasis is still associated with poor outcomes (22% with respiratory failure in a 6.6-year follow-up study).[23]

CLINICAL FEATURES

Presenting Clinical Features

The clinical case definition of bronchiectasis is imprecise, but the diagnosis should be considered when children have a chronic moist-sounding cough with or without exertional dyspnea, recurrent wheezing and chest infections, hemoptysis, growth failure, clubbing, and/or hyperinflation. The most common symptom is persistent (or recurrent) wet or productive cough of purulent or mucopurulent sputum. Sputum color reflects neutrophilic airway inflammation.[128,129] The frequency of chest wall deformity (hyperinflation) and digital clubbing varies among case series (5% to 60%).[20,31,114] Digital clubbing can disappear after medical or surgical treatment in association with disappearance of purulent sputum.[20,114] Although hemoptysis is much less common among children than in adults with bronchiectasis, a presenting finding of hemoptysis should raise the possibility of bronchiectasis. Chest auscultation may be entirely normal or reveal coarse inspiratory crackles over the affected regions. Reduced oxygen saturations and abnormal cardiac sounds associated with pulmonary hypertension are late signs in bronchiectasis. Like any other serious chronic respiratory illness, children with bronchiectasis may have growth failure[31] that is associated with delayed diagnosis of bronchiectasis.

The median age of diagnosis of bronchiectasis unrelated to CF in affluent countries is 4 to 5 years.[30,31] A New Zealand cohort[32] was older at 9 to10 years of age at diagnosis but also experienced more advanced disease. Idiopathic bronchiectasis is rare in infancy, but when present, it is likely to reflect congenital pulmonary malformations, such as cystic lung disease or tracheobronchomegaly,[130] or alternatively, primary ciliary dyskinesia. Only 50% of those with ciliary dyskinesia have the Kartagener triad of situs inversus, bronchiectasis, and sinusitis.[131]

Radiologic risk factors for development of bronchiectasis are the presence of atelectasis[49,132] and persistent lobar abnormalities.[51] In Alaska, children were more likely to develop bronchiectasis if chest radiographs obtained in children younger than 2 years of age showed lung parenchymal densities, persistent parenchymal densities of more than 6 months' duration, or repeated parenchymal densities.[51] Among Aboriginal Australian children hospitalized with lobar changes on admission chest radiographs, children with alveolar abnormalities were more likely to have bronchiectasis on follow-up.[132] In a prospective radiographic study of alveolar changes (179 lobes in 112 hospitalized children), the two most common involved lobes were the right upper lobe and left lower lobes.[132] Both lobes had similar rates of radiologic clearance on follow-up (22% and 27%, respectively). Most studies including those from the 1940s to 1960s described the left lower lobe as the most commonly affected lobe in children with bronchiectasis.[30,31,114]

Comorbid Conditions

Children with postinfectious bronchiolitis obliterans and CSLD share some common clinical features (airway obstruction, chronic cough, recurrent ALRIs) in addition to the same etiologic insult.[41,133] In a Brazilian study, clinical remission occurred in 23% of 31 children with postinfectious bronchiolitis obliterans (BO), 10% died, and the rest had persistent respiratory symptoms. In another study, a third of 19 children with postinfectious BO developed bronchiectasis.[41]

Phenotypes of childhood wheeze have been recognized, and airway hyperreactivity occurs in some individuals with bronchiectasis.[133] Undertreatment of asthma can lead to significant morbidity and contribute to the prevalence and morbidity of adult chronic obstructive airway disease.[134] Indeed the presence of features of asthma is a bad prognostic factor in both children[20,114] and adults[121] with bronchiectasis. The frequency of airway hyperreactivity in children with bronchiectasis varies from 26% to 74%.[31,30] As a corollary, clinicians must recognize that wheeze and cough may not be related to asthma but rather to increased airway secretions and airway collapse as features of bronchiectasis.

Gastroesophageal reflux disease (GERD) may coexist with any chronic respiratory illness and should be appropriately treated. There are published American and European pediatric guidelines on diagnosis and treatment of GERD.[135] However, data in adults indicate that GERD may resolve or significantly improve once the underlying respiratory disorder has been treated.[136] There is, however, no evidence-based approach to the management of GERD associated with bronchiectasis. Caution with regard to overdiagnosis and unnecessary treatment of GERD is necessary given the mounting evidence of increased risk of respiratory infections in children and adults receiving proton pump inhibitors in community and hospital cohorts.

Hypertrophic osteoarthropathy (clubbing, periostosis of the tubular bones, and arthritis-like signs and symptoms) may occur in children with bronchiectasis.[137] Systemic amyloidosis also has been reported as a complication or comorbidity in bronchiectasis.[138] Cardiac dysfunction, although rare, also has been reported and may not be accompanied by pulmonary hypertension. A study of 21 children with bronchiectasis showed that the ventricular systolic function was normal, but some patients had changes in left ventricular diastolic function indices.[139] The authors also found that isovolumetric relaxation time had a significant negative correlation with the clinical severity score. Other reported comorbid conditions associated with bronchiectasis are osteopenia,[140] scoliosis, chronic suppurative ear disease, social problems, past urinary tract infections, and developmental delay.[30,31]

DIAGNOSTIC EVALUATIONS

The goals of evaluating children with suspected bronchiectasis are (1) to confirm the diagnosis, (2) to define the distribution and severity of airway involvement, (3) to characterize extrapulmonary organ involvement associated with bronchiectasis (such as cor pulmonale), and (4) to identify familial and treatable underlying causes of bronchiectasis and contributors to its progression.

Diagnostic Criteria

Chest HRCT is the gold standard for diagnosis[84] and plain chest radiographs are insensitive. The c-HRCT protocol must be child appropriate to minimize risk.[141] Radiology centers inexperienced in dealing with children often use adult protocols that subject children to increased doses of radiation. Radiologic features of bronchiectasis also can occur in the absence of CSLD because they are present in pulmonary fibrosis, congenital lesions such as Mounier-Kuhn, and Williams-Campbell syndrome,[84] and can occur as a result of traction in nonsuppurative lung disease.[142]

The characteristic radiographic finding in bronchiectasis on HRCT is the presence of a "signet ring" where a dilated bronchus is greater than the diameter of the accompanying blood vessel in cross section (Fig. 30-3).[84,143]

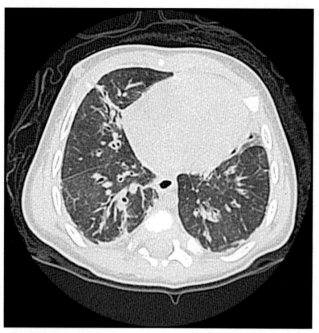

FIGURE 30-3. High resolution finding of bronchiectasis illustrating the "signet ring" appearance of a dilated airways adjacent to smaller associated pulmonary vessels.

However the current cutoff (>1 to 1.5), whereby the ratio is considered abnormal in children should be reduced to 0.8 in the presence of CSLD symptoms.[7] While this is generally appreciated by pulmonologists, most radiologists still use the adult criteria. Other HRCT findings of bronchiectasis are listed in Box 30-1.[84,143] The presence of bronchial dilatation relative to the accompanying vessel does not always equate to the presence of bronchiectasis because this finding also can be present in other conditions (Box 30-2). Abnormalities in the surrounding lung, such as parenchyma loss, emphysema, scars, and nodular foci, may be present.[143] Chest HRCT signs of bronchiectasis include "air-fluid levels in distended bronchi, a linear array or cluster of cysts, dilated bronchi in the periphery of the lung, and bronchial wall thickening due to peribronchial fibrosis."[144] Image quality and hence detection of bronchiectasis is dependent on the radiologic technique used (tube setting, radiation dose, collimation distance,

---

BOX 30-1 FEATURES OF BRONCHIECTASIS ON CHEST HRCT SCANS

1. Signet ring sign: internal diameter of bronchi is larger than accompanying vessel (diameters of both should be short axis)
2. Enlarged internal bronchial diameter
3. Failure of airway to taper normally while progressing to lung periphery
4. Presence of peripheral airways at CT periphery
5. Presence of associated abnormalities
   - Bronchial wall thickening
   - Mucoid plugging or impaction (seen as branching or rounded/nodular opacities in cross sections, tubular or Y-shaped structures, or tree in bud appearance)
6. Mosaic perfusion
7. Air trapping on expiration

*Compiled from references 84 and 234 to 236.

BOX 30-2 PITFALLS IN DIAGNOSIS OF BRONCHIECTASIS ON CHEST HRCT SCANS

False Positives
1. Physiologic constriction of pulmonary artery (creates relative bronchial enlargement)
2. Artifacts from cardiac pulsation and respiratory motion (creates pseudocystic pattern)
3. Pseudobronchiectasis or transient bronchial atresia (related to acute pneumonia or atelectasis)
4. Increased bronchoarterial ratio in patients considered normal, asthmatics, or at high altitude

False Negatives
1. Inappropriate HRCT protocol (wrong electronic windows and/or collimation)
2. Poor image due to movement artifacts
3. Nonuse of high resolution techniques

*Compiled from references 84 and 234 to 236.

---

and image intervals).[145] False-positive and false-negative situations that may occur are listed in Box 30-2. HRCT does not differentiate the etiologies of bronchiectasis.[146]

Etiologic Evaluation

Because most patients are usually diagnosed with bronchiectasis after many years of symptoms,[26] it may be difficult to define the etiologic role (such as infection or aspiration). Differentiating idiopathic from postinfectious bronchiectasis is particularly problematic. A common feature of many patients is impaired host defenses to infection (local or systemic).[147,148] However, often no cause is found even with extensive investigation, and many retain the label of idiopathic bronchiectasis.[38,148] Difficulties with ascribing the etiology of CSLD/bronchiectasis often arise from the availability of testing (such as functional tests for ciliary motility and extended immune testing), whether or not tests are performed and recorded systematically, the population studied, and the definitions used.

Identifying etiology and disease severity can influence surveillance frequency; management, including treatment intensity; and prognosis.[148,149] Investigations for specific causes of CSLD/bronchiectasis are recommended, even though many patients will not have an identifiable etiology.[2,25,26,29] Current best practices for investigating possible etiology are outlined in Table 30-3. Evaluation for primary ciliary dyskinesia syndrome is difficult to interpret in certain situations. Transient abnormal ciliary structure and orientation is commonly found in the presence of nasal space disease and infection.[150] This condition is addressed in another chapter in this textbook.

Bronchoscopic Findings

Bronchoscopy is indicated to identify obstructive bronchiectasis, which can be intraluminal (tumors and foreign body[151]), in the wall (e.g., underlying tracheobronchomalacia), or extramural from external airway compression. Bronchiectasis is a complication of inhaled foreign bodies and occurred among 25% of patients whose diagnosis of aspiration was delayed by more than 30 days.[152]

TABLE 30-3 EVALUATION FOR UNDERLYING ETIOLOGIES

INVESTIGATION TYPE	DETAILS	EVALUATION OF
Routine		
Baseline immune function	IgG, A, M, IgG subclasses, IgE, hemagglutinins, antibodies to vaccinations	Immune deficiency states
FBC	White cell count	Neutropenia
HIV status	HIV antibody, HIV PCR assay	HIV infection
Sweat test and consider genotype	Sweat chloride and CF genotype	Cystic fibrosis
Radiology	Chest HRCT scan Chest radiograph	Diagnosis, congenital malformation, and disease severity
Aspergillosis serology	Aspergillosis specific IgE Skin test, total IgE	Allergic bronchopulmonary aspergillosis
Cilial biopsy	Electron microscopy and ciliary beat function	Ciliary dyskinesia
Sputum	Microscopy, sensitivity, and culture	Number of polymorphs, microbiology
Additional Tests Depending on Clinical Characteristics		
Bronchoscopy	Airway abnormalities BAL	Obstructive bronchiectasis Congenital defect in bronchial walls
Investigations for GERD	Esophageal pH studies, manometry and/or upper endoscopy	GERD with or without aspiration syndromes
Barium meal		Tracheoesophageal fistula, esophageal abnormalities causing secondary aspiration such as achalasia
Mantoux	PPD tuberculin and atypical	Mycobacterium TB and atypical mycobacteria
Further immune tests	Neutrophil function, CH_{50}, etc	Immune function
Video fluoroscopy	Oropalatal function and assessment of laryngeal protection	Primary aspiration lung disease

BAL, Bronchoalveolar lavage; *FBC,* full blood count; *GERD,* gastroesophageal reflux disease; *HIV,* human immunodeficiency virus; *PCR,* polymerase chain reaction; *PPD,* purified protein derivative; *TB,* tuberculosis.

Bronchoscopic findings of major airways related to bronchiectasis have been classified into five types: Type I—mucosal abnormality/inflammation only, Type II—bronchomalacia (Fig. 30-4A), Type III—obliterative-like (Fig. 30-4B), Type IV—malacia/obliterative-like combination, and Type V—no abnormality.[153] The frequencies of these findings among 28 children with non-CF-related bronchiectasis were 58%, 17%, 17%, 4%, and 2% for Types I through V, respectively.[153] In the 33 children with postinfectious bronchiectasis and CSLD, structural airway lesions were present in 40%.[153] Bronchomalacia associated with bronchiectasis is related to chronic inflammation[154]; however it is unknown if bronchomalacia predates recurrent respiratory infections. Airway mucosal changes typical of chronic bronchitis are usually present in bronchiectatic airways at bronchoscopy. Bronchoscopic findings include atrophic mucosa, increased secretions, and airway friability. Airway flaccidity, hypertrophy of elements in wall, longitudinal corrugations, mucosal reddening, increased vascularity, dilated ducts and displacement due to lobar collapse also have been described in the proximal conducting airways (Fig. 30-5).[154]

Assessment of Severity

In children, spirometry is insensitive in detecting early structural lung damage, even during disease progression in CF[155] and non-CF-related bronchiectasis.[31,156] Spirometric values may be normal, but when a spirometric abnormality is present,[31,156] it is classically obstructive in the earlier stages and becomes a mixed obstructive and restrictive process later. Although FEV_1 has been shown to correlate to c-HRCT abnormalities in some populations,[32] it is not a sensitive measure, especially if bronchiectasis is localized.[31,156] In contrast, when bronchiectasis is diffuse, spirometric abnormalities, although insensitive to disease activity, better reflect disease severity.[157] Other pulmonary function test abnormalities described are a high residual lung volume, lower aerobic capacity, and lower maximal ventilation at maximal exercise.[158] Effort limitation (as determined by cycle ergometer exercise testing) does not relate to HRCT scores.[159]

There are at least eight radiographic scoring systems to assess severity of bronchiectasis using plain films. However, given the insensitivity of chest radiographs in

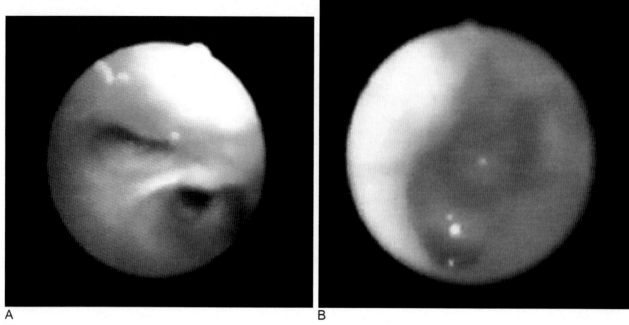

FIGURE 30-4. Major airway bronchoscopic findings in nonbronchiectasis. **A,** Bronchomalacia (airway Type II) of the right middle lobe. **B,** Obliterative-like lesion (airway Type III) seen in the segmental bronchi (middle of picture) while the adjacent bronchi is widely patent and more inflamed. (Reproduced[153] with permission from the BMJ Publishing Group. Chang AB, Boyce NC, Masters IB, et al. Bronchoscopic findings in children with non-cystic fibrosis chronic suppurative lung disease. Thorax. 2002;57:935-938.)

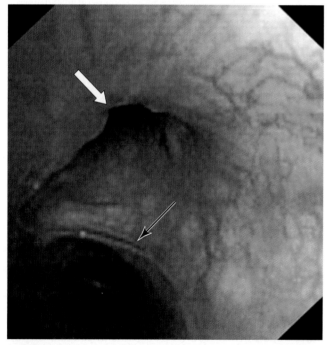

FIGURE 30-5. Airway mucosa abnormality in child with bronchiectasis, depicting mucosa erythema and irregularity, muscularis ridging (*black arrow*), and bronchomalacia (*white arrow,* right middle lobe).

detecting bronchiectasis, these scoring systems have been superseded by chest HRCT scoring systems described by Webb and colleagues,[84] Bhalla and colleagues,[160] and Reiff and colleagues.[146] These chest HRCT scoring systems are based on composite scores of multiple radiologic findings. Some systems use expiratory scans,[161] others do not.[84] The Webb composite score[84] is a summation score of severity, extent, and features of emphysema and consolidation/atelectasis. The Bhalla score[160] is derived from the sum of scores assigned to each of nine categories: severity of bronchiectasis, peribronchial thickening, extent of bronchiectasis, extent of mucous plugging, sacculations, generations of bronchi involved, number of bullae, emphysema, and collapse/consolidation. One study compared these three scoring systems in a group of 59 children with non-CF-related bronchiectasis.[31] The correlation between the scores ranged from 0.61 to 0.8 but none related to FEV_1 values. This lack of correlation is probably related to the focal or multifocal aspect of the disease and potential impairment of lung growth due to malnutrition and other factors.

Other evolving techniques to aid in diagnosis and assessment of severity of bronchiectasis include use of nitric oxide values,[162] breath condensate measurements,[163,164] nuclear medicine scans, and tests for heterogeneity of ventilation (e.g., lung turnover rates). The latter has been used in certain CF centers because these tests become abnormal before changes in FEV_1. Their role in non-CF-related bronchiectasis has not been studied, and to date, none of these assessment methods have defined roles in clinical practice. The role of exhaled nasal nitric oxide as a screening test for underlying ciliary dyskinesia is addressed elsewhere. In adults, outcome measures for short-term clinical research studies include 24-hour sputum volume, c-reactive protein (CRP), and St. George's Respiratory Questionnaire.[165] The last measure is relevant in children. Adult bronchiectasis studies also show that quality of life (QOL) measures,[166] particularly cough-specific QOL,[167] are relevant, important, and add to information provided by inflammatory data.[166] A validated pediatric cough-specific QOL[168] is available but has not been specifically studied in children with bronchiectasis.

Assessment of Disease Progression

To date there is little research on the most sensitive and appropriate method of assessing progression of bronchiectasis in children. Clinicians rely on frequency of respiratory exacerbations and on daily clinical symptoms, which may be perceived differently by children and their parents. In bronchiectasis, a disease-specific pediatric QOL measure does not exist but cough specific QOL surveys for children are available and relevant.[168]

The most sensitive objective assessment of disease progression is HRCT changes because these precede most pulmonary function changes.[31,156] However, repeated HRCT scans are generally not recommended purely for assessment of disease progression. Other assessments of disease progression include changes in chest radiographs, lung functions, markers of neutrophilic airway inflammation, and possibly assessments of airway proteases in stable outpatients. One small cross-sectional Turkish study showed significant correlation between HRCT severity scores and symptoms, FEV_1, sputum IL-8, and TNF-alpha levels (r = 0.64, r = −0.68, r = 0.41, r = 0.41).[97] However, there are no data relating these airway markers to imaging assessments of disease progression.

Assessment of Infection

Common respiratory pathogens in children with bronchiectasis are Streptococcus pneumoniae and Haemophilus influenzae non-type b. Other organisms include Moraxella catarrhalis and Pseudomonas aeruginosa. In pediatric bronchiectasis, the pathogen isolation rate from sputum or BAL is between 53% to 67%.[169] Pseudomonas is commonly found in adults with severe bronchiectasis, but it is uncommon in children until adolescence. Persistent Pseudomonas endobronchial infection is associated with more severe and progressive bronchiectasis and poorer QOL.[102] A number of patients with bronchiectasis are persistently colonized with potential pathogenic microorganisms, particularly among those with early onset disease, with varicose-cystic bronchiectasis, and $FEV_1 < 80\%$ predicted.[170] Sputum is the easiest method of obtaining an endobronchial microbiologic profile. In adults with bronchiectasis, sputum culture is generally reflective of lower airway organisms obtained by bronchoscopic protected brush brushings.[170] Other methods of identifying airway pathogens from children with bronchiectasis are oropharyngeal swabs, bronchoalveolar lavage, and induced sputum. Oropharyngeal cultures do not reliably predict the presence of bacterial pathogens in the lower airways of young children with CF.[171] In indigenous children with bronchiectasis, the sensitivity and negative predictive value (NPV) of nasopharyngeal cultures for individual respiratory bacterial pathogens causing lower airway infection (detected in BAL) ranged from 75% to 100%, and the specificity and positive predictive value (PPV) were lower (32% to 72%).[55]

Assessment and Importance of Exacerbations

Symptomatic exacerbations assumed to be infectious in nature are characterized by increased sputum expectoration; cough severity; change in cough quality (dry to wet); or sputum purulence, with or without reduction in exercise tolerance and energy.[169] Fever and hemoptysis are uncommon in exacerbations of pediatric bronchiectasis.[169] The endobronchial pathogens isolated during acute exacerbations have not been correlated with chronic endobronchial flora in children with bronchiectasis nor have bacterial concentrations in sputum. The only study to date that has examined exacerbations in pediatric bronchiectasis (limited for its retrospective nature) reported isolation rates of 62% during exacerbation and 48% during a stable state. Molecular techniques to examine bacteria type or viral identification were not performed.

Determinants of accelerated lung function decline in adults with bronchiectasis are frequency of hospitalized exacerbations, increased systemic inflammatory markers, and colonization with P. aeruginosa.[102] One study (52 children over 3 years of age) found that the only significant predictor of FEV_1 decline (over 3 years) was frequency of hospitalized exacerbations[5]; with each exacerbation, the FEV_1 % predicted decreased by 1.95% (p = 0.048), adjusted for time.[5] It is likely that interventions that can reduce exacerbations are also likely to be important for preventing adult lung dysfunction.[172] Furthermore, recurrent exacerbations is one of the strongest predictors of poor QOL in adults with bronchiectasis.[173] This finding is consistent with data for asthma that described exacerbations (requiring hospitalization or emergency treatment) in childhood, and adult asthma was associated with accelerated FEV_1 decline in participants not on preventative therapy.[174]

Despite the known importance of exacerbations in most chronic respiratory diseases (e.g., asthma,[174] COPD), data are scarce for the triggers, definitions, and effective treatment of bronchiectasis in both children and adults.[166,172,175] Whether or not viruses and other nonbacterial respiratory pathogens (mycoplasma and chlamydia spp.) trigger exacerbations has never been examined. In one retrospective cohort, 34% of exacerbations were preceded by an upper respiratory illness, but polymerase chain reaction (PCR) for viral studies were not done.[169]

▬ MANAGEMENT PRINCIPLES

As early as 1933, Roles and Todd emphasized the importance of early diagnosis and treatment in reducing mortality associated with bronchiectasis.[37] In bronchiectasis secondary to CF and primary ciliary dyskinesia, aggressive management of infections with antimicrobials; regular use of airway clearance methods; attention to nutrition, coupled with a vigilant monitoring of long-term clinical trends; and proactive care has lead to improved survival and preservation of lung function.[116,176] CF produces a specific type of progressive bronchiectasis that differs from other forms of bronchiectasis with respect to mucous rheology, airway surface lining abnormalities, salt contents, and extrapulmonary organ involvement. Nevertheless, management arguably should be as intensive in children with idiopathic bronchiectasis to minimize acute exacerbations, daily symptoms, and functional limitations, if not alter the natural history of the disease. Indeed more recent data have provided evidence that intensive treatment of children who either have bronchiectasis, or who are at risk of developing severe bronchiectasis, prevents poor lung function in adulthood.[5,8,9] Even among children with serious underlying conditions, such as congenital immunodeficiencies and bronchiectasis, comprehensive regular care and surveillance programs have delayed decline in lung function over a period of years.[9]

The aims of regular review include optimal postnatal lung growth, prevention of premature respiratory decline, maximal QOL, and prevention of complications due to bronchiectasis. Ideally a team approach with incorporation of allied health expertise (nursing, physiotherapy, nutritionist, social worker) should be used because this model has been shown to improve health outcomes for several chronic diseases.[177] Evidence-based guidelines of management of bronchiectasis have been published.[25,178-180] Issues that require regular monitoring are listed in Box 30-3.

Antimicrobials

There are few randomized, controlled treatment trials on childhood bronchiectasis, and only one trial that used antimicrobials for more than 4 weeks.[181] Brief antimicrobial interventions significantly improve the inflammatory profile in the airways[182,183] and blood ,[182,183] sputum production, cough frequency, and QOL measures.[183,184] In one study, 25 children were randomized to receive 12 weeks of roxithromycin (4 mg/kg twice a day) or placebo. A significant improvement in sputum markers and of airway responsiveness occurred after 6 weeks of treatment in the roxithromycin group but improvements in FEV$_1$ were not observed in either group.[181] A 12-month trial in adults with non-CF-related *Pseudomonas*-colonized bronchiectasis showed a reduced number of hospitalizations for those on the continuous treatment when compared with those in the symptomatic treatment arm.[185] Another 12-month randomized controlled trial demonstrated that the symptoms of cough expectoration, hemoptysis, and general disability were significantly less in the those adults treated with tetracycline compared with those treated with oral penicillin or placebo.[186] Long-term intervention trials have not been conducted in children with bronchiectasis. Comprehensive care programs for bronchiectasis have used both intermittent and chronic antibiotic treatment strategies.

The use of maintenance antimicrobials may be suitable in selected situations where frequent exacerbations occur.[187] In adults, regular use of macrolides and trimethoprim has been shown to be beneficial in reducing pulmonary inflammation, infective exacerbations, and improving lung function.[187,188] A Cochrane review[101] on the use of prolonged antibiotics for purulent bronchiectasis in both children and adults indicated a small improvement in symptoms but not in lung function or exacerbations rates.

Anti-inflammatory and Antioxidant Agents

In 18 children with CF and 15 children with idiopathic bronchiectasis, 6 months of beta-carotene supplementation reduced plasma levels of TNF-alpha and malondialdehyde, a marker of lipid peroxidation,[189] but did not change clinical status. In adults with bronchiectasis, nonsteroidal anti-inflammatory agents (NSAIDs) have a major effect on peripheral neutrophil function, significantly reducing neutrophil chemotaxis and fibronectin degradation by resting and stimulated neutrophils, but they have no effect on bacterial colonization of the airways or superoxide anion generation by neutrophils.[190] The Cochrane review on oral NSAIDs[191] reported no trials but did find a single trial on inhaled NSAIDs use in CSLD.[192] Tamaoki and colleagues reported a significant reduction in sputum production over 14 days in the treatment group (4 days of inhaled indomethacin) compared with placebo (difference −75.00 g/day; 95% CI −134.61 to −15.39) and a significant improvement in a dyspnea score (difference −1.90; 95% CI −3.15 to −0.65).[193] There was no significant difference between groups in lung function or blood indices.

Antisecretagogues and Mucoactive Agents

Mucoactive agents are treatments that enhance mucous clearance from the respiratory tract in conditions where mucous clearance is impaired.[90] Mucolytics reduce mucous crosslinking and viscosity by disruption of polymer networks in the secretions through severing disulfide bonds, depolymerizing mucopolysaccharides, liquefying proteins, and degradation of DNA filaments and actin.[90] In adults, high doses of bromhexine (not available in some countries) used with antibiotics eased difficulty in expectoration and reduced sputum production.[194] Recombinant deoxyribonuclease (rhDNAse) is efficacious in CF, but is contraindicated in non-CF-related bronchiectasis. In a double-blind, randomized clinical trial (RCT), multicenter study for 24 weeks in 349 adults with bronchiectasis, those given rhDNAse had higher exacerbation and hospitalization rates (relative risk of 1.35 and 1.85, respectively) and more rapid pulmonary decline (decrease in FEV$_1$ 3.6% in rhDNAse group; 1.6% in placebo group).[195] Inhaled osmotic agents, such as 7% hypertonic saline, improve airway clearance and lung

---

BOX 30-3 MANAGEMENT ISSUES FOR REGULAR REVIEW

Accurate diagnoses of underlying etiology and conditions that aggravate bronchiectasis
Philosophy of antibiotic use (maintenance, intermittent, regular hospitalizations)
Airway pathogens and drug-sensitivity profiles
Effectiveness of mucociliary clearance techniques
Nutritional state and support
Psychosocial support and adherence issues
Pattern and frequency of acute respiratory exacerbations
Presence of comorbid conditions
Education and promotion of self-management
Preventive measures (environment assessment, vaccines)
Indications for surgical resection of bronchiectatic regions
Complications related to bronchiectasis (e.g., hemoptysis, lung abscess, pulmonary hypertension, sleep disorders, reactive airway disease)
Review of new therapies and therapeutic strategies as they emerge (e.g., macrolide use for anti-inflammatory, anti-secretagogue effects)

function and reduce exacerbation frequency in people with suppurative lung disease (CF and non-CF).[196,197] Pretreatment with a short-acting bronchodilator is recommended to avoid bronchospasm, which occurs in a minority of patients. Inhaled mannitol is another promising osmotic agent that behaves like hypertonic saline.[198] It does this primarily by hydrating mucus (from water efflux into the airways), inducing cough, and reducing the surface tension of mucus.[199] Short-term studies[197,200] have confirmed laboratory-based findings of increased airway clearance. Preliminary analysis from a RCT in adults with bronchiectasis found that those randomized to 320 mg twice a day had improved QOL (difference of 2.4 units, p = 0.003), and required fewer antibiotics (16%) to treat exacerbations than the placebo group (27%) (p = 0.026).[200] No difference in microbiological outcomes was found between the groups, but the study was relatively short (3 months).[200]

Anti-secretagogues reduce airway mucous production and secretion. These agents include anticholinergic agents, macrolide antibiotics, and bromhexine. Fourteen-member-ring macrolides are antibiotics with anti-inflammatory activities, and they reduce mucous hypersecretion in adults with bronchiectasis.[201] Although its benefit also has been shown in children with CF, current evidence for universal recommendation is insufficient.[202] Similarly, there are no randomized controlled trials of anticholinergics in the treatment of acute or stable bronchiectasis.[203] Some anticholinergic agents such as atropine and glycopyrrolate slow mucociliary transport and predispose to further mucous stasis. An uncontrolled trial of tiotroprium in adults with hypersecretory states that are resistant to macrolides (including bronchiectasis) reduced daily symptoms and improved QOL with short-term use,[204] but it is not recommended in children.

Airway Clearance Methods

Although it is lacking a robust evidence-base, chest physiotherapy is used in children[205] and adults[206,207] to improve airway secretion clearance. Available studies suggest that chest physiotherapy is beneficial with improved QOL and exercise capacity and reduced cough and sputum volumes.[206,207] Thus daily chest physiotherapy is recommended in a form that maximizes potential benefit and minimizes burden of care.[179,206] In the past, postural drainage was standard therapy for children with CSLD/ bronchiectasis. However, this treatment may increase gastroesophageal reflux and possible aspiration.[208] Given the availability of various techniques for airway clearance and the lack of clear superiority of any one technique, specific choices should be individualized. In addition, children with bronchiectasis should be encouraged to uptake physical activity.

Asthma Therapy

Asthma in children with bronchiectasis should be treated on its own merits. Inhaled corticosteroids (ICS), at best, have a modest benefit in those with severe CSLD/ bronchiectasis and those with *P. aeruginosa*.[209] The updated Cochrane review (of six studies in adults, no pediatric studies) found that in the short term (ICS for <6 months' duration), adults on very high doses of ICS (2 g per day of budesonide equivalent) had significantly improved FEV_1, FVC, QOL, and sputum volume but not peak flow, exacerbations, cough or wheeze, when compared with adults in the control arm (no ICS). When only placebo-controlled studies were included in the review, there were no significant differences between groups in any of the outcomes examined (spirometry, clinical outcomes of exacerbation, or sputum volume). A single study on medium-term (>6 months) outcomes showed no significant effect of inhaled steroids on any of the outcomes.[209] There is no published RCT on the use of ICS for children with CSLD/bronchiectasis.[209] A recent withdrawal study reported that 12 week-withdrawal of ICS resulted in a significant increase in bronchial hyperreactivity and a decrease in neutrophil apoptosis but no change in clinical parameters or sputum inflammatory markers.[210] This suggest that ICS have little role in the management of CSLD/ bronchiectasis in children when asthma does not co-exist.

Short- and long-acting β-2 agonists also have an indeterminate role in the management in bronchiectasis[211,212] and their use must be individualized. Although the presence of asthma is associated with advanced bronchiectasis and a worse prognosis, treatment of asthma to alter long-term outcomes has not been studied. It may be that the asthmatic features associated with diffuse bronchiectasis reflect the disease itself rather than a concurrent condition. Whether published guidelines for asthma care pertain to patients with wheeze and airway reversibility, or hyperactivity, is unclear. Increased cough in children with bronchiectasis should be initially treated as an exacerbation of bronchiectasis.

Environmental Modification

In utero tobacco smoke exposure alters respiratory control and pulmonary development and physiology.[213,214] There is also emerging evidence that tobacco smoke can influence early immune function,[215] but its role in permanently altering local and systemic pulmonary immunity is unknown. Exposure to environmental tobacco smoke increases susceptibility to respiratory infections, causes adverse respiratory health outcomes, and increases coughing illnesses.[216] Cessation of parental smoking reduces children's cough.[217] Behavioral counseling for smoking mothers has been shown to reduce young children's ETS exposure in both reported and objective measures of ETS.[218]

Indoor wood smoke also increases acute respiratory infections, demonstrating an exposure-response effect.[219] Thus efforts to reduce smoke and biomass exposure including in utero exposure and children's exposure in the home must be maximized. Studies in NZ also have shown that retrofitting houses with insulation was associated with reduced odds for children taking time off school, adults taking time off work, visits to general practitioners, and hospital admissions for respiratory conditions, as well as energy savings.[220,221]

Prevention: Vaccines

Vaccination as per national schedule is recommended. Many of the diseases described as causing bronchiectasis (e.g., pertussis and measles) are now controlled in developed countries. Vaccinations for prevention of influenza are recommended in spite of the lack of evidence specific for bronchiectasis.[222,223] Although there is no specific evidence for influenza vaccine in those with CSLD/bronchiectasis,[222] indirect evidence suggests annual influenza vaccinations reduces morbidity, mortality, and health care cost in "at risk" groups.[224] For pneumococcal vaccination, limited evidence supports the use of the 23-valent pneumococcal vaccine in reducing acute infective exacerbations (number needed to treat for benefit [NNT] of 6, 95% CI 4, 32 over 2 years).[223] The 23-valent pneumococcal vaccine is recommended for high-risk children, including those with bronchiectasis.[225] The role of new 13-valent pneumococcal conjugate vaccine awaits further study in young children at risk for bronchiectasis.

Surgical Considerations

There are no controlled trials on the role of surgery in childhood bronchiectasis. Surgery is considered most often when bronchiectasis is focal and medical therapy has failed. Perioperative mortality for lobectomy and pneumonectomy has fallen dramatically over the last 30 years.[226] In several reviews of surgical therapy for bronchiectasis, the compiled group of adult and pediatric patients experienced 1% mortality (6/597) and an operative complication rate of 8.5% (51/597).[226,227] Complications included empyema, bronchopulmonary fistulas, hypotension, and bleeding. Surgical treatment of bronchiectasis was more effective in patients with localized disease.[227] Appearance of new bronchiectasis following surgical management has been described among Australian Aboriginal children.[31,228] Indications for surgical intervention are controversial and data from the 1940s and 1950s cannot be applied, given the major advances in antibiotics, airway clearance techniques, and nutrition supplementation, and possible changes in socioeconomic standards among underserved populations. Our suggested indications for surgical intervention are outlined in Box 30-4. Although lung transplantation has been reported widely for patients with cystic fibrosis, this option also has been used for adults with end-stage suppurative disease unrelated to CF.[229,230] Outcomes following lung transplantation in children without CF have not been reported.

Social Determinants and Health Care

Finally, health cannot be isolated from social, economic, environmental, and educational issues. Health is closely linked to socioeconomic factors,[231] and increased poverty (with its associated consequences such as poor housing and poor water supply) is an independent risk factor for increased respiratory infections.[232] To effectively reduce the morbidity and mortality from CSLD and bronchiectasis in children, a multifaceted approach encompassing good clinical care and public health concerns needs consideration. Although it is beyond the scope of this chapter to address this important issue, future work must focus on the public health issues predisposing to childhood bronchiectasis if the disparity between developed and developing countries is to be reduced.

Delivery of chronic disease programs requires comprehensive and highly-skilled primary health care services. Education of primary health care providers should ideally focus on identifying children for appropriate referral and high quality local management. Initial assessment requires specialist expertise. Specialist evaluation is recommended to confirm diagnosis, investigate etiology, assess baseline severity, and develop a management plan. Like other chronic illnesses, individualized and multidisciplinary case management operating within an interprofessional framework is optimal.[233] Similarly, clinical deterioration should prompt early referral for specialist care. Those with moderate or severe disease are best managed by a multidisciplinary team approach to chronic care.

■ ACKNOWLEDGMENT

We are grateful to Dr. Rosalyn Singleton for her expert comments and critique on the chapter published in the 6th edition of this textbook.

Suggested Reading

Chang AB, Bell SC, Byrnes CA, et al. Bronchiectasis and chronic suppurative lung disease in children and adults in Australian and New Zealand: Thoracic Society of Australia and New Zealand and Australian Lung Foundation Position Statement. *Med J Aust.* 2010;193:356–365.

Chang AB, Redding GJ, Everard ML. State of the art—chronic wet cough: Protracted bronchitis, chronic suppurative lung disease and bronchiectasis. *Pediatr Pulmonol.* 2008;43:519–531.

Fuschillo S, De FA, Balzano G. Mucosal inflammation in idiopathic bronchiectasis: cellular and molecular mechanisms. *Eur Respir J.* 2008;31:396–406.

Kapur N, Masel JP, Watson D, et al. Bronchoarterial ratio on high resolution CT scan of the chest in children without pulmonary pathology—Need to redefine bronchial dilatation. *Chest.* 2011;139(6):1445–1450. Epub 2010 Sept 23.

Pasteur MC, Bilton D, Hill AT. British Thoracic Society guideline for non-CF bronchiectasis. *Thorax.* 2010;65:i1–i58.

Redding GJ. Bronchiectasis in children. *Pediatr Clin North Am.* 2009;56:157–171.

Redding GJ, Singleton RJ, Lewis T, et al. Early radiographic and clinical features associated with bronchiectasis in children. *Pediatr Pulmonol.* 2004;37:297–304.

BOX 30-4 INDICATIONS AND CONTRAINDICATIONS FOR LOBECTOMY

Indications
1. Poor control of symptoms (purulent sputum, frequent exacerbations) despite optimal medical therapy
2. Poor growth in spite of optimal medical therapy
3. Severe and recurrent hemoptysis uncontrolled by bronchial artery embolization

Relative indications
1. Localized disease with moderate persistent symptoms

Contraindications
1. Widespread bronchiectasis
2. Young child (<6 years of age)
3. Minimally symptomatic disease

References

The complete reference list is available online at www.expertconsult.com

V

Infections of the Respiratory Tract Due to Specific Organisms

31 INFLUENZA

W. Paul Glezen, MD

Influenza imposes a substantial burden of disease in the United States.[1] Just before the 2009 influenza pandemic, influenza-associated mortality accounted for 610,660 years of life lost annually with an estimated cost to society of $87 billion each year. The deaths attributed to influenza during the pre-pandemic period occurred mainly in persons 65 years of age and older who, for the most part, were spared during the 2009 pandemic.[2] For persons dying in 2009, the mean age was 37 years and 85% were less than 65 years old. The preliminary estimate of years of life lost in 2009 due to the novel influenza A (H1N1) virus was 1,973,000 for all-cause mortality. The total burden has yet to be assessed, but it can be expected that the number of children hospitalized with severe complications of influenza will be high. Influenza virus infection is the most important cause of medically attended acute respiratory illness each year. The morbidity, mortality, and economic burden of influenza justify the recommendation for universal influenza immunization. The challenge will be to implement the recommendations effectively and efficiently.

■ PROPERTIES OF INFLUENZA VIRUSES

Influenza viruses belong to the family *Orthomyxoviridae*. Three types of influenza virus— A, B, and C—have been identified.[3] The viruses have segmented, negative-strand RNA genomes. Types A and B have eight different RNA gene segments and type C has only seven gene segments. The segmented genome permits reassortment within specific types and contributes substantially to the heterogeneity of influenza viruses, in general, and influenza A viruses specifically.

Influenza A viruses include 16 subtypes mainly infecting avian species. Subtypes are classified by the hemagglutinin (HA) and neuraminidase (NA) surface glycoproteins

(Table 31-1). Migrating wild aquatic birds (ducks and geese) have mild self-limited infections with influenza A viruses that are excreted from the cloacae. Transmission of infection to domestic fowl (chickens, turkeys, and quail) may result in mutation to highly pathogenic strains that produce devastating epizootics in commercial flocks. Avian influenza A (H5N1) has been spreading unabated in poultry flocks of Southeast Asia and the Middle East since 2003. By 2010, over 500 human infections have been recorded and approximately 60% have been fatal. The possibility of a mutation that would allow this virus to spread readily in human populations is a continuing threat. The great pandemic of 1918 was caused by an avian A (H1N1) virus that mutated to allow transmission in human populations (see Table 31-1). Other avian viruses, H7N7 and H9N2, also have caused sporadic infections in humans. Thus far, only influenza A subtypes H1, H2, and H3 have produced human pandemics with serologic evidence of recycling at 40- to 60-year intervals.[4]

The segmented genome allows facile reassortment of influenza viruses if two different influenza A viruses infect the same cell. Some animals, especially pigs, have receptors on respiratory epithelial cells for both avian and human influenza viruses. Thus, pigs are considered to be "mixing vessels" for emergence of reassortants that may be novel for human populations. The pandemic influenza A (H1N1) virus of 2009 is an example of this phenomenon.[5] The novel 2009 A (H1N1) virus has gene segments from avian, swine, and human viruses. The 1957 and 1968 pandemic viruses were human viruses that acquired 3 and 2 avian gene segments, respectively (see Table 31-1).

In addition to reassortment of gene segments, the surface glycoproteins of influenza viruses undergo point mutations that may alter the antigenicity of the viruses.[6] Changes in the HA are particularly important because the

TABLE 31-1 SOURCE OF INFLUENZA A GENE SEGMENTS FOR RECENT PANDEMICS

GENE SEGMENT	PANDEMIC YEAR			
	1918	1957	1968	2009*
PB1	Avian	Avian	Avian	Human
PB2	Avian	Human	Human	Avian
PA	Avian	Human	Human	Avian
HA	Avian	Avian	Avian	Swine
NA	Avian	Avian	Human	Swine
NP	Avian	Human	Human	Swine
M	Avian	Human	Human	Swine
NS	Avian	Human	Human	Swine

HA, Hemagglutinin; *M*, matrix proteins(2); *NA*, neuraminidase; *NP*, nucleoprotein; *NS*, nonstructural proteins (2); *PB1, PB2, PA*, viral polymerase complex.
*HA, NP, and NS from North American swine virus; NA and M from Eurasian swine virus.

HA is the attachment protein. Substitution of as few as four amino acids in at least two antibody combining sites near the receptor binding pocket of the HA may prevent antibody attachment that could neutralize the virus.[7] This means that antibodies developed from previous infection or vaccination may not protect from infection with the new variant, thereby requiring that the next vaccine include the new variant virus. As an example of frequency of antigenic variation due to mutations in the HA, a total of 21 H3N2 variants have been selected for influenza vaccines in the 42 years since the emergence of influenza A (H3N2) in 1968 through 2010. These mutations emerge more frequently for A (H3N2) viruses than for A (H1N1)

or B. Influenza B and C may have co-circulating lineages that are antigenically different; two influenza B lineages represented by B/Victoria/2/87 and B/Yamagata/16/88, produce sufficient morbidity to warrant representation in vaccines necessitating quadrivalent preparations.[8]

■ EPIDEMIOLOGY AND IMMUNITY

School-aged children have the highest influenza infection rate each year.[9] In the early stages of the epidemic, schoolchildren will comprise the majority of persons seeking medical care.[10] As the epidemic progresses, the proportions of preschool children and adults will increase. Longitudinal studies have shown that children in school introduce infection into the family and contribute to spread in the community. Infants and older adults with underlying conditions have the highest rates of hospitalizations and deaths due to influenza. However, the morbidity in schoolchildren is often overlooked; surveys of children hospitalized showed that older schoolchildren were more likely to have secondary bacterial complications and require ventilatory assistance than young children.[11] Over 70% of laboratory confirmed deaths due to the novel A(H1N1) virus were between 5 and 17 years of age (Fig. 31-1).[12] Asthma and chronic lung disorders were the most common underlying conditions, but many of the students had no chronic underlying condition.

In temperate zones, influenza usually occurs in the colder months of the year. Most epidemics peak in February but may begin as early as October. Transmission is enhanced when the absolute humidity is low because small particles will remain infectious for a longer period. Airborne infection is the most efficient mode of transmission although spread by direct contact and large particles is possible.[13] The incubation period is brief, 1 to 3 days, so that infection can spread rapidly. Children usually shed virus for 5 to 7 days and in quantities greater than adults who shed for 3 to 5 days.

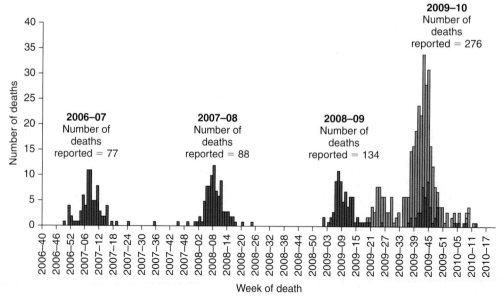

FIGURE 31-1. Number of influenza-associated pediatric deaths by week of death, United States, 2006-2010.[12] (Seasonal Influenza—Weekly Report: *Centers for Disease Control and Prevention,* May 23, 2010.)

Immunity to specific influenza antigens is long lasting. This is evident from the preexisting protection demonstrated by persons over 60 years of age against the 2009 pandemic virus.[14] The problem is that the surface antigens may change so that the upper age limit of susceptibility will increase with time as it did after the reemergence of influenza A (H1N1) in 1977.[15] Vulnerability of adults will vary from year to year, depending on the change in the surface antigens of the virus.[16] For children, the pool of susceptibles is supplemented each year so that when the virus is introduced into school or daycare populations, high infection rates are likely to ensue. Frequently, more than one influenza virus is prevalent, producing infection rates in the pediatric age groups of 40% to 50%.[17]

LABORATORY DIAGNOSIS

Several tests are available for diagnosis of influenza.[3] Nasopharyngeal specimens can be tested for conserved influenza antigens using commercial kits for enzyme immunoassay (EIA). These tests will not identify specific subtypes or variants and have variable sensitivity depending on quality of reagents. EIA may be valuable at point of care for diagnosis in young children (<5 years of age) who have a high frequency of febrile acute respiratory illness caused by multiple viruses. Young children usually have high concentrations of viral antigens in secretions that increase the sensitivity of EIA. Direct staining of shed epithelial cells with specific fluorescent-labeled antibodies (FA) will provide a diagnosis in the hospital setting but requires a skilled technician. Isolation of virus in tissue culture is important to provide the quantity of virus needed to characterize the isolates for antigenic change and sensitivity to antiviral drugs. Primary monkey kidney cells, MDCK cells, and LLC-MK2 cells will support the growth of most influenza viruses. Reverse transcription polymerase chain reaction (RT-PCR) is rapidly gaining favor for identification of influenza viruses. For this test, the influenza RNA is converted to DNA by reverse transcriptase. The 2009 pandemic A (H1N1) virus was not easily detected by EIA tests.[18] Identification was not possible for many laboratories until they received the specific primers for RT-PCR from the World Health Organization (WHO) Collaborating Laboratories (such as the Centers for Diseases Control and Prevention, Atlanta). Multiplex PCR methods are being developed for rapid identification of the common respiratory viruses in a single test. Measurement of serum antibody responses by hemagglutination inhibition and microneutralization tests are important for evaluation of immunity to vaccines.

CLINICAL MANIFESTATIONS

The clinical manifestations of influenza virus infection vary with the susceptibility of the host, the route of inoculation, and the dose of the infecting virus.[13,19] The typical influenza-like illness (ILI) with sudden onset, high fever, myalgia, cough, and sore throat probably results from an aerosol inoculation into the lower respiratory tract. Experimental aerosol infection of human volunteers required a very low dose (<10 $TCID_{50}$ [tissue culture infectious dose]) and resulted in a typical ILI. In contrast, a dose 10 to 30 times greater administered directly into the nose usually produces a mild upper respiratory illness in susceptible adult volunteers.[19] Nose drop inoculation would be equivalent to large droplet or direct contact infection.

Complications of influenza virus infection are common in children.[20] About 30% of young children will develop acute otitis media.[21] Croup and pneumonic infiltrates are common. Bacterial tracheitis is a life-threatening complication.[22] Febrile seizures may occur with the first fever spike,[23] and some children may develop encephalitis.[24,25] Acute myositis is a common complication of influenza B infection in children, and a rare complication is renal shutdown secondary to myoglobinuria.[20] Secondary bacterial pneumonia is more frequent in older children; the common pathogens are *Streptococcus pneumoniae* and *Staphylococcus aureus*.[26] Influenza infection will precipitate wheezing in children with asthma.[27] Even self-limited infections may not be benign. Young adults without underlying conditions who have recuperated from ILI may have pulmonary function abnormalities that persist for weeks after symptoms have subsided.[28,29] Alteration of function of respiratory epithelium may be evident with impaired clearance and increased mucous production.

PREVENTION

Annual influenza vaccination is now recommended for all persons 6 months of age or older.[30] Universal vaccination is a rational decision by policymakers observing that the previous recommendations targeted for those at high risk for complications and their contacts had expanded to include 85% of the total population. The province of Ontario introduced universal influenza immunization in 2000, and the program improved vaccine coverage for all and especially for those considered at high risk for complications.[31] Ontario has demonstrated lower rates for influenza-attributable mortality, hospitalizations, and emergency room visits than other Canadian provinces that have targeted programs.[32] Ontario uses many strategies to deliver vaccine; influenza vaccine is available free of charge in Canada. The United States faces a greater problem of implementing delivery of vaccine to over 300 million persons each year. Development of an infrastructure to deliver vaccines including school- and work-place based clinics should be considered.[33]

Currently two types of influenza vaccine—a live attenuated vaccine delivered by nasal spray and an inactivated subunit vaccine administered by injection—are available in the United States.[30] The two vaccines contain the same three viruses—influenza A (H1N1), A (H3N2) and B—that are updated each year. The live attenuated vaccine (LAIV) is licensed for healthy persons 2 to 49 years of age while the trivalent inactivated vaccine (TIV) is licensed for all over 6 months of age. Studies have shown that LAIV is superior to TIV for eligible children in the pediatric age group.[34] LAIV also was found to be safe and more efficacious for older children with asthma; in a direct comparison, children with asthma who received TIV had significantly more wheezing illness in the 14 days after vaccination than did those who received LAIV.[35] Younger children with mild intermittent asthma or recurrent respiratory infections tolerate LAIV well with no untoward reactions.[36] Future vaccines may contain antigens to both of the influenza B lineages; quadrivalent vaccines have been tested in clinical trials.[8]

Antiviral agents can be used for prophylaxis or treatment.[37] Two classes of antiviral drugs are available. The adamantanes —amantadine and rimantadine—are effective against influenza A viruses only. These drugs are classified as M2 inhibitors because they block the ion channel M2 protein that facilitates fusion of cell membranes at the time of virus entry.[3] Influenza A viruses readily become resistant to M2 inhibitors. The neuraminidase inhibitors (NA inhibitors), the second class of antiviral drugs, block the function of influenza neuraminidase that is important for release of virus particles from the infected cell. NA inhibitors are effective against both influenza A and B viruses. Oseltamivir is an oral preparation that is easily administered and effective for prophylaxis and treatment for children 1 year of age or older. If treatment is initiated within 48 hours after onset of illness, it is effective for shortening the course of illness, reducing complications, and limiting spread to contacts. Zanamivir is administered by inhalation and has the same effectiveness for prophylaxis and treatment for children 5 years of age or older. Some viruses may be resistant to oseltamivir because of a mutation that hinders a conformational change necessary for binding to neuraminidase. This conformational change is not necessary for binding of zanamivir; therefore, most of the viruses with oseltamivir resistance are still sensitive to zanamivir. Side effects of oseltamivir are the occasional occurrence of nausea and vomiting. Zanamivir

inhalation may be irritating to the airways and produce bronchospasm in persons with reactive airway disease.

Short-term prophylaxis with antiviral drugs can be used to protect persons who are immunodeficient at the time of exposure to infected contacts. If patients receive TIV when influenza is prevalent in the community, antiviral drugs may be indicated for prophylaxis for 10 to 14 days after vaccination to allow for an adequate antibody response. Antiviral prophylaxis is not necessary after LAIV and, in fact, is contraindicated.

Current recommendations suggest treatment only for those expected to have a serious illness or complications because of chronic underlying conditions. This includes all patients admitted to the hospital.[38,39] Treatment is most effective if initiated within the first 48 hours after onset.[39,40] It may not be possible to predict which patients will have a serious illness; therefore, a wiser course may be to treat all patients who present early. Not only will this shorten the course of the illness and reduce the risk of a complication, but also the risk that the patient will spread the infection to contacts is reduced. Rapid tests for influenza infection may be used to guide therapy but are not necessary after influenza is epidemic in the community, especially for those with ILI who are older than 5 years of age. Systematic early treatment has the potential to reduce secondary infection rates[41] and serious outcomes for the community as was demonstrated during the 2009 A (H1N1) pandemic.[42]

References

The complete reference list is available online at www. expertconsult.com

32 ATYPICAL PNEUMONIAS IN CHILDREN

L. Barry Seltz, MD, Misty Colvin, MD, and Leslie L. Barton, MD

Stedman's Medical Dictionary defines atypical as "not typical; not corresponding to the normal form or type." The term *atypical pneumonia* was first used by Reimann in 1938 when he described several cases of "severe, diffuse, atypical pneumonia" that were clinically different from other commonly described pneumonias.[1] In 1944, Eaton isolated an agent that was believed to be the principal cause of atypical pneumonia; this agent was later placed in the genus *Mycoplasma* and given the name *Mycoplasma pneumoniae*.[2] Subsequently, other pathogens have been grouped under atypical pneumonias because of similar clinical presentations. This chapter reviews the atypical pneumonias, many of which have received heightened attention in the last decade as a result of bioterrorism awareness.

HANTAVIRUS PULMONARY SYNDROME

Hantavirus pulmonary syndrome (HPS) was first described in 1993 when previously healthy young adults living in the southwestern United States developed an acute febrile illness complicated by diffuse pulmonary edema and cardiogenic shock with a high case fatality rate.[3]

Virology

Hantaviruses are single-stranded RNA viruses of the family Bunyaviridae. In cell culture, growth is slow and results in minimal, if any, cytopathic effects. At least 22 species are pathogenic in humans.[4] Sin Nombre virus causes most HPS in the western United States; eastern U.S. cases are generally caused by Black Creek Canal, New York, Monongahela, and Bayou viruses. Several other HPS-causing hantaviruses are found in Central and South America.

Epidemiology

In North, Central, and South America approximately 200 cases of HPS are reported each year.[4] In the United States, 20 to 40 cases occur annually (537 cases through December, 2009),[5] with the greatest number in the Southwest. HPS affects mainly adults; fewer than 7% of cases occur in children younger than 17 years.[5] Five children (6 to 14 years of age) were recently diagnosed with HPS during a 6-month period in 2009.[5] Infection is more common in males, with a male:female ratio of 2:1 to 3:1.[4]

Rodents are the reservoirs for hantaviruses[4]; the deer mouse *(Peromyscus maniculatus)* is the host for Sin Nombre virus (SNV). Approximately 10% to 15% of tested deer mice have antibodies against SNV.[6] Hantaviruses are primarily transmitted to humans through inhalation of infectious aerosols of rodent excreta. Transmission also may occur from direct inoculation into broken skin; infection resulting from rodent bites has been reported.[6] Andes virus (the cause of HPS in Chile) is unique because it can be transmitted from person to person.[7] The incubation period for HPS caused by SNV varies between 9 to 33 days.[7]

Pathophysiology

HPS results from changes in vascular permeability and immune activation. Hantaviruses infect vascular endothelial cells using discrete cell receptors, $\alpha_v\beta_3$ integrins, to gain entry.[8] Infection enhances endothelial cell permeability in response to vascular epidermal growth factor (VEGF), a cytokine that directs fluid across vascular barriers.[8] Increased permeability of the pulmonary capillaries leads to pulmonary edema. The secretion of pro-inflammatory cytokines by activated macrophages is also critical in the pathogenesis of HPS. High levels of IL-6, which has a depressive effect on myocardial function, have been associated with fatal outcomes.[9] Histopathologic features in fatal cases consist of an interstitial pneumonitis with a mononuclear cell infiltrate, alveolar edema, and focal hyaline membranes.[10]

Clinical Manifestations

The clinical course is divided into three stages: febrile prodrome, cardiopulmonary stage, and convalescence. The prodrome, lasting 3 to 6 days, is characterized by fever, headache, myalgias, malaise, and gastrointestinal symptoms.[4] A nonproductive cough heralds the cardiopulmonary phase, which progresses to severe dyspnea with the rapid development of pulmonary edema.[11] Significant myocardial depression occurs in severe cases and death may ensue within 2 to 4 days. In survivors, diuresis with resolution of pulmonary edema over 12 to 24 hours[11] is usually followed by a 1- to 2 week period of convalescence.[4]

In a recent series of 28 patients in Texas (mean age 35 years), the most common symptoms included fever, headache, and gastrointestinal symptoms.[11] Clinical illness in children are similar to those observed in adults; however, asymptomatic and mild forms of the disease may occur more frequently in the young.[5] Reported symptoms in children have included fever (100%), headache (100%), nausea/vomiting (90%), cough (90%), dyspnea (80%), and myalgia (80%).[12] Crackles or rales on lung examination are found in less than half of patients. Of 12 children with HPS, 67% required mechanical ventilation, 50% required inotropic support, and 17% received extracorporeal membrane oxygenation (ECMO). The mean hospital stay in survivors was 10 days; the case fatality rate was 33%.[12]

Laboratory Findings and Diagnosis

Typical laboratory findings include thrombocytopenia, leukocytosis, and elevated hematocrit. In five recently reported children, the maximum white blood cell count and minimum platelet count averaged 32×10^9/L and 36×10^9/L, respectively.[5] Other findings include elevated lactate dehydrogenase and transaminase levels, leukocyte band forms, and hypoalbuminemia.[12] Chest radiographs frequently show diffuse alveolar or interstitial infiltrates (Fig. 32-1).[5,12] Pleural effusions are common. Patients with initially normal chest radiographs can develop interstitial edema within 48 hours.[12]

Diagnosis is confirmed by evidence of hantavirus-specific IgM or IgG antibodies (generally measured by enzyme immunoassay), a positive reverse transcriptase polymerase chain reaction (PCR) in clinical specimens, or detection of hantavirus antigen by immunohistochemistry.[5]

Treatment

There is no specific therapy for HPS. Supportive management in an intensive care unit is critical. ECMO may benefit patients requiring both respiratory and circulatory support.[5] The utility of corticosteroids requires further evaluation.[4] Ribavirin has not been shown to improve patient outcomes.[13]

Prevention

Preventive measures include rodent-proofing homes, minimizing food sources, trapping around dwellings, and careful disposal of dead rodents. Protective gear should be used when disturbing areas of rodent infestation. Recommended cleaning agents include 10% bleach solution. No vaccines that protect against HPS are available.

■ LEGIONNAIRE'S DISEASE

The original description of Legionnaire's disease followed an outbreak of atypical pneumonia at an American Legion convention in 1976. Legionnaire's disease continues to be an elusive diagnosis because of its indistinct clinical course and radiographic findings, the failure to suspect *Legionella* and obtain appropriate diagnostic studies, and the imperfections of available diagnostic tests.[14] Though considered rare in otherwise normal children, the incidence of Legionnaire's disease may be higher than previously estimated in those who are immunocompromised, who have underlying lung disease, or who have hospital-acquired pneumonia.[15,16]

Microbiology

Legionella species are obligate aerobic, mobile, gram-negative, intracellular bacilli that require special staining (Dieterle stain) for visualization. Of the more than 50 recognized species, *Legionella pneumophila* type 1 causes 80% to 90% of clinical infections. *L. pneumophila* serogroups 2, 4, 6 and, uncommonly, other *Legionella* species also can cause Legionnaire's disease in both adults and children. The growth of *Legionella* requires 3 to 5 days' incubation on buffered charcoal yeast extract medium, enriched with both cysteine and ferric ions.

Epidemiology

Legionella are ubiquitous in the aqueous environment. Freshwater amoeba, such as Acanthamoeba and Hartmannella, are the natural hosts and probable reservoirs. Historically, epidemics have been linked to cooling towers, air conditioning, hot water tanks and plumbing, potable water devices, and air duct systems. Person-to-person transmission has not been documented. Legionnaire's disease is more common in adults than in children. Infection rates among men are twice those of women. Cigarette smoking, surgery, chronic lung disease, immunosuppression, and exposure to contaminated water sources are risk factors for Legionnaire's disease. A retrospective review of pediatric cases of Legionella pneumonia revealed that 38% of the documented cases occurred in children younger than 1 year of age, and 61% of the pediatric patients were male.[15] The incubation period for Legionnaire's disease is 2 to 14 days.

Pathology

Infection results from the inhalation of bacteria from an aerosolized contaminated water source or by microaspiration of a contaminated water source. Following phagocytosis by alveolar macrophages, *Legionella* multiply extensively causing cell lysis. The ensuing inflammatory response attracts polymorphonuclear cells, fibrin, macrophages, and erythrocytes to the site. This exudate fills

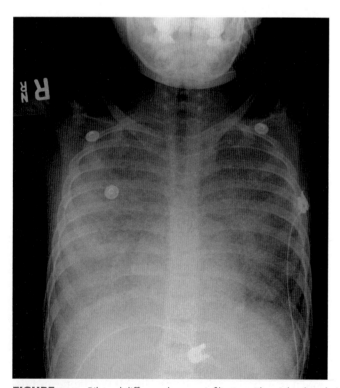

FIGURE 32-1. Bilateral diffuse pulmonary infiltrates with a right pleural effusion, prominent on anteroposterior radiograph of a school-age child with hantavirus pulmonary syndrome. (Courtesy of L. Barry Seltz, MD.)

the alveoli and terminal bronchioles. Hemorrhage and microabscesses are observed. Lymph nodes are involved occasionally. Bacteria also may be recovered from extrapulmonary sites such as the liver, spleen, and myocardium.

As with other intracellular organisms, the T cell–mediated response to infection confers immunity. Humoral immunity may aid in clearance of the organism by enhanced phagocytosis; otherwise, its role is limited. The risk of reinfection is unknown.

Clinical Manifestations

Infection with *L. pneumophila* results in two clinically distinct syndromes: Legionnaire's disease and Pontiac fever. Pontiac fever is an acute, self-limited, febrile illness without respiratory symptomatology. Legionnaire's disease is characterized by necrotizing multifocal pneumonia and a fulminant course. Asymptomatic and mild infections in children undoubtedly also occur.

Legionnaire's disease begins with a nonspecific prodrome of myalgias, fatigue, anorexia, malaise, headache, chills, vomiting, and watery diarrhea. The onset may be insidious or acute, but is usually followed by high fever. Relative bradycardia is well described in adults with Legionnaire's disease. Pleuritic chest pain and a dry cough ensue; the latter rarely becomes productive. Children with *Legionella* pneumonia may present with fever, cough, tachypnea, and hypoxia; chest pain may be absent.[15] Chest examination is universally consistent with a consolidating pneumonia: dullness to percussion, increased fremitus, bronchial breath sounds, and coarse crackles. A pleural friction rub may be heard, since nearly one third of patients with Legionnaire's disease will have pleural effusions.[15] The extrapulmonary manifestations of *L. pneumophila* infection include neuromuscular (e.g., meningoencephalitis, myositis), cardiac (e.g., myocarditis), gastrointestinal (e.g., hepatitis, pancreatitis), and renal (e.g., hypophosphatemia) abnormalities. Extrapulmonary manifestations are less common in children.[15,17] In more severe cases, patients become progressively ill, with confusion and delirium by the third to fourth day of illness. Shock, respiratory distress, or both develop by the fifth to sixth day of illness. Review of pediatric cases of Legionnaire's disease revealed an overall mortality rate of 33% although the mortality rates for immunosuppressed children and children less than 1 year of age were greater (84% and 58%, respectively).[15]

Laboratory Findings and Diagnosis

Legionnaire's disease must be considered in any patient with severe progressive pneumonia of unclear etiology. Leukocytosis, with a shift to the left, and lymphopenia are common. Thrombocytosis and disseminated intravascular coagulation also may occur. Legionnaire's disease often results in elevated liver transaminase levels, creatine kinase, bilirubin, and alkaline phosphatase. Hyponatremia and hypophosphatemia are more frequent in Legionnaire's disease than in other bacterial pneumonias. Hypoxia is often more severe than would be predicted by the extent of the pneumonia.[16] Chest radiographs characteristically demonstrate early interstitial or patchy infiltrates (unilateral or bilateral) described as an acinar filling pattern, followed by nodular consolidation and cavitation. The infiltrates often progress despite antibiotic therapy. Complete resolution of the lesions may take as long as 6 weeks.

Culture of sputum, and if available, lower respiratory secretions, pleural fluid, or lung biopsy specimens, is the definitive diagnostic modality. *Legionella* antigen also may be detected in urine specimens early in the course of the disease, but this method is only established for serogroup 1.[18] A combination of sputum culture and urine antigen detection may be the best diagnostic method.[14,18]

Indirect immunofluorescent antibody testing provides rapid results, requires specialized handling, and may yield false positives as a result of cross-reactions with other bacteria (e.g., *Pseudomonas*, *Bacteroides*, and *Flavobacterium*). Testing with monoclonal antibody improves the test's specificity. A positive immunofluorescent antibody test without other supporting evidence should not be considered diagnostic of legionellosis.[14] PCR testing is commercially available but should be interpreted cautiously.[18]

Serologic testing does not yield results rapidly enough to be useful as a diagnostic tool. An antibody titer of 1:256 or higher suggests a recent infection but is not confirmatory. Seroconversion may take 9 to 12 weeks. When obtaining serologic studies, it is important to request testing for IgM as well as IgG because some individuals will only demonstrate an IgM response. False-positive serologic results may occur because of cross-reactivity with other bacterial causes of atypical pneumonia (e.g., *Francisella tularensis*, *Coxiella burnetti*, *Mycoplasma pneumoniae*).

Treatment

Azithromycin has replaced erythromycin as the antimicrobial of choice for the treatment of Legionnaire's disease. Tetracyclines and trimethoprim-sulfamethoxazole are therapeutic alternatives. Although fluoroquinolones have demonstrated superior efficacy in adults, their use in children is restricted.[19] Rifampin has been recommended as adjunctive therapy in the presence of immunosuppression or severe illness, but it may offer little benefit.[19,20] Parenteral therapy should be administered until the patient responds clinically. The total duration of therapy is 5 to 10 days for azithromycin and longer when alternative therapies are used, or in the presence of severe disease or immunosuppression.

Prevention

Prevention of legionellosis is best achieved by identification and eradication of the environmental source. Culture-positive water may be superheated (70° C to 80° C), hyperchlorinated, or ionized by copper-silver units. Unfortunately, no method is particularly successful.

PSITTACOSIS

The first human outbreak of psittacosis (ornithosis) was reported in 1879. All seven patients had contact with sick parrots and finches and developed a febrile respiratory illness resulting in three deaths.[21] The term psittacosis derives from the Greek word for parrot, *psittakos*.[22]

Microbiology

Chlamydophila psittaci (formerly *Chlamydia psittaci*) is an obligate intracellular bacterium that contains both DNA and RNA within its cell wall. There are at least seven avian genotypes of *Cp. psittaci*.

Epidemiology

Psittacosis has a worldwide distribution and is generally sporadic. An epidemic, affecting 800 people, occurred in the United States in 1929 when a large shipment of infected parrots was exported from Argentina.[22] From 1985 to 1995, 1,132 cases of psittacosis were reported to the Centers for Disease Control and Prevention (CDC); from 2002 to 2007, 91 human cases were reported.[23]

Cp. psittaci infections occur in at least 465 bird species; it is most often found in psittacine birds (cockatoos, parrots, parakeets, and lories) and pigeons.[24] *Cp. psittaci* is now prevalent in turkeys in Belgium and other European countries.[24] Transmission generally occurs through inhalation of organisms aerosolized from feces or respiratory secretions from infected birds. Other modes of transmission include mouth to beak contact and handling infected birds' plumage and tissues.[23] Person-to-person transmission has not been proven.[23] The incubation period is approximately 5 to 14 days although it has been reported to have been as long as 1 month.

Pathophysiology

After inhalation, the organism establishes infection in the epithelial cells of the respiratory tract. Initial replication in respiratory epithelial cells is followed by spread of bacteria throughout the body, affecting multiple organs (heart, liver, gastrointestinal tract).[24] Noncaseating granulomas have been observed in the liver.[22]

Clinical Manifestations

Clinical features vary from an asymptomatic or mild influenza-like illness to systemic disease with severe pneumonia. Illness is generally of abrupt onset and is manifested by fever, headache, chills, myalgias, and a nonproductive cough; relative bradycardia is an unusual finding.[24,25] A pink maculopapular rash, Horder's spots, has been described.[25] Abdominal pain, vomiting, and diarrhea also have been noted.[24] Splenomegaly may be seen in up to a third of patients.[25] Rare complications include endocarditis, myocarditis, encephalitis, adult respiratory distress syndrome, and multiorgan failure.[24] Although still debated, *Cp. psittaci* has been associated with ocular lymphoma.[26] Before antibiotic therapy, 15% to 20% of patients died. Current mortality is less than 1% with appropriate treatment.

Laboratory Findings and Diagnosis

The white blood cell count is usually normal; leukopenia may develop in 25% of cases.[24] Anemia and elevated hepatic transaminase levels also have been observed. Chest radiographs are abnormal in up to 90% of hospitalized patients.[24] Lower lobe consolidation is the most common finding; nodular, military, and interstitial patterns also may be seen. A halo sign has been described on chest computed tomography.[27]

A confirmed case (CDC criteria) is a compatible clinical illness with laboratory evidence of *Cp. psittaci* infection by culture from respiratory secretions, a fourfold or greater increase in antibody by complement fixation or microimmunofluorescence (MIF) between acute and convalescent serum samples, or presence of IgM antibodies greater than or equal to 1:16 by MIF.[23]

Serology is limited by cross-reaction with other chlamydial species, including *Cp. pneumoniae*. PCR testing can determine the species and the genotype of the causative agent.

Treatment

Tetracyclines are the treatment of choice. For children younger than 8 years of age, a macrolide is recommended. Duration of therapy, for maximal efficacy and prevention of relapse, should be for a minimum of 10 days or for 10 to 14 days following defervescence. With widespread use of antibiotics in the poultry and bird industry, resistance to tetracyclines may emerge. Symptoms usually improve within 48 to 72 hours.

Prevention

Individuals handling potentially infected birds should wear protective clothing and respirator masks. Birds with suspected infection should be evaluated by a veterinarian. Deceased birds with possible infection should be sealed in an impermeable container and tested in a veterinary laboratory. Potentially contaminated cages should be disinfected using 1% Lysol, 1:1,000 dilution of quaternary ammonium compounds, or 1:32 dilution of household bleach.[23] Health care professionals and the public are in need of education to heighten awareness of the zoonotic potential of psittacine birds.

◼ CHLAMYDOPHILA PNEUMONIAE

In recent years, *Chlamydophila pneumoniae* has been recognized as an increasingly common respiratory pathogen in both children and adults. Formerly known as the Taiwan acute respiratory agent (TWAR) agent and placed in the same genus as *Chlamydia trachomatis*, it has now been placed in a separate genus, *Chlamydophila*, along with *Cp. psittaci*. As a result of improved diagnostic techniques and provider awareness, it has gained recognition as a distinct pathogen and has been implicated in many acute and chronic conditions.

Microbiology

Chlamydophila pneumoniae is a genetically, morphologically, and antigenically distinct member of the Chlamydiaceae family. *Chlamydiae* are obligate intracellular pathogens with a cell wall containing lipopolysaccharide, similar to gram-negative bacteria.[28,29] *Chlamydiae* exhibit two forms during their developmental cycle: an intracellular dividing form (reticulate body) and an extracellular, infectious, metabolically inactive form (elementary body).[28] *Cp. pneumoniae* exhibits a unique pear-shaped elementary body that distinguishes it from other *Chlamydiae*.[29]

Epidemiology

Chlamydophila pneumoniae infections are common. Initial infection peaks in children between the ages of 5 and 15 years of age in temperate, developed regions but may occur earlier in those residing in tropical or less developed areas. There is no evidence of seasonality, although epidemics occur every 4 to 5 years. The infection is probably transmitted via respiratory secretions from person to person or via fomites.[30] No animal reservoir exists, although the organism has been isolated from several species. An estimated 2% to 5% of adults and children are asymptomatic nasopharyngeal carriers of *Cp. pneumoniae*, but it is unclear whether carriers are a reservoir of infection. Concurrent infection with *M. pneumoniae* or *S. pneumoniae* occurs frequently. The incubation period is 21 days.[31]

Pathology

Following delivery to the respiratory mucosa, *Cp. pneumoniae* organisms are transported into the mucosal epithelial cells by endocytosis. Chlamydiae prevent fusion of the phagosome with lysosomes, thus inhibiting their own death. Within the phagosome, the elementary bodies differentiate into reticulate bodies and undergo binary fission.[28] At 36 to 48 hours following inoculation, multiplication ceases and the reticulate bodies return to infectious elementary bodies. The contents of the phagosome are released by cytolysis, exocytosis, or extrusion of the entire inclusion.[28]

Clinical Manifestations

Chlamydophila pneumoniae infections often begin with a nonspecific prodrome of sore throat, malaise, headache, low-grade fever, and cough. The course is prolonged (2 to 6 weeks) and often biphasic. Patients may demonstrate upper respiratory tract infections such as pharyngitis, laryngitis, or sinusitis. A significant number will develop pneumonia or bronchitis. *Cp. pneumoniae* is a potent trigger of inflammation and leads to an immunoglobulin E (IgE)–mediated bronchial reactivity.[32] Physical examination may reveal nonexudative pharyngitis, wheezes, and fine or coarse crackles.

Patient age often determines the severity of disease; adolescents more frequently develop lower respiratory tract infection.[33] Severe illness may affect previously healthy children and result in complications such as pneumatocele, pleural effusion, pneumothorax, interstitial fibrosis, or lung abscess. Other complications of *Cp. pneumoniae* infection include erythema nodosum, reactive arthritis, Guillain-Barré syndrome, meningoencephalitis, myocarditis, and endocarditis. *Cp. pneumoniae* also has been isolated from middle ear fluid in children with acute otitis media, generally with other pathogens. The organism has been linked to asthma, multiple sclerosis, chronic fatigue, and atherosclerotic heart disease; causation has not been confirmed. Mortality is often associated with comorbid conditions or secondary infections.

Laboratory Findings and Diagnosis

Although fairly ubiquitous, *Cp. pneumoniae* is diagnosed infrequently because of nonspecific radiographic and laboratory findings and a lack of reliable diagnostic tests. White blood cell counts are often normal or mildly elevated. Erythrocyte sedimentation rates are typically elevated. Chest radiography classically demonstrates a pattern of alveolar infiltrate or subsegmental pneumonitis without consolidation,[31,33-35] although a single subsegmental lesion of only one lobe is the most common lesion.[31,35] Pleural effusion is uncommon.

Serologic testing is the primary diagnostic modality. Detection of antibody by microimmunofluorescence is the only currently acceptable test to diagnose an acute infection.[36,37] Newer CDC criteria for serologic diagnosis require an IgM titer greater than 1:16 or a fourfold rise in the IgG titer.[37] As infection with *Cp. pneumoniae* may only lead to partial immunity, reinfections commonly occur. IgM antibody may be absent in disease associated with reinfection and may take up to 3 weeks to appear after primary infection related illness. Reliance on a single test for diagnosis is discouraged.[36,37] *Chlamydophila pneumoniae* may be cultured from the nasopharynx, sputum, or pleural fluid. Specimens must be placed in transport media, stored briefly at 4° C, and inoculated on cell-containing media. Identification of the bacteria by staining is difficult, since *Cp. pneumoniae*–specific reagent has limited availability. Polymerase chain reaction techniques have neither been standardized nor approved by the U.S. Food and Drug Administration (FDA) for commercial use.[37,38]

Treatment

Few studies have investigated the response of *Cp. pneumoniae* infection to antimicrobial therapy. *Cp. pneumoniae* is susceptible to macrolides, tetracyclines, and quinolones; however, the latter two are not routinely recommended in children. Young children may be treated with a 14-day course of oral erythromycin, a 10-day course of clarithromycin or a 5-day course of oral azithromycin.[36,38] Adolescent patients may be treated with a 5-day course of oral azithromycin, a 14- to 21-day course of oral doxycycline, or a 14- to 21-day course of oral tetracycline.[36,38] Prolonged antimicrobial therapy (up to 3 weeks) may be required.[36] Parenteral therapy may be required for patients with severe disease.

Prevention

Chlamydophila transmission may be decreased by avoidance of contact with persons with respiratory illness and their respiratory secretions. Antibiotics are not recommended either to eradicate carrier states or for postexposure prophylaxis. No vaccine exists for *Cp. pneumoniae* at this time.

MYCOPLASMA PNEUMONIAE

Mycoplasma were first identified in cattle over 100 years ago and in humans in 1937.[39] In 1944, Eaton recovered an organism now known as *Mycoplasma pneumoniae* from patients with atypical pneumonia.[2] Although more than 200 species of *Mycoplasma* are recognized, relatively few have been causally associated with disease in children; the best known is *Mycoplasma pneumoniae*.

Microbiology

Mycoplasma pneumoniae are small, double-stranded DNA, pleomorphic, cell wall-deficient organisms. *M. pneumoniae* grows relatively slowly; visible colony formation may take 3 weeks or longer.

Epidemiology

Infection occurs throughout the world and during all months of the year. *M. pneumoniae* is transmitted by respiratory droplets during close contact, with an incubation period of 2 to 3 weeks. The incidence of infection is about 4 per 1000 children per year.[40] *M. pneumoniae* causes between 9% and 42% of pediatric community-acquired pneumonia.[39] Lower respiratory tract infection is more common beginning at school age (5 years) but is being increasingly recognized in younger children. A recent study found 39/102 (38%) cases were in children younger than 5 years, including 8 infants 8 months of age or younger.[41] Reinfection may occur, although second episodes appear milder and reinfection is less common after pneumonia than after illness with milder symptoms.[40]

Pathophysiology

After secretions contact the respiratory epithelial surface, *M. pneumoniae* adheres to host respiratory mucosa through an attachment organelle. Peroxide and superoxide radicals are generated that induce oxidative stress in host cells. The production of cytokines and activation of lymphocytes may either minimize or exacerbate disease through immunologic hypersensitivity.[42] Toxin-mediated disease has recently been postulated with the identification of the community-acquired respiratory distress syndrome toxin (CARDS TX), which binds to surfactant protein A. Organisms reaching the lower respiratory tract are opsonized, and subsequent phagocytosis by activated macrophages contributes to the inflammatory exudate. Respiratory epithelial cells infected with *M. pneumoniae* typically lose their cilia and show a decrease in oxygen consumption, glucose utilization, and macromolecular synthesis that ultimately results in exfoliation.[42]

Clinical Manifestations

Approximately 20% of infections caused by *M. pneumoniae* are asymptomatic.[40] In symptomatic patients, the initial manifestation is usually pharyngitis followed by hoarseness. Fever and persistent cough are the predominant symptoms; rhinitis is less common.[43,44] Vomiting and diarrhea may affect up to 20% of patients.[41] On physical examination, children may have crackles (40% to 73%) or wheezing (35%).[41,44] Mean duration of illness is about 2 weeks, although cough has been reported to persist for 1 month or longer. More severe disease may be seen in normal children, as well as in certain high risk groups (e.g., those with sickle cell anemia, immunodeficiency, and chronic cardiorespiratory disease). *M. pneumoniae* also has been associated with several other disease processes including otitis media, sinusitis, mucocutaneous eruptions, myocarditis, pericarditis, hemolytic anemia, arthritis, glomerulonephritis, and nervous system disease (aseptic meningitis, encephalitis, cerebellar ataxia, transverse myelitis, peripheral neuropathy, psychosis, and Guillain-Barré syndrome).[39]

Laboratory Findings and Diagnosis

The white blood cell count is generally unremarkable,[41,45] and chest radiograph findings are variable (Fig. 32-2). In a study of children hospitalized with *Mycoplasma* pneumonia the most common radiographic findings were perihilar linear opacities (60%), reticulonodular infiltrates (40%), and segmental or lobar consolidation (28%).[45] Consolidation has recently been reported as the most common radiographic finding.[41,44] Pleural effusions are found in about 8% of patients.[41,44,45]

Several methods exist to detect *M. pneumoniae* infection including culture, serology, and molecular-based PCR testing. Serologic diagnosis involves detection of IgM antibodies, which generally appear 7 to 10 days after infection, and IgG antibodies, which appear approximately 3 weeks after infection.[40] Presence of IgM antibodies indicates recent infection, although they may persist for several months. Enzyme-linked immunosorbent assays (ELISA) are the most widely used assay. Serum cold agglutinins are nonspecific but may be present in about 50% of patients with pneumonia. PCR testing of nasopharyngeal or throat swab specimens is being increasingly utilized. Comparison of diagnostic techniques in 75 children with lower respiratory tract illness found evidence of *M. pneumoniae* infection by serology in 16/75 (21%) patients, PCR in 13/75 (17%) patients, and culture in 4/75 (5%) patients.[46] Of those with a positive serologic diagnosis, 11/16 (85%) patients had a positive PCR from nasopharyngeal aspirates.

Treatment

The antimicrobials of choice for *Mycoplasma* pneumonia are the macrolides and the tetracyclines administered for 10 days. A macrolide is the drug of choice for young children. In a retrospective study, children treated with a macrolide had a shorter duration of fever (4.9 days vs. 5.6 days) compared with those who did not receive

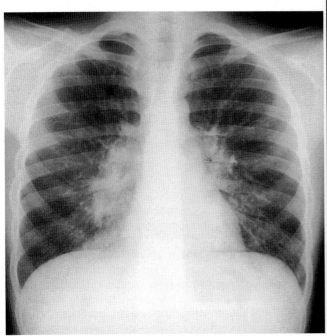

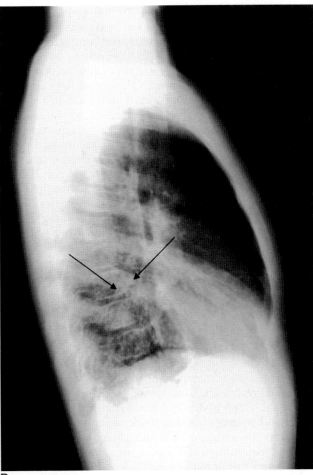

A   B

FIGURE 32-2. Bilateral perihilar infiltrates, prominent on anteroposterior radiograph **(A)**, and reticulonodular infiltrates, prominent on lateral radiograph **(B)** of an adolescent with *Mycoplasma pneumoniae*. (Courtesy of Rebecca Hulett, MD.)

a macrolide.[47] Macrolide resistance in *M. pneumoniae*, common in Asia, also has been documented in Europe and the United States.[48] Fluoroquinolones, while effective, are generally not used in children. Corticosteroids may be beneficial in children with severe pneumonia.[49]

Prevention

Vaccines have been developed with varying degrees of success. More severe illness has been reported in vaccinated subjects who did not have a significant immune response.[50] In certain circumstances (e.g., patients with sickle cell disease), prophylactic antibiotics may be prudent.

▄▄▄ INHALATIONAL ANTHRAX

Anthrax is a zoonotic disease that afflicts humans by causing three distinct disease patterns: dermatologic, gastrointestinal, and inhalational. The term *anthrax* is derived from the Greek word for coal *(anthrakos)* to depict the black eschar seen in cutaneous anthrax. Described in epidemics as woolsorter's disease, inhalational anthrax is rare but frequently fatal. The potential of anthrax as a biological weapon was realized in 2001 when the

distribution of the organism resulted in 22 human infections, 11 of which were inhalational anthrax. Five of the 11 inhalational cases were fatal.[51,52]

Microbiology

Bacillus anthracis is an aerobic, spore-forming, encapsulated, gram-positive, nonmotile bacillus. It grows optimally at 36° C and colonies may appear 15 to 24 hours after the inoculation of sheep blood agar. Following incubation, the spores form chains of rods that resemble bamboo and then sporulate. *B. anthracis* relies on three virulence factors: two exotoxins (lethal and edema toxins) and a specialized capsule. The lipopolysaccharide capsule blunts the immune response by inhibiting phagocytosis and activation of neutrophils. Lethal and edema toxins result in hemorrhage, edema, and necrosis.

Epidemiology

Bacillus anthracis and its extremely stable spores may be encountered worldwide. All domestic animals, including cattle, sheep and swine, may be infected subsequent to ingestion of spores and serve as hosts. Humans are infected following contact with infected animals or contaminated animal products. Animal products that have been associated with infection apart include hides, wool, hair, animal feces, bone meal, and commercial animal products. The majority of human anthrax infections from these sources are cutaneous; they show neither seasonality nor gender preference. Cutaneous lesions are considered potentially infectious but person-to-person transmission has rarely been reported. Gastrointestinal anthrax primarily occurs subsequent to the ingestion of raw or undercooked meat. Naturally occurring inhalational anthrax was considered rare; however, several cases have been reported in the last decade. In 2001, intentional contamination of the U.S. mail resulted in the aforementioned 11 cases of inhalational anthrax.[51-53] Inhalational and gastrointestinal anthrax cases have been reported in the Northeast resulting from animal hide exposure.[54,55]

The incubation period for anthrax is typically 1 to 7 days but has been reported as long as several months for inhalational anthrax due to spore dormancy and unpredictable clearance from the lungs.

Pathology

Following inhalation, spores are ingested by pulmonary macrophages and transported to hilar lymph nodes. Bacterial germination and toxin production occur in mediastinal lymph nodes. *B. anthracis* infection results in lymphatic dilatation, interstitial edema, and necrosis that cause local hemorrhage. Ultimately, hemorrhagic lymphadenitis, mediastinitis, and septicemia result.

Mechanisms of immunity are unclear. Humoral immunity against the toxin complex may play a role.

Clinical Manifestations

The cutaneous form of *B. anthracis* infection is characterized by painless eschar formation and surrounding edema at the site of inoculation of abraded skin and a rarely fatal course. Gastrointestinal anthrax may affect the oropharynx or the intestinal tract. While gastrointestinal anthrax is associated with significant morbidity and mortality, inhalational anthrax is the most lethal form of infection.

Inhalational anthrax begins with nonspecific symptomatology such as fever, myalgia, headache, cough, and abdominal and chest pain. The second phase of illness (second to fifth day) ensues rapidly, with severe chest pain and respiratory distress.[56,57] The course is often marked by hemorrhagic mediastinitis, hemorrhagic pleural effusion, and bacteremia leading to dyspnea, hypoxemia, cyanosis, and shock. Nearly half of patients presenting with inhalational anthrax demonstrate nuchal rigidity and obtundation.[56] Inhalational anthrax is usually fatal within 24 to 36 hours.[56]

The mortality of inhalational anthrax was previously estimated to be greater than 95%. The case fatality rate for the 2001 anthrax cases was 45%.[52]

Anthrax meningoencephalitis is a rarely reported complication of all forms of anthrax and follows dissemination of the organism via hematogenous or lymphatic routes. It is generally rapidly fatal.[57]

Laboratory Findings/Diagnosis

Chest radiography may reveal a widened mediastinum or prominent lymphadenopathy. Pulmonary hemorrhage and pleural effusions are frequently seen. Pulmonary infiltrates may be seen but should raise suspicion of superinfection. Computed tomography of the chest should be obtained in patients highly suspect for this infection to carefully evaluate the mediastinum and determine the presence of pleural fluid. Elevated transaminase levels were observed at the time of presentation in the 2001 cases.[58]

Identification of gram-positive bacilli on blood smear, in pleural fluid, cerebrospinal fluid, or on skin biopsy suggests the diagnosis of anthrax. The infection may be confirmed by culture of infected fluid or tissue and by serology. A single antibody titer greater than 1:32 measured by ELISA or a fourfold rise in titer is diagnostic. PCR, immunofluorescent, and immunohistochemical assays may be performed locally but are often sent to municipal, state, or CDC laboratories.

Treatment

Current regimens for treatment of inhalational anthrax are based on limited clinical experience; no controlled trial has been performed in humans. Although not routinely used in children, ciprofloxacin and doxycycline are the antimicrobials of choice as a component of a multidrug regimen for the treatment of inhalational anthrax in children.[58] One or two additional agents—rifampin, ampicillin or penicillin, vancomycin, clindamycin, imipenem, chloramphenicol, and clarithromycin—also are recommended for the treatment of inhalational anthrax.[59,60] Although active against *B. anthracis*, penicillin-resistant strains have been identified, and it should never be used as single-agent therapy. Clindamycin, an inhibitor of protein synthesis, is often used because it disrupts both the production and release of toxin by infected cells.[57] Parenteral therapy is given until the patient has improved; a minimum of 14 days is recommended. The recommended duration of therapy is 60 days. Corticosteroids have been used as adjunctive therapy for complications of inhalational anthrax such as severe edema, respiratory compromise, or meningitis.

Prevention

Anthrax vaccine (AVA) is commercially available and is administered to military personnel and those at high risk of exposure. The Advisory Committee on Immunization Practices (ACIP) currently recommends a five-dose series of AVA as preexposure prophylaxis for anthrax. Annual boosters are required to maintain immunity.[61] AVA is not approved for use in children.

The ACIP recommends that postexposure therapy include three subcutaneous doses of AVA in combination with antibiotics in previously unvaccinated people 18 years of age or older.[61] The use of AVA postexposure is not, however, contraindicated in children. In the event of a high-risk exposure, consultation with public health officials may result in immunization of an exposed child under the Investigational New Drug (IND) protocol held by the CDC.[61]

Ciprofloxacin and doxycycline are recommended as initial postexposure antimicrobials of choice for patients with confirmed or suspected aerosol exposure to anthrax spores.[55,59] Once proven susceptible, amoxicillin can be substituted for children.[55,59] Antibiotic prophylaxis should begin as soon as possible and continue for 60 days, followed by careful observation. Some authorities recommend a 100-day course of prophylactic antimicrobials based on prolonged persistence of the organism in the experimental animal model.[60]

Livestock in enzootic areas may be vaccinated annually. Contaminated carcasses should be incinerated to prevent the spread of disease.

TULAREMIA

McCoy first identified tularemia in 1911 in Tulare County, California, as an illness that resembled bubonic plague in ground squirrels; the causative agent was named *Bacterium tularense* for its site of discovery.[62] Edward Francis, a U.S. Public Health Service surgeon, identified several infections with *B. tularense* in humans and confirmed the deer fly as a vector for the disease. Following his many contributions to the study of tularemia and a nomination for a Nobel Prize, Francis was honored when the genus name for the causative organism was changed to *Francisella*.[63]

Microbiology

Francisella tularensis is an aerobic, nonmotile, pleomorphic, gram-negative coccobacillus. The bacterium does not produce any exotoxin but may contain endotoxin similar to other gram-negative bacilli. *Francisella tularensis* does not produce spores, yet it is resistant to freezing; the organism is readily killed by heat. Although it can be isolated on routine cultures, its growth is enhanced on glucose-cysteine-enriched blood agar. There are two distinct groups of *F. tularensis* responsible for the majority of human tularemia: type A (*F. tularensis* subspecies *tularensis*) denotes those strains that are highly virulent for humans and account for 90% of *F. tularensis* isolated in the United States and, less commonly, Europe; type B (*F. tularensis* subspecies *holarctica*) is a less virulent strain found throughout North America, Asia, and Europe.[63] *F. tularensis* subspecies mediasiatica and novocida are more rare causative agents of human tularemia.[63]

Epidemiology

Francisella tularensis is ubiquitous in northern latitudes. It has been isolated from contaminated soil and water, infected ticks, and over 200 species of animals. Although tularemia occurs throughout the year, it peaks during the winter months (hunting season) in the northern and eastern United States and during the summer months (tick season) in the southern and more central states. From 1990 to 2000, a total of 1,368 cases of tularemia were reported in the United States (only 59% were confirmed).[64] Four states accounted for 56% of all reported tularemia cases: Arkansas (23%), Missouri (19%), South Dakota (7%), and Oklahoma (7%).[64] The incidence of

tularemia was highest among males 5 to 9 years of age and those older than 75 years of age.[64] It occurred more frequently in American Indians and Alaskan Natives (0.5 per 100,000) than in Caucasians (0.04 per 100,000) or African Americans and Asians/Pacific Islanders (0.01 per 100,000 or less).[64] A more recent analysis of 190 tularemia cases in Missouri from 2000 to 2007 concluded that 78% occurred during the summer months and 66% were among males. Seventy-two percent of the 78 documented cases were associated with a tick bite.[65]

Contact with infected animals (or their carcasses) and bites by deer flies or ticks (primarily Dermacentor andersoni [wood tick], Dermacentor variabilis, [dog tick], and Ambylomma americanum [lone star tick]) are the most common means of human infection. The organism infects various species of animals naturally, yet fewer than a dozen species have been known to transmit the infection. Rodents (e.g., squirrels), and classically sheep, and lagomorphs (rabbits and hares) transmit the infection. Transmission of tularemia via cat and hamster bites has been reported, and it has been postulated that indirect transmission through a bite from a pet may be an important source of infection in children. Humans also have been infected by ingestion of contaminated water or food, or by aerosolization.[63,65,66] Person-to-person transmission has not been reported.

Pathology

Francisella tularensis may enter the body via the skin, mucous membranes, or respiratory or gastrointestinal tracts, but it typically infects the skin, lymph nodes, lungs, liver, and spleen. The bacterium spreads quickly to regional lymph nodes, causing a pattern of cellular changes characteristic of intracellular parasites. Organisms are rarely identified from lesions, which often demonstrate necrosis or granuloma formation. *Francisella tularensis* also may spread hematogenously, usually within the first week of infection. Reticuloendothelial hyperplasia is frequently observed. Although neutrophils are critical for the initial clearance of organisms, it is the T cell–mediated immune response, however, that is undoubtedly responsible for protective immunity.[63] Reinfection is rare.

Clinical Manifestations

Tularemia presents acutely with fever (typically higher than 103° F or 39.4° C), chills, myalgias, vomiting, headache, coryza, and sore throat often within 3 to 5 days following inoculation (range 1 to 21 days).[67] Relative bradycardia is frequently described.[68] Physical findings often include lymphadenopathy, skin lesions or rashes, hepatosplenomegaly, and pharyngitis. Subcutaneous nodules also may be noted. Untreated tularemia may cause persistent fevers. The six clinical syndromes of tularemia denote the site of organism entry: ulceroglandular, glandular, oculoglandular, oropharyngeal, typhoidal, and pneumonic.

Pneumonic tularemia is the most severe and lethal form of tularemia.[63,66,67] Although the disease is traditionally considered more common in adults, the number of reports in children have been increasing. Review of the tularemia cases from Missouri reveals that 24% were the pulmonic form; 4% of the patients with pulmonary disease were children.[65] The primary form of the syndrome is acquired by inhalation. A secondary form of pneumonic tularemia may occur during typhoidal or ulceroglandular disease. Signs and symptoms of pneumonic tularemia include sore throat, cough, dyspnea, chest pain, or pleuritic pain. Occasionally, a pleural effusion is present. These signs and symptoms of pneumonic tularemia are nonspecific and may be delayed. Thus, this disease is often confused with bronchiolitis, pneumonitis, or pharyngitis. Pneumonic tularemia is rare; a widespread outbreak should prompt concern for a bioterrorism event.[63,67]

Laboratory Findings and Diagnosis

The diagnosis of tularemia is confirmed by serologic testing. A single or initial titer of agglutinating antibody equal to or greater than 1:160 (by tube agglutination) or greater than 1:128 (by microagglutination) supports a presumptive diagnosis, and a fourfold increase in the IgG titer 14 days later (minimum) confirms the diagnosis. An ELISA that detects IgM, IgG, and IgA antibodies to *F. tularensis* has been developed.[63] Identification of the organisms in exudates and tissues may be accomplished by indirect fluorescent antibody, PCR, or immunohistochemical stains. Immunoblotting and antigen detection assays are not commercially available. Routine cultures of sputum or exudates must be directed to the appropriate laboratory facility to ensure proper handling and safety of laboratory personnel and to guide proper media selection.

The peripheral white blood cell count can range from 3000 to 15,000. Atypical lymphocytosis and sterile pyuria also have been reported. Nearly half of the patients have elevated transaminase levels.[62,68]

With pulmonic involvement, radiographic data may be difficult to interpret. Although a radiographic triad of findings (ovoid opacities, pleural effusion, and hilar adenopathy) associated with tularemic pneumonia has been well described, it is nonspecific.[62,66] Early radiographic findings may resemble peribronchial infiltrates that progress to bronchopneumonia in one or more lobes.[65] Radiographs of tularemia pneumonia in children may resemble community-acquired pneumonia, viral pneumonia, tuberculosis, fungal pneumonia, pneumonitis, and other atypical bacterial infections. In adults, lymphoma and carcinoma also may be diagnostic considerations.

Treatment

Aminoglycosides are the preferred antimicrobials for treatment of tularemia. Although streptomycin was the classic therapeutic choice, it has been superseded by gentamicin. Resolution of signs and symptoms of infection is prompt and usually occurs within days. The duration of therapy is 7 to 10 days but may be extended in severe or complicated disease.

The tetracyclines, chloramphenicol, and rifampin (bacteriostatic agents) also have been used to treat tularemia. However, these antimicrobials are not as effective as streptomycin or gentamicin and are associated with a high relapse rate. Fluoroquinolones have demonstrated clinical efficacy, but their use in children is restricted.

Beta-lactams are not effective. Surgical intervention may be required for suppurative lesions.

Prevention

Tularemia may be avoided by eliminating exposure to infected animals and the vectors of disease. Deceased rodents and lagomorphs should be incinerated or buried. Children should be instructed not to handle rodents and lagomorphs that appear ill or are deceased. Rubber gloves should be worn while preparing game animals, and the meat should be thoroughly cooked. Children and adults in endemic areas should wear protective clothing and use tick repellent. Following outdoor activities, inspection for ticks is mandatory, as is their careful removal.

A live vaccine, developed in 1960, remains unlicensed in the United States and for investigational use only. It has been successful in reducing the severity and incidence of tularemia in laboratory personnel, but its effect on naturally occurring disease is unknown. The vaccine is not recommended for postexposure prophylaxis. Doxycycline and fluoroquinolones have been used for postexposure chemoprophylaxis.

◼ Q FEVER

Q fever was first reported by E.H. Derrick in 1937 following investigation of a febrile illness in abattoir workers in Queensland, Australia. Initially named Q (for query) fever, this illness was characterized by fever, headache, malaise, anorexia, and myalgias lasting from 7 to 24 days.[69]

Microbiology

The etiologic agent is *Coxiella burnetti*, a gram-negative obligate intracellular bacterium. The bacterium was reclassified from the order *Rickettsiales* to *Legionellales*.

Epidemiology

Q fever is a zoonosis with a worldwide distribution. Humans are incidental hosts. The animal reservoir includes mammals, birds, and arthropods (mainly ticks). Common sources of human infection are cattle, goats, and sheep; pets, including dogs and cats, also have been implicated.

Q fever affects all age groups, although it is more prevalent in adults than in children.[70] The annual incidence in France has been estimated at 50 cases per 100,000 individuals. In the United States, the number of reported human cases increased from 21 in 2000 to 70 in 2004[70]; the overall seroprevalence in adults was recently reported at 3.1%.[71] In the Netherlands, possibly because of expansion of goat farming, more than 2300 human cases, including 6 deaths were identified in 2009.[72] In Greece, acute Q fever was diagnosed in 8 of 1200 (0.67%) hospitalized children over a 2-year period.[73]

Transmission usually occurs from inhalation of contaminated aerosols from parturient fluids of infected animals.[70] Infected mammals shed bacteria in urine, feces, milk, and birth products. Infection also has been reported from consumption of raw milk, blood transfusion, transplacental transmission, and sexual intercourse.[70] The incubation period is approximately 20 days.

Pathophysiology

C. burnetti exhibits antigenic variation; the wild virulent form, phase I, shifts to a mutant, avirulent form, phase II that is associated with a partial loss of lipopolysaccharide. *C. burnetti* can survive in the external environment for long periods of time. After inhalation, organisms enter host cells (macrophages) by phagocytosis.[26] Once internalized, organisms survive and multiply within acidic vacuoles. Phase I bacteria escape intracellular killing by inhibiting the final maturation of phagolysosomes.[74] Interleukin-10 appears to play a role in the development of chronic disease. Granulomas, consisting of a central lipid vacuole surrounded by a fibrinoid ring, form in infected organs.[74]

Clinical Manifestations

Following primary infection, about 60% of individuals remain asymptomatic.[74] Symptomatic illness is divided into acute and chronic forms, with chronic Q fever lasting at least 6 months. The most common presentation of acute Q fever in adults is a flu-like illness characterized by fever, fatigue, headache, and myalgias.[70] Other common presentations include pneumonia and hepatitis.

In a study of children, the most common manifestations of acute illness were fever (47%), pneumonia (18%), myocarditis (8%), central nervous system infection (8%), and influenza-like syndrome (5%).[75] Rare manifestations included pericarditis, hepatitis, hemophagocytosis, rhabdomyolysis, and hemolytic-uremic syndrome. Eight cases of chronic Q fever presented as either endocarditis (63%) or osteomyelitis (37%).[75]

Hospitalized children with Q fever have illness characterized by fever lasting 5 to10 days, headache, mild cough, abdominal pain, and vomiting.[73,76] Recovery was complete even without specific therapy directed against *C. burnetti*.[73,76] *C. burnetti* is thought to be a rare cause of community-acquired pneumonia.[69] Patients with Q fever pneumonia typically have fever, anorexia, and headache; cough is found in 60% to 70% of patients.[69] On examination of the chest, only about one half of patients have physical findings suggestive of pneumonia. Symptoms can last from 10 to 90 days.[70]

Laboratory Findings and Diagnosis

Laboratory findings are nonspecific. The white blood cell count is usually normal. Elevated hepatic transaminase levels and thrombocytopenia may be seen.[70] Autoantibodies, including antimitochondrial, anti–smooth muscle, and antiphospholipid, are commonly found.[70] Chest radiographic findings are nonspecific. Two children with Q fever pneumonia had unilateral segmental infiltrates.[73] The most common finding seen in 272 patients with Q fever pneumonia was lower lobe involvement (37%); other features included air bronchograms (26%), pleural effusion (10%), single or multiple rounded opacities (7%), and segmental consolidation (6%).[69]

Diagnosis rests on serologic testing, most commonly utilizing microimmunofluorescence, for antibodies (IgG, IgM, and IgA) to phase I and phase II antigens.[70] Seroconversion is usually noted 7 to 15 days after the onset of disease.[70] Antibody titers greater than 1:200 for IgG or 1:50 for IgM against phase II antigens suggest recent infection.[70] An IgG titer greater than or equal to 1:800 against phase I antigens is usually associated with chronic disease.[70] PCR may be useful in acute infection before the appearance of antibodies.

Treatment

Acute Q fever is usually a mild disease with spontaneous resolution within 2 weeks. Treatment is indicated in symptomatic patients and pregnant women. Doxycycline for 10 to 14 days is the treatment of choice for Q fever pneumonia. In a retrospective study of adult patients, the mean time to defervescence was 2.9 days with doxycycline, 3.3 days with clarithromycin, 3.9 days with erythromycin, and 6.4 days with beta-lactam antibiotics.[69] Antibody titers can be used to monitor the treatment course, particularly in cases of chronic infection.

Prevention

A whole cell vaccine developed in Australia has provided effective protection in occupational settings.[70] Ensuring that holding facilities for farm animals are located away from populated areas should decrease the risk of infection. In the Netherlands, use of an animal vaccine is planned to help curtail the spread of disease. In addition, 40,000 pregnant goats are being culled in an effort to halt the current Q fever outbreak.[72]

■ PNEUMONIC PLAGUE

Plague, a scourge since antiquity, has been the cause of at least three pandemics, including the "Black Death," which killed one third of Europe's population in the 14th century. The etiologic agent, *Yersenia pestis*, was first isolated by Alexandre Yersin in 1894 in Hong Kong following spread from China during the last pandemic.[77] Concerns regarding bioterrorism have renewed interest in plague.

Microbiology

Y. pestis is a gram-negative, nonmotile, coccobacillus that exhibits bipolar staining. It is a facultative anaerobe that recently (<20,000 years ago) evolved from *Yersenia pseudotuberculosis*.[78] The bacterium survives for up to 3 days at room temperature and for up to 11 months in the soil of rodent burrows.[78]

Epidemiology

Plague is enzootic in rodents in Africa, Asia, North America, and South America. Humans are usually infected through bites by rodent fleas; most fleas are infected by feeding on bacteremic domestic black rats, *Rattus rattus*, or brown sewer rats, *Rattus norvegicus*.[79] Domestic cats may become infected by eating rodents and serve as a reservoir of infection. Infection in humans may also occur by handling or eating contaminated animals, by exposure to aerosolized *Y. pestis,* and by inhalation of respiratory droplets from people or animals with pneumonic plague.[80]

Spread of pneumonic plague is believed to be inefficient because close contact is required with coughing patients in the final stages of disease.[81] The last documented person-to-person transmission in the United States occurred in 1924.[80]

The World Health Organization reported 28,350 cases of confirmed and suspected human plague in all countries from 1994 to 2003 with a case-fatality rate of 7.1%.[79] Plague was first identified in the United States in 1900; from 1947 to 2001, 421 cases of plague were reported to the CDC, of which 183 (44%) were in children 18 years or younger.[80] In 2006 in the United States, 13 cases (2 deaths) were reported.[79]

In the United States, human plague typically occurs between June and October, when rodent fleas are most active.[80] The incubation period is 2 to 10 days,[79] although it may be shorter (2 to 4 days) following direct infection of the airways.[81]

Pathophysiology

Yersenia pestis is inoculated into human skin via a flea bite, and organisms migrate via lymphatics to regional lymph nodes. *Y. pestis* has multiple virulence factors that enhance pathogen survival: plasminogen activator promotes bacterial spread; F1 antigen inhibits phagocytosis; type 3 secretion system translocates virulence factors into host cells; V antigen has anti-inflammatory activity; and Yops inhibits phagocytosis, platelet aggregation, and cytokine production.[77,79] The lipopolysaccharide envelope initiates inflammatory responses leading to septic shock.[79] After initial intracellular growth in mononuclear phagocytes, extracellular proliferation occurs, resulting in bacteremia and inflammation and necrosis in lymph nodes, spleen, and liver.[79] Pneumonic plague usually occurs from secondary hematogenous spread to the lungs following primary bubonic or septicemic plague. Primary pneumonic plague resulting from direct inhalation of *Y. pestis* is rare.[78]

Clinical Manifestations

Principal clinical syndromes include bubonic, septicemic, and pneumonic plague. The most common form is bubonic plague, an acute febrile illness associated with headache, weakness, chills, and malaise. A painful, swollen lymph node (bubo), which becomes fluctuant, arises proximal to the inoculation site. Lymph nodes in the groin are most frequently affected followed by axillary and cervical regions. Septicemic plague is characterized by endotoxemia with multiorgan system failure. Meningeal, pharyngeal, ocular, and gastrointestinal forms of the disease are rare.

Patients with pneumonic plague manifest sudden onset of fever, headache, chills, and malaise. Temperature is only slightly elevated initially but steadily rises during the course of disease.[82] Abdominal pain, nausea, vomiting, and diarrhea

may be present.[78] Cough generally develops after 20 to 24 hours; initially dry, it becomes increasingly productive.[81] Dyspnea that is out of proportion to findings on chest examination also appears.[82] In the final stages of illness, copious amounts of blood-stained sputum are produced.[81] In a series of 38 children (median age 8.5 years) diagnosed with plague (82% bubonic and 18% septicemic), the most common presenting symptoms were fever (95%), painful adenopathy (55%), vomiting (50%), lethargy/malaise/anorexia (39%), headache (29%), chills (29%), and abdominal symptoms (26%).[83] Six patients developed secondary pneumonic plague. The case fatality rate was 16%.

Laboratory Findings and Diagnosis

Laboratory findings are nonspecific. Leukocytosis, leukemoid reactions, disseminated intravascular coagulation, and fibrin degradation products may be seen.[78] In one study, the mean leukocyte count in children was 13,400; neutrophilia and/or bandemia (≥10% bands) was present in 88% of patients.[83] Chest radiographs typically show alveolar infiltrates,[80] which are often bilateral in cases of secondary pneumonic plague.[84] Mediastinal or hilar adenopathy and pleural effusions also may occur.[84]

Presumptive diagnosis of plague is made by Wright, Giemsa or Wayson stain showing a bipolar appearance of gram-negative bacilli from a bubo aspirate or sputum specimen.[77] Rapid diagnosis is made by detection of *Y. pestis* F1 antigen by immunofluorescence.[77] A dipstick test using monoclonal antibodies against the F1 antigen has been developed for use in the field.[79] PCR tests are available in some laboratories. Evidence of infection can be demonstrated by at least a fourfold increase (between acute and convalescent serum samples) in hemagglutinating antibodies against the F1 antigen; a single serum specimen with a titer of at least 1:16 is considered diagnostic. Enzyme-linked immunosorbent assays measure IgM (recent or current infection) and IgG (remote infection) antibodies against F1 antigen. Seroconversion occurs 2 weeks to 3 months after onset of illness. Diagnosis is confirmed by culturing *Y. pestis* from bubo aspirate, sputum, or blood.

Treatment

Streptomycin is considered the treatment of choice, but gentamicin is equally efficacious. Other agents include tetracycline and doxycycline. Oral doxycycline was reported to be as effective as intramuscular gentamicin (cure or clinical improvement found in 97% and 94% of patients, respectively).[85] Chloramphenicol is recommended for plague meningitis. Fluoroquinolones have been effective *in vitro,* in experimental animal infection, and in some human cases. Treatment is given for 7 to 10 days. Untreated bubonic plague has a mortality rate of 50% to 90%; untreated pneumonia or sepsis is fatal in most cases.[77] Appropriate therapy reduces mortality to 5% to 15%.[77] Fever abated an average of 6 days following the start of effective antibiotic therapy in pediatric plague[83]; temperatures also have been reported to normalize after just one day of therapy.[85] Immunotherapy, immune modulators, phages, and antiadhesion therapy require further study.[86]

Prevention

In outbreaks, flea control by insecticide application is important. Antimicrobial prophylaxis administered for 7 days is recommended for close, direct contacts of a patient with plague pneumonia. For children younger than 8 years of age, doxycycline, tetracycline, chloramphenicol, or trimethoprim-sulfamethoxazole are recommended agents. Older individuals may receive doxycycline or ciprofloxacin. Killed whole cell (which does not protect against plague pneumonia) and live attenuated vaccines have been limited by adverse reactions and short duration of protection; they are no longer available.[77] New subunit vaccines that protect against plague pneumonia are an area of current research.[79]

References

The complete reference list is available online at www.expertconsult.com

33 TUBERCULOSIS AND NONTUBERCULOUS MYCOBACTERIAL DISEASE

Anna M. Mandalakas, MD, MS, and Jeffrey R. Starke, MD

Despite the advances in diagnostic tests, availability of inexpensive curative treatment, and the nearly universal use of the bacillus Calmette-Guérin (BCG) vaccines, tuberculosis remains one of the three most important infectious diseases in the world in terms of mortality and morbidity. The World Health Organization (WHO) estimates that tuberculosis leads to 2 million deaths and over 9 million new cases annually. One million of these cases occur in children. As long as contagious tuberculosis persists in adults, children will be affected. However, many aspects of the epidemiology, pathophysiology, and natural history of childhood tuberculosis are fundamentally different from the features of the disease in adults. Thorough understanding of the disease is essential to treating individual children and designing effective interventions to control it.

While tuberculosis persists in many industrialized countries, disease caused by nontuberculous mycobacteria (NTM) represents an increasing proportion of all mycobacterial disease. The true incidence of NTM pulmonary disease likely is vastly underestimated because of the low sensitivity of available diagnostic techniques and the fact that there is no mandatory public health reporting of NTM infections. The most common site for NTM disease in normal children is the superficial lymph nodes of the neck; however, the most common site in adolescents and adults and in children with cystic fibrosis (CF) is the lungs. The accurate diagnosis of NTM disease can be challenging because of limitations of available diagnostic tests and a clinical presentation similar to tuberculosis.

MYCOBACTERIOLOGY

The genus *Mycobacterium* consists of a diverse group of obligate aerobes that grow most successfully in tissues with high oxygen content, such as the lungs. These nonmotile, non-spore-forming, pleomorphic rods range in length from 1 to 10 μm and in width from 0.2 to 0.6 μm. Their cell wall has a complex structure that includes a large variety of proteins, carbohydrates, and lipids. The mycolic acids are the most distinctive lipids. The lipid-rich cell wall makes them impermeable to many stains unless the dyes are combined with phenol. Once stained, the cells resist decolorization with acidified organic solvents, resulting in their hallmark trait of "acid-fastness." This property is demonstrated with basic fuchsin stain techniques, such as the Ziehl-Neelsen and Kinyoun methods, or the more sensitive fluorochrome method using auramine and rhodamine stains. It is not possible to distinguish one species of *Mycobacterium* from the others using only acid-fast staining.

Of the more than 60 species of *Mycobacterium* that have been described, about one half are pathogenic in humans.[1] The *M. tuberculosis* complex consists of five closely related species: *M. tuberculosis*, *M. bovis*, *M. microti*, *M. canetti*, and *M. africanum*. The most commonly encountered NTM are classified together as the *Mycobacterium avium* complex (MAC) and include the species *M. avium*, *M. intracellulare*, and *M. scrofulaceum*. In 1959, Runyon proposed a classification system of NTM based on rate of growth and pigmentation. However, more sophisticated methods of species identification have become readily available. Mycolic acid and genetic analysis have more clearly delineated the species.[2]

Methods used for the isolation of *M. tuberculosis* from clinical samples also have proven useful for the isolation of NTM. Unfortunately, the NTM are very susceptible to killing by NaOH and other alkaline agents used for the liquefaction and decontamination of sputum and gastric aspirates, which may lead to negative cultures even when the acid-fast stain of the specimen is positive. Solid culture media for the isolation of *M. tuberculosis* and most NTM are either egg-potato-based (Lowenstein-Jensen) or agar-based (Middlebrook 7H10) media that contain antibacterial additives to prevent overgrowth. Unfortunately, these additives have some antimycobacterial effect, lowering culture yields from samples with few mycobacteria.

All mycobacteria are obligate aerobes that grow best in the presence of 5% to 10% CO_2. Most species of NTM grow best at a neutral pH and a temperature of 35° C to 37° C, but *M. marinum* and *M. haemophilum* grow best at 28° C to 32° C. Isolation on solid media of slow-growing NTM takes 2 to 6 weeks; only the rapid growers *(M. fortuitum, M. chelonae, M. abscessus)* form visible colonies in less than 10 days. Automated systems using liquid media often lead to the isolation of all species of mycobacteria within 14 days. Sensitivity is increased and the time for isolation is decreased by a larger specimen size.

Traditional identification of NTM relied on statistical probabilities of a characteristic reaction pattern in a battery of biochemical tests. However, the slow speed of these tests has led to a search for more rapid methods of species identification. At present, many clinical laboratories use high-performance liquid chromatography analysis to speciate mycobacteria by determining the specific mycolic acid fingerprint of isolates grown in the laboratory. It is also common for laboratories to use genetic probes and/or polymerase chain reaction (PCR) to identify some common species of NTM, such as MAC and *M. kansasii*.

Drug susceptibility testing for *M. tuberculosis* can be performed either on solid or liquid media that contain standard concentrations of antimicrobial agents.[2] However, drug susceptibility testing for NTM is far more complicated. In general, *M. kansasii*, *M. marinum*, *M. xenopi*, *M. ulcerans*, *M. gordonae*, *M. malmoense*, *M. szulgai*, *M. haemophilum*, and some strains of MAC are susceptible to some or all standard antituberculosis drugs. For convenience, NTM organisms have been tested with the same methods, drugs, and critical concentration of drugs as are used for *M. tuberculosis*. However, the information generated is usually of little use in the management of NTM infections. For example, the drug concentrations used for testing susceptibility of *M. tuberculosis* are too low for use in testing MAC organisms. Drugs active against MAC and *M. kansasii* often have lower minimum inhibitory concentrations (MICs) in broth than on agar, so agreement between methods for these species has been poor. For the rapidly growing mycobacteria, routine susceptibility testing to antibiotics such as amikacin, cefoxitin, doxycycline, linezolid, sulfonamides, and the macrolides (erythromycin, clarithromycin, and azithromycin) should be performed on all clinically significant isolates. When and how MAC isolates should be subjected to susceptibility testing remains controversial.[3] Although determination of the MIC or synergy studies with various drugs may provide useful information, the meaning of these in vitro results and how to relate them to the testing of individual clinical isolates have yet to be determined in clinical trials. Because drug susceptibility testing of the NTM is not well standardized, interlaboratory variations in results are common and can be confusing for the clinician.

IMMUNOLOGY

The majority of studies on the human immune response to mycobacteria have centered on *M. tuberculosis*. Humans display a wide spectrum of immunologic responses to *M. tuberculosis*. The varied immunologic response is reflected in the diverse clinical manifestations ranging from asymptomatic infection with a positive tuberculin skin test to hematogenous dissemination with severe or fatal disease.[4–7]

Immunologically competent cells of the human host recognize *M. tuberculosis* by its antigens. An extraordinarily large number of these antigens have been described. In a few individuals, the innate immune system represented by macrophages, natural killer cells, and neutrophils control infection as part of the initial response to *M. tuberculosis*.[8] In the majority of infected persons, the acquired immune response is responsible for control of *M. tuberculosis* and the subsequent pathophysiologic events.

T cells, as antigen recognition units, have critical regulatory and effector roles in the immune response to *M. tuberculosis*. In the traditional model, macrophages present antigens from phagocytosed bacilli to T cells. Antigen-activated T cells secrete cytokines, which in turn stimulate macrophages, making them more effective at controlling mycobacterial growth. Recent advances in studies of the human immune response to mycobacteria have expanded on this simple model.[9] First, a large

variety of circulating and tissue-bound T-lymphocyte subsets (CD4$^+$, CD8$^+$, and γδT cells) have antigen receptors with high affinity for mycobacterial antigens.[5] Second, T cells also serve as cytotoxic effector cells against *M. tuberculosis*–infected macrophages. Third, after exposure to mycobacteria, macrophages produce a large number of cytokines in response to prior exposure to environmental NTM or a BCG vaccine. Of note, B lymphocyte–mediated humoral responses to mycobacterial antigens occur in patients, but they have no clearly demonstrated role in disease pathogenesis.

The course of infection is influenced largely by the host immune response to *M. tuberculosis*.[4–7] Most children infected with *M. tuberculosis* develop a latent tuberculosis infection (LTBI) characterized by a positive tuberculin skin test but no symptoms or radiographic abnormalities.[5] These children have an effective macrophage- and lymphocyte-activated response with a rapid expansion of T cells and production of protective cytokines and mediators. In children who develop disease, the most common manifestation is pulmonary disease, including a Ghon focus, enlarged lymph nodes, or bronchial disease. However, the immune system in these children contains the disease, which often resolves without chemotherapy.[10] A few children experience severe forms of disease, including progressive pulmonary tuberculosis, miliary tuberculosis, or tuberculous meningitis. These forms of disease result from an immune response that fails to contain the growth of the bacilli. The risk for disease development in childhood following primary infection is inversely related to age, suggesting an inadequate or immature immune response.[10,11]

Although children have classically been thought to progress from no infection to LTBI to TB disease in a linear, unidirectional fashion, a growing body of evidence suggests that a more complex, dynamic bidirectional continuum of responses exist leading to a spectrum of TB infection and disease states (Fig. 33-1).[12]

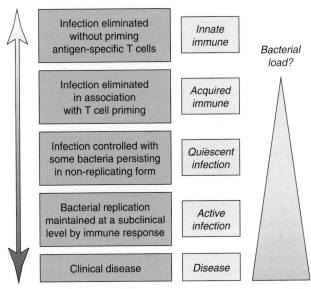

TRENDS in Microbiology

FIGURE 33-1. A spectrum of responses to tuberculosis infection.

Several lines of evidence suggest that the specific acquired host defenses against mycobacteria are genetically determined. Twin studies indicate that there is a higher concordance of tuberculosis among monozygotic compared with dizygotic twins.[13,14] Segregation analysis of tuberculosis in families indicates an oligogenic pattern of inheritance.[15] Homozygosity mapping of familial cases of NTM disease has identified mutations in the interferon-γ receptor 1 gene and IL-12 receptor that predispose to the serious and prolonged courses of disease.[16–18]

MYCOBACTERIUM TUBERCULOSIS

Epidemiology

Transmission

Transmission of *M. tuberculosis* is generally person-to-person and occurs via inhalation of mucous droplets that become airborne when an individual with pulmonary or laryngeal tuberculosis coughs, sneezes, speaks, laughs, or sings. After drying, the droplet nuclei can remain suspended in the air for hours. Only small droplets (<10 μm in diameter) can reach alveoli. Droplet nuclei also can be produced by aerosol treatments, sputum induction, aerosolization during bronchoscopy, and through manipulation of lesions or processing of tissue or secretions in the hospital or laboratory. Transmission occurs rarely by direct contact with infected body fluids or fomites.

Many factors are associated with the risk for acquiring *M. tuberculosis* infection, including[19] the extent of contact with the index case, the burden of organisms in the sputum, and the frequency of cough in the index case. Adults with pulmonary tuberculosis and bacilli present on acid-fast smear of sputum are more likely to transmit infection. In addition, the risk for transmission is directly correlated with the degree of contact with a contagious case. Most transmission to children occurs in the home. Markers of close contact such as urban living and overcrowding correlate with acquisition of infection.[20] An increased risk for infection has been demonstrated in several institutional settings, including nursing homes, schools, correctional institutions, and homeless shelters. A growing problem concerns tuberculosis transmission in refugee and orphanage settings.[21–23] There is some evidence that the risk for acquiring infection increases with age from infancy to early adulthood, likely because of increasing contacts with infectious persons. In many populations, men are more likely to be infected than women are. Although strains of *M. tuberculosis* show considerable variation in their virulence for guinea pigs, there is emerging evidence to suggest that strain virulence also may be an important factor in human infection.[24,25]

It has been noted for decades that children with tuberculosis rarely infect other children or adults.[26] In the typical case of childhood pulmonary tuberculosis, tubercle bacilli in endobronchial secretions are sparse. When young children with tuberculosis cough, they lack the tussive force of adults. Sputum production is rare in children, and collected specimens usually do not have acid-fast bacilli upon staining, indicating a low concentration of organisms. However, specimens from young infants with extensive tuberculosis infiltrates, children with cavitary lesions, or intubated children with tuberculosis should be handled as potentially infectious. The few documented cases of transmission from children have been in individuals with typical findings of adult-type tuberculosis, with lung cavities and sputum production, or infants with congenital tuberculosis, who have a large burden of organisms in the lungs. When transmission of *M. tuberculosis* has been documented in schools, orphanages, or children's hospitals, it almost invariably has come from an adult or adolescent with undiagnosed pulmonary tuberculosis. In fact, when a child is suspected clinically of having tuberculosis disease, the adults who accompany the child should undergo urgent testing (usually by chest radiograph) for tuberculosis to be sure they do not spread infection in the facility. A few classic studies have investigated the factors that influence whether or not an infected person will develop tuberculosis. It is clear that the risk for disease is highest shortly after initial infection and declines thereafter. From infancy to age 10 years, age is inversely associated with the risk for developing disease. Most young children who develop tuberculosis disease do so within the first year after infection, with most cases occurring within 6 months of transmission of the organism. For unknown reasons, there is a second peak in the risk for developing disease during late adolescence and early adult life.

Incidence and Prevalence

The World Health Organization (WHO) estimates that 2 billion people are infected with *M. tuberculosis (M. tb)*.[27] This reservoir of persons with latent *M. tb* infection (LTBI) is thought to lead to 9 million new TB cases and 2 million deaths annually. The WHO estimates that children account for 1 million of these deaths and carry 15% of the burden of disease. Seventy-five percent of childhood TB occurs in 22 high-TB-burden countries.[28] In these 22 high-burden countries, rates of tuberculosis range from 66 to over 600 cases per 100,000 population. Unfortunately, in many of these high-burden countries and most resource-poor countries, the only means used to diagnose pulmonary tuberculosis is acid-fast stain of the sputum, which is positive in up to 70% of adults with pulmonary tuberculosis but less than 10% of children with pulmonary tuberculosis. As a result, most national tuberculosis programs grossly underestimate the rate of childhood tuberculosis. In regions where improved case finding has been examined, children may represent up to 39% of all cases, with a skew toward more serious and complicated cases.[29]

Traditionally, the WHO required only reporting of smear-positive cases by age. Due to the high rates of smear-negative TB in children,[30] these reporting requirements led to a gross underestimation of the burden of TB in children. The WHO has recently mandated that pediatric cases and HIV co-infection be reported as well. These new mandates should support more accurate reporting of childhood TB.

It is instructive to examine the epidemiology of tuberculosis in the United States, where data collection and analysis are fairly complete. Because of effective public health strategies in the United States, the incidence of tuberculosis steadily declined from the 1950s to 1985. However, rates of tuberculosis began to dramatically increase in the late 1980s and early 1990s, resulting in a peak incidence of 10.5 per 100,000 population in 1992.[31] Of note, case rates were consistently highest in racial and ethnic minorities. Multiple factors contributed to the resurgence of tuberculosis in the United States, including a large influx of foreign-born persons in the late 1970s, the human immunodeficiency virus (HIV) epidemic, homelessness, crowded living conditions, decreased access to medical care, cutbacks in funding of tuberculosis control programs, and increased incidence of multidrug-resistant (MDR) tuberculosis.

During 1993 through 2002, the average year-to-year decrease in tuberculosis case rates was 6.8%, reaching 5.1 cases per 100,000 population in 2003.[32] The number of U.S. TB cases and the annual TB rate reached all-time lows in 2009, with TB rates from the 50 states and the District of Columbia ranging from 0.4 (Wyoming) to 9.1 (Hawaii) cases per 100,000 population (median: 2.7 cases per 100,000 population). Four states (California, Florida, New York, and Texas) reported more than 500 cases each for 2009. Similar to previous years, these four states combined accounted for half (50.3% [5801]) of all TB cases in 2009. Nevertheless, progress towards elimination has slowed over the past decade as compared to the prior decade (Fig. 33-2), and foreign-born persons and racial/ethnic minorities continue to have TB disease disproportionate to their respective populations. In 2009, the TB rate in foreign-born persons was nearly 11 times higher than in U.S.-born persons. The rates among Hispanics and blacks were approximately 8 times higher than among non-Hispanic whites, and rates among Asians were nearly 26 times higher. To help address the challenge of TB in foreign-born persons, in 2007, the Centers for Disease Control and Prevention (CDC) issued revised technical instructions for TB screening and treatment among persons applying for immigration to the United States.[33]

Childhood tuberculosis, defined as disease in children younger than 15 years, directly reflects the incidence of adult tuberculosis in a community. From 1992 through 2000, rates of TB declined in all U.S. age groups. Since 2000, the decline for overall rates in the United States has slowed, and the rate for the 15- to 24-year age group has declined at the slowest rate. From 1993 through 2006, approximately 16,000 cases of childhood TB were reported; 50% of these cases occurred in children 1 to 4 years of age. Analysis of all newly diagnosed, verified childhood tuberculosis cases reported to the National Tuberculosis Surveillance System from 1993 through 2001 offers important insight into the epidemiology of childhood tuberculosis in the United States.[34] A total of 11,480 cases of childhood tuberculosis were reported during this period. The highest annual case rates were consistently reported among those who were younger than 5 years of age, whose rates were 2.1 and 3.5 times higher than among children 5 to 9 and 10 to 14 years of age, respectively. Nearly 70% of all cases occurred in eight states (California, Texas, New York, Illinois, Georgia, Florida, New Jersey, and Pennsylvania). Urban areas reported over 70% of childhood tuberculosis cases, with one third of the total reported from New York City, Los Angeles, Chicago, San Diego, and Houston. Children who were racial or ethnic minorities comprised almost 90% of the cases. In 2001, the case rate for foreign-born children was 12.2 per 100,000 population compared with 1.1 per 100,000 population for U.S.-born children.[34] Sixty percent of all cases of tuberculosis reported in foreign-born children were diagnosed within 18 months of arrival in the United States. During that period, children who immigrated legally into the United States were not required to have a tuberculin skin test or a chest radiograph. Although some of these children may have been infected with *M. tb* after immigration, most were already infected at the time of immigration. Better screening of these children before immigration or access to medical care after immigration could have prevented many of these cases. From 2001 to 2006, pediatric case rates by age group have remained stable, with the population-adjusted rates being consistently greatest for

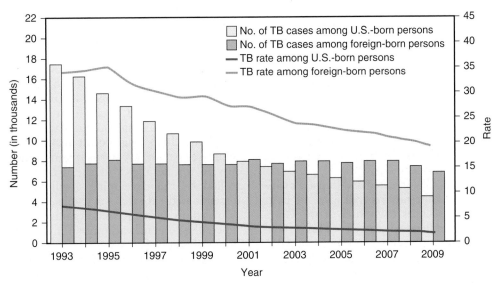

FIGURE 33-2. Number and rate of TB cases among U.S.-born and foreign-born persons, by year reported, United States, 1993-2009. (Data from *the Centers for Disease Control and Prevention,* Atlanta.)

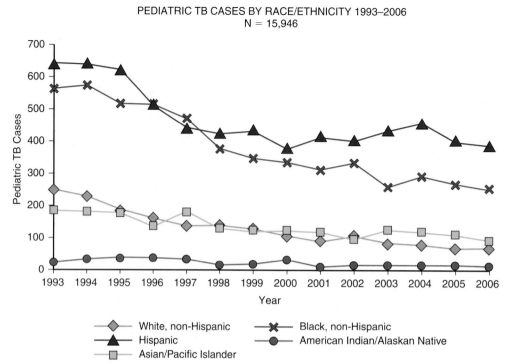

PEDIATRIC TB CASES BY RACE/ETHNICITY 1993–2006
N = 15,946

FIGURE 33-3. Pediatric TB Case Race by Race and Ethnicity, United States, 1992 to 2006. (Data from *the Centers for Disease Control and Prevention,* Atlanta.)

the toddler/preschool age group, followed by the infant group. Of note, using the standard categories of race and ethnicity, the greatest number of cases in recent years has been among Hispanic children (Fig. 33-3). Revised CDC guidelines that require intensified TB screening and treatment among children applying for immigration to the United States may improve these trends.[33]

TB-HIV Co-infection

The United Nations Program on HIV/Acquired Immuno-deficiency Syndrome (AIDS) estimates that every year 655,000 children are newly infected with HIV, and 450,000 HIV-infected children die. More than 90% of these children live in sub-Saharan Africa, where HIV is dramatically reversing gains made in child survival.[35] Although only 4% of HIV infections occur in children, children contribute to approximately 20% of AIDS deaths, reflecting the rapid progression to pediatric HIV disease seen in developing countries.[36] HIV-infected children are at increased risk of acquiring *M. tb* infection.[37] TB is a major cause of mortality in HIV-infected children, who have a high risk of progression to TB disease and death following *M. tb* infection.[38] Recent data suggest that HIV-infected infants and young children are at least 24 times more likely to develop culture-confirmed tuberculosis.[39]

Immune compromised, HIV-infected children are prone to developing disease manifestations indicative of poor organism containment, such as cavitation of the Ghon focus and disseminated (miliary) disease.[40–42] This presentation is notably similar to that of very young non–HIV-infected children.[43,44] The lack of an age-related difference in disease presentation suggests that immune maturation is less relevant in HIV-infected children.[40] Because of the common presence of other HIV-related lung pathology on

radiologic examination of the chest such as lymphocytic interstitial pneumonia (LIP), it is often challenging to diagnose TB accurately, particularly disseminated (miliary) disease. These tremendous diagnostic difficulties result in a tendency to overdiagnose TB in this vulnerable group of children.

Clinical Manifestations

Pathophysiology

After inhaling *M. tb*, the majority of children do not develop disease, but rather develop latent tuberculosis infection (LTBI). These children have a positive tuberculin skin test (TST) or interferon-gamma release assay (IGRA) result and no clinical or radiographic evidence of tuberculosis disease. It is presumed that these children are infected with a low number of viable tubercle bacilli that are dormant and do not cause clinical disease or pathologic changes. Before an adequate immune response is mounted, bacilli located in the regional lymph nodes enter the systemic circulation directly or via the lymphatic duct. This occult hematogenous spread disseminates bacilli to various organs where the bacilli may survive for decades.[45] If the dissemination is not controlled by the developing acquired immune response, disseminated tuberculosis results. The occult dissemination also provides the seed organisms for extrapulmonary tuberculosis, which accounts for 20% to 30% of childhood tuberculosis cases.

In some children, infection results in pathologic changes and associated clinical disease. In these children, tubercle bacilli reach a terminal airway and induce a localized pneumonic inflammatory process referred to as the parenchymal (Ghon) focus. Bacilli originating from this focus drain via local lymphatics to the regional lymph nodes. The triad of the parenchyma focus, local tuberculous lymphangitis and enlarged regional lymph nodes is referred to as the primary complex.

Evolution of Clinical Disease in Children

A review of information available from the prechemotherapy era provides a rich understanding of the natural evolution of clinical disease in children.[10,46] Following infection, all children progress through an asymptomatic incubation period generally lasting 3 to 8 weeks. The subsequent development of clinical disease is determined by the interaction of the host and the organism and is highly age dependent (Table 33-1).[46] In contrast to traditional theory, recent adult studies have demonstrated both conversion and reversion of measures of *M. tb* infection, including the tuberculin skin test and newer IGRAs.[47] These emerging data suggest that mycobacterial latency cannot be assumed following documentation of *M. tb* infection.[12] This has resulted in emerging theory that *M. tb* infection may be transient and/or cleared by the immune response. Similar data are lacking in children, but could provide useful insight to guide interventions for improved TB control.

Children younger than 2 years of age are at greatest risk for both the development of disease and severe manifestations of disease. After the age of 10 years, children are more likely to manifest adult-type disease. The most recent data available from the United States suggest that age-dependent disease presentation continues to persist despite available treatment for LTBI.[34] From 1993 to 2001, disseminated (1.4% of total cases) and meningeal (2.6%) tuberculosis were more frequently diagnosed in children younger than 5 years of age compared with children 5 to 9 years of age (miliary 0.4%, meningeal 1.4%) and children 10 to 14 years of age (miliary 1.4%, meningeal 1.4%). Children 5 to 9 years of age were more likely to have lymphatic tuberculosis (18.8%) compared with children younger than 5 years of age (14.1%) and children 10 to 14 years of age (15.6%). Among 190 children younger than 5 years in whom pulmonary and cavitary tuberculosis was reported, 54 (28%) were younger than 1 year and nearly all (90.5%) were U.S. born. Most adolescents (78%) had pulmonary disease and were more likely than adults and children to have pleural disease (5.2 % vs. 4.1% and 1.2%, respectively). More adolescents had cavitary disease on chest radiograph than adults or younger children.

The various manifestations of tuberculosis tend to occur in a predictable timetable.[45] Disseminated tuberculosis and tuberculous meningitis tend to be early manifestations, often occurring 2 to 6 months after initial infection has occurred. The primary complex and its complications occur most often 3 to 6 months after infection. It is not uncommon for untreated primary complex tuberculosis to result in calcification of the lung parenchyma and/or regional lymph nodes, a process that occurs at least 6 months after infection (Fig. 33-4).

TABLE 33-1	AVERAGE AGE-SPECIFIC RISK FOR DISEASE DEVELOPMENT FOLLOWING PRIMARY INFECTION[10]	
AGE AT PRIMARY INFECTION	**IMMUNE-COMPETENT CHILDREN (DOMINANT DISEASE ENTITY INDICATED IN PARENTHESES)**	**RISK OF DISEASE FOLLOWING URIMARY INFECTION**
<1 year	No disease	50%
	Pulmonary disease (Ghon focus, lymph node, or bronchial)	30%-40%
	TBM or disseminated disease	10%-20%
1-2 years	No disease	70%-80%
	Pulmonary disease (Ghon focus, lymph node, or bronchial)	10%-20%
	TBM or disseminated disease	2%-5%
2-5 years	No disease	95%
	Pulmonary disease (lymph node, or bronchial)	5%
	TBM or disseminated disease	0.5%
5-10 years	No disease	98%
	Pulmonary disease (lymph node, bronchial effusion, or adult-type)	2%
	TBM or disseminated disease	<0.5%
>10 years	No disease	80%-90%
	Pulmonary disease (effusion or adult-type)	10%-20%
	TBM or disseminated disease	<0.5%

TBM, Tuberculous meningitis.

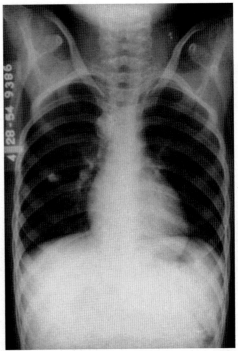

FIGURE 33-4. A calcified parenchymal lesion and lymph node in a child with tuberculosis infection. These lesions contain a small number of viable *M. tuberculosis.*

While pleural and lymph node tuberculosis often occur within 3 to 9 months after infection, other extrapulmonary forms of tuberculosis, especially skeletal and renal disease, may not occur for several years.

Intrathoracic Tuberculosis

Intrathoracic tuberculosis consists of pulmonary infection and pulmonary disease. The primary complex that occurs after inhalation of *M. tb* includes the parenchymal Ghon focus with associated tuberculosis lymphangitis and affected regional lymph nodes. Approximately 70% of the primary foci are subpleural. Lobes are equally affected, and 25% of children have multiple parenchymal foci. The combination of no clinical symptoms and a normal chest radiograph is referred to as tuberculosis infection. Pulmonary tuberculosis occurs when tuberculosis infection is complicated by clinical symptoms and/or radiographic abnormalities. Pulmonary disease may be associated with a diverse spectrum of pathology described in the following sections.

A Ghon focus with or without cavitation may accompany clinical disease, including weight loss, fatigue, fever, and chronic cough.[48] If the host is unable to contain the tubercle bacilli, progressive caseation occurs in the lung parenchyma surrounding the Ghon focus. The area of caseation may discharge into a bronchus, resulting in the formation of a primary cavity with possible endotracheal spread (Fig. 33-5). The tubercle bacilli disseminate further to other parts of the lobe and can involve an entire lung. On rare occasions, an enlarging primary focus ruptures into the pleural cavity, creating a pneumothorax, bronchopleural fistula, or caseous pyopneumothorax. Profound fever, cough, and weight loss accompany a severe progressive lesion. Before the advent of chemotherapy, 25% to 65% of children with progressive primary

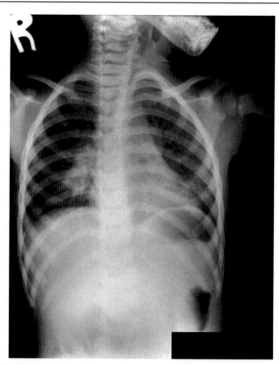

FIGURE 33-6. Hilar adenopathy in a child with early pulmonary tuberculosis. Most children with this radiographic appearance have few or no symptoms.

disease died. However, with appropriate therapy, the prognosis is excellent.

The hallmark of pulmonary tuberculosis is enlargement of the regional hilar, mediastinal, or subcarinal lymph nodes (Fig. 33-6).[49,50] Isolated thoracic adenopathy usually causes few or no clinical signs or symptoms. In some children, particularly infants, the lymph nodes continue to enlarge, resulting in lymphobronchial involvement, where the affected bronchus may become partially or totally obstructed because of nodal compression, inflammatory edema, polyps, granulomatous tissue, or caseous material extruded from ulcerated lymph nodes (Fig. 33-7). Although chest radiography rarely delineates the specific pathologic process causing the chest radiographic abnormalities, they are often apparent if bronchoscopy or a computed tomography scan of the chest is performed. The most frequently affected lobes are the right upper, the right middle, and the left upper lobe. Symptoms vary according to the degree of airway irritation and obstruction but frequently include a localized wheezing or persistent cough that may mimic pertussis. A common radiographic sequence is adenopathy followed by localized hyperinflation and then atelectasis of contiguous parenchyma, referred to as collapse-consolidation or segmental lesions (Fig. 33-8). The radiographic and clinical picture mimics foreign body obstruction and other obstructive disorders. Additional pathology that may accompany bronchial disease includes airway allergic consolidation, bronchopneumonia, and caseating consolidation. Children with allergic consolidation typically experience high fevers, acute respiratory symptoms, and signs of consolidation on chest radiograph. Children with caseating consolidation

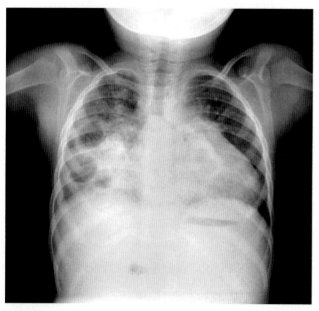

FIGURE 33-5. A young child with pulmonary tuberculosis has developed cavitation of the lung parenchyma.

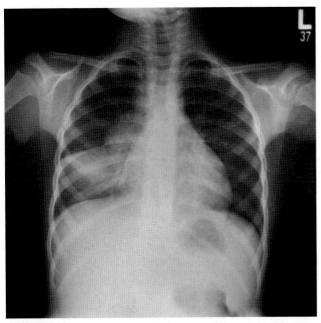

FIGURE 33-7. A classic collapse-consolidation lesion with hilar adenopathy in a child with pulmonary tuberculosis.

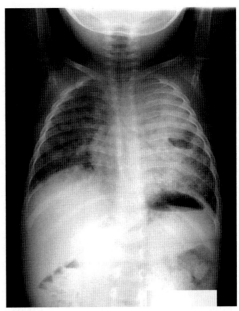

FIGURE 33-9. Pronounced caseating consolidation in a young child with pulmonary tuberculosis.

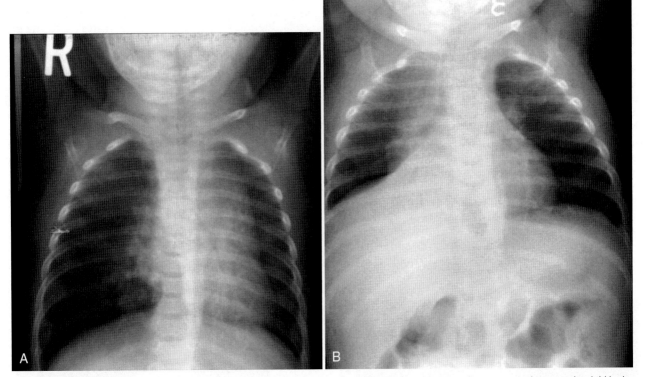

FIGURE 33-8. A, Hyperinflation of the right lower lobe in an infant with pulmonary tuberculosis and airway obstruction. At this point the child had respiratory distress. **B,** A chest radiograph from the same child several hours later shows complete collapse of the right lower lobe. At this point, the respiratory distress had ceased.

are very ill, with high undulating fevers, chronic cough, and occasional hemoptysis (Fig. 33-9).

In some children, an acute secondary bacterial infection that occurs distal to the obstructed bronchus plays a role in the clinical expression of disease. Children with secondary bacterial pneumonia often present with high fever, cough, and crackles. The clinical signs and symptoms often respond to antibiotics, but the chest radiographic findings do not clear because of the underlying tuberculosis.

Although segmental lesions and hyperaeration are the most common findings produced by enlarging thoracic lymph nodes, other problems may occur. Enlarged paratracheal nodes may cause stridor and respiratory distress. Subcarinal nodes may impinge on the esophagus and cause difficulty in swallowing, followed occasionally by the formation of an esophageal diverticulum, or the nodes may rupture directly into the esophagus and produce a bronchoesophageal fistula. Enlarged lymph nodes may compress the subclavian vein and produce edema of the hand and arm, or they may erode major blood vessels, including the aorta. They also may rupture into the mediastinum and point in the left, or more often the right, supraclavicular fossa. Compression of the left recurrent laryngeal nerve has been reported. Rupture into the pericardial sac causes tuberculous pericarditis. The late results of bronchial obstruction include the following possibilities: (1) complete reexpansion of the lung and resolution of the radiographic findings; (2) disappearance of the segmental lesion, with residual calcification of the primary focus or the regional lymph nodes; or (3) scarring and progressive contraction of the lobe or segment usually associated with bronchiectasis (Fig. 33-10). Permanent anatomic sequelae result from segmental lesions in approximately 60% of all cases, even though the abnormality usually is not apparent on plain radiographs. Cylindric (rarely saccular) bronchiectasis, sometimes stenoses, and elongation or shortening can be demonstrated on bronchography. Fortunately, most of these abnormalities are asymptomatic in the upper lobes. However, secondary infection may occur in the middle and lower lobes and cause the middle lobe syndrome.

Chronic pulmonary tuberculosis, often called adult type, or reactivation tuberculosis, is the type of disease that occurs in pulmonary tissue that was sensitized to tuberculous antigens by an earlier tuberculous infection that became dormant or latent. Chronic pulmonary tuberculosis rarely develops in children who acquired infection with *M. tb* before 2 years of age, but it is more common the closer infection occurs to the onset of puberty. It is rare in children younger than 10 years of age. The preponderance of evidence supports the concept that most cases of reactivation tuberculosis result from endogenous reinfection with the dormant bacilli. However, reinfection with a different strain of *M. tb*, leading to typical adult-type tuberculosis, has been documented.

Reactivation pulmonary tuberculosis arises from the small round foci of organisms in the apices of the lungs (often called Assmann or Simon foci) that resulted from the lymphohematogenous spread at the time of the initial infection.[51] Fibronodular infiltrates in one or both upper lobe apices are most common, but more extensive pulmonary involvement leads to diffuse consolidation or cavitation (Fig. 33-11). Involvement of thoracic lymph nodes is usually absent. Cough, remitting fevers, night sweats, chest pain, sputum production, and hemoptysis are the most common clinical manifestations.

Pleural tuberculosis results from direct spread of caseous material from a subpleural parenchymal or lymph node focus or from hematogenous spread.[52-54] Pleural tuberculosis is uncommon in children younger than 6 years of age and rare in those younger than 2 years of age. The presence of caseous material in the pleural space may trigger a hypersensitivity reaction, with the accumulation of serous straw-colored fluid containing few tubercle bacilli. This exudate has a high protein concentration and lymphocyte predominance; the amount of polymorphonuclear cells depends on the acuteness of onset. Although direct microscopy is usually negative, culture yields may be as high as 40% to 70%. Pleural biopsy often demonstrates caseating granulomas and increases the culture yield if ample tissue is collected. The clinical course associated with pleural involvement characteristically begins with acute chest pain, accompanied by high fever in the absence of acute illness, an ill-defined loss of vigor, and a dry cough. Active caseation in the pleural space may cause thick loculated pus, containing many tubercle bacilli (Fig. 33-12). The prognosis for children with tuberculous pleural effusion always has been good compared

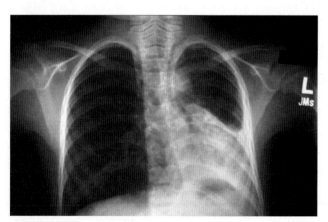

FIGURE 33-10. Bronchiectasis of the left lower lobe in a child with tuberculosis who was nonadherent to appropriate treatment.

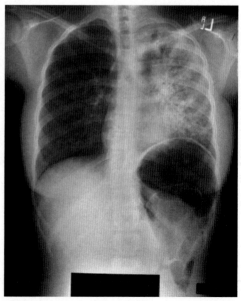

FIGURE 33-11. A chest radiograph of an adolescent girl with chronic pulmonary tuberculosis.

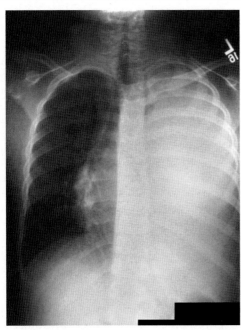

FIGURE 33-12. A large tuberculosis pleural effusion in an 11-year-old girl.

with other overt forms of tuberculosis, even before chemotherapy was available.

Tubercle bacilli from the lymphadenitis of the primary complex are disseminated during the incubation period in all cases of tuberculosis infection. The clinical picture produced by lymphohematogenous spread probably is determined by host susceptibility at the time of spread and by the quantity of tubercle bacilli released. Three clinical forms of dissemination are recognized:

1. The lymphohematogenous spread may be occult, in which case it usually remains so, or it may be occult initially with metastatic, extrapulmonary lesions appearing months or years later (e.g., renal tuberculosis).

2. So-called protracted hematogenous tuberculosis, rarely seen today, is characterized by high, spiking fever; marked leukocytosis; hepatomegaly and splenomegaly; and general glandular enlargement, sometimes with repeated evidence of metastatic seeding in the choroid plexus, kidney, and skin. Calcifications may appear subsequently, often in large numbers, in the pulmonary apices (Simon foci) and in the spleen, thus attesting to the earlier dissemination of tubercle bacilli via blood. The TST usually is strongly positive. Bone marrow biopsy may confirm the clinical impression, but treatment often must be started on a presumptive basis. Although this type of tuberculosis in past years often ended tragically in tuberculous meningitis, today it is completely treatable if diagnosed in time.

3. The third form of lymphohematogenous spread, analogous to sepsis with pyogenic bacteria, is miliary tuberculosis. It usually arises from discharge of a caseous focus, often a lymph node, into a blood vessel such as a pulmonary vein. It may be self-propagating, with repeated discharge arising at various sites. Most common during the first 2 to 6 months after infection in infancy, it can arise even in adults who have apparently well-healed, calcified lesions.

The clinical picture of miliary tuberculosis varies greatly, probably depending on the number of bacilli in the bloodstream.[44,55] Sometimes the patient is afebrile and appears to be well, and the condition is diagnosed by chance during contact investigation of another individual with infectious tuberculosis. The onset can be insidious, often occurring after the patient has had another precipitating infection. In rare cases, the onset is abrupt. Drowsiness, loss of weight and appetite, persistent fever, weakness, rapid breathing with a rustling sound on auscultation of the lungs, occasionally cyanosis, and almost always a palpable spleen are the clinical manifestations that lead the clinician to obtain a chest radiograph.

Usually within no more than 3 weeks after the onset of symptoms, tubercles, sometimes tiny and at times large, can be seen evenly distributed throughout both lung fields (Fig. 33-13). In the early stages, they often are detected best on a lateral view of the retrocardiac space. Recurrent pneumothorax, subcutaneous emphysema, pneumomediastinum, and pleural effusion are less serious but well-recognized complications of miliary tuberculosis. Cutaneous lesions, including painful nodules, papulonecrotic tuberculids, and purpuric lesions, may appear in crops.

The diagnosis usually is established by means of the clinical picture and a chest radiograph; sometimes by a liver or skin biopsy; by culturing *M. tb* from the gastric aspirate, urine, or bone marrow; or by fiberoptic bronchoscopy. Treatment usually is very successful.

Extrathoracic Tuberculosis

A complete description of extrathoracic tuberculosis is beyond the scope of this book. However, pulmonologists may encounter this possibility when evaluating children with pulmonary involvement and other manifestations. The most common forms of extrathoracic disease in children include tuberculosis of the superficial lymph nodes (scrofula) and the central nervous system. Other rare forms of extrathoracic disease in children are osteoarticular, abdominal, gastrointestinal, genitourinary, cutaneous, and congenital disease.

Tuberculosis of the superficial lymph nodes (scrofula) is the most common form of extrathoracic tuberculosis.[56,57] Although this disease historically was associated with *M. bovis* obtained by drinking unpasteurized cow's milk, most current cases occur after primary pulmonary infection with *M. tb* and occur within 6 to 9 months of initial

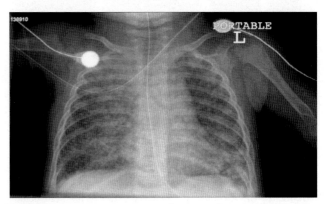

FIGURE 33-13. The appearance of miliary tuberculosis in the chest radiograph of an infant.

infection. Extension of primary lesions of the upper lung fields or abdomen leads to involvement of the supraclavicular, anterior cervical, tonsillar, and submandibular nodes. Rarely in children, tuberculosis of the skin or skeletal system can lead to involvement of the inguinal, epitrochlear, or axillary lymph nodes. Early during infection, lymph nodes are discrete, firm, and nontender. The lymph nodes become fixed to surrounding tissues and feel matted as the infection progresses. Low-grade fever may be the only systemic symptom. Although usually present, a primary pulmonary complex is visible radiologically only 30% to 70% of the time. TST results are usually reactive. Although spontaneous resolution is possible, untreated lymphadenitis frequently progresses to caseating necrosis, capsular rupture, and spread to adjacent nodes and overlying skin. Rupture through the skin results in a draining sinus tract that may require surgical removal. Excisional biopsy and culture of lymph nodes are often required to differentiate between *M. tb* and NTM disease.

Central nervous system disease is the most serious complication of tuberculosis in children and complicates approximately 0.5% of untreated primary infections. It is most common in children 6 months to 4 years of age and generally occurs within 2 to 6 months of primary infection.[58] Central nervous system disease arises from the formation of a caseous lesion in the cerebral cortex or meninges that results from early occult lymphohematogenous spread.[59] Lesions enlarge and discharge bacilli into the subarachnoid space, leading to an exudate that infiltrates the cortical and meningeal blood vessels. This results in inflammation, obstruction, and subsequent infarction of the cerebral cortex. The clinical onset of tuberculous meningitis can be rapid or gradual. Infants and children are more likely to experience a rapid progression to hydrocephalus, seizure, and cerebral edema over several days (Fig. 33-14). In most children, signs and symptoms progress over several weeks,

beginning nonspecifically with fever, headache, irritability, and drowsiness. Disease frequently advances abruptly with symptoms of lethargy, vomiting, nuchal rigidity, seizures, hypertonia, and focal neurologic signs. The final stage of disease is marked by coma, hypertension, decerebrate and decorticate posturing, and eventual death. Rapid confirmation of tuberculous meningitis can be extremely difficult with wide variability in cerebrospinal fluid characteristics and nonreactive TSTs in 40% of cases. Although some older studies reported normal chest radiographs in 50% of cases, more recent reports have indicated that 80% of young children with tuberculous meningitis have significant abnormality on the chest radiograph. Since improved outcomes are associated with early treatment, empirical antituberculosis therapy should be instituted for any child with basilar meningitis and hydrocephalus or cranial nerve involvement that has no other apparent cause.

Tuberculosis and HIV

Co-infection with HIV can change the clinical presentation of intrathoracic tuberculosis. In adults infected with both HIV and *M. tb*, the rate of progression from latent tuberculous infection to disease is increased greatly. Tuberculosis has typical clinical features when the patient's $CD4^+$ cell count is higher than 500/mm³. As the $CD4^+$ cell count declines, the clinical picture changes; pulmonary cavities are rare, but lower lobe infiltrates or nodules often accompanied by thoracic adenopathy are common. Sputum is produced less often, and more invasive diagnostic techniques are often required to establish the diagnosis.

Immune compromised, HIV-infected children have a higher risk of developing extrapulmonary disease manifestations indicative of poor organism containment, such as tuberculomas and disseminated (miliary) disease.[40–42] This presentation is notably similar to that of very young non–HIV-infected children. The lack of an age-related difference in disease presentation suggests that immune maturation is less relevant in HIV-infected children.[40] Because of the common presence of other HIV-related lung pathology on chest x-ray such as lymphocytic interstitial pneumonia (LIP), it is often challenging to diagnose TB accurately, particularly disseminated (miliary) disease. These tremendous diagnostic difficulties result in a tendency to overdiagnose TB in this vulnerable group of children. When pulmonary tuberculosis develops in an HIV-infected child, the response to standard short-course TB therapy is poor as evidenced by low cure rates and high mortality.[42,60] TB may further hasten the progression of HIV disease by increasing viral replication and depleting $CD4^+$ T lymphocytes.[61] The confirmation of TB disease in HIV-infected children is complicated by the low yield of culture and chronic HIV-related comorbidities.[41]

Diagnosis

Tuberculin Skin Test

The tuberculin skin test remains the most widely employed test for the diagnosis of tuberculosis and LTBI in children. The sensitivity and specificity of the tuberculin skin test

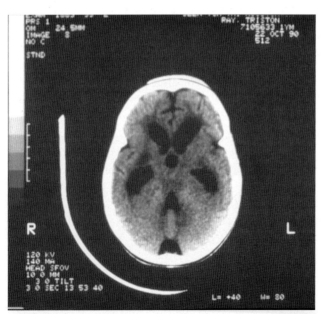

FIGURE 33-14. A computed tomography scan of the head demonstrating the communicating hydrocephalus that is typical of tuberculous meningitis.

are significantly affected by a number of factors that are reviewed in this section.

Infection with *M. tb* produces a delayed-type hypersensitivity reaction to specific antigenic components of the bacilli that are contained in extracts of culture filtrates called "tuberculins." A batch of purified protein derivative (PPD) called PPD-S, produced by Siebert and Glenn in 1939, serves as the standard reference material worldwide. All PPD lots are bioassayed to demonstrate equal potency to PPD-S. The standard test dose of a commercially available preparation is defined as the dose of that product that is biologically equivalent to 5 tuberculin units (TU) of PPD-S. A small amount of Tween 80 is added to the diluent of PPD to reduce adsorption by glass and plastic. To minimize adsorption and subsequent loss of potency, tuberculin should never be transferred between containers and should be delivered as soon as possible after transfer to the syringe. Tuberculin should be stored refrigerated and in the dark.

The tuberculin reaction is the classic example of a delayed-type hypersensitivity reaction. In response to the antigen, previously sensitized T cells release lymphokines that induce local vasodilation, edema, fibrin deposition, and recruitment of other inflammatory cells.[62] The reaction to tuberculin typically begins 5 to 6 hours after injection and reaches maximal induration at 48 to 72 hours. In some individuals, the reaction may peak after 72 hours, and the largest reaction size is considered the result. Vesiculation and necrosis rarely occur. In these cases, repeat tuberculin testing should be avoided.

Variability of the results of the TST may be reduced by careful attention to details of administration and reading. A one-fourth to one-half inch, 27-gauge needle and tuberculin syringe are employed to inject 0.1 mL of 5-TU PPD intradermally (Mantoux method) into the volar or dorsal aspect of the forearm. If done correctly, a discrete, pale wheal 6 to 10 mm in diameter is produced. If the first test is administered improperly, another test dose may be employed at once in a site several centimeters from the original site.

The TST should be read 48 to 72 hours following injection. The diameter of induration should be measured transversely to the long axis of the forearm and recorded in millimeters. Use of the ballpoint pen method developed by Sokal minimizes interobserver variability.[63] A dispassionate, trained health professional should interpret all skin tests.

A nonreactive TST does not exclude LTBI or tuberculosis. A number of factors can diminish tuberculin reactivity resulting in a false-negative reaction (Box 33-1) and decreased tuberculin test sensitivity. The administration of live-attenuated vaccines results in immune system suppression that appears more than 48 hours after vaccination. Tuberculin skin testing may be performed on either the same day as vaccination with live virus or 4 to 6 weeks later. Studies have demonstrated that up to 10% of immunocompetent children with reactive anergy tests and culture-confirmed tuberculosis have false-negative reactions to tuberculin testing.[51,64] In many of these children, TST conversion occurs after several months of treatment, suggesting that the infection was recently acquired or resulted in suppression of the immune response. Skin

---

BOX 33-1 FACTORS CAUSING FALSE-NEGATIVE TUBERCULIN SKIN TESTS

Factors Related to the Person Being Tested
Infections
Viral (measles, mumps, chickenpox, HIV)
Bacterial (typhoid fever, brucellosis, typhus, leprosy, pertussis, overwhelming tuberculosis, tuberculosis pleurisy)
Fungal (blastomycosis)
Live virus vaccinations (measles, mumps, polio, varicella)
Metabolic derangements (chronic renal failure)
Low protein states (severe protein depletion, afibrinogenemia)
Diseases affecting lymphoid organs (Hodgkin's disease, lymphoma, chronic leukemia, sarcoidosis)
Drugs (corticosteroids and other immunosuppressive agents)
Age (newborns, elderly patients with "waned" sensitivity)
Stress (surgery, burns, mental illness, graft-versus-host reactions)

Factors Related to the Tuberculin Used
Improper storage (exposure to light and heat)
Improper dilutions
Chemical denaturation
Contamination
Adsorption (partially controlled by adding Tween 80)

Factors Related to the Method of Administration
Injection of too little antigen
Subcutaneous injection
Delayed administration after drawing into syringe
Injection too close to other skin tests

Factors Related to Reading the Test and Recording Results
Inexperienced reader
Conscious or unconscious bias
Error in recording

HIV, Human immunodeficiency virus.

---

testing results were available in nearly all (95.4%) children reported to have newly diagnosed tuberculosis in the United States between 1993 and 2001. Eleven percent of these children had negative skin test results as defined by CDC guidelines.[34] Of note, children who were diagnosed with disseminated or meningeal tuberculosis were less likely to have a positive TST result (57.6% and 54.6%, respectively) than those with pulmonary tuberculosis (90.6%).

A number of factors have been associated with false-positive tuberculin reactions and decreased tuberculin test specificity. Because some antigens in PPD are shared with other mycobacteria, false-positive reactions can occur in children who have been infected with other mycobacteria, including BCG immunization. Exposure to NTM varies geographically and generally results in smaller, transient indurations than those of *M. tb*. There is no reliable method of distinguishing BCG-induced TST cross-reactivity from TST reactivity secondary to mycobacterial infection; IGRAs have the ability to make this distinction. The degree of BCG cross-reactivity is dependent on a number of factors, including strain of BCG employed, age and nutritional status at vaccination, frequency of skin testing, and years since vaccination.[65-68] In most studies of children who received a BCG vaccine during the newborn period, only 50% reacted to tuberculin testing at 12 months and 80% to 90% lose reactivity within 2 to 3 years. Although BCG vaccination of older children or adults results in greater initial and more persistent cross-reactivity, most of these individuals lose cross-reactivity within 10 years of vaccination. In general, the TST should be interpreted the same for patients who have not received a BCG vaccination; however, this will lead to some children with false-positive TST results being treated.

Interferon-Gamma Release Assays

The identification of genes in the *M. tb* genome that are absent from *M. bovis* BCG[69] and most NTM[70] has supported the development of more specific and sensitive tests for detection of *M. tb*.[71] *M. bovis* BCG has 16-gene deletions including the region of difference 1 (RD-1) that encodes for early secretory antigen target-6 (ESAT-6) and culture filtrate protein 10 (CFP-10).[70,72] ESAT-6 and CFP-10 are strong targets of the cellular immune response in patients with *M. tb* infection and disease.[73,74] In persons with *M. tb* infection or disease, sensitized memory/effector T cells produce IFN-γ in response to *M. tb* antigens, forming the biologic basis for both the TST and IGRAs. Research over the past decade[75-77] has resulted in the development of two commercial IGRAs that are approved for use in Europe and the United States. In brief, the latest generation Quantiferon TB Gold In-tube (QFT-GIT) (Cellestis Limited, Australia)[78] assay is an enzyme-linked immunosorbent assay (ELISA)–based whole blood assay measuring the amount of IFN-γ produced in response to three *M. tb* antigens. In contrast, the enzyme-linked immunospot (ELISPOT)–based T.SPOT.TB (Oxford Immunotec, United Kingdom)[79] uses peripheral mononuclear cells to detect the number of INF-γ–producing T cells. Manufacturer guidelines regarding test interpretation primarily are based on adults despite some data to suggest that test outcomes are age-dependent.[80]

A growing number of studies have compared the TST and IGRAs for the detection of *M. tb* infection and active TB in children. In the absence of a gold standard for infection, studies have measured sensitivity in populations with TB disease as a surrogate for *M. tb* infected persons. Other studies have used *M. tb* exposure as a surrogate of infection. Available data suggest that TST and IGRAs have similar accuracy for the detection of *M. tb* infection or the diagnosis of active TB in children. Nevertheless, the heterogeneous methodology of studies completed to date limits comparability of studies and interpretation of results. A rigorous, standardized approach to evaluating TB diagnostic tests in children is needed.[81]

IGRAs offer several pragmatic advantages as compared with the TST. Use of *M. tb*–specific antigens leads to improved specificity, which decreases the probability of false-positive responses, particularly in young, BCG-vaccinated children. Use of internal positive controls allows for the assessment of anergy, which can be useful in immune compromised and young children. Additionally, IGRAs do not require a second visit to measure the response and thus eliminate the chance of a missed reading. Although the direct cost of the assays is greater than that of the TST, evidence in adults suggests that IGRAs may be cost effective in certain populations and settings.[82-85]

Interpretation of Tests for *M. tuberculosis* Infection

The likelihood that a positive TST represents true infection (positive predictive value) increases as the prevalence of infection with *M. tb* increases in that population.[86] The same is true for IGRAs. The prevalence of LTBI is 5% to 10% in the general population of the United States and 0.1% to 1% for children entering school in many parts of the United States. Screening populations without a known or likely exposure to *M. tb* is likely to result in false-positive reactions. In contrast, the prevalence of LTBI in close contacts of individuals with infectious tuberculosis or immigrants from high-burden countries is much higher. Hence, TSTs and IGRAs have higher positive-predictive value in these target populations.

Interpretation of TST reactions is based on risk for infection (Box 33-2).[86] For children with the greatest risk for infection or developing tuberculosis after infection, or those with suspected tuberculosis disease, an induration greater than or equal to 5 mm is considered positive. For children with an increased risk for infection or progression to disseminated disease, an induration greater than or equal to 10 mm is considered positive. Children with low risk must have an induration greater than or equal to 15 mm to be considered positive. Varying interpretation of the TST based on a child's individual risk factors minimizes false-positive and false-negative readings. When considering treatment for LTBI in a child, it is also important to recognize that children have a low risk of adverse reactions to treatment. Children's low risk of adverse reactions to treatment coupled with their high risk of disease progression results in a more favorable risk-benefit ratio of treatment as compared with adults.

BOX 33-2 DEFINITIONS OF A POSITIVE TUBERCULIN SKIN TEST RESULT IN INFANTS, CHILDREN, AND ADOLESCENTS

Induration ≥5 mm
Children in close contact with known or suspected contagious case of tuberculosis disease
Children suspected to have tuberculosis disease:
- Findings on chest radiograph consistent with active or previously active tuberculosis
- Clinical evidence of tuberculosis disease
Children receiving immunosuppressive therapy or with immunosuppressive conditions, including HIV infection

Induration ≥10 mm
Children at increased risk for disseminated disease:
- Those younger than 4 years of age
- Those with other medical conditions, including Hodgkin's disease, lymphoma, diabetes mellitus, chronic renal failure, or malnutrition
Children with increased exposure to tuberculosis disease:
- Those born, or whose parents were born, in high-prevalence regions of the world
- Those frequently exposed to adults who are HIV infected, homeless, users of illicit drugs, residents of nursing homes, incarcerated or institutionalized, or migrant farm workers
- Those who travel to high-prevalence regions of the world

Induration ≥15 mm
Children 4 years of age or older without any risk factors

In the United States, it is preferable to screen children for LTBI risk factors with a questionnaire and complete TSTs or IGRAs when risk factors are identified.[86] For this approach to be effective, clinicians performing screening must be familiar with local tuberculosis case rates and community demographics. Local public health authorities should play an active role in determining interpretation of skin test reactions for individual communities. Unfortunately, there are no guidelines regarding age- or risk-specific interpretation of IGRAs.

Laboratory Diagnosis

Careful attention to the details of specimen collection and handling can optimize the isolation and identification of *M. tb*. A variety of specimens can be collected, including sputum, induced sputum, gastric aspirates, bronchial washings, bronchoalveolar lavage, transbronchial biopsy, urine, blood, cerebral spinal fluid, tissue, and other body fluids.[87,88] Because children cannot easily produce sputum, gastric aspirates are frequently obtained. Collection of gastric aspirates usually entails hospitalization to acquire about 50 mL of early morning gastric contents after the child has fasted for at least 8 to 10 hours, and preferably, while he or she is still in bed.[89] Alternatively, trained public health nurses may perform this procedure in the home. *M. tuberculosis* may be recovered from gastric aspirates in roughly 40% of children with radiographic evidence of significant pulmonary disease.[90,91] The culture yields are as high as 70% in infants. Because many specimens will contain an abundance of bacteria other than mycobacteria, specimens should be collected in a sterile fashion and held under conditions that minimize growth of contaminating organisms.

Diagnostic tests for tuberculosis either detect the presence of *M. tb* in a clinical sample or demonstrate a host response to the organism. Methods for diagnosis of tuberculosis are summarized in Table 33-2.

IGRAs are designed to measure the host immune response to *M. tb*, not the presence of the organism itself. Nevertheless, clinicians are increasingly using IGRAs for the diagnosis of tuberculosis disease. When trying to establish the diagnosis of tuberculosis, the value of a positive IGRA diminishes as the risk of *M. tb* infection increases in the patient. Thus, tests for the detection of *M. tb* infection, such as IGRAs and the TST, are most helpful as adjunctive tests to confirm disease in a patient with a high probability of active disease.[92]

Staining and Microscopic Examination

Acid-fast staining and microscopic examination are the easiest, quickest, and least expensive diagnostic procedures. Yield of microscopy is dependent on stain selection because the auramine-rhodamine fluorescent stain is more sensitive than the traditional Kinyoun of Ziehl-Neelsen stains. However, these methods can only provide physicians with preliminary confirmation of the diagnosis because of the inability to differentiate between *M. tb* and NTM. Additionally, there must be 5,000 to 10,000 bacilli present per millimeter of specimen to allow detection of the bacteria in stained smears, resulting in low sensitivity in children. Acid-fast staining of gastric aspirates is positive in fewer than 10% of children with pulmonary tuberculosis.

TABLE 33-2 SUMMARY OF LABORATORY METHODS FOR DIAGNOSIS OF TUBERCULOSIS

IDENTIFICATION METHOD	TEST SYSTEM	USE
Culture	Conventional media Colony morphology (3-5 weeks) Biochemical tests	Preliminary identification Species identification
Microscopic-observation drug-susceptibility (MODS)	Positive growth (1-2 weeks)	Identification and drug-susceptibility Easy, inexpensive, highly sensitive
Radiometric methods	Positive growth index (5-14 days)	Differentiates *Mycobacterium tuberculosis* from nontuberculosis mycobacteria species
Chromatography	HPLC mycolic acid profile Gas chromatography-fatty acid profile	Speciates all common mycobacteria
DNA probes	Gen-Probe ACCUPROBE Syngene SNAP probes	Identifies *M. tuberculosis* complex, *M. avium*, *M. intracellulare-avium* complex, *M. kansasii*, *M. gordonae* Identifies *M. tuberculosis* complex, *M. avium* complex
Rapid direct tests Direct smear	Acid-fast or fluorochrome stains	Easy, inexpensive, moderately sensitive
Antigen and antibody	EIA agglutination tests	Simple, low-cost, modestly specific, but not highly sensitive
Nucleic acid detection	PCR amplification	Moderately sensitive, highly specific, technically complex

DNA, Deoxyribonucleic acid; *EIA*, enzyme immunoassay; *HPLC*, high-performance liquid chromatography; *PCR*, polymerase chain reaction.

Culture

Culture is the most important laboratory test for the diagnosis and management of tuberculosis. A positive culture may result from as few as 10 organisms per milliliter of specimen. Growth of bacilli is necessary for precise speciation and drug susceptibility testing. Genotyping of the organism may be useful to identify epidemiologic links. Unfortunately, bacteriologic confirmation of tuberculosis in children is generally poor. For example, in the United States from 1985 to 1988, 90% of adult tuberculosis cases were bacteriologically confirmed, compared with 28% in children.[23] In three studies evaluating the role of bronchoscopy, only 13% to 62% of cultures in children with pulmonary tuberculosis were positive.[91,93,94] The yield from gastric aspirate was higher in these studies. Bronchoscopy can be useful to define anatomy or clarify the diagnosis, but it cannot be recommended solely to collect culture specimens in children.

Sputum smear or sputum culture were available for only 25% of children reported to have newly diagnosed tuberculosis in the United States between 1993 and 2001.[34] A small percentage of children were sputum smear or culture positive. Rates of positivity varied dramatically among age groups. Sputum smears were positive from 10.3% of 10 to 14-year-olds, 1.8% of 5- to 9-year-olds, and 1.6% of children under 5 years. Similarly, cultures were positive among 21.3% of 10- to 14-year-olds, 5% of 5- to 9-year-olds, and 4.2% of children under 5 years of age. Among all childhood tuberculosis cases, only 2.4% had positive gastric aspirate smears and 8.5% had gastric aspirate cultures positive for M. tb.[34] Because only positive gastric aspirate results were reported, it is impossible to know how many specimens were obtained or to determine the yield of this procedure.

It is clear that reliance on detection of M. tb using available methods will lead to misdiagnosis of the majority of cases of childhood pulmonary tuberculosis. Even in developed countries, the gold standard for diagnosis of childhood tuberculosis is a triad of (1) an abnormal chest radiograph and/or clinical findings consistent with tuberculosis; (2) a positive TST or IGRA result; and (3) a history of contact with an infectious TB case within the past year. If the results of drug susceptibility testing on the organism isolated from the contact case are available, obtaining a culture from the child adds little sensitivity or specificity to the diagnosis if the triad is present.[50,51]

DNA Methodologies

DNA probe methods use nucleic acid hybridization with specifically labeled sequences to rapidly detect complementary sequences in the test sample. Various systems are commercially available. Although the M. tb complex probe tests have been 99% to 100% specific, the methods' dependence on large numbers of bacilli means they can be used in the laboratory only on cultured organisms.[95]

Direct detection of the DNA of M. tb in clinical samples has been performed using nucleic acid amplification, most often utilizing polymerase chain reaction (PCR). Most techniques have used the mycobacterial insertion element IS6110 as the DNA marker for M. tb complex organisms.[96] Evaluation of PCR for childhood tuberculosis has been limited. When compared with the clinical diagnosis of pulmonary tuberculosis in children, the sensitivity of PCR on sputum or gastric aspirates has varied from 25% to 83%, and the specificity has varied from 80% to 100%.[97–99] A negative PCR never eliminates tuberculosis as a diagnostic possibility, and a positive result does not completely confirm it. The major use for PCR in children may be when the diagnosis of tuberculosis is not readily established on clinical and epidemiologic grounds, and perhaps, for children with HIV infection for whom a greater variety of causes of pulmonary disease must be considered.

Antibody and Antigen Detection

There has been some progress in the development of methods to detect M. tb antibodies and antigens. The use of enzyme immunoassay (EIA) has been reviewed extensively. Although a variety of serologic methods have been used to detect antibodies against M. tb, most of these tests lack sensitivity and specificity and are not available in the United States. Similarly, a large collection of techniques has been used to detect antigen, including competitive inhibition EIA, latex agglutination, reverse passive-hemagglutination, double-antibody sandwich EIA, and inhibition EIA. Three assays have been designed to detect specific protein antigen and offer the most promise with sensitivities and specificities ranging from 85% to 100% and 93% to 97%, respectively.[100–102]

Therapy

Latent Tuberculosis Infection

The majority of children with M. tb infection have LTBI. These children have a reactive TST or IGRA, normal chest radiograph, no clinical evidence of tuberculosis, and presumed infection with low numbers of viable tubercle bacilli. Children with LTBI should receive treatment for the following reasons: (1) infants and children less than 5 years of age have been infected recently, so risk for progression to disease is high; (2) risk for severe disease, including meningitis and disseminated disease, is inversely related to age; (3) children with LTBI have more years at risk for the development of disease later in life; and (4) children with LTBI become adults who may transmit organisms if they develop disease.[86]

Several large clinical trials have demonstrated the efficacy of isoniazid (INH) to reduce the risk for tuberculosis in children with LTBI. In 1958, the U.S. Public Health Service (USPHS) conducted a randomized trial to prevent tuberculosis disease in boarding schools in Alaska.[103] Two dosing regimens of INH were studied, 1.25 mg/kg/day versus 5 mg/kg/day given for 6 months to 1701 attendees 5 to 20 years of age either 5 days per week or daily. In 10 years of follow-up, participants who received the higher dose of INH had significantly less progression to tuberculosis (1.9%, 10 of 513) than participants receiving the lower dose (5.8%, 31 of 536). The study also demonstrated that an intermittent therapy course (5 days per week) was efficacious. Additional randomized controlled trials completed by the USPHS in the 1950s and 1960s found the protective efficacy of INH treatment of LTBI to be approximately 90% when analysis was restricted to compliant participants.[104] Secondary analysis of two USPHS household contact studies has suggested that the efficacy of INH treatment of LTBI plateaus at 9 to 10 months of therapy.[105] Similarly, in a study among the Inuit in Alaska, a second year of INH treatment did not result in additional benefit beyond that conferred by the first year of treatment.[106,107] Although the International Union against Tuberculosis and Lung Disease (IUATLD) has evaluated the efficacy of various durations of INH therapy in adults with LTBI, similar studies have not been conducted in children.[88] The current American Academy of Pediatrics (AAP) recommendation for treatment of LTBI in children is 9 months of INH given either daily (10 to 15 mg/kg, maximum 300 mg) usually under self-supervised administration, or twice weekly (20 to 30 mg/kg, maximum 900 mg) under directly observed therapy (DOT).[86] Recognizing the high risk of TB disease progression in childhood, the WHO recommends INH preventive therapy (IPT) in HIV-negative children who are younger than 5 years of age and in contact with an infectious adult source case, regardless of documentation of M. tb infection.[108]

There is limited and conflicting data on the effectiveness of treatment for LTBI in HIV-infected children.[109–111] The AAP currently recommends a 9-month INH regimen or at least a 6-month rifampin regimen in HIV-infected children. In most cases, treatment may be given daily without observation.[112] If compliance is inadequate, intermittent DOT may be instituted. The WHO has recently developed recommendations requiring national TB control programs to significantly scale-up TB screening, prevention, and treatment in HIV-infected adults and children.[113] These guidelines recommend IPT in HIV-infected children with a history of TB contact or one of the following symptoms: poor weight gain, fever, or current cough. Hence, lack of capacity to complete a TST cannot be a barrier to IPT delivery.

Despite international and national guidelines recommending IPT in children, delivery and monitoring of IPT to children remains poor. Existing data demonstrate that poor IPT delivery is due to missed opportunities for IPT,[39,114,115] poor uptake and adherence,[116,117] and limited administrative systems to support IPT delivery.[118] In order to improve IPT delivery in TB high burden settings, IPT must become a core intervention of both TB and HIV control programs that are supported by regionally appropriate tools, implementation, monitoring, and evaluation systems.

Rifampin has been used for the treatment of LTBI in children and adolescents when INH was not tolerated or the child was exposed to an INH-resistant, rifampin-susceptible source.[119] However, no controlled clinical trials have been completed. A 3- to 4-month regimen consisting of rifampin and INH has been used in England.[120] This observational study analyzing administrative data suggests that this regimen is effective, but no controlled trials have been reported.

LTBI treatment should be tailored according to host-immune factors, drug susceptibility, tolerance, and compliance (Table 33-3). If drug susceptibility is not available for either the child or source case, INH is recommended. Treatment of MDR tuberculosis infection must be individualized and should be delivered via DOT.

Window Prophylaxis

After infection with *M. tb*, children may take up to 3 months to develop an immune response sufficient to produce a positive TST result.[121] Children younger than 5 years of age have a short incubation period and may develop severe disease before developing skin test reactivity.[122] Because of this risk, children with a negative TST and known or suspected exposure to an adult with contagious tuberculosis should receive treatment for LTBI. Tuberculin skin testing should be repeated 3 months after initial exposure. If the second TST result is negative, therapy may be discontinued. If skin test conversion occurs, therapy should be continued for the full 9 months. Limited data suggest that young children may develop an immune response sufficient to produce a positive interferon-gamma reaction before a positive reaction to the TST.[123,124] Hence, in a TST-negative child, a positive IGRA reaction should be considered clinically relevant and prompt treatment for LTBI should be initiated.

TABLE 33-3 PREVENTIVE REGIMENS FOR LATENT TUBERCULOSIS INFECTION IN CHILDREN

RESISTANCE PATTERN OF SOURCE CASE	ANTIMYCOBACTERIAL AGENT DOSAGE AND DURATION	COMMENTS
INH susceptible or unknown	INH, 10 mg/kg as single daily dose ×9 mo (maximum 300 mg per dose) INH, 20-30 mg/kg twice weekly ×9 mo (maximum, 900 mg per dose)	Optimal duration for children is debated CDC and AAP recommend 9 mo Intermittent schedule should be given only by DOT
INH resistant or INH not tolerated	RIF, 10 mg/kg as single daily dose ×6 mo (maximum, 600 mg per dose)	
MDR-TB (resistant to INH and RIF)	Guided by susceptibility testing on a child or source case isolate	Should be provided in consultation with an expert DOT strongly recommended

AAP, American Academy of Pediatrics; *ATS*, American Thoracic Society; *CDC*, Centers for Disease Control and Prevention; *DOT*, directly observed therapy; *IDSA*, Infectious Disease Society of America; *INH*, isoniazid; *MDR-TB*, multidrug-resistant tuberculosis; *RIF*, rifampin.

Tuberculosis Disease

Principles of Treatment

Treatment of tuberculosis is designed to prevent the complications of disease in the host and the development of drug-resistance in the organism. Antimycobacterial agents should be bactericidal and effective against intracellular and extracellular organisms. Three or more drugs are used empirically for initial therapy and are adjusted when susceptibility testing is available. Initial use of a single agent will select for emergence of a dominantly resistant population of bacilli. Therapy is provided for extended periods via DOT. Length of therapy is dependent on the site of infection.

Pulmonary Tuberculosis

The first-line drugs used to treat tuberculosis in children are shown in Table 33-4.

Many therapeutic trials have been reported in children with pulmonary tuberculosis. A 6-month regimen consisting of INH and rifampin was effective in some patients with isolated hilar adenopathy.[125] Limited data are available to support a 6-month, INH-rifampin regimen for the treatment of pulmonary tuberculosis.[126] At least a dozen studies have examined the efficacy of 6-month regimens consisting of three or more drugs in children with pulmonary tuberculosis. The most common regimen studied consisted of INH and rifampin, supplemented with pyrazinamide during the first 2 months. Most trials used daily therapy for the first 2 months, followed by daily or twice weekly therapy to complete 6 months. In all of these trials, the overall success rate was greater than 95% for cure and 99% for significant improvement during a 2-year follow-up.

Although current guidelines recommend that all TB patients be started on a 4-drug regimen,[112] a 3-drug regimen may be used in children exposed to a source case with pan-susceptible TB. Hence, in children with suspected INH-susceptible pulmonary tuberculosis, the recommended treatment is a 6-month regimen consisting of INH and rifampin, supplemented during the first 2 months with pyrazinamide. Daily administration of the drug during the first 2 weeks to 2 months may be followed by twice-weekly therapy to complete 6 months. All treatment for tuberculosis disease should be administered by DOT unless there is a compelling reason to avoid it.

In children or adolescents with adult-type pulmonary tuberculosis or epidemiologic circumstances suggesting an increased risk for infection with drug-resistant organisms, the American Thoracic Society (ATS) recommends an initial 2-month treatment phase consisting of daily administration of four drugs: INH, rifampin, pyrazinamide, and ethambutol. This initial treatment is followed by 4 months of INH and rifampin twice-weekly therapy administered under DOT if the organism is susceptible to both drugs.[127] Although there have been concerns about the use of ethambutol in children because it can cause optic neuritis that is difficult to detect in children, this adverse effect is extraordinarily rare in children and should not preclude the use of ethambutol with extensive or drug-resistant disease.

The optimal treatment of pulmonary tuberculosis in children and adolescents with HIV infection is unknown. In children with TB-HIV co-infection who received 6 months of chemotherapy, a recurrence risk of 13% has been reported despite good adherence.[128] The AAP and ATS recommend initial therapy that should consist of 4 drugs for the first 2 months with a total duration of therapy that should last at least 9 months.[76] The WHO recommends that TB in HIV-infected children should be treated with a 6-month regimen similar to HIV-uninfected children, but treatment should not be delivered using intermittent schedules.[129,130] In TB-HIV co-infected adults, prolonged TB treatment duration[131-133] and use of highly active antiretroviral therapy (HAART)[133-136] reduce the risk of TB recurrence. In children, reduced TB incidence rates in those on HAART compared with those not on HAART are seen in retrospective and observational cohort studies.[137,138] The optimal timing for initiating HAART in HIV-TB co-infected children is not known.[108,139] When treating TB-HIV co-infected children, a number of special issues must be considered including drug-drug interactions, immune reconstitution inflammatory syndrome, and drug-resistant TB.[140]

TABLE 33-4 COMMONLY USED DRUGS FOR THE TREATMENT OF TUBERCULOSIS IN CHILDREN

DRUG	DOSAGE FORMS	DAILY DOSE (MG/KG)	TWICE WEEKLY DOSE (MG/KG/DAY)	MAXIMUM DOSE
Ethambutol	Tablets: 100 mg, 400 mg	20	50	Daily: 1 g Twice weekly: 2.5 g
Isoniazid*†	Scored tablets: 100 mg, 300 mg Syrup: 10 mg/mL	10-15	20-30	Daily: 300 mg Twice weekly: 900 mg
Pyrazinamide	Scored tablets: 500 mg	30-40	50	2 g
Rifampin*	Capsules: 150 mg, 300 mg Formulated in syrup from capsules	10-20	10-20	Daily: 600 mg Twice weekly: 600 mg
Streptomycin (IM administration)	Vials: 1 g, 4 g	20-40	20-40	Daily: 1 g

IM, Intramuscular.
*Rifamate is a capsule containing 150 mg of isoniazid and 300 mg of rifampin. Two capsules provide the usual adult (>50 kg body weight) daily doses of each drug.
†Most experts advise against the use of isoniazid syrup because of instability and a high rate of gastrointestinal adverse reactions (diarrhea, cramps).

Extrapulmonary Tuberculosis

Controlled trials have not been reported for children with extrapulmonary tuberculosis. In general, recommended treatment for extrapulmonary tuberculosis is the same as for pulmonary tuberculosis. Osteotuberculosis and tuberculous meningitis are exceptions. Recommended treatment of osteotuberculosis includes 9 to 12 months of INH and rifampin or 6 months of INH and rifampin supplemented by two other drugs during the first 2 months of therapy. There are inadequate data to support any 6-month treatment regimen for tuberculous meningitis. Recommended regimens consist of 4-drug treatment during the initial 2 months followed by 7 to 10 months of therapy with INH and rifampin.

Drug-Resistant Tuberculosis

The incidence of drug-resistant tuberculosis is increasing in the United States and the world because of poor patient adherence, the availability of some antituberculosis drugs in noncontrolled over-the-counter formulations, and poor physician management. In the United States, approximately 10% of *M. tb* isolates are resistant to at least one drug. Certain epidemiologic factors—disease in an Asian, Eastern European, or Hispanic immigrants to the United States; homelessness in some communities; and history of previous antituberculosis therapy—correlate with drug resistance in adult patients. Patterns of drug resistance in children tend to mirror those found in adult patients in the population.[141] Outbreaks of drug-resistant tuberculosis in children occurring at schools have been reported. Individual cases also have been recognized. Since it is difficult to isolate *M. tb* from children because of the paucibacillary nature of childhood TB, the determination of drug resistance in childhood TB usually is inferred from that of their source case. Hence, it is critically important to identify the adult source case that infected the child.

Therapy for drug-resistant tuberculosis is successful only when at least two bactericidal drugs are given to which the infecting strain of *M. tb* is susceptible.[142] If only one effective drug is given, secondary resistance will develop. When INH resistance is considered a possibility on the basis of epidemiologic risk factors or the identification of an INH-resistant source case isolate, an additional drug—usually ethambutol—should be given initially to the child until the exact susceptibility pattern is determined and a more specific regimen can be designed. Exact treatment regimens must be tailored to the specific pattern of drug resistance and the extent of disease. The duration of therapy usually is extended to at least 9 to 12 months if either INH or rifampin can be used and to at least 18 to 24 months if resistance to both drugs is present. Occasionally, surgical resection of a diseased lung or lobe is required. An expert in tuberculosis always should be involved in the management of children with drug-resistant tuberculosis infection or disease.

Adjunctive Therapy

Pyridoxine (25 to 50 mg/day) is recommended for infants, children, and adolescents treated with INH who have nutritional deficiencies, symptomatic HIV infection, and diets low in milk or meat products. Pyridoxine also is recommended for breastfeeding infants.

Corticosteroid administration is beneficial in the management of children when the host inflammatory reaction contributes significantly to tissue damage or impaired function. Administration of corticosteroids decreases mortality and morbidity in patients with tuberculous meningitis by reducing vasculitis, inflammation, and intracranial pressure. Corticosteroid administration may significantly reduce compression of the tracheobronchial tree caused by hilar lymphadenopathy, associated with miliary disease, and alveolar-capillary block, pleural effusion, and pericardial effusion.[127] Prednisone (1 to 2 mg/kg/day for 4 to 6 weeks) is most commonly employed.

Follow-up During Antituberculosis Therapy

The major goals of following children during treatment include promoting adherence, monitoring for toxicity and adverse effects of therapy, and assessing clinical response. Patients should be evaluated monthly and receive only enough medication for the interval between follow-up appointments. During the initial phase of treatment, clinicians should assess potential noncompliance. Children with missed appointments and poor compliance should be referred to the responsible public health agency that likely has programs incorporating incentives or behavioral modification.

Rates of adverse reactions caused by antituberculosis medications are low among children. INH and rifampin are associated with elevated serum alanine aminotransferase in less than 2% of children and rarely cause overt hepatitis. Elevated alanine aminotransferase levels are generally less than three times normal values, do not predict hepatotoxicity, and are not an indication for discontinuing treatment. Routine biochemical monitoring is not indicated if the child does not have liver disease and is not taking other hepatotoxic drugs. It is preferable to educate caregivers relative to potential adverse events and clinical symptoms (abdominal pain, vomiting, jaundice) necessitating medical evaluation and discontinuation of medication.

Frequent radiographic monitoring is not indicated. Because improvement of intrathoracic tuberculosis in children occurs slowly, chest radiographs are generally obtained at diagnosis, 1 or 2 months into therapy, and at completion of therapy. Radiographic resolution of hilar lymphadenopathy and associated pulmonary lesions may not occur for 2 to 3 years following treatment. A normal chest radiograph appearance is not necessary for completion of therapy. If resolution of radiographic abnormalities has not occurred by completion of therapy, radiographs may be obtained at 3- to 6-month intervals to assess continued improvement.

Control and Prevention

Bacillus Calmette-Guérin Vaccination

BCG vaccines have been administered to nearly 4 billion people and have been routinely administered to newborns in most countries except the United States and the Netherlands. Nevertheless, the immune response to BCG and its mechanism of action are not well understood. Large clinical trials have shown the efficacy of BCG vaccination to range from 0% to 80%. A number of factors contribute to the heterogeneity of results from these trials, including eligibility criteria, strain of vaccine employed, vaccine administration, diagnostic criteria, disease surveillance, and environmental factors.[143] Although BCG does not prevent primary pulmonary tuberculosis, studies have demonstrated that BCG vaccination decreases the risk for developing severe forms of disease in children, including meningitis and miliary tuberculosis.[144,145] The clinical presentation of tuberculosis disease in individuals who have received a BCG vaccination tends to be similar to that in nonimmunized persons.

BCG-induced immune responses in HIV-infected children are significantly lower compared with uninfected children.[146] Nevertheless, in the absence of antiretroviral therapy, HIV-infected infants have a significant risk of disseminated BCG disease that is associated with a case fatality rate exceeding 75%.[147,148] Following initiation of antiretroviral therapy, 5% to 10% of HIV-infected infants will experience BCG immune reconstitution inflammatory syndrome (IRIS).[149] The risk of serious BCG-related adverse events can be reduced by delaying BCG vaccination in HIV-exposed infants until their HIV status has been definitely established, and in HIV-infected infants by rapid initiation of antiretroviral therapy.[150] Based on the high risk of disseminated BCG disease in HIV-infected infants, the WHO has recommended that in infants where the HIV status has been established, BCG should not be given.[151] The practical feasibility of this recommendation has been questioned by tuberculosis experts in countries with high burdens of HIV and TB, where the feasibility of selectively deferred vaccination and potential disruption of general vaccination coverage is a concern.[152]

Public Health Involvement

Childhood tuberculosis, defined as tuberculosis in children younger than 15 years of age, is a direct reflection of the incidence of adult tuberculosis within a community. Childhood tuberculosis usually represents recent transmission from an infectious adult or adolescent and is considered a sentinel event in public health. In response to a case of childhood tuberculosis, health departments should conduct an investigation to identify the source of infection and additional cases.

Health departments conduct several different types of investigations. Contact investigations evaluate all contacts of an infectious adult or adolescent for tuberculosis disease or LTBI. Contact investigations have the highest yield for finding infected persons and are considered the cornerstone of reducing the incidence of tuberculosis in developed nations. Source case investigations evaluate all contacts of a child with tuberculosis to identify an infectious adult or adolescent and other infected persons. Source case investigations are less successful because source cases frequently do not reside in the United States if the child is foreign born or has lived abroad. It is the health department's responsibility to ensure that all persons with suspected tuberculosis are identified and evaluated promptly and that appropriate treatment is prescribed and successfully completed. These responsibilities are accomplished through a number of activities, including epidemiologic surveillance and investigations,

direct provision of diagnostic services and treatment, and monitoring of treatment decisions and outcomes. The health department should employ a tailored approach for each patient that accounts for individual needs to ensure completion of therapy. DOT is the preferred, core management strategy to ensure adherence and involves providing the antituberculous drugs directly to the patient and watching that he or she swallows the medications.

PULMONARY DISEASE CAUSED BY NONTUBERCULOUS MYCOBACTERIA

Epidemiology

Several problems compound the epidemiologic description of NTM infections in humans.[153] The NTM rarely cause fatal infection, so mortality statistics are not helpful. There is no public health mandatory reporting of NTM infection. Smaller laboratories that isolate NTM often do not refer isolates to reference laboratories for identification and drug-susceptibility testing, so statistics from even these laboratories grossly underestimate the incidence of NTM disease. Finally, isolating an NTM from a clinical specimen often is not sufficient for the diagnosis of disease. Distinguishing among saprophytes, colonizers, and truly pathogenic organisms requires clinical correlation not available from laboratory reports.

Transmission of NTM to humans occurs from environmental sources, including soil, water, dust, and aerosols. There is some evidence that MAC strains more commonly isolated from persons with disease tend to be aerosolized preferentially from standing water, suggesting that aerosols from natural water are a primary source of NTM causing human infection. MAC species are found frequently in animals, particularly birds and swine, which may be an important natural reservoir for the organisms. There is little evidence to suggest that animal-to-human transmission is a major factor in human infection. There is no evidence supporting human-to-human transmission of NTM.[153]

The number of reports of clusters of health care–associated disease caused by various species of NTM is growing. Most common are outbreaks by the rapid growers. Both clusters and sporadic NTM infections have been associated with a variety of surgical procedures, including sternal wound infections after open heart surgery, augmentation mammoplasty prostheses, corneal surgery, implantation of pressure equalizing tubes in the tympanic membranes, and insertion of central venous catheters. A number of outbreaks or pseudo-outbreaks of respiratory tract colonization caused by various NTM species have been associated with contaminated ice machines, showers, potable water supplies, infected laboratory supplies, contamination of topical anesthesia, or tap water in hospitals. Contamination of bronchoscopes or bronchoscopy supplies has been implicated in some of these outbreaks.[154] Isolation of the same NTM species from bronchoscopy samples in two or more patients in a short period should prompt an investigation to determine possible sources of contamination, especially if isolation of the NTM is a surprising finding.

The true incidence of disease caused by NTM is difficult to estimate. In the United States, there are marked geographic variations in rates and species. The best data come from a survey of state and major city health department laboratories conducted between 1981 and 1983.[155] Over 5000 patients diagnosed with NTM disease were investigated. The estimated annual prevalence of all NTM disease was 1.8 cases per 100,000 population, about 15% of the prevalence of tuberculosis. Rates were higher for MAC (1.3 per 100,000), *M. kansasii* (0.3 per 100,000), and the rapid growers (0.2 per 100,000).

The species of NTM causing infection and the anatomic site of disease vary by age. Among children, the majority of NTM infections are in the superficial cervical lymph nodes.[156] MAC is responsible for 95% of cases of NTM lymphadenitis in children. In contrast, the lung is the most common site of NTM disease in adults.[153] MAC organisms account for about 60% of the respiratory isolates, and *M. kansasii* constitutes about 25% of isolates. Early reports of MAC pulmonary disease found that most patients were males who had some form of preexisting lung disease such as emphysema and frequent alcohol abuse. In contrast, most recent reports have shown the majority of adults with MAC pulmonary disease to be women with no preexisting lung disease.[157] However, one recent study showed that adult patients with pulmonary NTM disease were taller and leaner than control subjects, with high rates of pectus excavatum, scoliosis, and mitral valve prolapse, but without recognized immune defects.[158] Up to 70% of adults with *M. kansasii* pulmonary infections have preexisting lung disease, while the majority of adults with pulmonary infection due to rapid grower NTM do not have chronic lung disease.[159] The majority of children with pulmonary infection by an NTM species have not had previous lung disease.[160,161]

An increasing number of cases of isolation of various NTM from the respiratory secretions of patients with CF has been reported recently.[162–172] It is difficult to compare these reports because the methods of ascertainment; culture methods; and definitions of colonization, infection, and disease differed widely. Because these patients have severe and progressive underlying pulmonary disease, it is difficult to assess the role of an NTM infection in an individual patient's clinical course. While the isolation of an NTM from a CF patient's sputum may be associated with a worsening clinical and radiographic course, in other patients the presence of an NTM may be an incidental finding. The CF patients from whom an NTM is isolated tend to be older and sicker, but there are an increasing number of reports of NTM affecting cystic fibrosis patients younger than 12 years of age.[173,174] The incidence of isolation of an NTM has ranged from as high as 24% to a low of 3% in CF patients. MAC is isolated most frequently, but *M. kansasii*, *M. gordonae*, and the rapid growers also may be encountered. Infection with *M. abscessus* has been associated frequently with a more rapid deterioration in clinical course.[164,175] Repeated isolation of the same species of NTM from a CF patient with an otherwise unexplained decline in clinical scoring, who responds to appropriate antimycobacterial therapy, represents the strongest clinical definition of NTM

lung disease in a CF patient.[163] However, a recent autopsy study showed that only two of six CF patients who had multiple respiratory cultures positive for an NTM had histologic evidence of disease (granuloma formation).[170]

Clinical disease due to NTM is common in adults and children with AIDS. Occasionally, the NTM pulmonary infection mimics tuberculosis. Although isolated pulmonary infection with an NTM in patients with AIDS has been reported, pulmonary involvement usually is part of a widely disseminated infection. MAC accounts for 85% of cases, followed in incidence by *M. kansasii* and *M. gordonae*. Disseminated disease with pulmonary involvement caused by NTM has been described rarely in patients with other immunodeficiency states (leukemia, lymphoma, and other malignancies) and in otherwise normal children.[176,177] NTM disease also has been reported in adults and children after organ transplantation.

Clinical Manifestations

The clinical manifestations of NTM infection depend on the species involved and the presence of underlying conditions in the patient. Although any organ system can be infected by NTM, certain organisms preferentially infect the lung (Table 33-5). This section presents the most common manifestations of pulmonary NTM infection in nonimmunocompromised hosts and then presents special considerations in patients with CF and immunocompromised hosts.

Mycobacterium Kansasii

Mycobacterium kansasii is a mycobacterium that produces pigment when grown on solid media. This organism is antigenically and clinically most closely related to *M. tb*. Infection with *M. kansasii* usually occurs in adults with underlying pulmonary disease, especially smoking-related chronic obstructive pulmonary disease (COPD). Other predisposing lung conditions include bronchogenic carcinoma, bronchiectasis, silicosis, and prior tuberculosis. In contrast, most of the children and adolescents reported with *M. kansasii* pulmonary disease have not had underlying chronic conditions. In the United States, *M. kansasii* is most common in midwestern and southwestern states, especially in Texas.[178] Moreover, the majority of cases of

TABLE 33-5	MOST COMMON SITES OF INFECTION FOR NONTUBERCULOUS MYCOBACTERIA
SITE	**MOST COMMON ORGANISMS**
Pulmonary	*M. kansasii, M. avium complex, M. xenopi, M. haemophilum, M. fortuitum, M. chelonae, M. gordonae* (rare), *M. szulgai* (rare), *M. malmoense* (rare)
Lymph node	*M. avium complex, M. kansasii, M. fortuitum, M. abscessus* (rare)
Disseminated	*M. avium complex, M. kansasii, M. fortuitum, M. chelonae, M. xenopi, M. haemophilum, M. gordonae* (rare)

tuberculosis occur among racial and ethnic minorities, while the majority of cases of *M. kansasii* pulmonary disease occur among whites.

In adolescents and adults, the most common signs and symptoms associated with pulmonary disease due to *M. kansasii* are similar to those found with tuberculosis. Most patients experience significant cough and sputum production. About one third of patients have hemoptysis and about one fourth experience chest pain. Fever, chills, and night sweats occur in a minority of patients but over half of the patients experience significant weight loss. Younger children with pulmonary disease due to *M. kansasii* tend to have fewer systemic signs and symptoms and may present with only a cough and failure to gain weight.

The typical radiographic findings of *M. kansasii* pulmonary disease in adolescents and adults are similar to those found with tuberculosis (Fig. 33-15). About half of patients experience cavitation with or without fibrosis. Pleural scarring and nonspecific pulmonary infiltrates also are common. Adenopathy is rare, and pleural effusion is exceedingly rare. Most pulmonary findings occur in the apical regions, but abnormalities may be found throughout the lungs. Almost 40% of patients experience bilateral disease.

The chest radiographic findings of *M. kansasii* disease in children are similar to those found with primary tuberculosis. Adenopathy is common, and many children experience the type of collapse-consolidation lesion seen in primary tuberculosis. Calcification of enlarged hilar lymph nodes is common. It is likely that some cases of *M. kansasii* pulmonary disease in children are misdiagnosed as tuberculosis because *M. kansasii* often causes a positive TST result, and cultures from children with either disease usually are negative. Fortunately, the treatment of pulmonary tuberculosis in children also is effective against most cases of *M. kansasii* disease.

Mycobacterium Avium Complex

Among immunocompetent hosts, pulmonary disease caused by MAC is much more common in adults than in adolescents or younger children. The average age of patients is about 60 years. About half the patients have preexisting pulmonary disease, including prior tuberculosis, COPD, silicosis, diabetes mellitus, or lung cancer. Patients without other pulmonary diseases tend to be younger and more frequently female.

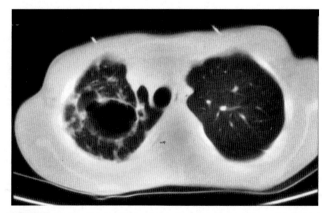

FIGURE 33-15. Computed tomography scan of an adolescent with pulmonary disease caused by *M. kansasii*.

Clinical features in adults tend to be similar in patients with or without predisposing conditions. Indolent productive cough with purulent sputum is the primary symptom in the majority of cases. It is common for patients to experience symptoms for up to 6 months or longer before the correct diagnosis is established. Hemoptysis is uncommon, and persistent fever is rare. Constitutional symptoms such as weight loss, night sweats, and malaise are uncommon.

The radiographic findings of MAC pulmonary disease in adults are similar to those with tuberculosis. About one third of patients have cavitation. However, a wide variety of radiographic findings can be seen, including lobar consolidation, interstitial disease, nodular or alveolar infiltrates, and involvement of multiple lobes. In one study among adults without preexisting lung disease, the most common presenting radiographic pattern was multiple discrete pulmonary nodules seen in 71% of patients.[157]

Because of the difficulty of proving the diagnosis by culture, the reported incidence of pulmonary MAC disease among children and adolescents is low.[179] Almost all reported patients have been younger than 5 years of age, and the clinical and radiographic patterns of disease have been similar to that of primary tuberculosis in children.[160,161] Many of the reported cases have been treated initially as tuberculosis but were further investigated because of unusual clinical or radiographic findings or failure to respond to the usual antituberculosis chemotherapy. The majority of affected children have been immunocompetent with no underlying pulmonary disease. Most infected children have come to clinical attention because of fairly mild but persistent symptoms, including cough and low-grade fever; more severe systemic signs or symptoms are rare. Localized wheezing has been noted occasionally, and the diagnosis of an aspirated foreign body considered. Systemic symptoms such as fever, night sweats, and weight loss are uncommon.

The most common radiographic presentation of MAC pulmonary disease in children has been enlargement of the hilar or mediastinal lymph nodes, sometimes with accompanying atelectasis. Some children have experienced repeated episodes of fever and cough, interpreted as recurrent pneumonia or bronchitis. They have more extensive radiographic involvement that is probably due to partial or complete obstruction of a bronchus caused by an enlarged lymph node. Several children have had the acute onset of pneumonia with extensive pulmonary infiltrates in one or several lobes, with a subsequent prolonged chronic course. Involvement of the pleura is exceedingly rare.

Several children with MAC pulmonary disease have undergone bronchoscopy, which generally demonstrates granulation tissue within one of the bronchi. Narrowing of the bronchus because of external compression from an enlarged lymph node can be seen occasionally. It is often the culture of this endobronchial material that leads to the isolation of MAC. Histologic examination of this tissue usually reveals caseating granulomas, which helps confirm the diagnosis of mycobacterial disease.

It becomes obvious that the diagnosis of pulmonary MAC disease in children is exceedingly difficult. MAC organisms can be isolated from the oral and gastric secretions of healthy children. Repeated isolation of the organism in association with an abnormal chest radiograph is suggestive but not diagnostic of significant infection. Definitive diagnosis usually requires invasive procedures such as bronchoscopy or pulmonary/endobronchial biopsy. It is likely that some cases of MAC pulmonary disease are misdiagnosed as tuberculosis on the basis of clinical and radiographic findings, a mild reaction to the TST, and spontaneous resolution over several months with or without appropriate chemotherapy. A key element in the differential diagnosis is the family investigation for tuberculosis. A case of "unusual" pulmonary tuberculosis in a child whose family has no risk factors for tuberculosis and whose other family members test negative for tuberculosis infection or disease should be investigated for the possibility of MAC pulmonary disease.[180]

Rapidly Growing Mycobacteria

Reports of pulmonary disease in children caused by the rapidly growing mycobacteria (M. fortuitum, M. chelonae, M. abscessus) are rare.[54] The importance of these infections among adults was not well recognized until the 1970s. Adult patients with this infection are predominantly white, female nonsmokers who have prolonged periods from the onset of symptoms to the correct diagnosis of their disease. Cough is an almost universal presenting symptom, whereas constitutional symptoms become important only with progression of disease. In one study, the mean length of time from onset of symptoms to the first positive culture was 26 months.[181] The most common symptoms at diagnosis are cough, sputum production, and malaise.[153,179] Fever eventually occurs in about one half of patients and hemoptysis occurs in about one third. About one third of patients have other pulmonary conditions, including preexisting tuberculosis, COPD, or bronchiectasis.

In contrast to other pulmonary mycobacterial infections, the most frequent patterns on chest radiograph of infections due to the rapidly growing mycobacteria are interstitial and alveolar densities. In many cases, the densities have a reticulonodular appearance. Cavitation is unusual, occurring in only 15% of patients. The upper lobes of the lung are involved in almost 90% of patients, but infiltrates may occur in any part of the lung.

Other Mycobacterial Species

Many other mycobacterial species have been associated with pulmonary disease. Pathogenic species of NTM that are rare causes of disease in the United States are M. xenopi, M. malmoense, and M. szulgai.[182] Most of the reported infections have been in adults; these infections appear to be exceedingly rare in children or not clinically detected. The pulmonary disease caused by these organisms tends to be similar to that caused by tuberculosis. The most common symptoms are productive cough, weight loss, and night sweats. The typical chest radiograph shows upper lobe densities, sometimes with cavitation. Pulmonary infections in children more often are similar to those caused by primary tuberculosis, including mild cough but a minimum of other signs and symptoms, and enlarged hilar or mediastinal lymph nodes, sometimes with associated pulmonary findings. The diagnosis

of pulmonary disease in children caused by these other mycobacteria is exceedingly difficult. However, if any mycobacterium is isolated from a gastric or bronchoscopy specimen from a child, consideration must be given to the mycobacterium as a cause of pulmonary disease.

Mycobacterial Infection in Cystic Fibrosis

The incidence of finding various NTM organisms in the sputum of patients with CF appears to be increasing. It is not clear whether the apparent increase is due to changing conditions or treatments, or whether CF patients are living longer and having a greater opportunity of becoming colonized. Early retrospective reports of NTM in CF sputum indicated it to be an infrequent problem. However, the true incidence of NTM colonization or infection was not evaluated because not all patients were tested. More recent prospective studies suggested a much higher incidence of NTM in some CF centers.[161,162]

A fundamental problem in caring for CF patients with NTM in the sputum is determining the difference between colonization and disease. The ATS has published guidelines for the diagnosis of NTM disease in normal hosts. For individuals without cavitary lesions on chest radiography, the criteria include (1) two or more sputum smears being acid-fast positive and/or resulting in moderate to heavy growth on cultures, (2) failure of the sputum cultures to convert to negative with either bronchial hygiene or 2 weeks of antimicrobial drug therapy, and (3) the exclusion of other reasonable causes for pulmonary disease. Unfortunately, these guidelines fail to differentiate among NTM species and are difficult to apply to CF patients with significant underlying pulmonary disease. The chronic suppurative lung disease present in patients with CF makes them likely hosts for NTM colonization. Malnutrition, diabetes mellitus, and frequent use of corticosteroids are additional risk factors for NTM infections in many CF patients. The signs and symptoms that may differentiate NTM colonization from disease in the healthy host include productive cough, dyspnea, hemoptysis, malaise, and fatigue. Older patients with advanced CF display these signs and symptoms much of the time, limiting the ability to use them as clinical indicators of NTM-related disease. Thus, in the CF patient, clinical indicators of tissue damage often cannot adequately differentiate between NTM colonization and disease. The differentiation can be made only at autopsy in some cases, and even patients with repeated positive sputum cultures for NTM may not have histologic evidence of mycobacterial disease.[170] The species of NTM found in the sputum of a CF patient may help in deciding whether colonization or disease is most likely present. Finding an unusual organism such as M. kansasii is more likely to reflect disease. While asymptomatic colonization with rapidly growing mycobacteria occurs, finding these organisms often is associated with a worsening course of pulmonary disease.[163] Of course, when a positive acid-fast stain of sputum from a CF patient is found, the possibility of disease caused by M. tb must be addressed immediately because of both personal and public health considerations. However, in general, patients with CF tend to have few risk factors for infection and disease caused by M. tb.

Because of the difficulty in distinguishing colonization from disease caused by NTM in CF patients, it is difficult to state specific clinical manifestations for NTM disease. Some patients experience an increase in cough and sputum production, weight loss, and other systemic symptoms such as night sweats or chronic low-grade fevers. Hemoptysis, which can occur in CF patients without NTM infection, appears to be no more frequent with NTM infection. Rarely, new cavitary lesions accompany the finding of an NTM in the sputum. Pleural involvement is exceedingly rare. There is some suggestion that NTM preferentially cause apical disease, but this is an inconsistent finding among various clinical reports. Some patients experience a decline in pulmonary function that is associated with the new acquisition of NTM in the sputum.

Unfortunately, a standard definition of NTM disease in CF patients using clinical, radiographic, and pulmonary function testing results, is probably not possible. It is fairly clear that a single isolation of an NTM in the sputum of a CF patient who is not experiencing a decline in pulmonary function probably represents colonization, and treatment is not necessary. Repeated isolation of the same species of NTM from the sputum in association with declining pulmonary function is more suggestive, but not diagnostic, of invasive NTM infection of the lung.[162] In many cases, a relatively short (1 to 2 months) trial of antimycobacterial therapy, directed at the specific species of NTM isolated, may help determine if significant infection is present.

Diagnosis

Nonspecific laboratory tests such as blood counts, erythrocyte sedimentation rate, urinalysis, and serum chemistry tests usually are normal in children with NTM infections and have no diagnostic value. The key to diagnosis is a high level of suspicion based on epidemiologic factors and the clinical presentation. Acid-fast stains of appropriate specimens may give an early clue to the presence of NTM infection. However, the number of NTM in most fluids and tissues is small, and acid-fast smears are frequently negative when an infection is present. In pulmonary disease among adults and adolescents, a positive acid-fast smear of sputum is much more likely to indicate tuberculosis than an NTM infection. A negative acid-fast smear never should dissuade the clinician from considering the diagnosis of NTM disease in an appropriate setting. Similarly, histologic studies of involved tissues are helpful if classic granulomatous changes are demonstrated, but many NTM infections in immunocompetent hosts cause only nonspecific acute and/or chronic inflammation without granulomas, especially with infections due to the rapidly growing mycobacteria.

Skin testing with PPD from *M. tb* and other mycobacteria has been used to detect infection with NTM. Infections caused by MAC commonly are associated with reactions to a standard TST from 0 to 10 mm. Larger reactions are seen but rarely exceed 18 mm. Infections by *M. marinum*, *M. kansasii*, and *M. fortuitum* frequently are associated with TST reactions of 10 to 20 mm. Of course, similar reactions may be caused by infection with *M. tb*. Determining the source of the skin reaction to tuberculin can be difficult and depends largely on epidemiologic factors, especially the likelihood that the child has been exposed to an adult with pulmonary tuberculosis. Investigation of adults in the child's environment usually is necessary to help determine if a moderate (8 to 15 mm) reaction is due to infection with *M. tb* or a cross-reaction that is due to infection by NTM; a negative skin test result never rules out NTM infection.

The most direct method for diagnosing NTM infection is appropriate mycobacterial culture of involved fluid or tissue specimens. Unfortunately, many NTM are plentiful in the environment and frequently are encountered as colonizers or agents that produce infection but not recognizable disease. The decision whether or not NTM disease requiring treatment is present rests with the clinician's judgment of the extent of tissue invasion associated with isolation of the organism. Wolinsky[183] suggested considering five clinical facts (Box 33-3). Disease in the respiratory tract usually is associated with moderate to heavy growth of NTM, not with just a few colonies on the plate. However, light growth in normally sterile body fluids or tissues—such as a lung biopsy or bronchoscopy specimen—may indicate invasive disease. Repeated isolation of the same species of NTM, particularly if it is one known to be associated with pulmonary disease, is much more likely to indicate invasive infection. Finally, the risk factors of the host for significant NTM disease are a strong consideration in determining the clinical significance of a positive culture.

Treatment[153]

Specific treatment of NTM disease depends on the location and extent of the infected tissue, the capability of the host's immune system, and the species of NTM involved.[184] In 2007, the ATS and the Infectious Disease Society of America published a lengthy guideline for the diagnosis, management and prevention of NTM infections that remains the best single source of information.[153] Surgery plays a more important role in the management of NTM disease than it does for tuberculosis because chemotherapy is relatively ineffective and most NTM infections are localized to one site. However, one important exception is the lung, where surgery is usually not employed, except in far advanced disease.

BOX 33-3 AIDS FOR DISTINGUISHING NONTUBERCULOUS MYCOBACTERIAL DISEASE FROM COLONIZATION

1. The amount of growth usually increases with disease.
2. Repeated isolation of the same organism is associated with invasive disease.
3. A site of origin from a closed anatomic site is more significant.
4. Is the species of mycobacterium a usual pathogen?
5. Does the host have other risk factors—an immunocompromised state, cystic fibrosis, or exposure to second-hand smoke?

Many infections due to NTM are similar in clinical presentation to tuberculosis. An important initial consideration in managing all mycobacterial infections is to be certain that *M. tb* is not the actual pathogen. Usually, until an NTM is identified by culture, treatment is directed at tuberculosis for both therapeutic and infection control/public health reasons. This principle is especially important for young children with pulmonary disease, immunodeficiency, or AIDS, since dissemination of tuberculosis in these patients may have disastrous consequences. Fortunately, the clinical progression of most NTM infections is slow enough that a period of several weeks to several months of treatment directed at tuberculosis will not have a significant deleterious effect on the outcome of the NTM infection.

Determining the species of NTM causing infection is critical for directing chemotherapy. In general, *M. kansasii*, *M. marinum*, *M. xenopi*, *M. gordonae*, *M. malmoense*, *M. szulgai*, and *M. haemophilum* are susceptible to one or more of the standard antituberculosis drugs. Treatment of the rapidly growing mycobacterial and most strains of MAC require other antibiotics. The drugs used most commonly to treat NTM infections are listed in Table 33-6. Multiple-drug therapy is used for all infections because of the propensity of mycobacteria to develop resistance to single drugs. The treatment regimens that have been developed are based on either limited clinical trials in adults or anecdotal evidence from small series or case reports.

There have been no clinical trials published concerning the treatment of pulmonary NTM infections in children and adolescents. Treatment regimens are derived from clinical trials in adults or the best opinions of "experts." However, pulmonary disease tends to be more extensive in adults than in children, and the number of infecting organisms is probably much larger in adults. There is general agreement on which drug regimens should be used for initial treatment of NTM infections, but it is unclear what the optimal length of therapy is for children with NTM infection. There is no consensus about the proper treatment of NTM pulmonary infections in patients with CF. Most clinicians begin an initial regimen of appropriate therapy for several months to determine if a clinical response will occur.

TABLE 33-6 COMMONLY USED DRUGS FOR NONTUBERCULOUS MYCOBACTERIAL INFECTIONS

DRUG	HOW SUPPLIED	DOSAGE (MG/KG/DAY) AND ROUTE OF ADMINISTRATION	SUSCEPTIBLE PATHOGENS
Amikacin	100-, 500-mg, 1-g vials	15-30 IM or IV in 3 doses; max: 1.5 g/day	*M. fortuitum, M. chelonae, M. ulcerans, M. avium* complex
Azithromycin	250-mg tabs, 20 mg/mL and 40 mg/mL suspensions	5 mg/kg/day	*M. avium* complex, *M. fortuitum, M. chelonae, M. abscessus*
Cefoxitin	1-, 2-, 10-g vials	100-200 IV in 4 doses; max:12g/day	*M. fortuitum, M. chelonae*
Ciprofloxacin	250-, 500-, 750-mg tabs	500-1500 total in 2 doses	*M. avium* complex
Clarithromycin	250-mg tabs, 25 mg/mL, 50 mg/mL suspension	10-30 PO in 2 doses	*M. avium* complex, *M. fortuitum, M. chelonae, M. abscessus, M. marinum*
Clofazimine	50-,100-mg caps	1-2 PO in 1 dose; max: 100 mg/day	*M. avium* complex
Doxycycline	100-mg tabs	2-4 PO in 2 doses; max: 200 mg/day	*M. marinum*
Erythromycin	250-, 500-mg tabs 250, 500 mg/mL suspensions	40 PO in 4 doses; max: 4g/day	*M. fortuitum, M. chelonae*
Ethambutol	100-, 400-mg tabs	15-20 PO in 1 dose; max: 1g/day	*M. kansasii, M. marinum, M. xenopi, M. ulcerans, M. gordonae, M. avium* complex
Isoniazid	100-, 300-mg caps	10-20 PO in 1 dose; max: 300 mg/day	*M. kansasii, M. xenopi, M. gordonae*
Rifampin	150-, 300-mg caps	10-20 PO in 1 dose; max: 600 mg/day	*M. kansasii, M. xenopi, M. marinum, M. ulcerans, M. gordonae, M. avium* complex
Streptomycin	1-, 4-g vials	20-40 IM in 1 dose; max: 1g/day	*M. avium* complex
Trimethoprim-sulfamethoxazole (TMP) TMP suspension	80-, 160-mg tabs 40 mg/5 mL	8-20 mg of TMP PO in 2 doses; max: 2 g/day	*M. marinum, M. fortuitum, M. chelonae, M. ulcerans*

IM, Intramuscular; *IV*, intravenous; *PO*, orally; *TMP*, trimethoprim.

Because *M. kansasii* is rarely a contaminant, all patients from whom *M. kansasii* is isolated in respiratory secretions should be considered to have disease and treated accordingly. There have been no randomized controlled trials of treatment for disease caused by *M. kansasii*. There have been, however, several retrospective and prospective studies of various treatment regimens.[9] A key drug for successful treatment has been rifampin. The current recommendation for treatment of pulmonary disease caused by *M. kansasii* is a regimen of INH, rifampin, and ethambutol given daily for at least 12 months after the sputum culture has become negative. Clarithromycin also can be used in multidrug regimens. Although pyrazinamide is used commonly for the treatment of tuberculosis, all isolates of *M. kansasii* are resistant to it. The use of intermittent drug regimens or shorter courses has not been adequately studied to permit their recommendation. Untreated strains of *M. kansasii* are always susceptible to rifampin, INH, ethambutol, and streptomycin. Because the concentrations of drugs used in susceptibility testing were chosen for their usefulness with *M. tb* and not *M. kansasii*, some *M. kansasii* isolates may be reported to be resistant to streptomycin or INH. However, these isolates are susceptible to slightly higher drug concentrations, and laboratory reports showing resistance to the lower concentrations have no clinical or therapeutic significance as long as a rifampin-containing regimen is being used.

Recommended regimens for treatment of MAC pulmonary disease are based entirely on results of clinical trials in adults.[185] The traditional recommendation for initial therapy of patients with MAC pulmonary disease was a 4-drug regimen consisting of INH, rifampin, ethambutol, and streptomycin. The usual recommendation for duration of therapy for the oral drugs was 18 to 24 months and for at least 12 months after sputum cultures became negative.

The advent of the macrolides, clarithromycin and azithromycin, and the successful use of these drugs for treatment of disseminated MAC infection in patients with AIDS have led to their use in the treatment of pulmonary MAC disease in patients without AIDS. Preliminary results of several trials have shown that substituting clarithromycin for INH in an initial three-drug regimen (streptomycin or amikacin is given only when cavitary or advanced disease caused by MAC is present) leads to a more rapid conversion of sputum to negative and higher cure and lower relapse rates. Resistance to clarithromycin emerges rapidly if the drug is used alone, but it does not occur frequently when combined with other drugs. Most experts now recommend inclusion of clarithromycin in the initial regimen for pulmonary disease due to MAC; the most commonly used other drugs are rifampin and ethambutol. It is not yet known if the inclusion of clarithromycin in the initial regimen leads to a shorter necessary total length of therapy, and treatment for at least 12 months after sputum cultures become negative is recommended. Although there is only anecdotal information available for treatment of MAC pulmonary infections in children, the regimens used in adults seem to be effective in children.

Treatment of deep-seated infections due to the rapidly growing mycobacteria can be especially difficult. There have been no randomized clinical trials of various combinations of antibiotics. Most treatment is based on susceptibility testing of the specific isolate because susceptibility patterns vary greatly even within a species.

The most commonly used drugs include amikacin, cefoxitin, azithromycin, doxycycline, linezolide, sulfonamides, and clarithromycin. Successful treatment of disease due to *M. fortuitum* often can be accomplished with chemotherapy alone. The adult patients with *M. abscessus* infection who were cured usually received amikacin and cefoxitin or imipenem for 1 to 3 months followed by surgical excision.

Unlike tuberculosis, NTM infections of the lungs in adults often require resectional surgery for complete cure, particularly infections caused by *M. abscessus*.[186] Even with optimal chemotherapy, eradication of the organism cannot be achieved in some patients. A combined approach with an initial period of chemotherapy to contain the infection followed by resectional surgery and a more prolonged course of chemotherapy leads to much higher cure rates. This is difficult surgery and it is important that the thoracic surgeon has some experience. There are no published guidelines about the need for resectional surgery in children with NTM pulmonary infection. In several case reports, excision of endobronchial lesions has been accomplished during bronchoscopy, but resection of lung parenchyma has seldom been performed and does not appear to be necessary in most cases.

Prevention

Little is known about the prevention of NTM infection in any group of individuals. Because these organisms are ubiquitous in nature, it is impossible to prevent exposure to them except under the most extreme circumstances. There has been no recommendation about the use of chemotherapy to prevent NTM infection in patients with CF. Until the risk factors for acquisition of NTM by CF patients are better delineated, chemoprophylaxis will not be a part of the management of these patients.

Suggested Reading

American Thoracic Society. Diagnosis, treatment, and prevention of nontuberculous mycobacterial diseases. *Am J Respir Crit Care Med.* 2007;367–417.

Colditz GA, Brewer TF, Berkey CS, et al. Efficacy of BCG vaccine in the prevention of tuberculosis. Meta-analysis of the published literature. *JAMA.* 1994;271:698–702.

Comstock G. Epidemiology of tuberculosis. In: Reichman LB, Hershfield E, eds. *Tuberculosis: A Comprehensive International Approach.* 2nd ed. New York: Marcel Dekker, Inc; 2000:129–148.

Cruz AT, Ong LT, Starke JR. Mycobacterial infections in Texas children: a 5-year case series. *Pediatr Infect Dis J.* 2010;29:772–774.

Daniel T, Boom W, Ellner J. Immunology of tuberculosis. In: Reichman L, Hershfield E, eds. *Tuberculosis: A Comprehensive International Approach.* 2nd ed. New York: Marcel Dekker, Inc; 2000:187–214.

Marais BJ, Gie RP, Schaaf HS, et al. The natural history of childhood intra-thoracic tuberculosis: a critical review of literature from the prechemotherapy era. *Int J Tuberc Lung Dis.* 2004;8:392–402.

Nelson LJ, Schneider E, Wells CD, et al. Epidemiology of childhood tuberculosis in the United States, 1993–2001: the need for continued vigilance. *Pediatrics.* 2004;114:333–341.

O'Brien RJ, Geiter LJ, Snider Jr DE. The epidemiology of nontuberculous mycobacterial diseases in the United States. Results from a national survey. *Am Rev Respir Dis.* 1987;135:1007–1014.

Pediatric Tuberculosis Collaborative Group. Targeted tuberculin skin testing and treatment of latent tuberculosis infection in children and adolescents. *Pediatrics.* 2004;114:1175–1201.

Starke JR. Transmission of *Mycobacterium tuberculosis* to and from children and adolescents. *Semin Pediatr Infect Dis.* 2001;12:115–123.

References

The complete reference list is available online at www.expertconsult.com

34 THE MYCOSES

JOSEPH J. NANIA, MD, AND PETER F. WRIGHT, MD

ENDEMIC MYCOSES

Histoplasmosis

Histoplasmosis is a fungus found in soil that is a significant cause of pulmonary and systemic disease in the geographic regions in which it occurs. In the United States, this area is broadly defined as the basins of the Mississippi and Ohio Rivers and their tributaries. The disease is acquired by airborne or dust transmission and is seen more frequently in people living in rural areas. In such areas, the majority of adults, at least historically, have had evidence of exposure to the microbe.

In many ways the disease mimics tuberculosis in its pathogenesis and clinical manifestations.[1] It was originally described in military recruits from the south central United States who had x-ray films interpreted as consistent with tuberculosis but negative tuberculin tests.[2] The acquisition of histoplasmosis is most often asymptomatic. Symptomatic histoplasmosis involves four major clinical scenarios. In infants, there can be a disseminated disease with hepatosplenomegaly, anemia, and a picture clinically most analogous to leukemia.[3] In the 1940s to 1960s there was rarely a time that such children were not hospitalized at Vanderbilt, an institution closely associated with the initial recognition of the disease. Clearly, the disease is less common now and, when found, may be associated with disorders in the innate immune system.[4] The second presentation, which can occur in all ages but most commonly in childhood, is of acute histoplasmosis with fever and pulmonary symptoms.[5] One classical pulmonary sign is unilateral wheezing with radiographic evidence of compression of a bronchus. A third presentation is with diffuse fibrosis of the mediastinum, occasionally with pericardial involvement.[6] This can be a life-threatening disease that is difficult to approach clinically. A fourth presentation is of recrudescent disease in children and adults in the face of malignancy, acquired or congenital immunodeficiency, or immunosuppression.

Histoplasmosis—The Microbe

Histoplasma capsulatum is a dimorphic fungus with a mycelial phase at ambient temperature and a yeast phase at body temperature. It is acquired by inhalation of spores from the soil. In the respiratory tract, the organism assumes an oval- to pear-shaped yeast form in infected tissue that is distinctive (2- to 4-μm organisms often in clusters with a large vacuole and condensed protoplasm at one end of the cell) and seen primarily in cells of the reticuloendothelial system (Fig. 34-1E and F). It can be recovered from sputum and gastric washings, but samples obtained at bronchoscopy or surgical biopsy offer the best diagnostic option. Histoplasma in the disseminated form of the disease can sometimes be seen in cells of the monocyte lineage on a peripheral blood smear. *H. capsulatum* is slowly growing and can be isolated on Sabouraud dextrose agar or on an agar incorporating a beef heart infusion. It is identified as a white, fluffy mold that darkens in color with age. Microscopically, the mold has long slender hyphae with round smooth microconidia. With further incubation, the large 7- to 25-μm distinctive tuberculate macroconidia are usually seen. Polymerase chain reaction (PCR)–based diagnosis of culture extracts and from tissue has been introduced but is not widely available.[7,8] Molecular hybridization to identify the mycelial phase is routinely used in clinical microbiology labs.

Epidemiology

Acquisition is obviously governed by the geographic distribution of the fungus. Within a known area of histoplasmosis prevalence, specific scenarios can be elicited that point to the possibility of histoplasmosis acquisition. The well-recognized association of the disease with exposure to blackbird and starling roosts relates to the bird droppings forming a fertile environment for growth of the fungus. Other scenarios include nearby soil disruption for farming or construction, cleaning poultry houses, spelunking, and cutting decayed wood. Globally, there are reports of histoplasmosis from a number of Caribbean countries and South and Central America (Costa Rica, Jamaica, and Brazil). Its impact as a tropical disease, particularly in the context of acquired immunodeficiency syndrome (AIDS), is not well defined.

Pathogenesis

As indicated, the pathogenesis of the disease parallels that of tuberculosis. The initial focus is in the peripheral lung, where the spores are taken up by macrophages and begin to replicate in the nonimmune host. They probably disseminate before there is a systemic immune response because recrudescent disease in adults can present far from the respiratory tract, for example, as tongue ulcers or epididymal thickening. As in tuberculosis, there is early transport to regional lymph nodes with formation of a primary complex. During this time, there may be persistent fever; respiratory symptoms; and, as the regional lymph nodes enlarge, compression of the major airways or pulmonary vessels. This is largely a tissue reaction to the microbe that may rarely progress to a diffuse fibrosis. Occasionally, if the initial inoculum is very large, there is diffuse pneumonia and, with resolution, a lung with a radiographic appearance resembling buckshot with multiple calcifications.

Clinical Manifestations

Pulmonary Histoplasmosis

The presenting signs in patients with acute histoplasmosis include fever, cough, and chest pain. The duration of fever is impressive, with over one half of the patients in a series

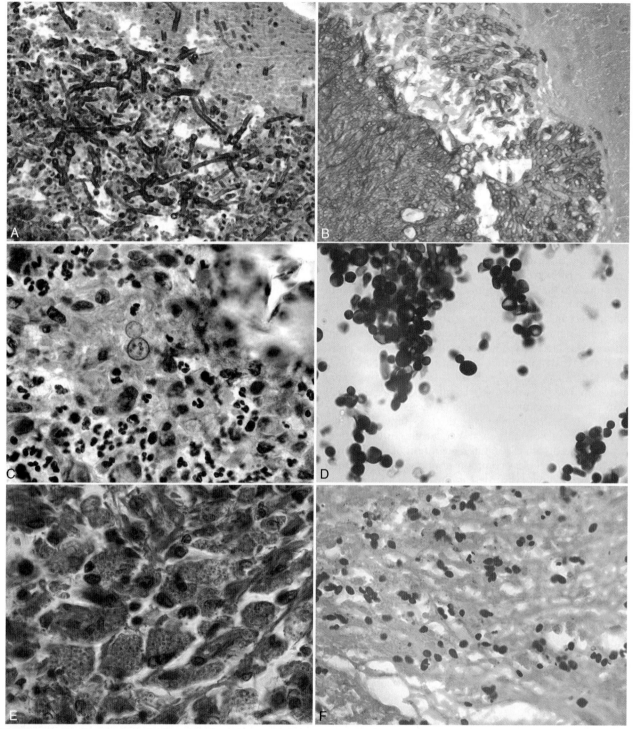

FIGURE 34-1. Panels showing the typical morphology of invasive aspergillosis (**A** and **B**), blastomycosis (**C** and **D**), and histoplasmosis (**E** and **F**). **A, C,** and **E,** Hematoxolyn and eosin. **B, D,** and **F,** Gomori's methenamine silver stain.

from Vanderbilt having fever of more than 2 weeks' duration.[5] On auscultation, more than 50% had wheezing that was often unilateral. The radiologic picture of acute histoplasmosis is well defined (Fig. 34-2A).[9] The diagnostic dilemma when there is mediastinal adenopathy is to distinguish it from lymphoma or tuberculosis (Fig. 34-2B).[10] Bronchial or vascular compression is best defined by a computed tomography (CT) scan (see Fig. 34-2B). Pericarditis can be appreciated by an enlarged cardiac silhouette. On

resolution of disease, there is often residual calcification. Pericardial involvement is seen, though not commonly. The fluid in these cases is often serosanguinous.

Acute Disseminated Histoplasmosis

There is an impression that disseminated histoplasmosis is on the decline. There were only 2 occurrences after 1970 in a series of 19 cases reported from Memphis.[3] Between 1932 and 1978 there were 84 cases of disseminated

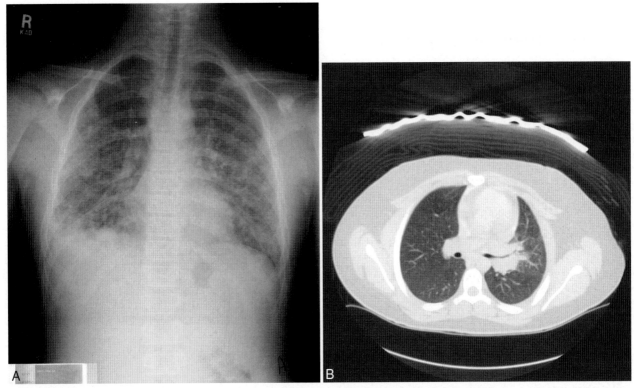

FIGURE 34-2. **A,** Chest x-ray in acute histoplasmosis showing a diffuse interstitial process. **B,** Cross-sectional CT with narrowing of the right main stem bronchus attributable to hilar adenopathy in histoplasmosis.

histoplasmosis documented at Vanderbilt.[5] In the following 30 years, there were less than a handful of cases. In the recent cases, we have had a child who clearly had an immune defect and another instance in which both a father and his daughter were hospitalized as neonates with disseminated histoplasmosis strongly indicative of a genetic predisposition. There are descriptions that histoplasmosis along with other granulomatous diseases may be associated with the delivery of tumor necrosis factor (TNF) antagonists, particularly infliximab (Remicade), a monoclonal antibody directed against TNF.[11] Inherited defects in innate immunity associated with granulomatous disease also are being described.[4] Disseminated histoplasmosis has been described as the presenting symptom in pediatric human immunodeficiency virus (HIV) infection[12] and in adult disease.[13]

Fibrosing Mediastinitis

Mediastinal disease in childhood differs from that in adults. In childhood, mediastinal involvement is an acute adenopathy. In the Vanderbilt experience, surgical intervention can be successful in relieving bronchial compression. In adults and occasionally older children, the diffuse fibrosis is a late complication of histoplasmosis and has no evidence of continued active replication of histoplasmosis.[6] Patients present with pulmonary ischemia and infarction with arterial involvement, pulmonary edema with venous involvement and hemoptysis, and hypoxemia with bronchial obstruction. There is little evidence of ongoing infection, and the surgical approach is extremely difficult because of loss of surgical

planes and little hope of relieving the vascular or bronchial compression. Steroids and other anti-inflammatories have no role, and until recently, there have been few options as vascular and airway compression set in. A recent promising development has been the insertion of stents in the pulmonary veins and/or arteries as described by Doyle and colleagues.[14] No effective way of relieving bronchial compression has yet been described. The description of a calcium-binding protein in histoplasmosis is proposed to contribute to the calcification of many older lesions.

Chronic Disseminated Histoplasmosis

The recrudescence of histoplasmosis is well recognized in adults with age, malignancy, or immunosuppression. Histoplasmosis is well recognized as confounding the diagnosis and care of pediatric patients with malignancy. St. Jude Children's Research Hospital has reported the largest series of histoplasmosis in the setting of malignancy.[15] These included cases of acute pulmonary disease,[10] disseminated disease,[15] and acute pulmonary disease mimicking malignancy.[10,15]

Rarer Clinical Presentations

Involvement of a number of organ systems besides the lung has been described in histoplasmosis. Joint involvement is seen in approximately 10% of cases of histoplasmosis and may be accompanied by erythema nodosum. Pericarditis is recognized both during the acute disease and as a complication of the fibrotic progression of the disease. Adrenal calcification and insufficiency can be seen. In AIDS, central nervous system (CNS) disease is seen frequently. Ocular involvement is described but uncommon. Transplacental transmission has been reported.

Diagnosis

The diagnosis of histoplasmosis is problematic. An intradermal skin test was available, and in the pediatric population, seemed very useful. A positive test read in a manner analogous to a tuberculin test was indicative of exposure. In an urban population in Nashville, a positive test was rarely (1 in 187 children tested) observed in children under 5 years of age. In contrast, it was positive in 22 of 23 children with documented histoplasmosis in an earlier pediatric series from Vanderbilt.[5] The skin test was taken off the market because of the high rate of positivity seen in adults from rural areas—for example, 80% positivity in naval recruits from middle Tennessee. This led to concerns that it was not indicative of current or recent infection and hence of little diagnostic value, although quite the opposite may be true in the pediatric age range. There are continued reports of the utility of the test from other countries.

The serologic diagnosis of histoplasmosis is fraught with dangers. A test does not become positive until 2 to 6 weeks after infection. A positive test may reflect disease at any point during life. There is cross reaction with other fungal diseases (blastomycosis, coccidiomycosis, and paracoccidioidomycosis) and a background rate of positivity in unexposed people. Two different types of assays are available: an immunodiffusion test that measures H and M bands and a complement fixation test. In acute infection, the complement fixation test is the most sensitive, and in the immunodiffusion assay, M bands are more common than H bands. The complement fixation test is usually interpreted as being positive when the result exceeds a cutoff of 1:32. The complement fixation test has been helpful in the differential diagnosis of a mediastinal mass between lymphoma and histoplasmosis.[10] It is concerning that in the Vanderbilt series, there were a number of children with histologically proven histoplasmosis whose complement fixation serology was negative.[5]

A uniquely important test in disseminated disease is the *H. capsulatum* antigen assay. Antigen is most consistently detected in urine but also may be positive in serum or bronchial lavage fluid.[16] The antigen test is usually not positive in localized pulmonary disease, but in primary disseminated disease in childhood or in the face of immunosuppression, it is both a strong indicator of disease and a useful parameter to follow as a measure of response to and duration of therapy once treatment is undertaken.

The most reliable way of making a diagnosis of histoplasmosis is with tissue histology or culture of tissue. The sample is incubated for up to 6 weeks at 30° C in Sabouraud dextrose agar or brain-heart infusion agar. The diagnosis in the mycelial phase can be confirmed by molecular hybridization (Gen Probe, San Diego). Tissue samples also should be stained using Grocott-Gomori methenamine–silver nitrate stain. The organism occasionally can be seen in the peripheral blood using a Wright-Giemsa stain in disseminated disease. In tissue, *H. capsulatum* has a narrow-necked budding yeast form in contrast to the broader-based blastomycosis (see Fig. 34-1*E* and *F*).

Treatment

Histoplasmosis in the normal host is usually a self-limited disease, and there are few indications for treatment. With prolonged fever, radiographic evidence of a large inoculum, or bronchial compression, we have instituted treatment with oral itraconazole in a dose of 5 to 10 mg/kg/day for 4 to 6 weeks. The newer extended spectrum-azole antifungals (voriconazole, posaconazole) are active against histoplasma but have not been studied systematically. In disseminated disease, the use of amphotericin B remains the gold standard with prolonged therapy to a total dose of 30 to 35 mg/kg over 2 to 3 months. Liposomal amphotericin has been shown to be comparable and less toxic though more expensive.[17] With AIDS, continued suppressive therapy with itraconazole is used, although recent evidence suggests it can ultimately be stopped.[13] As indicated, the urine histoplasma antigen if initially positive can be used to monitor the response to antifungal therapy, and treatment should be continued until the antigen is below the lower limit of detection. General recommendations for treatment of histoplasmosis in adults have been published by the Infectious Disease Society of America[18] and for all fungal infections by the American Thoracic Society.[19] Though primarily for adults, they form the best critical assessment of therapy for the pediatric patient as well.

Coccidioidomycosis

Coccidioidomycosis,[20] also referred to as "valley fever," is a disease caused by two closely related fungal species, *Coccidioides immitis* and *Coccidioides posadasii*. It is confined largely to parts of the southwestern United States. Geographically, infection is seen in regions of low rainfall, high summer heat, and alkaline soil. This defines its distribution in the central valleys of California, Arizona, New Mexico, and adjacent parts of Mexico. Coccidioides species are dimorphic fungi. In nature and in culture, the fungus grows in its mycelial form initially, eventually developing arthrospores or arthroconidia within the hyphae. These barrel-shaped spores serve as the infectious portion of the organism when they break off, become airborne, and are inhaled to the alveolar spaces of the lungs. Once in the lungs, the organism grows into larger round forms called spherules, which are the unique form seen in clinical specimens from infected patients. The spherules eventually rupture, releasing endospores that spread the infection to adjacent tissue. Occasionally, growth in infected humans reverts to the mycelial form, but there is not person-to-person spread. In many of the endemic regions, skin test positivity exceeds 50%, and there is an estimated 3% risk of acquisition of infection per year. Outbreaks of coccidioidomycosis are seen in connection with dust storms; thus, although the largest number of arthrospores is found in the soil at the time of rain, the greatest at risk of acquisition of disease is in the dry, dusty seasons of the year.

The majority of those infected develop subclinical infection or a mild self-limited influenza-like illness. Pulmonary coccidioidomycosis develops in about a third. The illness is characterized by an incubation period of 7 to 21 days, after which is the onset of cough, chest pain, and fever. About one third of sufferers will have clinically significant shortness of breath, and constitutional signs and symptoms, such as fatigue and weight loss, occur commonly. Skin eruptions often accompany acute infection. Although most commonly a fine papular rash can be seen, other eruptions occur in classic presentations, such as so-called "desert rheumatism" consisting of fever, arthralgia, and erythema nodosum. The presence of erythema nodosum is correlated with a low risk of extrapulmonary dissemination of the infection. Also, a dramatic eruption similar to erythema multiforme can be seen with acute pulmonary infection, more often in children than adults. Extrapulmonary manifestations are relatively rare but can involve bones, skin, and the central nervous system. The most severe and recalcitrant manifestation is meningeal disease, which is seen in less than 1% of patients; however, clinicians should have a low threshold for evaluating for the presence of CNS disease. More chronic forms of pulmonary infection are seen, often without a primary infection having been recognized. Nodules, calcification, cavitary lesions, and bronchiectasis are all late features of pulmonary coccidioides infection. Hemoptysis may often be the only symptom of a pulmonary cavity from coccidioides infection.

The diagnosis of the disease is most often made with specific serologic tests, although in acute disease, serology cannot rule out infection. Antibody detection by enzyme immunoassay (EIA) is readily available, and the IgG assay is quite reliable. Unfortunately the EIA IgM is less reliable, with both false-positive and false-negative results occurring. Confirmation by immunodiffusion (which detects both IgM and IgG) and complement fixation (which provides an IgG titer) are available and highly accurate.[21] An EIA to detect coccidioides antigens in the urine of infected patients has been developed and may prove useful in diagnosing coccidioidomycosis in patients who may not produce coccidioides-specific antibodies. A small retrospective study of mostly immunocompromised patients found *C. antigenuria* in about 70% of patients with culture-proven infection, mostly of a severe nature. The assay proved to have a very high negative predictive value except in patients who had infections with another endemic mycosis.[22] In the hands of pathologists experienced with the disease, direct identification of the organism in its spherule form in biopsy tissue or alveolar lavage fluid is diagnostic. *Coccidioides* is a rapidly growing fungus, with visible colonies of the mold forming in 5 to 7 days; so if culture material from an affected site can be obtained, the likelihood of recovering the organism is high (with the notable exception of cerebrospinal fluid [CSF], which rarely is culture positive). Radiographic findings in pulmonary coccidioidomycosis are variable. Lobar, nodular, and patchy bronchopneumonic infiltrates are all seen in acute disease, with or without hilar lymphadenopathy and pleural effusion. Chronic findings include nodules and thin-walled cavities, both of which may be minimally symptomatic. Rarely, rupture of a cavity may lead to severe disease with pyopneumothorax.

Treatment is not indicated for all patients.[23] Patients at higher risk for severe or disseminated infection should be treated, including those with HIV, organ transplants, prolonged use of corticosteroids, use of TNF inhibitors, or who are pregnant. Treatment is strongly considered for those of African or Filipino descent, given much higher rates of disseminated infection as compared with Caucasians. In addition, those lacking specific risk factors with severe disease also should be treated. Suggested criteria to indicate severe disease include weight loss of at least 10%, persistent night sweats, pulmonary infiltrates involving both lungs or most of one lung, prominent hilar lymphadenopathy, symptoms persisting over 2 months, or a complement fixation titer of at least 1:16. Other nonimmunocompromised patients with acute infection can generally be followed clinically for resolution of clinical and radiographic findings in the year following diagnosis. Chronic asymptomatic nodules or cavities do not require treatment, but patients with hemoptysis or pain from a cavitary lesion may benefit from antifungal therapy. No studies demonstrate the superiority of any of the available antifungal agents over another. With severe disease, amphotericin B is considered the drug of first choice, but the organism is sensitive to azole antifungal agents, including fluconazole and itraconazole. Fluconazole is well tolerated, highly bioavailable when given orally, and has the added advantage of excellent meningeal penetration. It is often used as first-line treatment. Itraconazole is equally effective, perhaps more so for bony infection, but requires serum drug level monitoring because of unreliable absorption. Voriconazole and posaconazole are not approved for treatment of coccidioidomycosis, but they have *in vitro* activity and anecdotally have proven effective in cases of disease recalcitrant to older triazole antifungals. Echinocandin antifungal agents (e.g. caspofungin) are active in animal models of coccidioidomycosis, but they should not be used for treatment of patients routinely because of variable in vitro activity. Length of treatment for pulmonary coccidioidomycosis has not been studied, but when initiated, antifungals are usually continued for 6 to 12 months.[23]

Blastomycosis

Blastomycosis[24] is another disease caused by a dimorphic fungus that exists in nature in a mycelial form and converts to a yeast at body temperature. The disease has an endemic geographic localization rather similar to histoplasmosis. It is found in the Ohio River Valley, with disease reported along the borders of the Great Lakes and the St. Lawrence River. It appears to grow best in warm, moist soil with decaying organic matter but has been difficult to isolate from nature. Spelunking has been identified as a particular risk factor.

Blastomyces dermatitidis is almost always acquired as a pulmonary infection, but hematogenous spread is seen quite frequently with involvement of the skin, osseous structures, and genitourinary tract among the most common sites of extrapulmonary disease. Approximately 50% of presentations are with pulmonary disease and the rest with extrapulmonary manifestations. The presenting pulmonary lesion is most frequently as an alveolar infiltrate or mass lesion. The presenting picture also may be that of a persistent pneumonia with a productive cough similar to that seen in histoplasmosis. The skin manifestations can include verrucous lesions and ulcerated lesions with friable granulation tissue. The bony lesions appear as osteolytic lesions. Involvement of the genitourinary tract in the male is seen as a prostatitis or epididymitis. The disease is considered relatively rare in children but is certainly seen. The diagnosis is based on visualization of the yeast in smears and in tissue specimens or by culture (see Fig. 34-1C and D). Growth of the organism is achieved by culture of the mycelial form at 30° C, with a shift to 37° C being used to see the more distinctive yeast forms. There is no reliable serology. Positive tests have considerable cross reaction with histoplasmosis. There is not a reliable skin test.

Treatment of acute pulmonary blastomycosis is generally recommended, although spontaneous resolution is frequent.[25] Once blastomycosis becomes a chronic or extrapulmonary infection, treatment is clearly indicated. No large controlled trials of therapy have been done, but amphotericin B is the drug of choice in life-threatening infections and itraconazole is considered the optimal azole drug for therapy of less severe illness. The duration of therapy is recommended to be at least 6 months, and levels of itraconazole should be followed.

OPPORTUNISTIC PULMONARY FUNGAL INFECTIONS

Despite recent promising advances in diagnosis and treatment, fungal infections continue to be a major cause of morbidity and mortality in immunocompromised hosts. Children with altered immunity constitute a growing proportion of pediatric patients. Great improvements in survival of patients with malignancies and other life-threatening conditions have been achieved through increased use and maximized intensity of therapies, such as transplantation and cytotoxic chemotherapy, which lead to altered host immunity. Such therapies lead to suppression of function and numbers of lymphocytes and phagocytes. Susceptibility to opportunistic fungi is further increased in these patients by frequent use of broad-spectrum antibacterial agents, disruption of normal mucosal barriers to infection, and frequent need for indwelling catheters and invasive procedures. Although rates of perinatally acquired HIV/AIDS have fallen in the United States with improved screening of pregnant women and the widespread availability of highly active antiretroviral therapy, HIV/AIDS continues to be a global health crisis and a major cause of immunosuppression in children worldwide.

The lungs are frequent sites of infection in immunocompromised patients. The respiratory tract is the portal of entry for most of the fungi that cause invasive disease including the opportunistic mycoses. Pulmonary fungal infections require a high index of suspicion. As is the case with most pulmonary infections in children, radiographic patterns lack etiologic specificity, and microbiologic diagnosis is seldom made without the use of invasive procedures to obtain a culture. Procedures such as bronchoscopy and lung biopsy have to be carefully timed because they may become too risky because of rapid progression of underlying disease.

Aspergillosis—Invasive Pulmonary Disease

The inflammatory syndrome of allergic bronchopulmonary aspergillosis and the superinfection of preexisting lung lesions with *Aspergillus* spp., commonly referred to as an aspergilloma, occur in patients without impaired host defenses. The invasive forms of pulmonary aspergillosis, however, occur almost exclusively in immunocompromised hosts. Only the invasive form of infection will be discussed in this section.

Aspergillus—The Microbe

Aspergillus is a ubiquitous environmental mold that lives primarily in the soil and decomposing plant matter. Exposures as varied as proximity to hospital construction/renovation and marijuana smoking have been implicated as sources of infection with *Aspergillus*.[26,27] The infective components of the organism are conidia, which are readily aerosolized from the end of hyphal stalks. Inhalation and subsequent germination of conidia leads to the formation of hyphae in the distal airways. Next, hyphal forms invade pulmonary blood vessels and parenchyma, with resulting pathology characterized by thrombosis and ischemic necrosis of the affected lung (see Fig. 34-1A and B). This sequence of events necessary to the pathogenesis of invasive *Aspergillus* infection may occur over a highly variable period of time because the incubation period is estimated to be between 2 days and 3 months.[23] After invasion of pulmonary tissue, spread to contiguous thoracic structures or hematogenous dissemination may occur.

Of about 180 species in the *Aspergillus* genus, 5 account for the vast majority of invasive disease reported. *A. fumigatus* causes the majority of invasive disease and is the species about which the most is known in terms of virulence factors and host immune response.[28] *A. flavus* is the principal species found in sinusitis and accounts for up to 10% of all invasive isolates. *A. niger, A. terreus*, and *A. nidulans* are less common causes of invasive disease. *A. terreus* is resistant to amphotericin B, and infection is associated with high rates of mortality.[26] *A. nidulans* is uncommon in patients with hematologic malignancies but is well described as a cause of invasive infections in patients with chronic granulomatous disease.[29] The varying pathogenicities of different species are thought to be related to variables such as the ability to grow at 37° C; conidial size; growth rate; and the production of enzymes, toxins, and other virulence factors.[28]

Immunity

Innate immunity is clearly an important part of the defense against *Aspergillus*. Anatomic barriers, including an intact mucosa, bronchial mucus, surfactant, and ciliated respiratory epithelium, eliminate conidia and prevent their germination after inhalation. Alveolar macrophages are responsible for ingestion of conidia, although killing after ingestion appears to be slow and incomplete. Although neutrophils do have some activity against conidia as well, their primary role is in adherence to and damage of hyphae. Oxidants are certainly important in hyphal damage, but neutrophils also have nonoxidative factors that are thought to contribute to an effective response. It appears that complement and platelets also have a role in the response to *Aspergillus*, albeit not as well characterized as the role of phagocytes. Although studies in humans are lacking, there is evidence from animal models to suggest a role for both T-cell and humoral immunity. The clinical observation has been made that AIDS patients without neutropenia or predisposing therapies such as corticosteroids are at risk for invasive aspergillosis, but whether or not impaired T-cell immunity is the key in the pathogenesis of invasive aspergillosis in these patients remains unclear.[28]

Predisposing Factors

The risk for developing invasive aspergillosis (IA) is associated with several immunocompromising conditions and therapies. The most common predisposing situations are neutropenia, corticosteroid therapy, cytotoxic chemotherapy, broad-spectrum antibiotics, and acute leukemia. A large multicenter review of 595 patients with IA reported the proportion of cases with various underlying diagnoses. Bone marrow transplant (BMT) was the diagnosis in 32% of patients, leukemia or lymphoma in 29%, solid-organ transplant in 9%, AIDS in 8%, solid-organ tumor in 4%, chronic granulomatous disease in 2%, and unspecified pulmonary or other miscellaneous underlying conditions in 14%. Only 2% had no identifiable predisposing risk factors.[30] In a more recent retrospective study comprised entirely of pediatric patients with invasive aspergillosis, underlying conditions were similar, although leukemia (63%) and chronic granulomatous disease (5%) accounted for larger proportions.[31] Among patients who have received BMT, IA occurs in roughly 5% to 10% of patients and is the leading cause of death. Recipients of allogeneic BMT were not neutropenic at the time of diagnosis of IA in 72% of cases in one large series.[32] Other risk factors for invasive disease in BMT included underlying diagnosis of hematologic malignancy, graft-versus-host disease, and corticosteroid therapy.

Whereas many patients with cancer undergo chemotherapy with cytotoxic agents, have periods of neutropenia, and receive broad-spectrum antibiotics, patients with leukemia carry a high risk of developing IA as a result of both the greater intensity of these factors in comparison with patients with other tumors and malignant transformation of immune cells. Patients with other tumors carry a lower risk of IA.

The risk of IA in recipients of solid-organ transplants varies depending on the type of transplant. Lung and heart transplant recipients have higher risks, with reported prevalence of 8.4% and 6.2%, respectively. Prevalence estimates in other organ transplants are lower: 1.7%, liver; 1.0%, pancreas; and 0.7%, kidney.[33] Precise rates specific to pediatric solid-organ transplant patients are not known.

Although later cases do occur, the period of 1 to 6 months after solid-organ transplantation is the time of highest risk of IA. Other than type of transplant and timing, risk factors in these patients include cytomegalovirus infection, smoking, poor graft function, and renal failure requiring hemodialysis. Receipt of the monoclonal antilymphocyte agent OKT3 is also identified as a risk factor.[33]

As mentioned earlier, HIV-infected patients are known to be at risk for IA. Although most cases occur in the setting of advanced AIDS, the well-known risk factors for IA are not consistently present. In one retrospective review of mostly adult HIV-infected patients with pulmonary IA, only 24% of patients had documented absolute neutrophil counts under 500/mm.[3,34] All patients with IA for whom clinical information was available, however, had other risk factors or comorbidities that have been proposed as predisposing to IA. Corticosteroids were being used in 15%, broad-spectrum antibiotics in 15%, and chemotherapy in 13%. Comorbid conditions included cytomegalovirus (63%), *Pneumocystis jiroveci* (previously *P. carinii*) (28%), bacterial and/or other fungal pneumonias (20%), lymphoma (13%), Kaposi sarcoma (10%), and atypical mycobacterial infection (10%).[33]

In a review of 473 HIV-infected children followed in the pediatric branch of the National Cancer Institute from 1987 to 1995, IA was diagnosed in 1.5% of patients.[35] Although five of the seven patients were neutropenic in the 4 weeks preceding diagnosis, two patients had no well-established risk factors. One of the two non-neutropenic patients had concurrent varicella and a history of lymphoid interstitial and recurrent bacterial pneumonia. The other had no comorbidities other than HIV infection.

Aspergillus infection is well described in premature neonates. In addition to commonly possessing risk factors such as therapy with broad-spectrum antibiotics and corticosteroids, low birth weight neonates have immature phagocyte and cellular immune function and often have compromised skin barrier function due to prematurity.[36,37] *Aspergillus* organisms more commonly gain entry in these patients via the skin and mucous membranes than is seen in other patient populations. Associations with *Aspergillus* infection in neonates include skin maceration from adhesive tape or venous arm boards, percutaneous catheter insertion sites, and necrotizing enterocolitis, all reflecting mucocutaneous portals of entry.[36,37] Although primary cutaneous aspergillosis occurs in neonates, IA with cutaneous dissemination is described, as is primary invasive pulmonary disease. A high index of suspicion for aspergillosis is necessary in these patients because diagnosis has commonly been made only after death.[36]

Of primary immunodeficiencies, chronic granulomatous disease has the best-characterized association with IA. There is a 33% lifetime risk of IA in chronic granulomatous disease.[38] Although *A. fumigatus* is the most common cause, *A. nidulans* occurs with unusually high frequency, was more likely to be fatal than *A. fumigatus*, and is rarely seen in patients without chronic granulomatous disease.[29] Severe combined immune deficiency is the other primary immunodeficiency for which the risk of IA is known to be significant. IA occurs in about 4% of severe combined immune deficiency patients and is usually fatal.[39]

Of immunosuppressive medications, corticosteroids are the agents whose administration is most clearly a risk factor for developing IA. Although the mechanisms are still incompletely understood, steroids have been shown to impair the anticonidial activity of macrophages and suppress neutrophils, both in recruitment and antifungal activity.[28] Steroids also are known to directly increase the growth rate of *A. fumigatus* and *A. flavus*. Less is known about the risk for IA conferred by immunosuppressant medications, such as cyclosporine A and tacrolimus, which act through the calcineurin pathway. Interestingly, these agents have been shown to enhance the effects of several antifungal medications in vitro, but the clinical implications of this observation remain to be seen.[40] Newer immunomodulating drugs with indications primarily for autoimmune diseases such as Crohn's and rheumatoid arthritis are known to predispose to a number of infections. Pulmonary aspergillosis has been reported in patients taking etanercept and infliximab, medications that interfere with the action of TNFs.[40,41] Further experience with these and similar immunosuppressive drugs will be needed to define[42] more precisely the risk of IA during therapy.

Clinical Presentation

Invasive aspergillosis can be classified into four clinical presentations: pulmonary aspergillosis, tracheobronchitis, rhinosinusitis, and disseminated disease.[26] Of these forms, pulmonary aspergillosis is the most common. In a study of aspergillosis in children with cancer, 70% of the 66 children with culture-proven disease had lung involvement.[43] In children with either chronic granulomatous disease or HIV/AIDS, pulmonary disease is also the most common manifestation.[35,38] Invasive pulmonary aspergillosis (IPA) has protean manifestations, presenting as hemorrhagic infarction, lobar pneumonia, lung abscess, solitary or multiple nodules, or pleural-based disease with effusion. The presenting symptoms are often nonspecific as well, with the most common complaints being fever, cough, and dyspnea. Findings that are more concerning for the diagnosis (albeit still not pathognomonic) are pleuritic chest pain and hemoptysis, both of which occur in the minority of patients with IPA.

Aspergillus tracheobronchitis associated with pseudomembrane formation and/or necrosis is a well-described entity in adults with HIV/AIDS, BMT, and lung transplant. This entity is thought to occur less commonly in children with the same underlying diagnoses.[44] The clinical presentation varies from hemoptysis, wheezing, and obstruction, or fever and cough to a lack of symptoms with findings on bronchoscopy.

Diagnosis

Diagnosis of IA is proven only by biopsy and culture. Morphologic identification of the mold in culture of tissue from a sterile site is definitive evidence, but microscopic morphology cannot identify the fungal species. Several genera of hyaline molds can have hyphae that resemble *Aspergillus*. Visualization of tissue-invasive hyphal forms typical of the mold in conjunction with positive culture from the same organ (e.g., lung tissue and culture of airway secretions) is also considered proof of aspergillosis

(see Fig. 34-1*A* and *B*).[43] When lung biopsy is performed, tissue from both the peripheral and central areas of the affected lung should be sampled.[44] Thoracoscopic biopsy for diagnosis of IPA has not been systematically studied in children but has been reported. Given that biopsy is often not possible in patients at risk for aspergillosis as a result of thrombocytopenia and other conditions related to their underlying diseases, alternate methods of diagnosis are often relied on.

The radiographic appearance of IPA is variable. Plain chest radiographs yield nonspecific findings: segmental consolidation, multilobar consolidation, perihilar infiltrates, pleural effusions, and/or nodular lesions.[45] The latter is more highly suggestive of fungal disease. Since plain radiographs can be completely normal in up to 10% of patients with IPA, CT is the imaging of choice for early diagnosis. Classic CT findings of the "halo sign" (distinct nodular lesion with surrounding area of decreased attenuation) and the "air crescent sign" (a late finding of nodular cavitation, usually occurring after recovery of neutrophil counts) appear to be less common in children with IPA than adults.[31,46] However, the presence of these findings is highly suggestive of the diagnosis of aspergillosis or other invasive mold infection.

Despite the angioinvasive nature of *Aspergillus* spp., positive blood cultures for the mold are rarely reported in IA. However, detection of galactomannan, a polysaccharide cell wall antigen of *Aspergillus* spp., in blood has been used in Europe and Canada for years in the diagnosis of IA and was approved for use in the United States in 2003. The antigen is detected by a double-sandwich enzyme-linked immunosorbent assay that recognizes circulating galactomannan in patients with IA. In some series, the sensitivity and specificity of the assay has been high, and detection of galactomannan has preceded the radiologic findings by 8 or 9 days in patients with IA. The sensitivity was 81% and the specificity was 89% in studies that led to Food and Drug Administration approval in the United States.[47] The galactomannan assay is best validated in neutropenic patients with hematologic malignancy, its sensitivity is significantly lower in other populations.[48] Although data are limited, poor sensitivity and positive predictive value have been documented in children.[48] Variables such as cutoff values for positivity, specimen treatment, preceding antifungal treatment, pretest probability of IA based on risk factors, and false-positive results in patients receiving piperacillin/tazobactam are thought to contribute to variability of results.[49] A number of assays (Fungitell and Fungitec) have been developed to detect another component of the fungal cell wall, (1-3)-β-D-glucan (BDG). As a nonspecific marker of invasive fungal infections, BDG assays have varying predictive values in studies of adult patients. However, the assay does not distinguish between the many fungi that contain BDG (*Aspergillus,* other molds, *Candida, Pneumocystis*), and performance of the assays in pediatric patients is largely unknown.[46] Diagnostic definitions have been proposed for IA, which include clinical, radiographic and microbiologic criteria to define the probability of IA in patients with hematologic malignancy.[50]

Detection of *Aspergillus* spp. in respiratory tract secretions has been used as a surrogate method of diagnosis in patients at risk for aspergillosis with clinical and radiographic findings consistent with the diagnosis. Both direct examination for hyphal elements (via staining with calcofluor or methenamine silver) and fungal culture should be performed on respiratory specimens. Although a negative culture of sputum or bronchoalveolar lavage fluid cannot rule out the diagnosis, a positive culture in a neutropenic or BMT patient with new pulmonary infiltrates is putative evidence of IPA.[51] In solid-organ transplant patients, non-neutropenic patients with chronic lung disease, and HIV-infected patients, however, the positive predictive value of respiratory tract cultures is much lower. Detection of *Aspergillus* spp. in bronchoalveolar lavage fluid by both galactomannan assay and PCR technology has been studied, but the precise role of these techniques in diagnosis remains to be seen. A pediatric study showed the galactomannan assay used on BAL fluid had a sensitivity of 78% and specificity of 100% for pulmonary aspergillosis in 85 children, 59 of whom were immunocompromised.[52] Bronchoalveolar lavage fluid PCR for *Aspergillus* spp. is prone to contamination by virtue of the ubiquitous nature of fungal conidia, and clinical performance of this test is not well validated.

Treatment and Prognosis

For over 40 years, amphotericin B was recommended as primary therapy for IA.[53] The toxicities of amphotericin B are well known, with nephrotoxicity being the most common dose-limiting side effect. Additionally, amphotericin B has only had modest success historically in the treatment of IA. Overall response rates to amphotericin B have been estimated at 55% and less than 40% in severely immunosuppressed patients.[30] Mortality with amphotericin B as sole therapy for IA was 65% in one large retrospective review.[30] Although the newer lipid formulations of amphotericin B offer reduced toxicity, they provide no proven increase in efficacy relative to the parent compound, amphotericin B deoxycholate.

Approved in an oral formulation in 1992, itraconazole was the first triazole antifungal with a spectrum of activity that included *Aspergillus* spp. and other filamentous fungi. Retrospective review has shown response rates to itraconazole, both as primary therapy and after an initial course of amphotericin B, to be better than those of amphotericin B as the sole therapy.[36] However, the number of severely immunosuppressed patients in the amphotericin B–treated group was markedly higher than those treated with itraconazole, probably reflecting the unwillingness of clinicians to use a relatively unproven new therapy on their patients at highest risk. Although itraconazole is certainly less toxic than amphotericin B, the dependence of oral absorption of itraconazole capsules on a low gastric pH limits its use in some patients. The availability of an oral solution of itraconazole with higher bioavailability and an intravenous formulation of the medication has circumvented this problem; however, the development and approval of other new antifungal agents that are effective against *Aspergillus* spp. have relegated itraconazole to a minor position in the treatment of aspergillosis.

In 2002, voriconazole was approved for use in the United States. It possesses broad activity against most *Aspergillus* spp. (including species such as *A. terreus* and *A. nidulans,* against which amphotericin B has been ineffective) and is available in both intravenous and highly bioavailable oral formulations. Shortly after approval of voriconazole, a landmark randomized comparative study, in 277 patients 12 years or older (including 240 patients with IPA), was published that established the agent as the treatment of choice for IA.[54] Compared with amphotericin B deoxycholate as primary therapy of IA, voriconazole showed a significantly higher rate of successful outcomes (52.8% vs. 31.6%), higher rates of survival (70.8% vs. 57.9%), and lower toxicity. Although no randomized trials have been published in pediatric patients, review of experience at the National Cancer Institute using voriconazole on a compassionate release basis offers the largest published series of children in whom the drug has been used. In the treatment of pediatric patients refractory to or intolerant of standard antifungal therapy given for aspergillosis and other invasive fungal infections, voriconazole was well tolerated and produced relatively satisfactory outcomes.[55] Posaconazole, another triazole antifungal, was approved in 2006 for the prevention of fungal infections in immunocompromised patients 13 years of age or older. It possesses potent anti-*Aspergillus* activity, and is expected to be effective for treatment of IA, as demonstrated in an open-label study of posaconazole for salvage therapy.[56]

Caspofungin acetate was approved for use in 2001 for salvage therapy of IA. It is the first echinocandin antifungal approved for use in the United States, and the mechanism of action targets the synthesis of β-1,3-D-glucan, an essential part of the fungal cell wall. Micafungin was approved in the United States in 2005 and anidulafungin in 2006, both for treatment of candidiasis, although both have activity against *Aspergillus* spp. that is similar to caspofungin. All echinocandin agents are available only for intravenous administration and have not been studied adequately to recommend them as an initial single-agent therapy for aspergillosis.[57]

Combination therapy for IA with previously listed agents and other antifungal agents such as 5-flucytosine has not been evaluated in randomized studies. *In vitro* and animal studies show promise for improved efficacy of a combination of an echinocandin and either a broad-spectrum triazole or amphotericin B in the treatment of IA. In a retrospective study of 47 patients with IA after cancer chemotherapy or BMT, patients receiving the combination of voriconazole and caspofungin for salvage therapy had a lower rate of mortality than historical controls who received voriconazole only.[58] A number of other similarly designed small studies have shown no clear benefit to combination therapy with echinocandins for IA.[59,60] Other than these small, nonrandomized studies, there are only anecdotal reports to support use of such combinations. Further investigations are needed before such combination therapy can be recommended.[53,61] Despite this lack of evidence, combination therapy has become the standard at some centers for initial therapy of IA.

Therapeutic surgical excision of IPA has been advocated by some for debulking of primary lesions and preventing disseminated infection or pulmonary hemorrhage. One retrospective review of 43 pediatric patients with IPA, most of whom were highly immunosuppressed, found a significantly higher survival rate in the 18 patients who underwent surgical intervention compared with those who received medical therapy only.[61] The retrospective nature of the study, high overall mortality rate in the series (91%), and limitations of medical therapy available at the time of the study (i.e., before approval of voriconazole) make it difficult to know if such findings can be generalized to current care. Although evidence is lacking, surgical resection of pulmonary aspergillosis is often performed in patients about to undergo stem cell transplantation, anticipating further immunosuppression afforded by conditioning regimens with possible progression of infection.

Adjunctive therapies such as colony-stimulating factors, interferon gamma (INF-γ), and infusions of granulocytes harvested from donors pretreated with granulocyte colony-stimulating factor (GCSF) have promise in the treatment of aspergillosis. Although these modalities have not yet been well studied, experience with certain patient populations has led to recommendations for their use. In severely neutropenic patients, GCSF and granulocyte transfusions can be considered as adjunct treatments for IA. In patients with CGD and IA, INF-γ is suggested.[50]

Optimal length of medical therapy for any form of IA, including pulmonary disease, is not known. Recommendations stress the need to determine length of treatment based on clinical and radiographic resolution of the disease, combined with consideration of the underlying immunosuppressive condition and the likelihood of its improvement or resolution.[50]

Cryptococcosis

Cryptococcosis—The Microbe

Cryptococcus neoformans var. *neoformans* and the related species, *C. neoformans* var. *gattii*, are encapsulated yeasts that have a worldwide distribution. Although *Cryptococcus* has been isolated from soil, trees, and fruit, there has long been recognition of a unique role of dried pigeon droppings as a naturally occurring culture medium for *Cryptococcus*.[62] Desiccated *C. neoformans* yeast and basidiospores from the organism's sexual state *(Filobasidiella neoformans)* are both about 2 μm. This size makes aerosolization and alveolar deposition the probable route of infection in humans. After inhalation, the organism initially grows in the alveoli without significant inflammatory response, probably because of the antiphagocytic effect of the polysaccharide capsule. Before development of cellular immunity, *C. neoformans* disseminates widely, most commonly manifesting as meningitis or parenchymal brain infection.[63] The reason for the tropism of *C. neoformans* for the CNS is not known.

Immunity

Cellular immunity is generally agreed to be the most important component of an effective immune response to *C. neoformans*. Pathologically, this is demonstrated by the formation of granulomatous inflammation in response to infection. T cells activate alveolar macrophages via cytokines such as INF-γ and promote transformation of macrophages into giant cells that are able to ingest the encapsulated yeast.[63] Humoral immunity plays a role in opsonization, activation of natural killer cells, and clearing of capsular polysaccharide. Although natural killer cells, neutrophils, and eosinophils are all thought to contribute to the immune response, patients with isolated defects in any of these components of immunity are not thought to be predisposed to symptomatic cryptococcosis. In contrast, conditions associated with defective cellular immunity are associated with an increase in symptomatic cryptococcal infections.

AIDS is clearly the underlying condition with which cryptococcosis has been seen most often and remains an AIDS-defining illness in HIV-infected persons. CD4+ lymphocyte counts are often fewer than 100 cells/μL. In adults with AIDS, *C. neoformans* disease occurs in about 5% of patients annually, but in children with AIDS, a considerably lower rate, not quite 1%, has been reported.[65] Reasons for the lower incidence in children with AIDS are not known, but it is not thought to be due to differential exposure to the organism.[66] In the pre-AIDS era, symptomatic cryptococcosis was a rare condition, occurring in less than one per million persons per year in the United States.[67] At that time, high-risk patients were those with defects in cellular immunity—patients with malignancies, particularly Hodgkin's disease and other hematologic cancers, and recipients of organ transplants. *C. neoformans* infection is also reportedly associated with sarcoidosis, diabetes mellitus, hyper–immunoglobulin M (IgM) syndrome, and hyper-IgE syndrome.[63] Disease due to *Cryptococcus gattii* in the Pacific Northwestern United States and adjacent parts of Canada in recent years has occurred more often in normal hosts.[68]

Clinical Manifestations

Although it is commonly thought of as an opportunistic infection that affects immunocompromised patients, particularly those with AIDS, *C. neoformans* infection may occur most commonly as subclinical or mild pulmonary disease in normal hosts. Evidence from a series of pediatric patients with pulmonary cryptococcosis[67] and a serologic survey of healthy urban children[66] support this notion. Cough, chest pain, and fever are common presenting complaints for symptomatic individuals. An isolated pulmonary nodule may be the only manifestation in immunocompetent individuals, at times associated with hilar adenopathy, but masslike and consolidative lesions with a particular predilection for the lower lobes also are well described.[63] Infections caused by *C. gattii* frequently affect normal hosts and the majority of cases described included either pneumonia or lung cryptococcoma as a clinical finding.[69]

Even in immunocompromised hosts, the pulmonary component of cryptococcosis may be mild or asymptomatic on presentation. Although the respiratory tract is the portal of entry for infection, it is estimated that less than 10% of patients with disseminated cryptococcosis have pulmonary symptoms at the time of diagnosis.[63] When symptoms are present, the presentation varies considerably, from a subacute cough with fever, chest pain, and weight loss, to rapidly progressive pulmonary disease with adult respiratory distress syndrome.[64] Highlighting the tendency for *C. neoformans* to disseminate, it is estimated that only about one third of HIV-negative patients with cryptococcosis have isolated pulmonary involvement.

Similarly, 90% of AIDS patients have concomitant meningitis or parenchymal brain lesions ("cryptococcomas") on presentation.[70] Virtually any organ can be infected in disseminated cryptococcosis, but in addition to the CNS, the skin, prostate, and eyes are particularly important sites of extrapulmonary infection. As with normal hosts, there is no typical radiographic pattern for pulmonary cryptococcal infection. Pulmonary nodules, mass lesions, lobar consolidations, and diffuse infiltrates with effusion have all been described in compromised patients.[71]

Diagnosis

Most clinical microbiology labs will not routinely identify *Cryptococcus* isolates to the species level. Although cultures may take up to a week to become positive, *Cryptococcus* spp. grow on most clinical media, including standard radiometric blood culturing systems. However, in the diagnosis of pulmonary disease, both the sensitivity and specificity of cultures of respiratory secretions are questionable.[63] The majority of cryptococcal isolates from sputum are thought to represent colonization.[69] Conversely, isolation of the organism from blood, cerebrospinal fluid (CSF), or other sterile body sites is reasonably sensitive and would be putative evidence of pulmonary cryptococcosis when clinical or radiographic signs are suggestive. It is important to note, however, that in immunocompromised hosts, other pulmonary (and nonpulmonary) opportunistic infections may be present simultaneously. *Mycobacterium tuberculosis*, nontuberculous mycobacteria, cytomegalovirus, *Nocardia*, and *P. jiroveci* (formerly *P. carinii*) have all been reported as co-pathogens, highlighting the need for appropriate studies to rule out such diagnoses in severely compromised patients.[69] Direct histopathologic identification of *C. neoformans* from biopsy specimens is both sensitive and specific for the diagnosis of pulmonary infection. Several different stains can be used to identify the yeast in tissue, including the nonspecific Grocott-Gomori methenamine–silver nitrate and others such as mucicarmine, which stains the polysaccharide capsule red.[70] Additionally, a monoclonal antibody against the main capsular polysaccharide antigen (GXM) has been used for specific identification of the yeast in tissue.[70] In examination of CSF, India ink has long been used to identify *C. neoformans*. The sensitivity is about 80% for AIDS patients and 50% for non-AIDS patients with cryptococcal meningitis, and it has been used on other clinical specimens as well.[70]

Detection of the capsular polysaccharide of *C. neoformans* in blood or CSF by latex agglutination or enzyme immunoassay is a reliable method of diagnosing disseminated infection. For the diagnosis of cryptococcal meningitis, CSF antigen detection assays are at least 90% sensitive and specific. However, these techniques are thought to be less sensitive in the patient with isolated pulmonary cryptococcosis.[71]

Antibodies to *C. neoformans* can develop in response to either colonization or infection and are not useful in diagnosis.[63]

As previously described, imaging of the chest by plain radiograph and CT is not diagnostic. Isolated or multiple nodules, pulmonary masses, lobar consolidation, cavitary lesions, pleural effusion, diffuse interstitial infiltrates, and adult respiratory distress–like appearance have all been described with pulmonary cryptococcosis.[64] If signs of increased intracranial pressure or other signs suggestive of CNS infection are present, magnetic resonance imaging or CT of the head to rule out hydrocephalus and cryptococcomas is indicated.

Given the limitations of noninvasive methods, invasive procedures are often necessary to confirm the diagnosis of cryptococcosis, especially when involvement is limited to the lungs. Either fine-needle aspiration or biopsy may be required to confirm the diagnosis. When pleural effusions are present, cultures of thoracentesis fluid are positive in about 40% of AIDS patients.[69] Some authors have questioned the need for examination of spinal fluid in nonimmunocompromised patients with pulmonary cryptococcosis, no overt signs of CNS infection, and a negative serum antigen.[70] However, given the frequency of concomitant meningitis, lumbar puncture with measurement of opening pressure, CSF India ink preparation, a cryptococcal antigen assay, and routine studies are generally recommended.[70]

Treatment

Because there is a paucity of data in children, recommendations for treatment[70] of cryptococcosis are extrapolated from studies and recommendations in adult patients. For asymptomatic patients with normal immunity and a positive culture for *C. neoformans* from the respiratory tract, fluconazole for 6 to 12 months or no treatment at all are both reasonable options. For normal hosts with mild-to-moderate symptoms, fluconazole (either intravenous or oral) is recommended for a period of 6 to 12 months. If fluconazole cannot be used, itraconazole, voriconazole, and posaconazole are effective alternatives. Patients with severe symptoms and all immunocompromised patients should be treated as CNS cryptococcal infection would be. Based on relatively large studies in both HIV-negative and HIV-positive patients, the preferred regimen is amphotericin B plus flucytosine for 2 weeks (or until CSF cultures are negative) followed by fluconazole to complete a course of approximately 12 months. In the appropriate epidemiologic setting, failure of fluconazole therapy may be due to infection with var. *gattii* and treatment may need to be changed. Fluconazole for primary therapy is discouraged for patients with severe disease because of unsatisfactory outcomes in preliminary studies. For HIV-infected patients, more studies have been done to justify alternative regimens. Induction therapy with amphotericin with flucytosine for 2 weeks (or without flucytosine for 4 to 6 weeks) followed by a prolonged course (minimum of a year, but longer as indicated by poor control of the patient's HIV infection) of fluconazole is preferred. Guidelines outline other options for those patients not tolerant of amphotericin B.[70] Outcomes for patients with cryptococcosis have been studied for those with CNS involvement, and mortality is predicted by several CSF parameters, such as organism load, opening CSF pressure, low CSF glucose or leukocyte count, and high titer of cryptococcal antigen in CSF or blood. Additionally, those being treated with corticosteroids or with an underlying diagnosis of lymphoreticular malignancy also have higher mortality with cryptococcosis. Persistent elevation in CNS pressure may require repeated lumbar puncture, and if CSF pressure remains elevated despite antimicrobial treatment, CNS shunts have been used. Prognosis for patients with isolated pulmonary cryptococcosis has not been studied thoroughly, but in the absence of dissemination, outcomes appear to be more favorable.[69]

Candidiasis

Candida spp. are yeast and common human commensals that most often colonize the gastrointestinal tract. Of about 150 known species of *Candida*, only about 10 cause human disease. *C. albicans* is by far the most common species, and it causes the majority of human infections. *Candida* spp. other than *C. albicans*, however, do account for almost half of isolates in some series.[73] Infections occur primarily via tissue invasion from endogenously acquired strains rather than by person-to-person spread. The immune response to *Candida* is complex, but the most important components in preventing invasive disease appear to be normal number and function of neutrophils and intact complement pathways.[74] T lymphocytes are clearly important in controlling mucosal and cutaneous candidiasis, but patients with defects of cellular immunity are not at increased risk for invasive infection.[73,74]

Although *Candida* spp. are the most common of fungal pathogens and a frequent cause of nosocomial infections, true pulmonary infection with *Candida* spp. is relatively rare. When pulmonary candidiasis does occur, it is usually in the setting of disseminated infection with hematogenous seeding or with aspiration of oropharyngeal secretions heavily colonized with *Candida*.[75] Neutropenic patients, low birth weight infants, or premature neonates whose mothers have *Candida* chorioamnionitis are the patients in whom pulmonary dissemination has occurred most often.[36]

The clinical manifestations and radiologic findings of pulmonary candidiasis are nonspecific. Fever, cough, and septic appearance are common. Patterns on chest radiographs have been described most often as multilobar consolidation, widespread bronchopneumonia, or nodular infiltrates. Rarely, cavitary lesions, adult respiratory distress syndrome, and pleural effusion have been encountered in histologically proven pulmonary candidiasis.[76]

It is clear that the diagnosis of pulmonary candidiasis cannot be made reliably in the absence of histopathologic confirmation.[76] Isolating *Candida* spp. from a culture of the airways has poor predictive value for the presence of true disease. In a large study of adult cancer patients, the positive predictive value of a culture of the sputum for pulmonary candidiasis was 42% and just 29% for bronchoalveolar lavage specimens, using histopathology from autopsy specimens as the gold standard.[76] Similarly, in a study of non-neutropenic patients, nearly 90% of bronchoalveolar lavage cultures positive for *Candida* spp. were judged to be probable or definite contaminants, despite the majority of the cultures having been done on protected brush specimens.[75]

It has even been reported that limiting identification of yeast in respiratory specimens to that by diagnostic microbiology laboratories has led to improved outcomes and reduced costs in patients.[77] The authors assert that fewer erroneous diagnoses of pulmonary candidiasis resulted in shorter length of stay and avoidance of unnecessary antifungal therapy.

When true pulmonary candidiasis occurs, high rates of mortality have been reported in neutropenic patients. Choice of antifungal agent and length of therapy for pulmonary disease specifically have not been well studied, but generally amphotericin has been used.[73] Echinocandins are likely to be effective, given good activity against most *Candida* species, but data regarding treatment of pulmonary candidiasis, in particular, is lacking. Consideration can be given to the use of flucytosine in combination with amphotericin or fluconazole as the primary agent, given a susceptible strain.[73] For *C. albicans*, 95% or more of strains are susceptible to fluconazole, but resistance is more common among strains of *C. krusei*, *C. glabrata*, and *C. tropicalis*. Standards for susceptibility to the triazole and echinocandin antifungals have been set for *Candida* spp., and testing is available commercially. In disseminated candidiasis, other sites of infection may dictate the type and length of treatment (e.g., endocarditis or endophthalmitis).

Zygomycosis

The causative agents of zygomycosis belong to the order Mucorales and class Zygomycetes.[78] Human disease caused by these filamentous fungi is most often due to *Rhizopus* but can also be due to *Mucor*, *Lichtheimia* (formerly *Absidia*), *Cunninghamella*, *Rhizomucor*, and a number of other species reported occasionally.[79] These environmental molds are found primarily in soil and organic matter in a near worldwide distribution. Although percutaneous and ingestional acquisitions are known to occur, the main route of transmission is inhalation of spores from an environmental source. Outbreaks of disease have been linked to construction, excavation, and contaminated air-conditioning filters.[80] The Zygomycetes share hyphal morphology characterized by sparse or absent septation and variable size (but wider than *Aspergillus* spp. hyphae). As with *Aspergillus* spp., angioinvasion is a typical finding on histopathology.

People with intact innate immunity are not at significant risk for invasive zygomycosis. Early observations of patients with impaired immune systems gave insight into the mechanisms of protection against these fungi. Diabetic patients have long been known to be at risk for developing rhinocerebral zygomycosis, most often during ketoacidosis. Dysfunctions of macrophage phagocytosis, neutrophil chemotaxis, and oxidative killing by neutrophils have been demonstrated in diabetic ketoacidosis. Similar to the response to *Aspergillus*, macrophages are primarily responsible for aborting the germination of spores through phagocytosis. Once germination has occurred, neutrophils are responsible for damaging fungal hyphae through attachment and oxidative damage without phagocytosis.[78] Given the importance of the innate immune response, it is not surprising that neutropenia is the single most common risk factor for developing zygomycosis. Other important risk factors include use of corticosteroids and broad-spectrum antibiotics and hematologic and organ transplantation. One must have a high index of suspicion for zygomycosis in a patient who develops a fungal infection while on voriconazole therapy because of intrinsic resistance to this medication. One other well-established at-risk patient group is that receiving iron chelation therapy.[78] It is thought that the Zygomycetes are able to use iron bound to chelators as a growth factor. Hemochromatosis itself also may be a minor risk factor for developing zygomycosis.

Zygomycosis can be classified into a few predominant forms: rhinocerebral, pulmonary, cutaneous, gastrointestinal, and disseminated disease. Pulmonary disease was the most common manifestation, found to account for 30% of zygomycosis, in a recent series from Europe.[79] It is clinically indistinguishable from pulmonary aspergillosis and associated with similarly high rates of mortality. Common factors predisposing to pulmonary zygomycosis include leukemia, lymphoma, BMT, and diabetes mellitus. The clinical presentation is commonly fever and pulmonary infiltrates that persist despite treatment for presumed bacterial pneumonia. In advanced disease, hemoptysis can occur because of angioinvasion and hemorrhagic infarction, which characterize this group of infections.[81]

Radiographic findings, as in aspergillosis, are quite variable. Isolated nodules, lobar consolidation, cavitary lesions, and disseminated pulmonary involvement have all been described.[78] The sensitivity of cultures of respiratory tract specimens is low, and fungemia is not usually detected with clinical cultures. Serology is not useful clinically, and antigen detection and molecular diagnostic techniques have not been developed for clinical diagnostic purposes.[78] These factors make early diagnosis of invasive zygomycosis very difficult, and in fact, the diagnosis is often preterminal or made at autopsy. This makes a high index of suspicion and aggressive, tissue-based approach essential, assuming the patient can tolerate the necessary procedure.

The treatment for zygomycosis is aggressive debridement and high-dose intravenous amphotericin B. In a retrospective review of 255 cases of pulmonary mucormycosis, mortality of patients treated surgically was significantly lower than those who received medical treatment alone.[81] These data must be interpreted, keeping in mind the potential for selection bias that exists in a retrospective analysis, but it supports strong consideration of surgical intervention for therapeutic reasons. This infection progresses rapidly and requires aggressive diagnostics and therapeutics.

In addition to attempting reversal of the predisposing condition leading to the infection, antifungal therapy with amphotericin B is indicated. Initial doses of amphotericin B deoxycholate should be 1.0 to 1.5 mg/kg/day and at least 5 mg/kg/day if using lipid formulations of amphotericin B.[82] Itraconazole has variable activity against this class of fungi. It is of note that newer triazole and echinocandin antifungals, including voriconazole and caspofungin, have no appreciable activity against the Zygomycetes.[82] In fact, an increase in zygomycosis in stem cell transplant patients receiving voriconazole as antifungal prophylaxis has been reported.[83] The triazole agent posaconazole has in vitro activity against Zygomycetes. Although there is

some published experience with posaconazole as salvage therapy,[84,85] clinical efficacy has not been demonstrated in a comparative trial. Nevertheless, this agent is very promising for treatment of zygomycosis infections. Length of treatment with antifungals has not been studied for pulmonary zygomycosis, but a course of therapy lasting many months is indicated for survivors, based on clinical response and reversal of the underlying immunocompromised state.

OTHER UNCOMMON PULMONARY MYCOSES

Sporothrix schenckii is a dimorphic fungus with a worldwide distribution in soil and decaying organic material. Sporotrichosis is most commonly a cutaneous or lymphocutaneous infection that manifests as a chronic, ulcerated skin lesion, often with regional lymphadenopathy.[86] In addition to cutaneous disease, sporotrichosis can occasionally occur as osteoarticular, meningeal, and pulmonary infection. Pulmonary disease and other forms of disseminated sporotrichosis are rare in children. Pneumonia occurs most commonly in middle-aged men with alcoholism and chronic obstructive pulmonary disease.[86] The presentation is subacute or chronic in most cases, and nonspecific. Signs and symptoms include cough, fever, weight loss, and hemoptysis. Radiographs often reveal chronic cavitary fibronodular disease, but no specific pattern is typical. The combination of surgical resection and amphotericin B is preferred for life-threatening or extensive pulmonary sporotrichosis. Itraconazole also has activity against *S. schenckii* and can be considered for less serious disease.[86]

Trichosporon spp. are yeasts related to *Cryptococcus* that cause an infection of the distal hair shaft called white piedra and a hypersensitivity pneumonia that occurs in summer months in Japan.[78] The yeasts of this genus also occasionally cause disseminated infections in immunocompromised hosts. *Trichosporon beigelii* (also referred to as *T. asahii*) has been reported as a cause of pneumonia in neutropenic patients, particularly in those with hematologic malignancies.[87] Although there are descriptions of isolated pulmonary infection (presumably from aspiration of the organism), most cases of pulmonary trichosporonosis have been reported as part of disseminated disease, including involvement of the bloodstream, kidneys, liver, skin, and retina.[87] Cough, dyspnea, and hemoptysis are typical. Radiographs often show diffuse alveolar infiltrates, but diffuse interstitial infiltrates, patchy reticulonodular infiltrates, lobar consolidation, bronchopneumonia, and cavitary lesions also have been described.[87] Diagnosis is based on isolation of the organism from the respiratory tract, but because *Trichosporon* spp. can colonize the oropharynx, sputum cultures are not by themselves diagnostic. It is also notable that, as a result of the relatedness of *Trichosporon* spp. to *Cryptococcus*, false-positive serum cryptococcal antigen tests have been reported in confirmed cases of trichosporonosis. Preferred treatment for invasive infection is fluconazole because decreased susceptibility to amphotericin B has been demonstrated.[88] The addition of flucytosine also may be considered.[36] Newer triazole antifungal agents, such as voriconazole, also have activity against *Trichosporon* spp., but the echinocandins do not.[80]

Fusarium spp. have been recognized as an infrequent but important cause of disseminated infection in neutropenic patients. This filamentous fungus, which is primarily a plant pathogen, has long been known to cause infections of the nails, skin, and cornea of humans. In recent years, it has been appreciated that *Fusarium* spp. such as *F. solani, F. oxysporum,* and *F. moniliforme* are important causes of infections of the lungs and sinuses, and of disseminated infection in patients undergoing leukemia chemotherapy, and hematopoietic stem cell transplant patients.[71] In addition to neutropenia, corticosteroid therapy seems to be an important predisposing factor in developing fusariosis. The clinical presentation is similar to other opportunistic mold infections in that sinusitis and pulmonary infiltrates are common; however, fusariosis differs in that metastatic skin lesions and isolation of the organism from blood culture are much more common. Diagnosis can be made with certainty only by isolation of the organism from culture of infected tissues or blood. Distinguishing *Fusarium* spp. from *Aspergillus* spp. or other septate hyaline molds by histopathology is unreliable.[19] Mortality from fusariosis has historically been greater than 50%, and amphotericin B treatment generally has been, at best, only modestly successful. Adjunctive treatment with colony-stimulating factors and/or granulocyte transfusions has been used as well.[19] Voriconazole has potent activity against *Fusarium* spp.; it is approved for treating fusariosis, and retrospective data of its use in successful treatment in immunocompromised hosts has been published.[89,90] In the latter of these reports, patients treated with combination antifungal therapy fared no better than those treated with monotherapy. Definitive data for the best therapeutic approach to fusariosis are lacking.

Phaeohyphomycosis is an invasive infection due to one of the dematiaceous molds, a group characterized by darkly pigmented cell walls.[71] As with many molds, the respiratory tract is the usual portal of entry for these fungi, and extrapulmonary dissemination is common. Infections generally occur in neutropenic hosts, as with the other opportunistic mold infections, and localize to the CNS, sinuses, and lungs. *Pseudallescheria boydii* and its teleomorph *Scedosporium* spp. are important causes of pulmonary infection, since they are difficult to treat and associated with high rates of mortality.[71] *Scedosporium apiospermum* has been reported as a cause of pulmonary infection in children with chronic granulomatous disease.[91] Another dematiaceous mold, *Bipolaris,* can cause pulmonary infection as well, although its most frequent manifestation is sinusitis. As with fusariosis, the diagnosis of phaeohyphomycosis must be established by culture because the activity of amphotericin B is not consistently fungicidal, and in some cases, depends on the specific species.[19] Newer triazole agents such as voriconazole have activity in vitro and have been used successfully in a small number of patients, including children intolerant or refractory to conventional therapy.[19] Surgical resection of fungal lesions and adjunctive colony-stimulating cytokine therapies can both be considered in difficult cases.[71]

Penicillium marneffei is a dimorphic fungus that has been identified as an important opportunistic infection in HIV-infected patients who live in or have traveled to eastern Asia. The lungs are the portal of entry, and it is thought that impaired cell–mediated and alveolar phagocytic function is the main predisposing factor in AIDS patients.[71] The clinical syndrome commonly includes fever, lymphadenopathy, hepatosplenomegaly, pulmonary infiltrate, weight loss, anemia, and generalized rash similar to that associated with molluscum contagiosum virus. Amphotericin B is favored for induction therapy, with itraconazole given long-term as maintenance/suppressive therapy.[71]

Acknowledgments

The authors wish to recognize the contributions of the following collaborators for their roles in obtaining radiographs and pathologic specimens used for the figures in this chapter: Richard M. Heller, Sharon M. Stein, and James D. Chappell. Dr. Richard Zuckerman and Dr. Joseph Schwartzman carefully reviewed late drafts of the manuscript.

References

The complete reference list is available online at www.expertconsult.com

35 PERTUSSIS AND OTHER *BORDETELLA* INFECTIONS OF THE RESPIRATORY TRACT

Ulrich Heininger, MD

Pertussis ("whooping cough") is an acute bacterial infection of the respiratory tract. The illness occurs worldwide and affects all age groups, but it is most serious in young, unprotected infants. It is caused by *Bordetella pertussis* (first described in 1906) and, less frequently, by *B. parapertussis* (1937).[1–3] The term *pertussis* was coined in 1670 and means "violent cough." The clinical picture was described for the first time in 1640 by Guillaume de Baillou, based on a 1578 epidemic in Paris.[3]

MICROBIOLOGY, PATHOGENESIS, AND IMMUNITY

Bordetella organisms are small, aerobic, gram-negative coccobacilli. Today, the genus comprises nine different species, of which six have been shown to cause respiratory tract illness in humans: *B. pertussis* and *B. parapertussis*, the causative agents of whooping cough; *B. bronchiseptica* and *B. holmesii*, which can cause variable respiratory symptoms; *B. trematum*, which has been found in ear and wound infections, and *B. petrii*, isolated from respiratory tract secretions in patients with cystic fibrosis and from a patient with mastoiditis.[1–6] However, the overwhelming majority of *Bordetella* infections are caused by *B. pertussis* and *B. parapertussis*, to which the following discussion pertains.

The organism is transmitted by aerosol droplets from infected to susceptible humans. After transmission, adhesion of the bacteria to ciliated cells of the upper and lower respiratory tract establishes colonization, followed by multiplication and spread on the epithelium, local mucosal damage, and finally, induction of respiratory symptoms. Invasiveness is extremely rare.[7] Asymptomatic, transient colonization frequently occurs during reinfection in immune individuals.[8] Animal studies suggest that a variety of virulence factors is involved in the various steps of infection of the respiratory tract (Table 35-1). Expression of these factors is regulated in response to environmental changes by BvgAS, a two-component signal transduction system.[9] The precise mechanisms during *B. pertussis* and *B. parapertussis* infection in the human host are unknown. Laboratory studies suggest that several factors working in concert allow adherence of the organisms to the epithelium, and filamentous hemagglutinin (FHA) inhibits phagocytosis. Later on, effects caused by adenylate cyclase toxin and pertactin expression allow effective phagocytosis and killing of the bacteria by the host. The popular belief that pertussis is a single-toxin illness caused by pertussis toxin (PT), exclusively produced by *B. pertussis*, is refutable by the observation that a similar illness results from infection with *B. parapertussis*, which

does not express PT.[10] Further insight into the pathogenesis of *Bordetella* infection will be gained now that several members of the genus have been sequenced.[11]

The pathology of pertussis has been characterized by studies of *B. pertussis* infection. It causes inflammation, congestion, and infiltration of the respiratory mucosa with lymphocytes and granulocytes and leads to accumulation of viscous secretions in the lumen of the bronchi, bronchiolar obstruction, and occasional atelectasis.[3] Later in the infection, necrosis of the midzonal and basilar parts of the bronchial epithelium result in necrotizing bronchitis (Fig. 35-1). Subsequently, bronchopneumonia may develop and is either caused by *B. pertussis* itself or by secondary infections with other pathogenic bacteria.

Infection with *B. pertussis* of a previously naïve host results in production of serum and salivary antibodies against a number of antigens such as PT, FHA, pertactin, and adenylate cyclase toxin.[12–14] Enzyme-linked immunosorbent assay techniques allow discrimination of class-specific antibodies, with IgG being more reliably detectable than IgA, IgE, and IgM. In individuals who have been "primed" by *B. pertussis* infection or immunization, reinfection will elicit a secondary immune response with or without concomitant symptoms.[8] Of note, infection with *B. pertussis* does not provide lifelong immunity, and apparently no cross protection between different species of *Bordetella* exists.[15,16] After natural infection, sustained IgG and IgA serum antibody levels against FHA, pertactin, and—though less—PT have been observed before returning close to baseline values after approximately 5 years.[17,18] Yet, the precise role of serum antibodies in immunity against pertussis is a matter of ongoing debate, and various studies show conflicting results.[19,20]

Cell-mediated immune responses to *B. pertussis* have been shown to play an important role in protection against pertussis. In mice, challenge with *B. pertussis* resulted in a predominant T helper 1 (Th1) cell–mediated immune response followed by complete bacterial clearance.[21] Specific protection could be conferred by adoptive transfer of immune spleen cells into immunosuppressed mice, further underlining the role of Th1 cells. Interestingly, persistent vaccine efficacy has been documented in young children several years after immunization despite significant antibody decline, and it was also preferentially mediated by Th1 cells.[22]

EPIDEMIOLOGY

Pertussis occurs worldwide, and humans are the only host of *B. pertussis*. Transmission occurs effectively by droplets, with secondary attack rates close to 100% in

TABLE 35-1 VIRULENCE FACTORS OF *BORDETELLA PERTUSSIS* AND THEIR SPECIFIC CHARACTERISTICS

FACTOR (GENE)	BVG REGULATION	MOLECULE	MAJOR ROLE	OTHER FUNCTIONS	COMMENTS
Pertussis toxin (PTX)	Yes	"A" protomer and "B" subunits	Toxin and first-line adhesion factor	Causes leukocytosis by lymphocytosis	Precise role in disease unknown
Filamentous hemagglutinin (FHA)	Yes	Large, filamentous protein (220 kd)	Major adhesin; predominantly in trachea	Not known	Need for inclusion in vaccine questionable
Fimbriae 2 and 3 (fim2, fim3, fimX)	Yes	Small, filamentous proteins (=23 kd)	Adhesion factor; predominantly in trachea	Agglutinogens; sustain infection	Important stimulator of host's immune response
Pertactin (prn1, prn2, prn3)	Yes	69-kd outer membrane protein	Adhesion factor, induces type-specific antibody	Major protective antigen (mouse model)	Important vaccine antigen, used for genotyping
Adenylate cyclase (cyaA)	Yes	Protein toxin	Toxin; inhibits phagocytosis by ↑ cAMP	Inhibits chemotaxis and induces apoptosis of macrophages	Candidate for future vaccines!
Tracheal cytotoxin (TCT)	No	Peptidoglycan derivative	Toxin; paralyzes mucociliary clearance system	Inhibits DNA synthesis and cell death	Nonimmunogenic → not suitable for vaccine
Dermonecrotic toxin (DNT)	Yes	Heat-labile toxin (140 kd)	Toxin; dermal necrosis and vasoconstriction	Effect only after injection in skin	Role in human disease unknown
Tracheal colonization (tcfA)	Yes	Proline-rich protein	Adhesion factor; predominantly in trachea	Not known	C-terminal homology to prn, factor brkA, and vag-8
Bordetella resistance to killing factor (brkA)	Yes	Outer membrane protein (32 kd)	Adhesion factor	Provides resistance to complement	C-terminal homology to prn, tcfA, and vag-8
Virulence-activated gene 8 (vag-8)	Yes	Outer membrane protein (95 kd)	Adhesion factor (?)	Not known	C-terminal homology to prn, tcfA, and brkA
Lipooligosaccharide (WLB)	Yes	Lipid A and trisaccharide	Presumably required for nasal colonization	Not known	Substantially species-specific structure within *Bordetella*
BVG intermediate-phase (bipA)	Yes	Outer membrane protein (137 kd)	Transmission (?) and adhesion factor	Not known	First of a new class of *Bordetella* protein A antigens ("intermediate phase")
Type III secretion system (bsc)	Yes	Several, not yet specified proteins	Secretes effector proteins into host cells	Downregulation of the host immune system	Appears to be functional only in *B. bronchiseptica* (and some *B. parapertussis* strains)
bteA (bteA)	Yes	Linked to type III secretion system (72 kDa)	Induction of cytotoxicity	Persistent infection (animal model)	Potential vaccine antigen

CAMP, Cyclic adenosine monophosphate.
Modified and updated from Heininger U. Recent progress in clinical and basic pertussis research. *Eur J Pediatr.* 2001;160:203-213.

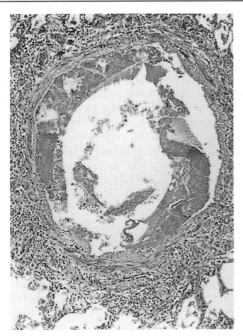

FIGURE 35-1. Necrotizing bronchitis (×100).

exposed susceptible individuals.[3] The incubation period is usually 7 to 10 days but may vary substantially. In a household contact study, secondary cases were noted to have their onset up to 6 weeks after the onset of illness in the primary case, especially when antibiotics were used.[23] Several studies have shown that females and males

are equally affected by pertussis in childhood, whereas a female preponderance (55% to 69%) is noted in adolescents and adults.[24-26] Most likely, this is due to more frequent contact of females with young children, from whom they acquire infection. The seasonal pattern of pertussis is variable between different geographic locations.[25,26]

The epidemiology of pertussis caused by *B. pertussis* infection is incompletely understood. Reasons for this are the lack of a uniform case definition, inconsistent use of diagnostic laboratory tests, variable surveillance systems, and incomplete case ascertainment due to underconsulting, underrecognition, underdiagnosis, and underreporting.[27] Furthermore, epidemiology is greatly influenced by pertussis immunization programs that, with high coverage rates, not only confer individual protection but also group (or herd) protection to some extent. In contrast to *B. pertussis*, *B. parapertussis* infections appear to occur independent of immunization activities, and their relative frequency varies considerably by geography and time.[10,28]

Although in most countries pertussis still mainly affects infants and young children, it is increasingly diagnosed in adolescents and adults who are also important sources of infection in young, unprotected infants in their families and households (Table 35-2).[15] A resurgence of cases and a gradual shift toward an increase of pertussis in adolescents and adults has been noted in North America and elsewhere.[24] Whether this increase is caused by waning vaccine immunity and a decreased chance for natural boosters, a consequence of increased awareness and diagnostic tools, or both is an ongoing debate. Of note, pertussis in adolescents and adults is frequently

TABLE 35-2 HOUSEHOLD MEMBERS AS THE SOURCE OF PERTUSSIS IN INFANTS

COUNTRY	INVESTIGATOR (YEAR)	STUDY POPULATION	OBSERVATION*
United Kingdom	Crowcroft (2003)[28a]	25 infants <5 months of age admitted to ICU because of proven pertussis	Primary case: Parent: N = 11 (44%) Sibling: N = 6 (24%)
United States	Bisgard (2004)[28b]	616 infants with proven pertussis	Source discovered in 264 (43%) cases: Parent: N = 123 (47%; 20% of total) Grandparent: N = 22 (8%; 4% of total) Sibling: N = 52 (20%; 8% of total)
France	Bonmarin (2007)[28c]	1668 hospitalized infants <6 months of age with proven pertussis	Source discovered in 892 (53%) cases: Parent: N = 491 (55%; 29% of total) Sibling: N = 223 (25%; 13% of total)
Multinational	Kowalzik (2007)[28d]	99 infants admitted to ICU because of proven pertussis	≥1 source (N = 30) discovered in 24 (24%) cases: Parent: N = 18 (60%; 18% of total) Other adult: N = 6 (20%; 6% of total) Sibling: N = 5 (17%; 5% of total)
Multinational	Wendelboe (2007)[28e]	95 infants <6 months of age admitted to hospital because of proven pertussis	≥1 source discovered in 44 (46%) cases: Parent: N = 27 (55%; ≈25% of total) Grandparent: N = 3 (6%; ≈3% of total) Sibling: N = 8 (16 %; ≈5% of total)
The Netherlands	de Greef (2010)[28f]	201 infants <6 months of age admitted to hospital because of proven pertussis	≥1 source discovered in 96 (48%) cases: Parent: N = 53 (55%; ≈25% of total) Sibling: N = 39 (41%; ≈19% of total)

*Restricted to household contacts; other sources, if any, were nonhousehold contacts

atypical, and true numbers of cases are probably higher than reported.[24,29] Furthermore, in support of a true change in epidemiology, a rise in fatalities due to pertussis has been observed in infants in the United States during the last decade. Whereas 1.67 deaths per million infants per year were reported in the 1980s, the rate increased to an average of 2.40 in the 1990s. The increased incidence almost exclusively affected infants under 4 months of age.[30]

The crucial role that mass immunization plays in controlling pertussis has been clearly demonstrated in countries such as Japan, England, and Sweden, where infant pertussis vaccination was either discontinued or markedly curtailed as a result of unsubstantiated concerns about vaccine-related adverse events.[3]

CLINICAL CHARACTERISTICS

Typical pertussis is a three-stage illness, comprising catarrhal, paroxysmal, and convalescent phases.[3] The catarrhal stage lasts for about 1 to 2 weeks and is characterized by flulike symptoms such as coryza, sneezing, lacrimation, conjunctival injection, malaise, nonspecific cough, and occasionally low-grade fever. It is followed by the paroxysmal stage, which in classical cases is marked by an increase of frequency and severity of cough with paroxysms as the most typical feature; characteristically, repetitive series of 5 to 10 or more hacking spells of cough occur during a single expiration. At the end of a paroxysm, a typical whoop, which is caused by the sudden rush of inspired air through a narrowed glottis, is noted. Cyanosis, neck vein distention, bulging eyes, tongue protrusion, salivation, lacrimation, sweating, and post-tussive vomiting of food or viscous mucus may occur. Fever is usually minimal or absent during this stage. Paroxysms may occur up to several times per hour, during both day and night, triggered by various stimuli such as eating and drinking and physical or emotional stress. The paroxysmal stage may last from a few days to several weeks, until the convalescent stage is reached; this phase is marked by a decrease in the frequency and severity of coughing spells. However, over a period of several months, similar coughing episodes may again occur, often associated with other respiratory tract infections. Notably, B. pertussis infections present with considerable variability that primarily depends on age, previous immunization, or infection. Other variables, including the presence of passively acquired antibody (in young infants), degree of exposure to the source of infection, specific bacterial inoculum, host genetic and acquired factors, and genotype of the organism, may contribute to attenuation of symptoms.

The variability of symptoms is exemplified by results from a study of 1860 culture-positive cases in unvaccinated children and adolescents in Germany. In that study, 38% of patients had a total coughing illness duration of 4 weeks or less, 18% had nonparoxysmal cough, 21% did not whoop, and 47% did not have post-tussive vomiting.[26] On rare occasions, B. pertussis infection has been found to cause otitis media and to be associated with unilateral hyperlucent lung (MacLeod's or Swyer-James syndrome) and the hemolytic uremic syndrome.[31–33]

There is a wide spectrum of complications of pertussis, most of which predominantly occur in young infants

(Table 35-3). Respiratory complications include bronchopneumonia with or without atelectasis, pulmonary hypertension, and otitis media mainly secondary to other respiratory tract pathogens. Pertussis also has been associated with activation of latent tuberculosis. Additional complications that have been observed as a consequence of pertussis include ulcer of the frenulum of the tongue, epistaxis, melena, subconjunctival hemorrhages, meningoencephalitis, encephalopathy with cerebral seizures, tetanic seizures caused by severe alkalosis as a result of loss of gastric contents due to persistent vomiting, subdural hematomas, spinal epidural hematoma, rupture of the diaphragm, rib fracture, umbilical hernia, inguinal hernia, rectal prolapse, dehydration, syndrome of inappropriate antidiuretic hormone secretion, apnea, and nutritional disturbances.[3] Death secondary to pneumonia, pulmonary hypertension, or sudden death, probably due to severe hypoxemia, occurs mainly in infants, for whom the mortality rate is 0.6%.[25,34] There is no evidence for long-term sequelae such as allergic sensitization after pertussis.[35]

Overall symptoms with B. parapertussis infection are similar to those caused by B. pertussis, but illness usually is less severe and of shorter duration.[8] Dual infections of B. pertussis and B. parapertussis have been observed.[36] Occasionally, B. bronchiseptica and B. holmesii have been isolated from children with pertussis-like illness.[37,38] The clinical role of Bordetella spp. isolated from sputum specimens in patients with cystic fibrosis is currently unknown.[8]

DIAGNOSIS AND DIFFERENTIAL DIAGNOSIS

In typical cases, a diagnosis of pertussis can be established on the basis of characteristic symptoms. However, several microorganisms other than B. pertussis or B. parapertussis can cause cough illnesses that can occasionally be confused with pertussis. In one study from Germany, the frequency of serologic evidence for an infection with microorganisms other than B. pertussis was assessed in children with pertussis-like illnesses.[39] Of 149 such children, a diagnosis of adenovirus ($n = 33$); parainfluenza viruses 1, 2, and 3 ($n = 18$); Mycoplasma pneumoniae infection ($n = 15$); and respiratory syncytial virus infection ($n = 14$) was made. In studies of concurrent outbreaks of Mycoplasma and B. pertussis infections it has been shown that clinical symptoms alone lacked adequate specificity to distinguish pertussis from mycoplasmal infection.[40] Moreover, in populations with high immunization rates, atypical presentations of B. pertussis may be more frequent than classical illness, and a high index of clinical suspicion is imperative in the diagnosis of pertussis.[26] These observations underscore the need for appropriate laboratory tests if there is any doubt about the diagnosis.

Isolation of B. pertussis or B. parapertussis from a person with a cough illness provides certainty of the diagnosis. Nasopharyngeal secretions, obtained by aspiration, or calcium alginate or Dacron swabs, and specific media (Regan-Lowe or Bordet-Gengou agar and modified Stainer-Scholte broth) are necessary to recover Bordetella spp. Alternatively, direct fluorescent antibody tests can be applied. Sensitivity of culture is optimal (≈95%) in

TABLE 35-3 COMPLICATIONS IN 1640 UNVACCINATED PATIENTS WITH *BORDETELLA PERTUSSIS* INFECTIONS BY AGE GROUP AS REPORTED IN FOLLOW-UP QUESTIONNAIRES

Complication	<6 Months (N = 63) N (%)	6-12 Months (N = 59) N (%)	1-4 Years (N = 610) N (%)	4-9 Years (N = 846) N (%)	>9 Years (N = 62) N (%)	Total (N = 1640) N (%)
Pneumonia	2 (3.2)	–	8 (1.3)	18 (2.1)	–	28 (1.7)
Apnea/cyanosis	10 (15.9)	1 (1.7)	–	1 (0.1)	–	12 (0.7)
Otitis media	–	–	6 (0.9)	4 (0.5)	–	10 (0.6)
Poor feeding/severe vomiting	2 (3.2)	–	2 (0.3)	2 (0.2)	1 (1.6)	7 (0.4)
Cardiopulmonary failure	1 (1.7)	–	–	–	–	1 (0.1)
Death	–	1 (1.6)	–	–	–	1 (0.1)
Others*	–	2 (3.4)	5 (0.8)	15 (1.8)	–	22 (1.3)
Unspecified	1 (1.6)	–	8 (1.3)	5 (0.6)	2 (3.2)	16 (1.0)
Any	15 (23.8)	3 (5.1)	29 (4.8)	45 (5.3)	3 (4.8)	95 (5.8)

AGE

*Includes cases of epistaxis, inguinal hernia, frequent paroxysms, and bronchitis.
From Heininger U, Klich K, Stehr K, et al. Clinical findings in *Bordetella pertussis* infections. Results of a prospective multicenter surveillance study. *Pediatrics.* 1997;100:e10.

unvaccinated, untreated individuals early in the course of the illness, when clinical suspicion of pertussis usually is low. During the paroxysmal phase, sensitivity of culture rapidly declines to 50% or lower. Over the last two decades, polymerase chain reaction (PCR) technique applied to nasopharyngeal specimens has markedly improved the diagnosis of pertussis. It is particularly useful in oligosymptomatic cases, in patients who have been started on antibiotics, and in patients with progressed illness. In addition, sensitivity of PCR in general is higher than that of bacterial culture and is therefore the preferred diagnostic tool. Advanced technology today allows discrimination between different species of the *Bordetella* genus, and recent developments such as real-time detection of the amplification products and LightCycler PCR now provide results within a few hours.[41,42]

Serologic tests are the most sensitive technique for the diagnosis of *Bordetella* infections. Enzyme immunoassays have been most widely applied, and although whole-cell preparations of *B. pertussis* can be used as antigens, purified proteins such as PT, FHA, and pertactin are preferable for their better specificity. IgG antibody assays provide sufficient sensitivity, but addition of IgA assays may be helpful. Although paired acute and convalescent phase serum samples are optimal, analysis of a single serum specimen is more appropriate for routine purposes. Unfortunately, however, serology tests are not standardized and interpretation of results is difficult in the presence of vaccine-induced preexisting antibodies.[43] Therefore, test results have to be interpreted cautiously, and cutoff values derived from age-matched control groups are required. IgA antibodies have traditionally been considered to be reliable indicators of recent or acute infection. A recent study, however, has shown persistently high IgA antibodies against FHA; pertactin; and, though less pronounced, PT for as long as 30 months after infection.[18] This observation further complicates the serologic diagnosis of *B. pertussis* infection in single-serum analyses.

Most cases of pertussis caused by primary *B. pertussis* infection in unvaccinated individuals will demonstrate leukocytosis due to lymphocytosis. This is caused by the effects of PT, which appears to reduce L-selectin expression by the T cells and thus prevents their homing to the lymphoid tissues.[44] In contrast, secondary infections and breakthrough cases of pertussis in vaccinated patients (with preexisting IgG antibodies to PT) frequently lack leukocytosis, as do patients infected with *B. parapertussis* (which does not express PT).[10]

The role of radiographic imaging in pertussis is limited. The most frequent abnormalities are consolidation, atelectasis, and hilar lymphadenopathy. In a case series of 238 hospitalized patients with pertussis, radiographic abnormalities were detected in 63 patients (26%). Pulmonary consolidation was seen in 50 patients (21%), atelectasis in 9 (4%), and lymphadenopathy in 22 (9%). Most consolidations were peribronchial (72%). For unknown reasons, both atelectasis and consolidation were more common on the right and predominantly involved the lower and middle lobes of the lung. Radiographic abnormalities were more common beyond infancy. Follow-up radiographs after 1 month demonstrated no significant radiographic

sequelae.[45] One can conclude that chest radiographs should be limited to severe cases and when pulmonary complications are suspected on the basis of clinical findings.

TREATMENT

Several antibiotics have proven *in vitro* activity against *B. pertussis* and *B. parapertussis*.[1] Sufficient minimal inhibitory concentrations have been demonstrated for macrolides and for fluoroquinolones. In contrast, minimal inhibitory concentrations of oral beta-lactam antibiotics, including cephalosporins, are unacceptable and render them unsuitable for treatment of pertussis. Oral erythromycin (succinate formulation at 50 mg/kg body weight/day given every 6 to 8 hours or estolate formulation at doses of 40 mg/kg/day in 12-hour intervals for 14 days) still is the preferred treatment in neonates and young infants. When given in the catarrhal or early paroxysmal stage of the illness, this will ameliorate the symptoms, eradicate the bacteria from the nasopharynx within a few days, and terminate contagiousness of the patient. Of the different formulations, erythromycin is favored by most experts. Erythromycin remains the first-line drug, although resistance has been observed in single isolates and ongoing surveillance of antibiotic susceptibility of isolated strains is advisable.[46] The mechanism underlying resistance is currently unknown. Seven days of treatment with erythromycin estolate was shown to be as effective as 14 days of treatment in a large Canadian study.[47] It should be noted, however, that this investigation was carried out in a highly vaccinated community, and results may have been different in unvaccinated children. Also noteworthy is that when erythromycin is used in young infants, the possibility of a hypertrophic pyloric stenosis occurring as an adverse event should be borne in mind, and parents need to be educated about the symptoms of this rare but significant risk.[48]

New macrolide antibiotics with improved gastrointestinal tolerability, such as clarithromycin or azithromycin, demonstrate efficiency comparable to that with erythromycin and are preferred in older children and adolescents.[49] In Canada, the microbiologic and clinical efficacy and the clinical safety of a 7-day course of clarithromycin (15 mg/kg/day in two doses for 7 days) was compared to a 14-day course of erythromycin (40 mg/kg/day in three doses for 14 days) in a prospective, randomized, single-blind (investigator) trial in children from 1 month to 16 years of age with culture-proven pertussis.[50] Nasopharyngeal cultures for *B. pertussis* were performed at enrollment and the end of treatment. Microbiologic eradication and clinical cure rates were equal: 100% (31/31) for clarithromycin and 96% (22/23) for erythromycin. Patients on clarithromycin had significantly fewer adverse events (45%) than those on erythromycin (62%).

In an open, uncontrolled study in the United States, 34 subjects (most of them children) with culture or PCR-proven *B. pertussis* infection received a 5-day course of azithromycin (10 mg/kg in a single dose on the first day and 5 mg/kg/day as single doses on the following 4 days). *B. pertussis* was eradicated from the nasopharynx in 33 (97%) of 34 patients after 72 hours, and all were negative on follow-up after 2 to 3 weeks.[51]

The role of intravenous anti-pertussis immunoglobulin treatment remains controversial. In one study, a hyperimmunoglobulin was prepared as a 4% IgG solution from the pooled plasma from donors immunized with inactivated pertussis toxoid, resulting in IgG PT antibody concentrations more than sevenfold higher than those in conventional intravenous immunoglobulin products.[52] Twenty-six children with laboratory-confirmed pertussis received one of three doses (1500, 750, or 250 mg/kg). All three treatment groups demonstrated a decrease of lymphocytosis ($p < .05$) and clinical improvement (paroxysmal coughing) by the third day after anti-pertussis immunoglobulin treatment. No serious adverse events occurred, but one patient experienced transient hypotension that responded to a decreased infusion rate. Unfortunately, no information on concomitant antibiotic treatment was provided. Prospective, controlled trials must be conducted before any firm conclusions on the value of immunoglobulin treatment of pertussis can be drawn.

Young infants, who are threatened by hypoxemia associated with apneic spells, should be hospitalized and their blood oxygen saturation closely monitored. Careful removal of respiratory secretions and oxygen supplementation may be necessary. Uncontrolled observations indicate that corticosteroids and/or β-adrenergic drugs adjunctive to antibiotics may ameliorate respiratory distress associated with pertussis, but evidence of efficacy is lacking.[3] Pneumonia, frequent apneic spells, and significant respiratory distress may require assisted ventilation, especially in neonates and young infants.[3] In young infants, extreme leukocytosis (>100,000/μl) and pulmonary hypertension carry a high risk for respiratory and cardiovascular failure. In spite of intensive treatment efforts, such as pulmonary artery vasodilators and extracorporeal membrane oxygenation, the outcome of these complicated courses is frequently fatal.[53,54]

General supportive medical treatment is important for patients with pertussis. Physical and emotional stress, which may trigger paroxysms, should be avoided. Furthermore, if post-tussive vomiting is present, careful attention should be paid to adequate fluid and food intake. Respiratory isolation precautions should be implemented until 5 days of effective antibiotic treatment have been received.

■ PREVENTION

Prevention of pertussis is possible by avoidance of exposure, postexposure antibiotic treatment, and immunization. Avoidance of exposure is usually impossible in clinical practice, given that contagiousness is highest during the early stage of illness in the primary case where a diagnosis of pertussis commonly has not yet been made. Prophylactic use of erythromycin (or clarithromycin or azithromycin) has been shown to protect from *B. pertussis* infection when given to close contacts and is most useful when administered before the occurrence of the first secondary case.[55] Recommended antibiotic dosage and duration is the same as for treatment and should be given to all close contacts regardless of age and immunization status according to recommendations by the American Academy of Pediatrics.[56] Postexposure active immunization also should be considered in unimmunized or incompletely immunized individuals by use of a dose of age-appropriate pertussis vaccine.

Active immunization is the most effective way to prevent pertussis. Over the last two decades, acellular pertussis vaccines (containing various numbers and quantities of *B. pertussis* antigens) have been developed, studied for safety, immunogenicity, and efficacy, and been implemented in most countries worldwide.[1] Virtually all countries recommend a primary series of two or three vaccine doses in infancy and usually also a reinforcing dose in the second year of life. Timely initiation of the immunization series, usually at 2 months of age, is crucial, because the risk for severe pertussis in immunized infants decreases from dose to dose when compared with unimmunized infants.[57] The optimal timing and number of further booster immunizations is a matter of ongoing debate.[27] Because vaccine-induced efficacy is sustained despite declining antibody values, observational studies are needed to answer these questions. Investigations conducted so far indicate ongoing efficacy after three or four doses of acellular pertussis vaccine for several years.[1] Today, most countries recommend booster doses at preschool age and/or in adolescents. Furthermore, several countries including the United States, Canada, France, and Germany have introduced a universal pertussis booster dose in adults, regardless of age.[58]

Overall, when compared with conventional whole-cell pertussis vaccines, acellular component vaccines have been shown to cause lower rates of local and systemic reactions such as fever.[3] Also, severe reactions such as febrile seizures and hypotonic-hyporesponsive episodes declined significantly (79% and 60%, respectively) with the broad dissemination of acellular pertussis vaccines.[59] Of some concern is that local reactions after pertussis immunization increase from dose to dose, and whole-limb swelling at the site of injection may occur. Yet, these side effects are only temporary, usually do not interfere with the child's well-being, and are without sequelae. Furthermore, they are considered to be less severe than those seen after five consecutive doses of whole-cell vaccine.[60] Providing timely and complete immunizations against pertussis for all infants and young children, followed by regular booster doses as needed throughout life, will be crucial to control pertussis better in the future.

Suggested Reading

Altunaiji S, Kukuruzuvic R, Curtis N, et al. Antibiotics for whooping cough (pertussis). *Cochrane Database Syst Rev.* 2007; CD004404.

Halasa NB, Barr FE, Johnson JE, et al. Fatal pulmonary hypertension associated with pertussis in infants: does extracorporeal membrane oxygenation have a role? *Pediatrics.* 2003;112:1274–1278.

Heininger U. Update on pertussis in children. *Expert Rev Anti Infect Ther.* 2010;8:163–173.

Henderson J, North K, Griffiths M, et al. Pertussis vaccination and wheezing illnesses in young children. Prospective cohort study. *BMJ.* 1999;318:1173–1176.

Mortimer EA. Pertussis and its prevention. A family affair. *J Infect Dis.* 1990;161:473–479.

Romano MJ, Weber MD, Weisse ME, et al. Pertussis pneumonia, hypoxemia, hyperleukocytosis, and pulmonary hypertension: improvement in oxygenation after a double volume exchange transfusion. *Pediatrics.* 2004;114:e264–e266.

References

The complete reference list is available online at www.expertconsult.com

36 TOXOCARIASIS, HYDATID DISEASE OF THE LUNG, STRONGYLOIDIASIS, AND PULMONARY PARAGONIMIASIS

AYESHA MIRZA, MD, and MOBEEN H. RATHORE, MD, CPE, FAAP, FIDSA, FACPE

TOXOCARIASIS (VISCERAL LARVA MIGRANS)

Toxocariasis is a soil-transmitted zoonotic infection that causes two main diseases in humans: visceral larva migrans (VLM) and ocular larva migrans (OLM). VLM results from an inflammatory response to the migration of immature, second-stage larvae through the viscera of a host that is not suitable for completion of the parasite's life cycle. The disease can involve many major organs and characteristically causes eosinophilia, hepatomegaly, and pneumonitis.

Etiology

Two species of *Toxocara* are primarily responsible for most cases of VLM: Dogs, wolves, and foxes are the definitive hosts for *T. canis*, whereas domestic cats are the host for *T. cati*. Other *Toxocara* spp. have been implicated in human infection, including *T. vulpis,* while the role of *T. lyncus* and *T. malaysiensis* in causing human infection is not clear. In addition, *Baylisascaris procyonis, Capillaria hepatica, Ascaris suum,* and rarely *Ascaris lumbricoides,* hookworm larvae, and *Strongyloides stercoralis* also can cause a VLM-like syndrome.

Epidemiology

Toxocara are found worldwide in domesticated and wild dogs and cats. *T. canis* is a common parasite of dogs found throughout the world. The prevalence of infected dogs varies from country to country, but levels above 40% are not uncommon. Infection with *Toxocara* is more prevalent than realized because many individuals do not express the complete VLM syndrome. Current seroprevalence data place toxocariasis among the most common zoonotic infections worldwide. In one study of children from different regions of the United States, the seroprevalence of *Toxocara* antibodies, as measured by enzyme-linked immunosorbent assay (ELISA), varied from 4.6% to 7.3%. One rural Pennsylvania community with poor sanitation had a 54% seropositive rate, versus 9% for a nearby community with better sanitation. The seroprevalence of *Toxocara* antibodies was 7% among young adults in Sweden. As in the United States, rural areas had a higher rate than urban areas. Puppies are especially dangerous because transplacental infection results in 77% to 100% of puppies becoming infected. By the time the animals are 3 weeks old, mature egg-laying worms can be present. Adult female worms shed 200,000 ova per day and are passed unembryonated onto the soil in the feces of the infected animal. Under suitable soil conditions, the ova become embryonated and infectious after a minimum of 2 to 3 weeks. Because of the thick shell, the embryonated ova can survive in moist soil for months. Most infections arise in children with a history of pica, or in individuals who have accidentally ingested contaminated soil. Animals are not directly infectious because of the time lag before the ova become infectious.

Pathogenesis

In the natural host, infectious ova are ingested and hatch in the upper alimentary tract. The second-stage larvae then migrate through the intestinal walls into the bloodstream and then into the liver and lungs of the infected animal. From the lungs, the larvae mature by migrating through the tracheobronchial tree and passing into the upper alimentary tract. There, the mature worm can begin laying eggs, which pass out in the feces to begin the cycle anew.

In aberrant hosts such as humans, the initial stages of infection are identical: infectious second-stage larvae hatch in the small intestine and then begin migrating through blood and lymphatics to the liver, lung, brain, and other organs such as the eye. However, before the larvae can complete their transtracheal passage and maturation to adult worms, host defenses block further migration of the larvae by encasing them within a granulomatous reaction, which is generally eosinophilic in nature. The pathogenesis of VLM is the direct result of the immunologic response of the body to the dead and dying larvae. Multiple eosinophilic abscesses may develop in the infected tissues. The larvae remain alive, infective, and antigenic for an indefinite period of time. The inflammation appears as an eosinophilic granuloma and an open biopsy of a granulomatous lesion will often show the *Toxocara* larva. Host antibodies are generated against excretory-secretory (ES) antigens of the larvae. These glycoprotein antigens contain protease, acetylcholinesterase, and eosinophil-stimulating activity. They also elicit Th 2 immune responses and high levels of interleukins 4 and 5.

Clinical Manifestations

Toxocara is mainly an infection of young children, since they have a greater opportunity to ingest the infectious ova. The classic case occurs in a male child, younger than 6

years, with a history of pica and exposure to dogs. A child with fever of unknown etiology and eosinophilia should be assumed to have *Toxocara* infection until proven otherwise. The extent of signs and symptoms depends on the number and location of granulomatous lesions and the host's immune response. The initial symptoms include a prodrome of anorexia, fever, and lassitude. More recently, the so-called "covert toxocariasis" has been implicated as responsible for many subtle clinical manifestations. In a study of children in Ireland, the most frequent clinical manifestations were fever, headache, anorexia, abdominal pain, nausea, vomiting, lethargy, sleep and behavior disorders, pharyngitis, pneumonia, cough, wheeze, limb pain, cervical lymphadenitis, and hepatomegaly. Another case-control study in French adults led to the term "common toxocariasis," a syndrome comprising chronic dyspnea and weakness; cutaneous rash; pruritus and abdominal pain, often with eosinophilia; elevated levels of immunoglobulin E (IgE); and high titers of *Toxocara*-specific antibodies. Both "covert" and "common" toxocariasis probably represent variations in the clinical spectrum of mild *Toxocara* childhood and adult disease.

It is the immediate hypersensitivity response to the larvae that manifests as symptoms of VLM. The specific signs and symptoms depend on the organ affected. Liver invasion is an early event; hepatomegaly of varying degrees is almost always present. With more severe involvement, various combinations of abdominal pain, arthralgias, myalgias, weight loss, high intermittent fevers, pulmonary disease, and neurologic disturbance may be seen. In addition to being an environmental risk factor for asthma, symptoms include idiopathic seizure disorder, functional intestinal disorders, skin diseases (prurigo and chronic urticaria), eosinophilic and reactive arthritis, and angioedema.

Pulmonary involvement has been reported in anywhere from 20% to 80% of infected children. Cough, if present, is generally nonproductive. Wheezing is the most frequent finding on chest examination, although rhonchi and crackles also have been described. Because of the wheezing, some patients are diagnosed initially as suffering from asthma. There is no typical chest radiograph. Descriptions of imaging studies range from patchy airspace disease with pseudonodular infiltrates on computed tomography (CT), to diffuse interstitial pneumonitis, to an asymptomatic pulmonary mass. A pattern similar to miliary tuberculosis has been reported in severe cases. The varied radiologic patterns may reflect whether direct larval invasion of lung tissue or a hypersensitivity reaction to larval antigens is the primary pathologic process present in that particular patient. Although pulmonary symptoms are generally mild, acute respiratory failure has been reported from *Toxocara* infection.

The time course for VLM may be quite prolonged. The initial stage of the illness lasts several weeks, beginning with low-grade fevers and nonspecific symptoms, and progressing to eosinophilia and hepatomegaly. Episodes of bronchitis, asthma, or pneumonia may occur. Over the next month, intermittent high fevers occur along with the major manifestations of the disease. Recovery may take as long as 1 to 2 years, during which time the eosinophilia resolves along with the hepatomegaly. Resolution of pulmonary infiltrates occurs more rapidly.

Complications

Neurologic disturbances have been described in severe cases because of invasion of the central nervous system by larvae. Seizures, encephalopathy, meningoencephalitis, and transverse myelitis have been reported. Ocular involvement occurs when a larva enters the anterior vitreous of the eye. This can be difficult to differentiate from retinoblastoma, especially when hepatomegaly and eosinophilia are absent. Manifestations of peripheral nervous system involvement include radiculitis and cranial nerve palsy. Renal, pancreatic, and cardiac invasion rarely occur. The few deaths described with VLM have resulted from myocardial, neurologic, or overwhelming systemic involvement.

Diagnosis

Neutrophilia occurs during the first few days but rapidly gives way to the eosinophilia classically seen in the disease. Eosinophilia can range up to 50% to 90% of the total white blood cell count. Levels above 30% were considered essential for the diagnosis in early studies. Leukocytosis is generally present, with extreme values of over 100,000 cells/mm³ occasionally reported.

Other laboratory findings also may be helpful in supporting a diagnosis of VLM. Serum IgE levels are above 900 IU/mm in 60% of patients tested. Hypergammaglobulinemia is frequently reported, characterized by elevations of any one or all of the immunoglobulin classes. Because of cross-reactivity between larval and blood group antigens, many patients will develop high anti-A and anti-B isohemagglutinin titers that persist for months after the initial infection. Bronchoalveolar lavage fluid also may exhibit a relative eosinophilia.

ELISA using the larval ES antigens to detect the host's antibodies is the most widely available and accepted test for confirmation. If a titer above 1:32 is considered, the diagnostic sensitivity is approximately 78%, with a specificity of over 92%. Because antibodies against *Toxocara* are present for years, an antigen-capture ELISA has been developed to separate acute from dormant infection; it is not commercially available.

Examination of the stool for ova and parasites is not helpful because the larvae rarely mature in humans. Before the ELISA against ES antibodies was developed, tissue biopsy to demonstrate the larvae in eosinophilic granulomas was the definitive test for diagnosis. Skin tests, other serologic testing, and fluorescent antibody techniques were troubled by low sensitivities and unacceptably high cross-reactivity with other parasitic infections.

Differential diagnosis should include the visceral lesions that may be produced by other nematode worms, as well as immature stages of certain spiroid nematodes and filarial worms. Invasion of the liver by *Fasciola hepatica*, a nematode worm, or *Capillaria hepatica*, a trematode, also might be included. *Toxocara canis* also may produce the PIE syndrome (pulmonary infiltrates and eosinophilia). Also to be considered in this diagnosis are trichinosis, hepatitis, leukemia, the many causes of intense eosinophilia, tuberculosis, asthma, lead poisoning, and the leukemoid reaction occurring in severe bacterial pneumonia.

Treatment

Albendazole or mebendazole are the treatments of choice for *Toxocara* infections. Albendazole is used at a dose of 10 mg/kg/day in two divided doses for 5 days and was superior to thiabendazole for the treatment of VLM in clinical trials. Most patients recover without specific anthelmintic therapy. Corticosteroids have been useful in patients with severe pulmonary involvement, possibly by treating the hypersensitivity component of the disease. Otherwise, treatment is symptomatic.

Prevention

Measures that decrease the ingestion of contaminated soil reduce the incidence of the disease. Anticipatory guidance should focus on the risks of pica and elimination of the behavior. Regular deworming of puppies and lactating or pregnant adult female dogs should be performed, and the risks of indiscriminate disposal of dog feces, especially in children's play areas, should be emphasized.

HYDATID DISEASE OF THE LUNG (PULMONARY HYDATIDOSIS)

The lung is involved in human hydatidosis caused by the cystic larval stage of the tapeworm *Echinococcus*; cystic hydatid disease is caused by *Echinococcus granulosus*, which is worldwide in distribution. Alveolar hydatid disease is associated with *Echinococcus multilocularis*, which is commonly seen in the Northern Hemisphere. Polycystic disease is caused by *E. vogeli* and is seen in Central and South America.[1]

The life cycles of *E. granulosus*, *E. multilocularis*, and *E. vogeli* are similar.[1] The first developmental stage is the tapeworm, which reaches sexual maturity only in the intestinal tract of its definitive mammalian host: dogs or other canines. Infectious ova are released during defecation, contaminating fields, irrigated lands, and wells. *Echinococcus* eggs are extremely resistant to climatic conditions, and in northern regions will survive for at least 2 years. When eggs are swallowed by humans, the outer shell is digested and the embryos penetrate the intestine and are hematogenously disseminated to various parts of the body, mostly to the liver and lung. In the lung, the embryos form hydatid cysts. Under ideal conditions, tapeworm heads, or protoscoleces, develop within the cysts.

Cystic Hydatid Disease

Classic, or pastoral, cystic hydatidosis is most commonly seen in the sheep- and cattle-raising areas of the Mediterranean, Middle East, South America, Russia, Eastern Europe, India, Australia, and Africa. In North America, it is seen among the Californian Basque sheep herders, and in Utah, New Mexico, and Arizona, particularly among the Native American populations.

Humans become infected from contaminated water and food or through close contact with infected dogs. Lung cysts develop when embryos pass through the liver, through lymphatic ducts bypassing the liver, by contiguous extension from the liver, or through the bronchi.

The hydatid slowly enlarges, and its rate of growth is dependent on the distensibility of the tissue and the age of the host. Pulmonary cysts grow faster in children. At a size of 1 cm, three layers can be identified within the cyst: (1) an inner layer of germinal epithelium or endocyst that is responsible for formation of daughter cysts by endogenous vesiculation; (2) a middle noncellular, laminated layer or ectocyst; and (3) an adventitia or pericyst, an outer capsule of fibrous tissue, vasculature, giant cells, and eosinophils resulting from a weak host reaction. With time, blood capsules and daughter cysts may develop and disintegrate, liberating free scoleces or "hydatid sand."

Echinococcus granulosus is known to affect all age groups and any body cavity, organ, or site; it most frequently affects the liver and the lungs, with the lung more commonly affected in children.[2] Infection occurs mostly during childhood, although years may elapse before manifestations are seen. There is no gender preference, and the slight differences in gender incidence are probably due to activity or occupation. Asymptomatic hydatidosis in family members is seen in 5% to 18% of cases.

In cystic hydatid disease, 17% to 75% of cases occur in children. After the age of 4 years, the distribution throughout childhood is even. In Tunis, of 643 children with pulmonary hydatid cysts, the mean age was 5 years (2 to 15 years).[2]

Involvement of the diaphragm and transdiaphragmatic extension into the lung has been described in patients with primary hydatid cysts of the liver. Other tissues that may be affected are the brain, eye, heart, mediastinum, blood vessels, pleura, diaphragm, pancreas, spleen, endocrine glands, bone, and genitourinary tract. The central nervous system is affected more often in children than in adults.

Clinical Features

Cyst size, location, and the potential for impairment of vital structures determine the clinical manifestations. A large proportion of pulmonary cases may be discovered incidentally on a routine chest radiograph. Most individuals harboring small lung cysts often remain asymptomatic 5 to 20 years after infection until the cyst enlarges sufficiently to cause symptoms. The slowly enlarging hydatid cyst is usually well tolerated. An awareness of symptoms is due to pressure from the enlarging cyst, secondary infection, and cyst rupture. The intact cyst is most commonly asymptomatic and may account for a third of all cases. This is more common in children.

The more common manifestations of pulmonary cysts are cough, chest pain, hemoptysis, fever, and malaise. Retarded growth patterns have been observed in many children. Other manifestations are sputum production, chest discomfort, loss of appetite, dyspnea, vomiting of cyst elements, dysphagia, and hepatic pain. Bronchospasm has been reported with relief of bronchial asthma after removal of the cyst.[3]

Children with echinococcosis may present as emergency cases because of complications of the disease. These complications may be mechanical, with hydatid growth affecting the bronchial tree or pleura; they also may result from hematogenous spread, infection, or allergic reaction. Cyst rupture, pneumothorax, atelectasis, bronchopleural fistula, empyema, residual cavity, bronchiectasis, secondary cysts, and superimposed infection including saprophytic mycosis have been reported. A rare complication is rupture into the cardiovascular system with dissemination or sudden death.

Up to 30% of lung cysts may be complicated by rupture into the pleural space or bronchus, precipitated by coughing, sneezing, trauma, or increased abdominal pressure. Chills, fever, increased cough, mild hemoptysis, and change in appearance on radiographs suggest rupture. The coughing up of hydatid cyst elements, described as "coughing up grape skins," is diagnostic. Secondary hydatidosis in the pleura, acute asphyxia by bronchial obstruction, and allergic reactions, including anaphylaxis, may follow cyst rupture and leakage.

Bronchobiliary fistula occurs in 2% of cases and is commonly, but not always, preceded by suppuration. The right side and posterior basal segment are most frequently affected. Pyrexia and weight loss may mimic malignancy, but bile expectoration is pathognomonic.

The cysts' unusual location is the cause of the following reported rarer complications: arterial emboli, portal hypertension, systemic venous obstruction, paraplegia, pleural effusion, phrenic nerve paralysis, transitory paralysis of cervical sympathetic chain, lower extremity thrombophlebitis, and stress ulcer.[4]

Diagnosis

Awareness of the disease is most important. Lung involvement is very likely if a cyst is present elsewhere in the body. Cystic hydatid disease is suspected based on a history of current or previous residence in an endemic area, clinical observations, and radiographic evidence. In 10% a diagnosis is suspected on routine radiographic study alone. A history of contact with possibly infected dogs may be obtained in only 29% to 48% of cases.

Physical examination is rarely definitive. Occasionally, a hydatid thrill (fluid wave) can be felt while percussing a large cyst. Demonstration of scoleces and hooklets of the parasite in vomitus, stool, urine, or sputum is pathognomonic but is rarely observed, and they may be seen only during surgery. Fine-needle aspiration under ultrasonographic or CT guidance may be successful with few complications in adults. However, observations in children are sparse, and the procedure carries a substantial risk because leakage may induce anaphylactic shock.

Hepatic function may be abnormal in one half of patients with liver cysts. An increased specific serum IgE may be observed, but eosinophilia is more often absent than present and is completely unreliable in areas endemic for other parasites.

The Casoni skin test involves injection of hydatid fluid in the dermis, which produces an erythematous papule in 50% to 80% of patients in less than 60 minutes. A Casoni test can be helpful if the results are strongly positive, but positive test results in known cases vary considerably, from 38% to 81%. False-negative results, sometimes due to infected cysts, and false-positive results occur in 30% of those tested. The Casoni test results remain positive for life.

Serologic tests include latex agglutination, indirect hemagglutination, complement fixation, agar gel diffusion, enzyme immunoassay, and immunoblot. Cross-reactivity between echinococcosis and cysticercosis (*Taenia solium* infection) is a problem with any test that employs whole-cyst antigens. Serum antibody testing by indirect hemagglutination is 91% sensitive and 83% specific at a titer greater than or equal to 1:128. Immunoblot is 86% sensitive and 99% specific. After surgical removal of the cyst, there is generally a rapid decline in antibody within 3 months. Failure to observe the decline suggests incomplete cyst removal. Antibodies may persist for years after surgical removal of a hydatid cyst. Serum antibody tests can be referred to the Centers for Disease Control and Prevention (CDC), Atlanta. False-negative results are more common in children and with pulmonary cysts. Up to 50% of patients with hydatid cysts in the lung or calcified cysts are seronegative. Laboratory tests may be more sensitive in complicated cysts, but at present, no single test is infallible, and there is still no serologic test that can effectively rule out the disease. Thus, disease awareness is most important.

The main diagnostic tool is the radiographic study, which is 98% to 100% accurate. However, with miniature screening radiographic studies, only 40% of cases are diagnosed. On occasion, inflammatory reactions and secondary infections may mask both closed and ruptured cysts.

On radiography, lung cysts are readily detected, and the possibility of a hydatid cyst in an endemic area should always be considered. An intact cyst is seen as a round or oval homogeneous lesion with a sharply defined smooth border surrounded by normal lung or a zone of atelectasis. It may be located in the periphery, center, or hilum; be single or multiple, and be unilateral or bilateral (Fig. 36-1). The final form depends on the location and neighboring structures. With an increase in size, bronchial dislocation occurs without obstruction, as has been demonstrated by tomography or bronchography. On fluoroscopy, good elasticity of the cyst wall is demonstrable, and there is no interference with movement of the diaphragm.

As the cyst grows, air passages and surrounding vessels are eroded, producing bronchial air leaks into the cyst adventitia. The bronchial connection is actually nonpatent before rupture because of pressure of the endocyst against bronchial passages, and it may be recognized only during surgery. With varying stages of air dissection into the cyst, different classic radiologic signs may be seen. A pericystic emphysema is seen before rupture. A "meniscus sign" or "crescent sign" is a crescentic radiolucency above the homogeneous cyst shadow on deep inspiration that is seen when air penetrates between adventitia and ectocyst. As air dissection continues, the parasite's membrane is torn, and some hydatid fluid flows out. An air-fluid level is seen within the cyst lumen as well as an air cup between ectocyst and adventitia, known as "double air-layer appearance" or the Cumbo sign. With free connection to a bronchus, the cyst wall is detached from

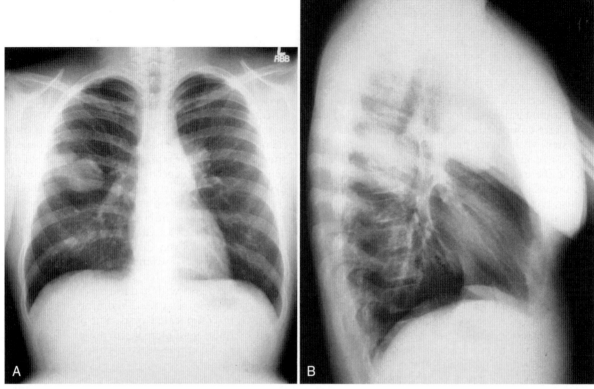

FIGURE 36-1. The posteroanterior **(A)** and lateral **(B)** chest radiographs from a 15-year-old boy with cough of several months' duration show bilateral circumscribed densities in the anterolateral right upper lobe and the superior left lower lobe. Histopathology after excision confirmed the diagnosis of hydatid cysts.

adventitia, crumbles, collapses, and floats on remaining cyst fluid. This result is seen on the radiograph as air between the collapsed floating cyst wall and the adventitia, known as the "water lily sign" or Camellote sign. The adventitial wall does not collapse at once, so the obliteration of the cyst cavity is not an immediate outcome.

Cystic hydatidosis of the lung occurs most often as a single unilocular cyst. Only about 7% to 38% occur as multiple unilocular cysts. The inferior lobes are most commonly affected. In children, the ratio of intact to ruptured cysts is 3:1, which is the inverse of that in adults. Unlike in spleen and liver hydatid cysts, calcification of lung cysts is rare. A high right hemidiaphragm and right basal bronchiectasis suggest bronchobiliary fistula. A tract on sinogram or bronchogram is diagnostic.

CT should be performed preoperatively to better define and localize the cysts. CT may aid in diagnosing pulmonary hydatid cysts (Fig. 36-2). CT can demonstrate the water density in the intact cyst and can differentiate pleural from parenchymal lung or chest wall pathology. CT is especially helpful in complicated lung disease when more than one compartment of the chest is involved.[5] The ability of CT to demonstrate characteristic hydatid anatomy, such as detached or collapsed membrane and daughter cysts, allows a specific diagnosis to be made.[6]

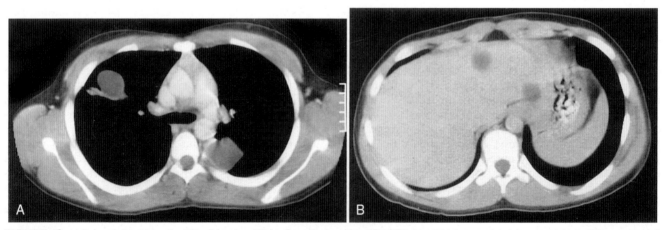

FIGURE 36-2. Computed tomography (CT) of the chest **(A)** confirms the location of fluid-filled cysts in the anterior right upper lobe and the superior left lower lobe (same patient as in Fig. 36-1), and liver involvement is seen on abdominal CT in this case **(B)**.

Ultrasonography helps distinguish cystic lesions from solid tumors. Pathognomonic signs on ultrasonography are multiple daughter cysts within a cyst, separation of the laminated membrane from the wall of the cyst, and collapsed cysts.[7] A simple cyst with a thick wall in patients from an endemic area is suggestive. Abdominal ultrasonography is also recommended for liver cyst detection. Angiography can sometimes demonstrate a characteristic halo effect around the cyst and may help determine the number and location of cysts.

Differential diagnosis of hydatid disease includes abscess, hamartoma, pulmonary arteriovenous fistula, benign granuloma, malignant tumor, metastases, and cysts of different origin. The presence of the Cumbo sign is confirmatory.

Histopathology

Histopathology depends on the size of cyst, the time after rupture, and the allergic reactivity of the host. With intact hydatid cysts, minimal atelectasis and compression are seen. A strong allergic eosinophilic reaction in surrounding lung tissue can be found with a recently ruptured cyst. Cysts ruptured for less than 10 days show reversible inflammatory infiltrates of lymphocytes or giant cell granulomata around parasite components. When the rupture is older than 10 days, severe fibrosis starts to develop, leading to dense scarring with subsequent tendency toward bronchiectasis and superinfection.

Treatment

There are currently three treatment options for cystic echinococcosis: surgery, ultrasound-guided aspiration, and chemotherapy. Each method has limitations depending on the specific case. Spontaneous cure is possible after coughing out the cyst and its contents, but more commonly, infection and toxemia follow from the residual cyst. Up to two thirds of symptomatic patients may die without intervention. When possible, surgery is the recommended treatment for all cases, although conservative management with benzimidazoles may be equally effective in asymptomatic patients. The success of surgery is dependent on the size and location of the cyst and on the skill of the surgeon. It is important to perform surgery immediately after diagnosis because a weak adventitial reaction and bronchial communications may lead to rupture with intrapulmonary dissemination. Only in the benign Alaskan-Canadian variant is conservative treatment recommended.

The aims of surgery are total eradication of the parasite with evacuation of the cyst and removal of the endocyst, prevention of cyst rupture and consequent dissemination during the operation, and extirpation of the residual cavity. The lung parenchyma should be preserved and resection should be avoided in children if possible because the damaged lung parenchyma has great capacity for recovery. Lung resection may be done in cases with bronchiectasis, severe inflammation, and large or multiple cysts that have destroyed lung parenchyma.

The posterolateral approach is favored. Surgical techniques to eradicate the parasite may include puncture and aspiration of cyst *in situ*, excision of the entire cyst by enucleation, wedge resection, segmentectomy, lobectomy, or pneumonectomy.

Such surgical procedures as enucleation with or without obliteration of the residual cavity by sutures (capitonnage) and cystectomy are mainly used for uncomplicated cysts. Lobectomy or segmental resection is reserved for lung destroyed by large cysts or bronchobiliary and biliary-pleural fistulas. One favored procedure is subtotal cystopericystectomy with total extirpation of the parasite or its rests in ruptured cysts, followed by closure of bronchial leaks and washing with a scolicidal solution. Subtotal extirpation of the pericyst or adventitia is then performed, leaving the hilar portion in place, because total resection of the adventitia in its hilar pole carries considerable risk. In many cases of cystic hydatid disease of the lung, Keystone[8] has found it possible to eliminate the intact cyst by positive-pressure ventilation to force the cyst from the surgical opening in the lung.

Rupture and spillage may occur and may lead to dissemination and anaphylaxis, which can be fatal. This complication, although uncommon even with spillage during surgery, is greatly feared. The differences in surgical techniques therefore reflect the desire to prevent spillage of viable cyst contents. Commonly, the operative field is protected with saline-moistened gauzes, and the cysts are gently manipulated.

After extirpation of the parasite, bronchial fistulas are closed. To prevent recurrence, the residual cavity is injected with scolicidal agents, such as formalin, hypertonic saline, povidone-iodine, or absolute alcohol. Because of extremely grave complications with the use of formalin and hypertonic solutions, others have used hydrogen peroxide with good results. The residual cavity is then either obliterated by sutures or left open to communicate with the pleural space. Alternatively, the pericystic membrane is resected with repair of bronchial leakage. With a bronchobiliary fistula, the usually accompanying biliary hypertension is corrected, and the hepatic cavity is obliterated or drained. In cases with bronchobiliary fistula, the operative mortality rate is between 5% and 50%.

The more common surgical complications in children include atelectasis, hydropneumothorax, wound infection, pleural reaction, and hemothorax. Other reported complications from surgery are chest infection, abscess, empyema, septic shock, bronchial rupture, pneumothorax, bronchobiliary fistula, biliary-pleural fistula, hemorrhage, massive aspiration, prolonged drainage, bronchiectasis, and allergic reactions, including anaphylactic shock and death with rupture. The perioperative morbidity rate is 3% to 10%, and the mortality rate is 0% to 5%. The recurrence rate is 0% to 5%.

According to the World Health Organization (WHO) guidelines, chemotherapy with benzimidazoles (i.e., mebendazole or albendazole) is indicated when surgery is impractical or impossible, when patients have multiple cysts in two or more organs, when peritoneal cysts are present, and for recurrent disease.[9,10] Presurgical use of albendazole or mebendazole can reduce the recurrence of cystic echinococcosis. Preoperative treatment also has been reported to reduce intracystic pressure and simplify removal.

The dose for mebendazole is typically 50 to 60 mg/kg/day, in three divided doses, for 3 to 6 months, often for up to a year. This medication interferes with uptake of glucose by cestodes and disrupts their microtubule system, but it is poorly absorbed and produces low blood concentrations. High-dose treatment with mebendazole 100 to 200 mg/kg/day for 3 months has been used in children successfully and without serious side effects. A peak therapeutic blood level of 80 ng/mL is recommended. Absorption is enhanced with meals. Repeated courses may be necessary. Cure of hydatid disease has been achieved in 35% to 75% of patients and recurrence rates have been low.

Adverse reactions to mebendazole may occur within the first month. Febrile and allergic reactions, alopecia, glomerulonephritis, and reversible leukopenia have been reported. With hepatobiliary disease, high blood levels and toxicity have been observed. Monitoring of clinical status, liver function, renal function, and complete blood count should be done weekly for the first month and biweekly thereafter.

In adult patients, albendazole has been as effective as or even better than mebendazole. High blood and tissue levels can be achieved Albendazole differs from mebendazole in two respects: it is absorbed at a higher rate and it undergoes almost total first-pass metabolism to its effective protoscolicide metabolite, albendazole sulfoxide. Its plasma concentration in hydatid-infested patients is about 10 to 40 times higher than that achieved with mebendazole. Cyst fluid concentrations also are higher than those achieved with mebendazole. Further enhancement of drug concentration in target tissues may be possible with the concurrent use of cimetidine or administration with a fat-rich meal. Only a few observations in children have been reported. For those who are 10 years of age and older, 28-day courses of 10 to 15 mg/kg/day in two divided doses, separated by 14-day drug-free periods, for several 1-month courses have been recommended. Albendazole is usually well tolerated. Liver function may be abnormal in 10% to 20% of patients during treatment but side effects are rarely severe. Presurgical and postsurgical treatment of cystic echinococcosis with albendazole prevents recurrences. In addition, praziquantel may be added, especially after surgery, when the risk of spillage is high. Praziquantel when given alone is not effective, but it does act synergistically with albendazole. Although limited data are available, the dose recommended is 40 mg/kg/wk. Use of albendazole has been shown to be a safe and effective alternative to surgery for treating uncomplicated liver cystic *Echinococcosis* and requires a shorter hospital stay.

Contraindications to chemotherapy with benzimidazoles include patients with large cysts that are at-risk for rupture and inactive or calcified cysts. Patients with chronic liver disease or bone marrow suppression also should not undergo benzimidazole treatment. Albendazole should not be used during the first trimester of pregnancy because it has teratogenic effects in animals, although these have not been observed in humans.

A newer benzimidazole compound oxfendazole that has been tested in animal models seems at least as effective as albendazole and is easier to administer. In addition to treatment with benzimidazole derivatives, percutaneous drainage of hydatid cysts under sonographic guidance with irrigation of the cavity using hypertonic saline and instillation of absolute alcohol has been successful in adult patients ineligible for surgery.

Prevention and Follow-up

Hydatid lung disease is preventable. Preventive measures include the use of veterinary taeniacides for dogs; the proper disposal of carcasses and entrails of animals to prevent dogs from gaining access; and the proper practice of hand, food, and drink hygiene to prevent contamination from dog excrement.

Follow-up abdominal ultrasonography should be done annually for 5 years or more. Chest radiographs and CT scans should be repeated after 2 or 3 years and at 5 years. A cyst cavity may remain, and serologic findings may be positive for several years.

Sylvatic Alaskan-Canadian Variant

The Alaskan-Canadian variety is clinically and morphologically distinct and has been named *E. granulosus* var. *canadensis*. It is seen in the tundra and northern coniferous forests of North America south to the Great Lakes, mainly among the native population, including the Eskimo, Aleut, and Native American Indians, 75% of whom live in areas where *E. granulosus* occurs. The wolf is the definitive host, and sometimes the dog, which ingests the tapeworm by eating the viscera of infected deer. Elk, reindeer, moose, and caribou also are intermediate hosts. Pig, sheep, and cattle resist the infection. Humans are not very suitable hosts.

The Alaskan-Canadian sylvatic infection is more benign; the cysts are smaller and more delicate, do not grow as rapidly, and produce fewer symptoms than the classic or pastoral *E. granulosus*. The risk of anaphylaxis with rupture is less, and the prospect for spontaneous cure without significant complications is excellent.

Most commonly affected organs are the liver and the lung, with lung involvement in 61% of the cases. Most cysts are simple, intact, and uninfected. For pulmonary cysts, the mean age is 22 years (5 to 77 years), and for liver cysts, it is 65.3 years (24 to 96 years). In patients with lung cysts, 71% are younger than 20 years.

Only 6% to 8% of cases are symptomatic, mostly because of cyst rupture, which occurs in some 26% of patients. Cough, purulent expectoration, and hemoptysis are usual complaints. Serious complications are rare, and no cases of anaphylaxis or seeding have been seen in the Alaskan[11,12] or Canadian experience.[13,14]

Diagnosis is based on a history of residence in an endemic area, and exposure to dogs, and routine radiographic study. Typically, a round or oval homogeneous water-like density with clear-cut borders and no surrounding reaction is seen. Classic signs such as water lily and crescent sign are rare. Laboratory tests are of little value. Eosinophilia is positive in only 29% of cases, hemagglutination in 10%, and the Casoni test in 56%. With cyst leak or rupture, test results are usually but not always positive.

The surgical risk is minimal. Extrusion of the intact vesicle is not appropriate, and an open wedge resection of adventitia with intact cyst is favored. Gentleness is very important. The bronchial stump should be closed, and the defect in the lung obliterated. Alternatively, cystectomy may be performed.

Quite commonly, the cyst evacuates into the bronchi, and the symptoms disappear. Thus, surgery is not recommended for asymptomatic patients who are managed by observation. No serious morbidity and mortality have been reported with this approach.

Alveolar Hydatid Disease

Echinococcus multilocularis is a cestode that differs morphologically and biologically in its larval and adult stages from *E. granulosus*. The usual definitive host is the fox, with dogs and cats acting as sources of human infection in endemic areas. Intermediate hosts are rodents and humans. The larval stage develops normally in rodents, but humans are unusual and poor intermediate hosts. The disease is usually found across much of the Soviet Union, central Europe, northern Japan, Alaska, and northern Canada. Human disease is rare in the Western Hemisphere, but the cestode is endemic in the north-central United States and Canada.

The infection usually occurs during childhood. A case-control study has identified the following risk factors: having a lifetime pattern of dog ownership, tethering dogs near the house, and living in a house built directly on the tundra rather than on gravel or permanent foundations, thus allowing contact with contaminated dog feces.[15] Other implicated factors are the drinking of unboiled melted snow and the skinning of foxes. The disease manifests usually between the ages of 19 and 40 years but has been seen in those as young as 5 years. The mean age at diagnosis in Alaska is 53 years. The disease favors neither sex.

The larval cestode persists in its proliferative phase because of the inability of humans to provide the conditions necessary for normal development. Instead of developing a thick, laminated layer and growing into large, single cysts, the parasite has a thin, deficient ectocyst that grows and infiltrates into the surrounding tissues. The growing cyst may have several small, fluid-filled pockets containing protoscoleces. Because of its structure, this larval form is called an alveolar or multilocular hydatid. It provokes a severe host reaction and becomes surrounded by an inflammatory or granulomatous reaction, instead of the fibrous host response seen with *E. granulosus*. A central area of necrosis is always seen.

The cyst is slow growing, behaves like a malignancy, and has been mistaken for carcinoma, which it can mimic clinically and microscopically. Untreated it can be just as devastating, with mortality rates as high as 80%. The primary site of infection is the liver, where a dense honeycomb of small, multilocular cysts is formed. The cyst appears as a solid cancerlike growth that may cavitate and attain massive size. Through the inferior vena cava it may metastasize to distant organs. Alveolar hydatid disease of the lung is invariably a metastatic focus.

Diagnosis is based on history of exposure, elevated serologic titers, and characteristic changes on radiographic studies. Physical signs are confusing, and subjective symptoms may be mild, vague, and ill defined. Patients present usually with asymptomatic hepatomegaly. When symptoms are present, they are commonly related to the abdomen: mild epigastric and right upper-quadrant abdominal pain or distress, intermittent fever, and jaundice.

On radiologic examination, hepatomegaly and hepatic calcification are the most common findings. Typically, the diagnosis is made with abdominal radiographs that show scattered radiolucent areas surrounded with calcification, sometimes referred to as the "Swiss cheese" liver calcification pattern. This finding is pathognomonic, but at least 5 years of illness must elapse before calcification can be demonstrated. Without the characteristic radiographic study, the diagnosis is rarely made preoperatively.

CT and ultrasonography will demonstrate an indistinct mass with a necrotic center. Serologic tests used are the same as those for *E. granulosus* but tend to produce more positive findings with high titers. Indirect hemagglutination titers decline markedly during the first year after radical surgical resection but not after chemotherapy. The EM2 ELISA, using a semipurified homologous antigen fraction, is more sensitive and specific than tests using heterologous *E. granulosus* antigen fractions.[16] Results may still be positive, however, even when the parasite is no longer viable.[17] Needle biopsy confirms the diagnosis. There is no risk for anaphylaxis or spillage of protoscoleces because the tumor is essentially solid.

Treatment is by surgery. Early diagnosis is very important to permit resection before infiltration becomes too extensive. However, many cases are undiagnosed until they are well advanced and the hepatic lesions are unresectable.

At surgery, liver invasion is often more extensive than suggested by the degree of calcification on the radiograph. Complete excision is the only hope. Cure is possible when partial hepatectomy or hepatic lobectomy can remove all multilocular cysts and still preserve enough organ function. Still, radical hepatic resection is curative in only 20% of cases. Palliative measures are designed to ensure adequate bile drainage.

If surgery is unsuccessful or impractical, mebendazole is recommended at 40 mg/kg/day in divided doses for life, which may prevent progression of the primary lesion and metastasis and prolong life. Benzimidazole compounds are parasitostatic rather than parasitocidal for *E. multilocularis*. Thus, treatment with these agents implies lifelong application. The overall success rate of such treatment ranges between 55% and 97%. Hepatic toxicity with the use of this drug can develop without warning, however, and does not seem to be dose related or likely due to hypersensitivity. Hepatic function should be monitored the entire time the drug is administered. Monitoring should be done weekly during the first month and monthly thereafter. Amphotericin B has shown to have some benefit as salvage treatment.

Though not fulminating, the disease is ultimately fatal unless early surgical intervention can remove the parasite cyst. Patients have survived at least 16 years after diagnosis. Death is due to liver failure; invasion of contiguous areas; and metastases to the lung, brain, and distant organs. The best means of preventing alveolar hydatid disease remains the control of the cestode in domestic animals, the primary source of human infection.

Polycystic Hydatid Cyst

Polycystic hydatid cyst disease is caused by *E. vogeli* and *E. oligarthrus*. Only *E. vogeli* causes pulmonary disease and it is polycystic in nature. Polycystic echinococcosis occurs only in Central and South America and because of that, it is also called neotropical echinococcosis. Ninety-nine human cases of polycystic hydatic cyst have been diagnosed in 11 countries.

Bush dog is the definitive host, and pacas and agoutis are intermediate hosts. Domesticated dogs also can get infected naturally and experimentally.[1] It is speculated that domesticated dogs play a role in transmission of the infection to humans.[18]

After liver, lung is the second most common organ involved in polycystic hydatid disease.[19] After establishing infection in the liver, the infection spreads to other organ systems, including the lungs.[20]

Clinically polycystic hydatid disease is similar to alveolar hydatid disease caused by *E. multilocularis*. The severity of the disease is between cystic and alveolar infections.[19] The typical clinical scenario is an infection lasting a long time and manifesting as chronic disease. The reported range before diagnosis is 1 month to 22 years. Clinical manifestations primarily include abdominal pain and a palpable abdominal mass, usually hepatomegaly. Patients may have jaundice, fever, weight loss, and anemia. Patients with pulmonary involvement will have hemoptysis and may have other chest symptoms depending on the size and location of the cyst. Eosinophilia is often present.

Serologic tests cannot differentiate between infections caused by *E. vogeli* and other echinococci.[21] Antibodies against *Echinococcus* can be detected in 75% of the infected individuals using indirect hemagglutination assay.[22] An ELISA in one study could specifically diagnose *E. vogeli* infection.[23] Pulmonary involvement can be diagnosed by the polycystic structures on chest radiography, ultrasonography, or CT. Identification of protoscoleces or rostellar hooks by the shape and dimension is diagnostic.[24]

Medical treatment is preferred over surgical intervention because of high risks associated with surgery. Albendazole is the drug of choice. Although experience in the treatment of polycystic hydatid disease is limited, it has shown success in small series. In operable cases, prolonged or even lifelong therapy with albendazole or mebendazole may be needed.

■ STRONGYLOIDIASIS

Strongyloidiasis is caused by the nematode *Strongyloides stercoralis*. The helminth is 2 to 3 mm long and 30 to 50 μm wide.[25] The life cycle of *S. stercoralis* is not completely understood. The female worm is infectious and it lays its embryonated eggs in the intestine; the rhabditiform larvae hatch in the mucosa and then bore through the epithelium and migrate into the intestinal lumen and are excreted in stool. The rhabditiform larvae, in the soil and under suitable warm and moist conditions, develop into filariform larvae (direct developmental cycle). However, the rhabditiform larvae can also develop into free-living (nonparasitic) adult male and female helminthes who can mate and lay eggs in the soil (indirect developmental cycle), and these eggs hatch into rhabditiform larvae that can develop into infectious filariform larvae. Similar to the hookworm, these infectious larvae can penetrate human skin, enter the bloodstream, and reach the heart and lungs. In the lung they molt, climb up the bronchi and trachea, and are swallowed. Once in the intestinal mucosa and crypts, they complete their life cycle.[26] Internal autoinfection can occur, when rhabditiform larvae in the lower bowel develop directly into filariform larvae that in turn penetrate the intestinal mucosa and gain access into lymphatic and hematogenous systems and reach the lung and bowel to complete their life cycle. Massive autoinfection can induce hyperinfection syndrome. Another phenomenon referred to as external autoinfection occurs when the filariform larvae penetrate the perianal skin.

Strongyloidiasis is present endemically in the tropical and subtropical parts of the world; the larvae are sensitive to dryness and extreme temperatures. It also occurs sporadically in temperate areas. Humans are the primary hosts, but primates, cats, and dogs also are frequently infested. Estimates of the global burden of strongyloidiasis range from 30 million to 100 million infected individuals. A prevalence of 0.4% to 4% has been estimated in the southern United States.[27,28] The infection occurs more frequently in rural areas and in lower socioeconomic groups.

Strongyloides stercoralis infection encompasses five clinical syndromes: (1) acute infection with Loeffler syndrome, (2) chronic intestinal infection, (3) asymptomatic autoinfection, (4) symptomatic autoinfection, and (5) hyperinfection syndrome (HS) with dissemination. The pathogenesis of HS may involve disruption in Th 2 cell-mediated, humoral, or mucosal immunity, which triggers conversion of the rhabditiform larvae into filariform larvae, which then migrate from the small intestines to other organs. The mortality of HS is 15% increasing to 87% when there is dissemination.[29] Because of the autoinfection phenomenon, patients may have symptoms for years.

Symptoms fall into three broad categories: cutaneous, intestinal, and pulmonary and can occur during acute or chronic disease and during HS.[30,31] The acute disease is often recognized by its cutaneous manifestations followed by pulmonary and intestinal symptomatology. The hallmark of cutaneous symptoms is pruritus at the site of larval entry, usually at the foot or ankle but sometimes also the perianal area. The site of entry has erythema and edema with a petechial or urticarial localized skin rash. Within a week or so the migration of larvae into the tracheobronchopulmonary tree causes itching of the throat, dry cough, and Loffler-like pneumonia with eosinophilia. This is followed by intestinal manifestations that include colicky abdominal pain (often epigastric), diarrhea, flatulence, and malaise.

Symptoms may be recurrent or continuous as the patient enters the chronic stage of the disease. This stage, if not treated, can last decades. With chronic infection the cutaneous features include stationary urticaria and larva currens (similar to larva migrans). Gastrointestinal symptoms are similar to those in the acute disease and can range from mild to severe. Burning or colicky abdominal pain can accompany diarrhea that can contain blood and mucus and alternate with constipation. In addition, patients may complain of anorexia, nausea, vomiting, flatulence, and perianal pruritus. There also may be epigastric tenderness. Chronic pulmonary manifestations include dry cough and wheezing. With worsening infection, patients may complain of fever, malaise, dyspnea, weakness, and weight loss. One half of affected patients with chronic strongyloidiasis may be asymptomatic.

HS occurs because of disseminated strongyloidiasis from massive autoinfection, resulting in an overwhelming larval burden and increased dissemination of the larvae to the lungs and other organ systems.[32,33] This results in severe pulmonary and extrapulmonary systemic symptoms. Although this syndrome can occur without a predisposing cause, it is usually associated with depressed cellular immunity caused by malnutrition, hematologic malignancies, or immunosuppressive therapy (e.g., steroids or anti-TNF-α). Human immunodeficiency virus (HIV)–infected patients do not seem to be at risk unless they are on steroids.[34] Pulmonary manifestations are increasing cough and dyspnea along with an odorless mucopurulent or blood-tinged sputum. Pulmonary changes include pneumonia, bronchitis, and pleural effusion. Rarely, miliary abscesses may form. Eosinophilia is usually absent in HS since use of corticosteroids reduces the levels of circulating eosinophils by inhibiting their proliferation and increasing apoptosis.

As for other helminthic infections, the diagnosis of strongyloidiasis is best made by visual identification. For S. stercoralis, identifying the characteristic rhabditiform larvae in stool, sputum, or duodenal fluid is diagnostic. However, a single stool specimen has a sensitivity of only 15% to 30%. Sensitivity increases to nearly 100% if seven consecutive daily stool specimens are examined in an expert laboratory.[35] This is of course not very practical. Serologic tests (gel diffusion and ELISA) are not useful. PCR of stool is under development and not commercially available at present.

The chest radiograph is normal in most infected patients. During pulmonary larval migration, there may be irregular and transient patches of pneumonitis or fine nodularity. Hyperinfection is accompanied by chest radiographic changes that range from focal to diffuse pulmonary infiltrates, to cavitation and abscess formation.

The combination of cutaneous, intestinal, and pulmonary symptoms, with eosinophilia on peripheral smear, and potential exposure in an endemic area provide essential clues for making the diagnosis. Pulmonary symptoms should be differentiated from pneumonitis caused by tuberculosis, mycoses, paragonimiasis, ascariasis, tropical pulmonary eosinophilia, and Loffler syndrome due to other causes.

The treatment is medical, and the goal is elimination of all the worms; therefore, repeated treatment is sometimes needed. Even after completion of treatment, patients must be followed for years to ensure complete eradication of all worms. Thiabendazole 25 mg/kg/dose twice a day for 2 or 3 days, or for 2 to 3 weeks for HS (if started early), is usually effective.[36] The duration of therapy should be determined by clinical response and worm burden. Ivermectin appears to be as effective as thiabendazole with fewer side effects. In fact, it is considered the drug of choice for most patients with strongyloidiasis, with thiabendazole and albendazole being alternatives.[37] Albendazole also appears to be as effective as thiabendazole.[38] Alternatives include mebendazole and pyrvinium pamoate. Pyrantel pamoate is not effective and should not be used for treatment.

PULMONARY PARAGONIMIASIS (LUNG FLUKE DISEASE)

Paragonimiasis, also known as lung fluke disease, benign endemic hemoptysis, oriental lung fluke, and pulmonary distomiasis, is caused by the genus Paragonimus. Most human disease is caused by Paragonimus westermani. Other species of Paragonimus, such as P. skrjabini, P. heterotremus, and P. miyazakii also can cause human disease. Paragonimiasis is a zoonotic infection of carnivorous animals, including those in the canine and feline families (which also serve as reservoir hosts). The animals are more likely the cause of infection than fresh water, although certain culinary habits (eating fresh or pickled crustaceans) also cause many infections. In humans the organism primarily infects the lungs, although brain and liver infections also have been reported.[39,40]

Paragonimus westermani is reddish brown in color, 7 to 16 mm long, 4 to 8 mm wide, and 2 to 5 mm thick.[41] Lung cysts have two adult flukes in them, and eggs reach the bronchi either by penetrating the intact cyst wall or after rupture of the cyst wall. From the bronchi, the eggs reach the mouth and are either spit out or swallowed and then excreted in stool. In the water, these eggs embryonate and hatch in approximately 3 weeks. The hatched miracidium invades the first intermediate host (one of several families of snails)[42] and after a protracted asexual cycle, they form sporocytes that turn into cercariae, which enter the second intermediate host (crustaceans), where they encyst and form the infectious metacercariae that reach the definitive host. Once eaten by the definitive host, the metacercariae encyst in the duodenum, penetrate the intestinal wall to reach the liver, and change into flukes. These flukes migrate through the diaphragm into the lung. Once in the lung, over a period of 5 to 6 weeks they mature into adult flukes and are encysted as a result of host immune response. Adult flukes begin to lay eggs 8 to 10 weeks after the infection.[43]

Paragonimiasis is seen in the Far East, Southeast Asia, the Indo-Pakistan subcontinent, some Pacific Islands, Africa, and parts of South and Latin America.[44]

As the life cycle of the fluke suggests, it can cause both pulmonary and extrapulmonary disease. The lesions are a result of direct mechanical damage by the flukes or their eggs, or by the toxins released by the flukes. The host response also adds to the damage in the lungs when the host immune response takes the form of eosinophilic infiltration and the subsequent development of a cyst of host granulation tissue around the flukes. Besides the adult flukes, the cyst also contains eggs and Charcot-Leyden crystals. The cysts are in the parenchyma of the lungs close to the bronchioles. The release of cyst contents can cause bronchopneumonia, and the cyst wall may fibrose and become calcified. In extrapulmonary infections, the flukes may form cysts, abscesses, or granulomata.

The symptoms depend on the site infected and the infectious burden. Some individuals may remain asymptomatic because of low inoculum burden. Pulmonary paragonimiasis has acute and chronic stages with different clinical manifestations. The main clinical manifestations of paragonimiasis are respiratory symptoms and eosinophilia. Once the flukes reach the lungs, the patient can have cough, dyspnea, and chest tightness or even pain; systemic symptoms of fever malaise and night sweats may be present. The patient may recall being sick days or weeks before their current illness with fever, diarrhea, and abdominal pain. Chills and urticarial rash may occur, leading to the diagnosis of a viral syndrome. A peripheral smear at this time shows eosinophilia. The diagnosis of paragonimiasis is frequently not made in the acute stage of the disease. The chronic stage usually follows 2 to 4 months later. Most patients look well, and the disease may resemble chronic bronchitis or bronchiectasis with a worsening cough that starts out dry and becomes productive and profuse. The sputum is gelatinous and blood streaked or rusty brown in color. Hemoptysis can be frequent and life threatening. Low-grade fever along with vague pleuritic chest pain may be present. Patients also may have weight loss and complain of muscular weakness. In uncomplicated pulmonary paragonimiasis, the chest examination may be remarkably normal. Children rarely have digital clubbing. Pulmonary paragonimiasis can be complicated by lung abscess, pneumothorax, pleural adhesions, empyema, and interstitial pneumonia. Pulmonary manifestations may be associated with abdominal (hepatic or peritoneal) and cerebral manifestations.[45]

Paragonimiasis is rare in children because they are less likely to indulge in consumption of exotic food and because this helminth is not transmitted by fecal-oral transmission, by person-to-person contact, or from consumption of infested water. In the United States the most likely patient is a refugee, a recent immigrant, or someone who has traveled to an endemic region.

Like other protozoal infections, the definitive diagnosis can be made by identifying the protozoal eggs. The characteristic operculated eggs can be identified in sputum or stool specimens although the sensitivity of the tests is low. Repeat examination may increase the sensitivity of these tests. Bronchoalveolar lavage also has been successful in identifying the eggs and making the diagnosis.[46] In complicated pulmonary paragonimiasis, the eggs can be identified in pleural fluid or lung abscess material. Rarely, adult flukes can be identified in the sputum. Serologic tests using various techniques (Immunoblot, counterimmunoelectrophoresis, complement fixation, and ELISA) are sensitive (96%) and specific (99%).[47] They are more useful in diagnosing extrapulmonary paragonimiasis. Skin testing cannot be used to make a diagnosis.

Chest radiography may be normal in acute pulmonary paragonimiasis, or it may show peribronchitis and hilar lymphadenopathy. However, in chronic paragonimiasis chest radiography may show various abnormalities, including patchy nodular or linear infiltration, well-defined homogeneous densities, pleural thickening, effusion, and calcification. The pathognomonic radiographic picture shows a ring shadow with a crescent-shaped opacity along one side of the border.[48-51] CT scan may define the cavities much better.[46,51]

Pulmonary tuberculosis is the major differential diagnosis because the same endemic areas have a high prevalence of tuberculosis. Other conditions to consider include pulmonary neoplasm and other parasitic infections endemic for the region.

Prevention efforts should be aimed at educating against the use of untreated fresh water for drinking or cooking (since this water may contain the infected crustaceans even though the water itself does not support the infectious metacercariae) and avoiding improperly prepared or raw crustaceans. Eradication of reservoirs is not practical.

Treatment is praziquantel 25 mg/kg/dose three times daily after meals for 3 days. Cure rates greater than 95% have been reported.[52] Bithionol (30 to 40 mg/kg over 10 days on alternate days) has been used with some success but has more adverse effects. Another drug used more recently with promising results is triclabendazole.

Suggested Reading

American Academy of Pediatrics. Red Book. 2009 Report of the Committee on Infectious Diseases. Elk Grove Village, Ill: American Academy of Pediatrics; 2009.

Bartelink AK, Kortbeek LM, Huidekoper HJ, et al. Acute respiratory failure due to toxocara infection. *Lancet.* 1993;342:1234.

Bastid C, Azar C, Doyer M, et al. Percutaneous treatment of hydatid cysts under sonographic guidance. *Dig Dis Sci.* 1994;39(7):1576.

Beaver PC. The nature of visceral larva migrans. *J Parasitol.* 1969;55(1):3.

Beaver PC, Snyder CH, Carrera GM, et al. Chronic eosinophilia due to visceral larva migrans. *Pediatrics.* 1952;9(1):7.

Beshear JR, Hendley JO. Severe pulmonary involvement in visceral larva migrans. *Am J Dis Child.* 1973;125(4):599.

Bhatia V, Sarin SK. Hepatic visceral larva migrans. Evolution of the lesion, diagnosis, and role of high-dose albendazole therapy. *Am J Gastroenterol.* 1994;89(4):624.

Borrie J, Shaw JHF. Hepatobronchial fistula caused by hydatid disease. The Dunedin experience 1952–79. *Thorax.* 1981;36(1):25.

Bouzid A, Nekmouche L, Benallegue S. Les kystes hydatiques multifocaux de l'enfant. *Chir Pediatr.* 1986;27(1):33.

Buijs J, Borsboom G, van Gemund JJ. Toxocara seroprevalence in 5-year old elementary school children. Relation with allergic asthma. *Am J Epidemiol.* 1994;140(9):839.

Burke JA. Visceral larval migrans. *J Ky Med Assoc.* 1977;75(2):62.

Cypress RH, Karol MH, Zidian JL, et al. Larva-specific antibodies in patients with visceral larva migrans. *J Infect Dis.* 1977;135(4):633.

de Savigny DH. In vitro maintenance of *Toxocara canis* larvae and a simple method for the production of *Toxocara* ES antigen for use in serodiagnostic tests for visceral larva migrans. *J Parasitol.* 1975;61:781.

Dogan R, Yuksel M, Cetin G, et al. Surgical treatment of hydatid cysts of the lung. Report on 1055 patients. *Thorax.* 1989;44(3):192.

Door J, Houel J, Dor V, et al. Le kyste hydatique du poumon considerations anatomo-chirurgicales. A propos d'une observation recente chez un enfant et d'une statistique de plus de 500 cas operes. *Ann Chir Thorac Cardiovasc.* 1967;6(2):369.

Elburjo M, Gani EA. Surgical management of pulmonary hydatid cysts in children. *Thorax.* 1995;50(4):396.

Feldman GJ, Parker HW. Visceral larva migrans associated with the hypereosinophilic syndrome and the onset of severe asthma. *Ann Intern Med.* 1992;116:838.

Gillespie SH, Bidwell D, Voller A, et al. Diagnosis of human toxocariasis by antigen capture enzyme linked immunosorbent assay. *J Clin Pathol.* 1993;46:551.

Glickman LT, Schantz PM, Dombroske RL, et al. Evaluation of serodiagnostic tests for visceral larva migrans. *Am J Trop Med Hyg.* 1978;27:492.

Gocmen A, Toppare MF, Kiper N. Treatment of hydatid disease in childhood with mebendazole. *Eur Respir J.* 1993;6(2):253.

Grunebaum M. Radiological manifestations of lung echinococcus in children. *Pediatr Radiol.* 1975;3(2):65.

Hartleb M, Januszewski K. Severe hepatic involvement in visceral larva migrans. *Eur J Gastroenterol Hepatol.* 2001;13:1245.

Horton RJ. Chemotherapy of *Echinococcus* infection in man with albendazole. *Trans R Soc Trop Med Hyg.* 1989;83(1):97.

Hotez PJ. Visceral and ocular larva migrans. *Semin Neurol.* 1993;13(2):175.

Jones WE, Schantz PM, Foreman K, et al. Human toxocariasis in a rural community. *Am J Dis Child.* 1980;134:967.

Lampkin BC, Mauer AM. Clinical manifestations of visceral larva migrans variability as related to duration of ingestion. *Clin Pediatr.* 1970;9:683.

Lamy AL, Cameron BH, Le Blanc JG, et al. Giant hydatid lung cysts in the Canadian northwest. Outcome of conservative treatment in three children. *J Pediatr Surg.* 1993;28(9):1140.

Lightowlers MV. Immunology and molecular biology of *Echinococcus* infections. *Int J Parasitol.* 1990;20(4):471.

Ljungström I, Van Knapen F. An epidemiological and serological study of toxocara infection in Sweden. *Scand J Infect Dis.* 1989;21(1):87.

Magnaval JF, Galindo V, Glickman LT, et al. Human Toxocara infection of the central nervous system and neurological disorders. A case control study. *Parasitology.* 1997;115:537.

Masuda Y, Kishimoto T, Ito H, et al. Visceral larva migrans caused by *Trichuris vulpis* presenting as a pulmonary mass. *Thorax.* 1987;42(12):990.

Mistrello G, Gentili M, Falagiani P, et al. Dot immunobinding assay as a new diagnostic test for human hydatid disease. *Immunol Lett.* 1995;47(1–2):79.

Mok CH. Visceral larva migrans. A discussion based on review of the literature. *Clin Pediatr.* 1968;7(9):565.

Mottaghian H, Mahmoudi S, Vaez-Zadeh K. A ten-year survey of hydatid disease *(Echinococcus granulosus)* in children. *Prog Pediatr Surg.* 1982;15:113.

Mutaf O, Arikan A, Yazici M, et al. Pulmonary hydatidosis in children. *Eur J Pediatr Surg.* 1994;4(2):70.

Nahmias J, Goldsmith R, Soibelman M, el-On J. Three- to 7-year follow-up after albendazole treatment of 68 patients with cystic echinococcosis (hydatid disease). *Ann Trop Med Parasitol* 1994;88(3):295.

Nelson S, Greene T, Ernhart CB. Toxocara canis infection in preschool age children Risk factors and the cognitive development of preschool children. *Neurotoxicol Teratol.* 1996;18(20):167.

Novick RJ, Tchervenkov CI, Wilson JA, et al. Surgery for thoracic hydatid disease. A North American experience. *Ann Thorac Surg.* 1987;43(6):681.

Oteifa NM, Moustafa MA, Elgozamy BM. Toxocariasis as a possible cause of allergic diseases in children. *J Egypt Soc Parasitol.* 1998;28:365.

Ozcelik C, Inci I, Toprak M, et al. Surgical treatment of pulmonary hydatidosis in children. Experience in 92 patients. *J Pediatr Surg.* 1994;29(3):392.

Ozer Z, Cetin M, Kahraman C. Pleural involvement by hydatid cysts of the lung. *Thorac Cardiovasc Surg.* 1985;33(2):103.

Patterson R, Huntley CC, Roberts M, et al. Visceral larva migrans. Immunoglobulins precipitating antibodies and detection of IgG and IgM antibodies against Ascaris antigen. *Am J Trop Med Hyg* 1975;24:465.

Perrin J, Boxerbaum B, Doershuk CF. Thiabendazole treatment of presumptive visceral larva migrans (VLM). *Clin Pediatr.* 1975;14:147.

Rubinsky-Elefant G, Hirata CE, Yamamoto JH, et al. Human toxocariasis: diagnosis, worldwide seroprevalences and clinical expression of the systemic and ocular forms. *Ann Trop Med Parasitol.* 2010;104:3.

Rausch RL, Wilson JF, Schantz PM, et al. Spontaneous death of *Echinococcus multilocularis.* Cases diagnosed serologically (by EM2 ELISA) and clinical significance. *Am J Trop Med Hyg.* 1987;36(3):576.

Roig J, Romeu J, Riera C, et al. Acute eosinophilic pneumonia due to toxocariasis with bronchoalveolar lavage findings. *Chest.* 1992;102:294.

Procop GW. North American Paragonimiasis (caused by *Paragonimus kellicotti*) in the context of global paragonimiasis. *Clin Microbiol Rev.* 2009;22(3):419.

Sadrieh M, Dutz W, Navabpoor S. Review of 150 cases of hydatid cyst of the lung. *Dis Chest.* 1967;52(5):662.

Saenz-Santamaria J, Moreno-Casado J, Nunez C. Role of fine needle biopsy in the diagnosis of hydatid cyst. *Diagn Cytopathol.* 1995;13(3):229.

Schantz PM. Toxocara larva migrans now. *Am J Trop Med Hyg.* 1989;41(suppl):21.

Seah SKK, Hucal G, Law C. Dogs and intestinal parasites. A public health problem. *Can Med Assoc J.* 1975;112(10):1191.

Snyder CH. Visceral larval migrans. *Pediatrics.* 1961;28:85.

Struchler D, Schubarth P, Gualzata M. Thiabendazole vs albendazole in the treatment of toxocariasis. A clinical trial. *Ann Trop Med Parasitol.* 1989;83(5):473.

Taylor MR, Keane CT, O'Connor P. The expanded spectrum of toxocaral disease. *Lancet.* 1988;1:692.

Teggl A, Lastilla MG, De Rosa F. Therapy of human hydatid disease with mebendazole and albendazole. *Antimicrob Agents Chemother.* 1993;37(8):1679.

Thompson WM, Chisholm DP, Tank R. Plain film roentgenographic findings in alveolar hydatid disease—*Echinococcus multilocularis. Am J Roentgenol Radium Ther Nucl Med* 1972;116(2):345.

Thornieporth NG, Disko R. Alveolar hydatid disease (*Echinococcus multilocularis*)—review and update. *Prog Clin Parasitol.* 1994;4:55.

Tuncel E. Pulmonary air meniscus sign. *Respiration.* 1984;46(1):139.

Wen H, Zhang HW, Muhmut M, et al. Initial observation on albendazole in combination with cimetidine for the treatment of human cystic echinococcosis. *Ann Trop Med Parasitol.* 1994;88(1):49.

Wilson JF, Rausch RL, McMahon BJ, et al. Albendazole therapy in alveolar hydatid disease. A report of favorable results in two patients after short-term therapy. *Am J Trop Med Hyg.* 1987;37(1):162.

Wilson JF, Rausch RL, Wilson FR. Alveolar hydatid disease. Review of the surgical experience in 42 cases of active disease among Alaskan Eskimos. *Ann Surg.* 1995;221(3):315.

Worley G, Green IA, Forthingham TE. *Toxocara canis* infection. Clinical and epidemiological associations with seropositivity in kindergarten children. *J Infect Dis* 1991;149:591.

References

The complete reference list is available online at www.expertconsult.com

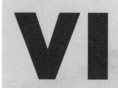

VI

Noninfectious Disorders of the Respiratory Tract

37 ATELECTASIS

Michelle Duggan, MB, MD, FFARCSI, and Brian P. Kavanagh, MD, FRCPC

Atelectasis, the reversible loss of aerated lung, is a key component of many acute lung disease states. Although, classically considered to be a depletion of lung volume through degassing of the alveoli, recent insights suggest an alternative explanation for atelectasis: that it represents accumulation of alveolar fluid. This chapter addresses a clinical diagnosis of atelectasis, effects of atelectasis and lung physiology, causes of atelectasis, new concepts about the nature of atelectasis, and its prevention or reversal.

▬ WHAT IS ATELECTASIS?

The answer to this is complex. Characteristically, atelectasis represents a radiologically apparent volume loss in a segment or lobe of a lung, or sometimes the whole lung. This situation is associated with impaired gas exchange, and usually with impaired lung mechanics. Studies in animals have directly visualized atelectasis occurring in the subpleural alveoli and have demonstrated the opening and closing of alveoli with positive-pressure ventilation, and the collapse of alveoli in the absence of end-expiratory pressure.[1] A more recent study using different imaging techniques concluded that lung volume increases by alveolar distension—rather than cyclic opening and collapse—in both normal and injured lungs.[2] Several studies using computed tomography (CT) have documented atelectasis related to general anesthesia and have categorized the densities, which appear radiologically, more reminiscent of tissue than of water,[3–4] which would suggest that atelectasis represents alveolar collapse, as opposed to fluid accumulation.

However, the nature of atelectasis may be more complex. Based on a variety of arguments, it has been suggested that instead of loss of alveolar volume,

atelectasis may represent replacement of alveolar volume by air spaces being filled with edema fluid.[5] There are three cardinal lines of reasoning that support such a hypothesis.

- *Pressure-Volume Characteristics*: Convincing evidence for this is derived from the pressure-volume characteristics of different lung conditions. When fluid is injected into a fluid-filled lung and when air is injected into an air-filled lung, there is a linear relationship between inflation pressure and lung volume. Relatively low pressures are required, and in both cases there is no hysteresis between the inflation vs. the deflation pressure-volume profile. However, when air is injected into a fluid-filled lung, the opening pressure is high, similar to that of the atelectatic lung, and there is a hysteresis between the inflation and the deflation phases; these characteristics make air inflation of a fluid-filled lung comparable to inflation of atelectatic lung.

- *Weight of the Lung*: The idea that atelectasis represents simple compression from heavier lung is unlikely because the weight of the lung accounts for only approximately one fifth of the vertical pleural pressure gradient. Thus, the forces acting to compress the lung are mostly derived from forces that are intrinsic to the lung (i.e., tissue recoil, surface tension) and not from compressive weight.

- *Interpretation of CT Images*: Conventionally, vertical gradients in the gray scale of pixels in a CT scan have been interpreted as evidence of steeper gradients in alveolar size. However, the correlation between gray scale and alveolar size holds only if the amount of water per alveolus is uniform. CT provides data on regional air content but not on regional volume or parenchymal strain, so it has limitations as a measurement tool of regional lung mechanics.

Thus, the exact nature of atelectasis is complex, and the answer appears to depend on the technique used.

WHY DOES ATELECTASIS OCCUR?

Theories of the development of atelectasis are traditionally based on the idea of maintenance of "opened lung" units, which are considered to reflect the balance of inward recoil of the lung tissue tending to collapse the lung, countered by outward recoil of the chest wall tending to expand the lung. The exact balance of these forces at the end of expiration represents the functional residual capacity (FRC) of the lung. The loss of lung volume is conventionally thought to reflect an imbalance of forces that usually keep the lung open, thereby allowing lung tissue to contract around empty air spaces.

Classification of Atelectasis

Atelectasis may be the result of one or more of the following mechanisms: inhibition of surfactant, resorption of alveolar gas, or compression of regional lung. It is possible that more than one of these influences is at play in any particular instance.

Surfactant Inibition

The composition of the surfactant involves phospholipids, natural lipids, and specific apoproteins as described elsewhere in this book. A major overall function is to stabilize the alveoli by reducing alveolar surface tension, thus preventing collapse. Many factors, including leakage of plasma proteins and vigorous ventilatory stretch, may alter the function of surfactant and its composition (e.g., the proportion of large aggregate fractions and tubular myelin, which are important for reducing surface tension, may be reduced). A lack of intermittent deep breaths, as is usually the case during mechanical ventilation, may result in a decreased content of active forms of alveolar surfactant.[6] However, two factors make this an unlikely sole explanation for the development of atelectasis. First, the lungs have a large reserve of surfactant (surfactant pool) and are therefore unlikely to become deficient except over a protracted period. Second, surfactant has a long turnover time (12 to 14 hours). Thus, it is unlikely that atelectasis commonly occurs on the basis of changes in surfactant, in the absence of other factors, in an otherwise healthy lung.

Gas Resorption

There are two means whereby gas absorption may result in atelectasis. First, in the presence of a patent airway, regions that have low ventilation compared to the perfusion will have low alveolar oxygen tensions when the fraction of inspired oxygen (FiO_2) is low. When the FiO_2 is increased (i.e., with supplemental oxygen), the alveolar oxygen tension (PAO_2) increases, and thus the rate at which gas transfers from the alveolus to the capillary blood is increased. In addition, as PAO_2 increases, alveolar nitrogen tension (PAN_2) decreases. Because nitrogen is insoluble, any increased absorption of oxygen will result in loss of alveolar volume. The second mechanism is thought to occur in the presence of an occluded airway. Here, ongoing gas uptake by the blood is not replenished by incoming gas from the airway, and the size of the lung unit becomes progressively smaller.

Compression Atelectasis

Compression atelectasis is defined as atelectasis that results when the forces causing the alveolus to collapse exceed the transmural pressure that distends and maintains the alveolus in an open state (Fig. 37-1). The pleural pressure is most compressive in the most dependent areas. During positive pressure ventilation, distension of the alveoli is enhanced, and during spontaneous ventilation it is dependent on the elastic recoil of the chest wall

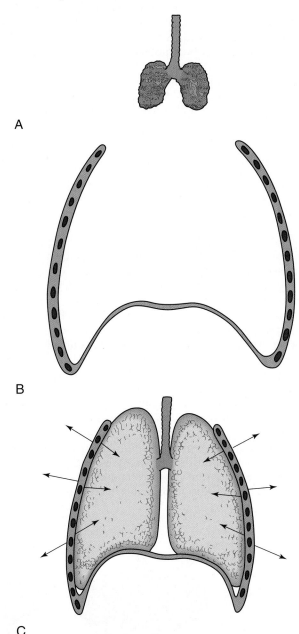

FIGURE 37-1. The balance of inward recoil of the lung tissue tending to collapse the lung countered by outward recoil of the chest wall tending to expand the lung. The exact balance of these forces at the end of expiration represents the functional residual capacity (FRC) of the lung. **A,** The resting state of the lungs when they are removed from the chest cavity, that is, total collapse. **B,** The resting state of the normal chest wall and diaphragm when open to the atmosphere and thoracic contents removed. **C,** The lung volume that exists at the end of expiration, the FRC. (From Shapiro BA, Harrison RA, Trout CA: The mechanics of ventilation. In: *Clinical Applications of Respiratory Care*, 3rd ed. Chicago: Year Book Medical, 1985, p 57.).

and the stability of the diaphragm. When in the supine position, the weight of the abdominal contents results in a net vector that tends to shift the dependent areas of the diaphragm into the chest.

During positive pressure ventilation, as in the operating room or in the intensive care unit, these changes may be compounded by several factors. First, use of sedation and neuromuscular blockade reduces the stability of the diaphragm, allowing its progressive shift into the chest. Second, positive pressure ventilation may result in a displacement of thoracic central blood from the chest into the abdomen, with further displacement of the diaphragm cephalad, which potentiates the development of atelectasis. These changes may account for the reduction in FRC associated with induction of general anesthesia, or in the critically ill child, where sedation and paralysis are being employed in an effort to facilitate positive pressure ventilation.

Consequences of Atelectasis

Atelectasis is associated with several important pathophysiologic alterations, which are addressed in the following sections.

Impaired Gas Exchange

Impairment of gas exchange, often the most obvious effect of atelectasis, will lead to worsened arterial oxygenation in the absence of supplemental oxygen. This concept was recognized following general anesthesia in the classic studies of Benedixen and colleagues.[7] The basis for impaired gas exchange in atelectasis is the absence of ventilation in the collapsed or filled alveoli, coupled with the perfusion of such non-ventilated lung units (Fig. 37-2). The latter issue results in shunting of intrapulmonary blood, and pronounced hypoxemia.

The consequences of impaired oxygenation are frequently unimportant in healthy lungs, but in diseased lung they may necessitate the application of higher FiO_2, or in mechanically ventilated children, greater elevations in either the inspiratory airway pressures or the pressure at end-expiration (positive end-expiratory pressure [PEEP]). The application of higher levels of FiO_2 can, as previously discussed, paradoxically worsen the situation through development of absorption atelectasis. In this situation, although the partial pressure of oxygen in arterial blood (PAO_2) may be improved, additional atelectasis develops over time, and the PAO_2 will become lower relative to the FiO_2. Thus, higher levels of FiO_2 will raise the PAO_2 (the immediate aim), but measures of oxygenation efficiency will be worsened (i.e., the alveolar-arterial oxygen gradient will be increased, or the ratio of PAO_2/FiO_2 will be decreased). The alternative therapies, increases in inflation pressure or PEEP, are associated with adverse effects of their own.

Impaired Lung Mechanics

A major consequence of atelectasis is impaired lung mechanics. This issue has been recognized since the 1950s before the effects on oxygenation were acknowledged.[8] It was demonstrated that spontaneous or mechanical breaths with the same tidal volume were associated with progressive impairment of respiratory system compliance. Normal compliance could be restored by a large breath at intervals, that is, three times the normal tidal volume. This phenomenon has been explored in detail in the perioperative setting through the use of fluoroscopy, which showed that lung volume decreases during general anaesthesia.[9] Importantly, the decrement in compliance resulting from progressive atelectasis is related to the lung volume lost and is reversed by recruitment maneuvers.

The major consequence of impaired lung mechanics is that compliance is worsened. This means that larger changes in transpulmonary pressure are required to generate a given tidal volume. Thus, for spontaneously breathing children, the work of breathing is increased, and for children receiving mechanical ventilation, increased ventilatory pressures are required.

Increased Pulmonary Vascular Resistance

Another complication associated with atelectasis is increased pulmonary vascular resistance. Early classic studies suggested that the pulmonary vascular resistance was minimal at ideal FRC, and whereas lung volume much above this notional value resulted in alveolar compression because of lung stretch, lung volume falling

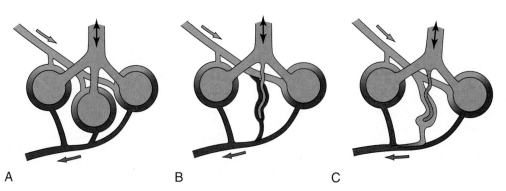

FIGURE 37-2. The basis for impaired gas exchange in atelectasis. The absence of ventilation in the collapsed or filled alveoli, coupled with the perfusion of such nonventilated lung units. This results in shunting of intrapulmonary blood and pronounced hypoxemia. **A,** The ideal relationship between alveolar ventilation and pulmonary circulation (V/Q ratio) is an even distribution of adequate ventilation and perfusion of pulmonary vessels. **B,** If alveolar collapse occurs but those alveoli are not perfused, then the overall relationship between ventilation and perfusion will remain unchanged and all venous blood will be oxygenated. **C,** If capillary blood flow is maintained through collapsed alveoli, venous admixture will occur, leading to hypoxemia. (Figure 1 in Bendixen HH, Hedley-Whyte J, Chir B, Laver MB: Impaired oxygenation in surgical patients during general anesthesia with controlled ventilation. *N Engl J Med.* 1963;269:991-997.)

below this value was thought to result in compression of extra alveolar vessels. Thus, this notion explained the changes in pulmonary vascular resistance on the basis of physical alteration of the pulmonary blood vessels—either stretching or narrowing because of increased lung volume or being compressed because of decreased lung volume. Subsequent work has changed that notion, however, and has demonstrated that increases in pulmonary vascular resistance associated with atelectasis result not from physical compression of the vessels but rather from regional alveolar hypoxia with reduced alveolar and mixed venous oxygen tension, leading to local hypoxic pulmonary vasoconstriction.[10] Indeed, recent studies have demonstrated that this significant increase in vascular resistance can occur in previously normal lungs in an experimental setting, resulting in right ventricular dysfunction and increased microvascular leakage.[11]

Worsening of Lung Injury

An important consequence of atelectasis is the potentiation of lung injury. While mechanical ventilation is designed as a supportive measure, its use can be associated with what is now termed ventilatory-associated lung injury. Most experimental studies have demonstrated that ventilator-induced lung injury occurs much more readily in the presence of low PEEP or low lung volume. Conversely, application of PEEP reduces or eliminates ventilator-associated lung injury, in some situations making it almost negligible.[12–13]

In experimental settings, this phenomenon is not restricted to ventilator-associated lung injury, and several studies have demonstrated that maintenance of lung volume (i.e., prevention of atelectasis) is associated with reduced injury secondary to reperfusion injury and possibly sepsis.[14–16] It was demonstrated that reducing atelectasis attenuated bacterial growth and translocation in a piglet model of streptococcal pneumonia.[17] This may be due to maintenance of lung volume reducing endothelial shear stress and optimizing vascular resistance, but the mechanism is incompletely understood.

Diagnosis

The diagnosis of atelectasis is most easily made bearing in mind the context of the patient, with for example, paralysis of a hemidiaphragm, known airway obstruction, or the presence of neuromuscular weakness.

Clinical Features

In such a setting, the clinical findings include dyspnea or tachypnea, asymmetric chest movement, and reduced breath sounds on the ipsilateral side. In cases of upper lobe atelectasis, instead of reduced or absent breath sounds, bronchial (tubular) breath sounds may be heard because of the proximity of the upper lobes to the major airways. Percussion of the affected lobes demonstrates increased dullness.

Radiological Features

The standard radiologic approach is a plain radiographic study of the chest. Segmental or lobar atelectasis, or atelectasis of the whole lung, is associated with increased density (i.e., opacification) of the atelectatic area. Indications of volume loss include hyperlucency of adjacent lung tissue and shift of adjoining structures. Hyperlucency occurs because the nonatelectatic lung is stretched to replace the lung volume that has become atelectatic. The shift of adjoining structures occurs because of the loss of lung volume inherent to the development of atelectasis. For example, atelectasis of a lower lobe can result in a downwards shift of the ipsilateral horizontal fissure or hilum, or an upward shift of the ipsilateral diaphragm. In addition, the mediastinum can be displaced towards an atelectatic side.

The presence of atelectasis also can be noted in a specific lobe because of the relationship to the heart or to the diaphragm. Lower lobe atelectasis, resulting in dense opacification of that lobe, can obliterate the normal contour of the adjacent diaphragm. Similarly, the presence of atelectasis in the right middle lobe or in the lingula can obliterate the normally visible right or left heart borders, respectively. In addition, obstruction of a main-stem bronchus, causing atelectasis, can sometimes be appreciated on the plain chest film.

Computed tomography (CT) can be used in the diagnosis of atelectasis with greater sensitivity than plain radiograph. However, CT-based diagnosis of atelectasis is usually made when performed for another indication, and CT is seldom indicated for the diagnosis of atelectasis per se. Nonetheless, atelectasis is an integral element of acute respiratory distress syndrome (ARDS), and some centers determine the distribution of atelectasis—usually in the dependent regions—through utilization of CT Scans. In such cases, CT is important because it may assist in directing the optimal position for care of the ventilator-dependent patient (e.g., prone vs. supine positioning). In addition to a response to prone positioning that can sometimes be predicted by CT, modern CT approaches can demonstrate relative overinflation of nonatelectatic areas induced by overly aggressive attempts to recruit atelectatic regions.[18]

A new approach is the use of ultrasonography. Several studies suggest that it is an extremely straightforward technique with higher sensitivity and ease of use than CT scanning in critically ill patients. The potential use for this technique is to distinguish between pleural fluid, consolidation, and atelectasis. Ultrasound allows imaging without the use of ionizing radiation. In addition, it can be done at the bedside quickly and with less cost. Soon it may become a new standard of care.

Factors Modifying the Development of Atelectasis

Several important factors modify the development of atelectasis, resulting in worsening of the condition where initiating factors were already present.

Posture

Changing from the upright position to the supine position reduces the functional residual capacity substantially.[19] The basis for this is that the abdominal contents tend to exert pressure on the diaphragm, especially upon its dependent (i.e., posterior) aspects (Fig. 37-3). The resultant diaphragmatic displacement coupled with the weight of the mediastinum, and to some extent, the weight of

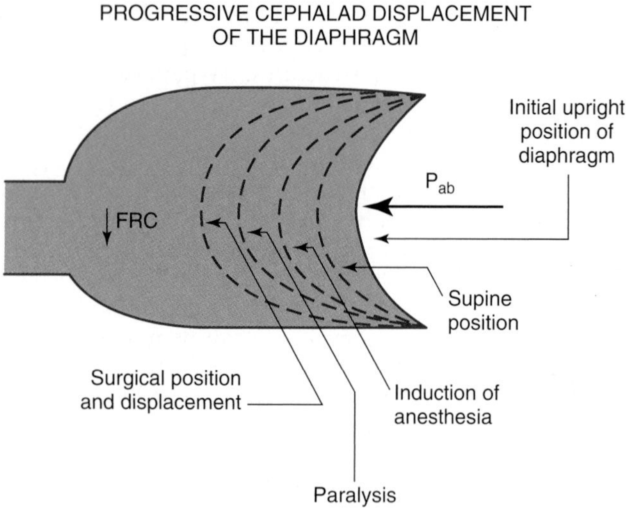

PROGRESSIVE CEPHALAD DISPLACEMENT
OF THE DIAPHRAGM

FIGURE 37-3. Several important factors modify the development of atelectasis. Anesthesia and surgery cause a cephalad displacement of the diaphragm, leading to a decreased functional residual capacity. The sequence of events includes assumption of the supine position, induction of anesthesia, muscle paralysis, surgical position, and displacement by surgical packs and retractors. *Pab,* Pressure of the abdominal contents. (From Benumof JL: General respiratory physiology and respiratory function during anesthesia. In: *Anesthesia for Thoracic Surgery.* Philadelphia: WB Saunders, 1987, p 100, Fig. 3-44.)

the overlying non-dependent lung combine to compress the dependent lung, thereby potentiating the development of atelectasis. Turning patients to the prone position during mechanical ventilation appears to largely reverse these effects.[20]

The effects of the supine position on atelectasis are exaggerated in obese subjects [21] because the influence of the mass of abdominal contents is significantly greater in obese compared with lean subjects. There is a correlation between body mass index (BMI) and atelectasis, and there also appears to be a correlation between vertical lung height and atelectasis. Morbid obesity is accompanied by increased atelectasis.[22]

Developmental Influences
Young children, up to 3 years of age, develop atelectasis more readily than older children. Several factors may contribute to this. The compliance of the thoracic rib cage is far higher in very young children. This results in less outward recoil of the chest wall, thereby causing less distending force on the lung and increasing the propensity of the lungs to develop atelectasis.[23] In addition to the reduced influence of the chest wall, young infants have an especially high closing volume (i.e., the lung volume at which the small airways begin to close). The greater closing volume means that airways, and subsequently lung units, become closed and set up conditions for development of atelectasis. One study examined the effect of continuous positive airway pressure (CPAP) before endotracheal intubation in children during anesthesia.[24] During induction of anesthesia, 6 cm H_2O significantly reduced atelectasis formation regardless of the Fio_2 used. Despite the potentially beneficial effect, the addition of CPAP reduces the margin of safety for patients by increasing the intragastric pressure, thereby predisposing the patient to

regurgitation and vomiting during anesthesia induction when vital reflexes are abolished; therefore, this practice has not become a standard of care.

Supplemental Oxygen
Use of supplemental oxygen, although sometimes necessary for treating the hypoxemia associated with atelectasis, can worsen the development of atelectasis per se for reasons previously outlined, despite augmenting the arterial oxygen tension. In this context, the arterial oxygen levels are increased but the efficiency of gas exchange in the lungs is worsened. The most important component of preoxygenation for general anesthesia is to build up a large oxygen store in the lungs before the induction of anesthesia to prevent hypoxemia in the event of a difficult intubation or a problem with ventilation. Dantzker and colleagues calculated the influence of inspired alveolar ventilation/perfusion ratio and inspired oxygen on alveolar stability.[25] They found that the critical V/Q ratio at which alveoli eventually collapsed was far higher while breathing 100% oxygen. The standard preoxygenation procedure is important in producing atelectasis; in fact, one study demonstrated the effect of increasing inspired oxygen concentrations during pre-oxygenation on atelectasis formation.[26] In clinical practice, avoiding the preoxygenation procedure and ventilation with 30% instead of 100% oxygen lessens formation of atelectasis during the induction and maintenance of anesthesia.[27] High oxygen concentrations also are used at the end of anesthesia to reduce the risk of hypoxemia during awakening.[28] A combination of airway suctioning to eliminate secretions and increasing Fio_2 increases the propensity toward atelectasis.

The concern about atelectasis during anesthesia has prompted studies on the use of recruitment maneuvers at the end of surgery and anesthesia. Recruitment maneuvers might best be followed by ventilation with moderate Fio_2; indeed the need for high Fio_2 also should be less where atelectasis has been prevented or reversed.

Pre-Existing Lung Disease
In addition, preexisting lung disease or acute lung disease will increase the likelihood of atelectasis formation and, if present, will worsen it.

Treatment of Atelectasis

Although no studies prove outcome benefits associated with the treatment of atelectasis, common sense suggests that in the presence of significant hypoxemia, increased work of breathing, or respiratory distress measures should be considered to reverse the effects of atelectasis. The feasibility of treating atelectasis depends on the balance between the physiologic burden caused by atelectasis, the risks of the intervention, and the potential for the therapy to work. The following approaches can be considered.

Recruitment Maneuvers
Recruitment maneuvers are designed to recruit atelectatic lung. The goals of any recruitment maneuver are to open up the lungs and keep them open,[29] and with ventilation,

opening is achieved by the inspiratory pressure and re-collapse prevented by PEEP. In the setting of mechanical ventilation, such maneuvers would usually take the form of either increasing PEEP in the setting of ongoing positive pressure ventilation or applying CPAP. It is not clear whether either of these approaches is superior, and the major issues for the clinician are the likelihood of there being recruitable lung (i.e., What are the chances of success?) balanced against the potential adverse effects associated with the maneuver. Gattinoni and colleagues conducted a study to examine the relationship between the percentage of recruitable lung in ARDS and the clinical and physiologic effects of PEEP.[30] They found that patients who had a higher percentage of potentially recruitable lung (i.e., lung tissue in which aeration could be restored,) had poorer gas exchange and respiratory mechanics, a greater severity of lung injury, and a higher mortality rate. A higher percentage of potentially recruitable lung may reflect the extent of inflammatory pulmonary edema in ARDS.[30-31]

The probability of success is difficult to predict, but in the postoperative state, for example, positive pressure can be expected to readily reverse the atelectasis. In lung injury, prediction of response may be possible on the basis of the topographical distribution of the injury, as evidenced by CT. Gattinoni and colleagues suggested that in daily practice, the level of PEEP should be limited to 15 cm H_2O in patients with a higher percentage of potentially recruitable lung and to 10 cm H_2O in patients with a lower percentage of potentially recruitable lung.[30] In addition, the timing of the lung injury also appears to be important. For example, recruitment maneuvers undertaken in early (i.e., approximately the first day of lung injury) ARDS had a far higher chance of success compared with those attempted later (i.e., approximately the seventh day of injury).[32] Finally, the cause of lung injury, for example whether the injury originates from pulmonary (e.g., aspiration injury, lung trauma, pneumonia) or nonpulmonary (e.g., systemic sepsis, pancreatitis) etiology, may have an impact in that nonpulmonary types of ARDS demonstrate recruitable lung potential that is not apparent in pulmonary types of ARDS.[33]

Chest Physiotherapy

Although randomized controlled trials of chest physiotherapy for pulmonary atelectasis are lacking, it is standard practice to attempt physiotherapy. For the older child, this involves deep breathing and coughing exercises, in addition to incentive spirometry. Percussion therapy is traditional and may be most effective in the context of coughing. In addition, vibration therapy also can be used. For younger children and infants, because of the lack of cooperation, the options are limited to percussion and vibration treatments. Techniques or devices that either encourage or force the patient to inspire deeply have long been recognized to be of clinical importance.[34]

Removal of Endobronchial Obstruction

Bronchoscopy and removal of an intraluminal obstruction (e.g., blood clot, inspissated secretions) are indicated in situations where atelectasis of a lobe or a whole lung is thought to be due to an obstruction that has not responded to conservative measures.

◼ SUMMARY

Atelectasis is generally a benign process, although, in the presence of preexisting lung disease or limited cardiopulmonary reserve, it may have significant consequences. Increasing understanding of the underlying nature of atelectasis and its contribution to acute lung injury will hopefully improve our approach to its prevention and management.

References

The complete reference list is available online at www.expertconsult.com

38 PULMONARY EDEMA

Hugh O'Brodovich, MD, FRCP(C)

Improvements in the intensive care and monitoring of patients with serious illnesses led to a greater appreciation of the significance of fluid movement into the lung as a complication of a variety of conditions. This, coupled with an improved understanding of the pathogenesis of pulmonary edema, has enhanced our ability to treat various illnesses in which pulmonary edema develops.

The chapter first outlines the relevant anatomy, factors that control fluid movement within the lung, mechanisms responsible for the genesis of pulmonary edema, and how this edema fluid is cleared from the lung's interstitium and airspaces. This background will enhance the reader's understanding of the pathophysiologic consequences of edema formation, including the clinical and laboratory findings. Common disorders associated with pulmonary edema are then described along with the approach to therapy, which is based on understanding the underlying pathophysiologic mechanisms.

ANATOMIC CONSIDERATIONS

Certain structural features of the lung are worth pointing out because they have a bearing on gas exchange during pulmonary edema. The capillaries are placed eccentrically within the alveolar septum (Fig. 38-1A). In some areas, the basement membranes of the capillary endothelium and the alveolar epithelium are fused with no additional space between them, even during edema formation. This situation is ideal for preserving gas exchange, at least until such time as the alveoli themselves are filled with liquid. In other areas, there is an interstitial space between the endothelial and epithelial basement membranes that contains secreted matrix. This matrix consists of structural proteins (e.g., collagens and elastin), attachment proteins for cells (e.g., laminin), and proteoglycans and glycosaminoglycans (e.g., hyaluronic acid, chondroitins, and heparan sulfate). In addition to supplying support to the capillary network, this widened portion of the alveolar-capillary membrane provides a channel for water and protein en route to the lymphatics and larger interstitial fluid spaces (Fig. 38-1B). As long as fluid can be confined to these channels, gas exchange can be preserved. Morphometric studies have shown that the majority of interstitial edema accumulates within the thick, and not the thin, portion of the alveolar-capillary membrane.[1]

Pulmonary capillaries, like muscle capillaries, have a continuous endothelium with relatively tight intercellular junctions. The bronchial microvasculature, much like visceral capillaries, is discontinuous, with intercellular fenestrations or gaps. Whether these gaps account for the greater fluid movement across the bronchial capillaries, but not the pulmonary capillaries, remains to be determined. The role of bronchial circulation in the genesis of pulmonary edema may have been underestimated, but it is certain that bronchial circulation plays an important pathophysiologic role in inflammatory airway diseases such as asthma or inhalational lung injury.

At the ultrastructural level, the available evidence from tracer studies indicates that the alveolar epithelial membrane contains tighter cellular junctions than does the capillary endothelial membrane. These epithelial tight junctions (zonulae occludentes) are estimated by both morphologic and physiologic studies to have an effective molecular radius of approximately 4 Å. This has two implications. First, that they markedly restrict the movement of small ions, thereby making ions most important in the genesis of osmotic pressure across the epithelial membrane. Second, that fluid leaking from the vascular spaces is likely to be confined initially to the interstitial and lymphatic spaces; alveolar edema results only when the volume that can be handled by these spaces are overwhelmed. In contrast to the epithelium, the pores between endothelial cells have an effective molecular radius of approximately 40 Å. This tenfold difference in interendothelial junction size allows the free movement of small ions and noncharged solutes, such as urea, but restricts the movement of larger macromolecules such as albumin and globulins. Thus, it is the protein concentration that is most important in the genesis of transvascular osmotic pressure. These large macromolecules move across the microvasculature; however, the relative contributions of movement via pinocytotic vesicles (vesicular shuttle) versus across pores that can enlarge ("stretched pores"), especially when there is increased intravascular pressure or injury, is unclear.

Although the alveoli are often portrayed as spherical, a polyhedral model is closer to reality (see Chapter 5). From the point of view of fluid movement in the lung, the importance of this shape is that the walls of the alveolar septa are flat, except at the corners where the septa meet. Thus, it is only at the corners, where the alveolar air-liquid interface is curved, that the force exerted by surface tension can lower alveolar fluid and interstitial fluid pressures as predicted by the Laplace relationship. The lower interstitial pressures at the corners favor movement of interstitial fluid that has traversed the alveolar capillary wall toward the corners of the alveolus. This is important from a lung fluid balance point of view. Alveolar type II epithelial cells are also predominately found in the corners of the alveoli.

Pulmonary blood vessels have been defined using both anatomic and physiologic criteria (see Chapter 5). Anatomically, the vessels have been classified traditionally by their morphologic characteristics as arteries, arterioles, capillaries, venules, or veins. Physiologically, these divisions are included under two broad classifications—alveolar and extra-alveolar vessels—based on their behavior relative to the hydrostatic pressures of the interstitium surrounding

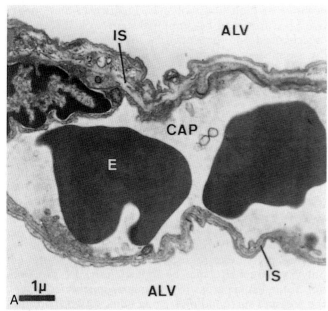

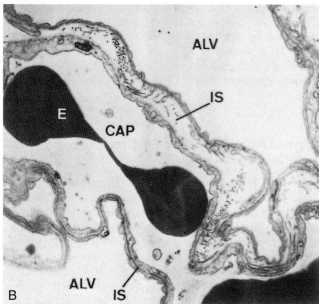

FIGURE 38-1. A, The normal alveolar septum in which the epithelial and endothelial basement membranes are fused in some areas and separated by an interstitial space of connective tissue in others. **B,** The alveolar septum in pulmonary edema. The areas where the basement membranes are fused remain thin; only the areas with a connective tissue interstitial space widen. *ALV,* Alveolar lumen; *CAP,* capillary; *E,* erythrocyte; *IS,* interstitial space. (From Mellins RB, Levine OR, Skalak R, et al. Interstitial pressure of the lung. *Circ Res.* 1969;24:197.)

alveolar septal walls (corner vessels) that are exposed to more negative pressures than the alveolar vessels. Unfortunately, there is no clear-cut correlation between the functional and the anatomic classifications. Fluid movement occurs at the level of the arterioles, capillaries, and venules; the bulk of fluid movement occurs at the level of the capillaries, with approximately three fourths arising from the alveolar vessels.[2]

Anatomically, the lung has two main compartments, each possessing markedly different potential volumes, into which edema fluid can move. The interstitial spaces of the alveolar capillary septae and peribronchovascular compartment can only accommodate small amounts of fluid. When this small interstitial safety reservoir, estimated to be a few hundred milliliters in an adult lung,[3] is filled with edema fluid, subsequent accumulation must take place in the alveolar space, which at functional residual capacity (FRC) has a volume of approximately 30 ml/kg body weight or approximately 2000 to 3000 milliliters in the adult lung. This anatomic difference, in part, explains why interstitial edema may resolve quickly, whereas alveolar edema takes significantly longer periods of time.

Juxtacapillary (J) receptors are distributed throughout the lung's interstitium and are stimulated by the presence of edema. They induce an increase in respiratory rate and their continued activation is responsible, in large part, for the continued tachypnea seen in pulmonary edema even when hypoxemia has been corrected through the use of supplemental oxygen and positive airway pressure.

FACTORS RESPONSIBLE FOR FLUID MOVEMENT

The factors responsible for fluid accumulation include intravascular and interstitial hydrostatic and colloid osmotic pressures, permeability characteristics of the fluid-exchanging membrane, and lymphatic drainage.

The equilibrium of fluid across fluid-exchanging membranes is generally expressed as the Starling equation:

$$Q_f = K_f[(Pmv - Ppmv) - \sigma(\pi mv - \pi pmv)]$$

wherein Q_f = the net transvascular flow; K_f = the hydraulic conductivity and filtration surface area of the fluid-exchanging vessels; *Pmv* = microvascular hydrostatic pressure; *Ppmv* = perimicrovascular (interstitial fluid) hydrostatic pressure; *πmv* = colloid osmotic pressure in the microvasculature; *πpmv* = colloid osmotic pressure in the perimicrovasculature, the interstitial fluid colloid osmotic pressure; and σ = the reflection coefficient, which is a measure of the resistance of the membrane to the movement of protein. Thus, σ influences the "effective" osmotic pressure of the protein. If the endothelium were completely impermeable to protein ($\sigma_{protein}$ = 1) then the 5 g/dL of plasma would yield approximately 28 mm Hg osmotic pressure (each 1 mOsm/L of solute yields 19 mm Hg pressure). The osmotic pressure resulting from proteins is also termed the "oncotic pressure."

the vessels, the interstitial fluid pressure. Alveolar vessels are in the alveolar walls and behave as if their outer walls were exposed to alveolar pressure. These vessels may collapse if airway pressures exceed vascular pressures, as is the case in Zone I perfusion conditions. Extra-alveolar vessels lie in the larger interstitial spaces and behave as if there outer walls were exposed to a pressure that is as negative as or more negative than pleural pressure and that tends to vary with pleural pressure. In addition, there are vessels lying in the intersections of

As discussed subsequently, the absolute values for the variables within the Starling equation may change during health and disease. However, it should be emphasized that in the normal lung, Q_f is positive and there is a continuous movement of fluid from the vascular to the interstitial spaces of the lung. Experimentally derived values are approximately: $Pmv = 20\,cm\,H_2O$, $Ppmv = -2\,cm\,H_2O$, $\pi mv = -33\,cm\,H_2O$, $\pi pmv = 20\,cm\,H_2O$, and $0.7 < \sigma < 0.95$.

The term *microvasculature* is used to describe the vessels from which fluid leaks because fluid exchange is not limited to the capillaries alone. In the following discussion, each of the above factors and the pathophysiologic influences on them are described in detail.

Vascular Forces

The pressure in the pulmonary microvasculature (Pmv) is frequently, but not precisely, referred to as pulmonary capillary pressure. For technical reasons, this pressure is extremely difficult to measure *in vivo*. The pulmonary artery wedge pressure (Pw), also known as the pulmonary artery occlusion pressure, reflects the pressure in the first pulmonary veins where there is flow from nonobstructed vascular routes. Pmv is higher than left atrial pressure by approximately 40% of the difference between left atrial (LA) pressure and pulmonary arterial (PA) pressure. The relative amounts of arterial and venular resistance within the pulmonary vasculature is altered during hypoxia, the infusion of vasoactive agents (e.g., catecholamines) or during disease (e.g., endotoxinemia). An increase in either PA or LA pressure will tend to increase the hydrostatic pressure, favoring movement out of the fluid-exchanging vessels. For example, Pmv may be increased by the elevation in LA pressures in left-sided heart failure or by increases in PA pressure as seen in large left-to-right shunts. Although both PA and Pw pressures increase in a linear relation to exercise-induced increases in cardiac output, the ratio is significantly less than 1:1 in healthy young adult humans.[4] Because the pulmonary vascular membrane is only slightly permeable to proteins and freely permeable to ions and small uncharged solutes, the plasma proteins normally are responsible for osmotic pressure (πmv). The πmv is significantly above the pulmonary microvascular hydrostatic pressure. The plasma colloid osmotic pressure may be markedly reduced in clinical conditions in which the plasma proteins are low (e.g., malnutrition, nephrosis, and massive burns) and thus may facilitate the formation of pulmonary edema.

Interstitial Forces

The interstitial hydrostatic pressure throughout the lung is normally negative relative to alveolar pressure,[5] and there is a positive alveolar-hilar pressure gradient[6] that facilitates the movement of interstitial fluid from alveolar to perihilar interstitial areas. The pressure surrounding the corner and extra-alveolar vessels is less than pleural pressure[5] and becomes considerably more negative at high lung volumes. In disease, these negative pressures may be amplified many fold because of "mechanical interdependence" of lung units.[7] When the expansion of some units of the lung lags behind surrounding lung units because of disease, the force per unit area distending the lagging unit is increased. Amplification of transpulmonary (distending) pressures by mechanical interdependence is seen in conditions characterized by increased respiratory resistance, decreased lung compliance, and expansion of the lung from the airless state. Mechanical interdependence can act on diseased areas of the lung to produce distending pressures that are exceedingly high. When transmitted to the interstitial space around blood vessels, these pressures can enhance edema formation and can cause the rupture of vessels. These considerations become especially important because various forms of constant distending pressures are used therapeutically. Although only 5 to 10 cm H_2O may be applied, if the pressure does not distend some areas of the lung as quickly as others, the pressure surrounding lagging units may be considerably greater because of amplification.

Surfactant alters the liquid pressure within the airspace and, by extrapolation, the alveolar interstitial pressure.[8] Thus increased air-liquid surface tension, whether as a result of inadequate or dysfunctional surfactant, will promote the movement of fluid from the vessels into the lungs.

Microvascular Filtration Coefficient and Vascular Permeability

There are significant technical difficulties in obtaining an accurate estimate of the K_f within intact lungs and, dependent upon the species and experimental approach, estimates had varied by more than three orders of magnitude. However, when the experimental protocol ensures that there is full recruitment of the pulmonary vascular surface area, there is remarkable consistency of the normalized baseline K_f values between species with widely varying body weights from mice to sheep.[9] Because there is a similar relation between alveolar surface area and body mass of different species, this feature optimizes gas exchange.

Experiments have shown that the walls of the pulmonary circulation are not a perfect semipermeable membrane and that the normal pulmonary vasculature has $0 < \sigma < 1$. The endothelial membrane has "pores" that are larger than some protein molecules. Fluid filtering through a pore will drag some protein with it. The larger the protein relative to the size of the pore, the less protein will be dragged. When the protein is the same size as or larger than the pore, the reflection coefficient σ is 1. As the size of the protein becomes progressively smaller, σ approaches zero.[10]

Early experimental evidence suggested that the microvascular permeability to protein is greater in the young than in the adult animal; however, subsequent work showed that there was no difference in lung microvascular permeability to protein between late term and postnatal animals and that the higher rate of fluid movement out of the newborn lung's microvasculature bed likely results from a greater portion of the younger smaller lung being in West's zone III perfusion status.[11]

Lymphatic Clearance

Whether there is fluid accumulation in the lung depends on the balance between fluid filtration into the lung and lymphatic clearance. Early in the onset of interstitial edema, lymphatic drainage of fluid is an important protective mechanism to prevent alveolar flooding. Although early work had indicated that increased motion or ventilation of the lung increased the lymphatic fluid drainage, suggesting a passive milking action, it is now known that there are active contractions of the lymphatic smooth muscle which can be further augmented by vasoactive agents. Indeed, rhythmic inflation and deflation is not required for normal lymphatic function in lungs that have normal or increased vascular permeability.[12] Lung lymph flow can increase up to tenfold acutely, and when there is chronic edema, the maximal ability of the lymphatics to clear fluid may increase many fold, presumably as the result of proliferation of the lymphatic vasculature. Because the lymphatics ultimately drain into the great veins, elevation of systemic venous pressure might be expected to increase fluid accumulation, not only by raising pressure in the fluid-exchanging vessels but also by opposing lymphatic drainage.

Surface Tension

Surface tension at the air-liquid interface on the inner surface of the alveolus tends to pull fluid away from the alveolar epithelium with a force of at least 2 mm Hg. This surface tension at the alveolar air-liquid interface would be expected to expand the perivascular space and to lower perimicrovascular pressure. As pulmonary edema fluid enters the airspace, it first collects in the corners, but as fluid continues to accumulate, the filling of an alveolus with fluid is self-accelerating once there is a critical amount of fluid in it.

Safety Factors That Oppose Edema Formation

A variety of clinical observations have indicated that transvascular hydrostatic pressures must be raised by 15 to 20 mm Hg before edema develops. Several factors provide this protection against edema formation. The interstitial fluid pressure, as previously described, is below alveolar pressure[13] and will rise when there is even minimal amounts of fluid accumulation within the lung[5,6] and thus oppose fluid movement. At the same time, the filtered fluid will dilute the interstitial plasma protein, thus lowering the interstitial colloid osmotic pressure and diminishing the movement of fluid out of the microvasculature. Lymphatic drainage of fluid and protein also contributes to this "margin of safety." The interstitial space itself, especially around the bronchi and blood vessels (bronchovascular cuffs), can sequester fluid (several hundred milliliters in the adult) and thus can provide an additional safety factor before fluid floods the alveoli.

▄ MECHANISMS THAT CAUSE PULMONARY EDEMA

There has been much effort to classify the different causes of pulmonary edema into cardiogenic and noncardiogenic pulmonary edema. Although this is useful to some degree, it should be remembered that in many lung diseases characterized by pulmonary edema, there are both increased transvascular pressure gradients and increased permeability to solutes. For example, 30% of patients diagnosed with acute lung injury have a pulmonary artery wedge (occlusion) pressure greater than 18 mm Hg.[14] The various etiologies of pulmonary edema are introduced by using the Starling equation as the basis for the discussion.

Increased Hydrostatic Pressure (Pmv) in the Pulmonary Microvasculature

Increased hydrostatic pressure in the pulmonary microvasculature is the most common and perhaps most easily understood cause of pulmonary edema in the pediatric and adult population. A variety of clinical conditions are associated with increased hydrostatic pressures in the pulmonary microvasculature, either as the result of elevation of vascular pressures distal to the lung's parenchyma, increased blood flow, increased blood volume, or pulmonary arterial or venular hypertension. In each case there would be an increase in the amount of water and solute leaving the microvasculature and entering the interstitium. Hypoxia increases pulmonary arterial pressures but does not increase vascular permeability to solutes.[15]

Decreased Plasma Colloid Osmotic Pressure (πmv)

If a patient has no other disorders, hypoproteinemia will not, by itself, cause pulmonary edema. Large pleural effusions may develop in diseases such as the nephrotic syndrome, but there is no evidence of lung edema as assessed by gas exchange and chest radiography. However, in patients where vascular pressure or alveolar capillary membrane permeability increases, pulmonary edema is more likely to develop and be more severe when the plasma protein concentration is low. This is seen with severe malnutrition, massive burns, protein-losing enteropathies, and nephrosis. Hypoproteinemia also can be seen in patients with a variety of other conditions when withdrawal of multiple blood samples for diagnostic purposes is coupled with the administration of large amounts of non–colloid-containing fluids.

Decreased Interstitial Hydrostatic Pressure (Ppmv)

As a result of mechanical interdependence of adjacent lung units, when inflation of some units lags behind that of others, large negative interstitial pressures can be generated around and within the lagging units. These negative pressures can be transmitted to the fluid-exchanging vessels (when there is airway closure), enhancing edema formation, especially in obstructive lung diseases such as asthma, bronchiolitis, and bronchopulmonary dysplasia (BPD), as well as in nonobstructive "stiff lung" disorders such as the respiratory distress syndrome (RDS).

Increased Pulmonary Vascular Surface Area

The normal adult lung usually has approximately one third of its microvascular bed perfused under resting conditions. Infants and young children have a greater percentage of their vascular bed distended with blood. Regardless of the absolute percentage, the lungs of all age groups can undergo significant recruitment and distention of the pulmonary vasculature. Although it had been suggested that various regions of the normal lung might have different permeability to solutes, most studies suggest that lung fluid movement simply increases in direct proportion to the increase in perfused pulmonary vascular surface area. Under normal conditions, the lung lymphatics can easily accommodate the threefold to fourfold increase in lung water and solute movement that is associated with full recruitment of the vasculature. However, when pulmonary vascular permeability is increased, similar amounts of recruitment can lead to marked increases in fluid movement as vessels with high permeability are recruited.[16,17]

Increased Vascular Permeability in Fluid-Exchanging Vessels

Increased alveolar-capillary membrane permeability to solutes can occur by different routes. Classic modeling of the pulmonary microvasculature uses the concept of various sized "pores" through which various sized solutes move under normal physiologic conditions. Thus, permeability could increase via an increase in the total number of pores, the diameter of the pores, or a combination of the two phenomena. For example, vasoactive agents could increase the size of the interendothelial junctions. Alternatively, or in addition, direct and extensive damage to the alveolar epithelium or endothelium occurring during over-ventilation lung injury[18,19] or stress-induced endothelial injury[20] will open up large nonphysiologic pathways for fluid and solute movement.

A variety of clinical conditions are believed to alter the permeability of the alveolar capillary membrane, presumably by damage to epithelial and endothelial cells. The cellular mechanisms for this injury can be divided into two major categories: direct and inflammatory-mediated lung injury.

Direct lung injury can occur when a toxic substance directly causes cell injury without a preceding inflammatory response. Direct lung injury is seen during the inhalation of a variety of noxious gases, including the oxides of sulfur and nitrogen, hydrocyanic acid, aldehydes, and so on. Similarly, the inhalation of gastric acid can directly damage lung epithelium. These produce denaturation of proteins, cellular damage, and pulmonary edema.

Inflammation-mediated lung injury, as occurs in acute lung injury (ALI) and acute respiratory distress syndrome (ARDS), most frequently arises from leukocytes and their

products. The unregulated release of leukocyte-derived toxic products occurs in response to direct injury or in response to various infective and inflammatory stimuli. These toxic products include reactive oxygen species (e.g., superoxide, hydrogen peroxide, hypochlorous acid, hydroxyl radical, peroxynitrite), proteolytic enzymes (e.g., elastase, collagenase, lysozyme), products of arachidonic acid (e.g., platelet-activating factor), and cationic proteins. Leukocytes have been implicated in animal models of acute lung injury induced by the administration of endotoxin, hyperoxia, microembolization, and mechanical ventilation. Non–leukocyte-derived vasoactive mediators also can increase vascular permeability. Examples include histamine, prostaglandins, cytokines, proteases, and reactive oxygen intermediates.

Increased permeability of the microvasculature also occurs in a variety of disorders characterized by aberrant regulation of the immune system. These include hypersensitivity pneumonitis and pulmonary vasculitis, which can occur in various disorders such as acute pulmonary systemic lupus erythematosus.

When there is increased pulmonary vascular permeability, an increase in microvascular hydrostatic pressure[16] or pulmonary blood flow[17] produces a much greater outward flow of fluid. As such, the combination of increased permeability and high left atrial pressures represents an especially difficult clinical challenge.

CLEARANCE OF PULMONARY EDEMA FLUID

Once the basic condition producing the edema is reversed, how quickly pulmonary edema resolves depends on whether the fluid is confined to the interstitium, from which it can be cleared in hours, or is also located in the alveolar space, from which it may take many hours or days to clear.

Interstitial fluid has two pathways for clearance. The lymphatics play the most important major role; however, a second site is the venular end of the microvascular bed where Pmv has decreased and the balance of Starling forces can favor reabsorption. Alveolar edema fluid, after being actively transported across the epithelium, is returned to the circulation either by direct entry into the pulmonary microvasculature across the thin side of alveolar capillary membrane or by the lymphatics after it has been translocated back to the interstitial space. Both of these potential pathways, however, require water and solutes to have first traversed the distal lung epithelium.

In both high-pressure and high-permeability pulmonary edema, there is a substantial amount of protein within the alveolar fluid that opposes protein osmotic reabsorption, and it has been shown that passive forces cannot explain the clearance of alveolar fluid from the intact lung.[21] Long-term studies have demonstrated that as edema fluid is reabsorbed, the protein concentration in the alveolar space actually increases to levels above those in the plasma. This suggested that an active transport of salt and water was involved in the clearance of air-space fluids. Numerous studies, as reviewed recently,[22] have demonstrated that nonprimate mammalian and human distal lung epithelium actively transports Na^+ with

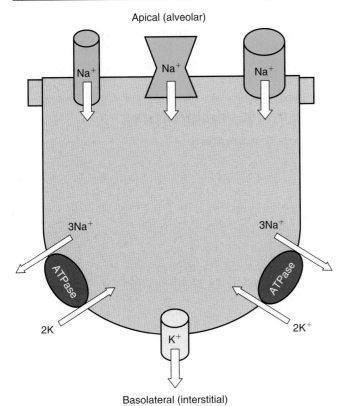

Apical (alveolar)

Basolateral (interstitial)

FIGURE 38-2. Model for Na+ transport by the alveolar epithelium. The Na+/K+ ATPase located on the basolateral membrane is responsible for the creation of the marked intracellular/extracellular (10:150 mM) Na+ concentration gradient. This chemical gradient along with the negative intracellular electrical potential arising from the permeability of the K+ channels attracts Na+ ions into the cell through Na+-permeant ion channels located in the apical membrane to be extruded across the basolateral membrane. There are different types of Na+ channels in the apical membrane, the most important of which is the amiloride sensitive epithelial Na+ channel (ENaC). The activity of these Na+-permeant ion channels represents the rate-limiting step in Na+ transport. Chloride (Cl−) follows both via the paracellular pathway past the tight junctions and also through the cell via the Cl− channel encoded by the cystic fibrosis transmembrane regulator (CFTR). Water follows in response to the osmotic gradient created by the active ion transport. For more details see reference 22.

Cl− and water following (Fig. 38-2). Although most research, for reasons of feasibility only, have focused on the alveolar type II epithelium's ability to actively transport salt, it is known that both the alveolar type I epithelium and clara cells play important roles in this active epithelial Na+ transport.[22] Studies in adult patients[23,24] have indicated that active alveolar fluid clearance rates in the human are in the range of 25 % per hour.

Protein clearance from the alveolar spaces is significantly slower than salt and water, and in animals, it is in the range of 1% per hour.[21] The relative amount of protein cleared by metabolic degradation and macrophage ingestion versus active transport by the pulmonary epithelium is unknown, but active transport is involved in the clearance of at least some proteins from the airspaces of the lungs.[25] Protein clearance from the interstitial space is believed to occur primarily by lymphatic clearance, but direct penetration into the circulation either before or after metabolic degradation also might occur.

The presence of protein in the alveolar and interstitial spaces may attract inflammatory cells. In acute lung injury syndromes, there is marked leakage of plasma protein into the alveolar space, and resultant activation of the coagulation cascade results in fibrin formation. The coagulum opposes the efficient reabsorption of fluid, and also fibrin and fibrin degradation products are potent stimuli for fibrosis within the lung. Circulating monocytes and alveolar macrophages likely play a major role in the clearance of inflammatory edema protein from the lung's airspaces.

In summary, a wide variety of mechanisms and sites exist for protein and electrolyte clearance and fluid removal, including pulmonary and bronchial circulations, lymphatics, active transport of ions, macromolecular metabolism and degradation, and mononuclear cell activity.

PATHOPHYSIOLOGIC CONSEQUENCES OF EDEMA

The pathophysiologic consequences and clinical findings in pulmonary edema are best understood by reviewing the sequence of events that lead from interstitial to airspace edema. Edema accumulates within the lung in a step-wise fashion (Fig. 38-3). Distal lung units in different regions of the lung will be at different stages of fluid accumulation because of their regional differences in pressure, alveolar-capillary integrity, and gravitationally dependent factors.

Increased pulmonary blood volumes, even without associated pulmonary edema, have been shown to cause a small decrease in lung compliance. Consistent with these findings, clinical studies have shown that infants with left to right congenital heart disease have low lung compliance that improves after correction of their shunt.[26]

In humans, the increase in airway resistance that occurs when there are small amounts of interstitial edema arises largely from a vagally mediated reflex.[27] Once interstitial edema worsens, the peribronchiolar cuffs of fluid would be expected to lead to increased closing volume and airway resistance, although this has been difficult to prove in morphometric studies of adult nonprimate lungs.[28] When small airways contribute a relatively greater proportion of the total airway resistance, as is the case in infants in contrast to adults, edema can lead to a greater increase in airway resistance. Small airway obstruction has been a presenting sign of a group of infants with ventricular septal defects and left-to-right shunts.[29] In addition, some children with interstitial edema as a result of left atrial obstruction (e.g., cor triatriatum) have also presented with a history of recurrent asthmatic attacks. To minimize the markedly increased work of moving their stiff lungs, a pattern of rapid, shallow breathing is used. The stimulation of vagal J receptors by the edema also contributes to the tachypnea and dyspnea so characteristic of early pulmonary edema.

For reasons previously outlined, the presence of edema increases airway resistance. As the airways narrow, closing volume increases and alveolar gas exchange is impaired because of the resultant low V/Q ratio. At this stage, hypocapnia results from the J receptor vagally

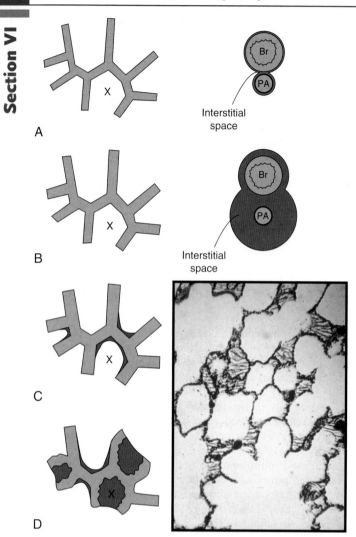

FIGURE 38-3. Schematic representation of the sequence of fluid accumulation during acute pulmonary edema. **A,** Normal alveolar walls and no excess fluid in perivascular connective tissue spaces. **B,** Initial fluid leak. Fluid flows to the interstitial space (at subatmospheric pressure) around the conducting vessels and airways. **C,** Tissue space fills, alveolar edema increases, and fluid begins to overflow into the alveoli, notably at the corners where curvature is pronounced. **D,** Quantal filling. Individual alveoli reach a critical configuration at which existing inflation pressure can no longer maintain stability. Note that the fluid filled alveoli are smaller in size than their adjacent air-filled alveoli. The insert is a photomicrograph of a flash frozen lung with pulmonary edema that illustrates the above scheme of fluid filling (From Staub NC, Nagano K, Pearce ML. Pulmonary edema in dogs, especially the sequence of fluid accumulation in lungs. *J Appl Physiol.* 1967;22:227-240.)

mediated reflex hyperventilation independent of the presence of hypoxemia. As edema worsens and alveolar flooding occurs, there is further hypoxemia as the blood shunts past nonventilating alveoli. Respiratory acidosis may supervene if the patient is depressed by sedation or if exhaustion develops. The extent to which bronchial mucosal edema intensifies the increase in airway resistance when pulmonary edema is accompanied by elevated systemic venous pressure is not known. With alveolar flooding and disruption of the normal alveolar lining, resistance to airflow increases, dynamic and static compliance are reduced, and there is increasing inhomogeneity

of airflow. Once the edema fluid floods into the airspaces, the proteins therein will impair surfactant function.[30] One can account for most of the clinical findings (e.g., crackles and diffuse wheezing) on the basis of interstitial, airway, and alveolar edema.

CLINICAL PRESENTATION

Physical Examination

In a general way, small increases in lung fluid are too subtle to be detected by currently available clinical methods and only when the extravascular fluid volume has increased considerably is the condition clinically obvious. The patient will be tachypneic, not just when hypoxemia stimulates ventilation, but also because of the stimulation of the J receptors. This latter point explains, at least in part, the continuing tachypnea even after correction of arterial hypoxemia by supplemental oxygen therapy. On auscultation, crackles occur when edema fluid is present in the terminal airways, and they are produced by the sudden opening of peripheral lung units (alveolar ducts or terminal bronchioli). When the fluid moves up to larger airways, rhonchi and wheezes are to be expected. The relative contribution of bronchial wall edema and bronchoconstriction to rhonchi and wheezes is not known. Chest wall retractions will be observed as the spontaneously breathing patient must generate more negative pleural pressures to overcome the markedly decreased total respiratory system compliance and mild increases in airway resistance. Grunting may be present in pulmonary edema and represents a useful maneuver to create a positive end expiratory pressure to prevent derecruitment of distal lung units.

Pulmonary Function Tests

Initially, vascular engorgement may lead to an *increase* in the diffusing capacity (DLCO) by increasing the amount of perfused vasculature within the gas exchanging regions of the lung. As interstitial edema increases, there will be an increase in closing volume, a decrease in maximum expiratory flow, an increase in V/Q inhomogeneity, and a decrease in arterial PO_2. With alveolar flooding, there is further air trapping, increased vascular resistance, decreased lung volumes, decreased dynamic lung compliance, decreased DLCO, and progressive hypoxemia arising from the increased intrapulmonary right-to-left shunting and rising $PacO_2$, the latter further decreasing alveolar PO_2. In patients with a patent foramen ovale, right-to-left shunting at the atrial level may occur as a result of the associated pulmonary hypertension and concomitant increase in right ventricular end diastolic pressure.

Imaging Studies

It has been shown that an infusion of 30 mL/kg of saline into healthy adult volunteers over 30 minutes increases extracellular fluid volume by 15% without altering the density of the lungs on computed tomography (CT) or the amount of Compton scattering; the only change on chest radiography and CT studies was an increase in the size of the azygos vein.[31] To this author's knowledge, human studies such as these have not been repeated, so it is unknown whether modern imaging techniques might be more sensitive.

The Chest Radiograph

Pulmonary edema can be detected in adult humans on a chest radiograph when extravascular lung water is increased by approximately 35%. Although most of the radiographic signs of pulmonary edema are nonspecific, improved radiographic techniques in conjunction with improved understanding of the pathophysiology of pulmonary edema have enhanced the usefulness of the chest roentgenogram in the diagnosis of pulmonary edema.

The Kerley lines represent interlobular sheets of abnormally thickened or widened connective tissue that are tangential to the x-ray beam (Fig. 38-4). These are more properly referred to as septal lines. Thickened septal lines may occur from a variety of processes, including fibrosis, pigment deposition, and pulmonary hemosiderosis. However, when they are transient, these lines are usually caused by edema. These septal lines of edema are more clearly visible in older children and adults with chronic edema than in infants, presumably because they are wider. Perivascular and peribronchial cuffing are also radiographic signs of interstitial edema fluid. For hydrostatic reasons, perivascular edema is greatest in the gravitationally dependent regions, and the normal tethering action of the lung is therefore less in this region. Increased resistance in the lower lobe vessels promotes the redistribution of blood to the upper lobes. This sign is, of course, of limited value in infants because they are most likely to be in the supine position, have smaller gravitational induced differences because of their size, and normally have only slightly increased pulmonary arterial pressures relative to children and adults.

More severe forms of pulmonary edema commonly produce a perihilar haze, presumably because the large perivascular and peribronchial collections of fluid are in this location. A reticular or lattice-like pattern also may be present and is more common inferiorly in an upright individual. Once the magnitude of pulmonary edema is sufficiently severe to lead to persistent airway closure or alveolar flooding, it is very difficult to separate edema, atelectasis, and inflammation on chest roentgenograms. Air bronchograms indicate airless distal lung units and not the underlying cause.

Because pulmonary edema can lead to airway obstruction in children from both vagal reflex[27] and bronchial froth,[32] airway closure can occur and produce air trapping.[29] Thus low diaphragms may be a useful sign of interstitial edema, provided there are no other reasons for airway obstruction. Although studies in children are limited, a summary of findings that allows separation of cardiogenic or hemodynamic edema, renal or overhydration edema, and injury or ARDS edema has been provided in adults.[33,34] There is an inverted base-to-apex redistribution of blood flow in patients with heart failure. The progressive recruitment of connective tissue spaces by edema fluid in both cardiac and renal disease gives rise to hilar blurring, peribronchial cuffing, and a hazy pattern of increasing lung density. In ARDS, there is more likely to be a patchy peripheral distribution of edema and a paucity of such findings as septal lines and peribronchial cuffing.

Computed Tomography (CT) and Magnetic Resonance Imaging (MRI)

Thin-section CT imaging of the thorax has provided new information regarding pulmonary edema (Fig. 38-5). For example, studies in ARDS have shown that the lung densities, presumably representing regional edema and microatelectasis, are very heterogeneous and shift with the position of the patient, with densities appearing in the most gravitationally dependent lung regions.[35-37] However, alterations in lung density have to be interpreted with caution. Increases in regional lung density can result from increases in extravascular lung water (i.e., edema), a decrease in regional gas volume, or both.

To date, MRI has had limited use in the management of patients with pulmonary edema. Its major advantage is that it does not require ionizing radiation. One major limitation is that despite obtaining excellent imaging of the larger pulmonary vessels, MRI provides very poor resolution of the lung's parenchyma. The safe transport to and the management of the patient within the MRI suite are also pragmatic limitations to this imaging modality. However, one center with a MRI within their critical care unit has used this approach to document that there is increased lung water content in premature babies with RDS.[38] Their findings are consistent with earlier studies of gravimetric measurement of lung water content in postmortem premature infants[39] and research studies on experimental respiratory distress syndrome in nonhuman primates (see Neonatal Respiratory Distress Syndrome).[40]

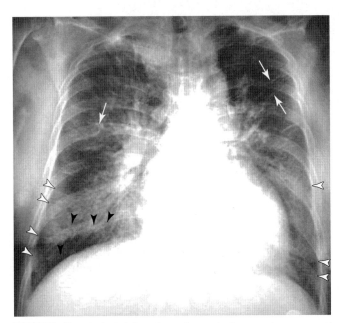

FIGURE 38-4. Kerley's A lines (arrows) occur in the upper lung zone and point towards the hilum and are directed toward, but do not extend to, the pleural surface. Kerley's B lines (white arrowheads) are usually in the lung base and are at right angles to, and in contact with, the pleural surface. Kerley's C lines (black arrowheads) are reticular opacities representing Kerley's B lines seen en face. (Reproduced from Koga T, Fujimoto K. Images in clinical medicine. Kerley's A, B, and C lines. N Engl J Med. 2009;360(15):1539.)

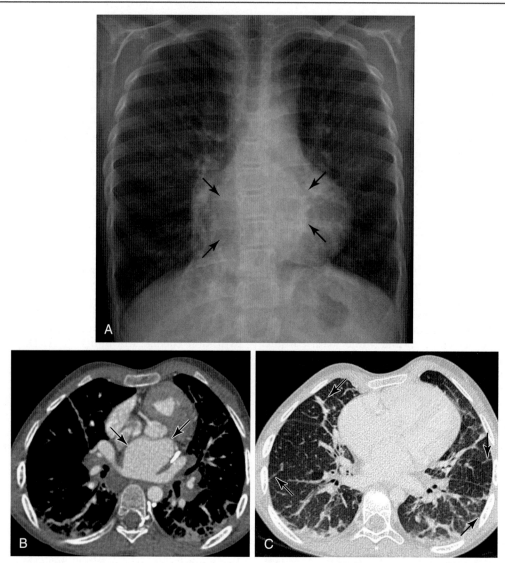

FIGURE 38-5. Images of a 7-year-old patient with Shone syndrome and longstanding mitral stenosis. **A,** Frontal chest radiograph reveals mild cardiomegaly with an enlarged left atrium *(arrows)*. There is vascular prominence of the upper lobes and features of the interstitial endema, including hyperinflation, perihilar prominence of vessels, and indistinct vascular margins. **B,** CT (mediastinal windows) illustrates the enlarged left atrium *(arrows)* and pulmonary veins. **C,** CT (lung windows) illustrates prominent vessels, areas of mosaic perfusion (darker and lighter regions) indicating small airway dysfunction and interlobular septal thickening *(arrows)*, which are the CT equivalent of Kerley B lines on plain chest radiographs. (Images courtesy of Dr. Beverley Newman, Stanford University.)

Distinguishing High Pressure from Low Pressure Pulmonary Edema

Direct measurements of Pmv would be useful in the differentiation of high-pressure from high-permeability edema. However, the use of pulmonary artery occlusion pressures to estimate Pmv has its limitations (see Vascular Forces), and patients with pulmonary edema often have both increased permeability and elevated pulmonary artery occlusion pressures.[14] Although B-type natriuretic peptide (BNP) has been found useful in identifying congestive heart failure (CHF), it does not reliably distinguish CHF-induced from ARDS- induced pulmonary edema.[41]

When patients with pulmonary edema have undergone endotracheal intubation, one can collect airway fluid that may reflect alveolar fluid. On this basis, investigators attempted to differentiate high-pressure from increased permeability pulmonary edema[42] by comparing the concentration of the protein in the airspace fluid with the simultaneously measured plasma protein concentration. Although this ratio was statistically significantly different between the two groups, there is such significant scatter that it is of little diagnostic utility for the individual patient. The reason for this variation and lack of clinical utility is now understood: the alveolar fluid's protein concentration not only depends on the leakiness of the alveolar-capillary membrane but also on the efficiency and amount of time available for the epithelium to actively pump salt and water out of the airspace with the resultant concentration of the protein that remains in the distal lung unit (see Clearance of Pulmonary Edema Fluid).

Endothelial cell injury has been assessed by the ability of the pulmonary circulation to remove or metabolize a variety of substances; however, these tests are neither sufficiently sensitive nor specific. Similarly, although the clearance rate of inhaled and deposited small solutes (e.g., ^{99m}Tc-DTPA) from the lungs provides an index of pulmonary epithelial integrity,[43] this approach is hampered by the inability to differentiate increased epithelial permeability from marked increases in regional lung volume.[44] Analysis of airspace fluid may be beneficial as proteomic analysis may reveal qualitative changes in the expression of some proteins and provide new markers for lung injury.[45] The receptor for advanced glycation end-products (RAGE) is an alveolar type I cell–associated protein and, although it is expressed in other organs, elevated levels in bronchoalveolar lavage reflect ALI.[46]

Quantitation of Pulmonary Edema in Patients

Indicator dilution techniques have been used to measure extravascular lung water (EVLW) content in humans. Traditional techniques have used a technique that depends on one tracer being confined to the vascular space and another tracer that diffuses into the perfused tissue. The difference in the sum of the two time concentration curves has been used to calculate the amount of EVLW. Measurements of EVLW are improved when results are normalized to lung volumes as predicted by height and gender rather than the previous approach of body weight, which is affected by obesity.[47] Useful information has been obtained using this approach. For example, EVLW correlates with mortality in critically ill adults[47,48] (Fig. 38-6). The major assumption, and limitation, of these techniques is that it can only measure that portion of the lung that is perfused; therefore, it may underestimate the total lung water or measurements may assess differing amounts of the lungs at different time points.[49]

▬ CLINICAL DISORDERS CAUSING PULMONARY EDEMA

High-Pressure Pulmonary Edema

This diagnostic label refers to conditions where there is a demonstrable increase in the forces promoting fluid movement out of the microvasculature. By far the most common cause is left-sided heart disease, which results in marked elevations of pulmonary venous and hence microvasculature hydrostatic pressure.

Obstructive lesions such as cor triatriatum, mitral stenosis, congenital obstruction of pulmonary venous drainage, and pulmonary veno-occlusive disease directly cause pulmonary venous hypertension. In contrast, other obstructive lesions such as coarctation of the aorta and severe aortic stenosis only cause pulmonary edema once left ventricular failure has occurred.

Myocardial failure with subsequent pulmonary venous hypertension may arise from either congenital or acquired heart disease. Examples of the former include hypoplastic left heart syndrome, and the latter includes intrinsic myocardial disease (e.g., cardiac glycogen storage diseases, endocardial fibroelastosis, viral and rheumatic myocarditis) and myocardial ischemia (e.g., anomalous left coronary artery or Kawasaki disease).

Markedly increased pulmonary blood flow occurs in patients with congenital arteriovenous fistulas or congenital heart defects that promote left-to-right shunting of blood (e.g., ventricular septal defect, patent ductus arteriosus). This leads to pulmonary vascular engorgement, especially in the case of anatomic left-to-right shunting. In either case, there is a marked increase in left ventricular output. When the burden on the left ventricle becomes too great and left-sided heart failure supervenes, pulmonary microvascular pressures are increased by both high flow and increased left atrial pressures.

Significant increases in blood volume can result in pulmonary vascular engorgement and edema. Fluid retention rapidly occurs in acute renal disease as a result of the expanded extracellular fluid volume. Nephrosis and chronic renal disease also may predispose an individual to pulmonary edema by the associated hypoproteinemia. Perhaps the most common cause of increased pulmonary blood volume is the overzealous administration of fluids. This will intensify the development of pulmonary edema by raising hydrostatic pressures and diluting plasma proteins. Finally, to what extent the inappropriate secretion of antidiuretic hormone, which occurs in disorders such as pneumonia, asthma and bronchopulmonary dysplasia, complicates and intensifies the development of pulmonary edema in these diseases is incompletely understood.

Airway Obstruction

Severe obstruction of the extrathoracic airways predisposes the patient to pulmonary edema (see Interstitial Forces). For example, croup and epiglottitis are associated with pulmonary edema.[50,51]

Diffuse small airway obstruction, as occurs in status asthmaticus, also promotes the development of pulmonary edema as a result of a lag in the expansion of the lung in spite of the development of very negative intrathoracic pressures.[52] Although airway inflammation is recognized as an important part of the pathogenesis of asthma, it is not clear to what extent edema of the airways, per se, plays in the airway obstruction. Certainly, any inflammation-induced increase in permeability would dramatically increase the amount of fluid moving across the vascular bed in response to a more negative interstitial pressure. Clinically, significant

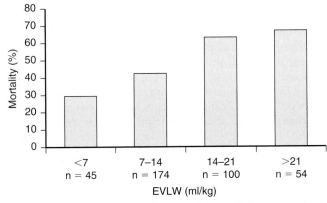

FIGURE 38-6. Mortality as a function of EVLW. Patients were classified into four groups according to their highest EVLW value. The asterisk indicates statistical significance to the next higher EVLW group (chi-squared). (Reproduced from Sakka SG, Klein M, Reinhart K, et al. Prognostic value of extravascular lung water in critically ill patients. *Chest* 2002;122(6):2080-2086.)

short-term improvements in gas exchange are often seen in some patients with asthma and bronchiolitis with the use of diuretics. Because these diuretics also change vascular compliance and pressures, the exact reason for the beneficial response is uncertain. Nevertheless, our improved understanding of how airway obstruction can promote the development of pulmonary edema led to the present therapeutic strategy of giving only maintenance, or less than maintenance fluids, to patients after they have had their deficits replaced. In the more distant past, it had been customary to advocate increased fluid intake for patients with asthma and bronchiolitis in the false hope that the increased fluid would loosen secretions and facilitate their expectoration; this has never been established, but it is certain that the increased amounts of fluid will promote the development of pulmonary edema.

Cardiac failure and pulmonary edema are also rarely seen in obstructive sleep apnea; in children, this condition is most frequently associated with hypertrophied tonsils and adenoids.[53,54] At the bedside, one can see severe intercostal retractions during inspiration. Indeed, this inspiratory pattern is similar to a Müller maneuver (i.e., a strong inspiration against a closed glottis or obstructed upper airway). The negative pressures would, in addition to promoting edema, also surround and restrain the left ventricle and create an increased afterload to the left ventricle (left ventricular afterload is equal to the mean aortic pressure minus the pleural pressure).

Reexpansion Pulmonary Edema

Reexpansion pulmonary edema is seen in some patients who have rapid lung reexpansion after drainage of a large pneumothorax or pleural fluid. Rarely, it causes systemic hypovolemia and shock as large volumes of fluid move from the space vascular to airspaces of the rapidly reinflated lung.

The reported incidence of reexpansion pulmonary edema varies considerably, and it has been speculated that the different incidence rates result from various factors. These include the duration of the atelectasis, characteristics of the collapsed lung, and the rate of evacuation of the pleural air or fluid. For example, in many of the case reports, the lung collapse had been present for some time before reexpansion. A prospective study revealed that 20% of adult patients treated with closed thoracostomy drainage for a spontaneous pneumothorax developed classic reexpansion pulmonary edema.[55] In contrast, another report found that the evacuation of pleural fluid was rarely associated with reexpansion pulmonary edema.[56] Regardless of the true incidence, it is irrefutable that this phenomenon does occur. Thus, caution must be exercised when draining large collections of fluid from the pleural space when there is associated collapse of a lobe or lung.

One of the mechanisms responsible for the syndrome is the sudden marked lowering of the interstitial fluid pressure. In addition, experimental studies of reexpansion pulmonary edema in rabbits[57] provide evidence that there is increased vascular permeability to protein. Although the mechanism for injury of the alveolar-capillary membrane is not known, there are at least two possibilities. The first is that there is increased and excessive stretch or tension of the alveolar septal walls during reexpansion of lungs that

have been collapsed for several days. Stress-related pulmonary endothelial injury[20] has been described in other experimental conditions, and overexpansion of lungs during positive-pressure ventilation is associated with increases in alveolar-capillary permeability.[18,19] Other mechanisms, such as reperfusion lung injury from reactive oxygen intermediates, also may play a role in the increased alveolar-capillary membrane permeability. Indeed, it has been shown that collapsed lung tissue has decreased mitochondrial superoxide dismutase (SOD) and cytochrome oxidase[58]; these changes could enhance oxygen free radical production.

Neonatal Respiratory Distress Syndrome

Studies in humans[38,39] and primates[40] prove that neonatal RDS (nRDS) in premature infants is associated with widespread airspace edema and that the well-described reduction in FRC results more from the excess fluid than from atelectasis.[40]

A number of factors contribute to airspace fluid in patients with nRDS. First, there is the fluid that had been secreted into the developing fetal lungs' airspaces during normal fetal lung development. This fluid must be cleared at birth so that effective gas exchange can occur, and clearance of airspace fluid results from active transepithelial Na^+ transport (see Fig. 38-2). Impaired clearance of this fetal lung liquid, arising from inadequate epithelial sodium transport[59,60] combined with an immature surfactant system,[61] results in nRDS.[62] Second, pulmonary edema fluid is generated during the course of nRDS by several mechanisms. These include the high pulmonary vascular pressures and blood flow, especially if there is a patent ductus arteriosus; low interstitial pressures, in part the result of high alveolar surface tension; low plasma protein concentration (and hence low plasma osmotic pressure)[63]; increased epithelial permeability[43]; lung endothelial injury from inflammation and, as a result of therapy, high airway pressures and high inspired oxygen concentrations.

Neurogenic Pulmonary Edema

Any acute cerebral insult, and rarely cervical spinal cord injury, can lead to neurogenic pulmonary edema (NPE).[64,65] Most frequently, it is seen with head trauma, subarachnoid hemorrhage, brain tumors, status epilepticus, and meningitis. The mechanisms responsible for pulmonary edema following lesions of the brain are not fully understood but appear to result from a combination of hemodynamic and permeability-altering factors. The hemodynamic response arises from a sympathetic storm that causes intense brief vasoconstriction from mediators such as norepinephrine, neuropeptide Y, and endothelin. Vascular permeability is also increased. This might occur by two mechanisms: pressure induced damage to the vascular bed or from the release of factors, such as TNF-α, IL-1β, and IL-6, from astrocytes and microglial cells, which may gain entry into the systemic circulation. These along with inflammatory processes arising from the sympathetic storm may induce a systemic inflammatory response.

The clinical signs of NPE are those of acute pulmonary edema, without evidence of left ventricular failure. There is no specific biologic marker for NPE, and it may develop acutely over minutes to hours or may be delayed. Evaluation of edema fluid suggests that patients may either have predominately high pressure or high permeability pulmonary edema.[66] In the treatment of NPE, it is important to remember that positive ventilatory pressures, especially positive end-expiratory pressure (PEEP), should be administered cautiously because they can interfere with cerebral venous return, thus promoting further cerebral edema. Depending on the severity of the primary result, NPE may resolve within the first 2 to 3 days and overall outcome relates to the neurologic outcome.

Acute Lung Injury and the Acute Respiratory Distress Syndrome

ALI and its most severe form, ARDS, frequently occur in critically ill patients. Regardless of the inciting event, the clinical and pathologic manifestations of ARDS are similar, indicating a final common pathway ultimately leading to severe endothelial and epithelial inflammatory injury. This causes a compromise of barrier and transport functions, which leads to high permeability pulmonary edema that is often compounded by increases in microvascular pressure from concomitant pulmonary hypertension and pulmonary venoconstriction.

An initiating event, such as sepsis, shock, head injury, or trauma triggers a systemic inflammatory response that promotes sequestration of polymorphonuclear leukocytes (PMN) within the lung. Histologically, ARDS is characterized by large numbers of PMN in the vascular, interstitial, and alveolar space in association with endothelial and epithelial injury. This, combined with the potential of PMN to induce tissue injury in diverse experimental systems, has led to the widely held concept that these potent phagocytes are central to the pathogenesis of ARDS, a notion supported by numerous human and animal studies. The clinical presentation, pathogenic mechanisms, and approaches to therapy are discussed in detail in Chapter 39.

High-Altitude Pulmonary Edema

High altitude pulmonary edema (HAPE) can occur when climbers are exercising intensively in hypoxic environments as they ascend to high altitudes. What are the relative contributions of exercise and hypoxia? Although pulmonary edema can occur during marathons conducted near sea level[67] or in elite swimmers,[68] it is extraordinarily rare for normoxic exercise to be associated with pulmonary edema. Similarly, moderate hypoxia by itself is not sufficient for the development of edema. Approximately one third of nonexercising children who rapidly ascend to modest elevations (from 568 to 3450 meters), develop acute mountain sickness (AMS) However, clinically obvious cerebral or pulmonary edema do not seem to occur.[69] Studies have shown that these symptoms of AMS can be prevented by the administration of acetazolamide, but not the herbal supplement ginkgo biloba, just before and during ascent.[70] Although exposure to even more modest hypoxia (equivalent to 2,438 meters altitude) is associated with small decreases in arterial saturation, it is not associated with AMS.[71]

Clinically important and severe HAPE may affect some sea-level dwellers soon after arriving at a high altitude. Arterial blood gas analyses suggest that there may be subclinical HAPE, or diffusion defect, even in asymptomatic climbers ascending Mt. Everest.[72] HAPE also may occur in some highlanders who return home after a brief stay at sea level.

Much of our initial understanding of HAPE came from observations of Indian soldiers transported to high altitudes during the Indo-China war of the past century.[73] Subsequent work has shown that the incidence of HAPE and acute mountain sickness is increased when the rate of ascent is rapid and subjects have little opportunity for acclimatization, whereas gender or previous altitude exposure have no effect.[74] Relevant to the previous discussion regarding pulmonary vascular recruitment, the incidence of HAPE is increased in children and young adults,[75] and in subjects with only one pulmonary artery.[76] Fatigue, dyspnea, cough, and sleep disturbances are common and may progress rapidly to severe tachypnea, shock, and death unless rapid descent to a lower altitude or administration of oxygen occurs.

The mechanisms leading to HAPE are still incompletely understood. Nonprimate animal studies show that although hypoxia increases pulmonary arterial pressures, it does not by itself increase vascular permeability to solutes.[15] However, the best available evidence suggests that HAPE is initiated by an excessive increase in Pmv. The cause of the Pmv is unknown, although the two favored hypotheses are an unequal pulmonary vasoconstriction with resultant overperfusion of remaining lung microvessels or an abnormal vasoconstriction of the pulmonary venules. Prospective studies suggest that first there is a noninflammatory leakage of fluid across the alveolar-capillary membrane followed by a secondary inflammatory reaction[77] as the disease progresses.[78] Some researchers have assumed that, in addition to a constitutional predisposition of some individuals to pulmonary hypertension with hypoxia, nonuniform increases in precapillary resistance are responsible for the very high pressures seen in at least some pulmonary capillaries. The observation that prophylactic administration of the calcium channel blocker nifedipine can diminish the incidence of HAPE[79] and that inhalation of nitric oxide (NO) decreases PA pressures and improves oxygenation[80,81] in such patients supports the speculation that HAPE is due in part to an inappropriate pulmonary vasoconstrictive response. The observation that salmeterol diminishes the frequency of HAPE[82] is intriguing; potential mechanisms include its effect on vascular resistance and the augmentation of lung epithelial Na+ transport.

Inhalation of Toxic Agents

Toxic lung injury can be induced by a wide variety of agents,[83] but only three examples are discussed here. The most common agent is smoke from fires, the toxicity of which will vary with the nature of the combustible product (e.g., plastics versus wood). In victims of fires, the auscultatory evidence of pulmonary edema resulting from inhalation of smoke with damage to the distal lung unit, including the alveolar capillary membrane is manifest within 24 hours and usually precedes roentgenographic changes.[84]

Chlorine gas inhalation is an example of a toxic gas that can cause severe lung injury. It is most frequently seen in industrial accidents but can occur following exposure to fumes from liquid chlorine used in swimming pools. Pulmonary edema is frequently seen; however, if the patient survives, there are no long-term sequelae.[85]

The inhalation of paraquat, a herbicide, results in the generation of reactive oxygen intermediates. This noxious agent causes pulmonary edema, presumably on the basis of a change in permeability. Even before morphologic evidence of alveolar injury is apparent, there is an increase in surface tension, presumably as the result of inactivation or impaired synthesis of pulmonary surfactant.[86]

Intravenous Agents

Infusion of any compound that can act as a microembolic agent can result in high-permeability pulmonary edema as demonstrated in animal models of lung injury[17] and humans who have accidently suffered from air microembolism.[87]

Narcotic-Induced and Medication-Induced Pulmonary Edema

Heroin and other narcotics also have been associated with pulmonary edema.[88,89] Pulmonary capillary wedge pressure has been elevated in some patients but has been normal in others. Whether hypoxia and acidosis or neurogenic pulmonary edema, as the result of cerebral edema, plays a role is not known. Clinical and roentgenographic signs of pulmonary edema have occurred following the intravenous administration of paraldehyde[90]; although a direct toxic action on the pulmonary vascular bed has been proposed, the cause remains obscure.

Salicylates also have been associated with the development of pulmonary edema in adults[91] and children.[92] Experimental studies in sheep suggest that salicylate pulmonary edema is not due to increased vascular pressure but rather to increased vascular permeability.[93] Insofar as these studies can be applied to the human, the researchers suggest that acetylsalicylic acid can cause pulmonary edema in doses considered therapeutic for some diseases. Although the mechanisms responsible for the altered vascular permeability remain unknown, at least two effects of salicylates could affect vascular integrity: alterations in platelet function and inhibition of prostaglandin synthesis.

■■THERAPY

It is not only biologically reasonable to maintain the postnatal airspace air-filled, and not fluid-filled; there is a substantial body of research that suggests that reduction or attenuation of pulmonary edema improves patient outcome. Decreasing pulmonary arterial wedge pressures[94] or avoiding positive fluid balances[95] are both associated with improved survival. EVLW correlates with mortality in adults[47,48] (Fig. 38-6). Similarly, a randomized study has shown that conservative fluid management improves lung function and shortens the duration of mechanical ventilation in acute lung injury.[96] Indirect assessments of

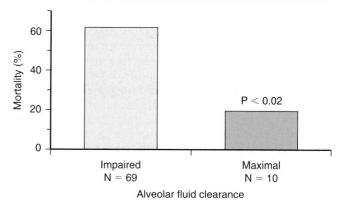

FIGURE 38-7. Plot of hospital mortality of two groups of patients with acute lung injury or the acute respiratory distress syndrome: those with maximal alveolar fluid clearance (≥14% per hour) and those with impaired or submaximal alveolar fluid clearance (<14% per hour). Columns represent percent hospital mortality in each group. Hospital mortality of patients with maximal alveolar fluid clearance was significantly less (π < .02). N = number of patients. (Reproduced from Ware LB, Matthay MA. Alveolar fluid clearance is impaired in the majority of patients with acute lung injury and the acute respiratory distress syndrome. *Am J Respir Crit Care Med.* 2001;163(1376):1383.)

the distal lung epithelium's ability to actively transport Na^+, with Cl^- and water following, from the airspace has been shown to correlate with survival and clinical outcome in both high pressure and high permeability pulmonary edema[24,97] (Fig. 38-7).

Therapy should be guided by the pathophysiologic consequences of the edema and how best to decrease further movement of fluid into, and promote liquid clearance from, the airspace.

Reversing the Hypoxemia

The first step is to reverse the hypoxemia. If pulmonary edema is mild and predominately interstitial in nature, then increasing the Fio_2 will treat the low V/Q ratios (0 < V/Q <1) arising from airway dysfunction. However, most patients in acute pulmonary edema have significant airspace pulmonary edema, which results in shunt (V/Q = 0), and requires an increase in transpulmonary pressures as the therapeutic approach. Positive airway pressures in general, and PEEP in particular, are beneficial for several reasons: (1) the recruitment (opening) of fluid-filled airspaces[35,36] so that they become partially filled with air and can then participate in gas exchange; (2) a reduction in the fluid filtration within the lung by impeding systemic venous return and therefore decreasing pulmonary vascular volume and pressure; and (3) the prevention of airway collapse, thus enhancing gas exchange. It is important to note that studies have shown that PEEP does not directly decrease lung water content[98] or lung lymph flow.[99]

An increase in transpulmonary pressures may be achieved using both noninvasive and invasive approaches. Although out of favor in the more distant past, it is now known that noninvasive ventilation can be effective in cardiogenic pulmonary edema.[100,101] Similarly, CT imaging has proven that when patients with ALI are placed in the prone position, there is recruitment of edematous lung units.[37] However, most frequently, intubation and assisted ventilation are required both for efficacy and to minimize potential side effects such as overdistention of the stomach and potential aspiration. Mechanical ventilation also reduces the oxygen consumption by reducing the work of breathing.

Reduce the Rate of Fluid Filtration

The second step is to reduce the rate of fluid filtration into the lung. Treating the disorder creating the pulmonary edema, for example CHF, is self-evident. Several therapeutic approaches are useful in treating the CHF-induced elevation of pulmonary microvascular pressures. They include measures that (1) improve cardiac contractility and allow the heart to achieve an increased stroke volume at a lower filling pressure (e.g., use of oxygen, digoxin, dopamine, or dobutamine); (2) reduce preload, including the sitting position and positive-pressure ventilation; (3) reduce both preload and afterload by relieving anxiety (e.g., use of morphine); (4) decrease plasma volumes with concomitant reduction of pulmonary microvascular and left atrial pressures (e.g., administration of diuretics); (5) decrease systemic or pulmonary vascular pressures, or both, using vasodilators such as prostacyclin, nitroprusside, or inhaled nitric oxide; and (6) reduce excessive salt and water intake.

Small changes in lung microvascular pressures can have profound effects on lung water accumulation[16] and lung lymph flow (Fig. 38-8) when there is increased permeability of the alveolar-capillary membrane. Similarly, when there is increased permeability of the alveolar-capillary

membrane, an increase in cardiac output, with minor changes in left atrial pressures, has a marked effect on lung lymph flow.[17]

A reduction in the rate of fluid leakage from the vasculature can also be achieved using other strategies based on the Starling equation (see Factors Responsible for Fluid Movement). For patients suffering from ARDS and its associated high permeability pulmonary edema our goal is to return the permeability of the alveolar-capillary membrane back to normal levels. Regrettably, despite decades of research, there is no proven way to modulate alveolar-capillary membrane permeability although low-dose corticosteroids[102] or activated protein C in the subset of ARDS patients with sepsis[103] may be beneficial to some degree in altering the course of the overall disease. A randomized double-blind clinical trial that excluded patients with sepsis showed that the administration of protein C did not improve clinical outcomes in ALI.[104]

Starling's equation indicates that altering intravascular osmotic pressure would lessen the flow of fluid out of the microvasculature. However, an increase in colloid osmotic pressure resulting from an infusion of colloid also would augment microvascular pressure as vascular volume is increased secondary to the movement of water from the systemic tissues to the vascular compartment and may undermine this effort. Indeed, studies in animals with high permeability pulmonary edema have shown that increasing colloid osmotic pressure had no effect on lung water content.[16]

Lowering systemic vascular pressures by use of diuretics and drugs that reduce vascular resistance or afterload are both advantageous for reasons previously described. However, diuretics such as furosemide are beneficial in pulmonary edema because of their ability to increase systemic venous capacitance and not because of the induced diuresis. Evidence for this statement includes the improvement in the patient's status, which is usually seen a few minutes after administering the diuretic before the diuresis. Similarly, furosemide can be beneficial in anuric patients suffering from pulmonary edema. It should be noted that the lung represents only 1% of the total body weight, so even a 1-L diuresis would only remove 10 mL from the lungs, with the remaining fluid coming from the remainder of the body. This 10 mL is trivial compared with the liters of fluid present in the airspaces of adult patients with florid alveolar edema (see Anatomic Considerations).

Minimize Treatment-Related Lung Damage

It is important to prevent or minimize treatment-related damage to the lung. This can occur through the use of very high concentrations of oxygen or the suboptimal use of mechanical ventilation with resultant distention of the lung and damage to the lung's epithelium and endothelium,[18,19] thereby increasing the permeability of the alveolar-capillary membrane to water and solutes. Attention to treatment of the underlying condition combined with excellent supportive care using "lung-protective" ventilatory strategies to minimize treatment-related lung damage have contributed to improved clinical outcomes.[105] This subject is discussed in greater detail in Chapters 22, 23, and 39.

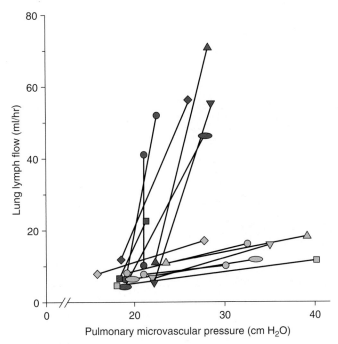

FIGURE 38-8. Relation of lung lymph flow to pulmonary microvascular pressures during hemodynamic edema (*green symbols.*) and during permeability edema produced by infusion of *Pseudomonas (blue symbols)*. For a given reduction in vascular pressures, there is a much greater reduction in lung lymph flow in permeability edema than in hydrostatic edema. (From Brigham KL, Wolverton WC, Blake LH, et al. Increased sheep lung vascular permeability caused by *Pseudomonas bacteremia. J Clin Invest.* 1974;54:792.)

Augment the Rate of Clearance of Airspace Fluid

The fourth step is to augment the rate of clearance of the airspace fluid. It has now been demonstrated that intact active fluid absorption from the airspaces correlates with improved survival and various important clinical parameters such as the length of assisted ventilation and oxygen requirements, regardless of whether the patients suffer from acute CHF-induced or ARDS-induced pulmonary edema[24,97] (see Fig. 38-7). Only 75% of patients with CHF-induced pulmonary edema have demonstrable alveolar fluid clearance, with approximately 40% being

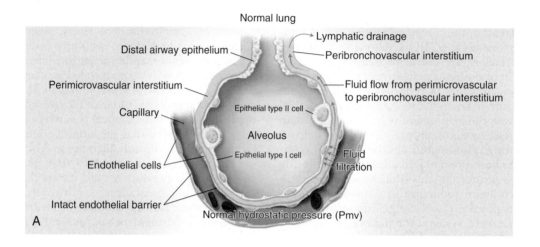

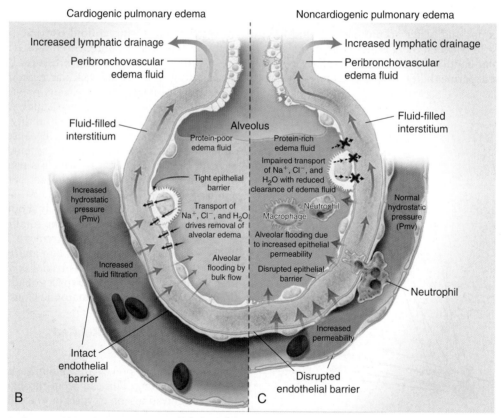

FIGURE 38-9. **A,** In the normal lung, fluid moves continuously outward from the vascular to the interstitial space according to the net difference between hydrostatic and protein osmotic pressures and to the permeability of the capillary membrane. **B,** When transvascular hydrostatic pressure increases in the microcirculation, the rate of fluid filtration rises. Since the permeability of the capillary endothelium remains normal, the filtered edema fluid leaving the circulation has a low protein content. The removal of edema fluid from the air spaces of the lung depends on active transport of Na^+ and Cl^-, with water following across the alveolar epithelial barrier. **C,** High permeability pulmonary edema occurs when the permeability of the microvascular membrane increases because of direct or indirect lung injury, such as the acute respiratory distress syndrome, resulting in a marked increase in the amount of fluid and protein leaving the vascular space. The pulmonary edema fluid has a high protein content because the more permeable microvascular membrane has a reduced capacity to restrict the outward movement of larger molecules such as plasma proteins. In edema due to acute lung injury, alveolar epithelial injury commonly causes a decrease in the capacity for the removal of alveolar fluid, delaying the resolution of pulmonary edema. (Reproduced from Ware LB, Matthay MA. Clinical practice. Acute pulmonary edema. *N Engl J Med.* 2005;353(26):2788-2796.)

capable of achieving maximal clearance rates.[24] The situation is even more grave for patients with ALI and ARDS because only 13% of these patients can achieve maximal rates of active airspace fluid clearance.[97] Active clearance of airspace fluid is impaired more frequently in men and when there is associated sepsis.[97]

Exogenous catecholamines augment fluid clearance from the airspaces in animals,[106] and a single center randomized controlled study showed that 7 days of intravenous salbutamol therapy is associated with a decrease in EVLW and ventilator pressures.[107] Consistent with these findings, aerosolized β agonists can decrease EVLW and improve clinical parameters in patients undergoing elective lung resections[108] and prevent HAPE in susceptible individuals.[82] However, studies in humans have not shown any correlation between the levels of circulating catecholamines and the rates of fluid clearance[24,97] and a multicenter trial did not show a beneficial effect of aerosolized albuterol in acute lung injury.[109] The lack of response in the multicenter study may have indicated the inadequate delivery of the aerosolized salbutamol to the airspace; that the epithelium is unresponsive; or alternatively, that more efficacious strategies may be required to augment airspace fluid clearance. A clinical trial using an intravenous infusion of salbutamol was discontinued when it became apparent that it did not improve patient outcomes and was an increase in mortality.[110] These clinical trials indicate that salbutamol should only be used to treat airway obstruction and not to increase the clearance of fluid from the alveolar spaces. New approaches are needed so that pulmonary edema fluid clearance can be increased without adverse side effects. Perhaps this may be developed from work showing that pulmonary edema fluid itself can modulate Na^+ and fluid transport by distal lung epithelium[111] or other studies where either mesenchymal stem cells (MSCs) or media conditioned by MSCs can restore effective Na^+ and water transport by injured human lung lobes.[112]

Suggested Reading

Figure 38-9 provides a schematic overview of the distal lung unit during health and during high pressure and high permeability pulmonary edema. More detailed information is available in the 111 references contained within the electronic version of this chapter, earlier versions of this book for classic references and review articles up to the mid-1980s that underpin some of the commentary within this chapter, and the following two recent review articles:

Eaton DC, Helms MN, Koval M, et al. The contribution of epithelial sodium channels to alveolar function in health and disease. *Annu Rev Physiol.* 2008.

Ware LB, Matthay MA. Clinical practice. Acute pulmonary edema. *N Engl J Med.* 2005;353(26):2788–2796.

References

The complete reference list is available online at www.expertconsult.com

39 ACUTE RESPIRATORY DISTRESS SYNDROME

Alik Kornecki, MD, Gavin C. Morrisson, MRCP, and Brian P. Kavanagh, MD, FRCPC

DEFINITION AND DIAGNOSIS

Acute respiratory distress syndrome (ARDS) is a diffuse, progressive inflammatory lung disease that was first reported in 1967 by Ashbaugh and colleagues in a cohort of 12 surgical patients.[1] They noted that their patients exhibited "...acute onset of tachypnea, hypoxemia and loss of compliance...." Further reports of patients with ARDS altered the acronym to indicate *adult* respiratory distress syndrome, in order to differentiate it from the respiratory distress syndrome of neonates, even though Ashbaugh's original description included an 11-year-old child. It is not until 1980 that regular reports[2] of ARDS in children established that it was also a pediatric syndrome and the 1994 North American–European Consensus Conference Committee (NAECC) recommended that the acronym "ARDS" revert to its original meaning (i.e., acute).[3] Although the pathophysiology of ARDS had been characterized soon after the original reports, definitive diagnostic criteria were lacking. Studies in adults throughout the 1970s and 1980s employed diagnostic criteria comprised of Pao_2/Fio_2 ratios, often including a minimum positive end expiratory pressure (PEEP) requirement and stipulating a minimum duration without clinical improvement.[4] The lack of uniformity in disease definition of ARDS was seen as one of the major obstacles to productive epidemiologic, interventional, and outcomes research. The aim of the NAECC was to rectify this situation with a simple, concise four-point definition (Table 39-1), and it distinguishes between two entities, ALI and ARDS, according to the severity of hypoxemia.

Over the years, it has been argued that the definition does not include the underlying disease, which may affect the outcome, and the clinical course; more importantly, the definition does not reflect the severity of lung disease because it does not incorporate any measure of airway pressure (e.g., level of PEEP). The requirement for bilateral pulmonary infiltrates on chest radiograph was intended to distinguish between the diffuse ALI/ARDS and focal processes such as lobar pneumonia or atelectasis; however, it is subject to considerable interobserver variability in both pediatric[5] and adult[6] patients.

Attempts to determine the applicability of the NAECC definition to the pediatric population has been made. In over 8000 consecutive admissions to a tertiary level pediatric center, investigators compared the NAECC definition of ARDS[3] to that of the Lung Injury Score (LIS)[4] and found good agreement.[7] The validity of the NAECC definition also has been tested against lung histopathology findings in children undergoing autopsy following an illness characterized by ARDS.[8] In that study of 34 children, 26 had ARDS defined as diffuse alveolar damage, with interstitial and intra-alveolar edema and hyaline

membranes. The investigators reported the NAECC definition had a sensitivity of 81% (95% CI, 60 to 92) and a specificity of 71% (95% CI, 70 to 98) and argued that adjustment of the NAECC threshold Pao_2/Fio_2 ratio to <150 would improve the specificity (86%, CI 42 to 99) of the definition. The main limitation of this study is in the selection bias because they obviously were limited to patients who died, whereas survivors may have had different pathophysiologic findings.

PATHOPHYSIOLOGY

ALI/ARDS arises as a consequence of an inflammatory process at the alveolar-capillary interface in the lung. The resultant endothelial and epithelial disruption leads to increased alveolar-capillary permeability and flooding of alveoli with protein rich edema fluid. Alveolar gas exchange is impaired and surfactant function is disrupted.[9] Classically, ARDS is described as a progressive clinical condition characterized by four stages, although these are rarely identified in pediatric cases. ARDS is triggered by an acute *direct* injury (e.g., aspiration) or *indirect* lung injury (e.g., sepsis) resulting in the onset of an *acute exudative* phase characterized by the production of pulmonary edema, cytokine release, and activated neutrophils. The acute exudative stage is associated with increased intrapulmonary shunting, reduced functional residual capacity (FRC), and a decrease in lung and chest wall compliance. Before the advent of computerized tomography (CT), the acute exudative stage was synonymous with the radiologic finding of bilateral homogenous parenchymal disease; however, pulmonary CT imaging changed our outlook of ARDS, revealing heterogeneity in the extent of regional lung injury, with the coexistence of severely injured (dependent) lung, and less injured lung and healthy lung regions. Gattinoni and colleagues suggested that the lung in ARDS be conceptualized as three functional regions: (1) fully aerated normal (usually nondependent) region(s), (2) poorly aerated injured but recruitable lung, and (3) nonaerated consolidated/atelectatic lung. This group also introduced the term *baby lung* to describe the small volume of normal aerated tissue in the nondependent lung regions of the lung that exhibits normal compliance.[10] During the acute phase of inflammation, abnormalities in coagulation may contribute to development of small vessel occlusion. In rare cases, pulmonary hypertension due to vascular obstruction and complicated by right ventricular failure has been described.[11]

The acute exudative phase may resolve within hours or days, and not all patients progress to the subsequent fibroproliferative—early repair—phase. Unfortunately

TABLE 39-1 NORTH AMERICAN-EUROPEAN CONSENSUS CONFERENCE COMMITTEE (NAECC)—ARDS/ALI

Onset: Acute

Chest radiograph: Bilateral infiltrates

Left atrial hypertension: No evidence (or PCWP <18 mm Hg, if known)

Acute lung injury (ALI) where Pao_2:$Fio_2 \leq 300*$

Acute respiratory distress syndrome (ARDS) where Pao_2:$Fio_2 \leq 300*$

PCWP, Pulmonary capillary wedge pressure.
*Regardless of PEEP level.

"repair" may not result in disease resolution in all patients but may presage the development of fibrosing alveolitis characterized by increased alveolar dead space, hypoxia, and reduced lung compliance; progression to this stage is associated with worse outcome. The fourth stage, the recovery stage, occurs within 10 to 14 days, with gradual improvement in lung compliance and oxygenation. The mechanism of resolution of the acute inflammatory process and fibrosis is not well established, and the rate of recovery is not well characterized; however, a return to normal lung function, in those patients without underlying chronic lung disease, is the norm.

PULMONARY (DIRECT) VERSUS NONPULMONARY (INDIRECT) ALI/ARDS

In the initial description of ARDS, Ashbaugh and colleagues observed that different insults appeared to induce a similar injury to the lung; therefore, they postulated that a common mechanism of injury must exist.[1] However, careful observation of the clinical progression and histological lung appearance in patients with ARDS suggested

that the pattern of lung injury might depend on the etiology. In 1994, the NAECC made a distinction between a direct or pulmonary injury (ARDSp), such as might occur following aspiration pneumonia, and contrasted this pattern with indirect or extrapulmonary (ARDSexp) injury associated with a systemic inflammatory response such as sepsis or acute pancreatitis[3] (Table 39-2).

Data provided by Flori and colleagues suggest that ARDSp constitutes 60% of pediatric ARDS cases,[12] similar to the reported incidence of ARDSp in adults (47% to 75%). The same authors also reported sepsis as the major cause (13% to 21%) of ARDSexp in children. Differences between ARDSp and ARDSexp may be most apparent in the acute exudative phase of the disease. One of the earliest attempts to characterize ARDS based on the mechanism of injury (i.e., direct vs. indirect), was made by Gattinoni and colleagues,[13] who reported differences in respiratory system mechanics. Subsequently, histologic[14] and morphologic[15] evidence supported the distinction between direct and indirect lung injury. These differences may impact the response to treatment and outcome; indeed, a recent study in children reported that ARDSexp had a greater mortality than ARDSp.[16]

Different mechanisms of injury to the alveolar-capillary unit have been postulated for ARDSp and ARDSexp. ARDSp is characterized by a primary injury to the alveolar epithelium resulting in intra-alveolar edema, and reduced lung compliance with preservation of the chest wall compliance.[13,14] In ARDSexp, the primary insult is systemic and the major injury is to the capillary endothelium; here the edema is predominantly interstitial, and the greater reduction of compliance occurs in the chest wall. Gross pathology of the lung in ARDSp suggests predominant consolidation, and in ARDSexp the striking finding is atelectasis.

Such differences in functional pathology may explain why in ARDSp there is a greater incidence of refractory hypoxemia and resistance to recruitment maneuvers and prone positioning[17-20] but a better response to surfactant administration[21] and iNO.[22] In the majority of patients,

TABLE 39-2 PULMONARY VS. EXTRAPULMONARY ACUTE RESPIRATORY DISTRESS SYNDROME (ARDS)

	DIRECT (PULMONARY) ARDS	INDIRECT (EXTRAPULMONARY) ARDS
Etiology	Pneumonia, bronchiolitis, near drowning, lung contusion, toxic inhalation	Sepsis, nonthoracic trauma, transfusion of blood products, cardiopulmonary bypass
Morphology	Consolidation	Atelectasis
Histology	Epithelial injury, alveolar edema	Endothelial injury, interstitial edema
Respiratory mechanics	Reduced lung compliance	Reduced chest wall compliance
Response to therapy		
Inhaled NO	↑Pao_2	→Pao_2
Prone position	↑Pao_2	→Pao_2
Surfactant	Possible improved outcome	No effect on outcome
Recruitment	→PaO_2	↑Pao_2

NO, Nitric oxide.

clinical differentiation between ARDSexp and the ARDSp is simple but of uncertain importance, while in other situations, it can be more complex (e.g., trauma complicated by sepsis).

Epidemiology and Outcome

The incidence of ALI in children is 3 to 5/100,000 per year,[16] about 5 to 10 times less than that in adults, and constituting 2% to 10% of all pediatric intensive care unit (ICU) admissions.[16,23] Approximately 80% of children with ALI will progress to ARDS,[24] and two thirds require early mechanical ventilation The majority of patients (60%) with ALI are less than 4 years of age and have an underlying chronic disease (e.g., prematurity, cardiac disease). The mortality among children with ALI/ARDS decreased from between 65% to 80% in the 1980s, to less than 20% now. The reduction in mortality can be attributed to improved management, including lower tidal volumes.[25]

In clinical trials, the reported mortality among children with ALI ranges from 7%[21] to 20%,[26] depending on the degree of hypoxemia, the country (28%[12] to 44%[16] in developed countries, 61%[27] in a developing country), the etiology (up to 40% to 60% in immunocompromised children,[28] minimal in bronchiolitis) and the presence of comorbidities (e.g., nonpulmonary organ dysfunction, central nervous system [CNS] dysfunction).[12]

Severity Score

Blood gas analysis, specifically oxygenation, is regarded as the standard for assessment of severity of ARDS. While the ratio (Pao_2/Fio_2) provides the threshold value for the definition of ALI/ARDS, the $(A - a)O_2$ difference (difference between "alveolar" vs. arterial Po_2) can express the degree of hypoxemia. Both indices should be used with caution because neither incorporate any measure of the *ventilatory* assistance being provided to the patient. In this regard the oxygenation index (OI) = [(mean airway pressure × Fio_2)×100]/PaO^2 attempts to correct that deficiency. However, even this may mislead if the ventilation strategy employed is not optimized, such as inappropriately high or low airway pressures or Fio_2 in the case of an intrapulmonary shunt that is minimally responsive to altered Fio_2 or airway pressure.

Although death in ARDS is usually attributable to multiorgan failure rather than persistent hypoxemia, the severity of oxygenation failure, expressed as the OI, does correlate with duration of mechanical ventilation and with mortality in children[29]; this is not the case in adults with ARDS.

In contrast to oxygenation, the ventilation index, VI[30,31]: [$Paco_2$ × peak airway pressure × respiratory rate]/1,000 has been employed to reflect the difficulty involved in clearing CO_2, (i.e., the pulmonary dead space). Murray and colleagues[4] proposed the lung injury score (LIS, incorporating chest radiograph, Pao_2/Fio_2, PEEP, and respiratory compliance) for the diagnosis of ARDS, as well as a measure of disease severity. This scoring system has been modified for use in children by altering the PEEP scoring ranges and correcting the total respiratory system compliance to account for variations in body weight (Table 39-3). Although physiologically sound, this scoring system is rarely used and performs less well than the Pao_2/Fio_2 in the current era of protective ventilation.[32] More recently the magnitude of dead space in the first days of ARDS has been shown to predict outcome in adult patients. In summary, indices of oxygenation impairment are more useful for prognostication in ARDS in children than in adults.

Genetic Modifiers of ALI/ARDS

Other than confirmation that high pressure, high volume ventilation is injurious to the lung, the history of ALI/ARDS research is replete with interventions that failed to demonstrate clinical benefit. These disappointments often occur against a background of sound physiologic reasoning and encouraging results from animal studies. It appears that part of the problem has been considering ALI a homogeneous disease process. It is already known that only a minority of patients exposed to recognized risk factors develop the ARDS syndrome. Increasingly, there is a recognition that heterogeneity exists in ALI with regard to the development and course of the disease, which is dependent on the interaction of the individual and the inciting event. Consideration of patient-derived factors likely to influence the manifestation of an inflammatory process leads inevitably to scrutiny of the genome. In 2002, Marshall and colleagues[33] were the first investigators to describe a preliminary association between a gene variant and ALI mortality. This group described the

TABLE 39-3 MODIFIED MURRAY LUNG INJURY SCORE

	SCORE 0	SCORE 1	SCORE 2	SCORE 3	SCORE 4
Alveolar consolidation (number of quadrants)	0	1	2	3	4
Pao_2 mm Hg/Fio_2	≥300	225-299	175-224	100-174	≤100
PEEP (cm H_2O)	≤4	5-6	7-8	9-11	≥12
Crs (mL/cm H_2O)	>0.85	0.75-0.85	0.55-0.74	0.3-0.54	<0.30

Crs, Total respiratory system compliance; *PEEP,* positive end expiratory pressure.

increased incidence of a high producer polymorphism of the angiotensin converting enzyme gene in patients with ARDS. Since this report, similar candidate gene studies have revealed a growing number of gene polymorphisms associated with the susceptibility to ALI/ARDS or its clinical course (e.g., genes encoding): pulmonary surfactant-associated protein B (SFTPB), interleukin-6 (IL-6), and coagulation factor V (F5). It is anticipated that an enhanced knowledge of the role of polymorphisms in ALI/ARDS will permit appropriate grouping of patients for investigation and facilitate personalized therapy.

DIFFERENCES BETWEEN CHILDREN AND ADULTS

The mechanical properties of the lungs of children and infants are different from those of adults. Chest wall compliance is inversely related to age, and with pressure preset ventilation, higher chest wall compliance may increase delivered tidal volume and thereby increase the risk for ventilator-associated lung injury (VALI) in young children. The infant lung has low inherent elastic recoil, which may protect against lung collapse, so lower PEEP levels may be required to maintain lung recruitment. The ratio of lung volume to body weight is greatest in the first 2 years of life, and this suggests that indexing the tidal volume (V_T) to body weight may result in a smaller fraction of lung volume being inflated in the young infant compared with the older child. Experimental data indicate that for a given level of inflation, the immune response to either sepsis or high V_T, as well as the propensity to structural injury, might be less in infant versus adult lungs. Finally, there are important outcome differences: the mortality for children with ARDS is less than in adults and high Fio_2 is associated with worse outcome in children but not in adults. These physiologic differences are important because adult guidelines for lung protective ventilation are predicated on the behavior of a respiratory system that is very different from that of the infant and young child.[34]

TREATMENT

Conventional Mechanical Ventilation

About 28% of patients with ALI do not require mechanical ventilation at the onset of the lung injury; however, almost half eventually require intubation and mechanical ventilation for worsening ALI and almost all children with ARDS require mechanical ventilation.[12]

Substantial clinical evidence indicates that the injudicious use of mechanical ventilation can initiate or exacerbate lung injury and contribute to the mortality associated with ALI/ARDS. Studies in animals have demonstrated that mechanical ventilation may induce lung injury through physical disruption of the alveoli (barotrauma); overdistension of the lung (volutrauma); recruitment and derecruitment of collapsed alveoli (atelectrauma); activation of the inflammatory process (biotrauma); and possibly, toxicity from high levels of oxygen.[35] Such factors may produce histologic damage and increased permeability of the alveolar-capillary interface that is indistinguishable from the lesions seen in other forms of acute lung injury.

The ventilation parameters associated with this iatrogenic lung injury are high levels of end-inspiratory airway pressure, large tidal volumes, low levels of end-expiratory airway pressure, and possibly high Fio_2. Understanding the roles of elevated levels of inspiratory pressure and V_T from laboratory[36] and clinical[37] studies informed the design of two important outcome studies that compared lower versus higher tidal volumes in patients with ARDS.[38,39] These studies demonstrated a clear association between higher V_T (or inspiratory pressures) and worse outcome. This approach, along with the belief from laboratory[40] and clinical trials[39] that higher levels of PEEP were protective, led to a gradual adoption of the idea that lung protective ventilation—lower tidal volumes, recruitment, and higher levels of PEEP—would ensure sufficient gas exchange while minimizing lung injury. Hence, we now employ lower V_T, up to 10 mL/kg; lower inflation pressure (<30 cm H_2O); higher PEEP (~5 to 12 cm H_2O); and lower Fio_2 than two decades ago.[25]

The physiologic goals of mechanical ventilation also have changed. It is no longer considered advisable to attempt to achieve normal blood gases values without regard for the V_T, Fio_2, or inflation pressures delivered to the patient. Mechanical ventilation is employed with regard to a risk/benefit estimation performed for each patient. If the achievement of normal pH, $Paco_2$, and Pao_2 levels require respiratory support strategies that may injure the lungs, then lower pH, Pao_2, and higher $Paco_2$ (permissive hypercapnia) are tolerated. Despite a lack of data regarding the effect of relative hypoxia on human organ systems in general, and on the developing infant brain in particular, the maintenance of $Sao_2 > 90\%$ (Pao_2 60 to 80 mm Hg) using the lowest oxygen concentration to achieve that result is considered by most pediatric intensivists to represent an optimal approach. Because the likelihood of lung injury is greater if the airway pressure, V_T, and concentration of inspired oxygen are elevated, many clinicians will reduce the target SaO_2 (85% to 88%) if necessary. Permissive hypercapnia ($Paco_2$ 60 to 80 mm Hg) with a pH > 7.2 appears to be well tolerated by most children (although it is avoided in the presence of raised intracranial pressure or pulmonary hypertension). The "protective" approach has not been validated in children, and the mechanical ventilation strategies used in children mirror the recommendations of the adult critical care community. This approach is physiologically sound, but given the increasingly recognized heterogeneity of ARDS, it is likely that some subtle disease features peculiar to pediatrics have been ignored.

Few studies regarding mechanical ventilation have been performed in children, and as a result, no specific approaches have been proved superior to others. Indeed most approaches for mechanical ventilation in children have been extrapolated from adult studies. Currently there are no data to support the superiority of one mode of ventilation over another (e.g., pressure control versus volume control). However, advocates of pressure control ventilation argue that it is more physiologic because of the decelerating flow, and that the V_T generated during each breath better reflects dynamic lung characteristics. Interestingly, Farias and colleagues[23,41] report that clinicians demonstrate a preference for pressure targeted ventilation and pressure regulated volume control (PRVC) ventilation when treating children.

Other Modalities of Ventilation

Noninvasive Ventilation

Driven by a desire to avoid the complications associated with endotracheal intubation, noninvasive ventilation has been the focus of various studies over the last decade. However, no data are available on the role of negative pressure ventilation in pediatric ALI/ARDS; therefore, we focus here on the use of noninvasive positive pressure ventilation (NIPPV) in adult patients presenting with respiratory failure, which has been described extensively.[42] The role of this modality of ventilation in the pediatric population is yet to be fully characterized, and although no randomized controlled studies of NIPPV in children have been performed, several case series describe its application in children with acute respiratory failure.[43-45] A trial of NIPPV may be attempted in any child with early respiratory failure; however, one should not persist with its use if there is no clinical benefit within 2 to 3 hours. It appears that patients who are hemodynamically unstable, have a greater severity of illness, or have ARDS[44] are less likely to benefit. Any ventilator may be used to provide NIPPV in volume or pressure modes, or a bi-level controlled or continuous positive pressure (CPAP) device can be used in children. The interface between the ventilation device and patient may be problematic when a facemask is used because of imperfect fitting and poor patient tolerance. In addition, facemask ventilation is unlikely to permit pressures greater than 15 to 20 cm H_2O on an ongoing basis. Novel interface devices such a helmet may circumvent some of these difficulties and have demonstrated efficacy in pediatric patients.[43]

High Frequency Oscillatory Ventilation (HFOV)

Although a variety of high frequency ventilation devices are available for clinical use, HFOV has achieved the greatest acceptance in neonatal, pediatric, and adult critical care practice. According to recent studies, between 5% and 52% of children with ALI/ARDS are ventilated using HFOV at some stage during their disease.[16,23,46] HFOV achieves effective gas exchange while avoiding high peak airway pressures and the inflation-deflation cycles characteristic of conventional ventilation. Lung volume (and hence oxygenation) is maintained by the application of a high continuous mean airway pressure. CO_2 removal is achieved despite small tidal volumes (2 to 4 mL/kg) by imposing a breath frequency of 300 to 900 (5 to 15 Hz) per minute, resulting in large minute volumes. HFOV therefore involves the application of the open lung strategy accompanied by small variation in airway pressure in the distal airways and alveoli. Hence, the cyclical application of high distending airway pressures (barotrauma) and the associated cyclical delivery of large tidal volumes (volutrauma) are avoided. In animal models of ALI/ARDS, HFOV has demonstrated comparable or superior gas exchange when compared with conventional ventilation and has incurred less lung injury. HFOV would appear

to represent a lung protective ventilatory device, but it has tended to be deployed when conventional mechanical ventilation (CMV) fails. Although there are no established criteria to define CMV failure, in general HFOV is considered when, despite a PIP of 30 to 35 cm H_2O and Fio_2 >0.6, inadequate oxygenation or hypercapnia develop. Only one prospective randomized controlled trial comparing conventional ventilation and HFOV has been performed in children. This study showed sustained improvement in oxygenation with HFOV but no significant differences in duration of ventilation or mortality.

Airway Pressure Release Ventilation (APRV)

APRV is a ventilator modality characterized by cyclical alternation between two levels (high and low) of positive airway pressure, while permitting spontaneous breathing activity at both levels of pressure support. Typically, 80% to 95% of the ventilatory cycle, is accounted for by the higher pressure (P_{high}, is usually 15 to 30 cm H_2O) and is only briefly interrupted by drops to a lower level of airway pressure (P_{low}, is usually 0 to 15 cm H_2O). The duration of both the P_{high} and P_{low} periods are time cycled and continue even when spontaneous breathing is not detected. In such a case, APRV will resemble inverse (inspiratory:expiratory) ratio pressure-control ventilation with a very long inspiratory time. APRV, facilitates an open lung ventilatory approach, avoids cyclical recruitment and derecruitment of alveolar units, permits homogenous gas distribution during inspiration, minimizes overdistension of healthy lung (volutrauma), and reduces the risk of low volume lung injury (atelectrauma). Few studies of the role of APRV in pediatric and adult ARDS have been performed. However, it has been shown that in children with mild to moderate lung disease, APRV provides good efficacy in ventilation and oxygenation compared with conventional ventilation with significantly lower peak and plateau airway pressures.[47] Because spontaneous breaths lower pleural pressure with this mode (i.e., do not trigger a cycled breath), it does not usually reduce cardiac output.[48]

Neurally Adjusted Ventilatory Assist (NAVA)

Patient-ventilator dyssynchrony is a major issue in the delivery of mechanical ventilation to patients capable of spontaneous breathing. More than 25% of adult patients exhibit dyssynchrony with the ventilator. Key considerations in patient-ventilator synchrony include signaling of the onset of the patient's inspiratory effort, the pressure/flow profile of gas delivery during the breath, and mechanisms to signal termination of the patient's inspiratory effort. NAVA is a relatively recent innovation in the quest to improve such synchrony. The NAVA system utilizes the electrical activity of diaphragmatic (right crural) muscle to signal the initiation of patient inspiratory effort. The signal is detected using electrodes embedded in the distal end of a gastric tube that is positioned astride the esophageal hiatus of the diaphragm. Because muscle electrical activity is proportional to the strength of the phrenic signal (which itself reflects the respiratory demands of the patient), the NAVA system offers both improved triggering and variable ventilatory support proportionate to the patient's respiratory demands. This is an improvement over circuit pressure or gas flow triggering systems and the use of a fixed amount of ventilatory support with each breath. Although there are few reports of NAVA use in either adults or children, it has been demonstrated that NAVA prevents excessive lung distension, efficiently unloads respiratory muscles, and improves but does not abolish patient-ventilator dyssynchrony.[49]

Adjuvants to Mechanical Ventilation

Prone positioning, surfactant, and nitric oxide administration have all been employed as adjuvant therapies in ventilated patients with ALI/ARDS. To date, none of these interventions has demonstrated an ability to improve patient outcome when employed as a routine part of care.

Prone Positioning

Prone positioning is safe and has been reported to produce a rapid and sustained improvement in arterial oxygenation in 90% of children with ALI/ARDS.[50] This response rate was superior to that reported in adults (60%). However, the improvement in oxygenation did not translate into a reduction in days of ventilation or patient mortality.[51] Prone positioning is best reserved for patients with persistent refractory hypoxemia when acceptable oxygenation cannot be achieved within the parameters of a lung protective ventilatory strategy. However, where it does not improve oxygenation, it should be discontinued.[52] A recent multicenter comprehensive study reported that 17.6% of children with ALI/ARDS receive prone positioning as part of their management at some time in the course of their disease.[23]

Inhaled Nitric Oxide (iNO)

Nitric oxide is a potent short-acting selective vasodilator. It has been shown to result in short-term improvements in oxygenation in some patients with ARDS/ALI, but it has no substantial impact on the duration of ventilator support or mortality when used as a routine part of care.[53] Currently only a minority (12%) of children with ALI receive iNO in the course of the disease.[23] Inhaled NO is best reserved for patients with refractory hypoxemia, with $Fio_2 > 0.6$, and in whom a trial of iNO demonstrated benefit. Where inhaled iNO is being used, some recommend that a daily trial be conducted to ensure that the minimal effective dose is being used because it has been shown that the iNO dose response usually falls during the course of the disease.[54]

Surfactant

The potential role of surfactant dysfunction in the pathogenesis of ARDS was suggested by Ashbaugh.[1] The concept of surfactant administration to patients with ARDS is very attractive, especially when seen in the context of its benefits in infantile respiratory distress. Despite several studies in adults and children with ALI/ARDS the role of surfactant administration has not been established. Comparison of results among studies is complicated by the differences in surfactant preparation and delivery methods. Walmrath and colleagues reported improvement in oxygenation when a high dose of bovine surfactant was administered to patients with ARDS

and sepsis.[55] Spragg and colleagues reported transient improvement in oxygenation when recombinant surfactant was administered to adult patients with ARDS in a phase III trial; in a post hoc analysis, they also reported a potential improvement in mortality in ARDSp but not in "extrapulmonary" ARDSexp.[56] A recent randomized trial in adults utilized natural porcine surfactant for patients with ALI, but this was not associated with improved outcome.[57] In children, a relatively small randomized controlled trial (RCT) reported a reduction in mortality following administration of natural calf surfactant[21]; however, no effect on ventilator-free days or length of hospitalization was reported. Although provocative, the study had significant methodological issues. In summary, the administration of surfactant in children with ALI/ARDS is not recommended as a routine. Whether the lack of effect on outcome is a matter of surfactant preparation, patient selection, or method of administration is unclear. Indeed, recent data from 59 centers indicated that surfactant was administered in only 4.2% of children who had ALI/ARDS.[23]

Corticosteroids

The use of corticosteroids for the treatment of ARDS was suggested by Ashbaugh in 1967.[1] Almost 50 years and several clinical trials later, it is still the subject of debate. ARDS is characterized by inflammation that may resolve within a short period; alternatively, it may progress to the unresolving inflammatory (i.e., fibroproliferative) stage. The anti-inflammatory properties of corticosteroids and the potential inhibition of both fibroblast proliferation and collagen deposition make corticosteroids an attractive option.

The use of corticosteroids has been examined (in adult patients) in different disease stages, including prophylactically (before development of ALI/ARDS),[38] during the early stages of disease(<7 days),[38] and in later stages of the disease (>7 or 14 days). Corticosteroids have been used for different durations and at different doses. Early studies focused on the prevention of ARDS after events that are known to potentially lead to ARDS (e.g., sepsis). High doses (≥30 mg/kg/day) of corticosteroids for a short period of time (≤24 hours) either had no impact on mortality[58,59] or, in one case, increased mortality.[60] A more recent study of early low-dose corticosteroids (1 mg/kg/day) for 25 days demonstrated a treatment benefit with improvements in lung injury score, days of ventilation, and mortality.[61] However, methodological issues provoked significant controversy.[61] Several studies that examined the role of corticosteroids late in the course of the disease (>7 days) reported contradictory results,[62,63] and there is some evidence that steroids introduced after 2 weeks of illness may result in increased mortality.[63]

In summary, current evidence from clinical trials does not support the use of corticosteroids in any phase of ARDS in adults. In children, no data are available. Further investigations are required to address the paucity of data in children and to specifically identify potential responders among the population of ARDS patients. A recent examination of adult patients with sepsis-induced ARDS who were nonresponders to adrenocorticotropic hormone

(ACTH) stimulation testing demonstrated improved lung function and decreased mortality with low-dose steroid use in early disease. This study underscores the importance of selecting groups likely to benefit from steroids when studying their potential use in ARDS.[64]

Neuromuscular Blocking Agents

No data are available regarding the use of neuromuscular blocking agents (NMBA) among ventilated children. In adults about 25% of patients receive such agents at some stage during the course of the disease. Clinicians tend to limit the use of NMBA because of the association with long-term muscle weakness.

A recent RCT in adults has suggested that continuous neuromuscular blockade (with cisatracurium besylate) in the first 48 hours of ventilation in ARDS significantly reduced mortality.[65] Mortality at 90 days in the NMBA group was 32% compared with 41% in the controls. This followed earlier mechanistic studies demonstrating that early administration of NMBA for the first 48 hours of ventilation improved oxygenation[66] and lowered inflammatory markers (IL-8 and IL-6) in the lung (bronchoalveolar lavage [BAL]) and serum of patients with ALI/ARDS.[67]

The mechanisms of benefit are speculative. Paralysis of ventilated patients may facilitate protective ventilation through optimization of patient/ventilator synchronization, through more accurate adjustment of V_T, or by reduction in inspiratory plateau pressure because of reduction in chest wall compliance. Moreover, the use of NMB may reduce the oxygen consumption, which in turn will reduce cardiac output and lung perfusion, which in turn may reduce lung injury.

Beta-Adrenergic Agonists

The alveolar edema in ALI/ARDS is mainly due to increased permeability and, to a lesser extent, to increased capillary hydrostatic pressure. The resolution of the alveolar edema is critical to recovery from lung injury. β agonists may reduce alveolar edema by different mechanisms. Alveolar fluid clearance is enhanced through upregulation of Na^+ transport in the alveolar epithelial cells. In addition, pulmonary vasodilatation and resulting reduction of pulmonary vascular pressure results in lowered capillary hydrostatic pressures, and β agonism may independently decrease endothelial permeability.

A recent RCT study in a small number (40) of adult patients[68] demonstrated that intravenous salbutamol reduced the extravascular lung water content and (perhaps as a result) lessened the inspiratory airway pressures required for ventilation. An observational review of children with ARDS suggested that inhaled bronchodilators were associated with a lower mortality.[12] Whether inhaled or IV treatment may affect outcome in patients with ALI/ARDS is still to be established.

Extracorporeal Life Support (ECLS) in Pediatric ARDS

Although pediatric ECLS is predominantly employed for cardiovascular support[69] it may have an important role in some pulmonary cases, especially where ARDS results from trauma. For pure respiratory failure in the absence of cardiovascular compromise, venovenous cannulation is appropriate. This provides oxygenated blood into the right ventricle but does not augment cardiac output. In contrast, venoarterial cannulation, providing oxygenated blood into the aorta under pressure, effectively augments the cardiac output while concomitantly increasing systemic oxygenation.

The survival rate (60%) for ECLS in ARDS has not substantially changed in the last 15 years.[70,71] in contrast to the improved outcomes associated with conventional management. Peters and colleagues[72] suggested that indices of oxygenation (Pao_2/Fio_2, alveolar-arterial oxygen gradient and OI) may overestimate the mortality in patients treated with modern conventional ventilatory strategies.[31,73] Because of the improvements in outcomes associated with conventional ventilation and because ECLS is used only when conventional ventilation has "failed," the efficacy of ECLS may be progressively underestimated because of "referral bias" of progressively more futile cases.

Tracheostomy

Ventilation via a tracheostomy tube has many purported benefits in facilitating weaning from mechanical ventilation: it improves patient comfort, reduces the work of breathing, facilitates bronchopulmonary toileting, reduces the incidence of pneumonia, and improves airway security. In addition, it may reduce the length of stay in the hospital or ICU and lower hospital costs, but most importantly, a tracheostomy facilitates patient weaning from mechanical ventilation and lowers patient mortality. For these reasons, tracheostomy has become a routine intervention in adult critical care, with 24% to 26% of all ventilated adult patients undergoing the procedure during their stay. Furthermore its role in the ventilatory management of the critically ill adult has been endorsed by the American College of Chest Physicians and the European Consensus in patients who are expected to require prolonged ventilation (>14 days). In contrast, there is no literature describing the preemptive use of tracheostomy in children in whom prolonged ventilation is anticipated, nor is it frequently employed in the pediatric population. A recently published study revealed that among ventilated children in Canada, the prevalence of tracheostomy was less than 1.5%.[74] These differences may be explained by the faster resolution of ARDS in children compared with adults, the introduction of a percutaneous dilatational tracheostomy technique that is performed at the bedside in adults but is not suitable for children, and the perception that tracheostomy is as an aggressive procedure with high complication rates in children.

References

The complete reference list is available online at www.expertconsult.com

40 LUNG INJURY FROM HYDROCARBON ASPIRATION AND SMOKE INHALATION

Ada Lee, MD, Michael R. Bye, MD, and Robert B. Mellins, MD

LUNG INJURY FROM HYDROCARBON ASPIRATION

Hydrocarbon toxicity resulting from the ingestion of petroleum solvents, dry-cleaning fluids, lighter fluids, kerosene, gasoline, and liquid polishes and waxes (mineral seal oil) continues to be a common occurrence in small children. It is estimated that 2% to 3% of exposures in children younger than 6 years of age reported to poison control centers are from these agents.[1] This is in addition to the potential harm from additives such as heavy metals, pesticides, and camphor, all of which have potential systemic toxicity.[2-4] Kerosene heaters, cleaning fluids, furniture polishes, and liquid floor waxes are present in homes, too frequently within the easy reach of toddlers, and they account for the persistence of hydrocarbon poisoning. In one series of hydrocarbon ingestions, the material was stored in a standard beverage container almost one third of the time.[5] The most commonly ingested materials are household cleaning products, solvents, and fuels; in some areas, kerosene ingestion is more common. In 2001, the U.S. Consumer Product Safety Commission required child-resistant packaging for products with low viscosity and a significant concentration of hydrocarbons (>10% by weight).[6] Similar attempts were made by the European Union in 1997. Unfortunately, these regulations do not seem to have had a significant impact on the frequency of such poisonings.[7]

Although central nervous system (CNS) abnormalities (i.e., weakness, confusion, and coma), gastrointestinal irritation, cardiomyopathy, and renal toxicity all occur, the most common and the most serious complication is pneumonitis. Deaths from hydrocarbon poisoning are almost always from respiratory insufficiency.

PATHOLOGY

Lung pathology in fatal cases includes necrosis of bronchial, bronchiolar, and alveolar tissue; atelectasis; interstitial inflammation; hemorrhagic pulmonary edema; vascular thromboses; necrotizing bronchopneumonia; and hyaline membrane formation.[8]

Experimental studies in rats reveal an acute alveolitis that is most severe at 3 days, subsides at 10 days, and is followed by a chronic proliferative phase that may take weeks to resolve.[9] Rats develop hyperemia and vascular engorgement of both large and small blood vessels within 1 hour of aspiration.[10] At 24 hours, there is a focal bronchopneumonia with microabscess formation. By 2 weeks, the process largely resolves, although some vascular engorgement and rare peribronchial inflammation persist. In humans, chest roentgenographic abnormalities persist for some time after physical findings have cleared, suggesting a similar prolonged recovery.

Dogs show different responses,[11] which also vary with the amount of kerosene ingested. A low dose causes destruction of alveolar cell linings and cells, resulting in emphysema but insignificant airway involvement. More intense airway obstruction is seen in a high-dose group. At 1 hour after high-dose ingestion, intra-alveolar edema and hemorrhage occur most prominently in the subpleural air spaces and those adjacent to large bronchi, suggesting induced interstitial inflammation. By 24 hours after ingestion, many airways show severe destruction and desquamation of the lining epithelium, resulting in near complete obliteration of the airways. The lumina are filled with degenerating neutrophils and scattered macrophages and lymphocytes. The surrounding lung parenchyma and the interstitium of the blood vessels show intense infiltration by macrophages and neutrophils, with microabscesses in the lung parenchyma. While most of the findings heal within a week, scattered bronchiolitis obliterans may persist. By 2 weeks, much of the lung tissue has returned to normal, with rare areas of bronchiolitis obliterans. The severity of these dose-related changes can be explained by two characteristics of kerosene. First, it is a solvent that can dissolve cell walls and/or lipid lining layers, resulting in the desquamation of cells and fluid influx into the airways. Second, as a foreign substance that can penetrate into the interstitium, it can provoke an intense inflammatory reaction. Since there are dose-related responses to kerosene with interspecies differences, accurate prediction of the process in humans is difficult.

PATHOPHYSIOLOGY

The risk for aspiration varies with the inherent properties of the hydrocarbon. Aspiration is much more likely to occur with a substance that has low surface tension, low viscosity, and high volatility. Low surface tension allows the substance to spread throughout the tracheobronchial tree. Low viscosity allows the substance to spread more readily, and to seep deeper into the tissues. High volatility increases the likelihood of CNS involvement, presumably due to more rapid absorption across the mucosa and into the bloodstream; highly volatile substances may also rapidly spread to the alveoli and immediately interfere with gas exchange.

Hydrocarbons increase surface tension by inhibiting surfactant,[12] which predisposes to alveolar instability and atelectasis. The instillation of artificial surfactant into the trachea of sheep following kerosene exposure resulted in significant improvement in oxygenation and mortality.[13]

There is one case report of a 17-month-old child with ARDS from hydrocarbon aspiration who survived after treatment with surfactant.[14]

Pulmonary lesions are believed to be caused by direct aspiration of the hydrocarbon into the airways. This may occur either during the initial ingestion or during subsequent emesis. Small amounts of aspirated hydrocarbons may produce more serious disease than larger amounts in the stomach. Evidence that hydrocarbons are removed by the first capillary bed they encounter[15,16] reinforces the notion that pulmonary damage occurs from aspiration. Indeed, the liver and the lungs filter out sufficient amounts of kerosene to help prevent CNS damage.[15] Fatalities are rarely attributed to CNS involvement per se.

CLINICAL FINDINGS

Cough may appear within 30 minutes of aspiration or may be delayed for hours. Initially, auscultation of the chest may be normal or may reveal only coarse or decreased breath sounds. When severe injury occurs, hemoptysis and pulmonary edema develop rapidly, and respiratory failure may occur within 24 hours. Radiographic signs of chemical pneumonitis, when present, will develop within 2 hours after ingestion in 88% of cases and within 6 to 12 hours in 98%.[17,18] The findings vary from punctate, mottled densities to pneumonitis or atelectasis and tend to predominate in dependent portions of the lung (Fig. 40-1A). Air trapping, pneumatoceles,[19] and pleural effusions may also develop (Fig. 40-1B). The radiographic abnormalities reach their peak within 72 hours and then usually clear within days. A review of 16 children showed that children whose chest radiographs were to become abnormal did so by 24 hours after the ingestion, and most cleared within 2 to 3 weeks.[20]

Occasionally, the radiographic findings persist for several weeks. There is a poor correlation between clinical symptoms, physical findings, and radiographic abnormalities. In general, the radiographic changes are more prominent than the findings on physical examination and persist for a longer period. When pneumatoceles occur, they are likely to do so after a patient has become asymptomatic. They require several months for spontaneous resolution.

Blood gas studies reveal hypoxemia without hypercapnia, suggesting ventilation-perfusion mismatch or diffusion block. Destruction of the epithelium of the airways together with bronchospasm caused by surface irritation adds to the ventilation-perfusion abnormalities. Displacement of alveolar gas by the hydrocarbon vapors add to the hypoxemia.

Long-term follow-up studies of pulmonary function in patients with hydrocarbon pneumonitis indicate residual injury to the peripheral airways. A study of 17 asymptomatic children 8 to 14 years after a hydrocarbon pneumonitis showed abnormal lung function in 14 (82%). The most common abnormalities were an elevated ratio of residual volume to total lung capacity, an increased slope of phase III, reduced forced expiratory volume in 1 second (FEV_1) and a high volume of isoflow[21]; these results indicate small airway obstruction and gas trapping. When radiographic changes accompany the ingestion of hydrocarbons, this same pattern of abnormal lung function is detected 10 years later, even in otherwise asymptomatic subjects. However, the frequency of airway reactivity appeared to be normal.[22]

MANAGEMENT

Initial management should comprise a history, physical examination, and chest radiograph. Because hydrocarbons do less damage when swallowed than when aspirated into the lungs, it is important to avoid emetics or gastric lavage. Some toxicologists recommend nasogastric lavage through a large bore tube in patients with a large amount of hydrocarbon with the potential for systemic

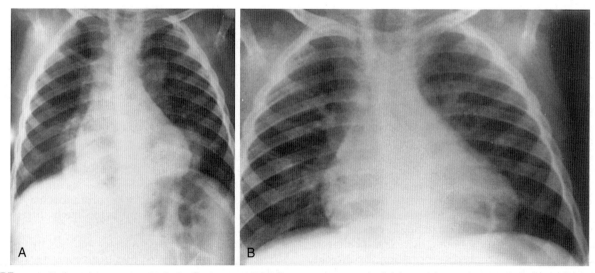

FIGURE 40-1. Hydrocarbon pneumonia. **A,** Confluent sequential infiltrate is present in the left lower lobe. **B,** Three weeks later, pneumatoceles are apparent; the large pneumatocele in the left lower lobe is at the site of the previous infiltrate. (From Felman AH. *Radiology of the Pediatric Chest.* New York: McGraw-Hill, 1987.)

toxicity, if the patient presents within 1 hour of ingestion.[23,24] If the child had no symptoms at the scene or in the emergency room and has a normal chest radiograph, observation for 6 to 8 hours is important. If no symptoms develop, the child may be safely discharged home.[18] If an abnormality is detected by history, examination, or radiography, arterial blood gas analysis should be performed. Even if no symptoms develop, a repeat chest radiograph at 24 hours is a prudent measure. If results of examination and radiography are normal at 24 hours and the child has no further symptoms, discharge can occur after providing education and reassurance. Supplemental oxygen must be given if the child is hypoxemic. Adequate hydration should be maintained, but excessive fluid administration may be counterproductive as pulmonary pathology evolves. Some have suggested a trial of bronchodilators if respiratory symptoms progress. Hypoxemic respiratory failure should be treated with mechanical ventilation and positive end-expiratory pressure. If the child fails conventional mechanical ventilation, both extracorporeal membrane oxygenation (ECMO)[25] and high-frequency jet ventilation[26] have been successful in improving oxygenation and allowing survival.

Although superimposed bacterial infection is a potential concern, there is no evidence that this is a common occurrence. Because leukocytosis and fever are common after hydrocarbon aspiration, it is often difficult to detect bacterial superinfection. One thoughtful review concluded that bacterial complications are rare.[27] Until there is further evidence to the contrary, antimicrobial therapy should be reserved for patients who are severely compromised by malnutrition, debilitation, or underlying disease or in whom the pneumonia is especially severe. Evolving evidence of infection on serial Gram stains of secretions from the endotracheal tube could be an indication for antimicrobials. Because airway closure and collapse are a significant part of the disease, continuous distending airway pressure is desirable to maintain FRC and to keep the concentration of inspired oxygen in safe ranges. Studies in animals and humans show no therapeutic or prophylactic role for corticosteroids.[28–30]

Prevention of the accidental ingestion of products containing hydrocarbons must be a high priority. Educating parents to keep potentially toxic materials out of the reach of young children seems obvious. Education about storage of such materials and avoiding containers that children associate with potable liquids must be stressed. If kerosene heaters are used in the home, the kerosene must be kept out of the reach of children.

HYDROCARBON "SNIFFING"

Deliberate inhalation of volatile hydrocarbons to induce a state of euphoria is common among adolescents. It is estimated that 13% of adolescents have used inhalants at one time or another.[31] Unlike other forms of drug abuse, this is more common among those in the seventh to ninth grades.[32,33] The euphoria of mild intoxication may be accompanied by mild nausea and vomiting. Prolonged exposure may lead to violent excitement followed by CNS depression, unconsciousness, and coma. Large doses

of halogenated hydrocarbons, especially when combined with exertion, excitement, and hypercapnia, may be associated with dysrhythmias and death. Medullary depression and respiratory paralysis are generally accepted as the mechanism of death in most gasoline inhalation fatalities. Strong psychological dependence may develop in some sniffers. Acute hypoxemia at the time of inhalation and shortly thereafter is not uncommon as a result of displacement of alveolar gas by the inhaled substance. However, this is usually transient and not significant. Lung injury per se from hydrocarbon sniffing has not been described. A toluene embryopathy has been described in infants born to mothers who sniffed toluene,[34] although the "polypharmacy" often used by the mothers may confound the data.[35]

RESPIRATORY COMPLICATIONS OF SMOKE INHALATION

Death from fire is the fifth leading cause of unintentional injury death in the United States. The United States ranks seventh out of 25 developed countries in fire deaths. Those at greatest risk are children younger than 4 years of age; African-Americans and Native Americans; those over 65 years of age, and the poor.[36] Fire accounts for approximately 3320 deaths per year in the United States.[36] A great deal of the morbidity and mortality in victims of fires results from pulmonary injuries due to smoke inhalation.[37] The severity of the lung injury depends on (1) the nature of the material involved in the fire and the products of incomplete combustion that are generated and (2) whether the victim has been confined in a closed space. The subject's minute ventilation also plays a role. The deeper and more rapidly the victim breathes, the greater the amount and degree of deposition of toxic materials into the airways and alveoli. The decreased inspired oxygen concentration that results from the fire stimulates compensatory hyperpnea in humans.

PATHOGENESIS

The pathogenesis of lung injury from smoke inhalation includes thermal and chemical factors. Because the upper airway is such an effective heat exchanger, most of the heat from inhaled smoke is dissipated before the inhaled material reaches the carina. Direct thermal damage, therefore, primarily affects the supraglottic airways. Only with steam, which is unusual in most fires, or with prolonged exposure to high ambient temperatures, will there be thermal injury to the intrathoracic airways.

Depending on the material involved in fires, a wide variety of noxious gases may be generated. These include the oxides of sulfur and nitrogen, acetaldehydes, hydrocyanic acid, and carbon monoxide (CO). Irritant gases such as nitrous oxide or sulfur dioxide may combine with lung water to form corrosive acids. Aldehydes from the combustion of furniture and cotton materials induce denaturation of protein, cellular damage, and pulmonary edema. The combustion of wood generates considerable quantities of CO and carbon dioxide. Plastics, if heated to sufficiently high temperatures, may be the source of very toxic vapors. Thus, chlorine and hydrochloric acid may be generated from polyvinyl chloride; hydrocarbons, aldehydes, ketones, and acids from polyethylene; and isocyanate and hydrogen cyanide from polyurethane.[39] Although the particulate matter carried in the smoke (soot) probably does not in itself produce injury, toxic gases may be absorbed on the surface of the particles and carried into the lungs; the soot particles may also be responsible for inducing reflex bronchoconstriction.

■ CARBON MONOXIDE POISONING

CO poisoning is an especially serious complication of smoke inhalation that occurs soon after exposure. While smoke inhalation is the most common cause of inadvertent CO poisoning, other causes include poorly functioning home heating systems; inadequate ventilation for fuel burning systems (e.g., gas grills, kerosene heaters and camp stoves); and motor vehicles idling in poorly ventilated areas. Some of these can also be the sources for intentional poisoning. The toxicity results from the combination of CO with hemoglobin to form carboxyhemoglobin (COHb), leading to severely impaired tissue oxygenation. The CO displaces oxygen from hemoglobin, reducing the delivery of oxygen to the tissues. CO not only has a higher affinity for hemoglobin than oxygen but also shifts the oxyhemoglobin dissociation curve to the left (Fig. 40-2).[40] For this reason, the toxicity of CO poisoning is greater at high altitude and in the presence of anemia. It is critical to remember that although the oxygen content of the arterial blood is low in CO poisoning, the Pao_2 is not reduced. Because the carotid body responds to Pao_2, ventilation may not be stimulated until acidosis develops. Together with the fact that COHb is bright red, this makes the clinical diagnosis very difficult. The bright red color of the blood also makes the currently available oximeters unreliable. If there is a suspicion of CO poisoning, an arterial blood gas must be obtained. The

reduction in hemoglobin available for oxygenation in CO poisoning is much more serious than an equivalent anemia because there is a left shift and a change in the shape of the oxygen dissociation curve, which decreases oxygen delivery to the tissues. CO also binds to myoglobin, resulting in anoxia of muscle cells. With prolonged exposure, CO binds to cytochrome oxidase, impairing mitochondrial function and reducing production of adenosine triphosphate. Both of these actions impair normal cellular function.

■ PATHOLOGY

Various pathologic lesions are found in smoke inhalation. Part of the variability in pathology may be attributed to differences in the toxic products generated in fires. However, many of the changes may not result simply from the direct chemical injury to the respiratory tract. Rather, they may reflect secondary circulatory, metabolic, or infectious complications of surface burns or may be induced by the administration of oxygen, the use of a mechanical ventilator, and the administration of excessive volumes of intravenous fluids.

Animal models of the pathology have been of limited value because steam rather than pure smoke was usually used, and the modifying effects of the upper air passages were eliminated by the use of tracheal cannulas. Experimental evaluation of the response to smoke has been carried out in anesthetized and intubated sheep, kept light enough to breathe spontaneously. Even in these animals, any protective effects of the upper airway were bypassed. Smoke was generated by burning material such as dyed cotton toweling. The smoke was then insufflated into the lungs. In sheep, a volume of 20 cc/kg for 12 breaths and an inspiratory time of 3 to 4 seconds produced physiologic effects similar to natural smoke inhalation, including mean COHb levels of 45%.[41]

The initial pathologic changes are tracheobronchitis. The greater the tidal volume of the insufflated smoke, the more intense the tracheobronchitis. With sufficient smoke quantity, denudation of intact ciliated cells of the trachea occurred, most likely from disruption of the cell-cell and the cell–basal layer adhesions.[42] With much larger volumes, an acute pulmonary edema caused by increased pulmonary vascular permeability occurred within 30 minutes.[43] The degree of atelectasis also correlated with the amount of smoke insufflated. Subsequent airway edema only occurred in those animals given large tidal volumes of smoke.[41] The degree of hypoxemia over the 24 hours studied did not correlate with the tidal breath size, but was constant for a given total smoke exposure. This suggests that the gas exchange deterioration was based more on the airway pathology than on the alveolar atelectasis or edema.

A group of infants carefully studied after exposure to smoke in a newborn nursery[44] were found to have necrosis of bronchial and bronchiolar epithelium with vascular engorgement and edema together with the formation of dense membranes or casts that partially obstructed the large and small airways. Bronchiolitis and bronchopneumonia were present in some, as were interstitial and alveolar edema. There was carbonaceous material in the alveoli, with alveolar hemorrhage.

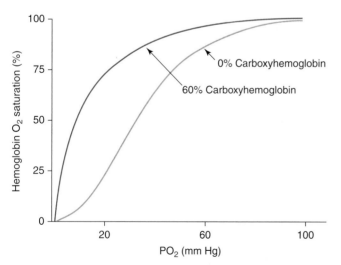

FIGURE 40-2. Oxygen–Hemoglobin Dissociation Curve. The presence of carboxyhemoglobin shifts the curve to the left and changes it to a more hyperbolic shape. This results in a decrease in oxygen-carrying capacity and impaired release of oxygen at the tissue level. (From Ernst A, Zibrak J. Carbon monoxide poisoning. *N Engl J Med.* 1998;339:1603-1608.)

Electron microscopic studies of 10 fatal cases of smoke inhalation following a hotel fire revealed interstitial and alveolar edema as well as engorgement of alveolar vessels.[45] Carbon particles were seen within alveolar macrophages. Type I pneumocytes showed more injury than was seen in the pulmonary endothelial cells. Patients who died after severe surface burns have had necrotizing bronchitis and bronchiolitis with intra-alveolar hemorrhage, hyaline membrane formation, and massive pulmonary edema. In these patients, it is difficult to know how much to attribute to direct pulmonary injury from smoke or to the complex metabolic, infectious, chest wall, and circulatory derangements that complicate surface burns and result in acute respiratory distress syndrome (ARDS). However, sheep exposed to surface burns plus smoke inhalation sufficient to raise the COHb levels to 25% to 30% fared much worse than those who received surface burns alone. The burn/inhalation group had greater amounts of lung lipid peroxidation products in bronchoalveolar lavage and at autopsy, even without evidence of pulmonary infection or ARDS.[46]

PATHOPHYSIOLOGY

Severe damage to the upper air passages leads to stridor, with increased extrathoracic resistance. Upper airway obstruction usually occurs within 24 hours of injury. This increases the work of breathing and can lead to alveolar hypoventilation. Inflammatory changes in the airways lead to ventilation/perfusion mismatch, exaggerating the hypoxemia. Depending on the severity and distribution of the airway obstruction, there may be atelectasis or air trapping. The latter is especially likely with premature closure of the small airways. Altered surfactant predisposes to atelectasis. Although reflex bronchoconstriction may contribute to the increase in airway resistance, it is difficult to assess the magnitude of its contribution because airway resistance is already high as a result of bronchial and bronchiolar edema and inflammation.

Smoke is a mixture of gases and particulate matter generated from the burning substances. The toxic effects of smoke are primarily seen when animals are exposed to whole smoke. When the particle phase of the smoke was filtered out, there were neither acute nor delayed toxic effects on lung function or gas exchange.[47] Since many of the oxidants are in the gas phase as well in whole smoke, it is possible that only those toxins carried on the smoke particles remain in the airway long enough to elicit the inflammatory response.

Pulmonary edema plays a prominent role in the pathophysiology of lung injury from smoke inhalation.[39] Studies in adults demonstrate increased extravascular lung water without a concomitant increase in pulmonary capillary wedge pressure. Studies in sheep reveal increased lung lymph flow and an increase in the lymph/plasma ratio of protein, suggesting increased permeability of the alveolar capillary membrane.[48] Increased bronchial circulation contributed to the pulmonary edema. Nitric oxide at extremely elevated levels acts as a free radical and potentiates the inflammatory response. Inhibition of inducible nitric oxide synthase reverses the loss of hypoxic pulmonary vasoconstriction and attenuates acute respiratory distress syndrome.[49,50]

Other products of combustion increase the damage. In dogs, acrolein results in delayed-onset pulmonary edema. Pure smoke, and smoke with added hydrochloric acid, did not have the same effects.[51] An animal model showed increased pulmonary vascular resistance and decreased cardiac output concomitant with increased secretion of leukotrienes C4, D4, and E4. Pretreatment with a leukotriene antagonist markedly attenuated and delayed those cardiovascular changes.[52] Additional studies in sheep suggest that the acrolein-induced pulmonary edema and pulmonary hypertension are mediated by cyclo-oxygenase products because pretreatment with cyclo-oxygenase inhibitors blocks the cardiorespiratory changes.[53] The acute pulmonary edema associated with very high-dose cotton smoke in sheep is blocked by a combined cyclo-oxygenase and leukotriene antagonist, but not by indomethacin, a cyclo-oxygenase inhibitor. Both agents block the elevated airway resistance and hypoxemia that presumably occur as a result of acute bronchoconstriction.[44] Prolonged exposure to acrolein in a kitchen resulted in severe respiratory distress in a previously healthy 27-month-old child who developed bronchiectasis 18 months after the initial exposure.[54]

Oxidants directly from the products of combustion also contribute to airway damage, closure, and atelectasis.[55] Early therapy with aerosolized deferoxamine-pentastarch in sheep exposed to cotton smoke attenuated these findings.[56] It is not clear whether the deferoxamine was acting directly as an antioxidant or reducing the free iron released in the airway, which could have been causing local oxidant release.

Neutrophil-mediated proteolytic activity has been implicated in the airway pathology. Sheep treated intravenously with the synthetic protease inhibitor gabexate mesilate after insufflation with cotton smoke had a significant reduction in transvascular fluid and protein flux and were able to maintain better gas exchange than a vehicle-treated control group.[57] Impaired chemotactic and phagocytic function of the alveolar macrophage after smoke inhalation increases the risk for pulmonary infection several days after the acute event.

Any inhaled cyanide binds to the intracellular cytochrome system, inhibiting cell metabolism and the production of adenosine triphosphate. While all cells contain the enzyme rhodanese, which is capable of converting hydrocyanide to thiocyanate, this capability will be outstripped by continued or high levels of cyanide. The thiocyanate will be excreted in the urine, assuming normal renal blood flow and urine output.[58]

CLINICAL FINDINGS

The initial assessment of a victim of a fire should focus on hypoxemia. Oxygen should be administered while blood gas studies, including CO levels, are drawn. The clinical manifestations of CO poisoning vary with the level of COHb. Mild intoxication leads to headache, diminished visual acuity, irritability, and nausea. COHb levels in excess of 40% produce confusion, hallucination, ataxia, and coma. CO may increase cerebral blood flow, the permeability of cerebral capillaries, and the cerebrospinal fluid pressure. CO may have long-term effects on the CNS. Myocardial dysfunction and irritability can result directly from CO, as well as from hypoxemia.

Patients immediately assessed at the scene of a fire have elevated blood cyanide concentrations. The cyanide levels of victims who die as a result of the smoke inhalation are significantly higher than the levels of survivors. Blood cyanide levels correlate with CO levels, and plasma lactate levels were better correlated with cyanide levels than with CO level. A plasma lactate concentration above 10 mM in the emergency department is a sensitive indicator of cyanide poisoning.[59]

Maximum inspiratory and expiratory flow-volume curves and flexible fiberoptic nasopharyngoscopy or bronchoscopy have been helpful in the early assessment of the extent of supraglottic or tracheobronchial injury and the likelihood of subsequently developing airway obstruction.[60] Although there may be some delay in the clinical evidence of respiratory tract injury resulting from smoke inhalation, manifestations of respiratory disease will usually develop within 12 to 24 hours. Absence of roentgenographic pulmonary disease is not very helpful in early diagnosis because abnormal findings may lag several hours or more behind auscultatory or physiologic evidence of damage.

Respiratory insufficiency may also occur as the result of airway obstruction anywhere from the supraglottic airways to the alveoli. It may be difficult to localize the level of obstruction; therefore, whenever there is clinical evidence of severe obstruction, the upper airways should be assessed by direct laryngoscopy before swelling of the head, neck, or oropharynx make this examination difficult. Fiberoptic bronchoscopy may be very useful to evaluate the extent of mucosal damage, but intense vasoconstriction in hypovolemic patients may mask the findings.[61]

Acute CO poisoning is also associated with acute myocardial injury and a delayed neuropsychiatric syndrome, which in children will lead to cognitive defects and sometimes to focal deficits. The mechanism of action of these complications has not been elicited.

◼ TREATMENT

The initial treatment should focus on reversing CO poisoning, if present, by the administration of high concentrations of humidified oxygen. CO levels may be reduced by half in about an hour when the patient breathes 100% oxygen. If severe CO poisoning is suspected, it is helpful to administer oxygen by non-rebreathing mask at flow rates higher than the victim's minute ventilation in order to achieve concentrations close to 100%. If results of clinical examination or arterial blood gas studies suggest alveolar hypoventilation, mechanical ventilation is necessary. Subsequently, the administration of oxygen may be important because of the hypoxemia resulting from bronchiolitis and alveolitis with premature closure of small airways. Constant positive distending airway pressure may also be necessary to maintain reasonable levels of Pao_2 without using excessively high and potentially toxic concentrations of inspired oxygen for prolonged periods of time.

Controversy exists regarding the importance of, and need for, hyperbaric oxygen in the management of CO poisoning. Hyperbaric oxygen at 2 to 3 atmospheres markedly hastens the decline of COHb levels, reducing the half-life of COHb to 20 to 25 minutes. However, the advantages of hyperbaric oxygen therapy may be offset by

complications during transfer to the hyperbaric chamber. While some clinicians claim that all patients with significant COHb levels should be sent to a hyperbaric chamber, there is scant evidence for this approach.[58] One review suggests using hyperbaric therapy for children with COHb levels of 25% or greater if symptomatic, and for any with levels of 40% or higher.[62] The potential risks of the hyperbaric chamber include oxygen toxicity to the lung, the fact that patients are not amenable to appropriate observation and intervention while they are in the chamber, and the need for tympanotomy. More data are necessary to adequately assess the risks and benefits of hyperbaric oxygen in the therapy of CO poisoning in children related to fires.[63] The incidence of cognitive deficits at 6 weeks and 1 year following acute CO poisoning has been reported to be reduced in adults treated with hyperbaric oxygen therapy.[64] However, a second slightly larger study over 2 years did not replicate these findings.[65]

Endotracheal intubation may be necessary for a patient with any of the following conditions: (1) severe burns of the nose, face, or mouth, because of the likelihood that nasopharyngeal edema and obstruction will develop; (2) edema of the vocal cords with laryngeal obstruction; (3) difficulty handling secretions; (4) progressive respiratory insufficiency requiring mechanical ventilation; and (5) altered mental status that decreases minute ventilation and diminishes the protective reflexes of the airway. Regardless of whether the glottis is bypassed by endotracheal tube or tracheostomy tube, constant positive airway pressure or positive end-expiratory pressure helps minimize edema and improve oxygenation. Noninvasive positive pressure ventilation may be attempted in patients with acute respiratory decompensation who are otherwise hemodynamically stable, conscious, and without extensive and deep facial burns or trauma. This mode of ventilation has been reported to be effective in avoiding intubation/re-intubation in a group of patients with burn-associated acute respiratory failure.[66] However, the risk of upper airway obstruction must be taken into account when selecting patients for noninvasive ventilation.

In addition to the increased airway resistance resulting from edema in and around the walls of airways, it is likely that some reflex bronchoconstriction occurs from irritation of airway receptors. This is more likely to occur in subjects with preexisting lung disease such as asthma or cystic fibrosis, or in cigarette smokers. For this reason, it seems reasonable to administer inhaled bronchodilators.

Airway obstruction by cast material containing fibrin often accompanies smoke inhalation injury. In sheep with acute lung injury following burn and smoke inhalation injury, a combination of nebulized heparin and recombinant antithrombin has been demonstrated to improve pulmonary gas exchange and lung compliance, with decreased pulmonary edema, and airway obstruction.[67] In children with burn and smoke inhalation injury, nebulized heparin and N-acetylcysteine resulted in a significant decrease in incidence of re-intubation for progressive pulmonary failure, decreased incidence of atelectasis, and reduced mortality.[68] Similarly, in adults with smoke inhalation injury, nebulized heparin and N-acetylcysteine reduced lung-injury scores.[69]

As in many other respiratory conditions, the role of chest physiotherapy is poorly defined. Nevertheless, mucociliary clearance is clearly impaired. The encouragement of deep breathing and cough, or gentle endotracheal suction in the presence of endotracheal intubation, coupled with postural drainage would seem to be reasonable.

Although corticosteroids are frequently advocated in the hope of suppressing inflammation and edema, most controlled studies fail to demonstrate a significant effect. Thus, it is difficult to marshal strong support for their use. Furthermore, long-term steroid therapy in victims of fires increases the susceptibility to infection. Until further evidence is available, the empirical use of corticosteroids is discouraged. One review suggests using corticosteroids only for evidence of peripheral airway obstruction, other illnesses requiring steroids, or recent use of steroids.[62] At the experimental level, ibuprofen (but not indomethacin) when given immediately after smoke inhalation injury prevented the development of pulmonary edema.[70] As animal studies further elicit the basic mechanisms of the events occurring within the airways and parenchyma, specific agents may become available to correct the pathophysiology.

Available evidence indicates that antimicrobial agents do not prevent subsequent infection and may only predispose to infection with resistant organisms. Because fever, elevated white blood cell count, and increased erythrocyte sedimentation rate may all result from smoke inhalation, and because the chest roentgenogram may show nonspecific opacities that represent either atelectasis or edema, it may be extremely difficult to establish the presence of an infection in the absence of positive blood cultures or a positive Gram stain of airway secretions. It would seem preferable to reserve antimicrobial therapy for patients in whom there is clinical deterioration despite supportive therapy. Changes in the amount, nature, or color of the secretions should raise the suspicion of a bacterial superinfection, which should be confirmed by Gram stain or culture. Because the prevention of infection is clearly an important part of the therapy in victims of fires, aseptic care of the trachea and humidifying equipment is essential. In a retrospective analysis of children, high-frequency percussive ventilation was associated with a lower incidence of pneumonia.[71]

While dogs benefited from surfactant after smoke exposure,[72] rabbits did not.[73] To our knowledge, there are no data in human subjects.

Smoke-exposed sheep did worse with ECMO support than with conventional mechanical ventilation. The ECMO was associated with pulmonary sequestration of leukocytes, increased pulmonary thromboxane B_2, increased blood-free wet/dry lung weight ratios, and more significant hypoxemia at 24 hours after identical degrees of smoke exposure.[74] Two children with inhalation injury and resultant respiratory failure refractory to conventional mechanical ventilation were successfully treated with ECMO.[75]

■ THE RELATIONSHIP OF PULMONARY INJURY FROM SMOKE INHALATION TO THE PULMONARY COMPLICATIONS OF SURFACE BURNS

Pulmonary damage from smoke inhalation generally declares itself during the first 24 hours. Individuals with widespread surface burns may develop pulmonary complications after several days, but these late complications are not the result of direct chemical or thermal injury. It is more likely that late pulmonary injury is attributable to metabolic, infectious, or circulatory derangements complicating the surface burns.[60]

Surface burns may be directly and indirectly related to pulmonary pathophysiology. The large amounts of intravenous fluids usually given to counteract ongoing surface and "third-space" losses in the tissues may increase pulmonary edema through two mechanisms. First, there may be pulmonary vascular engorgement from diminished myocardial function due to CO poisoning, the initial hypoxia, and other toxins involved in the fire. Second, the diffuse inflammation within the airways increases vascular permeability with fluid leak into the areas of gas exchange, worsening the hypoxemia and causing additional pulmonary edema. Careful monitoring of fluid balance is critical in these children.

A second indirect relationship between the surface burns and the lung is in the area of infection. Clearly, the postburn lung is at risk for pneumonia. Organisms may enter the body through the skin at the burn site. Scrupulous attention to the burn sites is necessary to reduce this possibility. The lung can be directly infected, in pneumonia, or as part of the sepsis syndrome.

The skin surface and lung may be directly related with severe skin burns of the thorax or upper abdomen. Chest wall edema or eschar formation, in addition to the pain at the skin site, all increase the risk for hypoventilation and atelectasis.[76] Attention must be directed to skin manifestations (e.g., eschars) and pain control. Pain control with narcotics may increase the risk for hypoventilation, but this can be easily monitored, and adequate pain control is important for children with burns.

Suggested Reading

Eade NR, Taussig LM, Marks MI. Hydrocarbon pneumonitis. *Pediatrics.* 1974;54:351–357.

Haponick E, Summer W. Respiratory complications in burned patients. Pathogenesis and spectrum of inhalation injury. *J Crit Care* 1987;2:49–54.

Horoz OO, Yilizdas D, Yilmaz HL. Surfactant therapy in acute respiratory distress syndrome due to hydrocarbon aspiration. *Singapore Med J.* 2009;50:130–132.

Lewander WJ, Aleguas A. Petroleum distillates and plant hydrocarbons. In: Shannon MW, Borron SW, Burns MJ, eds. *Haddad and Winchester's Clinical Management of Poisoning and Drug Overdose.* 4th ed. Philadelphia: Saunders Elsevier; 2007:1343.

Ruddy RM. Smoke inhalation injury. *Pediatr Clin North Am.* 1994;41:317–336.

Scharf SM, Prinsloo I. Pulmonary mechanics in dogs given different doses of kerosene intratracheally. *Am Rev Respir Dis.* 1982;126:695–700.

Vale JA, Kulig KAmerican Academy of Clinical Toxicology, European Association of Poison Centres and Clinical Toxicologists. Position paper: gastric lavage. *J Toxicol Clin Toxicol.* 2004;42:933–943.

Van Gorcum TF, Hunault CC, Van Zoelen GA, et al. Lamp oil poisoning: did the European guideline reduce the number and severity of intoxications? *Clin Toxicol (Phila).* 2009;47:29–34.

Weaver LK, Hopkins RO, Chan KJ, et al. Hyperbaric oxygen for acute carbon monoxide poisoning. *N Engl J Med.* 2002;347:1057–1067.

References

The complete reference list is available online at www.expertconsult.com

41 DROWNING

Andrew Numa, MBBS, FRACP, FCICM, Jürg Hammer, MD, and
Christopher Newth, MD, FRCPC, FRACP

DROWNING

Definitions

Traditionally, the definition of *drowning* has been death within 24 hours of an immersion event, and *near-drowning* is defined as any survivor from such an event. A new uniform definition of drowning was agreed upon during the World Congress on Drowning in Amsterdam, The Netherlands, in 2002.[1] Drowning is now defined as "a process resulting in primary respiratory impairment from submersion/immersion in a liquid medium." The term *drowning* now encompasses both fatal and nonfatal outcomes of immersion, and the term *near-drowning* is no longer used.

Epidemiology

Drowning occurs in all age groups and is responsible for approximately 4000 deaths per annum in the United States, with a mortality frequency of 12 to 18 deaths per million person-years.[2,3] The highest mortality rates of approximately 30 deaths per million person-years are observed in those who are 0 to 4 years of age and 15 to 19 years of age.[2,3] In the first year of life, drowning mortality in the United States is 63 per 100,000 live births.[3] Worldwide, drowning is the eleventh most frequent cause of death in children 0 to 4 years of age, the third most frequent cause of death in children 5 to 14 years of age,[4] and the second leading cause of injury-related death in childhood.[5] The vast majority of drowning deaths occur in non-Western countries; in Bangladesh more children 1 to 4 years of age die from drowning than from diarrhea or respiratory infection.[6] Even in a well-developed country such as Australia, where drowning accounts for less than 1% of all reported deaths, there is a disproportionate rate of death in children. The rate of drowning is 4.6 per 100,000 per year for children younger than 5 years of age, which is three times the rate for adults.[2] Nonfatal drowning episodes are believed to occur 3 to 10 times more frequently than fatal drowning episodes, worldwide.[7-11]

As with the majority of accidental deaths, there is a strong male preponderance with male-to-female incidence ratios ranging from 2:1 to 10:1.[2,3,5,10] Approximately one in three drowning fatalities occurs in accomplished swimmers.[12] Children can and do drown in any receptacle containing water, from buckets to bathtubs to the ocean. The majority of drowning events occur in swimming pools (usually the child's home pool) for children younger than 4 years of age and in open water for older children.[2,9,13]

Drowning is most frequently a primary event. However, the presence of underlying disease such as epilepsy or cardiac arrhythmia should always be considered, along with the possibility of drug or alcohol intoxication in older children. Approximately 6% to 10% of drowning victims have a previous history of a seizure disorder,[2,14] and it has been estimated that children with epilepsy have a relative risk for drowning of 96 in a bathtub and 23.4 in a swimming pool compared to nonepileptic children.[14] A primary arrhythmia such as prolonged QT syndrome should always be considered, particularly in patients who are capable swimmers.[15] Approximately 40% to 50% of adolescents who drown are intoxicated with drugs or alcohol.[13,16]

Drowning Sequence

Based upon studies in animals,[17] the sequence of events in drowning has been reported as (1) immediate struggle, (2) suspension of movement with frequent swallowing, (3) violent struggle, (4) convulsions and spasmodic inspiratory efforts, and (5) death.

Loss of consciousness is thought to be related to hypoxia, rather than hypercarbia.[12] Some observers have reported human victims who stop moving suddenly after swimming underwater, then float motionless on the surface of the water and subsequently quietly disappear.[7] The scenario of drowning without a struggle is probably due to a primary loss of consciousness secondary to other factors such as hypothermia[18] or cardiac arrhythmia.[9]

SEQUELAE OF SUBMERSION/ IMMERSION EVENTS

The drowning sequence has both pulmonary and nonpulmonary sequelae.

Pulmonary Injury

The majority of drowning victims aspirate water (saltwater or freshwater) at the time of drowning. However, in about 10% of cases, laryngospasm prevents the entry of water into the lungs.[10,19,20] The quantity of fluid aspirated is usually less than 22 mL/kg,[21] a volume that approximates the functional residual capacity (FRC). When aspiration occurs, local insult arises secondary to infection, surfactant depletion, aspiration of debris, and fluid shifts that depend on the relative tonicity of body fluids and aspirated fluid. While radiologic pulmonary edema is the most common finding, the incidence and degree appears to be the same irrespective of saltwater or freshwater immersion, although the mechanisms may be different. Seawater aspiration results in an osmotic gradient with fluid shifts into the alveolar spaces,[22-24] whereas aspirated freshwater is rapidly absorbed into the systemic circulation.[25,26] Pulmonary edema may arise in both seawater and freshwater aspiration secondary to neurogenic causes, forced inspiration against a closed glottis, and altered surfactant or pulmonary capillary permeability.[12,27]

Animal data suggest that 0.225% and 0.45% saline solutions are least injurious to the lungs in terms of gas exchange, possibly because they are rapidly absorbed from the alveolar spaces into the circulation along an osmotic gradient.[11,28-30] Freshwater will also be rapidly absorbed but causes rapid inactivation of surfactant and is probably the most injurious fluid to aspirate, followed closely by seawater, which is approximately 3% saline.[11] The presence of chlorine at 1 to 2 ppm in freshwater does not affect the pulmonary injury.[11]

Although it has been postulated that drowning in hypertonic fluid may lead to hypovolemia secondary to fluid shifts into the alveolar spaces,[22] animal data indicate that hemodynamic changes following drowning are entirely attributable to hypoxia and are independent of the tonicity of the aspirated fluid.[11,30]

Sepsis may occur, including with unusual and or atypical organisms,[31] and significant allergic reactions to aspirated materials have been described.[32] The incidence of pneumonia in adult patients requiring mechanical ventilation, as deduced from a retrospective study in the Netherlands, is around 50%.[33]

Pathologic findings are inconsistent and nonspecific. The most common finding in cases in which the drowning medium has entered the lungs is the presence of reactive edema, with hyperinflation of the lungs and increase in lung weight (emphysema acquosum), however these findings also may be seen in deaths from other causes including asphyxia and drug overdose.[34] Neurogenic pulmonary edema can occur, even when no water has been aspirated into the lungs.[27]

In severe cases of immersion/submersion accidents (with or without fluid aspiration), some patients will develop pneumonia and acute respiratory distress syndrome (ARDS). The management of this disorder is discussed in Chapter 48. However, in a database review of the 238 drowning patients admitted to the intensive care unit at Children's Hospital in Los Angeles over the past 24 years, only 24 (~10%) developed this serious complication. Figures 41-1 and 41-2 show the typical radiologic course of pulmonary injury in a drowning patient.

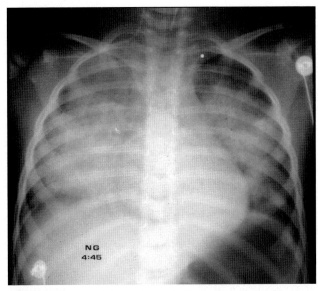

FIGURE 41-1. Initial chest radiograph of a drowning victim. The patient has an endotracheal tube in place and a right subclavian venous line going up into the internal jugular vein. Moderate pulmonary edema and some aspiration pneumonitis are seen, especially on the right.

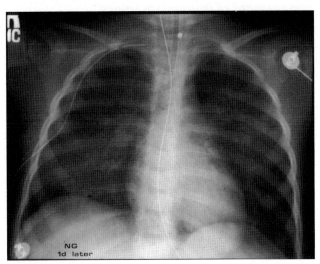

FIGURE 41-2. Chest radiograph of the drowning victim shown in Figure 41-1 taken 1 day after the event. Patient is still intubated and has a nasogastric tube into the stomach. The lung fields are almost clear again, but there is a chest tube on the right side that has drained a pneumothorax subsequent to right-sided aspiration pneumonia.

Nonpulmonary Sequelae

Hypothermia

Hypothermia is a common manifestation of drowning in water of almost any temperature. There is anecdotal evidence that rapid hypothermia in a submersion incident is neuroprotective, particularly in children. Conductive losses through the skin are compounded by rapid heat exchange across the pulmonary capillaries if a significant volume of water is inhaled. In a canine model, dogs breathing water at 4° C demonstrated a decrease in carotid artery blood temperature of 8° C within 5 minutes.[18] Cooling occurs most rapidly in small infants who have a relatively large surface area.[35] In cases of extreme hypothermia, rewarming is essential to allow return of cardiac function.[36,37] Hypothermia can also play a major role in facilitating aspiration in immersion victims. As the core temperature drops below 35° C, muscular incoordination and weakness occur, and this can interfere with

swimming. As the core temperature decreases further, obtundation develops. At core temperatures below 30° C, unconsciousness can occur and the myocardium becomes irritable. Atrial fibrillation can occur, and at temperatures below 28° C, ventricular fibrillation is likely.

Electrolyte Imbalances

Electrolyte imbalances may arise if a significant amount of non-isotonic water is aspirated, although this is unusual in regular seawater.[38] Although freshwater immersion victims have decreased serum sodium and saltwater immersion victims have elevated serum sodium and chloride levels,[19] these are rarely substantial or clinically significant. Even in the Dead Sea, which has electrolyte concentrations approximately 10 times higher than seawater, immersion victims rarely have severe abnormalities of sodium or chloride, although hypercalcemia and hypermagnesemia are common.[39,40] Hemolysis due to aspiration of hypotonic or hypertonic fluids appears to be an extremely infrequent complication.

Trauma

Traumatic injuries resulting from a fall into water must be considered but are generally of lesser importance than the immersion itself. Cervical spine injuries are the most critical to consider but are uncommon, occurring in only 0.5% of all nonfatal drowning cases, and only then in cases with a clear history of diving, motorized vehicle crash, or fall from a height.[41]

Hypoxic-Ischemic Damage

All organs are susceptible to hypoxic-ischemic injury following prolonged low cardiac output and inadequate oxygenation, and multiorgan failure is an almost inevitable consequence of severe submersion/immersion injury. Clinically, the brain is particularly susceptible, with the liver and the gastrointestinal tract being the most resistant.

Management of Pulmonary Injury

Management of the pulmonary injury will usually require supplemental oxygen and diuretic administration for pulmonary edema. In the most severe cases, the patient will require support with intubation and mechanical ventilation. In severe cases, the lung injury will comprise all the features of ARDS. The management of this disorder is addressed elsewhere.

Instillation of surfactant has been reported,[42-44] and it is an appealing therapeutic intervention given that the majority of victims aspirate a quantity of fluid that will denature and wash out existing surfactant. However, the temptation to administer surfactant should be considered in the light of recent randomized controlled trials demonstrating a lack of efficacy of surfactant in ARDS.[45-47] Administration of steroids appears to be effective in animal models of seawater aspiration,[48] and there is evidence to support the use of steroids in ARDS,[49] although this is by no means universally accepted.[50]

Broad-spectrum antimicrobials should be administered to treat likely bacterial contamination of the lungs, such as after drowning in stagnant water.[51] The incidence of neurologic infection is stated to be high, with a number of case reports in children.[52]

Most drowning victims will be hypothermic at the time of presentation. In cases of extreme hypothermia, rewarming is essential to allow return of cardiac function,[36,37] and if the core temperature is below 26° to 28° C or the patient is in cardiac arrest, rewarming is probably best achieved using cardiopulmonary bypass.[53] Given the potential benefits of hypothermia on hypoxic CNS injury, it is our view that 24 to 48 hours of modest hypothermia (core temperature 32° to 34° C) should be maintained immediately following the injury if there is any suspicion of the patient having sustained a hypoxic brain injury. Excellent neurologic outcomes have been reported after prolonged immersion in very cold water with several case reports indicating full neurologic recovery after periods

of up to 66 minutes in near-freezing water.[36,54,55] Children lose body heat more rapidly than adults do, and if significant brain cooling occurs prior to cessation of circulation, then some degree of neuroprotection may occur. It has been estimated that brain temperature needs to fall by at least 3° C within the first 5 minutes of immersion for cerebral protection to be effective.[35]

The role of induced hypothermia for neuroprotection following drowning remains less certain. Some recent studies have highlighted the beneficial effects of hypothermia on a variety of hypoxic CNS injuries in humans.[56,57] However, these studies had control arms of "usual care," and some patients became hyperthermic with potential harmful effects and the result of making the hypothermia group outcomes appear better.[58,59] In a Canadian trial using hypothermia in drowned children to reduce intracranial pressure and limit brain injury,[60] the death rate in the hypothermic group was higher than in the normothermic group, with most deaths attributed to neutropenic sepsis. However this trial was relatively small, and the hypothermia group was also managed with hyperventilation and high-dose phenobarbitone, which may have influenced the outcomes. Current Pediatric Advanced Life Support guidelines recommend consideration of cooling to 32° to 34° C for 12 to 24 hours in comatose children following cardiac arrest.[61] A randomized, controlled trial of therapeutic hypothermia versus normothermia after cardiac arrest is currently being undertaken by approximately 30 pediatric centers in the United States and Canada under the auspices of the National Institutes of Health, however this study excludes patients with cardiac arrest secondary to drowning in ice water who have a core temperature of ≤32° C on presentation.[62]

Other management comprises support of multiorgan failure that is beyond the scope of a respiratory text.

Outcome of Pulmonary Injury

Routine tests of pulmonary function have been reported as normal in adults[63] following a drowning accident. However, in a series of 10 functionally normal children[64] who were studied 6 months to 8.5 years (mean 3.3 years) after the submersion incident, only 1 had completely normal pulmonary function. Seven had abnormal methacholine challenges demonstrating a high incidence of bronchial hyperreactivity, and five had clear evidence of peripheral airways disease. It is possible that these children are at risk for developing chronic lung disease, especially if exposed to further airway or parenchymal irritants.

Outcome Prediction of Neurologic Injury

Biggart and Bohn[65] in Toronto conducted a retrospective review of 55 drowning victims (mean age 4.75 years) admitted to the intensive care unit during a 5-year period, to determine the factors that may influence survival both before and after hospital admission. Thirty-seven children survived, and 18 died; five survivors had profound neurologic damage resulting in a persistent vegetative state: the remaining 32 (58%) survived intact. The major factors that separated intact survivors from those who died, and from survivors in a persistent vegetative state, were the presence of a detectable heartbeat and hypothermia (less than 33° C) on initial examination in the emergency department.

In a subsequent review of 101 pediatric patients who had suffered an out-of-hospital respiratory or cardiac arrest over a 7.5-year span, Schindler and colleagues[66] confirmed these findings. Specifically, they noted that cardiac arrest as opposed to isolated respiratory arrest had a very poor prognosis, especially when efforts at resuscitation continued for more than 20 minutes and required more than two doses of epinephrine. They recorded nine patients with drowning, all of whom had cardiac arrest prior to reaching the emergency department and all of whom died.

Quan and coworkers[67] studied 77 children who had fatal or nonfatal drowning episodes in the Seattle area and concluded that advanced life support resuscitation efforts that continued for greater than 25 minutes were associated with a bad neurologic outcome and were therefore not warranted.

At this point, the best outcome predictors are observed in the field. Good outcomes are associated with sinus rhythm, reactive pupils, and neurologic responsiveness at the scene.[68]

The prediction of the neurologic outcome of children who survive the initial resuscitation event and arrive in the intensive care unit in a comatose state is highly relevant for parents and caregivers. It is difficult to provide early and accurate prognostic information on comatose children, especially if brainstem functions are intact. Severity of illness scores such as the Pediatric Index of Mortality (PIM2) and Pediatric Risk of Mortality (PRISM3) scores were developed to predict the risk of death in groups of patients, not individuals. However, PRISM has recently been applied to individuals, and it enables the prediction of either absence or presence of serious neurologic impairment or death in pediatric drowning patients, if they present at extreme values on this scale. However, in patients with intermediate PRISM scores, it is not possible to establish a reliable prognosis.[69] Electrophysiologic investigations, such as brainstem auditory evoked potentials and short-latency somatosensory evoked potentials (SSEP), are helpful to assess the likelihood of a permanent vegetative state or a higher level of cognition. Until now, the bilateral absence of SSEP is the only established predictor for a worse clinical outcome after cerebral hypoxia.[70,71] Today, diffusion-weighted MRI (DWI) provides a quick and reliable tool to detect early tissue injury in acute cerebral ischemia, because it is sensitive to water shifts between the extracellular and intracellular compartments, which conventional MRI often cannot detect. Preliminary results suggest that the extent of diffusion-weighted MRI pathology may serve as a reliable predictor for neurologic outcome after cerebral hypoxia[72] (Fig. 41-3). Magnetic resonance spectroscopy also shows promise as a diagnostic and prognostic tool in hypoxic/ischemic cerebral injury, with reduced N-acetyl aspartate and elevated lactate both associated with poor neurologic outcomes (Fig. 41-4).[73,74] Although CT is not a sensitive test for ischemic injury, the presence of any CT abnormalities suggestive of ischemia (typically loss of gray-white differentiation and/or basal ganglia edema or infarction) within the first 3 days of drowning is strongly correlated with poor a neurologic outcome, and the presence of CT abnormalities in the first 24 hours is associated with a very high risk of mortality.[75]

Prevention of Drowning

Drowning disproportionately affects children, and the majority are preventable. Drowning causes significant mortality and morbidity throughout the world,

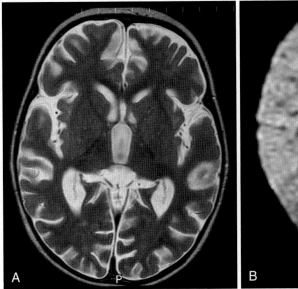
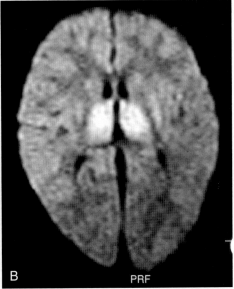

FIGURE 41-3. Magnetic resonance imaging (MRI) of the brain of a 3-year-old child 36 hours after a drowning accident. The child remained in a persistent vegetative state. **A,** The T2-weighted conventional MRI revealed no signs of hypoxia. **B,** Diffusion-weighted imaging shows hyperintensity bilaterally in the basal ganglia.

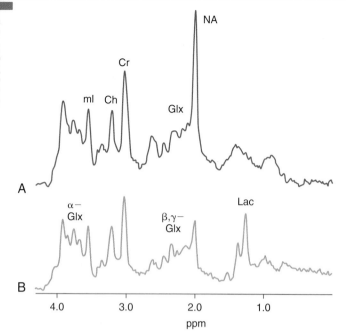

FIGURE 41-4. Cerebral Hydrogen 1 magnetic resonance (^{1}H-MR) spectroscopy of occipital gray matter in a 3-year-old boy 48 hours after drowning **(B)**, compared with a control spectrum in a healthy age-matched subject **(A)**. Note the loss of N-acetyl–containing metabolites (NA) and creatine (Cr), and the increase in lactate (Lac). (From Kreis R, Arcinue E, Ernst T, et al. Hypoxic encephalopathy after drowning studied by quantitative 1 H-magnetic resonence spectroscopy. *J Clin Invest.* 1996;97:1145.)

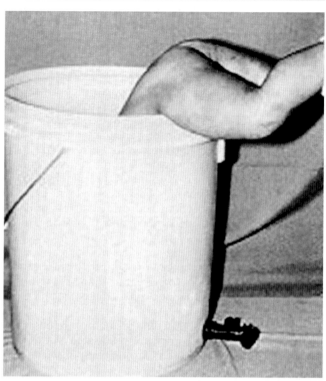

FIGURE 41-5. The body of a small child who had tipped headfirst into a bucket of water. The upper segment (torso and head) of a child is longer and heavier than the lower segment (unlike an older child or adult), and he could not extract himself. (From Moon RE, Long RJ. Drowning and near-drowning. *Emerg Med.* 2002;14:378.)

although modest decreases in the overall instances have been reported recently in the United States.[76] Factors that appear to have reduced the number of those drowned each year are legislative and public health interventions, such as pool fencing and public education campaigns, which have improved awareness of the dangers of leaving children unattended in bathtubs and of large commercial-type buckets into which smaller children can fall but not extract themselves (Fig. 41-5). Participation in formal swimming lessons has been demonstrated to be an effective preventive strategy in younger (1 to 4 years of age) but not older children.[77] Improvements in postresuscitation care have thus far not been shown to alter outcome significantly if there has been an out-of-hospital cardiac arrest.

References

The complete reference list is available online at www. expertconsult.com

42 TUMORS OF THE CHEST

Timothy A. Plerhoples, MD, and Thomas M. Krummel, MD

Tumors of the chest in children comprise a vast potpourri of pathology, congenital or acquired, benign or malignant. They may be found in any of the thoracic structures, from the lungs to the contents of the mediastinum. Such tumors may have their primary origins in the chest, or they may arise as primary tumors elsewhere with metastasis to the chest.

■DIAGNOSIS OF PULMONARY OR MEDIASTINAL TUMOR

Infants or children who have respiratory symptoms that do not disappear promptly when treated in the usual manner by expectorants, bronchodilators, and antibiotics must be suspected of having a space-occupying lesion. When symptoms persist, posteroanterior and lateral chest radiographs are an essential beginning.

Prenatal ultrasound, now routine, has led to a greater understanding of the natural history of lesions presenting in the fetus. Previously undiagnosed lesions are now seen with increasing frequency. When symptoms present after birth, radiographs should be the first step in the diagnostic workup. Only by such techniques can obstructive emphysema (Fig. 42-1), atelectasis (Fig. 42-2), and actual solid masses be seen at a stage of development when a resection may offer some hope of cure (Figs. 42-3 to 42-7).

In addition to undergoing an exhaustive history and physical examination, children with persistent symptoms and radiographic lesions should have other studies to rule out infections (e.g., mycobacterial or fungal) and genetic lung disorders. Examination of the bone marrow may give diagnostic evidence of a blood dyscrasia (e.g., leukemia or myeloma) or even metastatic malignancy.

Radiographic examination of the chest with special views such as apical lordotic and right and left oblique may be required. In addition, other imaging techniques such as fluoroscopy and cinefluoroscopy, ultrasound, or computed tomography (CT) may be necessary for final definition. Cinefluoroscopy allows repeated examination of the thoracic organs in motion (function) without subjecting the infant to excessive radiation exposure. During this examination and at the time of fluoroscopy, studies with barium in the esophagus will aid in determining any displacement of the posterior mediastinum. Ultrasonography is useful in locating and assisting in the needle aspiration of pleural fluid collections (Fig. 42-8). Mediastinal, pulmonary, and diaphragmatic densities are best detailed with axial CT of the thorax, which has added greatly to the accurate study of all these areas (Figs. 42-9 to 42-11).

Magnetic resonance imaging (MRI) has had a substantial impact on thoracic diagnostic workup in the last decade. It can distinguish masses in the mediastinum from vascular structures and is more sensitive than CT in detecting intraspinal extension. The two studies may be complementary, since CT demonstrates calcifications and bronchial abnormalities that are not seen on MRI. Thoughtful use and sequencing of these studies should be based on location of the abnormality and a provisional working diagnosis.

Diagnostic pneumoperitoneum (introduction of air into the peritoneal cavity, thereby outlining the diaphragm) may aid in the diagnosis of abnormalities adjacent to the diaphragm; congenital diaphragmatic hernias may also be visualized (Fig. 42-12). Given the sensitivity of CT and MRI, this technique's popularity is disappearing except as a last resort of the expert diagnostician.

Echocardiography and, occasionally, cardiac catheterization demonstrate any displacement of the heart due to masses in the lung, mediastinum, or pericardium. The use of aortograms assists in ruling out such vascular lesions as congenital aneurysm, vascular ring, congenital vascular malformations of the pulmonary tree, and sequestration. Aortograms are used to define bronchial arteries in patients with massive hemoptysis.

Bronchoscopy is an essential procedure for the study of the tracheobronchial tree. This procedure permits visual study of the vocal cords, larynx, trachea, and major bronchi and their segmental orifices. Congenital anatomic abnormalities may be visualized; prognosis in extensive lesions is evaluated by study of the carina and trachea. Bronchoscopy-guided transbronchial biopsy has been described in children for the diagnosis of chronic bronchiolitis, sarcoidosis, interstitial lung disease, and acute rejection in transplant recipients.[1,2] There are some reports of resecting mass lesions bronchoscopically with the aid of energy hemostasis (usually laser). Aspiration of secretions is an important therapeutic contribution. Bronchoalveolar lavage (BAL) allows sampling from distal airways and alveoli; investigation must include cytologic studies for malignant cells, routine bacterial smear, culture and sensitivity studies, acid-fast smear and cultures, and fungal smear and cultures (see discussion of bronchoscopy in Chapter 9).

Biopsy of palpable lymph nodes may aid in the diagnosis of abnormal processes in the lung. The scalene lymph nodes are usually the primary target because they drain the pulmonary parenchyma. Scalene lymph node biopsy, mediastinoscopy, or, now more directly, thoracoscopy with biopsy of available mediastinal nodes are of great help in the diagnosis of sarcoidosis, in lymphatic malignancies (e.g., Hodgkin's disease) and lymphosarcoma and in primary neoplasms of the lung and mediastinum. CT-guided percutaneous biopsy is now common in children, with a reported diagnostic rate of 85%.[3]

Lymph nodes obtained at the time of biopsy should be subjected to histologic study, and a portion must be sent to the bacteriology laboratory for routine bacterial smear and culture, studies for sensitivity of the organism to antimicrobials, acid-fast smear and culture, and fungal smear and culture (Fig. 42-13).

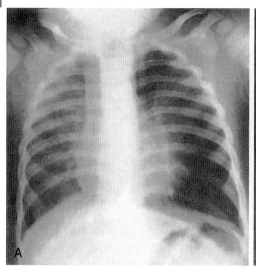

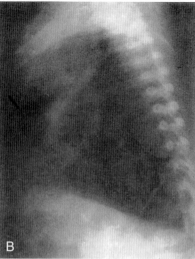

FIGURE 42-1. Chest radiograph revealing obstructive emphysema of the left lower lobe bronchus caused by partial occlusion of the lumen. **A,** Posteroanterior view. **B,** Lateral view. The left diaphragm is flattened, mediastinal and cardiac shadows are displaced toward the right, the left upper lobe is compressed, and there is increased radiolucency of the left lower lobe.

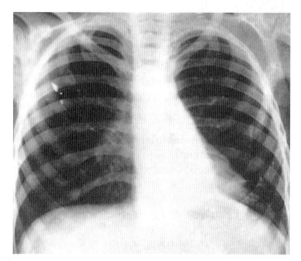

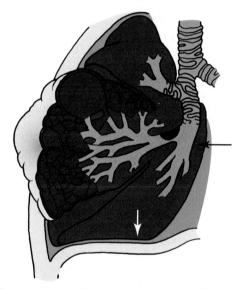

FIGURE 42-2. Chest radiograph revealing total atelectasis of the left lower lobe secondary to an inflammatory stricture of the left lower lobe bronchus. A retrocardiac position tends to confuse diagnosis in some cases.

FIGURE 42-4. Diagram illustrating obstructive emphysema. A partial obstruction leads to the retention of air in the pulmonary parenchyma distal to the obstructed bronchus. Retention of air will cause an ipsilateral compression of the adjacent normally aerated lung tissue, widening of intercostal spaces, descent of the diaphragm, a shift of the mediastinum away from the lung with the partially obstructing lesion, and a wheeze accompanied by decreased breath sounds over the affected lung.

Air bronchograms may show sufficient detail of the bronchial tree to dispense with any other diagnostic test for anatomy identifications (Fig. 42-14).

When all other methods have failed to produce a definitive diagnosis, thoracoscopy or thoracotomy should be considered. The use of single-lung ventilation (selective bronchial intubation or the use of balloon occlusion catheters) and preoperative placement of a radiologically guided blood patch can greatly facilitate the pursuit of tiny lesions. If the situation seems to present an inoperable problem, biopsy may still afford useful information (Fig. 42-15).

While thoracoscopy has been in use for a century, its use in children is a little over 3 decades old. Today it is the *primary mode of treatment* for not only limited procedures such as biopsy, decortication, and bleb resection, but also for more extensive operations such as lobectomy,

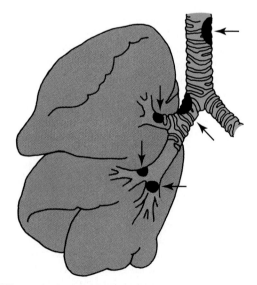

FIGURE 42-3. Diagram illustrating locations of lesions within the lumens of the major bronchi. The location of such lesions dictates the area of pulmonary involvement, unilaterality or bilaterality, and the extent of signs and symptoms.

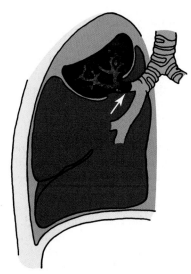

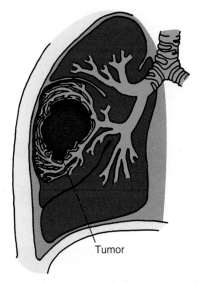

FIGURE 42-5. Diagram illustrating that persistence of a lesion with ultimate total obstruction gives rise to atelectasis, an absence of breath sounds over the affected lung tissue, an overexpansion of the surrounding lung tissue, and a shift of the diaphragm to a more normal position, with a return of the mediastinum to midline. Bronchial secretions may actually decrease in amount.

FIGURE 42-7. Diagram illustrating that if a tumor is within the pulmonary parenchyma, pressure on the adjacent lung and bronchi will give rise to a surrounding zone of pneumonitis that may actually show incomplete, temporary improvement with antimicrobial therapy.

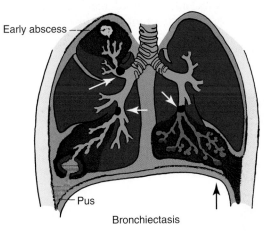

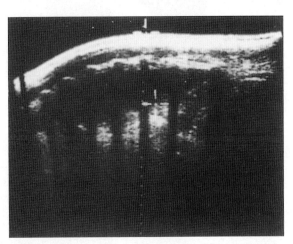

FIGURE 42-6. Diagram illustrating that persistence of an obstructing lesion leads to permanent destructive changes in the pulmonary parenchyma distal to the lesion, such as abscess formation, chronic pneumonitis with fibrosis, pleurisy, empyema, and bronchiectasis with parenchymal contracture secondary to fibrosis.

FIGURE 42-8. Typical ultrasonogram of pleural fluid. With such accurate localization, needle aspiration is easily carried out.

pneumonectomy, thymectomy, and repair of tracheoesophageal fistula.[4] Its rise has been facilitated by several technological improvements, including improved optics and light sources, and the development of specially designed instrumentation including hemostatic energy sources. Endoscopic linear staplers have made wedge biopsies and resections safe and simple procedures, leading many physicians to aggressively treat tumors that they may have just observed in the past.[5]

PULMONARY TUMORS

All forms of primary pulmonary tumors are unusual in children.

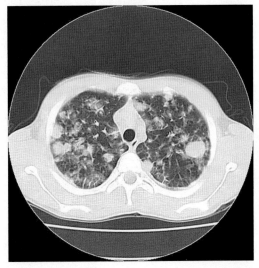

FIGURE 42-9. CT study of the chest showing metastatic pulmonary disease in a 14-year-old boy with testicular rhabdomyosarcoma.

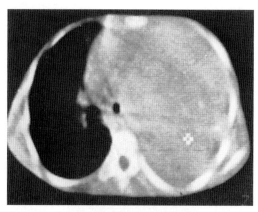

FIGURE 42-10. CT scan of a child with small-cell carcinoma.

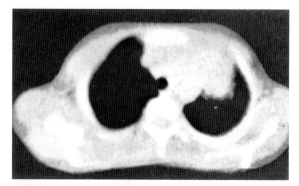

FIGURE 42-11. CT scan of the mediastinum and lung in a child with Hodgkin's disease.

Benign Pulmonary Tumors

Hamartoma

The term *hamartoma* was coined in 1904 by Albrecht, who defined it as a tumor-like malformation formed by an abnormal mixing of the normal components of the organ. Hamartomas of the lung consist largely of cartilage and may also include epithelium, fat, and muscle (Fig. 42-16). They are usually located in the periphery of the lung, but involvement of intermediate and primary bronchi has been reported. Developmental derangement is apparently responsible for their occurrence. Popcorn-like calcification is pathognomonic.

Unlike hamartomas in adults, which are usually asymptomatic and small, the rare tumor found in infancy can be large and symptomatic with significant mortality in the absence of prompt diagnosis and excision. The incidence of hamartoma is 0.25% among all patients,[6] but only six have been reported in children, with two successfully resected. The other four cases were discovered at autopsy. Hamartomas generally show obvious progressive intrauterine development and tend to attain considerable size at the time of birth. Recognition and prompt removal of such large intrapulmonic tumors are necessary for survival. Originally called *adenomatoid hamartoma*, congenital cystic adenomatoid malformation (CCAM), a cystic disease due to abnormal growth of normal lung components, may sometimes be mistaken for a true hamartoma (see Chapter 17).

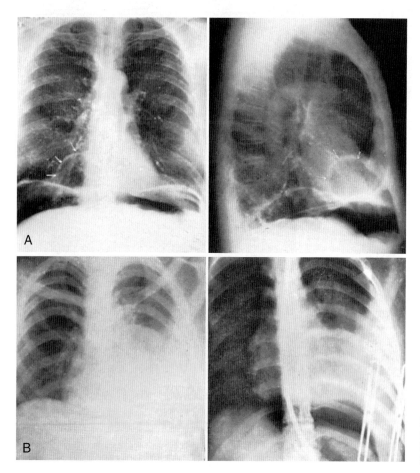

FIGURE 42-12. A, Diagnostic pneumoperitoneum showing congenital diaphragmatic Morgagni hernia. **B,** Outline of a normal diaphragm with intrapleural or pneumonic density above.

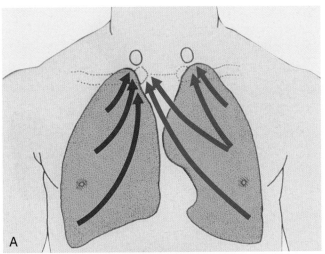

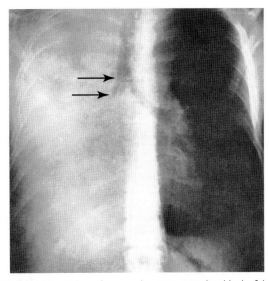

FIGURE 42-14. Air bronchogram showing a complete block of the right main bronchus in a patient with total right lung atelectasis.

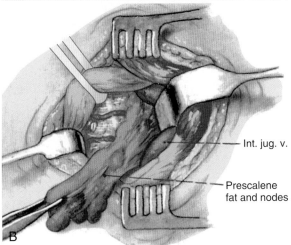

— Int. jug. v.

— Prescalene fat and nodes

FIGURE 42-13. A, Disease within the right lung usually drains into the right scalene lymph node group. Disease within the left lung may drain to either scalene node group in a pattern similar to that indicated on the illustration. Generally, left lung disease requires bilateral scalene node biopsy, whereas right lung disease requires only right scalene node biopsy. Regardless of the side of lung disease, all palpable nodes in the scalene node area should be examined by biopsy. **B,** The scalene group of nodes is contained in the fat pad bounded medially by the internal jugular vein, inferiorly by the subclavian vein, and superiorly by the posterior belly of the omohyoid muscle. The base of the triangle is formed by the anterior scalene muscle. Retraction of the internal jugular vein is essential to obtain access to all nodes in this group.

Mesodermal Tumors

Benign Parenchymal Tumors

Plasma cell granuloma (inflammatory pseudotumor) of the lung has been reported in children, with the greatest number between 8 and 12 years of age. Many patients are asymptomatic; others show signs of antecedent pulmonary infection. Radiographic appearance is typically that of a peripherally based lesion that may extend beyond the pulmonary parenchyma. The diagnosis is usually made histologically; lung-conserving resection should be performed if the diagnosis is suspected; however, gross resection is essential. Recurrence tends to occur in patients whose tumors involve more than one organ.[7]

Bronchial Adenoma

Bronchial adenoma is a neoplasm that arises from the mucous gland of the bronchi or the cells lining the excretory ducts of these glands.

Two histologic types are defined: carcinoid and cylindromatous. The carcinoid type (90%) has histologic resemblance to carcinoid tumor of the small bowel; it is composed of somewhat oval cells filled almost entirely by nucleus. The cells, which have barely detectable lumina, are arranged in a quasi-acinar fashion and are piled up in several layers. The tumor is very vascular and is surrounded by a thin capsule of fibrous tissue that is not invaded by the tumor cells. Metaplastic epithelium of the bronchial mucosa covers the intrabronchial component. The tumor is frequently shaped like a dumbbell, with the smaller component intrabronchial and the larger one intrapulmonic. The cylindromatous type (10%) is made up of cuboidal or flattened epithelial cells, arranged in two layers, which form corelike structures of the cylinders. Histologically, it closely resembles a mixed tumor of the salivary glands and basal cell carcinoma of the skin. There is a 40% incidence of malignancy. Though considered benign, bronchial adenomas have a definite malignant potential; lymph node metastasis is more frequent (15%) than distant blood-borne metastasis.

More than 100 cases of bronchial adenoma, all apparently of the carcinoid type, have been reported in the pediatric age group. There were metastases in 10% of the cases, and one case of carcinoid syndrome has been described.[8]

The most prominent symptoms and signs of a bronchial adenoma are recurrent and refractory pneumonitis, elevated temperature, cough, and chest pain due to bronchial obstruction with associated distal infection. Hemoptysis and wheeze are not as common in children as in adults. The right main bronchus is most commonly involved, and the diagnosis can usually be made by biopsy performed at bronchoscopy. The tumor occurs five times more commonly in males. The youngest

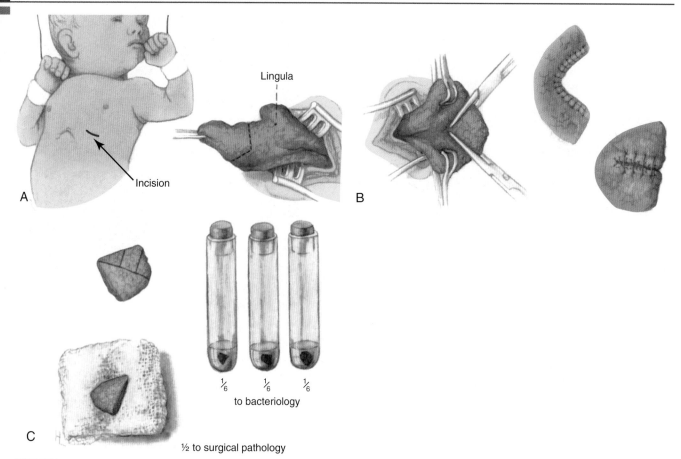

FIGURE 42-15. **A** to **C,** An adequate lung biopsy with specimens for bacteriology and pathology laboratories is essential. In general, a small open thoracotomy has many advantages over the blind needle biopsy technique.

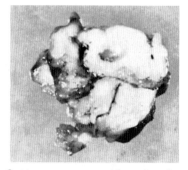

FIGURE 42-16. Hamartoma removed from the right upper lobe of an adult. Note the predominance of cartilage.

reported patient was a 10-month-old infant; all the other pediatric tumors were seen in children at least 4 years of age (Fig. 42-17).

Treatment consists primarily of resection of a segment, lobe, or total lung, according to the degree of involvement, which may be done thoracoscopically or via thoracotomy, depending on the location and extent of the lesion. Luminal excision by bronchoscopy should not be done because it does not permit complete removal of the tumor. Rarely, a bronchial adenoma can be removed by bronchial or sleeve resection, followed by airway reconstruction.

Tracheal Tumors

Papilloma of the Trachea and Bronchi

These lesions may be single but are more frequently multiple and often misdiagnosed as vocal cord nodules. The human papillomavirus (HPV) likely plays a role in pathogenesis, with types 6 and 11 predominantly found in recurrent papillomatosis. These lesions are usually seen in the larynx; tracheobronchial and pulmonary seeding has been reported.

Symptoms depend on the location and size of the tumor. Dyspnea, hoarseness, and stridor are the most common symptoms, occurring in two thirds of the cases. Cough, at first dry and later productive, is another common symptom. The lesions may be attached by a pedicle and may oscillate in and out of orifices during inspiration and expiration (flutter valve). Single, slow-growing, high lesions within the trachea may be asymptomatic for years.

Wheeze, audible at the open mouth, is the earliest sign of papilloma of the trachea. This eventually develops into stridor and is associated with slowly increasing dyspnea. Such secondary changes as obstructive emphysema, atelectasis, pneumonia, lung abscess, and bronchiectasis may occur in the distal parts of the tracheobronchial tree; empyema may also occur.

Unlike the adult variant, juvenile papilloma do not undergo malignant transformation. However, they should be removed because of their tendency to grow

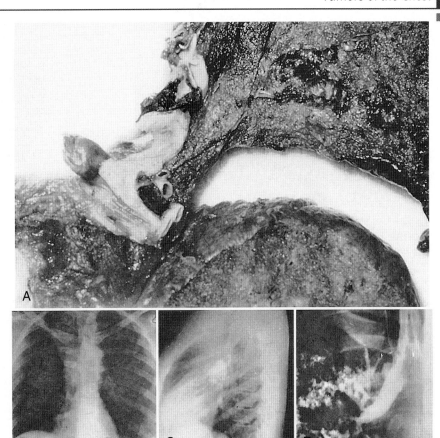

FIGURE 42-17. Bronchial adenoma (carcinoid type) **(A)** and total obstruction of the right upper lobe bronchus with resultant distal atelectasis **(B and C).** Recurrent pneumonitis, cough, and hemoptysis had occurred. Diagnostic biopsy at the time of bronchoscopy. **D,** Obstruction of the right upper lobe bronchus is demonstrated with bronchograms. The patient was treated by performing a right upper lobectomy.

progressively and obstruct the airway. Distal pulmonary infection or death from asphyxia may result. They tend to show multiple recurrences, although they often regress at puberty.[9]

Since papillomata are confined to the mucosal layer, surface destruction rather than full-thickness excision is warranted. Laser (CO_2) ablation is now used; interferon-α2a, retinoic acid, and indole-3-carbinol/diindolylmethane have been used as adjuvant therapies to expand the intervals between endoscopic laser treatments. Cidofovir has been used with success in selected patients. It is not yet clear whether vaccines against HPV will impact development of papilloma of the airway.

Fibroma of the Trachea
Nine cases of primary fibroma of the trachea have been reported in infants,[10] but no cases have been reported since 1953.

Hemangioma of the Trachea
Congenital hemangioma of the trachea is one of the most common tumors of the airway in children and may cause death by airway obstruction, bleeding complications, intractable cardiac failure (from atrioventricular shunting of blood within the tumor), or malignant change. In infants and children, these tumors are usually below the vocal cords, sessile, and flat, and they produce dyspnea. Among the reported patients, 90% have been 6 months of age at the time of onset of symptoms, suggesting a proliferative phase at that age, as seen in soft-tissue hemangiomas. Females predominate over males 2 to 1. More than half of infants have hemangiomas elsewhere.

The onset is insidious, with symptoms of respiratory obstruction such as stridor, retraction, dyspnea, wheezing, and sometimes cyanosis and cough. The symptoms tend to be intermittent and labile. Fever and leukocytosis are usually absent, but superimposed infection may produce fever and an elevated white blood cell count. The best diagnostic tool is bronchoscopy. Biopsy is not advisable; bleeding may be catastrophic and cause asphyxia or exsanguinating hemorrhage. Tracheostomy is necessary for severe obstructions; because many hemangiomas involute, observation can be undertaken once the airway is secure. Corticosteroids, both systemic and intralesional, have their champions and their skeptics. Recent data suggest that β blockers may help accelerate involution.[11]

Leiomyoma of the Lung
Grossly, these tumors cannot be differentiated from other benign tumors of the lung. Leiomyomas of the lung are usually asymptomatic unless there is partial or complete bronchial obstruction. In children, they tend to occur during immunodeficient states and Epstein-Barr viral infection. While exceedingly rare, their incidence does seem to be growing with the rise in HIV.[12]

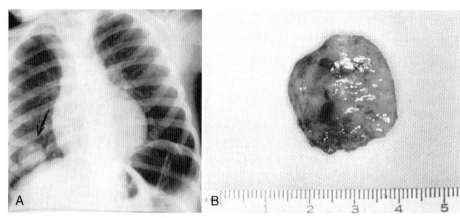

FIGURE 42-18. **A,** Three-year-old white male with an increasing mass in the right lower lobe of the lung. **B,** The shelled-out leiomyosarcoma after a lower lobectomy. There was no recurrence after 1 year.

Neurogenic Tumors

Of the more than 50 patients with proven primary intrapulmonic neurogenic tumors reported in the world literature, 9 were seen in children. Neurofibroma, schwannoma, and neurilemomas have been described. Resection was curative.

Malignant Pulmonary Tumors

Bronchogenic Carcinoma

Sixty cases of bronchogenic carcinoma are reported in children.[13] The youngest patient was a 5-month-old girl with cystic lung disease and malignancy in the left lung. Every cell type except alveolar cell carcinoma, giant cell carcinoma, and carcinosarcoma has been seen in the pediatric age group. Interestingly, squamous cell carcinoma is rare, with seven cases reported in the literature.[14] Usually asymptomatic, most cases present late, with mortality approaching 90% and mean duration of survival of 7 months. As in adults, prognosis is determined by histology, stage and response to therapy.

Despite the rarity of primary pulmonary neoplasms in children, this diagnosis should be considered in young patients with solitary pulmonary masses or persistent, atypical pulmonary symptoms. Localized lesions should be completely excised.

Fibrosarcoma of the Bronchus

Review of the literature reports 29 cases of primary fibrosarcoma of the bronchus in the pediatric age group.[15] Fever, probably due to bronchial obstruction and distal infection, is the most common symptom; hemoptysis is relatively uncommon. Diagnosis in these cases can be established by bronchoscopy. Resection is the treatment of choice, because recurrence is common when any other mode of therapy is used. These lesions tend to be low-grade with a relatively good prognosis, especially when in an endobronchial location.

Leiomyosarcoma

Fifteen cases of primary leiomyosarcoma of the lung have been reported in children.[16] Cough, fever, dyspnea, and signs of obstructive pneumonitis are usually present.

Surgical excision is indicated; bronchoscopic resection has been reported[16] (Fig. 42-18).

Multiple Myeloma

Multiple myeloma is usually limited to the medullary space. Extramedullary plasma cell tumors are relatively uncommon (myeloma or solitary plasmacytoma of the lung parenchyma). Only 19 cases have been reported, one of which was a plasmacytoma in a 3-year-old girl. Cytologic examination of sputum may be diagnostic.

Chorioepithelioma

A case of chorioepithelioma of the lung in a 7-month-old girl was reported in 1953 by Kay and Reed.[17] The presenting symptoms were fever, dyspnea, and anorexia; massive hemoptysis then occurred. A radiograph showed almost complete opacity of the right side of the chest. Pneumonectomy was performed, but the child died several hours postoperatively. This rare lesion has other scattered case reports in the literature.

Systemic Neoplasms Affecting the Lung

Myeloid and lymphatic leukemia may have a pulmonary component, but isolated pulmonary disease has not been reported. Similarly, Hodgkin's disease and lymphosarcoma may involve the lung during the course of the disease, but neither occurs as an isolated pulmonary lesion.

Metastatic Pulmonary Tumors

The majority of malignant lung lesions in children are metastatic. The principles of evaluation are standard; operative therapy should be based on the primary tumor, the characteristics of the metastatic lesion, and a full metastatic workup. Pulmonary metastases should only be resected after the primary site is eradicated and other sites are confirmed to be disease-free. Tumors most amenable to excision of pulmonary metastases include soft-tissue sarcomas and osteosarcomas.

Beyond the general principles outlined, there are disease-specific guidelines. With osteosarcoma, survival is considerably better in those with four or fewer lesions.

Even in those with many nodules, complete resection of all lesions correlates with survival; pleural invasion is ominous. Adjuvant chemotherapy is warranted only if there is a recurrence within a year.[18]

Because soft tissue sarcomas encompass a broad spectrum of sites of origin and cell type, rational resectional therapy of pulmonary metastases depends on both site and histology. Rarely does rhabdomyosarcoma come to metastatic resection, and resection has not shown increased survival in Ewing's sarcoma.

Resection of metastatic Wilms' tumor has shown no advantage compared to systemic therapy and radiotherapy, although biopsy may be warranted.[19]

Overall, resection of other lesions, single or multiple, unilateral or bilateral, has increased survival by 10% to 20%. Surgical approaches have been historically via thoracotomy, bilateral thoracotomy, or sternotomy; minimal access surgery via thoracoscopy is now a viable option. Preoperative mapping by CT scan, tattooing of small lesions by a blood patch, and single-lung ventilation all facilitate precise localization and wedge resection.

▬ MEDIASTINAL TUMORS

The mediastinum, the portion of the body that lies between the lungs, contains all structures of the thoracic cavity except the lungs and is bounded anteriorly by the sternum and posteriorly by the vertebrae. It extends superiorly from the suprasternal notch and terminates inferiorly at the diaphragm and is incapsulated by the parietal pleura. Cysts or tumors that arise within the mediastinum may originate from any of the structures contained therein or may be the result of developmental abnormalities.

For ease of definition of sites of disease, the mediastinum may be thought of as divided into four compartments (Fig. 42-19): (1) the superior mediastinum—the portion above a hypothetical line drawn from the junction of the manubrium and gladiolus of the sternum (angle) to the intervertebral disk between the fourth and fifth thoracic vertebrae; (2) the anterior mediastinum—the portion of the mediastinum that lies anterior to the anterior plane of the trachea; (3) the middle mediastinum—the portion containing the heart and pericardium, the ascending aorta, the lower segment of the superior vena cava bifurcation of the pulmonary artery, the trachea, the two main bronchi, and the bronchial lymph nodes; and (4) the posterior mediastinum—the portion that lies posterior to the anterior plane of the trachea.

Signs and Symptoms of Mediastinal Tumor

Many lesions (even very large ones) in the mediastinum remain asymptomatic for a considerable period. The patient becomes aware of lesions within the mediastinum only when pressure is exerted on sensitive structures or when the structures are displaced; therefore, the severity of symptoms depends on the size and location of the tumor, the rapidity of its growth, and the presence or absence of actual invasion of organs. Symptoms resulting from mediastinal lesions typically vary according to the degree of functional disturbance of mediastinal organs.

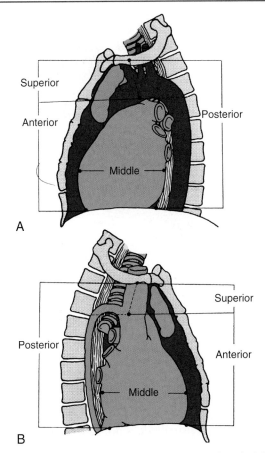

FIGURE 42-19. **A,** Mediastinal compartments as seen from the left hemithorax. **B,** Mediastinal compartments as seen from the right hemithorax.

Respiratory Symptoms

In a mediastinal lesion in a child, respiratory symptoms are the most prominent, resulting from direct compression on the respiratory tract. Such pressure causes narrowing of the trachea or bronchi or compression of the lung parenchyma (Fig. 42-20). Life-threatening tracheal compression represents an emergent need for intervention. Dry cough may be present; stridor or wheeze may occur simultaneously or may precede it. Compression may be sufficient to cause distal obstructive emphysema or atelectasis, pneumonitis, or chronic recurrent lower respiratory tract infections with associated fever and leukocytosis. The dry cough may be replaced by a productive one with mucoid sputum, which becomes purulent if infection occurs. The unilateral nature of the wheezing and respiratory complaints serves to rule out asthma, bronchiolitis, and chronic recurrent infections secondary to cystic fibrosis or hypogammaglobulinemia but does not eliminate the possibility of endobronchial or endotracheal lesions; nor can the possibility of a foreign body in the tracheobronchial tree be discarded. Bronchoscopy is necessary to make this differentiation.

Dyspnea is a common symptom of mediastinal tumors. Acute episodes of dyspnea with associated pneumonitis may occur when there is tracheal or bronchial obstruction, leading to distal infection. Hemoptysis occurs in fewer than 10% of mediastinal tumors in children. If the lesion in the mediastinum exerts pressure on the recurrent laryngeal nerve, hoarseness and a brassy cough result.

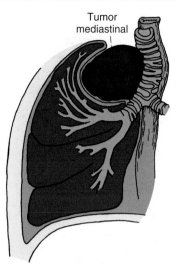

FIGURE 42-20. Diagram illustrating a large mediastinal tumor or cyst with pressure on the tracheobronchial tree as well as on the pulmonary parenchyma. Such a condition might possibly give rise to pulmonary symptoms.

Gastrointestinal Symptoms

Symptoms referable to the gastrointestinal tract result primarily from pressure on the esophagus. Regurgitation of food and dysphagia with a slight sensation of sticking in the lower esophagus are common. Displacement of the esophagus usually does not cause dysphagia; however, it may occur if there is fixation of the mass secondary to infection, hemorrhage, or malignant degeneration, thereby causing interference with the peristaltic activity of the esophagus.

Neurologic Symptoms

Older children often describe a feeling of vague intrathoracic discomfort, fullness, or ache caused by pressure on the sensitive intercostal nerves. Such pain may be mild or severe and is common in tumors of neurogenic origin. The appearance of herpes zoster may indicate involvement of an intercostal nerve, but this is not common in the pediatric age group. When lesions impinge on the pleura, the pain may be pleuritic. Erosion of vertebrae causes a boring pain located in the interscapular area. A malignant lesion that invades the brachial plexus causes severe pain in the upper extremities; the presence of Horner syndrome indicates involvement of the cervical sympathetic nerves. Inflammation, intracystic hemorrhage, or malignant degeneration causing pressure on the phrenic nerve may result in hiccups. Certain dumbbell tumors of the spinal cord and mediastinum may result in symptoms referable to spinal cord pressure.

Vascular Symptoms

Benign lesions of the mediastinum rarely cause obstruction of the great vessels in the mediastinum; however, obstruction is a common finding in malignant mediastinal tumors and carries a poor prognosis. Superior vena caval involvement gives rise to a dilatation of veins in the upper extremity, head, and neck. As the obstruction progresses, cyanosis of the head and neck area occurs in association with headaches and tinnitus. Either innominate vein may be involved, causing unilateral venous distention and edema of the ipsilateral upper extremity, head, and neck. Obstruction of the inferior vena cava is less common, but when present is associated with edema of the lower extremities.

Miscellaneous Symptoms

Fever is uncommon in mediastinal lesions unless there is secondary infection in the tracheobronchial tree; it is also seen with Hodgkin's disease, lymphosarcoma, and degeneration of malignant disease. Weight loss, malaise, anemia, and anorexia are uncommon unless there is malignancy.

Physical Findings

Often, there are no unusual physical findings; wheeze, rhonchi, or rales may occasionally be present. There may be dullness to percussion over the area of mediastinal enlargement, extending laterally from each sternal border or posteriorly between the scapulas and above the diaphragm. Occasionally, there is tenderness over the chest wall, when a mediastinal tumor exerts pressure on the parietal pleura in that area.

Diagnostic Procedures

The diagnostic procedures used for suspected lung lesions also apply for mediastinal tumors. The widespread use of and rapid improvements in CT scan and MRI have greatly aided the understanding of lesions and adjacent mediastinal structures.

A tumor or lesion of the mediastinum should not be aspirated preoperatively if an operation is clearly indicated. Needle aspiration should be reserved for inoperable tumors and for emergencies in which tremendous cystic enlargement may jeopardize the child's life, or may interfere with the induction of anesthesia.

Serum α-fetoprotein and β-human chorionic gonadotropin levels may aid with the diagnosis of germ cell tumors.

Hydatid disease is not common in the United States, and only when it is present in the lung adjacent to the mediastinum can mediastinal tumor be considered. The precipitin and skin test results are positive with an active hydatid cyst. Hooklets have been found in the sputum of patients so affected.

Mediastinal abscess is rarely confused with a neoplasm of the mediastinum. With abscess, there is usually a history of trauma, foreign body in the esophagus, or use of surgical or gastroscopic instruments in the area. High fever, tachycardia, dyspnea, extreme weakness, and prostration usually develop rapidly; thus, the signs and symptoms of acute infection are paramount. The development of an air-fluid level in the mediastinum is diagnostic of mediastinal abscess if the preceding physical findings are also present. Intensive antibiotic therapy and prompt surgical drainage are indicated. There may be masses in the neck secondary to extension from lesions within the mediastinum.

Primary Mediastinal Cysts

Lesions occurring within the mediastinum may be predominantly cystic or predominantly solid. Cystic lesions are usually benign; solid lesions have higher malignant

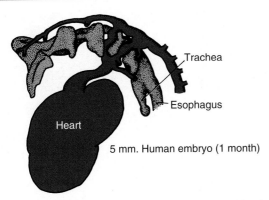

FIGURE 42-21. The foregut, which lies between the tracheal and esophageal buds, is the probable site of embryologic maldevelopment, which gives rise to the growth of foregut cysts.

potential. Primary mediastinal cysts likely represent abnormalities in embryologic development at the site of the foregut just when separation of esophageal and lung beds occurs (Fig. 42-21).

Structures that arise from the foregut are the pharynx, thyroid, parathyroid, thymus, respiratory tract, esophagus, stomach, upper part of the duodenum, liver, and pancreas; thus, abnormal development at this stage may give rise to bronchogenic cysts, esophageal duplication cysts, and gastroenteric cysts.

Bronchogenic Cysts

Maier[20] classified bronchogenic cysts according to location (Fig. 42-22) as tracheal, hilar (Fig. 42-23), carinal (Fig. 42-24), esophageal, and miscellaneous (Fig. 42-25). This classification remains useful. Modern nomenclature also uses the term *foregut duplication cysts,* a correct embryologic description of their developmental origin.

Bronchogenic cysts are usually located in the middle mediastinum but have been described in all mediastinal locations. Under microscopic examination, bronchogenic cysts may contain any or all of the tissues normally present in the trachea and bronchi (fibrous connective tissue, mucous glands, cartilage, smooth muscle, and a lining formed by ciliated pseudostratified columnar epithelium or stratified squamous epithelium). The fluid inside the cyst is either clear waterlike liquid or viscous gelatinous material.

Bronchogenic cysts are usually asymptomatic. There may, however, be frequent upper respiratory tract infections, vague feelings of substernal discomfort, and respiratory difficulty (cough, noisy breathing, dyspnea, and possibly cyanosis). Bronchogenic cysts may communicate with the tracheobronchial tree and show varying air-fluid levels accompanied by the expectoration of purulent material. If communication with the tracheobronchial tree is present, it may be visualized using bronchoscopy.

On radiographic examination, the bronchogenic cyst is usually a single, smooth-bordered, spherical mass (Fig. 42-26). It has a uniform density similar to that of the cardiac shadow. Calcification is unusual. Fluoroscopic examination of the cyst may demonstrate that it moves with respiration (due to attachment to the tracheobronchial tree); its shape may alter during the cycles of respiration. These lesions are occasionally identified on prenatal ultrasound.

When the bronchogenic cyst is located just below the carina, it may cause severe respiratory distress due to compression of either one or both major bronchi (Fig. 42-27). Early diagnosis and prompt removal are necessary.

There are no meticulous population-based studies of bronchogenic cysts, so incidence is conjecture. Phillipart and Farmer assembled perhaps the best composite review of all mediastinal masses; some 7% of mediastinal tumors were bronchogenic cysts.[21]

Bronchogenic cysts should be treated by surgical removal. Like most discrete lesions, most of these can be handled with thoracoscopic techniques. Regardless of approach, care must be taken when these lesions share a common wall with either the airway or the esophagus. If there has been antecedent infection, resection is complicated, as normal tissue planes may be obliterated.

Esophageal Cysts (Duplication)

Esophageal cysts are located in the posterior mediastinum; they are usually on the right side and are intimately associated in the wall of the esophagus (Fig. 42-28). They occur more frequently in males than in females.

There are two types of esophageal cysts; the more characteristic type resembles adult esophagus with the cyst lined by noncornified stratified squamous epithelium having a well-defined muscularis mucosae and striated

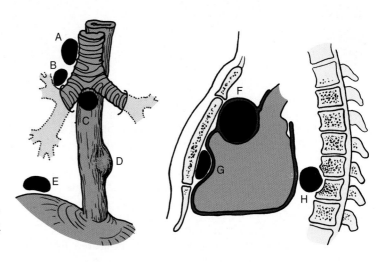

FIGURE 42-22. Diagram illustrating the location of bronchogenic cysts, as suggested by Maier.[20] Sites **B** and **C** are the ones most commonly reported. (From Maier HC. Bronchogenic cysts of the mediastinum. *Ann Surg.* 1948;127:476-502.)

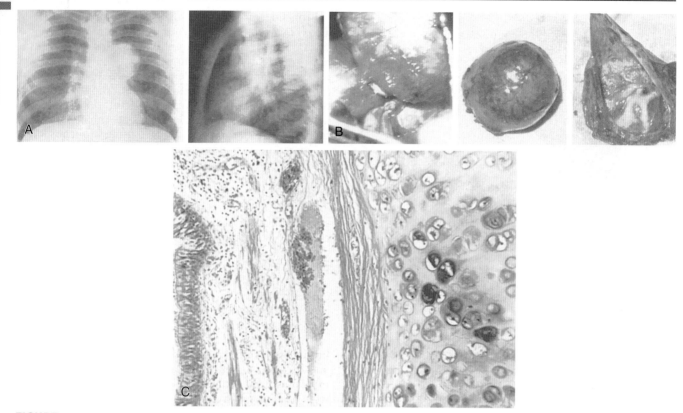

FIGURE 42-23. A, Typical left hilar bronchogenic cyst with a rounded, smooth border and a density similar to cardiac density. **B,** At the time of thoracotomy, a solid stalk was found attached to the left main bronchus. The cyst was unilocular and contained thick, yellowish mucoid material. The wall was thin with typical trabeculations. **C,** Microscopic study revealed cartilage, smooth muscle, and pseudostratified, ciliated, columnar epithelium.

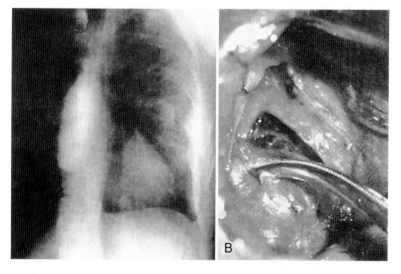

FIGURE 42-24. A, Overexposed posteroanterior chest radiograph shows a carinal bronchogenic cyst. **B,** At the operation, the location is clearly seen at the carina. A solid fibrous stalk is attached at the carina and is separated just beneath the instrument dissector.

muscle in the wall. Intimate association in the muscular wall of the esophagus is not, however, accompanied by communication with the lumen of the esophagus.

The second type is lined by ciliated mucosa, thus resembling the fetal esophagus. Esophageal cysts may be associated with mild dysphagia and regurgitation but usually are asymptomatic. Barium esophagram shows smooth indentation of the esophagus. On esophagoscopy, there is indentation of the normal mucosa by a pliable, movable, soft extramucosal mass. Removal is indicated for

the same reasons as bronchogenic cysts; thoracoscopic techniques are similar. Technically, these lesions may be more difficult to excise, especially if they are extensive or cross the diaphragm.

Gastroenteric Cysts

The third type of cyst arising from the foregut is the gastroenteric, which typically lies in the posterior mediastinum against the vertebrae. Such cysts are typically posterior or lateral to and free of the esophagus, with

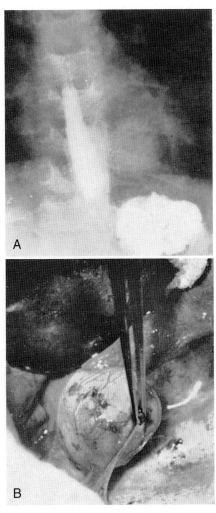

FIGURE 42-25. Bronchogenic cyst in a child. **A,** Radiograph. **B,** Photograph at surgery. The cyst is located retropleurally, overlying the distal thoracic aorta, and is not attached to the respiratory tract or esophagus.

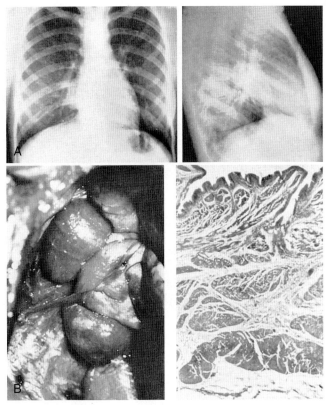

FIGURE 42-27. **A,** Bronchogenic cyst in a child whose mother had tuberculosis. The child was treated with anti-tuberculosis drugs for 1 year without change. **B,** A dumbbell-shaped bronchogenic cyst was found in the region of the inferior pulmonary vein during an operation. The microscopic section shows a wall with ciliated epithelium, no cartilage, and a smooth muscle wall of two layers.

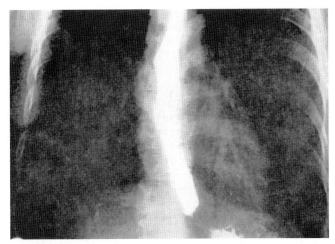

FIGURE 42-26. Esophogram of a hilar bronchogenic cyst with an esophageal indentation.

attachments posteriorly. The normal fetal esophagus is lined by columnar epithelium, much of which is ciliated, which only gradually converts to the stratified epithelium of the mature organ. The change is generally complete or almost complete at birth. Thus, if a cyst arises from the embryonic esophagus, it has a ciliated lining.

The enteric nature of a posterior mediastinal cyst is moderately certain if microscopic examination reveals a frank gastric or intestinal type of epithelium, but a better indication of the nature and origin is the presence of well-developed muscularis mucosae, and two or even three main muscle coats. Gastric glands are common, but esophageal, duodenal, or small-intestinal glands may also be found. At operation, the cyst sometimes seems grossly "stomach-like" or "bowel-like." Cysts encountered in the posterior mediastinum show a highly developed mesodermal wall and even the presence of Meissner's and Auerbach's plexuses, whereas the lining epithelium varies from columnar ciliated to typical small intestinal. Two types of gastroenteric cysts have been described: (1) acid-secreting cysts, which are functionally active, and (2) cysts in which the mucosa has no functional activity.

Males are predominantly affected with this abnormality. Unlike other foregut cysts, posterior gastroenteric cysts are usually symptomatic. The symptoms are usually due

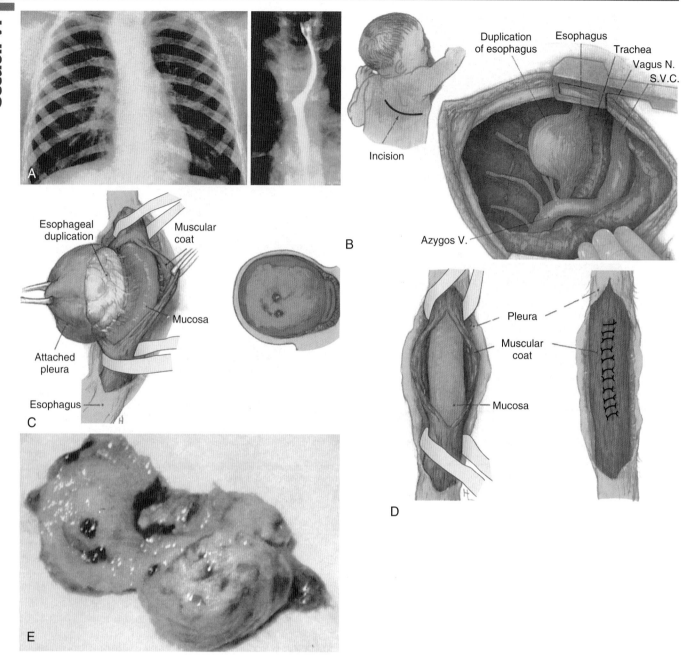

FIGURE 42-28. A, Posteroanterior chest radiograph taken of a child with an upper respiratory tract infection. A mass is seen in the posterior superior mediastinum presenting into the right hemithorax. At the time of an esophogram, the esophagus is seen displaced toward the left by a smooth mass. **B** to **D,** Drawings of findings at the operation. Note the plane of separation from the mucosa of the esophagus and the lack of communication with the esophageal lumen. **E,** An opened operative specimen, the cavity of which was filled with mucoid fluid. The lining of the duplication was typical squamous epithelium.

to pressure on thoracic structures or rupture into bronchi with massive hemoptysis and death. Actual peptic perforation of the lung with hemorrhage has been reported.

Hemoptysis in young infants is difficult to distinguish from hematemesis; it may follow ulceration of a gastroenteric cyst (with gastric lining) of the mediastinum, with subsequent erosion into the lung. Gastric epithelium associated with intestinal or respiratory epithelium is apparently less secretory. Many functional cysts may lose their functional activity when the secretory areas of the mucosa are destroyed. Renin, pepsin, chlorides, and free hydrochloric acid have been demonstrated in the contents of some of the cysts.

Posterior gastroenteric foregut cysts of the mediastinum are frequently associated with two other types of congenital anomalies: mesenteric abnormalities and vertebral abnormalities. When these are suspected, MRI is the preferred diagnostic test. Both types may occur in the same case. In the embryo, the notochord and the endoderm are at one time in intimate contact; thus, this combined developmental anomaly may result from abnormal embryonic development.

Penetration of the diaphragm by a cyst arising primarily from the thorax may occur; conversely, penetration of the diaphragm by the free end of an intramesenteric intestinal duplication is also possible.

A survey of the literature confirms that as many as two thirds of patients with mediastinal cysts have vertebral anomalies including hemivertebra, spina bifida anterior, or infantile scoliosis. Most of these vertebral lesions involve the upper thoracic and lower cervical vertebrae, and the cyst tends to be caudal to the vertebral lesion. MRI may be helpful in demonstrating these lesions. The presence of spina bifida anterior, congenital scoliosis, Klippel-Feil syndrome, or similar but less well-defined lesions in the cervical or dorsal vertebrae suggests enteric cysts in the mediastinum or abdomen.

Pericardial Coelomic Cysts

These mesothelial cysts are developmental in origin, and persistence is related to the pericardial coelom. The primitive pericardial cavity forms by the fusion of coelomic spaces on each side of the embryo. During the process, dorsal and ventral parietal recesses are formed. Dorsal recesses communicate with the pleuro-peritoneal coelom, and the ventral recesses end blindly at the septum transversum. Persistence of segments of the ventral parietal recess accounts for most pericardial coelomic cysts.

The cysts are usually located anteriorly in the cardiophrenic angles, more frequently on the right, and occasionally on or in the diaphragm (Fig. 42-29). They are usually asymptomatic and are discovered on routine chest radiograph. Rarely do they reach sufficient size to cause displacement of the heart or to produce pressure on the pulmonary tissue. Infection is unusual.

Pericardial cysts are usually unilocular. The walls are thin, and the intersurfaces are smooth and glistening, lined by a single layer of flat mesothelial cells. The mesothelium is supported by fibrous tissue with attached adipose tissue.

These cysts are very rare; only two have been reported in children. Because these cysts are benign, observation may be warranted. Alternatively, thoracoscopic excision can be undertaken.

Intrathoracic Meningoceles

Intrathoracic meningoceles are not true mediastinal tumors or cysts; they are diverticuli of the spinal meninges that protrude through the neuroforamen adjacent to an intercostal nerve and manifest beneath the pleura in the posterior medial thoracic gutter. The wall represents an extension of the leptomeninges, and the content is cerebrospinal fluid. Enlargement of the intervertebral foramen is common; vertebral or rib anomalies adjacent to the meningocele are also frequent. The most commonly associated anomalies are kyphosis, scoliosis, and bone erosion or destruction. The wall of these cysts is formed by two distinct components, the dura mater and the arachnoidea spinalis, with small nerve trunks and ganglia occasionally incorporated in it.

A syndrome of generalized neurofibromatosis (Von Recklinghausen's disease), kyphoscoliosis, and intrathoracic meningocele may occur, but thoracic meningocele as an isolated defect is much less frequent; four pediatric cases have been reported. This lesion is usually

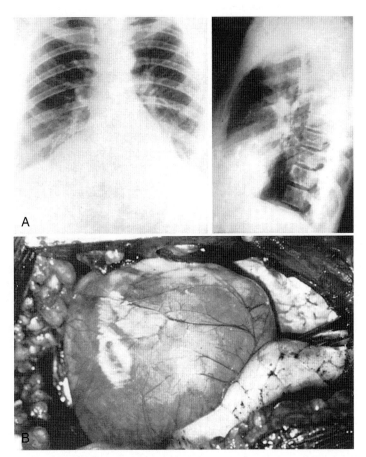

FIGURE 42-29. **A,** Typical location of a pericardial cyst in postero-anterior and lateral chest radiographs at the right cardiophrenic angle. **B,** A large cyst seen at the time of a thoracotomy.

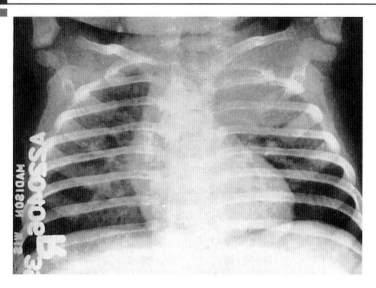

FIGURE 42-30. Mild respiratory distress in an infant with an enlarged thymus. Gradual improvement occurred with age and no specific therapy.

asymptomatic; it occurs on the right side approximately three times more often than on the left. Rarely, the lesion may be bilateral. In patients with neurofibromatosis, posterior sulcus tumors are usually meningoceles and rarely neurofibromas.

On radiograph examination, the lesion is a regular, well-demarcated intrathoracic density located in the posterior sulcus; associated congenital anomalies of the spine and thorax may be noted. On fluoroscopic examination, pulsations may be noted in the sac. Diagnosis may be confirmed by myelograms or MRI.

When diagnosis is securely established, no therapy is indicated unless the lesion is symptomatic. Operative complications such as empyema, meningitis, and spinal fluid fistula have been greatly reduced with appropriate antibiotic therapy.

Tumors of the Thymus

Normally, the thymus is located in the anterior superior mediastinum, but abnormalities of the thymus have been reported in all areas of the mediastinum. Abnormalities of the thymus in children are: (1) hyperplasia, (2) neoplasms, (3) benign thymomas, (4) cysts, (5) teratoma, and (6) tuberculosis.

Hyperplasia of the Thymus
Hyperplasia of the thymus is the most frequent of the thymic lesions. Because the normal thymus varies greatly in size and with age, *thymic hyperplasia* is a relative term. Steroids, infection, androgens, and irradiation may cause involution; those stimuli that cause hyperplasia are not well understood. As in other ductless glands, variations in size are probably related to patient individuality.

On chest radiograph of normal patients, a thymic shadow of variable size and shape is typically present during the first month of life. The mediastinal shadow in young infants is proportionally wider than in older children and adults because of the proportionally larger heart and thymic shadow. The thymic shadow typically disappears by 1 year of age. Among children older than 4 years of age, 2% still have a recognizable thymus on radiograph

examination. Calcifications are not present, and there are transmitted pulsations on fluoroscopy. Cervical extension of the thymus gland is common. If the thymus is located in the superior thoracic inlet, its enlargement may cause tracheal compression (Fig. 42-30).

In the unusual situation in which an enlarged thymus causes respiratory obstruction, treatment may be carried out in one of three ways. While the thymus does respond rapidly to small doses of irradiation (70 to 150 cGy), the concern of a carcinogenic effect has caused this method of treatment to be abandoned. Corticosteroids cause a rapid decrease in the size of the thymus, usually within 5 to 7 days. However, after cessation of corticosteroid therapy, the gland may reach a size greater than that before treatment was instituted. Such a response may also be used in distinguishing between a physiologic enlargement of the thymus and a neoplasm (Fig. 42-31). Excision may be indicated both for the treatment of respiratory obstruction and for diagnosis.

Neoplasm of the Thymus
Malignant thymic tumors in children are quite rare. Lymphosarcoma is more frequent; primary Hodgkin's disease of the thymus and carcinoma have both been described. In only one 19-year-old has there been an associated myasthenia gravis syndrome. An ectopic parathyroid carcinoma located in the thymus has been documented.[22]

Benign Thymoma
Rarely, benign thymic tumors have been reported in children, discovered after resection (Fig. 42-32).

Thymic Cysts
Multiple small cysts of the thymus are frequently observed in necropsy material, but large thymic cysts are rare (Fig. 42-33). While they are typically asymptomatic, manifesting themselves after 2 years of age, there have been reports of cysts causing respiratory failure in infants.[23] Techniques and operative approaches are site-specific. Thymic cysts have been resected from a cervical approach (Fig. 42-34).

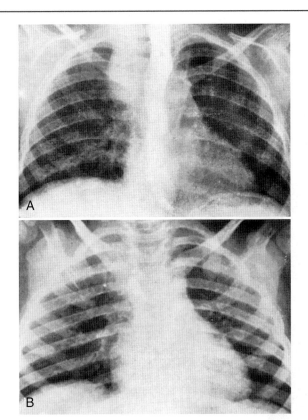

FIGURE 42-31. A, An enlarged thymus in an infant. **B,** A reduction in size can be seen after 7 days of steroid therapy.

Teratoma of the Thymus

Several cases of thymic teratoma have been reported. Patients typically have a good prognosis after resection.[24]

Tuberculosis of the Thymus Gland

A single case of tuberculosis involving only the thymus gland has been described in a stillborn infant.

Teratoid Mediastinal Tumors

Teratoid tumors of the mediastinum may be classified as: (1) benign cystic teratomas, (2) benign teratoids (solid), or (3) teratoids (carcinoma). They make up 10% to 12% of all teratomas and 20% of all mediastinal pediatric neoplasms.[25]

Benign Cystic Teratoma

Teratoma of the anterior mediastinum probably results from faulty embryogenesis of the thymus or from local dislocation during embryogenesis.

Benign cystic teratoma (mediastinal dermoid cyst) contains such elements of ectodermal tissue as hair, sweat glands, sebaceous cysts, and teeth. Other elements, including mesodermal and endodermal tissue, may also be found when benign cystic teratoid lesions are subjected to comprehensive examination; thus, such tumors are more properly classified as teratoid than dermoid cysts.

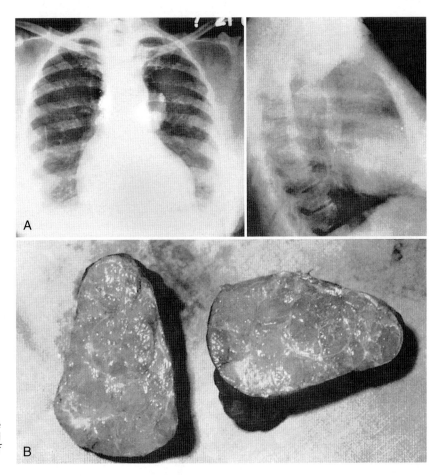

FIGURE 42-32. Benign thymoma located in the anterior superior mediastinum. **A,** Posteroanterior and lateral radiographs before surgery. **B,** Photograph of thymoma after excision.

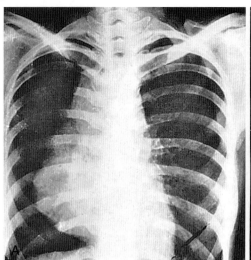
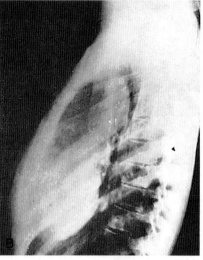

FIGURE 42-33. Large thymic cyst located near the diaphragm in an adult. Posteroanterior **(A)** and left lateral **(B)** radiographs.

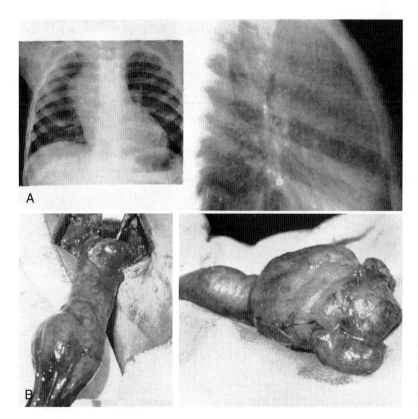

FIGURE 42-34. A, Large thymic cyst in a 4-year-old boy that was evident as a mass in the right side of the neck clinically as well as on a chest x-ray. Removal required a thoracotomy and a supraclavicular incision. **B,** Thymic cyst as seen after a thoracotomy and at the time of removal through a neck incision.

Cystic teratomas are more common than solid ones. These lesions are predominantly located in the anterior mediastinum and may project into either hemithorax, more commonly the right. In children, females are affected more often than males. Malignant degeneration is less common than in the solid form of teratoid tumor.

These cystic masses usually cause symptoms because of pressure on or erosion into the adjacent respiratory structures. Symptoms usually include vague chest discomfort associated with cough, dyspnea, and pneumonitis. Infection may cause a sudden exacerbation of symptoms, and rupture into the lung may occur with expectoration of hair; rupture into the pleura or pericardium may also occur.

On radiograph, the lesion is well outlined, with sharp borders; definite diagnosis on plain radiograph is not possible unless teeth can be demonstrated in the mass. Calcification, which is not unusual, appears as scattered masses rather than as diffuse stippling. Cystic swelling in the suprasternal notch may be visible.

Benign cystic teratomas should be removed. In cases in which infection, perforation, intracystic hemorrhage, or malignant degeneration has occurred, complete removal may be difficult or impossible, owing to adherence to surrounding vital structures.

Benign Solid Teratoid Tumors and Malignant Teratoid Tumors

Teratoma is the most common tumor occurring in the anterior mediastinum of infants and children (Fig. 42-35), and the mediastinum is the second most common location. The solid tumors in the teratoid group are much more complex and have a greater propensity for malignant change (Fig. 42-36). The incidence of malignancy has been reported from 10% to 25%. In addition to standard imaging studies, preoperative serum studies should include serum α-fetoprotein, carcinoembryonic antigen, and β-human chorionic gonadotropin, both as diagnostic markers and as baseline values to monitor disease burden. Patients present with chest pain, cough, dyspnea, and, rarely, hemoptysis.[26] Most mediastinal teratomas are present at birth; many are now detected prenatally. There are also multiple reports of large masses discovered only in adulthood.[27]

Benign solid teratoid tumors have well-differentiated structures that are rarely observed in malignant tumors. The connective tissue stroma of malignant teratoma is usually poorly arranged, but that of benign teratoma is dense and of the adult type. In the benign type, nerve tissue, skin, and teeth may be found. Skin and its appendages are usually present and remarkably well formed. Hair follicles preserve their normal slightly oblique position relative to the free surface and are always accompanied by well-developed sebaceous glands. Sweat glands, often of the apocrine type, are frequently located near the sebaceous glands. Smooth muscle closely resembling arrectores pilorum is occasionally encountered.

Mesodermal derivatives, such as connective tissue, bone, cartilage, and muscle arranged in organoid pattern, are frequently found. When present, hematopoietic tissue is found only in association with cancellous bone. Smooth muscle is most often observed as longitudinal or circular bundles in organoid alimentary structures. Occasionally, it is also seen in bronchial walls. Endodermal derivatives representing such structures as intestine and respiratory and pancreatic tissue are also present.

The final diagnosis of malignancy can be determined only after removal and histologic study of the tumor. Malignant degeneration typically involves only one of the cellular components. In general, the outcome is poor with malignant teratomas, chemotherapy and radiotherapy notwithstanding, which usually consists of etoposide, bleomycin, and cisplatin.[25]

Neurogenic Mediastinal Tumors

Neurogenic tumors, by far the most common tumors with posterior mediastinal origin, make up 25% to 35% of all mediastinal tumors. They have highly variable behavior, sometimes spontaneously regressing, undergoing differentiation, or proliferating to malignant disease. They may be classified as follows:

1. Neurofibroma and neurilemoma
   * Malignant schwannoma
2. Tumors of sympathetic origin
   * Neuroblastoma
   * Ganglioneuroma
   * Ganglioneuroblastoma
   * Pheochromocytoma
3. Chemodectoma

Benign neurofibromas, neurilemomas, and malignant schwannomas are extremely unusual in the pediatric age group, and when present they are most often asymptomatic (Fig. 42-37).

A neuroblastoma is a malignant tumor arising from a neural crest origin; the usual site is the adrenal medulla, but it may occur anywhere along the ganglia of the sympathetic nervous system from neck to pelvis. Although a primary neuroblastoma may cause the first clinical signs or symptoms (such as Horner's syndrome or respiratory distress), metastases in the bone, skin, or lymph nodes can also be the first indication of its presence. While most other childhood cancers have shown marked improvement in survival over the last 3 decades, neuroblastoma has not. Infants younger than 1 year of age do have a relatively better prognosis and respond better to chemotherapy, which tends to be ineffective for most patients. The International Neuroblastoma Staging System, adopted in 1988, relies on complete surgical resection along with lymph node and distal metastases to dictate treatment.[28] The ganglioneuroma is a benign tumor made up of mature ganglion cells, few or many, in a stroma of nerve fibers. Ganglioneuroblastoma is a tumor composed of various proportions of neuroblastoma and ganglioneuroma.

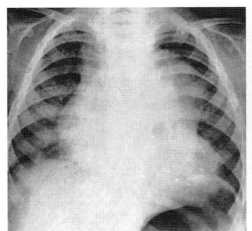 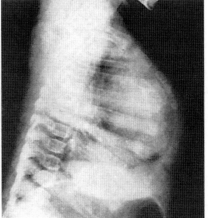

FIGURE 42-35. Large, solid, benign teratoma in an infant. Note the anterior mediastinal position and the forward displacement of the sternum.

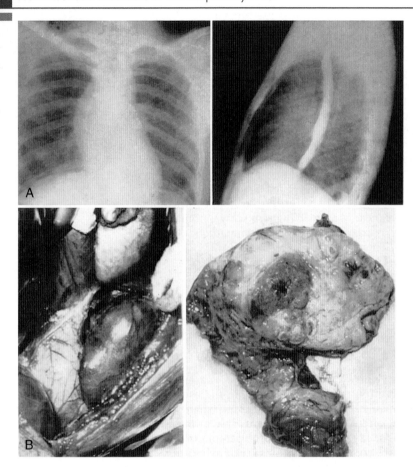

FIGURE 42-36. A, Posteroanterior and lateral radiographs of an anterior malignant teratoma in an older child. **B,** Note the anterior mediastinal position, with the teratoma wedged between the heart and the sternum.

Ganglioneuroma and ganglioneuroblastoma are more likely to present after 2 years of age. The more malignant forms, such as neuroblastoma, frequently become manifest before the age of 2 years. Ganglioneuroma is more common in children than in adults; respiratory symptoms are rare (Fig. 42-38).

Most of these tumors usually occur in the upper two thirds of the hemithorax and tend to extend locally. They may grow into the lower part of the neck and across the midline through the posterior mediastinum to the opposite hemithorax, descend through the diaphragm into the upper part of the abdomen or into the intercostal spaces posteriorly, and involve one or several of the vertebral foramina.

While some such tumors are discovered incidentally, symptoms such as radicular pain, paraplegia, motor disturbances, and Horner syndrome may be the presenting complaint. Upper respiratory tract infections, dyspnea, elevated temperature, and weight loss may occur. Neurogenic tumors of the neuroblastoma group usually occur in younger children, and respiratory symptoms, thoracic pain, and fever are more common (Fig. 42-39).

On radiographic examination, neurogenic tumors are round, oval, or spindle-shaped and are characteristically located posteriorly in the paravertebral gutter. On thoracic radiographs, a ganglioneuroma appears as an elongated lesion and may extend over a distance of several vertebrae. Typically, a neurofibroma tends to be more rounded in outline. Calcifications within the tumor may

be seen, more commonly in the malignant forms. Even though not demonstrated on radiographic examination, calcification may be found at the time of histologic examination. Bone lesions, such as intercostal space widening, costal deformation, vertebral involvement, and metastatic bone disease, are not uncommon. Staging with CT or MRI scans is routine and well proscribed in oncologic protocols.

The primary therapy for localized thoracic neurogenic tumors is surgical excision. Ganglioneuroma (benign) are generally amenable to resection. In malignant neurogenic tumors, all possible tumor should be excised and postoperative irradiation therapy initiated. Radiotherapy must be given judiciously because growth disturbances, pulmonary fibrosis, and other sequelae may develop. In the hourglass type of tumor, with intravertebral foramina extension, diagnostic CT myelogram is followed by laminectomy and excision of the extradural tumor to relieve spinal cord compression. Excision of the mediastinal component may be delayed for several days.

Mediastinal chemodectomas are usually located anteriorly; they are likely to be associated with similar tumors in the carotid body and elsewhere. There is a tendency for these tumors to be multiple. Mediastinal pheochromocytomas make up less than 1% of all mediastinal tumors; extra-adrenal pheochromoctyomas are more common in children than in adults. The tumor may be a cause of refractory hypertension in children as in adults.[29]

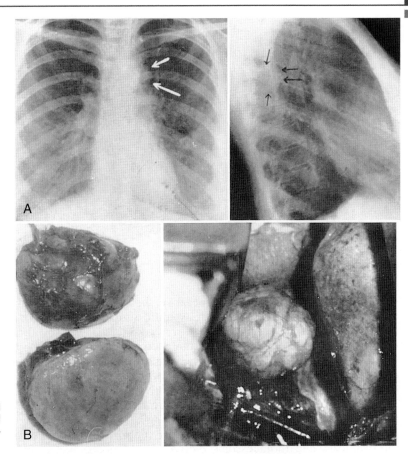

FIGURE 42-37. A, Neurofibroma seen posteriorly located in posteroanterior and lateral radiographs. **B,** Note the solid nature of the lesion, its round smooth outline, and its attachment to the intercostal nerve.

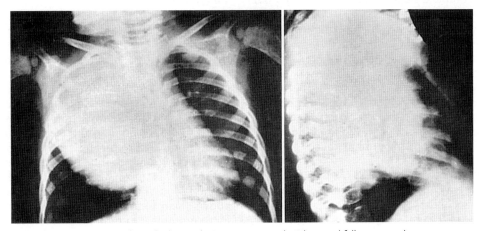

FIGURE 42-38. Large ganglioneuroma in an infant. The benign lesion was removed, with a good follow-up result.

Mediastinal Lymph Node Abnormalities

Abnormalities of the lymph nodes in the mediastinum may be classified as follows:
1. Leukemia
2. Hodgkin's disease
3. Lymphosarcoma
4. Sarcoidosis
5. Inflammatory disorders
   - Fungus
   - Nonspecific

Any lymph node enlargement in a child should be viewed with suspicion, since lymphatic tumors are one of the more frequently observed malignant growths in childhood. The diagnosis is made by biopsy. Hodgkin's disease, lymphosarcoma, and reticulum cell sarcoma group are found primarily in children older than 3 years of age, with a peak incidence from 8 to 14 years of age. More than 95% of children with primary lymphatic malignancy have lymph node enlargement as the presenting sign. Tonsillar hypertrophy and adenoidal hyperplasia, pulmonary hilar enlargement, splenomegaly, bone pain, unexplained fever, anemia, infiltrative skin lesions, and, rarely, central nervous system symptoms may also be present. The diagnosis should be sought through the study of peripheral blood smears, lymph node biopsy, pleural fluid examination, or bone marrow examination.

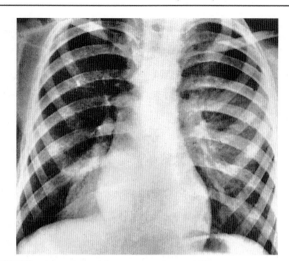

FIGURE 42-39. Neuroblastoma in a 6-year-old boy.

If all other diagnostic studies are negative, the mediastinal node can be biopsied. Fine-needle aspiration is usually not satisfactory, thus Tru-cut biopsy (directly, via mediastinoscopy, thoracoscopy, or anterior thoracotomy) is frequently required. Importantly, anesthetic management is complicated if there is greater than 50% tracheal luminal compression.

In most cases of mediastinal malignancy, bilateral hilar nodal involvement is present. Routine imaging studies, blood smear, and bone marrow studies may not provide the diagnosis, and thoracoscopic biopsy may be necessary. If localized, complete excision should be carried out if technically feasible.

Surgical excision has limited value in lymphosarcoma because the disease is usually widespread. However, when the lesions are apparently isolated in the neck, axilla, mediastinum, or gastrointestinal tract, removal makes sense. With few exceptions, all the tumors in this group are radiosensitive but not curable by radiation therapy. Chemotherapy for Hodgkin's disease currently relies on "tailored therapy" in which the goal is to limit the cumulative dose while maintaining maximum efficacy.[30]

Inflammatory Disorders

Lymph node enlargement in the hilus of the lung or mediastinum may be secondary to tuberculous, fungal, or bacterial lung disease. Diagnosis is usually confirmed by means of sputum culture, examination of bronchoscopic washings from the tracheobronchial tree, scalene node biopsy, and skin tests correlated with the general clinical picture. The same is true in sarcoidosis, where there may be involvement of the eye, skin, peripheral lymph nodes, mediastinal or hilar lymph nodes, and the lung parenchyma. Although nonspecific symptomatic or asymptomatic enlargement of the mediastinal lymph nodes may occur, a cause can usually be identified.

Castleman disease, or giant lymph node hyperplasia, was first described in 1954. Although this rare, benign, localized lymph node enlargement may occur in extrathoracic locations, it most often occurs as an isolated asymptomatic mediastinal or pulmonary hilar tumor. Grossly, the tumors are moderately firm and usually well encapsulated. Calcification may occur but is unusual.

On microscopic examination, the two main features of these lymphoid masses are a diffuse follicular replacement of the lymph node architecture and much follicular and interfollicular vascular proliferation. Sixty percent of patients with this entity are asymptomatic. When symptoms occur, they may include cough, fatigue, chest pain, and fever. Surgical excision is the treatment of choice and is usually curative.

Vascular-Lymphatic Abnormalities of the Mediastinum

Vascular-lymphatic abnormalities of the mediastinum may be classified as: (1) cavernous hemangioma, (2) hemangiopericytoma, (3) angiosarcoma, or (4) lymphangioma (cystic hygroma).

Vascular tumors isolated to the mediastinum in children are rare; they may occur at any level in the mediastinum but are more frequent in the upper portion of the thorax and in the anterior mediastinum. They are uniformly rounded in appearance and are moderately dense.

Though rare, *isolated* mediastinal lymphangiomas occur more often in infants and children than in adults. These tumors consist of masses of dilated lymphatic channels that contain lymph; they are lined with flat endothelium and are usually multilocular. They may appear to be isolated in the mediastinum (Fig. 42-40) but much more often have an associated cervical component. They may be rather large and unilateral, with lateral masses in the superior mediastinum.

Diagnosis of a cervicomediastinal lymphangioma is aided by physical examination of cervical swelling and radiographic examination of the chest. Periodic fluctuation in size frequently occurs in the cervical location. This is even more characteristic of the combined cervicomediastinal lesions; in these, the cervical component may increase in size during inspiratory movements. Radiographic and fluoroscopic examination may show descent of the mass into the mediastinum on inspiration with prominence in the neck during expiration.

Cystic hygroma confined to the mediastinum is usually discovered as an unanticipated finding on radiographic examination. The soft and yielding nature of the cysts allows them to attain considerable size without producing symptoms. On radiograph there is a somewhat lobulated, smoothly outlined mass; however, it is usually not possible to distinguish lymphangiomas from other benign tumors or cysts of the mediastinum from imaging.

When respiratory infections occur, lymphangiomas may become infected. Such infections are usually controlled by antibiotics or by drainage. Infection may be followed by local fibrosis and the disappearance of the mass. Spontaneous or posttraumatic hemorrhage into a cyst may result in extension of the cyst; this may cause sudden tracheal compression, which is a surgical emergency. Malignant change in lymphangiomas has not been reported.[31]

Surgical excision is the treatment of choice for localized lesions, although it may be challenging due to their tendency to grow around other structures. Incomplete resection assures almost certain recurrence. Extensive

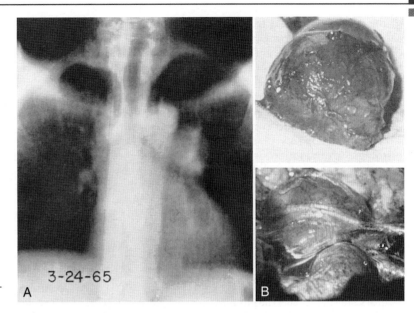

FIGURE 42-40. Large lymphatic cyst in the anterior mediastinum. **A,** Posteroanterior radiograph. **B,** Photographs.

disease remains an unsolved problem; for macrocystic variants, intralesional sclerotherapy has had some utility. Chylothorax may result when there is involvement of the thoracic duct. Anti-angiogenesis therapy has shown some promise in treating angiosarcoma, although further investigation is needed.[32] Sclerotherapy has gained favor in complex cervical lymphangiomas; the same principles should apply to thoracic locations.

Mediastinal Lipoma, Liposarcoma, and Lipoblastoma

Intrathoracic lipoma is rare in children. Lipomas of the mediastinum have been divided into three groups according to their location and form: (1) tumors confined within the thoracic cage, (2) intrathoracic lipomas that extend upward into the neck, and (3) intrathoracic lipomas with an extrathoracic extension forming a dumbbell configuration.

Of the mediastinal lipomas reported in the world literature, 76% were intrathoracic, 10% were cervicomediastinal, and 14% were of the dumbbell type. Only 15 occurred in the pediatric age group, and these were intrathoracic. They may grow to very large size; a mass weighing 7.9 kg has been reported.[33] Seven cases of liposarcoma of the mediastinum in children have been reported.[34] Although these tumors usually do not metastasize, their invasiveness and tendency to recur locally place them in the malignant group.

Lipoblastoma is a rare benign tumor that occurs in children and arises from fetal embryonal fat. Thirty-five cases have been reported in the world literature, only 1 of which was in the mediastinum. Nearly 90% of the tumors are detected in children younger than 3 years of age.[35] At surgery, the lipoblastoma appears as a soft, yellow-gray or white-gray mass that can be easily removed. Histologically, they may be confused for liposarcomas.

Complete surgical excision is the procedure of choice. Repeated surgical attacks may serve as a method of extended control, and radiation therapy may be added for palliative purposes.

THYROID DISORDERS

Substernal thyroid is a somewhat common anterior superior mediastinal tumor in the adult age group but apparently does not occur before puberty. Ectopic thyroid in the mediastinum does occur in children, and in such cases blood supply is derived from a mediastinal vessel.

PRIMARY CARDIAC AND PERICARDIAL TUMORS

Primary tumors of the heart in infants may cause cardiac enlargement or enlargement of the cardiac silhouette, giving rise to symptoms in the lungs or esophagus. Most frequently, the signs and symptoms of congestive heart failure are much more prominent than those of tumors of the respiratory system or esophagus.

Rhabdomyoma appears to be the only cardiac tumor showing a definite predilection for the younger age groups. This is particularly true of children with tuberous sclerosis, in whom rhabdomyoma of the heart is prone to occur. Such tumors are not considered true neoplasms and probably represent an area of developmental arrest in the fetal myocardium. It is not unusual for rhabdomyoma to regress spontaneously without having caused any appreciable impairment of cardiac function.

Myxoma is by far the most common primary tumor of the heart, accounting for slightly more than half of all primary cardiac tumors. It may be encountered at almost any age. The signs and symptoms vary widely but ultimately lead to cardiac failure that does not respond to the usual medical management. Most myxomas are located in the atria, more frequently on the left than on the right. They tend to proliferate and project into the chambers of the heart, preventing normal cardiac filling by obstruction to the mitral or tricuspid valve. The origin appears to be in the atrial septa. Excision on cardiopulmonary bypass is curative.

Primary sarcoma of the heart is less common than myxoma but may occur at any age. As a rule, it does not proliferate into the chambers of the heart; it infiltrates the wall of the myocardium and frequently extends into the pericardial cavity. Other primary tumors of the heart are angioma, fibroma, lipoma, and hamartoma. All are rare and usually produce prominent circulatory symptoms.

An aggressive surgical approach is advised in the management of these cardiac tumors using a variety of surgical techniques ranging from hypothermic circulatory arrest, on pump excision, and even cardiac autotransplantation.

Primary neoplasms of the pericardium are rare. On histologic examination, the predominant tumors are mesotheliomas (endotheliomas) and sarcomas, but leiomyomas, hemangiomas, and lipomas occasionally occur. A single instance of a large cavernous hemangioma of the pericardium has been described in an 8-year-old girl; it was successfully removed.

TUMORS OF THE DIAPHRAGM

Tumors involving the diaphragm may cause chest pain and discomfort or pulmonary compression; thus, they may simulate mediastinal or primary pulmonary neoplasms. Primary tumors of the diaphragm are extremely rare in the pediatric age group, with 41 cases reported in the world literature.[36]

Benign tumors of the diaphragm that have been reported, though not necessarily in children, are lymphangioma, hemangioma, lipoma, fibroma, chondroma, angiofibroma, neurofibroma, rhabdomyofibroma, fibromyoma, and primary diaphragmatic cyst.

Malignant tumors of the diaphragm that have been reported are rhabdomyosarcoma, fibrosarcoma, myosarcoma, leiomyosarcoma, and fibromyosarcoma. None of these tumors appears to have been reported in children.

PRIMARY TUMORS OF THE CHEST WALL

Figures 42-41 and 42-42 illustrate findings seen in two forms of chest wall tumors.

Lipoma of the chest wall is seen in adults but is rare in the pediatric age group. As noted previously, these may be dumbbell in shape, presenting on the chest wall with a large intrathoracic component. Chest radiographs, followed by CT scan, aid in its definition.

Extensive cavernous hemangiomas of the thoracic wall are seen in infancy or childhood. They may be isolated or associated with similar lesions in other tissues, including the lung. When multiple, the diagnosis of Osler-Weber-Rendu syndrome is suggested. Intrathoracic extension of these lesions may occur.

In Von Recklinghausen's disease, multiple cutaneous and subcutaneous nodules are present. Patients with this disease should be carefully studied for the possible coexistence of mediastinal neurofibromas or intrathoracic meningocele.

Rhabdomyosarcoma of the chest wall is often metastatic at presentation, and it carries a high mortality rate (25%) despite recent improvements in adjuvant therapy.[37]

Chondroma and chondrosarcoma are the principal bony tumors of the chest wall; 80% of these occur in the ribs or sternum, usually in the anterior extremity of a rib near the

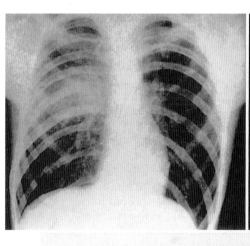
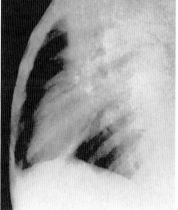

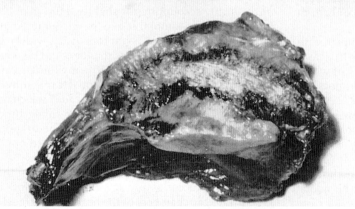

FIGURE 42-41. Reticulum cell sarcoma in the chest wall of an 8-year-old boy. He survived for more than 18 months.

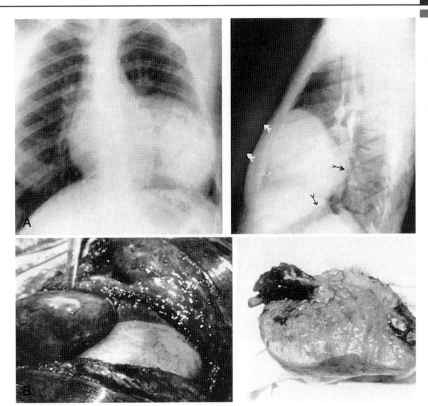

FIGURE 42-42. Desmoid tumor of the chest wall in a child 18 months after patent ductus surgery. The desmoid was in the line of the posterior lateral incision. **A,** Posteroanterior and lateral radiographs. **B,** Photographs.

costochondral junction. They may also occur in the sternum, scapula, clavicle, or vertebral bodies. There may be few, if any, symptoms. Radiographic examination reveals a discrete expansion of the bone with an intact, thinned-out cortex.

Chondrosarcoma of the rib occurs more frequently in males; it is usually seen in the posterior half and paravertebral portion of the rib, but it sometimes involves the transverse process and the vertebral body either primarily or secondarily. The direction of growth occasionally appears to be entirely internal, thus simulating the radiologic appearance of a primary pleural or mediastinal tumor. However, there usually is an externally visible and palpable mass.

Solitary plasmacytoma, a lesion histologically similar to multiple myeloma but localized to a single bone, may involve any part of the thoracic cage; it may involve the vertebrae, rarely invades the ribs, and may involve the lung itself. In solitary plasmacytoma, the bone is thinned and may be greatly expanded.

Ewing's sarcoma with a primary location in a rib is unusual before the second decade of life, with prognosis and treatment similar to tumors found in other sites. Recurrence is common.[38]

Suggested Reading

General

Adzick NS, Flake AW, Crombleholme TM. Management of congenital lung lesions. *Semin Pediatr Surg.* 2003;12:10.

Gushiken BD, Filly RA. Sonography for fetal thoracic intervention. In: Harrison MR, Evans MI, Adzick NS, et al, eds. *The Unborn Patient.* Philadelphia: Saunders; 2001:95.

Harrison MR, Evans MI, Adzick NS, et al, eds. *The Unborn Patient.* Philadelphia: Saunders; 2001.

Hebra A, Othersen HD, Tagge EP. Bronchopulmonary malformations. In: Ashcroft KW, ed. *Pediatric Surgery.* 3rd ed. New York: Saunders; 2000:273.

Rodgers BM, McGahren ED. Laryngoscopy, bronchoscopy, and thoracoscopy. In: Grosfeld JL, O'Neil JA, eds. *Pediatric Surgery.* 6th ed. Philadelphia: Mosby; 2006:971–982.

Rothenberg SS. Experience with thoracoscopic lobectomy in infants and children. *J Pediatr Surg.* 2003;38:102.

Shochat SJ. Tumors of the lung. In: Grosfeld JL, O'Neil JA, eds. *Pediatric Surgery.* 6th ed. Philadelphia: Mosby; 2006:640–648.

Sylvester KG, Albanese CT. Bronchopulmonary malformation. In: Ashcraft K, Murphy P, Holcomb GW, eds. *Pediatric Surgery.* 4th ed. Philadelphia: Saunders; 2004.

Tsao K, Albanese CT, Harrison MR. Prenatal therapy for thoracic and mediastinal lesions. *World J Surg.* 2003;27:77.

Benign Pulmonary Tumors

Adzick NS, Farmer DL. Cysts of the lungs and mediastinum. In: Grosfeld JL, O'Neil JA, eds. *Pediatric Surgery.* 6th ed. Philadelphia: Mosby; 2006:955–970.

Morini F, Quattrucci S, Cozzi DA, et al. Bronchial adenoma: an unusual cause of recurrent pneumonia in childhood. *Ann Thorac Surg.* 2003;76:2085–2087.

Rutter MJ. Evaluation and management of upper airway disorders in children. *Semin Pediatr Surg.* 2006;15:116–123.

Weldon CB, Shamberger RC. Pediatric pulmonary tumors: primary and metastatic. *Semin Pediatr Surg.* 2008;17:17–29.

Primary and Metastatic Malignant Pulmonary Tumors

Dishop MK, Kuruvilla S. Primary and metastatic lung tumors in the pediatric population: a review and 25-year experience at a large children's hospital. *Arch Pathol Lab Med.* 2008;132:1079–1103.

Kayton ML. Pulmonary metastasectomy in pediatric patients. *Thorac Surg Clin.* 2006;16:167–183, vi.

Mediastinal Tumors

Agrawal D, Suri A, Mahapatra AK, et al. Intramedullary neurenteric cyst presenting as infantile paraplegia. A case and review [Comment]. *Pediatr Neurosurg.* 2002;37:93.

Franco A, Mody NS, Meza MP. Imaging evaluation of pediatric mediastinal masses. *Radiol Clin North Am.* 2005;43:325–353.

Laberge J, Puligandla P, Flageole H. Asymptomatic congenital lung malformations. *Semin Pediatr Surg.* 2005;14:16–33.

Rizk T, Lahoud GA, Maarrawi J, et al. Acute paraplegia revealing an intraspinal neurenteric cyst in a child. *Childs Nerv Syst.* 2001;17:754.

Rothstein DH, Voss SD, Isakoff M, et al. Thymoma in a child: case report and review of the literature. *Pediatr Surg Int.* 2005;21:548–551.

Wright CD. Mediastinal tumors and cysts in the pediatric population. *Thorac Surg Clin.* 2009;19:47–61, vi.

Cardiac Tumors

Burke A, Virmani R. Pediatric heart tumors. *Cardiovasc Pathol.* 2008;17:193–198.

DeBusatmante TD, Azpeitia J, Mirailes M, et al. Prenatal sonographic detection of pericardial teratoma. *J Clin Ultrasound.* 2000;28:194.

Diaphragm and Chest Wall Tumors

Cada M, Gerstle JT, Traubici J, et al. Approach to diagnosis and treatment of pediatric primary tumors of the diaphragm. *J Pediatr Surg.* 2006;41:1722–1726.

van Aalst JA, Phillips JD, Sadove AM. Pediatric chest wall and breast deformities. *Plast Reconstr Surg.* 2009;124(suppl 1):38e–49e.

van den Berg H, van Rijn RR, Merks JH. Management of tumors of the chest wall in childhood: a review. J Pediatr Hematol Oncol. 2008;30:214–221.

References

The complete reference list is available online at www.expertconsult.com

43 CHEST WALL AND RESPIRATORY MUSCLE DISORDERS

JEAN-PAUL PRAUD, MD, PHD, GREGORY J. REDDING, MD, AND MARIE FARMER, MD

GENERAL CONSIDERATIONS

Since Lavoisier's stipulation in 1791 that respiration is essentially a phenomenon of oxygen (O_2) consumption and carbon dioxide (CO_2) production, the chest wall has been recognized as the vital pump responsible for the movement of gases between the atmosphere and the lungs. Today, much is known regarding the adaptability of this vital pump to satisfy changing metabolic needs under various physiologic and pathologic conditions (e.g., rest, exercise, and hyperthermia). Patients must overcome adverse conditions that affect chest wall function. These conditions range from the cartilaginous, pliable rib cage of the preterm infant to the scoliotic thorax of the adolescent, and from the weak chest wall in neuromuscular disease to the stiff rib cage in asphyxiating thoracic dystrophy or obesity. This vital pump also participates in numerous functions such as singing, talking, wind instrument playing, coughing, sneezing, load lifting, parturition, and hiccupping, all of which can interfere with lung ventilation.

In normal resting conditions, the diaphragm is the principal muscle used for inspiration while the accessory inspiratory muscles mainly stabilize the rib cage. When the inspiratory workload is increased, additional accessory inspiratory muscles are recruited, thereby producing an upward motion of the ribs resulting in a more pronounced thoracic expansion. Conversely, even during resting breathing, failure to fixate the rib cage will result (as it does in the case of chest wall muscle weakness) in an inward motion of the rib cage (i.e., rib cage paradoxical breathing). In normal resting conditions, expiratory muscles are inactive. During increased demands for air pumping, the expiratory muscles become activated during the second phase of expiration and decrease the end expiratory volume below functional residual capacity (FRC). Any decrease in the force of the expiratory muscles leads to an increased residual volume and decreased vital capacity.

Sleep is responsible for significant modifications in lung mechanics and respiratory muscle control. The passage to the supine position alone leads to a decrease in FRC, mainly caused by the cephalad movement of the abdominal content, and sleep leads to a decrease in tonic activity of intercostal muscles and upper airway muscles, a phenomenon further pronounced in REM sleep. These changes are responsible for paradoxical inward rib cage movement during inspiration in infants due to their compliant rib cage and in patients with neuromuscular disorders. Nocturnal hypoventilation with alteration of blood gases is often the first sign of chronic respiratory failure in progressive neuromuscular disorders such as Duchenne muscular dystrophy.

Respiratory Muscle Fatigue

The respiratory muscles may become fatigued when an imbalance develops between the energy supply to the inspiratory muscles and respiratory work. Loss of energy supply to the muscles results from a severe decrease in systemic arterial pressure or arterial O_2 tension. Alternatively, amyotrophy, rib cage deformity, or increased work to move the chest wall may lead to muscular fatigue and precipitate respiratory failure. In an attempt to avoid fatigue, a patient may opt to use less force per breath, thereby reducing tidal volume and compensating by taking more breaths per minute. Clinical and laboratory evaluation of the chest wall can provide essential information with regard to chest wall function in a particular patient (Table 43-1) and can lead to recognition of respiratory muscle fatigue or respiratory insufficiency. Acute respiratory muscle fatigue is characterized by progressive exhaustion of the respiratory muscles, leading to respiratory failure within minutes or hours. Careful bedside observation of the at-risk patient usually allows the recognition of signs indicating progression of fatigue. These include loss of nonbreathing functions of the respiratory apparatus, inappropriate respiratory rate and pattern of breathing, as well as other warning signs (Table 43-2). Chronic respiratory muscle fatigue is not as easily identified as the acute form, and respiratory symptoms may not correlate well with the degree of respiratory muscle fatigue. General fatigue and dyspnea on exertion can be the first symptoms of chronic respiratory impairment. However, the first manifestations of chronic respiratory muscle impairment often are symptoms of sleep hypoventilation, either nocturnal symptoms (i.e., parasomnias, enuresis, sweating) or daytime symptoms (morning headaches, hypersomnolence, chronic fatigue, decreased attention span, shortness of breath, right ventricular failure). Unfortunately, even a specific questionnaire fails to predict sleep-disordered breathing in children with advanced neuromuscular disorders.[1]

Assessment of Respiratory Function in Children with Chest Wall Dysfunction

Respiratory function must be assessed longitudinally in children with chest wall dysfunction. Routine measurements of lung function usually include spirometry, maximal inspiratory (at the mouth or sniff) and expiratory pressures, peak cough flow and gas exchange, and most often pulse oximetry and end-tidal CO_2. In addition, overnight assessment of respiratory function can be performed at any age via pulse oximetry and transcutaneous or end-tidal CO_2, or by polysomnography.

TABLE 43-1 ASSESSMENT OF CHEST WALL FUNCTION

Clinical Evaluation

Chest wall configuration (e.g., scoliosis, overdistention)
Pattern of spontaneous breathing
- Thoracic and/or abdominal breathing
- Paradoxical thoracoabdominal movements: inspiratory rib cage retraction, paradoxical inspiratory abdominal retraction (unilateral or bilateral)
Specific maneuvers
- Maximal variation in thoracic circumference
- Maximal excursion of diaphragm (inspection and percussion)
- Cough strength?

Laboratory Evaluation

Roentgenograms
- Cinefluoroscopic studies of diaphragmatic movements
- Plain roentgenograms in full expiration and inspiration
Real-time ultrasonography of the diaphragm
Pulmonary function tests
- Pressures: maximal inspiratory pressure (PI_{max}) at mouth, sniff inspiratory pressure, maximal expiratory pressure (PE_{max}) at mouth, transdiaphragmatic pressure
- Peak cough flow
- Lung volumes, forced spirometry
- Variations/coordination of rib cage and abdominal diameter (respiratory inductance plethysmography)
Electromyographic studies of respiratory muscles (magnetic stimulation of phrenic nerve)

TABLE 43-2 CLINICAL SIGNS OF RESPIRATORY MUSCLE FAILURE

Inability to Perform Nonventilatory Functions

Inability to eat/drink/cry
Reluctance to pause breathing voluntarily

Major Use of Accessory Muscles

Sternocleidomastoid muscles, pectoral

Increase in Respiratory Rate to Critical Level

Adolescents	55 breaths/min
Children 4-10 years	70-75 breaths/min
Infants 1-3 years	90 breaths/min
Neonates	120 breaths/min

Signs Reflecting Options Taken to Relieve Fatigue

Shallow breathing
Deep breaths with a brief pause to rest the muscles
Respiratory alternans

Signs Indicating Pending Respiratory Arrest

Cyanotic spell
Cyanosis with brief cough or brief pause
Recurrent apnea
Sustained paradoxical thoracic/abdominal movement
Drooling in absence of airway obstruction (cannot pause to swallow)
Central nervous system signs (confusion)

Other measurements such as muscle electromyography, measurement of esophageal pressure or mouth occlusion pressure, and cervical magnetic stimulation of the phrenic nerve are of interest in research but are not used in clinical practice.

International guidelines for patients with congenital neuromuscular disorders have been developed.[2] It is recommended that forced vital capacity (FVC) be measured annually in the sitting position. When abnormal (FVC <80% predicted), FVC should also be measured in the supine position to investigate for diaphragm weakness (a decrease in FVC >20% from the sitting position). While an FVC between 40% and 60% predicted indicates a low risk of nocturnal hypoventilation, an FVC <40% predicted or diaphragm weakness indicates a significant risk of nocturnal hypoventilation. Combined continuous overnight pulse oximetry and transcutaneous (or end-tidal) PCO_2 should be performed annually in children who are too young for FVC assessment or when the FVC is <60% predicted (and even more often when the FVC is <40% predicted). Full overnight polysomnography should be performed when overnight pulse oximetry + PCO_2 is not diagnostic in the presence of symptoms suggestive of sleep-disordered breathing. Arterial blood gas analysis can be considered in patients with clinical signs of respiratory failure, recurrent or current lower respiratory infection, abnormal overnight pulse oximetry or PCO_2, or an FVC <40% predicted. Peak cough flow should be measured annually during a steady state and during any episode of respiratory infection. While values less than 160 to 200 L/min in older teenagers and adults indicate that cough is ineffective and can place patients at risk of recurrent respiratory infections and respiratory failure, corresponding values are currently unknown in children.

Management of Children with Chest Wall Dysfunction

Adequate nutrition is essential for ensuring adequate functioning of the respiratory muscles. Patients with a chronic condition (e.g., cystic fibrosis, severe asthma, severe Duchenne muscular dystrophy) are commonly malnourished, a state that can lead to muscle atrophy and loss of respiratory muscle capacity to perform the work of breathing. An adequate O_2 supply and the correction of electrolytic imbalance (e.g., hypophosphatemia, hypocalcemia, hypokalemia, acidosis) are also needed for muscles to perform their work. Associated nonrelated respiratory problems (e.g., asthma, allergic rhinitis, enlarged adenoids or tonsils causing sleep-disordered breathing) must be carefully treated. Prevention of respiratory infections must be implemented by ensuring an optimal environment (e.g., avoiding passive smoking and large daycare centers) and by providing a 23-valent pneumococcal polysaccharide vaccine after 2 years of age and an annual flu vaccination. Respiratory muscle training is clearly beneficial in specific conditions in which respiratory muscles are intact, such as in quadriplegic patients following spinal cord injury. However, it must be used with caution in myopathies to avoid further muscle injury; in such cases, swimming and aquatic sports can be recommended without reaching the fatigue threshold, as long as it is physically possible. Assisted cough with lung recruitment techniques, either manually or through the use of the mechanical in-exsufflator

(Cough-assist), are of paramount importance in the management of patients with severe neuromuscular problems, especially during respiratory infections. Ventilatory support has finally become an essential tool for increasing quality of life and prolonging life in severely affected patients with neuromuscular disorders, by resting weakened respiratory muscles. The development of noninvasive intermittent positive pressure using BiPAP ventilation via nasal mask during nocturnal sleep has been especially instrumental in this regard. Current consensus suggests the indication of noninvasive nocturnal ventilatory support for patients with alveolar hypoventilation (e.g., current recommendations for Duchenne muscular dystrophy),[3] and this should be discussed in the presence of failure to thrive or recurrent chest infections (>3 per year). While most experts state that noninvasive mask ventilation is generally preferred, tracheostomy for ventilatory support should be considered in patients with bulbar involvement and severe retention of secretions despite assisted-cough techniques, and those with extreme ventilator dependency or ineffective noninvasive ventilation.[3] Note, however, that the use of tracheostomy can pose ethical dilemmas in patients with very severe disease and short life expectancy, when treatment burden must not outweigh the benefits.

Causes of Chest Wall Dysfunction

Chest wall movements should be envisioned as the result of a chain of effectors that successively transmit the drive to breathe from the respiratory centers to the upper motor neurons of the central nervous system, the lower motor neurons, and finally the respiratory muscle fibers. The central drive to breathe is transformed into a mechanical force resulting from contractions of respiratory muscles, which move the chest wall and generate inspiratory and expiratory pressures responsible for air movement into and out of the lungs. Table 43-3 illustrates the systemic conditions that cause disturbances at these various levels. Neurologic diseases at the level of the central nervous system (upper motor neurons) or at the level of peripheral innervation of the chest wall (lower motor neurons) may lead to secondary dysfunction of the muscular components of the chest wall. The best examples of these entities are hemiplegia, quadriplegia, infantile spinal muscular atrophy, and polyradiculitis (Guillain-Barré syndrome). Myopathies from various types of muscular dystrophy and myasthenia gravis result in failure of the respiratory muscles to produce an adequate contraction. In addition, systemic diseases associated with severe malnutrition may lead to a loss in respiratory muscle mass and force. Malformation of the chest wall architecture as seen in scoliosis, asphyxiating thoracic dystrophy, or advanced cystic fibrosis impairs the transformation of respiratory muscle contraction into adequate pressure because of the malposition of these muscles. Finally, obesity causes an additional mechanical load on both the thoracic and abdominal components of the chest wall and limits its performance capacity.

TABLE 43-3 CAUSES OF CHEST WALL DYSFUNCTION

SITE OF DEFECT	CAUSES
Central drive of breathing	Congenital or acquired
Upper motor neuron	Hemiplegia Cerebral palsy Quadriplegia
Lower motor neuron	Poliomyelitis Spinal muscular atrophies Guillain-Barré syndrome Tetanus Traumatic nerve lesions Phrenic nerve paralysis
Neuromuscular junction	Myasthenia gravis Congenital myasthenic syndromes Botulism Drugs
Respiratory muscles	Muscular dystrophies Congenital myopathies Metabolic myopathies Steroid myopathy Connective tissue disease Diaphragmatic malformation
Nonmuscular, chest wall structures	Scoliosis Congenital rib cage abnormality Overinflated rib cage in COPD Connective tissue disease Thoracic burns Obesity Giant exomphalos

COPD, Chronic obstructive pulmonary disease.

Despite their major differences in pathogenesis, the various entities that cause chest wall dysfunction share some clinical and physiologic features. Chest wall dysfunction leads to restrictive pulmonary disease with reduced lung volume, reduced absolute flow rate values, normal FEV_1/FVC ratio, reduced strength of respiratory muscles, and decreased ventilatory performance in response to exercise. Residual volume can be normal or augmented, depending on normal or decreased strength of the expiratory muscles, respectively. With respiratory muscle strength less than 50% predicted, the decrease in vital capacity is generally greater than expected because of decreased lung compliance (atelectasis) and rib cage compliance (costovertebral and costosternal joint ankylosis). Hypercapnia is usually present during wakefulness when respiratory muscle strength is less than 25% predicted but can occur when weakness is less profound if mechanical loads due to additional respiratory disorders coexist. With less severe disease, hypercapnia may be present during sleep, and patients are at risk of ventilatory failure during critical periods of their lives, such as in the neonatal period, during respiratory infections, following general anesthesia, and during the last trimester of pregnancy.

Finally, diagnosis of the cause of chest wall dysfunction in the floppy newborn/infant can be especially challenging.[4]

■ DISEASES OF THE MOTOR NEURONS

Spinal Cord Injury and Cerebral Palsy

Spinal Cord Injury

Spinal cord injury resulting in quadriplegia can occur at any age, including at birth or after cervical trauma in later childhood. Respiratory complications continue to be the major cause of morbidity and mortality in patients with cervical spinal cord injury.[5,6] The importance of respiratory impairment largely depends on the level of the spinal lesion and associated cerebral injuries, especially brainstem lesions leading to central hypoventilation. Ventilatory support is usually needed during the acute phase of cervical spine injury. Thereafter, patients with high cervical lesions (C1 to C3) invariably require long-term continuous ventilatory support. Younger patients are usually managed by positive pressure ventilation via tracheostomy, sometimes with bilateral diaphragm pacing for daytime ventilatory support, to free the child from the ventilator. In older patients, noninvasive positive pressure ventilation via the nose or mouth has become the first choice for nocturnal ventilatory support when possible, while daytime ventilation is provided either continuously by abdominal displacement ventilator (pneumobelt) or up to several hours by glossopharyngeal breathing. Nocturnal negative pressure ventilation is now used less frequently. On the other hand, patients with lower C5 to C6 spinal lesions can usually be weaned from the ventilator and do not have severe long-term respiratory impairment, despite alterations of intercostal and abdominal muscle function. Patients with C3 to C5 lesions (at the site of phrenic nerve emergence) will have variable respiratory dysfunction. Many patients can eventually be weaned from the ventilator. Breathing exercise programs have also been shown to be of crucial importance in the respiratory rehabilitation of these quadriplegic patients. In addition, assisted-cough techniques (either manually or mechanical in-exsufflation) are an essential addition in the management of quadriplegic patients, especially during respiratory infections.

Cerebral Palsy

The consequences of cerebral palsy on respiratory function are variable, depending on the extent of the cerebral lesions and can include respiratory muscle dysfunction and dystonia, abnormal breathing patterns, lung aspiration, and scoliosis. They are sometimes intermingled with abnormalities related to concomitant bronchopulmonary dysplasia. Upper airway muscle dysfunction can also be responsible for obstructive sleep-disordered breathing and swallowing disorders. Therapeutic options should be tailored to each patient and guided by ethical considerations, in close collaboration with the family.

Spinal Muscular Atrophies

Childhood spinal muscular atrophies (SMA) are a group of autosomal recessive neurodegenerative disorders classified as type I (Werdnig-Hoffman disease), type II, and type III (Kugelberg-Welander disease), based on the age of onset of muscle weakness and clinical severity. SMAs are caused by a mutation in the survival motor neuron (SMN 1) gene, which is responsible for production of the full-length SMN protein that is essential to motor neurons. This mutation is responsible for primary degeneration of the anterior horn cells of the spinal cord and often of the bulbar motor nuclei, which leads to skeletal muscle paralysis and atrophy. When suspected, SMA I, II, and III can be confirmed with a DNA blood test.

Werdnig-Hoffman disease is the most common monogenic cause of death in infancy and the most common severe neuromuscular childhood disorder after Duchenne muscular dystrophy. It has an incidence of about 1:10,000 live births. Clinical manifestations are apparent in the first 6 months of life and sometimes even at birth when the disease has begun *in utero* (which is recognized in retrospect by a reduction in fetal movements). Infants with Werdnig-Hoffman disease have impaired head control, with a weak cry and cough. Intercostal muscle weakness is responsible for paradoxical inward rib cage movement with each inspiration, with the diaphragm being relatively spared. Chest radiographs show a reduced intrathoracic volume and a bell-shaped thorax. Affected patients suffer from swallowing disorders and aspiration and are at risk of recurrent respiratory failure with viral respiratory infections. The prognosis is poor, with 95% of infants dying from respiratory failure by 18 months of age without intensive respiratory intervention. Respiratory management for SMA I patients raises important and unresolved ethical concerns and varies widely between countries and institutions; any therapeutic intervention must aim at increasing quality of life. Mechanical ventilation was traditionally denied by many physicians for fear that the burden of treatment outweighed the benefit. However, a growing number of publications recommend to thoroughly discuss the possibility of long-term mechanical ventilatory support, aiming at defining clear goals in partnership with parents. Thus, chronic, noninvasive ventilation can be used palliatively with the sole goal to facilitate discharge from hospital to home and reduce work of breathing. Otherwise, noninvasive ventilation with high-span BiPAP, often for at least 16 hours per day, can be used in an attempt to prolong life expectancy by improving rib cage deformity, pulmonary function, and lung development. Finally, the highly controversial option of long-term ventilation via tracheotomy may also be discussed with parents, yet underlining the usually associated complete loss of spontaneous breathing capability and the impossibility of language development. Most experts will clearly recommend noninvasive ventilation over tracheotomy in SMA I patients. Respiratory care must always include mechanical in-exsufflation, with the recommendation to use it at least twice daily, and as often as necessary during respiratory infections to maintain $SaO_2 \geq 95\%$, along with increased daytime noninvasive ventilation. Importantly, a written care plan must be decided with the parents in advance with regard to resuscitation and intubation/ventilation in case of a reversible event such as a respiratory infection.[7-11]

SMA Type II is an intermediate form and represents the largest group of SMA patients. Patients usually present with abnormal muscle weakness between 6 months and 1 year of age; they can sit, sometimes independently, but cannot walk. Swallowing disorders, gastric reflux, recurrent atelectasis, and respiratory infections vary in their degree of severity and carry the risk of respiratory failure. In older children, respiratory scoliosis can further aggravate respiratory function. Typically, recurrent pulmonary infections precede nocturnal hypoxemia, nocturnal hypoventilation, and then daytime hypoventilation. With adequate respiratory management tailored to respiratory involvement, including noninvasive ventilation, mechanical in-exsufflation, and prevention of respiratory infections, a good quality of life and lifespan into adulthood is expected for most patients.[7]

Patients with Kugelberg-Welander disease have onset of muscle weakness after 18 months of age and can walk. Respiratory involvement is usually minimal, and a normal lifespan is expected.

Perspectives for Drug Therapy in SMA Patients

In recent years, the availability of new animal models of SMA has significantly contributed to our understanding of the basic mechanisms, which has translated into several phase I and II clinical trials. The SMN protein is encoded by two adjacent and nearly-homologous genes, *SMN 1* and *SMN 2*. While all SMA patients retain one to four copies of *SMN 2*, the latter mainly encodes a truncated SMN protein, which cannot ensure motor neuron survival. Strategies aiming at upregulating SMN 2 promoter activity for higher expression of the SMN protein (e.g., histone deacetylase inhibitors) have generated some therapeutic hope. Unfortunately, phenylbutyrate did not show significant benefit in SMA II and III, and valproic acid showed only limited effects in SMA II. Efforts are now being made to use oligonucleotide technologies for modulating pre-mRNA splicing to get higher rates of inclusion of exon 7 into the processed SMN mRNA from the *SMN 2* gene. Other compounds with neuroprotective effects have been tried. While gabapentin and thyrotropin-releasing hormone have not shown any effect, preliminary data in SMA I suggest that riluzole, a glutamate antagonist, significantly increased life expectancy vs. controls; a larger trial is obviously needed. Overall, while there is no cure for SMA, recent progress in preclinical models offers hope for the development of drug therapy, which is a very active area of research.[12]

SMA with Respiratory Distress Type 1

Finally, an unusual variant of SMA (SMA with respiratory distress type 1 [SMARD1]) has been reported. SMARD1 usually presents at a few weeks of life with acute life-threatening respiratory distress caused by diaphragmatic paralysis.[13] SMARD1 has been retrospectively identified to be responsible for cases of sudden infant death syndrome in consanguineous parents. Peripheral weakness in SMARD1 patients is initially limited to distal lower limb muscles and is not the presenting symptom. Cranial involvement also appears later in the evolution. SMARD1 has been linked to mutations in the gene encoding for the immunoglobulin μ binding protein 2 on chromosome 11q13. This allows prenatal diagnosis and helps in decision making for initiating chronic ventilatory support, knowing the fatal issue of the disease.

Poliomyelitis

The acute disease induced by a poliovirus infection typically occurs in very young children. Destruction of the motor neurons of the spinal cord can result in asymmetrical, irreversible paralysis/paresis of thoracic muscles, with the risk of acute respiratory insufficiency. In addition, bulbar poliomyelitis can result in upper airway obstruction, aspiration, or respiratory failure. Various permanent sequelae, including scoliosis, restrictive pulmonary disease, and respiratory insufficiency can occur. Treatment is only supportive.

Diaphragmatic Paralysis

Diaphragm dysfunction can be due to a wide variety of disorders (Table 43-4), many of which are dealt with in other sections of this chapter or in other chapters of this book. This section will focus on diaphragmatic paralysis caused by phrenic nerve impairment.

Diaphragmatic paralysis generally results from injury to the phrenic nerve during thoracic or neck surgery. Tumors of the mediastinum, peripheral neuropathy, and agenesis of the phrenic nerve are less likely causes. In the newborn, stretching of the root C3 to C5 during breech delivery is a frequent cause, most often in association with brachial plexus injuries (Erb's paralysis). Most diaphragmatic paralyses are on the right side, with bilateral paralysis occurring in only 10% of cases. Diaphragmatic paralysis is responsible for abnormal elevation of the hemidiaphragm and decrease in the space available for the ipsilateral lung. It frequently causes respiratory failure in neonates, whereas it can be asymptomatic in older

TABLE 43-4 CLASSIFICATION OF DIAPHRAGMATIC DISORDERS

Disorders of Innervation

- Traumatic injury to the head or brainstem, cerebral stroke.
- Spinal cord disorders: spinal cord injury, syringomyelia, anterior horn disease (e.g., spinal muscle atrophy, poliomyelitis)
- Phrenic nerve injury: birth trauma, neck and thoracic surgery or trauma, demyelinating disease (e.g., Guillain-Barré syndrome), neoplasm, infectious neuropathies (e.g., tetanus, typhoid, diphtheria, measles, West Nile virus, cytomegalovirus), radiotherapy.

Neuromuscular junction

- Myasthenia gravis, congenital myasthenic syndromes
- Botulism

Muscle disorders

- Myotonic dystrophies, Duchenne muscular dystrophy, congenital muscular dystrophy
- Congenital and metabolic myopathies
- Polymyositis

Disorders of anatomy

- Congenital: congenital diaphragmatic hernia, congenital diaphragmatic eventration, diaphragmatic agenesis
- Acquired: traumatic rupture

Idiopathic

children. Prominent clinical features are unexplained tachypnea, hypoxia, or respiratory distress, which usually worsen in the supine posture, or failure to wean from ventilatory support after surgery. In less severe cases, recurrent atelectasis and infections, and failure to thrive can be observed. On chest radiograph, unilateral paralysis of the right hemidiaphragm should be suspected if it is more than two rib spaces higher than the left hemidiaphragm; on the left side, it results in an elevation of the hemidiaphragm of at least one rib space above the right hemidiaphragm. Contralateral mediastinal shift can also be observed in severe cases. Fluoroscopy with sniff test and ultrasonography performed in a spontaneously breathing patient show a paradoxical inspiratory upward motion of the hemidiaphragm. Electromyography in association with percutaneous stimulation of the phrenic nerve can confirm the paralysis. Repeated evaluations by fluoroscopy, ultrasonography, or electromyography can aid in improving diaphragmatic function.

Treatment depends mainly on the presence of respiratory symptoms. Asymptomatic diaphragmatic paralysis does not require any therapy. Treatment for symptomatic cases first consists of ventilatory support, when needed. Surgical plication is generally indicated in the presence of persistent or recurrent respiratory symptoms. Optimal timing for surgery in the neonate or child with diaphragmatic paralysis is controversial. Waiting for spontaneous recovery in symptomatic patients can be associated with significant morbidity, especially in high-risk patients on ventilatory support. Recommendations for such patients vary from immediate repair to waiting 2 to 4 weeks for signs of spontaneous recovery. The possibility of using video-assisted thoracoscopic surgery for diaphragm plication decreases the morbidity associated with traditional open thoracotomy. Long-term intermittent positive pressure ventilation, usually using BiPAP via nasal mask, is useful in the most severe cases of bilateral diaphragmatic paralysis.

Guillain-Barré Syndrome

Guillain-Barré syndrome (GBS) is an acute, inflammatory demyelinating disease of the peripheral nerves. Median annual incidence of GBS is about 1 to 3 cases per 100,000, with 30% of cases occurring in those younger than 20 years of age. It is considered to be an autoimmune disease often triggered by a preceding infection, including cytomegalovirus, Epstein-Barr virus, Varicella zoster virus, *Mycoplasma pneumoniae, Campylobacter jejuni,* and influenza vaccine. Diagnosis is mainly based on clinical criteria. Tingling paresthesia in distal extremities and proximal muscle weakness with aching pain usually develop over several days to 4 weeks, followed by a plateau period of 2 to 4 weeks and then progressive recovery. Polyradiculitis can involve various levels of lower motor neurons, including to the diaphragm and to other thoracoabdominal muscles, and cranial nerves. Respiratory failure caused by respiratory muscle weakness, aspiration pneumonia, and cough impairment can develop. Repeated measurements of vital capacity and blood gases are essential for appropriate decisions as to the need for mechanical ventilatory support, which is

required in 15% to 20% of affected children. Intubation must be considered when forced vital capacity is less than 20 mL/kg or maximal inspiratory/expiratory pressure is less than 30/40 cm H_2O or in the presence of dysphagia. While the duration of mechanical ventilation varies widely, recovery of adequate respiratory function is the rule. While not definitely proven, the early use of high-dose intravenous immunoglobulins or plasma exchange appears to induce a more rapid resolution of the disease.[14] On the contrary, corticosteroids do not hasten recovery.

MUSCLE DISEASES THAT AFFECT THE CHEST WALL

Muscular Dystrophies

Muscular dystrophies are a group of genetically determined diseases that primarily affect skeletal muscle and are characterized by progressive muscle wasting and weakness. Two types of muscular dystrophies commonly lead to respiratory insufficiency before adulthood: Duchenne muscular dystrophy and myotonic dystrophy. In addition, pulmonary function abnormalities and respiratory failure may occur in the childhood form of limb girdle muscle dystrophy, facioscapulohumeral dystrophy, and Emery Dreifuss syndrome, and in congenital muscular dystrophy.

Duchenne Muscular Dystrophy

Duchenne muscular dystrophy (DMD) is the most common and severe form of muscular dystrophy afflicting humans. Inherited as an X-linked recessive trait, it has an incidence of approximately 1:3500 male births. Almost one-third of cases results from new mutations. Becker muscular dystrophy is a milder form of the disease, with onset of muscle weakness in the second decade and slower progression; significant respiratory involvement, when present, usually occurs in adulthood. The gene responsible for DMD and Becker muscular dystrophy has been localized within the *dystrophin* gene located on the short arm of the X chromosome (Xp21). This *dystrophin* gene codes for dystrophin, a protein that links the normal contractile apparatus to the sarcolemma in skeletal muscle. *Dystrophin* gene mutations result in either a lack of dystrophin (usually DMD) or the expression of mutant forms of dystrophin (usually Becker muscular dystrophy).

The natural history of DMD is rather stereotyped. The disease presents in boys with proximal muscle weakness at 2 to 4 years of age. Fairly rapid progression results in loss of ambulation at around 10 years of age and premature death before 30 years of age. Death is due to respiratory failure in 80% of cases or to cardiac failure in 10% to 20% of cases. In the early phases of the disease, when gait is still preserved, respiratory function is essentially normal, although measuring inspiratory and expiratory pressures can readily show a loss in the strength of the respiratory muscles. Impairment of respiratory function is accelerated after loss of ambulation. DMD patients present a restrictive syndrome due to muscle weakness and contractures, spinal deformity, vertebrocostal joint ankylosis, and frequent obesity. Regular assessment of lung function (FVC, maximal inspiratory and expiratory pressures, peak cough flow, arterial or noninvasive assessment of blood gases, and overnight pulse oximetry) is essential in evaluating progression of the respiratory system disability (see the "Assessment of Respiratory Function in Children with Chest Wall Dysfunction" section earlier in the chapter). Serial measurements of FVC reported in absolute value have been found especially useful in DMD patients. Indeed, every DMD patient experiences a maximum plateau in absolute vital capacity between 10 and 12 years of age and a progressive decrease thereafter. Until the 1990s, before the regular use of nocturnal ventilatory support, the maximal vital capacity recorded and its rate of decline thereafter predicted survival time. Age when vital capacity was <1 liter reliably indicated a greater risk of dying in the next 3 years.

Natural history of the disease has been profoundly altered by treatment, particularly respiratory care and more recently the use of corticosteroids.

Long-Term Management of Respiratory Disability

Given that death is most often related to respiratory insufficiency, one key component of management of DMD patients is directed at slowing down the progression of respiratory insufficiency, while ensuring a good quality of life. In the first decade, prevention of respiratory infections, regular submaximal exercise, and treatment of any associated respiratory problems, (e.g., asthma or obstructive sleep apnea due to adenotonsillar hypertrophy) are mandatory and sufficient. Loss of ambulation coincides with the onset of progressively increasing respiratory problems. At some time in the second decade, loss of respiratory muscle strength will lead to recommending the use of lung volume recruitment maneuvers (either by self-inflating bag or mechanical in-exsufflation) and "respiratory aids," namely assisted-cough techniques (either manually or by mechanical in-exsufflation) and mechanical ventilation. The most recent consensus recommendations on when to use these techniques in DMD patients are detailed in Table 43-5.[3] While nasal mask ventilation with BiPAP is most often used for nocturnal ventilation, an oral interface with a volume-cycled ventilator is usually the most appropriate device for providing, on demand, daytime assisted ventilation. Many DMD patients are successfully managed with noninvasive ventilation 24 hours per day. Most experts now reserve tracheostomy for patients who cannot use noninvasive ventilation successfully or prefer tracheostomy, those with three failed attempts at extubation after acute respiratory failure despite optimal use of mechanical in-exsufflation and noninvasive ventilation, or when noninvasive assisted-cough techniques are not able to avoid lung aspiration of secretions with repeated SaO_2 drops <95%.[3]

Aside from back pain and difficulty in positioning, scoliosis contributes to the decrease in vital capacity, and preventing spinal curve progression is part of respiratory care. Early surgical correction is the treatment of choice because spinal bracing is not effective in DMD patients and may further reduce vital capacity. Ideally, surgery should be performed in DMD patients with a progressing Cobb angle of 20 degrees and a vital capacity of at least 40% of predicted values, to avoid postoperative respiratory failure. However, several reports have now shown that scoliosis surgery can be performed successfully in DMD patients with very severe respiratory disability (FVC <30% predicted), with careful preoperative and postoperative care.[15]

Obesity is frequent in DMD patients after loss of ambulation, and all obese patients should undergo a controlled weight-reduction program. Obesity in these patients increases the work of breathing and further compromises chest wall function. Conversely, patients with end-stage disease may suffer from severe weight loss with muscle wasting and bedsores, secondary to bulbar weakness (mastication and swallowing difficulties) and inability to feed themselves. Specialized dietary management must be implemented, and the use of gastrostomy for enteral feeding should be discussed with such patients and their families.

Management of Acute Respiratory Deteriorations

Respiratory infection is a serious complication in DMD patients because muscle weakness impairs both the ability to breathe and to clear airway secretions. Affected children should avoid contact with individuals with respiratory infections, and preventive immunization (influenza, pneumococcal pneumonia) should be performed. During respiratory infections, patients with DMD must increase their use of assisted-cough techniques and noninvasive ventilatory support to maintain an $SaO_2 \geq 95\%$. Oxygen therapy must be used with great caution and only in conjunction with respiratory aids to avoid masking and aggravating alveolar hypoventilation. Early appropriate antibiotic treatment is recommended when a lower respiratory tract infection is proven by culture or with an SaO_2 <95%. Inability to maintain $SaO_2 \geq 95\%$ in room air is an indication for hospitalization. When endotracheal intubation is necessary, results from a protocol specifically designed for extubating neuromuscular patients show a very high success rate.[16] An action plan for respiratory infections should be given to all DMD patients with significant respiratory involvement.

Using nocturnal and daytime noninvasive respiratory aids together with early, aggressive, and adapted management of respiratory infections, DMD patients can often live beyond 30 years, while usually ensuring an appreciable quality of life.

Corticosteroid Therapy

During the last decade, glucocorticoid treatment has been repeatedly shown to further improve the course of Duchenne muscular dystrophy. Early prescription of long-term corticosteroid treatment slows the decline in muscle strength and function, which in turn retards loss of ambulation, prevents the development of scoliosis, and retards the onset of significant respiratory disability.[17–19] In addition, limited data suggest that corticosteroids improve cardiac function. Current recommendations detailed by Bushby and colleagues and the DMD Care Considerations Working Group[20] propose that corticosteroid treatment be initiated as soon as the child reaches the plateau phase in motor skills (i.e., between 4 and 8 years of age). While it is further recommended to continue daily corticosteroid treatment after loss of ambulation, it is unknown if and when corticosteroids should be stopped.

TABLE 43-5 CONSENSUS ON RESPIRATORY CARE IN DUCHENNE MUSCULAR DYSTROPHY

Step 1: Volume Recruitment/Deep Lung Inflation Technique

- Volume recruitment/deep lung inflation technique (by self-inflating manual ventilation bag or mechanical in-/ex-sufflation) when FVC < 40% predicted

Step 2: Manual and Mechanically Assisted Cough Techniques

Necessary when:
- Respiratory infection present and baseline peak cough flow < 270 lpm*
- Baseline peak cough flow < 160 lpm or max expiratory pressure < 40 cm water
- Baseline FVC < 40% predicted OR < 1.25 liters in older teen/adult

*All specified threshold values of peak cough flow and maximum expiratory pressure apply to older teenage and adult patients

Step 3: Nocturnal Ventilation

Nocturnal ventilation** is indicated in patients who have any of the following:
- Signs or symptoms of hypoventilation (patients with FVC < 30% predicted are at especially high risk)
- A baseline SpO_2 < 95% and/or blood or end-tidal pCO_2 > 45 mmHg while awake
- An apnoea-hyponoea index > 10/hour on polysomnography OR four or more episodes of SpO_2 < 92% OR drops in SpO_2 of at least 4% per hour of sleep

Note: Optimally, use of lung volume recruitment and assisted cough techniques should always precede initiation of non-invasive ventilation.

**Recommended for nocturnal use: non-invasive ventilation with pressure cycled bi-level devices or volume cycled ventilators or combination volume-pressure ventilators. In bi-level or pressure support modes of ventilation, add a back-up rate of breathing. Recommended interfaces include: a nasal mask or nasal pillow. Other interfaces can be used and each has its own potential benefits.

Step 4: Daytime Ventilation

In patients already using nocturnally assisted ventilation, daytime ventilation*** is indicated for:
- Self extension of nocturnal ventilation into waking hours,
- Abnormal deglutition due to dyspnea, which is relieved by ventilatory assistance,
- Inability to speak a full sentence without breathlessness, and/or
- Symptoms of hypoventilation with baseline SpO_2 < 95% and/or blood or end-tidal pCO_2 > 45 mmHg while awake

Continuous non-invasive assisted ventilation (along with mechanically assisted cough) can facilitate endotracheal extubation for patients who were intubated during acute illness or during anesthesia, followed by weaning to nocturnal non-invasive assisted ventilation, if applicable.

***Recommended for day use: non-invasive ventilation with portable volume cycled or volume-pressure ventilators; bi-level devices are an alternative. A mouthpiece interface is strongly recommended during day use of portable volume-cycled or volume-pressure ventilators, but other ventilator-interface combinations can be used based on clinician preference and patient comfort.

Step 5: Tracheostomy

Indications for tracheostomy include:
- Patient and clinician preference****
- Patient cannot successfully use non-invasive ventilation,
- Inability of the local medical infrastructure to support non-invasive ventilation,
- Three failures to achieve extubation during critical illness despite optimal use of non-invasive ventilation and mechanically assisted cough
- The failure of non-invasive methods of cough assistance to prevent aspiration of secretions into the lung and drops in oxygen saturation below 95% or the patient's baseline, necessitating frequent direct tracheal suctioning via tracheostomy

****Note, however, that the panel advocates for the long-term use of non-invasive ventilation up to and including 24 hours/day in eligible patients.

(Reproduced with permission from Birnkrant DJ, Bushby KM, Amin RS, et al. The respiratory management of patients with Duchenne muscular dystrophy: a DMD Care Considerations Working Group specialty article. *Pediatr Pulmonol.* 2010;45:739-748.)

Side effects are obviously a concern, and a careful follow-up must be instituted. Taking into account the beneficial effect on muscle strength versus potential side effects, the most favorable treatment regime is 0.75 mg/day of prednisone (prednisolone) or 0.9 mg/day of deflazacort. When available, deflazacort appears to have somewhat different side effects, with less effect on weight and fewer behavioral problems.

Future Perspectives on Duchenne Muscular Dystrophy Treatment

DMD still remains an untreatable disease in humans. However, several novel therapeutic approaches are worth mentioning. Some approaches target the sarcolemmal defect secondary to lack of functional dystrophin. Upregulation of compensatory proteins such as utrophin, chemical repair of the weakened membrane, and increased glycosylation of the dystrophin complex to improve extracellular matrix attachment are still in the preclinical phase. More recently, mutation-specific therapies have been tested in phase I or II clinical trials. In "exon skipping," antisense oligonucleotides are used to skip unnecessary exons, bringing genetic code back into frame and allowing RNA processing and translation into a functional protein. In nonsense codon suppression, drugs are able to read through premature stop-codon mutations. While encouraging results have been obtained with some of the above mutation-specific therapies, substantial work remains to be done before they can be used to treat DMD patients effectively.[21] Finally, viral-based gene therapy and stem cell therapy are under investigation.[22]

Myotonic Dystrophy

Myotonic diseases are divided into nondystrophic types (hyperkalemic periodic paralysis, paramyotonia congenita, myotonia congenita) and dystrophic types such as myotonic dystrophy (Steinert disease).

Myotonic dystrophy is an autosomal dominant, inherited, and progressive disease that occurs at a frequency of 1:7500 to 1:18,500 individuals. The mutation responsible is an expansion of an unstable trinucleotide (CTG) in the region of the myotonic dystrophy protein kinase (DMPK) gene, on the long arm of chromosome 19. The degree of expression of this disorder is quite variable, leading to marked variation in clinical severity and age of onset. Myotonia and muscle weakness are the prominent clinical features, but many other organ systems can be affected (e.g., cataracts, cardiac dysrhythmias, hypersomnia, frontal balding, and endocrine disorders). Involvement of the respiratory system is the major factor contributing to morbidity and mortality.

Congenital Myotonic Dystrophy

Ten to fifteen percent of patients with myotonic dystrophy have a severe congenital form, which presents as generalized hypotonia without myotonia, along with respiratory and feeding difficulties.[4] Thin ribs and right diaphragmatic elevation can be observed on chest radiograph. Diagnostic suspicion is increased by examining the mother, who most often carries the mutation and presents mild weakness of eyelid closure and grip myotonia. DNA-based diagnostic tests confirm the diagnosis. Polyhydramnios, prematurity, hydrops fetalis with pleural effusions, and pulmonary hypoplasia can increase respiratory difficulties due to diaphragmatic weakness at birth. Fifty percent of neonates with congenital myotonic dystrophy require respiratory support at birth. The condition usually improves in early childhood but deteriorates in late childhood or adolescence, when features of the classic disease gradually appear. However, if ventilatory support is needed beyond 4 weeks of life in the neonatal period, prognosis is poor, with risk of sudden death in survivors, even without apparent respiratory exacerbations.

Classic Myotonic Dystrophy

The classic form of myotonic dystrophy begins in childhood. Although clinical signs of weakness of the expiratory muscles have been shown in children, a true restrictive syndrome is commonly reported in adult patients only, and respiratory failure is rare before late adulthood. However, weakness of the respiratory muscles and muscles of deglutition render myotonic dystrophy patients prone to postanesthetic respiratory failure, repeated aspiration pneumonias, and pulmonary infections. In addition, subjects with myotonic dystrophy are prone to sleep-disordered breathing, which may be either obstructive or central. Obesity can be an aggravating factor. Death in adults usually results from respiratory failure, and less commonly from heart failure.

Congenital Muscular Dystrophy

The term *congenital muscular dystrophy* refers to a group of rare genetic disorders in which weakness and an abnormal muscle biopsy are present at birth.[4] While muscle weakness tends to be stable over time, complications become more severe over the long run. Diagnosis is established from an observed increase in serum creatine kinase and a dystrophic or myopathic pattern on muscle biopsy. Abnormality in muscle immunostaining and abnormalities in brain MRI can distinguish some subtypes. Several forms of congenital muscular dystrophy can lead to respiratory compromise. Ullrich's congenital muscular dystrophy presents with kyphosis, proximal joint contractures, and distal joint hyperlaxity and brings about frequent respiratory failure near the end of the first decade. In rigid spine muscular dystrophy, characterized by rigid spine and scoliosis, severe nocturnal alveolar hypoventilation can present early and necessitate nocturnal noninvasive ventilatory assistance in the first years of life due to diaphragm weakness.[23]

Other Heritable Myopathies

Aside from muscular dystrophies, several other rare inherited myopathies can be responsible for respiratory function abnormalities of variable expression—from a severe neonatal form with acute bulbar weakness and respiratory failure to a more benign adult form.[24] A remarkable feature of these diseases is that the respiratory muscles can be severely impaired, causing respiratory failure, while the other skeletal muscles are relatively spared. Abnormal respiratory control can also cause respiratory failure in some cases. Nemaline myopathy can present as a severe neonatal form requiring full-time ventilation, or as a typical nemaline myopathy with progressive onset of respiratory insufficiency in later childhood. Severe respiratory insufficiency is also frequent in the neonatal period in myotubular myopathy. Respiratory failure has been reported in most patients with multiminicore myopathy, especially with the classic form beginning at birth, despite being ambulant, due to diaphragmatic weakness. Conversely, respiratory impairment is observed more rarely in central core disease. Patients with non-progressive respiratory abnormalities can be managed with intermittent positive pressure ventilation via nasal mask or tracheostomy. The decision to begin continuous mechanical ventilatory support in the most severe cases should take into account ethical considerations and the frequent lack of reliable prognostic factors.[2]

Hereditary metabolic myopathies constitute a heterogeneous group of muscular diseases that can present with respiratory failure.[25] Glycogenosis type II (Pompe's disease) is characterized by infiltration of all organs by glycogen, due to an inherited deficiency in acid maltase. While the neonatal form is fatal through cardiorespiratory failure, a milder form with primary alveolar hypoventilation due to respiratory muscle involvement has been reported in adolescence. Mitochondrial myopathies, a group of rare disorders with accumulation of abnormal mitochondria in skeletal muscle fibers, can affect both the peripheral and central nervous systems. Some forms present from infancy to young adulthood with respiratory insufficiency caused by skeletal muscle weakness or respiratory control abnormality.

Hereditary periodic paralyses are channelopathies characterized by recurrent attacks of muscle weakness with the possibility of severe respiratory muscle paralysis in the hypokalemic form. Management of the latter includes administration of potassium during attacks and prevention of recurrences by a low-carbohydrate, low-sodium diet, and drugs such as carbonic anhydrase inhibitors (acetazolamide, dichlorphenamide), spironolactone, and triamterene.

■ NEUROMUSCULAR JUNCTION DISEASES

Myasthenia Gravis and Congenital Myasthenic Syndromes

Juvenile Myasthenia Gravis
Similar to the adult form, juvenile myasthenia gravis is an autoimmune disorder of neuromuscular transmission most often associated with circulating autoantibodies against the acetylcholine receptor (AchR) or sometimes against the MuSK protein (muscle-specific kinase), a tyrosine kinase receptor, which is required for the formation of the neuromuscular junction.[26,27] The juvenile form may present at any age during childhood, even as early as 6 months of age. Myasthenia gravis is characterized by abnormal muscle fatigability. It is often restricted to ocular muscles in prepubescent children, with a high rate of spontaneous remission. Conversely, after puberty,

myasthenia gravis usually follows a progressive course with more generalized involvement of facial, upper airway, respiratory, or limb muscles. In addition, myasthenia gravis crises, which can lead to life-threatening respiratory failure, can be triggered by infection, fever, stress, or medications.

Diagnosis of myasthenia gravis relies on clinical symptoms, a transient improvement with the acetylcholinesterase inhibitor edrophonium chloride, electrophysiologic studies including repetitive nerve stimulation or stimulation single-fiber electromyography, and the presence of circulating anti-AchR or anti-MuSK autoantibodies. Long-term management is primarily based on anticholinesterase medication (pyridostigmine bromide). However, most patients require immunosuppressive agents, primarily prednisone. In the most severe patients, azathioprine, cyclosporine, cyclophosphamide, tacrolimus, or rituximab are used.[28] While thymectomy is indicated in case of thymoma and widely accepted in generalized AchR-myasthenia gravis, its role in the absence of thymoma is still questioned, especially in young children. During myasthenia gravis crises, noninvasive or endotracheal mechanical ventilation may be required, in association with plasmapheresis and high-dose prednisone.

Transient Neonatal Myasthenia
Transient neonatal myasthenia occurs in about 10% to 15% of infants born to mothers with autoimmune myasthenia gravis, due to transplacental transmission of maternal anti-AchR (or anti-MuSK) autoantibodies.[26,27] Clinical features are usually noted within 48 hours of birth and can include feeding difficulties, hypotonia, weak cry, facial weakness, ptosis, and, more rarely, respiratory difficulties. Antenatal onset of the disease with polyhydramnios or arthrogryposis multiplex congenita has also been reported. Diagnosis can be made on the presence of myasthenia gravis in the mother, a transient clinical improvement with intravenous edrophonium, or the presence of circulating anti-AChR (or anti-MuSK) antibodies. If necessary, management relies on pyridostigmine as well as adequate feeding and respiratory support until spontaneous remission of muscle weakness. If the response to anticholinesterase medication is negative, immunoglobulins, plasmapheresis, and exchange transfusion should be proposed. Total and definitive resolution occurs within 2 to 8 weeks. In fact, prevention through optimal disease control of all women of childbearing age diagnosed with myasthenia gravis is the real objective in transient neonatal myasthenia. In particular, prophylactic treatment with plasma exchange or steroids should be considered in a woman with a previously affected newborn, as the risk of recurrence is high.

Congenital Myasthenic Syndromes
Congenital myasthenic syndromes refer to a group of genetic disorders that result from various defects in neuromuscular transmission.[29] Congenital myasthenic syndromes are usually characterized by an autosomal recessive (less often dominant) inheritance, absence of myasthenia gravis in the mother, occurrence among siblings, and a wide spectrum in age of onset. With early

neonatal onset, clinical features can mimic neonatal myasthenia gravis and lead to respiratory failure with sudden apnea, or they can present with bilateral vocal cord paralysis. Other types beginning after the neonatal period are characterized by usually mild symptoms and sudden exacerbations of muscle weakness and respiratory failure, which can be triggered by infections or stress. Diagnosis relies on family history, clinical myasthenic findings, absence of circulating AchR antibodies, stimulation single-fiber EMG, positive response to pyridostigmine, or finding of one of the known mutations. As in neonatal myasthenia gravis, antenatal onset of congenital myasthenic syndrome has been reported. Management is based on pyridostigmine, or 3-4 diaminopyridine or epinephrine, depending on the specific type of congenital myasthenic syndrome. Subtypes of congenital myasthenic syndromes associated with mutations in *Dok-7* can also be treated with salbutamol. Feeding, respiratory support, or tracheotomy are used as needed.

Botulism

Botulism is a rare cause of neuromuscular transmission blockade in the pediatric population. The toxins produced by *Clostridium botulinum* are responsible for the impaired release of acetylcholine at the neuromuscular junction.

Infantile botulism is the most common form of botulism and occurs only in the first year of life (95% between 6 weeks and 6 months of age).[30] Infant botulism is caused by intestinal colonization by *Clostridium botulinum* followed by endogenous production and absorption of the toxin. Constipation is followed by cranial nerve palsies with prominent feeding difficulties and ptosis; a subacute, symmetric, and descending paralysis ensues. Progressive respiratory failure may follow, sometimes manifesting as acute respiratory arrest. Respiratory failure can be precipitated by aminoglycosides, which potentiate neuromuscular weakness caused by botulinum toxin, or by neck flexion during manipulation. Diagnosis is made using ELISA to identify *Clostridium botulinum* or the toxin in the infant's feces. The toxin may also be found in the serum. When necessary, EMG can provide rapid bedside support for the clinical diagnosis of infant botulism. Duration of ventilatory support is variable, but full recovery is expected with proper supportive treatment. Intravenous human-derived botulinum immune globulin was shown to decrease the average hospital stay from 5.5 to 2.5 weeks and must be administered as soon as infant botulism is suspected. Antibiotics against *Clostridium botulinum* are of no benefit and must not be given.

Food-borne botulism is related to the ingestion of the botulinum toxin, traditionally from home-canned food. Clinical signs are typical of botulism, with cranial nerve palsies followed by descending, symmetrical palsy of voluntary muscles, and the possibility of respiratory failure. Treatment consists of intensive care and early antitoxin therapy, optimally within the first 24 hours after onset of symptoms. Full recovery is the rule.

Wound botulism results from a wound infected with the bacteria and subsequent production of the toxin *in situ*.

SKELETAL ANOMALIES

Scoliosis

Scoliosis is the result of an underlying pathologic process leading to lateral and rotational curvature of the spine. The spinal deformity distorts thoracic cage structures, including respiratory muscles, and also intrathoracic organ orientation. The effects of scoliosis on pulmonary disability and reduced life expectancy have resulted in the development of screening programs in school-age children. The goal of such programs is to detect scoliosis and implement proper therapy early enough to avoid curve progression, subsequent chest wall deformity, and cardiopulmonary dysfunction.

Classification and Natural History

Etiology and age of onset determine the basis for the most commonly used classification of scoliosis (Table 43-6). Idiopathic scoliosis is defined as a structural scoliosis for which no specific cause can be established. Autosomal dominant, X-linked, and multifactorial patterns of inheritance have been reported to account for the hereditary factors of the disease. Idiopathic scoliosis, which accounts for 80% to 85% of cases, is further categorized into three types, according to the age at which the deformity is first noted: infantile, juvenile, and adolescent. Since numerous factors are known to cause scoliosis, the diagnosis of idiopathic scoliosis can be made only after exclusion of a

---

TABLE 43-6 CLASSIFICATION OF SCOLIOSIS

Idiopathic (85% of All Scoliosis)

- Infantile (<3 years of age)
- Juvenile (3-9 years of age)
- Adolescent (10 years of age to skeletal maturity)

Congenital (5% of All Scoliosis)

- Failure of formation (hemivertebra)
- Failure of segmentation
- Mixed

Neuromuscular (5% of All Scoliosis)

- Neuropathic
- Lower motor neuron (e.g., poliomyelitis)
- Upper motor neuron (e.g., cerebral palsy)
- Other (e.g., syringomyelia)
- Myopathic
- Progressive (e.g., muscular dystrophy)
- Static (e.g., amyotonia)
- Others (e.g., Friedreich's ataxia)

Associated with Neurofibromatosis (Von Recklinghausen Disease)

Mesenchymal

- Congenital (e.g., Marfan's syndrome)
- Acquired (e.g., rheumatoid disease)
- Others (e.g., juvenile apophysitis)

Traumatic

- Vertebral (e.g., fracture, radiation, surgery)
- Extravertebral (e.g., burns, thoracoplasty)
- Secondary to irritative phenomenon (e.g., spinal cord tumor)

primary etiology, such as Marfan syndrome, neuromuscular disease, chest wall surgery, or vertebral anomaly. In contrast, congenital scoliosis is caused by the presence of vertebral anomalies, which cause an imbalance in the longitudinal growth of the spine and abnormal growth patterns over time. While congenital scoliosis is often recognized at birth, diagnosis can be delayed until adolescence, when more subtle vertebral anomalies are present. Radiographic measurement of the severity of the curve (the Cobb angle), the level of the apex of the curve (i.e., cervical, high thoracic, thoracic, thoracolumbar, lumbar), and the number of curves (single or double) have all been used for comparison, prognostication, and development of treatment guidelines.

In the general school population, the prevalence of adolescent idiopathic scoliosis with curve greater than 10 degrees is 2% to 3%. The percentage drops to 0.5% and 0.2% for curves greater than 20 degrees and 30 degrees, respectively. Although the natural history of scoliosis is associated with curve progression, cardiopulmonary impairment, back pain, cosmetic deformity, and neurologic compromise, it varies greatly, depending on specific etiology, age of onset, genetic background, and curve pattern. Untreated adolescents with severe idiopathic scoliosis followed over a 50-year period were shown to have a mortality rate 2.2 times greater than controls. These deaths generally occurred in the fourth or fifth decade of life, due to cardiopulmonary insufficiency. Most of the survivors showed significant physical disability characterized by dyspnea, back pain, and exercise limitation. Similarly, adults whose scoliosis was first diagnosed before 8 years of age had greater mortality than the general population after age 40.[31] Untreated children with infantile scoliosis followed to maturity are often found to have severe and crippling deformities, with a spinal curvature usually exceeding 70 degrees; spontaneous regression of the scoliosis, however, has been reported in 10% to 60% of patients. Congenital scoliosis is usually progressive and results in severe spinal deformity if untreated. The ultimate severity of the curve depends on both the type of anomaly and the site at which it occurs. The most progressive of all anomalies is a unilateral unsegmented bar combined with single or multiple convex hemivertebrae on the contralateral side with or without associated fused ribs. In untreated infantile and congenital scoliosis, death may occur before adulthood as a result of cardiopulmonary insufficiency.

Pulmonary Function in Scoliosis

At an early stage of the disease, scoliosis is generally painless and asymptomatic. While restrictive lung disease is detectable when the Cobb angle is greater than 50 to 60 degrees, a Cobb angle greater than 90 degrees greatly predisposes to cardiorespiratory failure. A recent term, *thoracic insufficiency syndrome*, has been coined to identify children with spine and chest wall disorders that impair lung function or postnatal lung growth.[32] The syndrome encompasses early-onset scoliosis and scoliosis associated with underlying neuromuscular disease. As a result, lung function testing has been extended to infants where restrictive changes have been described.

Lung Function

The degree of restrictive lung disease is related to the severity of the three-dimensional deformity of the spine and chest wall produced by scoliosis. In adolescent idiopathic scoliosis, the features of the spinal deformity (i.e., the Cobb angle, number of vertebrae involved, cephalad location of the curve, and loss of the normal thoracic kyphosis) are the major determinants of reduced FVC and hence total lung capacity. Reduction of chest wall compliance and thus lack of chest wall excursion, impaired lung growth, or decreased inspiratory muscle strength from mechanical disadvantage from the chest deformity account for the effects of scoliosis on vital capacity and other lung volumes. Forced vital capacity is most sensitive to reductions in both thoracic cage size and reduced thoracic cage mobility. Residual volume reflects reduced size and is reduced less as a percent of predicted value than vital capacity. This may explain the elevated RV/TLC reported in patients with scoliosis. Airway resistance may be normal or slightly increased because of the mainstem bronchial distortion associated with chest deformity. This occurs in up to 10% of patients with adolescent idiopathic scoliosis. In children with obstructive lung disease and scoliosis, more common etiologies for airway obstruction (e.g., asthma) should be investigated. It is important to recall that height in children with scoliosis cannot be used to compare to predicted norms for spirometric indices and lung volumes. Multiple other methods, including arm spans or length of specific bones, have been proposed as surrogate estimates of height.[33] In some studies, ventilation-perfusion scans have shown that alveolar ventilation is greater in the lung on the convex side than in the (smaller) lung on the concave side. However, in others, ventilation and perfusion are greater where the lung volume, as measured by volumetric reconstructions from CT scans, is greater, regardless of convex or concave location.[34] While scoliotic individuals can present with exercise intolerance, there is seldom significant alteration of blood gases in patients with a Cobb angle less than 60 degrees unless additional lung disease is present. Nocturnal alveolar hypoventilation has been observed in patients with a Cobb angle greater than 60 degrees, and cardiorespiratory failure can be present in the most severe patients with a Cobb angle greater than 90 degrees. Both the apnea-hypopnea index and the arousal index are increased in children with early-onset scoliosis and thoracic insufficiency syndrome, irrespective of CO_2 elevation.[35] Patients with moderate to severe scoliosis should therefore be evaluated with oximetry and PCO_2 recordings during sleep and, if scoliosis is associated with muscle weakness or obesity, overnight noninvasive ventilatory support should be considered. Hypoventilation is more likely in patients with an upper thoracic curve, associated thoracic lordosis, structural vertebral anomaly, or associated respiratory muscle weakness.

Lung Growth

The consequences of scoliosis on lung growth remain unclear. Postmortem quantitative studies among adolescents suggest that alveolar multiplication is decreased in congenital or infantile scoliosis, whereas the alveoli may not enlarge normally in idiopathic juvenile or adolescent scoliosis. The number of pulmonary vessels in scoliotic children is also reduced in proportion to lung maldevelopment. Lung function studies have demonstrated a greater reduction in vital capacity for the same Cobb angle among children with early-onset scoliosis compared to adolescent onset, also raising the question of associated pulmonary hypoplasia in those with early-onset spine disease. Pulmonary hypoplasia has recently been produced in rabbits that undergo iatrogenic scoliosis with postnatal rib tethering.[36] The age of onset, rate of progression, and timing of progression may all contribute to development of postnatal pulmonary hypoplasia.

Management
Management of scoliosis depends on the age of the child and the degree of scoliosis, as well as the underlying condition that led to the scoliosis.

Adolescent Idiopathic Scoliosis
Management of adolescent idiopathic scoliosis should start with early detection, based on school screening programs before onset of the adolescent growth spurt. In skeletally immature patients with curves of less than 25 degrees, the risk of progression is low and a close follow-up may be sufficient. In patients with progressive curves greater than 25 degrees, bracing to stop spinal curve progression should be the first line of treatment. Such orthotic management is usually based on a full-time treatment regimen (more than 20 hours per day), but the Charleston brace is used during nighttime only. The weaning period begins when spine growth stops. Uncontrolled curve progression despite orthotic treatment, or curves greater than 50 degrees require surgery that is based on spinal fusion with pedicle screw instrumentation to correct for the three-dimensional deformation.[37] In younger adolescents, a new surgical treatment has been proposed using staples between vertebrae along the convex side of the scoliotic curve at the apex in order to promote unilateral vertebral growth on the concave side and maintain spinal flexibility.[38] Postoperative follow-up lung function measurements to evaluate this method have not been reported.

Juvenile Scoliosis
Children with nonprogressive spinal curves of less than 20 degrees usually require no other intervention than a close follow-up, especially at the time of the adolescent growth spurt. Children with a progressive spinal curve should be treated with a brace individualized to minimize further respiratory impairment with selective cutouts; those whose curve progression has not stopped or who have spinal curves greater than 40 degrees will require surgical treatment. Whenever possible, spinal fusion should be delayed until the onset of the adolescent growth spurt in order to maximize vertebral and hence thoracic cage growth.

Congenital and Infantile Scoliosis
Both congenital and infantile scoliosis should be considered very serious conditions. Indeed, it is difficult to stop the progression of the spinal curve in young children, and the consequences of a severely deformed and rigid chest can be catastrophic on a rapidly growing lung. Most cases of congenital scoliosis are progressive and do not respond to bracing. Surgical treatment for most patients was based on spinal fusion in the past. However, long-term follow-up studies on children fused while growing have demonstrated significant restrictive chest wall disease proportional to the length of spine that was fused and the location of the apex prior to surgery.[39] A totally different surgical approach, an expansion thoracoplasty on the concave side of the scoliosis by means of a vertical expandable prosthetic titanium rib (VEPTR) without spinal surgery, has been approved for use on a case-by-case basis for congenital scoliosis and underlying scoliosis related to neuromuscular disease. If fused ribs are present, the fusion is lysed and the ribs are separated with the VEPTR device to increase thoracic cage volume and minimize recurrent fusion of the ribs (Fig. 43-1). Additional methods of straightening the spine in young growing children (e.g., growing rods in the paraspinal region and then maintaining the spine curvature correction over years with repeated expansions of these devices) have been reported.[40] Expansion of the devices every 6 months increased vertebral height significantly more than expansions on an "as-needed" basis.[41] A new generation of expandable or "growing" titanium devices is emerging that will allow for expansion of the devices noninvasively. Preliminary results obtained a few years after surgery suggest that VEPTR promotes continued spine growth even for abnormal vertebrae, with no increase in curve amplitude. Postoperative studies with serial measures of vital capacity under anesthesia over 3 years demonstrated an improvement in absolute lung volume, but no change or a slight loss of lung function as a percentage of predicted norms.[42] Another study of 53 older children undergoing VEPTR insertion found no change in vital capacity but a small increase in residual volume, suggesting that the lung had been stretched as the thorax was expanded.[43] Importantly, there was a suggestion that lung function was better preserved when children underwent surgical correction of the scoliosis if they were younger than 6 years of age.[42]

Patients with nonprogressive juvenile scoliosis should be followed closely until skeletal maturity is attained. Active treatment is mandatory for progressive scoliosis. Failure to control the curve by bracing warrants surgical intervention. The type of surgery depends on the age of the child and estimates of further vertebral growth. Both spinal fusion and growing rods have been used for selected patients. Preoperative halo traction has also been used to minimize the severity of the spine curvature prior to surgery, particularly when the spine is flexible.[44] This approach may also delay more definitive intervention with a growing rod or VEPTR device and hence minimize the number of expansions and replacements of the instrumentation over time.

Spine Deformities in Neuromuscular Diseases
The problems in patients with neuromuscular diseases are more complex (e.g., severity of the deformity, involvement of the pelvis, and associated nutritional, neurologic, and cardiopulmonary problems). Although surgery provides significant benefit with regard to quality of life, the consequences on long-term pulmonary function depend on the underlying disease and the nature of the spine deformity.

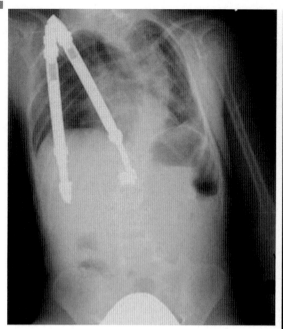
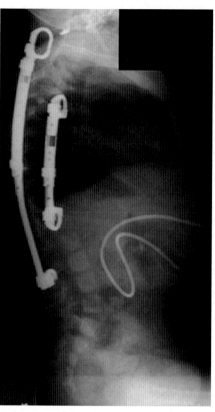

FIGURE 43-1. A pair of vertical expandable prosthetic titanium ribs (VEPTRs) in a child with early-onset thoracic scoliosis. The slide mechanism for expansion is located in the middle of each VEPTR. One device is attached from rib to rib (shorter device is on the lateral film), and one is attached from ribs to the spine.

New surgical devices are now being proposed to improve severe lordosis, which occurs in children with spina bifida. Of note, early treatment with corticosteroids largely prevents scoliosis development in DMD patients.

Postoperative Pulmonary Function in Scoliosis

Pulmonary complications are the principal cause of morbidity and mortality in the immediate period following surgery for scoliosis. Preoperative assessment of pulmonary function, including overnight oximetry and assessment of hypercapnea, should therefore be done as a guide to prevent and treat postoperative complications. The most frequent respiratory problems reported in the immediate postoperative course of surgery for scoliosis include atelectasis, hemothorax/pneumothorax, pneumonia, pulmonary edema, upper airway obstruction, pulmonary fat emboli, and, consequently, respiratory failure. Immediate pulmonary complications result from multiple factors such as the surgical procedure, the degree of preoperative pulmonary disability, the transient limitation of chest wall expansion as a result of pain, and effects of anesthetics and analgesics. The underlying pathologic conditions associated with scoliosis also contribute to the immediate postoperative course. In neuromuscular diseases, respiratory muscle weakness, cough impairment, and swallowing disorders increase the risk of immediate postoperative pulmonary complications. Noninvasive ventilation and mechanical in-exsufflation are a valuable aid for patients with and without neuromuscular weakness in the immediate postoperative period to reduce the duration of tracheal intubation.[16]

Surgical intervention corrects the spinal curvature, but improvement in lung volume and arterial oxygenation only becomes apparent late after surgery. Improvement may not be measurable for 2 years or more following surgery. In some cases, surgery can cause a deterioration of lung function, especially when an anterior fusion is added to posterior instrumented fusion and thoracoplasty.

Hypoplastic Thorax Syndromes

A variety of syndromes are associated with small thoraces leading to secondary respiratory failure in the first year of life and high mortality rates. These represent a separate category of *thoracic insufficiency syndrome*. Hypoplasia can occur as a result of a reduced circumference or a reduced thoracic vertebral height. There is a continuum of hypoplasia in most of these syndromes such that some patients live to adulthood without respiratory support. In addition, several syndromes are associated with multiorgan anomalies that impact prognosis as well. Recent development of expandable titanium devices has led to novel interventions with short-term respiratory improvements, but the long-term outlook remains unclear, even with new surgical interventions.

The most common hypoplastic thorax syndrome is asphyxiating thoracic dystrophy, also known as Jeune syndrome or thoracic-pelvic-phalangeal dystrophy.[45] It is an autosomal recessive disorder characterized by a narrow, hypoplastic rib cage, and generalized chondrodystrophy with short limb dwarfism. Pelvic and phalangeal abnormalities, polydactyly, renal and hepatic disorders, thrombocytopenia, and Shwachman syndrome have also been reported in conjunction with asphyxiating thoracic dystrophy, with renal disease emerging later in life as a serious concern. Estimates suggest that up to 600 patients per year are born worldwide with this disease. Asphyxiating

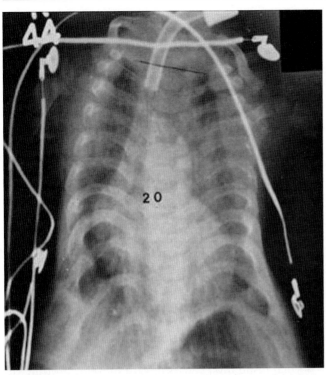

FIGURE 43-2. Chest radiograph of an intubated infant with asphyxiating thoracic dystrophy.

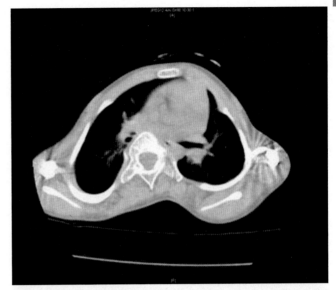

FIGURE 43-3. CT scan of a child with asphyxiating thoracic dystrophy. Note the shortened ribs that curve inward toward the cardiac borders in a "four-leaf clover" appearance.

thoracic dystrophy is usually diagnosed immediately after birth when the thoracic circumference is found to be <75% of head circumference and the infant is tachypneic. Characteristic chest radiograph findings reveal a narrow chest cage, with high-positioned clavicles, short horizontal ribs, and flaring of the costochondral junctions (Fig. 43-2). The CT scan is characteristic with a four-leaf clover appearance due to foreshortened ribs (Fig. 43-3). The lungs are constrained by the chest and are elongated in the process. If untreated, most infants with asphyxiating thoracic dystrophy die soon after birth due to respiratory failure. Less severe variants have been reported with clinical courses that vary from respiratory failure in infancy to few or no respiratory symptoms at all. In patients who survive the neonatal period, respiratory failure may occur during infancy and childhood because of chest constriction, impairment of lung growth, and superimposed pneumonia. Improvement in bone abnormalities may occur with age, however, thereby justifying life-support procedures (e.g., long-term mechanical ventilation) in early life. Several surgical procedures have been proposed and used clinically to increase thoracic cage size. These include the interposition of adjacent ribs with titanium connectors to make the existing ribs longer.[46] Alternatively, customized curved VEPTR devices have been used in conjunction with osteotomies of the ribs to enlarge the thoracic cavity. The latter can then be expanded regularly to increase the thorax as the child grows. Lung functions have not been reported following these surgical treatments, but mortality has been reduced to 50% in the first year of life in uncontrolled case series.[38]

An alternative type of chest wall hypoplasia is illustrated by patients with Jarcho-Levin syndrome. This syndrome is actually two distinct genetic disorders: spondylocostal dysostosis and spondylothoracic dysplasia. The former condition includes broadening, bifurcation, and fusion of the ribs; congenital scoliosis; and a shortened thoracic vertebral height (Fig. 43-4). It has both autosomal dominant and autosomal recessive inheritance patterns. In contrast, spondylothoracic dysplasia, which is inherited in an autosomal recessive manner, manifests as a shortened thoracic height caused by vertebral malformations, a fanlike rib configuration, and fusion of costovertebral junctions. This condition is more severe with a higher mortality in the first year of life due to respiratory failure.[47] Children have received titanium devices to further increase thoracic height, but lung functions following surgical intervention have not been reported.

Similar severe respiratory distress leading to death in infancy or early childhood has been reported in patients with other forms of thoracic cage hypoplasia, including thanatophoric dwarfism, achondroplasia, chondroectodermal dysplasia, and giant exomphalos.

MISCELLANEOUS DISORDERS THAT CAUSE CHEST WALL DYSFUNCTION

The Chest Wall in Obstructive Pulmonary Disease

In obstructive pulmonary disease, overinflation of the chest wall places the diaphragm and the other breathing muscles at a mechanical disadvantage for breathing. The diaphragm is flattened, and the inspiratory force generated by the contraction of muscle fibers is lower than that generated by the diaphragm when it is in its usual upward position with a normal dome. Because the ribs are in a more horizontal position, the inspiratory force generated by the intercostal muscles is also lower than that found with ribs in their normal oblique position. As a result, the maximal inspiratory and expiratory pressures generated in patients with severe forms of bronchopulmonary dysplasia, asthma, or cystic fibrosis are lower than in normal individuals. In addition, dysfunction of the chest wall may also be caused by

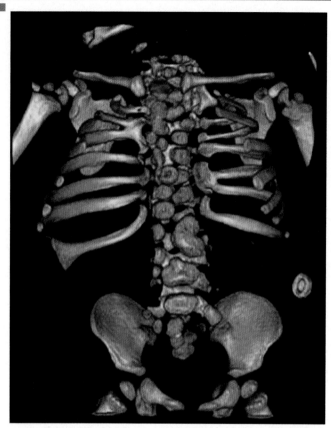

FIGURE 43-4. Vertebral and rib anomalies including fused ribs in a reconstructed image from a thoracoabdominal computerized tomographic study of a child with Jarcho-Levin syndrome. Note the foreshortened thorax with few normal thoracic vertebrae.

reduction in the mass of the respiratory muscles due to malnutrition and weight loss commonly found in patients with advanced forms of chronic obstructive pulmonary disease.

Obesity

Obesity in children is epidemic in developed countries. Consequences of obesity on pulmonary function in children have been examined in only a few studies. Results obtained primarily in adults show that the most consistent effect on lung volumes is decreased FRC caused by increased mass load of adipose tissue around the rib cage and abdomen, as well as periviscerally in the thoracic and abdominal cavity. In morbidly obese individuals, FRC decrease can be so important that it approaches residual volume. While total lung capacity is mildly decreased in proportion to the degree of obesity, residual volume is unchanged. Thus, obese individuals usually have an increased inspiratory reserve volume and a markedly decreased expiratory reserve volume. In addition, obesity is responsible for stiffening of the respiratory system, due to decreased lung compliance. The latter may be related to closure of dependent airways with atelectasis, increased pulmonary blood volume, or decreased FRC with an increase in alveolar surface tension. The presence of an associated decrease in chest wall compliance is more controversial.

Physical performance is decreased in obese children and adolescents. Compared to controls, obese children and ado-

lescents have similar ventilatory efficiency (minute ventilation/CO_2 production), but a higher absolute metabolic cost of exercise, an increased awareness of fatigue, and increased exercise-induced bronchospasm, even in nonasthmatic individuals.[48] Physical performance has been shown to be amenable to improvement, at least in the short term, by an intense management program, including dietary restriction, psychological support, and physical activity.[49]

Links between obesity and asthma, and between obesity and sleep apnea, are beyond the scope of this chapter.

The Chest Wall of the Newborn

The diaphragm and chest wall are immature at birth, especially in the preterm newborn. The insertion of the diaphragm to the rib cage is more perpendicular, which favors inward displacement of the lower ribs with any forceful diaphragmatic contraction. Moreover, the whole rib cage of the newborn is a highly pliable structure. This results in an inward movement of the ribs and the sternum with deep inspirations, such as with crying, hiccupping or sighing. In the absence of intercostal muscle activity to stiffen the rib cage (e.g., during REM sleep or in conditions with abnormal muscle weakness), even a normal inspiration causes inward movement of the rib cage with a proportional reduction of the inspired tidal volume. Excessive diaphragm contraction therefore has to be used to produce an adequate tidal volume. In addition, respiratory muscle mass and the proportion of fatigue-resistant fibers in the diaphragm are lower, resulting in less resistance to fatigue. This can be further amplified by nutritional difficulties or hypoglycemia, hypocalcemia, hypophosphatemia, or acidosis. To cope with these difficulties, the newborn in resting conditions breathes rapidly, with limited excursion of the diaphragm. In disease conditions, rather than increasing the depth of each breath, the newborn further increases respiratory rate, thereby preventing diaphragmatic fatigue by decreasing duration of the inspiratory contraction. In addition, the newborn often prevents respiratory failure by increasing resting alveolar gas stores (i.e., the end expiratory lung volume). This is accomplished by increasing respiratory rate, hence decreasing the time devoted to lung deflation, or by braking the expiratory flow, through active glottal closure and progressive postinspiratory decontraction of the diaphragm. However, in situations of extreme prematurity, newborns are prone to respiratory muscle fatigue, sometimes even in resting, normal conditions. Respiratory muscle fatigue is more often the cause of respiratory failure in the newborn than at any other time in life.

Acknowledgments

Jean-Paul Praud is supported by Le Fonds de recherche du Québec and the Canadian Institutes for Health Research and is the holder of the Canada Research Chair in Neonatal Respiratory Physiology.

References

The complete reference list is available online at www.expertconsult.com

44 THE EPIDEMIOLOGY OF ASTHMA

M. Innes Asher, BSc, MBChB, FRACP, Jacob Twiss, BHB, MBChB, PhD, DipPaed, FRACP, and Eamon Ellwood, DipTch, DipInfo Tech

Asthma is one of the most common noncommunicable diseases in children. Studies of the epidemiology of asthma have burgeoned in the last 2 to 3 decades. This reflects worldwide concern that asthma is increasing in prevalence and is an important cause of morbidity not only in developed, but also in developing countries.[1] The hope of finding factors that influence asthma in populations that are amenable to interventions has not yet been fulfilled. This chapter gives an overview of key advances in epidemiologic knowledge that have public health and clinical relevance.

DEFINITION AND MEASUREMENT IN EPIDEMIOLOGIC STUDIES

Definitions

When a child presents to a clinician, the diagnosis of asthma is made in clinical practice by characteristic findings on history of episodic wheeze, cough, or breathlessness and usually a normal physical examination in the interval phase. Wheeze is the most frequent symptom of the variable airway obstruction that occurs in asthma. Clinical definitions are described in all pediatric asthma guidelines. For example, the British Thoracic Society and Scottish Intercollegiate Guidelines Network[2] and Global Initiative for Asthma guidelines[3] emphasize the exclusion of other conditions causing wheeze, cough, or breathlessness, especially in the very young child. More recently, there has been a focus on clarifying the definition of wheezing in preschool children with two categories proposed: episodic viral wheeze and multiple trigger wheeze.[4]

Epidemiologic studies investigate populations rather than individuals, and thus the methods of assessment need to be appropriate for this task. Measurements are made in individuals from which the presence or absence of asthma is determined, and thus the population prevalence or incidence is estimated, sometimes with characterization by severity or some other parameter. When comparisons are made between populations (and within populations at different points in time), it is vital that the same standardized methods are used to ensure confidence in the estimates obtained.

The most common approach in epidemiologic studies is the use of written questionnaires completed by the parent for younger age groups and self-reported by adolescents. The latter may report a higher rate of symptoms than reported by the parent for the same adolescents.[5-7] This may be caused by a greater awareness of milder symptoms in the adolescent, or symptoms occurring when the parent is not present and not reported to the parent. An asthma symptoms video questionnaire was developed in 1992 in response to possible translation problems with written questionnaires used between populations who speak different languages, some of whom have no word for *wheeze*. The video shows scenes of young people with asthma, thereby avoiding the need to describe symptoms verbally. The validity of the video has been investigated by comparison with bronchial hyperresponsiveness (BHR),[8-13] and most studies show a close relationship. Its relationship to the written questionnaire is close between populations,[14] but within populations the prevalence estimates are lower with the video questionnaire,[15] and its relationship within individuals is not clearcut.[10,16-19]

Questions about more recent symptoms (in the last 12 months) are more reliable than questions about symptoms in the past because they reduce errors of recall. The most commonly used standard question is "Have you (has your child) had wheezing or whistling in the chest in the last 12 months?" When the answer is yes, the term *current wheeze* is commonly used. Parental report of wheeze over the past 12 months has been shown to have a range of sensitivity of 0.58 to 0.88 and a specificity of 0.64 to 0.95 for physician diagnosis of childhood asthma.[20-22] Provided that the information has been collected in a standardized manner, any information biases are expected to be in both directions, thus enabling reliable comparisons between populations.[23]

In view of some of the potential limitations of questionnaires, there has been a search for an objective "asthma test" from which the diagnosis can be made with certainty. In the late 1970s, a test of nonspecific BHR was suggested as an objective test for diagnosing asthma and assessing its severity.[24,25] BHR is measured using a nonspecific inhaled challenge such as methacholine, histamine, or hypertonic saline challenge, or a standardized exercise test.[26] Its usefulness in children is limited, as the test cannot be reliably performed in epidemiologic studies in the field with children younger than 6 years of age.

The initial inclusion of BHR as a diagnostic test for asthma was based on subjects who were attending hospital clinics and were not representative of the community at large. In 1990, Pattemore and colleagues reported a study of an unbiased community sample in New Zealand in which they found that the level of BHR was a poorer predictor of doctor diagnosis of asthma than responses to the question "Has your child had wheezing in the last 12 months?" on written questionnaires.[27] Although there was a trend for greater BHR among children with more severe symptoms, the confidence intervals showed a large overlap between groups. Similar observations have been made in subsequent population-based studies.[28,29] Thus BHR, while related to asthma, is not equivalent to asthma.

Study Designs

Several designs are commonly used in studies of asthma epidemiology. Care must be taken in the interpretation of study findings because of the many factors that may influence asthma.[23] The randomized trial has rarely been used in epidemiologic studies. Cross-sectional studies are most suitable for estimating the prevalence of asthma symptoms, diagnosis, and severity; relating these to other measured factors, and generating hypotheses. Most such studies have been within populations, but in 1985 the first study between centers in different countries was completed.[30] This was followed by several other comparisons between populations, and then in 1992 the International Study of Asthma and Allergies (ISAAC) was established, a multiphase cross-sectional study that became the largest epidemiologic study of asthma in children ever undertaken.[31] ISAAC used a simple standardized methodology with written and video questionnaires about asthma symptoms in Phases One and Three[14,32,33] with a conventional cross-sectional study design. Phase Two, which used more intensive standardized modules to make comparisons between populations (centers), followed the cross-sectional design with case control analyses.[34,35] Case control studies identify children with asthma and a control group of children without asthma, and then follow with a comparison of exposure of cases and controls to factors of interest (e.g., environmental tobacco smoke).

Ecological studies can be used to compare cross-sectional population data with environmental data, but they have recognized limitations compared with individual-level studies.[36,37] In particular, the estimated ecological effect may not reflect the biological effect at the individual level. However, ecological analyses are appropriate for attempting to explain why prevalence varies between populations and for putting the results of individual-level epidemiologic studies within populations in context.[38] ISAAC has therefore used ecological studies to identify associations that may be worthy of further investigation.[39]

Longitudinal studies (cohort studies) involve repeated observation of participants over time and may also include a series of cross-sectional measurements. These studies are particularly useful in identifying determinants

of asthma and its expression over the life course. See the Natural History section later in the chapter for several examples of these studies. Caution is needed in comparing one cohort study with another, as a recent analysis found 60 different definitions of asthma from 122 publications from cohort studies.[40] Studies that measure the incidence of asthma (number of new cases per year) involve long periods of time and especially large resources.

◼ THE PREVALENCE OF ASTHMA

Variation of Prevalence Between Countries and Regions

Until the mid-1980s, most studies of asthma had been undertaken within developed countries whose populations originated from the British Isles, and thus the global distribution of asthma was largely unknown. From the mid-1980s to the mid-1990s, there were a few studies of asthma in children between regions of the world.[30,41–48]

ISAAC developed a standardized and coordinated approach with simple inexpensive standardized methodology that enabled the collection of comparable data from children throughout the world (including non-English language populations and countries in the developing world).[14,49–53] ISAAC Phase One collected information concerning symptoms of asthma on more than 700,000 children (6 to 7 years of age) and adolescents (13 to 14 years of age) in 156 centers located in 56 countries around the world.[49,54] Wide variation in the prevalence of asthma was found around the world, even within genetically similar groups.

Further study of the global prevalence and severity of asthma symptoms was undertaken in ISAAC Phase Three, conducted between 2000 and 2003, involving 798,685 adolescents from 233 centers in 97 countries, and 388,811 children from 144 centers in 61 countries.[32] In this more comprehensive study (as in ISAAC Phase One), striking variations in prevalence were again found around the world. In adolescents, self-reported prevalence of wheeze in the past 12 months (current wheeze) varied from 32.6% in Wellington (New Zealand) to 0.8% in Tibet (China). Thirty-five centers (15%) had a prevalence of current wheeze ≥20%, and these were mostly from the English language countries and Latin America. Twenty-two centers (9.4%) had a prevalence of <5%, and they were mostly in the Indian subcontinent, Asia Pacific, Eastern Mediterranean, and Northern and Eastern Europe (Fig. 44-1). In children, parent-reported current wheeze ranged from 37.6% in Costa Rica to 2.4% in Jodhpur (India). Twenty-one centers (14.6%) had a prevalence of current wheeze ≥20%, and all but two were English language countries or Latin America. Seventeen centers (11.8%) had a prevalence of <5%, and these were mostly from the Indian subcontinent, Asia-Pacific, and Northern and Eastern Europe (Fig. 44-2). The size and location of these differences suggests that environmental factors are the most likely explanation for the global variations.

Indicators of asthma at the population level are prevalence of asthma symptoms, hospital admission, and mortality, and the rates for these vary greatly throughout the world. A recent report showed consistently positive associations

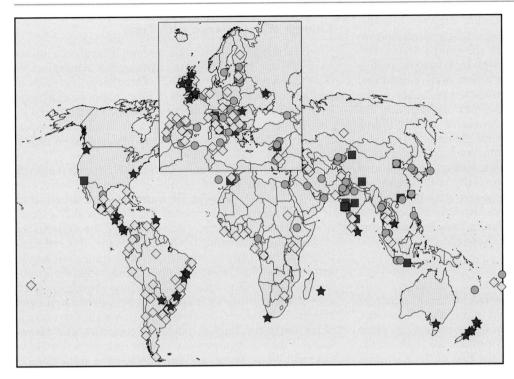

FIGURE 44-1. Prevalence of current wheeze* according to the written questionnaire in the 13- to 14-year age group. Symbols indicate prevalence values of <5% *(blue square)*, 5% to <10% *(green circle)*, 10% to <20% *(yellow diamond)*, and ≥20% *(red star)*. *Wheeze in the past 12 months. (Lai CKW, Beasley R, Crane J, et al. Global variation in the prevalence and severity of asthma symptoms: Phase Three of the International Study of Asthma and Allergies in Childhood (ISAAC). *Thorax.* 2009;64:478.)

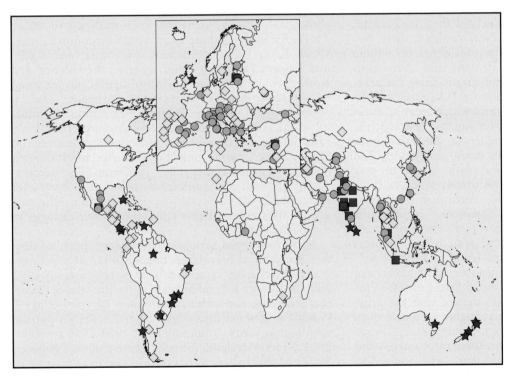

FIGURE 44-2. Prevalence of current wheeze* in the 6- to 7-year age group. Symbols indicate prevalence values of <5% *(blue square)*, 5% to <10% *(green circle)*, 10% to <20% *(yellow diamond)*, and ≥20% *(red star)*. *Wheeze in the past 12 months. (Lai CKW, Beasley R, Crane J, et al. Global variation in the prevalence and severity of asthma symptoms: Phase Three of the International Study of Asthma and Allergies in Childhood (ISAAC). *Thorax.* 2009;64:480.)

between national data on severe wheeze symptom prevalence from ISAAC Phase One, national hospital admissions for asthma, and national data on mortality admissions.[55]

Differences Between Rural and Urban Settings

Comparisons between urban and rural areas in the same country, with most reports coming from Africa, have shown consistent differences, with asthma prevalence being higher in the urban locations. For example, in Ghanaian children, exercise-induced bronchospasm was found more commonly in urban rich than in urban poor or rural children.[56] In Zimbabwean children, urban living and higher material standards were associated with higher prevalence of reversible airways obstruction.[57] In Kenyan children, exercise-induced bronchospasm and symptoms of asthma were found more commonly in urban children than in rural children.[58,59] Wheeze and asthma are especially rare in rural subsistence areas in Ethiopia.[60] Authors of these studies suggest that wealth, lifestyle, housing, and urban environmental exposures may contribute to increasing asthma prevalence. In the United States, two studies have found differing results. In Arkansas, asthma prevalence was similar between representative rural and urban groups, but asthma morbidity was higher in the rural group.[61] However, in Wisconsin, asthma was less commonly reported among farm-reared rural children than among non–farm-reared rural children.[62] Thus different aspects of the rural environment need exploration. Other studies of the effect of the farming environment on the occurrence of asthma, especially in European settings, suggest that microbial exposure may be a potentially protective effect resulting in low asthma prevalence in rural environments (see Infection, Immunization, and Microbial Exposure later in the chapter).[63]

Changes with Migration

Studies of migration have provided further evidence of powerful environmental influences on the occurrence of asthma, generally demonstrating an increase in prevalence when children migrate from low to high prevalence areas. In 1975 to 1976 in the first of these studies, Tokelauan children were observed in two environments. Asthma was more than twice more common among Tokelauan children in New Zealand than in Tokelau. Among children examined in New Zealand, there was no significant difference in the prevalence of asthma between those born in New Zealand and those born in Tokelau.[64] Among Asian immigrants from Pakistan, India, and East Africa in Blackburn, U.K, there was an increasing rate of asthma symptoms with increasing duration of stay in the U.K.[65] In Melbourne, Australia, the prevalence of wheeze was higher in Australian-born Asians and non-Asians than in Asian immigrants, and it was also strongly associated with length of stay in Australia.[43] In the ISAAC Australia study, asthma prevalence was higher among Australian-born children than among those born elsewhere.[66] In teenagers in Melbourne, Australia, there was an effect of length of residence on the prevalence of symptoms in subjects born outside Australia and now living in Melbourne.[67] Children born in the United States were more likely than children born outside of the United States to have current asthma.[68] A study in Israel showed that the prevalence of asthma symptoms was higher in native-born Israelis compared with Ethiopian immigrants, lower compared with immigrants from Western countries, and similar to immigrants from the former Soviet Union. The younger the age at which immigrants from the former Soviet Union and Ethiopia arrived in Israel, the higher their prevalence of asthma at 17 years of age.[69] Among Mexican Americans in the United States, children who were born in the United States had higher rates of asthma than their Mexican-born peers, and most were influenced by where they were born, age at immigration, and duration of U.S. residence.[70–72] Most recently, in ISAAC Phase Three (a global study), adolescents who were immigrants had fewer symptoms of asthma than those born in their new country. The effect diminished with increasing duration of residence in the adopted country.[73]

Change of Prevalence with Time

Many studies showed that asthma prevalence increased during the 1990s in Britain,[74–78] Australia,[79,80] New Zealand,[81,82] and Japan.[83] These large increases in prevalence over short periods of time cannot be explained by genetic variation and therefore are likely to be caused by environmental factors, but epigenetic factors may operate. These time-trend studies were undertaken in only a limited number of countries.

Therefore ISAAC Phase Three, which undertook an extensive study of time trends in asthma prevalence in over 100 centers in over 50 countries after a period of at least 5 years,[84] contributed the first "world" picture of changes in prevalence. As these were the majority of centers who undertook ISAAC Phase One, this reflected the large worldwide interest in time trends of prevalence. Following reports from English language countries in the 1990s of increases in asthma prevalence from the 1980s, continuing increases in prevalence had been expected. However, in most high-prevalence countries, particularly the English language countries, the prevalence of asthma symptoms changed little between Phase One and Phase Three, and even declined in some cases.[33] In contrast, a number of countries that had high or intermediate levels of symptom prevalence in Phase One showed significant increases in prevalence in Phase Three. Examples include Latin American countries (e.g., Costa Rica, Panama, Mexico, Argentina, and Chile) and Eastern European countries (e.g., the Ukraine and Romania). Other countries with significant increases in symptom prevalence included Barbados, Tunisia, Morocco, and Algeria. With the exception of India, all of the countries with very low symptom prevalence rates in Phase One reported increases in prevalence in Phase Three, though only the increases for Indonesia and China were statistically significant. The percentage of children and adolescents reported to have ever had asthma increased significantly, possibly reflecting greater awareness of this condition and/or changes in diagnostic practice.

There have been several other recent reports of time trends in asthma prevalence, outside of ISAAC, that generally reflect these same trends. In Germany from 1992 and 2001, there was no increase in the prevalence of current wheezing and asthma in children 10 years of age.[85] Canadian national data showed a fall in the proportion with high-severity symptoms from 1994-1995 to 2000-2001.[86] In Switzerland, four consecutive surveys between 1992 and 2001 suggest that the increase in prevalence of asthma in children 5 to 7 years of age living in Switzerland may have ceased.[87] A study of Swedish children between 1985 and 2005 suggested that the increase in asthmatic symptoms in schoolchildren has peaked, and the percentage of children with questionnaire-reported wheezing and severe symptoms has declined.[88] A non-ISAAC study of children 12 to 15 years of age in Taiwan between 1995 and 2001 showed that most of the 12-month prevalence of asthma symptoms decreased among boys but stabilized among girls.[89] In Turkey in the 9-year period from 1995 to 2004, the prevalence of asthma symptoms increased in schoolchildren 6 to 12 years of age in Istanbul.[90]

In children 7 to 8 years of age in London, there was evidence of an increase in the prevalence of asthma between 1991 and 2002.[91] Five surveys in Aberdeen from 1964 to 2004 showed a decrease in asthma symptoms most recently.[92] In the United Kingdom, trends in asthma indicators were reviewed from 1955 to 2004. The prevalence of asthma increased in children 2- to 3-fold, but it may have flattened or even fallen recently while current trends in adult prevalence were flat. The prevalence of a lifetime diagnosis of asthma increased in all age groups. The incidence of new asthma episodes presenting to general practitioners increased in all ages to a plateau in the mid-1990s and declined since then. During the 1990s, the annual prevalence of new cases of asthma and of treated asthma in general practice showed no major change.[93]

There have been other aspects of time trends studied. In the first report of ethnic-specific time trends of asthma prevalence within a country using ISAAC data, the prevalence in children increased in Māori and Pacific populations and decreased in European populations over a 10-year period, but there were no significant differences in adolescents.[94] In a gender-related time-trend study in Aberdeen, Scotland, from 1989 to 2004 in children 9 to 11 years of age, the male-to-female ratio significantly narrowed for wheeze.[95]

Prevalence by Age, Gender, and Ethnicity

Age
The prevalence of asthma increases from the preschool years to school age and from preadolescence to adolescence. However, there needs to be caution about comparing parent-reported symptoms in younger children to self-reported symptoms in adolescents, as the latter may report a higher rate of symptoms than the parent for the same adolescents.[5-7]

Gender
Gender differences in asthma symptom prevalence are present throughout the childhood years, but the pattern changes with age. In preschool children in Sweden, the age-specific asthma prevalence from 1 to 6 years of age showed somewhat higher levels for boys than for girls.[96] There are consistent reports of higher asthma symptom prevalence in school boys than girls. In adolescents, there is a mixed picture with considerable variation between countries, but, on average, prevalence in teenage girls is slightly higher than in teenage boys. These reports come from the United States,[97] the United Kingdom,[98] and from ISAAC Phase One in 156 centers in 56 countries in children 6 to 7 years of age and 13 to 14 years of age.[14] In a cross-sectional study in Rio de Janeiro State, Brazil, asthma prevalence was more frequent and severe among girls than boys.[99] A recent review of the literature confirmed these observations; they found that boys were consistently reported to have more prevalent wheeze and asthma than girls. In adolescence, the pattern changes and onset of wheeze is more prevalent in females than in males. A further recent study found that asthma, after childhood, is more severe in females than in males and is relatively underdiagnosed and undertreated in female adolescents.[100] However, in contrast a very large study of Californian adolescent males and females exhibited nearly the same patterns of prevalence.[101] The factors that influence the differences in gender-related expression of disease are not known, but suggestions include parental atopy,[102] and hormonal changes with maturation.

There has been recent work demonstrating differences in time trends between genders. In children 7 to 8 years of age in Sweden studied 10 years apart, the prevalence of current wheeze increased in boys, whereas in girls the prevalence tended to decrease, seemingly explained by observed increases in the prevalence of risk factors for asthma in boys compared with girls.[103] In a longitudinal study in New Zealand, males more often developed childhood wheeze and females more often developed adolescent-onset wheeze. Paternal history was a stronger risk factor for wheeze in females than in males.[102] In Aberdeen, Scotland, in four repeated cross-sectional studies over a 15-year period, the male-to-female ratio significantly narrowed for wheeze, partly caused by disappearance of the bias to diagnose asthma in symptomatic males but not in females, suggesting that other environmental factors enhancing the expression of asthma and atopy in females could be explored in future research.[95]

Ethnicity
Until the last decade, relatively few studies investigated the comparative prevalence in indigenous children compared with the colonizing populations and more recent immigrants. A range of differences has been found, generally showing a more clinical symptoms among indigenous children. In ISAAC Phase One in New Zealand, greater severity among Māori (indigenous) and Pacific children (Polynesian not indigenous) was found.[104] In ISAAC Phase Three 8 to 10 years later, the prevalence of current wheeze was higher in Māori and Pacific children compared with European/Pakeha children, and it was higher in Māori and European/Pakeha adolescents than in Pacific adolescents. Māori populations had a higher prevalence of almost all severe symptoms compared with European/Pakeha populations.[94] In a study of Canadian children living in northern and remote communities, Aboriginal children had significantly lower prevalence of asthma ever, while the prevalence of wheeze was similar to non-Aboriginal children.[105]

Studies in children of different ethnicities (non-indigenous) within countries have shown ethnic differences. In nationally representative U.S. samples among currently symptomatic children 3 to 17 years of age, Mexican children had a lower prevalence and Puerto Ricans had a higher prevalence of asthma symptoms than non-Hispanic African-American and white children.[106,107] Among children from different Asian-American subgroups, a wide variation occurred in asthma prevalence.[68]

The causes of ethnic differences in prevalence are complex. It is not straightforward to separate socioeconomic influences from ethnicity, as commonly indigenous people and non-white ethnic groups are usually relatively socioeconomically disadvantaged compared with white groups. To illustrate this in a nationally representative U.S. sample of children 3 years of age, asthma prevalence declined with increasing income for non–African-American but not African-American children.[108] In New York children 4 to 13 years of age, asthma prevalence within different ethnic and income groups was consistently lower in neighborhoods of greater socioeconomic status, except among Puerto Rican children, who had high asthma prevalence, regardless of school attended or income.[109] Differences in symptomatology may reflect differences in disease management,[104] inequalities in access to care,[94] or other factors. In the U.K. millennium cohort at 3 years of age, more Black Caribbean children and fewer Bangladeshi children reported ever asthma and recent wheeze compared with white children. After adjustments, the disadvantage in asthma and recent wheeze for Black Caribbeans was mostly explained by socioeconomic factors. However, for Bangladeshi children, asthma and wheezing illnesses appeared to be underreported, accounted for by the recentness of migration and low English language use, suggesting that potential explanations for observed differences may be different between ethnic groups.[110] In a very large study of Californian adolescents, an increased risk was observed for asthma and BMI, and there were no substantial differences in this basic pattern found between the six examined racial/ethnic groups.[101] Different types of risks may contribute to variations in asthma morbidity for urban children from specific ethnic groups with asthma whose health outcomes lag far behind their non-Latino white counterparts.[111] These findings are reinforced by a conceptual model related to four main domains that has been developed to explain asthma health disparities in Latino children in the United States: the individual and family, the environment or context in which the child lives, the health care system, and provider characteristics (with potential mechanisms).[112]

THE BURDEN OF ASTHMA

Childhood asthma imposes a tremendous burden on children, families, caregivers, society, and health care providers. Precise quantification is difficult due to differences in definition, geographical prevalence, asthma severity, and the complexity of its impact. Asthma burden is also changing. While it has been high in the developed world for some time, it is increasingly being felt in developing countries where prevalence is rising. Asthma's burden has multiple components that act at different levels (child, family, and society), as shown in Table 44-1.

Perception of burden is highly individual and influenced more by health care utilization than objective measures. Parents may perceive high burden, even in children with objectively mild intermittent asthma.[113] On the other hand, high medication use and frequent health care visits are associated with higher perceived burden yet better control (as defined by hospital bed days). Studies consistently demonstrate disparities in both objective and perceived asthma burden according to ethnicity and socioeconomic status, likely a reflection of capacity to access and implement effective therapy.[113] Baydar and colleagues found that ethnic disparity in burden all but disappeared when comparing families with the same health care access and degree of asthma control.[113] Uniquely they also examined

TABLE 44-1	COMPONENTS OF THE BURDEN OF ASTHMA
COMPONENT	**LEVEL**
Direct physiologic impairment (e.g., lung function)	Child
Direct asthma symptoms (e.g., cough, wheeze, dyspnea)	Child
Sleep disturbance leading to daytime impairment	Child, family
Missed schooling and reduced educational achievement	Child, society
Missed socializing opportunities	Child
Functional limitations (e.g., sports, recreation)	Child
Psychosocial impact/quality of life for child and family	Child, family
Exacerbations and hospitalizations	Child, family, society
Work absenteeism for caregivers	Child, family, society
Direct and indirect economic costs	Child, family, society
Mortality	Child, family, society

how perceived and actual burden changed over time. Those engaged in "asthma control activities" including high levels of effort toward medication adherence and non-emergency health care visits had more favorable perceived and actual burden levels. Despite the advent of effective pharmaceuticals and management guidelines emphasizing proactive care, a large proportion of children with asthma have poor control and reactive health care.[114] An estimated one third of the direct economic costs and up to three quarters of the total economic costs are caused by inadequate treatment resulting in poor control.[115] Indicators of asthma burden will be reviewed later in the chapter.

Sleep Disturbance, School Absenteeism, and Quality of Life

Sleep disturbance caused by nocturnal asthma symptoms is common and a central feature in classifying asthma severity. In ISAAC Phase One, nearly 2% of children 13 to 14 years of age had at least weekly wheeze-induced sleep disturbance worldwide.[14] The rates in children 6 to 7 years of age were similar. In those who wheezed at any time, over 12% had at least weekly wheeze-induced sleep disturbance. The rates were even higher in another multinational study.[114] Rabe and colleagues[114] surveyed over 3000 children and nearly 8000 adults with asthma across 29 countries including North America, Europe, and Asia. They reported at least weekly sleep disturbance in 20% to 50% of respondents (adults and children combined). Three other recent pediatric studies (United States and Australia) found rates of 20% to 50% over a 4-week period.[116–118] Desager and coworkers sought to better characterize the ISAAC findings by combining a common pediatric sleep questionnaire with the ISAAC survey in Antwerp.[119] They that found children with wheeze were much more likely to experience restless sleep (OR 5.0, p <0.001), daytime sleepiness (OR 3.8, p <0.001), and daytime tiredness (OR 5.1, p <0.01) compared with non-wheezers. Stores and colleagues studied sleep in children with asthma compared with matched controls utilizing questionnaires, neurocognitive testing, and polysomnography.[120] They found that children with asthma had significantly more disturbed sleep with lower sleep efficiency and greater daytime sleepiness. In addition, they performed poorer at memory recall tasks and scored higher on depression and psychosomatic symptom scores. Many of these measures improved following adjustments in asthma therapy.

In the United States, asthma is the leading cause of school absenteeism due to a chronic illness and accounts for over 6 million school absence days per year (a mean of 1.5 to 2.5 days per child with asthma).[121–123] The mean absenteeism for children with asthma is 30% higher than average.[122] Those with nocturnal symptoms are nearly 4 times as likely to miss school as those without.[123] The impact may be even greater in the developing world. A prospective study of children with mostly mild persistent asthma in Kathmandu found nearly three quarters missed more than 7 days of schooling *per month* caused by illness.[124] An asthma education program reduced this proportion to 12%. The impact on learning will be even greater when impaired school performance is considered in addition to absenteeism.

Children with asthma are at greater risk of psychological problems, especially those involving internalization. Many studies have suggested a bidirectional relationship between mental and physical health in asthma operating at internal (psychoneuroimmunologic) and external (behavior and therapy adherence) levels.[125] Children with asthma are more likely to experience anger, fear, frustration, anxiety, loneliness, and guilt than controls.[126] It frequently restricts participation in sporting and social activities and may even limit choices such as family pets.[126] Gender differences have been observed in both quality of life scores and how children adapt to the burden of asthma. Consistent with many reports, a recent Swedish study of children attending a specialist clinic found that quality of life scores were significantly poorer in girls than in boys, despite severe asthma being twice as common among the boys.[126] Girls appear more likely to incorporate asthma and asthma therapy into their personal identities, while boys attempt to exclude or deny it.[126]

While quality of life measures are seen as important indicators in chronic disease, quality of life is not necessarily lower in those with chronic illness than in healthy controls.[125] In children, the relationship between asthma severity and quality of life has been inconsistent. Studies comparing diseases have found that childhood asthma fairs better than diabetes, cystic fibrosis, or rheumatoid arthritis in quality of life scores.[127] In fact, children in the aforementioned Swedish study scored toward the top end of the quality of life range despite having frequent symptoms.[126]

Nevertheless, maintaining quality of life, particularly in the emotional parameters, may be an important marker for successful management of and adaption to asthma. Goldbeck and colleagues found that psychological factors were greater determinants of quality of life in asthma than asthma severity.[125] They found no correlation between asthma severity and emotional or behavioral symptoms but did find that psychological problems impaired asthma management. Another study reported that symptoms of mild to moderate depression were common in adolescents with asthma and strongly associated with disease activity.[128] The authors speculated that the emotional symptoms caused the increased asthma activity, not the reverse. Over one third of parents also scored in the depressive range. While there was correlation between child and parental depression scores, there was no correlation between parental depression and child asthma severity.

Hospitalization

Asthma is one of the most common reasons for children requiring inpatient care in the developed world, and admission rate is commonly used as a measure of asthma severity and morbidity. Clearly admission has a large impact on health services, children, and their families, however care needs to be taken when interpreting rates and trends over time. Asthma hospital admission rates vary considerably between hospitals within the same city, regionally within a country, and between neighboring countries.[129–131] Although some of this variability is caused by differences in disease prevalence and severity, other factors also contribute, including variability in primary care, admitting practices, and the organization of acute inpatient facilities. Also, rates from different centers and countries often are obtained through different methodologies. Nevertheless, published figures are high and demonstrate substantial geographic variation, with recent rates of 60 to 450 admissions per 100,000 children per year (Table 44-2).

TABLE 44-2   RECENTLY PUBLISHED GLOBAL ASTHMA ADMISSION RATES

COUNTRY	CHILDHOOD RATE (PER 100,000 PER YEAR)	YEAR(S)
Australia[55,144]	274-450*	2002, 2006
New Zealand[145,598]	~200	2006
United States[55,143]	190-210	2002, 2006
United Kingdom[55,599]	170-260	2001, 2002
Sweden[599]	180	2000
Taiwan[146]	105	2002
Spain[599]	60	2000

*The higher estimate included children admitted with asthma in the 0- to 1-year age group.

Trends Over Time in Asthma Hospitalizations: 1960 to 1990

Asthma hospital admission rates increased dramatically from the mid to late 1960s into the 1980s. These increases were evident in several countries including Australia, Canada, England and Wales, New Zealand, and the United States.[132] The size of the increase was significant and ranged from a 3-fold increase in the United States to a 10-fold increase in New Zealand over an approximate 15-year period.[132] In New Zealand, admission rates increased in both the 0- to 4-year and the 5- to 14-year age groups.[132] In England, Wales, and the United States, the largest increase in hospitalization rates occurred in children younger than 5 years of age.[133,134] Increase in both prevalence and severity of asthma were thought to be the main contributing factors to the increase in hospitalization rates.[75,135] An increase in the number of children hospitalized and, to a lesser extent, the number of hospitalizations per child contributed to the increase in asthma hospitalization rates in England, Wales, and New Zealand from the 1960s to the 1980s.[136,137] Evidence of increased severity includes an increase in the proportion of patients hospitalized with asthma who then required intubation.[135] The increase in hospital admission rates in New Zealand was substantially greater than the 2-fold increase in asthma prevalence over this time period.[132] Neither diagnostic transfer nor increases in admissions for less severe asthma were contributory.[132,135,136]

Trends Over Time in Asthma Hospitalizations: 1990 to 2007

Pediatric asthma hospital admission rates stabilized or decreased during the 1990s in several countries including England, Wales, Australia, New Zealand, and the United States.[133,138-145] This is not a universal phenomenon, even in the developed world. In Taiwan, for example, a substantial increase has been seen since 1996.[146] In England, hospital admission for wheeze between 1990 and 2000 decreased by 52% in children 0 to 4 years of age and by 45% in children 5 to 14 years of age.[147] Over a longer period in Australia (1993 to 2007), the childhood admission rate for asthma decreased by 42%.[144] While a similar decrease has been described in New Zealand, there has been an upswing in admissions since 2003, though it is still much lower than the 1990 rate.[145] There is considerable variability between states and populations in the United States, however overall admission rates have been stable since 1991.[143]

Given admissions are the result of asthma prevalence, severity, asthma management, and the influences of risk and protective factors, it is unlikely that any single factor explains the variable hospitalization rate. It is certainly not solely attributable to parallel changes in asthma prevalence. More effective proactive management of chronic asthma or more effective out-of-hospital care of exacerbations are likely important factors. Similarly asthma severity may have changed as a result of social and environmental factors.

However, in Australia and the United Kingdom at least, primary care visits for childhood asthma have also decreased substantially (~40%), so reduced hospitalization does not appear to be the result of higher admission thresholds or of a shift of care from the secondary to primary sector.[144,148] Asthma severity or control may have changed as a result of social and environmental factors, and large reductions in primary care visits for viral respiratory infection has led to speculation that reduced respiratory infection is behind apparent improvements in asthma control.[148] In Australia, the average length of stay in hospital with childhood asthma has decreased by 24% from 2 days in 1998 to 1.5 days in 2006.[144] It is not clear whether this represents reduced asthma severity, changes in asthma management, or both.

Risk and Protective Factors for Hospital Admission

Prehospital Care

Effective asthma management reduces the risk and severity of exacerbations, thus leading to a reduction in hospitalization. Effectiveness depends on many factors such as access, education, understanding, adherence, affordability, and treatment efficacy. The introduction of medications (e.g., inhaled corticosteroids) together with management strategies (e.g., asthma action plans) has been shown to affect the risk of admission and re-admission. Variability in hospital admissions between populations, regions, and over time is likely to be strongly influenced by the uptake and quality of prehospital care. Quality of ambulatory care, implementation of guidelines, written action plans, and inhaled corticosteroid usage all affect hospitalization rate.[149-153]

Socioeconomics/Poverty and Ethnicity

Living in poverty remains one of the major factors that increase the likelihood of a child being hospitalized with asthma and modify the impact of other factors. Access to regular nonemergency care is associated with improved control. Poverty and ethnic minority status is often associated with poorer health care access, poorer quality health care, less health care continuity, poorer housing, living in polluted areas, tobacco smoke exposure, poorer education, premature birth, and higher risk of respiratory infection—which are all in turn associated with asthma hospitalization.[154-157] In the United States, private health insurance versus public insurance has been associated with higher continuity, improved asthma education, better control, and lower hospitalization.[113] Importantly, poverty also appears to modify the potency of other risk factors such as air pollution.[158] Low parental literacy has been found to increase hospitalization.[159]

Asthma hospital admission rates vary with ethnicity; they are usually higher in indigenous or disadvantaged populations. The New Zealand Māori, U.S. African-American, and Australian Aborigine populations all have substantially higher hospitalization rates, although some data suggests that this disparity has been decreasing.[144,145,160,161]

Climate and Environmental Exposures

Asthma hospitalization rates vary with season. Temperature changes, other weather phenomena (e.g., thunderstorms, pollens, fungi), and prevalence of respiratory viral infection likely explain this.[162,163] Autumn is the peak season in both hemispheres.[164–166] In England and Wales, a second asthma hospitalization peak in spring is described for children 5 to 14 years of age that may reflect pollen activity.[166] Peaks in pollen activity and air particulate matter have been associated with admission rate.[158,167,168] Air pollution from road traffic near housing has also been associated with repeated hospital encounters.[169] Environmental tobacco smoke exposure is an important and modifiable risk factor for hospitalization.[170]

Age, Gender, and Obesity

Children younger than 5 years of age are at highest risk of hospital admission.[144,145,160,161] An earlier age of onset of symptoms is associated with an increased risk of hospitalization.[171] Gender differences in asthma hospitalization rates vary with age. In the 5- to 14-year age group, boys are more likely than girls to be hospitalized with asthma, and in the 15- to 24-year age group, girls are twice as likely as boys to be hospitalized with asthma.[134,157] Children who are overweight or obese are more likely to have more severe asthma, more exacerbations, and more admissions, and they are more likely to require intensive care.[172] The exact mechanism remains unclear.

Disease Severity

Hospitalization is frequently used as a marker of severity and even to define "difficult" asthma. It is therefore potentially circular to describe severity as a risk factor for admission. Nevertheless, children with chronic severe asthma, defined by a range of measures including frequency of respiratory symptoms, medication use, lung function, and airway hyperresponsiveness, are at greater risk.[173,174] Children with mild or intermittent asthma still have significant exacerbations however, even requiring intensive care (see later in the chapter), so chronic phenotypes may not reliably predict exacerbation severity.[175,176] Atopy, particularly as evidenced by an elevated IgE or rhinitis, also increases the risk of hospitalization.[171]

Viral Infection

As many as 85% of exacerbations are associated with viral infection in school-age children.[177] Indeed, virus infection may be the most important modifiable risk factor for hospitalization.[178] While rhinoviruses are most commonly implicated, coronaviruses, respiratory syncytial virus, parainfluenza viruses, and influenza (especially, in 2009, H1N1 influenza) are all implicated.[148,177,179,180] Urquhart and colleagues demonstrated that the decreasing rates in asthma hospitalizations and physician visits in the United Kingdom have occurred in parallel with decreasing rates of viral respiratory infections, and they argue that infection may be the most important explanation for the decrease in hospitalization.[148] In contrast, in the United States, where hospitalizations have stabilized rather than decreased, asthma-related community visits have increased.[143]

Risk Factors for Admission to Intensive Care

Children who are admitted to intensive care with life-threatening asthma are more likely to have severe asthma, be older, have a longer history of asthma, have a longer duration of symptoms prior to admission, be atopic, and/or be overweight or obese.[172,181] While they are also more likely to be under the care of a respiratory specialist, be on more than one regular medication (including inhaled corticosteroids and long-acting beta agonists), have asthma management plans, and have a history of previous hospital admission, these are all likely markers of asthma severity rather than causative factors. An important proportion have a history of only mild asthma and may have recurrent intensive care admission with few or no interval symptoms, which indicates that chronic asthma severity phenotypes do not necessarily predict severity of exacerbations.[175] Tobacco smoke exposure, while more common in children with asthma and associated with poorer control, has not been shown to be a risk factor for intensive care admission.[174]

Mortality

An estimated 250,000 people die from asthma every year. The majority are adults in low- to moderate-income countries.[182] In the context of such a prevalent condition, death from asthma during childhood is very rare, with many factors influencing its rate. These include overall asthma prevalence, pharmaceutical use, management guidelines, environmental factors, and health care access/delivery. Most asthma deaths are preventable with appropriate and timely medical intervention. Estimating asthma mortality is made difficult by the lack of universal definitions for both *asthma* and an *asthma death*. Further, a lack of reliable prevalence data may impair case fatality rates.

Asthma mortality increases with age and peaks during adolescence in the childhood age range and in the elderly among adults.[183] Most epidemiologic comparisons are made in the 5- to 34-year age group because the classification of both asthma and cause of death is more reliable in this age range.[139] In a systematic review of asthma mortality (5- to 34-year-olds) in 20 countries, Wijesinghe and colleagues found recent asthma mortality to be very low, with rates ranging from 0.1 to 0.5 per 100,000 per year.[184] For comparison, the "any-age" asthma mortality was recently estimated at 2 per 100,000 in the United States.[183] Estimates reflect single–cause of death data, which may underestimate the true contribution asthma makes to mortality. French and American studies utilizing multiple-cause models reported "asthma-related deaths" to be at least two times the "asthma as underlying cause of death" rate.[183,185] The impact is likely to be greatest in the elderly, where comorbidities are very common. However, the concept that asthma may contribute to mortality causation without being the single cause is relevant in childhood.

Trends in Asthma Mortality Over Time

Revisions of the International Classification of Diseases have made the interpretation of temporal trends more difficult, although this effect has been less marked for children than for adults. For example, in the United States, introduction of the tenth revision in 1998 was estimated to have accounted for approximately 25% of the decrease in asthma deaths that occurred from 1998 to 1999.[186] Nevertheless, the examination of international time trends is valuable in considering asthma burden and also the effectiveness or risks of asthma management.

Data from Australia, England and Wales, New Zealand, and the United States show that asthma mortality rates between 1910 and 1940 were low (less than 1 per 100,000 per year in people 5 to 34 years of age) and were relatively stable.[187] Starting with Australia and New Zealand, endemic mortality rates gradually increased until the 1980s, when they started to gradually decrease to record lows.[184,187] Epidemics of asthma deaths were observed in many countries during the 1960s and particularly in New Zealand in the late 1970s and 1980s. Figure 44-3 shows the asthma mortality rates (deaths per 100,000 persons 5 to 34 years of age) in 20 countries between 1960 and 2005.

While asthma mortality is complex, trends can be viewed as resulting from changes in asthma prevalence and changes in asthma case fatality. In the 1960s, asthma mortality rates increased 2- to 10-fold within a 2- to 5-year period in Australia, England and Wales, New Zealand, Norway, and Scotland, but there was no increase observed in Canada, Denmark, Germany, or the United States. Peak mortality rates during these epidemics were from 2 to 3 per 100,000 persons 5 to 34 years of age,

lasting 10 to 15 years in affected countries.[187] Considering asthma prevalence, these epidemics resulted from a rapid increase in case fatality. While there may not be a single explanation, pharmaceutical usage and in particular the introduction of isoprenaline forte inhalers likely played a major role.[93,187]

A further epidemic of asthma deaths occurred from 1976 to 1989, most noticeably in, but not confined to, New Zealand.[184] During this period the asthma mortality rate in New Zealand was the highest in the world, peaking in 1979 at 4.1 per 100,000 persons 5 to 34 years of age (see Fig. 44-3).[184,188,189] The use of the potent and less selective β_2 agonist fenoterol is considered the major factor.[184,190–192] Asthma mortality rates decreased rapidly in New Zealand following warnings and subsequent restrictions of the sale of fenoterol.[193]

Unlike the asthma mortality epidemics, the rising endemic asthma mortality seen until the 1990s does not appear to be caused by a single predominant factor and may reflect rising overall prevalence rather than increased case fatality. Mortality, hospitalization, and incidence rates all increased over this same time period.[187] The increases were substantial, with a median increase in mortality of 45% in 15 developed countries from 1975-1977 to 1985-1987.[187] The increases occurred in a wide range of countries with differing lifestyles, and they were variable in countries with similar lifestyles. A wide range of age groups was affected. For example, in the United States, from 1980 to 1993, increases were evident in the 0- to 4-year, 5- to 14-year, and 15- to 24-year age groups.[194]

Although the trend across developed countries for asthma mortality to increase was consistent, there was considerable variability between countries in pediatric

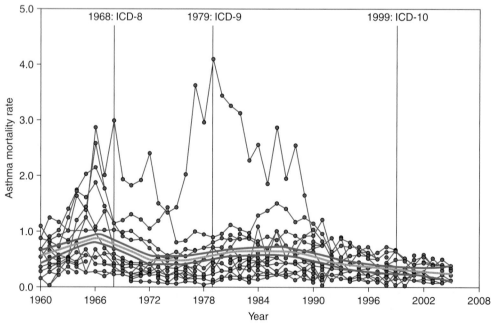

FIGURE 44-3. Asthma mortality rates (deaths per 100,000 persons 5 to 34 years of age) in 20 countries between 1960 and 2005 *(blue circles and interpolation)* and the smoothed fit *(green line)* with 90% confidence intervals *(orange lines)*. Countries included are Australia, Austria, Belgium, Canada, Denmark, England and Wales, Finland, France, Germany, Hong Kong, Italy, Japan, the Netherlands, New Zealand, Norway, Republic of Ireland, Scotland, Spain, Sweden, and the United States. The ICD codes introduced during this period were ICD, 8th revision in 1968, ICD, 9th revision in 1979, and ICD, 10th revision in 1999. (Wijesinghe M, Weatherall M, Perrin K, et al. International trends in asthma mortality rates in the 5- to 34-year age group: a call for closer surveillance. *Chest.* 2009;135:1046.)

asthma mortality rates. For example, from 1981 to 1990, in the 5- to 14-year age group, mortality rates ranged from 0.38 per 100,000 per year in Sweden to 1.75 per 100,000 per year in New Zealand.[194]

Asthma mortality rates have decreased in both children and adults since the late 1980s in New Zealand, Australia, Canada, England, Wales, Spain, and West Germany and since the mid-1990s in the United States.* Over the same time period as this decrease in asthma mortality, asthma prevalence and severity has been stable or has increased. This suggests that improved management of asthma has contributed to the reduced mortality and the introduction of inhaled and systemic steroids, together with consensus guidelines, have been credited.[93,186,200-202]

Simplistically, increasing asthma mortality prior to the mid-1990s may be attributed to increases in underlying prevalence, epidemics caused by particular pharmaceuticals, and the subsequent decrease in mortality caused by improved treatment, in particular inhaled and systemic steroids.

Mortality Risk Factors

Numerous risk factors for fatal asthma have been identified. The most important are asthma severity, age, ethnicity, and poverty, although patterns of health behavior, including therapy adherence, are likely also important. Two patterns of presentation are often observed. The most frequent is one of delayed presentation in someone known to have severe asthma, but in whom the severity of the fatal attack is underestimated or escalation in treatment is delayed. The second pattern is rapid, unexpected deterioration and death, and this may occur in an individual who was previously identified as having only mild asthma.[203,204]

Genetic, Ethnic, and Socioeconomic Determinants

Genes, environment (including exposures, lifestyle, and health behaviors), and gene by environment interactions encompass all the potential determinants of disease severity and risk of fatality. Asthma mortality is greatest in low-to moderate-income countries and countries where access to asthma medications (particularly "controller" medications) and health care are limited.[182,205] Within individual countries, asthma fatality is higher in those from the lowest socioeconomic households.[144,206,207] Socioeconomics and ethnicity are often difficult to disentangle, however, at least one U.S. study found both to be independent risk factors for asthma death.[206] Socioeconomic disadvantage is likely through both increased adverse exposures and poorer health care access.[142,208] Poorer educational achievement is also associated with increased mortality, as both a consequence of poverty and as an independent risk factor.[206] While there is considerable interest in the genetic influences for asthma, there is little evidence of specific genetic risk factors for fatality at the time of this writing. Asthma case-fatality varies greatly by ethnicity. However, it is more likely a reflection of environmental factors such as health behaviors, health care access, and the

influence of poverty rather than a reflection of race-based genetics.[192] The New Zealand Māori, the United States African-American, and the Australian Aborigine populations all have considerably higher asthma mortality (RR 2-5) than the European ethnicities and were more greatly affected during asthma death epidemics.[144,206,207,209,210]

Nevertheless, important biological and genetic differences may exist. Steroid therapy is thought to have been influential in reducing asthma mortality, and African-American individuals may be less sensitive to glucorticoid action.[211] Genetic polymorphisms for the β_2-adrenergic receptor influence beta agonist therapy efficacy. For example, significant differences in bronchodilator responsiveness, probability of wheeze, and exacerbation rates have been seen comparing those homozygous for *Arg16* with those homozygous for *Gly16*.[212,213] Another gene, *RANTES* (regulated upon activation normal T cell expressed and secreted) causes chemotaxis and activation of several cell types involved in the asthmatic airway inflammatory response including eosinophils, monocytes, basophils, and T cells. A polymorphism for this gene has been described that is present at increased frequency in Taiwanese children with near-fatal asthma compared to those with mild to moderate asthma and compared with Taiwanese non-asthmatic children.[214] Gene by environment interaction is likely to be important and is poorly accounted for in current research. For example, tobacco smoke exposure appears to influence the impact of the *Arg16* and *Gly16* alleles.[212] While allele frequency does vary between ethnicities (e.g., the β_2-adrenergic receptor polymorphism *Glu27* is much less common in African-American individuals), it remains unclear how much influence this has on ethnic differences in asthma severity, hospitalization, and mortality.[212,215]

While not specifically addressing the question of genetics versus environment, asthma mortality risk is heritable. Teerlink and colleagues found that the risk of dying from asthma was proportionate to "relatedness" with others who had died of asthma.[216] The relative risk was 1.7 for a first-degree relative and 1.3 for a second-degree relative. In addition, they utilized a genealogic index of familiarity to index familial aggregations, showing an "excess of relatedness" in fatal asthma.

Mortality risk by gender varies with age. In childhood, boys with asthma have a 1.5- to 2-fold increased risk of an asthma death, largely the result of higher prevalence.[143] However this reverses in late adolescence or early adulthood, and, considering the whole lifespan, studies variously report no gender difference or an increase in female mortality.*

Season

The impact of season on asthma mortality varies with age, region, and perhaps ethnicity. Interestingly, mortality peaks at different times to hospitalization. For the 5- to 34-year age group living in the United States, England, Wales, or New Zealand, asthma mortality is highest in spring or summer.[164,183,209,218] A more complex pattern with peaks associated with school holiday periods has also been described.[164] While reduced supervision or health care access over summer and while on holiday has been a possible explanation, very few of the summer

---

*References 93, 142, 184, 186, 187, and 195–199.

*References 143, 183, 185, 194, 197, 206, and 217.

asthma deaths occur while actually away on holiday.[218] Among those younger than 5 years of age or older than 34 years of age, mortality is higher during winter, perhaps an indication that infection is a more important precipitating factor for them.[183] Sensitization to a specific aeroallergen accounts for part of the seasonal and regional clusters of sudden, life-threatening asthma.[219] In some countries (Germany and Sweden), there may be no seasonal variability at all.[220]

Asthma Severity, Setting, and Psychological Factors

Children with more severe asthma are at increased risk of an asthma death. Cohort studies of children with a near fatal asthma episode have demonstrated that such children are at increased risk of subsequent fatal episodes. One study found a more than 1000-fold increased risk of a subsequent fatal episode.[221] However, in children, some of the risk factors for near-fatal asthma and fatal asthma differ. Male gender, high rate of regular short-acting β2-agonist use, and poor adherence are risk factors for both; however, those with near-fatal asthma tend to be younger, have a slower onset of asthma symptoms, and are more likely to have concurrent infection and use more inhaled corticosteroids.[220]

Psychological factors appear to make a significant contribution of the risk of death in children with severe asthma.[222] A case control study compared children hospitalized with severe asthma who died over the subsequent months to years with a control group of children with asthma of similar severity. Factors apparent during the hospital admission that were associated with an increased risk of subsequent fatal asthma included conflict about asthma management between parents and hospital staff, age-inappropriate self-care of asthma, depressive symptoms, and disregard of asthma symptoms.[223]

While exercise may precipitate asthma symptoms, a diagnosis of asthma is not uncommon in children and young people participating in sports at recreational and competitive levels. While death caused by asthma during sporting activities has been described, it is poorly defined. Becker and colleagues found, in the United States, that European ethnicity, male gender, and age between 10 and 20 years were risk factors for sports-related asthma deaths and that individuals generally had only mild, if sometimes persistent asthma.[224] As with exercise, physiologic changes at night and during sleep also precipitate asthma symptoms. While a diurnal pattern in asthma mortality has not been reported, exacerbations that begin during the night are more likely to be fatal in children.[225] This may be the result of physiology; however, these children were slower to receive "rescue" therapy, perhaps caused by lower parental supervision at night.

Fatal asthma often occurs in the setting of concurrent respiratory infection. A U.S. study found asthma-related deaths were over four times more likely than non-asthma deaths to have respiratory infection, except pneumonia, listed on the death certificate.[183] The study also found that while most asthma deaths occurred in hospital, compared with non-asthma deaths a greater proportion occurred in the community.

Disability-Adjusted Life Years Lost

Disability-adjusted life years (DALYs) attempts to describe the years of healthy life lost, providing a measure that incorporates both loss of life and loss of quality life (i.e., the burden of both fatal and nonfatal disease). In 2001, asthma was ranked the 25th leading cause of DALYs with an estimated 15 million DALYs lost worldwide—a similar result to diabetes, bipolar disorder, schizophrenia, and cirrhosis of the liver.[182] There are no DALY data specifically for children.

Economic Burden

The economic cost of asthma is immense, composing up to 2% of total health care expenditure in developed countries—an astonishing figure for a single disease.[226,227] Considering just school-age children, the direct U.S. medical expenditure for asthma in 1996 was just over 1 billion dollars ($401 per child with asthma), including payments for prescribed medicine, hospital inpatient stay, hospital outpatient care, emergency room visits, and office-based visits.[121] Hospitalization accounted for a substantial proportion of this cost. Parents' loss of productivity from asthma-related school absence days accounted for a further $720 million. When the lifetime lost earnings caused by asthma mortality are included, the total economic impact of asthma in school-age children was nearly $2 billion (in 2003 dollars) per annum ($791 per child with asthma). A similar, if more limited, study in the European Union estimated the annual cost of childhood asthma there to be 2.5 to 4.5 billion Euros (2004).[228] Similarly high economic burdens have been reported in Taiwan, Turkey, Singapore, and Canada.[229-231] An employer-based study utilizing health insurance data in the United States compared employees with asthmatic children to those without.[232] Those with asthmatic children had higher health costs and more sick leave. Interestingly, it was not just the children's health care costs that were increased but also their parents'—perhaps an indication of the impact of asthma burden on parental health or, alternatively, of uncontrolled confounding factors including familial asthma.

The majority of asthma-related costs (direct and indirect) reflect the management of exacerbations—whether at home by parents or in health care facilities. Despite effective pharmaceuticals and consensus guidelines, a large proportion of childhood asthma is poorly controlled through undertreatment. It has been estimated that more than 30% of the direct and possibly up to 75% of the total economic costs are caused by inadequate treatment resulting in poor control.[115] An important implication for health policy is that improving control through education, health care access, and perhaps targeting those worst affected, can reduce overall cost.[233,234]

ETIOLOGY OR "PREDISPOSING, PRECIPITATING, PERPETUATING, AND PROTECTIVE" FACTORS

Evidence from population studies over time, between countries and regions of the world, and of migrants suggests that variations in population prevalence of asthma are too large to be explained by genetic variation and are therefore likely caused by environmental factors. But which are the important environmental factors? Do some protect against asthma starting up in the first place, and do others increase risk? What does genetics contribute?

The Genetic Determinants of Asthma

Genes and gene by environment interaction have major roles in determining whether an individual develops asthma, its phenotype and natural history, and how it responds to therapies. Unlike monogenic diseases such as cystic fibrosis (where alterations in a single gene explain much of the disease's development and which has simple Mendelian inheritance), the genetic determinants of asthma are much more complex. Multiple genes are involved (polygenetic inheritance), different combinations of genes act in different families (genetic heterogeneity), and the same gene or set of genes influences multiple traits (pleiotropy) (e.g., asthma and eczema). Furthermore, gene by gene and gene by environment interaction appears to be very important.

Like other aspects of asthma, genetic research is complicated by a lack of consistent diagnostic criteria or definition for asthma. Investigation has often focused on atopy, elevated IgE, and evidence of BHR. The varying asthma phenotypes, including age of onset, further complicate the exploration of associated genes. Outside the laboratory, evidence for genetic influence on asthma comes from family studies, ethnic and geographical disparity, and twin studies. Some caution needs to be taken with inheritance data because children inherit not just genes but environmental exposures and health behaviors. Exposure to environmental antigens begins antenatally.[235]

Nevertheless a recent review, sourcing studies from over 20 countries from all geographical regions of the world, found that a family history of asthma was consistently associated with increased asthma risk.[236] Odds ratios for a first-degree relative ranged from 1.5 to 9.7. While individual studies varied, overall the risk associated with maternal, paternal, or sibling history of asthma was similar. The risk increased if more than one parent was affected. Similarly, a family history of atopy elevated asthma risk. An extension of family history studies, segregation analysis can yield more detailed relationships. Unsurprisingly, given current understandings of asthma genetics, segregation studies have come to varying conclusions regarding inheritance: mixed, co-dominant, single locus, and polygenic.[235] Among the phenotypic characteristics examined, total IgE appears most likely to be majorly influenced by a single gene, although the inheritance remains unclear.[235] As noted, substantial differences in prevalence exist by region, by ethnicity, and over time. While it is unlikely that genetics explains the rapid changes observed in the last half century, it may contribute to some of the ethnic disparity given different frequencies of gene polymorphisms. Numerous twin studies in asthma have been published utilizing self-report diagnosis, IgE and allergy testing, and lung function tests.[235] They attribute 36% to 75% of the variance in asthma risk to genetics.

Advances in technology and techniques have allowed increasingly sophisticated investigation of genetic determinants. *Candidate gene association, genome-wide linkage,* and, most recently, *genome-wide association (GWA)* studies, largely utilizing case-control cohorts, have identified single nucleotide polymorphisms associated with asthma and/or aspects of asthma control. Well over 100 genes have been associated with asthma or atopy-related phenotypes, with at least 40 replicated in two or more independent samples.[237–241] For example, *ADAM33* is thought to alter the hypertrophic response of bronchial smooth muscle to inflammation. While the associations may be strong, the individual effects sizes (~odds ratio) are generally small (OR 0.5 to 1.5), and future research will need to determine not only the functions of identified polymorphisms but also how they interact with each other and the environment.[237] It remains to be seen how many of these prove to be true susceptibility genes. In contrast to the linkage studies, GWA permits research that is not hypothesis-driven and therefore the potential discovery of totally novel genes and/or pathophysiology. In these studies, the genomes of large numbers of individuals within a case-control cohort can be examined seeking associations between asthma phenotypes and individual genes. The first GWA study in childhood asthma, published in 2007 lead to the discovery of three polymorphisms (including *ORMDL3*) on Chromosome 17p21. These findings have been confirmed in other studies across diverse ethnic populations.[242] While the mechanisms are still to be elucidated, they are strongly associated with an early-onset asthma that remits in early adulthood.[243] As asthma phenotypes are age-related, achieving understanding of its genetic etiology may prove difficult with cross-sectional studies, and long-term longitudinal genetic studies will likely be required.[244]

Similarly studies will need to carefully examine environmental exposures. Investigations on a polymorphism in the promoter of CD14 have shown that the same variant may lead to distinct transcriptional patterns if the gene is expressed at different times and/or different cell types.[241] It exhibits a protective effect against increased IgE levels in children with intermediate exposure to farm animals, whereas high levels of IgE were observed in children with high animal exposure. The same polymorphism can therefore be linked to different and even opposite phenotypes, depending on environmental conditions.

ORMDL3, ADAM33, and *CD14* are merely examples of the many polymorphisms being identified. As yet, they have limited clinical utility, however research methods and findings are progressing very rapidly. While asthma genetics are complex, they hold great promise, potentially yielding new opportunities in prevention, prognostication, and therapeutics.

The Relationship Between Asthma, Atopy, and Allergy

Atopy

Atopy (from Greek "strangeness") is defined as "a personal, and/or familial tendency to produce IgE antibodies in response to ordinary exposure to allergens, usually proteins."[245] Asthma in children is commonly described as an allergic, IgE-mediated, atopic disease. The proposed process is that allergen exposure produces allergic sensitization and that continual exposure leads to clinical asthma through the development of airways inflammation, BHR, and reversible airflow obstruction. Various measures of atopy (e.g., positive skin-prick tests, elevated serum IgE levels, parental history of asthma) are associated with an increased risk of developing asthma.[246] For example, in the Tucson Children's Respiratory Study (Arizona, U.S.), when compared with children who had not wheezed, a larger proportion of children with persistent wheezing were more likely to have mothers with a history of asthma, elevated serum IgE levels at 9 months of age, or positive skin skin-prick tests for aeroallergens. Positive skin-prick tests for aeroallergens were also associated with an increased risk of late-onset wheezing.[246] In Avon, U.K., in the ALSPAC study, at 7 years wheezing onset after 18 months was most strongly associated with atopy and airway responsiveness.[247] Atopy causes an increased risk for persistence and severity of asthma, and this is discussed in the Natural History section later in the chapter.

There may be an interaction between atopy and infections. In a small study of asthmatic children, the duration of BHR after a single natural cold was 5 to 11 weeks. However, an increased rate of symptomatic cold and asthma episodes in atopic children was associated with considerable cumulative prolongation of BHR, which might help explain the role of atopy as a risk factor for asthma persistence.[248] Sly has proposed a two-hit model for asthma in which airway inflammation triggered by viral infection or allergy during postnatal lung growth disrupts underlying tissue differentiation programs, leading to anomalies in respiratory function, which last for long periods later in life. Although both allergy and respiratory infections during early life are independently associated with risk for subsequent development of asthma, the highest odds ratios for persistent asthma are seen in children who have both.[249]

ISAAC confirmed a strong correlation between symptoms of asthma and allergic rhinoconjunctivitis, and also atopic eczema.[50] However, in this cross-sectional study most children had current symptoms of only one condition, and less than 1 in 10 symptomatic children had current symptoms of all three diseases. Some of this lack of concurrent symptoms may be explained by the "atopic march," with eczema occurring in the youngest children, followed by asthma and later by allergic rhinitis. However, the lack of overlap—even for "symptoms ever"—was less than expected if the explanatory mechanism were the same for all three conditions. A recent systematic review found that although there is an increased risk of developing asthma after eczema in early childhood, only one in three children with eczema develops asthma during later childhood.[250] This is lower than previously assumed. Furthermore, recent evidence suggests that the risk of subsequent childhood asthma is not increased in children with early atopic dermatitis who are not also early wheezers, suggesting that a co-manifestation of phenotypes rather than a progressive atopic march may be the explanation.[251]

However, atopy does not explain the many children with asthma who do not have an atopic constitution. In 1999,

Pearce and colleagues challenged the closeness of the relationship between asthma and atopy.[252] The epidemiologic evidence suggests that only 50% of the child and adult population with asthma have IgE-mediated disease. Comparisons across populations or time periods showed only a weak and inconsistent association between the prevalence of atopy and asthma. Nonallergic asthma may be a separate entity from allergic asthma, and a different set of preventive strategies may be required for this type of asthma. The etiology of and risk factors for non–IgE-mediated asthma therefore need to be explored further.[252] Comparatively little research has been done in this direction.

The World Allergy Organization has articulated the distinction between allergic and nonallergic asthma in their recommendations on nomenclature.[253] In their summary and guideline on the prevention of allergy and allergic asthma, Johansson and Haahtela state that individuals with a family history of atopy have an increased risk of allergic sensitization, and that this represents a high risk for allergic asthma.[254] However, the distinction between allergic and nonallergic asthma may be difficult in clinical practice, especially as the measurement of total serum IgE and skin-prick testing is not routine in many countries, and in much of the world it is unavailable to most of the population due to cost.

In a recent systematic review of 36 articles that studied 48 populations of unselected children and reported prevalence rates for asthma and atopy, no difference was found in the prevalence of asthma cases in the quartiles of childhood populations subdivided for the prevalence of atopy. In addition, atopy did not increase significantly in the subgroups of populations subdivided by asthma quartiles. In both subgroups, however, atopic asthma increased with increasing atopy or with increasing asthma.[255]

Further evidence of the diminished agency of atopy for asthma came from a recent study of bronchial biopsies obtained from 55 children 2 to 10 years of age undergoing bronchoscopy for appropriate clinical indications (not asthma). This showed that the airway pathology typical of asthma is present in non-atopic wheezing children just as in atopic wheezing children. These results suggest that, when multitrigger wheezing responsive to bronchodilators is present, it is associated with pathologic features of asthma, even in non-atopic children.[256]

The role of atopic sensitization in determining asthma prevalence in children was explored further in ISAAC Phase Two, a multicenter cross-sectional study of 9- to 11-year-old school children in randomly sampled schools in 30 centers in 22 countries. Skin-prick test reactivity was used as the measure of atopy. The mean effect size (odds ratio) for skin-prick test reactivity on current wheeze in affluent countries was about double that of nonaffluent countries, which is where most of the world's children live.[35] Thus the relationship between atopy and asthma is important, but it may have been overemphasized to the detriment of exploration of the nonallergic mechanisms of asthma.

Allergens

The concept of allergen exposure causing asthma dates back to the seventeenth century, and clinical studies date back to the first part of the twentieth century.[257] The major airborne allergens associated with the risk of asthma differ within and between communities and may alter with climate, season, housing, and hygiene. How important then are they in the cause of asthma and its maintenance? Are they triggers that just exacerbate asthma, or are they a cause?

Numerous studies demonstrate a relationship between risk for sensitization and the level of exposure to allergen.[257] The relation between the incidence of sensitization to house dust mite (HDM) and cat allergens during the first 3 years of life has been clearly demonstrated by a West German study.[258] Increasing exposure, both in a group of infants with atopic parents and in a group with non-atopic parents, was associated with increasing incidence of sensitization. Wahn and colleagues concluded that allergen intervention needs to begin in early life. However, it is still being clarified whether this applies in other parts of the world and to what extent sensitization leads to clinical disease. In ISAAC Phase Two, in non-affluent countries a higher proportion of children with positive skin-prick tests had no detectable specific IgE than in affluent countries. Total serum IgE was associated with asthma symptoms among children with both positive skin-prick tests and specific IgE.[259]

Many studies show that persistent asthma is associated with exposure to allergens in the indoor environment. Also, typical outdoor allergens such as pollens are also regularly found indoors, but they are rarely an independent risk factor for persistent asthma.[260]

In many temperate and humid regions, the greatest risk for asthma has been associated with allergy to HDM.[261] In Australia, the association between exposure to HDM, sensitization, and asthma is very strong. Increased use of nonfeather pillows, which have less tightly woven encasements and more allergens, appeared to explain a modest rise in prevalence of wheeze over a 13-year period in London.[262] In some dry climates, the strongest risk factor is allergy to the fungus *Alternaria* spp.[263,264] In other urban communities, allergy to cockroach appears to be the dominant allergen and is strongly associated with asthma risk, but it is not clear if this is independent of socioeconomic status[265,266]

Allergy to cats and dogs appears to be important in many places,[267] but in a study of children in the Netherlands, pet ownership (cats, dogs, birds, and/or rodents in the home) was associated with a lower prevalence of respiratory allergy and symptoms. However, past, but not current pet ownership was associated with a higher prevalence of symptoms and pet allergy. These results suggest that selective avoidance and removal of pets leads to distortion of cross-sectional associations of pet ownership and respiratory allergy and disease among children.[268] In a prospective study in Oslo, Norway, in children 10 years of age, no risk modification was seen for dog allergens.[269] In adolescents in Norway, sensitization to pet allergens (i.e., cat, dog, and horse) was associated with increased BHR in children with asthma, but it did not increase the risk of being sensitized to pet allergens.[270] In Sweden, early exposure to cats and dogs appeared to have a protective effect on the development of IgE sensitization.[271] However, in a study in New Delhi,

India, dogs and cats at home were significant risk factors associated with the symptoms of asthma in schoolchildren.[272] Nonallergic effects of exposure to animals are discussed in the Housing, Animals, and Climate section later in the chapter.

In ISAAC Phase One, exposure to allergenic pollen was assessed by exposures around the dates of early life[273] and did not appear to increase the risk of acquiring symptoms of respiratory allergy, and may even give some protection. Other studies have found that the symptom prevalence of hay fever and asthma tends to be lower in rural areas than in urban areas, and tends to be lowest among people living on farms,[274-277] but this has not been consistently found outside Europe and the United States. The degree of consistency in the inverse associations suggests the possibility of a protective effect of pollen on allergy.

If allergen exposure is important in the etiology of asthma, it seems probable that it will be involved in its persistence rather than its initial occurrence. In the setting of occupational asthma in adults, continuing exposure to the relevant occupational allergen is generally associated with a higher risk of persisting asthma, although the relationship may be more complex than this.[278] Exposure-response relationships may be influenced by properties of the allergen or route of exposure, the genotype of the exposed individual, and environmental agents (e.g., endotoxin). Recommendations have been made to reduce exposure for young children already sensitized to HDM, pets, or cockroaches to prevent the onset of allergic disease, and to eliminate or reduce the exposure of asthma patients who are allergic to indoor allergens (e.g., HDM, cockroaches, and animal danders) to improve symptoms and to control and prevent exacerbations.[254] This might be achieved by chemical, physical, and combined methods of reducing mite allergen levels. However, a recent Cochrane Systematic Review that assessed the effects of reducing exposure to house dust mite antigens in the homes of people with mite-sensitive asthma found no effect of the interventions on number of patients whose asthma improved, asthma symptom scores, or medication usage. If any further trials are done, they need to be larger and more methodologically rigorous and must use other methods than those used so far, with careful monitoring of mite exposure and relevant clinical outcomes.[279] These findings suggest that reducing allergen exposure is unlikely to make an important impact on the burden of asthma in populations.

Birth Weight, Growth, Physical Activity, and Obesity

Birth Weight and Growth

Studies have found associations between low birth weight and increased risk of asthma. These associations could be caused by confounding genetic or environmental factors. The risk of childhood asthma increased with reduced birth weight both in a cohort of twins and within monozygotic twin pairs, supporting the hypothesis that fetal growth per se influences the risk of asthma later in life.[280]

In a prospective British cohort, low birth weight was found to be a risk factor for early childhood wheezing, independent of maternal smoking.[281] They suggested that this effect may be mediated through intrauterine undernutrition causing small airways. In a study from Israel 17-year-old adolescents had a higher risk of asthma if they had birth weights less than 2500 grams, but the mechanisms were not clear.[282] In a U.S. nationally representative sample, the prevalence of childhood asthma decreased as birthweight increased.[283] The relationship between low birth weight and asthma needs to be explored further, especially with studies from developing countries.

Physical Activity

There is recent interest in whether physical activity could be an independent risk factor for asthma. In a prospective community-based study of Danish children, there was a weak correlation between physical fitness, and reduced risk for the development of asthma.[284] In a cross-sectional Norwegian study, children with asthma who exercised less had more BHR than those who exercised more.[285] However in children 9 to 10 years of age from a rural district in northern Tanzania, aerobic fitness was not associated with asthma symptoms.[286] Not undertaking enough physical activity is also being explored as potential risk factor. In a large Italian study of children 6 to 7 years of age, spending a lot of time watching television independently increased the risk of asthma symptoms.[287] In Kaohsiung, Taiwan, schoolchildren who had more sedentary time had increased risk of respiratory symptoms and asthma.[288] In schoolchildren in Taipei, Taiwan, greater TV-watching time increased the risk of respiratory symptoms, while habitual physical activity decreased the risk of respiratory symptoms.[289]

The relationship between physical fitness and possible protection from the development of asthma is worthy of further exploration.

Obesity

The prevalence of obesity among children and adolescents has increased in Western countries due to changes in diet and physical activity associated with environmental changes that influence these. The method of defining obesity needs consideration. Body mass index (BMI), percent body fat, and skinfold thickness produce relatively comparable results when analyzing the interaction between obesity and asthma.[290] Prospective studies consistently support a link between obesity and reported wheezing or asthma diagnosis in children. However, there are still no clear explanations for such a link, and many different mechanisms may underlie the association. Obesity can be associated with symptoms commonly attributed to asthma, such as wheezing, dyspnea, and sleep apnea. Obese subjects are less fit and may have more frequent bouts of breathlessness on exertion accompanied by an exaggerated symptom perception. Some authors suggest that physicians should be cautious about diagnosing asthma in obese children on the basis of self-reported symptoms alone and should confirm the diagnosis by using objective measurements and evaluations of markers such as lung function parameters, bronchial hyper-reactivity, atopic sensitization, and indices of

lung inflammation that can better identify asthma phenotype and exclude overdiagnosis.[291] It is unclear, however, whether obesity merely exacerbates the asthmatic symptoms, creates susceptibility to onset of asthma, or develops concurrently with the respiratory disease. Obesity could have potential biological effects on lung function and systematic inflammation while also sharing certain comorbidities and etiologies with asthma.[292] Atopic sensitization and bronchial hyperreactivity do not explain the observed associations. After puberty, the association between asthma and obesity tends to be stronger in girls than in boys. It is conceivable that severe obesity in adolescent females may aggravate asthma through mechanisms different from those linking prepubertal obesity to unremitting asthma in males.[293]

Several single cross-sectional studies have reported an association between asthma and obesity, and in several longitudinal studies an increased incidence of asthma has also been reported in subjects who are overweight. Cross-sectional studies in the same population repeated after a period of time in the United Kingdom[294] and New Zealand[295] found that increases in prevalence of wheeze were not associated with concurrent increase in obesity. However, in the more recent New Zealand study, increasing BMI standard deviation score was significantly associated with current wheeze.[295] In a recent report of a cross-sectional study, increased BMI was found to influence asthma prevalence.[296] More recent studies have confirmed a relationship between obesity and asthma. In a very large study of Californian adolescents, an increased risk of asthma was observed for individuals as low as the 45th to 55th percentile of BMI, and the risk increased with increasing BMI.[101] In a large Italian study of children 6 to 7 years of age, high body weight independently increased the risk of asthma symptoms in children.[287] In a very large U.S. national study in children 13 to 17 years of age, obesity was positively associated with diagnosed asthma.[297] In a very large population-based survey of schoolchildren in southern Taiwan, higher BMI was associated with higher asthma incidence in both sexes.[298] In Kaohsiung, Taiwan, schoolchildren who were overweight or at risk of being overweight had an increased risk of respiratory symptoms and asthma.[288] In schoolchildren in Taipei, Taiwan, overweight increased the risk of respiratory symptoms, while habitual physical activity decreased the risk of respiratory symptoms.[289] For boys and girls, extremes of annual BMI growth rates increase the risk of asthma.[299,300] In southern California, being overweight is associated with an increased risk of new-onset asthma in boys and in nonallergic children.[301]

There is a stronger association between obesity and asthma in females. In Tasmania, higher BMI in nonasthmatic young females at 7 years of age predicts risk of asthma developing in adult life.[302] The Tucson Children's Respiratory Study (Arizona) found that in females, becoming overweight or obese between 6 and 11 years of age increases the risk of developing new asthma symptoms and increased bronchial responsiveness during the early adolescent period.[303] A New Zealand longitudinal study found that 28% of asthma developing in women after 9 years of age was caused by overweight.[304] However in

U.S. African-American youth, gender modified the association between BMI and asthma-related morbidity among adolescents with asthma, with effects found in males but not females.[305]

The mechanism relating obesity to asthma is not clear. However, when it was found that in 11- to 19-year-old children in Tehran, Iran, asthma was significantly more frequent in both girls and boys with abdominal obesity, it was hypothesized that visceral fat may produce proinflammatory mediators that have been shown to cause subepithelial fibrosis and airway remodeling in animal models.[306,307] In a national study in the United States, higher BMI and elevated serum CRP levels were associated with asthma of greater severity, requiring further exploration.[308] In a cross-sectional study of Mexican adolescents 11 to 24 years of age, the association between obesity and asthma seems to be greater among girls with early puberty, suggesting the role of female hormones.[309] As sleep-disordered breathing and obesity each are associated with asthma and wheeze, it has been suggested that the relationship between obesity and wheeze may be partly mediated by factors associated with sleep-disordered breathing.[310] In adolescents, obesity may complicate asthma management by interfering with the ability to accurately perceive symptoms for some patients. More remains to be learned about the role of sociodemographic factors underlying this relationship.[311]

Underweight

Surprisingly, there are recent reports that suggest a relationship between asthma and being underweight. For boys and girls, extremes of annual BMI growth rates increase the risk of asthma.[299] In 9- to 10-year-old children from a rural district in North-Tanzania where more than every fifth child reported asthma symptoms, lower body fat was associated with higher occurrence of asthma symptoms.[286] In a very large population-based survey of schoolchildren in southern Taiwan, it was shown that underweight male children may have lower expiratory flow rates and thus potentially have more asthma symptoms.[298] These studies demonstrate that the relationship between growth and asthma is complex.

Diet

It is not surprising that diet may be linked to asthma as it has been for many noncommunicable diseases. Over the past few decades, "Westernization" has seen many countries moving away from the traditional diet of locally grown foods to a more Western diet. Dietary patterns have changed rapidly with modernization or Westernization, and the associated move away from plant-based foods and the addition of manmade fat. Rapid changes have occurred in association with Westernization, including changes to the production and availability of food, changing food preferences, increased supply of processed foods for consumption as well as supplies for food aid, use of fertilizers and pesticides, reduced land availability, increased prices of staple foods, urbanization, migration, economic factors, and market fluctuations. Most of the dietary studies to date have a cross-sectional design, and therefore they are more suited for raising questions

and hypotheses than in proving causative relationships. A recent review summarized some of the key hypotheses and research findings.[312]

Fish

The low prevalence of asthma among populations with a high fish intake[64] suggested that there may be a protective factor in fish. Oily fish is rich in Omega-3 fatty acids, which potentially reduce the synthesis of proinflammatory cytokines, which, it is speculated, could either prevent the development of asthma or reduce its severity by altering airway inflammation and BHR. Regular consumption of fresh oily fish was observed to be associated with reduced risk of asthma symptoms in Australian children.[313] In ISAAC Phase Two, consumption of fish in affluent countries was associated with a low prevalence of current wheeze.[314] Clinical trials of fish oil or Omega-3 and Omega-6 fatty acid supplements have shown no effect,[315-317] an increase in fatty acid levels,[318,319] a positive effect on FEV_1,[320] a decrease in BHR,[319] and a reduction in occurrence of cough in atopic children at 3 years of age, and of wheeze at 18 months (but not 3 years) of age.[321] Supplementation of Omega-3 and Omega-6 fatty acid exposure from early life did not affect atopy and asthma at 5 years of age.[322]

Vegetables, Fruit, and Antioxidants

Several cross-sectional studies suggest that fresh vegetables and fruit may be protective against the development of asthma in children, possibly through the antioxidant properties of vitamins A, C, E, and β carotene.[321,323,324] Antioxidant studies have focused on vitamin C, vitamin E, carotenoids, flavonoids, and antioxidant nutrients such as selenium and zinc. A wide range of cross-sectional studies has been done on the relationship of antioxidants with asthma. Vitamin C, β carotene, magnesium, and selenium were associated with a reduction in asthma prevalence[325-329] and may prevent or limit an inflammatory response in the airways by reducing reactive oxygen species and inhibiting lipid peroxidation. Flavonoids also may be potential antiallergic substances,[330] and a recent study on enzymatic and nonenzymatic antioxidant systems in childhood asthma suggested that antioxidant defenses (e.g., glutathione peroxidase and superoxide dismutase) were lowered in asthmatic children.[331] However, not all studies on the role of antioxidants have been positive. A meta-analysis determined that dietary intake of antioxidants vitamins C and E and β carotene does not significantly influence the risk of asthma.[332] The potential role of antioxidants as supplements has been explored[333] but a number of studies have been inconclusive.[334] Overall, supplementation studies have suggested a minor role for individual antioxidants in asthma prevention.[335] Several cross-sectional studies have indicated an inverse association between consumption of fruits and vegetables and symptoms of asthma, though the particular foods and symptoms varied.[336-341] However, a smaller study of Dutch children found no clear association between fruit and vegetable intake and asthma symptoms.[342] Ecological analysis of ISAAC Phase One data involving 53 countries found an inverse association between asthma symptoms and food of plant origin.[343] In ISAAC Phase Two, fruit intake was associated with a low prevalence of current wheeze, and in nonaffluent countries with cooked green vegetables.[314]

The possible protective value of antioxidants is supported by an ecological study of exposure to paracetamol (which depletes the antioxidant glutathione), which was associated with an increase of asthma symptoms,[344] and subsequent ISAAC cross-sectional studies in younger and older children where paracetamol use was reported.[345,346] In a large cross-sectional study of youth (NHANES III), serum vitamin C and β carotene but not vitamin E were inversely associated with asthma.[329] Interventions with antioxidants have not been shown to be effective, and further studies are needed in this area.

Other potential constituents of fresh fruit and vegetables that may be protective also need consideration. In another large cross-sectional study of more than 10,000 Chinese schoolchildren recruited from Hong Kong, Beijing, and Guangzhou, the prevalence of asthma and wheeze was two times higher in Hong Kong than in the other two cities from Mainland China.[347] Frequent consumption of raw vegetables was one of the factors explaining the disparity of asthma prevalence between Hong Kong and Mainland China.[348] In Taipei, Taiwan, schoolchildren's consumption of fruit was associated with reduced risk of respiratory symptoms.[341,349]

Cereals and Rice

Many of the protective compounds in whole grains (i.e., wheat, rice, and corn) are also found in fruit and vegetables, but some plant compounds are more concentrated in whole grains. The ISAAC ecological analysis showed a consistent negative association between calories from cereal, rice and protein from cereal and nuts, and symptoms. It was speculated that if the daily per capita amount of calories from cereal and rice consumed were increased by 10% of total energy consumption, it may be possible to achieve a 3.2% decrease in the prevalence of current wheeze and a 0.4% decrease in severe wheeze.[343]

Polyunsaturated Fat

As intake of saturated fats and cholesterol is reduced in Western societies, more polyunsaturated fatty acid (PUFA) is consumed. In 1997, Black and Sharpe cited evidence that contradicted the antioxidant hypothesis, instead proposing that the increase in asthma prevalence may have stemmed from an increased consumption of polyunsaturated fatty acids (PUFAs) and a decreased consumption of saturated fat.[350] The Omega-6 PUFAs may particularly have a role in regulating immune response and inflammation. These PUFAs are found largely as linoleic acid in foods such as margarine and vegetable oils, which have risen in consumption with Westernization.[351] Linoleic acid is a precursor of arachidonic acid that is converted into prostaglandin E_2 (PGE_2), which inhibits interferon-γ (IFN-γ) and promotes an inflammatory environment that favors asthma development. Meanwhile, Omega-3 PUFAs may have an anti-inflammatory role. Thus, the increase in Omega-6 PUFA consumption and the decrease in Omega-3 PUFA consumption may immunologically increase the susceptibility of the population, although PUFAs may have other immunosuppressive

mechanisms that require further study.[352] Investigation of the lipid hypothesis found mixed results. A number of cross-sectional studies showed beneficial associations between foods containing Omega-3 PUFAs and asthma,[353] but studies on cord blood PUFA composition and development of atopic disease have been inconclusive.[354] There have been conflicting reports on the relationship between levels of PUFAs and wheeze. PUFA derived from vegetables in the ISAAC ecological analysis was associated with decreased symptom prevalence,[343] supporting the hypothesis that it is industrially-derived PUFA that is responsible, rather than naturally derived PUFA from vegetables.[322,355] Disappointingly, intervention studies have not found consistent results nor provided sufficient support for dietary supplementation with PUFAs.[322,352,356–358]

Trans Fatty Acids

Trans fatty acids are found in industrially hydrogenated fats used in spreads, dairy products, and the fat of ruminant animals. These fatty acids may influence the desaturation and chain elongation of Omega-6 and Omega-3 fatty acids into precursors of inflammatory mediators, such as leukotrienes. A European ISAAC investigation found a significantly positive association between trans fatty acids and the prevalence of childhood asthma, and the hypothesis that they may play a part in the development of childhood asthma seems worth pursuing.[359]

Vitamin D

In 2007, Litonjua and Weiss hypothesized that vitamin D deficiency can increase the incidence of asthma in young children.[360,361] Vitamin D does not occur naturally in humans and is acquired through supplements and exposure to sunlight. The higher prevalence of asthma in Westernized countries might be linked to the fact that people spend much more time indoors and away from sunlight. Observational studies in the United States and the United Kingdom have reported that maternal intake of vitamin D during pregnancy was associated with lung function, suggesting that increased vitamin D in maternal diet may reduce risk of wheeze and other symptoms of asthma.[362,363] As with other hypotheses, further investigation would be appropriate, especially in pregnancy.

Chemicals and Trace Elements

A sodium hypothesis was proposed in 1987 based on a correlation between table salt purchases and asthma mortality.[364,365] Several studies have investigated the relationship between sodium intake and asthma, demonstrating little effect of increased sodium intake on bronchial reactivity and clinical symptoms of asthma.[317,366] A more recent trial in which participants adopted a variable sodium diet found no benefit for asthma either.[367] In a large Italian study of children 6 to 7 years of age, data support the hypothesis that a salty diet independently increases the risk of asthma symptoms in children.[287]

Selenium is an essential component of the antioxidant enzyme glutathione peroxidase (see the Vegetables, Fruits, and Antioxidants section earlier in the chapter) and can also up-regulate immune responses that characterize allergic asthma—a more complex effect that cannot be explained just by case-control studies.[368] However, many studies have shown no association between selenium and asthma,[369] and no beneficial effect of selenium supplementation.[317] Magnesium has been implicated through its possible effects on bronchial smooth muscle. Low magnesium intake has been correlated with decreased lung function in children.[370] Although intravenous magnesium is recommended to control acute severe asthma (by enhancing bronchial smooth muscle relaxation) in many emergency departments,[371] magnesium deficiency has not been shown in asthma patients.[317] Nevertheless, due to a paucity of studies on magnesium and asthma prevalence, its importance remains to be seen.

Food Preservatives and Additives

The changes of dietary habits with migration include the addition of preservatives, traces of pesticides, and food additives such as metabisulfites, benzoate, and tartrazine, which have also been implicated in asthma exacerbations.[372] There have been no studies of the separate effect of food preservatives and additives on asthma and allergy. However, the consumption of fast food has become a feature of some more affluent societies. In ISAAC Phase Two, higher lifetime prevalence of asthma was associated with high burger consumption.[314] Within this cross-sectional study, in children in Hastings, New Zealand, hamburger consumption was shown to be positively associated with asthma symptoms, while takeaway consumption had a marginal effect on BHR.[373] In a Canadian study of selected children 8 to 10 years of age, the children with asthma were more likely to consume fast food than the children without asthma.[374]

Mediterranean Diet

The Mediterranean diet, on the other hand, has been suggested as a healthy dietary pattern that may reduce the risk of asthma. In ISAAC Phase Two, food selection according to the Mediterranean diet was associated with a lower prevalence of current wheeze and asthma ever.[314] In fact, ISAAC data indicated lower asthma prevalence in Mediterranean countries with diet as a possible variable to explain this disparity.[14] There is a consistent relationship between a Mediterranean diet and asthma symptoms,[336,375,376] but not for current wheezing in all studies.[377] Further investigation of this association and possible mechanisms would be of interest.

Breast Feeding

Patterns of breast feeding have changed in the last few decades, particularly in affluent countries, where rates became particularly low 3 to 4 decades ago, but have gradually increased since.[378] The relationship between breast feeding and the development of asthma is unclear because of the conflicting outcomes of longitudinal studies. These show either no beneficial effect,[281,379–381] or a beneficial effect.[382–384] A 2004 cohort study showed exclusive breastfeeding for more than 4 months reduced the risk of asthma at the child's age of 4.[385] One study found an increased risk of asthma in those who were breast fed.[386] The lack of consistency of research findings makes it difficult to make any recommendations. Controversy about the interpretation of the evidence has been appraised.[387,388] More recently, several studies in affluent countries have found no clear association (positive or negative) from breast feeding,[389–391] even when the mother is asthmatic,[392,393] or small protective effects.[283,394–396] In susceptible infants, the risk of developing allergic symptoms, but not the risk of sensitization, was modified by intake of Omega-3 long-chain polyunsaturated fatty acids through breast milk.[397] Breast feeding has other child health benefits, and thus its encouragement until 4 to 6 months of age is recommended. To date, there is no evidence demonstrating that high-risk infants benefit from modulation of maternal diet during lactation. Currently no special diet for the lactating mother has been recommended.[254]

In an analysis from ISAAC Phase Two, any breast feeding was associated with less wheeze in countries of all income levels.[398] However, when types of wheeze and income of country were explored, breastfeeding was associated only with non-atopic wheeze in low- and middle-income countries, and it showed no protective association for atopic wheeze in countries of all income levels. The lack of inclusion of nonaffluent countries in most breastfeeding studies to date may explain some of the conflicting evidence. To illustrate this, a study in India in children who live with close animal contact and mud flooring and who were exclusively breast fed were less likely to develop asthma than those who were not breast fed.[399]

Maternal Diet in Pregnancy

The intrauterine environment is thought to play an important part in the development of chronic disease in later life,[400] although there is no documented direct effect of maternal diet during pregnancy on asthma.[379] Maternal diet during pregnancy could potentially influence asthma protectively (for example through antioxidant intake) or alternatively adversely, with antigens passing through the placenta and amniotic fluid leading to programming of the developing immune system by stimulating T-cells and cytokines. In 2002, no advantages were found in a randomized controlled trial eliminating cow's milk and eggs in the last trimester.[401,402] Devereux and colleagues found that increased maternal intake of vitamin E was associated with decreased proliferation of cord blood mononuclear cells in response to allergens, suggesting a potential beneficial effect of maternal nutrition against atopy.[403] Two maternal antioxidant studies showed an inverse relationship of antioxidants vitamin E, vitamin C, and zinc with wheeze.[404,405] The selenium status of a cohort of 2000 pregnant mothers was also inversely associated with wheezing in the child,[406] but this disappeared after the 5 years of age. One study of maternal PUFA intake found that maternal oily fish consumption during pregnancy was protective for childhood asthma, particularly in children who have asthmatic mothers.[407] In keeping with many other diet studies, however, a longitudinal study of maternal consumption of various food types found no association between fish intake and asthma outcomes in children,[408] despite another study suggesting an association.[409] There was also no association between asthma and maternal consumption of foods such as vegetables, egg, and dairy. In contrast to the more specific antioxidant and vitamin D studies, the effect of broader food groups on asthma outcomes seems less significant.[410] However a protective effect of a high level of adherence to a Mediterranean diet during pregnancy was found against asthma-like symptoms at 6 years of age.[411] There is an obvious need for more randomized controlled trials of interventions on maternal diet using nutrients and factors that have the potential to impact the intrauterine environment and fetal immune and lung development.[412]

Toxins And Pollution

Environmental Tobacco Smoke

Environmental tobacco smoke (ETS) exposure is undoubtedly an important risk factor for asthma. Both active smokers and non-smokers exposed to ETS have been found to be affected adversely. ETS consists of mainstream smoke that has been inhaled and exhaled by the primary smoker and sidestream smoke that arises directly from a burning cigarette. It contains many agents that have pathologic effects on human tissues.[413] Children can be exposed to tobacco smoke before or after birth. It has been difficult to isolate the effects on asthma of intra-uterine exposure per se, as postnatal exposure continues in many instances. Does prenatal ETS cause allergic sensitization? No correlation was found between cord blood IgE of newborns and an active smoking history of either mothers or fathers.[414,415] However, cord blood eosinophil counts were found to correlate with the urinary cotinine levels of mothers.[416] In the Tucson Children's Respiratory Study (Arizona), maternal prenatal but not postnatal smoking was associated with current wheeze at 3 years of age only.[417] A recent Taiwanese study found that prenatal and household ETS exposure had significant adverse effects on respiratory health in Taiwanese children.[418] Passive exposure of pregnant women to ETS during the third trimester in a Greek study was positively associated with asthma- and allergy-related symptoms in their preschool-age children.[419]

The effect of tobacco smoke on BHR and asthma, apart from lung size and lung function, has also been studied. In a large meta-analysis, the pooled odds ratio for maternal smoking on BHR was 1.29.[420] Four studies of circadian variation in peak expiratory flow found increased variation in children exposed to ETS. A clear effect of exposure to ETS on BHR in the general population has not been established. While the meta-analysis suggested a small but real increase in BHR in school-age children, limited evidence suggests greater variation in peak expiratory flow in children of smoking parents.[420]

In 1998 Strachan and Cook undertook a systematic quantitative review of case-control and longitudinal studies investigating the effects of ETS on wheezing and asthma after the first year of life. Maternal smoking was associated with an increased incidence of wheezing illness up to 6 years of age (pooled odds ratio 1.31), but less strongly thereafter (1.13). The pooled odds ratio for asthma prevalence from 14 case-control studies was 1.37 if either parent smoked. Four studies suggested that parental smoking is more strongly associated with wheezing among "non-atopic" children. Indicators of disease severity, including symptom scores, attack frequency, medication use, hospital attendance, and

life-threatening bronchospasm were, in general, positively related to household smoke exposure. The excess incidence of wheezing in smoking households appears to be largely in early wheezers with a relatively benign prognosis, but among children with established asthma, parental smoking is associated with more severe disease. These studies suggest that ETS is a cofactor provoking wheezing attacks, rather than causing the underlying asthmatic tendency.[421]

In a cohort study of 6000 children, maternal smoking was found to be an additional risk factor for wheeze, primarily in low socioeconomic status groups.[422] Similarly, asthma severity in children whose mothers stopped smoking was found to decrease.[423] In a subsequent study investigating the effect of intrauterine and postnatal ETS exposure in high-risk infants in the first 3 years of life, ETS exposure increased the risk of wheezing in the first year of life, but it had little effect on the development of atopy.[424] In ISAAC Phase One, the picture that emerged for tobacco was mixed, with no association observed with country tobacco consumption.[425] However, there was generally a positive relationship between women smoking and asthma symptoms.

A literature review found that exposure duration may be a more important factor in the induction of asthma than previously understood and suggests that secondhand smoke could be a more fundamental and widespread cause of childhood asthma than some previous meta-analyses have indicated.[426] About half of the world's children may be exposed to ETS, exacerbating symptoms in 20% of children with asthma. However, it is reassuring that favorable health outcomes can be attained with reduced exposure. Community opinion may need to shift further in favor of protecting children and others from ETS before minimal interventions can be successful. This will require continued efforts by the medical and public health establishments, combined with legislation mandating tobacco-free public places and ETS-related media campaigns.[427]

Is there evidence that stopping ETS exposure is beneficial? A recent U.S. study has demonstrated an association between ETS exposure reduction and fewer episodes of poor asthma control, respiratory-related emergency department visits, and hospitalizations. These findings emphasize the importance of ETS exposure reduction as a mechanism to improve asthma control and morbidity.[170]

What about adolescents who take up smoking? Asthma and active cigarette smoking interact to cause more severe symptoms, decline in lung function, and impaired short-term therapeutic response to corticosteroids. Clinical and public health programs should encourage asthmatics who smoke to quit.[428] However, in Latin America a recent study found that the prevalence of tobacco smoking in the last 12 months was 16%, with significant female predominance. More than 27% of asthma symptoms were attributable to active tobacco consumption, suggesting that potent and more effective campaigns against tobacco smoking should be implemented in developing countries, where active tobacco smoking is dramatically increasing in children.[429] Public health measures have been beneficial in Scotland where, after adoption of comprehensive smoke-free legislation in 2006, there was a reduction in the rate of hospital admissions for asthma in preschool and school-age children.[430]

Outdoor Air Pollution

There is a great deal of interest in the relationship of air pollution and asthma that needs clarification.[431] Urban air pollution comprises several factors that may affect respiratory illness: ozone (O_3), NO_2, sulfur dioxide (SO_2), acid aerosols, and particulates. Many children with asthma experience deterioration of their symptoms associated with increases in outdoor air pollution.[432] However, there is no evidence for increased air pollution contributing to increased prevalence of asthma.[433] In ISAAC Phase One, a weak inverse relationship was demonstrated between city-level air pollution with particulate matter ≤ 10 microns (PM_{10}) and symptoms of asthma, even after controlling for GNP, which has a strong inverse association with air pollution.[434] Meta-analyses of data from countries with multiple centers found by contrast a consistent pattern of weak positive associations. These generally weak associations were in line with existing ecological evidence on the association between particulate air pollution and asthma. This finding is not incompatible with the extensive evidence from individual-level studies that air pollution may aggravate existing asthma, since this may not have an important effect on prevalence. The effects of air pollution may be modulated by stress. In a prospective cohort study in southern California, children from stressful households were more susceptible to the effects of traffic-related pollution and *in utero* tobacco smoke on the development of asthma.[435] Short-term fluctuations in pollutant levels may have different effects from chronically high concentrations. Neither does it exclude a causal role for roadside exposure for which there is limited evidence. Thus there is little evidence that outdoor air pollution increases the risk for development of asthma and allergy.

To the contrary, studies in Germany found lower rates of the prevalence of asthma in the more polluted East Germany compared with West Germany. During 1989 to 1991, there was a lower prevalence of asthma in Leipzig (in the former East Germany) compared to Munich (in the former West Germany).[46,351] A study of children in Dresden, Germany, using the ISAAC Phase Two protocol[34] showed that benzene, NO_2, and carbon monoxide were associated with increased prevalence of morning cough and bronchitis. However, IgE-sensitization, symptoms of IgE-mediated diseases, and BHR were not associated with these pollutants.[436] In a study in Swiss schoolchildren, there was no association between long-term exposure to air pollution and asthmatic and allergic symptoms.[437] On the other hand, a cohort study of children in Japan identified increasing prevalence of bronchitis, wheeze, and asthma with increasing indoor NO_2 exposure among girls, but not boys. Increased incidence of asthma was also identified among children living in areas with high outdoor NO_2 concentrations.[438] In Latin America, a high prevalence of asthma was found in heavily polluted São Paulo, Brazil, with symptom rates comparable to less polluted cities in Australia and New Zealand.[439] Accurately modeled urban air pollution in France was associated

with some measures of childhood asthma.[440] Although the current U.S. standard for ozone is based on short-term exposure, a recent cross-sectional study suggests that chronic (12-month) exposure to ozone and particles is related to asthma outcomes among children in metropolitan areas throughout the United States.[441] In South Durban, South Africa, increased lower respiratory symptoms (cough, wheezing, chest tightness or heaviness, and shortness of breath) were strongly and consistently associated with prior-day fluctuations in ambient levels of both SO_2 and PM_{10}.[442] In western Morocco, air pollution was a determinant factor but is not the only factor increasing the risk of asthma in children; other factors (e.g., respiratory diseases, infectious diseases, genetics, and passive smoking) present a high-risk threat.[443] In a study in Puerto Rico, proximity to some air pollution sources was associated with increased risks of asthma attacks.[444] In Argentina, a relationship was found between higher exposure to photochemical pollutants and high prevalence or risk of asthma symptoms.[445] In southern California communities, respiratory health in children was adversely affected by local exposures to outdoor NO_2 or other freeway-related pollutants.[446]

Society is experiencing a transition from classical pollution dominated by SO_2 and particulates generated by coal and oil combustion (with the effects primarily on cough and bronchitis) to pollution mixtures dominated by traffic exhausts represented by NO_2 (with effects on wheeze).[447] Motor vehicle traffic has increased greatly during the last decades, and its role in the development of asthma has been investigated. Diesel exhaust may have a particularly strong influence.[448,449] A positive association between self-reported truck traffic in the street of residence and reported asthma symptoms in adolescents was observed in German cities.[450,451] There were similar findings in the Netherlands.[448] In Italy, exposure to exhaust from heavy vehicular traffic in metropolitan areas increased the occurrence of wheezing.[452] In Kenya, children from an urban area were exposed more frequently to motor vehicle fumes on the way to school than rural children, and this partially explained observed differences in prevalence.[59] In asthmatic children in the Netherlands, black smoke, particulates, and O_3 were associated with acute respiratory symptoms and medication use.[449] A study of children younger than 5 years of age in Birmingham, U.K., showed an increased risk of hospitalization for asthma for children living in areas with high traffic flow.[453] One study in Germany found no association with traffic pollution and BHR.[454] In Taiwan, long-term exposure to traffic-related outdoor air pollutants such as NOx, CO, and O_3 increased the risk of asthma in children.[455] Children experiencing the highest burden of emissions in Nicosia Cyprus seem to be at a higher risk of reporting asthmatic symptoms.[456] Higher self-reported exposure to truck traffic on the street of residence obtained as part of ISAAC Phase Three was associated with higher reports of asthma symptoms in many locations of the world.[457] In the United States, children 4 to 12 years of age with asthma were more likely to have symptoms with exposure to traffic-related fine particles.[458] However, in Oslo there were no associations of long-term traffic-related exposures with asthma onset or with current respiratory symptoms in children 9 to 10 years of age.[459] Traffic-related pollutants (e.g., NO_2) are associated with asthma without overt evidence of other atopic disorders among female children living in a medium-sized Canadian city. The effects were sensitive to the method of exposure estimation. More refined exposure models produced the most robust associations.[460] In Lima, Peru, the prevalence of asthma was significantly related to traffic flow density.[461]

There is some new evidence that exposure to traffic-related air pollution may cause asthma in children. In the Netherlands, the association between traffic-related air pollution and the development of asthma in a prospective birth cohort study with a unique 8-year follow-up was studied with $PM_{2.5}$ levels, NO_2, and soot. Associations were stronger for children who had not moved since birth.[462] In a large Canadian study, there was a significantly increased risk of asthma diagnosis with increased early life exposure to CO, NO, NO_2, PM_{10}, SO_2, and black carbon, and proximity to point sources. Traffic-related pollutants were associated with the highest risks. These data support the hypothesis that early childhood exposure to air pollutants plays a role in development of asthma.[463] In children from participants in the Southern California prospective cohort, markers of traffic-related air pollution were associated with the onset of asthma. The risks observed suggest that air pollution exposure contributes to new-onset asthma.[464]

In Cape Town, South Africa, community concern about asthma prompted an epidemiologic study of children living near a petrochemical refinery. The results supported the hypothesis of an increased prevalence of asthma symptoms among children in the area as a result of refinery emissions and provided a substantive basis for community concern.[465] In La Plata, Argentina, exposure to particulate matter and volatile organic compounds arising from petrochemical plants but not from high traffic density was associated with worse respiratory health in children.[466] In Leicester, U.K., a study examining the exposure to PM_{10} at or near each child' home address found a dose-dependent inverse association between the carbon content of airway macrophages and lung function.[467]

Infection, Immunization, and Microbial Exposure

Infection

The relationship between infection and asthma symptoms has intrigued clinicians and epidemiologists for decades. The "hygiene hypothesis" was first proposed by Strachan in 1989: that allergic diseases could be prevented by infection in early childhood.[468] This hypothesis was suggested by the observation that hay fever (but not asthma) at 11 and 23 years of age was inversely related to the number of children in the household at age 11 years, with the number of older children being more influential than birth order. Strachan proposed that allergic diseases could be "prevented by infection in early childhood transmitted by unhygienic contact with older siblings or acquired prenatally from a mother infected by contact with her older children. Later infection or reinfection by younger siblings might confer additional protection against hay fever."[468]

The hypothesis that was proposed about hay fever has been widely applied to asthma, with little evidence. The first decade of the hygiene hypothesis was twice reviewed by Strachan.[469,470] Let Strachan have the last word on the hygiene hypothesis:

> "The hygiene hypothesis remains a credible but nonspecific explanation for observed variations over time, place and persons at risk for developing atopic allergic disorders. More prospective studies are needed to unravel which infectious agents exert a protective effect and the time period of importance for sensitization. The clinical implications of these advances in our understanding of the etiology of atopic allergic disorders are currently limited."[470]

A 1995 review of infants with wheeze suggested two groups: those who have lower-than-normal lung function shortly after birth, who will become symptom free during the preschool years, and those who persist with wheezing.[471] The factors that determine which group will be persistent wheezers are not well understood, but the potential role of rhinovirus is being explored.[471,472] Because of limitations in the existing literature, a comprehensive review of asthma and respiratory infections cannot provide a clear answer to the central question of whether respiratory viral illness causes asthma, exacerbates underlying asthma, or both.[473] The more children an individual is exposed to at an early age, the less likely that child will have development of persistent or late-onset asthma, and the timing of this exposure matters; exposure to other children during the toddler years is more protective. More frequent respiratory tract illnesses may not be the only factor in this observed relationship.[474]

A further analysis of the Tucson study showed that daycare during the first 6 months of age was protective against the development of asthma. Daycare during the first 6 months also increased the risk of frequent wheeze (more than 3 episodes in the previous year) at 2 years of age, but decreased the risk of frequent wheeze at 6 to 13 years of age.[475] The mechanism was thought to be exposure to infection.

In a very large prospective study in Tennessee, timing of birth in relationship to winter virus season conferred a differential and definable risk of developing early childhood asthma[476] A prospective cohort study in Germany showed that children with 2 or more episodes of runny nose before 1 year of age were less likely to have been diagnosed as asthmatic by a doctor or have wheeze by 7 years, and they were less likely to be atopic by 5 years of age. One or more viral infections of the herpes type before 3 years of age were also inversely associated with asthma at 7 years of age. Conversely, repeated lower respiratory tract infections in the first 3 years was associated with increased risk of wheeze at 7 years of age.[477] Viral infections are the major precipitant of asthma exacerbations, leading to a complex of inflammatory processes. Although knowledge of the mechanism underlying infection-induced asthma exacerbations has increased substantially since the late 1990s, a great deal of further work is still clearly warranted. Moreover, the interactions between viruses, other pathogens, air pollution, and allergen sensitization and exposure are not completely understood.[478]

Respiratory syncytial virus (RSV) has warranted special consideration because it is the most common cause of bronchiolitis, an acute wheezy illness of infants. A study of children enrolled in the longitudinal cohort study, the Tucson Children's Respiratory Study (Arizona) showed that RSV lower respiratory tract infections before 3 years of age were associated with an increased risk of infrequent wheeze and frequent wheeze at 6 years of age. Risk decreased with age and was not observable at 13 years of age.[479] RSV-positive children younger than 5 years of age with asthma had a longer duration of illness prior to hospital presentation than RSV-negative children but were not more likely to be admitted or to have a longer duration of ongoing symptoms.[180] The relationship between RSV lower respiratory tract infections in early childhood and asthma has been the subject of much debate. Some cohort studies have failed to identify a link between early RSV infection and atopic asthma. Cohort studies focusing on wheezing in early childhood have indicated that this is associated with an increased incidence of atopic asthma, but that this risk is not increased by RSV infection. Indeed, wheeze associated with rhinovirus infection may be a better marker for possible asthma. In contrast, there is no increased risk of atopic disease in infants with RSV acute bronchiolitis. These studies confirm earlier suggestions that the phenotype of respiratory illness and hence the host response rather than the infecting organism is the best predictor of the future pattern of respiratory illness.[480]

Rhinovirus infections are nearly universal in children with asthma during common cold seasons, likely because of a plethora of new strains appearing each season. Illnesses associated with viruses have greater duration and severity. Finally, atopic asthmatic children experienced more frequent and severe virus-induced illnesses.[481] Symptomatic rhinovirus infections are an important contributor to asthma exacerbations in children 2 to 17 years of age from a selected population in Atlanta.[482] A recent review has identified mechanisms by which rhinovirus lower respiratory tract infection, particularly in a susceptible host, could promote the development of childhood asthma. Further studies are needed to elucidate the mechanisms underlying the link between rhinovirus wheezing in early childhood and subsequent asthma development.[483]

A number of other infectious agents have been studied. Although a cross-sectional study in Finland showed a positive association between measles infection and asthma,[484] this finding has not been replicated. In an Italian population, a history of pertussis or pneumonia was not associated with asthma.[485] In a randomized double-blind controlled trial of pertussis vaccine in Sweden, there was a positive association between whooping cough disease and asthma by 2½ years of age.[486] An increased incidence of asthma has been found in children with HIV1 on highly active antiretroviral therapy. This might be driven by immunoreconstitution of CD41 T cells.[487] In a prospective study in Germany, there was an inverse correlation between Chlamydia pneumoniae infection of the upper airways and the later development of asthma, suggesting that this organism may be a potentially protective factor.[488]

There has been interest in the relationship between parasitic infections, IgE, and asthma. It has been suggested that high degrees of parasitic infections could prevent asthma symptoms in atopic individuals in Ethiopia in a comparison of urban and rural areas.[489] However studies in Latin America demonstrate high prevalence of asthma symptoms in areas with higher endemic parasite load.[439] A cross-sectional study of 1320 children 4 to 14 years of age from two Cuban municipalities found that asthma and atopy were unrelated to helminth infections.[490] In southern Brazilian children 8 to 12 years of age, most asthma and wheeze is non-atopic, suggesting that some helminths may exert an attenuating effect on the expression of the atopic portion of the disease, whereas viral bronchiolitis predisposes more specifically to recurrent airway symptoms.[491] In Thailand, hookworm infection was an independent risk factor for childhood wheeze.[492]

Experimental evidence suggests that exposure to Mycobacterium tuberculosis may reduce the risk of developing asthma. In a partly longitudinal study of children in Japan, an inverse relationship was found between tuberculin skin response and symptoms of asthma. However, it is unclear whether Bacille Calmette Guerin (BCG) vaccination, primary TB infection in childhood, or sensitization to harmless environmental mycobacteria were responsible[493] (BCG vaccination is discussed further in the Immunization section that follows).

An ecological analysis of ISAAC Phase One data showed an inverse association between TB notification rates[494] and estimated TB incidence,[495] and the lifetime prevalence of wheeze and asthma and the 12-month prevalence of wheeze assessed from a video questionnaire, adjusted for GNP. A decrease in tuberculosis notifications of 25 cases per 100,000 was associated with a 4.7% increase in the prevalence of wheeze ever. These findings support other evidence that exposure to Mycobacterium tuberculosis may reduce the risk of developing asthma. This may occur through induction of Th1-type immune responses. The implications of this relationship in the changing world of TB disease (the increase in AIDS and the concomitant increase in TB cases in Africa, and the decrease of TB in other regions such as Latin America) need further study.

Immunization

It has been postulated that immunization in early life may either promote or protect against asthma. The balance of evidence from studies to date suggests no effect. A large cross-sectional study in the United States found that DTP or measles vaccine appeared to increase the risk of asthma ever, but not wheezing in the last 12 months.[496] Other studies have found that immunization has no effect or even a protective effect on IgE-mediated disease. In a large prospective cohort study in the United Kingdom, there was no increased risk for wheezing illnesses in pertussis-vaccinated children.[497] In a randomized double-blind controlled trial of the pertussis vaccine in Sweden, the cumulative incidence of IgE-mediated disease was similar in the three vaccination and placebo groups.[486] In a large Canadian study, a negative association between delay in administration of the first dose of whole-cell

DPT immunization in childhood and the development of asthma was found; the association was greater with delays in all of the first three doses. The mechanism for this phenomenon requires further research.[498] A U.K. study provided no evidence of an association between vaccination against pertussis in infancy and an increased risk of later wheeze or asthma, and it does not support claims that vaccination against pertussis might significantly increase the risk of childhood asthma.[499] American ecological data do not show associations between changes in childhood vaccine exposures and asthma prevalence.[500] A meta-analysis of observational studies did not support an association, provocative or protective, between receipt of the BCG or whole-cell pertussis vaccine and risk of asthma in childhood and adolescence.[501] However in a historical cohort in England, a potentially protective effect of neonatal BCG vaccination and asthma symptom prevalence was found.[502] Moreover a meta-analysis of BCG vaccine in early life supported the hypothesis that exposure to the BCG prevents asthma, possibly through a modulation of the immune maturation process.[503]

An ecological analysis of the ISAAC Phase One data using immunization rates for the year of birth of the ISAAC participants, adjusted for GNP, undertook two levels of immunization analyses: country level and center level. The country-level analyses showed no associations between symptoms of asthma and national immunization rates for DTP, measles, and BCG.[504] The more powerful center-level analyses showed small inverse relationships between DTP and measles in the older age group only, with no associations with BCG. In view of earlier reports that immunization might be a risk factor for asthma, this mainly null result is reassuring for population immunization programs, given their importance for child health.

Other Microbial Exposure

The concept that live microbial food constituents may have a beneficial effect on human health was first proposed in the early 1900s by Metchnikoff.[505] In the last century, the dominance of *Bifidobacteria* and *Lactobacillus* in the initial gut flora of the developing world infant has been increasingly replaced by a variety of other organisms in the developed world, and this has been an intriguing area for further exploration.[506-508] However, in two double-blind randomized placebo-controlled trials in Finland, there was no difference in the prevalence of asthma symptoms following *Lactobacillus* administered in pregnancy and for 6 months after birth.[509,510] Further study, possibly large-scale birth cohort analyses using molecular methods to test for microbiota,[511] is required before any recommendations can be given about probiotic administration for asthma prevention.

Does antimicrobial usage have any effect through the unwanted effects of antimicrobials causing major depletion of the commensal microflora of the gut? Most relevant studies are retrospective or cross-sectional, and one of the largest potential problems is the concept of self-selection. For children who wheeze with lower respiratory infections, prescription of antimicrobial treatment may be a marker for children who

are more likely to wheeze in the first place. In ISAAC Phase One, the relationships between symptom prevalence and antimicrobial exposure were not clearcut. A mixture of weak inverse and positive effects was found between symptom prevalence and total antimicrobial sales and broad-spectrum antimicrobial sales.[512] In a further cross-sectional study with parental responses on individual questionnaires in ISAAC Phase Three, an association was found between antimicrobial use in the first year of life and current symptoms of asthma.[513] The Boston birth cohort study[514] followed infants at high risk for atopy, from birth to 5 years, excluding children who were treated with antimicrobials for wheezing. There was no association seen between antimicrobial use and asthma 5 years of age.

Increased exposure to bacterial compounds in stables where livestock is kept may prevent the development of allergic disorders in children. The consumption of "raw" unpasteurized milk may contain a higher microbial load, particularly of *Lactobacillus*, than industrial processed skim milk.[515] Increased concentrations of bacterial compounds such as endotoxin and its purified derivative lipopolysaccharide have been found in stables where livestock has been kept.[516] Endotoxin levels are also high in stables of farming families in the European Alps, and also in the dust from their kitchen floors and children's mattresses compared to non-farming families.[517]

Endotoxin levels are also likely to be particularly high in developing countries where poultry and livestock are kept in close proximity to human housing. One study from Africa found a significantly decreased development of IgE-sensitization in children in whose homes pigs were kept.[518] Bacterial endotoxin is known to induce production of Th1-associated cytokines, interferon γ, and interleukin 12 and therefore has the potential to decrease allergen sensitization. Reductions in allergen sensitization and IgE-mediated disease have been found in children of farmers; children with pigs, dogs, or cats in their homes; children raised in daycare from an early age; and children of large families. An intriguing notion for further exploration is whether endotoxin could reduce the clinical expression of atopy. To date there is no evidence to support this, but observational studies and randomized trials to test this hypothesis would be of interest.[519] In the Boston Home Allergens and Asthma Study,[520] a longitudinal analysis of wheezing in young children and the independent effects of early-life exposures to house dust endotoxin, allergens, and pets suggests that the timing, dose, and other environmental factors may be important. In this study, the investigators found that higher levels of endotoxin were associated with increased risk of wheezing initially, but this risk rapidly decreased with time. The protective effects of cat and dog ownership were independent of the endotoxin level.

An inner-city study in the United States showed that outdoor and indoor fungi, particularly *Penicillium* spp, worsened asthma morbidity in inner-city children.[521] On the other hand, in a cross-sectional study in five European countries, the protective effect of being raised on a farm was largely unexplained by the mattress microbial agent levels of bacterial endotoxin, fungal b(1,3)-glucans and fungal extracellular polysaccharides.[522] In a small study in

Palestine, a nested case-control found mostly negative results, but suggested that that endotoxin on living room floors might protect against atopic wheeze.[523]

In the United States among children at risk of atopy, early exposure to high levels of dust mite allergen is associated with increased risks of asthma and late-onset wheeze. In these children, endotoxin exposure is associated with a reduced risk of atopy but an increased risk of wheeze. Early endotoxin exposure may be a protective factor against atopy but a risk factor for wheeze in high-risk children.[524] In a prospective study of children 10 years of age in Oslo, Norway, no risk modification was seen for endotoxin and b(1,3)-glucans.[269] In a recent study in the urban United States, both Gram-negative and Gram-positive bacterial exposures in the bed were associated with decreased asthma symptoms, but may act through different mechanisms to confer protection. It was proposed that endotoxin exposure in later childhood has independent protective effects on allergic disease.[525]

Housing, Animals, and Climate

There is growing recognition of the importance of the indoor environment in asthma. An increasing body of evidence suggests that indoor pollutants contribute to asthma morbidity, but the amount of research on indoor air pollution and asthma is small compared with outdoor pollutants. While a number of indoor ultrafine particle sources have been identified and thoroughly characterized, the potential health effects of these exposures remain largely unexplored.[526] Experimental and epidemiologic studies, however, suggest that pollutants, such as NO_2 and ozone, may potentiate the effect of allergen exposure in atopic individuals.[527] More detailed epidemiologic studies comprehensively evaluating indoor pollutants and allergen exposures are warranted. Characteristics of the housing itself may be relevant too. The relationships between housing type and asthma were explored in a New York study. Markers of housing deterioration, especially roaches, rats, and water leaks, were found in all types of housing and among residents with a wide range of socioeconomic levels, but residents of public housing had higher odds of current asthma than residents of private housing, after adjusting for individual disease risk factors and markers of housing quality.[528]

Damp and Mold

There is a common belief that damp housing is bad for respiratory health, including asthma. Cross-sectional and longitudinal cohort studies that have been conducted in children show a small increased risk of having asthma symptoms if the home has damp or mold. However the potential benefits of reducing mold in the home have not been investigated. In a study in the Netherlands, sensitization to HDM and possibly mold allergen is related to living in a damp home and childhood respiratory symptoms.[529] In a study of U.S. children, dampness in the home was common and a predictor of wheeze and asthma.[530] In a population study in Israel, viable molds were common but IgE-sensitization to molds was a poor predictor of development of allergic symptoms. However, allergy to molds in atopic subjects increases the risk of symptomatic allergic disease.[531] In a study in children in London, there was no significant difference in the degree of bronchospasm measured from children in homes with or without mold, but wheeze in the last year was associated with reported dampness and mold.[532] In a small study of children in southern California, the degree of atopy and reactivity to mold and pollens played a significant role in asthma severity in asthmatic children.[533] In a cohort study in Taiwan with assessment of exposure before the onset of asthma, exposure to molds had independent influence on the development of asthma.[534] In another Taiwanese study, visible mold on the walls was associated with seasonality of childhood asthma in Taiwan.[535] In a small study in Turkey, indoor molds had no effect on the symptoms of patients with asthma and/or rhinitis monosensitized to molds.[536] However, simultaneous estimation of relative humidity in bedrooms and recordings of ambient temperature and humidity showed no association with respiratory symptoms.[537] Nevertheless, it seems prudent to reduce or avoid damp housing conditions.[254]

Animals

The role of the farm environment and close human contact with animals in the development of asthma has captured a lot of interest.[538,539] Although the first report from Switzerland showed no protective effect,[275] the next cross-sectional study of Finnish children showed that the childhood farm environment reduced the risk of asthma and wheezing.[276] Among Austrian children living in a rural area, children living on a farm had less asthma than those in a nonfarming environment.[277] In Bavaria, Germany, farmers' children had a lower prevalence of asthma and wheeze than their peers who did not live in an agricultural environment.[538] However, in a large cross-sectional study of Chinese children of a wide age range, pet keeping and parental atopy increased the risk of asthma in children.[540,541]

In a subsequent study of Austrian, German, and Swiss farmers' children, current wheeze was lower among children who spent time in the stables. This effect was stronger for children who spent time in the stables during the first year of life (OR 0.36 and 0.33, respectively) than for those who spent time there from 2 to 5 years of age (OR 0.73 and 0.87), compared with nonfarming children. Similar reductions were found with those who drank unpasteurized farm milk. Time spent in the stables and consumption of farm milk in the first year was independently associated with asthma outcome. Among farmers' children who spent time in the stables in the first year of life, drank farm milk, and whose mother spent time in the stables while pregnant, there was only one case of asthma (expected 19 cases).[515] These results suggest that exposure to the farming environment influences the development of asthma and IgE-sensitization in a potently protective way. A protective effect of the farm environment has since also been found in Finland,[276,542] four European centers and New Zealand in the ECRHS study,[543] Nepal,[544] Crete,[545] Canada,[546] and Australia,[547] but not in a further New Zealand study.[548] However in a cohort of rural

Iowa children, a high prevalence of asthma health outcomes was found among children living on farms that raise swine and add antimicrobials to feed, despite lower rates of atopy and personal histories of allergy, suggesting the need for more population-based studies to further assess environmental and genetic determinants of asthma among farm children.[549]

The relationship with animals is thus complex. For example, in a study in rural Austria, Germany, and Switzerland, although pet exposure was very frequent, the inverse relation between current dog contact and asthma was mostly explained by simultaneously occurring exposure to stable animals or was restricted to farm children. In addition, bias due to pet avoidance in asthma-susceptible families may contribute to the apparent protective effect of pets.[550]

Other Indoor Factors

Outdoor particles readily penetrate indoors. This partially explains why epidemiologic time series studies consistently find associations between health outcomes and PM measured at outdoor fixed sites, despite the fact that people spend most of their time indoors.

Exposure to NO_2 through the use of unvented gas cookers in homes is associated with respiratory symptoms. Over half of U.S. households contain a source of NO_2.[551] There are limitations in the studies because they often do not control for volatile organic compounds.[552] In addition NO_2 may aggravate respiratory symptoms in the presence of coexistent infection.[553] A study of children in Victoria, Australia, showed that NO_2 was a marginal risk factor for respiratory symptoms, with a dose response association present. Gas stove exposure was a significant risk factor, even after controlling for personal NO_2 exposure, suggesting an additional risk. No difference was noted between atopic and non-atopic children.[554] A study of asthmatics in Port Adelaide, Australia, demonstrated associations between personal NO_2 exposure measured by lapel sensors, and asthmatic symptoms such as chest tightness, breathlessness on exertion, and daytime and nighttime asthma attacks in children.[555] Higher indoor NO_2 concentrations were associated with increased asthma symptoms in preschool inner-city children.[556] In a study in the United States, exposure to indoor NO_2 at levels well below the Environmental Protection Agency outdoor standard (53 ppb) was associated with respiratory symptoms among children with asthma in multifamily housing.[551]

In a study in Bavaria, Germany, coal or wood heating in children's homes reduced the risk of becoming sensitized to pollen and developing hay fever, BHR, and asthma.[557]

Indoor exposure to mixtures and single components of volatile organic compounds can be related to asthma symptoms, but there is no evidence that increasing exposure of a population to these compounds initiates asthma and allergic disease. Although gasoline is a common volatile organic compound and can contaminate the indoor environment in motor vehicles and buildings, there is no evidence to link this to asthma.[558]

Microbial volatile organic compounds and plasticizers (used in water-based paints and polyvinyl chloride) at school may be a risk factor for asthmatic symptoms in children. In Sweden recently, amounts of plastic material in dwellings have been found. Airborne microorganisms, volatile organic compounds of possible microbial origin, selected plasticizer compounds, and formaldehyde were found in school classrooms and outside the building.[559]

Formaldehyde is one of several volatile organic compounds now commonly found indoors in homes in western environments. Sources are particle board, plywood, fiber board, paneling, urea formaldehyde foam insulation, and some carpets and furniture, as well as some household chemicals. Formaldehyde exposure may increase the risk of IgE-sensitization to common aeroallergens.[560] Frequent use of chemical-based products is associated with persistent wheezing in preschool children.[561] A significant positive association was found between formaldehyde exposure and childhood asthma. Given the largely cross-sectional nature of the studies underlying this meta-analysis, further well-designed prospective epidemiologic studies are needed.[562]

In Kenya, the higher prevalence of asthma symptoms in urban than rural localities has been related to the home environment.[59] Urban homes tend to have different structures from rural homes, and carpets are exclusively found in the urban setting. Urban homes use gas and electricity as the major domestic fuel, and also use kerosene and charcoal, whereas rural homes use firewood as the major domestic fuel. In Germany, wood and coal heating and feather bedding were negatively associated with symptoms, whereas exposures such as truck traffic in a residential street and active smoking were positively associated with symptoms.[47]

There has been recent interest in chlorinated swimming pools and asthma. An ecological analysis in Europe found that the prevalence of childhood asthma and the number of indoor chlorinated swimming pools in Europe were linked through associations that are geographically consistent and independent of climate, altitude, and socioeconomic status of the country.[563] A recent review suggested an association between childhood swimming and new-onset asthma, but exposure measurement needs attention.[564]

Climate and Weather

A potential role of climatic conditions in the etiology of asthma and allergy has often been suspected and is of particular interest for the future because of climate change. Most studies on the effects of climate have looked at short periods of variations in the occurrence or severity of symptoms. Little is known about the effect of long-term climatic conditions on the prevalence of asthma symptoms. Studies on the long-term effect of climate have been limited to comparisons of areas within countries.[565] A study in Bermuda related emergency department acute asthma visits with relative humidity, average daily temperature, and northeasterly winds.[566] In a comparative study in the United Kingdom, Australia, and New Zealand, the prevalence of asthma among children was greater in the warmer regions.[567] In London, new episodes of asthma in adults during a 2-day thunderstorm were associated with a decrease in air temperature and an increase in grass pollen concentration.[162] A larger study in England of the effect of thunderstorms and airborne grass pollen over a 4-year period showed that thunderstorm-associated increases in hospital admissions for acute asthma were amplified after a run of high pollen counts.[163] An inverse association between the prevalence of BHR and altitude of the study area has been observed in mountaineering expeditions in Italy and Nepal.[568]

As climate affects whole populations, ecological studies are ideally suited to examine the relationship between prevalence of diseases and climatic conditions between populations. In the worldwide ISAAC analyses few significant associations were seen.[569] However, in studies in two large continents with quite marked climate differences—Latin America[439] and Africa[570]—no relationship was observed for asthma symptoms prevalence with respect to latitude, altitude, humid/dry climate or other geographical aspects, suggesting that meteorologic and geographic factors, individually, would not be able to explain the wide variability in the prevalence of asthma, rhinitis and eczema in the world. As the world becomes more affected by climate change there may be some regions such as western Europe where prevalence of disease is affected by potentially modifiable factors including humidity and temperature,[569] but at a global level our ecological analyses showed little effect.

Economic Factors

Early reports of increasing prevalence of asthma in Western countries suggested that asthma may be associated with the economic development occurring with Westernization. This hypothesis was explored in an ecological analysis of ISAAC Phase One data from 52 countries using Gross National Product (GNP) as a marker of economic development of countries. A weak positive association was found between GNP and symptoms of asthma; an increase of $10,000 per capita was associated with a 3% increase in the prevalence of wheeze.[571] However within Latin America, ISAAC suggested a reverse trend, with prevalence of symptoms of asthma tending to be higher in poorer areas.[439] Further supportive evidence of this association was found recently in ISAAC Phase Three, where data from 98 countries showed that the prevalence of asthma symptoms showed a positive relationship with Gross National Income (GNI), although the prevalence of severe symptoms correlated inversely with GNI.[32] However caution should be used in interpreting the findings because of the great inequalities in income distribution within almost all countries in developing regions of the world. GNP represents the total economic activity of the country, reflecting mean wealth rather than median wealth. Thus countries with a highly skewed income distribution caused by concentration of wealth in the hands of a small fraction of the population may have a relatively high per capita GNP, while the majority of citizens have a relatively low level of income.[572] A further consideration is that GNP does not measure factors that affect quality of life, such as the quality of the environment.

Within countries, some studies have shown that severe asthma symptoms in developed countries are more frequent in poorer sections of society.[573] However in a prospective British cohort, high socioeconomic status was related to persistence of wheeze at 16 years of age.[281] In a national birth cohort study from England, Wales, and Scotland, the prevalence of asthma showed no social class gradient.[574] In Cardiff, Wales, social deprivation was not related to asthma prevalence, but was related to admission to hospital.[575] A South African study had a similar finding with severity measured by high symptom occurrence.[576] In a cross-sectional study in Italy, socioeconomic conditions were associated with hospitalization for asthma and were severity and weakly associated with prevalence, with the association being strongest for individual indicators (parental education) rather than area-based indicators.[577] Poorer disease management is the postulated mechanism. In Auckland, New Zealand, there were higher lifetime and current prevalence rates of wheeze in children in lower socioeconomic status groups.[578] In Brazil, the prevalence of asthma increased with poorer sanitation and with higher infant mortality at birth and at survey year, Gini coefficient (as a measure of income inequality within the country) and external mortality, and in contrast, asthma prevalence decreased with higher illiteracy rates.[579] However, another study in Brazil found that the prevalence of asthma and related symptoms is quite variable and independent of socioeconomic status.[580] In Santiago, Chile, a higher maternal education level was associated with lower prevalence of wheeze in the last 12 months.[581] In Canada, disparities in asthma control between children from families of different socioeconomic status persist, even with adjustment for utilization of primary care services and use of controller medications.[582] In a nationally representative U.S. sample of children 3 years of age, asthma prevalence declined with increasing income for non–African-American but not African-American children.[108] Among New York children 4 to 13 years of age, children living in predominantly low socioeconomic status communities had a 70% greater risk of current asthma, independent of their own ethnicity and income level. Asthma prevalence within different ethnic and income groups was consistently lower in neighborhoods of greater socioeconomic status, except among Puerto Rican children, who had high asthma prevalence regardless of school attended or income.[109] In another study, U.S. non-Hispanic African-American children were at substantially higher risk of asthma than non-Hispanic white children only among the very poor. The influence of neighborhood environment on childhood asthma in a non–inner-city setting (Rochester, Minnesota) was small to modest.[583]

The concentration of racial/ethnic differences only among the very poor suggests that patterns of social and environmental exposures must overshadow any hypothetical genetic risk.[584]

The ecological economic analysis undertaken in the ISAAC Phase Three global study of asthma prevalence[32] revealed a significant trend toward a higher prevalence of current wheeze in centers in higher-income countries in both age groups, but this trend was reversed for the prevalence of severe symptoms among children with current wheeze, especially in the adolescents. Although asthma symptoms tended to be more prevalent in high-income countries, they appeared to be more severe in low- and middle-income countries. In a recent publication, Wilkinson and Pickett[585] describe the far-reaching effects of income inequality on indicators of societal health and well-being. The measure of income inequality used was the ratio of the income share of the richest 20% of country population to the poorest 20%. The effect of this measure is being examined in ISAAC Phase Three.

Explanations for these gradients have been explored. The positive association between socioeconomic status and prevalent childhood asthma might be explained by differential access to medical care that remains unmeasured, by the hygiene hypothesis (e.g., lower socioeconomic status may associate with higher protective exposures to endotoxin in early life), or by socioeconomic status acting as a proxy for unmeasured neighborhood characteristics.[586] A psychobiological explanation for the epidemiologic relationship between low SES and poor asthma outcomes has been proposed, suggesting that the experience of stress, particularly among lower socioeconomic status children, has implications for childhood asthma morbidity.[587]

■ NATURAL HISTORY

Asthma is commonly described as a chronic reversible obstructive airways disease. However for many children, asthma is a transient rather than chronic condition. Equally, while intermittent bronchospasm and mucus hypersecretion lead to acute exacerbations and much of the disease's early burden, asthma is now also being characterized by persistent inflammation and airway remodeling. As this chapter has noted, numerous environmental and genetic factors act in concert, resulting in a very heterogeneous condition in terms of age of onset, symptoms, severity, response to therapy, and course. As a result, it is not possible to define a single natural history for asthma, but some important aspects can be highlighted.

Preschool Asthma

In 1995, Martinez and colleagues published a highly influential work based on the first 6 years of the Tucson Children's Respiratory Study.[246] This study involved a birth cohort of some 1200 infants with close respiratory follow-up. They found that wheeze was a very common experience such that one third of children had at least one episode before 3 years of age. Wheeze prevalence was 32% in the first year, 17% in the second year, and 12% in the third. Of those who wheezed before 3 years of age, 60% were wheeze-free at 6 years of age. The authors grouped children as "never wheezed" (52%), "transient early wheezing" (20%), "persistent wheezing" (14%), and "late-onset wheezing" (15%).

Transient wheezers were more likely to have mothers who smoked, had evidence of early airway narrowing, and generally wheezed in association with viral infection. Persistent wheezers were more likely to have a family history of asthma, elevated IgE, and normal early airway caliber. In contrast, others subsequently found early airflow limitation at 4 weeks of age was associated with an increased risk of childhood airway responsiveness and wheeze.[588] The Tucson study reinforced the concept of different childhood asthma phenotypes, that many children "grow out of" asthma, and that the different phenotypes may be predictable based on risk factors. Other cohort studies have had similar findings.[589] Children in the Tucson study with persistent wheezing have significantly reduced lung function at 6 years of age. The authors believed that the poorer lung function was not congenital, but rather the result of persistent airway inflammation.

As a result of these observations, it is common to see descriptions of childhood asthma in terms of phenotypes that have different ages of onset, different characteristics, and different natural histories (Fig. 44-4). While the cohort studies found statistically significant differences in family history, allergic sensitization, and lung function between groups, on an individual basis these are insensitive and nonspecific.[246,589]

School-Age Asthma and Beyond

The Melbourne Asthma Study enrolled a random cohort of children 7 years of age with a history of wheeze in 1964 and has reviewed regularly since.[590] While there are methodological problems for a study of such long duration and with evolving therapies, particularly the introduction of inhaled corticosteroids that may have influenced the results, this study found that individuals generally tracked according to their early status. Those with infrequent very mild symptoms at 7 years of age were often asymptomatic during adolescence, although some had ongoing mild symptoms later in adulthood. Alternatively, those with more frequent or persistent asthma tended to have ongoing symptoms. At 42 years of age, 90% of those with severe childhood asthma continued to have troublesome symptoms.

Lung function was also reviewed. Those who had wheezed only in association with viral infection at enrollment and those whose symptoms had resolved at review were found to have lung function similar to the control group at 14 years of age and at subsequent reviews. Those initially classified with frequent or persistent asthma at the initial or subsequent review conversely had evidence of airway obstruction at 14 years of age. At subsequent reviews up until 42 years of age, there was no evidence of any further divergence in lung function between those with ongoing symptoms, frequent or severe symptoms, and those without. Authors speculated as to whether the initial fall followed by stability was the result of the introduction of regular inhaled corticosteroid therapy. Further, they concluded that their data showed those with mild or infrequent symptoms did not require steroid therapy to avoid progression. Follow-up of children in

Wheezing phenotypes in children

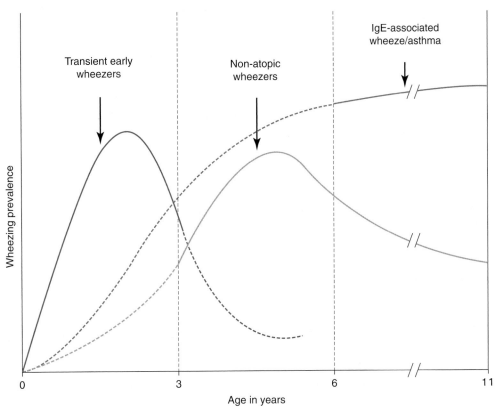

FIGURE 44-4. Epidemiologic wheeze phenotypes of early and mid-childhood. (From Stein RT, Holberg CJ, Morgan WJ, et al. Peak flow variability, methacholine responsiveness and atopy as markers for detecting different wheezing phenotypes in childhood. *Thorax.* 1997;52:951.)

the Tucson study had similar results. Those characterized as persistent wheezers at 6 years of age had poorer lung function at both 6 and 16 years of age than the those who had never wheezed. However, again there was no evidence of progressive divergence between the groups during childhood. In contrast, a quarter of the children enrolled in the Childhood Asthma Management Program did have evidence of progressive deterioration in lung function independent of treatment arm over the 4- to 6-years follow-up.[591] Inflammatory markers were measured in a subset of participants. Those with evidence of progression had more prominent eosinophilic inflammation.[591] It is worth noting that several studies in adulthood asthma have demonstrated abnormal decline in lung function.[592]

The Melbourne study also considered allergic features and found that the presence of atopy or allergic sensitization during childhood increased the risk of more severe asthma in adulthood. Other cohort studies have reinforced the roles of allergic sensitization, early environmental exposures, and early lung function deficits in the prediction of asthma persisting into adulthood.[592–594]

At the same time as cohort studies began demonstrating early and persistent lung function abnormalities in children with asthma, pathology studies have demonstrated persistent airway inflammation and remodeling.[592] Airway remodeling refers to thickening of the reticular basement membrane (RBM), epithelial fragility, hypertrophy and

hyperplasia of smooth muscle, deposition of extracellular matrix, and hypertrophy of mucus glands. These changes begin early. RBM thickening, absent at 12 months, is present by a median of 29 months in those with recurrent wheeze.[592,595,596] It is a consistent finding in children with severe or difficult asthma. It is not clear whether remodeling is reversible. These findings are of concern and lead to a different model for asthma with persistent and potentially progressive airway changes rather than simply reversible bronchospasm. Adding to this concern, the latest review of the Melbourne cohort reported that at 50 years of age, individuals who had been classified with severe asthma at 6 years of age had 37 times the risk of developing chronic obstructive pulmonary disease (COPD) compared with controls.[597] The risk was also elevated for those with original diagnoses of persistent asthma (OR 9) and intermittent asthma (OR 3) but was not elevated for those with mild viral-induced wheeze. Again, they reported no acceleration in lung function decline.

In summary, while the majority of early childhood wheeze has a benign course, for those with frequent/persistent wheeze there is evidence of airway inflammation and remodeling, impaired lung function, and persistence of troublesome symptoms into adulthood. Recent reports raise the possibility that childhood asthma, persisting into adulthood, may predispose to COPD. This subject is reviewed in detail in Chapter 17.

■CONCLUSION

In the last 20 to 30 years, epidemiologic studies have advanced knowledge about the worldwide prevalence and variation in asthma and its natural history. The roles of atopy and allergens have received considerable emphasis, but it is now time to focus more on environmental risk and protective factors such as diet, the human microbial environment, obesity, and air pollution. Observational studies are effective at generating hypotheses, however randomized controlled trials of environmental factors are required. The need for such evidence is even greater when one considers that the asthma epidemic experienced in the developed world is now affecting developing countries, with their very large populations and more limited health resources, as they become more urbanized. Future research should study the underlying causes of non-atopic asthma in low- and middle-income countries with a particular emphasis on urban versus rural prevalence and severity gradients to unravel the environmental risk factors associated with urbanization and demographic change. In addition to these environmental influences, it is anticipated that new tools in genetic investigation will permit much greater understanding into how genes and gene by environment interaction influences the etiology, response to therapy, and overall course of childhood asthma.

Over the same period, changes in management including new pharmaceuticals have demonstrated our ability to modify disease burden at individual and population levels. While inhaled corticosteroids appear to have been highly beneficial, the potential role of pharmaceuticals in mortality epidemics provides a cautionary tale. Asthma continues to exert a very high burden on the child, family, and society, and in many populations existing therapies are not employed to optimal effect. This explains some of the disparity in burden seen between countries, ethnicities, and socioeconomic groups. Mortality, hospitalization, and emergency visits are highly visible asthma burdens, yet asthma also exerts a high toll in school and work absenteeism, sleep disruption, lifestyle limitations, and psychosocial impact. The overall economic impact of asthma is enormous.

While much of what we thought we knew about asthma is being brought into question, the next few decades hold great promise in developing a greater understanding of the role of genetics and gene by environment interactions, leading to new models for prevention, prediction, and management. There is also considerable opportunity to better implement existing therapies across both the developed and developing world and therefore reduce the disparities in burden that are currently evident.

Suggested Reading

Prevalence
Lai CKW, Beasley R, Crane J, et al. Global variation in the prevalence and severity of asthma symptoms: Phase Three of the International Study of Asthma and Allergies in Childhood (ISAAC). *Thorax*. 2009;64:476–483.

Environmental Factors
Asher MI, Stewart AW, Mallol J, et al. Which population level environmental factors are associated with asthma, rhinoconjunctivitis and eczema? Review of the ecological analyses of ISAAC Phase One. *Respir Res*. 2010;11:8.

Global Burden
Masoli M, Fabian D, Holt S, et al and the Global Initiative for Asthma (GINA) Program. The global burden of asthma: executive summary of the GINA Dissemination Committee report. *Allergy*. 2004;59:469–478.

Mortality
Wijesinghe M, Weatherall M, Perrin K, et al. International trends in asthma mortality rates in the 5- to 34-year age group: a call for closer surveillance. *Chest*. 2009;135:1045–1049.

Genetics
Moffatt MF. Genes in asthma: new genes and new ways. *Curr Opin Allergy Clin Immunol*. 2008;8:411–417.

Obesity and Asthma
Peroni DG, Pietrobelli A, Boner AL. Asthma and obesity in childhood: on the road ahead. *Int J Obesity*. 2010;34:599–605.

Natural History
Panettieri RA, Covar R, Grant E, et al. Natural history of asthma: persistence versus progression—Does the beginning predict the end? *J Allergy Clin Immunol*. 2008;121:607–613.

References

The complete reference list is available online at www.expertconsult.com

45 THE IMMUNOPATHOGENESIS OF ASTHMA

Thomas A.E. Platts-Mills, MD, PhD, and Peter W. Heymann, MD

Wheezing in childhood has become progressively more common as a cause for visits to physicians, emergency rooms, and hospitals.[1-3] Some of this increase may reflect misdiagnosis, overanxious parents, or shortness of breath in unfit children. However, the large majority of children receiving treatment have objective evidence of asthma, such as audible wheezing on chest examination, reversible changes in expiratory flow, or bronchial hyperreactivity (BHR). A large proportion of these children also have indirect evidence of inflammation, which includes elevated exhaled nitric oxide (NO), lowered pH of lung condensate, and peripheral blood eosinophilia, as well as evidence of allergic sensitization.[4-7] The general acceptance that asthma is an inflammatory disease came partly from biopsy studies but, more significantly, from the evidence that steroid treatment is effective, and the reversibility of BHR with prolonged allergen avoidance.[8,9] The fact that lung inflammation and attacks of asthma can be caused by allergen exposure is undoubted. Many children are aware of acute episodes related to visiting a house with an animal. In addition, bronchial challenge can induce both eosinophil infiltration of the lungs and prolonged increases in BHR as well as acute changes in forced expiratory volume in 1 second (FEV_1). Indeed, the most consistent method of inducing "inflammation" in the lungs is to put allergen into the lungs of an allergic subject. However, bronchial challenge or segmental challenge is not the same as natural exposure. Not only is the quantity of allergen inhaled much greater, but the number of particles and the size of particles is dramatically different. The natural form of exposure to allergens is as a relatively small number of particles that are 2 to 20 µm in diameter. These are inhaled over prolonged periods (i.e., seasonally or all year round). Only a small proportion of naturally occurring attacks of asthma appear to be directly related to increased exposure. It appears more likely that allergen exposure plays a chronic role in maintaining bronchial inflammation and reactivity.

Although many different foreign proteins can give rise to sensitization, a select group dominates the epidemiology of asthma. This group includes mites, cat, dog, cockroach, and the fungus *Alternaria*. The main characteristic of these protein sources may be the fact that exposure is perennial. However, recent evidence suggests that the allergens are not equal; either the properties of the protein or the nature of the particles may influence the immune response sufficiently to influence both the prevalence and titer of immunoglobulin E (IgE) antibody responses.

Understanding the immunopathogenesis of asthma is important intellectually because it has to be taken into account in hypotheses about the increase in asthma. In addition, understanding the immunopathogenesis is important as part of the rationale for allergen-specific treatment and pharmacologic anti-inflammatory treatment. Although short-term increases in allergen exposure are not thought to be an important precipitant of acute episodes of asthma, there is a very strong association between immediate hypersensitivity and acute episodes. In part, this may reflect the increased BHR associated with elevated IgE and IgE antibodies. More significant may be recent evidence that the impact of rhinovirus infections on the lungs is strongly related to elevated IgE and elevated IgE antibodies, especially among asthmatic children who will have a greater risk for an exacerbation when they experience a rhinovirus infection during periods of increased allergen exposure.[10-12]

THE RELATIONSHIP BETWEEN ALLERGENS, ALLERGEN SENSITIZATION, AND ASTHMA

The evidence that allergens play a causal role in asthma comes from a wide variety of experiments (Box 45-1).[13] However, the primary evidence concerns the association between sensitization and asthma. These studies are case control, population based, and prospective, but in all cases the evidence for sensitization comes from measurement of IgE antibodies or immediate responses to skin testing. Although the implication of these studies is that allergen entering the lungs plays an important role in lung inflammation, only a minority of studies show a clear dose response between exposure and asthma symptoms. On the other hand, there are no studies showing a relationship between inhaled allergens and asthma in nonallergic individuals. The most likely explanation of dose-response data (i.e., lack of simple dose response to relationship) comes from (1) the effect of sensitization, (2) the inaccuracy of the measurements of allergen exposure, (3) the differences between allergen sources, and (4) the fact that most acute episodes and probably most episodes of wheezing are also triggered by viral infections and aggravated by one of the many nonspecific factors that can contribute to symptoms (Fig. 45-1). Additionally, the clinical relevance and host response to aeroallergens are known to vary among individuals with similar skin tests (or serum titers of allergen-specific IgE antibody) and allergen exposures.

THE ALLERGENS ASSOCIATED WITH ASTHMA

Dozens if not hundreds of sources of allergens have been associated with asthma. However, there are only a few that are sufficiently common to play a role in epidemiologic studies, and most of these are either perennial indoor allergens or outdoor allergens that have a long season (Table 45-1). The first studies used "house dust" to skin test, but because it was impossible to define what was in the extract, it was difficult to evaluate the results.[14] The discovery or definition of *house dust mites* was a critical event in understanding the pathogenesis of asthma. Voorhorst and Spieksma identified *Dermatophagoides pteronyssinus* in dust and developed skin test reagents. It rapidly became obvious that dust mites were an extraordinarily important cause of sensitization in all countries where the humidity was high enough to support their growth.[9,15] The reasons why dust mites are so important are still not clear. It could reflect their presence in bedding, the nature of the particles that become airborne, the biochemical/immunologic nature of the allergens

(some of which are proteolytic enzymes), or some other factor present in the particles (e.g., endotoxin).[16,17]

The other allergens that appear to play an important role in asthma include cats, dogs, rodents, and cockroaches, all of which are predominantly inside the house. Although pollens are an important source of sensitization and can cause asthma, seasonal asthma is generally less severe (with the exception of young children who may experience a severe exacerbation triggered by rhinovirus during a spring pollen season)[11] and often is not consistent from one year to the next. Sensitization to fungi is also observed in children with asthma. However, there are great problems with the consistency of the fungal extracts, and there is no consistent method for measuring mold allergens indoors. Molds that are thought to play an important role in all but the rarest cases of childhood asthma are *Alternaria* and *Aspergillus*, of which the latter can also colonize the lungs and rarely lead to symptoms of allergic bronchopulmonary aspergillosis (ABPA) (see Chapter 59).[18,19]

The obvious common feature of the allergens listed in Table 45-1 is that they are perennial. While in most cases this means indoor, it may not be true for the fungi or prolonged seasonal exposures to the combination of tree and grass pollen allergens. Inhalation of dust mite and cockroach allergens is thought to be largely in the patients' house. For many years it was assumed that all significant exposure to the indoor allergens occurred at home. This concept has had to be revised, because it is now clear that significant exposure to cat and mite allergens can and does occur outside the child's home. For cat and dog, significant allergen is present in schools and also most houses that do not have a cat. Furthermore, there is extensive evidence that the quantities found away from animals are sufficient to sensitize.[20,21] Indeed, in a recent study, 80% of the children who were skin test–positive to cat allergen had never lived in a house with a

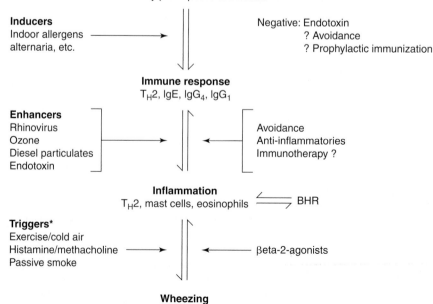

ROLE OF ALLERGENS IN THE DEVELOPMENT OF SENSITIZATION, INFLAMMATION AND REVERSIBLE AIRWAY OBSTRUCTION
Genetically predisposed individuals

FIGURE 45-1. The immune response to allergens requires exposure, but the time course and the dose response are variable. On its own, this response is asymptomatic. Continued exposure to allergen gives rise to inflammation, and this response can be enhanced by diesel particulates, endotoxin, or rhinovirus infection. Inflammation is not necessarily associated with symptoms, but most patients have increased BHR, so that bronchospasm can easily be triggered.

TABLE 45-1 PROPERTIES OF INDOOR ALLERGENS: 2011

AIRBORNE PARTICLES	SIZE/WEIGHT	ALLERGEN	HOMOLOGY
Dust Mite (Demlatophagoides pteronyssinus)			
Feces	10–40 μm/25 kd	Der p 1	Cysteine protease
	13 kd	Der p 2	Epididymal protein
German Cockroach (Blattella germanica)			
Frass saliva	>5 μm/36 kd	Bla g 2	Aspartic protease
		Bla g 5	
Cat (Felis domesticus)			
Dander particles	23 kd		Glutathione S-transferase
	36 kd	Fel d 1	Uteroglobin
Dog (Canis familiaris)			
	2–15 μm/21 kd	Can f 1	
Mouse (Mus domesticus)			
Urine on bedding, etc.	2–20 μm/22 kd		Lipocalin MUP
Rat (Rattus norvegicus)			
	Rat n 1	19 kd	Pheromone binding
Grass			
Grass pollen	30 μm/29 kd	Lol p 1	Cysteine proteinase

For details of properties of allergens, see www.allergen.org.

cat. The message is that preventing primary exposure to animal dander is not possible. Dust mite allergens are not widely distributed away from the sites of mite growth, but children may get high exposure in daycare centers or in a relative's (e.g., grandparent's) home.[22] The effects of exposure to mite outside the child's house for a week or two, or of exposure in daycare several days a week, are not known. However, one explanation of the lack of success of primary avoidance studies is that sensitization can occur outside the house. Some of the recent studies suggest that avoidance measures at home can limit the lung effects caused by allergen exposure, even if they cannot prevent sensitization.[22]

The importance of cockroaches as a source of allergen in the United States has become obvious.[5,23] Most of the published data relate to cockroach-derived allergens in the patients' home or own bedroom.[24] On the other hand, it is well recognized that many children spend time living in the houses of friends or relatives, and this is particularly common among children in cities.

The implication is that exposure outside the child's normal home could be relevant to both sensitization and ongoing symptoms.

ALLERGEN PROTEINS

Over the past 20 years, a large number of proteins have been identified and cloned. In many cases, the proteins show sequence homology with other proteins that have a defined function (e.g., proteinases, transport proteins, and profilins).[25,26] It is important to remember that sequence homology does not define function; enzymatic activity in particular can be completely lost with minor changes in structure.[27] On the other hand, the mite allergen Der p1 is a cysteine protease and can act on many proteins including CD-25 and CD-23.[26] Although this protein can cleave biologically relevant surface antigens and can open up tight junctions in vitro, it is much more difficult to establish that these activities are relevant to its allergenicity.[25] Certainly, enzymatic activity is not a necessary property of allergens since many major allergens are not enzymes (e.g., Fel d 1, Der p 2, Bla g 2). The recent evidence about mechanisms of tolerance to cat allergens suggests that the structure of the allergen is significant. However, it is not clear whether this reflects the primary structure, the tertiary structure, or the biologic properties of the allergens. The allergen proteins do have some physical properties in common. In particular, the molecular weight is generally between 15 and 40 kd. In addition, the proteins are almost all freely soluble in aqueous solution and are antigenically foreign. Thus, the simple view had been that all proteins that were soluble and were inhaled could give rise to an IgE antibody response in children and thus could become an allergen. However, in the past 5 years it has become clear that all allergens are not "created equal."

AIRBORNE PARTICLES CARRYING FOREIGN PROTEINS, RELEVANCE TO EXPOSURE, AND DEPOSITION IN THE CHEST

The saturated vapor pressure of molecules that are the size of allergens is close to zero. Thus, airborne exposure to allergens is only in the form of particles, and these are dramatically different from one source to another. In the outdoor air, most particles can be identified under a microscope (e.g., pollen grains and fungal spores). Most areas have regular counts of pollen grains and mold spores reported to the public. By contrast, the particles on which mite, cat, dog, and cockroach allergens become airborne cannot be reliably identified microscopically (Fig. 45-2). Because of this, the science of indoor allergens is dependent on sensitive assays for the major allergens (see Table 45-1). The situation is made more difficult because the particles that have been defined for two of the major indoor allergens are only airborne transiently after disturbance. Airborne behavior, particle size, and allergen content have been estimated for many allergens (Table 45-2).

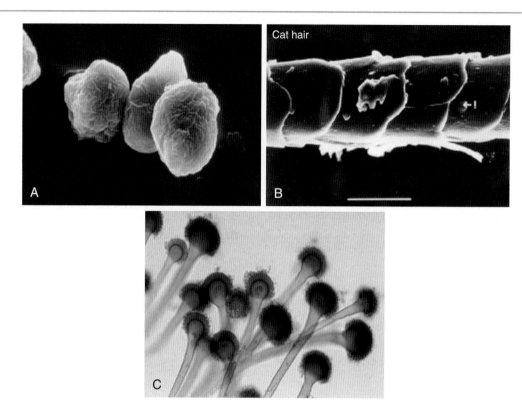

FIGURE 45-2. A, Mite fecal particles seen with scanning electron microscopy, approximate size 25 μm in diameter. **B,** Cat hair showing pattern of hair and dander particles. **C,** Aspergillus sporing bodies with multiple spores forming on the endospore.

TABLE 45-2 CONTRAST BETWEEN DIFFERENT ALLERGENS

	DUST MITES	**CATS**	**ASPERGILLUS**
Species	*D. pteronyssinus*	*F. domesticus*	*A. fumigatus*
Particles	Fecal pellets	Dander	Spores
Size	15–30 μm	2–20 μm	1–4 μm
Airborne	10 min post disturbance	Many hours	Fall slowly outdoors
Allergens	Der p 1, Der p 2	Fel d 1	Asp f 1–Asp f 6
Mass per particle	0.2 ng	0.01 ng	<0.001 ng
Mass inhaled per day	~10 ng	0.5 μg	No estimates

The aerodynamic size of particles not only defines the speed at which the particles fall in still air (i.e., indoors) but is also relevant to the deposition of particles in the respiratory tract. Traditionally, it was considered that particles larger than 5 μm in diameter were *nonrespirable*. However, this term came out of research in the mining industry, and *nonrespirable* meant that particles would not reach the alveoli. For many inorganic particles, it is thought that deposition in the alveoli causes the maximum damage. In contrast, larger particles can reach the tracheobronchial tree. Here the situation is complex because the size of particles is inversely related to the proportion of the particles that enters the lungs; on the other hand, the quantity of allergen per particle increases by the cube of the diameter. Thus, although only 5% of particles of 20 μm in diameter enter the lungs, this may be a more effective method of delivering protein to the

bronchi. For a particle of 1 μm, approximately 30% will enter the lungs, but the volume and thus the quantity of protein is only 0.05% of a particle of 20 μm. Thus, although mite fecal particles and pollen grains are large, they may be an effective method of delivering allergen to the lungs, particularly during quiet mouth breathing.

Although mold spores are generally considered to be "outdoor" allergens, indoor exposure may also be relevant because of the long periods of time spent indoors— on average, 23 hours per day. Thus, 200 spores/m³ indoors may be more significant than 2000 spores/m³ outdoors. And, again, particle size may be important. Strikingly, *Alternaria* spores are larger than most other fungal spores and have been associated strongly with asthma in the Southwest and Midwest of the United States.[18,19] Mold spores are different from pollen grains, mite fecal particles, cat dander, or cockroach debris in that they have a firm outer surface that is designed to resist desiccation. As a result, they do not release proteins rapidly. Indeed, some of the major allergens *of Aspergillus* are not expressed until the spores germinate. The importance of these differences in particles can be appreciated by comparing (1) mite fecal particles, (2) cat dander, and (3) *Aspergillus* spores (see Table 45-2 and Figure 45-2).

The characteristics of the particles carrying allergens dictate not only the total quantity inhaled, but also the speed of release locally and the quantity of allergen released at each site of deposition. Whether these properties contribute to differences of immune response remains to be determined. However, there are major differences between the allergens that are relevant to (1) the prevalence of sensitization and (2) the nature of symptoms.

THE PARADOXICAL EFFECTS OF CAT OWNERSHIP

Children raised in a house with a cat are not at increased risk for sensitization and, indeed, in many studies the presence of a cat in the house leads to a decreased risk for sensitization to cat allergens. This can be seen in case-control studies or by comparing population-based studies.[28–31] The studies on populations show that children raised in countries with the highest percentage of cat ownership have a lower prevalence of skin sensitivity, or IgE antibody, to cats. This becomes particularly obvious when comparing IgE antibody to cat with IgE antibody to mite.[32] On the other hand, in countries where cat sensitization is the most important correlation with asthma, cat ownership can decrease the risk for asthma.[33]

There are important differences between studies in relation to cat ownership that may reflect differences in dose or timing of exposure. However, there may also be more complex issues of the relationship between different allergens and the concomitant effects of endotoxin exposure.[34,35] There have been three major proposals to explain the cat paradox:
1. That the effect is due to reverse causation (i.e., that allergic families avoid owning cats).
2. That the presence of cats or dogs or both increases levels of bacterial contamination in the house, and that this can be measured as endotoxin.[34,35]
3. That high-dose exposure to the cat allergen Fel d 1 (i.e., the presence of a cat in the house) can induce an allergen-specific form of immunologic tolerance.[28,36]

Investigation of the cat paradox has been carried out in countries with different climates, housing conditions, and furnishing. The extremes may be the most instructive. In northern Scandinavia cat allergen is the most important cause of sensitization, and there is virtually no sensitization to mites or cockroaches. Most of the children who become allergic to cats and become asthmatic have never lived in a house with a cat. In this environment, cat ownership leads to decreased allergy, decreased prevalence of asthma, and decreased incidence of asthma.[33,37] In contrast, in an environment with high concentrations of mite allergen in most houses (i.e., the United Kingdom, Australia, New Zealand, or southeastern United States), sensitization to dust mites dominates over other forms of

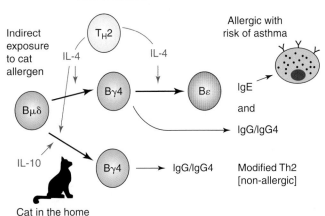

THE IMMUNE RESPONSE IN ALLERGIC INDIVIDUALS AND THE MODIFIED Th2 RESPONSE

FIGURE 45-3. The immune response to cat allergens may take a traditional T helper 2 (Th2) response with immunoglobulin G4 (IgG4) and IgE antibodies. Alternatively, among children living with a cat, a significant number produce IgG1 and IgG4 antibodies to Fel d 1 without IgE (modified Th2 response). The T cells are thought to control IgE production both in nonallergic and allergic children.

sensitization in childhood.[4,6,28,32,38,39] As a result, the presence of a cat has no effect on the prevalence of asthma. In addition, the presence of a cat has no effect on the prevalence of sensitization to dust mite. Thus, cat exposure can induce an allergen-specific form of tolerance. The implications of this phenomenon go beyond the relevance of cats in the house:
1. That allergens are distinct not only in their ability to sensitize but also in their ability to tolerize at high dose.
2. That producing IgG and IgG4 antibodies to the cat allergen Fel d 1 after chronic exposure does not create a risk for symptoms on exposure to cat allergen; this argues very strongly that IgE antibodies are essential for the response that gives rise to asthma (Fig. 45-3).
3. That the effects of cat ownership cannot be ascribed to a nonspecific effect on sensitization or IgE antibody production, because cat ownership does not decrease IgE antibody to dust mites.

RELEVANCE OF DIFFERENT ALLERGENS TO TOTAL SERUM IGE AND THE ASSOCIATED RISK FOR ACUTE ASTHMA

When comparing IgE antibody responses to dust mite and cat, not only is the prevalence of IgE antibody to mite higher, but the titer of IgE antibody to mite can be much higher. In addition, the mean total IgE is higher in some cohorts of children. This raises the question of whether specific IgE responses can increase the levels of total IgE. At the time of this writing the evidence is unclear, but the prevalence of wheezing children with a total IgE greater than 200 IU/mL is far higher in countries where dust mite is the dominant source of allergens. The relevance of an elevated total IgE is clear from prospective studies, emergency room, and hospitalization data.[5,11] In several different studies, increased risk for acute episodes of asthma can be seen with either total serum IgE or elevated specific IgE antibody greater than 10 IU/mL.

Given the apparent effect of total IgE on the risk for asthma and the different effect of some allergens on total IgE, we could ask whether these allergens increase the risk for acute episodes. Preliminary evidence suggests that acute episodes and hospitalization for asthma are less common in countries where the houses do not have dust mite allergens. Equally, children who make an IgG and IgG4 antibody response to cat allergens without IgE antibody have very low mean levels of total IgE (i.e., ~25 IU/mL) and no associated risk for wheezing.

THE INTERACTION BETWEEN VIRAL INFECTION AND ALLERGIC RESPONSES IN CHILDREN WITH ACUTE EPISODES OF ASTHMA

Viral infection is a precipitant of asthma both in a prospective study on wheezing children and in case-control studies in an emergency room or in a hospital.[5,11,40,41] The results show unequivocally that viral infections are an important precipitant of acute episodes. However, the data for children younger than 3 years of age is strikingly different from the data on older children. For children younger than 3 years of age, it is possible to identify one or more viruses in a very large proportion of children presenting with or admitted to the hospital with acute episodes of asthma or bronchiolitis (Fig. 45-4). This includes not only respiratory syncytial virus (RSV) and influenza, but also rhinovirus and the newly described metapneumovirus.[11,42] At this age, the symptomatic children are no more allergic than age-matched children without respiratory symptoms admitted to the same emergency room or hospital. Indeed, in one study the mean total IgE of children admitted to the hospital was only 8 IU/mL. Among children older than 2 (or 3) years of age and in young adults, the data are completely different because rhinovirus is the main virus that has been shown to be associated with acute episodes, and the children are highly

allergic.[11,40] Indeed, the mean total IgE of children 3 to 11 years of age admitted to the hospital for asthma was approximately 330 IU/mL, while the value for controls was approximately 35 IU/mL. Very similar data have been seen from a study in the United Kingdom.[41] The question is: How does rhinovirus precipitate acute episodes of wheezing, and why is this response so strongly associated with allergy?

Understanding of the mechanisms by which rhinovirus induces acute episodes of asthma in allergic children has been obtained from observational studies or challenge studies. The evidence from emergency room studies is that when the children present, they have elevated peripheral blood and nasal eosinophils, as well as elevated exhaled nitric oxide and lower pH of exhaled condensates.[7,10,11,41] All of these features can be induced to some degree with rhinovirus challenge of a nonsymptomatic asthmatic.[10,43] These studies are done in children using the NIH definition of children (i.e., up to 21 years of age). However, it is striking that the response to rhinovirus challenge is much more marked among asthmatics with total IgE of greater than 200 IU/mL.[10] Rhinovirus challenge has been investigated experimentally for approximately 40 years, primarily in nonallergic or nonasthmatic individuals, to study the pathogenesis of the common cold. The results are absolutely clear that this virus does not induce asthma in a nonasthmatic individual. Of course, the rhinovirus is primarily a pathogen of the nose and is an extremely unusual cause of pneumonia. Thus, there are two possible explanations. The first explanation is that rhinovirus enters the lungs sufficiently to cause increased symptoms and pathology in allergic individuals. The second explanation is that events in the nose can trigger events in the lungs by a neurologic, cellular, or cytokine-mediated effect. Studies from Madison, Wisconsin, have established beyond doubt that a rhinovirus infection can alter response of the lungs to an allergen challenge.[43,44] Other studies indicate that the virus can be identified in the lung using reverse transcriptase polymerase chain reaction in subjects (asthmatic and nonasthmatic) infected experimentally with rhinovirus.[45,46] Whether rhinovirus infects

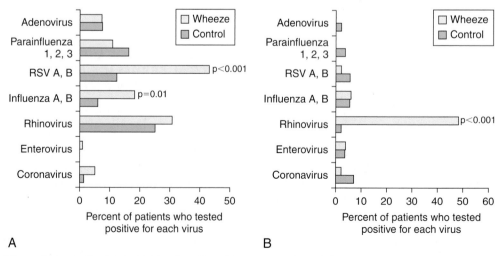

A

B

FIGURE 45-4 Evidence of recent viral infection obtained from nasal secretions on children admitted to the hospital with or without wheezing. The results are shown for children younger than 3 years of age (**A**) and 3 to 18 years of age (**B**). (From Heymann PW, Carper HT, Murphy DD, et al. Viral infections in relation to age, atopy, and season of admission among children hospitalized for wheezing. *J Allergy Clin Immunol.* 2004;114:244.)

the lower airway during natural rhinovirus infections has been more difficult to establish. Moreover, it is unclear whether direct infection of the lower airway is required to induce an exacerbation of asthma, or whether other mechanisms are at play. Based on other experimental rhinovirus challenge data, it is also controversial whether allergen challenge given prior to viral inoculation increases the risk for an asthmatic response. Surprisingly, repeated nasal allergen challenge administered prior to rhinovirus challenge in one study did not increase either the severity of the "cold" or the lung response.[47] Mechanistically, more recent studies suggest that viral infections in atopic children may initiate an atopy-dependent cascade that then amplifies and sustains airway inflammation among children who may experience loss of symptom control or an exacerbation of their asthma provoked by infection.[48] Understanding more about this process is critical for the development of new treatments.

More puzzling are the effects of and interactions between viral infections and allergen-induced airway inflammation during early childhood and the development of asthma. Initially, prospective studies focused predominantly on RSV bronchiolitis, especially among infants who required hospitalization, as a risk factor for developing asthma.[49] More recent studies indicate that this problem is not likely to be virus specific, because wheezing illnesses provoked by rhinovirus have been reported to impart a stronger risk for subsequent wheezing by 6 years of age than wheezing caused by RSV.[50] In contrast, studies in support of the hygiene hypothesis indicate that presumed exposure to more frequent infections at daycare may protect against asthma, especially if daycare attendance occurs during the toddler years (which is also when sensitization to aeroallergens, judged by skin testing or serum IgE, is detected more frequently).[51] Taken together, these studies suggest that host factors, which would include atopy, may be important determinants for virus-induced wheezing that begins in early life and persists as children grow older. However, the relationship between viral infections and predisposing host factors in the genesis of asthma remains a conundrum, and future studies to decipher this relationship are of great interest in furthering our understanding of the development of pediatric asthma phenotypes.[52,53]

Mechanisms of inflammation in the respiratory tract

There is little doubt that inflammation in the lungs contributes to asthma symptoms and to reversible changes in lung function. It has become increasingly clear that the respiratory tract epithelium plays a critical role in responding to the environment, initiating inflammatory events, and influencing Th2 inflammatory events thought to be critical in the pathogenesis of airway inflammation in the asthmatic host.[54] From a clinical perspective, it has been shown that prolonged allergen avoidance, or steroid treatment, can decrease inflammation of the lungs in parallel with improvement of asthma. Thus, both allergen avoidance and steroids can decrease symptoms, improve lung function, and decrease BHR. What is not clear is

how much the different elements of the predominantly allergen-induced inflammation contribute to BHR or changes in lung function. The most convincing association with symptoms is the presence of peripheral blood eosinophils and the presence of eosinophils in the nose. Given the evidence that eosinophil granule contents (e.g., major basic protein [MBP] or eosinophil cationic protein [ECP]) are toxic to bronchial epithelium, it seemed logical that eosinophils played a major role in the inflammation of asthma. Surprisingly, treatment with anti-interleukin-5 (anti-IL-5), which successfully reduced peripheral blood eosinophil counts, did not improve asthma symptoms or bronchial mucosal eosinophils significantly.[55] Considerable attention has been focused on the sequence of events that leads to deposition of collagen below the basement membrane in children with asthma. This and other changes have been associated with the term *remodeling*; however, one should avoid using this term because it is widely misinterpreted. *Remodeling* has been used to imply (1) progressive decline in lung function; (2) collagen deposition, increase in goblet cells, and fibroblast activity; and (3) changes in the elasticity of the lung. Unfortunately, there are no clear studies that connect any of the inflammatory changes with decreases in lung function. Furthermore, there is little evidence that progressive decline in lung function is an important feature of asthma in childhood. In most studies, those patients who present with lower than average lung function will maintain decreased lung function over long periods of time. In the Childhood Asthma Management Program study, there was little evidence for decline in lung function over 4 years, although approximately 25% did experience a decline in lung function, irrespective of treatment. Furthermore, the beneficial effects of inhaled steroids in controlling the disease that were highly significant did not result in any significant difference in lung function 1 month after stopping treatment. Thus, the evidence that inflammatory changes can lead to progressive changes in lung function is not clear, thus one should avoid using the term *remodeling*. On the other hand, the fact that inhaled steroids provide effective control for mild or moderate asthma argues strongly that inflammation plays an ongoing role in the symptoms. However, steroids have such a wide range of actions that their efficacy does not provide evidence about which part of the inflammatory response is relevant.

▬ RELATIONSHIP BETWEEN IMMUNE RESPONSES, INFLAMMATION, AND SYMPTOMS

The primary epidemiologic evidence linking allergens to asthma relates to skin tests or serum IgE antibodies. However, IgE antibody production is T-cell dependent, and the immune response to allergens also includes IgG, IgG4, and IgA antibodies. It could be argued that the association with IgE is seen most clearly because this form of sensitization is easy to detect (i.e., tests for allergen-specific IgE antibody *in vitro* or skin tests *in vivo*). There are many studies, however, in which T-cell responses or IgG antibodies to allergens have been found in nonallergic and nonwheezing children. Thus, there are good reasons to focus on the role of immediate (i.e., IgE-mediated) hypersensitivity. Allergen challenge of the lungs of an allergic subject produces immediate (i.e., within 15 minutes) declines in FEV_1, late responses, eosinophil infiltration, and prolonged increases in BHR. Mast cells can release not only histamine, cystinyl leukotrienes, and platelet-activating factor (PAF), but also cytokines including IL-5 and chemokines. The following are several recent developments that relate directly to understanding the role of the immune response in inflammation and symptoms:

1. The response of the lungs to intradermal injections of allergen-derived peptides that will react directly with T cells.
2. The clinical efficacy of anti-IgE treatment in patients with moderate to severe asthma.
3. The evidence that children who make IgG and IgG4 antibodies to cat allergen without IgE antibodies do not have an increased risk for asthma.

T CELL PEPTIDE RESPONSES

Although not currently available as a treatment, there is extensive evidence that injections of peptides derived from Fel d 1 can induce a delayed (i.e., within hours) response in the lung and can have a beneficial effect on symptoms.[56,57] These results strongly support the view that T cells in the lung can contribute to the pathology of asthma. However, as of the time of this writing, the studies have all been conducted in allergic subjects. Thus, there are two questions: First, are the quantities of peptides reaching the lungs a realistic model of what could happen during natural exposure; and second, how do the T cells get to the lungs? Lymphocytes are recruited to sites of local "inflammation" following the presence of a foreign antigen. Thus, an attractive argument is that in children with IgE antibody, the local deposition of an allergen particle can trigger mast cell degranulation, which leads to the recruitment of a variety of cells, including lymphocytes. Most of these cells are short-lived in the tissues. However, T cells recruited to the tissues may persist locally. The presence of T cells in the lungs of allergic patients could explain many features of the chronicity of asthma. However, the hypothesis is that these cells will only accumulate locally in children who already have immediate hypersensitivity.

TREATMENT WITH MONOCLONAL ANTIBODIES TO IMMUNOGLOBULIN E

Monoclonal antibodies to the antigenic site on human IgE that binds to the receptor for IgE (Fc-ε-R1) only bind to free IgE that is not bound to a mast cell or basophil. Thus, treatment with monoclonal antibodies to IgE would seem to be a logical treatment for allergic disease and, indeed, the success of anti-IgE treatment in clinical trials has been encouraging.[58] Indeed, some children derive major benefit from this form of treatment. The implication is that IgE antibodies play a role in the persistence of inflammation and BHR in the lungs. This finding is not only significant clinically but also because it provides proof of the concept that IgE antibodies play a direct role in asthma.

A MODIFIED TH2 RESPONSE TO CAT ALLERGEN IS NOT ASSOCIATED WITH SYMPTOMS OF ASTHMA OR LUNG INFLAMMATION

Atopic children raised in a house with a cat are less likely to develop IgE antibody to cat allergens, but as many as 50% of these children have made an IgG antibody response to the cat allergen Fel d 1 without IgE antibody.[9,33] What is relevant to the present discussion is that this IgG antibody response on its own does not create a risk for wheezing. Thus, children living in a house with a cat and very high exposure to cat allergen do not develop symptoms unless the immune response includes IgE antibody. Furthermore, the nonallergic subjects mount a T-cell response that is similar to the response observed in allergic children. The implication is that T cells only play a role if there is also an IgE antibody response, which could mean either that the T cells have a subtle difference or that IgE antibody is necessary for T cells to be recruited to the lungs.

Changes in the lungs of children with asthma include a cellular infiltrate, excess mucus production, collagen deposition, and irritability of smooth muscle. The mechanism of this response includes a cascade of leukotrienes, prostaglandins, cytokines, and chemokines. Many of these have been identified as potential targets for treatment. However, given the number of molecules identified, it has been difficult to establish their role in the lung response. Many different approaches have been used, including measurement of cytokines, in samples obtained from the lungs, gene expression studies, detailed studies in murine models, and the development of antagonists or monoclonal antibodies suitable for clinical trials. Ultimately, it is clinical trials that provide the most convincing evidence. Thus, the efficacy of leukotriene antagonists, albeit not as effective as inhaled corticosteroids in reducing lung inflammation and symptoms, strongly supports a role for these molecules in asthma. The results of the studies with anti-IL-4 or IL-4 receptor antagonists have been positive in moderate to severe asthma but were unconvincing in mild persistent asthma. Some years ago, the results with antagonists for PAF were consistently negative. Several other targets have been investigated and abandoned by the pharmaceutical industry. The continuing success of corticosteroids either as a local or a systemic drug may reflect the fact that they influence the expression of multiple genes as well as dramatically reducing circulating and tissue eosinophils. If, as seems obvious, corticosteroids are clinically effective because they have multiple actions, other agents may need to be combined (e.g., anti-IL-5 and an IL-4 antagonist). However, experiments of this kind would be difficult to carry out as clinical trials, and the associated costs and risks of side effects would be significant.

■ SUMMARY

The treatment of asthma in children older than 3 years of age is focused on long-term anti-inflammatory treatment. This strategy recognizes that the large majority of these children have inflammation in their medium and large bronchi, and that this response is a major cause of reversible airflow obstruction. In addition, many or most of these children are allergic to one or more of the allergens that are found in homes in the area where they live. It is well established that inhaling allergen in an allergen challenge can induce an eosinophil-rich cellular infiltrate and prolonged increases in nonspecific BHR. Thus, there is a logical case that inhaling allergens is a cause not only of sensitization but also of the disease. This view is supported by some but not all results of allergen avoidance studies.[9,59] On the other hand, it is difficult to establish a simple dose response between allergen exposure and the prevalence or severity of asthma. However, the complexity of the relationship between allergens and asthma (see Fig. 45-1) would tend to obscure the dose response. Simple relationships between exposure in the patient's home and wheezing could be obscured by (1) genetics, (2) the inaccuracy of floor dust assays as a measurement of inhaled exposure, (3) exposure to "indoor" allergens in buildings other than the child's home, and (4) tolerance to allergens at high dose.

Viral infections are important in provoking wheezing exacerbations throughout childhood. In children younger than 3 years of age, many different viruses can induce bronchiolitis. At this age, RSV, influenza, metapneumovirus, and rhinovirus may all play a role. The major defined risk factor for viral-induced wheezing episodes in children younger than 3 years of age is small lung size at birth, and at this age, allergy does not play a significant role. Many of the children who have early viral-induced episodes will go on to have persistent asthma. However, early wheezing episodes are common, and it is not clear whether the early infections associated with these episodes influence the subsequent development of allergy or persistence of asthma. After 3 years of age, the role of viral infections changes, in part because of the development of protective, acquired immunity to many of the viral pathogens that cause wheezing during infancy. As children grow older, the virus that appears to play an important role and is detected most frequently in asthma exacerbations during the school-age years is rhinovirus, and this effect is predominantly seen in asthmatic children who are allergic. More significantly, these children are not simply skin test–positive, but they have major elevations of total serum IgE (geometric mean value for 53 children age 3 to 18 years of age was 390 IU/mL).[11] This result is consistent with other studies and suggests that conditions that increase total IgE could be a risk factor for severe episodes of asthma.

Elevated total IgE is strongly associated with asthma. Burrows and colleagues[60] reported that the higher the total IgE, the greater the prevalence of asthma. It has been clearly shown that total IgE is strongly influenced by genetics; however, recent studies suggest that some allergens can contribute more than others. In particular, dust mite, cockroach, grass pollens, and the fungus *Alternaria* have been shown to induce high-titer IgE antibody (i.e., 10 IU/mL) and in some instances to increase total serum IgE. In contrast, for cat and dog allergens, not only are positive skin tests less common, but the titer of IgE antibody is generally lower. Thus, some allergens, but not others, can increase total IgE to a level that is associated with acute episodes. This effect may contribute to the higher prevalence and severity of asthma in some communities (e.g., New Zealand, the United Kingdom, and the North American inner city) compared with others (e.g., Scandinavia).

The relevance of immunopathogenesis to treatment can be seen in three ways. First, controlling the inflammatory response has become a mainstay of treatment using inhaled steroids, leukotriene antagonists, and anti-IgE, the latter given to a smaller subset of children with more severe asthma. Second, allergen-specific treatment using avoidance or immunotherapy can influence inflammation in the lungs. Third, some future approaches to therapy could focus on altering the immune response using peptides or recombinant molecules that can influence T-cell responses and IgE antibody production. Given the complexity of the immune response to allergens and its relationship to symptoms, it is no surprise that analysis of the genetics of asthma has provided inconsistent results. Presumably, environmental effects related to both the time course and the dose of different allergens and viral pathogens, as well as the modulating effects of endotoxin exposure, can alter the association with different genes. In addition, the effects of many different changes in lifestyle may also influence these relationships. The implication is that we should continue to focus on interpreting and altering the inflammatory response to the environment.

References

The complete reference list is available online at www.expertconsult.com

46 ASTHMA IN THE PRESCHOOL-AGE CHILD

Miles Weinberger, MD, and Mutasim Abu-Hasan, MD

ASTHMA IN THE PRESCHOOL-AGE CHILD

What Is Asthma?

What is asthma? This question is of particular importance in evaluating respiratory disease in the young child where euphemisms for asthma have been common, including *reactive airway disease (RAD), wheezy bronchitis, obstructive bronchitis, recurrent bronchiolitis,* and so on. Sometimes describing or defining asthma is like the parable of the blind men describing the elephant who felt it was like a tree, a snake, or a rope depending on whether they were feeling a leg, the trunk, or the tail. Like the blind men examining only one part of the elephant, asthma is sufficiently diverse in its presentation that its perception depends on the experience of the observer. Some have suggested that, like love it cannot be defined, but it is recognizable when confronted.[1]

The complexity and challenge of defining asthma has been discussed extensively by Sears.[2] In examining the 12 definitions and references in his review, a common theme to all is the presence of airway disease that varies over time either spontaneously or as a result of treatment. A committee of the American Thoracic Society agreed upon the definition that "Asthma is a disease characterized by an increased responsiveness of the trachea and bronchi to various stimuli and manifested by a widespread narrowing of the airways that changes in severity either spontaneously or as a result of therapy."[3] This definition was expanded by a subsequent committee of the American Thoracic Society to include "The major symptoms of asthma are paroxysms of dyspnea, wheezing and cough, which may vary from mild and almost undetectable to severe and unremitting..."[4] This definition and others, most notably that of Simon Godfrey, added to the definition that the airflow obstruction and clinical symptoms are largely or completely reversed by treatment with bronchodilators or corticosteroids.[5]

Inflammation was introduced into the definition by Hargreave[6] and subsequently incorporated into the National Asthma Education Program Expert Panel Reports from the U.S. National Institutes of Health.[7,8] However, a definition based on inflammation is not helpful in differential diagnosis or early disease identification because noninvasive measures of inflammation are neither readily available nor well validated. This is especially true for young children, where even the ability to make physiologic measurements is limited. For a definition of a disease to be useful, it should provide a basis for making the diagnosis. While airway inflammation is certainly a component of asthma, the value of including this as a major component of the definition has also been challenged by McFadden and Gilbert, who commented, "Airway inflammation and hyperresponsiveness...are not unique to this illness. The usefulness of these characteristics in defining asthma is unclear."[9] This issue is discussed further by Brusasco and colleagues, who argued that the airway narrowing in asthma is not necessarily related to airway inflammation.[10] Asthma has thus proved to be challenging to define because of the diversity in its clinical presentation, the variability of its clinical course, and the absence of a specific diagnostic test.

The ability to define asthma is essential for both the study of the disease and for diagnosis. The reported prevalence of asthma varies greatly depending on how asthma is defined for the purpose of diagnosis in epidemiologic studies.[11,12] Similarly, attempts to study the genetics of asthma have struggled with the definition.[13–15] The challenge of defining asthma becomes greatest in the very young child. While there is an absence of internationally accepted criteria for the definition of asthma in early childhood, birth cohort studies have nonetheless been attempted using various criteria to define asthma or potential asthma.[16] Martinez has emphasized the heterogeneity of asthma and the identification of specific phenotypes based on patterns of natural history and presence of early allergic sensitization.[17] Others have further categorized asthma by clinical phenotype in both children and adults.[18–20] This recognition of different, yet often overlapping clinical patterns of disease certainly complicates epidemiologic and natural history studies. Nonetheless, it is essential to appreciate and identify these differing clinical patterns that share primarily the end-organ responsiveness that we identify as asthma. Treatment decisions and family counseling regarding the expected outcome often relate to the early phenotype in the preschool-age child.

THE EPIDEMIOLOGY OF EARLY CHILDHOOD ASTHMA

When Does Asthma Start?

While asthma can begin at almost any age, it most commonly begins in infancy with a viral respiratory infection that causes the lower airway inflammatory disease with consequent wheezing and coughing that is commonly known in the United States as bronchiolitis. The most common cause of this initial wheezing episode is respiratory syncytial virus (RSV). Rhinovirus, although less commonly the cause of the initial episode, may be even more likely associated with subsequent recurrent wheezing.[21] Other viruses that cause similar acute respiratory symptoms include human metapneumovirus, coronavirus, and others.[22] As many as 3% of infants in the United States are hospitalized annually because of lower respiratory illness from these infections.[23] While it is premature to call the first episode of such symptoms *asthma*, this initial viral respiratory infection–induced lower airway obstruction in infancy is often the harbinger of more to come, consistent with a diagnosis of asthma. In fact, when the onset of symptoms consistent with asthma was examined in an epidemiologic study of the population in the vicinity of Rochester, Minnesota, by investigators at the Mayo Clinic, the majority of those with asthma had their onset during the first year of life (Fig. 46-1).[24]

Thus, when a healthy baby becomes infected with RSV (or rhinovirus), as virtually all of them eventually do, most get only the symptoms of a common cold with coryza. A substantial minority experience bronchiolitis, the most common cause of hospitalization during the first year of life. Of those who experience bronchiolitis, approximately 25% to 50% subsequently have symptoms of an intermittent pattern of asthma manifested by recurrent wheezing in association with subsequent viral respiratory infections.[25,26] While clinical experience and natural history studies suggest that remission is common later in childhood, some continue to have recurrent or chronic symptoms consistent with a diagnosis of asthma throughout childhood, and some recur or continue into adult life[27] (Fig. 46-2).[28]

Who Gets Asthma?

An asthma phenotype is present in approximately 25% of the offspring of a parent with asthma.[29] Further evidence for a genetic influence on the asthma phenotype is seen in twin studies, where there is a higher concordance in monozygotic twins compared to dizygotic twins, even though both twins share the same environment.[30,31] But even in identical twins, the concordance is not much over 50%. Both genetics and environment therefore appear to contribute to asthma.

WHEN AN INFANT GETS RSV

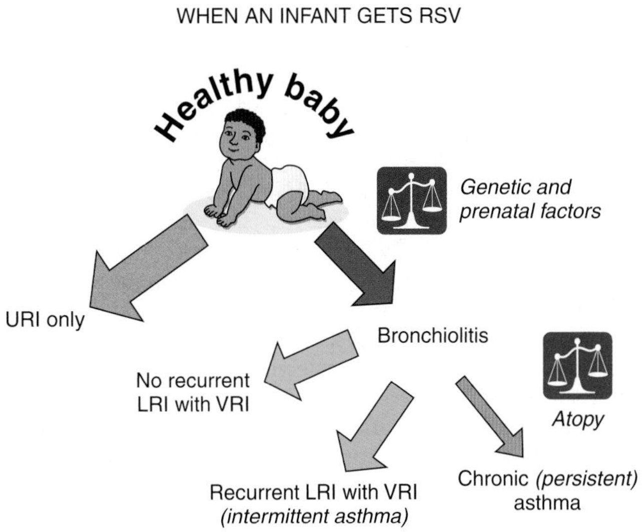

FIGURE 46-2. Clinical consequences of initial infection following respiratory syncytial virus in infancy. *URI,* Upper respiratory illness; *LRI,* lower respiratory illness; *VRI,* viral respiratory infection. (Reproduced with permission from Weinberger M. Clinical patterns and natural history of asthma. *J Pediatr.* 2003;142:S15-S20.)

The genetics are complex. Airway hyperresponsiveness and IgE-mediated sensitivity to inhalant allergens appear to be independent characteristics.[32] Airway reactivity or hyperresponsiveness is considered a hallmark of asthma.[33] Persistence of asthma beyond the preschool years has been found to be associated with increased airway responsiveness in early life.[34] However, airway hyperresponsiveness is not diagnostic of asthma. Airway hyperresponsiveness to a cholinergic stimulus is found with increased frequency in nonasthmatic parents of children with asthma at a frequency that suggests that such responsiveness is transmitted as an autosomal dominant trait, which is a necessary but not sufficient biologic variable to cause clinical asthma.[35,36]

Total IgE production appears to have strong genetic determination based on the observations of very high concordance in monozygotic twins and lesser concordance in dizygotic twins, both of whom should have similar environmental exposures.[37] However, less well studied is the genetics of antigen-specific IgE. Other genetic variables that can affect the phenotypic manifestations of atopic sensitization include the affinity of IgE receptors on target cells, the interaction of IgE with receptors, IgE-induced release of mediators, and end-organ responsiveness. Despite their clinical usefulness as an aid in the assessment of diseases affected by atopic sensitization, neither the size of allergy skin tests nor the titer of antigen-specific IgE can reliably predict disease or severity.

Although inhalant sensitivity tends to develop later than ingestant sensitivity in early childhood, Wilson and colleagues found sensitivity to cockroach in 29%, dust mite in 10%, cat in 10%, and *Alternaria* in 4% of 49 asthmatic infants younger than 1 year of age.[38] Arshad and Hyde examined the development of atopy in a prospective study of 1167 infants.[39] They found that dust mite–positive skin tests were more prevalent in formula-fed infants. While positive skin tests to animal danders were more prevalent among infants exposed to the respective

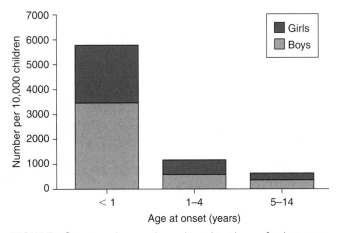

FIGURE 46-1. Annual age- and sex-adjusted incidence of asthma onset in a population-based epidemiologic study in Rochester, Minnesota. (From Yunginger JW, Reed CE, O'Connell EJ, et al. A community-based study of the epidemiology of asthma. Incidence rates, 1964-1983. *Am Rev Respir Dis.* 1992;146:888-894.)

animals, they did not find that exposure to animal dander influenced the prevalence of clinical disorders. However, in a case control study of 193 children with asthma 1 to 4 years of age, Lindfors and coworkers found that high-dose exposure to cat or dog resulted in increased risk of asthma, with indoor dampness and exposure to environmental tobacco smoke having apparent synergistic effects.[40] In a subsequent report, they described a dose-response relationship between cat exposure and sensitization to cat but not to dog.[41] Sears and colleagues found a relationship between children born in winter and sensitization to cats and house dust mites.[42] In a prospective longitudinal study in Tucson, Sherrill and coworkers found an association between sensitization before 8 years of age as determined by skin testing and symptoms of asthma, whereas those who developed positive skin tests only after 8 years of age did not differ in frequency of asthmatic symptoms from those never sensitized.[43] While Nelson and colleagues found an association of many positive skin tests among 1041 school-age children with "mild to moderate" asthma, these investigators found that only dog, cat, and *Alternaria* mold correlated independently with increased lower airway hyperresponsiveness measured by methacholine challenge, although there was no correlation with decreased pulmonary function.[44] Although this latter study did not involve preschool-age children, it indicates that some inhalant allergens are more asthmagenic than others. In an English birth cohort study, Cullinan and coworkers found no linear relationship between early allergen exposure, sensitization, and asthma.[45]

Thus, developing asthma is a function of genetic and environmental variables, not all of which are known. While those with a viral respiratory infection–induced intermittent pattern appear to have a familial predisposition, the genetics of that pattern are not well studied. Both airway hyperresponsiveness and IgE-mediated sensitivity to inhalant allergens in infancy appear to be predictors of the eventual development of persistent symptoms.

THE PATHOPHYSIOLOGY OF EARLY CHILDHOOD ASTHMA

There are only limited studies of the pathophysiology of asthma in preschool-age children. Such studies are obviously hindered by the ethical dilemma of subjecting nonconsenting and vulnerable children to intrusive pathologic and physiologic assessment procedures.[46] Autopsy and bronchial biopsy data are rare in infants and young children because of the rare occurrence of death in this age group and the evident difficulty of obtaining endobronchial biopsies in children.[47–49] One study examined mucosal biopsies in a small number of highly selected children 1 to 3 years of age with severe, recurrent wheeze, most of whom were atopic. They observed in those children increased thickness of reticular basement membrane and increased eosinophil density consistent with the characteristic pathologic features of asthma in adults and older children.[50] In contrast, another highly selected group of much younger infants referred for severe wheeze at a median age of 12 months had no evidence of airway

inflammation or structural change on bronchial biopsy,[51] which implies that these changes develop between 1 and 3 years of age.

Because of the paucity of data, there has been a tendency to discuss the pathophysiology of asthma as if it were a homogeneous entity across age groups. However, concepts and models of asthma derived from adult studies may not be applicable to common phenotypes of asthma in the young child.[52] This is particularly evident for the non-atopic intermittent viral respiratory infection–induced asthma that predominates in infants and children. This seems to be distinct from the chronic atopic asthma found more commonly in older children and adults.[18,28,53] Bronchoalveolar lavage studies, for instance, show no evidence of airway inflammation in children with a history of intermittent non-atopic asthma during their symptom-free periods,[54] while airway inflammation seems to persist in patients with atopic asthma, even when they are asymptomatic.[55,56] Symptomatic preschool-age non-atopic asthmatic children have predominantly noneosinophilic airway inflammation compared to the eosinophilic airway inflammation characteristic of atopic children with asthma, which suggests different inflammatory mechanisms between these asthma phenotypes.[57–62]

RSV bronchiolitis has been associated with an increased incidence of subsequent episodes of wheezing and asthma.[63–65] Studies in twins investigated whether RSV bronchiolitis alters airway reactivity and creates recurrent wheezing and asthma or whether it is just a marker of infants who are genetically predisposed to respond to RSV and other common viral respiration infections with lower airway inflammation and bronchospasm.[66,67] Evidence from these studies supports the latter hypothesis. Recent investigations have provided evidence that the predisposition relates to a defect in innate immunity that permits common respiratory viruses to propagate in the lower airway. The result is profuse inflammatory response of the airways, resulting in narrowing and obstruction to air flow rather than just causing upper respiratory inflammation with coryza (as occurs in nonasthmatics).[68–71] For the preschool asthmatic, this is of particular importance because of their high frequency of viral respiratory infections.

While there are many strongly held opinions and anecdotal reports for gastroesophageal reflux causing wheezing and cough, evidence supporting this hypothesis is largely absent.[72–74] Similarly, arguments for sinusitis and postnasal drainage as a cause of cough are not based on sound data.[75,76] A systematic approach permits the identification of the causes of wheeze and cough, which, when recurrent, will most frequently be a manifestation of asthma.[77]

THE NATURAL HISTORY OF EARLY CHILDHOOD ASTHMA

Viral respiratory infections are a major cause of asthma exacerbations at all ages[78–81] and appear to be the major risk factor for the large increase in hospital admissions for asthma that occurs in the fall months.[82] Preschool-age children have a particularly high frequency of viral respiratory infections, with most getting 3 to 8 infections per year and

10% to 15% getting 12 or more per year.[83] This is a likely explanation for the frequency of asthma hospitalization in the preschool age group exceeding that of older children and adults. The smaller airways in the young child are also more easily obstructed by inflammation associated with a viral respiratory infection, which is a likely contributing factor to increased hospitalization. The hospitalization rate for asthma among U.S. children 1 to 4 years of age has been approximately 1 in 200 compared with 1 in 500 among children 5 to 14 years of age, and 1 in 1000 for individuals 15 to 24 years of age (Fig. 46-3).[84]

While most preschool-age children with asthma remit or greatly improve by school age, those with evidence for atopy (i.e., the predisposition to make IgE antibody to major inhalants) are most likely to continue having a substantial frequency of asthmatic symptoms (Fig. 46-4).[85] The long-term clinical course of asthma in young children has been examined in a prospective study with repeated evaluations for up to 35 years.[86] In 1963, all children entering the first grade in Melbourne, Australia, had a medical examination that included a short questionnaire and interview. As part of the questionnaire, parents were asked if their child had experienced episodes of wheezing or asthma during their preschool years and whether it had been associated with a viral respiratory infection. Based on this survey, an overall community prevalence for asthma symptoms in childhood was estimated to be about 20%, a rate similar to that described more recently in the United States.[87–89]

A stratified sample was then randomly selected the following year from the approximately 30,000 7-year-old children previously surveyed. This sample included 105 second graders who had never wheezed to serve as controls, 75 with less than 5 episodes of wheezing with viral respiratory infections, 104 with 5 or more episodes of wheezing with viral respiratory infections, and 113 with recurrent wheezing not limited to association with viral respiratory infections. Three years later, the investigators entered 83 children from the same population who had severe chronic asthma since before 3 years of age. These children, then 10 years of age, had persistent symptoms at the time of entry with a barrel chest deformity and/or forced expiratory volume in 1 second (FEV_1) that was ≤50% of the forced vital capacity (FVC). All of the groups of children were reevaluated at ages 14, 21, 28, 35, and 42 years of age.[90–93]

When the subjects were examined at 42 years of age, a correlation between the nature of the symptoms in childhood and the subsequent outcome was apparent (Fig. 46-5). Over 50% of those with asthma symptoms limited to an association with viral respiratory infection prior to 7 years of age were asymptomatic at 42 years of age. A substantial number were still having episodic asthma,

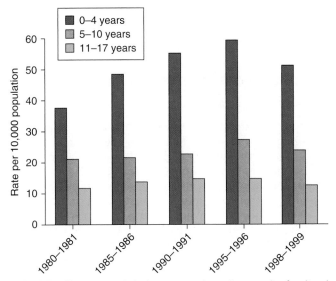

FIGURE 46-3. Hospital discharge rates for asthma as the first-listed diagnosis, by age group and year—United States, 1980-1999. Data from the National Center for Health Statistics, Center for Disease Control. (Adapted from Akinbami LJ, Schoendorf KC. Trends in childhood asthma: prevalence health care utilization, and mortality. *Pediatrics.* 2002;110:315-322.)

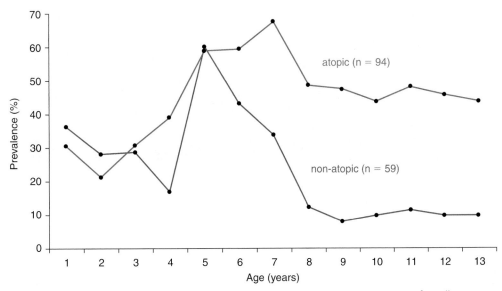

FIGURE 46-4. Prevalence of symptoms by age in atopic and non-atopic asthma. (Reproduced with permission from Illi S, von Mutius E, Lau S, et al. Perennial allergy sensitization early in life and chronic asthma in children: a birth cohort study. *Lancet* 2006;368:763-770.)

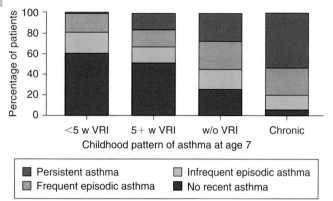

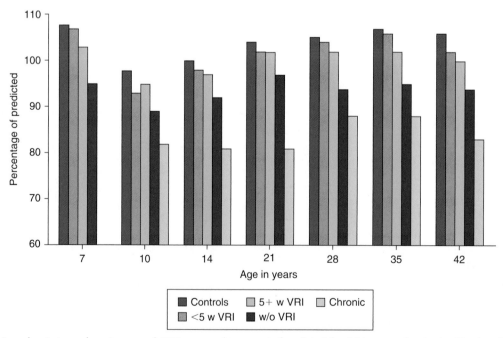

FIGURE 46-5. Clinical expression of childhood asthma at age 42 years among a stratified random sample from a population of 30,000 children surveyed at entry to first grade, about 20% of whom had symptoms consistent with asthma. The sample included 105 second graders who never wheezed, 75 with less than 5 episodes of wheezing with viral respiratory infections (<5 w VRI), 104 with 5 or more episodes of wheezing with viral respiratory infections (5+ w VRI), 113 with recurrent wheezing not associated with viral respiratory infections (w/o VRI), and 83 from the same population who had severe chronic asthma (chronic). (Adapted from Phelan PD, Robertson CF, Olinsky A. The Melbourne asthma study: 1965-1999. *J Allergy Clin Immunol.* 2002;109:189-194.)

and a few had developed persistent asthma. Nevertheless, the frequency of all patterns of active asthma at 42 years of age was greater among those in whom wheezing without viral respiratory infection had been reported in childhood. About 50% of those with chronic asthma as children continued to have persistent symptoms at 42 years of age with only 11% reporting no recent asthma. Repeated measurements of FEV$_1$ to 42 years of age did not differ significantly from controls among the two groups of children

who had only wheezing with viral respiratory infection. Those with chronic asthma generally had significant decrements in FEV$_1$ that persisted but were not progressive (Fig. 46-6).

It is notable that the subjects in this 35-year study who began with asthma in their preschool years had, for the most part, little in the way of what today would be considered optimal treatment. The initial identification of these patients occurred prior to the introduction of inhaled corticosteroids, cromolyn, or even optimal use of oral theophylline. The investigators did not intervene in the patients' care, limiting their involvement to the interval assessments and recommendations communicated only to the subjects' physicians. However, the authors commented that the recommendations were rarely followed. This longitudinal study therefore provides unique data regarding the natural history of asthma, beginning in the preschool years.

■ DIAGNOSIS AND ASSESSMENT

Clinical Presentation

The typical symptoms of asthma include cough, expiratory wheezing, and dyspnea. Wheezing, the classical finding associated with asthma, is defined as musical, continuous sounds that originate from oscillations in narrowed airways. However, parental reporting of wheezing is confounded by their conceptual understanding of the term.[94] In a survey of parents whose infants had noisy breathing, 59% initially used *wheeze* to describe the respiratory noise their infant made. However, after being shown video clips

FIGURE 46-6. Forced expiratory volume in 1 second (FEV$_1$ expressed as percent of predicted) for children over time by classification of childhood asthma at the time of recruitment. The categories of asthma at the time of entry into the study included those with <5 wheezing episodes with viral respiratory infections (<5 w VRI), those with >5 episodes with VRI (5+ w VRI), those with episodic wheezing without VRI (w/o VRI), and those with severe persistent asthma (chronic), and controls from the same cohort. (Adapted from Phelan PD, Robertson CF, Olinsky A. The Melbourne asthma study: 1965-1999. *J Allergy Clin Immunol.* 2002;109:189-194.)

illustrating wheezing and an upper airway *rattle* (*ruttle* is the British term), only 36% still described the respiratory sound of their infant as *wheezing,* whereas the use of the word *ruttle* doubled.[95] In another report using video clips, 30% of parents labeled other sounds as wheeze, while 30% used other words to describe wheezing.[96] Confusion regarding terminology for respiratory sounds is also seen among health care professionals.[97] This illustrates the importance of reliable physician observation of the respiratory sounds to distinguish polyphonic expiratory wheezing from other respiratory sounds. This confusion should be borne in mind when interpreting epidemiologic studies of the prevalence of "wheeze."

Troublesome cough is a characteristic of asthma,[98] and in our experience cough is as frequent a symptom as wheezing. In one report, where children with chronic cough as the only symptom were followed for 3 years, 75% were subsequently diagnosed with classic asthma as the cause of the cough.[99] Shortness of breath and recurrent dyspnea, especially with exertion, are other typical symptoms of asthma, but they are rarely present alone in the absence of wheezing or cough. However, isolated cough, especially of recent onset, should not be too readily diagnosed as asthma.

During an acute severe exacerbation of asthma, labored breathing with intercostal and suprasternal and substernal retractions may be present. Physical findings commonly include polyphonic expiratory wheezing as a manifestation of diffusely narrowed small airways. Coarse crackles can be present from mucous in the larger airways. Hypoxemia from ventilation-perfusion mismatching is common early in the course of acute asthma with a somewhat decreased PCO_2 resulting from the increased hypoxic ventilatory drive. A rising PCO_2 is an indication of impending respiratory failure. At other times, physical signs of asthma may be absent. This may mean that the asthma is quiescent at the time, but symptoms present hours before or a nightly cough may still be occurring in the absence of any physical signs when seen by the physician.

Chest radiographs of infants and young children with asthma often show varying patterns of opacification. Common observations include areas of atelectasis from mucous plugging of the airways. Peribronchial thickening by inflammation may appear as "rings" and "tram tracks" when airways are cut on cross-section or linearly, respectively. These radiologic abnormalities and the presence of coarse crackles on auscultation are a likely explanation for the frequent diagnoses of pneumonia made in infants and young children with asthma.[100,101] Obtaining chest films in nonfebrile wheezing children therefore results in no useful clinical information and has the adverse effect of encouraging inappropriate use of antibiotics.[102] In our own survey of school-age children with unequivocal asthma referred to our clinic, 30% had prior diagnoses of pneumonia associated with symptoms identical to those subsequently associated with diagnoses of asthma.[103]

Therefore, in the preschool-age child who is not symptomatic at the time seen, the diagnosis is dependent on a careful history of previous symptoms consistent with the

definition of asthma. Specifically, children with recurrent lower airway symptoms manifested by wheezing, cough, or labored breathing should be considered to potentially have asthma. A family history of asthma or recurrent lower respiratory disease in early childhood is supportive evidence. Confirmation of the diagnosis requires a convincing history of completely symptom-free periods either spontaneously or as a result of treatment. If encountered when symptomatic, a complete response to an inhaled bronchodilator is strong supportive evidence. However, commonly a short course of relatively high-dose systemic corticosteroid is needed to reverse the inflammation contributing to the airway obstruction. This is a particularly efficient and safe method to test the reversibility of the airway disease. Persistence of symptoms not responsive to such a diagnostic trial of systemic corticosteroid requires consideration of alternative diagnoses.

Wheezing and Cough: When Is It Asthma, and When Is It Not?

Asthma is often underdiagnosed[11] because recurrent lower respiratory symptoms are attributed to bronchitis or pneumonia. Since acute exacerbations of asthma are associated with airway inflammation that causes similar symptoms, signs, and radiologic changes to an acute viral or *Mycoplasma pneumoniae* infectious process, misdiagnosis is understandable if the episode is observed in isolation. However, true pneumonia is uncommon in wheezing children, especially if they are afebrile.[103] Moreover, recurrence with repeated viral respiratory infections distinguishes the hyperresponsive airway of asthma from the normal airway, where similar lower respiratory symptoms occur only rarely. Asthma is also overdiagnosed when symptoms characteristic of but not confined to asthma (e.g., wheeze, cough, and dyspnea) are too readily attributed to asthma, even when other characteristics of asthma are not present (see Table 46-1).[104–106]

TABLE 46-1	DIAGNOSES TO CONSIDER WHEN COUGH, WHEEZE, OR LABORED BREATHING IN THE PRESCHOOL-AGE CHILD IS NOT CONSISTENT WITH ASTHMA

Aspiration syndromes
Bronchomalacia
Bronchopulmonary dysplasia
Protracted bacterial bronchitis (see Chapter 26)
Compression of the airway from aberrant great vessels (e.g., vascular ring)
Cystic fibrosis
Foreign body in the airway
Foreign body in the esophagus (compressing the airway)
Primary ciliary dyskinesia
Pertussis
Tracheal polyps
Tracheomalacia
Vocal cord dysfunction

The Clinical Patterns of Asthma

Three rather distinct clinical patterns of asthma can be seen in childhood: intermittent, chronic, and seasonal allergic. By far the most common, particularly in the preschool child, is an intermittent pattern in which symptoms occur exclusively following the viruses that cause the common cold; these children are completely free from symptoms during the intercurrent periods. Although it is an intermittent pattern, the symptoms may range from mild to severe. They are, in fact, the major contributors to the high hospitalization rate in this age group (see Fig. 46-3).[84] Because children in this age group have a particularly high frequency of acquiring viral respiratory infections (especially if they are in daycare or have older siblings in school), it can be difficult during peak times of seasonal viral respiratory illnesses to distinguish this pattern from the less common chronic pattern of asthma. Moreover, children with persistent symptoms from chronic asthma also experience exacerbations from viral respiratory infections, and this compounds the diagnostic difficulty. At this age, an absence of specific IgE to major inhalant allergens is generally predictive of a viral respiratory infection–induced pattern.[86,107] When the pattern is unclear during the peak of the viral respiratory disease season, the marked decrease in the frequency of acute exacerbations during summer months when viral respiratory illness is less common can eventually make it more apparent that the pattern is indeed intermittent from viral respiratory infections.[82]

The chronic pattern of asthma is associated with persistent symptoms. While exacerbations may occur with viral respiratory illnesses as is seen in the more common intermittent pattern, these children have daily or near daily symptoms of asthma, even between such exacerbations. Such children most commonly, though not always, have evidence for specific IgE to inhalant allergens. Demonstration of the chronic pattern of asthma may require close clinical monitoring following complete clearing of symptoms with a short course of systemic corticosteroids to determine if symptoms return spontaneously soon after discontinuation of the systemic corticosteroids. If the patient remains well until an apparent viral respiratory illness, then this is consistent with an intermittent pattern of asthma.

Less common in this age group but nonetheless important to recognize are children with a seasonal allergic pattern. Diagnosis of this pattern requires demonstration of specific IgE to seasonal inhalant allergens associated with asthma in patients whose symptoms occur with exposure to those seasonal inhalant allergens. These allergens vary geographically and therefore require some knowledge of the aerobiology of the region where the child lives. Examples of major allergens that contribute to seasonal allergic asthma are grass pollen, which peaks in May and June in the California and Pacific Northwest valley areas,[108] and *Alternaria* in the Midwest farm country, which is variably present throughout the growing season but peaks when the farmers are stirring up decaying vegetation during harvest time.[109]

Evaluation of the Preschool Child with Asthma

A detailed history is the major tool for evaluating asthma, and this is particularly true for the preschool child. Recurring lower respiratory symptoms consisting of cough, labored breathing, and expiratory wheezing are consistent with a diagnosis of asthma. Since the major event preceding these symptoms is commonly that of a viral respiratory infection, sometimes with an initial fever at the onset of the illness, diagnoses of bronchitis or pneumonia might have been made previously for these symptoms. It therefore becomes essential in the history to query the specific symptoms that have occurred rather than to accept prior diagnoses of bronchitis or pneumonia uncritically. The history is essential for both diagnosing asthma and identifying the clinical pattern. When the history is unclear or the duration of symptoms has been brief, a prospective history can be useful by utilizing parent-maintained diaries of symptoms and responses to bronchodilators and corticosteroids.

The physical examination in the preschool child with asthma may be normal at the time seen since an intermittent pattern is common at this age. If symptomatic at the time of examination, physical findings may include varying degrees of respiratory distress with retractions, tachypnea, and use of accessory muscles of respiration. Even if such findings are present, a diagnosis of asthma can only be made if there have been recurrences of lower respiratory tract symptoms. In infancy, only a first episode should be called *bronchiolitis*. While such an initial presentation identifies a child at risk for having recurrences consistent with a diagnosis of asthma, it is the pattern of recurrences that characterizes asthma.

A chest radiograph is not generally helpful but may be useful if the diagnosis of asthma is questionable and other diagnoses need to be considered. Pulse oximetry provides a useful screen for oxygenation. Low oxygen saturation justifies blood gases to determine if the PCO_2 is low or elevated, which identifies whether the desaturation is a manifestation of ventilation-perfusion mismatching or a sign of respiratory failure that requires prompt admission to an intensive care unit capable of providing assisted ventilation. Pulmonary function testing, which is so valuable in the evaluation of asthma, is not readily obtainable in the preschool-age child. However, carefully and patiently instructed older preschoolers have the potential to perform spirometry, and the effort can lead to useful information.[110]

Confirmation of the asthma diagnosis sometimes requires a therapeutic trial. When a child is seen with expiratory wheezing and increased work of breathing and he or she has an impressive response to a bronchodilator, this is obviously supportive of the diagnosis. But with viral respiratory infection–induced symptoms where the inflammatory component of airway obstruction with mucous secretion and mucosal edema predominates, bronchodilator responses may be equivocal. For children with troublesome and persisting symptoms, a therapeutic trial of systemic corticosteroids becomes an effective means for assessment. Persistence of respiratory

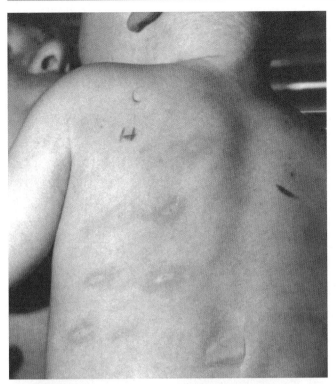

FIGURE 46-7. This 11-month-old infant was hospitalized at 9 months of age with severe acute asthma preceded by rhinoconjunctivitis during the peak of the grass pollen season in a northern California valley area. The typical wheal and flare of the multiple related species of grass pollen native to that area are seen on the left side of the infant's back. They are much larger than the histamine control (H) with no reactivity to the diluent control (C). Skin tests on the right side of the back to other common inhalant allergens were all negative. While immunotherapy using injections of allergenic extracts is rarely indicated at this age, this infant illustrates a striking exception where benefit could reasonably be expected.

symptoms, despite a high dose of oral or parenteral corticosteroids, warrants reconsideration of the diagnosis and further evaluation.

Allergy skin testing is a quick and useful means of assessing the potential role for specific IgE to inhalant allergens in a child with asthma (Fig. 46-7). There is a common belief that allergy skin testing is not useful in this age group. However, there is extensive documentation of positive skin prick tests in the preschool-age child and even in infancy.[38-43] The presence of allergen-specific IgE to inhalant allergens can identify the occasional young child with asthma who has an allergic component to his or her disease. Intradermal tests provide greater sensitivity than prick testing, though with less specificity for correlations with clinical symptoms for most allergens. Clinical correlation for an intradermal test has been reported to be better than prick testing for Alternaria,[111] a major outdoor mold, and it is our clinical impression that the greater sensitivity of intradermal testing provides clinical relevance for other molds, epidermals, and dust mites. Even when results do not correlate with symptoms, in a child with the common pattern of viral respiratory infection–induced asthma at the time initially evaluated, the presence or absence of allergen-specific IgE to inhalant allergens provides prognostic information regarding a greater risk for developing persistent symptoms.[112,113]

From the history, physical findings, response to treatment, and allergy skin testing, the diagnosis can be confirmed, the pattern of asthma identified, and the likelihood of decreasing versus persistent symptoms can be determined.[114] When the evaluation raises doubts about the diagnosis of asthma, alternative diagnoses should be considered and appropriate diagnostic tests undertaken (see Table 46-1).

Recognizing an Exacerbation of Asthma

Asthma is typically characterized by a fluctuating course. While many increases in symptoms readily respond to administration of a bronchodilator, the most severe episodes, commonly referred to as *exacerbations*, require more vigorous treatment, and often lead to hospitalization. Since early treatment may prevent the need for emergency visits and hospitalization, recognition of an impending exacerbation is an important part of evaluation. Since wheezing is commonly associated with labored respiration, a yearlong study examined the antecedent symptoms and signs that precede wheezing in children with a pattern of intermittent exacerbations. The most reliable indicator of subsequent wheezing was troublesome cough.[115] Examining specifically the clinical characteristics of an asthma exacerbation, defined as requiring an oral corticosteroid, in children 2 to 5 years of age, the combination of increased daytime cough, daytime wheeze, and nighttime requirement for use of bronchodilators preceded the need for oral corticosteroids by 1 day.[116]

Treatment

There have been many therapeutic options available for asthma.[117] Epinephrine by injection was introduced for treatment of asthma in the early twentieth century. Ephedrine, an oral agent with epinephrine-like properties, was isolated from the ancient Chinese herb, Ma Huang, in the 1920s. Subsequent evolution of pharmaceutical development led to inhalational adrenergic bronchodilators with progressively more β_2-specific agonist activity and longer duration of action. Theophylline had been used as a bronchodilator for the relief of acute asthmatic symptoms since the 1930s, initially in patients unresponsive to injected epinephrine,[118] and subsequently as an oral agent in fixed dose combination with ephedrine.[119] The most important use for theophylline eventually became maintenance therapy for controlling the symptoms of chronic asthma.[120] Studies of the pharmacodynamic and pharmacokinetic characteristics of theophylline, the development of reliably absorbed slow-release formulations, and the availability of rapid, specific serum assays improved both the efficacy and safety of this drug. Identification of anti-inflammatory effects for theophylline increased interest in this medication.[121] However, inhaled corticosteroids have largely replaced its use.

Corticosteroids were introduced for treatment of asthma in the 1950s, initially for systemic use and in the 1970s as inhalational agents. Cromolyn, a mast cell stabilizer, also became available in the 1970s. Leukotriene modifiers are the newest class of medications available for the treatment of asthma. Other agents described in the medical literature as having a role for asthma treatment are anticholinergic bronchodilators, magnesium sulfate, and nedocromil. Injections of allergenic extracts have been used for many years as treatment for inhalant allergen–induced rhinoconjunctivitis and asthma. An anti-IgE monoclonal antibody, omalizumab, is available as another means of treating allergic asthma. Since there is little data for use of omalizumab in the preschool asthmatic, it should rarely be considered for use in this age group, and even then only by an experienced specialist. Environmental manipulation has long been a nonpharmaceutical approach to treatment. The availability of so-called "alternative therapy" and folk remedies further confound choices for both physician and patient.

Consideration of strategies for treatment selection provides a more focused selection of therapeutic options. Essentially, treatment can be divided into *intervention*, which are the measures used to stop acute symptoms of asthma, and maintenance medication, which are the measures used to prevent asthma symptoms.

Intervention Measures

Virtually all children with asthma will need occasional intervention for acute symptoms. Bronchodilators and systemic corticosteroids are the major medications used for acute symptoms of asthma. A β_2-adrenergic bronchodilator, such as albuterol (salbutamol), provides rapid airway smooth muscle relaxation. However, viral respiratory infection–induced exacerbations commonly result in progression of symptoms leading to an exacerbation that could result in requirement for unscheduled urgent medical care and hospitalization. A typical pattern of such a viral respiratory infection–induced exacerbation is initial rhinorrhea, followed within a day or so by troublesome cough, with another day resulting in respiratory distress manifested by labored breathing, chest retractions, and wheezing. Examining the most reliable signs of an impending major exacerbation, coughing was found to be the most predictive.[115,116] Bronchodilators provide quick relief from the bronchospastic component of the airway obstruction of asthma but have no effect on the progression of the process that results from inflammation. Identification of progression by increasingly troublesome cough permits consideration for early use of a systemic corticosteroid. It is important to consider that much viral respiratory–induced wheezing in young children runs a brief, benign, and self-limited course. However, for those with a history of prolonged symptoms or for those with a pattern of urgent care requirements or hospitalization, early use of adequate doses of corticosteroids provides substantial clinical benefit.[122]

Acute symptoms generally can be relieved by an inhaled β_2 agonist. Infants, toddlers, and preschool-age children can receive this bronchodilator effectively from a metered-dose inhaler (MDI) delivered through a valved holding chamber (Fig. 46-8). Efficacy generally matches or exceeds that from a nebulizer with more rapid delivery and convenience for home care.[123–125] The addition of aerosolized ipratropium to albuterol, while not routinely of added benefit, does have a clinically important additive

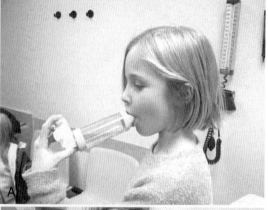

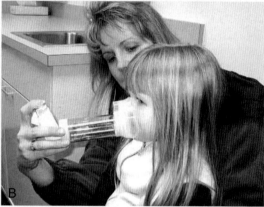

FIGURE 46-8. Demonstration of inhaled medication from a metered-dose inhaler (MDI) with a valved holding chamber in a preschool-age child **(A)** and with a facemask in a toddler **(B).** The MDI injects aerosol into the chamber with one-way valves that permits inhalation of the medication from the chamber while exhalation is into the ambient air. Three to six actuations of albuterol (90 mcg/actuation) in this manner with at least three to four breaths after each actuation to evacuate the chamber provides bronchodilator effectiveness equivalent to 2.5 mg of albuterol by open nebulizer with greater convenience and lower cost.

effect for those with more severe acute airway obstruction.[126] Theophylline, magnesium, and intravenous β_2 agonists are additional agents of potential clinical value when severe airway obstruction is not rapidly relieved by an inhaled β_2 agonist even with ipratropium.

Systemic corticosteroids are potent anti-inflammatory agents for asthma and have long been recognized as effective for treating acute exacerbations. However, the tradition for many years was to use them only when it was apparent that more conservative measures had failed. Several studies over the past 15 years have demonstrated that earlier aggressive use of systemic corticosteroids in children with an acute exacerbation of asthma decreases the likelihood of requiring urgent medical care and hospitalization.[127] While there is concern that the high frequency of viral respiratory infection–induced asthma in the preschool-age child will, at least for periods of time, result in an excessive frequency of oral corticosteroid use, the risks of this effective strategy appears minimal.[128]

Storr and colleagues examined the effect of oral prednisolone in children who were hospitalized with acute asthma.[129] In a randomized double-blind placebo-controlled trial, 67 children received prednisolone and 73 received placebo shortly after admission. Mean age of the children was 5 years. Those younger than 5 years of age received 30 mg of prednisolone, and those 5 years of age or older received 60 mg. At a 5-hour decision time, about 20% of those who received prednisolone could be discharged compared with only about 2% of those who received placebo. Among those not discharged at 5 hours, more rapid improvement and earlier discharge occurred in the prednisolone-treated patients than in those in who received placebo.

Tal and coworkers examined the value of systemic corticosteroids in children ranging from 0.5 to 5 years of age seen in an emergency room for acute asthma.[130] Using 4 mg/kg of IM methylprednisolone, or normal saline, in a double-blind placebo-controlled trial, the decision to admit to hospital at 3 hours after medication administration was reduced from over 40% of the 35 children given placebo to about 20% of the 39 given the methylprednisolone.

Scarfone and colleagues examined the effect of oral prednisone in children with a mean age of 5 years seen in an emergency room.[131] In a randomized double-blind trial, 36 received 2 mg/kg of prednisone and 39 received placebo. No differences were seen in a mock decision to admit at 2 hours, but at 4 hours, about 50% of the placebo-treated children were admitted, compared with only about 30% of the prednisone-treated children. The differences were substantially larger for a subgroup judged most sick in which over 70% of the placebo-treated children were admitted, compared to less than half that number for the prednisone-treated children.

These studies suggest that an adequate dosage of systemic corticosteroids administered early in the course of an asthma exacerbation has the potential to prevent the need for unscheduled medical care or hospitalization.[122] Some studies examining the early use of systemic corticosteroids in primary care, and in children with relatively mild symptoms admitted to the hospital, have demonstrated that many preschool-age children have sufficiently rapid improvement during exacerbations that the addition of a systemic corticosteroid may be superfluous.[132,133] An additional confounding factor in the decision for early use of a systemic corticosteroid during an acute exacerbation of asthma is the lack of information regarding optimal dosage in pediatrics. However, a study in adults with acute asthma in an intensive care unit demonstrated progressive benefit from 15-, 40-, and 125-mg doses.[134] Thus, higher doses are likely to provide more benefit than lower doses, but we have only empirical experience by which to make optimal dosage selection.[135]

The response to systemic corticosteroids for bronchiolitis has been controversial.[136,137] In an attempt to reconcile conflicting data regarding corticosteroids for bronchiolitis, a review of existing studies suggested that high doses early in the course *may* have the potential to favorably influence the clinical course.[138] However, this still remains speculative.

The use of inhaled corticosteroids for acute symptoms of asthma has been examined in the emergency department and at the onset of exacerbations at home. Such attempts have been only marginally successful with (at best) some amelioration of symptoms at very high doses.[139] Only one study, in which fluticasone 1500 mcg/day was initiated at the onset of a respiratory tract infection and continued for 10 days, was associated with a decrease in oral corticosteroid use, but there was no significant decrease in hospitalization, acute care visits, or albuterol use.[140] The authors expressed concern regarding the adverse effects on growth resulting from prolonged courses of high-dose fluticasone and did not recommend the strategy studied.

Maintenance Therapy

Maintenance medication, sometimes called *controller therapy*, has evolved considerably over the years. These are medications used to prevent daily or frequently recurring symptoms. Cromolyn sodium, nedocromil, theophylline, montelukast, and the various inhaled corticosteroids have been the major maintenance medications. Cromolyn and nedocromil generally have become of historical interest only. They are weakly potent, require frequent administration, and if an aerosol medication is to be given, low doses of inhaled corticosteroids are more effective and equally safe. Theophylline, while more effective than cromolyn and nedocromil, has a narrow therapeutic index and is still less effective than a low-dose inhaled corticosteroid.[120]

Montelukast appears to be no more effective than cromolyn or nedocromil but has the convenience factor of being a once-daily oral medication that is very safe, although there has been a recent warning about behavioral side effects added to the U.S. package insert because of postmarketing case reports. However, extensive analysis of available data from clinical trials in 8827 subjects who received montelukast and 4724 who received placebo found no difference in behavior-related adverse experiences.[141,142] Montelukast is less effective than an inhaled corticosteroid.[143] While there has been some suggestion that montelukast decreases viral respiratory infection–induced wheezing in children 2 to 5 years of age,[144] the high frequency of atopy in that study makes it likely that the small decrease in symptoms was simply a consequence of the modest effect previously documented for montelukast in young children with mild persistent asthma.[145] Another study in children 2 to 14 years of age showed modest reductions when used episodically for intermittent asthma,[146] but again a high frequency of atopy confounded the interpretation that the effect was on viral respiratory infection–induced asthma rather than just influencing a worsening of the allergic component of asthma. Montelukast was also examined to see if the increase in troublesome symptoms during fall in children 2 to 14 years of age could be attenuated with seasonal use of montelukast. Beneficial effect was limited to boys 2 to 5 years of age and girls 10 to 14 years of age.[147] Montelukast has also been examined for its effect to prevent the recurring respiratory symptoms following bronchiolitis and was found ineffective for this purpose.[148,149]

Inhaled corticosteroids have become the maintenance medication with the greatest degree of efficacy. In preschool-age children with persistent asthma, these agents can be effectively delivered either by MDI via a valved holding chamber or by nebulizer, with a decrease in asthmatic symptoms.[150–152] Although there is evidence for dose-related systemic effects,[153] conventional low doses have a well-established safety record.[154,155] A minimal degree of hypothalamic-pituitary axis suppression and a small degree of transient growth suppression is detectable at modest doses, but neither clinically detectable adverse effects nor sustained effect on growth are apparent except at higher doses.[156] A newer inhaled corticosteroid appears not to have dose-related systemic effects.[157]

Limitation of Maintenance Medication

There is considerable emphasis currently on maintenance medication, with inhaled corticosteroids demonstrably and unequivocally the most effective medication for eliminating the daily symptoms and signs of chronic (persistent) asthma. However, convincing data have demonstrated that these agents, at least in conventional doses, do not prevent exacerbations of asthma from viral respiratory infections.[158–160] There are no currently available therapeutic measure that can, as safe maintenance therapy, prevent viral respiratory infection–induced asthma.[161] Since viral respiratory infections are the major contributors to acute care requirements for asthma,[78–82] especially in young children who have a high frequency of these common cold viruses,[83] providing effective intervention measures for the family to treat viral respiratory infection–induced asthma is critically important in current efforts to stem the endemic tide of asthma morbidity.

Environmental Aspects of Treatment

Environmental factors that influence the course of asthma in young children include both irritant and immunologic (i.e., allergic) stimuli. By far the most important and well-documented factor that worsens asthma and increases the risk of emergency care requirements and hospitalizations is environmental tobacco smoke.[162–164] The greatest effect appears to be in younger children, although many asthmatic children readily relate an increase in symptoms from even casual exposure to cigarette smoke. While parents may state that they do not smoke around the child, such partial measures appear to have little effect in decreasing exposure in the young child. In a cross-sectional survey, only banning smoking from the home was found to be associated with reduction in urinary cotinine levels in infants.[165] Particulate-producing indoor fires such as wood-burning stoves and fireplaces are potential offenders. Strong odors such as perfume, incense, and other airway irritants such as burning leaves can also act as environmental triggers for asthma.[166] Leaf burning, with its release of toxic and irritating smoke, can cause considerable problems in communities that continue to permit the practice in populated areas.[167]

Questions have been raised about other environmental substances and their role in asthma. Natural gas from range-top burners or nonventilated room heaters releases substances that at least have the potential to be airway irritants and have been associated with some increase in the frequency of respiratory illness in children.[168] Areas of controversy relate to low levels of naturally occurring chemicals. Formaldehyde has been a topic of concern. While formaldehyde and many other chemicals have potentially toxic effects on the airway at high concentrations (as may occur during occupational exposure),[169] it is not apparent that normal household exposure to trace amounts of formaldehyde that leach from some manufactured products actually causesproblems.[170,171] Because asthma is commonly triggered by multiple factors, with common cold viruses causing some of the most severe symptoms in children and accounting for the majority of emergency room visits and hospitalizations, the mere presence of low levels of chemical substances (e.g., formaldehyde) does not necessarily imply an etiologic role.

House-dust mites have been identified as a major factor in increasing symptoms in known asthmatic children living in humid areas such as the southeast United States. They are probably a less significant problem in dry climates or cold northern climates, where central heating results in very low humidity during winter. Airborne particles from cockroaches have been identified as an environmental factor triggering asthma in northeastern inner-city areas.[172] Indoor molds can be a major trigger for asthma, depending upon the indoor environment. Indoor molds thrive in high-humidity situations and particularly when there is water seepage (e.g., in basements or bathrooms).[40] Outdoor molds that grow on decaying vegetation are a major seasonal allergic trigger for asthma in many parts of the country, particularly in the U.S. farm belt.[109] Animal danders can be triggers for asthma in sensitized children.[41]

Environmental manipulation as treatment of asthma in young children therefore requires identification of the major offenders. Tobacco smoke and other indoor lung irritants should obviously be avoided. Traditional environmental control measures for allergens require documentation that the child has specific IgE to those factors. Creating homeless dogs and cats, or compulsive cleaning, for a nonallergic child with predominantly viral respiratory infection–induced asthma is unlikely to provide clinical benefit. When specific IgE to a household inhalant is found, measures to decrease exposure should be undertaken if the history supports those inhalants as risk factors for worsening the disease. There are no rigid guidelines for making these decisions, which require a clinical judgment that is complicated by the multiple factors that can worsen asthma. Placing dustproof casings on the mattress and pillow, the major sources of exposure to dust mites, is a prudent measure for those with large positive skin tests to dust mites, as is using a vacuum cleaner with a HEPA filter. These and other dust mite measures have the potential to be effective for selected patients.[174,175] Reducing humidity in the home to below 60% has the potential to decrease indoor molds and thereby potentially decrease symptoms for those demonstrated to be clinically sensitive to these common aeroallergens.

Immunotherapy (Allergy Shots) for Environmental Aeroallergens

There has long been controversy regarding the potential for clinical benefit from administration of allergenic extracts, either as subcutaneous immunotherapy (SCIT) or the more recently considered sublingual immunotherapy (SLIT).[176] The issue is not whether or not injections of some allergenic extracts can reduce symptoms of inhalant allergy; this evidence is well supported with controlled clinical trials.[108] The problem relates to the complexity of asthma, the multiple factors that contribute to symptoms (not all of which are allergic), and the limitations of evidence from controlled clinical trials. The major precipitants for asthma in young children are viral respiratory infections, for which there is little reason to expect benefit from immunotherapy with allergenic extracts, even among those with some positive allergy skin tests. When aeroallergens are judged to contribute to the asthma of a young child, some of the most potent asthmagenic aeroallergens such as the molds have little evidence for the efficacy of immunotherapy.[177] Thus, while the clinical indications for administration of allergenic extracts are extremely limited for asthma, especially for preschool-age children, there will be occasional exceptions where it should be considered (see Fig. 46-7).

Family Education

Many families who have young children with asthma lack knowledge of their disease[178,179] and fail to recognize and respond appropriately to symptoms and signs that precede severe attacks.[180,181] The recognition that patient self-management skills needed to be upgraded led to the development of several self-management programs.[182] Most cover similar topics: discrimination of symptoms, explanations of how different medications work and when to use them, recognition of situations that require emergency care, discussions of asthma triggers and how to avoid them, and the importance of effective communication between the patient or family and health care workers.[183] These programs are based on social and behavioral theories that suggest education can improve understanding of asthma and thereby provide motivation to take an active part in one's own asthma management.[184] Social learning theory suggests that cognitive factors, memory or retention, motivation, and self-efficacy are crucial links between initial training and subsequent performance of the desired tasks in asthma self-management programs.[185] However, the results of these programs have often been equivocal at best.[186,187]

Since asthma is a heterogeneous disease with various clinical patterns, generic family education has limited value. Once the diagnosis is made and the asthma in the individual child is characterized regarding clinical pattern and precipitating factors, the information should be shared with the family. Because the most common pattern of asthma in young children is a viral respiratory infection–induced pattern, an explanation of this mechanism and the frequency of viral respiratory infections in the preschool-age group prepares the family for

TABLE 46-2	PATIENT INSTRUCTION INTERVENTION ACTION PLAN FOR ACUTE SYMPTOMS OF ASTHMA

Asthma symptoms include cough, wheeze, and labored breathing. Symptoms are particularly likely to begin or increase with a viral respiratory infection (common cold).

Increasing cough is often the first sign of asthma triggered by a viral respiratory infection and can be used to identify when an oral corticosteroid may be indicated to prevent progression to wheezing and labored breathing.[115,116]

When you observe asthma symptoms in your child, do the following:

First: use an inhaled bronchodilator.

If symptoms stop completely: Repeat inhaled bronchodilator when necessary.

If symptoms are not completely relieved: Repeat inhaled bronchodilator.

If symptoms still are not completely relieved or if a third dose for acute symptoms is needed within 8 hours or if more than four doses in 24 hours: a short course of oral corticosteroids may be needed; call for advice if you have questions, or give the first dose and then call so that frequency of courses and response can be monitored.

anticipated events. Whether or not maintenance medication is used for an element of persistent symptoms unrelated to viral respiratory infections, an explanation that exacerbations are likely to occur with colds prepares the family for the need to utilize intervention measures at these times. Further, explaining the limitation of bronchodilators with regard to the inflammatory component of airway disease in asthma prepares the family for the need to recognize bronchodilator subresponsiveness as a sign of progressive airway inflammation and the need to intervene with an oral corticosteroid. These principles should be outlined in a very simple written action plan (Table 46-2).

■ SUMMARY

The controversies and confusion regarding defining asthma are greater in the preschool-age child than later in childhood. This is caused, at least in part, by the varying clinical patterns of asthma, with the predominance of viral respiratory infection–induced asthma in the early years. While the persistent pattern of asthma in later childhood typically has its origins in the early years, spontaneous improvement with age is common for the intermittent viral respiratory infection–induced pattern. The genetics of asthma in young children is complex, with components of both airway hyperresponsiveness and atopic allergy for those who eventually develop persistent asthma. However, even the intermittent viral respiratory infection–induced pattern appears to have a familial tendency, although this has been less well studied. The inflammatory component of asthma is different for asthma associated exclusively with viral respiratory infections from that seen in the allergic model of asthma. The natural history of asthma in the preschool years has been well studied. While more than half of those with the common viral respiratory infection–induced pattern will remit, most with severe chronic asthma will continue into adult life. Despite the benign course of the intermittent pattern in the early years, this age group has the greatest frequency of hospitalizations because of the frequency of viral respiratory infections in this age group. Maintenance therapy, even with inhaled corticosteroids, does not prevent viral respiratory infection–induced exacerbations in these patients. Early intervention with a short course of relatively high-dose oral corticosteroids is essential to minimize the need for urgent care and hospitalization for acute severe exacerbations from viral respiratory infections. Inhaled corticosteroids are the most effective agents for maintenance in those with persistent asthma, and they can be effective when given by nebulizer or more conveniently by MDI with a valved holding chamber for infants and young children. Allergic evaluation may provide information for therapeutic environmental elimination measures in this age group, however it is primarily of prognostic value, with the absence of specific IgE to common inhalant allergens predictive of less likelihood for persistent symptoms later in childhood.

Suggested Reading

Busse WW, Lemanske Jr RF, Gern JE. Role of viral respiratory infections in asthma and asthma exacerbations. *Lancet.* 2010;376:826–834.

Phelan PD, Robertson CF, Olinsky A. The Melbourne asthma study: 1965-1999. *J Allergy Clin Immunol.* 2002;109:189–194.

Weinberger M. Pediatric asthma and related allergic and non-allergic diseases: patient-oriented evidence based essentials that matter. *Pediatric Health.* 2008;2:631–650.

Weinberger M, Abu-Hasan M. Pseudo-asthma: when cough, wheezing, and dyspnea are not asthma. *Pediatrics.* 2007;120:855–864.

Weinberger M, Solé D. The natural history of childhood asthma. In: Pawankar R, Holgate S, Rosenwasser L, eds. *Allergy Frontiers: Therapy & Prevention.* Vol. 5. Springer; 2010:511–530.

References

The complete reference list is available online at www.expertconsult.com

47 WHEEZING IN OLDER CHILDREN: ASTHMA

Carolyn M. Kercsmar, MD, MS

INTRODUCTION

Wheezing is a musical high-pitched, largely expiratory sound made through the partially obstructed larger airways, most commonly caused by asthma in school-age children. A number of other conditions can cause both acute and chronic wheezing in children, but many causes are associated with other symptoms that generally distinguish them from asthma (Box 47-1). The major focus of this chapter will be on the diagnosis and treatment of asthma.

As defined in the National Heart, Lung, and Blood Institute (NHLBI) guidelines, asthma is characterized by variable, reversible obstruction of air flow (but not completely so in some patients), which may improve spontaneously or may subside only after specific therapy.[1] Airway hyperreactivity, defined as the inherent tendency of the trachea and bronchi to narrow in response to a variety of stimuli (e.g., allergens, nonspecific irritants, or infection) is also a prominent feature. Both the airway obstruction and hyperreactivity may be associated with chronic, dysregulated airway inflammation that involves many cell types (e.g., eosinophils, lymphocytes, neutrophils, epithelial cells, airway smooth muscle, fibroblasts) and mediators (e.g., cytokines, chemokines, enzymes, growth factors, IgE). Symptoms of wheeze, cough, and shortness of breath are generally episodic in most patients but may occur daily in some. Asthma is now viewed as a complex, heterogeneous disorder with numerous phenotypes that differ in children and adults. Although all asthma phenotypes demonstrate airway obstruction, the pathophysiological processes, genetics, natural history, and response to treatment differ widely. The underlying pathophysiology, obstruction of the airways, is similar in all but the pathologic processes, genetics, natural history and response to treatment differ widely.

Although there has been an increased awareness of the prevalence of childhood asthma, substantial physical, psychological, and socioeconomic morbidity continue to occur. Among the 7 million children younger than 18 years of age in the United States with asthma, it is estimated that more than 14 million schooldays are lost, 3 million sick visits are made to a health care provider, and 200,000 hospitalizations occur because of asthma each year.[2] The annual direct and indirect health care costs for treatment of asthma were recently estimated at nearly $20 billion per year in the United States. Poor, disadvantaged minority children who reside in central urban areas have both the highest prevalence and greatest morbidity. Nevertheless, both acute health care utilization and mortality rates from asthma appear to have stabilized in recent years, following a steady rise in the period from 1980 to the mid-1990s. Mortality remains rare and is declining, and less than 150 children and adolescents younger than 15 years of age in the United States die annually from asthma.

PATHOLOGY

Examination of postmortem lung specimens of patients who died of asthma shows marked hyperinflation with smooth muscle hyperplasia of bronchial and bronchiolar walls, thick tenacious mucous plugs often completely occluding the airways, markedly thickened basement membrane, and variable degrees of mucosal edema and denudation of bronchial and bronchiolar epithelium[3] (Fig. 47-1). Eosinophilia of the submucosa and secretions is prominent whether or not allergic (IgE-mediated) mechanisms are present. Mucous plugs contain layers of shed epithelial cells and eosinophils, as well as neutrophils and lymphocytes. Although the exact role of airway eosinophils in causing and perpetuating the asthma phenotype remains controversial, eosinophil products (e.g., major basic protein and other proteases) may play an important role in the destructive changes observed. The mucosal edema with separated columnar cells and stratified nonciliated epithelium, which replaces ciliated epithelium, results in abnormal mucociliary clearance. Mast cells are increased in airway smooth muscle of asthmatics. In addition, there is increased mast cell degranulation, which is often worse in those with more severe asthma. Submucosal gland hypertrophy and increased goblet cell size are not constant features of asthma, being more characteristic of chronic bronchitis. The thickened basement membrane caused by submucosal deposition of type IV collagen and various other materials is a striking feature of asthma and has been reported even in mild asthmatics. Basement membrane thickening is thought to occur early in the disease, but its pathogenetic significance remains to be determined. All of these findings have been observed in symptom-free asthmatic individuals who died accidental deaths as well as in transbronchial biopsy specimens from research subjects (Fig. 47-2). Significant basement membrane thickening in airway mucosal biopsies taken from pediatric patients with severe asthma has been observed in the absence of active eosinophilic or neutrophilic infiltrate.[4,5] Moreover, normal lung function as measured by forced expiratory volume in 1 second (FEV_1) can be achieved by patients with severe remodeling. These observations call into question the role of inflammation and remodeling in asthma that is difficult to control. Although an occasional patient may show localized bronchiectasis and small focal areas of alveolar destruction, these are not characteristic of asthma, and there is little evidence that asthma leads to destructive emphysema. However, the incomplete reversibility of air flow limitation seen in some asthmatics suggests that a phenotype exists that may be considered a form of chronic obstructive pulmonary disease.

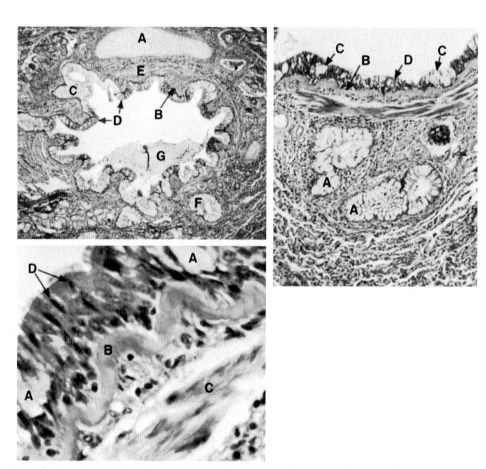

FIGURE 47-1. Sections of asthmatic lung. *Top left,* Cross-section of bronchus (original magnification ×66) showing cartilage *(A),* thickened basement membrane *(B),* epithelium containing many goblet cells *(C),* area of many ciliated epithelial cells *(D),* connective tissue *(E),* mucous gland *(F),* and mucous plug *(G). Top right,* Bronchial epithelium (original magnification ×136) showing mucous glands *(A),* hyaline basement membrane *(B),* goblet cells *(C),* and ciliated cells *(D). Bottom left,* Bronchial epithelium (original magnification ×700) showing goblet cell *(A),* basement membrane *(B),* connective tissue *(C),* and ciliated respiratory epithelial cells *(D).*

PATHOPHYSIOLOGY

Air flow limitation in asthma results from a combination of obstructive processes, principally mucosal edema, bronchospasm, and mucous plugging. The relative roles of these processes in producing obstruction may differ, however, according to the age of the child, the size and anatomy of various portions of the airway, the type of agent precipitating obstruction, and the duration and severity of asthma.

Airway obstruction results in increased resistance to air flow through the trachea and bronchi and in decreased flow rates due to narrowing and premature closure of the smaller airways. These changes lead to a decreased ability to expel air and result in hyperinflation. Although

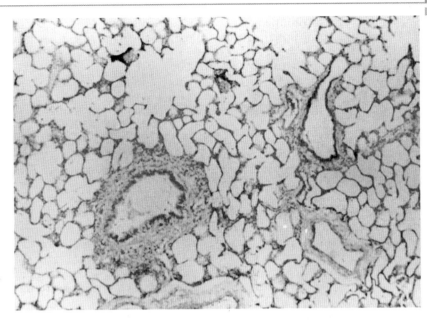

FIGURE 47-2. Autopsy specimen from an asthmatic child who died from toxic ingestion. Note the infiltration of cells around the bronchus with sloughing of epithelial cells into the bronchial lumen. The alveoli all appear normal.

pulmonary overdistention benefits respiration by helping to maintain airway patency, the work of breathing increases because of the altered pulmonary mechanics. To a certain extent, increasing lung volumes can compensate for pulmonary obstruction, but compensation is limited as tidal volume approaches the volume of pulmonary dead space, with resultant alveolar hypoventilation.

Changes in resistance to air flow are not uniform throughout the tracheobronchial tree, and because of regional differences in this resistance, the distribution of inspired air is uneven, with more air flowing to the less resistant portions. In most patients with asthma, both larger and smaller airways are obstructed, but some patients may have small airway obstruction primarily, or even exclusively.[6] The pulmonary circulation also is affected by hyperinflation, which induces increased intrapleural and intra-alveolar pressures and uneven circulation to the alveoli. The increased intra-alveolar pressure, decreased ventilation, and decreased perfusion (the last through hypoxic vasoconstriction) lead to variable and uneven ventilation-perfusion relationships within different lung units. The ultimate result is early reduction in blood oxygenation, even though carbon dioxide is eliminated effectively because of its ready diffusibility across alveolar capillary membranes. Thus, early in acute asthma, hypoxemia occurs in the absence of CO_2 retention. The hyperventilation resulting from the hypoxemic drive causes a fall in partial pressure of carbon dioxide in alveolar gas (PA_{CO_2}). However, as the obstruction becomes more severe and the number of alveoli being adequately ventilated and perfused decreases, a point is reached at which CO_2 retention occurs.

Alterations in pH homeostasis result from respiratory and metabolic factors. Early in the course of acute asthma, respiratory alkalosis may occur because of hyperventilation. Metabolic acidosis occurs because of the increased work of breathing, increased oxygen consumption, and as a result of excessive β-adrenergic agonist treatment. When respiratory failure is superimposed, respiratory acidosis may result in a precipitous decrease in pH.

In short attacks of acute asthma, bronchospasm, mucosal edema, or both can occur. In a minority of asthmatics, acute severe episodes are characterized by neutrophilic, not eosinophilic infiltration; and bronchospasm occurs with little mucus secretion. These episodes may have an abrupt onset and cause severe or life-threatening symptoms. Mucous secretions become far more important as a cause of obstruction as the inflammation becomes more intense and prolonged, and when damage to and sloughing of epithelial cells impairs mucociliary function and increases reflex bronchoconstriction.

INFLAMMATORY CELL BIOLOGY AND ASTHMA ETIOLOGY AND PATHOPHYSIOLOGY

Although tremendous strides have been made in the cellular and molecular biology of asthma in the past decade, a complete understanding of the causative factors and those responsible for perpetuating the asthmatic state remain inadequately explained. Current data support the hypothesis that inflammation underlies the pathophysiology of asthma, and multiple immune cells, the airway epithelium, inflammatory leukocytes, and other airway structural cells may all play a role. In recent years, the role of the eosinophil as the primary effector cell in producing the asthma phenotype has been called into question.[7,8] The mechanisms producing airway inflammation are legion, and the role of each component is only partially understood. Certain processes appear to initiate inflammatory cascades, others perpetuate the response, and some do both. Gene by environment interactions also are critical to the development of the asthmatic phenotype. The propensity to develop IgE-mediated sensitization to environmental allergens coupled with subsequent exposure is one of the strongest predictors for the development of childhood asthma. Recruitment of leukocytes from the microvasculature to the airways, their activation, and subsequent release or synthesis of inflammatory substances may be a primary means for initiating the asthmatic state. The persistence and chronic activation of mast cells, dendritic cells, eosinophils, and lymphocytes in the airways as a result of Th 2 cytokine-mediated events (e.g., interruption of apoptosis) may be important in producing chronic asthma. In addition, innate immune responses modulated by toll-like receptor recognition and Th17 cells also may be operative in some asthma phenotypes.[9] Impaired production of natural airway defense mediators such as lipoxins, resolvins, and protectins (all important in the active resolution of airway inflammation) may also promote a proinflammatory state in the asthmatic airway. Prolonged or recurrent episodes of inflammation are associated with progressive structural and functional changes in the airway epithelium, musculature, and connective tissue. The continued dysregulation of the cytokine networks perpetuates inflammation in what now may be the structurally altered airways of chronic asthma. Several specific effector mechanisms (e.g., IgE, arachidonic acid metabolites, mast cell proteases, numerous cytokines, nitric oxide, the β-adrenergic receptor, growth factors, and intrinsic muscular abnormalities) appear to play key roles in airway inflammation and are discussed further in Chapter 6.

◼◼NATURAL HISTORY AND PROGNOSIS

Knowledge of the natural history of asthma remains incomplete, but several longitudinal studies have added substantial insight. The widespread notion that most children "outgrow" their asthma in adolescence is only partially true. Between 30% and 70% of children with episodic asthma have less severe or absent symptoms by late adolescence, and some features of childhood presentation and course seem to predict clinical outcome. Several studies indicate that disease severity in childhood usually determines disease severity in adolescence and adulthood. Data from the Melbourne Asthma Study suggested that mild asthma or infrequent wheezing associated with viral infections in childhood was not likely to progress to severe disease in adulthood. In this longitudinal cohort of approximately 500 subjects, data have been collected on the symptoms, growth, and lung function for almost 40 years.[10] Subjects were entered in the study at 7 years of age and were classified as never wheezed (controls), mild wheezy bronchitis, wheezy bronchitis, and asthma; a cohort with more severe asthma was added a few years later. The loss of lung function seen in the groups with asthma and severe asthma by 14 years of age did not worsen over time. Asthma exacerbations and symptoms did continue in over half of the patients. Data from the Childhood Asthma Management Program (CAMP) also indicate that outcomes in children initially diagnosed with moderate asthma vary and are predicted by certain features. During a 7- to 10-year follow-up period of 909 children initially enrolled in a 4-year-long clinical trial of placebo versus budesonide versus nedrocromil, 6% remitted, 39% had periodic asthma, and 55% had persistent disease. Prestudy factors associated with disease remission

included lack of allergen sensitivity and exposure to indoor allergens, milder asthma, older age, less airway responsiveness (methacholine PC_{20}), and higher pre-bronchodilator FEV_1. Moreover, there was no effect on disease outcome by treatment. These results also highlight the lack of current anti-inflammatory treatments' ability to alter disease natural history.

Studies of children with asthma based both on history and on assessment of pulmonary function indicate that many children who lose overt symptoms have persistent airway obstruction. Nonspecific airway hyperreactivity associated with asthma is present in formerly asthmatic patients who are free from clinical asthma.[11] Individuals who had asthma as children have significantly a lower FEV_1, more airway reactivity, and more frequent persistence of symptoms than those with infection-induced wheezing or the controls. In addition, 88% of the adults with childhood asthma who had persistent symptoms had positive methacholine challenge test results, as did 42% of the asymptomatic former asthmatics. The recurrence of overt asthma after years of freedom from symptoms is not unusual. Thus, asthma is often a lifelong disease with periodic exacerbations and remissions, although laboratory evidence of decreased pulmonary function and airway hyperresponsiveness may persist even when symptoms are quiescent.

In children and adolescents, asthma frequently is a completely reversible obstructive airways disease, and indeed no abnormalities in pulmonary functions can be detected in many asthmatic patients when they become symptom free. However, recent studies that examine not only symptoms and pulmonary function but also indices of airway inflammation and bronchial hyperresponsiveness suggest that airway inflammation may persist in the absence of symptoms. In a study of 54 young adults (18 to 25 years of age) with atopic asthma or asthma in clinical remission (absence of symptoms for at least 12 months, median duration 5 years), subjects in remission were found to have evidence of airway inflammation and remodeling.[11] When compared with normal healthy controls, the subjects in remission had increased epithelial and subepithelial major basic protein and reticular basement membrane thickness; values were close to those of subjects with active asthma. Peripheral eosinophil counts were also elevated in the remission patients, and there was a significant correlation between basement membrane thickness, exhaled nitric oxide, and hyperresponsiveness to adenosine monophosphate. These findings indicate that the airways of some asymptomatic asthmatics, seemingly in clinical remission, may still show significant abnormalities and evidence of active inflammation. Such changes could result in disease reactivation later in life; however, evidence suggests that current anti-inflammatory treatments are not likely to prevent disease recurrence but will improve symptom control during use. It is unclear that continued treatment in the face of absent symptoms will alter natural history of the disease in these patients.[12]

Asthma does progress to chronic obstructive disease in some, but not all, individuals. The functional and structural causes of this irreversible airway obstruction variant of asthma are not understood. A process referred to as *airway remodeling* is often suggested as the cause of chronic obstruction and severe asthma, but data to conclusively support this hypothesis are lacking. It is believed that chronic mucous plugging, tracheobronchial ciliary dysfunction, smooth muscle and goblet cell hyperplasia, and collagen deposition in the lamina reticularis of the basement membrane occur as a consequence of persistent inflammation. Genetically determined dysregulation of inflammatory mediator production with or without repeated exposure to certain environmental stimuli may also play a role. As mentioned earlier in the chapter, some of these pathologic changes can be seen in the airways of children with mild asthma and reversible obstruction. In addition, data from animal models demonstrate that even when inflammation is suppressed and changes consistent with remodeling are reduced markedly, airway hyperresponsiveness persists.[13] Taken together, these data suggest that airway remodeling alone is probably not responsible for severe, irreversible airway obstruction or bronchial hyperresponsiveness.

The natural history of childhood asthma and the effects of aggressive long-term management on outcomes remains incompletely understood, but a great deal of data have come from the CAMP study.[14] CAMP was a well-designed comprehensive longitudinal study in which the primary objective was to compare the effects of long-term treatment (4 years) with an inhaled steroid (budesonide [BUD]) and a nonsteroidal treatment (nedocromil) to placebo in school-age children (n = 1041) with mild to moderate asthma. The hypothesis was that treatment with an inhaled steroid would result in better lung growth compared to no or lesser treatment. Primary outcome was postbronchodilator FEV_1, but a wealth of other data on atopy, airway reactivity, symptoms, exacerbations, and linear growth was obtained. After a brief improvement in FEV_1 in the BUD group, there was no difference in FEV_1 between the groups over the last 3 years of the study. However, patients in the BUD group had decreased hospitalizations and urgent care visits compared with the placebo group. Patients in the nedocromil group also had fewer emergency visits but not hospitalizations, and both groups had less oral prednisone use. There was a small, transient decrease in growth velocity in the budesonide group compared to the placebo and nedocromil groups. These data suggest that long-term treatment with inhaled steroids in school-aged asthmatics does not alter pulmonary function over time, even though the symptom control improved. Failure to alter the natural history of asthma, as measured by lung function, in the CAMP study was thought in part to be caused by beginning treatment too late after the onset of disease. However, subsequent studies of inhaled steroid treatment (Fluticasone 88 mcg twice a day) in younger children (2-3 years of age) who had recurrent wheezing and were at very high risk for developing asthma showed improvement in clinical symptoms and exacerbations compared to those receiving placebo. However, the treatment did not prevent clinical symptoms or alteration in lung function (measured by impulse oscillometry) in the subsequent year

when treatment was stopped.[15] These data again indicate the inability of inhaled corticosteroids (ICSs) to modify long-term disease state.

ASTHMA MORTALITY

Despite the relatively high prevalence of asthma, mortality rates for childhood asthma are extremely low and have stabilized and actually decreased over the past decade.[2] Overall, fewer than 4000 individuals (of whom fewer than 150 are children) die of asthma in the United States each year. However, death rates are significantly higher in African Americans of all ages. Analyses of causes of death in children with asthma suggest that the major causes are the failure of the physician, parent, or patient to appreciate the severity of asthma, which results in inadequate or delayed treatment, poor access to health care, and the use of inappropriate medications (e.g., overreliance on β-adrenergic agonists and avoidance of use of corticosteroids).[16] Labile asthma, regardless of severity, also is a risk factor, as are respiratory infections, nocturnal asthma, history of respiratory failure, and marked diurnal variation in air flow limitation. Some patients cannot perceive severe air flow obstruction, especially when it occurs gradually, and a small number may have sudden profound bronchospasm, which is fatal. Other factors, such as exposure to allergens (mold), psychosocial disturbance, poverty, previous episodes of respiratory failure, history of hypoxic seizure, previous admission to an intensive care unit, and psychological factors in both the patient and family have been implicated in deaths from asthma.

DIAGNOSIS OF ASTHMA

An asthma diagnosis requires demonstration of episodic symptoms of air flow obstruction or airway hyperresponsiveness. In addition, the airway obstruction must be at least partially reversible, and alternative diagnoses should be excluded. The methods to establish these criteria include a detailed medical history, a physical examination with focus on the respiratory system, and performance of spirometry in children who are at least 5 years of age or older. A number of ancillary tests (e.g., allergy skin tests, inhalation challenge tests) may also be useful and, in some cases, necessary.

Although patients with asthma may present in a variety of ways, most have certain common historical features, such as intermittent or recurrent wheezing, an expiratory, musically high-pitched, whistling sound produced by air flow turbulence in the large airways below the thoracic inlet. Many parents and even older children cannot accurately describe wheezing and may actually report stridor (from upper airway obstruction), stertor, snoring, or rhonchial breathing. Careful explanation or even demonstration of wheezing is often necessary to obtain an accurate history. Wheezing can also be generated by adduction of the vocal cords and forceful inspiration and expiration. Inspiratory wheezing per se is not characteristic of asthma and suggests obstruction in the laryngeal area, such as that induced by croup or vocal cord dysfunction. However, wheezing also occurs during inspiration when asthma worsens and may disappear altogether as obstruction becomes more severe and air flow is limited. Asthma can occur without wheezing if the obstruction involves the small airways predominantly. Coughing or shortness of breath may be the only complaint. So-called "cough-variant asthma" may be overdiagnosed. Probably no more than 5% of asthmatic children have cough as the only or primary symptom, and the cough should resolve with appropriate asthma medications and recur when the medications are stopped. Older children often complain of a "tight" chest with colds, recurrent "chest congestion," or bronchitis. Usually, symptoms are more severe at night or in the early morning and improve throughout the day. A history of symptomatic improvement after treatment with a bronchodilator suggests the diagnosis of asthma, but a failure of response does not rule out asthma. When asymptomatic, many asthmatic children will have normal lung function (FEV_1). Reduction of the FEV_1/FVC is considered to be a more reliable indicator of airway obstruction in children. An inhalation challenge test (e.g., methacholine) should be performed when asthma is suspected but spirometry is normal or near-normal.

Family history is often positive for asthma or allergy (allergic rhinitis, eczema) in a first-degree relative. A history of personal allergy is found in more than two thirds of children with asthma.

Physical Examination

The physical examination should focus on overall growth and development; the condition of the entire respiratory tract including the upper airway, ears, and paranasal sinuses as well as the chest; and other associated signs of allergic disease. Weight and height should be recorded and plotted on a growth percentile chart. Although severe asthma can adversely affect linear growth, it is not a common feature and its presence should suggest alternative diagnoses.

Unless acutely ill, examination of the lungs frequently is normal in children who are ultimately diagnosed as having asthma. In some cases, auscultation reveals coarse crackles or unequal breath sounds, which may clear at least partly on changing position or coughing. Although wheezing can be elicited frequently with a forced expiratory maneuver, occasionally there is only prolongation of expiration without wheezing. The older child or adolescent may resist exhaling forcefully to induce latent wheezes, because such a maneuver may induce coughing that can increase bronchospasm. Some patients with severe asthma do not wheeze because too little air is exchanged to generate the sound. Wheezing from the lower respiratory tract should be differentiated from similar sounds that can emanate from the laryngeal area in (normal) children with sufficient forced expiration.

A variety of extrapulmonary signs indicating the presence of complicating factors (e.g., allergy or cystic fibrosis) should be sought in all children being evaluated for asthma. Nasal polyps occur rarely in the child with uncomplicated asthma, and their presence suggests cystic fibrosis. Digital clubbing is not a feature of asthma; although clubbing may be a nonpathologic familial trait, its presence suggests cystic fibrosis, congenital heart disease, inflammatory bowel disease, or other chronic lung disorder. The conjunctivae should be examined for edema, inflammation, and tearing, suggesting allergy. Flexor creases and other areas of skin should be examined for active or healed atopic dermatitis.

Hyperventilation and/or vocal cord dysfunction (VCD) syndrome should be considered in the differential diagnosis of the child with asthma apparently refractory to all therapy. Both conditions are more likely to occur in adolescence or later childhood and may be mistaken for asthma or may coexist with it. Typically, the patient with hyperventilation is anxious and complains of marked dyspnea and difficulty getting enough air to breathe in spite of excellent air exchange on auscultation and an absence of wheezing. Often, there are associated complaints of headache and tingling of the fingers and toes. Pulmonary function tests are helpful in differentiating hyperventilation syndrome from asthma; a normal spirogram during or around the time of symptoms is inconsistent with asthma. Immediate therapy consists of giving reassurance and having the patient re-breathe into a paper bag to elevate $Paco_2$. VCD is another condition that must be differentiated from true asthma.[17] In these patients, wheezing is often a prominent feature, may occur on inspiration and expiration, and is typically loudest over the trachea or central, anterior chest. This condition is more common in older children, adolescents, and females, and it may also be seen in elite athletes. One small study estimated that VCD was involved in more than 10% of patients presenting to an emergency room for treatment of acute asthma[11] Most patients with VCD cannot voluntarily induce an episode, although in some patients, including highly trained athletes, exercise can precipitate an attack. Although VCD was originally described in adults with psychiatric disorders, this condition in children is less frequently associated with serious psychological disturbances and should not be labeled as such. The etiology in children remains poorly understood. The mechanism involves holding the anterior third of the vocal cords in a position of relative adduction during inspiration, but also in expiration. There may also be inward deflection of the supraglottic structures as well. The result is loud wheezing in a patient who has normal oxygen saturation and responds poorly to inhalation of a bronchodilating aerosol. Patients may appear comfortable or anxious in the face of loud wheeze. Pulmonary function testing may reveal a pronounced flattening of the inspiratory loop; however, since most patients with VCD also have true asthma, there may be some evidence of large and/or small airway obstruction on the expiratory loop as well (Fig. 47-3). An increase in the mid–vital capacity expiratory/inspiratory flow ratio from the normal value of about 0.9 to a value of greater than 2 indicates extrathoracic obstruction consistent with VCD. It should be noted that most patients with VCD will have normal pulmonary function testing when asymptomatic. The diagnosis is confirmed by direct observation of paradoxical vocal cord movement via flexible laryngoscopy during an acute episode. Upper and lower airway examination with

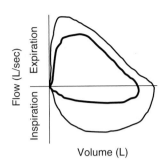

FIGURE 47-3. Flow-volume curve from a patient with vocal cord dysfunction. The thin line represents the flow at normal baseline. The thick line represents the flow during an obstructive episode and depicts a slight decrease in expiratory flow and a marked decrease in and flattening of the inspiratory loop.

a flexible bronchoscope should be considered in patients with atypical reports of wheeze, dyspnea on exertion, or stridor to identify anatomic lesions such as cysts, hemangioma or laryngotracheomalacia. Older children with both VCD and asthma often can distinguish the "site" of the wheezing when the source of the problem is explained to them. The absence of nocturnal symptoms may also be a diagnostic clue that VCD rather than asthma is causative. Effective treatment consists of appropriate asthma medication (when an asthma diagnosis has been confirmed) and referral to a speech therapist or psychologist specializing in behavior modification in order to learn relaxation techniques.

Asthma Triggers

Most older children will identify more than one precipitating factor responsible for asthma. Moreover, patterns of reactivity may change. Thus, exercise-induced asthma (EIA) may not be viewed as a problem in many adults with asthma who have learned in childhood that exercise induces symptoms and consequently have developed a lifestyle that avoids exercise. Allergic factors that precipitated asthma in childhood may no longer cause symptoms in adolescence or adulthood, even though the patient continues to have asthma. Patterns also may change with treatment or the institution of environmental control measures. The use of quality of life questionnaires can help uncover latent symptoms and provide information that may be useful in identifying more subtle triggers.

Allergens

In the majority of children with asthma, it is possible to induce an asthmatic reaction to substances in which IgE-mediated reaction is involved. Allergens that can induce asthma include animal allergens, mold spores, pollens, insects (cockroach), infectious agents (especially fungi), and, occasionally, drugs and foods. Cockroach allergen appears to be a potent factor, particularly in inner-city children, and it has been associated with increased health care utilization in children who are both sensitized and exposed to allergen.[18] Allergic reactions may induce

bronchoconstriction directly, may increase tracheobronchial sensitivity in general, or may be obvious or subtle precipitating factors. Bronchoconstrictor responses to allergens via IgE antibody–induced mediator release from mast cells generally occur within minutes of exposure, last for a relatively short period of time (20 to 30 minutes), and resolve. Such reactions are often termed *early antigen* or *asthmatic response*. It is the "late asthmatic response" (which occurs 4 to 24 hours after antigen contact) that results in more severe and protracted symptoms (lasting hours) and ultimately contributes to the chronicity and severity of the disease. The late response is due to inflammatory cell reaction and release of multiple mediators including IL-4, IL-5, and IL-13. Such allergen-induced dual responses can only be demonstrated in approximately half of all asthmatics challenged in a laboratory setting. It is unclear why mast cell degranulation that should induce an inflammatory infiltration in all patients does not induce late symptoms in all patients.

Irritants

Numerous upper and lower respiratory irritants have been implicated as precipitants of asthma. These include paint odors, hairsprays, perfumes, chemicals, air pollutants, diesel particulates, tobacco smoke, cold air, cold water, and cough. Some allergens may act as irritants (e.g., molds). Some irritants such as ozone and industrial chemicals may also initiate bronchial hyperresponsiveness by inducing inflammation, yet they do not produce a late-phase response. Active and passive exposure to tobacco smoke, in addition to acting as a precipitant and aggravator of asthma, also can be associated with an accelerated irreversible loss of pulmonary function.

Weather Changes

Atmospheric changes commonly are associated with an increase in asthmatic activity. The mechanism of this effect has not been defined but may be related to changes in barometric pressure and alterations in the allergen or irritant content of the air.

Infections

By far, the most common infectious agents responsible for precipitating or aggravating asthma are viral respiratory pathogens. It is estimated that up to 85% of asthma exacerbations in school-aged children are due to viral infections, and rhinovirus has emerged as a prominent pathogen in causing acute asthma.[19] In some instances, bacterial infections (e.g., pertussis or mycoplasma), and, more rarely, fungal infections or colonization (e.g., bronchopulmonary *Aspergillosis*) and parasitic infestations (e.g., *Toxocariasis* and *Ascariasis*) can be triggers. The mechanisms of viral-induced exacerbations are incompletely understood, but probably involve some direct respiratory epithelial injury caused by infection, alteration of host inflammatory responses driven by the infection, and influence of other cofactors (concomitant allergen exposure or mediator production). For instance, it is clear that children who have significant respiratory viral–induced wheezing are more likely to have elevated IgE and allergen sensitization.[20] In addition, asthmatics may have decreased production of interferon α and interferon γ, which can be associated with decreased airway function.

Exercise

Strenuous exercise (i.e., exercise sufficient to cause breathlessness and hyperventilation) may induce bronchial obstruction in as many as 90% of individuals with persistent asthma; this phenomenon is termed *exercise-induced bronchospasm (EIB)*. In addition, exercise can cause significant bronchospasm in up to 40% of individuals with allergic rhinitis who do not have persistent asthma. When otherwise normal individuals develop bronchoconstriction in response to exercise with hyperventilation, it is often termed *exercise-induced asthma (EIA)*; this may occur in 10% to 13% of the general population. Symptoms induced by exercise may be subtle (mild dyspnea) to significant coughing, wheezing, and/or excessive breathlessness. Symptoms typically begin after 5 to 10 minutes of vigorous activity and are most prominent after activity ceases. The mechanisms underlying EIA remain somewhat uncertain. Recent data indicates that hyperventilation of cold, dry air causes heat and water loss from the airways, producing a hyperosmolar lining fluid and injuring the airway epithelium. Induced sputum obtained from individuals with EIB demonstrates columnar epithelial cells, eosinophils, and increased concentrations of leukotrienes. There is also cytokine release from neutrophils.[21] Cooling of the airways has also been described to result in vascular congestion and dilatation in the bronchial circulation. The subsequent mucosal swelling as a result of vascular congestion and edema produces airway narrowing. Symptoms of EIB usually resolve spontaneously within 1 hour after ceasing exercise, but may require treatment with a short-acting β agonist (SABA) for complete resolution. There is typically a refractory period of 1 to 3 hours following an episode of EIA/EIB during which further exercise will not cause significant bronchospasm. Although studies are conflicting, there is generally not a late-onset response (8 to 12 hours postexercise) following the immediate reaction. EIA may be both underdiagnosed when symptoms are subtle, or it may be overdiagnosed or misdiagnosed due to a number of masquerading conditions (e.g., vocal cord dysfunction, poor conditioning, or cardiac dysfunction).

Emotional Factors

Emotional upsets clearly trigger asthma in some individuals; however, there is no evidence that psychological factors are the basis for asthma. Coping styles of patients, their families, and their physicians can intensify or lead to more rapid amelioration of asthma. Conversely, denial of asthma by patients, parents, or physicians may delay therapy to the point that reversibility of obstruction is more difficult. Psychological factors have been implicated in deaths from asthma in children. The influence of psychosocial factors on compliance is yet another important factor related to treatment failure or success. Asthma itself can strongly influence the emotional state of the patient, the family, and other individuals associated with the patient. In addition, recent work indicates that psychosocial stressors, both internal (lack of parental support) and external (witnessing violence), may modulate immune responses, increase inflammation, or decrease steroid responsiveness, leading to poorer asthma control.[22]

Gastroesophageal Reflux

Reflux of gastric contents into the tracheobronchial tree can aggravate asthma in children and is one of the causes of nocturnal asthma. Typical symptoms of gastroesophageal reflux (GER)—heartburn, chest pain, regurgitation, sour brash—may be absent in many children with asthma; estimates are that reflux may be "silent" in over 50% of asthmatic patients.[23] Pediatric studies have reported a prevalence of GER between 19% and 80% with a mean of about 22%.[24] However, due to methodologic flaws and absence of longitudinal studies, a clear association between GER and asthma symptoms in children remains unclear. Although the exact extent to which reflux exacerbates asthma remains controversial, it is clear that acid (or even nonacid) reflux of gastric contents into the distal esophagus can lead to cough and bronchospasm, presumably via increased vagal activity. Aspiration of gastric contents in even micro amounts is also presumed to cause bronchial irritation and bronchospasm. A recent large trial of proton pump inhibitors in adults with asymptomatic GER did not show any benefit to asthma control.[25]

Allergic Rhinitis and Sinusitis

Acute or chronic sinusitis can be associated with aggravation of asthma and can be a cause of recalcitrant asthma. In some patients, asthma and sinusitis occur at the same time; the nasal symptoms from the sinusitis may make cough and other symptoms of asthma worse and less responsive to bronchodilator therapy alone. The upper airway may be viewed to some extent as a continuum of the lower airway; inflammatory mediator release in the lower airway may be triggered as a response to sinus infection. This subject is discussed in more detail in Chapter 49.

Nonallergic Hypersensitivity to Drugs and Chemicals

Aspirin and nonsteroidal anti-inflammatory drugs (NSAIDs), such as ibuprofen, can exacerbate asthma in selected individuals by increasing production of 5-lipoxygenase metabolites, including leukotrienes. The typical aspirin-sensitive asthmatic has nasal polyps, urticaria, and chronic rhinitis. Aspirin ingestion may diminish pulmonary function and produce wheeze, cough, rhinitis, conjunctivitis, urticaria, and angioedema in 10% to 20% of adults with asthma. Although more common after the third decade of life, the prevalence in children (as determined by a decrease in FEV_1 of at least 20% from baseline following aspirin or NSAID ingestion) has been reported to be as high as 5% when determined by direct challenge testing.[26] Although aspirin in particular is rarely given to children and adolescents because of the risk of Reye's syndrome, there is a very high cross-reactivity to common NSAIDs in aspirin-susceptible patients. High-dose acetaminophen may also cause wheezing in a small portion (<2%) of aspirin-sensitive asthmatics. Some (but not all) recent studies suggest that early-life use of acetaminophen may increase the risk of developing asthma, and one large trial found a reduced risk of an acute care visit for asthma following treatment with ibuprofen compared to treatment with acetaminophen.[27] The absence of a history of increased symptoms following NSAID ingestion in asthmatic children is generally sufficient to warrant safe use of NSAIDs as needed. However, aspirin/NSAID sensitivity should be considered in children and adolescents with severe or difficult-to-control asthma, who also have chronic rhinitis, urticaria, and nasal polyps.

Metabisulfite has been reported as a precipitant or aggravator of asthma, both by allergic and nonallergic mechanisms. Sensitive individuals should avoid foods containing or preserved using sulfites (e.g., shrimp, dried fruit, beer, and wine).

Endocrine Factors

Aggravation of asthma and increased pulmonary function variability occurs in some adolescent and adult women in relation to the menstrual cycle, beginning shortly before menstruation and ending shortly after the onset of menses. Whether this reflects changes in water and salt balance, irritability of bronchial smooth muscle, or other factors is unknown. The use of the oral contraceptive pill has been reported to both aggravate and ameliorate premenstrual asthma. Hyperthyroidism has been reported to worsen or precipitate asthma in an occasional patient, and treatment of hyperthyroidism usually ameliorates the asthma.

Vitamin D deficiency has gained increasing attention as a possible contributor to both the development of asthma and a contributor to its control. Data from the NHANES study indicated an inverse relationship between serum vitamin D concentration and FEV_1/FVC. In addition, several studies demonstrate lower vitamin D levels in African Americans, Hispanics, and obese individuals, all groups with increased risk for higher asthma morbidity. Among asthmatic children, vitamin D insufficiency (defined as serum concentration ≤30 ng/mL) occurs in approximately one third of those studied.[28] Among 1024 participants in the CAMP study, 35% were vitamin D insufficient at study entry. This group had an increased risk of severe asthma exacerbation (OR 1.5, 1.1 to 1.9, P = .01) during the 4 years of the study, after adjusting for numerous factors (i.e., age, sex, BMI, and

treatment group). Those in the budesonide treatment group had an even greater effect (OR 1.8, 1.0 to 3.2, P = .05). These results are similar to those described for a cohort study (n = 616) of asthmatic Costa Rican children, 28% of whom were vitamin D insufficient. Serum vitamin D was inversely associated with serum IgE and peripheral eosinophil count. In addition, higher vitamin D levels were associated with a significant decrease in risk of hospitalization in the previous year, a decrease in use of anti-inflammatory medicines, and increased airway responsiveness. The mechanisms by which vitamin D influences asthma expression remains unclear, but there are many possibilities. Vitamin D suppresses RANTES secretion in bronchial smooth muscle, and it can inhibit mast cell differentiation and maturation. Vitamin D treatment of T reg cells from steroid-resistant asthmatics resulted in increased production of the anti-inflammatory cytokine IL-10 with steroid stimulation.[29] Moreover, it has also been speculated that polymorphisms in the vitamin D receptor play a role in asthma, but data are thus far inconsistent. These data suggest that steroid resistance may be related to vitamin D deficiency, but large-scale clinical trials to demonstrate efficacy of vitamin D in asthma treatment have not been performed. Further research is needed to substantiate the role of vitamin D in asthma pathophysiology.

Nocturnal Asthma

There is a circadian variation in airway function and bronchial hyperresponsiveness in most patients with asthma. In individuals with a normal sleep-wake cycle, the worst peak expiratory flow rate (PEFR) and the most pronounced reactivity occur at approximately 4 AM, and the best occur at 4 PM. Nocturnal asthma is a risk factor for asthma severity and even death in some asthmatics. Although nocturnal asthma may result from late-phase reactions to earlier allergen exposure, GER, or sinusitis in some patients, these conditions are not present in most patients with severe nocturnal asthma. Another explanation is an increase in inflammatory cell infiltrate as an exaggerated normal circadian variation. Abnormalities in central nervous system control of respiratory drive, particularly with defective hypoxic drive and obstructive sleep apnea, as well as enhanced melatonin release resulting in increased inflammation, may also be present in some patients with nocturnal asthma.

LABORATORY DIAGNOSIS

A number of laboratory studies may be useful in confirming the diagnosis of asthma, and objective measures of pulmonary function are among the most important.

LUNG FUNCTION TESTS

Pulmonary function tests (PFTs), particularly spirometry, are objective, noninvasive, and extremely helpful in the diagnosis and follow-up of patients with asthma.

Examination of the forced vital capacity (FVC), FEV_1, and forced expiratory flow rate over 25% to 75% of the forced vital capacity (FEF_{25-75}) is a reliable way to detect baseline airway obstruction. Examination of the volume-time curve and shape of the flow-volume loop provides an estimate of the adequacy of the patient effort in performing the test. A PFT should be attempted on all children older than 5 years of age when considering the diagnosis of asthma. In children, measurement of FEV_1 alone also may miss airway obstruction; the FEV_1/FVC has been proposed as a more sensitive measure of obstruction. It has recently been proposed that FEF_{25-75} is a more sensitive indicator of response to bronchodilator and indicator of airway hyperresponsiveness than either FEV_1 or FVC.[30] However, FEF_{25-75} is a highly variable measure that is readily influenced by expiratory time and change in FVC. Larger and longer-term studies will be necessary to validate the utility of this measure in asthmatic children.

Documentation of reversibility of air flow obstruction following inhalation of a bronchodilator is central to the definition of asthma. If obstruction is demonstrated on a baseline PFT, a bronchodilating aerosol (albuterol) should be administered and the PFT repeated in 10 to 20 minutes. An improvement of at least 12% and 200 mL in the FEV_1 is considered a positive response and is indicative of reversible air flow obstruction. A 10% improvement in the % predicted FEV_1 is also considered a positive response.

Use of a peak flow meter in the office setting may provide some useful information about obstruction in the large central airways, but the test should not be used to diagnose asthma. PEFR is extremely effort dependent and is reflective of obstruction only in the large central airways.

Although the standard spirometry has long been considered the gold standard for use in diagnosing and monitoring change in airway function in patients with asthma, other modalities may have particular application in both younger and older children. Forced oscillation capitalizes on the resonant oscillation properties of the airways to measure conductance and reactance and, indirectly, airway resistance.[31] The technique requires only tidal breathing on a mouthpiece for 30 seconds in order to obtain a measurement. Response to a bronchodilator can also be detected.

BRONCHIAL CHALLENGE TESTS

Airway hyperreactivity to substances such as methacholine, histamine, hypertonic saline, adenosine monophosphate, or mannitol forms the basis of an adjunctive diagnostic test for asthma. However, the sensitivity and specificity of the tests vary widely, and bronchoprovocation testing cannot serve as the sole determinant of an asthma diagnosis. Methacholine and histamine are considered direct bronchoprovocation agents because they react directly on smooth muscle. Direct bronchoprovocation challenge testing with methacholine is very sensitive and has a better negative than positive predictive value. As such, it is generally more helpful in excluding than diagnosing asthma because positive results may be seen in disorders such as cystic fibrosis, chronic obstructive pulmonary disease, chronic bronchitis, allergic rhinitis, and even in some normal individuals. FEV_1 is the primary measure used to assess response, and the concentration of methacholine at which a 20% decrease in FEV_1 occurs is recorded (PC_{20}); other methods use the cumulative dose (PD_{20}). A PC_{20} of ≤4 mg/mL is considered a positive test result indicative of airway hyperreactivity. However, there is no universally accepted threshold PC_{20} value that is considered diagnostic of asthma (Table 47-1). Accurate interpretation must account for degree of baseline obstruction (if any), the pretest probability of asthma, the presence of current symptoms, and the degree of recovery in postchallenge FEV_1. Mild transient adverse effects (i.e., cough, wheezing, chest tightness, and dizziness) are uncommon and occur in less than 20% of patients receiving either histamine or methacholine challenge. Delayed or prolonged reactions are extremely rare, and fatalities after methacholine have not been reported. However, methacholine (or any bronchoprovocation test) should not be performed if the baseline FEV_1 is low, (generally less than 60% predicted).[32]

Indirect bronchoprovocation agents (i.e., hypertonic saline, AMP, mannitol) act by inducing release of inflammatory mediators in the airway, which then cause bronchoconstriction. In addition, indirect testing is well-correlated with the degree of airway inflammation. Inhalation testing with dry-powder mannitol recently has good validity, and a commercial kit is currently approved for use in Europe, Australia, and the United States. Mannitol has the advantage of being safe and easy, and it requires no special equipment apart from a spirometer. A cutpoint of 15% decrease in FEV_1 from baseline had a specificity of 98% but a sensitivity of 58%.[33] If confirmed in further studies, mannitol may become a valuable diagnostic aid for confirming asthma diagnosis.

Other agents such as allergens and occupational sensitizers have been used for inhalation challenge tests, but such challenges may pose significant risk and should only be performed by experienced physicians and investigators in the context of specific clinical or research settings. Indeed, bronchial challenge tests with any inhaled

TABLE 47-1	INTERPRETATION OF METHACHOLINE CHALLENGE TEST RESULTS*	
PC_{20} (MG/ML)	**SUGGESTED INTERPRETATION**
<1.0	Moderate to severe reactivity (asthma likely)
1-4	Mild reactivity
4-16	Borderline reactivity
>16	Normal (no significant reactivity; asthma unlikely)

*Assumes that there is no baseline airway obstruction and that postchallenge improvement to baseline FEV_1 occurs.

agents should only be performed in certified pulmonary function laboratories under the direct supervision of a trained specialist.

EXERCISE CHALLENGE TEST

In individuals 6 years of age through adulthood, a treadmill or bicycle ergometer exercise test provides useful information about the presence of EIB or EIA. In children with histories suggestive of EIB, an exercise challenge test is a more useful diagnostic aid than a methacholine challenge test. Although the inhaled air should be dry, it is probably not necessary to use subfreezing air as was suggested in the past. The child should exercise at maximal level for 4 to 6 minutes and for a total time of 6 to 8 minutes. Maximal exercise is usually determined by heart rate (80% to 90% of age maximum) or ventilation (FEV$_1$ × 35); the target should be reached relatively quickly. Pulmonary function should be measured 5 minutes before exercise. Following exercise, serial pulmonary function measurements should be obtained for at least 20 minutes (at 5, 10, and 20 minutes postexercise) to determine the severity of EIA. A decrease in FEV$_1$ of more than 10% to 15% is diagnostic of exercise-induced bronchoconstriction.

OTHER TESTS

Complete Blood Cell Count

Often the complete blood cell count is normal and offers little information in the diagnosis or management of asthma. However, eosinophilia, if present, most commonly suggests asthma, allergy, or both. Although there are other causes of peripheral eosinophilia in children (i.e., gastrointestinal or systemic eosinophilic disorder, parasitic infection, malignancy, human immunodeficiency virus infection), asthma and allergy are the most likely causes. The complete blood cell count may be most useful when searching for other complicating conditions (e.g., immunodeficiency states) rather than as a primary diagnostic aid.

Cytologic Examination of Sputum

Obtaining induced sputum by inhaling hypertonic saline aerosols generated by an ultrasonic nebulizer is a useful technique for helping identify active inflammation in the airways characteristic of asthma.[28] The presence and number of eosinophils and other inflammatory cells can provide useful information about disease phenotype, activity, and response to therapy. Improved asthma control and reduced exacerbations were noted when there were less than 3% eosinophils in the induced sputum of adult asthmatics.[34] Neutrophilic inflammation predominates in some patients, while others have a paucity of inflammatory cells. Response to treatment and adjustment of drug doses may be guided by induced sputum cellularity. Although the technique of obtaining induced sputum is relatively simple, it does require trained personnel, use of an established protocol, specimen processing, and children that are at least 10 years of age.

Exhaled Nitric Oxide

Nitric oxide (NO) is an important and widespread regulatory molecule that has diverse biological functions. NO is synthesized from L-arginine by three different forms of the enzyme NO synthase (NOS): constitutive forms—endothelial NOS (eNOS) found in endothelial cells and nNOS in neuronal tissue—and an inducible form, iNOS. Although the precise role of NO in the asthmatic airway remains uncertain, NO can function as a bronchodilator, has antimicrobial properties, has antiproliferative action on fibroblasts, and is involved in regulation of ciliary beat frequency and epithelial ion transport.[35] Although it does not occur in all individuals, high exhaled NO concentrations in the asthmatic compared to the normal patient and a reduction with inhaled steroid treatment suggests an active or counterregulatory role in the development or persistence of asthma. Most data support direct correlation between clinical markers of eosinophilic airway inflammation and fractional exhaled NO (FeNO) including the degree of airway hyperresponsiveness as measured by methacholine challenge.[36-38] Other measures (e.g., FEV$_1$, bronchodilator response, and symptom report) correlate only weakly with FeNO.[39] Other weaknesses of FeNO include poor ability to identify non-eosinophilic inflammation and lack of specificity for asthma. Elevated FeNO also occurs in individuals with allergic rhinitis, eosinophilic bronchitis, chronic obstructive pulmonary disease (COPD), lung allograft rejection, and GERD.

If other clinical conditions associated with elevated FeNO are excluded, a FeNO above documented clinical cutoffs (Table 47-2) can be useful in differentiating asthma from other similar conditions. In a recently published study of 150 children (5 to 18 years of age, mean 12.5 years) referred to a specialty clinic for evaluation of respiratory symptoms suggestive of asthma, FeNO values >19 ppb yielded a sensitivity of 80%, a specificity of 92%, a PPV of 89%, and an NPV of 86% for the diagnosis of asthma.[40] Although somewhat easier to perform than standard spirometry, it is still unlikely that children much younger than 6 or 7 years of age will consistently be able to perform an online FeNO measure; however, offline collection methods using tidal breathing and Mylar collection bags have been used in younger children

TABLE 47-2 RANGE AND INTERPRETATION OF FeNO VALUES IN ADULTS AND CHILDREN

	LOW	NORMAL	HIGH
Adult	<5	5-33	>35
Children 4-10 years	<5	5-20	>20
Children 10-17 years	<5	5-25	>25

and infants. Commercial devices are now available that permit the rapid, noninvasive, and easy measure of eNO and are priced in the same range as a desktop portable spirometer.

A number of studies have demonstrated the presence of a variety of inflammatory mediators in the liquid condensate from cooled exhaled air collected over a number of minutes. Cytokines, leukotrienes, nitrates, and other substances all have been reported in exhaled breath condensate (EBC), and some may correlate with asthma disease activity.[41,42] In addition, an acid pH in the EBC has also been reported to be a marker of airway inflammation. However, there is still great controversy over standardization of the technique, the derivation of the measured substances (sampling of airway lining fluid rather than volatilized molecules), and the measurement of mediators. Although EBC may prove useful as a noninvasive measure of airway inflammation in the future, it is currently a research tool.

Serum Tests

Determining quantitative levels of immunoglobulin G (and subclasses), M, and A is useful only to rule out immunodeficiency syndromes in children with recurrent or chronic infection. In children with asthma, IgG levels usually are normal, IgA levels occasionally are low, and IgM levels may be elevated. Systemic steroids, however, can depress IgG and perhaps IgA levels. IgE is likely to be elevated in the child with asthma, atopy, or both; however, a normal IgE does not rule out asthma as a cause of symptoms. In addition, in the child with shifting pulmonary infiltrates, a marked elevation of serum IgE (>1000 IU) should prompt tests for both IgG and specific IgE antibody to *Aspergillus* to evaluate for allergic brochopulmonary aspergillosis.

Sweat Test

A sweat test should be performed on children with chronic respiratory symptoms, including recurrent wheezing, to rule out cystic fibrosis. Associated signs and symptoms that should prompt a sweat test include poor weight gain and short stature, steatorrhea, nasal polyps, pansinusitis, hemoptysis, and digital clubbing. Newborn screening for cystic fibrosis is now universal in the United States, and most cases of cystic fibrosis are diagnosed in infancy or the preschool years. However, mutations conferring pancreatic sufficiency are typically associated with milder pulmonary disease and may present much later.

Radiographs

All children with suspected asthma should have a chest radiograph at some time to rule out parenchymal disease, congenital anomaly, and (direct or indirect) evidence of a foreign body. A chest radiograph should be considered for the child admitted to a hospital with asthma, particularly if there are localized findings on physical examination (i.e., crackles, egophony, diminished breath sounds). Radiographic findings in asthma may range from normal to hyperinflation with peribronchial interstitial markings and atelectasis. The following abnormalities are most commonly seen in hospitalized children with asthma: hyperinflation with increased bronchial markings (Fig. 47-4*A*); infiltrates, atelectasis, pneumonia, or a combination of the three (Fig. 47-4*B*); and pneumomediastinum (Fig. 47-4*C*), often with infiltrates. Pneumothorax occurs rarely (Fig. 47-4*D*).

Paranasal sinus radiographs also should be considered for children with persistent nocturnal coughing, nasal symptoms, and headaches. Screening sinus computed tomography cuts are a more desirable study because they provide a more thorough examination of the paranasal sinuses than plain films, for a similar cost and radiation exposure.

Allergy Testing

Allergy testing (skin testing or *in vitro* serum allergen-specific IgE measure) is indicated in patients in whom specific allergic factors are believed to be important and probably in all children with severe asthma. Numerous allergic factors that might contribute significantly to the asthma (e.g., pollen, mold, dust mite, cockroach, or dander from domestic animals) occur in the home or at school. After taking a detailed environmental history, skin testing should be performed (usually percutaneous or scratch) limited to the most likely allergens as suggested by the history.

Skin test results may vary with age, drug therapy, and inherent skin factors. Drugs that affect skin test results include H_1 antihistamines (which may inhibit skin reactions for up to 72 hours or longer), tricyclic antidepressants, and some histamine (H_2) blockers. Topical and systemic corticosteroids or montelukast do not affect skin reactions. Positive (histamine) and negative (saline) control tests should be included to detect inherent skin factors that may affect the reaction to allergen, such as dermatographism and extensive dryness or eczema.

The *in vitro* measure of allergen-specific IgE (s-IgE) makes use of the affinity of serum IgE antibody for antigen that has been bound to a solid phase substrate. An enzyme-linked anti-IgE detects the quantity of specific IgE bound to the disk. The s-IgE is no more specific than the antigen employed, but it can produce a quantitative result, thus allowing degree of sensitization to be measured. The s-IgE test is significantly more expensive, but it can be done in commercial laboratories and is useful for special situations in which skin tests are impractical (e.g., for the patient with generalized dermatitis and the rare patient who is too ill for direct testing or must continue to receive medications with antihistaminic activity).

◼ THERAPEUTIC CONSIDERATIONS

Both the most recent U.S. guidelines for the diagnosis and management of asthma (Expert Panel Report 3) and the international Global Initiative for Asthma (GINA)

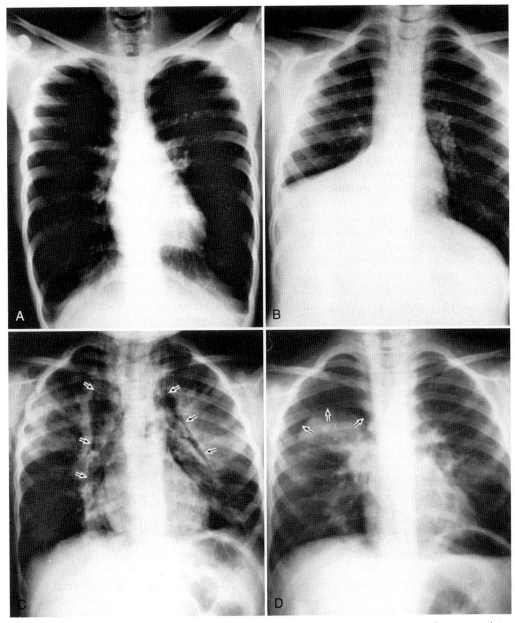

FIGURE 47-4. Radiographic findings in asthma. **A,** Hyperinflation with increased bronchial markings. **B,** Atelectasis involving a complete lobe. **C,** Massive pneumomediastinum complicating asthma. **D,** Pneumothorax secondary to paroxysmal coughing in asthma. Arrows mark air in **C,** lung margin in **D.**

guidelines stress the importance of asthma control as compared to severity.[1,43] Asthma severity refers to the intrinsic intensity of the disease and is typically assigned prior to beginning treatment with controller medications, and is also reassessed at intervals after treatment to determine degree of responsiveness. As a result, severity becomes defined by the level of treatment necessary to achieve and maintain adequate control. Identifying children and adolescents with severe or refractory asthma is probably important because the need for close monitoring and aggressive treatment will be significant. For most other patients, accurate assessment of control is more important than severity assignment in order to adequately manage asthma.

Asthma control is divided into two components: impairment and risk. The *impairment* domain refers to preventing chronic daytime and nighttime symptoms (i.e., cough,

wheeze, exercise limitation), reducing the need for rescue medication (SABA) for the treatment of symptoms, maintaining normal levels of activity (i.e., playing, sleeping, attending work or school), preserving normal or near-normal lung function, and meeting patient and parent expectations. The *risk* domain refers to preventing severe exacerbations that require emergency medical treatment or hospitalization, loss of lung function or impairment normal lung growth, and adverse effects caused by medication use. This strategy draws attention to management of current symptoms and functional impairment as well as future effects of asthma and its treatment on lung function and severe exacerbations. It also highlights the very important observation that asthma treatment strategies that improve symptoms may not always result in prevention of significant exacerbations.

Asthma is best managed in a continuous fashion by forming a partnership with a knowledgeable physician. The concept of expecting a near symptom-free lifestyle (for all but the most severely affected patients) should be instilled in patients and their families. Unnecessary restrictions of the child's and family's lifestyles should be avoided. Participation in recreational activities, sports, and school attendance should all be expected. Psychosocial factors such as the child's behavior, social adjustments in the family and at school, and attitudes toward managing asthma should also be addressed. Parents should understand that asthma is a chronic disease with acute exacerbations that with currently available treatments can be controlled, but not cured. As we obtain more insight into the nature of the inflammatory process in the asthmatic airway and develop newer noninvasive monitoring techniques, control of airway inflammation and prevention of airway remodeling and progressive obstructive pulmonary disease may also become a realistic goal of asthma management.

CLASSIFICATION OF ASTHMA

Over the past several years, increasing awareness has been focused on the broad heterogeneity of asthma, both with respect to its causes, manifestations, and response to treatment. Identification of specific asthma phenotypes is in its infancy, although the use of biomarkers, molecular phenotyping, and cluster analysis based on symptoms and lung function can help to identify specific subtypes. Age of onset of symptoms, lung function, inflammatory patterns in induced sputum (e.g., eosinophilic versus neutrophilic), and atopic versus non-atopic are all markers used to characterize disease severity, symptom pattern, and response to treatment. Considerable research is needed to accurately identify asthma phenotypes and to determine clinically useful methods for classification.

Although the clinical utility is somewhat questionable, asthma severity may be classified into broad categories based on frequency of daytime and nighttime symptoms (i.e., cough, wheeze, shortness of breath), functional impairment (i.e., sleep disturbances, play disruption, school absenteeism), need for SABA rescue/reliever treatment, and objective measures of pulmonary function (PEFR or FEV_1) that are typically present *before* the patient is treated. In addition, the number, frequency, and intensity of severe exacerbations—defined as an increase in symptoms sufficient to warrant treatment with oral corticosteroids or treatment in the emergency department or inpatient hospital unit—should be considered. Some patients who have relatively well-controlled symptoms and good functional status may have frequent or intense exacerbations. Although the correlation between the number and intensity of exacerbations with severity levels is less clear, the greater the number and severity (e.g., need for hospitalization, intensive care treatment), the higher the severity. Such designations are helpful to select appropriate initial management strategy.

However, the degree of severity of asthma often changes in a given individual with time, response to treatment,

airway or injury growth, the development of newly acquired allergic sensitivities, or change in exposure to recognized triggers. As a result, determination of *control* after treatment has been instituted is of greater significance than assigning a severity level. Using very similar criteria, asthma is determined to be well controlled, not well controlled, or very poorly controlled (Table 47-3). Control is determined at every visit, and appropriate treatment adjustments are made. The frequency of physician office visits for assessment of asthma control is variable and depends on disease activity but typically is every 1 to 6 months. Those with poor control or recent exacerbation may require more frequent visits for treatment adjustment and monitoring of response and lung function. The determination of asthma control in the impairment domain may be facilitated by using a validated questionnaire. There are several short, office based, self-administered instruments (e.g., the Asthma Control Test, Asthma Control questionnaire, Asthma Therapy Assessment Questionnaire) that provide a score indicative of well controlled, not well controlled, and poorly controlled asthma.[1] These tools do not assess the risk domain, which must also be factored into treatment decisions. It is important to remember that asthma is a chronic disorder that may become clinically obvious only periodically—one in which the severity of airway obstruction, intensity of symptoms, and degree of impairment is frequently underestimated by physicians and patients alike.

The most recent NHLBI guidelines classify asthma as either *intermittent* or *persistent*; and within the persistent category as *mild, moderate, or severe.*[1]

Intermittent Asthma

When symptoms are mild, easily controlled, and occur no more often than twice per week and the baseline pulmonary function is normal, asthma is classified as intermittent. In addition, patients with intermittent asthma do not require chronic administration of anti-inflammatory medications, but they may be treated with a SABA alone. EIA also may be considered intermittent disease. Individuals with only EIA rarely have symptoms triggered by other agents. Although children with intermittent asthma have little daily morbidity due to asthma, it is important to remember that severe attacks can occur, particularly in response to certain viral infections or profound allergen exposure. Children with intermittent disease usually have between 0 and 1 exacerbations per year. These features also indicate asthma that is well-controlled.

Mild Persistent Asthma

Children and adolescents with mild persistent asthma have cough or wheeze more than twice per week, but less than daily. Nocturnal symptoms of cough or wheeze occur no more often than 3 to 4 times per month, and pulmonary function (FEV_1 and FEV_1/FVC) is in the normal range. Overt asthmatic symptoms are generally

TABLE 47-3 ASSESSING ASTHMA CONTROL AND ADJUSTING THERAPY IN CHILDREN 5 TO 12 YEARS OF AGE

COMPONENTS OF CONTROL		Classification of Asthma Control (5–11 years of age)		
		WELL CONTROLLED	**NOT WELL CONTROLLED**	**VERY POORLY CONTROLLED**
Impairment	Symptoms	≤2 days/week but not more than once on each day.	>2 days/week or multiple time on less than 2 days/week	Throughout the day
	Nighttime awakenings	≤1x/month	≥2x/month	≥2x/week
	Interference with normal activity	None	Some limitation	Extremely limited
	Short acting beta-agonist use for symptom control (not preventionof EIB)	≤2 days/week	>2 days/week	Several times per day
	Lung function • FEV or peak flow	>80% predicted/ personal best	60-80% predicted/ personal best	<60% predicted/ personal best
	• FEV1/FVC	>80%	75%-80%	<75%
Risk	Exacerbations requiring oral systemic corticosteroids	**0-1/YEAR**	**≥2/YEAR (SEE NOTE)**	
		Consider severity and interval since last exacerbation		
	Reduction in lung growth Treatment related adverse effects	Evaluation requires long term followup Medication side effects can vary in intensity from none to very troublesome and worrisome. The level of intensity does not correlate to specific levels of control but should be considered in the overall assessment of risk.		
	Recommended action for treatment (See Figure 4-1B for treatement steps)	• Maintain current step • Regular followup every 1–6 months • Consider step down if well controlled for at least 3 months	• Step up at least 1 step and • Reevaluate in 2–6 weeks • For side effects consider alternative treatment options	• Consider short course of oral systemic corticosteroids • Step up at least 1 step and • Reevaluate in 2 weeks • For side effects consider alternative treatment options

EIB, Exercise-induced bronchospasm; *EFV$_1$,* forced expiratory volume in 1 second; *FVC,* forced vital capacity.
- The stepwise approach is meant to assist, not replace, the clinical decisionmaking required to meet individual patient needs.
- The level of control is based on the most severe impairment or risk category. Assess impairment domain by patient's/caregiver's recall of previous 2–4 weeks and by spirometry/or peak flow measures. Symptom assessment for longer periods should reflect a global assessment such as inquiring whether the patient's asthma is better or worse since the last visit.
- At present, there are inadequate data to correspond frequencies of exacerbations with different levels of asthma control. In general, more frequent and intense exacerbations (e.g., requiring urgent, unscheduled care, hospitalization, or ICU admission) indicate poorer disease control. For treatment purposes, patients who had ≥2 exacerbations requiring oral systemic corticosteroids in the past year may be considered the same as patients who have persistent asthma, even in the absence of impairment levels consistent with persistent asthma.
- Before step up in therapy:
  — Review adherence to medications, inhaler techinque, environmental control, and comorbid conditions.
  — If alternative treatment option was used in step, discontinue it and use preferred treatment for that step.
From EPR 3, NIH Publication 08-4051.

mild and resolve more or less completely with a dose or two of albuterol. There are relatively few of these brief episodes with no symptoms or functional impairment between episodes. Mild asthmatics may also have two or more exacerbations per year. This form of asthma probably represents at least one half of all cases of childhood asthma.

Moderate Persistent Asthma

There is evidence of mild airway obstruction, with some functional impairment and noticeable asthmatic symptoms between overt episodes. Patients have symptoms during most to all days and nocturnal symptoms at least weekly, and they may report frequent slowed play and missed schooldays. FEV$_1$ and FEV$_1$/FVC measures are often in the range of mild obstructive lung disease (60% to 80% of predicted). As with mild asthmatics, those categorized as moderate also may have two or more serious exacerbations per year.

Severe Persistent Asthma

Individuals with true severe or refractory asthma are uncommon; it is estimated that no more than 5% to 10% of the adult and pediatric asthma population meets a definition of severe asthma. In several clinical trials attempting to enroll severe patients, most were no longer classified as severe once issues of accurate diagnosis, adherence, proper treatment and medication device use, treatment of co-morbid conditions, or allergen avoidance were addressed.[44]

Severe persistent asthma has been defined in a variety of ways. The U.S. Expert Panel 3 report uses a symptom and lung function–based system that describes children and adults with severe asthma as having symptoms that recur throughout the day, and having obvious functional impairment on most days. Exercise tolerance is quite limited. Night awakenings occur during most nights, and school or work attendance may be poor (>20 days missed per year). Spirometry reveals the FEV_1 and FEV_1/FVC to be less than 60% and <75%, predicted for age, respectively, and there may be greater than 30% diurnal variation in PEFR measurement. A subgroup of severe asthmatics has refractory disease. These individuals have troublesome symptoms that require high doses of medication to control, or they have persistent symptoms, frequent exacerbations, or residual air flow obstruction on spirometry despite substantial medication use.[45] Specific features may include high PEFR variability, severe and chronic airways obstruction, rapidly progressive loss of lung function, and variable but less than expected response to treatment with corticosteroids. Patients with severe or refractory disease may in fact exhibit good clinical control of symptoms, but at a high treatment burden. In patients for whom other conditions have been ruled out, refractory asthma has further been defined as requiring treatment with continuous or near-continuous oral corticosteroids or high-dose ICSs in order to maintain control. Alternatively, such patients will exhibit at least two of the following criteria: treatment with at least one other controller medication in addition to ICS, daily use of SABA, persistent air flow obstruction (FEV_1 <80% predicted), one or more acute care visits per year, three or more short courses of oral steroids in 1 year, rapid deterioration with ≤25% reduction in oral or inhaled steroid dose, or a previous near-fatal asthma episode. There are likely to be several severe phenotypes with distinct pathophysiology, or environmental exacerbating factors. Refractory or severe disease is more common among those who report an early age of onset of symptoms (before 12 years of age), in African Americans, and in women. Use of cluster analysis techniques shows promise in further stratifying severe asthma phenotypes into more discrete subtypes that will help with prospective identification and long-term follow up and treatment.[46] Children with life-threatening asthma may exhibit most or all of the symptoms mentioned earlier in the chapter, but in addition they have experienced an extremely severe asthma episode leading to respiratory failure and/or the need for endotracheal intubation and mechanical ventilation. Such an event places them at risk for future severe episodes and death caused by asthma. Although serious exacerbations may be more common in those with severe disease, even patients with mild or intermittent asthma can experience a life-threatening episode. Some studies have identified an association of asthma disease severity with genetic polymorphisms such as in the $β_2$-adrenergic receptor, TNF-α, and *RANTES/CCL5*.[47] However, the complex inheritance of asthma, the influence of epigenetic factors, and modifying genes distinct from the asthma disease susceptibility locus all confound the accurate identification of genetic influences. See Chapter 48 for a detailed discussion of severe asthma.

Other Measures for Assessing Asthma Severity and Control

Biomarkers that provide more information on disease activity and severity could better guide asthma treatment and improve control and/or reduce exacerbations. However, currently available tests are limited in both availability and utility or practicality. Determining degree of airway reactivity based on methacholine responsiveness and adjusting treatment to decrease airway reactivity has been shown to achieve better pulmonary function and fewer exacerbations than monitoring symptoms and pulmonary function alone.[48] Patients treated using the hyperresponsiveness strategy received a higher dose of ICS throughout the course of the study. Repeated methacholine challenge testing is expensive, time-consuming, and generally impractical in the clinical setting. Green and colleagues demonstrated that using the number of eosinophils found in an induced sputum sample to adjust level of treatment resulted in fewer acute exacerbations and hospitalizations than reliance on symptoms and pulmonary function alone.[34] Again, in pediatric patients, obtaining induced sputum samples is usually restricted to those older than 9 years of age and is also labor-intensive and somewhat uncomfortable for the child. Measurement of FeNO has been proposed as a more direct and easily obtainable measure of airway inflammation[36] and therefore can be used to titrate treatment to achieve better control. Although in steroid-naïve asthmatics FeNO is elevated and in most patients the levels decrease within 1 week of instituting inhaled steroid treatment, FeNO remains essentially unchanged in as many as 30%, even when clinical improvement occurs.[38,49] Moreover, two recent large randomized, controlled trials that used either daily home or intermittent in-office FeNO measures to adjust treatment failed to find a difference in improvement in the number of symptom-free days and a reduction in ICS dose when compared to standard treatment using symptom report and pulmonary function measures.[50,51] However, FeNO may be useful when there is discordance between patient-reported symptoms and airway inflammation.[46] For instance, some obese asthmatics have high symptom report, but little airway eosinophilia; in such patients, FeNO measures could permit safe ICS dose reduction and use of other treatments that may be more effective.[51] In spite of its limitations, FeNO may be useful in some settings, such as a diagnostic aid for asthma, identification of steroid-responsive patients and (to a lesser extent) adjusting the dose of controller medications, and predicting relapse during medication taper. Further studies are needed to determine clinical utility and effectiveness.

PHARMACOLOGIC MANAGEMENT OF ASTHMA IN CHILDREN OLDER THAN 5 YEARS OF AGE

The medical treatment of asthma involves the administration of controller medications designed to prevent asthma symptoms and the use of rapid-acting reliever medications that act quickly to abort acute exacerbations. Controller

TABLE 47-4A USUAL DOSAGES FOR LONG-TERM CONTROLLER MEDICATIONS

MEDICATION	YOUTH >12 YEARS	CHILD DOSE
Systemic Corticosteroids		
Methylprednisolone (chronic control)	7.5-60 mg Once daily or every other day as needed for control	0.25-2 mg/kg[1]
Prednisolone, Prednisone (short-course for exacerbation)	40-60 mg Administer for 3-10 days once or in 2 divided doses	1-2 mg/kg maximum 60 mg/day
Dexamethasone	12-16 mg Give oral or IM for 1-2 days	0.6 mg/kg, maximum 16 mg
Long-Acting Inhaled β-2 Agonists*		
Salmeterol 50 mcg/puff Formoterol 12 mcg/ capsule	50 mcg q 12 hours 1 capsule q 12 hours	50 mcg q 12 hours 1 capsule q 12 hours
Combination Medication		
Fluticasone/Salmeterol DPI 100, 250, 500 mcg/50 mcg MDI 45/21, 115/21, 230/21 mcg	1 inhalation bid 2 inhalations bid	1 inhalation bid 1-2 inhalations bid
Budesonide/formoterol MDI 80/4.5; 160/4.5 mcg	1-2 inhalations bid	1-2 inhalations bid
Mometasone/formoterol MDI 100/5 mcg; 200/5 mcg	1-2 inhalations bid Adjust dose strength to achieve control	1-2 inhalations bid
Leukotriene Modifiers		
Montelukast	10 mg daily 5 mg daily (6-14 yrs) 10 mg daily (>14 yrs)	4 mg daily (2-5 yrs)
Zafirlukast	20 mg twice daily	10 mg twice daily (7-11 yrs)
Methylxanthines		
Theophylline, sustained release	300 mg daily Adjust dose to serum concentration 5-10 mg/mL	10/mg/kg daily, max 300 mg

*Should not be used for symptom relief or for exacerbations. Use with inhaled corticosteroids.

medications are administered to all asthmatics other than those with intermittent disease and are typically, but not uniformly, anti-inflammatory in nature (Table 47-4A). Reliever medications are short-acting β_2 agonists or anticholinergics. Several new classes of immunomodulatory drugs are under development, and one anti-IgE (omalizumab) is currently available for treatment of severe persistent asthma.

RELIEVER MEDICATIONS: SHORT-ACTING β AGONISTS

Short acting β_2-adrenergic agonists (SABAs) constitute the most potent bronchodilators currently available for treatment of asthma[1] and are used to relieve bronchospasm and its attendant symptoms of cough, wheeze, and shortness of breath. SABAs bind to the widely distributed β-adrenergic receptors (primarily those located on the bronchial smooth muscle, airway epithelial cell, or mast cell) and result in the intracellular conversion of adenosine triphosphate (ATP) to adenosine 3',5' cyclic monophosphate. The result is relaxation of airway smooth muscle and improved air flow. Onset of action is generally within a few minutes, peak action occurs at approximately 30 minutes, and duration of action occurs from 4 to 6 hours.[1] Preferred route of administration is via inhalation because this method results in the most rapid onset and duration of action while minimizing adverse effects. Inhalation of SABAs can be accomplished with the use of a small-volume jet nebulizer, metered-dose inhaler (MDI) usually with a spacer, or dry-powder inhaler (DPI).

Several selective SABAs are available for use in treating acute asthma, such as terbutaline, pirbuterol, and albuterol. Racemic albuterol, the predominant bronchodilator in current use, is a 50:50 mixture of (R)-enantiomers and (S)-enantiomers. Levalbuterol, the (R)-albuterol isomer, has 100-fold more potent β_2 receptor binding than (S)-albuterol, and it is responsible for the bronchodilator effects of the racemate. *In vitro*, (S)-albuterol has been demonstrated to increase intracellular Ca^{2+} to stimulate eosinophil recruitment and degranulation and recruit other inflammatory cells.[52]

TABLE 47-4B ADJUNCT MEDICATIONS FOR SEVERE EPISODES

MEDICATION	CHILD (<12 YEARS)	ADOLESCENT
Magnesium Sulfate		
Intravenous (IV)	Bolus: 50 mg/kg/dose (25 to 75 mg/kg/dose; max 2 g) Administer over 20 min	
Systemic (Injected) β₂ Agonists		
Epinephrine		
Intramuscular (IM) 1:1,000 (1 mg/mL)	0.01 mg/kg (max 0.3-0.5 mg) every 20 minutes for 3 doses	0.3 to 0.5 mg every 20 minutes for 3 doses
Terbutaline		
Intravenous (IV) Subcutaneous (SQ) (1 mg/mL)	0.01 mg/kg bolus (max 0.4 mg) over 10 minutes 0.01 mg/kg (max 0.25 mg) May repeat every 15 min for 3 doses	0.01 mg/kg bolus (max 0.75 mg) over 10 minutes 0.01 mg/kg (max 0.25 mg) May repeat every 15 minutes for 3 doses

- No advantage has been found for higher-dose corticosteroids in severe asthma exacerbations.[1]
- There is no advantage for intravenous administration over oral therapy, provided gastrointestinal function is intact.
- Therapy following a hospitalization or emergency department visit is typically 5 days but may last from 3 to 10 days. Studies indicate that there is no need to taper the systemic corticosteroid dose when given up to 10 days. Dosages in excess of 1 mg/kg of prednisone or prednisolone have been associated with adverse behavioral effects in children, whereas 1 mg/kg provides equivalent pulmonary benefit without the adverse effects.

The *in vivo* effects of (S)-albuterol remain controversial; however, it has no bronchodilator activity and has a prolonged plasma half-life, but it does not cause bronchoconstriction or interfere with the binding of (R)-albuterol to its receptor. When administered in equivalent doses based on concentration of (R)-albuterol, there does not appear to be any consistent clinical advantage to using levalbuterol versus racemic albuterol as measured by improvement in clinical symptoms, pulmonary function testing, or adverse effect profile. However, one large randomized controlled trial comparing (R)-albuterol versus racemic albuterol found 10% fewer hospitalizations in the (R)-albuterol group.[53] Other smaller studies could not replicate these results on hospital admission but confirmed the lack of differential clinical benefit and adverse event profile. A recent trial comparing the utility of continuously nebulized racemic or levalbuterol also failed to show an advantage of levalbuterol.[54] Since levalbuterol is typically more expensive than the racemic drug, the routine use of levalbuterol generally is not recommended.

Typical adverse effects of SABAs include muscular tremor, tachycardia, irritability, and, with more excessive doses, hypokalemia, hypertension, and tachyarrhythmia. Adverse effects are greater with systemic administration (oral, IV, IM) compared to the inhaled route. Moreover, the dose delivered by an MDI is substantially less than that from a small-volume nebulizer, and since most of the inhaled dose is swallowed and absorbed by the gastrointestinal tract, annoying side effects are best minimized by using the MDI.

The clinical significance of serious adverse events that develop as a result of the chronic administration of inhaled SABAs is, in most instances, probably less than was once believed. The current recommendation is for the as-needed use of a SABA for relief of symptoms or for protection against EIA.

The increase in asthma deaths reported in the United Kingdom in the late 1960s was initially related to overuse of high-dose isoproterenol inhalers, and the increase in asthma deaths reported in New Zealand was believed to be associated with the use of inhaled fenoterol. Removal of these drugs from the market correlated with a decline in asthma deaths. A retrospective review of prescription records in patients in Canada found an increased risk for asthma death or near-death in patients who used more than one canister of a SABA per month. However, an association with the use of a number of other asthma medications was also noted, suggesting that disease severity might actually be more causative than overuse of SABAs alone.

Other reports have suggested that repeated use of a SABA may result in an increase in airway hyperresponsiveness or a decrease in protection from allergen-induced bronchospasm. The reduction in beneficial effects of SABA following chronic use may result in part from receptor desensitization. The decrease in response may be the result of uncoupling of the receptor from its signaling G protein, inactivation of receptors, or reduction in receptor number caused by increased degradation or decreased synthesis. Although these actions occur *in vitro*, the *in vivo* biological correlates and clinical importance are questionable. A well-designed randomized double-blind placebo-controlled study performed in adults with mild asthma examined the effects of regularly administered albuterol versus intermittent administration compared with placebo. There was no significant difference in any outcome measures between the groups, including exacerbations, treatment failures, lung function, symptoms, or methacholine responsiveness.[55] However, regular use of albuterol was also not beneficial to the patients. Finally, there may be specific subgroups of patients who are at risk for developing adverse effects as measured by worsening pulmonary function with chronic use of SABAs, and this may be related to genetic variability in the β-adrenergic receptor. Nine polymorphisms in the β-adrenergic receptor *(BAR)* gene have been described, and several of the more frequent types may have biological significance. One of interest involves the beta 2AR-16 region, with replacement of arginine (Arg16) for glycine (Gly16). In a study involving bronchodilator response in children, those with the *Arg/Arg* polymorphism had the highest prevalence (60%) of bronchodilator response to a single dose of albuterol, whereas fewer than 30% of those with the *Arg/Gly* polymorphism responded and only 13% of those with the *Gly/Gly* polymorphism were responders.[56] In contrast, data from a prospective study of chronic albuterol administration to patients segregated by BAR genotype found that those with the Arg16 homozygous polymorphism had steadily declining PEFR as compared with those receiving intermittent treatment or treatment with ipratropium.[57] This effect did not occur in those with the *Gly/Gly* genotype. Chronic administration of ipratropium to the *Arg/Arg* group did not result in PEFR deterioration. Although further work is necessary to accurately identify at-risk polymorphisms and haplotypes in the BAR, these data suggest that in the future, pharmacogenetic profiling may aid in prescribing SABA use in the most effective and safe manner.

ANTICHOLINERGIC AGENTS

Ipratropium bromide is a quaternary ammonium congener of atropine and is an anticholinergic compound approved for use as a bronchodilator. Anticholinergic agents produce bronchodilation by antagonizing the activity of acetylcholine at the level of its receptor, particularly those found on airway smooth muscle located in the large, central airways. The onset of action of ipratropium is relatively slow (20 minutes), and the peak effect occurs at 60 minutes.[1] Ipratropium, unlike atropine, is poorly absorbed across mucous membranes and has little toxicity at the usual doses. In particular, ipratropium does not inhibit mucociliary clearance. Data from several studies conducted in children presenting to the emergency department for treatment of acute asthma indicates that when combined with a β-adrenergic agonist, ipratropium improves pulmonary function and relieves symptoms better than either drug alone.[1] The effect is modest and appears to be most evident in those who present with the most severe airway obstruction; this may be a marker for patients who have increased cholinergic tone in the large central airways. Ipratropium has not been shown to be effective in the treatment of children hospitalized with acute asthma, particularly if ipratropium failed to induce improvement when administered in the emergency department.[58]

Tiotropium bromide is another long-acting anticholinergic that is currently approved in the United States for the treatment of COPD, but not asthma. It has a duration of action that exceeds 24 hours and can be administered once a day from a dry-powder inhaler. A recently published study of adults (older than 18 years of age) with asthma not adequately controlled with an ICS alone demonstrated that the addition of tiotropium to ICS was superior to doubling the dose of ICS and was non-inferior to the addition of a LABA, as measured by change in morning PEFR, as well as symptom days, quality of life, and asthma control score.[59] Other studies examining the role of tiotropium in asthma, including its long-term safety and use in children, are underway or under consideration.

CONTROLLER MEDICATIONS

Inhaled Corticosteroids

Inhaled corticosteroids are currently considered the most effective controller medication available for the treatment of chronic asthma. Most ICSs have a high topical potency and relatively low systemic effects, either as a result of poor absorption or rapid and effective metabolism to inactive compounds. However, all ICSs are absorbed through the respiratory epithelium, resulting in the potential for systemic effects.

The ideal ICS should demonstrate excellent clinical efficacy and minimal to no toxicity in combination with a convenient and easy-to-use inhaler device. To achieve such a profile, an ICS should have the following properties: a high affinity for and potency at the glucocorticoid receptor; prolonged retention in the lung; a high level of serum protein binding for the systemically absorbed fraction; a high volume of distribution; minimal or no oral bioavailability; and rapid, complete systemic inactivation (e.g., high first-pass hepatic inactivation, or inactivation in the lung before systemic absorption).[60] These properties confer a higher therapeutic index with prolonged anti-inflammatory activity in the lung and relatively few systemic adverse effects. Pharmacologic properties alone are not sufficient for optimum clinical effect. Inhalation devices should provide maximal deposition in the lung in both large and smaller airways with little to no deposition or absorption in the oropharynx or gastrointestinal tract. Once-daily administration is also likely to improve patient adherence. Delivery devices should be simple to use, should be acceptable to a wide age range, and should deliver a consistent dose throughout the life of the inhaler.

Fluticasone Propionate

Fluticasone propionate (FP) is a potent and poorly absorbed (oral) topically active corticosteroid that is extensively metabolized in the liver to an inactive compound. This highly lipophilic drug demonstrates an extremely high affinity for lung glucocorticoid receptors (GRs) compared to beclomethasone (BDP) and shows a slow rate of dissociation from its receptor.

As a result, FP has a negligible oral bioavailability, and the topical–to–systemic activity ratio is exceptionally favorable and better than most currently available ICSs. However, FP is readily absorbed through the respiratory mucosa and can enter the systemic circulation in this fashion (without hepatic metabolism). FP is more likely to produce sore throat and hoarseness. In addition, there have been reports of adrenal suppression in children younger than 12 years of age who receive more than 400 mcg/day of FP, but the data are inconsistent. FP is therefore considered a high-potency ICS with the potential to effectively control symptoms and improve lung function, but at higher doses it has greater potential to cause adverse effects. *In vivo*, FP appears at least twice as potent as BDP and BUD on a milligram-per-milligram basis. Comparative trials indicate that fluticasone at half the dose of BUD and BDP results in a slight improvement of some pulmonary function measures such as morning PEFR and end of treatment trial FEV_1.[61]

FP is currently available in MDI and dry-powder inhaler form in three strengths (Table 47-5). FP is approved in the United States for use in children 4 years of age and older.

Budesonide

BUD has been widely studied and used clinically for many years. It has moderate potency *in vitro* and *in vivo* with well-documented clinical efficacy and safety. In addition, the presence of a free C21 hydroxy group on the BUD molecule results in formation of esters with long-chain fatty acids. This results in an inactive depot of drug within the airway epithelial cells that is released slowly into an active state. BUD is currently available in a dry powder inhaler and a nebulizer suspension. BUD is approved in the United States for use in children 1 year of age and older.

Beclomethasone

Although clearly less potent than FP and slightly less so than BUD, BDP is effective in reducing symptoms and improving pulmonary function. However, BDP is readily absorbed from the gastrointestinal tract, and the parent compound (beclomethasone dipropionate) is metabolized to the more potent monopropionate. As a result, BDP has a less favorable topical-to-systemic potency ratio. However, concerns about its ability to cause adverse effects such as growth and adrenal suppression have not been substantiated. BDP is currently available as a fine-particle aerosol dispensed by a hydrofluoroalkene propellant. This propellant system permits greater deposition into the lower and smaller airways and a reduction in the effective dose. The clinical advantage of these properties remains to be clarified. BDP is approved in the United States for use in children 5 years of age and older. In low- and middle-income countries, the low cost of BDP makes it a very attractive medication.

Mometasone

Mometasone is a potent, highly topically active steroid that has long been used to treat allergic rhinitis and dermatologic disorders. It has the advantage of poor systemic absorption and has been shown to be effective in improving lung function and controlling symptoms in children with asthma who were previously treated with other ICSs and SABAs. Mometasone is similar to FP in its high receptor affinity and half-life. It appears to have a similar safety profile to other ICSs. Mometasone is approved

TABLE 47-5 ESTIMATED COMPARATIVE DAILY DOSAGES FOR INHALED CORTICOSTEROID IN OLDER CHILDREN AND ADULTS

DRUG	LOW DAILY DOSE		MEDIUM DAILY DOSE		HIGH DAILY DOSE	
	5-11 YR	>12 YR	5-11 YR	>12 YR	5-11 YR	>12 YR
Beclomethasone HFA 40 or 80 mcg/puff	80-160 mcg	80-240 mcg	>160-320 mcg	>240-480 mcg	>320 mcg	>480 mcg
Budesonide suspension for nebulization dry powder (90, 180, or 200 mcg/inhalation)	0.5 mg 180-400 mcg	180-600 mcg	1.0 mg 400-800 mcg	>600-1200 mcg	>2.0mg > 800 mcg	>1200 mcg
Flunisolide HFA 80 mcg/puff	160 mcg	320 mcg	320 mcg	320-640 mcg	≥640 mcg	>640 mcg
Fluticasone HFA/MDI: 44, 110, 220 mcg/puff DPI: 50, 100, 250 mcg/puff	88-176 mcg 100-200 mcg	88-264 mcg 100-300 mcg	>176-352 mcg 200-400 mcg	264-440 mcg 300-500 mcg	>352 mcg >400 mcg	>440 mcg >500 mcg
Mometasone DPI 110, 220 mcg/puff	110 mcg	220 mcg	110-220 mcg	400 mcg	>400 mcg	>400 mcg
Ciclesonide MDI 80, 160 mcg/puff	NA	160 mcg	NA	320 mcg	NA	640 mcg

HFA, Hydrofluoroalkane; *NA*, not approved for this age group. Adapted from NAEPP Expert Report 3.

in the United States for use in children 4 years of age and older. It is available as a dry-powder inhaler for treatment of asthma and is labeled for once-a-day dosing.

Ciclesonide

Ciclesonide is a prodrug that must be metabolized to active form in the lung, where its metabolite has approximately 100 times greater receptor affinity. It has essentially no oral bioavailability and is tightly bound to plasma proteins. Ciclesonide is converted at the airway epithelial cell into its active metabolite, des-ciclesonide. (Des-CIC); the enzyme responsible for the conversion is only found in the lower respiratory tract. A recent meta-analysis concluded that ciclesonide was probably as effective as fluticasone, budesonide, and beclomethasone in equivalent doses at improving pulmonary function and controlling mild symptoms. Incidence of oral candidiasis was lower in groups treated with ciclesonide. A single long-term (12-month) safety study in children compared two doses of ciclesonide to placebo and concluded that there was no significant effect on linear growth or adrenal suppression.[62] The study was somewhat flawed in that there was no active comparator, no clinical effect of drug was seen, and adherence was indirectly measured. Further studies in children are necessary to assess dose responsiveness and safety. Ciclesonide is approved in the United States for use in children 12 years of age and older.

OTHER INHALED CORTICOSTEROIDS

Triamcinolone and flunisolide are relatively less potent steroids that, while effective, are less commonly used. Both must be given in fairly high microgram amounts, resulting in a bitter unpleasant taste.

Mechanism of Action and Clinical Use

The action of corticosteroids begins as passive diffusion across the cell membrane and into the cytoplasm where binding to the glucocorticoid receptor (GR) occurs. The GR exists in the cytoplasm as a large heterodimeric complex that includes two 90-kd heat shock protein molecules. After hormone binding, the heat shock proteins are shed, the complex is translocated to the nucleus, and then the complex binds as a dimer to a glucocorticoid response element (GRE) on steroid-responsive genes.

The GR acts to regulate transcription of target genes either directly or indirectly by interaction with other transcription factors. The binding of GR to GRE results in either induction or repression of the gene. The number of GREs and the proximity to transcriptional start sites results in increased steroid inducibility of the gene. GRs may also act independently of binding to GRE by acting as a coactivator of other transcription factors (e.g., STAT5) or by modulating chromatin structure by recruiting histone deacetylase and effecting gene silencing.[63] Because topical steroids can also cause rapid

effects (e.g., skin blanching), it is likely that a nongenomic mechanism of action for ICSs occurs that is characterized by a rapid cellular mechanism of action and transient vasoconstriction on the microcirculation. This action could involve the generation of vasoconstrictive mediators at the point of GC binding to certain membrane receptors or at the time of dissociation of the HSP from the cytoplasmic receptor complex.

A major target of corticosteroids is the nuclear transcription factor NFκB. Corticosteroids block NFκB signaling by preventing it from binding to DNA and decreasing transcription of proinflammatory cytokines. Corticosteroids may also inhibit NFκB by directly increasing inhibitory (IκB) production. IκB proteins bind to NFκB and keep it anchored in the cytoplasm.

Corticosteroids inhibit the transcription of a number of cytokines and chemokines implicated in the pathogenesis of asthma, such as interleukin-1 (IL-1) through IL-6, TNFα, granulocyte-macrophage colony-stimulating factor, IL-13, IL-8, RANTES (released on activation, normal T cell expressed and secreted), and eotaxin. Steroids may also inhibit the synthesis of some cytokine receptors, such as the IL-4 receptor, intracellular adhesion molecule (ICAM), and vascular cell adhesion molecule (VCAM). In addition to the action on cytokines, steroids also inhibit the inducible form of nitric oxide synthase, cyclo-oxygenase, phospholipase A2, and endothelin, all important factors in the inflammatory cascade relevant to asthma. Corticosteroids also increase the synthesis of β-adrenergic receptors by increasing gene transcription.

ICSs are currently recommended as first-line therapy for children 5 years of age and older with other than intermittent asthma. ICSs are the most effective chronic treatment for asthma and reduce airway reactivity, reduce acute symptoms and exacerbations, attenuate the late allergen response, and decrease the need for rescue bronchodilators. In addition, ICSs decrease deposition of collagen and tenascin in the subepithelial basement membrane. For these reasons, ICSs alone should be used as the initial treatment for persistent asthma; it is not appropriate, in the vast majority of cases, to use a fixed-dose combination of ICS plus a long acting β-agonist as initial treatment. Withdrawal of ICS treatment is usually accompanied by a rapid return of airway hyperresponsiveness and decreased symptom control within several weeks.

A small but substantial proportion of patients do not have a significant response to ICS. The mechanisms of this relative steroid resistance is not yet fully understood. Children and adolescents who are obese, smoke cigarettes, and have significant and continuous exposure to certain allergens are relatively refractory to the beneficial effects of ICSs on symptoms and lung function. Recent data suggest that vitamin D deficiency is associated with worse asthma control, and the mechanism may involve induced steroid resistance.[29] Studies to further examine this relationship are ongoing.

The dose-response curve for ICS treatment reaches a plateau at a fairly low dose in most patients, and there is little added benefit to pulmonary function or airway reactivity when doses are as much as quadrupled. A study performed in adults to evaluate the efficacy and safety of escalating doses of ICS demonstrated that for the majority of patients, maximal improvement in FEV_1 and methacholine responsiveness occurred at low to moderate doses of FP and BDP, with no added benefit of extremely high doses.[64] However, a substantial linear increase in cortisol suppression was seen as ICS dose increased. It is likely that most of the clinical benefit with the least risk will occur at low to medium doses of ICS. Patients receiving higher ICS doses require more careful monitoring for both response to therapy and emergence of systemic side effects. However, higher doses of ICS may be required to effectively decrease serious exacerbations.

Local adverse effects, such as oral candidiasis and dysphonia, are the most common but least severe complications of ICS treatment. They are dose-related with some variability depending on steroid type, and they only occur in a small minority of patients (1% to 3%). Reducing the dose, using a spacer device, and rinsing the mouth with water after use may minimize both these side effects. The more serious systemic adverse effects for children include adrenal suppression and depression of linear growth. Adrenal suppression has been extensively studied, although the results are often difficult to interpret owing to flawed design, previous use of oral corticosteroids, or inappropriate tests used to assess adrenal function. Nonetheless, adrenal suppression is unlikely in children receiving less than 400 mcg/day of inhaled BUD, or fluticasone 200 mcg/day, even after long-term use.[1,14] Adrenal suppression can be measured in children receiving higher doses, as indicated by impaired adrenocorticotropic hormone stimulation tests. However, in most patients, even these impairments are of no or uncertain clinical significance when the patient is well. A significant stress (e.g., major illness, surgery) could warrant administration of exogenous corticosteroids to prevent an Addisonian response.

The effect of ICSs on linear growth in most patients is minimal, even after long-term administration of low-dose ICSs. Moreover, most of the decrease in growth velocity appears in the first few months after initiating steroid treatment. Although it was initially feared that each year of treatment (even with low-dose inhaled ICSs) would result in over 1 centimeter of lost height, longer-term studies have not confirmed this. Data on the growth of children in the 4-year-long CAMP trial demonstrated that there was indeed a significant decline in growth velocity over the first year of the study, but the growth rate returned to normal thereafter. Children in the BUD group were on average 1.1 cm shorter than those in the placebo and nedocromil groups at the end of the 4-year treatment period.[14] In addition, Agertoft and Pedersen showed that there was no reduction in final predicted adult height in a group of 142 children treated with a mean dose of 400 mcg/day of BUD for an average of 9.2 years.[65] These longer-term studies of chronic low-dose ICSs point to an excellent safety profile and the potential to reach final predicted adult height, in spite of short-term decline in height velocity. Since there is interindividual variability in clinical response to corticosteroids and predisposition to develop adverse effects, careful monitoring of each individual patient's growth during ICS treatment should be performed, and the dose should be adjusted to the lowest necessary to achieve good symptom control.

SYSTEMIC CORTICOSTEROIDS

The therapeutic benefits of systemic corticosteroids are marred by their potential adverse effects, which include excessive weight gain, hypertension, osteoporosis, decreased linear growth, metabolic derangement, and cataracts. Adverse effects from long-term steroid therapy may be reduced, but not eliminated, by using steroids with shorter half-lives (e.g., prednisone, prednisolone, methylprednisolone) at the lowest possible dose administered in the morning in a single dose and given every other day.

LONG-ACTING β AGONISTS

β-adrenergic agonists that have a prolonged duration of action (8 to 12 hours) occupy a unique niche in the asthma treatment armamentarium, somewhere between that of a controller and a reliever medication. There are currently two long-acting β agonists (LABAs) available on the U.S. market and approved for use in children: salmeterol (approved for patients 4 years of age and older) and formoterol (approved for patients 12 years of age and older); others, such as indacaterol, are in clinical trials. The two available agents differ in structure, potency, efficacy, and selectivity for the beta receptor. Salmeterol is a partial agonist, has a relatively slow onset of action (10 to 30 minutes), and has extremely high selectivity for the β_2 receptor. Salmeterol is more than 10,000 times more lipophilic than albuterol, and it also has three to four times the affinity for the β_2 receptor of albuterol. However, salmeterol diffuses out into the cell membrane somewhat slowly to approach the β_2 adrenoceptor active site. This process results in a slower onset of action (~30 minutes). Salmeterol has a long side chain that interacts with an exosite domain of the β_2 receptor. This side chain attachment allows the head to associate and dissociate with the active receptor site for a prolonged time period and results in the long duration of drug action.[66] It is currently only available as a dry powder in a Diskus device in the United States, but it is also available in MDI form in other countries.

Formoterol is a moderately lipophilic, highly effective full agonist with a very different molecular structure to salmeterol. It is taken up into the cell membrane to form a dose-dependent depot, from where it progressively diffuses out to interact with the active site. It has a rapid onset of action (~5 minutes) comparable to albuterol, but duration of activity is 12 hours. Formoterol is also dispensed as a dry-powder inhaler (U.S.), MDI, or nebulizer solution; the latter is labeled for use in COPD only.

The continued use of LABAs can lead to an alteration in its biologic effects. Although mechanisms of action of this tolerance to the bronchoprotective effect are unclear, down-regulation of beta-receptor number or lack of receptor sensitivity are possibilities. Following a single dose of salmeterol (25 to 50 mcg), there is sustained improvement in bronchodilation for at least 12 hours, as well as a bronchoprotective effect to both methacholine and exercise. However, after repeated doses, within a few days or weeks there is loss in degree of bronchoprotection to methacholine, and exercise. For methacholine, there is a smaller increase in doubling doses, but it is unclear if this is clinically significant. When used as monotherapy, protection from EIB persists after daily dosing for 2 to 4 weeks, but in several studies the duration of action decreases from 9 to 12 hours to as little as 1 hour. Chronic use of LABAs may also decrease the responsiveness and time to recovery with SABA administration after exercise induced bronchoconstriction. The bronchodilator effect is more resistant to decrease following repeated dosing, and the decline is usually most apparent after a few days of use followed by stabilization. Formoterol is likely to behave in a fashion similar to salmeterol.[67]

The LABAs are not generally considered anti-inflammatory agents, but studies show that salmeterol has either no effect on airway inflammation or reduces inflammatory cells in the airway mucosa. It has also been proposed that LABAs may enhance the actions of ICSs, although the mechanisms are controversial.

Past and recent concerns persist about the use of LABAs as monotherapy and the risk of adverse events. A study performed by the Asthma Clinical Research Network demonstrated that the combination of triamcinolone and salmeterol was effective in controlling asthma in patients 12 to 65 years of age.[68] However, complete withdrawal of the ICS and continuation of the LABA resulted in significant deterioration in asthma control as measured by asthma exacerbations, deterioration in pulmonary function, and need for oral corticosteroid treatment. These data and those from similar studies all suggest that LABAs cannot be used as a replacement for ICSs and should never be used as monotherapy for treatment of chronic asthma.

Deaths have also been reported in patients chronically using inhaled salmeterol. It remains uncertain if there is a direct link between medication use and death, or if the increase in deaths is a reflection of inappropriate use of a LABA (e.g., attempt to use it as an acute bronchodilator and/or in place of a controller medication). A recent large trial (>26,000 enrollees) compared the safety of daily salmeterol or placebo added to usual treatment for chronic asthma over a 28-week period.[69] The Salmeterol Multicenter Asthma Research Trial (SMART) trial was stopped early when an interim analysis showed futility in reaching the required enrollment numbers as well as an association between salmeterol use and severe or fatal asthma. The risk for asthma-related death, albeit small (13 of 13,174) in the salmeterol group was significantly greater than that in the placebo group (4 of 13,179); $RR = 4.37$ (95%, CI 1.25 to 15.34) for combined asthma deaths or life-threatening experiences. This translates into a death rate of 1.98 per 1000 person-years and is significantly greater than the expected death rate in the United States asthmatic population of 0.48/1000 person-years. Importantly, the increased risk for death was stronger in African-American subjects. The African-American

participants were also more likely to have more severe asthma and less likely to be treated with an ICS. However, the study was not designed or powered to accurately examine the effects of race or concomitant use of an ICS on modulating the effect of salmeterol. Although there were a number of flaws in this trial, the data resulted in a "black box" warning being placed on the salmeterol package insert advising of the potential risk of life-threatening asthma. The results of several subsequent pooled analyses of adverse effects of LABA have also supported the conclusion that unopposed LABA use is associated with asthma deaths. As a result, the U.S. FDA now recommends that (1) LABA not be used as monotherapy; (2) LABA not be used in patients whose asthma is well-controlled on ICS alone; (3) LABA be used in combination with another controller medication; and (4) LABA be discontinued as soon as possible after asthma control is achieved. In addition, a recent meta-analysis that used reports of events provided by the drug manufacturers to the FDA suggests that there is an increased risk of death with LABA use even with the use of an ICS.[70] These data remain controversial, and further large-scale trials are planned to determine the actual risk.

Some of the risk attributable to chronic LABA use may be attributed to polymorphisms in the *BAR* at the 16 position. Similar to the results obtained with chronic administration of SABA to those with the *Arg/Arg* polymorphism, it was suspected that a similar deterioration in pulmonary function and symptom control might occur with LABA use, even when given in conjunction with an ICS. In a prospective randomized cross-over 18-week study of ICS treatment plus LABA or placebo in adult patients stratified by *BAR* 16 polymorphisms *(Arg/Arg or Gly/Gly)*, there was no difference in the degree of improvement in PEFR or FEV_1 with the addition of LABA, regardless of genotype. However, those with the *Gly/Gly* polymorphism had a higher PC_{20} with LABA treatment compared to placebo; there was no difference in PC_{20} in the *Arg/Arg* group between placebo and LABA.[71] No difference in adverse effects were seen in either group. These data suggest that chronic use of LABA in combination with an ICS is safe in patients with either genotype. However, longer-duration treatment and larger-scale studies will be necessary to determine continued efficacy and safety.

A major benefit of LABAs is use in combination with an ICS to improve asthma control without increasing the steroid dose. A number of studies that included older children and adults have demonstrated that the addition of a LABA to a regimen that includes an ICS results in improved asthma control and improved pulmonary function compared to doubling the dose of ICS.[72] More importantly, the ICS dose can often be reduced by as much as 50% and still maintain asthma control when the LABA is added. Although the data are striking and consistent in studies on adults, there are fewer pediatric studies. An early study performed in 177 schoolchildren 6 to 16 years of age compared 400 mcg/day of BDP alone to 400 mcg BDP plus salmeterol 50 mcg/day to 800 mcg/day BDP for 52 weeks. The children, however, had extremely well-controlled asthma at enrollment in the study. All patients improved with respect to pulmonary function, symptom score, and airway reactivity, with no significant differences among the groups during the 1 year of treatment.[73] These data suggested that addition of a LABA to an ICS in pediatric patients may not have the same steroid-sparing effect or enhancement of steroid effect as that seen in adults. However, the participants all had relatively mild asthma and likely reached maximum treatment benefit at even the lowest dose of BDP tested. Therefore, the addition of a LABA or higher-dose ICS conferred no further benefit, but growth suppression occurred at the higher ICS dose. A more recent large multicenter trial (VIAPAED) compared the effect of salmeterol 50 mg plus fluticasone 100 mg combination (given in a single inhaler) compared to fluticasone 200 mg given twice daily for 8 weeks in 441 children 4 to 16 years of age whose asthma was not well controlled while taking an ICS alone.[74] The primary outcome was change in morning PEFR, and secondary outcomes examined asthma control. Children in the salmeterol plus fluticasone group had a significantly higher morning PEFR (30.4 ± 34.1 L/min combination versus 16.7 ± 35.8 L/min fluticasone) and a longer duration of asthma control (approximately 1 week longer, favoring combination). A recently published study conducted by the Childhood Asthma Research and Education Network in asthmatic children 6 to 17 years of age who were not well controlled on ICS alone examined the response to addition of LABA, doubling the dose of ICS, or adding montelukast.[75] Using a double-blind randomized triple-crossover design and a composite of three outcomes (exacerbations, asthma-control days, and FEV_1), this study demonstrated a differential response to the treatment steps in 161 of the 165 children enrolled. Although all treatments improved asthma control in most patients, the response to LABA step-up was most likely to be the best option compared to LTRA (1.6 relative probability) or double the dose of ICS (1.7 relative probability). White race or Hispanic ethnicity predicted a better response to LABA; African Americans were as likely to respond to LABA and double the dose of ICS and least likely to respond to LTRA. Neither baseline methacholine sensitivity nor FeNO predicted treatment response, but those with a higher ACT score (>19) and without eczema were more likely to respond to LABA. Last, genotype at the 16 position of the BAR receptor also did not predict best treatment response. Although all step-up options provided good symptom control during the trial, 120 courses of prednisone were prescribed to treat exacerbations, indicating that none of the step-up options eliminated acute asthma flares. However, the duration of this trial was relatively short (16 weeks), and issues of safety or long-term maintenance of effect remain unanswered. Although some would argue that doubling the dose of ICS may be safer and less expensive than adding a LABA or LTRA, the more important issue is to carefully and frequently monitor the patient with poorly controlled asthma who requires any step-up therapy to ensure both safety and efficacy. Failure to improve or the development of any adverse effect or medication intolerance warrants further medication adjustment and re-evaluation.

There are currently three fixed-dose combination inhaled steroid and LABA medications available; the dosing interval for all is every 12 hours. It is also possible to administer each medication separately from individual inhalers; however, this is less convenient for the patient, may be more expensive, and runs the risk of inadvertent overuse of LABA. Although use of separate inhalers does allow more flexibility in adjusting the dose of ICS, this strategy is not recommended because of the risks associated with unopposed LABA use. Salmeterol is combined with fluticasone in a dry-powder inhaler or MDI; the dose of salmeterol is fixed at 50 mcg per inhalation, while the fluticasone component is available in three different concentrations to allow for flexibility in dosing the ICS while avoiding excessive LABA use. A combination of formoterol and budesonide or mometasone is also available in dry-powder inhaler or MDI forms.

When the LABA combined with an ICS is formoterol, a different dosing strategy is possible because of the rapid onset of action of formoterol. When taken in combination with an ICS for relief of symptoms at the first sign of deterioration, the additional dose of ICS helps to prevent serious exacerbation. This strategy was examined in a large multicenter trial that evaluated 2760 asthmatics 4 to 80 years of age who were randomized to treatment with budesonide 320 mg twice daily and terbutaline as reliever, budesonide/formoterol 80/4.5 mg twice daily and terbutaline as reliever, or budesonide/formoterol 80/4.5 mg twice daily both as maintenance and reliever. The child treatment arm (4 to 11 years of age) was dosed at once a day.[75a,76] Both adults and children in the budesonide-formoterol as maintenance and reliever arm had significantly reduced risk of exacerbation compared to the other two treatment arms. The child study showed a significant reduction in severe exacerbations (defined as sustained fall in morning PEFR, need for oral corticosteroid, acute care visit or hospitalization); 14% of those in the combined maintenance plus reliever group had a severe exacerbation, compared to 38% in the budesonide/formoterol plus SABA group and 26% in the budesonide plus SABA group. In addition, the overall exposure to oral corticosteroids and exacerbations requiring medical attention was also significantly reduced in the maintenance plus reliever group. Last, linear growth over the year was approximately 1 cm greater in the groups receiving budesonide formoterol compared to the higher-dose budesonide group. Although this treatment approach has found acceptance in Europe, Australia, and Canada (but not in the United States), some concerns remain about safety and long-term effectiveness. Overuse of the budesonide/formoterol combination can occur, leading some patients to mask progressing symptoms or delay seeking medical attention. Overuse (or possibly any use) of LABA could also be detrimental to some patients, as suggested by recent systematic review of adverse events associated with LABA plus ICS use.[77] More studies are needed before the long-term safety and effectiveness, particularly in children, is established.

■ LEUKOTRIENE ANTAGONISTS

Leukotrienes are lipid mediators produced by the metabolism of arachidonic acid via a complex cascade, including the action of phospholipase A_2. The enzyme

5-lipoxygenase catalyzes the production of leukotrienes; LTB_4; and the cysteinyl members LTC_4, LTD_4, and LTE_4 from arachidonic acid. Arachidonic acid can also be a precursor for the cyclo-oxygenase pathway and results in the production of prostaglandins and thromboxane. However, it is the cysteinyl leukotrienes (cysLTs) that are the potent mediators that induce smooth muscle constriction, vascular permeability, mucus hypersecretion, edema formation, and inflammatory cell recruitment into the airways. Elevated levels of cysLTs are recovered from bronchoalveolar lavage fluid, and urinary LTE_4 levels are elevated following airway allergen challenge in atopic asthmatics. CysLTs are produced by a number of cell types found in the airways, including mast cells, eosinophils, basophils, macrophages, and neutrophils. Corticosteroids do not directly inhibit the synthesis or block the action of leukotrienes.

Two basic strategies targeting cysLTs include inhibition of 5-lipoxygenase and leukotriene receptor antagonism. Because of the nature of the lipoxygenase synthetic cascade, interruption at an early level (e.g., at the 5-lipoxygenase) could diminish overall cysteinyl LT and LTB production, both of which are generally elevated in biological fluids (i.e., blood, bronchoalveolar lavage fluid, urine) from symptomatic asthmatics. The 5-lipoxygenase inhibitor Zileuton blocks the bronchoconstrictor response to inhaled allergen or cold air challenge, exercise, and aspirin ingestion in sensitive individuals. However, because the drug must be given four times per day and reversible elevation of liver function tests are noted in some patients, it has limited clinical use and has largely been replaced by leukotriene receptor antagonists.

There are two clinically available leukotriene receptor antagonists: zafirlukast and montelukast. When administered orally, zafirlukast resulted in significant reduction in daytime and nighttime symptoms and the need for SABA compared with placebo. Zafirlukast has modest efficacy at best, must be given twice daily, and in some patients also results in elevated hepatic enzymes. Montelukast is a LTD_4 receptor antagonist and is administered once a day. It has been shown in a number of studies to decrease urinary excretion of LTE_4, reduce both circulating and sputum eosinophil counts, and decrease exhaled nitric oxide.[1] Clinical effects include improvement in FEV_1 and protection from EIB and allergen-induced bronchospasm. Improvement in pulmonary function can be detected after the first dose and reaches a peak after a few weeks of treatment. However, the montelukast effect on asthma control is not as great as that from an ICS, as measured by improvement in FEV_1, symptom control, and reduction in inflammatory markers. Treatment with montelukast results in more treatment failures than use of low-dose fluticasone. Other trials in children with slightly more significant disease based on lower FEV_1 also showed significantly greater improvement in pulmonary function measures, symptom reduction, and need for rescue SABA with fluticasone compared to montelukast.[78] Predicting which patients will have a more favorable response to montelukast versus ICSs has proven difficult. However, a study examining the rate of response of children with mild asthma to ICS, montelukast, or both demonstrated that 23% responded to fluticasone alone, 5% responded to montelukast alone, 17% responded to both, but 55% responded to neither drug.[79] However, children who are older and have had asthma for a longer duration, have a parental history of asthma, have a higher exhaled nitric oxide, and have a lower PC_{20} are more likely to respond favorably to ICS treatment compared to LTRA treatment.[80] Montelukast may provide improved asthma control when combined with other controller medications, such as inhaled steroids. Although study results are somewhat conflicting, most show that the addition of montelukast to an ICS results in modest improvement that is not quite as efficacious as adding an LABA, particularly on pulmonary function outcomes. One pediatric trial demonstrated a small improvement in FEV_1 (6.0% montelukast, 4.1% placebo, $P < .01$) and in the need for rescue bronchodilator use (1.65 puffs/day montelukast, 1.98 puffs/day placebo, $P < .013$) when montelukast was added to a regimen of low-dose BUD.[81] Adverse effects of montelukast have been relatively minor and mainly consist of headache, abdominal pain, vivid dreams, and sleep disruption. Recent reports of behavioral changes (e.g., moodiness, depression) and an unsubstantiated association with a suicide report have led to a label change including behavioral changes as a possible side effect of treatment with montelukast. There are several case reports of adults who developed Churg-Strauss syndrome when treatment with montelukast was instituted and ICS treatment withdrawn. Since the majority of these patients had what was considered to be severe steroid-dependent asthma, it is believed that the development of systemic vasculitis was actually the emergence of an underlying disease as a result of steroid withdrawal and less likely a result of the direct action of montelukast. Care should be taken, however, if montelukast is used in an attempt to decrease or discontinue oral steroids in a patient with presumed severe asthma.

OTHER DRUGS

Methylxanthines: Theophylline

Although methylxanthines have been used for the treatment of asthma since the early part of the twentieth century, their role in managing acute and chronic asthma has become very restricted. Theophylline is now considered a second- or third-line medication, largely because it is a poor acute bronchodilator, it has a narrow therapeutic index and significant adverse effects, and other anti-inflammatory drugs have replaced it. It does have the advantage of being inexpensive and can be administered in a long-acting oral formulation.

Theophylline is a phosphodiesterase inhibitor that causes smooth muscle relaxation and bronchodilation. However, theophylline can also act centrally as a respiratory stimulant and may also increase diaphragmatic contractility and help prevent diaphragmatic fatigue. In addition, more recent data suggests that it blocks histone deacetylation, which may be important to the action of corticosteroids and modulation of inflammatory mediators; further work is necessary to confirm the clinical relevance of this action. Low-dose theophylline (amounts sufficient to cause a serum level between 5 to 10 mg/mL) may be helpful in some patients for chronic management. The addition of theophylline to ICSs may have a steroid-sparing effect in some patients, but it is less effective than adding a long-acting β agonist. Use in the intensive care unit in patients with severe exacerbation has been reported to improve resolution of the acute episode and shorten stay in the intensive care unit.

However, adverse effects, such as tremor, gastric irritation, gastrointestinal hemorrhage, agitation, and convulsions, may occur at even relatively low serum concentrations. Many commonly used medications can interfere with theophylline metabolism resulting in clinically significant elevation (e.g., some macrolide and fluoroquinolone antibiotics) or lowering (carbamezipine) of serum concentrations. Febrile viral illnesses may also substantially increase serum concentrations. Careful monitoring of serum concentration is mandatory when doses above 10 mg/kg/day are administered to children and adolescents.

CROMOLYN SODIUM AND NEDOCROMIL

Inhaled cromolyn has a mild anti-inflammatory action and clinical benefit in children and adolescents with mild to moderate asthma. Comparative studies and a recent meta-analysis suggest that cromolyn has minimal effect on controlling chronic asthma, and previous reports of efficacy may have been confounded by publication bias. Cromolyn is effective in preventing EIB, but less so than a SABA. Cromolyn MDI is no longer available in the United States, and the nebulizer formulation must be used three to four times a day.

Nedocromil sodium, another NSAID agent, was compared to placebo and inhaled BUD in the CAMP study. It was effective in reducing symptoms and exacerbations compared with placebo, but less so than BUD.[14] Nedocromil is no longer available in the United States. Both drugs have an excellent safety profile, with cough, unpleasant taste (nedrocomil), and throat irritation being the most common adverse events.

A number of medications currently used for other indications have been utilized in the treatment of severe, refractory asthma with varying degrees of success. Gold salts, methotrexate, and cyclosporine all have anti-inflammatory properties and have had some efficacy in ameliorating severe, steroid-resistant asthma. However, these medications have significant untoward effects, limited efficacy, or both, and they are rarely used.

Several other novel approaches to asthma therapy involve immune modulation, which may be useful for both the prevention and treatment of asthma. Use of a humanized monoclonal anti-IgE antibody (omalizumab) to complex with and lower the circulating concentration of IgE has demonstrated efficacy in select patients. This drug is approved by the U.S. Food and Drug Administration for use in patients 12 years of age and older and in Europe (but not the United Kingdom) for children 6 years of age and older. Omalizumab is a recombinant DNA-derived human monoclonal antibody that binds to serum IgE to form complexes that prevent IgE from binding to high-affinity sites (FcεRI) on mast cells and basophils. The IgE-mediated cross-linking of allergen and subsequent inflammatory mediator release and production is thereby prevented. Omalizumab has multiple immunomodulatory effects that include reducing sputum eosinophils; downregulating FcεRI on basophils, mast cells, and dendritic cells; and reducing both early- and late-phase asthmatic responses after allergen challenge. Omalizumab is administered subcutaneously every 2 to 4 weeks, and the dose and interval of administration is determined by serum IgE level and patient weight. The dose is based on the amount of drug necessary to reduce serum-free IgE to about 10 IU/mL. Because it is not recommended to administer more than 375 mg of omalizumab per treatment, individuals who have circulating IgE levels above 700 IU/mL are not generally considered candidates for treatment; however, in the UK at least, the upper limit of IgE has been raised to 1300 IU/mL.

Current U.S. and European guidelines restrict recommending treatment with omalizumab to patients with moderate to severe allergic asthma who continue to have poorly controlled asthma while receiving step 5 or 6 treatment.[1,43] Treatment with omalizumab (when administered with inhaled and/or oral corticosteroids plus LABA) reduces the ICS dose required to maintain asthma control, decreases exacerbations (including emergency visits and hospitalizations), decreases the need for rescue medication, decreases reported symptoms, and improves quality of life. The data on improving lung function are somewhat conflicting, although airway hyperresponsiveness may be improved. The degree of improvement in most studies has been modest and offset by the substantial effects in the placebo groups. In one large trial in adults comparing omalizumab to ICS plus LABA, there was a reduction in the exacerbation rate during a 28-week treatment trial.[82] However, the effect was modest (0.68 versus 0.91; $P = 0.042$) and significant only after posthoc adjustment for exacerbations occurring in the previous year. Trials in children 6 to 12 years of age treated with moderate to high doses of ICS also showed modest improvement in exacerbation rates and symptom measures during both constant and tapering doses of ICS.[83] However, due to safety concerns, particularly regarding development of malignancy, cardiovascular events, and anaphylaxis, the U.S. FDA has not approved the drug for use in children younger than 12 years of age.

Adverse effects have been mild and comparable with those receiving placebo. Reports of anaphylactic or serious allergic reactions occurring hours to days after initial or subsequent injections occur infrequently but must be anticipated. Treatment is extremely expensive (~$12,000 per year) and is likely to be cost-effective only when used in patients who respond well and have had frequent serious exacerbations in the past. In addition, not all patients respond favorably to omalizumab, and predicting who will respond remains difficult. Among those receiving treatment with omalizumab, only about 60% will demonstrate a clinical response. Baseline patient characteristics (e.g., serum IgE level, lung function, height, or weight) were not consistently useful in predicting responder status. Patients should be observed for at least 16 weeks of treatment before determining if a positive response to treatment has occurred.

Treatment with monoclonal antibodies targeting important proinflammatory cytokines have yielded mixed results. An early study examining the administration of anti-IL-5 antibody resulted in significant reduction in circulating and airway eosinophils without significant improvement in asthma symptoms or pulmonary function. However, a more recent study that targeted patients with severe eosinophilic asthma showed a significant reduction in exacerbations and improvement in quality of life with mepolizumab treatment compared to placebo.[84] Preliminary studies using the combined IL-4/IL-13 antagonist, pitrakinra, has demonstrated the ability to block allergen-induced bronchospasm in allergic asthmatics. These studies highlight the importance of careful asthma phenotype characterization in order to target treatments to patients most likely to accrue benefit.

Immunotherapy for asthma may afford some promise, particularly with the use of newer antigens, such as immunostimulatory DNA sequences and CpG DNA vaccines. Sublingual vaccines against single allergens such as grass pollen have also shown promise in both treating and preventing asthma. Larger-scale trials with other allergens including cockroach are currently underway.

MANAGEMENT OF CHRONIC ASTHMA

The effective management of chronic asthma should focus on (1) identification and elimination of exacerbating or aggravating factors, (2) pharmacologic therapy, and (3) education of the patient and family about the disease and the management skills necessary to avoid and treat acute exacerbations. The goals of effective management of chronic asthma in children include minimizing symptoms and exacerbations, maintaining normal activities of daily living, maintaining normal or near-normal pulmonary function, and avoiding adverse effects from asthma medications. To achieve these goals, a combination of pharmacologic and nonpharmacologic modalities must be utilized.

Successful asthma management includes appropriate grading of disease control (see Table 47-3). Asthma severity, or the intrinsic intensity of the disease, should be distinguished from asthma control. Patients may have relatively mild asthma that is poorly controlled due to multiple factors, such as inadequate treatment, impaired adherence, or excessive exposure to allergens or irritants. Once appropriate medical and environmental measures are instituted, the asthma may become "mild" in terms of absence of symptoms and normalization of pulmonary function while taking low doses of a controller medication. Patients who demonstrate a progressive decline in pulmonary function, frequent exacerbations, and persistent or recurrent symptoms in spite of regular use of controller medication and environmental controls have more severe disease.

The emphasis in most guidelines is now placed on establishing asthma control, which includes minimizing impairment (symptoms) and avoiding risk of serious exacerbations, medication adverse effects, loss of lung function, and (in the case of children) reduction in lung growth. As discussed earlier in the chapter, other biomarkers of airway inflammation (eNO, sputum eosinophils, markers of oxidative stress in exhaled breath condensate) in some circumstances add additional useful data for grading asthma severity and guiding treatment to improve control. Several brief, validated questionnaires can be used in most clinical or community settings to provide a rapid assessment of asthma control. The Asthma Control Test, Asthma Control Questionnaire, and Asthma Therapy Assessment Questionnaire all provide a numeric score based on answers to questions about daytime symptoms, nighttime symptoms, activity limitation, SABA use, and a global question about perceived asthma control.[1] The scores equate to well-controlled, not well-controlled, and poorly controlled asthma, and they provide an easy, rapid assessment of the impairment domain of asthma control. Although the utility of the scores as a point in time measure is established, the responsiveness to change over time, collection of data in relation to recent exacerbation, and seasonal variability all need further evaluation.

The risk domain of control includes exacerbations that are severe enough to warrant treatment with oral corticosteroids, emergency medical care, or hospitalizations. There are limited data that are useful in predicting future exacerbations; however, there is an inverse relationship between FEV_1 and the risk of developing an exacerbation in the subsequent year. In addition, having one severe exacerbation is a strong risk for a subsequent episode in the same year. Data are lacking to accurately correlate the number and severity of exacerbations with degree of asthma control, More than one exacerbation per year indicates asthma control is inadequate and the frequency and severity of exacerbations increases with worsening control. Patients should start treatment at the step most appropriate to the initial severity grading (or control level for those already receiving treatment) of their asthma.

The most recent National Asthma Education and Prevention Program (NAEPP) guidelines continue to list four severity classifications: intermittent, mild, moderate, and severe persistent, but have expanded the stepwise treatment algorithm to 6 steps (Fig. 47-5). Immunotherapy continues to be recommended for children who are at steps 2 to 4, have documented allergy, and have persistent symptoms. However, immunotherapy is most likely to be effective for those with single allergen sensitization, and this evidence for efficacy is strongest for animal dander, house dust mites, and pollen. The two added treatment steps for adolescents and adults are aimed at those who are allergic, have refractory symptoms in spite of high-dose ICSs plus another anti-inflammatory controller. At these steps 5 and 6, recommended additional treatment includes oral corticosteroids and omalizumab for those older than 12 years of age who are also allergic. The treatment steps are used in conjunction with control levels. Patients who achieve good control are maintained at the lowest step level possible. Those with not well-controlled or poorly controlled asthma receive step-up

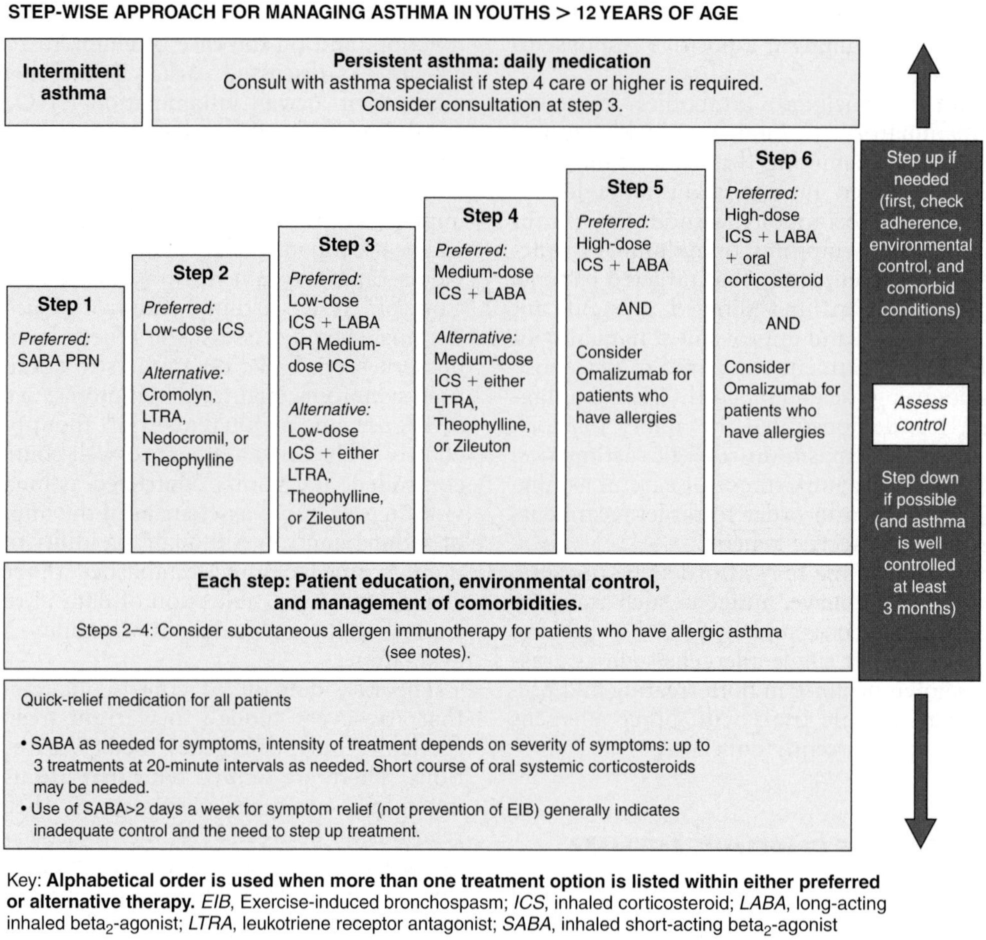

STEP-WISE APPROACH FOR MANAGING ASTHMA IN YOUTHS > 12 YEARS OF AGE

FIGURE 47-5. Stepwise treatment algorithm for chronic treatment of children and adolescents with asthma.

treatment until control is achieved. Step-down to a lower treatment level should be attempted once control is maintained for at least 3 months and no other contraindications for reducing medication exist (e.g., persistent allergen exposure, entry into high-risk season). Patient education, environmental controls, and management of co-morbid conditions are stressed at all steps. In addition, it is critical that all patients and their adult caregivers be thoroughly trained in the appropriate use of the specific medication delivery devices and monitoring tools prescribed (e.g., MDI, DPI, nebulizer, PEFR meter).

INTERMITTENT ASTHMA

Children with intermittent asthma or EIA have brief episodes of wheeze or cough that are easily relieved with SABA treatment and occur no more frequently than once or twice per week. Treatment is with the as-needed use of an inhaled SABA agonist.[1] The usual dose of inhaled racemic albuterol is 2 to 6 puffs (90 mcg/puff) every 3 to 4 hours or 0.15 mg/kg (usual dose 2.5 mg, maximum 5 mg) nebulized from a small-volume nebulizer in 2 mL of saline. Other SABAs (e.g., pirbuterol, levalbuterol, and terbutaline) may also be used, and it is unlikely that there is any significant difference in efficacy among the drugs.

Numerous studies have demonstrated that administration of albuterol by MDI is equally effective as that given by nebulizer.[1,43] Moreover, use of an MDI by older children (with or without a valved holding chamber) is far more convenient and less expensive than a nebulizer. EIA may be prevented to large extent with inhalation of albuterol (or formoterol) 5 to 20 minutes before exercise. Montelukast taken 1 to 2 hours before exercise may also help prevent EIB.

MILD PERSISTENT ASTHMA

The majority of asthmatics are classified as having mild persistent asthma, based on symptoms that occur several times per week, but not daily; infrequent nocturnal symptoms; and normal pulmonary function. The primary treatment of mild persistent asthma is a low-dose ICS. Data from multiple studies support the superior efficacy of ICSs compared with other treatments in improving pulmonary function, reducing symptoms and need for rescue medications, and improving bronchial hyperreactivity. As outlined previously, the safety profile for ICSs given at low dose is excellent. There are few data to suggest that one type of ICS will offer significantly greater benefit than the others, but the dose equivalency and ranges for low, medium, and high doses differ (see Table 47-5).

Beclomethasone, fluticasone, and budesonide have been extensively studied in children for many years, are available in easy-to-use devices (MDIs or dry-powder inhalers), are well-tolerated by most patients, and the adverse event profile is well understood. Large comparative effectiveness trials, particularly in children, are sparse. However, a recent retrospective observational study that used a large general practice research database in the United Kingdom examined asthma control in newly treated asthmatics 5 to 60 years of age. Using a matched cohort analysis, over 2600 patients, including 773 children age 5 to 12 years of age who were prescribed HFA, BDP, or FP, were followed for 2 years. Although more than 80% of the patients in each group achieved control, patients who were treated with or received step-up treatment with BDP were more likely to be controlled (adjusted odds ratio 1.30 (95% CI, 1.02 to 1.65).[85] However, the control measure used was a composite of largely risk domain elements (i.e., exacerbation, oral steroid use, hospitalization) and likely missed impairment domain measures (symptoms). Older inhaled steroids (e.g., flunisolide, triamcinolone) with lower topical potency are used less frequently. Newer inhaled steroids, such as ciclesonide, are currently labeled for use in the United States for children 12 years of age and older.

Although chronic daily dosing of ICS is the general recommendation to maintain good asthma control, other strategies have been investigated and hold promise as valid alternatives. There are a few studies that have compared chronic daily inhaled steroid use with intermittent treatment. In a study of 225 adults (18 to 65 years) with mild persistent asthma but no history of unscheduled visits or hospitalizations in the previous year, participants were randomized to treatment with 200 mcg of budesonide twice a day, zafirlukast twice a day, or placebo for 12 months.[86] Using a symptom-based action plan, participants who developed an exacerbation were instructed to begin treatment with 800 mcg twice daily of budesonide for 10 days or 0.5 mg/kg of prednisone for 5 days if symptoms worsened. There was no difference among groups in the primary outcome of change from baseline morning PEFR, or in the secondary outcome of exacerbations. However, those in the daily budesonide group had fewer symptom days (26 over 12 months), higher asthma control scores, lower FeNO and sputum eosinophils, but not asthma-related quality of life scores, than those in the other two groups. Interestingly, among the 76 patients in the placebo (intermittent ICS use) group, 1 used a single short course of ICS and 9 used 2 courses, resulting in an average per-patient use of ICS of only 0.48 week during the yearlong study. Although this study has not yet been replicated, it suggests that mild asthmatics who do not have frequent severe exacerbations could be successfully managed with intermittent ICS treatment initiated at the onset of an exacerbation. This strategy appears to benefit the risk domain more than the impairment (daily symptom) domain preferentially; therefore, if daily symptom burden reduction is more important that infrequent and mild exacerbation reduction, a daily treatment strategy may be preferable. Implications for pediatric asthma management with intermittent steroid use may be even greater, since the risk, albeit minor, of growth suppression is higher in children. A study examining the intermittent use of budesonide compared to daily budesonide or cromolyn use also demonstrated that good control could be achieved in some patients with intermittent treatment.[87] Children with mild asthma who were diagnosed within the previous year were randomized to receive treatment with 400 mcg budesonide twice daily for 1 month then 400 mcg daily for the next 2 to 6 months or cromolyn sodium 10 mg nebulized 3 times a day. Children in the budesonide group were further divided after 6 months of continuous treatment; one group received 200 mcg per day for 7 to 18 months and the other received placebo. All participants began treatment with 400 mcg bid of budesonide for 2 weeks to treat any exacerbation. Those who required oral corticosteroids or other treatment were withdrawn from the study. There was no difference among the groups in the primary outcome of improvement in morning PEFR at any point in the study. Those in the budesonide group had fewer exacerbations while receiving continuous treatment compared to those in the cromolyn or intermittent group (mean 0.97), compared with 1.69 in group 2 and 1.58. The number of asthma free days did not differ between the continuous and intermittent budesonide groups. Growth velocity and total linear growth was reduced (~ 1.0 cm) in the continuous group compared to intermittent and cromolyn groups. However, growth velocity improved during the placebo period. These data suggest that some patients with mild asthma of relatively new onset may achieve adequate control after a period of stabilization with continuous ICS treatment, with intermittent ICS use, and with less risk of minor growth suppression. However, daily use of an ICS, even when tapered to low dose, provides the best overall control, particularly in the exacerbation risk domain.

An alternative treatment is a leukotriene receptor antagonist, such as montelukast. This drug has the advantage of once-a-day oral administration and only uncommon mild adverse effects (i.e., nausea, headache, vivid dreams). However, numerous comparative studies indicate that ICSs provide superior asthma control. Although the current NAEPP guidelines still list cromolyn, nedocromil, and theophylline as alternative treatments, nedocromil and cromolyn have limited availability and efficacy, and theophylline is less well tolerated.

MODERATE PERSISTENT ASTHMA

Children who have daily symptoms, nocturnal symptoms more than weekly, and mild obstruction on pulmonary function have moderate persistent asthma. Children who continue to experience symptoms or exacerbations while being treated with low-dose ICSs should have a step up in treatment. Current recommendations for treatment include increasing the ICS dose to the moderate range, or continuing the low-dose ICS and adding a second controller drug with a complimentary mechanism of action. As discussed earlier in the chapter, the dose response curve for ICSs reaches a plateau at relatively modest doses, as determined by pulmonary function and bronchial hyperreactivity measures. However, certain patients may derive benefit in both the impairment and risk domains when the ICS dose is increased to the moderate range. LABAs are the current add-on drugs of choice because of the large body of evidence from randomized controlled trials that indicate efficacy and effectiveness. In older children and adults, the addition of a LABA to a low-dose ICS results in greater improvement in pulmonary function and reduction in symptoms than a further increase in steroid dose. The availability of a fixed-dose combination of fluticasone and salmeterol or BUD and formoterol in a single dry-powder inhaler make this combination attractive. An alternative is to raise the dose of the inhaled steroid alone to the medium range; this is the current recommended strategy (US EPR 3) for children younger than 4 years of age, but is a secondary option in older children. When concerns exist about the use of LABA or medium-dose ICSs, addition of a leukotriene receptor antagonist (e.g., montelukast) should be considered. Although the additive effect of LTRA is more limited, the safety profile may be viewed as more favorable. LTRA when added to inhaled BUD in one study resulted in a modest improvement in PEFR and a reduction in need for SABA.[81] Low-dose theophylline is another low-cost add-on medication that may also help improved symptom control.

Data indicate that the latter two add-on medications are also effective in improving asthma control, but less so than with the addition of the LABA. Use of theophylline as a single daily dose of a time-release preparation can be well tolerated and is typically less expensive than using a LABA or LTRA. Any patient who has deterioration of lung function while using a LABA chronically should have an alternative medication prescribed. Whatever combination of medications is used, attempts should be made at regular intervals to decrease the ICS dose to the lowest level that adequately controls symptoms and maintains normal pulmonary function. Children in this category will benefit from referral to a pulmonologist and may also require ongoing specialty care.

SEVERE PERSISTENT ASTHMA

Approximately 5% to 10% of patients will have severe persistent asthma as described by persistent daily symptoms, frequent nocturnal awakenings, and a moderate or severe obstructive pattern on pulmonary function testing. These symptoms may occur in spite of treatment with high-dose ICSs, LABAs, and/or a LTRA or low-dose theophylline. Patients with the most severe disease have inadequate response to even high doses of ICS in combination with other available controller medications. If there is no response, oral corticosteroids are the next recommended treatment step. It may be necessary to administer a short course (<10 days) of daily dosing (40 to 60 mg/day) and then a longer every-other-day course at the lowest effective dose (0.5 mg/kg every other day). Before instituting such therapy, a thorough search for remediable exacerbating factors or co-morbid conditions (e.g., sinusitis, persistent allergen exposure, poor compliance, GER, vocal cord dysfunction) should be sought. As soon as symptoms are controlled, the lowest possible oral steroid dose at which symptom control is maintained should be administered. Although a single morning dose is generally preferred to minimize systemic side effects, some

patients with severe or refractory symptoms may benefit from twice-daily dosing. Children receiving chronic oral corticosteroid therapy should be carefully monitored for development of adverse effects, such as hypertension, cataract formation, hyperglycemia, loss of bone mineral content, and impaired linear growth. Systemic corticosteroids may be given in the presence of acute viral infections, otitis media, or pneumonia and will not result in worsening infections. However, patients who develop varicella while taking systemic corticosteroids or take the medication during the incubation period should have the steroid dose reduced to the minimum tolerable to control the asthma and be provided adrenal replacement. In addition, consideration should be given to administering acyclovir for 5 to 7 days. The patient should also be carefully observed for signs of severe or disseminated disease. If there has been a significant exposure to varicella identified within the previous 96 hours, passive immunization with varicella zoster immune globulin can be offered. Children with persistent asthma should receive varicella vaccine if they have not previously contracted the disease.

A proportion of severe asthmatics may be steroid resistant; in one series of patients with refractory asthma, 25% were determined to be steroid resistant. Such patients may have altered steroid metabolism or receptor dysfunction. A careful evaluation and specialized pharmacokinetic and cellular studies may be needed to ascertain the etiology of the defect. Patients deemed to be steroid resistant may be candidates for alternative therapies, such as omalizumab or other immunosuppressants.

Children with severe asthma should receive routine care from a specialist. Frequent visits to assess symptom control, pulmonary function testing, quality of life, patterns of medication use, presence of comorbid conditions, adverse effects caused by treatment, and adherence to treatment regimen are essential.

HOLDING CHAMBERS AND SPACER DEVICES

A number of studies indicate that as many as 80% of patients use MDIs incorrectly even after appropriate instruction, and many residents, physicians, and nurses are unable to teach patients correctly. Proper steps are given in Table 47-6. Although there is a relatively small difference in the amount of medication that reaches the lower respiratory tract from a properly used MDI alone compared with an MDI plus a valved holding chamber (10% for MDI alone, 15% for MDI plus holding chamber), valved holding chamber use helps ensure that the maximum possible dose reaches its target. The holding chamber also minimizes deposition of the medication in the mouth and oropharynx, a particularly important feature when ICSs are prescribed. There are several important points to remember when using a VHC. The child should take a slow deep inspiration and try to hold his or her breath for 5 to 10 seconds. Only one medication should be dispensed into the chamber at a time, although the same chamber may be used for other medications. A holding chamber that is of at least 150 mL volume and

TABLE 47-6 DIRECTIONS FOR USE OF A METERED-DOSE INHALER, WITH AND WITHOUT A SPACER

MDI USE WITHOUT SPACER DEVICE	MDI USE WITH SPACER DEVICE
1. Shake canister for 5 seconds.	1. Shake canister for 5 seconds.
2. Position finger on top of canister for support.	2. Attach canister to spacer.
3. Patient exhales normally (to FRC).	3. Patient exhales normally (to FRC).
4. Place mouthpiece 2 cm in front of open mouth around tube (may place in mouth if coordination is a problem).	4. Place mouthpiece in mouth and close lips.
5. Begin slow inspiration.	5. Activate canister.
6. Activate canister.	6. Begin slow inspiration.
7. Complete inhalation over several seconds.	7. Complete inhalation over several seconds.
8. Hold breath for 10 seconds.	8. Hold breath for 10 seconds.
9. Wait 30-60 seconds, and repeat steps 2-8 for prescribed number of inhalations.	9. Wait 30-60 seconds, and repeat steps 2-8 for prescribed number of inhalations.

that accommodates the MDI canister in its original boot is preferable to one that requires the canister to be inserted into an adapter. The latter chambers may not result in accurate dispensing of medication because of a mismatch between the adapter and the actuator. Newer holding chambers are made of antistatic plastics or metal that minimize static charge, which can cause excessive retention of medication in the chamber. Washing the chamber with a mild detergent and air drying can also help prevent static charge.

PEAK EXPIRATORY FLOW RATE MONITORING

Home monitoring of PEFR has been advocated for optimal management of the patient with moderate to severe persistent asthma, but the utility remains somewhat limited. PEFR is only moderately correlated with FEV_1, and other measures such as such as FEF_{25-75}, FEF_{50}, or MMEF can be used as a valid measure of obstructive ventilatory defect. The degree of diurnal and day-to-day PEFR variability has been proposed for years as a marker of asthma severity and airway hyperreactivity. However, the correlation between PEFR variability and AHR is only moderate. Moreover, the correlation of PEFR variability with other clinical markers of asthma disease activity or severity remains unclear. PEFR probably has its greatest value when used repeatedly to indicate severity of an acute asthma exacerbation and the subsequent response to treatment. Normal PEFR ranges are determined by the patient's age, sex, and height and are readily available. Some patients have PEFR readings well above, or in some cases below published standards. For this reason, an individual patient's personal best reading is often used as a target. It is important that the personal best be determined only when efforts have been made to ensure that asthma is optimally managed at the time the measure is made; this may require short courses of oral corticosteroids and other anti-inflammatory medications.

Small portable handheld PEFR devices can provide an objective measure of lung function in the home or school setting. Newer devices record measurement electronically and some also measure FEV_1 and FEV_6. Patients may use the PEFR reading to alter medications according to a predetermined plan. Patients and families must know when and how to use the PEFR meter, how to interpret the measurement and respond to the reading, and when to communicate with their physician. Some of these steps can be obviated with the use of a commercial system that uses a recording PEFR meter capable of transmitting via phone line or the Internet, a longitudinal collection of readings synthesized into a report to the managing physician. Although earlier guideline recommendations were that all patients with asthma use a PEFR-driven asthma action plan, studies suggest that routine use of PEFR monitoring is more likely to benefit those with more severe or unstable disease and is more likely to be used intermittently (around the time of increased symptoms, seasonally) rather than continuously.[1,43]

After determining the target, normal, or personal best PEFR reading, a care plan incorporating the measure can be made. Sample plans may be obtained in readily available sources (Fig. 47-6).[1]

The zones are generally defined as follows:

Green: PEFR 80% to 100% predicted/personal best; all clear, no symptoms.

Yellow: PEFR 50% to 80% predicted/personal best; indicates worsening airway obstruction or an impending attack. Symptoms include slowed play, intermittent cough, wheeze, and dyspnea.

Red: PEFR less than 50% predicted/personal best; indicates significant airway obstruction and need for immediate medical attention. Symptoms include severe dyspnea, retractions, continuous wheeze, or cough.

There are limitations to PEFR monitoring efficacy. The PEFR is effort dependent; some children learn how to deliberately adjust the reading artificially high or low by the effort used. In addition, PEFR only measures obstruction in the large central airways; many asthmatics have a normal or near-normal PEFR, but significant obstruction

ASTHMA ACTION PLAN

PLAN FOR: _____ Date: _____ Nurse: _____ Doctor: Dr. _____

Hospital/Emergency Phone Number: _xxx-xxx-xxxx/ 911 Doctor's Phone: _xxx-xxx-xxxx (weekdays) / xxx-xxx-xxxx (night and weekend)

GREEN ZONE: Doing Well

Take these control medicines every single day. They work to keep your lungs healthy and prevent asthma symptoms.

- No cough, wheeze, chest tightness, or shortness of breath during day or night

- Can do usual activities

PEAK FLOW between _____ and _____

(80%–100% of my best)

Medicine	How much to take	When to take it

Before running or sports:

☐ _____ ☐ 2 puffs ☐ 4 puffs ☐ 1 aerosol ☐ 5 to 20 minutes ☐ 60 minutes
before exercise

YELLOW ZONE: Asthma Getting Worse

- Cough, wheeze, chest tightness, or shortness of breath, or
- Waking at night due to asthma, or
- Can do some, but NOT all activities

PEAK FLOW between _____ and _____

(50%–80% of my best)

First: **Add quick-relief medicine:** Albuterol, ventolin, proventil, maxair, or xopenx
Inhaler ☐ 2 to 4 puffs   **OR**   ☐ **aerosol machine** (1 vial) once

Next: AFTER 1 hour
- IF your symptoms return to the GREEN ZONE:
  ☐ Take the quick-relief medicine every 6–8 hours for 1–2 days

- IF your symptoms **DO NOT** return to the GREEN ZONE:
  ☐ Repeat quick-relief medication NOW and then every 4–6 hours for 1–2 days
  ☐ ADD/DOUBLE inhaled steroid: _____ puffs/vial twice daily for 7–10 days
  ☐ **Advair:** stop 100/50 and start higher strength preparation: 250/50 or 500/50
  ☐ Add
  ☐ Call doctor for more advice

Remember: Continue all green zone medications.

RED ZONE: Medical Alert!

- Very short of breath, or
- Quick-relief medicines have not helped, or
- Cannot do usual activities, or
- Symptoms are the same or worse after 24 hours in the yellow zone

PEAK FLOW less than _____

(less than 50% of my best)

Add this medicine (In addition to green and yellow zone medicines):
☐ **Albuterol or** _____ ☐ 4 puffs or ☐ aerosol machine

☐ **Repeat albuterol or** _____ **in 20 minutes if NOT better**

☐ **Oral steroid: one dose a day for 3–5 days**
   Take _____ pills (_____ mg) prednisone **OR** Take _____ cc/mL Prelone or Orapred

Then: • **Call your asthma doctor (xxx-xxx-xxxx) or pediatrician** *NOW.*
      • Go to the hospital or call an ambulance if your child is still in the RED ZONE after 20 minutes **AND** you have not reached the doctor.

FIGURE 47-6. Sample treatment plan form for management of chronic asthma. Instructions may use peak expiratory flow rate monitoring in addition to symptoms to assess the need for additional treatment.

in the small airways or as measured by FEV_1 or FEV_1/FVC. Moreover, it is unclear that long-term PEFR use as part of an asthma action plan results in better outcomes than monitoring symptoms without PEFR and adjusting therapy accordingly.[14] Studies indicate similar outcomes with asthma action plans with or without PEFR use.

NONPHARMACOLOGIC MEASURES

Nonpharmacologic interventions necessary for successful management include formation of an effective partnership with a knowledgeable health care provider, frequent monitoring of asthma symptoms and response to therapy, objective measures of pulmonary function, and avoidance of asthma triggers. Trigger avoidance is important, yet patients are often unaware of specific triggers or how to put environmental controls in place. Environmental exposures (e.g., diesel particulates, ozone, sulfur dioxide) are likely to be more pronounced in those living near highways, on bus lines, or near certain industrial plants. For the indoor environment, dust mites, cat and dog dander, mold, and, in the inner city, cockroach antigen all have been strongly linked to asthma exacerbations and morbidity. Removal of these allergens can result in reduced symptoms and airway hyperresponsiveness. However, it is difficult to reduce indoor allergen burden below the threshold likely to induce symptoms without a multifaceted approach. The use of room air filters and special cleaning agents have some appeal but are not as effective as keeping ambient humidity low (30% to 40%), putting plasticized covers on pillows and mattresses, washing bedding weekly in hot water, and removing carpeting. A recent study suggested that application of dust covers alone is not effective in improving airway function. Removing pets from the bedroom and ideally from the household is also desirable. Exterminating roaches is difficult, but use of integrated pest management strategies and eliminating water sources can be effective. For all asthmatics, avoidance of passive exposure to cigarette smoke is of paramount importance. The Inner-City Asthma Study utilized a multidimensional environmental intervention that instructed families on providing a "safe sleeping zone" for the asthmatic child. Pets, dust, and other irritants were barred from the sleeping area, and HEPA room filters and vacuums were provided to all. In addition, specific strategies to reduce mold and roaches were implemented in households where dust sampling revealed high levels. This integrated and individualized strategy resulted in significant allergen reduction and improvement in symptom-free days over the yearlong intervention and beyond.[88] Another trial optimized asthma medical care and control and then provided a mold and moisture remediation program that removed existing mold and repaired construction defects and leaks that promoted the mold problem. Compared to those who lived in homes not remediated, the children in the intervention group had more symptom-free days and fewer serious exacerbations.[89]

Use of ancillary personnel (e.g., a social worker who can conduct formal risk assessment of psychosocial, economic, and school-related risks) may be of great benefit

in improving asthma control. Social determinants of chronic disease management often relate to, or operate through, poverty. Substandard housing, limited access to high-quality medical care, and transportation and child care barriers can all contribute to poor asthma control in patients from lower socioeconomic groups. Impaired maternal mental health, lack of social supports, and child behavior problems may all contribute to poor adherence and asthma control.

Adherence to a treatment regimen is key to successful asthma management. Adherence differs from compliance, in that adherence stresses the role of the patient and family in helping to develop a treatment program and contributing to the strategies necessary to utilize the treatment plan. Compliance implies that a patient must utilize a plan derived by the physician; failure to do so indicates that the patient is at fault and irresponsible. The factors that contribute to adherence are complex and incompletely understood. It is difficult to predict which patients will have good adherence, and it is not well correlated with race, gender, or intelligence. Moreover, many patients overreport good adherence in an attempt to please the physician. Adherence to suggested medical treatment for asthma often ranges from 30% to 70% use of prescribed medicine. Families should be encouraged to identify areas of a treatment regimen that might offer difficulty, concerns they have about medications, and lifestyle issues that might impair adherence. Physicians must be willing to provide suitable alternatives (e.g., medications, dose schedules). Regularly scheduled office visits should be conducted to evaluate the success of the treatment plan and offer the patient the opportunity to voice concerns and ask for help. When a child or the parents fail to adhere, the physician should try to find out the reasons and to work out a practical solution that is acceptable to the patient and family. Use of motivational interviewing techniques and shared decision-making strategies can often provide better results that direct reminders.

Patients must be given ready access to medical advice, for example, over the telephone, including how to deal with school-related asthma management and behavior problems. Other technologies, such as text messaging, email, videoconferencing, and social networking are also gaining popularity as ways to communicate with patients. Most importantly, parents and patients must learn that frequent symptoms and limitation of lifestyle due to illness should not be accepted; a symptom-free existence should be the goal.

MANAGEMENT OF AN ACUTE EPISODE

Acute asthma in children can occur as a mild illness that responds promptly to bronchodilators, or it can develop into a medical emergency over a matter of a few hours or days. Failure to respond to aggressive home treatment mandates further evaluation and treatment in the physician's office or a hospital emergency department. Use of treatment algorithms and guidelines provide useful infrastructure on which to base treatment, referral, and admission decisions (Fig. 47-7).

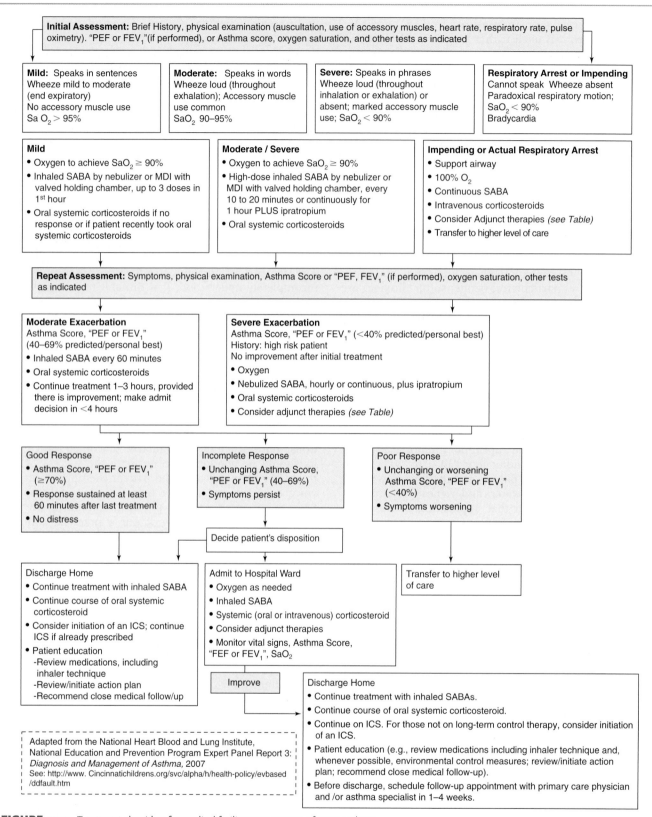

FIGURE 47-7. Treatment algorithm for medical facility management of acute asthma.

For mild acute asthma (cough, wheeze without dyspnea; PEFR between 50% and 80% predicted) treatment can begin at home or in the physician's office, and the drug of choice is an inhaled SABA, most commonly albuterol, 0.15 to 0.3 mg/kg/dose (or 2.5 to 5 mg) given once from a small-volume nebulizer, or preferably, 2 to 6 puffs (90 mcg/puff) of albuterol (using a valved holding chamber if necessary) every 20 minutes for 1 hour. If symptoms resolve, PEFR (if used) improves, and the patient remains well for 3 to 4 hours, the albuterol can be repeated as necessary, routine medications continued, and contact with the physician considered. Doubling the dose of inhaled steroids at the onset of an exacerbation is no longer recommended because most studies have not found a clear benefit. Higher (quadruple) doses of inhaled steroids for acute exacerbations may benefit some patients, but the data are thus far limited.[90] However, initiating ICSs as a chronic treatment for a steroid-naïve patient during an acute episode is appropriate, but other treatment with a SABA and systemic corticosteroids should still be used as necessary. If symptoms persist and PEFR improves little, the dose of inhaled albuterol should be repeated and a dose of oral steroid (1 to 2 mg/kg, maximum 60 mg prednisone) should be given. Physician contact is necessary at this point.

For the patient with progressive symptoms in spite of all of the listed measures, care should be sought in a medical facility. In the emergency department, further administration of nebulized albuterol (2.5 to 5.0 mg) or 4 to 6 puffs every 20 minutes may be continued for another hour, and an oral corticosteroid dose may be given if not done earlier. There is no benefit to giving intravenous steroids unless the patient cannot tolerate or will not take the oral form. Ipratropium (250 or 500 mcg) should also be given every 20 to 30 minutes by nebulizer for three doses; this may most likely benefit patients with more severe exacerbations of airway obstruction. A subcutaneous injection of epinephrine (or terbutaline) can be given if the patient is in severe distress and unable to comply with aerosol therapy. Studies of continuous albuterol nebulization (10 to 15 mg/hour) have yielded mixed results, although most favor continuous nebulization over intermittent administration. Significant adverse side effects during continuous nebulization protocols in severe acute pediatric asthma are rare, suggesting that this mode of delivery is safe, if not necessarily more effective, and may be more convenient for patient and staff. A recent study compared continuously nebulized levalbuterol to racemic albuterol and found no significant efficacy or safety advantage, using pharmacologically equivalent doses.[54]

Other treatments that may be used in the acute hospital setting include intravenous magnesium sulfate ($MgSO_4$) and heliox. $MgSO_4$ can act as a smooth muscle relaxant, possibly by blocking calcium-mediated contraction, decreasing acetylcholine release from neuromuscular junctions, and reducing histamine-induced airway spasm. $MgSO_4$ has been utilized for patients who fail to improve significantly following administration of inhaled SABA and systemic corticosteroids. Several studies demonstrate improved pulmonary function, decreased symptoms, and decreased rate of hospitalization following a single infusion of 40 to 75 mg/kg (maximum 2 g) over a 20-minute period. $MgSO_4$ should strongly be considered in severely ill patients who are in a monitored unit in an emergency department and are failing conventional therapy. Adverse events include flushing, headache, decreased blood pressure, and weakness; the more significant effects are infrequent unless the serum magnesium level rises above twice normal.

Heliox, a mixture of helium (80%) and oxygen (20%), is a specialty gas that is less dense than nitrogen. When administered to the acutely ill asthmatic, heliox can decrease airway resistance by restoring laminar flow in obstructed airways where flow has become more turbulent. Work of breathing is decreased, and the patient is less likely to fatigue. However, there is no direct curative action of heliox, and its effect occurs only while in use. It may also be used to drive a small-volume nebulizer to deliver albuterol, but this requires a specialized closed delivery system. Current data do not support the routine use of heliox in the emergency department. Heliox may be a useful bridge therapy for the severely ill patient in the intensive care unit who is tiring. It becomes less effective if concentrations lower than 70% helium are used, making it less useful in significantly hypoxemic patients.

Montelukast administered intravenously or orally as an adjunct treatment for status asthmaticus in addition to standard treatment with a SABA and systemic corticosteroids has not proven useful in improving symptoms, pulmonary function, or need for hospital admission in children.[91] However, a study in adults with acute severe exacerbations showed improvement in FEV_1 with intravenous montelukast, but there was no decrease in need for hospitalization. The routine use of montelukast for treatment of status asthmaticus cannot be recommended at this time.

Failure to clear symptoms (particularly dyspnea, chest wall retractions, or use of accessory muscles); reverse persistent hypoxemia (O_2 saturation <92% while breathing room air); and improve air exchange and (if measured) PEFR to above 40% to 50% predicted are some indicators for hospital admission.

HOSPITAL MANAGEMENT OF ASTHMA

Status asthmaticus, or acute severe asthma that is resistant to appropriate outpatient therapy, is a significant medical emergency that requires prompt, systematic, and aggressive management in the hospital. The initiation of early appropriate therapy shortens hospitalization and reduces complications for the vast majority of acutely ill patients. In spite of improved efforts at diagnosing and treating asthma, status asthmaticus continues to be the one of the most common discharge diagnoses from children's hospitals, accounting for 15% to 30% of all admissions. The increase in hospitalizations for asthma reported in all age groups during the previous decade now appears to have slowed.

GENERAL TREATMENT

A physician, nurse, respiratory therapist, and consultant pulmonologist team should manage the child with status asthmaticus in a closely monitored inpatient unit. Although the management of each child with status asthmaticus must be individualized, certain general principles apply to all patients with this disease.

Humidified oxygen should be administered (2 to 3 L/min by nasal cannula or 30% fraction of inspired oxygen [FIO_2] by facemask) to maintain oxygen saturation in arterial blood (SaO_2) greater than 93% at sea level.

The appropriate use of oxygen helps relieve dyspnea, aids in bronchodilation, supports the myocardium, and helps to prevent arrhythmias. Failure of improvement in hypoxemia with modest amounts of oxygen suggests either severe airway obstruction and impending respiratory failure or a complicating factor, such as pneumonia, atelectasis, or another diagnosis besides asthma. Intravenous infusion of fluids is generally not required unless the patient is unable to take or tolerate oral fluids or requires IV access for steroids or antimicrobials (if needed for concomitant infection). Pulmonary function tests (FEV_1 or PEFR) may be performed at the bedside if the child can cooperate; however, most acutely ill children cannot do acceptable spirometry. Pulse oximetry (or arterial or capillary blood gas if hypercarbia or acidosis is suspected) should be measured as soon as possible and repeated as the patient's condition warrants. Although not needed on all asthmatics, a chest radiograph provides information on other pulmonary problems that might complicate management in patients who do not respond rapidly to treatment (e.g., pneumonia, atelectasis, pneumomediastinum, or pneumothorax).

Details about the acute illness (its duration, progression, manifestations, and initiating factors), information on the duration and the reports of previous acute episodes, and level of functional morbidity and medication use at the patient's stable baseline should be noted. The patient's medication (including the names, dosages, and exact time of all medications administered within 24 hours) and any systemic corticosteroid drugs administered within 12 months should be documented. These data will be useful in constructing a treatment plan upon hospital discharge.

On physical examination, the general appearance and level of activity, respiratory effort, presence or absence of wheezing, tachycardia, tachypnea, air exchange, adventitious breath sounds, use of accessory muscles, dyspnea, and color are important clinical parameters that provide information about pulmonary dysfunction.

Although the number of pharmacologic agents for treatment of status asthmaticus is relatively limited, management strategies are inconsistent among and within institutions (see Table 47-4A and B). Evidence-based practice is often replaced by physician personal experience and preference. Elimination of treatment that adds risk and cost but does not improve quality of care should be a primary goal. Status asthmaticus readily lends itself to treatment by the standardized clinical pathway, and several published studies have demonstrated shortened hospital stays using such care paths.[92]

Medical management of the hospitalized asthmatic should include aggressive use of inhaled bronchodilators, most commonly albuterol and systemic corticosteroids. The frequency of treatment should be guided by the patient's condition. In most inpatient, non–intensive care unit settings, inhalations may be administered as frequently as every 1 to 2 hours. In some settings, where close monitoring is available outside the intensive care unit, consideration may be given to administering albuterol continuously (10 to 15 mg/hour)

for short time periods (1 to 4 hours). Treatments should be administered only if the patient's respiratory status indicates need; studies have shown that such assessment-driven administration of SABAs is as effective as scheduled treatments. Moreover, patients who are treated on an "as-needed" basis are likely to receive fewer treatments at less cost. If the patient cannot tolerate oral therapy, intravenous administration of corticosteroids should be ordered. Solumedrol, 1 to 2 mg/kg (maximum 125 mg) may be given daily. Failure to improve significantly after a maximum of 12 hours of such therapy should prompt a search for other complicating factors and impending respiratory failure and indicates a need for more aggressive monitoring and treatment. If at any time the patient's condition deteriorates, consideration should be given to administering immediate intensified treatment, such as subcutaneous epinephrine (0.01 mL/kg, maximum 0.3 mL) or terbutaline, or 500 mcg aerosolized ipratropium with 5 mg albuterol. If a favorable response is observed, the aerosol treatment may be repeated every 20 minutes over the next hour. Patients who fail to sustain improvement after such treatment should be transferred to the intensive care unit.

The asthmatic child requiring intensive care should be monitored carefully for the development of respiratory failure. Physical findings such as severe dyspnea, inability to lie flat, poor air exchange, severe wheezing, and use of accessory muscles of respiration are all indicators of impending respiratory failure. Continuous cardiorespiratory monitoring and pulse oximetry with intermittent determination of arterial or venous blood gas measurement to assess oxygenation, ventilation, serum electrolyte, and acid-base status is necessary. Treatment should consist of continuously nebulized albuterol (0.15 mg/kg/hour, maximum 15 mg), ipratropium 500 mcg nebulized every 4 to 6 hours, and solumedrol 1 to 2 mg/kg (maximum 125 mg) every 24 hours. A few studies suggest that intravenous aminophylline may result in more rapid resolution of symptoms compared with placebo, although overall intensive care length of stay was not affected. For the patient who fails to respond, treatment with a bolus and possible continuous intravenous infusion of a β-adrenergic agonist (e.g., terbutaline) can be considered (intravenous albuterol or salbutamol is not available in the United States). Delivery of the medication via the circulation may provide relief of bronchospasm in areas not receiving medication via the inhaled route due to severe airway obstruction. However, most studies do not report significant improvement compared with use of continuous nebulized SABA treatment. The starting dose of terbutaline is 5 mcg/kg, followed by a continuous infusion of 0.4 mcg/kg/min. The dose is increased by 0.2 mcg/kg/min to a maximum dose of 12 to 16 mcg/kg/min, although higher doses may be necessary. Baseline and twice-daily cardiac isoenzymes and continuous electrocardiograms must be monitored because myocardial toxicity has been reported. Serum potassium concentration should also be closely monitored because frequent SABA administration may deplete levels.

Although every effort should be made to avoid intubation and mechanical ventilation, a small percentage of severely ill patients (<10%) may require invasive ventilatory support. It is difficult to mechanically ventilate an asthmatic, and the complication rate may exceed 30%. Indications for intubation have become more conservative and should be reserved for patients who have apnea, unstable vital signs, impaired level of consciousness, severe acidosis, extreme fatigue, and failure of noninvasive ventilation. A trial of noninvasive ventilation using continuous positive airway pressure (CPAP) or bilevel positive airway pressure (Bi-Pap) may be successful in some patients. Low levels of H_2O pressure (5 to 10 cm) may be helpful in reducing work of breathing and improving oxygenation over a several-hour trial. Some patients become anxious using the tight-fitting facemask necessary for effective CPAP and may require a modest dose of a short-acting benzodiazepine to comply with treatment. Risks include gastric distention, vomiting, aspiration, or air leak.

A skilled intensivist or anesthesiologist using rapid-sequence induction anesthesia should perform intubation when necessary. It is important to make certain the patient is adequately hydrated prior to intubation and not given excessive positive pressure bag ventilation immediately after. Asthmatic patients are at risk for significant hypotension following intubation because of extreme hyperventilation leading to auto-PEEP, which impedes systemic venous return; this can be further exacerbated by volume depletion and application of aggressive positive pressure ventilation. Continuous sedation usually is required during mechanical ventilation. High peak inspiratory pressure is often noted, and efforts should be made to reduce it to less than 45 mm Hg. Use of selective hypoventilation must be practiced, and attempts to immediately normalize ventilation should be avoided. Relief of hypoxemia, respiratory distress, and muscle fatigue are the goals. Volume ventilation with a square wave form and the lowest volume and flow to minimize peak pressure and volume damage while maximizing expiratory time is usually recommended, but there are reports of successful use of pressure-controlled ventilation as well. Relatively low respiratory rates (8 to 10/min) and low tidal volumes (6 to 8 mL/kg) should be tried. Decreasing the minute ventilation can maximize expiratory time; this can be best accomplished by using a lower respiratory rate or tidal volume. Shortening the inspiratory time by increasing the inspiratory flow rate can work, but it may be less effective and may contribute to airway injury caused by high shear forces. As long as metabolic acidosis is not present, a pH as low as 7.2 can be tolerated. Intravenous infusion of sodium bicarbonate for more profound acidosis is controversial and generally not recommended. All medications should be continued while the patient is mechanically ventilated. Delivery of aerosolized bronchodilators through the endotracheal tube using an MDI and spacer device should be continued as well. Extubation should be considered and attempted using standard criteria, such as normoxemia with an FIO_2 of <0.40, spontaneous tidal volume >5 mL/kg, vital capacity >15 mL/kg, maximum inspiratory pressure >−25 cm, and ability to protect the airway and handle secretions. Most patients can be successfully weaned and extubated within 72 hours.

Several other therapies for the severely ill asthmatic have been tried, but they are still considered unproven or experimental. Intravenous $MgSO_4$ should be tried, particularly if not administered previously. Heliox has been reported to decrease pulsus paradoxus and improve air flow in acutely ill, nonintubated asthmatic children and can also be administered during mechanical ventilation. However, this therapy is unproven, and the less-dense gas alters ventilator function, requiring careful ventilator adjustment and a knowledgeable respiratory therapist. Administration of inhaled general anesthetic agents (e.g., enflurane and sevoflurane, which are bronchodilators) has also been used with some success; however, reports are anecdotal, and no controlled trials have been conducted. These agents are also myocardial irritants and may precipitate serious arrhythmias in the acidotic, hypoxemic asthmatic. Ketamine infusions can be considered for sedation of the intubated patient, since the drug also has some bronchodilator properties. However, the psychoactive adverse effects of ketamine can be problematic in older children and may only be partially obviated by the concomitant administration of a benzodiazepine.

Of note, most patients who develop life-threatening asthma and respiratory failure do so outside the hospital or shortly after arriving at a medical facility. Most asthma deaths occur prior to reaching an intensive care unit and institution of successful airway management. Once successfully stabilized in an intensive care unit that is familiar with the management of acute severe asthmatics, patients who have not experienced respiratory arrest or prolonged hypoxia are likely to survive intact.

Suggested Reading

Allakhverdi Z, Comeau MR, Jessup HK, et al. Thymic stromal lymphopoietin is released by human epithelial cells in response to microbes, trauma, or inflammation and potently activates mast cells. *J Exp Med.* 2007;204:253–258.

Cockcroft DW. Direct challenge tests: Airway hyperresponsiveness in asthma: its measurement and clinical significance. *Chest.* 2010;138:18S–24S.

Fitzpatrick AM, Teague WG, Meyers DA, et al, for the National Institutes of Health/National Heart, Lung, and Blood Institute Severe Asthma Research Program. Heterogeneity of severe asthma in childhood: Confirmation by cluster analysis of children in the National Institutes of Health/National Heart, Lung, and Blood Institute Severe Asthma Research Program. *J Allergy Clin Immunol.* 2011;127:382–389.

Holgate ST. Epithelium dysfunction in asthma. *J Allergy Clin Immunol.* 2007;120:1233–1244.

Kim HY, DeKruyff RH, Umetsu DT. The many paths to asthma: phenotype shaped by innate and adaptive immunity. *Nat Immunol.* 2010;11:577–583.

Mackay D, Haw S, Ayres JG, et al. Smoke-free legislation and hospitalizations for childhood asthma. *N Engl J Med.* 2010;363:1139–1145.

O'Byrne PM, Pedersen S, Lamm CJ, et al, START Investigators Group. Severe exacerbations and decline in lung function in asthma. *Am J Respir Crit Care Med* 2009;179:19–24.

Wenzel SE, Barnes PJ, Bleecker ER, et al, T03 Asthma Investigators. A randomized, double-blind, placebo-controlled study of tumor necrosis factor-alpha blockade in severe persistent asthma. *Am J Respir Crit Care Med.* 2009;179:549–558.

References

The complete reference list is available online at www.expertconsult.com

48 SEVERE ASTHMA

ANDREW BUSH, MD, FRCP, FRCPCH

Most children with asthma respond to low doses of properly used inhaled corticosteroids (ICSs). Occasionally an additional medication such as a long-acting β_2 agonist (LABA) is required. Worldwide, the most common reason for poorly controlled asthma is that the medications are not accessible in the community. The issues of defining severe asthma in a uniform manner were addressed in a recent WHO document.[1] The document addresses the problem of "nightmare asthma" in the context of communities with access to modern asthma therapy. Estimates of the prevalence of such children are hard to come by, but they probably account for up to 5% of all childhood asthmatics.[2] However, this group consumes a huge proportion of health care resources and is associated with considerable morbidity and even premature mortality. This chapter summarizes a possible approach that specialist pediatrics pulmonologists might employ when referred such children. Although insights can be gained from adult practice, adult data must not be extrapolated directly to children. There is too little evidence about the management of severe preschool wheezing disorders, so they are not discussed in this chapter; most of this chapter is based on personal practice and is not evidence-based.

PEDIATRIC AND ADULT SEVERE ASTHMA: SIMILARITIES AND DIFFERENCES

Children with severe asthma are predominantly highly atopic. If anything, there is a male preponderance. Complete steroid responsiveness is unusual. We initially reported on a group of "difficult" asthmatics who had undergone evaluation in the clinic, but not the detailed multidisciplinary assessment described later in the chapter.[3] There were baseline data on 102 children, mean age 11.6 years (SD: 2.8) in a cross-sectional study, and longitudinal prospective assessment of corticosteroid responsiveness in 89. The median dose of ICSs was 2 mg/day; 14% had been intubated and ventilated at least once, and more than a third were prescribed maintenance systemic steroids. 86% were atopic, 59% were male, and 23% had persistent air flow limitation. 51% had additional or alternative diagnoses, although it was not possible to determine how much they contributed to the morbidity, because there were no protocol-driven interventions. 24% reported one or more food allergies; these were not verified by double-blind challenges, but allergic sensitization by specific IgE was common. Forty-seven patients (46%) had a high-resolution computed tomography (HRCT) performed; three patients (6%) had bronchiectasis. The majority underwent bronchoscopy as part of their evaluation. Positive bronchoalveolar lavage (BAL) cultures were seen in 19/76 (25%), of which neutrophilia was present in 10/15 (67%). BAL eosinophilia was present in 25/68 (37%), and neutrophilia was present

in 30/68 (44%), including 11/68 (16%) with mixed cellularity. Endobronchial biopsy could be analyzed in 68 patients. Mucosal eosinophilia was present in 53% and neutrophilia in 53%, including 17/36 (47%) with mixed cellularity. Increased reticular basement membrane thickening was present in 73%. A pH study was completed in 55/102 (54%) of children, 75% of which showed evidence of gastroesophageal reflux (GER); in most cases, treatment of reflux did not change the symptoms. Corticosteroid responsiveness either to 40 mg prednisolone orally for 2 weeks, or a single intramuscular injection of triamcinolone, was assessed by symptom score, spirometry including bronchodilator responsiveness, and noninvasive measurements of inflammation (FeNO and sputum cytology, where available). Only 11% normalized all these parameters after a steroid trial; partial responsiveness was common; steroid responsiveness could not be convincingly predicted from baseline data. This is in marked contrast to adult studies. The ENFUMOSA study reported that severe asthma was dominated by women who had a lower prevalence of atopy and more neutrophilic inflammation.[4] The SARP group also reported that there was less skin-prick test positivity in severe asthmatics.[5] Analysis of the Brompton cohort of severe adult asthmatics also demonstrated a female preponderance (75%), with 70% demonstrating evidence of atopy.[6] Sixty-nine percent of this cohort reported that their asthma first manifested before they were 20 years old. The relationship between childhood and adult phenotypes is unclear; recall bias is such that without longitudinal studies, it is impossible to know what sort of problems the adult with severe asthma had as a child.[7] However, our data suggest that many children continue with a severe phenotype,[8] and the TENOR study reported that over a 2-year period, few severe asthmatics achieve control of their disease.[9] The longest follow-up of severe asthmatics, the Melbourne cohort (now from 10 to 50 years of age) showed that severe asthmatics continued to have low lung function over the decades in which they have been studied, and that nearly half developed COPD.[10] Obviously most if not all would not have received modern state-of-the-art treatment, but nonetheless, this underscores the poor long-term prognosis of severe asthma.

THE INITIAL LABEL: PROBLEMATIC SEVERE ASTHMA

Numerous patterns of symptomatology may lead to referral for a specialist opinion. These include one or more of the following:

1. Persistent (most days, for at least 3 months) chronic symptoms of airway obstruction (prompting short-acting β_2 agonist use ≥3 times/week) despite high-dose ICS (beclomethasone equivalent 800 mcg/day) and trials of add-on medications (long-acting β_2 agonist,

leukotriene receptor antagonist, and oral theophylline in the low, anti-inflammatory dose). Although for mild asthma the plateau of the ICS dose response curve is low (perhaps even 200 mcg/day),[11] it may be higher in those with relative steroid resistance.[12] It should be noted that there is a poor correlation between symptoms and parental administration of β_2 agonists.[13]

2. Type 1 brittle asthma[14] (chaotic swings in peak flow). Definitions and virtually all data are in adults.

3. Recurrent severe asthma exacerbations that have required:
   - *either* at least one admission to an intensive care unit
   - *or* at least two hospital admissions requiring intravenous medication(s)
   - *or* ≥2 courses of oral steroids during the last year, despite the above therapy.

4. Type 2 brittle asthma[14] (sudden and catastrophic attack on a base of apparently good control); again, most data come from adults.

5. Persistent air flow limitation (PAL): postoral steroid, postbronchodilator Z score <−1.96 for forced expiratory volume in 1 second (FEV_1) using appropriate reference populations.[15]

6. The necessity for alternate day or daily oral steroids.

It should be noted that these are not mutually exclusive categories, and that all numbers and definitions are arbitrary.

Problematic severe asthma is an umbrella term for three different categories,[16-19] and it is the initial job of the specialist to place the child in the correct group.

Group 1: Wrong Diagnosis (Not Asthma)

Misdiagnosis is quite common, and a full history, physical examination, and diagnostic workup is mandatory. The tests performed will depend on clinical suspicion and the prevalence of particular diagnoses in the area in which the specialist practices. I will not discuss this topic in this chapter.

Group 2: Co-Morbidities (Asthma Plus)

If it has been shown that the child genuinely has asthma, one should consider conditions that may co-exist or worsen asthma.[20] These include obesity, GER, dysfunctional breathing patterns, food allergy, and rhinosinusitis. Some of these areas are controversial; it is not known whether food allergy is causally related to asthma severity or is merely a marker. GER frequently co-exists with severe asthma, but the evidence that treating it improves the asthma is scant to nonexistent. The relationship between upper and lower airway disease is debated,[21] but because rhinosinusitis may have such profound effects on quality of life,[22] it should be treated on its own merits, and any improvement in asthma control should be regarded as a bonus. Obesity is associated with a pauci-inflammatory form of asthma,[2] and nonspecific respiratory symptoms related to obesity may be incorrectly diagnosed as asthma; however, it is a long step between identifying obesity as a problem and actually persuading the child to lose weight. Dysfunctional

breathing syndromes, including vocal cord dysfunction, frequently co-exist with asthma, and, unless correctly identified as such, may lead to inappropriate escalation of asthma therapy.[24-26]

Group 3: The Real Deal, But What Is the Deal?

Children who have genuine asthma and in whom co-morbidities have been addressed as far as possible either have *difficult asthma* or *severe therapy-resistant asthma*. The term *difficult asthma* as used here means that the basics have not been gotten right. This is common; in one study comparing two add-on therapies in children uncontrolled on ICS and LABA, only 55 of 292 children could be randomized; most of the rest either did not have asthma or were not taking treatment.[27] In another study in which the benefit of exhaled nitric oxide (FeNO) measurements to protocol-driven asthma therapy was evaluated, the improvements during the run-in period, when correct management was stressed, were so great that there was no scope for any additional benefit of FeNO.[28] By contrast, children with severe therapy-resistant asthma have ongoing problems even when the basics have been gotten right. This group should be considered for "beyond the guidelines" innovative therapies. Of course, it needs to be acknowledged that identifying a problem such as adherence is one thing, and dealing with it effectively is quite another! However, it makes no sense to be using invasive or toxic medications (e.g., omalizumab and methotrexate) just because a child will not take a moderate dose of ICS with an appropriate device.

▬ THE NEXT EVALUATION: DOES THE CHILD HAVE DIFFICULT OR SEVERE THERAPY-RESISTANT ASTHMA?

We recommend a nurse-led, multidisciplinary evaluation as the next step.[29] The key component of this is the home visit. Four areas are addressed: adherence and other medication issues, cigarette smoke exposure, allergen exposure, and psychosocial issues.

Adherence and Other Medication Issues

These issues were thought to be important in around half of our patients. It should be noted that clinic-based assessments of adherence are little better than flipping a coin. Issues included the following:

- Failure to collect sufficient prescriptions to cover medication needs.[30] It is accepted that merely collecting a prescription does not ensure adherence, but failure to collect a prescription guarantees that the medication is not being taken
- Medications stockpiled, particularly in their original wrappings, obviously unused
- Medications out of date, or empty canisters being used
- Inaccessible medications (e.g., at the back of a cupboard or behind a sofa) obviously never accessed

• Medications not supervised. Even very young children (20% of children 7 years of age, 50% of children 11 years of age) may be left to be responsible for taking medications without adult supervision.[31] Very often the mother believes she is supervising the child, but detailed probing reveals that she is merely calling upstairs and relying on the accuracy of the child's response.

• Wrong inhaler device or poor technique with an inappropriate device, despite repeated training.[32-34] Often adolescents will discard the spacer as "babyish" and use a metered-dose inhaler straight into the mouth.

Cigarette Smoke Exposure

Passive smoke exposure, and indeed active smoking, is all too common. Measurement of urinary or salivary cotinine may be illuminating. In adults, active smoking leads to a pauci-eosinophilic, steroid-resistant phenotype.[35-38] There is mounting evidence that passive smoke exposure in children has a similar effect. Most parents who smoke swear they never smoke inside the house, but clear evidence that this is not the case is frequent on a home visit.

Allergen Exposure

Particular attention is paid to allergens to which the child is sensitized, and for which avoidance is practical. The relevance of allergen avoidance, in particular house dust mite allergen, has been disputed.[39-41] Problems with studies include recruitment of relatively mildly affected children, short-term duration, and failure actually to achieve allergen reduction or measure whether this has happened. There are no studies in severe asthma, a group in which perhaps commitment to reducing allergens may be greater because of the severity of symptoms and intensity of treatment. Our practice is to advise allergen avoidance, in particular furry pets, if the child is sensitized, for the following reasons:

• There is biological plausibility. Allergen exposure in the sensitized patient leads to IL-2– and IL-4–mediated steroid resistance.[42,43]

• The natural experiment of school exposure to cat allergens on classmates in a sensitized child who does not have a cat at home leads to a pattern of symptoms similar to occupational asthma, with progressive deterioration during the week, getting better at weekends and during the holidays.[44]

• Subclinical allergen exposure, if the patient is sensitized, can cause worsening airway inflammation and bronchial responsiveness, even in the absence of any acute clinically detectable change in lung function.[45]

• Very high levels of antigen (soya bean, grass pollen during a thunderstorm) can themselves trigger asthma exacerbations.[46,47]

• The combination of viral infection, allergen sensitization, and exposure to that allergen is strongly predictive of an exacerbation severe enough for hospital admission[48]; of the three factors, only allergen exposure is amenable to intervention.

• The greater the number of allergic triggers, the more likely is the child to exacerbate.[49] This finding confirms the view that atopy is not an "all or none" phenomenon.[50]

• Many if not all allergen avoidance studies have been carried out in relatively mildly affected children who have less potential to benefit and therefore less incentive to stick to very demanding regimes.

Ongoing allergen exposure is common in these children. The allergens may show global variation. Fungal exposure is also explored, particularly if a diagnosis of severe asthma with fungal sensitization (SAFS) is being considered (see later in the chapter).

Psychosocial Issues

There are numerous potential interactions between the brain and the airway.[50-53] Psychological stress may affect the airways by poorly understood probably neural reflexes. In a study of high school students, there was a much more marked airway eosinophilic response at the high-stress time of examinations as compared to normal term time.[53] Unsurprisingly, anxiety and depression are common in both parents and children. Most referrals to clinical psychology are made after a discussion in the home, where parents are more likely to be able to discuss sensitive issues.[29]

It is important when addressing these issues to ensure that all concerned realize that no one believes the symptoms are being fabricated, or are "all in the mind." Our approach is to treat both asthma and psychological issues in parallel, rather than become involved in futile discussions about whether asthma caused the stress, or the stress caused the asthma; both should be treated on their individual merits.

Multidisciplinary Team Assessment

The above data are discussed in detail at the severe asthma team meetings. Typically, less than half of the children referred go on to a more detailed evaluation. For the rest, interventions such as improvement of adherence, attention to psychological issues, and environmental measures are put in place. These may not be successful, but failure to improve adherence, for example, does not mean the child needs a bronchoscopy or cyclosporine therapy.

▰▰ THE FINAL EVALUATION: DISCORDANT PHENOTYPES, PATTERN OF AIRWAY INFLAMMATION, STEROID RESPONSIVENESS, AND PERSISTENT AIR FLOW LIMITATION

Having as far as possible reduced the referred group to the true severe therapy-resistant asthmatics, we next proceed to an invasive evaluation[18] with the aim of answering the following four questions:

1. Does this child have a discordant phenotype? In other words, is there dissociation between inflammation and symptoms? There seems little point in prescribing more powerful anti-inflammatory medication if the airways are not inflamed.[23]

2. What is the pattern of any airway inflammation: is it eosinophilic, neutrophilic, or mixed type? For example, a neutrophilic phenotype might suggest that a trial of macrolides may be helpful.

3. Is the child corticosteroid-responsive?

4. Does the child have PAL? Again, there seems little point in escalating therapy to try to reverse the irreversible.

Our protocol requires two visits, 4 weeks apart, and the tests are summarized in Table 48-1. In summary, noninvasive and invasive assessment of airway pathology is carried out, and the noninvasive assessment is repeated after a single intramuscular injection of triamcinolone. We perform BAL and endobronchial biopsy, but not transbronchial biopsy for distal inflammation because of safety issues.[54] We do not perform HRCT to measure, for example, airway wall thickness as a biomarker, because there is yet insufficient evidence to justify this. Of course, HRCT is performed if there is a diagnostic indication. Bronchial responsiveness is also not routinely measured; it would be deemed unsafe in many children who have very impaired spirometry. If spirometry is normal, and symptoms and objective findings are very different, failure to elicit any evidence of bronchial responsiveness to methacholine is a strong pointer that symptoms are being overreported. In terms of determining steroid responsiveness, there is no evidence in pediatrics as to the optimal dose, duration, and route for the steroid trial. We use triamcinolone 40 to 80 mg as a single intramuscular dose, depending on age and body weight, which means that adherence is not an issue.

Assessment of Phenotype Discordance and the Pattern of Airway Inflammation

The weakness of our approach is the failure to determine whether there is peripheral airway inflammation in the absence of distal inflammation,[55-57] and also a lack of understanding as to whether mucosal or luminal inflammation is important.[58,59] Distal inflammation is not assessed for want of a tool; transbronchial biopsy has been rejected as unsafe,[54] and the overlap between groups of alveolar nitric oxide production[60,61] means this is not a useful clinical tool.[62] The final option, video-assisted thoracoscopic lung biopsy, is deemed too invasive on present evidence. Luminal and mucosal inflammation are frequently discordant, and the evidence as to which is most important is conflicting and unresolved.[63]

Assessment of Steroid Responsiveness

The adult definition of steroid resistance (<15% increase in FEV_1 after 2 weeks of oral prednisolone in a patient who can bronchodilate >15% with acute use of β_2 agonists)[64] is not appropriate for children with severe asthma, who may have normal spirometry.[65-67] In addition to the lack of consensus about steroid dosing, there is no pediatric agreed definition of steroid responsiveness. We assess this in the domains of symptoms (ACT), spirometry, and inflammation (induced sputum eosinophils or FeNO), as summarized in Table 48-2. Partial response in one or more domains is most common; both complete response in all domains and total nonresponse is each seen in 10% to 15% of children we have studied.[3] Note that more than half the children have steroid unresponsive eosinophilic inflammation[68]; this underscores that true severe pediatric asthma really does exist, albeit being less common than is sometimes thought.

TABLE 48-2 POSSIBLE CRITERIA FOR STEROID RESPON-SIVENESS IN CHILDREN WITH SEVERE ASTHMA

PARAMETER ASSESSED	REQUIREMENT FOR RESPONSE	NUMBER (PERCENT) RESPONDERS*
Symptom response	Asthma control test[120] increases to >20/25 or by at least 5 points	23/47 (49%)
Lung function response	FEV_1 increases to normal (>−1.96 Z-score) or by >15% No acute response to bronchodilator	29/52, (56%)
Inflammatory response (if paired induced-sputum samples are available)	Sputum eosinophil count normal (<2.5%)[121]	22/42 (52%)
Inflammatory response (if paired induced-sputum samples are not available)	FeNO* normal (<24 ppb)[122]	22/52 (42%)

*Exhaled nitric oxide measured at flow 50 mL/s
Nonresponse, no improvement in any dimension; partial response, one or two domains improve; complete response, all three domains normalizes.
From Bossley CJ, Saglani S, Kavanagh C, et al. Corticosteroid responsiveness and clinical characteristics in childhood difficult asthma. *Eur Respir J.* 2009;34: 1052–1059.

TABLE 48-1 INVASIVE ASSESSMENT OF SEVERE ASTHMA*

	ACT	SPIROMETRY, BDR	INDUCED SPUTUM	FeNO (MULTIPLE FLOW RATES)	BRONCHOSCOPY, BAL, EBX	INTRAMUSCLAR TRIAMCINOLONE
Visit 1	√	√	√	√	√	√
Visit 2	√	√	√	√	X	X

*The quadruple aim is to identify children with discordant symptoms and inflammation; to determine the pattern of airway inflammation; to determine if the child is corticosteroid-responsive; and to evaluate whether there is persistent airflow limitation.
BAL, Bronchoalveolar lavage; *BDR,* bronchodilator response; *EBX,* endobronchial biopsy; *FeNO,* fractional exhaled NO.
From Bush A, Saglani S. Management of severe asthma in children. *Lancet.* 2010;376:814-825.

These data do beg the question as to whether a larger dose or a longer duration of therapy would result in all children except those with PAL eventually becoming asymptomatic. There are no data to answer this question. Clearly, the definition of steroid sensitivity must include a component of risk; the distinction between absolute steroid unresponsiveness (which is probably very rare) and responsiveness only to such high doses of steroids that serious side effects are inevitable is of little practical value. This is yet another area in which further work is necessary.

Does the Child Have PAL?

The lung function definition of PAL (mentioned earlier in the chapter) is straightforward. However, there is no evidence to guide the dose, duration, and route of administration of the steroid trial. We do know that 40 mg daily oral prednisolone prescribed (and taken) for a 2-week period is insufficient to diagnose PAL as well as steroid responsiveness.[69] Anecdotally, probably a single dose of triamcinolone is also insufficient. As with the determination of steroid responsiveness, safety must be a factor.

▄▄ OPTIONS FOR PHENOTYPE THERAPY

Underpinning this whole approach is the yet unproven belief that trying to understand the underlying pathophysiology of severe therapy-resistant asthma and using this knowledge to guide treatment is better than a succession of blind therapeutic trials. This section reviews the actions resulting from a phenotype-based approach.

Persistent Air Flow Limitation

Perhaps least controversial is to ensure that children with PAL are not overtreated because of poor lung function. The typical picture is a substantially reduced FEV_1 at all visits, with no bronchodilator response (BDR) and no evidence of inflammation. The most likely diagnosis is obliterative bronchiolitis. HRCT shows patchy air trapping, but unless there is also frank bronchiectasis, the HRCT appearances may be impossible to distinguish from those of poorly controlled asthma.[70] Treatment is reduced until the appearance of either airway inflammation, judged by FeNO or induced sputum, or BDR. Often therapy can be discontinued completely, although it should be remembered that obliterative bronchiolitis and asthma might coexist, particularly in the atopic child.

Steroid-Sensitive and Steroid-Resistant Eosinophilic Inflammation

The child who has evidence of airway eosinophilia at the time of the visit for bronchoscopy, which disappears at the follow-up visit, should initially be treated with the lowest oral steroid dose that controls symptoms. It may be possible to minimize the oral steroid dose by using high- dose ICSs, up to 2 mg/day fluticasone equivalent. If this dose is potentially unsafe or causes intolerable side effects, then the options are as for the child with steroid-resistant eosinophilic inflammation; these are discussed later in the chapter. In both cases, it is essential to ensure that every effort has been made to exclude environmental causes of secondary steroid resistance, in particular ongoing exposure to allergens.

Omalizumab

This is the only therapy for which there is any evidence of safety and efficacy,[71–73] and it would thus be the first choice in most cases, provided the IgE is less than 1300 IU. Before starting treatment, we insist that every effort is made to reduce the burden of allergen in the home, including the removal of offending pets. We perform a 16-week trial and continue therapy if there is a response. The long-term efficacy and safety of omalizumab is not known. In the United Kingdom, this treatment is not available for children younger 11 years of age; there is no rational basis for this decision by the regulatory authorities.[74]

Immunomodulatory Agents

There is limited evidence in children to support trials of cyclosporine[75] and methotrexate[76] as steroid-sparing agents with close attention to detailed monitoring to prevent side effects. There is no evidence on which to recommend azathioprine.

Gold Salts

There is no evidence to support a trial of gold salts in this setting.[77]

Macrolide Antimicrobials

We mainly use macrolide antimicrobials for neutrophilic asthma (discussed later in the chapter), however there is no reason why they cannot be trialed in eosinophilic phenotypes. They are potentially safer than the other immunomodulatory agents, although evidence is lacking in pediatric asthma.

Immunoglobulin Infusions

There is limited evidence of efficacy in pediatric asthma, and the treatment is invasive and inconvenient. However, a 6-month trial of treatment may be worthwhile in resistant cases.

Neutrophilic Asthma

Persistent neutrophilic inflammation in a child who is symptomatic with asthma should prompt a further review for alternative diagnoses characterized by airway neutrophilia (e.g., cystic fibrosis, primary ciliary dyskinesia and persistent bacterial bronchitis), co-morbidities that might be contributing (e.g., GER) and environmental factors (particularly cigarette smoke exposure). Options for pharmacological therapy include macrolide antimicrobials and theophyllines.

Macrolide Antimicrobials

There is considerable evidence of benefit in children with other neutrophilic airways diseases, especially CF and diffuse panbronchiolitis.[78–87] There is limited evidence of benefit in adults with neutrophilic asthma.[88,89] There are no good data to inform choice of macrolides, dose, and duration of therapy. By analogy with CF, we use azithromycin in a daily dose of 250 mg in children under 40 kg body weight, and 500 mg in heavier children. We trial therapy for 6 months, reducing to the same dose 3 times per week if the benefits justify continuing therapy. Even in CF, however, there is no agreement as to the optimal dosing regimen.

Theophyllines

In theory, low-dose theophyllines (aiming at plasma levels of 5 to 10 mg/L rather than 10 to 20 mg/L, as for conventional therapeutic doses) have anti-inflammatory properties. They accelerate neutrophil apoptosis and may restore steroid responsiveness by histone deacetylase–dependent mechanisms.[90–94] In our hands, however, therapeutic benefit is rare.

Pauci-Inflammatory Asthma

These children typically have chronic symptoms or exacerbations despite having no evidence of airway inflammation on standard asthma therapy. The first necessity is to document objectively that the symptoms are really caused by variable air flow obstruction. The next is to be as certain as possible that there is no residual airway inflammation, and we always resort to bronchoscopy if there is any doubt. We would reduce anti-inflammatory medication to the lowest level that controls inflammation. For children with chaotically variable peak flow, we have used a continuous infusion of subcutaneous terbutaline with some anecdotal success.[95] We admit the child to hospital and carry out a double-blind trial, with only the ward pharmacist knowing whether the syringe of medication supplied is terbutaline or placebo. We use four treatment periods with a washout between. Often, the child improves in hospital irrespective of the infusion because adverse environmental effects have been removed and basic medications are being given! For a few children, terbutaline infusions can be dramatically successful. The mechanism is unclear, and concerns about safety remain (given the worries about long-acting β_2 agonists.[96,97] For those with single really severe acute exacerbations on the background of apparent good control, we again first ensure that all evidence of airway inflammation has been treated. It may be wise to give the child a source of injectable adrenaline for instant relief, for use while inhaled or nebulized medication is obtained.

The "Exacerbating" Phenotype

Exacerbations are part of the lives of virtually all asthmatics. There is often confusion in the literature between exacerbations and loss of baseline control,[98] (Table 48-3). The distinction may sometimes be difficult; if peak flow measurements have not been made, then a mild viral exacerbation may mimic a transient loss of control due to unsuspected increased allergen exposure. The presence of coryzal symptoms may be a helpful pointer to a viral exacerbation. The distinction is important. Loss of control usually is treated easily with an increased dose of ICSs, whereas uncritically increasing ICSs in a well-controlled child between exacerbations does not merely

TABLE 48-3 DIFFERENCES BETWEEN EXACERBATIONS OF ASTHMA AND LOSS OF BASELINE CONTROL

EXACERBATION	LOSS OF BASELINE CONTROL
Abrupt decrease in peak flow, little diurnal variability	Marked diurnal variability, baseline relatively stable
Usually viral, occasionally overwhelming allergen exposure	Usually related to adverse environmental exposures (e.g., allergen or tobacco smoke)
Very difficult to prevent	Usually easily abolished by low-dose inhaled corticosteroids

From Reddel H, Ware S, Marks G, et al. Differences between asthma exacerbations and poor asthma control. *Lancet.* 1999;353:364-369.

fail to prevent exacerbations, but has led to severe side effects including profound hypoglycemia and adrenal failure.[99,100]

Exacerbations are mostly due to viral infection[48]; however, a really severe and overwhelming exposure to allergens can give rise to an acute attack indistinguishable from a viral exacerbation, at least clinically. Examples are the Barcelona Soya Bean epidemic, and the grass pollen thunderstorm outbreaks.[46,47] There are differences in sputum cytology; the viral exacerbations are neutrophilic,[101] and it is becoming clear that there are important interactions between viral infection and eosinophilic airway inflammation.[102]

In adult practice, acute exacerbations on the basis of apparent good control is associated with eosinophilic airway inflammation between exacerbations and may respond to the anti–IL-5 monoclonal antibody, mepolizumab.[103,104] However, there is no evidence for either proposition in children. In children, the following measures should be trialed; mepolizumab has not been used, and indeed, there is no convincing evidence that IL-5 is pivotal in the pathophysiology of the inflammatory infiltrate between exacerbations.

- Ensure at least that a low-dose ICS is being taken.[48] There is no evidence that increasing the dose between exacerbations is helpful, and careful monitoring is mandatory if a higher dose is being tried. If there is no response to an increased dose, dose reduction, not exacerbation, is mandated. Low ICS doses are associated with a reduction in exacerbations.
- Is there evidence of eosinophilic airway inflammation between exacerbations that is best assessed using induced sputum? This would be an indication to increase the dose of ICS.
- Baseline control should be optimized as far as possible because the TENOR study has shown that persistent very poor control is associated with exacerbations.[105]
- Baseline lung function should be optimized as far as possible. The TENOR study also showed that low baseline lung function is associated with exacerbations.[105]
- Allergen exposure should be minimized. The combination of viral infection, allergic sensitization (neither of which are amenable to modulation), and allergen

exposure was associated with risk of a severe asthma exacerbation leading to hospital admission.[48] In the TENOR study, a greater number of allergic triggers was also associated with exacerbations.[5]

• In difficult exacerbations, invasive assessment to determine whether there is untreated eosinophilic airway inflammation between exacerbations may be worth considering. This is routine for us for every child who has been admitted to the intensive care unit with acute severe asthma.

One should pay particular attention to children who have already had an admission to intensive care (because this is predictive of future admissions)[106,107] and those who are food allergic (which is at least a marker of risk of admission to intensive care).[108] It has to be stated that, whereas all of the measures discussed have been shown to be associated with exacerbations, no study has shown prospectively that modulating any of them reduces exacerbations. As in so many situations, good outcome data are lacking.

Severe Asthma with Fungal Sensitization

The severe asthma with fungal sensitization (SAFS) phenotype has largely been described in adults,[109] and its existence is controversial— even in this age group. Definition is severe asthma on standard grounds (see earlier in the chapter) and sensitization by either skin-prick test or specific IgE to any of seven fungi (*Aspergillus fumigatus, Alternaria alternata, Cladosporium herbarum, Penicillium chrysogenum, Candida albicans, Trichophyton mentagrophytes,* and *Botrytis cinerea*) without evidence of allergic bronchopulmonary aspergillosis. This last is not usually a consideration in pediatric asthma, where this diagnosis is very rare. One adult proof-of-concept study suggested that treatment with oral itraconazole may be valuable.[110] In children, the evidence for this phenotype is restricted to anecdotal case reports.[111] However, it would seem sensible if SAFS is suspected that fungal exposure in the household is minimized (including checking the cleanliness of the child's nebulizer if applicable) and a trial of itraconazole given. This approach has the merit of being safer and less invasive than most if not all of the therapeutic options listed earlier, but one must remember the interaction between budesonide and itraconazole through the Cytochrome P-450 enzyme system.[112]

■ SEVERE ASTHMA IN LOW- AND MIDDLE-INCOME COUNTRIES

Worldwide, severe asthma is most common in low- and middle-income countries, and the WHO has defined the category "untreated severe asthma." This is asthma that is untreated either because of failure to make the diagnosis or because basic access to care or to medications and spacers is not available or affordable. It is clear that more good could be achieved for children with asthma by ensuring that all have access to a cheap basic asthma kit

(salbutamol, beclomethasone, prednisone, and a plastic bottle spacer) than all the cytokine-specific treatments put together. Untreated severe asthma is an important group in low- and middle-income countries.[113–115] In addition to treatment access issues, there may be other environmental factors. These may be common to those in high-income countries (e.g., exposure to tobacco) or specific to low- and middle-income countries (e.g., biomass fuel usage), both of which worsen asthma.[116] Another issue may be lack of locally applicable asthma guidelines, failure to apply basic principles of asthma treatment, and lack of asthma education for families. It would be naïve to suggest that medications alone are the answer, but equally wrong to think that the problem cannot be tackled without medications. Sadly, much money is wasted on useless medication (e.g., expectorants) in low- and middle-income countries rather than on asthma kits of proven efficacy. Untreated severe asthma may also be found in parts of the so-called *developed* world in which the costs of medications are prohibitive and reimbursement of health care costs is inadequate. Children in whom compliance with the medication regime is very poor despite access to medications can also be placed in this category; we in fact place them in the *difficult asthma* category and reserve the term *untreated severe asthma* for those in whom most of the primary problem is inability to access medications.

■ FUTURE WORK

It is clearly essential that we ensure access of medication in the poorest areas, with educational material that is appropriate for those areas, and continue to reinforce the message of education. Housing issues must be tackled as far as possible, and the pernicious activities of the tobacco industry must be exposed and ruthlessly tackled.

Difficult Asthma

The evidence marshaled above and elsewhere has shown clearly that much of the problem is related to failure to get the basics right. Renewed attention to detail and intensive monitoring at the first sign that things are not going well is essential. Unfortunately, it is easier and quicker to prescribe more medications without asking why the existing medications are not working.

Severe Therapy-Resistant Asthma

Sadly, there are no randomized controlled trials of any treatment in well-characterized groups of children with severe therapy-resistant asthma. Since these children are rare and are a very heterogeneous group, we can only remedy this by international collaboration. Even the superb CARE network was reduced to futility when trialing a comparison of two add-on medications in severe asthma.[27] Collaboration will mean ensuring assessment by uniform protocols, similar to those set out above, so we can ensure that homogeneous groups are being studied. This will also enable basic mechanisms to be studied, including genetics and gene by environment interactions. The next challenge is to try to enroll such children in therapeutic trials of novel therapies such as bronchial thermoplasty[117] and cytokine-specific treatments.[118] The tension is to try to get children any benefits of these treatments while balancing the risks of severe adverse reactions.[119] There is no easy way forward.

SUMMARY

This chapter has proposed a systematic way of approaching the child referred with *nightmare asthma*. This approach allows the identification of those whose underlying asthma is not in fact severe, but is manageable if one gets the basics right. A detailed protocol is suggested to investigate those children thought to have severe therapy-resistant asthma and try to produce an individualized treatment plan. Sadly, despite this, many children in this category continue to have substantial morbidity both from asthma and the treatment, and some die from the disease. The long-term outlook is little studied, but the current evidence is that the prognosis for remission is not good.

Suggested Reading

Adams NP, Bestall JC, Jones P, et al. Fluticasone at different doses for chronic asthma in adults and children. *Cochrane Database Syst Rev.* 2008;(4): CD003534.

Bousquet J, Mantzouranis E, Cruz AA, et al. Uniform definition of asthma severity, control, and exacerbations: document presented for the World Health Organization Consultation on Severe Asthma. *J Allergy Clin Immunol.* 2010;126:926–938.

Bracken M, Fleming L, Hall P, et al. The importance of nurse-led home visits in the assessment of children with problematic asthma. *Arch Dis Child.* 2009;94:780–784.

Bush A, Hedlin G, Carlsen KH, et al. Severe childhood asthma: a common international approach? *Lancet.* 2008;372:1019–1021.

Bush A, Saglani S. Management of severe asthma in children. *Lancet.* 2010;376:814–825.

de Groot EP, Duiverman EJ, Brand PL. Comorbidities of asthma during childhood: possibly important, yet poorly studied. *Eur Respir J.* 2010;36:671–678.

Haselkorn T, Fish JE, Zeiger RS, et al. TENOR Study Group. Consistently very poorly controlled asthma, as defined by the impairment domain of the Expert Panel Report 3 guidelines, increases risk for future severe asthma exacerbations in The Epidemiology and Natural History of Asthma: Outcomes and Treatment Regimens (TENOR) study. *J Allergy Clin Immunol.* 2009;124:895–902. e1-e4.

Haselkorn T, Zeiger RS, Chipps BE, et al. Recent asthma exacerbations predict future exacerbations in children with severe or difficult-to-treat asthma. *J Allergy Clin Immunol.* 2009;124:921–927.

Hedlin G, Bush A, Lødrup Carlsen K, et al. Problematic Severe Asthma in Childhood Initiative group. Problematic severe asthma in children, not one problem but many: a GA2LEN initiative. *Eur Respir J.* 2010;36:196–201.

References

The complete reference list is available online at www. expertconsult.com

49 THE INFLUENCE OF UPPER AIRWAY DISEASE ON THE LOWER AIRWAY

JONATHAN CORREN, MD

During the past century, practicing clinicians have frequently observed that allergic rhinitis, sinusitis, and asthma coexist in the same patients. Despite a wealth of data supporting an association between the upper and lower airways, not until recently have reliable data emerged that suggest that upper airway disease is a risk factor for the development of asthma and that experimentally induced nasal dysfunction causes asthma to worsen. In addition, there is a growing body of literature demonstrating that appropriate treatment of nasal allergy and chronic sinus disease results in improvements in asthma symptoms and lower airway function. In this review, data from a variety of epidemiologic, clinical, and laboratory studies will be highlighted to help clarify our understanding of these complex and important relationships.

ALLERGIC RHINITIS AND ASTHMA

The Epidemiologic Relationship Between Allergic Rhinitis and Asthma

The first population-based studies that explored the relationship between allergic rhinitis and asthma were cross-sectional surveys, which demonstrated that rhinitis and asthma commonly occur together. Many of these studies reported that nasal symptoms occur in 28% to 78% of patients with asthma[1] as compared with approximately 5% to 20% of the general population.[2] Generally, these data were drawn from a variety of epidemiologic studies and clinical settings in which patients were not interviewed in a standardized fashion and insensitive instruments were used for detecting rhinitis. In a study that utilized a standardized and detailed questionnaire in 478 patients across all age groups, rhinitis was found to be a nearly universal phenomenon in patients with allergic asthma, occurring in 99% of adults and 93% of adolescents.[3] Conversely, asthma has been shown to affect up to 38% of patients with allergic rhinitis,[1] which is substantially higher than the 3% to 5% prevalence noted in the general population.

While these studies demonstrate that rhinitis and asthma frequently occur in the same patients, longitudinal studies are required to accurately assess the actual risk for developing asthma in patients with rhinitis alone. Settipane and colleagues[4] published the first prospective study regarding the relationship between allergic rhinitis and the development of asthma. In a study that spanned 23 years from entry to completion, 690 adolescents who had allergic rhinitis (without chest symptoms) developed asthma 3 times more often (10.5%) than individuals without rhinitis (3.6%). In another prospective study, Burgess and coworkers[5] enrolled 8583 children, beginning at 7 years of age, and evaluated them at 13 and 43 years of age. Children diagnosed with allergic rhinitis at the beginning of the study had a 2- to 7-fold increased risk of developing asthma at both 13 and 43 years of age. In the most recent study, Rochat and colleagues[6] followed 1314 healthy children from birth to 13 years of age. Allergic rhinitis present at 5 years of age was found to be a significant predictor for developing wheezing between 5 and 13 years of age, with an adjusted relative risk of 3.82. These longitudinal studies, taken together, strongly support the role of allergic rhinitis in childhood or adolescence as a risk factor for developing subsequent asthma.

In children younger than 2 years of age, it has been more difficult to prospectively assess the progression of allergic rhinitis to asthma, in part due to the high prevalence of viral upper respiratory tract infections in this age group. In the study by Rochat,[6] children with allergic rhinitis diagnosed by 2 years of age were not at increased risk of developing wheezing between 5 and 13 years of age. The authors noted that rhinitis at 2 years of age is usually not a persistent condition and will often remit as the child grows older.

Studies dating back over 20 years have demonstrated that adults and adolescents with allergic rhinitis are more likely to have increased bronchial hyperresponsiveness than children without rhinitis.[7] More recently, airway hyperresponsiveness has also been shown to be increased in children who have allergic rhinitis but no asthma. Choi and colleagues.[8] performed bronchial methacholine challenges in a group of 115 nonasthmatic children, 4 to 6 years of age. Bronchial hyperresponsiveness (BHR), assessed as a methacholine dose required to produce wheezing or oxygen desaturation <8 mg/mL, was significantly more common in children with allergic rhinitis compared with non-rhinitis children (32.5% vs. 9.4%, respectively). Among the children with allergic rhinitis, serum total IgE, the number and pattern of skin-prick test responses, blood eosinophil markers, and parental history of allergic rhinitis and atopic dermatitis were not different between the BHR-positive and BHR-negative groups, whereas the persistent type of rhinitis and parental history of asthma were more frequent in the BHR-positive group than in the BHR-negative group.

While nonspecific bronchial hyperresponsiveness appears to be more common in children with allergic rhinitis, a second and equally important question is whether this characteristic predisposes them to the development of asthma. A 12-year follow-up study of 291 randomly selected children and adolescents (7 to 17 years of age) examined a number of historical and laboratory features, including bronchial responsiveness to inhaled histamine.[9] Increased airway responsiveness to histamine was a powerful independent predictor of future lower airway disease, with an approximate 4-fold increased risk of developing symptomatic asthma during this period of observation. In a second study, Ferdousi and colleagues[10] followed up a much smaller group of children (n = 28) for only 2 years. Sixteen of the 28 children were found to have an increase in BHR (assessed by isocapnic hyperventilation of cold air or inhaled methacholine challenge), and 8 of these 16 developed asthma after 2 years.

These studies support the theory that bronchial hyperreactivity may represent an intermediate phase between nasal allergy and symptomatic asthma and may help identify children and adolescents at highest risk for developing asthma.

Pharmaco-economic studies from the past decade have attempted to correlate the presence of rhinitis with asthma severity and health care costs attributable to asthma. In an analysis of a database of 1261 children with asthma, Huse and colleagues[11] compared patients with significant nasal allergy with those who had mild or no symptoms of nasal disease. These investigators noted that patients with more severe rhinitis were much more likely to have nocturnal awakening caused by asthma (19.6% vs. 11.8%, respectively), "moderate to severe asthma" as defined by the National Asthma Education Program (60.2% vs. 51.2%, respectively), or work loss related to asthma (24.1% vs. 21.1%, respectively). Similarly, Halpern and co-workers[12] observed that patients with symptomatic rhinitis used more asthma medications, particularly more inhaled and supplemental oral corticosteroids. Judging from these recent investigations, one can postulate that allergic rhinitis may also be related to increased asthma severity and the use of more potent anti-asthma medications. Although these data suggest that rhinitis may be contributing to asthma, an alternative explanation for this association may be that nasal inflammation is a marker for increasing dysfunction of the entire respiratory tract. The possibility of a cause-and-effect relationship is better addressed by therapeutic studies of rhinitis therapy in patients with asthma.

It has been speculated that allergic rhinitis may add a significant burden of disease to patients with asthma. A survey of approximately 800 parents of children with asthma attempted to determine the impact of nasal disease upon their quality of life.[13] In three-quarters of children, rhinitis symptoms preceded the diagnosis of asthma. The concomitant presence of nasal allergy and asthma disrupted the ability to get a good night's sleep (79%), to participate in leisure and sports activities (75%), to concentrate at work or school (73%), and to enjoy social activities (51%). Importantly, most patients (79%) reported worsening asthma symptoms when nasal symptoms were most active. Many (56%) avoided the outdoors during the allergy season because of worsening asthma symptoms. The majority of patients (60%) indicated difficulty in effectively treating both conditions, and 72% were concerned about using excessive medication. Information collected from this study and other similar data indicate that allergic rhinitis does impose a significant additional symptomatic burden on patients with asthma.

COMMON IMMUNOPATHOLOGY OF ALLERGIC RHINITIS AND ASTHMA

During the past decade, we have learned that the immunologic processes leading to allergic rhinitis and atopic asthma are the same. A large number of studies have examined the composition of inflammatory cell infiltrates in the nasal and bronchial mucosa of patients with allergic rhinitis and asthma. Critical cells that have been consistently identified in both upper and lower airway tissue include eosinophils, mast cells,[14] and T helper (Th) lymphocytes expressing the Th 2 type.[15]

Allergen provocation studies have also demonstrated striking similarities between immunopathologic processes in the nasal and bronchial mucosa, including allergen-induced infiltration by inflammatory cells, cellular activation, and cytokine and chemokine expression or production.[16] In addition, the development of early- and late-phase reactions and the acquisition of airway hyperresponsiveness have been convincingly demonstrated in both the nasal and the lower airways after allergen provocation.[17]

Histologic studies of individuals with allergic rhinitis and no evidence of clinical asthma consistently demonstrate abnormalities of the bronchial mucosa, including thickening of the lamina reticularis and mucosa eosinophilia. These abnormalities are generally less pronounced than those of asthmatic patients,[18] but sometimes the findings in subjects with rhinitis are indistinguishable from those in subjects with mild asthma.[19] These findings are compatible with the above-mentioned studies of bronchial responsiveness in patients with allergic rhinitis and suggest that both the upper and lower airways are histologically and functionally abnormal in patients with rhinitis and no asthma.

EFFECTS OF RHINITIS THERAPY ON ASTHMA

Physicians often note anecdotally that treatment of allergic nasal disease results in improvements in asthma symptoms and pulmonary function. However, there have been relatively few well-controlled, large-scale clinical trials that have attempted to quantify this effect.

Intranasal Corticosteroids

Several small studies have examined the efficacy of topical intranasal corticosteroids in patients with allergic rhinitis and mild asthma. Two of these trials addressed the role of prophylactic, preseasonal treatment with nasal corticosteroids in patients with primarily seasonal symptoms. Welsh and coworkers[20] compared the effects of intranasal beclomethasone dipropionate, flunisolide, and cromolyn versus placebo in adolescent and adult patients with ragweed-induced rhinitis. Both of the topical corticosteroids were significantly more effective in reducing nasal symptoms than was either cromolyn or placebo. Unexpectedly, in 58 of the subjects who also had mild ragweed asthma, lower airway symptoms were also significantly improved in the patients receiving intranasal corticosteroids. Corren and coworkers[21] later examined the effects of seasonal administration of intranasal beclomethasone dipropionate on bronchial hyperresponsiveness in adolescent and adult patients with fall rhinitis and mild asthma. Compared with baseline values, bronchial responsiveness to inhaled methacholine worsened significantly in the placebo group but did not change in the group using active treatment. Together, these two small trials suggest that prevention of seasonal nasal inflammation with topical corticosteroids reduces subsequent exacerbations of allergic asthma.

Other studies have examined the effects of intranasal corticosteroids in patients with chronic perennial allergic rhinitis and mild asthma. The first study to document these effects used intranasal budesonide in children with severe allergic rhinitis and concomitant asthma.[22] Four weeks of active therapy significantly reduced the objective measures of nasal obstruction as well as daily asthma symptoms and exercise-induced bronchospasm. In a subsequent study of children with perennial rhinitis and asthma, Watson and colleagues[23] evaluated the effects of intranasal beclomethasone dipropionate on chest symptoms and bronchial responsiveness to methacholine. After 4 weeks of active treatment, asthma symptoms were significantly reduced, as was airway reactivity to methacholine. As an adjunct to this study, the investigators performed a radiolabeled deposition study of the beclomethasone aerosol and found that less than 2% of the drug was deposited into the chest area. These studies demonstrate that intranasal corticosteroids are effective in improving lower airway symptoms and bronchial hyperresponsiveness in patients with chronic, established nasal disease, and asthma. In view of the fact that the corticosteroid spray did not penetrate into the lungs, the study by Watson and colleagues[23] also asserts that the reduction observed in asthma was caused by improvements in nasal function rather than direct effects of the medication on the lower airways.

Antihistamines

The presence of histamine in the lower airways has been correlated with bronchial obstruction,[24] and histamine has long been thought to play a role in bronchial asthma. However, early studies of first-generation antihistamines in adolescents and adults showed minimal improvements in bronchial asthma, and initial small trials of second-generation antihistamines yielded mixed results.[25,26] However, two recent large-scale clinical studies using an antihistamine alone and an antihistamine-decongestant combination both resulted in significant improvements in asthma control. Grant and colleagues[27] demonstrated that seasonal symptoms of rhinitis and asthma were significantly attenuated in patients treated with cetirizine 10 mg once daily in a large group of adolescents and adult patients. In a second study using loratadine 5 mg plus pseudoephedrine 120 mg twice daily in patients with seasonal allergic rhinitis and asthma, Corren and colleagues[28] demonstrated that asthma symptoms, peak expiratory flow rates, and forced expiratory volume in 1 second (FEV_1) were all significantly improved in patients

taking active therapy. In reviewing data from these and similar trials, it is difficult to determine whether the salutory effects of antihistamines in asthma can be attributed to direct effects on lower airway physiology or are due to improvements in rhinitis. Because many of the currently available agents appear to have weak or transient effects on resting airway tone, benefits to the lower airway may in fact be due to modulation of upper airway function.

These studies have shown that treatment of rhinitis may result in improvements in asthma symptoms, lower airway caliber, and bronchial hyperresponsiveness and suggest that nasal disease contributes to the pathophysiology of asthma. Based on the data in these studies, treatment of rhinitis may reduce symptoms of mild asthma to such an extent that the requirement for asthma therapy may be reduced. It is uncertain whether these findings are applicable to patients with more severe asthma. Larger, longer-term studies of intranasal corticosteroids and H_1 antihistamines will need to be performed in well-defined populations of asthmatics before firm conclusions can be made.

■ PATHOPHYSIOLOGIC CONNECTIONS BETWEEN ALLERGIC RHINITIS AND ASTHMA

Although there is increasing evidence that allergic rhinitis may influence the clinical course of asthma, the mechanisms connecting upper and lower airway dysfunction are not entirely understood. A variety of theories have been invoked, including both direct and indirect effects of nasal dysfunction on the lower airways.

Systemic Effects of Nasal Inflammation on the Lower Airways

Research over the past few years has demonstrated that several inflammatory mediators produced during allergic reactions may enter the systemic circulation. Experimental nasal allergen challenge has been shown to induce both peripheral blood eosinophilia[29] and activation of peripheral blood leukocytes.[30] It has been postulated that the net result of these various factors on the systemic circulation is the promulgation of inflammation in other sites. Clinical research that supports this hypothesis was recently completed by Braunstahl and colleagues,[29] in which nasal allergen provocation was performed in subjects with allergic rhinitis. Prior to and 24 hours after the nasal challenge, bronchial mucosal biopsies were performed that demonstrated that the number of eosinophils in the lower airway mucosa, as well as the expression of adhesion molecules, increased after nasal allergen challenge. Further supporting this interaction between the upper and lower airways, Braunstahl and colleagues[31] also found increased inflammatory markers in the nasal mucosa following the instillation of allergen into the lower airways of subjects with allergic rhinitis. Given this emerging evidence, it is likely that systemic factors do play a critical role in the interaction between the upper and lower airways.

Impaired Mucosal Function

It has been shown that allergic inflammation in the respiratory mucosa results in impairment of the barrier function of the epithelium.[32] It has been hypothesized that this alteration in epithelial integrity might then lead to increases in allergen uptake, synthesis of IgE, and ultimately involvement of the lower airways. Alternatively, impaired nasal mucosa may be more susceptible to viruses, resulting in an increase in allergic sensitization and subsequently more asthma.[33]

Nasal-Bronchial Reflex

Early mechanistic studies investigated the effects of several mucosal irritants on lower airway function in normal human subjects. In 1969, Kaufman and Wright[34] applied silica particles onto the nasal mucosa of individuals without lower airway disease and noted significant, immediate increases in lower airway resistance. Bronchospasm induced by nasal silica was blocked by both resection of the trigeminal nerve[35] and systemic administration of atropine. Fontanari and coworkers[36] recently reevaluated the possibility of a neural connection between the upper and lower airways by using cold, dry air as the nasal stimulus. These investigators demonstrated that nasal exposure to very cold air caused an immediate and profound increase in pulmonary resistance that was prevented by both topical nasal anesthesia and cholinergic blockade induced by inhalation of ipratroprium bromide. Both these studies strongly suggest the presence of a reflex involving irritant receptors in the upper airway (afferent limb) and cholinergic nerves in the lower airway (efferent limb).

Subsequent studies used challenge materials considered to be more biologically relevant to allergic rhinitis, including histamine, whole pollen particles, and allergen extracts. Yan and Salome[37] performed nasal histamine challenges in subjects with perennial rhinitis and stable asthma and observed that FEV_1 was reduced by 10% or more immediately after provocation in 8 of 12 subjects. Importantly, radiolabeling studies were performed as part of this study that demonstrated that histamine was not deposited into the lower airways. However, other studies that used histamine[38] or allergen[39] failed to demonstrate bronchoconstriction after nasal provocation. This discrepancy in results may be partly explained by the type of patients who participated in these studies. Whereas Yan and Salome[37] investigated subjects with perennial, symptomatic nasal disease, the majority of other studies examined asymptomatic patients outside their pollen season. Certainly, a substantial degree of heterogeneity exists between patients in their lower airway response to nasal stimulation.

In addition to neurally mediated bronchospasm, it has been postulated that a nasal allergic reaction might result in an alteration in lower airway responsiveness. Corren and colleagues[39] investigated the effects of nasal allergen provocation on nonspecific bronchial responsiveness to methacholine. Ten subjects with seasonal allergic rhinitis and asthma were selected for study; all patients related worsening of their asthma to the onset of hay fever symptoms. Nonspecific bronchial responsiveness was significantly increased 30 minutes after nasal challenge and persisted for 4 hours.

Because radionucleide studies demonstrated no evidence of allergen deposition into the lungs, it seems unlikely that these increases in airway reactivity can be attributed to direct effects of allergen. In addition, the rapidity with which these changes occurred suggests the possibility of a reflex mechanism.

Mouth Breathing Caused by Nasal Obstruction

Nasal blockage resulting from tissue swelling and secretions may cause a shift from the normal pattern of nasal breathing to predominantly mouth breathing. Previous work has shown that mouth breathing associated with nasal obstruction resulted in worsening of exercise-induced bronchospasm, whereas exclusive nasal breathing significantly reduced asthma after exercise.[40] Improvements in asthma associated with nasal breathing may be the result of superior humidification and warming of inspired air before it reaches the lower airways.[41] Similarly, it would be expected that airborne allergens and pollutants would also be less likely to enter the lungs during periods of normal nasal function.

Postnasal Drip of Inflammatory Material

Patients frequently complain that postnasal drip triggers episodes of coughing and wheezing. Early studies investigating the possibility of aspiration of nasal secretions demonstrated that substances placed in the upper respiratory tract could later be recovered from the tracheobronchial tree.[42] More recently, Huxley and colleagues[43] investigated pharyngeal aspiration during sleep both in healthy subjects and in patients with depressed sensorium. With the use of a radiolabeled marker that was intermittently released into the nose, pulmonary aspiration was detected in a significant number of both the normal and the ill subjects. In a more recent and definitive investigation, however, Bardin and colleagues[44] were unable to document significant aspiration of radionuclide in a study of 13 patients with chronic rhinosinusitis and asthma.

It is difficult to determine which of these experimental mechanisms is most important in linking the nose to the lower airways. In all likelihood, however, several of these phenomena may contribute in some way to alterations in lung physiology in patients with allergic rhinitis and asthma.

DIAGNOSTIC AND THERAPEUTIC IMPLICATIONS

Diagnosis

The previously discussed data suggest that all patients with asthma be evaluated to exclude concomitant allergic rhinitis. The patient should be questioned regarding types of symptoms, focusing on the presence of nasal congestion, sneezing, itching, discharge, and postnasal drip. Other associated symptoms (e.g., snoring, poor sleep quality, and ear congestion or popping) should also be investigated and kept in mind when choosing therapy. The upper airway should then be carefully examined, with an emphasis on the size and vascularity of the nasal turbinates, type and presence of nasal secretions, tonsillar size, and color and elasticity of the tympanic membranes.

With regard to diagnostic testing in patients with persistent rhinitis and asthma, allergy skin tests or *in vitro* measures of specific IgE should be performed using a panel of common airborne allergens. At a minimum, these should include house dust mite (*Dermatophagoides farinae* and *D. pterynissinus*), cockroach, animal danders (cat and dog), indoor and outdoor molds (*Penicillium, Aspergillus, Cladosporium,* and *Alternaria*) and regional pollens. This information is critical in establishing an appropriate program of environmental control measures. Other tests, including total serum IgE level, microscopic analysis for nasal cytology, and total circulating blood eosinophils, have not proven helpful in either differentiating allergic rhinitis from other nasal disorders or in assessing the severity of the problem.

Allergen Avoidance

Once allergy testing is complete, the physician may devise a comprehensive program of allergen avoidance. The effects of environmental control strategies have been most heavily studied with regard to dust mites and furry pets (Box 49-1).[45] Compliance with these measures may be difficult but will certainly be helpful in many patients with hypersensitivity to these allergens.

Pharmacotherapy

While carefully designed allergen avoidance strategies may reduce symptoms to varying degrees, most patients will still require pharmacotherapy. In patients with persistent

---

BOX 49-1 ALLERGEN AVOIDANCE STRATEGIES

House Dust Mites
Weekly washing of all bedding in hot water (>130° F)
Weekly vacuum cleaning of all floor surfaces, using HEPA-type vacuum cleaner or standard vacuum cleaner with double-thickness reservoir bag
Removal of carpeting, or treatment of carpeting every 2 to 3 months with acaricidal spray or powder

Animal Danders (Any Furry Pet)
Optimal—Removal of the animal from indoor environment, followed by replacement of carpeting and aggressive housecleaning
Possibly effective—Keeping the cat indoors and instituting the following measures:
   Noncarpeted floors
   Plastic or leather furniture
   Frequent vacuum cleaning of floors
   High-flow air filtration
   Frequent cat bathing

Indoor Mold
Thorough eradication of infestation
Repair of source of water intrusion

Cockroach
Appropriate handling and storage of food and garbage

---

symptoms, particularly if nasal congestion is present, intranasal corticosteroids should be considered as first-line therapy. A large number of studies have established that there are no differences in efficacy between all of the available compounds,[46] and most (including budesonide, mometasone furoate, and fluticasone propionate) have been shown to have no significant effects on linear growth velocity in young children. These drugs should be used on a regular basis in patients with daily symptoms, or as long as symptoms dictate in children with intermittent problems.

Oral H_1 antihistamines have long been a mainstay of therapy for allergic rhinitis and are most effective in relieving sneezing, itching, and rhinorrhea, with minimal effects on nasal congestion. For this reason, they are often combined with oral decongestants, such as pseudoephedrine. A number of newer oral antihistamines that cause minimal or no sedation have been approved for use in young children, including cetirizine, fexofenadine, and loratadine.[47] Because they are available in a number of different formulations (i.e., tablets, rapidly dissolving pills, and liquids), patient preference may dictate choice of medication.

Recently, montelukast, a leukotriene D_4 receptor antagonist, has gained approval as treatment for allergic rhinitis in children.[48] Montelukast has been shown to reduce all of the symptoms of rhinitis, including nasal congestion. Because montelukast also has been shown to be effective in treating concomitant asthma, this medication may be very effective as a solo treatment for children with mild persistent allergic rhinitis and concomitant asthma.

Specific Allergen Immunotherapy

Many children will continue to have persistent symptoms of rhinitis despite employing environmental control measures for indoor allergens and a combination of drugs, often including an intranasal corticosteroid with an antihistamine or montelukast. Occasionally, children may experience adverse effects that necessitate discontinuation of some or all of their rhinitis medications. In these children, specific allergen immunotherapy should be strongly considered. Studies performed over the past decade have demonstrated that subcutaneous specific allergen immunotherapy to a wide range of allergens, including dust mites; cat dander; selected outdoor molds; and numerous grass, tree, and weed pollens, had a high rate of clinical efficacy, with approximately 75% of children manifesting a good clinical response. Other studies have documented multiple salutory immunologic effects of immunotherapy, including a reduction in allergen-induced early- and late-phase allergic responses and attenuation of cytokine (e.g., Interleukin-4) production. An important potential benefit of immunotherapy is its effect on progression of allergic airway disease. A recent large prospective study in children with seasonal allergic rhinitis demonstrated that a 3-year course of subcutaneous immunotherapy (SCIT) reduced the development of asthma symptoms and improved bronchial responsiveness compared with an open control group.[49] In a follow-up of this group 7 years after stopping SCIT, 24 of 53 (45%) children treated with placebo had developed asthma, compared with 16 of 64

(25%) who received active immunotherapy, representing a 44% reduction in asthma cases.[50] Regarding duration of treatment, once initiated, SCIT should be continued for at least 3 years.

More recently, investigators have turned their attention to other modes of administering allergen immunotherapy to both children and adults, particularly sublingual immunotherapy (SLIT). In a meta-analysis of clinical trials of SLIT in children with allergic rhinitis and asthma, SLIT caused a significant reduction in both symptoms (SMD −1.14; 95% CI −2.10 to −0.18; p = 0.02) and medication use (SMD −1.63; 95% CI −2.83 to −0.44; p = 0.007).[51] SLIT does have advantages compared with SCIT, including the absence of a buildup phase, fewer systemic reactions, and the convenience of home administration. However, it is unknown whether SLIT is as effective as SCIT, whether the effects are sustained after stopping treatment, and whether it can prevent the development of lower airway disease. Future trials will be essential in answering these questions.

Given the ability of SCIT to cause long-term modifications in nasal allergic disease as well as reduce the risk of developing asthma, allergen immunotherapy should be a strong consideration in all children with moderate to severe allergic rhinitis.

SUMMARY

Allergic rhinitis is virtually ubiquitous in children with asthma. In adolescents, allergic rhinitis may in fact serve as a risk factor for developing asthma. Intranasal corticosteroids appear to significantly modulate lower airway reactivity and have been shown in a number of small studies to have beneficial effects on mild asthma. Current research suggests that the upper and lower airways are most importantly connected via the systemic circulation, which likely distributes products of inflammation throughout the respiratory tree. Allergic rhinitis should always be considered in patients with asthma and should be treated aggressively once it has been identified. Immunotherapy may be particularly useful in children with allergic rhinitis and new-onset asthma because it may modify the long-term prognosis of their airway disease.

CHRONIC SINUSITIS AND ASTHMA

Epidemiologic Relationship Between Chronic Sinusitis and Asthma

Since the early twentieth century, physicians have noted that chronic sinus disease and asthma frequently coexist in the same patients. In 1925, Gottlieb[52] noted that 31 of 117 adolescent and adult patients with asthma suffered from severe symptoms of sinusitis. Other investigators reported similar findings in both children and adults during the next decade, with an incidence of symptomatic sinusitis as high as 72% in patients with asthma.[53] Conversely, a large retrospective study of pediatric, adolescent, and adult patients with chronic sinusitis noted a 12% incidence of asthma.[54] Only one third of the patients with both sinus disease and asthma in this study reported that sinusitis preceded their lower airway symptoms.

Attempts to define the incidence of sinus disease in patients with asthma again lay dormant until the early 1970s. These more recent reports have emphasized the role of radiography in diagnosing sinusitis. Several studies have demonstrated that 31% to 53% of asthmatics across all age groups have abnormal sinus radiographs, with 21% to 31% of patients demonstrating significant findings (defined as opacification of one or both maxillary sinuses, air-fluid levels, or mucosal thickening >5 mm).[55-58] In a more recent study that examined the utility of sinus computed tomography (CT) scanning in children with asthma, it was noted that 58% of the children had varying abnormalities of all of the sinuses[59] (Table 49-1).

Although the incidence of radiographic sinus abnormalities is universally high in asthmatics, others have questioned whether these changes have clinical significance. Fascenelli[60] prospectively performed sinus radiography on 411 asymptomatic adolescent and adult male volunteers and noted a 28% incidence of maxillary sinus abnormalities. Most of these changes, however, consisted of minimal thickening, and only 5% of the group demonstrated significant thickening (>5 mm) of the maxillary antrum. In a similar prospective study of young children, Kovatch and colleagues[61] noted that 8 of 22 (36%) asymptomatic children younger than 1 year of age demonstrated either thickening greater than 4 mm or opacification of the maxillary sinuses. Only 2 of 31 (6%)

TABLE 49-1 PREVALENCE OF RADIOGRAPHIC SINUSITIS IN ASTHMATICS

STUDY	SAMPLE SIZE	AGE RANGE (YR)	TOTAL ABNORMALITIES (%)	SIGNIFICANT ABNORMALITIES (%)*
Berman et al.[55†]	52	19-80	62	NA
Rachelefsky et al.[56†]	70	3-16	52	27
Schwartz et al.[57†]	217	9-70	47	21
Zimmerman et al.[58†]	138	6-19	31	31
Chen et al.[59‡]	53	4-14	58	NA

*Opacification, air-fluid level, or >5 mm mucosal thickening.
†Plain films only.
‡Plain films and computed tomography.
NA, Not assessed.

children older than 1 year of age, however, demonstrated these same changes. These two studies demonstrate that it is unusual to detect significant radiographic abnormalities of the maxillary sinuses in normal, healthy individuals older than 1 year of age. Significant abnormalities of sinus radiographs are much more common in patients with asthma than in healthy, nonasthmatic individuals, suggesting that these radiographic findings most likely reflect pathologic changes of the sinus tissue rather than radiologic artifact.

UNIQUE FEATURES OF CHRONIC SINUSITIS IN ASTHMATICS

Although a large proportion of asthmatics have abnormal sinus radiographs, it remains controversial whether these changes are caused by bacterial infection or represent chronic, noninfectious inflammation or both. Clinical and histologic studies suggest that the paranasal sinuses of these patients may be affected by a process that is clinically and pathogenetically distinct from sinusitis in nonasthmatics.

Clinical Features

Chronic sinusitis in children is often an indolent illness, usually characterized by one or more of the following symptoms: nasal congestion, purulent anterior or posterior nasal drainage, or cough.[62] Although headache may also be a prominent complaint in adolescents and adults, it is uncommon in children with chronic sinusitis. Additionally, fever is most unusual. Because cough may be the most prominent presenting symptom of chronic sinusitis in children, the physician must maintain a high index of suspicion regarding this possibility. Therefore, any child with symptomatic asthma and cough who has responded poorly to conventional asthma treatment (e.g., inhaled corticosteroid plus a long-acting β_2 agonist, a leukotriene D_4 receptor antagonist, or both) should be evaluated thoroughly for chronic sinus disease, particularly if nasal congestion or postnasal drip are present.

Histopathology

More than 60 years ago, Hansel[63] studied the histology of nasal and sinus mucosa in patients with asthma, allergic rhinitis, or both conditions. Pathologic examination of sinus tissue in these patients revealed infiltration with a large number of eosinophils, hyperplasia of mucus-producing cells, and stromal edema. Moreover, these findings were remarkably similar to the pathologic features of bronchial asthma.

More recently, Harlin and colleagues[64] explored the role of the eosinophil and eosinophilic granular proteins in chronic sinusitis by assessing sinus tissue specimens obtained at surgery from 26 patients ranging from 13 to 74 years of age. Sinus tissue was examined by routine histology as well as immunofluorescent staining for major basic protein, a principal granule-stored protein of the eosinophil. All 13 sinus specimens from patients with asthma (allergic and nonallergic) and 6 of 7 specimens from patients with allergic rhinitis demonstrated significant

numbers of eosinophils and tissue deposition of major basic protein. In 6 patients with chronic sinusitis and no history of asthma or nasal allergy, however, none demonstrated significant sinus tissue eosinophilia, and only 1 of 6 showed significant tissue staining for major basic protein. In a study limited to children (mean age 9 years), Baroody and colleagues characterized the histopathology of chronic sinusitis in patients with and without asthma.[65] Sinus tissue in all patients with chronic sinusitis contained large numbers of eosinophils and was highest in those children with concomitant asthma. Additionally, the presence of allergy was not predictive of sinus eosinophilia in these patients.

While these studies reveal the nature of the inflammatory infiltrate in chronic sinusitis, Hisamatsu and colleagues[66] examined the effect of eosinophilic proteins on the ciliary activity of sinus mucosa in vitro. The investigators found that eosinophil-derived major basic protein damaged the mucosal epithelium and caused ciliostasis at concentrations that may be achieved in vivo. These findings have great clinical importance because ciliary dysfunction may be one of the key factors contributing to persistent bacterial infection of the paranasal sinuses.

These studies indicate that there is significant eosinophil invasion and deposition of eosinophilic granule–derived proteins into the tissues of the paranasal sinuses in both children and adolescents with concomitant sinusitis and asthma. Additionally, eosinophil infiltration of sinus mucosa causes epithelial alterations, which may predispose to recurrent or chronic infection.

Microbiology

In 1974, Berman and colleagues[55] studied 21 adolescent and adult patients with asthma and radiographic abnormalities of the maxillary sinuses. Bacterial cultures of sinus aspirates demonstrated positive bacterial growth in only 5 of 25 aspirates. Eighty percent of the subjects in this study, however, had minimal evidence of sinusitis (mucosal thickening <2 mm and no sinus polyps). Therefore, conclusions from this study are most relevant to patients with mild sinusitis and may not be applicable to individuals with evidence of more severe disease. In children with asthma and chronic sinusitis, several bacteriologic studies have been conducted. In 1983, Adinoff and colleagues[67] published a report regarding 42 asthmatic children with sinusitis. Only 12% of maxillary sinus aspirates had positive bacterial cultures; however, many of the studies involving children showed only mild radiographic abnormalities with <5 mm mucosal thickening. Friedman and colleagues[68] in 1984 and Goldenhersh and colleagues[69] in 1990 performed maxillary aspirates in groups of 8 and 12 asthmatic children, respectively, with significant radiographic evidence of sinusitis (i.e., opacification, air-fluid levels, or mucosal thickening >5 mm). These two groups demonstrated that 60% and 75% of these children, respectively, had positive bacterial cultures, and the organisms were the same as those found in acute sinusitis, including *Streptococcus pneumoniae,* *Haemophilus influenzae,* and *Moraxella catarrhalis.* Taken together, the above studies demonstrate that the majority of children with sinusitis and asthma appear to have a chronic inflammatory disease of the sinus mucosa that is prone to persistent infection with predominantly aerobic bacteria. Data from the radiographic studies also suggest that minor degrees of mucosal inflammation observed on sinus radiograph are usually not associated with active bacterial infection.

Allergic Fungal Sinusitis

An unusual type of chronic sinusitis in children is caused by an allergic reaction to fungi, referred to as allergic fungal sinusitis (AFS). A recent retrospective review characterized 20 patients (7 to 18 years of age) with AFS and determined that 90% had nasal polyps, 55% had a prior history of asthma, and 50% had proptosis. Laboratory analyses revealed that all patients had abnormal sinus CT findings and positive skin tests to fungi, 90% had an elevation of total IgE, and 70% had peripheral eosinophilia.[70] Surgical specimens demonstrated allergic-type mucin in 55% of patients and positive fungal cultures in 85%. Importantly, relapse was seen in 55% of patients at 1-year follow-up.

◼ EFFECTS OF SINUS THERAPY ON ASTHMA

For the past century, otolargyngologists have cataloged the effects of sinus therapy on asthma symptoms. Because most of the earliest data were based on postsurgical observations, we will review those studies first.

Surgical Treatment

In the early twentieth century, physicians observed that surgical treatment of nasal and sinus disease resulted in variable improvements in asthma symptoms. In 1936, Weille[71] published his study of 500 asthmatic patients of varying ages, 72% of whom had chronic sinus disease. Following sinus surgery in 100 of the patients, 56 reported that their chest symptoms were improved, and 10 experienced complete resolution of asthma. Improvement in asthma symptoms, however, also occurred in 40% of the patients who did not undergo sinus surgery. In 1969, Davison[72] reported that 23 of 24 adolescent and adult patients with chronic sinusitis and asthma experienced a 75% or greater improvement in asthma symptoms after surgical drainage of the sinuses. Werth[73] presented the results of sinus surgery in children, noting that 20 of 22 pediatric patients with severe asthma and sinusitis experienced a marked improvement in asthma after sinus surgery.

To date, there have been no randomized, controlled trials examining the effects of sinus surgery on lower airway symptoms or function. The study by Weille does indicate that asthma symptoms may improve spontaneously in the absence of surgical intervention. Collectively, however, these reports suggest that long-term control of asthma symptoms may improve after surgical sinus procedures.

Medical Treatment

During the past decade, multiple investigators have studied the effect of medical therapy on asthma symptoms, primarily in children. In 1981, Businco and

colleagues[74] reported that 10 of 12 children with chronic asthma had an improvement in lower airway symptoms after medical therapy, although no objective measures of pulmonary function were performed. In 1983, Cummings and colleagues[75] performed a double-blind, placebo-controlled study of sinus therapy in asthma. Active treatment (i.e., antimicrobials, nasal steroids, and oral decongestants) of children with opacification or marked thickening of the maxillary sinuses resulted in significantly fewer asthma symptoms and a reduced requirement for inhaled bronchodilator and oral steroid therapy. Neither pulmonary function results nor measures of bronchial reactivity were significantly improved with active treatment. In 1984, Rachelefsky and colleagues[76] studied 48 children with a 3-month or longer history of sinusitis and wheezing. After 2 to 4 weeks of antimicrobials with or without antral lavage, 38 of the patients were able to discontinue daily bronchodilator therapy, and 20 of 30 patients demonstrated normalization of pulmonary function tests. During the same year, Friedman and colleagues[68] studied eight children experiencing asthma exacerbations associated with sinusitis. After 2 to 4 weeks of antimicrobial therapy, seven of eight patients reported improvement in lower airway symptoms. Although baseline indices of pulmonary function were not changed after the completion of antimicrobials, there was a significant improvement in FEV_1 following inhaled bronchodilator therapy.

Similar to the surgical observations, these studies suggest that medical treatment of sinusitis may result in improvement of bronchial asthma. Although only one randomized, placebo-controlled trial has been done, both chest symptoms and lower airway function do appear to improve significantly after aggressive medical therapy.

◼ PATHOPHYSIOLOGIC LINKS BETWEEN CHRONIC SINUSITIS AND ASTHMA

As noted in the section entitled Allergic Rhinitis and Asthma, a number of potential mechanisms may help explain the connection between upper and lower airway dysfunction. Specifically, with respect to the relationship between sinus inflammation and asthma, an animal model has provided some promising insights into this interaction. Brugman and colleagues[77] created an experimental model of sinus inflammation in rabbits using complement fragment C5a. Although induction of sterile sinus inflammation in rabbits caused no changes in baseline lung function, bronchial responsiveness to inhaled histamine was significantly increased. Because these changes could be prevented by strategies that blocked drainage of inflammatory exudates beyond the larynx, the researchers postulated that postnasal drip was most likely responsible for the alteration in airway reactivity. Importantly, however, there was no evidence of lower airway inflammation by either histologic examination or bronchoalveolar lavage. This association of hyperresponsiveness with morphologically normal airways is difficult to explain but again suggests the possibility of a neurally mediated response.

DIAGNOSTIC AND THERAPEUTIC IMPLICATIONS

In children with moderate to severe asthma, we believe that chronic sinusitis should always be considered as a possible provocative factor. The clinical history and physical examination, however, are neither sensitive nor specific for chronic sinus disease. Therefore, we evaluate all children with poorly controlled or steroid-requiring asthma with a Waters' view (occipitomental) sinus radiograph, which is primarily useful for examining the maxillary sinuses. Although CT of the paranasal sinuses has proven to be considerably more sensitive than plain radiographs in detecting subtle mucosal disease,[78] we believe that plain radiographic examination has an important role as an initial imaging study. First, plain radiographs are simple, convenient, and relatively inexpensive to perform. Second, in contrast to CT imaging, plain radiographs do not require sedation in infants or young children. Finally, the significance of subtle sinus CT changes is unclear because such abnormalities may be present in up to 50% of children[79] who have no clinical evidence of either sinusitis or asthma. We reserve CT imaging of the sinuses for patients with clinical histories strongly suggestive of sinusitis who have normal plain radiographs and patients with persistent, severe sinus disease before surgical intervention.

Flexible fiberoptic rhinoscopy has been suggested as an alternative to plain radiographs because purulent drainage may be visualized in the vicinity of the middle and superior meatus.[80] In our experience, however, the absence of pus does not rule out active infection because sinus drainage may be obstructed by ostial edema or obstructing lesions of the nasal airway. Additionally, rhinoscopy will not detect significant hyperplastic changes in the sinuses, which may play an important pathogenic role in asthma. In the context of sinus disease, we generally use rhinoscopy for identifying anatomic lesions (e.g., adenoidal hypertrophy) that may predispose the patient to sinusitis.

Patients who demonstrate significant radiographic abnormalities of the maxillary sinuses (i.e., opacification, air-fluid levels, or thickening >5 mm, or more than 50% of the maxillary antrum) are treated with medical therapy. We classify medical treatment modalities for chronic sinusitis into three categories: antimicrobials to eliminate possible concomitant infection, medications to reduce swelling, and measures to thin and evacuate secretions (Box 49-2).

Because up to 25% of the bacterial isolates found in chronic sinusitis are β lactamase producers, we prescribe amoxicillin-clavulanate potassium as a first-line antimicrobial for a period of no less than 3 weeks. In children who are allergic to penicillin, clarithromycin is employed as an alternative agent. For nasal swelling, we often use topical decongestants (e.g., oxymetazoline) for the initial 3 days of therapy and continue oral decongestants (either phenylpropanolamine or pseudoephedrine) for an additional 7 to 10 days. If nasal swelling does not respond to these measures, we prescribe a 5- to 7-day tapering course of oral corticosteroids. All patients are also started on a topical nasal corticosteroid, which is usually continued on a long-term basis. We have found that evacuation of secretions, particularly dried crusts, is enhanced by performing nasal irrigations with saline or increasing humidification using a free-standing humidifier or hot shower. Nasal saline irrigations have been evaluated in a

---

BOX 49-2 MEDICAL TREATMENT OF CHRONIC SINUSITIS IN ASTHMATICS

Antimicrobials
Amoxicillin-clavulanate potassium for a minimum of 21 days (or clarithromycin in penicillin-allergic patients)
If the patient does not respond, alternative use of β-lactamase–resistant antimicrobial (e.g., cefuroxime) for 21 additional days

Medications to Reduce Swelling
For severe swelling, topical oxymetazoline for 3 days
If swelling persists, continue with oral pseudoephedrine on a regular basis for 7 to 10 days or longer if needed
Use of intranasal corticosteroid spray for 3 to 6 weeks
If swelling does not respond, use of prednisone 0.5 mg/kg body weight, tapered over 5 to 7 days

Measures to Enhance Evacuation of Secretions
Use of saline irrigations
Use of hot steam inhalations

---

number of clinical trials, and a recent Cochrane review concluded that this treatment modality is helpful to patients with chronic sinusitis, either when used alone or as an adjunct to other treatments.[81] If no improvement in nasal symptoms occurs and the patient's asthma remains poorly controlled, we institute a second 3-week course of another β lactamase–resistant antimicrobial (e.g., cefuroxime axetil). If patients fail to respond adequately to the aforementioned regimen, we consider sinus CT and refer them to an otolaryngologist for consideration of endoscopic sinus surgery.

SUMMARY

A great deal of data support an association between chronic sinusitis and asthma. We have developed a better understanding of the pathogenesis of sinus disease in asthmatic patients and now realize that eosinophilic sinus infiltration plays a direct role in chronic mucosal inflammation that may predispose the paranasal sinuses to recurrent or chronic bacterial infection. Long-term blinded, placebo-controlled trials need to be completed before we can reliably predict the effect of sinus therapy on clinical asthma. Until then, we recommend that sinus disease be considered in all patients with moderate to severe asthma and treated aggressively when it is identified.

Suggested Reading

Braunstahl G-J, Overbeek S, Kleinjan A, et al. Nasal allergen provocation induces adhesion molecules expression and tissue eosinophilia in upper and lower airways. *J Allergy Clin Immunol*. 2001;107:469–476.

Burgess JA, Walters EH, Byrnes GB, et al. Childhood allergic rhinitis predicts asthma incidence and persistence to middle age: a longitudinal study. *J Allergy Clin Immunol*. 2007;120:863–869.

Jacobsen L, Niggemann B, Dreborg S, et al. Specific immunotherapy has long-term preventive effect of seasonal and perennial asthma: 10-year follow-up on the PAT study. *Allergy*. 2007;62:943–948.

Kusel MM, de Klerk NH, Kebadze T, et al. Early-life respiratory viral infections, atopic sensitization, and risk of subsequent development of persistent asthma. *J Allergy Clin Immunol*. 2007;119:1105–1111.

Platts-Mills TA. Allergen avoidance. *J Allergy Clin Immunol*. 2004;113:388–391.

References

The complete reference list is available online at www.expertconsult.com

50 GENETICS AND PATHOPHYSIOLOGY OF CYSTIC FIBROSIS

GARRY R. CUTTING, MD, AND PAMELA L. ZEITLIN, MD, PhD

The genetic basis of cystic fibrosis (CF) has been recognized by the medical community since the 1940s.[1] A genetic etiology and autosomal-recessive inheritance was suggested by the recurrence of CF in siblings and the absence of the illness in parents. Genetic linkage analysis confirmed that a single locus was responsible for classic CF.[2,3] In 1989, technical breakthroughs allowing identification of disease-causing genes on the basis of position rather than function enabled Tsui and colleagues to clone the gene responsible for this disorder.[4] The identified gene was aptly named the cystic fibrosis transmembrane conductance regulator (CFTR).[5] During the past 20 years, our understanding of the molecular basis of CF has exploded. We now recognize that mutations in CFTR give rise to a range of phenotypes extending from classic CF to single-organ pathology. The successful use of therapies directed at the complications of CF has raised the question as to potential efficacy in disease phenotypes that mimic CF, including idiopathic bronchiectasis,[6,7] chronic Pseudomonas aeruginosa airways colonization in tracheostomy patients,[8] or chronic obstructive pulmonary disease.[9] The assumption that all carriers of a single mutation in CFTR are asymptomatic also has been questioned. The consequences of many mutations on the function of the encoded protein have been determined, allowing correlation of altered function of CFTR with CF pathophysiology. Novel molecules capable of repairing several different classes of CFTR mutations are in clinical trials in North America, Europe, and Israel, raising the very real possibility of treatments directed at the primary cause of CF.

CFTR GENE

Structure

The CFTR gene resides on the long arm of human chromosome 7 and encompasses approximately 189,000 base pairs of DNA.[10] The coding portion of the gene is divided into 27 exons that are transcribed into a messenger RNA (mRNA) of approximately 6500 base pairs.[5] The exon and intron structure of the CFTR gene is well conserved among mammals and evolutionarily distant species such as amphibians (Xenopus) and fish (killifish and dogfish).[11]

Transcription of CFTR is initiated 80 base pairs upstream from the start site of translation.[12,13] The CFTR gene demonstrates exquisite temporal and spatial differences in expression. For example, specific cell types within the human lung express high levels of CFTR, while surface epithelial cells have a very low level of CFTR expression.[14] CFTR expression is also regulated during development.[15,16] Despite considerable evidence that the expression of CFTR is highly selective, the precise elements that regulate CFTR expression have not been identified. Sequences immediately upstream of the transcriptional start site of CFTR generate low-level expression in most tissues. This pattern of expression is consistent with the presence of basal promoter elements.[17,18] A cyclic adenosine monophosphate (cAMP) response element has been identified within this region of CFTR, but this element does not appear to account for the spatial and temporal expression patterns.[19] Assays that search for binding of protein to DNA have identified several regions elsewhere in the CFTR gene that may be involved in transcriptional regulation.[20-23] Furthermore, cross-species analysis has identified regions of the CFTR gene that are highly conserved, suggesting a possible role in regulation of gene expression.[11] Strain-specific differences in CFTR expression in mice have been mapped to sequences about 700 base pairs upstream of the CFTR gene, indicating the existence of regulatory elements in this region.[24] Finally, epigenetic mechanisms such as methylation do not appear to play a major role in regulating CFTR expression.[25,26] Thus, despite extensive efforts to locate transcriptional elements, the molecular mechanisms regulating CFTR expression are incompletely understood.

Splicing

Variations in *CFTR* splicing patterns have been identified by the reverse transcription–polymerase chain reaction technique.[27,28] There are relatively few alternatively spliced transcripts that create functional isoforms of *CFTR*.[29] However, RNA transcripts resulting from alternative splicing of exon 5 *CFTR* have not been identified in other species or in other tissues. Transcripts missing a portion of exons 13 and 14a encode a functional isoform of *CFTR* expressed in mouse and human kidney.[30] Neither the heart nor the kidney appears to be primarily involved in CF pathophysiology; thus, the role of these alternatively spliced forms of *CFTR* is unclear.

In contrast to alternative splicing, many aberrantly spliced versions of *CFTR* have been identified. Aberrantly spliced *CFTR* RNA transcripts do not produce functional *CFTR*. Aberrant splicing occurs as a result of variation in intronic or exonic sequences required for normal splicing of *CFTR*. The aberrant splicing of exon 9 is a notable example.[31,32] Variation in the length of the polythymidine tract, an element in the 3′ splice site of intron 8, is correlated with the amount of properly spliced *CFTR* mRNA.[33] Longer versions of this tract called 9T and 7T are common in the population and are associated with high levels of normally spliced CFTR mRNA. A shorter version of this tract called 5T is associated with a substantial reduction in full-length *CFTR* RNA.[34] While abbreviated polythymidine tracts in 3′ splice sites do not usually cause missplicing of the subsequent exon, it appears that a special situation occurs in the *CFTR* gene. Sequence surrounding exon 9, including unusual variation in splice sites surrounding exon 9 and splice-silencing sequences in intron 9, appear to make exon 9 vulnerable to missplicing.[35-37] Thus, alterations in secondary splicing signals of this exon such as the polythymidine tract have an exaggerated effect on splicing. The splicing efficiency of *CFTR* genes bearing 5T also varies by tissue. The vas deferens splices *CFTR* genes bearing the 5T variant less efficiently than respiratory epithelia, which explains the existence of congenital bilateral absence of the vas deferens without other symptoms.[38,39]

Individuals carrying the 5T mutation in their other *CFTR* gene manifest a variety of phenotypes ranging from healthy to nonclassic CF (see later). The latter phenomenon is due to the variable effect that 5T has on splicing of *CFTR* exon 9. This splicing variability is caused by variation in the number of TG dinucleotides adjacent to the polythymidine tract.[40] The role of the TG tract in splicing of 5T alleles is controversial. It may serve as a site for binding of a splicing repressor, or the RNA may form a secondary structure such as a hairpin that affects gene expression.[41,42] Either way, there is a robust correlation between the length of the TG tract and the phenotypes associated with a 5T variant.[43]

Many other *CFTR* transcripts derived from aberrant splicing of exons 9 through 12 have been reported, yet none appear to be correlated with phenotype.[28,44-47] Another example of aberrant *CFTR* splicing involves exons 23 and 24, resulting in a prematurely truncated CFTR protein that is nonfunctional.[48] The many mutations that affect *CFTR* splicing and result in disease are summarized in the following section.

Mutations

More than 1500 mutations in the *CFTR* gene associated with disease have been reported to the Cystic Fibrosis Genetic Analysis Consortium (http://www.genet.sickkids. on.ca/cftr/). The Consortium website has implemented mutation nomenclature according to Human Genome and Variome Society (HGVS) guidelines. Mutations are now provided in legacy and HGVS format (http://www. genet.sickkids.on.ca/cftr/). Legacy names are used in this chapter, and the HGVS nomenclature is provided with the first mention of a mutation. The vast majority of *CFTR* mutations reported to be associated with disease involve only one or a few nucleotides. Nearly 50% of mutations change an amino acid, while mutations that affect splicing or introduce a nonsense codon account for approximately 25%. Deletion and insertion mutations that alter the reading frame and usually result in the introduction of a premature termination codon account for about 20%. Deletions and insertions involving multiples of three nucleotides are much less common (2%). The latter mutations do not shift the reading frame, so a protein missing one or more amino acids is usually produced (e.g., *CFTR* with the ΔF508 (HGVS p.Phe508del) mutation). Most of the remaining disease-associated mutations (3%) involve the deletion of larger regions of DNA involving hundreds to thousands of base pairs. Finally, a few mutations (1%) have been purported to have occurred in sequences thought to be involved in transcriptional regulation of the *CFTR* gene, although a convincing case has been made in only a few cases.[49] In addition to the disease-associated mutations, almost 270 mutations in *CFTR* have not been associated with disease. These mutations have been termed *sequence variants* or *polymorphisms*. However, there are some polymorphisms in *CFTR* (e.g., *M470V* HGVS p.Met470Val) wherein an effect on phenotype has been suggested.[40,50] Mutations that are "silent" (that do not change an encoded amino acid or known splicing signal) are not predicted to alter *CFTR* function. However, the elucidation of intronic and exonic signals that enhance or repress exon splicing raises the possibility that some "silent" changes may affect *CFTR* splicing.[51,52]

The distribution of disease-associated mutations in the *CFTR* gene among human populations has been extensively reviewed.[53,54] One mutation, a deletion of three nucleotides that leads to loss of a single phenylalanine residue at codon 508 (ΔF508), accounts for approximately 70% of CF alleles in northern European Caucasians. The frequency of the ΔF508 mutation varies on the European continent from lower than 50% of CF alleles in southern Europe to as high as 88% of CF alleles in Denmark. The ΔF508 mutation is quite rare in native Africans and native Asians. However, the ΔF508 mutation is found in racially admixed populations. For example, 30% of the *CFTR* genes in American CF patients of African descent have the ΔF508 mutation.[55] On the other hand, the second most common mutation in African Americans with CF (3120 + 1G>A; HGVS c.2988+1G>A) appears to be a common CF allele in native Africans.[56,57] Deleterious CF alleles also have been found in CF patients of Asian ancestry.[58,59] These mutations have not been observed in white or native African populations. Thus, rare deleterious mutations in the *CFTR* gene occur in all human populations. However, it is the commonness of the ΔF508 mutation in Europeans that accounts for the high incidence of CF in whites.

In addition to ΔF508, only about 25 other mutations occur with a frequency of 0.1% or greater in the white CF population.[55,60] Other mutations are seen with some frequency in African Americans.[56] Finally, some ethnic groups have one or several mutations that reach a frequency of 1% or greater that are rare in the general population. The higher frequency of the latter mutations is probably the consequence of a founder effect.[61] The remainder of the reported mutations (~1000) has been reported in only a small number of individuals. Screening for the ΔF508 mutation and 22 mutations that have a frequency of >0.1% detects about 85% of mutations in white CF patients.[62] Mutation screens involving 50 to 100 CF mutations produce a minimal increase in detection rate in the general CF population (1% to 3%). Because there are so many rare mutations, in order to achieve a detection rate for classic CF over 95%, screening of the entire coding region of the *CFTR* gene is required.[63,64]

CFTR Protein

Characteristics
The CFTR protein is composed of a linear stretch of 1,480 amino acids that form an integral membrane glycoprotein. A comparison of the nucleotide sequence across available databases places this protein as a member of the ABC transporter superfamily. The topology of the protein contains the common features of twofold symmetry with six transmembrane domains and an intracellular nucleotide-binding fold. The CFTR is unique in the presence of a central intracellular R domain enriched in phosphorylation sites used by the protein kinases A and C. Although most members of the superfamily are transporters (e.g., the multidrug resistance transporter MDR transports chemotherapy agents), the CFTR is a cAMP-regulated chloride and bicarbonate channel that must function for the outwardly rectifying chloride channel (ORCC) to transport chloride. Functional CFTR also downregulates the epithelial sodium channel (ENaC) in those cells in which both reside. More controversial functions have been reported, including transport of nucleotides and fatty acids.

Biogenesis

The CFTR polypeptide is translated from the mRNA in the endoplasmic reticulum (ER) as a linear chain of amino acids with hydrophilic (water-soluble) and hydrophobic (lipid-soluble) domains. The nascent polypeptide is assisted by interactions with chaperone proteins within and outside the ER to assume a tertiary or folded structure that buries the membrane-spanning domains in the ER membrane. The process is relatively slow, taking approximately 10 to 15 minutes to complete, and is followed by two different fates. Depending on the cell type making the CFTR, the wild-type chain could be ubiquitinated and sent to the proteasome for degradation,[65] or it could continue along the trafficking pathway to the Golgi apparatus. Chloride transport through the CFTR can be detected in the ER using patch-clamping techniques, but it is not known whether the immature functional channel is the one protected from proteasomal degradation. The successful CFTR is packaged into vesicles for transport.[66] Adequate anion channel transport through cell surface CFTR depends not only on the characteristics of the channel pore or degree of phosphorylation and ATP hydrolysis but also on numbers of CFTR proteins and residence time at the surface. CFTR is actively recycled from the plasma membrane, and some mutants are much less stable than WT-CFTR.[67]

Function

The three-dimensional topology of CFTR is under investigation. The two nucleotide binding domains (NBDs) and the R domain probably interact such that phosphorylation of the R domain is required for chloride channel opening and probably affects the affinity of the NBDs for adenosine triphosphate (ATP).[68] ATP hydrolysis at NBD1 is associated with opening the channel, but hydrolysis at NBD2 is associated with closure. The chloride pore is formed by transmembrane domains, and the single-channel conductance is low at 6 to 10 picosiemens. The current-voltage relationship is linear, meaning that it is just as easy for chloride to leave as to enter the cell, depending on the direction of the voltage applied across the membrane. This bidirectionality is possible because ATP is the ligand that is hydrolyzed to gate the channel.

The most common mutation in CFTR, the ΔF508 deletion of the code for phenylalanine at position 508, has two consequences. First, the channel has a low open time for chloride—about 10% of normal.[69,70] Second, the newly translated CFTR is unstable in the ER, leading to premature proteolysis and a reduced half-life in the cell. The mutation appears to affect intermolecular interactions within CFTR rather than NBD1 folding.[71,72]

Cellular Distribution and Function

Developmental Expression and Function
CFTR mRNA is detectable in many fetal tissues in the first trimester. Data have been collected for fetal lung, intestine, pancreas, and kidney from humans, rats, rabbits, and mice. During early mammalian embryonic tissue development, *CFTR* may be more important as a regulator of other ion channels rather than as a pathway for chloride transport.[73] CFTR protein becomes detectable in the second trimester, still quite early in development. *CFTR* expression declines in postnatal lung, and this decline begins even earlier in the rat in the last trimester. There is a bronchial centrifugal expression gradient and a developmental shift from apolar localization to apical localization, with a timing

that matches that of *CFTR* regulation of the epithelial sodium channel ENaC. In other words, since ENaC function is required to resorb fetal lung fluid at birth as an adaptation to air-breathing, *CFTR* expression, a downregulator of ENaC function, declines and ENaC expression increases.

Postnatal Expression and Function

Regulated airway fluid and ion composition becomes more important for the air-breathing mammal than it was during lung development. CF lungs are morphologically normal at birth, in part because there are sufficient alternative chloride transport pathways in fetal lung to support tissue expansion and differentiation.[73] After birth, airway mucociliary clearance is affected by the depth and characteristics of the periciliary fluid layer, which in turn is dependent on ENaC function.[74-76] Over time, the human infant with pancreatic-insufficient CF is increasingly vulnerable to infection and inflammation in the airways, which lead to the classic lung phenotype of airways obstruction.

Tissue Distribution

Absent or reduced function of CFTR can be measured quantitatively in the sweat duct, where the reabsorptive coil is designed to conserve chloride, sodium, and water to protect the mammal from dehydration. The diagnostic sweat test takes advantage of the cholinergic pathway for generation of sweat by the sweat gland coil. CFTR is only responsible for at most 1% of sweat generation but is required for chloride reabsorption in the duct, thus leading to elevated sweat chloride concentrations.

CFTR plays a vital role in several other organs, tissues where epithelial proteins are secreted along with electrolytes. The most important organs are the airways, bile ducts, pancreatic ducts, and vas deferens. Interestingly, although CFTR is highly expressed in the kidney, its absence is not detrimental. The simplified scheme in which CFTR plays an electrophysiologic role to control the ion and water content of luminal secretions is insufficient to explain the nature of CF lung disease. In CF lungs, additional abnormalities of fluid are associated with chronic inflammation and infection.

Genotype-Phenotype Correlations

Molecular Consequences of Mutations

The effect of disease-associated mutations on CFTR function has been investigated for a small fraction of CF alleles. Mutations that have been studied include those that are common in CF patients (e.g., ΔF508, G551D; HGVS p.Gly551Asp), those that occur in patients with mild forms of the disease (e.g., A455E HGVS p.Ala455Glu), and those that occur in known or putative functional domains of CFTR (e.g., R347H; HGVS p.Arg347His and R347P; HGVS p.Arg347Pro). The functional consequences of these mutations can be grouped into five classes.[77,78] Mutations that have consequences that do not fall into one of the five classes are discussed at the end of this section.

Class I mutations cause changes in the synthesis of CFTR by affecting CFTR transcription. These mutations manifest their effect within the nucleus and usually involve the processing of transcripts. In most cases, the introduction of a premature termination codon, whether by a change of a codon to a nonsense mutation or by frameshift, results in degradation of the transcript by a nonsense-mediated mRNA decay mechanism.[79] G542X (HGVS p.Gly542X) is an example of this type of mutation.[80] In some cases, the premature termination codon does not lead to nonsense-mediated decay, and a truncated but nonfunctional protein is produced (e.g., R1162X [HGVS p.Arg1162X]).[81,82] A third consequence of nonsense mutations is that they can cause skipping of the exon in which they occur.[83] An example of this phenomenon is seen with the R553X (HGVS p.Arg553X) mutation.[84] Mutations in the highly conserved splicing signals 5′ and 3′ of exons invariably lead to a loss of full-length transcript due to exon skipping.[85] Loss of exons also can cause a shift in the reading frame leading to the introduction of a premature termination codon and subsequent RNA degradation. In each case, these types of mutations lead to complete, or almost complete loss of functional CFTR protein and produce a classic form of CF (Fig. 50-1). Some of the nonsense mutations in CFTR have been shown to be rescued with application of a compound, ataluren, derived from aminoglycoside antibiotics that can induce read-through of premature termination codons. This investigational drug is in phase III clinical trials in CF worldwide. The premature termination codon mutants are relatively frequent in Israel, where early phase clinical trials have shown some promise.[86,87]

The second class of mutations involves those that affect the processing of CFTR[88] (see Fig. 50-1). A prime example of a class II mutation is ΔF508. Loss of the phenylalanine residue at codon 508 within the first nucleotide-binding fold leads to a misfolding of CFTR.[89] Misfolded CFTR is recognized by chaperones that shunt the misfolded protein to degradation pathways.[90] The folding defect can be partially overcome by reduction in temperature. Cells grown at 21° C instead of 37° C can produce properly folded CFTR.[91] Folded CFTR bearing ΔF508 is functional in the cell membrane, but it is not stable and is more rapidly removed from the membrane than its wild-type counterpart.[92] Because ΔF508 is found in at least 70% of CF patients, the mechanisms underlying CFTR degradation have been studied intensively in hopes of finding approaches that permit CFTR bearing the ΔF508 mutation to evade degradation (see the Molecular Therapy chapter). Other class II mutations have been found that reduce folding efficiency, resulting in a small amount of properly folded functional CFTR at the cell membrane.[93,94] Two new molecules have been developed for correction, VX809, and potentiation, VX770, of the ΔF508 mutant protein.[95,96] Each investigational drug alone, and then the two in combination, are in clinical trials.

Disease-associated mutations in class III affect the regulation of CFTR (see Fig. 50-1). Binding of ATP to the NBDs is required to activate CFTR. Mutations that affect CFTR interaction with ATP have been shown to alter its function.[69,97] An example is the G551D mutation in

CLASSIC CF GENOTYPES

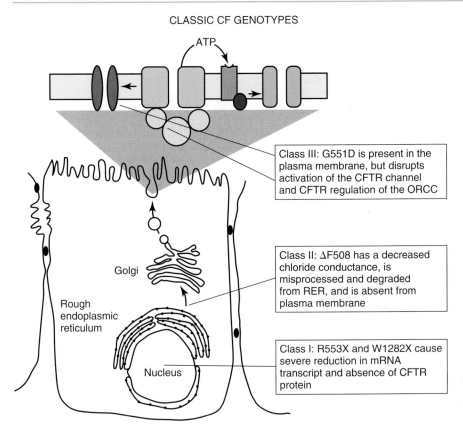

Class III: G551D is present in the plasma membrane, but disrupts activation of the CFTR channel and CFTR regulation of the ORCC

Class II: ΔF508 has a decreased chloride conductance, is misprocessed and degraded from RER, and is absent from plasma membrane

Class I: R553X and W1282X cause severe reduction in mRNA transcript and absence of CFTR protein

Golgi

Rough endoplasmic reticulum

Nucleus

FIGURE 50-1. Functional consequences of severe classic mutations leading to pancreatic insufficiency. *ORCC,* Outwardly rectifying chloride channel; *RER,* rough endoplasmic reticulum.

which the glycine (G) at codon 551 is substituted with aspartic acid (D). The G551D mutation severely affects interaction with ATP, creating a form of CFTR that is properly folded and inserted in the cell membrane, yet unable to be activated.[89,98] Intriguingly, a second mutation has been reported to the same residue in which serine replaces glycine. This substitution reduces but does not eliminate function, so a mild CF phenotype is created.[99] Some of the class III mutants respond to VX770 by increasing chloride transport. Early phase clinical trials in CF suggested safety and biologic efficacy.[100]

Class IV mutations alter the chloride conduction properties of CFTR, and in some cases, affect the magnitude and the ion selectivity of the channel pore.[101,102] Most class IV mutations occur in the transmembrane domains. Since class IV mutations may reduce but not eliminate the flow of ions, some CFTR function is preserved (Fig. 50-2), which in turn leads to a milder phenotype or a nonclassic form of CF. However, by the same token, it is recognized that altering this property of CFTR produces CF. Thus, loss or alteration of the chloride channel function of CFTR is key to the development of the CF phenotype, demonstrating that a defect in chloride transport is the primary abnormality in cells of CF patients.

Class V mutations also are associated with a milder form of CF, because they can also result in the production of a reduced amount of normally functional protein (see Fig. 50-2). An example of the latter type of mutation is 3849 + 10 kbC > T (HGVS c.3717 + 12191C > T). This mutation occurs within intron 19, approximately 10 kilobases from the nearest splice site of exon 19, and leads to the aberrant splicing of CFTR, a nonfunctional protein.[103] However, the aberrant splicing mechanism is incomplete, and a small amount of normally spliced CFTR transcript is made, leading to the synthesis of some normal CFTR and a CF phenotype that is moderate in severity.

Cystic fibrosis–causing mutations have been shown to affect other functions of CFTR. CFTR regulates other ion channels such as the ENaC and the ORCC.[104] Mutations in the first NBD have been shown to variably affect CFTR regulation of these channels.[105,106] Mutations in the N terminus or in the C terminus of CFTR can affect the trafficking, membrane insertion, or stability of CFTR.[107,108] These genotypes are sometimes classified as class VIA or VIB. Finally, mutations in ENaC have been shown to cause cases of atypical CF.[109,110]

Clinical Consequences of Mutations

Correlation of CFTR genotype with CF phenotype has been investigated using three methods. In genotype-driven studies, patients are grouped according to genotype and clinical features are compared. When patients who were homozygous for the ΔF508 mutation were compared with patients who carry one copy of ΔF508 and a different CF mutation, it was shown that a number of the less common mutations produce the same degree of disease severity as the ΔF508 mutation.[111] Some mutations cause less severe organ disease, or disease in a subset of organ systems affected in classic CF, resulting in a "nonclassic" CF phenotype.[112] CFTR genotype demonstrates

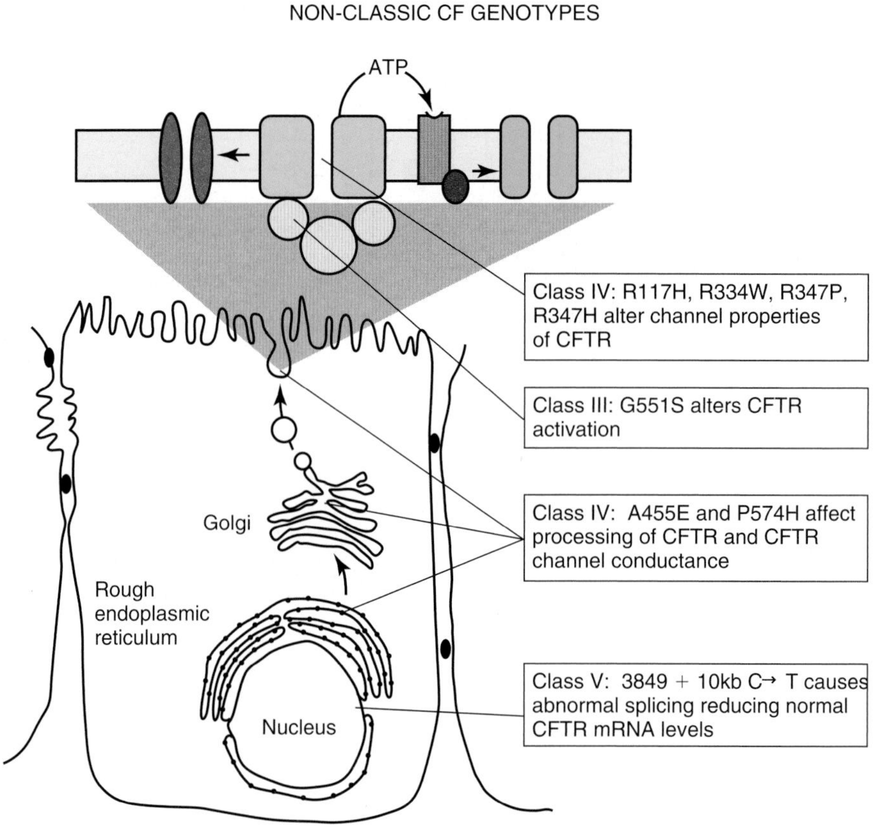

FIGURE 50-2. Functional consequences of mutations leading to nonclassic (mild) forms of CF.

a consistent association with the severity of pancreatic disease.[113] A less consistent correlation has been noted with abnormalities in sweat chloride concentration.[114] However, only one mutation, A455E, has been unequivocally correlated with severity of lung disease.[115,116] A few other mutations, particularly those in class IV and V, may associate with less severe lung disease.[117] In the phenotype-driven method, CFTR mutations are identified in patients grouped according to disease severity. This approach has identified relatively uncommon mutations that are associated with nonclassic forms of disease.[118–121] A third approach has been to correlate the class of mutation with the severity of disease. Those who carry mutations that cause a complete or nearly complete loss of function, such as class I, II, and III mutations, usually manifest classic CF. Mutations that permit some residual function, such as those in classes IV and V, have been associated with milder phenotypes usually associated with pancreatic sufficiency.[114,117,122] However, it is important to recognize that many exceptions exist. For example, CFTR bearing A455E affects processing of CFTR (class II) but is associated with pancreatic-sufficient CF and milder lung disease.[93,94]

Diagnosis of atypical forms of CF can be difficult, especially when one or more alleles fails to demonstrate a disease causing mutation.[123,124] Sweat chloride may be normal in some combinations of CF genotypes, making the test less reliable for nonclassic CF. Standardization of protocols to measure nasal epithelial chloride and sodium transport has proven useful in the diagnosis of CF.[125,126] The Nasal Potential Difference test (NPD) can detect both classic and nonclassic forms of the

disease,[127] and has been a secondary outcome measure in clinical trials of ataluren, VX809, and VX770.

PATHOPHYSIOLOGY

CF is caused by reduction or dysfunction of the CFTR, a cAMP-regulated chloride and bicarbonate channel and a master regulator of other ion channels that co-exist in the apical membranes of cells lining the airways, sweat glands, hepatobiliary system, and reproductive tracts. In the absence of disease, CFTR activity downregulates or tempers the sodium absorption through ENaC.[128,129] In CF, the combination of a reduction in chloride transport and unregulated excessive sodium transport leads to the classic ion and water hydration defects that occur in the pancreas and vas deferens *in utero,* and the airways, biliary tract, intestines, reproductive tracts, and sweat glands after birth. CFTR is also expressed in other organs that do not succumb to disease such as the heart and kidneys. Abundant alternative channels exist in those tissues to compensate for lack of CFTR-mediated chloride transport.[30,130,131]

Airways Dehydration and Disruption of Mucociliary Clearance

Airway surface liquid bathes the cilia of the upper airway and the depth and composition of this fluid is regulated by CFTR and ENaC. In CF, the ASL height is reduced and cilia are less efficient at moving particles and mucus.[132] Secondary effects of CFTR function include abnormal mucus secreted by the submucosal glands and epithelial cells. The blanket of airway surface mucus becomes excessive, but does not help to eradicate bacteria that colonize and inflame the CF airways.

CFTR controls both the ENaC and the outwardly rectifying chloride channel (ORCC). When CFTR is absent, the ORCC cannot secrete chloride, amplifying the secretion defect.[133] The calcium-activated chloride channel (CaCC) and the pH-activated ClC-2 co-exist and are independent of CFTR.[134–140] The latter are therapeutic targets in CF. Recently, a phase III program testing aerosolized denufosol, which activates the CaCC through binding to P2Y2 receptors and increasing intracellular calcium, failed to improve lung function over 1 year. It is yet unclear whether activation of an alternative chloride secretion pathway will be sufficient to overcome the defects associated with classic CF.

CF airways quickly become colonized with bacteria after birth. Defective mucociliary clearance likely plays a major role, but additional defects in bacterial clearance related to the importance of CFTR in the lipid raft region of the plasma membrane are emerging.[141–144] Inflammation in response to bacterial colonization is excessive and ineffective.[145,146] The ASL becomes infiltrated with neutrophils that respond to IL-8 secretion. As the neutrophils die, they liberate their DNA, which contributes to the viscosity of the mucus. Aerosolized DNase thins this mucus and improves lung function. Aerosolized hypertonic saline also facilitates clearance and improves lung function by a different mechanism.

■ CHARACTERISTICS OF SYSTEMIC DISEASE

Airways, Upper and Lower

Lung disease remains the major expression of morbidity and mortality in CF. Infants with CF are born with normal lungs, and pulmonary disease develops over a variable time course. The earliest lesion is obstruction of the small airways by abnormally viscous airway mucus. A secondary bronchiolitis with plugging of the airways invariably follows and develops into bronchiectasis as the respiratory epithelium becomes chronically infected. A striking feature of CF lungs is that the parenchyma is virtually untouched for much of the course, while the airways are severely afflicted. The airways become a reservoir for chronically infected mucopurulent secretions, first by *Staphylococcus aureus* and *Haemophilus influenzae,* and later by a distinctive mucoid form of *P. aeruginosa.* Once mucoid *P. aeruginosa* colonizes the lungs, it is virtually impossible to eradicate. Emergence of methicillin-resistant strains of *S. aureus* (MRSA) is increasing and a cause for concern.[147] Respiratory failure is the major cause of death, with the median life span now increased to 37 years in the United States (Cystic Fibrosis Foundation Registry Data).

The respiratory disease is usually progressive, with superimposed acute exacerbations. Cough is an early symptom and may be nonproductive and mistaken for asthma. Production of sputum develops and is an indicator of chronic inflammation and infection. A typical course is characterized by intermittent acute pulmonary

exacerbations in which there is an increased volume of sputum, a change in the color of sputum, decreased exercise tolerance, and weight loss. Digital clubbing is a universal finding with progression of the lung disease. The chest radiograph becomes abnormal early in the course of the disease and demonstrates hyperinflation (Fig. 50-3) and patchy atelectasis (Fig. 50-4). The chest computed tomography (CT) scan is even more sensitive to

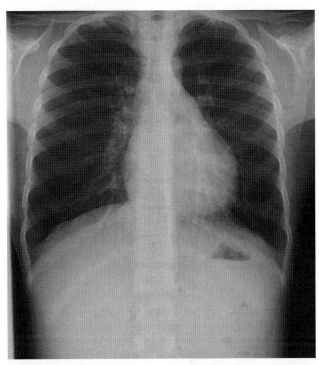

FIGURE 50-3. Chest radiograph of a 10-year-old female with CF (genotype ΔF508 homozygous) who complained of increasing cough and sputum production. Both lung fields are hyperinflated, and there are increased lung markings. Expectorated sputum culture grew nonmucoid *P. aeruginosa.*

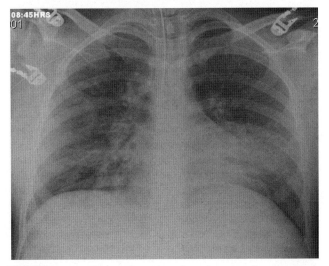

FIGURE 50-4. Chest radiograph at bronchoscopy of an adolescent female with CF (genotype ΔF508/621 + 1G) who complained of sudden and transient chest pain on the left side, followed by an increase in cough. There are lingular, right lower, and right middle lobe infiltrates and atelectasis. Lung fields improved after 14 days of intravenous antibiotics directed against the *S. aureus* and mucoid *P. aeruginosa* that grew from bronchoalveolar lavage cultures.

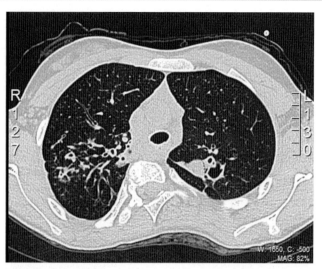

FIGURE 50-5. Spiral chest CT scan of an adolescent female with CF (genotype ΔF508 homozygous) and a slight decline in forced expiratory volume in 1 second. There is bilateral upper lobe bronchiectasis. Her sputum cultures grew *P. aeruginosa* and MRSA.

changes (Fig. 50-5) and may be preferred over the chest radiograph for a quantitative assessment of progression of lung disease.[148] Bronchiectasis develops from progressive chronic infection and destruction of the airways (Fig. 50-6). Pulmonary function tests early in the disease reflect small airways obstruction but then progress toward a decrease in the FEV$_1$ (forced expiratory volume in 1 second) and increases in residual volume, functional residual

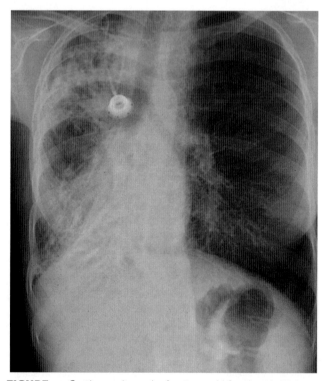

FIGURE 50-6. Chest radiograph of a 16-year-old female with CF (genotype ΔF508 homozygous) and recurrent pulmonary exacerbations. The left lung shows hyperaeration and bronchial wall thickening. The right lung shows decrease in volume, bronchial wall thickening, and bronchiectasis. Sputum cultures grew *Achromobacter xylosoxidans*.

capacity, and the ratio of residual volume to total lung capacity. The vital capacity is eventually reduced. With treatment of the acute exacerbations, small improvements in some of these lung functions can be documented.

The upper airway is also severely affected in CF. Chronic pansinusitis is found in more than 99% of patients with CF, due in part to mucous gland hyperplasia, abnormal chloride ion transport by the sinus epithelial cells, and colonization with bacteria. Chronic sinusitis may contribute to infection of the lower respiratory tract by acting as a reservoir of infection. CT scans of the sinuses are useful in assessing the extent of sinus involvement and in the selection of patients who might benefit from a surgical drainage procedure.

Sinus involvement is complicated by nasal polyposis in 6% to 40% of patients. Nasal polyps should be suspected if nasal air flow is obstructed, the nasal bridge widens, or there is persistent epistaxis or loss of taste and appetite. Polyps appear in childhood and can recur after initial resection. If the disease is left untreated, serious bony erosions can occur. Medical management consists of topical glucocorticoids, macrolide antibiotics for anti-inflammatory action, antibiotics to cover the organisms in the sinuses, and surgical approaches.[149]

Inflammation

A particularly intense inflammatory state appears early in the CF airways. Konstan and colleagues[150] demonstrated that the inflammatory infiltrate is predominantly neutrophilic. Bronchoalveolar lavage studies in infants suggest that inflammation may even precede colonization with bacteria, although this is controversial.[151,152] If inflammation is both a primary defect related to dysfunctional CFTR and a result of infection, then anti-inflammatory therapy may be helpful.

Immune-mediated inflammation contributes significantly to the lung damage present in patients with CF. Specific anti-pseudomonal antibiotics do not eradicate the organism permanently. Despite aggressive intravenous therapy with large doses of increasingly more potent agents, colonization proceeds. Chronic infection then elicits recruitment and activation of neutrophils in the airways. The neutrophils release proteases such as granulocyte elastase and cathepsin G. This protease burden has been associated with both destruction of the lung matrix and cleavage and inactivation of a variety of opsonins. There is also evidence of immune complex formation in CF patients that correlates with disease severity and prognosis.

Infection

Nonencapsulated *H. influenzae* often colonizes the oropharynx of the young child with CF. Although it is not considered a serious pathogen, rising antibody titers to *H. influenzae* have been detected.[153] *S. aureus* is the most frequent organism detected initially on oropharyngeal cultures, and it is still debated whether chronic antibiotic prophylaxis against this organism is useful. The acquisition of MRSA is increasing and emerging as a potential pathogen in communities of healthy children, as well as the CF clinics. *P. aeruginosa*, nonmucoid, is acquired at varying times after birth, and transformation to a mucoid phenotype is associated with increased inflammatory burden and sputum volume. Early intervention strategies and chronic antibiotic protocols are aimed at eradicating or reducing the infection for as long as possible. *Burkholderia cepacia* complex (composed of nine different species) is particularly feared. Genomovar III is highly virulent and transmissible and can be associated with a sepsis-like condition that markedly reduces survival. Transient colonization with a *B. cepacia* spp. is becoming more common.

With more aggressive antibiotic strategies in place and frequent sputum and oropharyngeal cultures, a number of multiply resistant organisms are being identified. *Stenotrophomonas maltophilia, Alcaligenes xylosoxidans,* and nontuberculous mycobacteria alone or in combination with *P. aeruginosa* or *S. aureus* are challenging clinicians.

Additional details pertaining to bacterial, viral, and fungal pathogens in CF are discussed in Chapter 61. An extremely important message to learn from this work is that infection control strategies in the acute care setting, ambulatory clinics, and the home are mandatory if we are to contain the spread of transmissible organisms.[154]

Gastrointestinal Disease

Gastrointestinal disease begins in utero in the pancreas, where dysfunctional CFTR produces a deficiency in exocrine pancreatic secretions because of progressive plugging of the pancreatic ducts by viscous secretions. The combination of the *in utero* deficiency of proteolytic enzymes with secretion of abnormal mucoproteins by the goblet cells of the small intestine leads to obstruction of the distal ileum by inspissated, tenacious meconium. About 15% of infants with CF are born with intestinal obstruction called meconium ileus. There are associated intestinal complications including small bowel atresia, volvulus, perforation, and peritonitis; alternately, there may simply be delayed passage of meconium and distal colonic obstruction secondary to the meconium plug syndrome.

The loss of pancreatic enzyme activity leads to intestinal malabsorption of fats and proteins and, to a lesser extent, carbohydrates, after birth. Pancreatic function is lost incrementally until complete loss is seen in 85% of patients. Infants manifest poor or absent weight gain, chronic abdominal distention, absence of subcutaneous fat and muscle tissue, steatorrhea, and rectal prolapse. Paradoxically, the untreated child often has a voracious appetite, but the caloric intake is insufficient to meet daily needs.

In older individuals, intestinal mucous gland hyperplasia is associated with abnormal mucins and slowing of intestinal transit time. If pancreatic enzyme replacement is inadequate, fecal impaction or distal intestinal obstruction syndrome can result.

Children, adolescents, and adults with residual pancreatic function may develop recurrent episodes of pancreatitis. Serum and urine amylase and serum lipase are elevated. Attacks can be precipitated by a fatty meal, alcohol, or tetracycline. Patients with one or more class IV or V mutations tend to have residual pancreatic function.

Liver disease can result from biliary tract obstruction and inflammation. Normally, CFTR is found on the apical membranes of biliary tract cells where chloride transport facilitates bile flow. In CF, focal biliary cirrhosis appears in 10% to 20% of infants by 1 year and in up to 80% of adults.[155,156] Little is known about the pathogenesis of liver failure in CF, or why some individuals escape significant injury. Therapeutic intervention is limited to dietary bile salts to reduce biliary sludging.

Sweat Gland Effects

The gold standard for diagnosis of CF for many years has been the demonstration of elevated Cl^- and Na^+ in sweat collected by quantitative pilocarpine iontophoresis. Although no histopathologic changes can be found in the CF sweat gland, the function is abnormal as a result of inadequate reabsorption of salt by the distal collecting duct. The CF sweat is isotonic with plasma, and the skin of affected infants has been described as tasting "salty." Heavy exercise in hot, humid climates can lead to increased salt losses and profound clinically significant dehydration.

Sweat production occurs in all individuals primarily by cholinergic stimulation. Cyclic AMP-mediated sweat secretion is present but insignificant. That is why sweat can be produced in CF individuals using the cholinergic pathway. Sweat chloride concentrations can sometimes be normal or borderline in people with a mild *CFTR* mutation. Thus, genetic mutation analysis or nasal potential difference testing may be required to make the diagnosis of CF.

Reproductive Tissues

The male reproductive tract is exquisitely sensitive to defects in CFTR function. Even carriers of one CF gene can present with isolated male infertility. Azoospermia results from an atretic or absent vas deferens that begins *in utero*. Most males with CF are infertile by this mechanism.

Disorders Related to the Cystic Fibrosis Transmembrane Conductance Regulator
Congenital Bilateral Absence of the Vas Deferens
Male infertility due to obstructive azoospermia is a consistent feature of CF. It has been estimated that 98% of all males with CF have this condition.[157] One notable exception has been males who carry the 3849 + 10 kbC > T mutation, where a substantial fraction are fertile.[158] Male infertility is due to malformation of structures derived from the Wolffian duct reproductive tract manifesting as atrophy of the vas deferens. The seminal vesicles and associated structures also can be involved.[159] Abnormal development of the male reproductive tract begins *in utero* and continues in the first year of life.[160] On occasion, only one of the vas deferens is destroyed while the other remains patent. This reduced-fertility condition is termed unilateral absence of the vas deferens. Males with CF produce sperm, although spermatic morphologic abnormalities have been reported.

Congenital bilateral absence of the vas deferens (CBAVD) also has been reported in healthy males as an isolated cause of male infertility.[161] It has been estimated that approximately 1 in 5000 males are affected with this condition. Because of the phenotypic overlap between CBAVD and male infertility seen in CF males, investigators analyzed the *CFTR* genes in males with isolated CBAVD and discovered that a high proportion carried CF mutations.[162] More recent studies with extensive analysis of the *CFTR* gene indicate that approximately 86% of CBAVD patients carry at least one deleterious mutation.[163] ΔF508 is the most common mutation occurring in approximately 44% of the cases.[163] The second most common *CFTR* mutation in CBAVD males (32%) is the 5T polymorphism of the intron 8 splice acceptor.[164] The frequency of 5T in the general population (10% carrier rate) posed a question as to how it could be associated with male infertility. Pedigree studies revealed that 5T is inconsistently associated with CBAVD, suggesting that other variables contribute to the disease. The dinucleotide TG tract immediately adjacent to the T tract (see earlier) determines whether the 5T variant produces male infertility in an individual who carries a mutation in his other *CFTR* gene.[40,43] The mutation R117H (HGVS p.Arg117His) is also quite common in males with CBAVD. Approximately 10% of CBAVD males carry this mutation, yet less than 1% of CF patients carry this mutation. The 5T variant in intron 8 also plays a role in this phenomenon. The R117H mutation has occurred at least twice in human evolution—once in association with the 5T variant and once in association with the more common 7T variant.[165] Males and females who have a CF mutation paired with R117H and the 5T variant invariably have a CF phenotype, while those males who have R117H with the 7T variant usually develop CBAVD, although some cases of CF have been observed.[163,165] Notably, females with this combination of mutations have presented with pancreatitis and with a normal phenotype.[166,167]

Pancreatitis

Pancreatitis is a rare presenting sign of CF in patients with residual pancreatic function.[168] Isolated pancreatitis does not present with similar clinical features to CF. However, the concept that CFTR dysfunction may play a role in idiopathic pancreatitis is supported by two observations. First, sweat electrolyte concentrations have been found to be elevated in a subset of chronic pancreatitis patients.[169] Second, CFTR is known to be expressed in pancreatic ducts, a major site of disease in pancreatitis. In 1998, two studies of patients with idiopathic pancreatitis found an increased frequency of mutations in the CFTR gene.[166,170] In both studies, the frequency of CFTR mutations in the patients with pancreatitis was significantly higher than in the control population and higher than the expected frequency in the general population. Several other reports have since confirmed that CF mutations occur at a higher frequency in patients with isolated pancreatitis.[171–174] However, it appears that additional genetic or environmental influences are required for the development of pancreatitis.[175] Mutations in other genes known to give rise to monogenic forms of pancreatitis such as the secretory trypsinogen inhibitor gene *ST8SIA4 (PST1)* can combine with *CFTR* mutations to increase the risk of developing pancreatitis.[171,172] While nonalcoholic chronic pancreatitis has been associated with CF mutations, it is not clear that the risk of developing pancreatitis in the case of alcohol abuse is increased in the presence of *CFTR* mutations.[176]

Sinusitis

Chronic sinusitis is a consistent feature of CF, including mild forms of the disease.[168] In addition, some males with CBAVD and *CFTR* mutations also have chronic rhinosinusitis.[177,178] Because the sinus epithelium is reliant on *CFTR* function for fluid and electrolyte transport, alterations in *CFTR* could play a role in isolated cases of chronic rhinosinusitis. Indeed, patients who presented with chronic rhinosinusitis to an otorhinolaryngology clinic were found to have a higher frequency of CF mutations than disease-free control populations, suggesting that deleterious mutations in *CFTR* predispose to the development of sinusitis.[50] Two other studies have found that patients with chronic rhinosinusitis have an increased frequency of CF mutations,[179,180] while one study did not find this association.[181] More recently it has been demonstrated that the prevalence of chronic rhinosinusitis in CF carriers is approximately twice the population prevalence.[182] Thus, reduction of *CFTR* function by approximately 50% appears to increase the risk of developing chronic forms of sinus disease.

References

The complete reference list is available online at www.expertconsult.com

51 DIAGNOSIS AND PRESENTATION OF CYSTIC FIBROSIS

Colin Wallis, MD, MRCP, FRCPCH, FCP, DCH

A diagnosis of cystic fibrosis (CF) has lifelong implications for affected individuals, their families and their acquaintances; consequently it needs to be made accurately and early. A late diagnosis is often preceded by a catalogue of doctor's visits, family anguish, and anger with a delay in the initiation of treatment that may have an impact on long-term outcome. Equally disturbing is a small but increasingly documented experience of children who are diagnosed as having CF, but on review—often years later—they are found not to meet diagnostic criteria.

For the majority of children, the diagnosis is easy. A clinical suspicion of CF is confirmed by a positive sweat test, and further diagnostic support is provided by the identification of two disease-causing mutations in the gene for the cystic fibrosis transmembrane regulator (CFTR) on chromosome 7. A classic phenotype is either present at the time of diagnosis or presents soon thereafter, and a relatively predictable clinical course unfolds.

For many regions and nations with a high incidence of cystic fibrosis, newborn screening (NBS) for CF has been introduced. Screened infants still require a diagnostic workup, but NBS provides the opportunity for a CF diagnosis and treatment in infancy before the onset of symptoms.

Over the last decade, several developments have led to the question, "What makes a diagnosis of CF?"[1-4] These include: (1) the recognition of an ever-widening phenotype for an individual with two CFTR mutations ranging from completely normal via atypical forms to a classic CF phenotype; (2) The development of newborn screening programs, whereby a newborn, on the basis of genetic information alone or an intermediate sweat test result, could be given the CF label without necessarily having or even developing clinical disease; (3) the recognition that a CF phenotype can emerge over time presenting de novo in adulthood or moving from "atypical" forms to more classic CF; and (4) the development of sophisticated clinical investigations that allow detection of subtle changes in end organs that hitherto would have gone undetected (e.g., detailed computed tomography scanning and the measurement of epithelial potential difference [PD]).

DIAGNOSTIC CRITERIA FOR CYSTIC FIBROSIS

A possible definition for CF disease could involve the following sequence of pathologic events:
- Disease usually arises from two disease-causing mutations in the gene encoding for CFTR.

- Mutations result in changes to the fluid and electrolytes on cell surfaces.
- Changes lead to abnormal secretions and inflammatory responses.
- These manifestations predispose to obstruction and infection
- Obstruction and infection may produce end organ disease in tubular structures such as the upper and lower airways, vas deferens, gut, liver, and pancreas with secondary impact on growth and nutrition.

In more than 90% of cases, the diagnosis of CF arises from a clinical suspicion supported by a positive sweat test and genetic confirmation.[5] A Cystic Fibrosis Foundation Consensus Panel (USA) synthesized diagnostic criteria for CF.[6] The key features are summarized in Box 51-1. The basic premise of the consensus statement is that CF is a clinical and not a genetic diagnosis, although it acknowledges that genetic testing may have a role in sorting out atypical clinical situations. Any such document must be considered a work in progress to accommodate new developments[7] and acknowledged shortcomings.[8]

MAKING THE DIAGNOSIS OF CF

A clinician may need to confirm a diagnosis of CF in various settings such as when (1) a patient has one or more suspicious clinical features, (2) a newborn screening program has identified a child at risk for CF, (3) an individual is being examined after the diagnosis of CF in a family member, or (4) postnatal confirmation is required when an antenatal test has proven suspicious for CF. Evidence for the diagnosis of CF can be accumulated from a number of sources.

Clinical Suspicion

The majority of children with CF present with a history of bulky fatty stools, failure to thrive, and recurrent chest infections.[9] Shortly after birth 10% to 15% will present with meconium ileus. However, a wide range of less common presenting features is highlighted in Box 51-2. Any child or adult presenting with these signs and symptoms of CF should be investigated further. A possible diagnosis of CF in a child with suggestive clinical findings should not be discounted just because the child appears too well or is thought to be too old. Although the diagnosis is established in most children by the age of 1 year,[10] in approximately 10% of children, the diagnosis is delayed until after 7 years.[9,11] Patients with pancreatic sufficiency and non-Caucasian patients are vulnerable to delays in diagnosis.[12,13]

BOX 51-1 DIAGNOSTIC CRITERIA FOR CYSTIC FIBROSIS (CF FOUNDATION CONSENSUS PANEL)

One or more characteristic phenotypic features consistent with CF:
- Chronic sinopulmonary disease
- Gastrointestinal and nutritional abnormalities
- Salt loss syndromes
- Male urogenital abnormalities resulting in obstructive azoospermia

OR

A history of CF in a sibling

OR

A positive newborn screening test result

AND

An increased sweat chloride concentration

OR

Identification of two CF mutations

OR

Demonstration of abnormal nasal epithelial ion transport

BOX 51-2 CLINICAL FEATURES OF CF AT DIAGNOSIS IN UNSCREENED POPULATIONS—GROUPED ACCORDING TO AGE AND APPROXIMATE ORDER OF FREQUENCY

0 to 2 Years
Failure to thrive
Steatorrhea
Recurrent chest infections including bronchiolitis/bronchitis
Meconium ileus
Rectal prolapse
Edema/hypoproteinemia/"kwashiorkor" skin changes
Severe pneumonia/empyema
Salt depletion syndrome
Prolonged neonatal jaundice
Vitamin K deficiency with bleeding diathesis

3 to 16 Years
Recurrent chest infections or "asthma"
Clubbing and "idiopathic" bronchiectasis
Steatorrhea
Nasal polyps and sinusitis
Chronic intestinal obstruction, intussusception
Heat exhaustion with hyponatremia
CF diagnosis in a relative

Adulthood (Often Atypical CF)
Azoospermia/congenital absence of the vas deferens
Bronchiectasis
Chronic sinusitis
Acute or chronic pancreatitis
Allergic bronchopulmonary aspergillosis
Focal biliary cirrhosis
Abnormal glucose tolerance
Portal hypertension
Cholestasis/gall stones

The Sweat Test

The sweat test was first described in 1959 and remains a gold standard for the diagnosis of CF.[14] In the appropriate clinical setting, whether the child has entered the diagnostic algorithm via clinical suspicion or newborn screening, a positive sweat chloride test is diagnostic of CF. A number of other rare conditions (sometimes single case reports) have been associated with a positive sweat test, but these are usually clearly distinguishable by their clinical features. Examples are listed in Box 51-3.

BOX 51-3 EXAMPLES OF NON-CF CAUSES OF A POSITIVE SWEAT TEST

- Adrenal insufficiency or stress
- Anorexia nervosa
- Ectodermal dysplasia
- Eczema
- Fucosidosis
- G6PD deficiency
- Glycogen storage disease type 1
- Human immunodeficiency virus (HIV) infection
- Hypoparathyroidism
- Hypothyroidism
- Malnutrition from various causes
- Nephrogenic diabetes insipidus
- Pseudohypoaldosteronism

The standard sweat test (Gibson and Cooke technique) requires skill and care and should be undertaken by accredited laboratories. Localized sweating is stimulated by the iontophoresis of pilocarpine on the skin. Sweat is collected on filter paper or gauze or in microduct tubing over a controlled period of time to ensure that the rate of sweating and the total sweat collected are sufficient and standardized. Guidelines for sweat testing procedures and precautions are available in published[15-17] and electronic format at www.acb.org.uk/docs/sweat.pdf.

Chloride is the analyte of choice.[18,19] The sodium levels and osmolality of sweat are less reliable and should never be used in isolation. A sweat chloride concentration of more than 60 mmol/L is considered positive, and levels below 40 mmol/L are likely to be in the normal range; however, a normal sweat test does not necessarily exclude CF in rare situations. Some CF-causing mutations such as A445E, R117H (with 7T) and 3849 + 10C > T produce symptoms including sinopulmonary disease and infertility, but they may have normal sweat chloride levels.[20]

Results lying between 40 to 60 mmol/L have traditionally been considered intermediate and require further evaluation. A proportion of patients with chloride concentrations in the intermediate range will have two *CFTR* mutations, a situation found with increasing frequency with the advent of more detailed *CFTR* mutation testing.[20]

In infants under the age of 6 months, the lower limit of the intermediate range may include levels between 30 and 39 mmol/L. Some diagnostic algorithms now consider the intermediate range as 30 to 60 mmol/L range, especially in infants younger than 6 months of age.[7,21]

Following the introduction of NBS for CF, sweat tests are increasingly performed on infants. It is recommended that sweat chloride testing in asymptomatic newborns with a positive NBS test be performed when the infant is at least 2 weeks of age and more than 2 kg[22,23] The majority of affected infants will have a chloride level greater than 60 mmol/L. A sweat chloride value between 30 and 59 mmol/L in infants younger than 6 months of age should be considered intermediate and trigger further patient evaluation, including repeat testing when older.[24-26]

Some normal adolescents and adults can have sweat chloride values in the intermediate range, and sweat chloride levels alone may be insufficient to diagnose CF in the older adolescent.[25] A false-positive sweat test in the severely malnourished child or the critically ill child in intensive care needs cautious interpretation and follow-up.

Research continues to explore the development of an easier sweat test. Collecting systems such as the macroduct[28] and nanoduct[29] simplify collection, and the role of sweat conductivity as a diagnostic tool in CF is also gaining credence.[30,31] In one large trial, the best conductivity cutoff value to diagnose CF was ≥90 mmol/L and the best conductivity cutoff value to exclude CF was <75 mmol/L.[32] However, most clinicians and laboratories will choose to confirm a positive sweat conductivity result with a formal measurement of chloride concentration.

Mutation Analysis

The 1989 identification of the CF gene[33] and the characterization of its protein product (CFTR) held the promise that the diagnostic dilemmas for the condition were over. If you had two *CFTR* mutations, you had CF; if not, you didn't. Unfortunately it has not worked out that simply.

First, there are over 1600 different CF gene mutations associated with CF disease. Techniques now available do not allow a full screen of the entire CF genome, and most laboratories will only search routinely for the commonest mutations within their region. Examples of *CFTR* mutations are listed in Table 51-1, highlighting the dominance of the ΔF508 mutation (present in >70% of CF alleles in Caucasian populations).[9] The majority of the mutations are rare, and the functional consequences of these rare mutations are not always known (Table 51-2). Customizing mutation panels to match the patient's ethnic background and clinical presentation can enhance the sensitivity of deoxyribonucleic acid (DNA) testing in CF.

Second, there is a range of mutation types that have been classified into groups according to the functional impact on the CFTR.[34] The final protein product may be incomplete, complete but incorrectly packaged and processed, or produce a final CFTR molecule that is unstable or incapable of reaching the cell surface in sufficient numbers to be physiologically effective. In addition to the "disease-causing" mutations, there are also recognizable polymorphisms that do not necessarily result in a clinical phenotype but may influence the structure of the final protein product when associated with another mild mutation. The number of thymidine repeats in intron 8 is a well-described example, where the 5T allele leads to a substantial reduction in functional protein compared with the 9T allele; the 7T allele is intermediate in its effect.

Even though the presence of two mutations is very supportive of the diagnosis of CF in the appropriate clinical setting, two alterations in the gene that encodes *CFTR* does not necessarily mean that classic CF disease develops. The clinical phenotype associated with two *CFTR* mutations is far broader than could ever have been anticipated.[35] Examples are listed in Box 51-4.

TABLE 51-1 COMMON MUTATIONS THAT CAUSE CYSTIC FIBROSIS LISTED ACCORDING TO FREQUENCY*

TRADITIONAL NAME	HGVS† NOMENCLATURE	FREQUENCY IN CAUCASIANS(%)
ΔF508	p.Phe3508del	75.0
G551D	p.Gly551Asp	3.4
G542X	p.gly542X	1.8
R117H	p.arg117His	1.3
621 + 1G>T	c.489+1G>T	1.3
1717-1G>A	c.1585-1G>A	0.6
1898+1G>A	c.1766+1G>A	0.6
ΔI507	p.Ile507del	0.5
N1303K	p.Asn1303Lys	0.5
R560T	p.arg560Thr	0.4
Q493X	c.1477C>T	0.3
R1162X	p.Arg1162X	0.3
R533X	p.Arg553X	0.3
W1282X	p.Trp1282X	0.3
3659delC	c.3527_3528delC (p.Lys1177Serfs)	0.3
1154insTC	c.1021_1022dup (p.Phe342HisfsX28)0.3	
E60X	p.Glu60X	0.2
G85E	p.Gly85Glu	0.2
P67L	c.200C>T (p.Pro67Leu)	0.2
R347P	p.Arg347Pro	0.2
V520F	p.Val520Phe	0.2
1078delT	c.946_947delT (p.Phe316Leufs)	0.1
2184delA	c.2052_2053delA (p.Lys684Asnfs)	0.1
A455E	p.Ala455Glu	0.1
R334W	p.Arg334Trp	0.1
S549N	p.Ser549Asn	0.1
2789+5G>A	c.2657+5G>A	0.1
3849+10kbC>T	c.3717+10kbC>T	0.1
711 + 1G>T	c.579+1G>T	0.1

*In Caucasian populations, variations in frequency occur among between different ethnic groups and geographic regions.
†"New" Human Genome Variation Society nomenclature.

TABLE 51-2 EXAMPLES OF *CFTR* MUTATIONS WITH REGARD TO THEIR CLINICAL CONSEQUENCES

MUTATION GROUP	EXAMPLES
A. CF-causing	F508del, R553X, R1162X, R1158X, 2184delA, 2184insA, 3120+1G>A, I507del, 1677delTA, G542X, G551D, W1282X, N1303K, 621+1G>T, 1717-1G>A, A455E, R560T, G85E, R334W, R347P, 711+1G>T, 711+3A>G,* 1898+1G>A, S549N, 3849+10kbC>T, E822X, 1078delT, 2789+5G>A, 3659delC, R117H-T5,* R117H-T7,* D1152H,* L206W,* TG13-T5*
B. CFTR-related associated disorders	R117H-T7,* TG12-T5,* R117H-T5,* D1152H,* TG13-T5,* S997F, R297Q,* L997F, M952I, D565G,* G576A,* TG11-T5,† R668C-G576A-D443Y, R74W-D1270N
C. No clinical consequences	I148T, R75Q, 875+40A/G, M470V, E528E, T854T, P1290P, 2752-15G/C, I807M, I521F, F508C, I506V, TG11-T5†
D. Unknown or uncertain clinical relevance	Mainly missense mutations‡

* Mutations that may belong to either Group A or Group B.
† Mutations that may belong to either Group B or Group C.
‡ Certain common sequence (missense) variants with subclinical molecular consequences (e.g., M470V) may co-segregate on the same chromosome and exert more potent, cumulative phenotypic effect. Such polyvariant haplotypes could be potentially disease causing.[67]

BOX 51-4 EXAMPLES FROM THE RANGE OF CLINICAL FEATURES THAT CAN BE ASSOCIATED WITH TWO MUTATIONS IN THE CF GENE

- "Classic CF" with pancreatic insufficiency
- Sinopulmonary disease, pancreatic sufficiency and positive sweat test
- Sinopulmonary disease and male fertility with a normal sweat test
- Severe sinusitis and congenial bilateral absence of the vas deferens
- Male infertility only
- Chronic pancreatitis only
- Allergic bronchopulmonary aspergillosis
- Sclerosing cholangitis
- Positive sweat test only[27]
- No clinical features including normal sweat chloride

Failure to find two CF mutations from a selective or extended search does not exclude the diagnosis of CF. To exclude a patient with symptoms of CF and a positive sweat test from potentially beneficial treatment because the laboratory cannot detect two CF mutations would clearly be misguided. There are also rare reports of patients with classic CF symptoms and signs and a positive sweat test who do not appear to have any mutations in the *CFTR* gene, even when the entire gene has been sequenced, screening all 27 exons and the intron-exon boundaries.[36]

These findings suggest that, on these rare occasions, CF may be caused by mutations within the promoter region of the *CFTR* gene, in one of the introns, or even in a distant controlling gene from an unrelated locus.[37]

Assessment for End Organ Involvement

To determine the presence of end organ disease in a patient with the genetic predisposition to develop CF disease but in whom there are few clinical indicators, more detailed end organ assessment is sometimes suggested. Examples include the following:

1. Testing for pancreatic function testing can involve sophisticated tests or timed stool collections for fecal fat analysis. A simple test for quantification of fecal elastase 1 to diagnose pancreatic sufficiency[38,39] has shown considerable sensitivity and reliability and is not contaminated by exogenous enzyme administration. Caution is required in the interpretation of early stool samples, especially in the premature infant or newborn within the first few days of life.[40]
2. Sputum, bronchoalveolar lavage fluid, oropharyngeal swabs, or sinus aspirates can be cultured for known CF pathogens. If a child with "idiopathic" bronchiectasis is found to be infected with typical CF pathogens such as *Staphylococcus aureus* or mucoid *Pseudomonas aeruginosa*, then reevaluation for the possibility of a CF diagnosis is necessary.
3. Computed tomography scanning can be used to evaluate subtle pulmonary changes not readily visible on plain radiography.
4. Computed tomography also can be used to evaluate the sinuses.
5. Postpubertal males can have semen analysis, or younger males can be assessed with ultrasound for congenital bilateral absence of the vas deferens.[41]
6. Valuable information can be obtained with spirometry, including assessment of small airways even in young children, using such newer techniques as the multiple breath washout test.[42]

Transepithelial Potential Difference Measurements

In rare instances where the diagnosis of CF remains unclear or the evidence is equivocal, further evidence of CFTR dysfunction is sometimes sought. Patients with CF demonstrate a more negative potential difference across respiratory epithelium than normals.[43] Nasal potential difference (PD) can be measured in the mucosa or the inferior turbinates, and further diagnostic accuracy is ensured by documenting a bioelectric profile of change to the basal reading in the presence of amiloride perfusion with the addition of a chloride-free solution and isoproterenol[44,45] (Fig. 51-1). PD measurements are difficult to perform, especially in young children, and the technique is generally confined to specialist centers.[46,47] Results are influenced by recent viral infections, the presence of rhinitis, the precise anatomic localization of the measuring catheter, and polyps and the genotype. Not infrequently, atypical forms of CF with borderline sweat chloride levels produce a nasal PD that is also equivocal.[48,49]

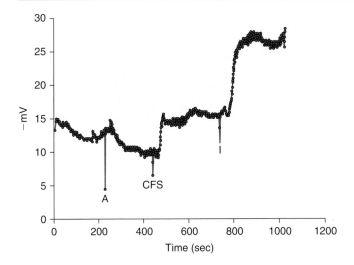

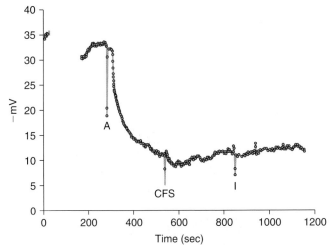

FIGURE 51-1. Nasal PD in a normal subject *(top)* and a CF patient *(bottom)* illustrating the response to perfusion with amiloride *(A)*, followed by the addition of a chloride free solution *(CFS)* and then isoproterenol *(I)* .

Recent publications on the diagnostic value of rectal potential difference done either *in vivo* or on biopsy specimens have considered the advantages in assessing CFTR function in gut epithelium.[50–52]Although these techniques are not yet widely available, they show promise.[53]

■ ANTENATAL TESTING FOR CF

Parents with an increased risk of having a child with CF, either because their own carrier status is known or they already have an affected child, may request antenatal testing. The diagnosis can be confirmed or excluded with a high degree of accuracy by direct mutation analysis performed on fetal cells obtained by chorionic villus sampling (10 weeks of gestation) or cultured amniotic fluid cells (15 to 18 weeks of gestation).

Preimplantation diagnosis is an alternative for at-risk couples. After *in vitro* fertilization, a cleavage-stage biopsy is carried out on day 2 or 3, and normal or carrier embryos are then transferred to establish pregnancy. Further postnatal confirmation is still recommended.

Occasionally routine fetal anomaly scans may detect evidence of a meconium ileus by abnormal bowel

echogenicity or evidence of perforation. Although such findings are usually available too far into the second trimester to enable decisions regarding the fate of the pregnancy, a positive scan will help in providing optimal facilities for the delivery and subsequent medical and surgical care. Hyperechoic bowel often occurs as a benign variant and is usually distinguished by spontaneous resolution, usually before the third trimester.[54]

■ NEONATAL SCREENING FOR CYSTIC FIBROSIS

Although CF is not a model disease for a newborn screening program, the ability to identify CF in infants as early and accurately as possible has advantages that outweigh any potential disadvantages.[55–57] Over the last decade, newborn screening has been widely adopted by many regions and countries and is now emerging as a common method leading to the diagnosis of CF and sharply altering the traditional diagnostic paradigm of symptom-led investigations.[58–60] A range of screening algorithms have been developed, often to suit local resources and conditions.[61,62]

CF neonatal screening is based on the immunoreactive trypsin assay, which is relatively inexpensive to perform on the newborn heel prick sample.[63] Increased immunoreactive trypsinogen (IRT) concentrations can be observed in healthy newborns, but in newborns with CF, they tend to remain raised for weeks to months without returning to normal. A repeat IRT 2 weeks after birth further improves the specificity of the screening algorithm. Infants with raised or persistently raised IRT proceed to further testing. This may consist of a panel of common *CFTR* mutations for the region or a sweat test. The sweat test remains very useful in identifying affected individuals who carry one identified mutation. An example of the algorithm currently adopted by the United Kingdom is illustrated in Figure 51-2.

Screened babies may have early manifestations of pulmonary or gastrointestinal disease at the time of diagnosis, but they also may be completely asymptomatic. CF teams have had to acquire special skills in conveying information to the families of these seemingly well children.[64] Many teams are now working on guidelines for the early management of the screened well child.[65]

Although the screening program is designed to pick up all cases of classic CF who will benefit from early therapy, and exclude healthy carriers, many centers find that increasing numbers of atypical forms are also identified. Infants identified by hypertrypsinogenemia on NBS may have sweat chloride values <60 mmol/L and up to 2 *CFTR* mutations, at least 1 of which is not clearly categorized as a "CF-causing mutation."[66] These infants are invariably pancreatic sufficient. The term CFTR-related metabolic syndrome (CRMS) is proposed to describe these atypical cases. The natural history of CRMS is unknown. It may emerge with time to adopt a more classic phenotype or take the clinical course of the atypical form. Equally they may enjoy trouble free lives. Standards for diagnosis, monitoring, and treatment are being developed for this increasingly common CF phenotype.[66]

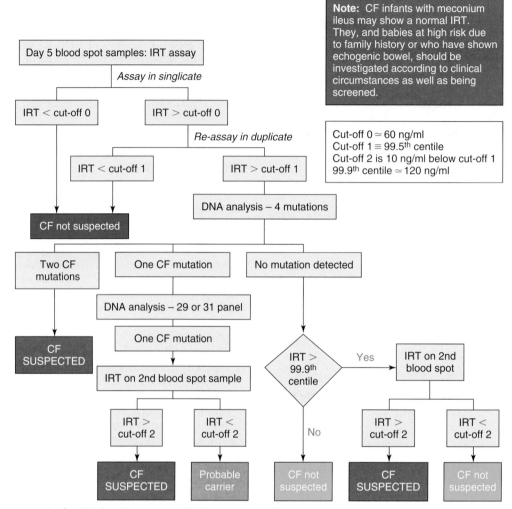

FIGURE 51-2. An example of a NBS algorithm using an IRT/IRT/DNA protocol.

GENOTYPE-PHENOTYPE CORRELATIONS

Although an abnormal CF genotype is likely to give a positive sweat test and result in end organ disease, the road from genotype to phenotype is highly unpredictable. Mutations may be both mild and severe, and mild mutations may be dominant over severe ones, but the final effect on the phenotype is far more complex.[35,67–70] A few possible exceptions exist:

1. Pancreatic sufficiency has been linked to certain mutations such as R117H and A445E, although insufficiency may emerge with time.
2. Homozygosity for the ΔF508 mutation generally (but not exclusively) produces a more severe phenotype in all affected organs when compared with CF patients carrying one ΔF508 mutation or none.[71]
3. Mutations carrying a milder pancreatic phenotype (e.g., R117H, R334W, 3849 + 10kbC > T) may be associated with less abnormal sweat tests[72] and perhaps a similarly mild effect on nasal potential difference responses.[73]
4. The male reproductive tract appears to have the highest demand for fully functioning CFTR, but splice mutations such as 3849 + 10 kbC > T allow for the production of sufficient CFTR to make fertility possible (although not guaranteed).[74]

5. Caregivers should avoid making prognostic predictions based on genotype alone.[67] There are four major contributing factors that influence the path from genotype to end organ involvement and an individual's eventual phenotype[75]:
6. The severity of the individual *CFTR* mutations: "mild" mutations may cause milder phenotypic effects but when there is a mixture of mild and severe mutations the final impact is unpredictable. Sometimes mild mutations may have a dominant effect on severe mutations with a "corrective" effect. Similarly, co-existent polymorphisms hitchhiking within the *CFTR* gene may influence the final protein product.
7. Modifying genes: Genes lying elsewhere in the genome have significant influence on the behavior of the CFTR protein. These genes and their protein products can correct or exacerbate influencing pathologic processes such as the biochemistry of the cell surface liquid, the innate and acquired immunity of the lungs, and they may even influence the predisposition to meconium ileus.[76] Each individual with CF is likely to have an immense orchestra of modifying genes and proteins unique to themselves and influential in their clinical outcome.
8. Environmental factors: the environment in which a patient with CF lives and grows has central bearing on the outcome of their disease. Treatment and adherence

to therapy, social circumstances and diet, exposure to infections such as *Pseudomonas*,[77] or viral infections in infancy can produce a sustained negative influence on the clinical course.

9. The passage of time is an important influence on outcome. CF is not necessarily an all or nothing disease. A clinical phenotype can emerge with time, especially in some of the atypical forms. Effective therapies and adherence to treatment can help stall the disease progression. Patients with documented pancreatic sufficiency in childhood can become pancreatic insufficient in later life. Some, but not all, patients with CF will develop diabetes, liver disease, and osteoporosis.

▄▄▄ CYSTIC FIBROSIS PHENOTYPES

Classic CF

The diagnosis of classic CF needs to be made early and confidently. No racial group is exempt and children of ethnic minorities or mixed heritage are at greatest risk of a delayed or missed diagnosis. The clinical features of recurrent chest infections, malabsorption with pancreatic insufficiency in the majority (but not all), salt-losing syndromes, or an infant presenting with meconium ileus or rectal prolapse requires investigation. A positive sweat test and/or two *CFTR* mutations is diagnostic. Appropriate therapy should be introduced without delay.

Atypical CF (with Symptoms)

There is a growing group of children and adults who do not present with the full spectrum of clinical features associated with classic CF. The terms "equivocal CF" or "CFTR-related disorders" or "variant CF" have all been used to describe these atypical forms.[78–80] Frequently there is single organ involvement. Sweat testing can be normal, intermediate, or positive, and mutation analysis may reveal two, one, or no mutations. Examples of such conditions are listed in Box 51-5. Caregivers have recognized that it is inappropriate to label individuals with these atypical forms as having classic CF.[4] Both the diagnostic labeling and management needs to be tailored to the patient's individual phenotype and requirements.[81] The introduction of arduous therapies aimed at the patient with classic CF does not seem appropriate or beneficial. The negative connotations of a CF label can be avoided with a more considered approach to diagnostic categorization.

The concept of classic and atypical forms has been useful in countering the "all-or-nothing" approach to the diagnosis of CF. However it should be recognized that careful monitoring and timely management are crucial for all affected children, even those with atypical forms. Terms such as "atypical" or "mild" should not lead to complacency in care and follow-up.[7]

Atypical CF (Without Symptoms)

NBS infants with hypertrypsinogenemia are being identified with two *CFTR* mutations (one of which may not be characterized as "disease-causing") or one identified mutation and an equivocal sweat test who do not fit the criteria for a CF diagnosis. Frequently there is no evidence for end organ CF disease. Previously, this scenario was rarely encountered and was considered a form of genetic "pre-CF."[3] However, the advent of widespread NBS has revealed increasing numbers of these infants, and the term "CFTR metabolic syndrome" has now been proposed.[82] It is possible that clinical features may emerge with time, but evidence is insufficient to label these asymptomatic infants as having CF. Most clinicians would advise a program of careful surveillance, including repeating the sweat test at 6 months of age. Therapy is reserved for early end organ changes.[65] The role of prophylactic therapy, such as physiotherapy or antibiotics, is unclear.

Suggested Reading

Borowitz D, Parad RB, Sharp JK, et al. Cystic Fibrosis Foundation practice guidelines for the management of infants with cystic fibrosis transmembrane conductance regulator-related metabolic syndrome during the first two years of life and beyond. *J Pediatr.* 2009;155(suppl 6):S106–S116.

Castellani C, Southern KW, Brownlee K, et al. European best practice guidelines for cystic fibrosis neonatal screening. *J Cyst Fibros.* 2009;8(3):153–173.

Comeau AM, Accurso FJ, White TB, et al. Guidelines for implementation of cystic fibrosis newborn screening programs: Cystic Fibrosis Foundation workshop report. *Pediatrics.* 2007;119(2):e495–e518.

De Boeck, Wilschanski M, Castellani C, et al. Cystic fibrosis: Terminology and diagnostic algorithms. *Thorax.* 2006;61(7):627–635.

Farrell PM, Rosenstein BJ, White TB, et al. Guidelines for diagnosis of cystic fibrosis in newborns through older adults: Cystic Fibrosis Foundation consensus report. *J Pediatr.* 2008;153(2):S4–S14.

Goubau C, Wilschanski M, Skalicka V, et al. Phenotypic characterisation of patients with intermediate sweat chloride values: Towards validation of the European diagnostic algorithm for cystic fibrosis. *Thorax.* 2009;64(8):683–691.

Green A, Kirk J. Guidelines for the performance of the sweat test for the diagnosis of cystic fibrosis. *Ann Clin Biochem.* 2007;44(Pt 1):25–34.

Groman JD, Karczeski B, Sheridan M, et al. Phenotypic and genetic characterization of patients with features of "nonclassic" forms of cystic fibrosis. *J Pediatr.* 2005;146(5):675–680.

LeGrys VA, Yankaskas JR, Quittell LM, et al. Diagnostic sweat testing: The Cystic Fibrosis Foundation guidelines. *J Pediatr.* 2007;151(1):85–89.

Mayell SJ, Munck A, Craig JV, et al. A European consensus for the evaluation and management of infants with an equivocal diagnosis following newborn screening for cystic fibrosis. *J Cyst Fibros.* 2009;8(1):71–78.

Rosenstein BJ, Cutting GR. The diagnosis of cystic fibrosis: A consensus statement. Cystic Fibrosis Foundation Consensus Panel. *J Pediatr.* 1998;132(4):589–595.

Sermet-Gaudelus I, Mayell SJ, Southern KW. Guidelines on the early management of infants diagnosed with cystic fibrosis following newborn screening. *J Cyst Fibros.* 2010;9(5):323–329.

Solomon GM, Konstan MW, Wilschanski M, et al. An international randomized multicenter comparison of nasal potential difference techniques. *Chest.* 2010;138(4):919–928. Epub May 14, 2010.

Southern KW, Merelle MM, Dankert-Roelse JE, et al. Newborn screening for cystic fibrosis. *Cochrane Database Syst Rev.* 2009;(1): CD001402.

References

The complete reference list is available online at www. expertconsult.com

---

BOX 51-5 CONDITIONS THAT MAY BE ASSOCIATED WITH AN INCREASED INCIDENCE OF *CFTR* MUTATIONS BUT INSUFFICIENT EVIDENCE TO FULFILL A CF DIAGNOSIS

- Pancreatitis—acute or recurrent
- Disseminated bronchiectasis
- Isolated obstructive azoospermia
- Allergic bronchopulmonary aspergillosis
- Diffuse panbronchiolitis
- Sclerosing cholangitis
- Neonatal hypertrypsinogenemia
- Rhinosinusitis
- Heat exhaustion

52 PULMONARY DISEASE IN CYSTIC FIBROSIS

ALBERT FARO, MD, PETER H. MICHELSON, MD, MS, AND THOMAS W. FERKOL, MD

Cystic fibrosis (CF) is the most common, life-shortening inherited disease of Caucasians. Based on data from neonatal screening, this autosomal recessive defect occurs in approximately 1 in 3500 live births. The life expectancy of a child born with CF has gradually improved and is now approaching 38 years in the United States.[1] Nevertheless, much of the morbidity and mortality from CF continues to result from progressive airway involvement. The CF lung is susceptible to infection; endobronchial infection induces an intense inflammatory response that leads to bronchiectasis and eventually respiratory failure, thus shortening the life of the patient. In this chapter, we build on earlier sections and relate the pulmonary manifestations and complications of CF lung disease to its pathophysiology and describe current and emerging therapies to address this progressive lung disease.

PATHOGENESIS OF LUNG DISEASE

Cystic fibrosis is caused by defects in the cystic fibrosis transmembrane conductance regulator (CFTR), a cyclic adenosine monophosphate (cAMP)-regulated chloride channel expressed on the surface of airway epithelial cells and the serous cells of the submucosal glands.[2] CFTR is functionally linked to other apical chloride channels, such as the calcium-dependent chloride channels (ClCa) and the epithelial sodium channel (ENaC), which reabsorbs sodium in the airways. Aberrant expression or function of the CFTR in the airway leads not only to reduced chloride conductance but also to dysregulation of epithelial sodium channel activity. Failure of chloride secretion and massive sodium hyperabsorption result in dehydration of the airway surface. The desiccated secretions obstruct the airways and reduce mucociliary clearance, permitting bacterial infection to become established and allowing the inflammatory response to be amplified.[3–5] Investigators have proposed other gaps in innate airway defenses that could contribute to bacterial persistence and chronic infection in the CF airway, including impaired antibactericidal factors produced by airway epithelia, excessive bacterial binding to the airway surface, and possibly reduced bacterial uptake by the epithelium[6–8] (Fig. 52-1).

Respiratory infections are not a consequence of altered or abnormal pulmonary development. The lungs of neonates with CF appear histologically normal with the exception of plugging and distension of submucosal gland ducts. Bacterial cultures of respiratory secretions from infants often fail to yield a specific pathogen. There is a period of time early in disease when the airway has not been chronically colonized, but various bacteria may be found intermittently. As intrabronchial mucous stasis evolves, the respiratory tract becomes persistently infected with common patterns of bacterial species. Bacterial infection is highly localized to the endobronchial spaces.[9–12]

Initially, *Staphylococcus aureus* and *Haemophilus influenzae* are isolated from patients with CF. *S. aureus* is often found in the respiratory tract of infants and young children with CF[13] and the prevalence of methicillin-resistant *S. aureus* strains has greatly increased. Though its significance in the pathogenesis of CF lung infection has been questioned,[14] there is mounting evidence that methicillin-resistant *S. aureus* contributes to pulmonary deterioration and worse survival.[15] The significance of *H. influenzae* in the progression of CF lung disease is uncertain; however, it is a recognized and often treated pathogen in other forms of bronchiectasis.[9,16]

P. aeruginosa emerges as the predominant organism over time[1] and most children with CF have had lung infection with *P. aeruginosa* by 3 years of age. Early *P. aeruginosa* isolates have planktonic, motile, nonmucoid phenotypes. Most patients eventually become chronically infected with mucoid *P. aeruginosa* that survives in the lung as biofilms, and these anaerobic, sessile communities of bacteria contribute to antibacterial resistance in the CF airway.[9,17,18] Approximately 80% of adults with CF in the United States are chronically infected with mucoid *P. aeruginosa*[1]; the isolation of mucoid strains of *P. aeruginosa* from the lungs of a patient is characteristic but not pathognomonic for CF. Acquisition of mucoid strains of *P. aeruginosa* from the lungs of a patient is associated with a poorer prognosis. Encouragingly, recent studies have reported that persistent infection with *P. aeruginosa* can be delayed or avoided with antibiotic treatment, which may lead to slower decline in pulmonary function.[19–20]

Antibiotic-resistant strains of *P. aeruginosa* are found increasingly in CF respiratory secretions. Other resistant, gram-negative bacteria, including *Stenotrophomonas maltophilia* and *Achromobacter xylosoxidans*, are opportunistic organisms that can be acquired later in life, but their involvement in progression of CF lung disease is unclear.[21] *Burkholderia cepacia complex*, however, can have profound effects on the clinical course of the disease, being associated with rapidly progressive necrotizing pneumonia and mortality.[22] The prevalence of *B. cepacia* complex varies markedly among care centers, with a nationwide prevalence of about 3%.[1] Most *B. cepacia* complex infections are caused by genomovar II *(B. multivorans)* and genomovar III *(B. cenocepacia)*. These organisms are transmissible and infection control policies are critical to limiting exposures and spread. Epidemic infections have been linked to *B. cenocepacia*,[23] but other genomovars have been associated with severe disease.[24] Other bacteria also can be transmitted between

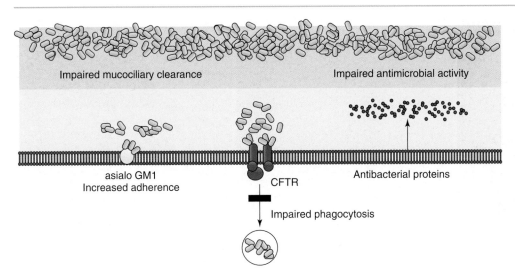

FIGURE 52-1. Proposed pathologic mechanisms for initial infection of the CF airway, including ineffective mucociliary clearance, impaired bactericidal proteins, excessive bacterial binding to glycolipids (asialo GM1) on the airway surface, and reduced bacterial uptake by the epithelium via the CFTR protein.

CF patients. Infection control guidelines have been developed and applied to patients in both clinical settings and social activities.

Invasive fungal infections are rare, but nontuberculous mycobacteria, typically *M. avium-intracellulare* complex or *M. abscessus*, can infect the CF lung. About 13% of patients nationwide harbor nontuberculous mycobacteria in their lung.[25] Therefore, patients with CF should be screened at least annually for mycobacterial colonization.

In patients with respiratory symptoms refractory to antibiotic therapy, viral infections should be considered. Indeed, there is evidence indicating that viruses play a significant role in the pathogenesis of pulmonary exacerbations and are associated with progressive clinical deterioration.[26] Respiratory viruses have the potential for injuring or altering the airway and can induce secretion of inflammatory mediators from respiratory epithelium. Moreover, viral infections result in a damaged epithelial barrier, leading to acquired ciliary dyskinesis, disruption of cell-cell connections, and cell death.[27] A breach in the airway epithelium potentially allows pathogens to reach the basolateral surface, provoking a greater inflammatory response.[28] More recently, investigators have shown that viral infections can affect airway surface fluid levels

in CF epithelial cell cultures.[29] In particular, influenza can complicate CF disease, but immunization and chemoprophylaxis have lessened its clinical impact.

Although pulmonary infection contributes to the morbidity of patients with CF, the intense host inflammatory response hastens the progressive, suppurative pulmonary disease. Inflammation in the CF lung is remarkably compartmentalized, with infection and inflammation primarily contained in the airway lumen, while the alveolar space is relatively spared. The airway is filled with mucopurulent secretions. Large numbers of neutrophils are found in the airway, even in toddlers and older children with CF.[30,31] Bronchoalveolar lavage (BAL) from CF patients has remarkably high concentrations of pro-inflammatory mediators, including interleukin-1 (IL-1), tumor necrosis factor-alpha (TNF-α), and IL-8[32,33] (Fig. 52-2). Infection and local mediators stimulate epithelial cell secretion of IL-8, a potent neutrophil chemoattractant and activator that perpetuates airway inflammation. Complement-derived chemoattractants and leukotriene B₄ also contribute to neutrophil influx.[34,35] Both IL-1ß and TNF-α are macrophage-derived cytokines that contribute to the local inflammatory response in the CF airway by mediating neutrophil chemoattraction and degranulation. More recently, IL-17 pathways have been

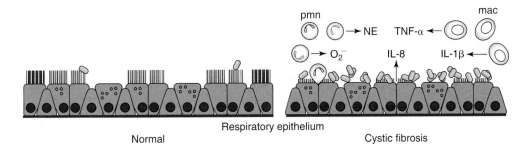

FIGURE 52-2. Inflammatory response in the CF airway. In the CF airway, IL-1ß and TNF-α are macrophage-derived cytokines that contribute to the local inflammatory response by mediating neutrophil chemoattraction and degranulation, inducing epithelial cell secretion of IL-8, and increasing surface expression of the adhesion molecules. The combination of chemoattractants and adhesion molecules induces neutrophils to migrate into the airway, where GM-CSF prolongs their survival. Degenerating neutrophils release oxidants and proteases, such as neutrophil elastase, which lead to epithelial injury, stimulate secretion of IL-8, and interfere with airway defenses.

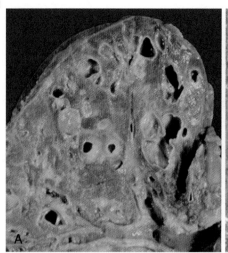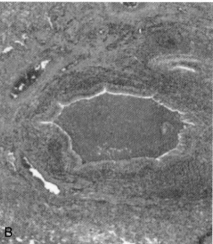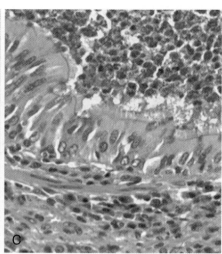

FIGURE 52-3. Gross and histopathology of the CF lung. **A,** Photograph of CF lung explant from an adolescent CF patient showing bronchiectatic changes and mucous plugging, primarily involving the upper lobe. **B** and **C,** Photomicrographs of a section of CF lung explant (40× and 400×, magnification), demonstrating intense endobronchial and peribronchial inflammation with plugging of airways by exudate, degenerating neutrophils, bacteria, and mucus. (**A,** Image generously provided by Carlos Milla, MD, Stanford University.)

increasingly recognized as key molecules for proinflammatory gene expression in the airways that are involved in the pathogenesis of CF lung disease.[36]

Inflammation in the CF lung is primarily driven by local stimuli, mediators, and chemoattractants and is not a local effect of a systemic inflammatory reaction. Systemic indicators of inflammation are often normal or only modestly increased, even during acute exacerbations. Several lines of evidence suggest that airway inflammation in CF may be excessive to the threat posed by bacteria, possibly mediated through dysregulation of the transcription factor NF-κB or other signal transduction molecules.[37–42] Though not a universal finding, infants and children with CF have high levels of proinflammatory cytokines and neutrophils in BAL fluid,[11] even in the absence of detectable infection.[10] It is possible that inflammation may occur independent of infection or that a relatively minor infection may induce a robust inflammatory reaction in the CF lung that does not subside. However, not all *in vitro* models and clinical studies have demonstrated an exaggerated inflammatory response in the CF airway.[43,44] It is possible that this phenomenon may be related to reduced apical surface fluid volume.[45]

The inflammatory response in the CF airways is characterized by a massive influx of neutrophils across the respiratory epithelium, even in individuals with mild pulmonary involvement. The phagocytic system affords protection against bacterial invasion, and neutrophil-derived proteases, such as neutrophil elastase, participate in the intralysosomal degradation of engulfed bacteria.[46] However, these proteases are released during phagocytosis and neutrophil death. With disease progression, the protease burden in the CF airway overwhelms the existing antiprotease defense.[31,47] Neutrophil elastase plays several roles in the pathogenesis of CF lung disease. It digests diverse substrates, including structural proteins, which weakens the airway and results in bronchiectasis and bronchomalacia. Uninhibited neutrophil elastase can enhance the inflammatory response in the bronchi[48] and paradoxically interfere with nonspecific airway defenses.[49–50]

As disease progresses, the airway lumen is filled with neutrophil exudates, acute and chronic inflammation, and bacteria. Mononuclear cell infiltration of the submucosa, goblet cell hyperplasia, and submucosal gland dilatation are also features of the CF airway. Respiratory cilia are normal or have nonspecific changes secondary to epithelial injury. Bronchiectasis is the predominant pathologic feature, more severe in the upper lobes (Fig. 52-3). Despite high bacterial concentrations in the CF lung, bacteremia and sepsis are rare. Tissue invasion is uncommon, and as a rule seen with particular organisms, such as *B. cepacia* complex and *S. aureus*, which are associated with necrotizing pneumonias. Segmental hyperinflation or atelectasis results from airway obstruction. Lung overinflation, postinflammatory blebs, and bronchiectatic cystic lesions increase susceptibility to pneumothorax. Over time, bronchial arteries become hypertrophied and can cause pulmonary hemorrhage. Chronic alveolar hypoxia and inflammatory changes contribute to pulmonary hypertension and cor pulmonale.[51]

CLINICAL MANIFESTATIONS AND COMPLICATIONS

The onset and progression of clinical manifestations of CF lung disease is highly variable. Mucociliary clearance is impaired throughout the conducting airways, and the CF patient depends on cough to mobilize purulent endobronchial secretions and reduce bacterial burden. However, it is unusual for neonates to have respiratory symptoms, but older infants can present with tachypnea, wheezing, and cough, often precipitated or exacerbated by respiratory viral infections. Before neonatal screening, these respiratory symptoms were often misdiagnosed as asthma or recurrent bronchitis and appropriate therapy was delayed.

At some point, cough becomes both the prominent symptom and increasingly productive. As the lung disease progresses, CF patients can experience exercise intolerance, dyspnea, and shortness of breath. Persistent airway infection and inflammation cause bronchiectasis, an acquired anomaly that is defined as the irreversible, abnormal dilatation of affected segmental and subsegmental bronchi.[52] Typically, bronchiectasis begins in the upper lobes in CF patients, then progresses to involve the whole lung. The treatment of bronchiectasis is the treatment for the CF lung disease. With few exceptions, lobar resection is seldom indicated because the disease will ultimately progress to involve all lobes.

Caused by the accumulation of purulent secretions and airway obstruction, atelectasis often coexists with bronchiectasis. Segmental and lobar atelectases most often involve the upper lobes early in disease. Atelectasis also generates negative intrapleural pressure and dilates the associated bronchus, already weakened by the lytic enzymes released from the neutrophils in the purulent material in the airway. Typically, treatment involves airway clearance techniques, bronchodilators, inhaled recombinant DNAse or other mucolytic agents, and antibiotics.

Altered homeostasis between airway pathogens and local host defenses leads to acute changes in respiratory signs and symptoms; this phenomenon is termed a *pulmonary exacerbation*.[55] Clinically, a pulmonary exacerbation is manifested as increased respiratory symptoms such as cough, dyspnea, and sputum production, often accompanied by systemic symptoms such as fatigue, anorexia, and weight loss. Pulmonary function values usually decrease during exacerbations, and a therapeutic goal is to restore the best baseline of pulmonary function, regardless of the patient's symptoms. Pulmonary exacerbations are treated with aggressive airway clearance techniques and antibiotic therapy based on bacterial isolates from sputum or oropharyngeal cultures.[53,54]

CF patients have chronic upper respiratory tract involvement, clinically manifested as nasal congestion and rhinorrhea. Pansinusitis is almost universally present in affected individuals. If nasal symptoms develop or worsen, systemic antibiotic therapy may be indicated. The percentage of CF patients who have features consistent with clinical sinusitis varies widely.[55,56] Bacteria isolated from the paranasal sinuses parallel those found in the lower respiratory tract, though distinct strains may colonize different anatomic sites in the CF airway.[57] Occurring in 7% to 56% of CF patients,[56] nasal polyposis is a common complication leading to nasal obstruction and congestion, which can require surgical intervention. Surgical management is usually successful, but sinusitis and polyps often recur and repeated procedures may be required.[58]

Digital clubbing is a sign of long-standing pulmonary involvement and develops in virtually all CF patients. Hypertrophic pulmonary osteoarthropathy, a syndrome characterized with clubbing, long bone periostitis and synovitis that usually flares during acute pulmonary exacerbations, has been described in CF patients but is relatively rare.

Hemoptysis is common in older CF patients, particularly during pulmonary exacerbations, and is usually treated with antibiotics and, depending on the volume, withholding airway clearance. As CF lung disease progresses, bronchial arteries or collateral vessels enlarge and may rupture into an inflamed airway, producing massive hemoptysis, defined as more than 240 mL in 24 hours. Roughly 4.1% of all patients with CF will suffer massive hemoptysis, a medical emergency, in their life.[59,60] These episodes can be fatal. Pulmonary hemorrhage can be worsened by coagulopathy secondary to hypovitaminosis K or underlying CF liver disease. Though patients can be stabilized with intravenous vasopressin, selective bronchial artery embolization is the definitive treatment.[61] Recurrent hemoptysis does occur and repeated embolization may be indicated.

Airway hyperreactivity is often diagnosed in patients with CF, as evidenced by routine treatment with inhaled albuterol and corticosteroids. Roughly half of children and adults with CF have a bronchodilator response, even if they do not have asthma-like symptoms.[62,63] In several studies, airway hyperresponsiveness to exercise, histamine, or methacholine was found in 22% to 54% of children with CF.[64,65]

Allergic bronchopulmonary aspergillosis (ABPA) is an inflammatory complication, clinically manifested by wheezing and cough refractory to standard therapies. ABPA is an intense immunologic response to surface colonization with the fungus *Aspergillus fumigatus*, characterized by (1) clinical deterioration that is not explained by other etiologies, (2) elevated serum quantitative immunoglobulin (Ig) E concentrations (>500 IU/mL), (3) positive skin test to *Aspergillus fumigatus* or elevated in vitro *Aspergillus*-specific IgE levels, and (4) *Aspergillus*-specific IgG levels or precipitins. Other features include pulmonary consolidations and central bronchiectasis.[66] The incidence varies greatly, and it should be considered in instances of persistent airway obstruction and atelectasis. A high index of suspicion is required. Serum quantitative IgE concentrations should be measured annually to monitor for this complication. Once the diagnosis is made, patients are treated with extended courses of high-dose corticosteroids. Antifungal therapy is a therapeutic option to reduce the antigen burden in the lung, but few studies have shown that this strategy reduced the duration of corticosteroid treatment or improved outcome.[67]

Cor pulmonale is a complication of hypoxemia that is most commonly seen in patients with advanced disease. Early pulmonary hypertension can be managed by aggressive treatment of the underlying pulmonary disease and administration of supplemental oxygen. However, diuretics may be indicated in patients with right-sided heart failure.

■ PROGNOSIS

Survival of patients with CF has improved dramatically since it was first described over 70 years ago. While gastrointestinal signs and symptoms tend to predominate early, sinopulmonary manifestations increase with age. The progressive lung disease leads to considerable morbidity and respiratory failure and accounts for the vast majority of CF deaths.[1] In the United States, the predicted survival has steadily increased and is now 37.4 years (Fig. 52-4). This improvement is related to advances in monitoring and better, more aggressive treatment strategies.

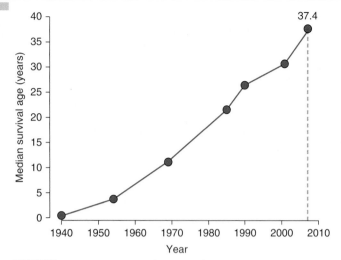

FIGURE 52-4. Increasing median survival age in CF patients over time, modified from CFF Patient Registry.[1]

Thus, routine surveillance studies are recommended in the care of children with CF, which include regular spirometry to monitor lung function, chest radiographs, and sputum or oropharyngeal cultures to assess lower respiratory tract flora.

Factors that negatively affect prognosis include malnutrition,[68] diabetes mellitus,[69] infection with *P. aeruginosa*[70,71] and *B. cepacia* complex,[22,72] and frequency of pulmonary exacerbations.[70] There is a gender gap in CF, with males tending to do better than female counterparts.[73,74] Socioeconomic status can influence survival of CF patients, and environmental factors such as exposure to tobacco smoke and airborne pollutants have detrimental effects.[75,76] Conversely, patients with atypical or pancreatic-sufficient forms of the disease have slower decline in pulmonary function when compared with those with classic CF and their prognosis and long-term survival are better.

It is thought that progression and extent of lung disease can be slowed with early diagnosis and intervention, which was used as a rationale for the introduction of newborn screening. By 2010, all 50 states of the United States have CF newborn screening universally required by law or rule, although the screening approaches used by individual states vary.

■ EVALUATIONS

The United States Cystic Fibrosis Foundation (CFF) has established Clinical Practice Guidelines that outline standards for routine monitoring and intervention to slow progression of lung disease. Evaluations include regular radiologic examinations, pulmonary function testing, and microbiologic cultures of airway secretions. Clinical evaluations also are important. Weight loss, anorexia, exercise tolerance, and school attendance are important measures of pulmonary morbidity. Indeed, the child's nutritional health is relevant to pulmonary outcomes. Younger children who have maintained their body weight had better pulmonary function at 6 years of age, showing the relationship between nutrition and lung disease.[77]

Chest imaging studies are useful tools to assess disease progression. Standard chest radiographs are often normal early in life, but as disease evolves, lung hyperinflation, peribronchial thickening, mucous plugging, and atelectasis develop. The progressive bronchiectasis, characteristic of CF lung disease, is usually a later finding on plain chest films. High-resolution computed tomography of the chest is more sensitive and provides greater anatomic detail, showing abnormalities well before detection on plain radiographs or changes in pulmonary function. Chest tomography can be performed on infants and small children, and may reveal unsuspected airway wall thickening, segmental overinflation, and early bronchiectasis (Fig. 52-5).[78–80] Recently, several investigators have developed scoring systems to measure the extent of lung disease and response to therapy. Despite its advantages, there are still no consensus guidelines regarding the use of computerized tomography, and there are concerns about long-term consequences of radiation exposure.[81]

Pulmonary function testing is routinely used to assess CF lung disease in children and adolescents with CF. Spirometric measurements permit assessment of progression of airway disease and are routinely used to diagnose pulmonary exacerbations and response to antibiotic therapy. Most CF children are able to perform reproducible spirometric maneuvers by 6 years of age. The forced expiratory volume in one second (FEV_1), or more accurately, the rate of FEV_1 decline, is a useful index of disease severity. Deteriorating FEV_1 is a key marker for disease progression.[82–84] Pulmonary function decline varies greatly among patients, but this decade, the average annual reduction in FEV_1 is approximately 2% per year in the United States. The 2-year morbidity of CF patients with a baseline FEV_1 30% of predicted for age is 50%.[82] Blood gas measurements are remarkably normal until late in the course, but they may reveal gas exchange abnormalities related to worsening ventilation-perfusion inequalities in patients with more advanced lung disease or clinical deterioration. Finally, infant pulmonary function testing has emerged as an evaluation tool in young children; however, the predictive value of these studies for later measures of disease severity has not been clearly demonstrated.

Because progression of CF lung disease is inextricably linked to airway infection, regular comprehensive microbiological assessments of specimens from the lower respiratory tract (e.g., sputum) are important.[9] Younger patients may not be able to expectorate, and in those cases respiratory secretions can be collected using post-tussive oropharyngeal swabs or bronchoalveolar lavage. Investigations have shown that negative oropharyngeal cultures may exclude lower airway infections, but a positive culture is not reliable to make the diagnosis of *P. aeruginosa* endobronchitis.[85] It is essential that respiratory cultures be processed and performed in laboratories with expertise in the handling of CF specimens and that recognize the difficulties in speciation of infecting pathogens. The CFF has established guidelines for the handling and processing of respiratory tract specimens and supports reference laboratories for confirmatory identification of certain organisms such as *B. cepacia* complex.

Hypertonic saline has been used to induce sputum for lower airway sampling for both microbiological

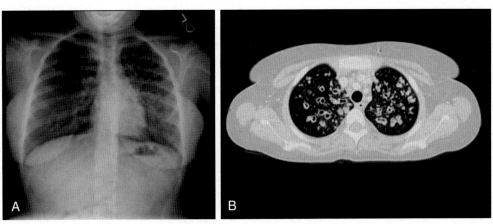

FIGURE 52-5. Chest imaging of an adolescent CF patient. Standard posteroanterior radiograph **(A)** and high resolution computerized tomography **(B)** of the chest show lung overinflation, bronchiectasis, and airway wall thickening.

and inflammatory markers in older pediatric patients.[86] Cytokines, chemokines, oxidation species, and neutrophil products are elevated in the CF lung, and they also may be increased in the sputum and bronchoalveolar lavage fluid during exacerbations. However, such measures can have significant interpatient and intrapatient variability, even in those with seemingly stable lung disease. It is unclear whether these markers reflect or predict disease progression. Inflammatory markers in the blood, such as peripheral leukocyte counts and C-reactive protein levels, have not been useful in the assessment of lung disease.

TREATMENT

Treatment for CF lung disease is evolving, incorporating the newer therapies developed over the last two decades.[87,88] Current management incorporates antibiotics, anti-inflammatory agents, inhaled mucolytics, vigorous airway clearance, and nutritional support (Fig. 52-6)[89] in an attempt to forestall progression of CF lung disease.

Airway Clearance

Effective airway clearance is a critical component of CF therapy.[90] In order to maintain lung health, physical removal of airway secretions is needed not only to relieve airway obstruction but also to reduce infection and airway inflammation.[91] Numerous airway clearance therapies (ACT) have been used and remain one of the most fundamental therapies for individuals with CF.[92] Additionally, novel agents aimed at restoring airway surface liquid and changing mucous viscosity have provided new opportunities to clear mucus and sustain normal lung function.[93,94]

Many passive and active methods of ACT are used in CF care. Active therapies include positive expiratory pressure, active-cycle-of-breathing technique, and autogenic drainage.[92,95–98] The most common passive methods are percussion and postural drainage and high-frequency chest wall oscillations. No specific ACT has been definitively shown to be superior, so an individual's choice should be based on age, experience, effectiveness, and adherence.[87,92,99,100]

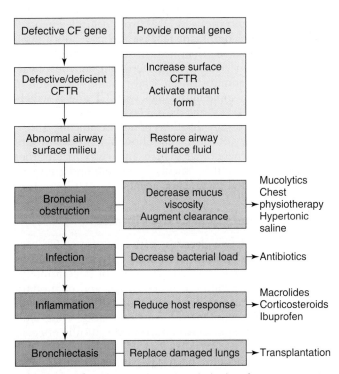

FIGURE 52-6. Pathophysiologic cascade leading from mutant CFTR gene to bronchiectasis in the CF lung, interventions, and current treatment strategies.

As an adjunct to airway clearance techniques, one must consider the benefit offered by aerobic exercise to mobilize secretions. In a recent systematic review of exercise for children with CF, both improved pulmonary function and aerobic fitness were demonstrated.[101] In addition to increased aerobic fitness, exercise programs may confer both short- and long-term protection against pulmonary function decline.

Any discussion of ACT would not be complete without discussing the recent advances in agents aimed at rehydrating secretions.[93] Reduced mucous viscosity and associated increased mucociliary clearance is achieved by improved airway surface hydration offered by these agents.[102,103] Working as a surface-acting osmotic agent, inhaled mannitol resulted in improved lung function in a small, short-term, placebo-controlled trial.[104] A larger, multicenter, randomized phase III trial examining these effects is presently underway. Hypertonic saline acts directly as an osmotic agent and increases airway surface liquid volume. In older CF patients, hypertonic saline resulted in reduced frequency of pulmonary exacerbations and enhanced airway clearance.[105] As a result, tolerability was established in younger children,[106] prompting a larger, multinational investigation of the benefit of hypertonic saline in infants and younger children. Finally, inhaled bronchodilators are often used before ACT to maintain airway patency and facilitate mucous removal.[107]

Inhaled Mucolytics

Aerosolized mucolytics have been incorporated into CF care to facilitate airway secretion clearance. The inspissated secretions in CF are predominately composed of pus with high concentrations of DNA from degraded neutrophils. Inhaled recombinant DNAse (dornase alfa) has a significant role in the treatment of CF lung disease[108] by reducing sputum viscosity and increasing mucous clearance. Regular administration leads to improvement in lung function in some individuals with CF and is widely used. N-acetyl-L-cysteine is a classic mucolytic agent because it hydrolyzes disulfide bonds in mucins, and it has a long history of use in CF[109]; however, little data support its effectiveness other than as an airway irritant that induces cough.[110] Other mucolytics remain under investigation as potential therapeutic agents.[108]

Antibiotic Therapy in Cystic Fibrosis

During the past two decades, antibiotic use in CF care has witnessed a strategic revolution in both indications for usage and modes of delivery. Antibiotics continue to be used in the setting of acute infections and pulmonary exacerbations but are now also routinely used to eradicate organisms in otherwise asymptomatic young children or to reduce bacterial burden in chronically infected patients.

CF patients acquire bacterial pathogens in an age-dependent manner that over time will chronically colonize their airways. Chronic infection with P. aeruginosa portends a worse prognosis, and once established, is virtually impossible to eradicate.[9,18,19] However, recent studies treating initial acquisition of P. aeruginosa have shown that the organism can be eradicated with aggressive antibiotic therapy.[20,21,111,112] Although patients reacquired the organism later, the realization that early P. aeruginosa infection can be effectively eradicated led to a change in how antibiotics are prescribed in CF. No longer are antibiotics solely used to treat symptomatic disease; now they are used to treat early positive P. aeruginosa cultures, even in the absence of symptoms. Unfortunately, data demonstrating that early eradication significantly impacts later lung function are lacking at this time. In addition, there is insufficient evidence to state whether one antibiotic regimen is superior to another in achieving eradication.[113-115]

Although there is no consensus as to what defines a pulmonary exacerbation, most clinicians would agree that increase in cough, increase in sputum production,

decline in lung function, shortness of breath, weight loss, and new adventitious sounds on auscultation warrant further investigation or therapy. Antibiotic treatment during an exacerbation, depending on the circumstance, may be delivered intravenously, orally, or by nebulization. The severity of the symptoms and the patient's available resources will assist the clinician in determining the appropriate course of therapy. Antibiotic therapy is typically guided by the findings of previous sputum or deep oropharyngeal culture and the susceptibility testing of the identified organisms. These cultures typically reflect the airway flora in older children and adolescents, but that may not be the case in infants.[85] Bronchoalveolar lavage (BAL) fluid cultures may be necessary to more accurately direct therapy. Antibiotics may be changed during the course of treatment based on more recent culture and susceptibility results or the patient's clinical response. It is important to note, however, that susceptibility testing in vitro does not necessarily correlate with clinical response.

Infections caused by P. aeruginosa in patients with CF are usually treated with two antibiotics of different classes in an attempt to prevent the emergence of resistance and also in the hopes of achieving synergy (Table 52-1). However, it is important to note that using the results from testing for susceptibility to multiple drug combinations does not confer any advantage to clinician-selected combinations of antibiotics, and multiple drug combination synergy testing is no longer routinely recommended.[116] The most common combination of intravenous therapy for P. aeruginosa involves the use of an aminoglycoside with a β-lactam antibiotic. Higher doses of systemic aminoglycosides are required in patients with CF because of increased clearance and altered pharmacokinetics,[117] so drug concentrations must be monitored and maintained in the therapeutic window. For CF patients with multidrug resistant P. aeruginosa, colistin may be used intravenously, but requires close monitoring for neurologic symptoms and renal toxicity. Concurrent intravenous aminoglycoside therapy should be avoided with intravenous colistin. Oral fluoroquinolones are frequently used, but P. aeruginosa can develop resistance rapidly.[118] Inhaled antibiotics can be used in conjunction with either intravenous or oral therapy, depending on the microbiological results.

Length of antibiotic therapy is determined by resolution of symptoms and return of lung function to its previous baseline or to a new plateau. Concern for emergence of resistant organisms limits extending courses beyond these endpoints. Complete eradication of organisms in the chronically infected patient is not achievable. Typically, return of lung function to baseline and resolution of symptoms can be achieved with 10 to 21 days of therapy with the majority of patients receiving 2 weeks of antibiotics; however, the data to define adequate length of therapy are lacking.[119]

Suppressive or maintenance therapy with inhaled antibiotics is appropriate for the majority of patients who are chronically infected with P. aeruginosa. Inhaled tobramycin administered on an alternate monthly basis led to a significant improvement in lung function.[120]

TABLE 52-1 APPROPRIATE ANTIBIOTICS FOR TREATMENT OF CYSTIC FIBROSIS PATHOGENS

PREVALENT BACTERIA	ANTIBIOTIC OPTIONS	PEDIATRIC DOSE*	ADULT DOSE*	NOTES
Staphylococcus aureus	Cefazolin	30 mg/kg IV q8h	1 g IV q8h	
	Nafcillin	25–50 mg/kg IV q6h	2 g IV q6h	
Methicillin-resistant *S. aureus*	Vancomycin	15 mg/kg IV q6h	500 mg IV q6h OR 1 g IV q12h	Administer slowly to avoid histamine release
	Linezolide	10 mg/kg q12h		
Pseudomonas aeruginosa	**Beta-lactam**	50 mg/kg IV q8h	2–4 g IV q8h	Usual strategy is one beta-lactam and one aminoglycoside or colistin
	Ceftazidime	100 mg/kg IV q6h	3 g IV q6h	
	Ticarcillin	100 mg/kg IV q6h	3 g IV q6h	
	Piperacillin	15–25 mg/kg IV q6h	500 mg–1 g IV q6h	
	Imipenem	40 mg/kg IV q8h	1–2 g IV q8h	
	Meropenem	50 mg/kg IV q8h	2 g IV q8h	
	Aztreonam			
	Aminoglycoside			
	Tobramycin	10 mg/kg q24h	10 mg/kg q24h	Serum concentration peak 8–12 µg/mL, trough <2 µg/mL are sought
			5–7.5 mg/kg IV q8h	
	Amikacin	5–7.5 mg/kg IV q8h	50–80 mg IV q8h	Serum levels peak 20–30 µg/mL, trough <10 µg/mL are sought
	Colistin	1 mg/kg IV q8h		
Burkholderia cepacia complex	Meropenem	40 mg/kg IV q8h	1–2 g IV q8h	
	Minocycline	2 mg/kg IV or PO q12h	100 mg IV or PO q12h	Should not be given to those <8 years of age
	Amikacin	5–7.5 mg/kg IV q8h	5–7.5 mg/kg IV q8h	
	Ceftazidime	50 mg/kg IV q8h	2 g IV q8h	
	Chloramphenicol	15–20 mg/kg IV q6h	15–20 mg/kg IV q6h	Serum level peak 15–25 µg/mL, trough <5–15 mg/mL are sought
	Trimethoprim/ Sulfamethoxazole	4–5 mg/kg of trimethoprim component IV q12h	4–5 mg/kg of trimethoprim component IV q12h	
Stenotrophomonas maltophilia	Ticarcillin/clavulanate	100 mg/kg of ticarcillin component IV q6h	3 g of ticarcillin component IV q6h	
	Trimethoprim/ Sulfamethoxazole	4–5 mg/kg of trimethoprim component IV q12h	4–5 mg/kg of trimethoprim component IV q12h	
	Aztreonam	50 mg/kg IV q8h	2 g IV q8h	
Achromobacter xylosoxidans	Chloramphenicol	15–20 mg/kg IV q6h	15–20 mg/kg q6h	Serum level peak 15–25 µg/mL, trough <5–15 µg/mL are sought
	Minocycline	2 mg/kg IV or PO q12h	100 mg IV or PO q12h	Should not be given to those <8 years old
	Ciprofloxacin	15 mg/kg IV or PO q12h	400 mg IV or 500–750 mg PO q12h	
	Imipenem	15–25 mg/kg IV q6h	500 mg–1 g IV q6h	
	Meropenem	40 mg/kg IV q8h	1–2 g IV q8h	

*Most doses are expressed as milligrams per kilogram of body weight. The dose given to children should not exceed that for adults.

Additionally, emergence of tobramycin resistance is low when employing this strategy. Similar improvement in FEV_1 was recently described with inhaled aztreonam.[121] Aerosolized colistin has been used and this route minimizes the risk of systemic toxicity.[122]

Infection with nontuberculous mycobacteria is a growing concern.[123] Finding "atypical" mycobacteria presents a perplexing problem for the CF clinician trying to determine whether this organism is colonizing the airway or is acting as a pathogen; many of the presenting symptoms and radiographic findings can be explained by the more commonly isolated bacteria. In addition, therapy for nontuberculous mycobacteria involves prolonged treatment with multiple antibiotics, each of which has associated toxicities and variable tolerability. The recommended approach is to first treat the other organisms found on culture and closely monitor the patient's response to this therapy. When nontuberculous mycobacteria are cultured from a patient with CF, it is recommended that routine macrolide therapy be discontinued to prevent the emergence of resistance. The long-term implication of the presence of nontuberculous mycobacteria in the CF airway is unclear.[124]

Anti-inflammatory Therapy in Cystic Fibrosis

Approximately 30 years ago, CF caregivers noted that patients with CF who were hypogammaglobulinemic tended to have less severe lung disease than those with elevated serum IgG concentrations,[125] which supported the hypothesis that an overzealous immune response in patients with CF may be deleterious and provided rationale for early trials with anti-inflammatory therapy. Two studies using systemic corticosteroids demonstrated an improvement in lung function over placebo.[126,127] However, excessive side effects were noted during the larger second study, including diabetes, cataracts, and growth failure, during alternate-day dosing. Multiple studies have examined the potential use of inhaled corticosteroids in patients with CF but failed to show benefit.[128]

High-dose ibuprofen slows the annual rate of decline in lung function with the greatest effect seen in school-aged children.[129] Yet the risks associated with its use, such as gastrointestinal hemorrhage and renal failure, though small, are so dramatic that few CF centers have adopted this treatment.

Azithromycin is known to possess anti-inflammatory effects, but its exact mechanism of action in CF is unclear. Studies in CF patients over 6 years of age infected with *P. aeruginosa* in whom azithromycin was administered thrice weekly demonstrated better lung function, weight gain, and fewer pulmonary exacerbations compared with placebo.[130] A recent study in patients not chronically infected with *P. aeruginosa* failed to demonstrate a difference in lung function, but did show a 50% reduction in pulmonary exacerbations compared with placebo.[131] Adverse effects have been minimal, and this agent has gained widespread acceptance.

Other novel approaches include addressing the depletion of antioxidants in the neutrophils and airway surface liquid in patients with CF. N-acetylcysteine, a glutathione prodrug, given orally in high doses decreased sputum elastase activity in patients with CF.[132] A large multicenter study to better evaluate this agent is presently underway. Also in the drug development pipeline are protease inhibitors such as recombinant alpha$_1$-antitrypsin, which have been tested previously in clinical trials with modest clinical effect.[133]

Use of anti-inflammatory therapy in CF is the proverbial double-edged sword and must be approached cautiously because the immune system does contain infection within the lung. A clinical trial with a leukotriene B4 antagonist had to be terminated early because the treatment group had more pulmonary exacerbations requiring hospitalizations.[134] Another trial examining the efficacy of nebulized interferon-γ1B also increased hospital admissions.[135] Identifying a safe and effective anti-inflammatory treatment will continue to be an active area of research in CF.

Preventative Care

Prevention of complications remains a priority for CF clinicians. The adoption of newborn screening in the United States has had a significant impact on care and expanded traditional prophylaxis to include presymptomatic identification of nutritional and respiratory complications. While preventing illness with immunization remains a significant focus, avoiding nutritional deficiencies and

eradicating *P. aeruginosa* have become active areas of both research and quality improvement.

Immunization against measles and influenza is an important component of CF care. Though systematic reviews have failed to demonstrate long-term benefit of immunization,[136] the impact of influenza can be substantial,[137] and yearly vaccination continues to be recommended. Similarly, respiratory syncytial virus infection is associated with more severe respiratory complications; thus, prevention using palivizumab should be considered in all children younger than 2 years of age, and it is recommended in high-risk patients.[138]

Nutritional interventions have resulted in improved outcomes. Better growth parameters at age 3 are associated with improved lung function at 6 years of age.[77] Furthermore, with earlier recognition by newborn screening, the risk of being more severely malnourished and having more lung disease was noted in the controls versus the screened cohort.[139] Unfortunately, the advantage provided by screening is not undisputed because studies to date have not demonstrated a long-term pulmonary benefit.[140] However, a reduced treatment burden may result from earlier diagnosis and an overall improvement in outcome.[141]

Anti-bacterial prophylaxis remains a controversial topic. A trial with cephalexin to prevent early *S. aureus* infection did not improve health outcomes and unexpectedly increased *P. aeruginosa* colonization.[142,143] However, the latter effect has not been reported elsewhere. Several antipseudomonal vaccines have been developed but failed to show clinical effectiveness in protecting against *P. aeruginosa* infection.[144] Although its benefit to CF patients is unclear, antipneumococcal vaccination should be performed as a routine childhood immunization.[145]

Pseudomonas eradication strategies have been developed as a means to delay acquisition and improve pulmonary outcomes. Although studies remain ongoing, recently published data from the ELITE trial demonstrated greater than 90% effective eradication of *P. aeruginosa* with a median time to recurrence of more than 2 years following a 28-day course of inhaled tobramycin.[115] Data from the EPIC[20] trial and other studies will shed more light on choice and duration of therapy recommended for early antipseudomonal therapy.[146]

Lung Transplantation in Cystic Fibrosis

Although we have witnessed great improvements in median survival over the past decade, there are still patients with CF who progress to advanced lung disease and respiratory insufficiency at a very young age. For these children and adolescents, replacement of their damaged lungs with new lungs is their only hope to prolong survival and improve their quality of life. In 2008, a total of 157 adults and children with CF underwent bilateral lung transplantation in the United States. Unfortunately, lung transplantation is not a panacea, with 5-year survival rates remaining at approximately 50%.[147] Although many factors are associated with success, if lung transplantation is to truly extend life, appropriate timing of the procedure is paramount. During the last 20 years, several models have been proposed to predict survival with CF, but none are substantially better than the others.[82,148]

Transplant physicians grasped the importance of these predictor models early in determining the appropriate time to list patients for transplantation. Before 2005, the lung allocation system in the United States was based on time spent waiting on the list. Since then, donor lungs have been allocated using the lung allocation score (LAS),[149] derived from variables that include forced vital capacity (FVC), body mass index (BMI), age, renal function, diabetes, supplemental oxygen, and assisted ventilation, among others. Consequently, those CF patients 12 years of age or older who are highest on the waiting list in the United States are those who are the sickest, not those who have waited the longest. Nevertheless, despite this new, more equitable system of organ distribution, patients still die waiting for lungs.

Contraindications to lung transplantation for CF vary, based on individual center experience or emergence of new information. Because of very poor posttransplant outcomes, some centers will consider the presence of *B. cenocepacia* or *B. dolosa* as absolute contraindications. The need for invasive positive pressure ventilation before transplant is no longer considered an absolute contraindication to transplantation at most centers. Short-term outcomes in regard to morbidity and mortality are worse in patients requiring ventilatory support, but long-term outcomes do not appear to be impacted.[150] Multiorgan failure is a contraindication to lung transplantation, but for CF patients with both advanced liver disease and end-stage lung disease, simultaneous liver-lung transplantation is feasible with outcomes just as good as, if not better than, lung transplantation alone.[151]

It is worth briefly mentioning the importance of adherence to a strict posttransplant regimen. Patients with a history of nonadherence to CF care tend to do poorly posttransplant. In general, adolescents do worse posttransplant than any other age group despite the fact that they tend to have fewer comorbidities than either transplanted infants or adults.[152] Referring centers must take responsibility in beginning the dialogue concerning a history of nonadherence with the family before referring the patient to the transplant center, so that both centers can effectively work together in addressing these issues. The strict posttransplant regimen, lifelong immunosuppression, and disappointing long-term outcomes only reinforce the need to choose not only the appropriate candidates but also the optimal timing of lung transplantation so as to provide patients with improved survival.[153] In a controversial study, performed pre-LAS, it was found that the majority of children with CF did not derive a survival benefit. However, since the study was performed at a time when patients were listed years before needing a transplant to accrue time, the covariates that were studied may not have been appropriate.[154-155] In the United Kingdom, with a different allocation system, a study did find that transplantation provided children with

CF a survival benefit.[156] Most studies to date seem to suggest that patients do derive a clear benefit in terms of quality of life.[157]

Emerging Therapies in Cystic Fibrosis

Improved clinical outcomes in CF patients are encouraging. Between 2000 and 2008, the number of adults with CF has increased by 50%, a testament to the progress being made with the widespread institution of conventional therapies alone. Although there are many therapies in the CFF drug development pipeline to ameliorate symptoms, our focus in this section is to describe agents that have the potential to more proximally correct the basic ion transport defect, including modulation or correction of defective CFTR and activation of other ion channels.

Several small molecule therapeutics have the potential to activate or modulate mutant forms of CFTR. These therapeutic agents have allele- or mutation-specific effects. Class I mutations are nonsense mutations resulting in the absence of CFTR production; several agents allow the ribosome to read through the premature stop codon but not through normal termination codons. A phase II study using a candidate drug (atalauren) demonstrated improvement in nasal potential difference, lung function and body weight.[158] A much larger multinational, multicenter study is ongoing.

For class II mutations, such as the common $\Delta F508$, a small molecule corrector designed to chaperone the defective CFTR protein partially restored cAMP-mediated chloride secretion in human bronchial epithelia from patients homozygous for $\Delta F508$.[159] However, it is likely that the restoration of adequate CFTR function will require the addition of a potentiator, allowing the mutant CFTR to gate appropriately. Studies *in vitro* have indicated that such potentiators (VX770) can enhance gating of G551D CFTR.[160] Initial clinical trials showed improvement in pulmonary function and a marked reduction in sweat chloride levels, making potentiators the first therapeutic agents to ever affect this physiologic outcome. A larger 1-year clinical trial is presently under way.

Another potential strategy is to modulate non-CFTR ion channels at the apical surface. A UTP analogue (denufosol) has been shown to activate non-CFTR chloride channels by stimulating $P2Y_2$ receptors on epithelial cells. The agent also appears to inhibit sodium absorption. A phase III, placebo-controlled study in patients with mild lung disease showed modestly improved FEV_1,[161] but a subsequent, large clinical trial failed to show an effect. Another modulating agent increases free intracellular calcium concentrations that activate an alternative chloride channel, and a single center phase II trial with this aerosolized drug demonstrated a change in FEV_1.[162]

Finally, somatic gene therapy is a potential strategy for correcting CF. More than 20 clinical gene therapy trials were conducted in the United States with disappointing results. Many obstacles to airway gene therapy need to be overcome, including airway obstruction that prevents vector delivery to the epithelial or submucosal gland cells,

Section VIII

incitement of acute inflammatory and immune responses that interfere with repetitive dosing, and inefficiency of gene delivery to the airway epithelium. Nevertheless, this research continues.

CONCLUSIONS

Pulmonary disease in CF is the consequence of defective function of apical ion channels and impaired mucociliary clearance, which renders the airway susceptible to endobronchial bacterial infection and induces an intense inflammatory response that leads to bronchiectasis and, ultimately, respiratory failure. Children with CF born today have greater potential to live longer, primarily because of earlier diagnosis and multidisciplinary, center-based care, where children can benefit from treatments for downstream consequences of defective ion transport, such as inhaled mucolytics, antibiotics, anti-inflammatory agents, and airway clearance techniques. More recently, newer therapeutics have emerged that target the basic defect and have shown promise in early clinical trials. If successful, these treatments are poised to profoundly change the course of CF lung disease.

Suggested Reading

Chmiel JF, Berger M, Konstan MW. The role of inflammation in the pathophysiology of CF lung disease. *Clin Rev Allergy Immunol.* 2002;23:5–27.

Davis PB. Cystic fibrosis since 1938. *Am J Respir Crit Care Med.* 2006;173:475–482.

Elizur A, Cannon CL, Ferkol TW. Airway inflammation in cystic fibrosis. *Chest.* 2008;133:489–495.

Ferkol T, Rosenfeld M, Milla CE. Cystic fibrosis pulmonary exacerbations. *J Pediatr.* 2006;148:259–264.

Flume PA, O'Sullivan BP, Robinson KA, et al. Cystic fibrosis pulmonary guidelines: chronic medications for maintenance of lung health. *Am J Respir Crit Care Med.* 2007;176:957–969.

Gibson RL, Burns JL, Ramsey BW. Pathophysiology and management of pulmonary infections in cystic fibrosis. *Am J Respir Crit Care Med.* 2003;168:918–951.

Knowles MR, Boucher RC. Mucus clearance as a primary innate defense mechanism for mammalian airways. *J Clin Invest.* 2002;109:571–577.

O'Sullivan BP, Freedman SD. Cystic fibrosis. *Lancet.* 2009;373:1891–1904.

Rowe SM, Miller S, Sorscher EJ. Cystic fibrosis. *N Engl J Med.* 2005;352:1992–2001.

References

The complete reference list is available online at www.expertconsult.com

53 NONPULMONARY MANIFESTATIONS OF CYSTIC FIBROSIS

Najma N. Ahmed, MD, MSc, FRCP(C), and Peter R. Durie, MD, FRCP(C)

Cystic fibrosis is characterized by the abnormal secretion of fluid, electrolytes, and macromolecules by exocrine glands. In 1989, Tsui and colleagues isolated the CF gene on chromosome 7, and this led to the discovery of its gene product, the cystic fibrosis transmembrane conductance regulator (CFTR), which functions as a cAMP-dependent chloride channel.[1] The pathophysiologic basis of CF centers on the defective function of this protein in various tissues. In the gastrointestinal (GI) tract, CFTR is expressed in the crypt and villous cells of the intestine, the apical membrane of cholangiocytes, and the apical membrane of the pancreatic ductal epithelium. CFTR also is expressed in the reproductive tract, resulting in altered fertility in patients with CF. The absence or dysfunction of CFTR in various tissues results in a broad spectrum of disease manifestations involving the bronchopulmonary tree, exocrine pancreas, hepatobiliary system, and the male reproductive system. The spectrum of clinical manifestations is summarized in Box 53-1. This chapter presents a summary of the current knowledge of the extrapulmonary manifestations of cystic fibrosis.

▄ PANCREATIC DISEASE

Pathobiology

Quantitative pancreatic stimulation testing shows that patients with CF have abnormal ductal chloride and bicarbonate secretion.[2] Under normal conditions, the pancreas secretes 2.5 L/day of a bicarbonate-rich fluid. In patients with cystic fibrosis, impaired electrolyte transport results in a reduction in fluid secretion, which leads in turn to protein hyperconcentration and ductal obstruction by viscous secretions (Fig. 53-1).[3] Impaired ductal secretion of Cl^- by dysfunctional or absent CFTR was proposed to reduce the amount of Cl^- available for transport via the ductal apical Cl^-/HCO_3^- exchanger, resulting in low levels of pancreatic bicarbonate secretion.[4] However, it is now understood, that pancreatic bicarbonate secretion can also occur in the absence of luminal chloride.[5] CFTR-mediated Cl^- transport results in the depolarization of the ductal epithelial cell, which stimulates entry of bicarbonate via basolateral electrogenic Na/HCO_3^- cotransporters. Bicarbonate is then secreted via a predominantly conductive pathway.[6] CFTR is also permeable to bicarbonate but at a level of only 25% compared with its chloride permeability, and the role of CFTR-mediated HCO_3^- transport under physiologic conditions is unclear.

In its most severe form, pancreatic disease begins *in utero*. There is rapid progression of acinar damage within the first year of life in patients with pancreatic insufficiency. Morphologic evaluation of the pancreas in infants dying with CF has shown a marked lack of development of acinar tissue. Duct obstruction by proteinaceous secretions is thought to lead to duct dilatation and acinar loss. Histologically, there is extensive destruction of pancreatic acini, with replacement by fat and fibrous tissue. It is important to note that in order to develop pancreatic insufficiency, over 95% of pancreatic function must be lost.

Pancreatic Phenotype

Cross-sectional data indicate that approximately 85% of CF patients are pancreatic insufficient (PI) and require enzyme supplementation. The remaining patients have adequate pancreatic reserve to allow for adequate nutrient digestion and do not require enzymes. This group of patients is termed pancreatic sufficient (PS). Studies have shown that PS patients are diagnosed at a later age, have lower mean sweat chloride concentrations, and better pulmonary function than patients with pancreatic insufficiency. Moreover, the PS patients, as a group, have better survival. In contrast, PI patients are more likely to have meconium ileus, distal intestinal obstruction syndrome, and severe liver disease.

Newborn screening programs have shown that approximately 60% of patients are PI at diagnosis. Infants with PI have high serum trypsinogen levels at diagnosis that decline to undetectable levels by 7 years of age. The majority of the PS infants progress to PI within the first 2 to 3 years of life. Such patients show a progressive but delayed decline in serum trypsinogen levels. As we later describe, the remaining PS patients show prolonged retention of their pancreatic sufficient status.

Genotype-Phenotype Correlations

Over 1700 different mutations or putative mutations have been identified in the *CFTR* gene, most of which are rare. Genotype-phenotype studies have shown that the strongest association between the *CFTR* genotype and the clinical phenotype is in the exocrine pancreas. The PI and PS phenotypes are associated with distinct "severe" or "mild" mutations in the *CFTR* gene, respectively. Patients who are PI at diagnosis, or who progress to PI, carry "severe" mutations on both alleles, whereas patients who are PS, carry at least one "mild" mutation. The "mild" allele confers a dominant effect over the "severe" allele. This subject is covered in more detail in Chapter 50.

The pancreatic phenotype has been shown to correlate with the functional consequences of *CFTR* mutations. Over 95% of patients with *severe* class I, II, and

BOX 53-1   CLINICAL MANIFESTATIONS OF CYSTIC FIBROSIS

Systemic
- Failure to thrive
- Malnutrition/Kwashiorkor
- Micronutrient deficiencies

Esophagus
- Gastroesophageal reflux
- Esophagitis/stricture
- Esophageal varices

Pancreas
- Pancreatic insufficiency
- Pancreatitis
- CF-related diabetes

Intestine
- Meconium ileus
- DIOS
- Constipation
- Rectal prolapse
- Fibrosing colonopathy

Hepatobiliary
Extrahepatic
- Microgallbladder
- Distended Gallbladder
- Cholelithiasis
- Common bile duct stenosis
- Cholangiocarcinoma
- Sclerosing cholangitis

Intrahepatic
- Neonatal cholestasis
- Steatosis
- Focal biliary cirrhosis
- Multilobular cirrhosis

Reproductive
- Infertility due to obstructive azoospermia in men
- Impaired fertility in women

DIOS, Distal intestinal obstruction syndrome.

III mutations, are pancreatic insufficient or progress to pancreatic insufficiency after diagnosis. In contrast, most patients with *mild* class IV and V mutations are consistently pancreatic sufficient.[7]

Clinical Presentation

Pancreatic Insufficiency

The vast majority of patients present in infancy or early childhood with classic manifestations of CF such as meconium ileus, malnutrition/growth failure, steatorrhea, and rectal prolapse. Even patients diagnosed by newborn screening at 6 to 8 weeks of age may have signs and symptoms of malnutrition with or without respiratory symptoms. Stool testing shows microscopic evidence of undigested triglyceride, increased fecal fat losses following a 72-hour balance study, or low fecal enzymes (elastase-1 or chymotrypsin). There may be biochemical evidence of fat-soluble vitamin deficiencies. At presentation, up to 50% of conventionally diagnosed patients may be hypoalbuminemic. Infants can present with hypoproteinemia, edema, growth failure, and ascites.[8,9] A small minority of CF patients with PI manage to elude diagnosis until later childhood, and rarely, adolescence.

Pancreatic Sufficiency

Patients with the "nonclassic" PS phenotype usually present later in childhood and early adulthood. Clinical manifestations are frequently quite subtle, usually involving a single organ, and unlike patients with the pancreatic insufficient form of CF, patients usually experience relatively normal growth and do not have symptoms of maldigestion. Sweat chloride measurements are, on average, lower in PS patients than those observed in the PI CF patient population, and in many cases, individual values may be within the normal or borderline range.

Cross-sectional data from Toronto indicate that approximately one fifth of nonclassic CF patients develop pancreatitis, and in one third of PS patients, the diagnosis of pancreatitis preceded the diagnosis of CF.[10-12] Liver disease also may be an isolated presenting feature of CF disease, although this is extremely uncommon.

Assessment of Pancreatic Function

An accurate assessment of pancreatic function is essential in the management of patients with CF. Pancreatic function should be objectively assessed at the time of diagnosis, and furthermore, patients who are PS should be monitored regularly for evidence of progression to pancreatic insufficiency. Pancreatic function may be assessed using several methods. Most commonly 72-hour fecal fat balance studies are used to identify patients with the PI phenotype. Accurate measurement of fat intake is critical in obtaining a valid result. Pancreatic insufficiency is defined by fat losses of more than 15% of intake in infants less than 6 months of age, while in older infants a cutoff of more than 7% of intake is used. Serum trypsinogen can distinguish PI from PS in patients older than 7 years of age. At birth, serum levels are usually elevated, but then decline to low or undetectable levels in PI patients by 5 to 7 years of age. In contrast, PS patients show fluctuating levels both within and above the normal range at all ages. In patients who are PS at diagnosis and progress to PI, there is a delayed decline in serum trypsinogen levels.

Fecal pancreatic elastase-1 is a useful alternative test for the assessment of pancreatic function, although it does have some limitations. The test is not influenced by the concurrent ingestion of pancreatic enzymes. A negative test result (>100 µg/g stool) had a 99% predictive value for ruling out pancreatic insufficiency. In patients with CF, the sensitivity and specificity were 100%. However, in other conditions causing steatorrhea, including short gut and Shwachman-Diamond syndrome, fecal elastase-1 measurements had lower specificity.[13]

Quantitative pancreatic function testing, using duodenal intubation and a marker perfusion technique, is useful to quantify pancreatic reserve, as well as fluid and anion secretion. However, this test is limited by its invasive nature, cost, and complexity. Quantitative exocrine pancreatic function has been shown to correlate with the functional consequences of *CFTR* gene mutations. Patients with class I, II, or III mutations have severely impaired

NORMAL ACINAR AND DUCTAL SECRETION

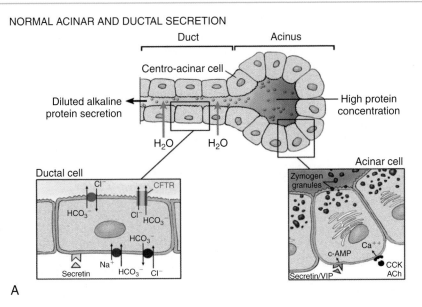

A

CYSTIC FIBROSIS

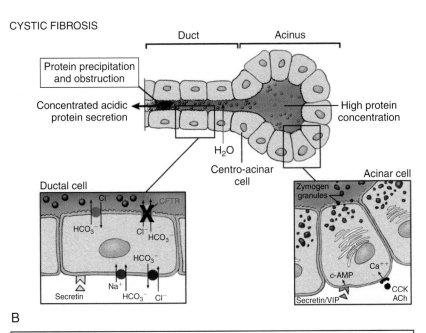

B

Under normal circumstances (A) Cl^- and HCO_3^- secretion provides a driving force for the movement of fluid into the lumen of the duct, which maintains the solubility of secreted proteins in a dilute, alkaline solution. In CF (B), impaired anion transport results in decreased secretion of more acidic fluid, which leads to precipitation of secreted proteins. Intraluminal obstruction of the ducts then causes progressive pancreatic damage and atrophy.

FIGURE 53-1. Pathophysiology of pancreatic disease in CF.

acinar and ductular function compared with controls. In contrast, those with class IV or V mutations have a wide range of enzyme output extending from just above the threshold for developing PI into the normal range.

Management of Pancreatic Insufficiency

Only patients who have documented pancreatic insufficiency should receive pancreatic enzyme supplementation. There is a wide variety of commercial pancreatic enzymes available in tablet, powdered, or microencapsulated forms.

Enteric-coated pH-resistant microsphere preparations are most commonly used. These preparations were developed to protect the enzymes from degradation by acid and pepsin in the stomach. They allow for release of the enzymes at a pH of 5.5 to 6, and in theory, the enteric coating of the microspheres should dissolve in the proximal small intestine. Ideally, the dose of enzyme should be determined by nutrient intake of fat, protein, and carbohydrate. However a simplified approach based on the patient's age and weight has been established (Table 53-1). Usually, half the standard dose is used for snacks. Current

TABLE 53-1 DOSING GUIDELINES FOR PANCREATIC ENZYMES

AGE	DOSE OF ENZYMES
Infant	2,000–4,000 units lipase/120 mL formula or breastfeeding
< 4 years	1,000–2,500 units lipase/kg/meal
> 4 years	500–2,500 units lipase/kg/meal

guidelines recommend a dose of 1000 U lipase/kg/meal for children under 4 years of age or at 500 U lipase/kg/meal for children over 4 years of age. The dose should not exceed 10,000 U lipase/kg/day. The total daily dose should reflect three meals per day and two to three snacks per day. Patients should be maintained on a high-energy diet that is rich in fat, and growth should be monitored closely.

The response to pancreatic enzymes is extremely variable from patient to patient; consequently, dosing requirements may vary. If response to enzyme therapy is poor, growth is poor, or symptoms persist, the patient should be reevaluated for other contributing factors (Box 53-2). Patients should not arbitrarily increase enzyme dosing without consulting their CF team. The dose should not exceed 10,000 lipase U/kg/day because of the increased risk of fibrosing colonopathy, which is discussed later.[14] Children who are unable to swallow whole capsules may open the capsule and the contents may be mixed with a small amount of apple sauce or other acidic food. The microspheres should not be crushed or allowed to sit in food. Enzymes should be stored in a cool dark place and expiration dates should be followed

One factor that can interfere with the efficacy of pancreatic enzymes is the inability of the CF pancreas to produce the normal alkaline secretions that help neutralize acidic gastric contents entering the small bowel. The lower intestinal pH results in impaired enzyme release,

BOX 53-2 FACTORS AFFECTING RESPONSE TO ENZYME SUPPLEMENTS

Enzyme Supplements
- Inappropriate storage
- Expiration of product

Poor Compliance
- Refusal of medication
- Incorrect administration
- Desire to lose weight

Dietary Issues
- Excessive juice intake (carbohydrate malabsorption)
- Inappropriate eating behavior (i.e., frequent small meals)
- High fat " fast foods"

Low Intestinal pH
- Inadequate breakdown of enteric coating
- Contents released all at once

Concurrent Gastrointestinal Disorder

Adapted from Borowitz D, Baker RD, Stallings V. Consensus report on nutrition for pediatric patients with cystic fibrosis. *J Pediatr Gastroenterol Nutr.* 2002;35(3):246-259.

and/or reduced enzyme activity. Acid-suppression therapy may therefore be useful to raise the intestinal pH. Furthermore, severe cholestatic hepatobiliary disease can contribute to malabsorption in CF. Investigations should be pursued to identify other comorbid conditions if patients do not respond to therapy. A poor response to therapy also may result from a concomitant gastrointestinal disorder, including chronic giardiasis, celiac disease, inflammatory bowel disease, and bacterial overgrowth.

Complications of Therapy

Fibrosing Colonopathy
The first description of colonic strictures in CF patients occurred in 1994. In fibrosing colonopathy, there is colonic narrowing with circular intramural fibrosis that may be limited to the ascending colon or may extend to involve the entire colon. Barium enema may demonstrate a localized apple core–like lesion in the ascending colon, or the entire colon may appear contracted and featureless. Bowel wall thickness is increased on two-dimensional imaging. However, evidence of bowel wall thickening should be interpreted with caution because unaffected patients with CF have colonic wall thickening on ultrasound.[15,16] Histology may show evidence of severe fibrosis in the lamina propria, and superficial inflammation with eosinophils, cryptitis, or apoptosis (Fig. 53-2).

Although the precise cause is unknown, retrospective case-control studies showed a strong risk association with high-dose pancreatic enzyme use. Patients at higher risk for this complication include children under 12 years of age who have been taking enzymes with lipase intake exceeding 6000 U/kg/meal for more than 6 months. Other risk factors may be a history of distal intestinal obstruction syndrome, meconium ileus, or prior intestinal surgery.[17] Clinically, patients may have obstructive symptoms, abdominal pain, bloody diarrhea, or poor weight gain.

A significant subgroup of patients with fibrosing colonopathy has required surgical intervention. Patients with this condition need to be monitored closely because they may develop strictures. Management of patients with fibrosing colonopathy also includes immediate reduction of the dose of enzyme supplements to within the recommended range.[14] The long-term prognosis for patients with this condition remains unclear.

Allergy
Immediate hypersensitivity reactions to pancreatic extracts have been reported in patients, caregivers, and parents of patients with CF. Clinical symptoms often mimic asthma, but severe anaphylactic reactions have been reported. This reaction is an IgE-mediated phenomenon and is a rare occurrence.[18,19]

CYSTIC FIBROSIS–RELATED DIABETES MELLITUS (CFRD)

Pathobiology

Glucose intolerance in CF was first described in 1938 by Andersen.[20] However, it was not until 1962 that diabetes mellitus (DM) was established as a secondary

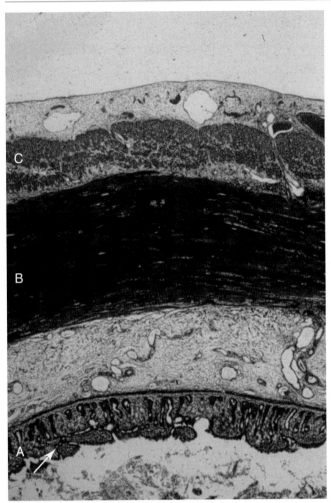

FIGURE 53-2. Histologic findings in fibrosing colonopathy. Classification system for *CFTR* mutations (see text for details). Intestinal cross-section from a patient with fibrosing colonopathy illustrating **(A)** nonspecific acute and chronic inflammation in the mucosa *(arrow)*, **(B)** hypertrophy of the muscularis mucosa, and **(C)** a ring of fibrous tissue.

complication of CF. Only patients with pancreatic insufficiency are at risk for this complication. Approximately one third of CF patients have CFRD, although this varies based on the age and ethnicity of the population, and also depends on the rigor of screening. Children with CF who are under 10 years of age appear to have a similar risk of insulin-requiring DM compared with that of the general population. Beginning in adolescence, the overall incidence of CFRD is 3% to 4%. During adolescence and adulthood, the incidence of CFRD progressively increases, with the median age of onset being 20 years of age. As many as 45% to 50% of patients over the age of 30 have CFRD.[21] In addition, a family history of type 2 diabetes increases the risk of CFRD threefold.

The pathogenesis of CFRD is unclear but is thought to result from the accumulation of viscous secretions in the pancreatic duct leading to duct obstruction, progressive pancreatic fibrosis, fatty infiltration, and amyloid deposition. A reduction in islet cell mass also has been described. Recently, it has been suggested that an increase in oxidative stress and the accumulation of misfolded CFTR in the endoplasmic reticulum (ER) of islet cells may result in ER stress leading to beta cell apoptosis. Basal insulin secretion appears to be maintained in CF patients with or without CFRD. However, there is a reduction in insulin secretion in response to stimulation. While insulin resistance is not involved in the pathogenesis of CFRD, it may exacerbate hyperglycemia because of a reduction in peripheral and hepatic insulin sensitivity.

There has been some debate regarding the impact of CFRD on morbidity and mortality. However, a recent multicenter study showed that patients with CFRD had worse lung function and nutritional status and concluded that CFRD reduces survival. Treatment with insulin appears to reverse the decline in pulmonary function and restore nutritional status. Long-term morbidity from microvascular complications including diabetic retinopathy and nephropathy was initially thought to be low, but recent studies have shown high incidence, which appears to be similar to type-2 diabetes mellitus.[22] In contrast, macrovascular complications appear to be rare, likely because of steatorrhea and loss of lipoproteins.

Diagnosis

Rarely, patients may present with overt symptoms such as polydipsia and polyuria. More frequently patients are asymptomatic or present with subtle symptoms such as impaired growth or delayed puberty. There also may be an unexplained decline in lung function. CFRD may be intermittent at first and may occur in association with physical stress such as infection, nocturnal enteral feedings, or steroid treatment.

The recommended diagnostic tool for CFRD is the oral glucose tolerance test (OGTT). The CF diabetes consensus conference proposed a classification system for CFRD, which is shown in Table 53-2.[23] Studies have shown that a subgroup of CF patients may have diabetic glucose tolerance as illustrated by an OGTT without fasting hyperglycemia. Moreover, there is no consensus on whether such patients should be treated with insulin. In type 1 and 2 DM, fasting glucose is the diagnostic test of choice; however, in CFRD a number of patients will be missed if this is used as the sole screening test. Thus, an OGTT may be required. Hemoglobin A1c (HbA1c) is not a reliable diagnostic screening test because it may be falsely low. Recently, continuous glucose monitoring has been suggested as a potential diagnostic tool[24]; patients who had a blood glucose of >7.8 mmol/L at least 4.5% of the time were more likely to have a decline in FEV_1 than nondiabetic CF controls.

Management

Nutritional management of CFRD is aimed at maintaining normal nutritional status. A multidisciplinary approach that includes members of the CF and endocrine teams is essential. Strong evidence-based data for the management of CFRD is lacking; therefore, current management is based on extrapolation from standard CF and diabetes care. It is vitally important to maintain normal growth in adolescents or to maintain an acceptable body mass

TABLE 53-2 CLASSIFICATION OF GLUCOSE INTOLERANCE IN CYSTIC FIBROSIS

GLUCOSE TOLERANCE	FASTING BLOOD GLUCOSE (MMOL/L)		2-HOUR BLOOD GLUCOSE (MMOL/L)
CFRD with fasting hyperglycemia	≥ 7.0		N/A
CFRD without fasting hyperglycemia	< 7.0	AND	≥ 11.1
Impaired glucose tolerance	<7.0	AND	7.8-11.1
Normal glucose tolerance	<7.0	AND	<7.8
Indeterminate	<7.0	AND	Mid-OGTT >11.1 or postprandial hyperglycemia by continuous glucose monitoring

CFRD, Cystic fibrosis–related diabetes mellitus; *OGTT,* oral glucose tolerance test.

index (BMI) (20 to 25 kg/m²) in adults. Therefore, instead of adjusting nutrient intake to maintain euglycemia, insulin therapy should be adjusted to permit an appropriate energy intake for the CF patient. As with all patients with CF, 35% to 40% of calories should be derived from fat. Carbohydrate intake should not be excessively restricted, and patients should follow a daily diet consisting of three meals and three snacks.[21]

Approximately 15% of patients with CFRD have fasting hyperglycemia, and this group will require insulin therapy.[21] Studies have documented that the initiation of treatment results in a stabilization of lung function and nutritional status. At the present time, there is no evidence of a defined role for oral hypoglycemic agents. Insulin therapy is tailored on an individual basis because there are no data on specific insulin regimens in patients with CFRD. Most regimens combine a basal bolus schedule with intermittent doses of short-acting insulin at mealtimes. HbA1c measurements should be done to monitor long-term glycemic control. Patients also should be screened annually for the development of microvascular complications with an eye exam and urinalysis for microalbuminuria.

Patients with CFRD without fasting hyperglycemia are at risk of progression to fasting hyperglycemia and should be monitored carefully. Recent data suggest that these patients also may benefit from insulin therapy. A recent study compared the effect of insulin vs. oral hyperglycemic therapy vs. placebo. Patients treated with insulin had an improvement in the rate of BMI loss at 1 year, while no change was seen in the placebo group.[25] Patients treated with the oral hypoglycemic agent had an initial improvement, but this was not sustained at 1 year.

Patients with impaired glucose tolerance should also be closely monitored for progression and the development of clinical symptoms but there is no evidence for the initiation of treatment in this group.

◼ INTESTINAL DISEASE

Pathobiology

CFTR is localized to the apical surface of intestinal crypt and villous cells. At the cellular level, mutations give rise to impaired chloride and bicarbonate secretion by epithelial cells, resulting in decreased fluid content in the intestinal lumen. In the CF intestine, the consequences of impaired fluid and electrolyte transport are demonstrated clinically by meconium ileus (MI) in the infant and distal

intestinal obstruction syndrome in the older child and adult. CF meconium has a lower water content and a high protein concentration that is thought to result in more viscous, adherent meconium on the ileal surface, leading to luminal obstruction.

Meconium ileus occurs in about 15% to 20% of patients and is almost exclusively seen in individuals who carry two severe mutations (class I, II, or III). Concordance studies have shown that the risk of developing MI in affected siblings is increased if the index case has MI; conversely, the risk is decreased if the index case does not have MI. Given that only a subset of patients develops MI, the effect of secondary genetic factors on intestinal disease has been evaluated. Using a CF mouse model, a modifier locus for the intestinal phenotype was identified on murine chromosome 7.[26] Subsequently, a modifier locus for meconium ileus was identified on human chromosome 19q13[27] (CFM1), in a region that is syntenic to the murine locus. However, further studies were unable to replicate these findings in other populations. Nonetheless, it remains possible that CFM1 is a genetic modifier in the French-Canadian population in which it was studied initially. Recently another potential modifier locus has been identified on chromosome 12p13.3. Further study of this region identified that the *ADIPOR2* gene plays a role in the development of MI.[28] This gene encodes one of two adiponectin receptors; however, the mechanism by which this may influence the development of MI remains unclear.

Although CFTR plays a major role in fluid and electrolyte transport in the intestine, more recent studies have suggested that other chloride channels also play a role and may therefore have an impact on disease manifestations.[29,30]

Clinical Manifestations of Intestinal Disease

Intestinal disease in CF can present with various manifestations, and it appears that both genetic factors other than CFTR and environmental factors contribute to a specific phenotype.

CFTR-related Intestinal Diseases
Meconium Ileus
Meconium ileus (MI) may be the earliest clinical manifestation of CF. In patients with this condition, one should have a high index of suspicion for CF. However, patients

without CF may also present with MI, especially premature infants; therefore, further diagnostic testing is required to confirm the diagnosis.[31] MI can be *simple,* in which there is bowel obstruction, or *complicated,* which is characterized by both intrauterine complications and bowel obstruction. Approximately, 50% of patients with MI develop complications that include ileal atresia, necrosis, intestinal volvulus, or meconium peritonitis secondary to bowel perforation.

Clinically, the infant presents with signs and symptoms suggestive of intestinal obstruction, including abdominal distension and bilious vomiting without the passage of meconium. X-rays may show multiple dilated bowel loops with a ground glass appearance, with or without calcification, in the right lower quadrant. Contrast studies with non-ionic contrast material, which should be avoided in patients with suspected perforation, show an unused microcolon and ileal obstruction (Fig. 53-3).

In simple MI, nonsurgical intervention using a hypertonic contrast medium such as Gastrografin[32] will often relieve the obstruction by allowing for dissolution and subsequent passage of the inspissated meconium. Because the hypertonicity of these agents may induce dehydration or fluid and electrolyte disturbances, intravenous fluid and electrolyte therapy is recommended. Failure of enema therapy or complicated MI is an indication for surgical intervention. In some cases, the inspissated material can be manually disimpacted or irrigated and removed. A T-tube ileostomy may be placed for instillation of N-acetylcysteine or Gastrografin. Surgical resection is hardly ever required in cases with simple MI, but

it is common in those with the complicated form. Patients with complicated MI have a higher incidence of surgical complications. A recent evaluation in an animal model suggests that surfactant may be considered as an alternative therapy for the treatment of MI[33] Survival of patients with MI is over 90% and long-term survival is similar to CF patients without this complication.[34]

Distal Intestinal Obstruction Syndrome

Because of the viscous nature of intestinal contents, some CF patients develop symptoms of partial or complete bowel obstruction at an older age. This is a result of inspissated material in the ileum, cecum, and proximal colon. Previously, this condition was termed MI equivalent; however, it has been renamed distal intestinal obstruction syndrome (DIOS). More recently, definitions have been proposed to clearly separate DIOS from constipation, and a further distinction has been suggested between complete and incomplete DIOS.[35] Complete DIOS is defined as (1) complete intestinal obstruction as evidenced by bilious vomiting or fluid levels in the small bowel on abdominal x-ray; (2) a fecal mass in the ileocecum; and (3) abdominal pain, distension, or both. Incomplete DIOS is defined as (1) a short history of abdominal pain or distension or both and (2) fecal mass in the ileocecum but without signs of complete obstruction. Approximately 4% to 5% of patients with CF will develop DIOS, most of whom are PI. DIOS appears to be more common among patients who had MI in infancy. In addition, the incidence of DIOS appears to increase with age, occurring most commonly in adolescents and adults.

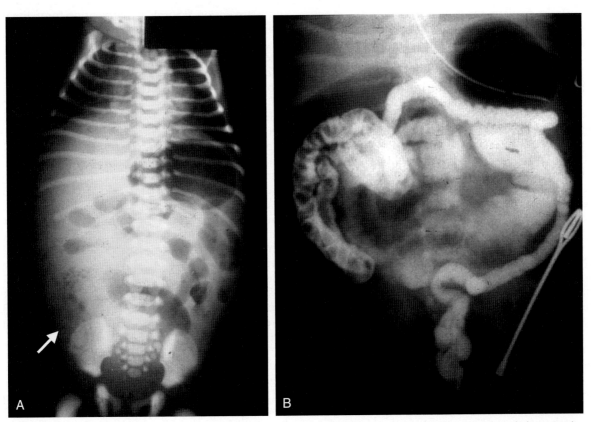

FIGURE 53-3. Meconium ileus. **A,** Abdominal x-ray showing air-fluid levels in the small bowel and granular material in the right lower quadrant with an absence of air in the colon. **B,** Barium enema showing the presence of inspissated material in the small bowel and a microcolon.

Clinically, patients present with abdominal pain that may be associated with a palpable fecal mass in the right lower quadrant. In most cases, there is no associated vomiting. However, on the rare occasion that there is vomiting, complete bowel obstruction should be entertained. It is important to consider other entities that may present with similar features, including appendicitis, appendiceal abscess, intussusception, Crohn's disease, and fibrosing colonopathy. Plain x-rays are helpful if they demonstrate a fecal mass in the right lower quadrant, with or without evidence of obstruction. Sonography or computed tomography may be important to rule out other causes for the patient's symptoms.

A number of options for managing DIOS can be tailored to the severity of symptoms. In milder cases, mineral oil or other laxatives may be of benefit. Patients who fail treatment with mineral oil should be considered for oral or nasogastric lavage using a balanced electrolyte and polyethylene glycol solution.[36] The lavage solution is usually administered at a rate of 750 mL to 1000 mL/hr (20 mL/kg/hr for younger children with a maximum volume of 100 mL/kg) to a total volume of 4 to 6 L. Contraindications to lavage include complete obstruction or signs of peritonitis. Gastrografin enemas, or enemas with other hyperosmolar contrast media, also may be useful, both to provide further imaging and to help relieve the obstruction, particularly if complete bowel obstruction is suspected. Adequate volumes of contrast are required to enter the ileum. Gastrografin should not be used if the patient is dehydrated or has symptoms and signs of peritonitis. N-acetylcysteine, a mucolytic agent, also may be of benefit. Patients with recurrent DIOS can be considered for the placement of a button gastrostomy or gastrostomy button in the appendix to allow for regular irrigation.[37]

Constipation

Patients with CF are much more likely to have constipation than true DIOS. The history is often helpful in distinguishing the two problems because patients with DIOS usually have normal stool frequency and consistency. In contrast, patients with constipation may have abdominal cramping, altered frequency of bowel movements, and difficulty passing stool. Unlike the findings in DIOS, x-rays show diffuse distribution of fecal material throughout the colon. Patients with constipation should be evaluated for evidence of a poor compliance or inadequate response to enzyme therapy. Treatment involves long-term laxative use, such as mineral oil. Severe cases may require colonic lavage with a balanced electrolyte solution.

Rectal Prolapse

Rectal prolapse occurs in approximately one fifth of patients with CF and in about 50% of cases; it may be the presenting feature of CF disease. Most cases present at a young age between 1 month and 3 years of age. Rectal prolapse is more common in PI patients and may be related to the bulky stools. In most cases, it resolves spontaneously after 3 years of age. In patients for whom this is the presenting feature of CF, the institution of enzyme supplementation may result in improvement, but some patients will continue to prolapse for some time. In patients with constipation, treatment of the constipation is also of benefit. Surgical intervention is rarely indicated.

Appendicitis

Appendicitis is often difficult to diagnose in patients with CF. Symptoms may be mild and other diagnoses such as DIOS are often considered first. It is therefore important to have a high index of suspicion for this condition to avoid a delay in diagnosis and an increased risk of complications, which include abscess formation, perforation, and portal vein thrombosis. The incidence of acute appendicitis is reported to be lower in patients with CF than in the general population (1% vs. 7%). Clinical symptoms may be mild or severe, and the milder presentation may be tempered by concurrent antibiotic use. The presence of peritoneal signs or fever should lead to further evaluation either by ultrasound or CT. Data from Toronto covering a 10-year period show that 9/803 patients with CF underwent an appendectomy. In all patients, an initial diagnosis of DIOS had been made. Five out of the 9 patients had surgery within 3 days of symptom onset. In the remaining patients, the diagnosis was delayed and all developed appendiceal abscesses.[38]

Intussusception

Intussusception occurs in patients with CF with an estimated prevalence of 1%. Patients may present with classical colicky abdominal pain, vomiting, and a palpable mass with rectal bleeding.[39] However, the symptoms can be quite nonspecific and may resemble DIOS. Most intussusceptions are ileoileal or ileocolic, and the lead point for the intussusception is thought to be mucoid fecal material that is adherent to the intestinal mucosa. The diagnosis is made by ultrasound, single contrast enema, or air enema. The latter two interventions can be used to reduce the intussusception.[40] Surgical intervention for manual reduction or resection is rarely required.

Secondary Intestinal Complications
Pseudomembranous Colitis

Up to 50% of patients with CF are colonized with *Clostridium difficile*.[41] This high colonization rate may be related to chronic antibiotic use. However, pseudomembranous colitis is considered to be rare, according to case report data.[41–43] Despite its rare occurrence, *C. difficile*–related colitis has been fatal in patients with CF.[43] In our experience, CF patients with *C. difficile* colitis may not present clinically with diarrhea or bloody diarrhea but may present dramatically with toxic megacolon. Other patients may have subtle symptoms that mimic other clinical diagnoses. Stool testing for *C. difficile* toxin should be performed if the clinical diagnosis is unclear. In addition, patients with CF who have undergone lung transplantation, appear to be at higher risk for developing *C. difficile*–associated diarrhea.[44] Treatment should be instituted with metronidazole or oral vancomycin if indicated. Patients with toxic megacolon may need emergency subtotal colectomy as a lifesaving intervention.[43]

Gastroesophageal Reflux Disease

Gastroesophageal reflux is common in both children and adults with CF. The etiology is likely multifactorial and may be related to respiratory disease, physiotherapy, and transient relaxation of the lower esophageal sphincter. Based on pH monitoring, there is an estimated 20%

incidence of gastroesophageal reflux in infants with CF; however, the proportion of patients reporting symptoms is higher.[45] In some patients with CF, postural drainage may exacerbate symptoms, and alteration of the physiotherapy technique may be beneficial. Some reports suggest that gastroesophageal reflux is more frequent in patients with severe lung disease.[46] There have been several case reports of complications, including esophageal stricture and Barrett's esophagus.[47]

The diagnosis is usually established by symptoms such as heartburn, regurgitation, dysphagia, or anorexia. Esophagogastroscopy and esophageal biopsy may be useful if the diagnosis is in doubt, or if the response to therapy is poor. Treatment with H_2-receptor antagonists or proton-pump inhibitors usually results in symptomatic improvement.

Associated Conditions
Inflammatory Bowel Disease (IBD)
Crohn's disease has been reported in patients with cystic fibrosis.[48–50] In one study, the prevalence of Crohn's disease was shown to be eleven times that observed in a non-CF population.[51] Symptoms of inflammatory bowel disease may mimic CF-associated symptoms, such as DIOS. Investigations should be initiated, if despite appropriate management of CF, there is continued abdominal pain, anemia, hypoalbuminemia, and poor weight gain or growth disturbance. Furthermore, any extraintestinal features suggestive of IBD should prompt further investigation.

Gastrointestinal Malignancies
There are reports of an increased risk of gastrointestinal malignancy in patients with CF. This trend is becoming more evident as patient survival increases. A large population-based study has shown an approximately sevenfold increased risk of GI-related malignancy. Cholangiocarcinoma has been reported,[52,53] as well as early onset colon cancer,[54] pancreatic adenocarcinoma,[55] and intestinal adenocarcinoma.[56] Furthermore, patients undergoing transplantation may be at even higher risk because of the use of immunosuppressive medication. It is therefore important to be vigilant for these complications because the symptoms may mimic other CF-associated manifestations.

▰ HEPATOBILIARY DISEASE

Liver disease was described in the earliest reports of cystic fibrosis by Andersen.[20] The presence of bile duct plugging in the livers of CF patients led to the hypothesis that bile duct obstruction by viscous secretions was the trigger for progressive liver damage. Liver disease in CF is characterized by abnormalities of the intrahepatic and extrahepatic biliary tract. There is a spectrum of liver abnormalities ranging from mild elevation of liver enzymes to focal biliary cirrhosis; multilobular biliary cirrhosis with portal hypertension; and rarely, liver failure. Because the development of liver disease is often not accompanied by clinical symptoms, early identification of CF-associated liver disease is difficult.

Pathobiology
CFTR is expressed exclusively at the apical surface of cholangiocytes and the epithelium of the gallbladder but not in hepatocytes. It plays a role in ductal secretion by creating both osmotic and electrogenic driving forces for the passive movement of sodium and water. The apical chloride gradient also is thought to facilitate HCO_3^- secretion via CFTR and the Cl^-/HCO_3^- exchanger. CFTR also may be involved in the regulation of other ion channels in bile duct epithelium.

Histologic evaluation of the liver demonstrates ultrastructural abnormalities of cholangiocytes, suggesting that injury to these cells may be the first step leading to portal fibrosis. Dysfunction of CFTR leads to an alteration in bile composition with increased concentrations of bile acids and other biliary constituents, resulting in inspissations and obstruction of small bile ducts. This in turn may lead to the release of pro-inflammatory cytokines and the activation of hepatic stellate cells.

Almost all patients with CF have minor focal hepatobiliary manifestations of disease. However, only a subset of patients with CF (5%) develops severe liver disease with cirrhosis and portal hypertension (CFLD). CFLD is more common in males and usually manifests early with a median age at diagnosis of about 10 years. In a recent cross-sectional evaluation of a large number of patients with CFLD (N = 260), more than 90% of subjects were diagnosed before 20 years of age.[57] There is no correlation between specific CFTR mutations, but CFLD patients carrying severe mutations on both alleles carry a greater risk of having liver disease.[58] The early age of onset of CFLD and the low prevalence, even in subjects with the same mutations, suggest that additional genetic factors play a role in its pathogenesis. In a recent study, a candidate gene association study of a number of genes identified was used to interrogate for potential genetic modifiers of the hepatic phenotype, including those that were associated with CFLD in previous studies that used very small numbers of patients. Following replication analysis in a replication cohort, the alpha-1-protease inhibitor (SERPINA1) Z allele was the only gene that conferred an increased (five-fold) risk of CFLD.

Clinical Presentation
A wide variety of intrahepatic and extrahepatic manifestations of disease have been described in CF patients. (Table 53-3) Despite the relatively low prevalence of CFLD, it remains the most important nonpulmonary cause of mortality in CF. Identifying patients at risk of severe liver disease is not straightforward because hepatic biochemistry is a poor predictor of CFLD. Given the recent findings that the SERPINA1 gene is a genetic modifier in CFLD, if additional genetic modifiers of CFLD are identified, genotyping has the potential for identifying those at higher risk for severe disease.

A careful physical examination should be done at each clinic visit to monitor for evidence of hepatosplenomegaly. The presence of a firm liver that may be enlarged, or splenomegaly, strongly suggests the presence of significant liver disease. With disease progression, the liver may shrink and no longer be palpable.

TABLE 53-3 HEPATOBILIARY MANIFESTATIONS OF CYSTIC FIBROSIS

	INCIDENCE (%)
Extrahepatic	
Microgallbladder	30
Distended gallbladder	20
Cholelithiasis	1-10
Common bile duct stenosis	Rare
Cholangiocarcinoma	Rare
Sclerosing cholangitis	Rare
Intrahepatic	
Neonatal cholestasis	<2
Steatosis	20-60
Focal biliary cirrhosis	11-70
Multilobular cirrhosis	5-15

TABLE 53-4 ASSESSMENT FOR LIVER DISEASE

HISTORY	PHYSICAL EXAMINATION	LABORATORY INVESTIGATION
Jaundice (including neonatal history)	Liver span, texture	AST, ALT, GGT, ALP
Pruritus	Splenomegaly	Bilirubin (total and direct)
Hematemesis/ melena	Ascites	Albumin
Bruising/bleeding	Chronic liver disease	INR, PTT
Medication use	Nutritional status	CBC, differential, platelets
Alcohol intake Family history of liver disease		Screen for other causes of liver disease if indicated

ALP, Alkaline phosphatase; *ALT,* alanine aminotransferase; *AST,* aspartate aminotransferase; *CBC,* complete blood count; *GGT,* gamma glutamyl transpeptidase; *INR,* international normalized ratio; *PTT,* partial thromboplastin time.

Annual blood tests are often done in patients with CF (Table 53-4), and in our experience, approximately 40% of patients have biochemical abnormalities that generally are one-fold to two-fold higher than the upper reference limits. These values tend to fluctuate with time in each individual. In those with cirrhosis, coagulation status and albumin should be monitored to assess liver synthetic function. There is no association between elevated transaminase values and the severity or progression of liver disease. However, if biochemical tests are more than four-fold above the upper reference limits, it is important to consider biliary tract obstruction with stones or sludge or another cause of liver disease. Other etiologies include viral hepatitis, metabolic liver disease, autoimmune liver disease, drug toxicity, structural abnormalities, and hepatic congestion secondary to right heart failure. It should also be noted, that normal biochemical hepatic tests do not exclude severe CF-associated liver disease.[2,59,60]

Ultrasound is a useful monitoring tool for assessing CF patients suspected of liver disease. It can show the presence of extrahepatic abnormalities (gallbladder abnormalities, cholelithiasis, and bile duct dilatation) and define the size and texture of the liver and spleen. In more advanced liver disease, Doppler studies can document the direction of flow in the portal vein and sometimes detect varices. Sonography also may be useful in documenting hepatic abnormalities in the absence of biochemical abnormalities. Recently, hepatic elastography (Fibroscan) has been evaluated as a screening tool in patients with CFLD.[61] This technique uses sonography to assess the degree of liver stiffness and has been shown to be useful in the identification of fibrosis in other chronic liver diseases. However, further study is required to determine the utility of this test in CFLD.

Liver biopsy is not recommended as a routine procedure for the evaluation of CF-associated liver disease. It may be helpful if a diagnosis of non-CF-related liver disease is suspected, or it may be useful to assess whether there is predominantly steatosis or focal biliary cirrhosis. Because of its focal nature, a normal biopsy does not exclude the presence of CF-associated liver disease. From a technical perspective, if a biopsy is to be performed, it should be done using ultrasound guidance to determine a safe location because the lungs may be hyperinflated. Ultrasound guidance also can be useful to target a specific affected region of the liver. Contraindications to percutaneous liver biopsy include an uncorrectable coagulopathy, thrombocytopenia (<80,000/uL), dilated intrahepatic ducts or hepatic veins, significant ascites, or concerns regarding patient cooperation. If a biopsy is warranted in such patients, a transjugular or laparoscopic approach should be considered.

Disease Manifestations

Extrahepatic Complications
Microgallbladder
Microgallbladder is present in up to 30% of patients with CF of all ages. Twenty percent of patients less than 5 years of age have gallbladder anomalies, and this increases to 40% by 5 and 10 years of age, and to 60% between 15 and 20 years of age. Gallbladder dysfunction also has been reported. The underlying cause of these abnormalities is unclear.

Cholelithiasis
The incidence of gallstones in patients with CF appears to be decreasing. Early studies indicated that between 8% and 12% of children with CF had gallstones. The incidence appears to increase with age, and a separate study showed that among adults, 24% to 33% had gallstones. However, recent studies suggest that prevalence figures may be as low as 1%.

The development of cholelithiasis is likely related to the presence of lithogenic bile secondary to increased losses of bile acids.[62] Patients with pancreatic insufficiency have increased bile acid losses in the stool, which does not appear to occur in PS patients. There are multiple mechanisms by which malabsorption leads to the development of gallstones, including interference with the binding of bile salts to ileal receptors, as well as bile acid precipitation. Defective chloride transport by biliary epithelium also may play a role by altering the viscosity of bile and allowing for stone formation.

Gallstones may be identified as an incidental finding on imaging. The majority of patients remain asymptomatic and no intervention is required. Laboratory investigations may show elevation of gamma glutamyl transpeptidase (GGT), alkaline phosphatase, and bilirubin in those who present with biliary colic. If symptoms are persistent or recurrent, a laparoscopic or open cholecystectomy should be considered. At the time of cholecystectomy, an intraoperative cholangiogram and liver biopsy also should be performed.[63] Ursodeoxycholic acid is not useful in the management of gallstones in CF patients.[64]

Abnormalities of the Biliary Tree

Biliary tree abnormalities, which were first described at autopsy in CF adults, identified focal dilatation and fibrosis of the biliary tree, cholelithiasis, and solitary paraductal mucous cysts. Subsequently, it has become apparent that the intrahepatic and extrahepatic bile ducts can be obstructed with sludge or mucus. Endoscopic retrograde cholangiopancreatography (ERCP) or percutaneous transhepatic cholangiograms (PTC) often reveal images that appear identical to sclerosing cholangitis. Distal common bile duct stenosis was first described in case reports, which identified extrinsic compression of the distal common bile duct by the fibrotic head of the pancreas.[65,66] A prospective study using hepatobiliary scintigraphy and transhepatic cholangiography showed that 96% of patients with CF-related liver disease had evidence of biliary tract obstruction suggestive of bile duct stenosis, whereas this was not seen in any of the patients without CFLD.[60] However, other ERCP studies[67,68] suggest that the prevalence of this complication is less than 10% among patients with CF-associated liver disease.

Patients with common bile duct stenosis or intrinsic common bile duct obstruction with stones or sludge may present with right upper quadrant pain or jaundice.[60] These patients also appear to have more severe steatorrhea. If this condition is suspected, an abdominal ultrasound and hepatobiliary scintigraphy should be performed. If these tests are suggestive of biliary obstruction more detailed imaging by ERCP or PTC should be performed. Such procedures can be diagnostic and therapeutic because sludge or stones can be removed, strictures can be dilated, biliary stents can be placed, or a sphincterotomy can be performed. If the problem is persistent or recurrent, surgical intervention may be required to relieve the obstruction.

Cholangiocarcinoma

Cholangiocarcinoma has been reported rarely in adult patients with cystic fibrosis.[53,69] Although rare, this complication should be considered in adult CF patients who present with obstructive jaundice, abdominal pain, or weight loss.[69]

Intrahepatic Complications

Neonatal Cholestasis

The exact incidence of neonatal cholestasis in CF infants is unclear. Some believe that this complication is rare, while other studies have shown that up to 68% of infants may have evidence of cholestasis[70] An association between the presence of MI and the development of neonatal cholestasis has been suggested,[71] although this has not been confirmed.[59]

Clinically, infants may present with jaundice or acholic stools. Consequently, CF should always be considered in the differential diagnosis of neonatal cholestasis. The clinical picture can sometimes be difficult to distinguish from extrahepatic biliary atresia (EHBA). Hepatobiliary scintigraphy may not distinguish between CF and extrahepatic biliary atresia. Similarly, the histologic findings of bile duct proliferation and plugging may be similar in both conditions. Characteristic inspissated, eosinophilic material within the bile ducts of CF liver biopsies is not a feature of extrahepatic biliary atresia. It is important to differentiate between CF and EHBA because most infants with CF have spontaneous resolution of their cholestasis, while those with biliary atresia need to undergo a Kasai portoenterostomy in a timely fashion. There have been occasional reports of patients with both CF and extrahepatic biliary atresia.

The long-term prognosis of patients with neonatal cholestasis is not well defined, but it appears that most of these patients do well.[72] While the occasional infant with neonatal cholestasis has developed multilobular cirrhosis at an older age, there is no clear evidence of an association between the two entities.

Hepatic Steatosis

Many patients with CF also develop hepatic steatosis; however, it is unclear as to whether this entity progresses to fibrosis. Autopsy studies have documented steatosis in 60% of liver biopsy specimens. Steatosis may be focal or involve the entire liver and may occur in isolation or in association with fibrosis and cirrhosis. While the pathogenesis of CF-associated steatosis is not understood, malnutrition, essential fatty acid deficiency, increased cytokine release, and concomitant medication use have all been implicated as risk factors.

Clinically, patients may or may not have an enlarged, soft liver. Ultrasound may be helpful to determine the presence of steatosis, but magnetic resonance imaging (MRI) may be required. Careful nutritional assessment should be performed, documenting dietary intake and enzyme use. A thorough history also should be performed, specifically regarding alcohol and medication use. Diabetes mellitus also can be associated with steatosis, and OGTT should be performed if clinically indicated.[63]

Focal Biliary Cirrhosis

Focal biliary cirrhosis is the pathognomonic hepatic lesion of CF. It occurs with variable frequency, but the incidence appears to increase with age. One autopsy study indicated that 72% of patients who died after the age of 24 had focal biliary changes.[73] A subset of patients with focal biliary cirrhosis may progress to multilobular biliary cirrhosis. Grossly, the liver may show fibrotic changes, which may be superficial or may create a furrowed appearance.

Histologically, there are varying degrees of focal portal fibrosis and bile duct obstruction with bile duct proliferation, and adjacent areas may appear normal. Periodic acid-Schiff positive material may be seen obstructing the ducts. Most patients with focal biliary cirrhosis are asymptomatic and do not develop any significant hepatic complications. Liver enzymes may be normal or moderately elevated.

Multilobular Biliary Cirrhosis

Multilobular biliary cirrhosis is the most severe form of CF-related liver disease. The time frame for development of this complication is variable, but the median age of diagnosis is 9 years. The primary complications are related to portal hypertension and hypersplenism. Most patients show stable hepatocellular function for many years, even decades.

On examination, a nodular liver may be appreciated, often on palpation of the left lobe. Splenomegaly, which can be massive, is an indication of the development of portal hypertension. Abdominal distension, with dilated abdominal wall veins, spider nevi, and palmar erythema may become evident with progressive liver disease. Evidence of hypersplenism can be seen on laboratory testing with thrombocytopenia and/or anemia or neutropenia. With the development of cirrhosis and portal hypertension, patients may present with secondary complications, including variceal hemorrhage. Ultrasonography may suggest fibrosis and cirrhosis, but it is not very sensitive. However, it can help document the direction of portal venous flow and may reveal the presence of varices, although it is not a reliable diagnostic tool. Deterioration in nutritional status also may be noted as liver function worsens, and fat-soluble vitamin levels may be low and difficult to correct. The development of jaundice, hypoalbuminemia, and coagulopathy are usually late and ominous signs, indicative of hepatic failure.

Management of Liver Disease

Pharmacologic Interventions

No specific therapy has been shown to alter the course of cirrhosis in CF. Ursodeoxycholic acid (UDCA), has been shown to improve bile flow.[74] It also may displace toxic bile acids[75] and improve bicarbonate secretion by cholangiocytes.[75] Treatment does result in improvement of routine biochemical tests,[76,77] but there is no evidence that it alters the long-term outcome. Furthermore, there does not appear to be any beneficial effect on nutritional status or when advanced liver disease is already present.[78] In theory, if there were a method to identify which patients with CF were at risk for severe biliary cirrhosis, it would be possible to assess the long-term prophylactic potential of UDCA. Pharmacokinetic studies indicate that the therapeutic dose of UDCA is 20 mg/kg/day divided twice daily.[76]

Taurine therapy has been recommended for patients with CF-associated liver disease, either alone or in addition to UDCA. CF patients with liver disease may be deficient in taurine secondary to bile acid malabsorption. UDCA also may increase the taurine required for bile acid conjugation.[79] However, a randomized controlled trial did not show any significant effect on liver function

or fecal fat excretion.[77] At present, there is no evidence to support the routine use of this agent.

Nutrition

Patients with CFLD are at higher risk of malnutrition, and special attention should be paid to their nutritional requirements. Energy requirements may be higher as a result of increased intestinal fat losses. Protein intake should not be restricted unless encephalopathy develops. Fat-soluble vitamin levels should be monitored closely and doses increased as necessary. Guidelines for vitamin supplementation in the setting of liver disease are shown in Table 53-5. Following a change in dose, levels should be repeated in 1 to 2 months.[80]

Portal Hypertension and Hypersplenism

Patients with portal hypertension should be counseled regarding the risk for variceal bleeding. Appropriate precautions should be taken to prevent blunt abdominal trauma, which could lead to splenic rupture. Gastrointestinal bleeding also can occur as a result of portal gastropathy or portal colopathy. Patients are also at increased risk of bleeding because of thrombocytopenia related to hypersplenism.

At present, there is insufficient evidence for prophylactic treatment of portal hypertension in patients with CF before the first variceal bleed. Studies in adults with known varices have shown that beta-blockade is useful in the prevention of first variceal hemorrhage.[81] However, there have not been any randomized controlled trials in children. Furthermore, the possibility of bronchospasm as a side effect makes these agents less appealing for patients with CF.

The treatment of variceal bleeding is no different from patients with other causes of portal hypertension. Emergent treatment with packed red blood cells and platelets, as well as fresh frozen plasma to correct the coagulopathy, may be required. Adjuvant treatment with intravenous octreotide and proton pump inhibitors also should be instituted.[82] If the bleeding does not respond to conservative measures interventional endoscopy should be undertaken. Endoscopic intervention with sclerotherapy or variceal band ligation may be required, depending on the age of the patient and the size and nature of the varices. These procedures usually are performed serially until varices are ablated. Annual follow-up should then be done to screen

TABLE 53-5	FAT-SOLUBLE VITAMIN DOSAGE IN PATIENTS WITH LIVER DISEASE	
	DOSE	LAB MONITORING
Vitamin E	15-25 IU/kg/day	Vitamin E levels
Vitamin D	800-1,600 IU/day vitamin D2 or D3	25-hydroxyvitamin D
Vitamin K	2.5 mg/day (infants)	INR
Vitamin A	5,000-10,000 IU/day (adolescents/adults) Optimal dose not clear: 2-4× RDA	Retinol, retinol-binding protein

INR, International normalized ratio; *RDA*, recommended daily allowance.

for recurrence. Some patients may require a transjugular intrahepatic portosystemic shunt or a surgical shunt procedure if bleeding cannot be controlled with endoscopic therapy. Unlike other patients with cirrhosis who have a high 1-year mortality rate, median survival after the first episode of variceal bleeding in CF is 8.4 years.

Liver Failure

Patients with CFLD often remain stable with adequate hepatocellular reserve for years and even decades. However, referral to a transplant centre before the onset of end-stage liver failure is important, given the long waiting times for cadaveric donors. Once hepatocellular dysfunction develops, initial treatment is supportive and includes correction of the coagulopathy; treatment of ascites; and management of hypoglycemia, fluid and electrolytes, and hepatic encephalopathy. Treatment of ascites often results in symptomatic improvement, and maintenance therapy with spironolactone may be useful in managing fluid retention. If hepatic encephalopathy develops, treatment with lactulose should be instituted along with dietary protein restriction.

Five-year survival following liver transplant approaches 90% and is similar to that of patients undergoing liver transplantation for other reasons.[83] There is no evidence that immunosuppressive therapy adversely affects pulmonary disease. In our experience, patients with CFLD are more likely to die of end-stage lung disease (or require a lung transplant) before hepatocellular failure occurs. In fact, CFLD patients with stable hepatocellular function can tolerate sole lung transplantation with no worse prognosis or lung function than CF patients without CFLD.[84]

This affects the timing of transplantation because CF patients listed for lung-liver transplant are likely to face a significantly longer wait for multiple organs to become available. If they were listed for sole lung transplantation, their chances of surviving to transplantation potentially would be much improved. Nonetheless, there are several reports of a few patients who have undergone successful combined transplants of the lung and liver with 1- and 5-year actuarial survival rates of 85% and 64.2%, respectively.

NUTRITION

Pathobiology

Malnutrition has been an important concern in CF since early descriptions of the disease. Both impaired weight gain and linear growth are seen in CF patients; however,

over the past decade, aggressive nutritional support has resulted in improved nutritional status and survival. Nutritional support is an integral part of comprehensive care of individuals with CF, with the target being to maintain normal growth.

The impact of nutrition support on survival is most strikingly shown by a comparative study of two CF clinics (Boston and Toronto). The major difference between these two clinics at the time of the study was the approach to nutrition, with the Toronto clinic having a more aggressive approach to nutritional intervention. The patients attending the Toronto clinic were taller, and the Toronto male patients also were heavier. In this study, Corey and colleagues[85] showed marked differences in patient survival despite no other differences in the patient population and their pulmonary function. This study therefore suggests that improved survival is linked to better nutritional status.

The pathogenesis of malnutrition in CF is complex. It is likely the result of a number of factors that ultimately lead to energy imbalance (Fig. 53-4). Firstly, there are increased energy losses in CF patients with pancreatic insufficiency because of maldigestion/malabsorption. Despite adequate enzyme supplementation, persistent fat and protein maldigestion occurs as a result of multiple factors (see Box 53-2). Furthermore, increased energy losses can occur in the setting of CF-related diabetes and CF-related liver disease. Energy intake also plays a role in the development of the energy imbalance in CF. Oral intake may be limited for multiple reasons, including anorexia secondary to respiratory disease, gastroesophageal reflux, DIOS, and advanced liver disease. There are variable reports regarding energy intake in CF patients, with some studies showing increased intake in those with normal growth compared with those with growth retardation. However, other studies have found nutrient intakes to be close to the normal range. Resting energy expenditure (REE) in CF patients is increased, which correlates with worsening pulmonary status. The precise basis for the increase in REE in patients with CF however is not clear; the relationship to the severity of lung disease suggests that it is due to inflammation or increased work of breathing. While it has been suggested that a component of increased REE is due to the underlying CF defect, not all studies have demonstrated evidence that the primary CF defect results in increased cellular energy expenditure.

 Needs

 Intake

- Increased intestinal losses
  - Pancreatic insufficiency
  - Bile salt metabolism
  - hepatobilary disease
  - GE reflux
- Increased energy expenditure
  - Pulmonary disease
- Increased energy losses
  - CF related diabetes

- Anorexia (due to severe lung disease)
- Cytokine release (due to inflammation)
- Esophagitis
- Iatrogenic fat restriction
- Distal intestinal obstruction syndrome
- Psychosocial issues
  - Feeding disorders
  - Depression

FIGURE 53-4. Model for the development of energy imbalance in cystic fibrosis.

Ultimately, it is the imbalance between energy needs, losses, and intake that results in an energy deficit in patients with CF. Furthermore, over time, with progression of lung disease, there may be an increasing energy deficit and weight loss. Loss of muscle mass in turn impacts respiratory status, resulting in a vicious cycle with progressive nutritional and pulmonary deterioration. It is important to emphasize that this imbalance can be corrected with adequate caloric intake.

Nutritional Management

A multidisciplinary approach to nutritional therapy is imperative. Patients should have anthropometrics done at diagnosis and each visit and should have their diet and enzyme intake reviewed. Patients with CF should follow a high energy diet with supplemental fat. This is done in an attempt to optimize caloric intake and prevent an energy deficit. Because of impaired fat absorption, patients with PI do not appear to be at risk of hyperlipidemia. However, lipid levels should be monitored if the patient has pancreatic sufficiency, if there is a family history of hyperlipidemia, or if the patient has undergone a lung or liver transplant and is on immunosuppressive agents that are known to affect lipid metabolism.

In patients who are losing weight, it is important to review all three components that contribute to energy balance, namely, energy intake, losses, and expenditure. Dietary records can be used to assess intake, and fat absorption can be assessed using 72-hour fat balance studies. If available, indirect calorimetry can be used to estimate energy expenditure. Alternatively, energy requirements can be estimated using the following equation: basal metabolic rate × 1.1 (for malabsorption) × activity factor (1.5 to 1.7) + 200 to 400 kcal/day. Intervention is then targeted appropriately to increase caloric intake and optimize enzyme supplementation.

In some patients, nutritional therapy with nasogastric or gastrostomy feedings is needed to improve nutritional status or maintain energy balance. Several studies have examined the benefit of enteral feeding in patients with CF.[85-87] Short-term supplementation is generally of no long-term benefit. Although there is an initial improvement in nutritional status with supplementation, this effect is lost when supplementation is ceased. However, studies have shown that long-term nocturnal enteral supplementation results in improvements in growth and body composition. Although there is no direct evidence that nutritional intervention results in improved long-term survival, several studies have shown a decrease in the rate of deterioration of pulmonary function following improvement in nutritional status.

Vitamin Supplementation

Fat-soluble vitamin deficiency is common in patients with CF because of pancreatic insufficiency and hepatobiliary dysfunction A prospective study of patients identified by newborn screening indicated that 35% of patients had vitamin A, D, or E deficiency.[80] Follow-up of these patients showed that while vitamin A and D deficiency resolved with supplementation, vitamin E deficiency was still common. Vitamin E deficiency can lead to hemolysis and, if prolonged, to peripheral neuropathy. Vitamin A deficiency can result in night blindness, keratomalacia, pigmentary retinopathy, and even permanent corneal damage. Moreover, it also may result in immune dysfunction and may predispose to infection. Prepubertal children with CF do not appear to have osteopenia, although this has been well documented in adolescents and adults.[88] Osteopenia in patients with CF is likely caused by many factors. Vitamin D supplementation is important to maintain normal bone mineralization because it has been shown that bone demineralization occurs in these patients. Adults with CF are at a high risk of complications secondary to vitamin D deficiency, including the development of fractures. This is of even more importance in patients living in areas with reduced sunlight exposure.

Subclinical vitamin K deficiency, measured by serum PIVKA-II (prothrombin-induced in vitamin K absence) has been shown to be almost universal in PI patients with CF who do not receive supplementation.[89] However, supplementation does not appear to return PIVKA-II levels to normal in all patients.[90] This may be related to inadequate dosing because there is little evidence regarding appropriate dosing of vitamin K. Subclinical vitamin K deficiency may be important in the development of metabolic bone disease in patients with CF because of its role in the carboxylation of the bone matrix protein osteocalcin. Serial monitoring of fat-soluble vitamin levels should be performed in patients with pancreatic insufficiency, and doses of supplements should be adjusted if necessary (Table 53-6).

TABLE 53-6 RECOMMENDED DOSAGE OF FAT-SOLUBLE VITAMINS FOR CF PATIENTS WITH PANCREATIC INSUFFICIENCY

	0-12 MONTHS	1-3 YEARS	3-8 YEARS	>8 YEARS
Vitamin A (IU)	1,500	5,000	5,000-10,000	10,000
Vitamin D (IU)	400	400-800	400-800	400-800
Vitamin E (IU)	40-50	80-150	100-200	200-400
Vitamin K (mg)*	0.3-0.5	0.3-0.5	0.3-0.5	0.3-0.5

*Objectively determined dosing guidelines are not available for vitamin K, and dosage should be adjusted according to coagulation parameters and PIVKA-II (prothrombin-induced in vitamin K absence) levels
Adapted from Borowitz D, Baker RD, Stallings V. Consensus report on nutrition for pediatric patients with cystic fibrosis. *J Pediatr Gastroenterol Nutr.* 2002;35(3):246-259.

SINGLE ORGAN MANIFESTATIONS OF CFTR DYSFUNCTION

Male Infertility

The vast majority of adult men with CF are infertile due to obstructive azoospermia.[91,92] While earlier studies attributed CF male infertility to congenital bilateral agenesis of the vas deferens (CBAVD), more detailed evaluation of the reproductive tract has revealed a variety of obstructive anatomic abnormalities.[93]

It is also recognized that 1% to 2% of otherwise healthy males who are infertile also have obstructive azoospermia. Phenotype evaluation of these men reveal that more than two thirds of them carry at least one *CFTR* gene mutation, and on extensive mutation analysis, up to 50% carry *CFTR* gene alterations on both alleles.[94,95] All have at least one mild class IV or class V mutation on at least one allele. A subset of these patients may fulfill diagnostic criteria for CF. These findings suggest that the male genital tract is exquisitely sensitive to even minor losses of CFTR function, because the majority of healthy men with CBAVD do not appear to have any evidence of clinically significant CF-associated disease in other organs.

CFTR and Pancreatitis

As mentioned previously, patients with CF may present with pancreatitis. However, there is increasing evidence of a role for CFTR in the pathogenesis of recurrent acute and chronic pancreatitis. A number of studies have shown that approximately 40% of patients with recurrent acute or chronic pancreatitis carry *CFTR* mutations on one or both alleles.[12,96] However, this does not necessarily imply that they have CF. Many of the mutations found in this group of patients are rare, and the functional consequences are unknown. Careful clinical evaluation at a specialized CF clinic is required to determine if such patients fulfill the diagnostic criteria for CF.[97] At present, identification of *CFTR* mutations on one or both alleles alone is not sufficient to establish a diagnosis of CF.

CONCLUSION

The discovery of the *CFTR* gene has provided great insight into the pathogenesis of cystic fibrosis. However, it has become clear that it is a complex disease and that there are probably a number of genetic and environmental factors that contribute to the development of disease heterogeneity. With continuing improvement in survival, many other complications such as gastrointestinal malignancies, CFRD, and issues concerning fertility are now becoming evident. Comprehensive care addressing all aspects of CF, in childhood and adulthood, continues to be central to optimizing the health and well-being of these patients.

References

The complete reference list is available online at www.expertconsult.com

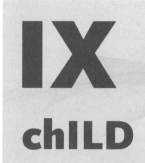

IX
chILD

54 NEW CONCEPTS IN CHILDREN'S INTERSTITIAL LUNG DISEASE AND DIFFUSE LUNG DISEASE

ROBIN R. DETERDING, MD

The field of children's interstitial lung disease (chILD) and diffuse lung disease has undergone tremendous development over the past decade, driven by new genetic discoveries, improved techniques in imaging and lung biopsy, and organized efforts to better define clinical phenotypes.[1] This progress has resulted in recognition of new disorders, the definition of a diffuse lung disease pediatric classification system, and formation of the chILD Foundation (www.childfoundation. us) and chILD Research Network. Chapters in this section have been organized to align with these new developments and to provide the reader with a new frame work to care for these children.

The cliché that "children are not little adults" is a good paradigm to explain the confusing early literature on children with ILD.[1,2] Though adult patients with desquamative interstitial pneumonitis (DIP) were found to have a good prognosis, children with DIP had high mortality.[3,4] DIP in children is now a recognized pathologic phenotype consistent with congenital surfactant mutations that have significant mortality.[5,6] Conversely, children with severe ILD were frequently labeled as cases of idiopathic pulmonary fibrosis (IPF),[7,8] which is synonymous histologically with usual interstitial pneumonia (UIP), a leading cause of mortality in adult ILD.[9] However, on further review the histologic diagnostic criteria for UIP characterized by fibroblast foci have not been seen in infants and young children and have been seen in only one older adolescent.[10] New disorders in young children less than 2 years of age, not previously described in adult patients, also were reported. There were disorders such as neuroendocrine cell hyperplasia of infancy (NEHI),[11,12] pulmonary interstitial glycogenosis (PIG),[13] and alveolar capillary dysplasia with misalignment of pulmonary veins (ACDMPV).[14] The differences in diagnosis highlighted that forcing children with ILD into adult classification systems did not serve their interests and signaled the need to reorganize thinking in this area and create a pediatric-specific diffuse lung disease classification system.[6,9]

NEW CONCEPTS, TERMINOLOGY, AND CLASSIFICATION

The field of diffuse lung disease is large and includes commonly recognized pediatric diseases. For example, diffuse lung diseases such as cystic fibrosis, chronic lung disease of prematurity, and pulmonary infections have recognized clinical presentations and diagnostic testing. However, once these more recognized disorders have been ruled out, some children remain undiagnosed and are labeled with the general term ILD, as if this were a final diagnosis, or listed as having unknown lung disease. The concept of chILD syndrome was created to further define this subset of poorly diagnosed children with diffuse lung disease.[15] chILD syndrome is defined as a child who has three to four of the following findings without a known underlying lung disease to fully explain the clinical condition: (1) respiratory symptoms, coughing, rapid breathing, or exercise intolerance; (2) physical signs such as crackles, adventitial breathing sounds, digital clubbing, or intercostal retractions; (3) a low blood oxygen tension or hypoxemia; and (4) diffuse parenchymal abnormalities on chest imaging.[16] chILD syndrome is a constellation of findings that should signal the clinician that further diagnostic evaluation is indicated to reach a definitive diagnosis. Using this definition, Van Hook reviewed two large data sets of young children with biopsy-proven diffuse lung disease and found this definition to be sensitive to make the diagnosis of chILD syndrome.[17] Furthermore, if a child with a known diagnosis has symptoms out of proportion to the recognized disease, they may still have chILD syndrome and require further evaluation for a secondary diagnosis. This is an important nuance as some chILD diseases occur in conjunction with other known conditions such as congenital heart disease and chronic lung disease of prematurity.[6] (See Chapter 55 for further discussion.)

The designation of a pediatric-specific classification system for diffuse lung disease was essential. Based on the expertise of Dr. Claire Langston and her extensive experience reviewing lung biopsies in children with diffuse lung disease, she proposed a new clinical and pathologic classification system that incorporated features unique to children, especially the category "disorders more common in infancy" (Table 54-1).[5] A landmark study published in 2007 reported on the application of this classification system by a multidisciplinary cooperative that reviewed more than 180 lung biopsies over a 5-year period in children less than 2 years of age at 11 children's hospitals in North America.[6] This review further established that the Langston classification system could realistically be applied and was appropriate for infants and young children. Chapters in the chILD section are organized loosely around these categories and should provide a diagnostic framework for children with diffuse lung disease. Minor refinements of this classification system are evolving, especially related to the category "disorders of the normal host" that deals mostly with environmental insults.

Three large retrospective studies illustrate that children with chILD syndrome are overly represented in infants and younger children.[5,6,8] The application of the Langston classification system also demonstrated that over half the patients reviewed could be classified in the category "disorders more prevalent in infancy."[6] It is less clear if the Langston pediatric classification system is appropriate for older children. Preliminary data from a review of more than 180 lung biopsies in children older than 2 years of age at multiple centers in North America, using the same methodologies as the previous under 2 years of age retrospective review, suggest that the classification system does work well for these older children.[18] Biopsies in older children were rarely classified in the category "disorders more common in infancy"; older children had significantly more biopsies classified in the categories "disorders related to system disease" (see Chapters 57 and 58) and "disorders related to the immunocompromised host" (Section 10).[18] This is further illustrated in the chapters that deal with these categories.

GENERAL DIAGNOSTIC APPROACH

Any newborn or child presenting with diffuse lung disease should have a complete history and physical (H&P) performed.[19] Although most diagnoses are not established with an H&P, specific clues can be uncovered that may be suggestive. Important history questions should include: birth history, a complete family history for use of oxygen or pulmonary deaths in any age family member to suggest genetic disease, previous pulmonary infections to suggest lung injury, family history of autoimmune disease, and a thorough environmental history to evaluate for hypersensitivity pneumonitis.[15,20] A complete physical examination should evaluate evidence of nutritional indices, sinopulmonary disease, chest wall deformities, skin rash, clubbing, and neurologic disorders.

Other noninvasive testing should then be completed to rule out known causes of lung disease such as cystic fibrosis, primary ciliary dyskinesia, aspiration, immunodeficiency,

TABLE 54-1 DIFFUSE PEDIATRIC LUNG DISEASE CLASSIFICATION

CLASSIFICATION CATEGORY	SPECIFIC DISORDERS	COMMON AGE PRESENTATION
Disorders more Common In Infancy		
Developmental Disorders	Alveolar Capillary Dysplasia with Misalignment of Pulmonary Veins (ACDMPV)	Birth
Growth Abnormality Disorders (Alveolar simplification)	Pulmonary hypoplasia, chronic neonatal lung disease associated with chromosomal disorders, associated with congenital heart disease	Birth
Specific Conditions of Unknown Etiology	Neuroendocrine Cell Hyperplasia of Infancy (NEHI), Pulmonary Interstitial Glycogenosis (PIG)	Birth – 1 month (PIG) Infancy – 24 months (NEHI)
Surfactant Dysfunction Mutations	*Surfactant protein B (SFTPB), Surfactant protein C (SFTPC), ATP-binding cassette A3 (ABCA3); NKX2.1* (thyroid transcription factor-1); and histology consistent with a surfactant mutations	Birth (*SFTPB*) Birth – Adulthood (*SFTPC, ABCA3 NKX2.*)
Disorders Related to Systemic Disease	Immune-mediated collagen vascular disease, storage disease, sarcoidosis, and Langerhans cell histiocytosis.	Childhood - Adolescences
Disorders of the Normal Host / Environment Exposure	Infectious or post infectious process, hypersensitivity pneumonitis, aspiration, eosinophilic pneumonia.	Infancy - Adolescences
Disorders of the Immunocompromised Host	Opportunistic infections, transplantation and rejection, therapeutic interventions	Infancy - Adolescences
Disorders Masquerading as Interstitial Lung Disease	Pulmonary hypertension, cardiac dysfunction, veno-occlusive disease, lymphatic disorders	Birth - Adolescences
Unknown	Pulmonary biopsy tissue that cannot be classified	

hypersensitivity pneumonitis, pulmonary infections, or autoimmune disease.[15] An echocardiogram should be completed to rule out masqueraders of lung diseases such as congenital heart disease and pulmonary vein abnormalities and to identify the presence of pulmonary hypertension, which may require more aggressive treatment and may be associated with a worse prognosis.[21,22]

Imaging is often ordered to determine the pattern of diffuse lung disease. Chest radiographs are nonspecific and not helpful for specific diagnoses. Volume-controlled inspiratory and expiratory high resolution computerized topography (HRCT) has been the most helpful way to obtain quality images for children with chILD syndrome and may suggest bronchiolitis obliterans, pulmonary alveolar proteinosis, hypersensitive pneumonitis, and neuroendocrine cell hyperplasia.[23–25] The lowest amount of radiation possible should always be used. In children less than 4 years of age or those neurologically impaired, HRCTs will require sedation for optimal scans and some children may require prone positioning if atelectasis is seen posteriorly.[25] Though HRCT scanning is available at most hospitals around the country, it is highly recommended that scans in newborns, infants, and young children be completed at centers with expertise and protocols developed to optimize HRCTs for children with chILD using the lowest radiation dose possible.

Infant pulmonary function testing is currently used to evaluate children with cystic fibrosis and chronic lung disease of prematurity. Limited but important data exist for children with chILD syndrome. Infant pulmonary functions can be completed reliably in children with NEHI at centers experienced in these techniques and may be helpful because a classic pattern of airway obstruction and gas trapping has been reported in infants and young children.[26] Data suggest that the severity of small airway obstruction may correlate to the prominence of bombesin staining (a marker for neuroendocrine cells) in the lung tissue[27] and that measures of small airway obstruction also may trend toward correlation with lower weight.[26] Some experienced chILD centers currently use infant pulmonary function data in conjunction with other testing (HRCT imaging, bronchoscopy, and clinical findings) to determine the need for a diagnostic lung biopsy in a child with classic findings for NEHI.[15]

Genetic testing has emerged as a significant consideration in the evaluation of children with chILD, especially for inborn errors in surfactant metabolism. Any child with chILD syndrome without a clear etiology, and especially those who present with a family history of infant deaths, prolonged oxygen use, or family members with IPF, should have testing for abnormalities in surfactant metabolism.[28] Clinical testing is available through CLIA-certified laboratories. The type of genetic testing is related to clinical presentation such that those who present immediately in the newborn period with respiratory failure and pulmonary hypertension may be more likely to have *surfactant protein B (SFTPB)* and *ATP-binding cassette A3 (ABCA3)* mutations, while those who present later may be more likely to have *surfactant protein C (SFTPC)* mutations.[29] For those infants who present with respiratory failure and congenital hypothyroidism, investigations for mutations in the *NKX2.1* or *thyroid*

transcription factor-1 (TTF-1) gene should be evaluated because this is a more recently recognized gene that regulates surfactant proteins.[30] As the time to sequence these genes has decreased and test results can become available in weeks and not months, many centers wait for test results before proceeding to lung biopsy if the child's clinical status is stable. If test results are unclear or if testing is negative, a lung biopsy may then be indicated. There is still a great deal to learn about both genetic and environmental modifiers for these genes that contribute to disease. Chapter 56 provides a more detailed discussion of disease associated with abnormal surfactant metabolism. Recently, the forkhead box transcription factor *(FOXF)* gene has been associated with familial cases of children with ACDMPV and testing may be indicated for this fatal disorder.[31] Finally, more genetic mutations are likely to be found in the future in children with chILD, such as NEHI, which has been shown to occur in families,[32] and some surfactant genetic abnormalities may be important modifiers of more common diseases such as respiratory distress of the newborn[33–35] and adult disease such as chronic obstructive pulmonary disease (COPD).[36–38]

Bronchoscopy and bronchoalveolar lavage (BAL) remain important diagnostic tools in the evaluation of children with chILD syndrome. This is particularly true in children who have pulmonary hemorrhage who are immunocompromised to diagnose infection.[39–41] Bronchoscopy also may be important to rule out anatomic abnormalities and to suggest alveolar proteinosis,[42] pulmonary histiocytosis,[43] sarcoidosis,[44] and Niemann-Pick disease.[45] Active research is currently underway to identify diagnostic BAL biomarkers that may aid diagnosis, provide prognostic information, and shed insight into the pathophysiology of chILD syndrome.[46,47] More specific information about the use of bronchoscopy and BAL is addressed in each chapter.

Lung biopsy still remains the gold standard for diagnosis when the less invasive testing is negative or inconclusive.[19,48] The pediatric classification system relies heavily on histologic diagnosis, and the application of this classification system to lung biopsies is likely to provide a classification category or the diagnosis of the chILD syndrome.[6] At this time, only lung biopsies can accurately establish a diagnosis of pulmonary hemorrhage with diffuse capillaritis,[40] pulmonary interstitial glycogenosis,[6,13] alveolar simplification,[6] and ACDMPVs[5]; lung biopsies also will likely provide the final diagnosis for infections in the immunocompromised patient, NEHI, unclear genetic testing for surfactant mutations, hypersensitivity, follicular bronchiolitis, and other lymphocytic disorders in chILD syndrome.[5,6,49,50]

When weighing the decision to pursue a lung biopsy, many factors that relate to severity of illness, progression of disease, and the skill of the surgical and pathology team are considered. Any surgical approach should include the least invasive approach for the patient, and many centers now consider this to be a video-assisted thorocoscopy (VATS).[51] Centers experienced in chILD and VATS have shown that a chest tube may not be needed outside the operating room and may be pulled in the operating room if the procedure was done in a child with a simple lung biopsy that does not require positive pressure postoperatively.[52] This is particularly important in chILD syndrome where splinting and pain may create scenarios that derecruit lung and prolong the hospital course. Selecting and processing the tissue is critical to making the correct diagnosis and this must include selecting the best site for the biopsy, inflating the lung tissue, saving tissue for electron microscopy, and freezing tissue for future evaluation. Choosing a biopsy location is frequently aided by an HRCT and a recent study in NEHI suggests that more than one biopsy site may be required to make this diagnosis.[27] Guidelines for tissue handling have been published by the chILD research pathology working group and should be followed.[53] Because experience reviewing the lung tissue in these rare conditions may be limited, sending the slides for expert review is sometimes indicated.

RESOURCES FOR FAMILIES AND PHYSICIANS

The pursuit of improved care and cures for children with rare diffuse lung disease requires partnerships between families, clinicians, and foundations. Private foundations frequently must provide the advocacy and resources for family education and support, as well as funding to move these fields forward through research. Throughout each chapter we have identified associated foundations to serve as a resource for physicians and families as they struggle to find information and support for children with these diseases.

Suggested Reading

Deterding RR. Infants and young children with children's interstitial lung disease. *Pediatr Asthma Immunol Pulmonol.* 2010;23(1):25–31. www.liebertonline.com/doi/pdfplus/10.1089/ped.2010.0011.

Deutsch GH, Young LR, Deterding RR, et al. Diffuse lung disease in young children: Application of a novel classification scheme. *Am J Respir Crit Care Med.* 2007;176(11):1120–1128.

Dishop MK. Diagnostic pathology of diffuse lung disease in children. *Pediatr Allergy Immunol Pulmonol.* 2010;23(1):69–85. www.liebertonline.com/doi/pdfplus/10.1089/ped.2010.0010.

Guillerman RP. Imaging of childhood interstitial lung disease. *Pediatr Allergy Immunol Pulmonol.* 2010;23(1):43–68. www.liebertonline.com/doi/pdfplus/10.1089/ped.2010.0010.

Langston C, Patterson K, Dishop MK, et al. A protocol for the handling of tissue obtained by operative lung biopsy: recommendations of the chILD pathology co-operative group. *Pediatr Dev Pathol.* 2006;9(3):173–180.

References

The complete reference list is available online at www.expertconsult.com

55 CHILDHOOD INTERSTITIAL LUNG DISEASE DISORDERS MORE PREVALENT IN INFANCY

Lisa R. Young, MD, and Gail H. Deutsch, MD

Although there are areas of overlap, childhood interstitial lung diseases (chILD) frequently include differing entities and histologic patterns than those described in the literature addressing ILD in adults. The areas of distinction are particularly apparent for ILD in infants and young children; therefore, this chapter reviews specific forms of chILD that are more prevalent in infancy.

One factor prompting the need for distinct consideration of chILD in infants is the occurrence of a prominent case clustering in infancy. In a series reported by Fan and colleagues, the median age of onset was 8 months.[1] Two subsequent large multicenter studies also have shown a predominance of cases in young children. In The European Respiratory Society task force survey of chronic ILD, children younger than 2 years of age comprised 31% of cases.[2] Because this study's inclusion criteria required symptom duration of at least 3 months, neonates with a rapidly progressive course would have been excluded, and the proportion of cases in young children is likely underestimated. In ongoing studies using lung biopsy ascertainment, The Children's Interstitial Lung Disease Research Network (ChILDRN) has identified that approximately 50% of lung biopsies for diffuse lung disease are performed in children younger than 2 years of age.[3,4] Furthermore, within the cohort of young children, infants represent a large proportion of cases. Of 187 cases reviewed in the ChILDRN infant study, 30% underwent biopsy by 3 months of age and 52% by 6 months of age.[3]

Furthermore, from a practical clinical standpoint, it is useful to separately consider the differential diagnosis of ILD in an infant versus an older child. Certain entities are either not seen in older children or clearly have symptom onset in infancy. Finally, there is high variability in morbidity and mortality associated with infant ILD disorders, highlighting the critical need for accurate diagnosis. This chapter highlights several disorders that present in infancy or within the first year of life, including alveolar capillary dysplasia with misalignment of pulmonary veins (ACDMPV), pulmonary interstitial glycogenosis (PIG), and neuroendocrine cell hyperplasia of infancy (NEHI). Additionally, although bronchopulmonary dysplasia is discussed in Chapter 23, lung growth abnormalities are included in this chapter because they manifest in infancy, and their clinical and radiographic presentation frequently overlaps with other forms of infant ILD. Disorders of surfactant production and homeostasis, more prevalent in infancy but also present in older children, are discussed separately in Chapter 56.

ALVEOLAR CAPILLARY DYSPLASIA WITH MISALIGNMENT OF PULMONARY VEINS

Clinical Presentation

Alveolar capillary dysplasia with misalignment of pulmonary veins (ACDMPV) is a rare and generally lethal developmental disorder of the lung that typically causes very early postnatal respiratory distress and persistent pulmonary hypertension unresponsive to supportive measures.[5,6] The name of the disorder is largely based on distinctive abnormalities of the pulmonary vasculature and is also variably termed alveolar capillary dysplasia (ACD) and congenital alveolar capillary dysplasia. The majority of affected infants with ACDMPV have additional malformations with cardiac (commonly hypoplastic left heart), gastrointestinal (intestinal malrotation and atresias), and renal abnormalities being the most frequent.[7–9]

Affected infants are usually term or near-term, and the initial presentation is indistinguishable from persistent pulmonary hypertension of the newborn, which typically develops within a few hours after birth; however, delayed onset by weeks or even months has rarely been described.[10–12] Infants with ACDMPV do not respond, or respond only transiently, to extensive therapeutic interventions, including inhaled nitric oxide and extracorporeal membrane oxygenation (ECMO).

Radiographic Findings

Per case reports, the initial chest radiograph is often normal with subsequent development of diffuse hazy opacities. Findings also are dependent on concurrent anomalies.

Histologic Findings

ACDMPV is defined by a characteristic constellation of features, of which anomalously situated pulmonary veins running alongside small pulmonary arteries is essential (Fig. 55- 1A-D). Normally, pulmonary veins are in the interlobular septa, arising from small veins that drain pulmonary lobules. In addition to aberrant placement of the veins in ACDMPV, there is reduction or absence of veins in interlobular septa. Muscularization of small pulmonary arteries and arterioles is often striking, and capillary density in alveolar walls is reduced (Fig. 55- 1E, F). Simplification of the lobular architecture with lymphangiectasia is variably present.

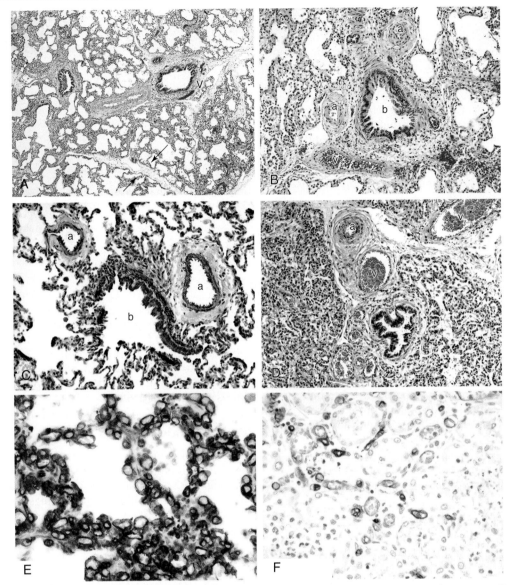

FIGURE 55-1. Alveolar capillary dysplasia with misalignment of pulmonary veins. **A, B,** and **D,** Pulmonary veins (v) that are normally in the interlobular septa (arrows) are malpositioned and accompany pulmonary arteries (a) and bronchioles (b). There is lobular maldevelopment with no alveoli and interstitial widening (**A,** H&E, 40×; **B,** H&E, 100×; **D,** 10×, Movat pentachrome stain). **C,** Normal airway for comparison (Movat pentachrome stain, original magnification 100×). **E** and **F,** The marked decrease in alveolar wall capillaries is highlighted by the endothelial cell marker CD31 (400×).

Epidemiology

Approximately 200 cases of ACDMPV have been reported in the literature to date. Some cases (~10%) are familial, usually with affected siblings.[8,13,14] No sex predilection has been identified.

Etiology and Pathogenesis

Stankiewicz and colleagues recently identified overlapping microdeletions encompassing the *FOX* transcription factor gene cluster on chromosome 16q24.1 in 10 patients with ACDMPV and concurrent anomalies.[15] The same study found de novo heterozygous mutations in the coding sequence of *FOXF1* in 18 additional patients with sporadic ACDMPV. Based on the phenotype of patients with microdeletions versus point mutations, the authors hypothesized that ACDMPV results from haploinsufficiency of *FOXF1*, while the frequently associated cardiac and gastrointestinal anomalies are due to haploinsufficiency for the neighboring *FOXC2* and *FOXL1* genes. *Foxf1* in mice is regulated by hedgehog signaling and encodes a transcription factor involved in murine vasculogenesis, lung, and foregut development.[16,17] Mice with reduced levels of pulmonary *FOXF1* die of pulmonary hemorrhage with deficient alveolarization and vasculogenesis but do not have malposition of pulmonary veins.

It is currently unclear whether the prominent arterial and lobular abnormalities in this disorder are primary or secondary to the vein misalignment. Medial hypertrophy of small pulmonary arteries may result from deficient lobular development with poor gas exchange and resultant hypoxemia.

Diagnostic Approach

The diagnosis of ACDMPV should be considered in infants who present with severe hypoxemia and idiopathic pulmonary hypertension for which no anatomic cause can be established. Although the disorder may be suspected clinically, currently, the diagnosis can only be established by lung biopsy or autopsy; however, genetic testing may play a greater role in the future. On histologic examination, the characteristic constellation of findings may be subtle, particularly when the lung sample is limited with few bronchovascular bundles for evaluation. Patchy distribution rarely has been reported,[18] and multiple lung sections may be required for confirmation.

Differential Diagnosis

The presentation of ACDMPV with persistent pulmonary hypertension of the newborn overlaps with other etiologies of severe idiopathic neonatal lung disease, including genetic abnormalities in surfactant metabolism (particularly *SFTPB* and *ABCA3* mutations), diffuse pulmonary interstitial glycogenosis, and lymphangiectasia. Histologically, ACDMPV should be distinguished from other disorders that demonstrate a similar arrest in lung development, including congenital alveolar dysplasia and advanced pulmonary hypoplasia. Although these disorders also demonstrate lobular simplification and, frequently, vascular changes, they do not have malpositioned veins in the lobules.

Treatment and Prognosis

Standard therapy is supportive and includes mechanical ventilation, inhaled nitric oxide, and ECMO. These therapies prolong life by days to weeks but have not led to long-term survival. The longest reported survival is 101 days.[10] Lung transplantation rarely has been attempted. Given the grim prognosis and recent identification of genetic abnormalities, achieving the correct diagnosis on lung biopsy or seeking autopsy evaluation in suspected cases is recommended.

◼◼◼ LUNG GROWTH ABNORMALITIES PRESENTING AS CHILDHOOD ILD

Clinical Presentation

Although not traditionally considered a classic form of ILD, abnormalities of lung growth represent a prominent proportion of cases that undergo lung biopsy to define the nature of the diffuse lung disease.[3] Furthermore, the features of tachypnea, retractions, hypoxemia, and often diffuse radiographic abnormalities overlap with other forms of chILD.

Although lung growth abnormalities are traditionally considered in the context of prematurity and prenatal onset pulmonary hypoplasia, they also occur in the setting of congenital heart disease, chromosomal abnormalities (particularly trisomy 21), and otherwise normal term infants with early postnatal lung injury (Box 55-1).

BOX 55-1 CONDITIONS ASSOCIATED WITH DEFICIENT LUNG GROWTH

Factors Limiting Prenatal Lung Growth
- Oligohydramnios (e.g., premature rupture of membranes, bladder outlet obstruction)
- Restriction of thoracic volume from space-occupying lesions or thoracic deformities
- Central nervous system neuromuscular disorders and other agents resulting in decreased fetal breathing

Prematurity-related Chronic Lung Disease (Classically Termed *Bronchopulmonary Dysplasia*)

Congenital Heart Disease
- Disorders with poor pulmonary blood flow (e.g., Tetralogy of Fallot)
- Cyanotic heart disease impairing postnatal alveolarization

Chromosomal Abnormalities
- Trisomy 21 with deficient postnatal alveolarization
- Other chromosomal abnormalities

While difficult to objectively define, most infants diagnosed with lung growth abnormalities by lung biopsy were reported to have clinical severity deemed out of proportion to their known comorbidities or circumstances.[3] In other words, typically an additional form of ILD is suspected, leading to the decision to pursue surgical lung biopsy in these patients.

Radiographic Findings

Radiographic findings are variable based on the etiology, age of the infant, and severity of the growth abnormality (Fig. 55-2). Subpleural cysts may be present and are frequently seen in pulmonary hypoplasia associated with Down syndrome.[19]

Histologic Findings

The ratio of lung weight to body weight is the most reliable parameter of lung growth, especially in preterm infants.[20,21] Obviously, this criterion is not useful for lung biopsies; therefore, microscopic criteria are employed. The simplest method is the radial alveolar count, which is the number of alveoli transected by a perpendicular line drawn from the center of a respiratory bronchiole to the nearest septal division or pleural margin. The radial alveolar count in a full-term infant should average five alveolar spaces. Although this method is a valuable tool to evaluate lung complexity and growth, it requires standardized inflation of the lung because the radial alveolar count is substantially reduced in uninflated lungs.[22,23] In prenatal onset pulmonary hypoplasia, there is a reduction of alveolar spaces for gestational age, which is often accompanied by prominence of the bronchovascular structures and a widened interstitium. Lobular simplification with alveolar enlargement, often accentuated in the subpleural space, characterizes deficient alveolarization of postnatal onset (Fig. 55-3A, B). Following the widespread use of surfactant replacement and other therapies, the histology of "new bronchopulmonary dysplasia (BPD)"/chronic neonatal lung disease is characterized by less fibrosis and more uniform inflation

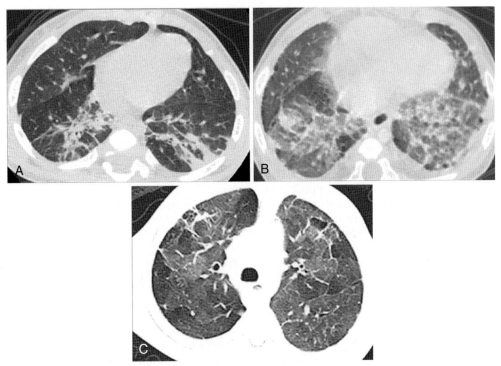

FIGURE 55-2. Imaging appearance of lung growth abnormalities. **A,** Chest HRCT from a 22-month-old child shows thickened irregular scarlike densities bilaterally, most pronounced in the lower lobes. Other findings (not shown) included mild airspace consolidation, mild air-trapping, and peribronchial cuffing without definite bronchiectasis. These findings were thought to be consistent with bronchopulmonary dysplasia in this former 27-week preterm infant with history of prolonged need for ventilatory support. **B,** Chest HRCT from a 5-month-old, former 32-week preterm infant with trisomy 21 and atrioventricular (AV) canal defect shows diffuse irregular opacities, architectural distortion, septal thickening, and numerous small subpleural cysts. **C,** Chest HRCT from a 3-year-old former 30-week preterm infant shows mosaic appearance with irregular ground-glass opacities and geometric areas of hyperlucency that are predominately peripheral in location and consistent with dilated secondary pulmonary lobules. Other findings included scattered small cysts, few dilated bronchi, and air-trapping on the expiratory images (not shown).

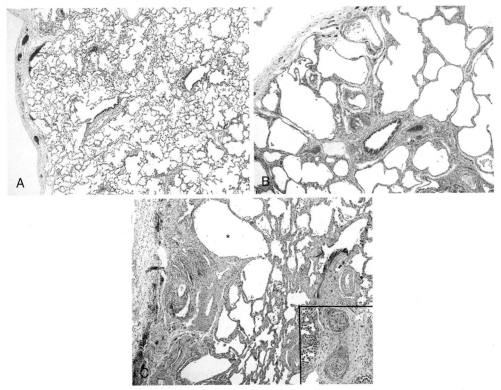

FIGURE 55-3. Abnormal lung growth. Lung biopsy from a 3-year-old former 32-week preterm infant. **(B)** demonstrates the characteristic abnormalities of impaired postnatal alveolarization, with reduced and markedly enlarged airspaces; compare with a normal term infant at the same magnification **(A)**. **(B,** H&E, 40×.) In Down syndrome **(C)** deficient lung growth is often most prominent in the subpleural space with cystic dilatation of alveoli *(asterisk)* and invariably accompanied by prominent hypertensive changes of the pulmonary vasculature *(inset)*.

than the classic form of BPD.[24] Hypertensive changes of the pulmonary arteries are commonly seen and are especially prominent in infants with a severe lung growth abnormality or Down syndrome (Fig. 55-3C).[3,25] As subsequently discussed, PIG is a frequent histologic finding in biopsies demonstrating impaired lung growth.

Epidemiology

The epidemiology of lung growth abnormalities is best considered in the context of associated conditions, including prematurity, oligohydramnios, congenital heart disease, and trisomy 21. Whereas only a small portion of cases undergo lung biopsy, it is important to acknowledge that lung growth abnormalities are recognized as a principal cause of diffuse lung disease in young children that prompts surgical lung biopsy. In the ChILDRN study, lung growth abnormalities represented the primary diagnostic category, with 25% of lung biopsies from children younger than age 2 years of age being classified in this category. Furthermore, this was the leading diagnostic category for 5 of the 11 participating centers.[3]

Etiology and Pathogenesis

Lung growth is a continual process that occurs well into the postnatal period. As such both prenatal and postnatal insults can impact lung maturation and growth. Distension of the lung with liquid and fetal respiratory movements is required for normal fetal lung growth, so any mechanism that interferes with these processes can result in a prenatal growth disorder. Prenatal onset pulmonary hypoplasia ranges from mild to severe, depending on the mechanism of hypoplasia and timing of the insult in relation to the stage of lung development. Early insults that take place before 16 weeks gestation (renal anomalies, congenital diaphragmatic hernia) may interfere with airway branching and acinar development, while later events (premature rupture of membranes) will impact acinar development only. Postnatal onset growth abnormalities impact late alveolarization, which is most evident in the subpleural space. Multiple factors likely lead to deficient alveolarization in infants with congenital heart disease, including hypoxia and abnormal pulmonary blood flow.

Diagnostic Approach

Clinical context provides high pretest probability of this diagnosis, and consideration of the clinical setting may obviate the need for lung biopsy in many cases. Infant pulmonary function tests may suggest pulmonary hypoplasia but do not exclude concurrent processes. For infants with respiratory morbidity out of proportion to their clinical context, lung biopsy may still be required for diagnosis and to exclude alternative diagnoses. Proper tissue handling is essential, and expert pathologic review may be required.[26]

Differential Diagnosis

The clinical differential diagnosis is broad and may include other abnormalities in lung development such as lymphangiectasia, ACDMPV, pulmonary interstitial glycogenosis, and genetic disorders of surfactant production and metabolism. From the pathology perspective, the presence of alveolar enlargement and simplification is often misinterpreted as emphysematous change or a consequence of lung remodeling after injury. However, unlike these processes, there is no evidence of a destructive process in a lung growth abnormality such as inflammation, type II cell hyperplasia, or significant fibrosis. Nonetheless, without proper orientation and handling, alveolar simplification may be overlooked or difficult to recognize. Indeed, in the ChILDRN study, the majority of lung growth abnormality cases were not suspected clinically or recognized histologically at the initial institution, especially when occurring outside the setting of prematurity.[3]

Treatment and Prognosis

Lung growth and maturation are key determinants of postnatal outcome, especially in premature infants or those with chromosomal or congenital abnormalities. Management is focused largely on supportive care and underlying conditions, and the latter largely drives prognosis. Recognition of this category of diagnosis may have important clinical implications, particularly because corticosteroids may not be indicated in this setting. Lung growth abnormalities are associated with considerable morbidity and mortality when compared with other causes of diffuse lung disease. In the ChILDRN study, mortality was 34% for lung growth abnormality cases, a proportion similar to the entire study cohort. However, among lung growth abnormality cases, prematurity and pulmonary hypertension were independent clinical predictors of mortality. On lung biopsy, severe lung growth abnormality, as judged by degree of alveolar enlargement and simplification, was associated with a high mortality (80%).[3]

◼ PULMONARY INTERSTITIAL GLYCOGENOSIS

Clinical Presentation

Pulmonary interstitial glycogenosis (PIG) is a form of chILD unique to neonates and young infants.[3,27] Most infants with PIG are symptomatic in the first days to weeks of life, which may follow an initial period of well-being after birth. There is clinical and pathologic evidence to support that PIG is often a self-limited disorder, and the diagnosis is typically made by 6 months of age.[3,27,28] The clinical presentation can be highly variable, ranging from indolent tachypnea and hypoxia to neonatal acute respiratory failure and pulmonary hypertension. PIG can occur in either term or preterm infants and may be an isolated disorder or a component of other congenital conditions. PIG commonly occurs in the setting of lung growth abnormalities (see previous discussion), such as chronic neonatal lung disease of prematurity and pulmonary hypoplasia.[3] It also has been observed in infants with congenital heart disease; pulmonary hypertension; meconium aspiration; and rarely, other developmental anomalies.

Radiographic Findings

Case series have reported that chest radiographs have diffuse infiltrates or hazy opacities, but no common high-resolution computed tomography (CT) scan pattern has been identified (Fig. 55-4A-D).[3,27,29–32]

Histologic Findings

Also known as cellular interstitial pneumonitis and histiocytoid pneumonia,[33] the term *pulmonary interstitial glycogenosis* was coined by Canakis and colleagues, based on the histologic finding of increased glycogen-laden mesenchymal cells in the alveolar interstitium. Lung biopsy shows a patchy or diffuse expansion of the alveolar walls by bland spindle-shaped cells with pale or bubbly cytoplasm (Fig. 55-4E, F). Patchy distribution is common when there is a concomitant lung growth abnormality.[3] Associated inflammation or fibrosis in the interstitium is absent. The cells are strongly immunopositive for vimentin, a mesenchymal marker, and periodic acid Schiff (PAS) stain may demonstrate PAS-positive diastase labile material within the cytoplasm of the cells (Fig. 55-4G, H). Because the preservation of glycogen is influenced by the use of aqueous fixatives (i.e., 10% formalin), the presence of PAS positivity may be difficult to demonstrate on routine sections. Electron microscopy is considered the best approach to reveal the accumulation of monoparticulate glycogen in these interstitial cells; treating ultrathin sections with tannic acid enhances visualization of glycogen.[27]

Epidemiology

The initial report of PIG included seven neonates, five of whom presented in the first 24 hours of life.[27] In the ChILDRN study,[3] six cases (3.2% of infant lung biopsies) were identified in which PIG was the only significant histologic finding. All but one case presented with hypoxia at birth, and the mean age at biopsy was 1.3 ± 0.4 months. Although PIG is a rare disorder, recent experience indicates that PIG occurs more frequently and in a broader clinical spectrum than previously recognized. Expert pathologic review of lung biopsies from the multi-institutional ChILDRN study found that patchy PIG was present in over 40% of cases classified as having a lung growth abnormality. This included not only chronic neonatal lung disease due to prematurity, but also pulmonary hypoplasia and lung growth abnormalities in the setting of trisomy 21 and congenital heart disease. Patchy PIG also was present in 22% of cases classified as vascular disorders masquerading as ILD. Published and personal experience indicates that it is very unusual to observe PIG in lung biopsies of patients older than 6 months of age.

Etiology and Pathogenesis

The etiology of this condition is poorly understood. Some authors propose that accumulation of immature mesenchymal cells within the interstitium may represent a selective delay or aberration in the maturation of pulmonary mesenchymal cells.[27] Others have suggested that PIG might reflect a nonspecific feature of several conditions that transiently alter lung growth and development in the neonatal period.[34] These mesenchymal cells have been demonstrated to have transient proliferative capacity,[28] similar to interstitial fibroblasts in animal models of lung development and injury.[35–37] Within these models, coordinated control of fibroblast proliferation and apoptosis is necessary for septation of the distal airspaces during alveolarization.[38]

Diagnostic Approach

Currently, lung biopsy is the only way to diagnose PIG. The diagnosis may be suspected in the context of a neonate with respiratory compromise, particularly when the severity is disproportionate to the degree of coexisting conditions, including prematurity and congenital heart disease.

Differential Diagnosis

Disorders to be considered in the clinical differential diagnosis include sepsis, congenital heart disease, lung developmental disorders (e.g., alveolar capillary dysplasia with misalignment of the pulmonary veins), pulmonary hypoplasia, pulmonary vascular disease, lymphangiectasia, and genetic disorders of surfactant production and metabolism. Primary ciliary dyskinesia (PCD) also could mimic milder cases of PIG because of the frequent occurrence of neonatal tachypnea in PCD.[39] From the perspective of the pathologist, careful attention is required to identify potential concurrent histologic findings, such as lung growth abnormalities or structural alterations of the pulmonary vasculature.

Treatment and Prognosis

The natural history is unknown, but mortality is overall rare and largely related to complications of prematurity or pulmonary hypoplasia.[3,27,32] Patients may remain symptomatic for months, and supportive care is a mainstay of therapy. Most children will require supplemental oxygen, and some will require aggressive support, including mechanical ventilation and therapy for pulmonary hypertension. When present, comorbidities such as congenital heart disease or complications of prematurity are often the focus of management. In the original report by Canakis and colleagues, six of the seven infants improved over time, with mortality occurring in one infant born at 25 weeks gestation.[27] Similarly, in the ChILDRN study, no mortality occurred among the six cases of diffuse PIG,[3] and clinical improvement also has been reported in the small number of published case reports.[28,29,31] However, high mortality has occurred when significant pulmonary conditions are present along with PIG, particularly lung growth abnormalities.[28,32] High-dose pulse corticosteroids have been reported to have benefit in case reports and case series,[27–30] but no controlled studies have been

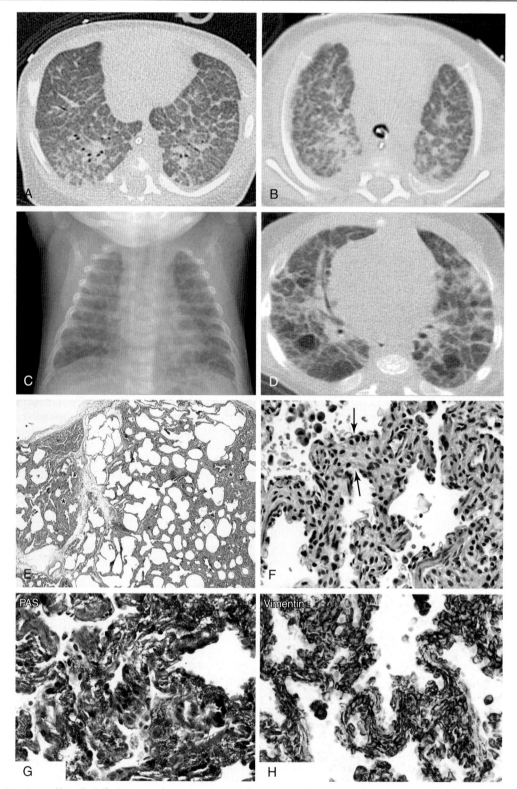

FIGURE 55-4. Imaging and histologic findings in pulmonary interstitial glycogenosis. Chest HRCT (**A** and **B**) from a 2-week-old infant shows diffuse interstitial markings and interlobular septal thickening present bilaterally throughout all lung zones. This infant with a 38-week estimated gestational age had no respiratory difficulties at birth, but required supplemental oxygen in the first days of life, intubation on day of life 5, and nitric oxide for severe pulmonary hypertension. Chest radiographic (**C**) and HRCT (**D**) images from a 5-month-old, former 34-week preterm infant show diffuse coarse interstitial and parenchymal abnormalities including architectural distortion and cystic change. This infant had persistent tachypnea and hypoxemia without need for mechanical ventilation; lung biopsy (**E**) (H&E, 40×) performed at 5 months of age showed patchy pulmonary interstitial glycogenosis *(asterisks)* and moderate deficient alveolarization, consistent with a lung growth abnormality. **F,** On higher power (H&E, 200×), the bland spindled cells of pulmonary interstitial glycogenosis are seen to widen the alveolar septa *(arrows)*. These cells contain glycogen (**G**) (periodic acid Schiff stain, 200×) and show strong immunoreactivity with vimentin (**H**) (200×).

performed, and there is little evidence to guide therapeutic recommendations. It has been suggested that consideration for use of corticosteroids should be assessed in the context of clinical severity and the potential detrimental impact on postnatal alveolarization and neurodevelopment in this patient population.[32]

NEUROENDOCRINE CELL HYPERPLASIA OF INFANCY

Clinical Presentation

Neuroendocrine cell hyperplasia of infancy (NEHI) is a rare disorder previously termed *persistent tachypnea of infancy*.[40] Reported in 2005 by Deterding and coworkers, NEHI occurs in otherwise healthy term or near-term infants who present with tachypnea and retractions, generally of insidious onset, in the first few months to one year of life. Crackles are prominent and hypoxemia is common, while wheezing is rare.[41] Many patients develop failure to thrive, and upper respiratory infections may lead to exacerbation of symptoms. Infant pulmonary function testing in NEHI patients has been reported to reveal a mixed physiologic pattern, including profound air-trapping and proportionate reductions in the forced expiratory volume in 0.5 seconds (FEV0.5) and forced vital capacity (FVC), with particularly reduced FEF75 and FEF85 and markedly elevated functional residual capacity (FRC), residual volume (RV), and RV/TLC.[42,43] Pulmonary function testing has not been systematically studied in older children, although personal experience suggests that this physiologic pattern can persist in at least some cases.

Radiographic Findings

Chest radiographs may be normal or may reveal hyperinflation.[41] High-resolution CT (HRCT) findings are distinctive with geographic ground-glass opacities centrally and in the right middle lobe and lingula (Fig. 55-5A-C). Air-trapping is often demonstrated when expiratory images are performed. Brody and colleagues evaluated chest HRCT scans from 23 children with biopsy-proven NEHI and 6 children with other forms of ILD. Although HRCT specificity for the diagnosis of NEHI was 100% in this study, when two expert radiologists reviewed the CTs, the sensitivity of HRCT was incomplete, as readers did not suggest NEHI in up to 22% of the cases.[44]

Histologic Findings

In contrast to the clinical severity of the disorder, lung biopsies in NEHI often show minimal to no pathologic alterations and may be initially interpreted as normal (Fig. 55-5D). Patchy mild inflammation or fibrosis (bronchiolitis) may be present, especially following a viral

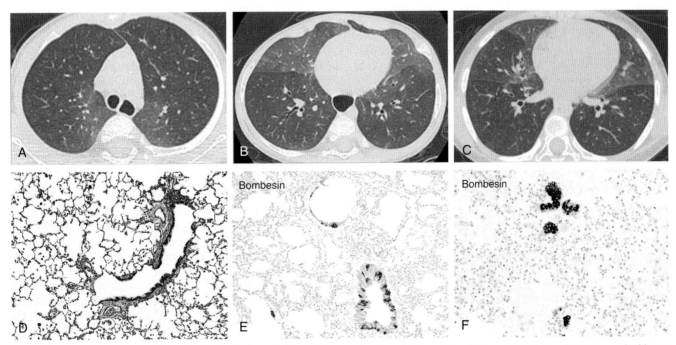

FIGURE 55-5. Characteristic radiographic and pathologic findings in Neuroendocrine cell Hyperplasia of Infancy (NEHI). **A** and **B,** A 13-month-old term infant presented at age 6 months with chronic tachypnea, retractions, and hypoxemia, but had chronic indolent respiratory symptoms since the first month of life and poor weight gain since 5 months of age. HRCT images obtained at total lung capacity under general anesthesia show well defined regions of apparent ground glass opacity in the medial portions of the upper lobes **(A)** and in the right middle lobe and lingula **(B)**. Diffuse air-trapping was seen on expiratory images (not shown). **C,** HRCT shows a similar pattern of apparent regional ground glass opacity in a 3-year-old with chronic tachypnea, retractions, and crackles since infancy being treated for recurrent pneumonia and refractory asthma. No additional radiographic abnormalities were identified. **D.** Lung biopsies from NEHI patients typically show essentially normal histology. Mild non-specific changes that may be present in the biopsy include mild periairway lymphocytic aggregates and increased alveolar macrophages (H&E, 100×). **E,** Increased neuroendocrine cells within bronchioles is best visualized by bombesin immunostaining (100×). **F,** Neuroepithelial bodies (NEBs) around alveolar ducts are frequently prominent (200×).

infection, but these findings are not sufficient to support an etiology for the patient's significant symptomatology. Pathologic diagnosis of NEHI rests on finding an increased proportion of neuroendocrine cells within distal airways, best seen by bombesin and serotonin immunohistochemistry.[41] Neuron-specific enolase, calcitonin, synaptophysin, and chromogranin have been shown to be less reliable in demonstrating this increase in neuroendocrine cell numbers. Immunohistochemical assessment of this disorder requires an adequate biopsy, with at least 10 to 15 airways for evaluation. Because wide intrasubject and intersubject variability in neuroendocrine cell number that does not relate to imaging appearance of the region biopsied has been reported, more than one biopsy site is recommended.[43] Currently, formal criteria for defining neuroendocrine cell excess in NEHI are lacking, and outside the setting of a pathologist experienced with the disorder, morphometric quantification of bombesin staining may be required. In general, bombesin immunopositive cells in NEHI are prominent in the distal respiratory bronchioles and as clusters (neuroepithelial bodies) in the alveolar ducts (Fig. 55-5E, F).[43] Two individual airways with more than 10% bombesin-immunopositive areas or cell numbers of the airway epithelium also suggest the diagnosis. A minor degree of airway injury does not alter pathologic confirmation of the diagnosis.[43]

Epidemiology

The incidence and prevalence of NEHI are unknown. The original series of 15 cases had a slight male predominance, which was not observed in a subsequent series.[41,43] In the ChILDRN study, NEHI cases represented 10% of all lung biopsies from children younger than 2 years of age.[3] A recent study from a large referral center identified 19 cases (14%) from among 138 lung biopsy cases accrued over a 10-year period.[43] The number of cases suspected solely on the basis of clinical and imaging criteria is unknown but represents a growing proportion of cases as the diagnostic approach has evolved over recent years.

Etiology and Pathogenesis

The etiology of NEHI is unknown, but familial cases with affected siblings have been identified, suggesting there may be a genetic predisposition.[45] It is currently unclear whether pulmonary neuroendocrine cells are simply a marker of NEHI or are directly involved in the pathogenesis of the disorder. A recent study correlating neuroendocrine cell prominence and the severity of small airway obstruction on infant pulmonary function tests (iPFT) in NEHI patients suggests a potential causal role.[43] Based on the role of pulmonary neuroendocrine cells and bombesin in oxygen sensing and airway and arterial tone, it has been hypothesized that neuroendocrine cells may lead to ventilation/perfusion mismatch within the lung.[41] The physiologic abnormalities observed on iPFT in NEHI suggest that the disorder is not fully explained on this basis.[42,43] The absence of active neuroendocrine cell proliferation in lung biopsies

and lack of correlation with airway injury suggest that neuroendocrine cell prominence in NEHI is not due to injurious stimuli.[43]

Diagnostic Approach

The initial diagnostic approach should be to exclude more common causes of the clinical symptoms such as infection, cystic fibrosis, and congenital heart disease. Lung biopsy (via video assisted thorascopic surgery [VATS]) is currently considered the definitive diagnostic approach. Pathologic interpretation should be performed by a pediatric pathologist experienced in this diagnosis and placed in context with the clinical and radiographic findings. Increasing clinical experience with the disorder and the characteristic constellation of patient findings, radiographic appearance, and iPFT data have led many clinicians to confidently suggest the diagnosis without a lung biopsy. The presence of an increased number of neuroendocrine cells on lung biopsy is not sufficient for the diagnosis because neuroendocrine cell prominence is associated with various other pulmonary conditions, including BPD, sudden infant death syndrome, pulmonary hypertension, and cystic fibrosis.[46–51] Nonetheless, recent data indicate that neuroendocrine cells are more prominent in NEHI than in other lung disorders associated with increased numbers of neuroendocrine cells.[43]

Differential Diagnosis

Disorders to be considered in the clinical differential include acute or chronic infection, asthma, and airway injury, including bronchiolitis obliterans. In addition, other infant lung disorders such as pulmonary hypoplasia, pulmonary interstitial glycogenosis, and genetic disorders of surfactant production and metabolism should be considered. As discussed previously, neuroendocrine cell prominence on lung biopsy should be correlated with other potential pathologic findings, and other entities associated with increased neuroendocrine cells should be excluded.

Treatment and Prognosis

There is no known definitive therapy for NEHI, and management largely consists of general supportive and preventative care. Most children will require supplemental oxygen, and many will require nutritional supplementation. Because corticosteroids are not helpful in most cases,[41] establishing the diagnosis of NEHI helps avoid the complications of long-term steroids. Although long-term outcomes are not well-established for this recently recognized disorder, a diagnosis of NEHI brings a cautious but welcomed prognosis relative to other forms of chILD. No deaths have been reported, and no patients have required lung transplantation.[3,41,43] The clinical course is prolonged, but most children demonstrate gradual improvement. The need for supplemental oxygen is variable and may be many years in duration.[41,43] Patients may remain symptomatic with respiratory infections or exercise intolerance.[45,52]

TABLE 55-1 FORMS OF CHILDHOOD ILD 'MORE PREVALENT IN INFANCY'

DISORDER*	ALVEOLAR CAPILLARY DYSPLASIA WITH MISALIGNMENT OF THE PULMONARY VEINS	LUNG GROWTH ABNORMALITIES	NEUROENDOCRINE CELL HYPERPLASIA OF INFANCY (NEHI)	PULMONARY INTERSTITIAL GLYCOGENOSIS (PIG)
Common age of presentation	Birth	Birth	Infancy with most in first year of life Rare at birth	Early neonatal
Hereditary basis	Yes *FOXF1*; autosomal dominant	Uncertain Frequent in association with chromosomal abnormalities	Suspected Not established	Unknown
Associated features	Other congenital anomalies PHTN	Prematurity Congenital heart disease Trisomy 21 PHTN	None known	Prematurity Congenital heart disease PHTN
Common imaging pattern	Uncertain	Variable May include architectural distortion, cystic change	CXR: Hyperinflation, normal, or mild perihilar infiltrates HRCT: GGO in RML and lingula Air-trapping	Variable Frequent diffuse interstitial infiltrates
Diagnostic approach	Lung biopsy; emergence of genetic testing	Clinical context, lung biopsy	Lung biopsy definitive; HRCT and iPFT may strongly suggest	Lung biopsy
Outcome	Fatal without lung transplant†	Variable	Gradual improvement (years)	Variable

CXR, Chest x-ray; *FOXF1*, Forkhead box F1 gene; *GGO*, ground-glass opacities; *HRCT*, high-resolution computed tomography; *iPFT*, infant pulmonary function test; *PHTN*, Pulmonary hypertension; *RML*, right middle lobe.
*Genetic disorders of surfactant production and metabolism also are more prevalent in infants and young children. (See Chapter 56.)
†Variable penetrance and phenotype data are emerging.

SUMMARY

Forms of chILD most prevalent in infancy include entities with overlapping clinical features but often distinct imaging and histologic findings (Table 55-1). Recognition of these disorders informs diagnostic approach, enables timely diagnosis, and has implications for management and prognosis.

Suggested Reading

Brody AS, Guillerman RP, Hay TC, et al. Neuroendocrine cell hyperplasia of infancy: Diagnosis with high-resolution CT. *AJR Am J Roentgenol.* 2010;194(1):238–244.

Canakis AM, Cutz E, Manson D, et al. Pulmonary interstitial glycogenosis: a new variant of neonatal interstitial lung disease. *Am J Respir Crit Care Med.* 2002;165(11):1557–1565.

Deterding RR, Pye C, Fan LL, et al. Persistent tachypnea of infancy is associated with neuroendocrine cell hyperplasia. *Pediatr Pulmonol.* 2005;40(2):157–165.

Deutsch GH, Young LR. Pulmonary interstitial glycogenosis: words of caution. *Pediatr Radiol.* 2010;40(9):1471–1475.

Deutsch GH, Young LR, Deterding RR, et al. Diffuse lung disease in young children: application of a novel classification scheme. *Am J Respir Crit Care Med.* 2007;176(11):1120–1128.

Langston C, Patterson K, Dishop MK, et al. A protocol for the handling of tissue obtained by operative lung biopsy: recommendations of the chILD pathology co-operative group. *Pediatr Dev Pathol.* 2006;9(3):173–180.

Stanewicz P, Sen P, Bhatt SS, et al. Genomic and genic deletions of the FOX gene cluster on 16q24.1 and inactivating mutations of FOXF1 cause alveolar capillary dysplasia and other malformations. *Am J Hum Genet.* 2009;84(6):780–791.

Young LR, Brody AS, Inge TH, et al. Neuroendocrine cell distribution and frequency distinguish neuroendocrine cell hyperplasia of infancy from other pulmonary disorders. *Chest.* 2011;139(5):1060–1071.

References

The complete reference list is available online at www.expertconsult.com

56 LUNG DISEASES ASSOCIATED WITH DISRUPTION OF PULMONARY SURFACTANT HOMEOSTASIS

LAWRENCE M. NOGEE, MD, AND BRUCE C. TRAPNELL, MD, MS

Pulmonary surfactant is a mixture of specific lipids and proteins that reduces surface tension at the air-liquid-tissue interface, thereby preventing alveolar collapse at end expiration. This critical function requires tight regulation of alveolar surfactant composition and quantity, that is, surfactant homeostasis, which is achieved through coordinated expression of multiple genes, resulting in balanced production and clearance of surfactant.

The most common lung disorder associated with disruption of surfactant homeostasis is the respiratory distress syndrome (RDS), which occurs mainly in premature infants. Surfactant deficiency is the primary pathogenic driver and results from insufficient production by alveolar epithelial cells secondary to immaturity. Surfactant augmentation is now standard therapy for RDS and has markedly reduced the associated morbidity and mortality. Another disorder of surfactant homeostasis is pulmonary alveolar proteinosis (PAP), a syndrome (not a disease) characterized by the slow, progressive accumulation of surfactant lipids and proteins within alveoli, resulting in displacement of air and impairment of oxygen uptake. The most common cause of the PAP syndrome is an autoimmune disease mediated by neutralizing autoantibodies against the cytokine granulocyte-macrophage colony-stimulating factor (GM-CSF). High levels of GM-CSF autoantibodies block GM-CSF stimulation of alveolar macrophages, which is critical for enabling surfactant catabolism in these cells. While autoimmune PAP occurs most commonly in adults and adolescents, it has been seen in children as young as 8 years of age.

Although the causal role of surfactant deficiency in RDS was established over 50 years ago, in the past 15 to 20 years, lung disorders caused by single-gene mutations that disrupt the production of normal surfactant have been identified. Similarly, single gene disorders that impair GM-CSF–dependent surfactant clearance by alveolar macrophages also have been identified. These genetic disorders of surfactant homeostasis can be usefully categorized as disorders of surfactant production or surfactant clearance.

The clinical presentation and features, pathogenesis, natural history, therapeutic responses, and prognosis of individual disorders of surfactant homeostasis vary widely. While RDS usually occurs in premature infants and can be treated by surfactant replacement, infants with genetic disorders of surfactant production are usually full-term and can have a more severe course that is often fatal. Secondary metabolic disturbances in surfactant-producing epithelial cells can injure them, exacerbating the abnormality in surfactant production. Milder forms of surfactant production disorders comprise the molecular basis for some interstitial lung diseases (ILDs) observed in older children and adults. In contrast, disorders of surfactant clearance are associated with the gradual accumulation of surfactant in alveoli and terminal airspaces, resulting in slowly progressive dyspnea of insidious onset that can be treated by whole lung lavage. Although effective in most cases, this therapy is highly invasive and requires general anesthesia, independent intubation of each lung, and mechanical ventilation of one lung concurrent with repeated filling and draining of the other lung to physically remove surfactant. In some patients this is performed every 2 months. While rare, disorders of surfactant homeostasis are associated with significant morbidity and mortality. A heightened awareness can improve early recognition and accurate diagnosis and facilitate counseling about prognosis and the risk of disease recurrence in future pregnancies. Understanding the pathophysiology of these disorders provides insights into normal surfactant metabolism and how genetic mechanisms contribute to more common diseases such as neonatal RDS.

This chapter summarizes current knowledge concerning the clinical and laboratory findings associated with lung disorders involving surfactant production and catabolism that cause acute and chronic lung disease. It is highly likely that advances in the understanding of lung development and surfactant metabolism combined with technological advances and data derived from the human genome project will allow for identification of additional genetic mechanisms for neonatal and pediatric lung disease.

▰ OVERVIEW OF SURFACTANT COMPOSITION AND METABOLISM

Pulmonary surfactant is a complex mixture of phospholipids, neutral lipids, and specific proteins; it is produced by the alveolar type II epithelial cell (AEC2), stored in intracellular organelles known as lamellar bodies, and secreted by exocytosis into the alveolar lumen. The major lipid present in pulmonary surfactant is phosphatidylcholine (PC), a large fraction of which contains two palmitic acid side chains that are fully saturated (dipalmitoyl or disaturated phosphatidylcholine, DPPC or DSPC); its presence is critical for surfactant to function in reducing surface tension. A member of the ATP-binding cassette family of membrane transporters, ABCA3 is located on the limiting membrane of lamellar bodies and has an important role in the transport of phospholipids into lamellar bodies during the biosynthesis of surfactant.

The effective lowering of surface tension also requires the presence of one or both of two extremely hydrophobic surfactant proteins (SP), SP-B and SP-C. Addition of either SP-B or SP-C to isolated surfactant lipids yields a surfactant preparation that lowers surface tension *in vitro* and effectively treats surfactant deficiency in animal models.[1-3] Both SP-B and SP-C are present in varying amounts in the mammalian derived exogenous surfactant preparations used to treat infants with RDS. Pulmonary surfactant also contains two larger glycoproteins, SP-A and SP-D, which are members of the collectin family, having both a collagenous domain and a carbohydrate binding domain. The principal roles for SP-A and SP-D appear to be in local host defense because both molecules can bind to a wide variety of microorganisms and facilitate their uptake and killing by alveolar macrophages.[4] SP-A also interacts with surfactant phospholipids, calcium, and SP-B in order to form tubular myelin. Mice genetically engineered to be unable to produce SP-A lack tubular myelin in their lungs, but they do not develop RDS or spontaneous lung disease with age and have increased susceptibility to infection with a number of different microorganisms.[5] Genetically engineered mice unable to produce SP-D are also more susceptible to infection with certain organisms and develop an accumulation of surfactant lipids in their lungs and emphysema as they age.[6-8] SP-A

and SP-D also may have immune modulatory roles.[9] Mutations in one of the genes encoding SP-A *(SFTPA2)* have been reported as a cause of pulmonary fibrosis and lung cancer in adults.[10] Mutations in the gene encoding SP-D *(SFTPD)* as a cause of human lung disease have not yet been reported.

The production of ABCA3 and surfactant proteins A, B, C, and D is developmentally regulated and increases during gestation. Specific transcription factors that bind to DNA sequences in the promoter regions of each gene are important for the proper expression of each protein, including the transcription factor NKX2.1 (also called thyroid transcription factor 1).[11,12] After secretion, pulmonary surfactant is both recycled into AEC2s and is catabolized by alveolar macrophages. In order for macrophages to properly mature and efficiently catabolize surfactant, GM-CSF must bind to a specific receptor at the cell surface and initiate specific signaling events. The receptor is composed of two chains: a specific ligand-binding α chain (CD116) and a β chain (CD131) that enhances affinity and is shared with the receptors for IL-3 and IL-5.[13,14] Binding of GM-CSF to its receptor initiates intracellular signaling cascades and activates the transcription factor PU.1, which regulates multiple alveolar macrophage functions including the ability to catabolize surfactant components[15] (Fig. 56-1).

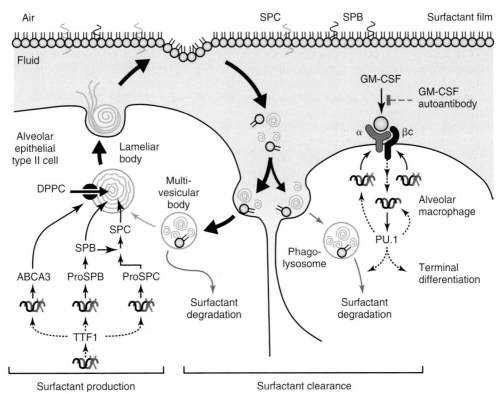

FIGURE 56-1. Simplified overview of surfactant production and catabolism. Surfactant lipids and proteins are synthesized by alveolar type II cells, with thyroid transcription factor 1 (TTF1) needed for transcription of SP-B, SP-C, and ABCA3. SP-B and SP-C are synthesized as proproteins and processed in lamellar bodies. The lamellar bodies fuse with the apical cell membrane and the surfactant complex is secreted by exocytosis, with SP-B and SP-C helping enhance adsorption to the air-liquid interface and organize surfactant lipids. Surfactant material is recycled through type II cells by endocytosis and taken up in multivesicular bodies. Surfactant is internalized and its components broken down in phagolysosomes of alveolar macrophages. Binding of GM-CSF to its receptor initiates signaling pathways leading to nuclear binding of the transcription factor PU.1 to regulatory pulements in genes needed for macrophage maturation and functions, including catabolism of surfactant.

DISORDERS OF SURFACTANT PRODUCTION

Surfactant Protein B (SP-B) and Hereditary SP-B Deficiency

SP-B is a 79–amino acid, hydrophobic protein that facilitates adsorption to the air-liquid interface and enhances the surface tension–lowering properties of surfactant phospholipids.[2] SP-B is encoded by a single gene (SFTPB) that spans approximately 10,000 base pairs on human chromosome 2 and contains 11 exons, the last of which is untranslated. The gene directs the production of a 381–amino acid preproprotein, which undergoes proteolytic processing to yield the mature peptide found in the airspaces, with the mature peptide domain corresponding to exons 6 and 7 of the gene.[16,17] SP-B is produced primarily by AEC2s, routed to lamellar bodies, and secreted along with surfactant phospholipids into the airspaces. The gene also is expressed within the lung in nonciliated bronchiolar epithelial cells, although only AEC2s fully process the proprotein (proSP-B) to mature SP-B.

Hereditary SP-B deficiency was the first recognized genetic cause of surfactant deficiency.[18] The index case was a full-term infant who presented with clinical and radiographic signs of RDS, but who did not improve despite maximal medical support, including extracorporeal membrane oxygenation (ECMO). A family history of a previous full-term child who had died in the neonatal period from lung disease supported a genetic mechanism. A frameshift mutation in the SP-B gene was subsequently identified on both alleles in affected infants, establishing an inherited deficiency of SP-B as the basis for their lung disease.[19]

SP-B deficiency is an autosomal recessive disorder with affected infants having loss-of-function mutations on both alleles. The first identified mutation remains the most frequently identified and involves a net 2 base insertion in codon 121 (termed 121ins2), which results in a frameshift and premature codon for the termination of translation. The 121ins2 mutation has been found principally in individuals of Northern European descent, and likely has resulted from a common ancestral origin.[20] Over two dozen other SP-B mutations have been identified as well as a deletion spanning exons 6 and 7.[21-27] Most of these mutations are unique to a given family, although several mutations have been identified in apparently unrelated families in certain ethnic groups.[22] Complete deficiency of SP-B is lethal, with the only therapeutic option being lung transplantation.[28,29]

Partial SP-B deficiency can be associated with intermediate survival, suggesting that a critical level of SP-B is needed for normal lung function.[30,31] Mice who were genetically engineered to be able to turn off their SP-B production developed lung disease when their SP-B levels fell below 20% to 25% of normal adult levels.[32] Having a loss of function SP-B mutation on only one allele could thus be a risk factor for the development of lung disease if other factors further reduce SP-B expression. This hypothesis is supported by the observation that genetically engineered mice with one null SP-B allele were more susceptible to pulmonary oxygen toxicity than their wild-type littermates.[33] In a population-based study, carriers for the 121ins2 mutation were found to be at risk for reduced lung function as adults, particularly in conjunction with smoking.[34]

Pathology findings in lung tissue from SP-B-deficient infants include nonspecific findings of interstitial fibrosis and AEC2 hyperplasia. These findings also are observed in other disorders of surfactant production (Fig. 56-2). While findings of alveolar proteinosis were prominent in the lungs of some of the first infants identified with this disorder, this finding has not been universal in the lungs of SP-B-deficient infants. Moreover histopathologic findings of alveolar proteinosis are observed in other genetic abnormalities of surfactant production and catabolism. Histologic finding of alveolar proteinosis may thus be suggestive of an inherited surfactant abnormality, but the term congenital alveolar proteinosis should not be used synonymously with SP-B deficiency.

Inactivation of the SP-B gene in genetically engineered mice resulted in a neonatal lethal respiratory phenotype, further supporting an essential role for SP-B in normal lung function.[35] Both SP-B-deficient infants and animals have secondary changes in the metabolism of other surfactant components, indicating a role for SP-B beyond lowering surface tension in the airspaces. These secondary changes include markedly abnormal lamellar bodies and accumulation of aberrantly processed SP-C peptides that result from incomplete processing of the SP-C precursor (proSP-C) to mature SP-C.[36-38] This block in SP-C processing may result in SP-B-deficient infants also being deficient in mature SP-C, and the partially processed proSP-C peptides are not very surface active, further contributing to surfactant dysfunction in these infants.[39] The lamellar bodies in SP-B-deficient mice and infants are poorly organized, with loosely packed lamellae and vacuolar inclusions, having the appearance more of multivesicular or composite bodies (Fig. 56-3). This appearance is consistent with a role for SP-B in membrane fusion of smaller vesicles in order to pack and organize lipid bilayers into lamellar bodies.[40] The final processing steps for mature SP-C occurs in lamellar bodies, and the failure to properly form this intracellular organelle is thus likely related to the SP-C processing abnormality.

The incidence of SP-B deficiency is unknown, although it is likely that the disease is rare. The carrier frequency of the 121ins2 mutation in the U.S. population was estimated to be approximately 1 in 1000 individuals.[41,42] Combining this finding with the observation that the 121ins2 mutation has accounted for approximately two thirds of the mutant SFTPB alleles identified to date, this would predict a disease incidence of 1 in 1.5 million live births. The relative incidence in other countries and subpopulations may differ; the carrier rate for the 121ins2 mutation in Denmark was found to be 1 in 560 individuals, which would still predict a very low incidence of disease.[34]

Surfactant Protein C Genetic Abnormalities and Lung Disease

SP-C is an extremely hydrophobic 35–amino acid peptide that is encoded by a single gene (SFTPC) spanning approximately 3500 base pairs on human chromosome 8, containing 6 exons, of which the sixth is untranslated.

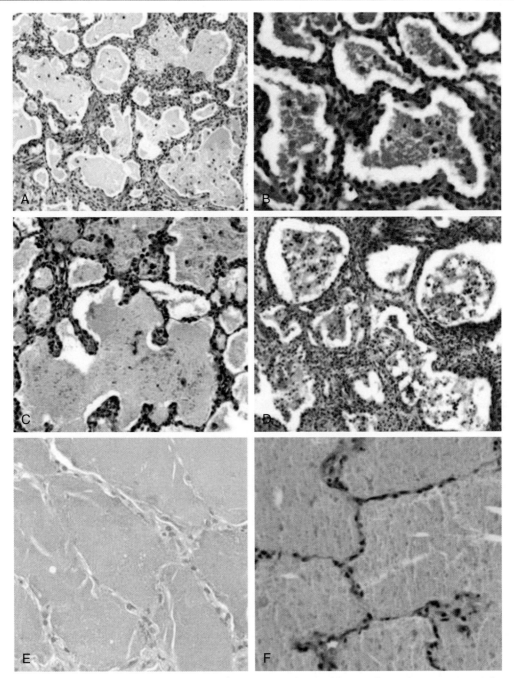

FIGURE 56-2. Variable and overlapping histology associated with genetic disorders disrupting surfactant homeostasis. **A** is from an SP-B-deficient infant, demonstrating marked accumulation of granular proteinaceous material with entrapped macrophages filling distal airspaces. **B,** Similar pathology is demonstrated in a patient with ABCA3 deficiency and from a patent with an SP-C mutation **(C)**, although with better preservation of the alveolar architecture in **C. D** is from a patient with a different SP-C mutation, demonstrating interstitial thickening and accumulations of foamy macrophages in the airspaces but with scant amounts of proteinaceous material. **E** and **F** are from patients with *CSF2RA* and *CSFR2B* mutations, respectively. Although the airspaces are totally filled with granular material, the alveolar walls remain thin without thickening with mesenchymal or inflammatory cells or fibrosis. (Pictures courtesy of Susan Wert, PhD.)

Alternative splicing at the beginning of exon 5 would result in translation products of 191 or 197 amino acids. SP-C, like SP-B, enhances the surface tension lowering properties of surfactant lipids and is present in mammalian derived exogenous surfactant preparations used to treat infants with RDS[2,16,17,43] Whereas SP-B deficiency generally results in neonatal-onset lung disease that is rapidly fatal, the phenotype associated with *SFTPC* variants is much more variable.

The first identified subject with an *SFTPC* abnormality was a 6-week-old infant whose family history was notable for a 3-generation history of interstitial lung disease (ILD) characterized as desquamative interstitial pneumonia inherited in an autosomal dominant fashion.[44] Lung biopsy findings were interpreted as consistent with nonspecific interstitial pneumonitis or chronic pneumonitis of infancy (CPI).[45] Mature SP-C was not detected in lung tissue, and DNA sequence analysis of *SFPTC* revealed a

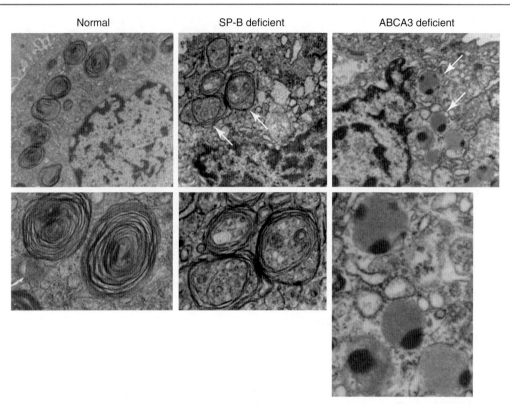

FIGURE 56-3. Ultrastructural findings associated with SP-B and ABCA3 deficiency. A portion of a type II cell with normal lamellar bodies is shown in the top left panel. In the top middle panel, a type II cell from an SP-B-deficient patient contains abnormally formed lamellar bodies with large whorls and vacuolar inclusions *(arrows)*. In the top right panel the lamellar bodies in the type II cells of a patient with ABCA3 deficiency are small and dense, with eccentrically placed inclusions *(arrows)*. The bottom panels show higher power views of normal *(left)*, SP-B-deficient *(middle)* and ABCA3-deficient *(right)* lamellar bodies. (Pictures courtesy of Susan Wert, PhD.)

single base substitution in the first base of intron IV that resulted in the skipping of exon 4 (with the mutation subsequently referred to as Δexon 4) and a shortened proprotein. The same mutation was identified in the child's mother, who along with the child also had reduced levels of proSP-C expression as evaluated by immunohistochemical staining. A mutation was identified on only one allele of the *SP-C* gene, which was consistent with the autosomal dominant inheritance pattern, but did not readily explain the reductions in proSP-C protein and mature SP-C protein. However, SP-C self-associates in the secretory pathway and thus a dominant negative effect on SP-C production from the abnormal proSP-C that resulted from the mutation could have accounted for the lack of mature SP-C.[46] Subsequent studies in which the *SFTPC* Δexon4 mutation was expressed in *in vitro* systems provided support for this mechanism because the abnormal proSP-C was neither processed to mature SP-C nor routed appropriately in the cells and was rapidly degraded.[47,48]

Multiple other reports of familial lung disease inherited in an autosomal dominant pattern and sporadic lung disease due to *de novo SFTPC* mutations have since been published.[49–66] One mutation, a predicted substitution of isoleucine by threonine in codon 73 (p.Ilet73Thr or p.I73T), has accounted for 35% to 50% of the mutant *SFTPC* alleles reported to date from multiple unrelated families.[49–54,59,66] This mutation has arisen on genetically diverse *SFTPC* alleles, suggesting recurrent mutation as the mechanism for a common mutation.[52,66] The majority

of other reported mutations are located in the region encoding the carboxy-terminal domain of proSP-C. This domain has homology to a group of proteins known as BRICHOS that have been mutated in familial dementias.[67] SP-C lung disease may thus represent a conformational disease with accumulation of misfolded protein in the cell causing secondary cellular toxicity.[68] Proper folding of this domain may provide an important chaperone function in terms of moving the hydrophobic proSP-C protein through the cell.[69,70]

The incidence and prevalence of lung disease associated with *SFTPC* mutations are unknown. The population frequency of the p.I73T mutation was examined in a samples obtained from neonatal screening programs, but this mutation was not found on any of the almost 9000 alleles examined, precluding a reliable estimate.[42] Sequence analysis of *SFTPC* in 760 individuals in Denmark with abnormal pulmonary phenotypes, only 31 of whom had ILD, identified two novel *SFTPC* coding variants. Thirty-nine individuals with one these variants were then identified from almost 48,000 screened, approximately 1 in 1200. However it is not clear that the variants identified represented disease-causing mutations. None of the individuals with these variants had ILD, although one variant (p.Ala53Thr) was associated with a slightly increased risk for asthma.[71]

The pathophysiology of lung disease due to *SFTPC* mutations is complex and incompletely understood. Lack of mature SP-C could plausibly contribute to the lung disease. Mice unable to produce SP-C because of targeted inactivation of their *SP-C* gene develop progressive air space enlargement and interstitial inflammation as they age in a strain-dependent fashion.[72,73] The variability depending on the genetic background of the null mice indicates that genetic modifiers are likely important in the development of SP-C-related lung disease. Mutations in other genes important in surfactant metabolism, such as *ABCA3*, may modify the severity of lung disease caused by *SFTPC* mutations.[51] Human lung disease resulting from null mutations on one or both alleles of the *SP-C* gene has not been reported. Familial ILD associated with markedly reduced *SP-C* expression in lung tissue and undetectable SP-C in bronchoalveolar lavage fluid (BALF), but without any identified *SFTPC* mutations in affected individuals to account for these findings, has been observed.[74] These observations both support a role for SP-C deficiency in the pathogenesis of ILD and indicate that genes other than *SFTPC* may result in SP-C deficiency (i.e., locus or genetic heterogeneity).

Alternatively *SFTPC* mutations may cause lung disease due to toxicity from abnormal proSP-C, a "gain of toxic-function" mechanism. All of the *SFTPC* mutations associated with human lung disease reported to date are predicted to result in the production of an abnormal proprotein, which is likely misfolded.[68] The exposure of hydrophobic epitopes in the misfolded proprotein may be directly toxic to AEC2s, especially if produced in sufficient amounts to be unable to be efficiently degraded through the proteasome pathway. Proteasome dysfunction also may inhibit expression of other surfactant proteins, further contributing to surfactant dysfunction.[75] Accumulation of misfolded protein within the endoplasmic reticulum may trigger the unfolded protein response (UPR), and eventually, caspase activation and apoptosis of AEC2s.[47,48,76–78] Increased levels of UPR components and caspase activation also have been observed in lung tissue from patients with pulmonary fibrosis not caused by *SFTPC* mutations, suggesting that protein misfolding may be a more general mechanism for AEC2 injury.[79,80]

Clinical features in children and adults with *SFTPC* mutations have been summarized in several clinical studies and include chronic respiratory symptoms (dyspnea, cough) and signs (tachypnea, crackles), as well as failure to thrive, digital clubbing, and the need for supplemental oxygen.[49,81] The age of onset of symptoms is variable, with some infants developing respiratory distress immediately after birth, and other individuals remaining asymptomatic well into adulthood.[44,62,64,81] Infants and children with severe disease who require aggressive supportive measures, including mechanical ventilation, may show gradual improvement over time. Lung disease in some children appears to have been triggered or exacerbated by viral infections.[64,81] Cells in culture that stably expressed the *SFTPC* Δexon 4 mutation at low levels did not have overt signs of cellular toxicity, but they died when exposed to RSV, providing a potential mechanism for such a genetic-environmental interaction.[82] Radiographic findings depend on severity of disease, but ground-glass opacities are common as are peripheral cysts seen on high resolution computed tomography (HRCT).[83]

There are currently no specific therapies for patients with *SFTPC* mutations. Treatment has included corticosteroids, hydroxychloroquine, and azithromycin, but the efficacy of these agents in lung disease due to *SFTPC* mutations is unknown and is complicated by the variability in the natural history of the disease.[61,81] The generation of an animal model of the disease will be important in order to test both existing and novel therapies. Finally, if accumulation of misfolded proteins other than SP-C within AEC2s and triggering of the UPR is a general mechanism for cellular injury and eventual pulmonary fibrosis, future therapies for SP-C-related disease may benefit patients with more common forms of ILD.

ABCA3 Deficiency

ABCA3 is a member of the adenosine triphosphate (ATP) binding cassette family, transmembrane proteins that hydrolyze ATP to transport substances across biologic membranes.[84] A single gene for ABCA3 *(ABCA3)* spans more than 80 kb on human chromosome 16 and contains 33 exons, of which the first 3 are untranslated. The gene encodes a 1704 amino acid protein with two membrane-spanning and two nucleotide-binding domains. ABCA3 expression is developmentally regulated, with expression increasing in later gestation, and its expression also is increased by glucocorticoids.[85–87] ABCA3 is primarily expressed within AEC2s in the lung where it is localized to the limiting membrane of lamellar bodies and expressed at low levels in a number of other tissues, including kidney, intestine, thyroid, and brain.[85–88]

ABCA3 deficiency was first recognized as a cause of lung disease with the identification of disease-causing mutations in multiple unrelated infants who had clinical and/or radiographic signs of severe neonatal surfactant deficiency.[89] A family history of severe neonatal lung disease or consanguinity, or both, was suggestive for a genetic mechanism. The lung histology findings were similar to what had been observed in patients with *SFTPB* or *SFTPC* mutations, which were excluded by a combination of protein expression and genetic studies. Abnormal lamellar bodies in lung tissue from affected infants (described below) supported a role for ABCA3 in lamellar body formation and surfactant metabolism.

ABCA3 deficiency is inherited in an autosomal recessive fashion and disease results from loss-of-function mutations on both alleles. Genetically engineered mice lacking ABCA3 do not inflate their lungs and die from respiratory failure perinatally.[90–93] The phospholipid profile of the lungs of such animals is markedly abnormal, with very low levels of DSPC and phosphatidylglycerol.[90,92] Similarly bronchoalveolar lavage fluid (BALF) from ABCA3-deficient infants who underwent lung transplantation in infancy had diminished surface-tension lowering properties and was markedly reduced in DSPC content compared to controls.[94] These observations support an essential role for ABCA3 in the transport of lipids important for surface-tension reduction and account for the severe RDS-like phenotype observed in some infants.

While initial reports focused on children with severe neonatal disease, it has since been recognized that ABCA3 deficiency may result in milder lung disease and prolonged survival.[95–98] Affected children do not always have symptoms in the neonatal period and may present later with findings similar to children with *SFTPC* mutations.[83,95,96] The precise mechanisms whereby some children do not exhibit findings of neonatal surfactant deficiency are unknown, but the relatively milder phenotype in these children is likely due to retained ABCA3 function. A mutation predicted to result in the substitution of valine for glutamic acid in codon 292 (p.Glu292Val or p.E292V) has been found in multiple unrelated subjects with ILD, and *in vitro* studies of this mutation demonstrated partially impaired lipid transport compared with wild-type ABCA3, supporting a correlation between genotype and phenotype.[99] Some mutations also may be associated with endoplasmic reticulum (ER) stress and trigger the UPR, contributing to AEC2 injury and chronic lung disease.[100] Over 100 *ABCA3* mutations have been reported scattered throughout the gene[51,89,94–98,101–112] Type I mutations are not properly routed to distal cellular compartments, and type 2 mutations result in reduced ATP hydrolysis or impaired lipid transport.[99,113,114] This classification scheme does not incorporate nonsense and frame-shift mutations, which are likely associated with unstable transcripts, and is likely to evolve as our understanding of normal ABCA3 cell biology increases. Finally, heterozygosity for an *ABCA3* mutation may modify the course of both rare (*SFTPC*-related) and common (RDS) lung diseases.[51,115]

Absent or abnormal lamellar bodies have been observed in the lungs of ABCA3-deficient infants.[89,101,104,116,117] AEC2s in affected infants contain small, dense-appearing inclusions that have densely packed membranes upon higher magnification. Eccentrically placed electron-dense inclusions within the abnormal lamellar bodies give them a "fried-egg" appearance.[117] Similarly abnormal lamellar bodies were observed in genetically engineered ABCA3 null mice.[91,93] This ultrastructural appearance was distinct from that of SP-B deficiency, in which the abnormal lamellar bodies are larger and loosely packed with vesicular inclusions, often with the appearance of composite or multivesicular bodies.[36,37,101] (Fig. 56-3). Ultrastructural examination of lung tissue obtained at biopsy or autopsy may thus be helpful in establishing the diagnosis of ABCA3 deficiency and distinguishing it from other inborn errors of surfactant metabolism. A caveat is that most of the reported ultrastructural studies were in children with the most severe form of the illness, and ultrastructural findings may be more variable in children with milder disease.

The incidence and prevalence of ABCA3 deficiency are unknown. The relative frequency with which ABCA3-deficient infants have been identified compared with those with SP-B deficiency or *SFTPC* mutations suggests that it may be the most frequent cause of genetic surfactant dysfunction.[107] This would not be surprising given the relatively large size of the *ABCA3* gene. One study examined the population frequency of ABCA3 p.E292V and found that the carrier frequency was 1 in 275 individuals in the U.S. population.[42] As this mutation has accounted for approximately 10% of the mutant *ABCA3* alleles reported to date, this could translate to a carrier rate as high as 1 in 27 individuals, which would predict a disease incidence of 1 in 3000. This seems likely to be

an overestimate given available data on the incidence of neonatal respiratory failure in term infants and childhood interstitial lung disease.[118–120] Population-based studies of the frequency of *ABCA3* mutations will be needed to resolve this question.

Currently there is no specific treatment for ABCA3 deficiency. *ABCA3* gene transcription is increased by glucocorticoids *in vitro*, providing a rationale for treatment with steroids to augment any remaining gene function, but clinical evidence for the efficacy of steroids for this condition is lacking. As with ILD due to *SFTPC* mutations, hydroxychloroquine and azithromycin have been used, but it is currently unknown whether these agents alter the course of the disease. Lung disease may be progressive and lung transplantation has been performed in children with end stage lung disease due to ABCA3 deficiency, with results comparable to those of similarly age-matched subjects.[121]

NKX2.1 Haploinsufficiency

NKX2.1 (also known as thyroid transcription factor 1 or TTF1) is a member of the homeodomain-containing family of transcription factors.[11,122] It is encoded by a single, 3-exon gene spanning 3 kb on human chromosome 14q13.3. NKX2.1 is expressed in the thyroid, where it is important for development of that gland; in the central nervous system (CNS), primarily basal ganglia; and in the lung, where it is critical for the expression of surfactant proteins A, B, and C, as well as ABCA3.[86,122,123] Initial case reports of near-term infants with an RDS phenotype and heterozygous chromosomal deletions encompassing the location of *NKX2.1* supported that loss of one *NKX2.1* allele (haploinsufficiency) could result in lung disease.[124,125] As other genes were involved in these deletions, it could not be definitely concluded that the phenotype resulted from the loss of the *NKX2.1* locus alone. Subsequently loss-of-function mutations in *NKX2.1* were identified as the cause of the disorder benign familial chorea.[126] Patients with mutations in *NKX2.1* who had combinations of neurologic symptoms, hypothyroidism, and acute and chronic lung disease were then identified; thus, "brain-thyroid-lung syndrome" has been used to encompass the constellation of findings in patients with *NKX2.1* mutations or deletions.[127–130] Approximately 50% of reported patients with *NKX2.1* deletions or mutations had some pulmonary disease, but detailed evaluation of lung function was not performed in all subjects.[129] Affected individuals need not have abnormalities in all three organ systems and may have normal thyroid function, or chemical hypothyroidism may be present without clinical symptoms. The neurologic findings may be subtle in infants, consisting of nonspecific hypotonia or developmental delay, and attributed to the severity of the lung disease. The more specific finding of chorea may not manifest until later in life.

As NKX2.1 is essential for the expression of SP-B, SP-C, and ABCA3, it is not surprising that reductions in the amount of this transcription factor could result in the phenotypes of RDS (surfactant deficiency) and ILD (surfactant dysfunction). Complete loss-of-function of one

NKX2.1 allele has been demonstrated both by complete gene deletions and *in vitro* studies of mutations demonstrating impaired DNA binding or decreased transcription of reporter genes.[127,128,131] It is unknown whether lung disease results primarily through the reduction of one surfactant component (such as SP-B or ABCA3) below a critical level needed for normal lung function or a combination of reduced levels of more than one protein. Surfactant protein expression has been evaluated in a single patient with an *NKX2.1* deletion, with diminished immunoreactivity for SP-A and ABCA3, but robust staining for SP-B and proSP-C observed.[132] Because SP-A also is regulated by NKX2.1, reductions in this pulmonary collectin may account for the observation of recurrent pulmonary infections observed in some subjects. Lung pathology findings may include those observed with other causes of surfactant dysfunction, as well as alveolar simplification.[130,132,133] The mechanisms for the variable severity of the disease are unknown, but they may relate to either genetic variants in *NKX2.1*, affecting expression level of the remaining functional allele, or factors controlling the expression and function of the multiple other transcription factors (including GATA6, FOXA2, C/EBPα, NFAT) needed for surfactant protein and *ABCA3* gene expression.

The incidence of lung disease due to *NKX2.1* mutations or deletions is unknown. Such mutations appear to be a rare cause of congenital hypothyroidism,[134] but studies focusing on the frequency of the pulmonary phenotype have not been performed. Familial disease due to *NKX2.1* mutations and deletions has been reported but the majority of reported cases appear to have resulted from *de novo* events.[129,135] Thyroid hormone replacement is indicated in those patients with evidence of hypothyroidism, but specific therapies for the lung disease due to *NKX2.1* mutations have not been evaluated.

DISORDERS OF SURFACTANT CLEARANCE

PAP is a syndrome that occurs in a heterogeneous group of diseases and is defined histopathologically by the presence of a finely granular, lipoproteinaceous material filling pulmonary alveoli and terminal airspaces. The accumulated material stains with eosin and periodic acid-Schiff reagent, has biochemical and ultrastructural features identical to surfactant, and frequently contains cholesterol "needles" and cellular debris. Depending on the underlying causative disease, alveolar distortion and fibrosis may or may not be present. The relative proportions of these specific histologic features vary markedly among the diseases causing PAP, that is, the histopathologic pattern depends on the pathogenesis involved.

Pathogenesis

The pathogenesis of PAP remained obscure for nearly four decades after its initial description in 1958 because research was hampered by its rarity and the heterogeneity of diseases associated with its development.[136,137] The vast majority of cases occurred in previously healthy individuals without significant environmental pulmonary exposure other than smoking, referred to as idiopathic or acquired PAP. However PAP also occurred in association with various underlying diseases, termed *secondary PAP* (see below).

A serendipitous but critical pathogenic clue for the common idiopathic form was the observation that mice deficient in GM-CSF or a component of its receptor developed a phenotype virtually identical to idiopathic PAP in humans.[13,14,138,139] Although PAP caused by GM-CSF deficiency has not yet been reported in humans, a second pathogenic clue was the observation that idiopathic PAP is specifically associated with high levels of neutralizing autoantibodies against GM-CSF.[140–142] Passive transfer studies established that GM-CSF autoantibodies cause PAP by blocking GM-CSF signaling to alveolar macrophages,[143] which is required to stimulate surfactant catabolism.[143] Additional pathogenic insight was provided by the identification of hereditary PAP in children due to genetic mutations that impair GM-CSF receptor function.[144–148]

Nomenclature

A plethora of different terms has been used to report on PAP, resulting in inconsistent use of overlapping terminology; some brief definitions are useful here. Elucidation of the pathogenic mechanism of the most common PAP-associated disease (idiopathic PAP) was the basis for recommending use of the term *autoimmune PAP*.[149] Genetic diseases causing hereditary PAP can be specified by the affected gene (i.e., *CSF2RA* or *CSF2RB*, encoding the GM-CSF receptor alpha or beta chains, respectively). These autoimmune and genetic diseases share strikingly similar features including clinical presentation (though age of presentation may be different), radiographic appearance, histopathology (alveolar filling without marked distortion), pathophysiology, overlapping pathogenesis (loss of GM-CSF signaling), and response to whole lung lavage therapy. Consequently, they are usefully considered together and sometimes called primary PAP reflecting their occurrence in previously healthy individuals.

PAP occurring as a consequence of another underlying disease is referred to as secondary PAP. Diseases associated with the development of secondary PAP include hematologic disorders (e.g., myelodysplasia, hematologic malignancies, aplastic anemia), certain chronic infections (e.g., HIV), toxic inhalation exposures (e.g., silica fibers, metal dusts), other genetic diseases not involving disruption of GM-CSF signaling (lysinuric protein intolerance), and generalized myelosuppresion caused by chemotherapy and hematopoietic stem cell transplantation.[137,142]

PAP also can occur in disorders of surfactant production as previously described. Pulmonary surfactant in these disorders is deficient in one or more critical components of surfactant, resulting in deficiency of functional surfactant that causes marked alveolar distortion, a spectrum of acute and chronic interstitial lung diseases, and varying degrees of accumulation of abnormal surfactant (PAP). The clinical presentation, response to whole lung lavage (which is poor), and therapeutic approaches are quite different from primary PAP, in which the primary abnormality is the accumulation of biochemically and functionally normal surfactant without alveolar distortion.

Autoimmune PAP

This disease is caused by an immune attack directed at GM-CSF that blocks signaling to alveolar macrophages (and other cells), thereby impairing their ability to catabolize surfactant lipids and proteins. Neutralizing, polyclonal immunoglobulin (Ig)G (primarily IgG1 and IgG2) is associated with the development of PAP when levels exceed a critical threshold required to eliminate GM-CSF signaling *in vivo* (estimated to be approximately 5 μg/mL). Disruption of GM-CSF signaling blocks the terminal differentiation of alveolar macrophages, impairing surfactant catabolism and a number of host defense functions. Loss of GM-CSF signaling also impairs neutrophil host defense functions, which together with impairment of macrophage host defense functions resulting from maturational arrest provides a molecular explanation for the increased morbidity and mortality from infection seen in this disorder.[150] Impaired pulmonary surfactant clearance caused by reduced catabolism in alveolar macrophages results in a slow net accumulation of surfactant within alveoli, which blocks the entry of air and transfer of oxygen into the blood, eventually resulting in hypoxemia and respiratory insufficiency. Alveolar distortion is not a prominent histopathologic feature in most patients, but lymphocytosis can be present and fibrosis has been reported.

Autoimmune PAP accounts for roughly 90% of all PAP cases with a respective incidence and prevalence of 0.42 and 6 to 7 per million in the general population.[137,151] The disorder affects all races and ethnic groups, is globally distributed, and is twice as common in men as women (and in smokers as nonsmokers). The disease usually presents in the third to fifth decade of life with progressive dyspnea of insidious onset, and diffuse bilateral lung infiltrates on radiological evaluation. The presentation is similar in younger adults, adolescents, and children as young as 8 years of age. Clubbing is not a feature, although occasionally fever and hemoptysis may be present and usually indicate the presence of a secondary infection.

Whole lung lavage is currently the standard therapy for autoimmune PAP; it works well in most patients and improves survival and quality of life. Occasionally, or possibly late in the course of disease, whole lung lavage therapy can become less effective. Over the past decade, a series of small clinical studies has demonstrated that GM-CSF augmentation can be effective in treating this disease. However, none of the indications for use or route or timing of administration, dosage, or duration of therapy have been evaluated in prospective clinical trials. Thus, further studies are needed. Anti-CD20 therapy using rituximab has been successful in a very limited number of patients with this disease and more studies are needed to evaluate the safety and efficacy of this promising potential therapy.

PAP Caused by Autosomal Recessive *CSF2RA* Mutations

In 2008, two groups independently reported children with the phenotype of PAP who had deleterious variants in the gene encoding the α-chain of the GM-CSF receptor *(CSF2RA)*, which is located within the pseudoautosomal

regions of the X and Y chromosomes. In one report, two sisters were found to be compound heterozygotes for a complete deletion of the *CSF2RA* locus and a missense mutation that was demonstrated *in vitro* to produce nonfunctional GM-CSF receptors[146] The proband developed progressive dyspnea apparent by age 4, was diagnosed with PAP on lung biopsy at age 6, and responded well to whole lung lavage therapy. Her 8-year-old sister had the same genotype and evidence for mild PAP by HRCT but was asymptomatic at the time of the report and had not needed any therapy for PAP. These two genetically similar siblings illustrate the phenotypic variability of this disorder. In another report, a child with Turner's syndrome (45 XO) was diagnosed with PAP at 3 years of age, confirmed on biopsy, and found to have a partial deletion of *CSFR2A* accounting for the lack of receptor expression and GM-CSF signaling.[144] The child died of a respiratory infection following a bone-marrow transplant before engraftment.

A subsequent study expanded on these initial observations with the identification of five additional patients with deleterious *CSF2RA* genetic variants from three families of differing ethnicity and geographic origin, indicating that this disorder is not confined to one ethnic group or geographic location.[147] The age of onset of symptoms ranged from 1.5 to 9 years; one patient was asymptomatic. Usual presenting symptoms included dyspnea and fatigue. None of the subjects had auto-antibodies to GM-CSF, but all had elevated serum levels of GM-CSF compared with family members and healthy control subjects. A variety of *CSF2RA* genetic defects were identified; CSF2RA protein was absent in all but one patient with a missense mutation, but all affected patients had reduced signaling induced by GM-CSF in isolated mononuclear cells. Symptomatic patients had undergone multiple whole lung lavages with intervals ranging from every several months to over 2 years. All were alive at the time of the report, ranging in age from 4 to 13 years.[147]

PAP Caused by Autosomal Recessive *CSF2RB* Mutations

A genetic defect of the GM-CSF receptor was first suggested as a mechanism for PAP in four infants who had undetectable amounts of the common β-chain (βc) shared with IL-3 and IL-5 receptors as determined by immunologic methods.[152] Deficient response to exogenous stimulation by GM-CSF also was observed in monocytes obtained from affected infants. However, no convincing genetic mechanism was identified to account for the lack of βc, and the only genetic variant identified in its gene *(CSF2RB)* was subsequently found to be a polymorphism.[145]

Function-altering mutations in *CSF2RB* have since been reported in two unrelated patients.[145,148] Both presented with the typical symptoms and signs of PAP, one at age 9 and the other at age 36. Both had elevated levels of serum GM-CSF, and antibodies to GM-CSF were not detected. One patient was homozygous for a missense mutation that was confirmed in *in vitro* studies to be non-functional; the other was homozygous for a single base deletion in exon 6 and had no detectable βc protein. In contrast to the earlier report involving infants with absent βc protein expression, these reports provided convincing evidence that genetic defects in *CSF2RB* can cause the phenotype of PAP. The mechanism(s) for decreased βc expression in the infants in the earlier study and whether it contributed to the pathophysiology of their lung disease remain unknown. It is interesting that the age at presentation of patients with *CSF2RB* mutations was older than those with *CSF2RA* genetic variants, but additional patients will have to be identified to determine if there is a true difference in age of onset of disease, depending on the gene involved.

Genetically determined primary defects in GM-CSF production have not been reported as a cause of PAP in humans, although this mechanism is expected based on observations in experimental animals.[138,139] PAP develops in some but not all children with lysinuric protein intolerance (LPI), a disorder of cationic amino acid transport caused by mutations in the gene *SLC7A7*, a member of the solute carrier family.[153–155] The mechanism of PAP in children with LPI is unknown, but appears likely to involve macrophage dysfunction rather than surfactant production because defects are present in mononuclear phagocyte lineage cells,[156] and PAP recurred in a child with LPI who had undergone heart-lung transplantation,[157] consistent with alveolar macrophages and not alveolar epithelial cells comprising the site of pathogenic disruption of surfactant homeostasis.

The number of patients with PAP caused by GM-CSF receptor defects identified to date is small; thus, information regarding the natural history of these disorders remains unclear. Whole lung lavage has been successfully used to ameliorate the severity of the pulmonary symptoms, but as the underlying defect persists, in most cases, therapy is required on a periodic basis.[147] As serum GM-CSF levels are already elevated, and patient macrophages do not respond to GM-CSF *in vitro*, exogenous GM-CSF seems unlikely to benefit most of these patients because components of the GM-CSF receptor are absent. However, in cases where impaired GM-CSF signaling is due to decreased GM-CSF binding affinity rather than the absence of the receptor itself, GM-CSF augmentation therapy to increase the GM-CSF concentration may overcome the signaling defect and restore surfactant clearance by alveolar macrophages.[145,146] Clinical trials to evaluate inhaled GM-CSF as a potential therapy thus warrant consideration. As alveolar macrophages are bone-marrow derived based on experiments in βc receptor–deficient mice, bone marrow transplantation may be curative for this group of disorders.[158] Cell and gene transfer based therapeutic strategies are also in development.

▄ DIAGNOSTIC APPROACH

The identification of genetic abnormalities as causes of disorders of surfactant production and clearance provides the means for diagnosis of these rare conditions through noninvasive genetic testing. Although specific therapies may not be available for all these disorders, timely diagnosis is important to provide accurate counseling regarding prognosis, assessment of risk for other family members, and recurrence risk for future pregnancies. Clinical algorithms for a diagnostic approach to suspected genetic causes of surfactant production and catabolism have not been formally evaluated, but the typical clinical presentations of each disorder may provide guidance as to which patients to evaluate for these disorders (Fig. 56-4).

Genetic Testing

Diffuse lung disease in a full-term infant with radiographic features of surfactant deficiency should prompt consideration of a genetic disorder of surfactant production.

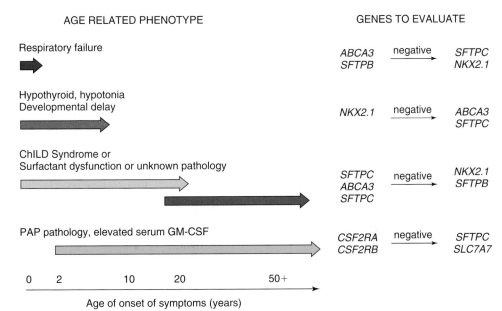

FIGURE 56-4. Genetic evaluation based on age of onset and clinical presentation. Ages of different clinical presentations from newborn to adult are represented by *arrows* on the left, and primary genes to be evaluated for each phenotype and age-of-onset are listed on the right. If initial studies are negative, than additional genes also may be evaluated, listed on the far right.

Gestational age of more than 38 weeks, male gender, operative delivery (especially elective), and white race are known risk factors for RDS in near-term infants.[119,159] Absence of these risk factors or failure to improve after the first 7 to 10 days of life, or a family history of severe neonatal lung disease should increase suspicion for a genetic mechanism for the lung disease. ABCA3 deficiency is likely the most frequent cause of this phenotype; evidence for hypothyroidism should prompt consideration of an NKX2.1 deletion or mutation. SP-B deficiency is extremely rare, but because the disease is usually progressive, severe, persistent disease should prompt evaluation of SFTPB. Because SFTPC mutations usually result in disease later in life, evaluation for SFTPC mutations should be considered if mutations in other genes have been excluded or if there is a family history of ILD or pulmonary fibrosis inherited in an autosomal dominant pattern.

The diagnosis of genetic disorders of surfactant production and catabolism should be considered in older children and young adults who present with chronic diffuse lung disease of unknown etiology. Particular clinical and radiographic findings that have been associated with some of these disorders and that would increase suspicion include digital clubbing, pectus excavatum, failure to thrive, diffuse ground glass infiltrates on HRCT imaging, and peripheral lung cysts. The absence of a family history of lung disease should not preclude evaluation as de novo SFTPC and NKX2.1 mutations may cause sporadic disease, and ABCA3 deficiency is inherited as an autosomal recessive disorder. Whereas most children with ABCA3 deficiency have neonatal lung disease, there is sufficient overlap between the later-onset clinical presentations of ABCA3 deficiency and SFTPC mutations to warrant analysis of both genes. SFTPB analysis can usually be deferred in older children because most SP-B-deficient children have very severe lung disease and survival beyond the first year of life is rare. Neurologic findings, including hypotonia or developmental delay, should prompt consideration of an NKX2.1 mutation or deletion, as should hypothyroidism. NKX2.1 mutations and deletions also should be considered in children in whom there is a strong clinical suspicion or lung pathology findings of surfactant dysfunction in the absence of positive genetic findings for SFTPC, ABCA,3 or SFTPB. Finally, children or adolescents with insidious onset of disease and diffuse alveolar infiltrates after the neonatal period or who have biopsy findings consistent with alveolar proteinosis should be evaluated for CSF2RA and CSF2RB mutations.

There are important limitations to genetic testing. Such testing is not 100% sensitive; functionally significant variants in untranslated regions that affect gene expression or mRNA splicing will not be detected. Gene deletions, insertions, duplications, and rearrangements may be missed unless specific methods are used to look for such variants. Additionally, interpretation of results may be difficult, particularly in the case of missense mutations, for it may not be possible to determine whether an identified novel variant represents a disease-causing mutation or a rare yet benign sequence variant. It may be difficult to determine whether subjects in whom only one ABCA3 mutation is identified are affected with a mutation that escaped detection on the other allele or are simply carriers, and the finding of an ABCA3 mutation is therefore unrelated to the cause of their lung disease. Full analysis of all of the genes of interest may take several weeks, which may be inadequate in a patient who is unstable or has rapidly progressive disease. Finally, genetic testing is expensive; the costs for such testing may not be covered by insurance, and it may be impractical for most patients to pay for the testing out of pocket.

Lung Histopathology

Lung biopsy is sometimes considered to be the gold standard in diagnosis of interstitial lung diseases but has distinct limitations. Lung histopathology can help distinguish disorders of surfactant clearance from disorders of surfactant production, based in part on the presence and level of disruption of alveolar architecture. However, lung histopathology does not distinguish the relatively common form of autoimmune PAP from hereditary PAP caused by CSF2RA or CSF2RB mutations; nor can it distinguish between the latter two. Sampling error can be an important limitation for diagnosis based on lung histopathology even when tissues are obtained based on surgical biopsies. This is particularly true in diseases with a heterogeneous, 'geographic' involvement of the lungs. When lung biopsies are indicated, the tissues should be obtained and handled appropriately, according to published guidelines in order to optimize diagnostic yield and should include obtaining tissue for electron microscopy and frozen tissue.[160]

Lung and Serum Biomarkers

Serum GM-CSF autoantibody testing, while not yet commercially available, is particularly useful in identifying individuals with autoimmune PAP and has a sensitivity and specificity approaching 100%. This test is available at centers currently conducting test validation studies and is recommended for all adults, adolescents, and older children with the typical history and radiographic findings of PAP. Identification of specific biomarkers in blood or lung fluid could provide useful tools for diagnosis or disease progression.[147,161] For example, increased levels of surfactant protein in either lung fluid or serum may provide a simple and useful means to monitor lung disease severity in these disorders. However, such tests are currently available only in research protocols, and are of uncertain sensitivity and specificity for surfactant-related lung diseases.[102] In contrast, the finding of an elevated serum GM-CSF level and a negative serum GM-CSF autoantibody level in patients with hereditary PAP caused by CSF2RA or CSF2RB mutations appears to be a useful screening diagnostic test.

■ SUMMARY

Single gene defects have been identified that disrupt surfactant production and metabolism (ABCA3, SFTPB, SFTPC, NKX2.1), as well as surfactant catabolism

TABLE 56-1 GENETIC DISORDERS ASSOCIATED WITH DISRUPTION OF SURFACTANT HOMEOSTASIS

	TTF1 HAPLOINSUFFICIENCY	SP-B DEFICIENCY	ABCA3 DEFICIENCY	SP-C GENE MUTATION	GM-CSF RECEPTOR A CHAIN DEFICIENCY	GM-CSF RECEPTOR B CHAIN DEFICIENCY
Gene	NKX2.1	SFTPB	ABCA3	SFTPC	CSF2RA	CSF2RB
Chromosomal location	14q13.3	2p11.2	16p13.3	8p23.3	Xp22.32 Yp11.3	22q13.1
No. of Exons	3	11	33	6	13	14
Age of onset	Newborn to childhood	Newborn	Newborn to adolescent	Newborn to adult	Infancy to adolescent	Childhood to adult
Pulmonary presentation	nRDS ILD	nRDS	nRDS ILD	ILD nRDS	Dyspnea	Dyspnea
Extrapulmonary involvement may include	Hypothyroidism Hypotonia Developmental delay Chorea	None	Failure to thrive	Failure to thrive	Poor growth	None (?)
Inheritance	Sporadic or AD	AR	AR	AD or sporadic	AR*	AR
Pathogenesis	Loss of function	Loss of function	Loss of function	Gain of toxic function or dominant negative	Loss of function	Loss of function
Pathology		PAP CPI	PAP DIP CPI NSIP	CPI NSIP DIP PAP UIP	Alveolar surfactant accumulation without Alveolar wall disruption	Alveolar surfactant accumulation without Alveolar wall disruption
Course/outcome	Variable	Fatal	Variable	Variable	Variable	Variable

AD, Autosomal dominant; *AR*, autosomal recessive; *CPI*, chronic pneumonitis of infancy; *DIP*, desquamative interstitial pneumonia; *ILD*, interstitial lung disease; *nRDS*, neonatal respiratory distress syndrome; *NSIP*, non-specific interstitial pneumonia; *PAP*, pulmonary alveolar proteinosis; *UIP*, usual interstitial pneumonia;
*Pattern is autosomal recessive because the locus is on the pseudoautosomal region of X chromosome.

(CSF2RA, CSF2RB). The phenotypes of these disorders include acute neonatal respiratory failure; progressive diffuse childhood lung disease; pulmonary fibrosis in adults; and dyspnea and respiratory failure from surfactant accumulation in children, adolescents, and adults. There is considerable overlap in the clinical features and lung pathology findings associated with these disorders, which are summarized in Table 56-1. Genetic testing is needed for specific diagnosis, which may obviate the need for lung biopsy in some patients. Specific therapies for these disorders are not currently available. Lung transplantation has been performed for disorders of surfactant production. Disorders of surfactant catabolism result from macrophage dysfunction, and bone marrow transplantation would be needed. Given the complexity of the surfactant system, it is likely that other genetic disorders disrupting surfactant metabolism will be identified as causes of rare lung disease, providing new insights into normal surfactant metabolism, and suggesting candidate genes contributing to the pathogenesis of more common lung diseases such as neonatal RDS.

ACKNOWLEDGEMENTS

The authors gratefully acknowledge the collaboration and contributions of Jeffrey Whitsett, Susan Wert, Timothy Weaver, and Takuji Suzuki, Cincinnati Children's Hospital and University of Cincinnati College of Medicine, Cincinnati, OH; Aaron Hamvas and F. Sessions Cole, St. Louis Children's Hospital and Washington University, St. Louis, MO; and Michael Dean, NCI, Frederick, MD. We are also grateful for the support of grants from the National Institutes of Health, HL-54703 (L.M.N), HL-085433 (B.C.T), National Center for Research Resources, RR019498 (B.C.T.), the Division of Pulmonary Biology, Cincinnati Children's Hospital Research Foundation (B.C.T.) and the Eudowood Foundation (L.M.N.).

References

The complete reference list is available online at www.expertconsult.com

57 PULMONARY INVOLVEMENT IN THE SYSTEMIC INFLAMMATORY DISEASES OF CHILDHOOD

Sharon D. Dell, BEng, MD, FRCPC, and Rayfel Schneider, MBBCh, FRCPC

In this chapter we highlight pulmonary manifestations of the systemic inflammatory diseases of childhood, with a focus on the diseases that are either common in the pediatric rheumatology clinic or those that commonly involve the lungs. These include juvenile idiopathic arthritis (JIA), the connective tissue diseases (systemic lupus erythematosus [SLE], scleroderma [SSc], juvenile dermatomyositis [JDM], and mixed connective tissue disease [MCTD]), vasculitides (especially Wegener's granulomatosis [WG]), and sarcoidosis. Clinically significant pulmonary involvement due to systemic inflammatory disease is rare in the pediatric setting. However, it is important for the pediatric pulmonologist to be familiar with this topic for two reasons: (1) pulmonary involvement may be associated with high morbidity and mortality in this population, and (2) pulmonary disease may be the predominant initial clinical presentation in a subset of these patients. The systemic inflammatory diseases most frequently encountered by the pediatric pulmonologist include WG, SLE, SSc, and MCTD. Symptom patterns along with specific autoantibody serologic tests are most useful for diagnosing the underlying systemic inflammatory disease (Table 57-1). Pulmonary involvement in these cases often can be a difficult diagnostic dilemma because lung toxicity due to potent pharmacotherapies and opportunistic infections must be considered alongside the possibility of the lung being a target organ of the underlying inflammatory disease. Lung disease may involve any compartment of the lung (chest wall, pleura, airways, parenchyma, and vasculature), and often concurrent pulmonary etiologies may be present (e.g., pulmonary fibrosis and chest wall restriction). Although there is certainly overlap in the pulmonary manifestations among different diseases, certain patterns are recognized with greater frequency in some entities (Table 57-2). For example, interstitial lung disease (ILD) and pulmonary arterial hypertension (PAH) are characteristic of systemic sclerosis, while pleuritis and pleural effusions are characteristic of JIA and SLE and would be very unusual in the context of JDM. For the purposes of classifying lung disease in this chapter, ILD is defined as a clinical diagnosis of "pulmonary fibrosis" or a lung biopsy histopathologic pattern of nonspecific interstitial pneumonitis (NSIP), usual interstitial pneumonitis (UIP), lymphocytic interstitial pneumonitis (LIP), bronchiolitis obliterans organizing pneumonia (BOOP, also known as cryptogenic organizing pneumonia), or diffuse alveolar damage (DAD).[1] Treatment of lung disease is specific to the underlying systemic disease and is often effective at reducing pulmonary morbidity. Prognosis is variable and dependent on the severity of the disease and

its response to therapy. Disease progression is monitored by following symptoms, particularly dyspnea, the use of routine pulmonary function and exercise testing, and high-resolution computed tomography (HRCT) imaging. The role of serologic biomarkers, particularly SP-D and KL-6, is an area of active investigation. As prognosis for the systemic inflammatory diseases improves, increasing emphasis is being placed on early detection and treatment of lung disease.

JUVENILE IDIOPATHIC ARTHRITIS (JIA)

Epidemiology

JIA is the most common chronic rheumatic disease in childhood with a prevalence of 16 to 150 per 100,000.[2] The term *juvenile idiopathic arthritis* includes a heterogeneous group of diseases that have in common the following characteristics: arthritis that begins before the age of 16 years, persists for at least 6 weeks, and for which no specific cause can be found. Overall, girls are affected approximately twice as commonly as boys, but this varies considerably with the different subtypes. The age of onset ranges from less than 1 year of age to 16 years of age with a peak between 1 and 3 years for the most common subtypes. The onset of JIA in the first 6 months of life is rare and should raise suspicion of another diagnosis. In a large, multiethnic cohort of JIA patients, children of European descent had an increased risk of JIA, and there were significant differences in the frequency of different subtypes of JIA in different ethnic groups.[3]

Etiology and Pathogenesis

The cause of JIA remains unknown, and the pathogenesis has not been clearly elucidated. Given the heterogeneity of the disease phenotypes, it is not surprising that the different subtypes have different genetic predispositions and associations, different autoantibody profiles, and differences in immune dysregulation. JIA is a complex genetic disease with multiple genetic associations. HLA-A2 is associated with early onset JIA, especially in the oligoarticular subtype. There are strong HLA associations with oligoarticular JIA (HLA-DRB1*08, 11 and 13 and DPB1*02). HLA-DRB1*08 also is associated with rheumatoid factor (RF)-negative polyarticular JIA, and RF-positive JIA is associated with *DRB1*04, DQA1*03*, and *DQB1*03*.[4] There is also a significant association of HLA-B27 with enthesitis-related arthritis and juvenile

TABLE 57-1 COMMONLY REQUESTED SEROLOGIC TESTS FOR SELECTED PEDIATRIC SYSTEMIC INFLAMMATORY DISEASES WITH POSSIBLE PULMONARY INVOLVEMENT

AUTOANTIBODY SEROLOGIC TEST	DISEASE ENTITY	COMMENTS
ANA	Nonrheumatic disease	Present in 10% of normal children; may occur with infection, drug, malignancy
	SLE	Present in virtually 100% of SLE, but not specific
	Oligoarticular JIA	Present in 60% to 80%, marker for uveitis
	JDM	Present in 50% to 75%
	SSc	Present in 90% systemic sclerosis, 50% of localized scleroderma
	MCTD	Present in 100%, speckled pattern and very high titer
Anti-dsDNA	SLE	Present in 60% to 90%; very specific; titer correlates with disease activity
Anti-Sm	SLE	Present in 25% to 40%; very specific; correlates with renal disease
Anti-Ro/anti-La	SLE, Sjögren's syndrome	
Anti-RNP	SLE, MCTD, scleroderma	When present in very high titer, suggests MCTD
Anticardiolipin	SLE, antiphospholipid antibody syndrome	May also occur in infection and malignancy; IgG isotype associated with thrombosis
Anti-Jo-1	Myositis	Rare in children; marker for ILD in adult dermatomyositis
Anti-Scl-70	SSc	Marker for severe lung disease
Anticentromere	Limited SSc	Rare in children; marker for late development of pulmonary hypertension
ANCA	Vasculitides	May also occur with SLE and inflammatory bowel disease
c-ANCA	Wegener's granulomatosis	Sensitive and specific, especially when associated with anti-proteinase 3 antibody
p-ANCA	MPA	Sensitive and specific, especially when associated with anti-myeloperoxidase antibody
Rheumatoid factor	RF + polyarticular JIA	Poor sensitivity and specificity for JIA; when present in patients with JIA, it is associated with severe disease (usually adolescent females); also positive in 50% WG

ANA, Antinuclear antibody; *ANCA*, antineutrophil cytoplasmic antibody; *anti-dsDNA*, anti–double-stranded deoxyribonucleic acid; *anti-Sm*, anti–smooth muscle antibody; *ILD*, interstitial lung disease; *JDM*, juvenile dermatomyositis; *JIA*, juvenile idiopathic arthritis; *MCTD*, mixed connective tissue disease; *MPA*, microscopic polyangiitis; *RF*, rheumatoid factor; *RNP*, ribonucleoprotein; *SLE*, systemic lupus erythematosus; *SSc*, systemic sclerosis; *WG*, Wegener's granulomatosis.

ankylosing spondylitis.[5] A number of polymorphisms have been associated with JIA, including a polymorphism involving the protein tyrosine phosphatase N22 gene.[6] The systemic subtype is characterized by a lack of auto-antibodies and by significant elevations of interleukin-6 (IL-6) and dysregulation of interleukin-1 production. Recent studies using biological agents that block the actions of both IL-6 (tocilizumab) and IL-1 (anakinra) have proven to be effective in treating patients with active systemic disease. The dysregulation of IL-1 in systemic JIA and the efficacy of IL-1 inhibitors in reversing manifestations of the disease suggest that it is more likely an autoinflammatory disease than an autoimmune disease. Antinuclear antibodies (ANA) are frequently found in children with oligoarticular disease and are seen somewhat less frequently in polyarticular JIA. The presence of ANA is clearly associated with a higher risk of uveitis, the most common extra-articular manifestation of both oligoarthritis (occurring in 21%) and RF-negative polyarticular arthritis (14%).[7]

Clinical Manifestations

The clinical manifestations of JIA depend on the subtype, which is defined by the presenting features within the first 6 months of disease onset (Table 57-3). The most common subtype in Europe and North America is oligoarticular JIA, which primarily affects large joints. This can remain oligoarticular or extend after the first 6 months to involve additional joints. Both oligoarticular and RF-negative polyarticular JIA most commonly affect young preschool age girls. Asymptomatic anterior uveitis occurs in oligoarticular JIA, RF-negative polyarticular JIA, and psoriatic arthritis. If undetected by routine slit lamp examination, uveitis can result in blindness. Rheumatoid factor–positive polyarticular JIA most commonly first manifests in older girls; is phenotypically similar to adult rheumatoid arthritis, where arthritis affects small and large joints in a symmetrical pattern; and is sometimes associated with rheumatoid nodules. Enthesitis-related arthritis (ERA) typically develops in boys over the age of 8 years and is characterized by

TABLE 57-2 SUMMARY OF PULMONARY MANIFESTATIONS OF SYSTEMIC INFLAMMATORY DISEASE IN CHILDREN

	JIA	SLE	JDM	SSC	MCTD	SARCOIDOSIS	WG	MPA
Frequency at initial presentation[a]	+	++	+	+++	+	+++	+++	+
Frequency during disease course[b]	+	+++	+	+++	+++	+++	+++	++
Chest wall/diaphragm[c]	+	+	+++	+	+	–	–	–
Pleural disease[d]	++	+++	–	+	++	+	+	–
Large airway lesions[e]	–	–	–	–	–	++	++	–
Bronchiectasis	+	+	–	+	–	+	+	–
Acute pneumonitis[f]	+	++	+	–	–	–	–	–
Interstitial lung disease (ILD)[g]	+	+	+	+++	++	+	–	–
Pulmonary granulomas	–	–	–	–	–	+++	+++	–
Vasculitis/DAH	+	+	–	+	+	–	++	+++
Pulmonary hypertension	–	+	+	++	++	–	–	+
Thrombosis	–	++	–	–	–	–	+	–

DAH, Diffuse alveolar hemorrhage; *JIA,* juvenile idiopathic arthritis; *MCTD,* mixed connective tissue disease; *MPA,* microscopic polyangiitis *SLE,* systemic lupus erythematosus; *SSc,* systemic sclerosis; *WG,* Wegener's granulomatosis.
[a]Pulmonary involvement at initial presentation of systemic inflammatory disease.
[b]Frequency of pulmonary involvement during disease course.
[c]Includes respiratory muscle weakness and diaphragm dysfunction.
[d]Pleuritis and/or pleural effusion.
[e]Upper airway and endobronchial lesions and/or stenosis visible on bronchoscopy.
[f]A clinical diagnosis with acute onset of fever, tachypnea, hypoxia, and pulmonary infiltrates with or without pleural effusion on chest imaging, in the absence of infection and usually responding quickly to anti-inflammatory treatment.
[g]Includes clinical diagnosis of "pulmonary fibrosis" and histopathologic diagnosis of usual interstitial pneumonia (UIP), nonspecific interstitial pneumonitis (NSIP), lymphocytic interstitial pneumonitis (LIP), bronchiolitis obliterans organizing pneumonia (BOOP), and diffuse alveolar damage (DAD).

predominantly lower limb arthritis in association with enthesitis, inflammation where ligaments, tendons, or joint capsules attach to bone. The heel and knee are the most commonly involved entheses. This may be the forerunner of ankylosing spondylitis in adult life. ERA may be accompanied by symptomatic anterior uveitis with a painful, red eye in a proportion of patients. Systemic arthritis is distinct from the other subtypes because the systemic manifestations of fever, rash, hepatosplenomegaly, lymphadenopathy and serositis (particularly pericarditis) are usually prominent at onset. Arthritis may occur at disease onset but sometimes only develops after weeks or even months. The diagnosis of psoriatic arthritis in children may depend on arthritis associated with psoriatic nail changes, dactylitis, or a family history of psoriasis because arthritis frequently precedes the development of psoriatic skin lesions by many years.

Classification and Diagnosis of JIA

The International League of Associations for Rheumatology (ILAR) criteria for the classification of JIA are now widely accepted. The inclusion criteria for the different subtypes are listed in Table 57-3. There are also a number of exclusions for each category that are beyond the scope of this chapter

Pulmonary Involvement in JIA

Pulmonary involvement in JIA is uncommon, and significant pulmonary manifestations, except for pleuritis, are sufficiently rare to warrant thorough evaluation for other conditions such as infections, systemic vasculitis, SLE, and other connective tissue diseases. Pleuritis is a well-reported manifestation of systemic JIA, but it is usually accompanied by pericarditis. One should be particularly careful to exclude the diagnosis of SLE in an older girl who presents with isolated pleuritis and arthritis. There are few reports of pulmonary disease in JIA. One of the earliest studies, completed 30 years ago, found pulmonary disease in 4% of patients. The radiologic abnormalities included pneumonitis, interstitial reticular and nodular infiltrates, and pleural effusions. Pathologic correlates of these finding were pulmonary hemosiderosis, lymphoid follicular bronchiolitis, and lymphocytic interstitial pneumonitis. Some patients with parenchymal disease

TABLE 57-3 SUBTYPES OF JIA

SUBTYPE	SUBTYPE INCLUSION CRITERIA[269]	PERCENTAGE OF ALL JIA[2]	SEX RATIO[2]
Systemic	Arthritis PLUS fever for 2 weeks, daily for at least 3 days PLUS at least one of the following: Rash Serositis Generalized lymphadenopathy Hepatomegaly or splenomegaly	4%–17%	F = M
Oligoarticular	Four or fewer affected joints within first 6 months Persistent: remain with ≤4 joints Extended: >4 joints after 6 months	27%–56%	F>>>M
Polyarticular RF negative	≥5 joints in first 6 months	11%–28%	F>>M
Polyarticular RF positive	≥5 joints in first 6 months	2%–7%	
Enthesitis-related arthritis	Arthritis PLUS enthesitis OR Arthritis OR enthesitis PLUS at least 2 of the following: Sacroiliac joint tenderness and/or inflammatory spinal pain Presence of HLA-B27 Family history of HLA-B27–associated disease Anterior uveitis (usually symptomatic) Onset of arthritis in a boy >8 years	3%–11%	M>>F
Psoriatic arthritis	Arthritis PLUS psoriasis OR Arthritis PLUS at least 2 of the following: Dactylitis Nail pitting or onycholysis Psoriasis in a first-degree relative	2%–11%	F>M
Unclassified	Does not meet criteria for one of the above OR Meets criteria for >1 of the above	11%–21%	

developed radiographic evidence of interstitial fibrosis.[8] There are additional reports of pulmonary hemosiderosis in JIA[9,10] and a report of lymphocytic interstitial pneumonitis that actually preceded the diagnosis of RF-positive JIA by 10 years.[11]

The most severe pulmonary manifestations have been seen with the systemic and polyarticular subtypes. Pulmonary hypertension has been reported in a patient with systemic JIA in the absence of any documented pulmonary parenchymal disease. This patient responded well to treatment with cyclosporine and systemic corticosteroids.[12] Severe, potentially fatal, endogenous lipoid pneumonia in children with systemic JIA, not secondary to aspiration, is a rare complication associated with severe, refractory disease. A 5-year-old girl who developed radiographic features suggestive of progressive pulmonary fibrosis had interstitial and intra-alveolar cholesterol granulomas identified on lung biopsy. Although she appeared to stabilize on immunosuppressive treatment with methotrexate and etanercept, she subsequently succumbed with respiratory failure.[13] We have seen an additional systemic arthritis patient with a similarly refractory disease course who developed fatal pulmonary lipoid pneumonia (Fig. 57-1). A 21-year-old male, following a long history of severe systemic JIA with persistent systemic symptoms and damaging arthritis, developed endogenous lipoid pneumonia that was ultimately treated with double lung transplantation.[14]

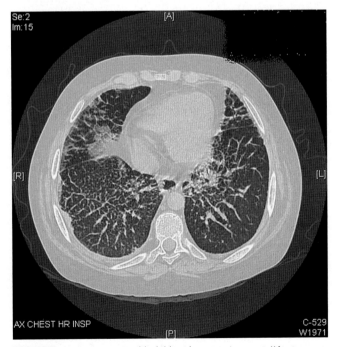

FIGURE 57-1. A 12-year-old child with systemic onset JIA at age 15 months who developed gradual onset of dyspnea, cough, and crackles on auscultation. HRCT scan showed bilateral diffuse interstitial changes, including thickening of the interlobular septa, nodules, and areas of fibrosis and ground-glass densities. A lung biopsy confirmed the diagnosis of endogenous lipoid pneumonia with interstitial and intra-alveolar cholesterol granulomas.

Bronchiolitis obliterans organizing pneumonia (BOOP) has been described in adults with rheumatoid arthritis,[15] but there are few reports of this complication associated with JIA.[16] Bronchiolitis obliterans (BO) was described in a 12-year-old girl following treatment of her arthritis with intramuscular gold injections. Despite immunosuppressive treatment and subsequent lung transplantation, the BO was progressive and fatal.[17] BO also has been reported in a patient with JIA whose first symptoms were those related to pneumomediastinum.[18]

Studies of pulmonary function in JIA have detected abnormal pulmonary function tests (PFTs) in more than 50% of asymptomatic patients. Restrictive disease patterns have been more commonly identified than obstructive abnormalities.[19] Results of diffusing capacity of the lung for carbon monoxide (DLCO) measurements have been more variable, with reductions in DLCO reported in 3.7% to 45%.[20-22] Reductions of maximum inspiratory and expiratory pressures, suggestive of respiratory muscle weakness, may influence PFTs in these patients, but there also may be a correlation of impaired pulmonary function with disease severity, as measured by the erythrocyte sedimentation rate (ESR) and requirement for treatment with methotrexate. Because methotrexate is the most commonly used second-line drug for the treatment of JIA, it is important to consider whether it has any impact on the development of lung disease. Low-dose weekly methotrexate has been reported to cause an acute pneumonitis associated with fever, cough, and dyspnea. There also have been concerns raised about methotrexate-induced chronic, progressive pulmonary fibrosis.[23,24] However, several studies suggest that methotrexate does not increase the risk of pulmonary disease in children with arthritis.[20,25,26]

Macrophage activation syndrome (MAS) is a severe, potentially life-threatening complication of JIA, occurring in approximately 10% of children with the systemic subtype. Characteristic clinical features are sustained, high fever, hepatosplenomegaly, lymphadenopathy and sometimes bleeding, bruising and encephalopathy. Characteristic laboratory features include a sudden drop in white blood cell counts, platelet counts, and hemoglobin with elevated transaminases, LDH, coagulopathy, and very high levels of serum ferritin. A significant proportion of patients develop myocardial dysfunction and require intensive care support. One large series reported pulmonary involvement in 50% of patients and one third of all patients required ventilatory support.[27] Pulmonary manifestations include lung infiltrates, pneumonitis, pulmonary edema, and pulmonary hemorrhage.

Treatment

Nonsteroidal anti-inflammatory drugs (NSAIDS) and intra-articular corticosteroid injections[28] are considered first-line treatments for children with JIA and may be all that is required to treat oligoarticular involvement or mild disease. Those children, for whom arthritis does not respond adequately, especially those with a polyarticular course, are treated with low-dose weekly methotrexate. The advent of new biologic agents has dramatically improved outcomes for children whose arthritis is refractory to methotrexate.[29] Tumor necrosis factor-alpha (TNF-α) inhibitors, such as etanercept,[30] adalimumab,[31] or infliximab usually are used if there is an inadequate response to methotrexate or if there is intolerance to methotrexate. Different treatment algorithms are followed for different subtypes: neither methotrexate nor TNF-α inhibitors are particularly effective for systemic JIA. Children who have persistent systemic symptoms and arthritis despite NSAIDS usually respond to systemic corticosteroids. New evidence supports the use of IL-1 antagonists such as anakinra[32] or the IL-6 antagonist, tocilizumab,[33] for patients who are steroid dependent. Pediatric rheumatologists are starting to treat patients with IL-1 inhibition even before corticosteroids are used. Acute symptomatic serositis, especially pericarditis, may require intravenous pulsed methylprednisolone. A similar approach is taken for MAS with early use of cyclosporine or IL-1 inhibitors if there is not a rapid response. Enthesitis-related arthritis does not respond as well as other subtypes to methotrexate but may respond to treatment with sulfasalazine.[34] Axial spine involvement may need early institution of TNF-α inhibitors.

Prognosis

The mortality in JIA is well below 1%,[35] with a disproportionate mortality risk in the systemic subtype, largely because of the associated MAS and infections associated with immunosuppressive therapy. Overall, active arthritis persists on long-term follow-up even into adult life in more than 50% of patients. Poor prognostic features of the systemic subtype include persistent systemic symptoms, marked thrombocytosis, and polyarticular arthritis in the first 6 months of disease.[36] For the other subtypes, positive rheumatoid factor, marked and persistent elevation of inflammatory markers, involvement of the hip joint, and early joint space loss and erosions predict poor outcome.[37,38] Acute pleuritis usually responds well to treatment without sequelae, but some rare pulmonary manifestations such as lipoid pneumonia and pulmonary fibrosis may do poorly in the long term.

■ SYSTEMIC LUPUS ERYTHEMATOSUS (SLE)

Epidemiology

SLE predominantly affects young women, but in approximately 15% to 20% of individuals, the disease presents before 18 years of age. SLE is relatively rare in children, with an estimated incidence of 10 to 20 per 100,000 that is considerably higher in black, Hispanic, South and Southeast Asian, and North American First Nations populations. In postpubertal adolescents, females are clearly more commonly affected than males (approximately 6:1), but in the younger age groups, the female predominance is much less marked.[39]

Pathogenesis

SLE is the prototypic autoimmune disease, characterized by the presence of autoantibodies in virtually all patients. There is substantial evidence of both innate and adaptive immune dysregulation and also of immune activation and autoimmunity resulting from the interaction of lupus-associated genes with environmental triggers. Environmental triggers include ultraviolet radiation, infections, drugs, and chemicals. The activation of the immune system is amplified by lupus autoantibodies and their associated nucleic acids, together with cytokines and chemokines, resulting in inflammation and tissue damage.[40] Autoantibodies actually can be detected many years before the development of clinically symptomatic SLE.[41]

Clinical Features

Common presenting symptoms of SLE in children are rash, joint pain, and constitutional symptoms such as fatigue, fever, and weight loss. The most common presenting features in a large cohort of pediatric lupus patients were arthritis (67%), malar rash (66%), nephritis (55%), and central nervous system disease (27%).[42]

The American College of Rheumatology criteria for the classification of lupus in adults appear to apply well to children with SLE (Box 57-1) and have been reported to achieve a sensitivity of 96% and specificity of 100% for the diagnosis of SLE in a pediatric population.[43] Although the classification criteria require that 4 or more of the 11 criteria are present, there are no published diagnostic criteria, and the diagnosis of SLE in children can certainly be made when fewer than 4 criteria are present.

BOX 57-1 CLASSIFICATION CRITERIA FOR SLE*

1. Malar rash
2. Discoid rash
3. Photosensitivity
4. Nasal or oral ulcers
5. Arthritis involving at least two joints
6. Serositis
   Pleuritis, or
   Pericarditis
7. Renal disorder
   Proteinuria > 0.5 g/day, or
   Cellular casts in the urine
8. Neurologic disorder
   Seizures, or
   Psychosis
9. Hematologic disorder
   Hemolytic anemia, or
   Leukopenia (< 4,000/mm), or
   Lymphopenia (< 1,500/mm), or
   Thrombocytopenia (< 100,000/mm)
10. Immunologic disorder
    Anti-DNA antibody, or
    Anti-Sm antibody, or
    Anti-phospholipid antibody
11. Positive antinuclear antibody

Adapted from Hochberg MC. Updating the American College of Rheumatology revised criteria for the classification of systemic lupus erythematosus. *Arthritis Rheum.* 1997;40(9):1725.

*A person is classified as having SLE if at least 4 of the 11 criteria are present serially or simultaneously.

Pulmonary Involvement

Pulmonary involvement in pediatric SLE has been reported to occur in 18% to 40% of patients within the first year of diagnosis and in 18% to 81% of patients at any time during the disease course.[44] It occurs more frequently in Afro-Caribbeans.[45] Studies that report higher rates of pulmonary involvement include abnormal PFTs or abnormal imaging studies even in the absence of symptoms. Pulmonary involvement can indeed be very mild, or even asymptomatic, but it also can be life-threatening with respiratory failure. Pulmonary lupus has been reported to be more severe when SLE begins within the first 2 years of life.[46] Pleuritis with pleural effusion is the only pulmonary manifestation to be included among the criteria for the classification of SLE[47] and occurs in 9% to 32% of patients[48–50] and may even be the initial clinical manifestation of SLE. In a large cohort of adult lupus patients, pleuritis was found to occur more frequently in patients with a younger age at disease onset, longer disease duration, who manifested more cumulative disease-related damage, and in those who had positive anti-Sm and anti-RNP antibodies.[51] Pleural effusions are exudative and may be unilateral or bilateral. These must be differentiated from infectious exudative effusions and also from transudative effusions related to renal or cardiac disease. SLE is associated with an increased risk of a wide range of infections, including bacterial, viral, mycobacterial, fungal, and parasitic infections with the respiratory tract as one of the common sites.[52] In addition, immunosuppressive treatments to control the disease confer an increased risk of opportunistic infections such as pneumocystis, cytomegalovirus, and fungal infections. Inflammatory pulmonary lesions may be difficult or even impossible to differentiate from pulmonary hemorrhage or pulmonary infections. Because infection is the leading cause of death in children with lupus,[53] rigorous exclusion of potential infections is necessary before attributing pulmonary manifestations to disease activity. Cultures of sputum (if obtainable), nasopharyngeal secretions, blood, and pleural fluid should be performed, but bronchoalveolar lavage and lung biopsy may be necessary. Children at risk should be carefully evaluated for tuberculosis.

Acute pneumonitis is uncommon in adults with lupus and even less common in pediatric lupus. The presentation includes fever, nonproductive cough, dyspnea, pleuritic chest pain, and tachypnea. Chest radiographic findings are nonspecific with infiltrates that can mimic infections or hemorrhage and that may be accompanied by pleural effusions (Fig. 57-2). Chronic ILD due to SLE is extremely rare; in a necropsy series of 90 lupus patients, none had acute or chronic pneumonitis.[54] If chronic pneumonitis does occur, Sjögren's syndrome, infection, or drug toxicity should be excluded. Chronic ILD can follow acute lupus pneumonitis[55] but also can develop in a more insidious manner with exertional dyspnea, chronic cough, pleuritic chest pain, and basal rales.[56] Patients tend to have multisystem manifestations of SLE. Pulmonary function studies typically follow a slowly progressive course with a restrictive pattern, but they may improve or at least stabilize. Histopathology demonstrates alveolar

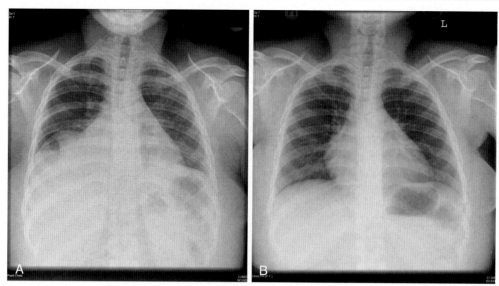

FIGURE 57-2. Chest radiographs of a 10-year-old girl diagnosed with systemic lupus erythematosus who presented with acute onset of fever, dyspnea, chest pain, malaise, weight loss, malar skin rash, and arthralgias. **A,** Initial presentation with pleuritis and acute interstitial pneumonia. Radiograph shows bilateral pleural effusions and lower lobe opacification, worse on right side. **B,** Rapid resolution of symptoms and imaging abnormalities after pulse steroid therapy.

wall thickening, interstitial fibrosis, interstitial lymphocytic infiltrates, and granular deposits of immunoglobin and complement.

Pulmonary hemorrhage is a rare but potentially life-threatening complication of SLE in children that has been reported to occur at disease onset[57] or during the course of the disease. Significant acute pulmonary hemorrhage is accompanied by severe dyspnea with or without hemoptysis and a sudden drop in hemoglobin and may progress rapidly to respiratory failure. Lupus nephritis is present in a high proportion of patients. The mortality resulting from pulmonary hemorrhage in an adult series of SLE has been as high as 50%.[58] Chest radiographs show diffuse alveolar opacities indistinguishable from fluid or infection. A recent report strongly recommends that lupus patients with acute pulmonary hemorrhage should be carefully investigated for pulmonary infections[59] since more than 50% of patients had an infection identified within 48 hours of presentation with pulmonary hemorrhage. Infections identified included *Pseudomonas*, cytomegalovirus, and *Aspergillus*. Empiric treatment with antibiotics may improve survival. Thrombotic thrombocytopenic purpura (TTP) should be ruled out, particularly in the presence of fever, thrombocytopenia, and renal dysfunction because these may be associated with SLE.

Pulmonary hypertension is rare in children with SLE, but it has been reported in 14% of adult patients followed at a tertiary care center.[60] In a large series of adult patients followed at nontertiary care centers, the prevalence of pulmonary hypertension determined by echocardiography was found to be 4.2 %.[61] The presence of a lupus anticoagulant was the only risk factor identified for the development of pulmonary hypertension in this cohort. Raynaud's phenomenon occurs more frequently in lupus patients with pulmonary hypertension than in other lupus patients. Potential causes of pulmonary hypertension in SLE include pulmonary vasculitis, pulmonary thromboembolism, ILD, and valvular heart

disease. Serum endothelin levels have been found to be higher in patients with pulmonary hypertension than in other lupus patients, and antiendothelial cell antibodies are elevated in patients with active lupus and pulmonary hypertension.[62]

Antiphospholipid antibodies are found more frequently in SLE than other connective tissue diseases with a prevalence of 44% for anticardiolipin antibodies, 40% for anti-β2 glycoprotein I, and 22% for the lupus anticoagulant.[63] Anticardiolipin titers correlate with lupus disease activity. Several studies have confirmed a strong association with antiphospholipid antibodies and vascular thromboses in children with SLE. Lupus anticoagulant appears to confer the highest risk of thrombosis, but there is also a clear association of thrombosis with anticardiolipin and anti-β2GPI.[64,65] Pulmonary embolism is the most frequent pulmonary manifestation of the antiphospholipid antibody syndrome and recurrent pulmonary embolism can result in pulmonary hypertension.[66]

Shrinking lung syndrome occurs predominantly in adults with SLE but also has been reported in children. It typically presents with progressive dyspnea, pleuritic chest pain, and tachypnea. Chest radiographs may demonstrate reduced lung volumes, raised hemidiaphragms, and basal atelectasis (Fig. 57-3), and PFTs are usually restrictive. Chest computed tomography (CT) scans do not reveal significant pleural or parenchymal lung disease. The cause of this syndrome in SLE remains unclear but diaphragmatic dysfunction with poor diaphragmatic movement demonstrable on fluoroscopy have been reported in some pediatric cases.[67] Diaphragmatic dysfunction with subsequent shrinking lung syndrome has been linked to symptomatic pleuritis.[68] Although the optimum treatment is not clear, some patients appear to respond to immunosuppressive therapy.[69]

Studies in pediatric SLE patients without clinically or radiographically apparent lung disease have found PFT

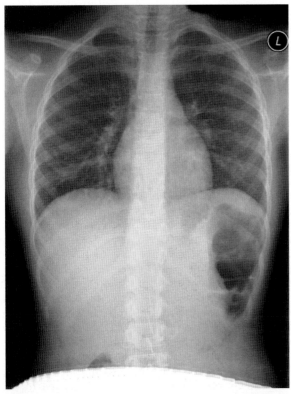

FIGURE 57-3. Chest radiograph of an 11-year-old child diagnosed with lupus and "shrinking lung syndrome." Child presented with fever, muscle weakness, weight loss, malaise, and severely restricted PFTs. Chest radiograph showed an elevated left hemidiaphragm while HRCT scan showed only subtle nonspecific changes out of keeping with pulmonary function. PFTs normalized over a period of 6 months with high-dose prednisone treatment.

abnormalities in at least one third, with a range of 38% to 84%.[70] PFT abnormalities most frequently seen are restrictive with or without a diffusion abnormality. Most studies have not shown any correlation between PFT abnormalities and lupus disease activity. It is important to note that isolated abnormal PFTs in children with lupus do not predict progressive lung disease.[71]

HRCT imaging in a cohort of 60 Norwegian patients with childhood-onset SLE revealed that 8% had abnormal findings, including micronodules and bronchiectasis, but none had ILD.[72] These findings did not correlate with PFT abnormalities. Although CT imaging is more sensitive than plain chest radiography, routine screening of asymptomatic pediatric lupus patients with CT is not recommended.

Treatment

Because infection is the major cause of mortality in pediatric SLE, children with pulmonary manifestations require rigorous investigation and treatment of infectious complications. It also is important to exclude other causes of pulmonary pathology in SLE such thromboembolism, drug toxicity and the impact of cardiac or renal disease. Corticosteroids are highly effective in treating lupus pleuritis and pleural effusions and remain the mainstay of treatment for moderate to severe pulmonary manifestations of SLE in children. The majority of children with SLE are treated with hydroxychloroquine, which is particularly

effective for cutaneous disease, arthritis, and mild constitutional symptoms and in reducing the risk of disease flares.[73] Immunosuppressive drugs such as azathioprine[74] and mycophenolate mofetil[75] frequently are used to prevent organ damage and as corticosteroid-sparing agents. There also may be a role for methotrexate[76] and cyclosporine.[77] For the most severe manifestations, such as pulmonary hemorrhage, pulse methylprednisolone (30 mg/kg/dose up to 1000 mg) may be administered daily for 3 days, followed by high-dose daily oral systemic corticosteroids. Although there are no controlled clinical trials for the treatment of pulmonary hemorrhage, intravenous pulse cyclophosphamide is also frequently used.[78] Although plasmapheresis is not of proven benefit, it has been used in life-threatening pulmonary hemorrhage. Certainly, in patients with TTP and catastrophic antiphospholipid antibody syndrome, plasmapheresis can be a life-saving therapy.[79] Rituximab, a B-cell depleting biologic agent, is assuming an increasing role in the treatment of pediatric SLE, but its role in the treatment of pulmonary manifestations remains to be defined.[80,81] Vascular thromboses associated with antiphospholipid antibodies require anticoagulation.

Prognosis

Disease severity is greater in children with SLE than in adults, and the majority of children develop organ damage within 5 to 10 years of diagnosis. Long-term morbidity includes premature atherosclerosis and osteoporosis.[39] Five-year survival rates in pediatric SLE range from 85% to 95%, but this may be improving with a recent study reporting a 99.6% survival rate. Renal disease and infections were the most common causes of death.[35]

JUVENILE DERMATOMYOSITIS

Juvenile dermatomyositis (JDM) is a rare autoimmune inflammatory myositis in which a capillary vasculopathy causes characteristic cutaneous and muscle manifestations, although other organs can be affected. In children, symptomatic lung involvement is infrequent, which is distinct from adult dermatomyositis (DM) where symptomatic lung involvement occurs in more than half of patients.

Epidemiology

JDM is the most common inflammatory myopathy in children, accounting for approximately 85% of cases,[82] with an incidence of 0.2 to 0.4 per 100,000 children.[83–86] It is a distinct disease entity from adult DM. Peak incidence occurs from 5 to 10 years of age,[85,86] and females are 2 to 5 times more likely to develop the disease than males.[84,86,87] A case report in monozygotic twins has suggested a genetic predisposition to JDM in some families.[88]

Pathogenesis

Although the etiology of JDM is unknown, genetics, environmental exposure, and infections are thought to be related to disease development.[82] No specific causative gene has been found but certain HLA alleles (HLA-B8, HLA-DQA1*0301 and HLA-DQA1*0501) and polymorphisms in TNF-α and IL-1 receptor antagonists have been reported as risk factors for the development of JDM and for certain phenotypes.[89] There is increased type I interferon gene expression[90] and upregulation of MHC class I expression on the surface of muscle fibers. JDM is characterized by various degrees of vasculopathy with immune complex deposition and the development of calcinosis in the later stages of disease.

Clinical Manifestations

JDM has a relatively homogeneous presentation in children with mainly cutaneous and muscle manifestations.[87,91] The initial symptoms are usually skin rash (often with heliotrope rash over the eyelids and Gottron's papules over extensor surfaces of joints), fever, and proximal muscle weakness. Characteristic changes in the nail fold capillary bed are common, and measuring the density of capillaries/mm may be a useful tool for monitoring clinical activity in JDM.[92] Other disease manifestations include skin ulcerations, soft tissue calcification, arthritis, lipodystrophy, and insulin resistance. Serious gastrointestinal and lung involvement occur only occasionally.

Diagnosis

According to the traditional criteria of Bohan and Peter,[93,94] the diagnosis of JDM is based on the following five criteria: proximal muscle weakness, characteristic rash, elevated muscle enzymes, characteristic myopathic findings on electromyography, and typical muscle biopsy findings. Criteria for definite JDM are the pathognomonic rash and three other criteria, while the diagnosis of probable JDM requires the rash and two other criteria.[91] Most children with JDM do have both proximal muscle weakness and rash, and elevated serum muscle enzymes are usually, but not always, present. Newer proposed criteria include the presence of nail fold capillary abnormalities,[92] magnetic resonance imaging (MRI) that demonstrates the presence of muscle inflammation, calcinosis, and dysphonia.[95] In cases where the diagnosis remains uncertain, the more invasive muscle biopsy may be necessary. JDM must be differentiated from other noninflammatory causes of muscle weakness (muscular dystrophies and metabolic myopathies), transient postviral myositis, and myositis due to other rheumatologic diseases (systemic scleroderma, systemic lupus erythematosus, mixed connective tissue disease, and systemic juvenile idiopathic arthritis). An elevated C-reactive protein level and ESR and the presence of antinuclear antibodies are common but nonspecific findings that have limited diagnostic value. Myositis-specific antibodies, which are commonly associated with adult forms of DM and polymyositis, are uncommon in JDM; hence, they are not usually helpful in making the diagnosis.[96] However, the presence of anti-Jo-1 and antisynthetase antibodies are associated with ILD in adults[97] and also may be associated with more severe disease in children that more closely resembles adult DM.[89,96]

Pulmonary Involvement

ILD is a common cause of morbidity and mortality for adult onset DM and polymyositis, occurring in up to 65% of cases.[98] In adults, ILD may precede, appear concomitantly with, or develop after the onset of skin and muscle manifestations.[98] In contrast, symptomatic pulmonary involvement is infrequent in children with JDM. In the largest case series of JDM presented to date, only 1 of 105 patients (<1%) at the Hospital for Sick Children in Toronto, Canada, developed symptomatic ILD.[91] (Fig. 57-4). Other case series have reported higher rates of ILD detected by pulmonary function testing and HRCT scanning; however, most of these cases were not histologically confirmed.[99,100] Although symptomatic ILD is rare enough that its description is mainly limited to case reports,[101–104] it is important to recognize its onset because it can be rapidly progressive and fatal[102–104](Fig. 57-5). Pneumomediastinum is a characteristic complication of adult DM with interstitial pneumonitis[105] and also has been reported in JDM[101–104] (Fig. 57-6). Aspiration pneumonia and hypoventilation also are frequently reported pulmonary complications in adult DM.[98] In adult studies, the strongest predictive factor for ILD in patients with myositis is the presence of anti-Jo-1 antibodies.[97]

The most common presenting symptoms of ILD are cough and dyspnea; however, ILD is reported to occur without symptoms. PFTs show a restrictive ventilatory defect, with decreased lung volumes, reduced diffusing capacity for carbon monoxide, and a normal or elevated FEV1:FVC ratio. Decreased DLCO is not specific for ILD because it also may occur with pulmonary hypertension, which can occur in patients with a variety of connective tissue diseases. Chest radiographs may have changes suggestive of ILD, but a HRCT of the lungs is considered the standard procedure for initial evaluation of patients

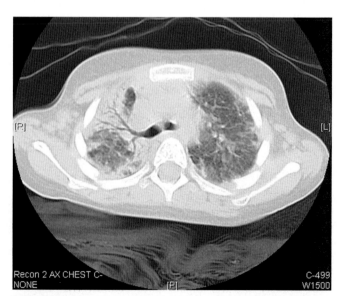

FIGURE 57-4. A 2-year-old child who presented with fever, hypoxia, and persistent chest infiltrates. HRCT showed bilateral patchy airspace consolidation with air bronchograms. A lung biopsy confirmed the diagnosis of bronchiolitis obliterans organizing pneumonia (BOOP). Six months later the child developed myalgias and heliotrope rash and was diagnosed with JDM.

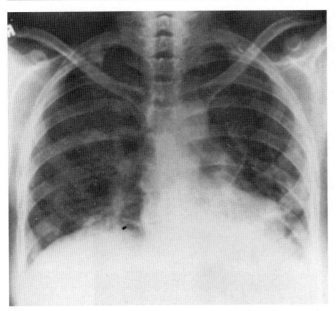

FIGURE 57-5. Chest radiograph of a 21-year-old female diagnosed with juvenile dermatomyositis at 12 years of age and onset of slowly progressive pulmonary fibrosis at 18 years of age. The heart is normal in size, and soft tissue calcifications are present in both axillae. Interstitial thickening and cystic changes are bilateral and most pronounced at the bases.

with suspected ILD. The most common pattern observed in adult DM is irregular linear opacities with areas of consolidation and ground-glass attenuation, suggesting active inflammation.[98] Honeycombing occurs uncommonly. The differential diagnosis for ILD always includes infection and drug-induced lung disease. Bronchoalveolar lavage can help rule out infection. Although lung biopsies are not routinely performed in adult DM, in children where ILD is uncommon and there are no data on the role of HCRT in predicting histologic patterns, a lung biopsy may be required to obtain a diagnosis. Pulmonary fibrosis,[103] acute interstitial pneumonitis,[102] and BOOP[91] (see Fig 57-4) have all been reported as lung histologic findings in JDM.

Many observational studies have reported asymptomatic pulmonary function abnormalities in 30% to 40% of children with JDM.[91] A small longitudinal case series reported pulmonary function abnormalities in 5 of 12 patients with JDM who had no respiratory symptoms, but these abnormalities were generally of a mild nature and nonprogressive, showing a restrictive defect.[106] More recently, a larger case-control study of 59 JDM patients from Oslo showed a restrictive ventilatory defect in 26% compared with 9% of controls.[107] These mild nonprogressive restrictive pulmonary defects generally have been attributed to respiratory muscle weakness or calcinosis in the chest wall and need to be differentiated from the reduced lung compliance that occurs with ILD. Findings of reduced maximal inspiratory and expiratory pressures, reduced maximal voluntary ventilation, normal DLCO, and an increased residual volume without decreased FEV1:FVC ratio help distinguish respiratory muscle weakness from ILD.

Treatment

The mainstay of treatment is high-dose corticosteroids, usually weaned slowly over a 1- to 2-year period. Intravenous pulse methylprednisolone frequently is used for children with more severe weakness. Immunosuppressive therapy is used to treat JDM, based on results reported in observational studies and clinical experience because no randomized controlled trials exist to evaluate treatment in this population.[108] The most commonly used immunosuppressive agent is methotrexate, which is administered weekly. Since reports of the benefits of methotrexate in reducing the duration and cumulative dose of systemic corticosteroids have emerged, in many centers methotrexate is routinely added to systemic steroids at the initiation of treatment.[109] There are also reports of the efficacy and steroid-sparing effects of cyclosporine in JDM,[110] and some clinicians use cyclosporine as initial therapy together with prednisone.[111] Cyclosporine also has been reported to be effective in combination with systemic corticosteroids in the treatment of a small series of children with JDM-associated ILD.[112] Controlled trials of intravenous immunoglobulin in adults[113] and uncontrolled trials in children support its use.[114] In patients with severe or life-threatening disease, such as ILD, chronic skin ulceration, or gastrointestinal involvement, intravenous cyclophosphamide (500 to 750 mg/m^2 every 4 weeks) is used in combination with high-dose corticosteroid therapy.[115] Rituximab has been shown to be associated with clinical improvement in a single small case series of JDM.[116]

Prognosis

Mortality rates for JDM declined from more than 30% in the 1960s before routine glucocorticoid therapy was given, to less than 3% in the 2000s with the advent of early combination immunosuppressive therapy.[108] Patients with typical disease who are treated with early immunosuppressive therapy now usually have an excellent prognosis.[117] Long-term morbidity is generally related to disease complications, such as calcinosis and other complications related to drug toxicity, including growth retardation and osteoporosis[118] Acute onset and rapidly progressive ILD with associated air leak is only very occasionally a cause of mortality in JDM.[102–104] Small defects in pulmonary function should be followed over time to ensure that slowly progressive ILD, which is well described in adult DM, does not develop.

▄ SCLERODERMA (SSC)

Epidemiology

Systemic scleroderma, also known as systemic sclerosis (SSc) is rare in childhood. One study of Finnish children found an incidence of juvenile SSc of 0.05 per 100,000,[119] but there are no reliable prevalence data. It has been estimated that up to 10% of adults with SSc have the onset of their disease in childhood.[120] In a large series of children from multiple countries, juvenile SSc was almost four times more common in females and began at a mean age of 8 years.[121]

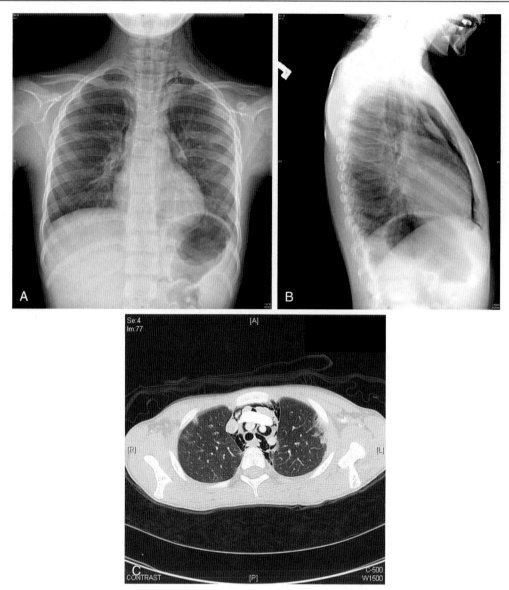

FIGURE 57-6. Posteroanterior **(A)** and lateral **(B)** view of chest radiograph of 9-year-old child presenting with JDM, showing extensive pneumomediastinum and blunting of right CP angle. **C,** HRCT scan of chest also shows multiple pleural-based wedge-shaped opacities with interstitial thickening and cystic areas consistent with early ILD (usually NSIP pattern).

Clinical Features

Systemic sclerosis can be divided into limited and diffuse forms. More than 90% of children with juvenile SSc have the diffuse form,[121] which is a multisystem connective tissue disease that involves thickening and hardening of the skin, as well as multiple organ involvement. A higher proportion of children than adults with the disease have features of an overlap connective tissue disease syndrome.[122]

Although there are no validated diagnostic criteria for juvenile SSc, the 1980 criteria for adult SSc[123] have been widely used for children. These rely on the presence of either the major criterion of sclerodermatous changes proximal to the metacarpophalangeal or metatarsophalangeal joints or the presence of at least two of the following minor criteria—sclerodactyly, digital pitting scars, or bibasilar pulmonary fibrosis. New classification criteria

for juvenile SSc have been proposed for children whose disease begins before the age of 16 years. These criteria require the presence of the major criterion of proximal sclerodermatous changes and at least 2 of the minor criteria, which have been expanded to 20 items, including involvement of other organ systems and some serologic abnormalities.[124] The proposed minor criteria include sclerodactyly, peripheral vascular disease (Raynaud's phenomenon, nail fold capillary abnormalities, digital tip ulcers), gastrointestinal (dysphagia, reflux), cardiac (arrhythmia, heart failure), renal (renal crisis, hypertension), neurologic (neuropathy, carpal tunnel syndrome), and musculoskeletal disease (tendon friction rub, arthritis, myositis). The proposed pulmonary criteria have been expanded to include reduced DLCO of <80% and PAH in addition to pulmonary fibrosis seen on chest radiography or HRCT.

The skin abnormalities often are heralded by a phase of edema, which is then followed by the development of skin tightening and sclerosis, and as this becomes more prominent, contractures develop. When sclerosis affects the face, loss of wrinkling of the skin results in the pathognomonic expressionless facies. The skin subsequently can atrophy and develop telangiectasia. The vasculopathy is reflected in abnormalities easily seen in the nail fold capillaries with drop-out, dilatation, tortuosity, and hemorrhages. The most common, nondermatologic clinical features of juvenile SSc in the two largest series reported to date were Raynaud's phenomenon (72% to 84%), followed by joint (64% to 79%), gastrointestinal (65% to 69%), and pulmonary (42% to 50%) involvement. Cardiovascular (29% to 44%), renal (10% to 13%), and neurologic disease (3% to 16%) occurred less frequently. Calcinosis developed in 18% to 27%.[121,125]

Pathogenesis

SSc is characterized by inflammation, excessive fibrosis, and vasculopathy affecting the skin and multiple organs with evidence of immune, endothelial, and fibroblast dysfunction. While the etiology and exact pathogenetic mechanisms remain elusive, endothelial cell injury appears to be an early and important event. Endothelin-1 has emerged as an important mediator of the vascular changes, and serum levels correlate with disease severity markers.[126] There are features of autoimmunity with the following SSc-selective autoantibodies included in the new proposed minor criteria: anticentromere, antitopoisomerase I (Scl-70), antifibrillarin, anti-PM-Scl, antifibrillin, and anti-RNA polymerase I or III. ANA is found in approximately 80%, extractable nuclear antigen (ENA) in 40%, and anti-Scl-70 in approximately one third of pediatric patients.[121]

Pulmonary Involvement

Pulmonary disease is seen in approximately 50% of children with SSc. The major forms of lung involvement are ILD and PAH (Figs. 57-7 and 57-8). ILD is more common and has been reported in more than 80% of patients in one study,[127] while PAH is seen in 4% to 9%.[121,128] The typical form of ILD (seen in 77.5% of adult cases) has a histologic pattern of nonspecific interstitial pneumonitis.[129] SSc also is associated with pleuritis, pleural effusions, bronchiectasis, BOOP, and alveolar hemorrhage. Spontaneous pneumothorax with severe fibrosis and aspiration pneumonia associated with esophageal reflux also may be seen.[130] ILD and progressive decline of pulmonary function have been associated with more severe esophageal dysmotility in adults with SSc.[131]

Pulmonary involvement is often asymptomatic. Although dyspnea is the most frequent symptom in children with lung involvement, it only occurs in 10% to 26% of children with SSc at presentation or during the disease course.[128] Dry cough is even less frequent. Abnormal chest radiography is seen in 12% at presentation and in 29% during the disease course.[121]

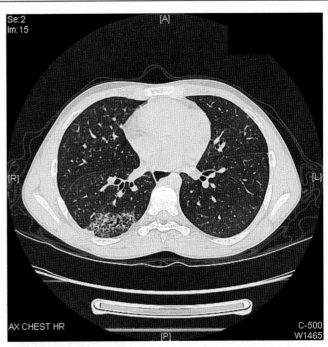

FIGURE 57-7. Early ILD in teen with scleroderma. HRCT shows typical changes of peripheral interlobular septal thickening with fibrosis and traction bronchiectasis.

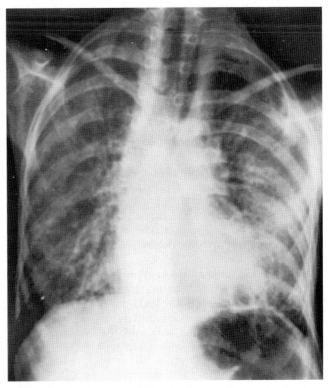

FIGURE 57-8. An 18-year-old female who was diagnosed with scleroderma at 6 years of age and had onset of ILD at 10 years of age. This chest radiograph shows an advanced case of scleroderma lung with chronic pulmonary fibrosis in a reticulated honeycomb pattern more prominent in the lower lobes. The heart is minimally enlarged, gaseous distention of the proximal and distal thirds of the esophagus is present, and there is a moderate right convex scoliosis.

Ground-glass opacities are suggestive of ILD, and a reticular pattern and traction bronchiectasis may be seen.[130] HRCT is a more sensitive method of detecting these findings than routine radiography and may detect additional abnormalities, such as pleural micronodules.[132] Patients with normal HRCT scans on initial assessment are likely to have normal HRCT scans after a follow-up period of 5 years.[133] One study in adults with SSc found that ground-glass opacity was the most common finding on HRCT and was only reversible in a small minority of patients who had sequential scans,[134] suggesting that ground-glass opacity may actually indicate fine fibrosis.

PFTs are important in the initial assessment and ongoing monitoring of patients with SSc. Reduced DLCO may be an early marker of ILD or PAH and also correlates with the severity of these disease manifestations.[130] Children with SSc most often have reduced forced vital capacity with a restrictive PFT pattern (42% to 65%). It is important to note that almost half of those with abnormal PFTs do not have lung imaging abnormalities.[128] Serial PFTs in adults with SSc and severe pulmonary fibrosis demonstrate that most of the lung volume loss occurs in the first 4 years of the disease.[135]

The best way to monitor pediatric SSc patients for the new onset of ILD or progression of ILD is not clear. A study of serial PFTs and HRCT in children with SSc found that PFTs, particularly lung volume studies, correlate with findings on HRCT, suggesting that monitoring with PFTs can identify which patients require follow-up HRCT. The authors acknowledge, however, that PFTs do not completely exclude mild pulmonary involvement, and they therefore entertain the notion of a surveillance low radiation dose HRCT at some point during follow-up for lung disease.[136] More extensive disease on HRCT correlates with poor prognosis in adult SSc patients.[137]

In adults, anti-Scl-70 antibodies are associated with ILD while anticentromere antibodies are protective.[138] In children, serum KL-6 has been reported as a potentially useful biomarker of ILD in juvenile SSc and correlates with PFT abnormalities and the severity of ILD.[139] Lung biopsy is generally not required when the clinical features, PFT results, and imaging findings are typical for ILD. Moreover, pathologic findings do not reliably predict disease course and outcome.[129] BAL has not been found to reliably predict disease course or response to treatment.[140]

PAH may occur as an isolated phenomenon or in association with ILD. Right heart catheterization may be the gold standard for identifying PAH, but Doppler echocardiography is effective and noninvasive. Anticentromere antibodies are associated with isolated PAH, and anti-U3 RNP antibodies are associated with PAH in adults with SSc.[141]

Treatment

There have been no controlled treatment trials in juvenile SSc. Treatment approaches for juvenile SSc-related lung disease have therefore drawn heavily on reports of successful treatment in adults. Both daily oral cyclophosphamide[142] and monthly intravenous cyclophosphamide[143] have demonstrated some degree of efficacy in ILD associated with SSc, with only modest benefits on respiratory function. There are only uncontrolled studies using mycophenolate mofetil, azathioprine, and rituximab in adults. Lung transplantation has been successful in carefully selected patients who have limited involvement of other major organs.[144] Autologous hematopoietic stem cell transplantation also has been shown to stabilize major organ disease and is currently being evaluated in controlled trials.[145]

Prognosis

Antitopoisomerase I (anti-Scl-70) antibodies and anti-U3RNP antibodies are associated with pulmonary fibrosis and poor prognosis.[146] The mortality risk in adults with SSc is dramatically higher with PAH, and survival is also negatively impacted by lung disease, even without PAH.[147] Survival in pulmonary hypertension associated with ILD is significantly worse than isolated PAH.[148] Similarly, in children with a fatal outcome, pulmonary involvement occurs more frequently and earlier in the disease course. Overall, the survival is better in children than in adults with SSc, with a 95% 5-year survival reported in one study.[125] However, some children with early organ involvement have a rapidly progressive course. Scleroderma-related heart disease is a frequent cause of death among children with SSc.[122]

■ MIXED CONNECTIVE TISSUE DISEASE (MCTD)

MCTD is a rare diagnosis in children that can have life-threatening pulmonary involvement. It is characterized by the presence of high titer anti-U1 ribonucleoprotein (RNP) antibodies in combination with clinical features of SLE, SSc, and/or dermatomyositis and was first described as a distinct clinical phenotype in 1972.[149]

Epidemiology and Pathogenesis

MCTD accounts for only 0.1% to 0.5% of pediatric rheumatology cases.[150] Median age of childhood onset is approximately 11 years (4 to 16 years), with girls diagnosed 3 times more often than boys.[150] More commonly, MCTD presents in women in the second to third decade of life, although pediatric onset accounts for 25% of cases.[151]

The etiology of MCTD is unknown. Complex interactions occur between the innate and adaptive immune systems, and there is evidence that anti-RNP antibodies are involved in pathogenesis of the disease.[152]

Clinical Manifestations and Diagnosis

Children usually have an insidious onset of disease, with Raynaud's phenomenon, constitutional symptoms (malaise, fatigue, and low grade fever), and polyarthritis as initial clinical symptoms in combination with a high titer of speckled ANA pattern.[153–156] A high titer of anti-RNP antibodies is a strong predictor of the eventual evolution to MCTD.[157] Classic clinical manifestations of other connective tissue diseases (often the skin rash of SLE or JDM, SSc skin, swollen hands, proximal muscle weakness, esophageal dysmotility, pericarditis, leukopenia, and pulmonary dysfunction) develop sequentially over time but not in any predictable manner or time frame. A clear diagnosis of MCTD may not be evident for years, and the initial presenting syndrome may be referred to as "undifferentiated CTD."

Several sets of diagnostic criteria for MCTD exist; however, Kasukawa's criteria are used most frequently in children and are the most restrictive.[158] Three criteria must be fulfilled for diagnosis of MCTD: (1) Raynaud's phenomenon or swollen fingers or hands; (2) anti-RNP antibody positive; and (3) at least one abnormal sign or symptom from two or more of these categories: SLE, SSc, or dermatomyositis. Almost any organ can be involved in MCTD; however, four clinical features are distinctive for MCTD: (1) the presence of Raynaud's phenomenon and swollen hands or fingers, (2) the absence of severe renal or central nervous system disease (differentiates MCTD from SLE), (3) more severe arthritis with insidious onset of pulmonary hypertension (without pulmonary fibrosis), and (4) autoantibodies with specificity to ant-U1 RNP.

Pulmonary Involvement

Pulmonary disease is a major source of morbidity and mortality in adults with MCTD, occurring in about 75% of adult patients.[159] Case series of MCTD in children suggest a similar frequency of pulmonary involvement in children, although pulmonary hypertension seems to be less common and lung disease is generally mild.[156] Pulmonary disease onset is often initially asymptomatic and develops insidiously. Common symptoms include dry cough, dyspnea with exertion, and chest pain. Pulmonary fibrosis, pleural effusions, and PAH are the most common manifestations. Other findings include thromboembolic disease, pulmonary hemorrhage, diaphragmatic dysfunction, and aspiration pneumonitis.[160]

PAH is due to a pulmonary vasculopathy with intimal proliferation and medial hypertrophy of pulmonary arterioles. Unlike SSc, the lung parenchyma is not fibrotic.[151] One case of pulmonary hypertension due to veno-occlusive disease has been reported in the literature.[161] PAH should be suspected with symptoms of exertional dyspnea, increased second heart sound, or dilatation of pulmonary arteries on chest imaging.

Treatment and Prognosis

No controlled trials are available to guide therapy of MCTD, so that treatment is based on case series experience and conventional therapies that are known to be effective for manifestations of disease common to other CTDs (SLE, SSc, PM/DM). Because the clinical course of disease in MCTD is variable, therapy should be individualized to address specific organ involvement and disease severity. Most clinical manifestations of MCTD, with the exception of Raynaud's phenomenon, are steroid responsive. Low-dose glucocorticoids, nonsteroidal anti-inflammatory drugs, hydroxychloroquine, or combinations of these medications are used for early non-aggressive disease. Vasodilating drugs are used for Raynaud's phenomenon, with nifedipine the most commonly used. High-dose systemic corticosteroids, methotrexate, or cytotoxics may be added for more severe disease, particularly organ-threatening disease.

PAH may require treatment with the same classes of drugs used to treat idiopathic PAH (prostacyclin analogues, endothelin receptor antagonists, phosphodiesterase type 5 inhibitors; see Chapter 72 for management of PAH). PAH can be fatal but is not always progressive and sometimes resolves.[151,162] Multiple case reports in adults[151,159,163] and children[162,164,165] also report successful treatment of PAH with immunosuppressive therapy (corticosteroids and cyclophosphamide), considering the PAH as part of a "disease flare." Heart and lung transplantation is an option for end-stage PAH.

MCTD is considered incurable, and outcomes are variable depending on organ involvement; however, most children have a favorable prognosis. Ten-year mortality is reported at 16% to 28% in adults and 7.6% in children.[162] Deaths most often are due to rapid onset pulmonary hypertension in adults[151] and infection in children.[162]

▰ SARCOIDOSIS

Sarcoidosis is a chronic multisystem disorder of unknown etiology affecting mostly young adults and rarely, children. It is characterized by noncaseating epithelioid cell granulomas, which have a predilection for thoracic lymph nodes and lung tissue. Children with sarcoidosis who present to the pulmonologist commonly have a similar disease to adult sarcoidosis with bilateral hilar adenopathy (BHL) with or without parenchymal infiltrates. Most disease will spontaneously resolve within 2 years without any specific therapy; however, progression to pulmonary fibrosis and blindness are two potential long-term morbidities that call for careful consideration for treatment and follow-up of the sarcoidosis patient.

Early onset sarcoidosis (EOS), with symptom onset at the age of 4 years or younger and a unique phenotype of skin rash, uveitis, arthritis, and absence of lung disease, was previously described to be a rare presentation of sarcoidosis.[166] However, it is now believed that EOS is the sporadic form of Blau's syndrome, a familial autoinflammatory disease with autosomal dominant inheritance caused by mutations in the NOD2/CARD15 gene.[167,168] With increasing recognition of EOS, previously unidentified visceral involvement, including interstitial pneumonitis, has now been reported[169] EOS tends to present to the pediatric rheumatologist and is not discussed further in this chapter.

Epidemiology

The incidence of sarcoidosis varies by geographic location, race, and age, but it usually develops before the age of 50 years and peaks in incidence between 20 and 39 years. The highest incidence of disease has been reported in northern European countries (5 to 40 cases per 100,000 people) and amongst black Americans (35.5 cases per 100,000 compared with 10.9 per 100,000 in white Americans).[170] The incidence in children is less well described but is generally felt to be much lower than in adults. Data from the Danish national patient registry show an overall incidence of 0.29 per 100,000 children-years (15 years of age and younger) compared with the overall Danish incidence of 7.2 per 100,000 person-years. Incidence in children increases with age and peaks at 1.02 per 100,000 in 14- to 15-year-old children.[171] In the two largest American pediatric case series from Virginia[172] and North Carolina,[173] 75% of children with sarcoidosis were black and most were over the age of 10 years. Males and females are equally affected. There is some familial clustering of cases, but no inheritance pattern has been established.[174]

Etiology and Pathogenesis

The etiology of sarcoidosis remains largely unknown; however, a variety of environmental, occupational, and genetic risk factors have been associated with the disease.[170,175] In particular, the mycobacterium tuberculosis catalase-peroxidase protein has been identified as a potential sarcoidosis antigen.[176] Gene-environment interactions are believed to be important in the development of disease, and to date, one such interaction has been identified: an association between an HLA class II antigen susceptibility gene (the HLA-DQB1 allele) and exposure to humidity in the workplace.[177]

Granulomatous lesions are the hallmark of sarcoidosis, and they may occur in any organ of the body. These are typically noncaseating, which distinguishes them from the necrotizing granulomatous lesions of tuberculosis and Wegener's granulomatosis. The granulomas consist of tightly organized collections of predominantly CD4+ T lymphocytes and mononuclear phagocytes (epithelioid cells, macrophages and multinucleated giant cells). The epithelioid and giant cells may contain Schaumann or asteroid inclusion bodies. In the lung, most granulomas are located in the perilymphatic areas, including near bronchioles, in the subpleural space, and the perilobular spaces (Fig. 57-9). In more mature granulomas, fibroblasts and collagen may encase the ball-like cluster of cells. Special stains for fungi and mycobacteria are negative. The granulomatous lesions usually heal with preservation of lung parenchyma; however, in 20% to 25% of patients, fibroblasts proliferate at the periphery of the granuloma and produce fibrotic scar tissue.

Clinical Manifestations

Children older than 8 years of age tend to present with similar manifestations as adults, with pulmonary findings predominating. Granulomatous lesions may occur

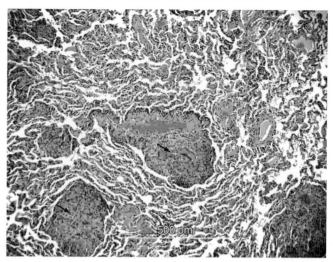

FIGURE 57-9. Biopsy of the apex of the left lung from a 15-year-old African American boy with a history of skin lesions, bilateral ankle swelling, a painful red eye, and lung infiltrate (see Fig. 57-10). Biopsy shows non-necrotizing interstitial granulomas *(arrows)*. Special stains for acid-fast bacillus and fungi were negative, as were stains for vasculitis. Similar results were found on biopsy of axillary lymph nodes.

in any organ, but the lungs, lymph nodes, eyes, skin, and liver are the most commonly involved. Occasionally joints, bone, spleen, central nervous system (neurosarcoidosis), heart, or kidneys are involved. Nonspecific and often minor symptoms of general malaise, weight loss, fatigue, and fever are common. Other symptoms are related to local tissue injury caused by granulomas and hence depend on the organs involved. Cough, dyspnea with exertion, and chest pain are common symptoms of lung involvement.[171,178,179] Common skin lesions include papules, plaques, nodules, changes in old scars, erythema nodosum, hyperpigmented lesions, and hypopigmented lesions. Lupus pernio, erythroderma, and ichthyosis are less common skin lesions in children. Central nervous system involvement may present with headache, seizures, cranial nerve palsies, motor signs, hypothalamic dysfunction, and hydrocephalus.[180] Physical exam findings may include peripheral lymphadenopathy, eye changes, skin rashes, hepatosplenomegaly, abnormal chest sounds, neurologic deficits, and parotid gland enlargement. Cardiac disease is rare but may present with heart block, arrhythmias, or dilated cardiomyopathy. Asymptomatic patients may be identified by routine screening chest radiographs. Löfgren's syndrome, a triad of acute arthritis, bilateral hilar adenopathy (BHL), and erythema nodosum is a common presentation in 9% to 34% of adults[181] but is less common in children.[171] A diagnosis of sarcoidosis should prompt slit-lamp examination of the eye to look for asymptomatic uveitis because blindness is one of the described morbidities of sarcoidosis.

Frequent laboratory abnormalities include an increased ESR, anemia, hypergammaglobulinemia, cutaneous anergy (>40% of adults), hypercalciuria (19% to 30%), hypercalcemia (8 to 12%), eosinophilia, leukopenia, and increased angiotensin-converting enzyme (ACE) (60% to 80%). Rheumatoid factor is occasionally positive (14% of adults).

Pulmonary Involvement

Pulmonary involvement occurs in more than 90% of adult[181] and pediatric[182] cases, commonly affecting the intrathoracic lymph nodes and the pulmonary parenchyma (Fig. 57-10). Presenting symptoms of pulmonary sarcoidosis may include dyspnea, wheezing, and cough. Physical examination of the chest may be normal or include crackles and wheezing. Radiographic findings can be divided into the following stages: stage 0 = normal radiograph; stage I = bilateral hilar adenopathy (BHL); stage II = BHL with parenchymal infiltrates; stage III = parenchymal infiltrates without BHL. Some authors also define pulmonary fibrosis as stage IV disease. In a recent Danish pediatric cohort study, 10% of children presented with stage 0 disease, 71% with stage II, and 8.3% with stage III disease. Parenchymal infiltrates may be nodular, fibrotic, or alveolar and tend to occur in the upper lobes. Pleural effusion, pneumothorax, pleural thickening, calcification, and atelectasis also have been reported. PFTs may be normal, particularly with stage 0 or I disease. The most common abnormality is a restrictive pattern with a reduction in DLCO, and occasionally, an obstructive pattern may be seen.[178,179,183]

Airway involvement is well described in adults with sarcoidosis.[184] Airway changes are best appreciated with bronchoscopy and include specific changes of waxy yellow mucosal nodules and non-specific changes such as erythema, edema, granularity, and cobblestoning of airway mucosa and bronchial stenosis, typically in the lobar and segmental bronchi. In our experience, these typical airway lesions also may be observed in children with sarcoidosis (Fig. 57-11). Airway hyperreactivity is well documented in adult studies and is associated with the presence of visible airway involvement on bronchoscopy.[185]

Progression of granulomatous lung lesions to pulmonary fibrosis and end-stage lung disease may be a fatal complication of pulmonary sarcoidosis. Pulmonary disease also may be complicated with the development of bronchiectasis and chronic infections, including development of an aspergilloma in damaged tissue. Hemoptysis may occur secondary to bronchiectasis or aspergilloma development.[181]

Diagnosis

Box 57-2 describes the clinical evaluation that should be considered for a patient with suspected sarcoidosis. Diagnosis is established when typical clinical features are supported by a tissue biopsy showing noncaseating granulomas. One also must be careful to exclude other causes of noncaseating granulomas, including immunodeficiency syndromes (especially chronic granulomatous disease), fungal and mycobacterial infections, berylliosis, ulcerative colitis, and Wegener's granulomatosis. Any organ that is involved and accessible may be used

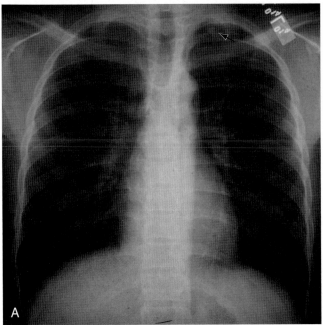

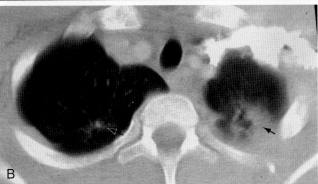

FIGURE 57-10. Chest radiograph **(A)** from the adolescent described in Figure 57-9 that shows an 8-mm density in the left lung apex *(arrow)*. Chest CT image **(B)** shows parenchymal opacifications in the lung apices *(arrows)* and axillary adenopathy on the right (not shown). The patient was diagnosed with sarcoidosis after lung and axillary lymph node biopsies revealed typical sarcoid granulomas (see Fig. 57-9).

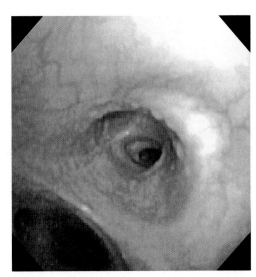

FIGURE 57-11. Bronchoscopy picture of sarcoid airway: right upper lobe (RUL) airway involvement with hypervascularity and waxy nodules

BOX 57-2 CLINICAL EVALUATION FOR THE PATIENT WITH A SUSPECTED DIAGNOSIS OF SARCOIDOSIS*

Initial Evaluation

- Complete history and physical examination, including careful examination of lungs, peripheral lymph nodes, skin, eyes, parotid glands, liver, spleen, nervous system, and joints
- Chest radiograph, both posteroanterior and lateral views
- PFTs, including spirometry, lung volumes, and DLCO
- Tuberculin skin test
- Biopsy of affected organ, with special stains and culture of specimen
- Electrocardiogram
- Complete blood count with white cell differential, ESR, serum calcium, creatinine, alkaline phosphatase, alanine and aspartate aminotransferases
- Serum level of angiotensin-converting enzyme (if elevated, may be useful to monitor patient compliance)
- 24-hour urine collection for calcium:creatinine ratio
- Complete ophthalmologic evaluation (slit-lamp, tonometric, and funduscopic)
- Other tests as indicated for assessment of involved organs (e.g., MRI with gadolinium and cerebral spinal fluid analysis if central nervous system involvement)
- Consider referral to pediatric rheumatologist for comanagement of disease, depending on local experience
- Consider genetic analysis for CARD15 mutations, especially if young or no pulmonary involvement

Follow-up Monitoring

- Occurs every 3 months initially and for at least 3 years after discontinuation of therapy
- Assessment for decline in physiologic function based on initial organ involvement (for lung involvement follow chest radiograph and PFTs)
- Tests to monitor side effects of therapy (e.g., bone densitometry and blood pressure for steroid use, semiannual eye exam for hydroxychloroquine use)
- Further testing as indicated if new symptoms or physical findings develop

*Summarized from recommendations in the following publications: Statement on Sarcoidosis. Joint Statement of the American Thoracic Society (ATS), the European Respiratory Society (ERS) and the World Association of Sarcoidosis and Other Granulomatous Disorders (WASOG) adopted by the ATS Board of Directors and by the ERS Executive Committee, February 1999. *Am J Respir Crit Care Med.* 1999;160:736-755. Pattishall EN, Kendig EL Jr. Sarcoidosis in children. *Pediatr Pulmonol.* 1996;22:195-203. Iannuzzi MC, Rybicki BA, Teirstein AS. Sarcoidosis. *N Engl J Med.* 2007;357:2153-2165.
DLCO, Diffusing capacity of the lung for carbon monoxide; *ESR,* erythrocyte sedimentation rate; *MRI,* magnetic resonance imaging; *PFTs,* pulmonary function tests.

for a tissue diagnosis. In children, biopsies are often performed from peripheral lymph nodes, skin lesions, salivary glands, lung lesions, and the liver.[179] It is generally accepted that young adults presenting with Löfgren's syndrome do not require a biopsy to confirm the diagnosis.[183] The Kveim-Siltzbach test is no longer used as a diagnostic test in routine clinical practice.

When mediastinal nodes or lung tissue are the obvious site for biopsy, several options for tissue diagnosis exist. Transbronchial lung biopsy (TBLB) has a relatively high yield (40% to 90% sensitivity) in adults with at least stage I disease, but there are no data on its utility in children.[183] In one adult study, endobronchial biopsy (EBB) in addition to TBLB was safe and increased the diagnostic yield of bronchoscopy by 20%. When abnormal airway mucosal lesions were

visualized, 75% of EBB were positive, whereas only 30% of EBB specimens were positive in those with normal appearing airways.[186] If TBLB does not yield a diagnosis, which occurs in about 58% of unselected adult patients,[187] surgical biopsy of mediastinal nodes or peripheral lung lesions is the next step.[183] Hilar and mediastinal nodes may be assessed with mediastinoscopy, or alternatively, with the newer and minimally invasive technique of endobronchial ultrasound-guided transbronchial needle aspiration (EBUS-TBNA), which has been reported to have a sensitivity of 71% to 85% for diagnosing sarcoidosis.[187,188] Although technical issues limit the application of this technique to younger children, EBUS-TBNA has been reported to be successful in the diagnosis of sarcoidosis in a 13 year old with BHL, as well as hypercalcemia, nervous system, and eye involvement.[189] CT-guided transthoracic fine-needle aspiration with core needle biopsy also may be used as an alternative to surgical biopsy to access peripheral pulmonary infiltrates in centers with sufficient experience.[190]

Bronchoalveolar lavage (BAL) cell profiles are not specific for sarcoidosis, but they may help to narrow the differential diagnosis. BAL shows a lymphocytosis in > 85%; neutrophils are normal or low except in late disease; CD4:CD8 ratio is increased (opposite to findings in ILD associated with connective tissue diseases) in 50% to 60%. BAL cell profile is not helpful in monitoring disease progression or response to therapy.[179,183]

Treatment

The decision to treat pulmonary sarcoidosis is often difficult because disease spontaneously remits in many patients. If therapy is needed, corticosteroids are the mainstay. Efficacy data on treatments for pulmonary sarcoidosis are mainly based on adult data, which are well summarized in two Cochrane reviews.[191,192] Limited observational data from a pediatric cohort suggest similar outcomes of corticosteroid therapy in children.[179] Indications for treatment of lung disease are generally based on data about the natural history of spontaneous remission of different forms of lung disease: stage 1, 60% to 80%; stage II, 50% to 60%; and stage III, 30% remit.[170,181,183]

The following criteria should prompt consideration for corticosteroid treatment:

1. Pulmonary sarcoidosis: Worsening pulmonary symptoms, deteriorating lung function, progressive radiographic changes (worsening of interstitial opacities, cavitation, progression of fibrosis with honeycombing, development of pulmonary hypertension)
2. Cardiac, neurologic, ocular, renal involvement or hypercalcemia, even with mild symptoms, because fatal arrhythmias, blindness, and renal failure may develop
3. Severe debilitating symptoms from any organ involvement

Therapy is not indicated in asymptomatic children with stage I or II pulmonary disease with normal or mildly abnormal lung function. However, stage III disease needs to be followed closely because adult data suggest that the majority do not resolve, it may progress to pulmonary fibrosis, and most patients will require therapy in the future.[183,191] The limited pediatric data also support this concept.[178,179,182]

Corticosteroid dosing typically is started at a relatively high dose (1 mg/kg/day depending on severity of disease) for 4 to 6 weeks and then is tapered. A response to therapy is usually seen within 6 to 12 weeks of initiation of therapy, with improvement in symptoms, pulmonary infiltrates, and lymphadenopathy on imaging and variable improvement in pulmonary function. Steroid therapy typically needs to be continued for 12 to 18 months in order to prevent relapse of disease. Relapses are treated with increasing doses of corticosteroids. Alternative immunosuppressive and/or cytotoxic therapies may be added if disease is steroid resistant or as steroid-sparing agents in relapsing disease; however, data on efficacy of these agents are very limited.[192] Low-dose methotrexate is the most commonly used alternative therapy that has been shown to have a steroid-sparing effect in one adult randomized controlled trial[193] and in a small case series of children.[194] Hydroxychloroquine has been reported to be successful in treating patients with hypercalcemia and neurologic involvement.[195,196] Infliximab, a TNF inhibitor, has a strong pathophysiologic basis for use, but side effects of therapy are a concern, and randomized controlled trials do not support its routine use. It has been shown to have limited efficacy in severe pulmonary disease refractory to steroid therapy.[197] Successful lung transplantation has been reported in many young adults with end-stage lung disease, and candidate selection criteria specific to sarcoidosis have been published.[198]

Prognosis

In adults, spontaneous recovery occurs in about two thirds of patients with sarcoidosis within 2 years of diagnosis without therapy. Another one third to one half of patients are treated with corticosteroids and most improve with treatment, but relapse occurs in many as the drug is tapered or discontinued. The clinical course is chronic or progressive in 10% to 30%, and fatalities occur in 1% to 5% of patients, typically because of progressive pulmonary fibrosis or central nervous system or cardiac involvement.[183] Limited long-term pediatric outcome data from the United States,[199] France,[179] and Denmark,[182] suggest that most children with sarcoidosis also have a good prognosis because most have a complete recovery. Chronic active disease with impaired lung function occurs in a small proportion, and there are few deaths (mainly patients with neurosarcoidosis). The data from Denmark, which is population-based, is particularly informative for white children with sarcoidosis, showing that 78% of children show complete recovery, 11% have chronic active disease with multiorgan involvement and impaired lung function, and 7% die of their disease.[182] Pulmonary involvement may lead to progressive pulmonary fibrosis and end stage chronic lung disease; this seems to be more likely with

stage III pulmonary disease at the onset in both adults and children.[182,183,199] Eye involvement may lead to blindness.

Löfgren's syndrome (i.e., BHL, erythema nodosum, fever, and polyarthritis) has an excellent prognosis with greater than 85% spontaneous remission rates within 6 to 12 months. Clinical factors associated with a worse prognosis in adults include black race, hypercalcemia, lupus pernio, splenomegaly, pulmonary infiltrates on chest radiograph (stage II and III disease), chronic uveitis, cystic bone lesions, nasal mucosal sarcoidosis, neurosarcoidosis, cardiac involvement, and low family income.[183] In children, where prognostic data are much more limited, erythema nodosum has been associated with a good prognosis while central nervous system involvement is associated with a poor prognosis.[182]

CHILDHOOD VASCULITIDES

Vasculitis is defined as the presence of inflammation in a blood vessel. Vasculitis syndromes are generally classified according to their clinical manifestations, the size and type of blood vessels involved, and the pathologic features found within the vessel walls. Clinical manifestations and epidemiologic features are different in childhood vasculitides compared with adult vasculitides.[85] Recently, a pediatric classification scheme has been developed by the European League against Rheumatism and the Paediatric Rheumatology European Society that includes classification criteria for the more common childhood vasculitis syndromes (Table 57-4).[200,201] The clinical presentation of vasculitis depends on the size of the vessel involved. When predominantly large- or medium-sized vessels are affected, arterial insufficiency to the affected organ results in infarction, necrosis, and end-organ dysfunction. Smaller vessel (arterioles, venules, capillaries) inflammation may result in leakage of blood into the tissues. In the lung, this causes diffuse alveolar hemorrhage (DAH), which is characterized by diffuse alveolar infiltrates and a drop in hemoglobin with or without hemoptysis. Other clinical features suggestive of vasculitis are associated acute glomerulonephritis, pulmonary-renal syndrome, ulcerating or deforming upper airway lesions, cavitary or nodular disease on chest imaging, palpable purpura, and multisystem disease.

Pulmonary involvement has been reported in association with most vasculitis syndromes; however, clinically significant pulmonary involvement occurs mainly with vasculitis associated with antineutrophil cytoplasmic antibody (ANCA). ANCA-associated vasculitis (AAV) syndromes are characterized by necrotizing vasculitis of small vessels, frequent pulmonary and renal involvement, and a paucity of immune deposits in the blood vessel wall. The AAV syndromes with frequent pulmonary involvement are Wegener's granulomatosis (WG), microscopic polyangiitis (MPA) and Churg-Strauss vasculitis (CSS) (see Table 57-4). MPA is recognized mainly as a rare pauci-immune small vessel vasculitis of adults involving the skin, joints, kidneys, and lungs, but it may present in childhood

TABLE 57-4 CLASSIFICATION OF CHILDHOOD VASCULITIS AND ASSOCIATED PULMONARY INVOLVEMENT*

CLASSIFICATION CATEGORY	PULMONARY INVOLVEMENT
I. Predominately Large Vessel Vasculitis	
• Takayasu arteritis	Rare: Pulmonary arteritis[270,271]
II. Predominately Medium Size Vessel Vasculitis	
• Childhood polyarteritis nodosa	Rare: Isolated case reports of pulmonary arteritis in adults[272,273]
• Kawasaki disease	During acute phase cough is common and chest radiograph changes occur in 15%[274]
	Unresolving pneumonia is a rare presentation of atypical disease[275]
III. Predominately Small Vessel Vasculitis	
Granulomatous	
• Churg-Strauss syndrome[†]	Nonfixed pulmonary infiltrates in 85%; prior history of asthma almost universal (see text)
• Wegener's granulomatosis[†]	Almost universal: upper and/or lower airways and/or parenchymal (see text)
Nongranulomatous	
• Microscopic polyangitis[†]	Pulmonary hemorrhage in 30% to 50% and may have clinical presentation identical to idiopathic pulmonary hemosiderosis (see text)
• Henoch-Schönlein purpura	Rarely may have pulmonary hemorrhage[276]
IV. Other Vasculitides	
• Behçet disease	Infrequent (1% to 8%); pulmonary artery aneurysms, hemoptysis, thrombi reported in adults[277]
• Vasculitis secondary to infection, malignancy, and drugs, including hypersensitivity vasculitis	Rarely may have pulmonary hemorrhage or thrombosis
• Vasculitis associated with connective tissue diseases (SLE, SSc, JIA)	See Table 57-2
• Unclassified	Isolated pulmonary arteritis case report[278]

JIA, Juvenile idiopathic arthritis; *SLE,* systemic lupus erythematosus; *SSc,* scleroderma.
*Table includes only vasculitides with reported pulmonary involvement.
[†]ANCA-associated vasculitides that commonly have pulmonary involvement

and is often (10% to 30%) associated with pulmonary hemorrhage.[202,203] It is distinguished from WG by the presence of high titers of anti-myeloperoxidase (MPO)-ANCA and the absence of granulomatous inflammation pathologically. It may present initially to the pulmonologist as a case of idiopathic pulmonary hemosiderosis with isolated pulmonary capillaritis, with the subsequent development of pauci-immune glomerulonephritis.[204] MPA is discussed in detail in Chapter 58 (Diffuse Alveolar Hemorrhage in Children). CSS, or allergic angiitis and granulomatosis, is a small vessel vasculitis that is exceedingly rare in children, and most of the published literature is limited to single case reports.[205–207] It is characterized by fever, peripheral eosinophilia, migrating pulmonary infiltrates, and anti-MPO-ANCA antibodies in patients with concomitant severe atopic asthma or allergic rhinitis. Sinusitis, skin, and cardiac involvement are also common while renal disease is uncommon.[208,209] In the largest pediatric case series report of 117 children with new diagnoses of AAV from 30 different North American centers from 2004 to 2008, 2 children had CSS compared to 76 with WG and 17 with MPA.[206]

The differential diagnosis for DAH and pulmonary-renal syndrome includes ANCA-associated vasculitides, Goodpasture syndrome, SLE, thromboembolic disease, and infections, and is discussed separately in Chapter 58. The remainder of this section focuses on WG because it is the most common vasculitis syndrome presenting to the pulmonologist, and it may initially present with isolated airway or lung involvement.

GRANULOMATOSIS WITH POLYANGITIS (GP)

"Granulomatosis with polyangitis (GP)" has recently replaced the older nomenclature "Wegener's granulomatosis."

Epidemiology

Vasculitis is rare in children. One English survey of family clinicians estimated an annual incidence of 53.3 per 100,000 children younger than 17 years of age, with Henoch-Schönlein purpura and Kawasaki disease being the most common vasculitides. All other primary vasculitides, including ANCA-associated vasculitides, had an incidence together of 0.24 per 100,000.[85] Population-based studies of GP from America and Norway specifically suggest that incidence is less than 1 per million in children, and the disease incidence peaks in the fourth to sixth decades of life.[211,212] The multicenter ARChiVe (A Registry for Childhood Vasculitis: e-entry) study suggests that GP accounts for most (65%) new pediatric ANCA-associated vasculitis cases. The GP patients had a median age at diagnosis of 14.2 years (range 4 to 17 years); 69% were Caucasian and 63% female.[206]

Pathogenesis

The etiology of GP is largely unknown; however, the almost universal presence of ANCAs and response to immunosuppressive therapy provide strong rationale for an autoimmune basis.

Many recent studies examining the effects of ANCA-neutrophil and neutrophil-endothelial cell interactions have provided evidence supporting a pathogenic role for ANCAs. ANCAs are directed against the neutrophil granule components proteinase 3 (PR-3-ANCA) and myeloperoxidase (MPO-ANCA). ANCAs interact with these target antigens on cytokine-primed neutrophils. This causes neutrophil activation and interaction with endothelial cells via multiple signaling pathways. The end result is tissue inflammation and damage as the neutrophils migrate through the endothelial cells and undergo respiratory burst and degranulation with release of toxic products. Failure of adaptive immune system regulation mechanisms results in a loss of self-tolerance so that T helper and B cells assist in this autoantibody reaction.[213] The histopathology of all AAV is thus marked by necrotizing vasculitis of the small blood vessels without immune complex deposition (i.e., pauci-immune vasculitis). GP is distinguished among the AAV by the anti-PR-3-ANCA specificity and by the presence of granulomas (Fig. 57-12).

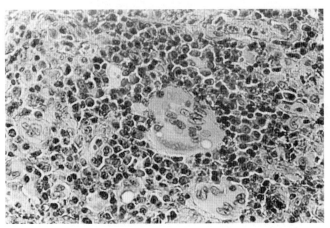

FIGURE 57-12. Photomicrograph of a lung biopsy from a patient with WG, showing a dense pleomorphic infiltrate, numerous mononuclear cells, scattered neutrophils, and several giant cells. This aggregate of cells would be considered a granuloma.

What is still poorly understood is why and how ANCAs develop in the first place. It has long been recognized that some drugs and infectious agents may trigger the development of ANCAs and a clinical syndrome of secondary vasculitis that is similar to the clinical presentation of primary vasculitis.[214] Some studies have suggested a triggering role for infections, particularly bacteria colonizing the upper airway like *Staphylococcus aureus*.[215] This has led to a clinical trial investigating the role of prophylactic cotrimoxazole in preventing GP relapses.[216] In addition, other autoantibodies have recently been described as having a potential role in the disease pathogenesis, including lysosomal membrane protein 2[217] and anti-endothelial cell antibodies.[218]

Clinical Manifestations

Four large pediatric case series describe the typical clinical presentation of GP with a triad of upper airway, lower respiratory tract, and renal disease manifestations.[206,219-221] Symptom onset is most often insidious, with dyspnea or chronic cough along with constitutional symptoms, but it also may be dramatic, presenting with pulmonary hemorrhage, upper airway obstruction, or renal failure. The median interval from symptom onset to diagnosis is 2.7 months (range 0 to 49 months).[206] Most children present with multiorgan involvement. The most frequent presenting features are constitutional (fever, malaise, fatigue, weight loss) (89%); pulmonary (80%); ear, nose, and throat (80%); and renal (75%). Less commonly, eyes (37%), skin (35%), gastrointestinal (42%), musculoskeletal (57%), and nervous systems (25%) may be involved.[206] In a series of 25 patients from Toronto, Canada, 16% experienced venous thrombosis associated with antiphospholipid antibodies during the disease course.[221] Case reports describe involvement of the heart, spleen, and pituitary gland. Contrary to the adult experience, limited GP without renal involvement is uncommon in children. Laboratory abnormalities include elevated white blood cell counts; normochromic normocytic anemia; thrombocytosis; elevated ESR or C-reactive protein levels; abnormal urinalysis with proteinuria, hematuria, and red blood cell casts; and elevated serum creatinine. ANCAs are present in 89% of children with a cytoplasmic immunofluorescence staining pattern (cANCA) in 86%, and 68% are positive for anti-PR3,[206] which is comparable to serology results in adults with GP.[222]

Pulmonary Involvement

Presenting pulmonary symptoms include dyspnea or chronic cough in over half of affected children.[206,220] Hypoxia requiring oxygen therapy is present in 19%.[206] Hemoptysis may signal necrotizing mucosal airway involvement or DAH. Symptoms of dyspnea with hoarseness and stridor suggest subglottic stenosis. Subglottic stenosis has been reported in one series to occur with higher frequency in pediatric-onset GP compared with adults[219]; hence, this feature has been included in the new EULAR/PReS classification criteria.[201] Frequent upper airway findings include sinusitis; nasal septal ulceration or perforation; otitis media; mastoiditis; hearing loss; oral ulcers; and nasal cartilage damage, characteristic of long-standing disease, with resultant saddle-nose deformity (which must be distinguished from the diagnosis of relapsing polychondritis). About half of children will have abnormalities on chest radiographs. The most common findings are nodules, followed by fixed infiltrates. Cavitations, mediastinal lymphadenopathy, pleural effusions, and pneumothoraces also may occur. Chest CT is more sensitive in detecting small nodules and ground-glass abnormalities than plain radiography. The largest case series (n = 18) of chest CT findings in children with WG showed pulmonary involvement in 90% of newly diagnosed patients with nodules (90%), ground-glass opacification (52%) and air space opacification (45%) being the predominant findings. Nodules tended to be multiple (69% had more than five nodules), larger than 5 mm in diameter, and cavitating in 17%. (Fig. 57-13) Air-space opacification usually correlated with clinical evidence of pulmonary hemorrhage.[223] Chest CT findings in children were similar to findings in adults, except that the frequency of identified bronchial narrowing seems to be lower in children (6.7%) compared with adults (59%) (Figs. 57-14 and 57-15).[223,224] Sinus CT may be useful

to identify upper airway involvement, particularly sinus opacification and bony destruction. PFT abnormalities are seen in 42% of cases, and these may show obstructive or restrictive defects, depending on the tissues involved.[206,225]

It is important for the pulmonologist to recognize the bronchoscopy findings of GP because they may provide the first clue to the diagnosis for a child presenting with nonspecific symptoms of cough (Fig. 57-16). Mucosal erythema, edema, ulceration, hemorrhage, cobblestoning, nodules, polyps, submucosal tunneling, synechial bands, and airway stenosis have all been described in airways from the oropharynx down to the bronchi, in case series that include mostly adults and a few children.[225–228] Endobronchial findings are nonspecific because similar findings may be encountered with infections and sarcoidosis.

Diagnosis

The diagnosis of GP is based on a combination of clinical findings (e.g., pulmonary-renal syndrome), supportive serology (i.e., anti-PR-3 ANCA-positive), and characteristic histopathology (pauci-immune granulomatous inflammation of predominantly small to medium sized blood vessels or pauci-immune glomerulonephritis). If GP is suspected, it is important to examine the urine and to obtain chest imaging to rule out asymptomatic renal

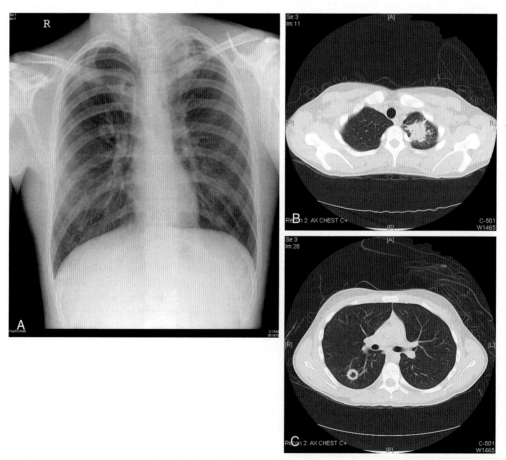

FIGURE 57-13. A 15-year-old teen with GP who presented with renal failure, pulmonary infiltrates, and ANCA-positive serology. **A,** Chest x-ray shows air space infiltrate in the left upper lobe and near the right hilum. **B** and **C,** HRCT scan confirms a cavitating lesion in right lower lobe and multiple bilateral nodules and areas of air space disease.

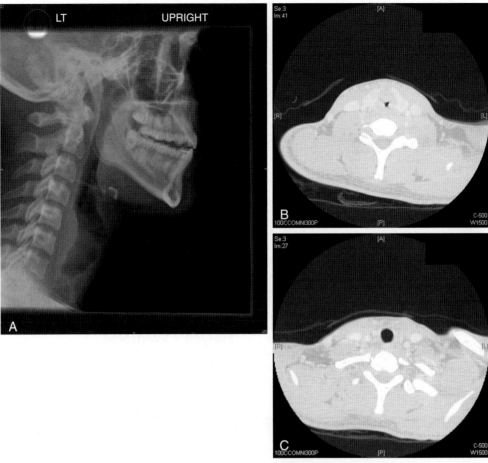

FIGURE 57-14. A 15-year-old teen with GP, presenting with a hoarse voice, hemoptysis, weight loss, and ANCA-positive serology. **(A)** Soft-tissue radiograph of neck shows narrowing of trachea at the level of the seventh cervical vertebrae. **B** and **C**, CT scan of neck shows severe stenosis of the upper trachea (15 mm in length and narrowing to a diameter of 4 mm **[B]** from 14 mm **[C]** above the stenotic area) secondary to circumferential soft tissue thickening. Stenosis improved with pulse steroid therapy and local airway laser ablative therapy.

or pulmonary disease. The differential diagnosis often includes infections (especially mycobacterial, fungal or helminthic infections), other causes of pulmonary-renal syndrome (other ANCA-associated vasculitides, SLE, MCTD, Goodpasture syndrome), sarcoidosis, ulcerative colitis with pulmonary involvement, malignancy, and chronic granulomatous disease. Kidney biopsy has a high yield for identifying pauci-immune glomerulonephritis if there are urinary abnormalities. Diseased upper respiratory tract tissues (e.g., ears, nose, sinuses, trachea) and endobronchial airway lesions offer relatively noninvasive access for tissue diagnosis, but they often have low yields for diagnosis. Lung biopsy yield also may be low because disease is often patchy, but open lung biopsy procedures may offer a better yield than less invasive fine needle aspiration or transbronchial techniques.

Treatment

Standard treatment for GP at diagnosis is a combination of glucocorticoids and cyclophosphamide (CPA). This therapy has changed GP from a rapidly fatal disease to a manageable chronic illness with frequent relapses in most adults and children.[229,230] CPA may be used as a daily oral therapy or pulse intravenous therapy, which results in a less cumulative dose but may be associated with an increased relapse risk. Disease remission may be maintained with low-dose weekly methotrexate or daily azathioprine.[231] Methotrexate also may be effective in inducing remission when the disease is localized or has milder manifestations.[232] Rituximab, a monoclonal antibody against B cells, has been used effectively for severe refractory disease that does not respond to conventional cytotoxic therapy and is emerging as an excellent option for treating disease relapses.

Obstructing airway lesions, including tracheal and bronchial stenosis, may not respond to cytotoxic therapy. These lesions should be managed by a specialized airway team with expertise in the area. They may require intralesional injections of glucocorticoids, endoscopic dilatation, stent placement, or tracheostomy.[225–228] Intralesional corticosteroids may be most effective when used before other surgical interventions that may result in scarring[233]

Patients with GP are at increased risk of infection because of the immunosuppressive therapy they are receiving and the presence of vulnerable damaged tissues.[234] Prophylaxis against *Pneumocystis jiroveci* pneumonia is recommended while receiving CPA[235] and should be considered for children receiving high-dose corticosteroids with methotrexate and also those receiving rituximab.[236]

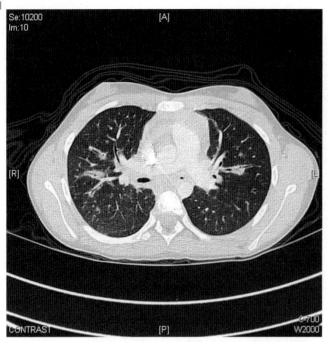

FIGURE 57-15. A 15-year-old girl with granulomatosis with polyangitis (GP) presenting with hemoptysis and ANCA-positive serology. CT scan shows pericardial effusion, diffuse bilateral irregular peribronchial soft tissue thickening and an 11-mm nodular-like mass surrounding the left main-stem bronchus causing pinhole narrowing; no cavitary lesions are present.

Prognosis

GP was almost universally fatal in both adults and children at an average of 5 months after diagnosis before the advent of cytotoxic therapy.[229,230] With current induction therapy, over 90% of patients will be expected to respond partially or completely; however, about half will relapse within 5 years.[229] Fatalities reported in children are due to lung disease or sepsis[219] while malignancy, renal failure, and cardiac disease are additional reported causes of death in adults with GP.[229] Long-term morbidity may result from persistent airway obstruction, renal insufficiency, or treatment-related side effects including cystitis or infertility (due to CPA) and cataracts, glaucoma, vertebral compression fractures, and growth effects (due to steroids).[219,221,229]

■ OTHER SYSTEMIC INFLAMMATORY DISEASES WITH SIGNIFICANT PULMONARY INVOLVEMENT

Sjögren's Syndrome

Sjögren's syndrome (SS) is a chronic inflammatory autoimmune disorder that is characterized by lymphocytic infiltration of the exocrine glands. It is often associated

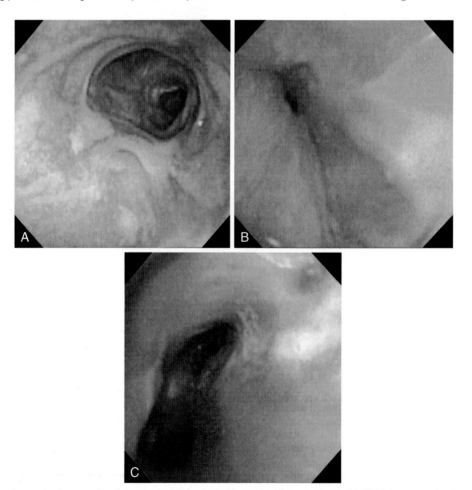

FIGURE 57-16. Bronchoscopic photographs of the airways of a 15-year-old teenager diagnosed with GP **(A)** Main carina showing mucosal erythema. **B,** Left main stem bronchus showing pinhole stenosis. **C,** Left secondary carina showing erythematous friable mucosa.

with other CTD including JIA, SLE, SSc, and JDM. The classic symptoms are keratoconjunctivitis sicca (dry eyes), and xerostomia (dry mouth) along with a high prevalence of ANA, RF, anti-Ro and anti-La antibodies. SS is rare in children, with most major pediatric rheumatology centers only reporting a few cases. There is a lower frequency of sicca symptoms and a higher frequency of parotitis with childhood onset compared with adult onset SS.[237–239] Pulmonary involvement occurs in up to 75% of adult patients but is usually mild and nonprogressive.[240–242] Dryness of the airways resulting in "sicca" cough occurs in up to half of adult patients. Small airways obstructive disease and airway hyperreactivity also are common and are thought to be caused by lymphocytic inflammation around the bronchioles and bronchi (follicular bronchiolitis). ILD occurs infrequently, usually with the histopathologic changes of lymphocytic interstitial pneumonitis (LIP), a finding generally not seen with other CTDs in the absence of SS.[243,244] Chest radiograph imaging changes include diffuse reticular or reticulonodular infiltrates and bronchiectasis while CT scan may have a variety of additional findings including ground-glass attenuation, subpleural nodules, and cysts.[241] Pulmonary hypertension responsive to steroid and cyclophosphamide therapy has also been reported in a 9-year-old child with SS.[245] Prognosis is generally very good, but a poor outcome may be related to progression of LIP to lymphoma in adults.[246]

Inflammatory Bowel Disease

Inflammatory bowel disease (IBD), including Crohn's disease (CD) and ulcerative colitis (UC), is commonly associated with extraintestinal manifestations, but it is only rarely (<1%) associated with clinically significant pulmonary manifestations.[247,248] Subclinical pulmonary involvement is probably common as latent pulmonary function abnormalities have been demonstrated in case series of children with CD[249] and adults with both CD and UC[250,251] who have no respiratory symptoms and normal chest radiographs. The main abnormality is a reduction in DLCO that tends to be worse during active disease. Children with CD also have been demonstrated to have bronchial hyperreactivity.[252] The etiology of these pulmonary function abnormalities is likely secondary to a subclinical airway or alveolar inflammatory process, as BAL samples in CD show hypercellularity with lymphocytosis.[253–255]

Symptomatic lung disease associated with IBD has been reported in two large case series,[256,257] as well as multiple case reports, and is summarized well in recent reviews.[248,258] Bronchiectasis is the single most common disorder described in adults although a range of rare pulmonary manifestations have been reported, including tracheal stenosis, colobronchial and ileobronchial fistulae, chronic bronchitis, bronchiolitis obliterans, BOOP, granulomatous pulmonary nodules (including necrobiotic[259]), ILD, pulmonary vasculitis, and pleural effusions.[248,260] Descriptions of pulmonary disease in children with IBD are limited to isolated case reports of granulomatous nodules, bronchiolitis obliterans and BOOP in CD[261–263] and vasculitis, and BOOP and ILD in UC.[264–266] HRCT findings include

air trapping with mosaic perfusion pattern, tree-in-bud appearance, bronchiectasis, and multiple pulmonary nodules.[257] Pulmonary involvement in IBD usually responds to corticosteroid therapy, with systemic therapy for more severe or interstitial disease and inhaled therapy for mild airways disease.[258] Infliximab therapy (monoclonal antibody to TNF-α) has been used successfully in children with granulomatous lung disease.[263] The differential diagnosis for pulmonary manifestations associated with IBD also must include drug-induced disease (especially hypersensitivity pneumonitis associated with sulfasalazine[267] and mesalamine[268]), opportunistic infection, malignancy, and thromboembolism. When significant lung disease and IBD co-exist, consideration also should be given to distinguishing between CD and sarcoidosis or UC and WG because these diseases may have striking similarities; however, management strategies may differ.[248]

CLINICAL APPROACH TO DIAGNOSIS AND MANAGEMENT OF PULMONARY INVOLVEMENT IN THE SYSTEMIC INFLAMMATORY DISEASES OF CHILDHOOD

The clinical presentation of pulmonary involvement is highly variable. The most common presentation for ILD is slowly progressive dyspnea with or without a dry cough. Dyspnea due to ILD must be distinguished from the dyspnea due to muscle weakness, deconditioning, thromboembolic disease, and cardiac causes. Patients also may present with pleuritic chest pain. Infection and drug toxicity always must be considered in the differential diagnosis of pulmonary involvement.

Following a detailed history and physical examination, pulmonary function testing may be very helpful for further elucidating the type of pulmonary involvement. Patterns of pulmonary function impairment are suggestive of certain diagnoses (Table 57-5). Abnormal PFTs are best followed up with HRCT. The anatomic distribution of pulmonary involvement varies with the type of disease (see Table 57-2). Patterns of HRCT findings have been much better described and correlated with pathologic changes in the adult literature; however, some generalities can be extrapolated to the pediatric population. Ground-glass densities generally correlate with parenchymal lung disease while peribronchovascular changes and air trapping correlate with airways disease. Pleural inflammation is manifested as pleural thickening with effusion.

Bronchoscopy with bronchoalveolar lavage (BAL) may be very helpful for distinguishing autoimmune lung disease from opportunistic infection, alveolar hemorrhage, and cancer. BAL cytology patterns may suggest specific disease etiologies, although BAL for monitoring CTD-ILD is still investigational. There also may be characteristic airway changes of WG or sarcoidosis noted during bronchoscopy, and endobronchial biopsy may yield additional diagnostic information (see previous disease sections in this chapter).

Lung biopsy is reserved for a small subset of patients where a diagnostic dilemma remains, despite investigation using previously suggested modalities. If lung biopsy is required, it is best to do so expeditiously before clinical deterioration of the patient makes it too risky or even impossible to undertake. It may be needed to rule out an opportunistic infection or to confirm a diagnosis of inflammatory lung disease that will require a change in the management strategy, particularly the addition of a cytotoxic or biologic agent with potential significant side effects.

Occasionally, patients may present with sudden onset of new respiratory symptoms. Progression to respiratory failure can occur rapidly. Multiple etiologies of disease need to be considered as the potential cause of acute respiratory deterioration (Table 57-6). Prompt recognition and treatment of the cause of respiratory symptoms in this scenario may be lifesaving.

See Box 57-3 for key messages in the approach to pulmonary involvement in the systemic inflammatory diseases of children.

TABLE 57-5 PATTERNS OF PULMONARY FUNCTION AND GAS EXCHANGE IMPAIRMENT IN LUNG DISEASE ASSOCIATED WITH SYSTEMIC INFLAMMATORY CONDITIONS

	PATTERN OF VENTILATORY IMPAIRMENT	DIFFUSING CAPACITY FOR CARBON MONOXIDE	GAS EXCHANGE CHARACTERISTICS
Chest wall restriction (muscle weakness or chest wall deformity)	Restrictive defect with low MIPS/MEPS* (especially with associated muscle weakness) and low peak flow in more severe disease	Preserved until severe loss of volume	With severe disease, hypoventilation results in hypercapnia and hypoxia with a normal a-A gradient[†]
Pulmonary fibrosis	Restrictive defect	Reduced	With severe disease, hypoxia at rest
Bronchiectasis	Obstructive defect	Preserved until severe end stage disease	With end-stage disease, hypoxia at rest
Diffuse alveolar hemorrhage	Variable—often restrictive	Increased if hemorrhage is recent[‡]	During active bleeding, hypoxia, often profound with a wide a-A gradient[†]
Pulmonary vascular disease	Normal pulmonary function tests	Reduced	Hypoxia at rest even with moderate pulmonary hypertension
Mixed disease: pulmonary fibrosis and muscle weakness	Restrictive defect, often severe	Less reduced than expected for degree of restrictive defect	Hypoxia at rest or with exercise is frequent

*MIPS/MEPS refers to maximal inspiratory pressures and maximal expiratory pressures as measured at the mouth opening.
[†]a-A gradient = alveolar-arterial oxygen gradient.
[‡]Within the past 24 to 36 hours.

TABLE 57-6 CAUSES OF ACUTE RESPIRATORY DETERIORATION IN CHILDREN WITH SYSTEMIC INFLAMMATORY DISEASES

ETIOLOGY	DISTINGUISHING FEATURES
Infection	Fever, tachypnea, change in cough, increase in sputum volume, change in sputum color, malaise, new areas of consolidation on chest imaging; may be difficult to distinguish from disease flare
Air leak: pneumothorax or pneumomediastinum	Sudden onset of chest pain or shoulder tip pain and dyspnea, tracheal shift in the presence of tension pneumothorax, absence of fever and cough, more common in dermatomyositis/polymyositis
Upper airway obstruction	Stridor and dyspnea of subacute onset caused by progressive tracheal circumferential soft tissue thickening in Wegener's disease
Acute pneumonitis or pleuritis	Fever, new nonproductive cough and/or chest pain, dyspnea, basal coarse crackles on chest examination, hypoxia, diffuse interstitial infiltrates on chest imaging, more common in lupus and JIA
Diffuse alveolar hemorrhage	Anemia, tachypnea, and hypoxemia, hemoptysis usually absent, diffuse alveolar infiltrates on chest imaging, more common with ANCA positive serology and lupus
Pulmonary embolus	Sudden onset chest pain, dyspnea, hypoxemia, no change in chest radiograph or rounded or wedge-shaped opacity with apex directed to hilum, more common with hypercoagulable states like lupus
Progression of chronic lung disease	End-stage lung disease before deterioration, absence of fever or viral prodrome, rapid increase in dyspnea and oxygen need over a period of 1 to 2 weeks, mild (or no) changes on chest imaging out of keeping with severity of symptoms
Cardiac dysfunction	Low blood pressure, poor perfusion, may have wheezing, signs of left or right heart failure, cardiomegaly and/or pulmonary venous congestion on chest imaging, abnormal electrocardiogram

BOX 57-3 KEY MESSAGES IN THE APPROACH TO PULMONARY INVOLVEMENT IN THE SYSTEMIC INFLAMMATORY DISEASES OF CHILDHOOD

- Pediatric pulmonologists must work closely with the rheumatologist to diagnose and manage lung disease associated with systemic inflammatory diseases of childhood.
- The differential diagnosis of respiratory symptoms includes generalized muscle weakness, deconditioning, cardiac disease, thromboembolic disease, opportunistic infection and drug toxicity effects, as well as inflammatory lung disease.
- Recognize that pulmonary disease may sometimes be the predominant initial presentation of a systemic inflammatory disease.
- Specific inflammatory diseases are associated with probable patterns of pulmonary involvement (Table 57-2).
- Pulmonary function testing, including measurement of lung volumes and diffusing capacity for carbon monoxide, are helpful in refining the differential diagnosis, measuring the severity, and following the progression of lung disease (see Table 57-5).
- Bronchoscopy may reveal recognizable airway abnormalities associated with specific conditions (e.g., Wegener's granulomatosis and sarcoidosis).
- Bronchoalveolar lavage is helpful in ruling out infection, and the cytology count also may help to refine the differential diagnosis of lung disease.
- High morbidity and possible mortality are associated with pulmonary involvement of some systemic inflammatory diseases; hence, it is important to diagnose and treat early.
- Pulmonary involvement may require specific drug therapies for some diseases (e.g., cyclophosphamide for vasculitis).
- Most treatment protocols in pediatrics are extrapolated from results of clinical trials in adult patients.
- Early identification of pulmonary involvement may lead to application of new therapies, including biologic agents and therapies for pulmonary arterial hypertension

Suggested Reading

Black H, Mendoza M, Murin S. Thoracic manifestations of inflammatory bowel disease. *Chest.* 2007;131(2):524–532.

Cabral DA, et al. Classification, presentation, and initial treatment of Wegener's granulomatosis in childhood. *Arthritis Rheum.* 2009;60(11):3413–3424.

Fathi M, Lundberg IE, Tornling G. Pulmonary complications of polymyositis and dermatomyositis. *Semin Respir Crit Care Med.* 2007;28(4):451–458.

Iannuzzi MC, Rybicki BA, Teirstein AS. Sarcoidosis. *N Engl J Med.* 2007;357(21):2153–2165.

Levine D, et al. Chest CT findings in pediatric Wegener's granulomatosis. *Pediatr Radiol.* 2007;37(1):57–62.

Lilleby V, et al. Pulmonary involvement in patients with childhood-onset systemic lupus erythematosus. *Clin Exp Rheumatol.* 2006;24(2):203–208.

Milman N, Hoffmann AL. Childhood sarcoidosis: long-term follow-up. *Eur Respir J.* 2008;31(3):592–598.

Polychronopoulos VS, et al. Airway involvement in Wegener's granulomatosis. *Rheum Dis Clin North Am.* 2007;33(4):755–775, vi.

Polychronopoulos VS, Prakash UBS. Airway Involvement in Sarcoidosis. *Chest.* 2009;136(5):1371–1380.

Wells AU, Steen V, Valentini G. Pulmonary complications: one of the most challenging complications of systemic sclerosis. *Rheumatology (Oxford).* 2009;48(suppl 3):iii, 40–44.

References

The complete reference list is available online at www.expertconsult.com

58 DIFFUSE ALVEOLAR HEMORRHAGE IN CHILDREN

Timothy J. Vece, MD, Marietta M. de Guzman, MD, Claire Langston, MD, and Leland L. Fan, MD

The lungs receive blood from two separate systems, the bronchial circulation and the pulmonary circulation. The bronchial circulation is a high-pressure, low-volume circuit supplied by the bronchial arteries, which vary in number and origin, but most often arise directly from the aorta or one of its branches. These vessels provide blood to the conducting airways from the mainstem bronchi to the terminal bronchioles. Because the bronchial circulation is subject to high pressures, bleeding from this system has the potential to be profuse, sometimes resulting in massive hemoptysis and even death.[1-4] In contrast, the pulmonary circulation is a low-pressure, high-capacitance circuit that arises from the right ventricle and provides blood flow to the acinar units involved with gas exchange. Disruption of this system results in alveolar hemorrhage, which is often low-grade, chronic, and more diffuse. Although massive hemoptysis is rare, uncontrolled alveolar hemorrhage can be fatal at times.[3]

Pulmonary hemorrhage arising from either the systemic or pulmonary circulation has multiple causes and can be localized or diffuse (Box 58-1). Bleeding from the nasopharynx, oropharynx, or upper digestive tract is common and must be ruled out as a source of "simulated" hemoptysis, or true hemoptysis when the blood is aspirated.[3] Bleeding from the upper airway can occur from internal sources such as a subglottic hemangioma or tumor, or from external sources such as a foreign body or intubation.[5-10] Intubation may induce ulceration and granuloma formation of the airway wall that predisposes to hemorrhage. More serious iatrogenic causes capable of inducing massive and fatal hemoptysis include erosion of a chronic tracheostomy tube into the aorta or innominate artery and perforation of the pulmonary artery by a Swan-Ganz catheter.[11-14]

In children with advanced cystic fibrosis, hemoptysis is relatively common because severe chronic airway inflammation leads to progressive bronchiectasis and increased dilatation and fragility of bronchial vessels in the airway walls.[2,9,15,16] Bleeding can also occur in bronchiectasis related to primary ciliary dyskinesia or immunodeficiency.[17,18] Infection of the airways or lung parenchyma from viruses, fungi, and bacteria, particularly *Streptococcus pneumoniae* and *Staphylococcus aureus*, is a common cause of hemoptysis in children. In these cases, mechanical trauma from forceful coughing may contribute to bleeding. Finally factitious hemoptysis should be considered in a child with unusual symptoms and a negative evaluation.

This chapter focuses mainly on diffuse alveolar hemorrhage (DAH) arising from the small vessels and capillaries of the pulmonary circulation. A cardinal feature of DAH is the presence of hemosiderin-laden macrophages in the acinar units because macrophages are responsible for clearing free erythrocytes from the lung. In a simulated alveolar hemorrhage model, hemosiderin-laden macrophages first appeared 3 days following a single episode of simulated hemorrhage, peaked at days 7 to 10 with hemosiderin staining in 60% of macrophages, and were still found at 2 months in 10% (Fig. 58-1).[19] The etiology of DAH includes both immune-mediated and non-immune-mediated disorders (Box 58-2).

ETIOLOGY OF DIFFUSE ALVEOLAR HEMORRHAGE

Immune-Mediated Alveolar Hemorrhage

A subgroup of children and adolescents with DAH has the pathologic findings of pulmonary capillaritis (PC). Though a histologic diagnosis, PC usually defines an underlying systemic vasculitis or an immune-mediated disease process. PC can occur as an isolated disorder or as part of a pulmonary-renal syndrome or a more systemic disorder. The more common causes are antineutrophil cytoplasmic antibody (ANCA)–associated vasculitis and systemic lupus erythematosus (SLE). Of the ANCA-associated vasculitides, DAH from PC has been reported in 12% to 55% of patients with microscopic polyangiitis[20,21] and in 7% to 45% of patients with Wegener's granulomatosis.[22] In contrast, SLE, a more common disease, has a lower incidence of pulmonary hemorrhage, but the hemorrhage can be life threatening and should be treated aggressively. (Chapter 57 reviews SLE in detail.) PC also has been reported in Henoch-Schönlein purpura, Behçet's disease, cryoglobulinemic vasculitis, and juvenile idiopathic arthritis.[23,24]

Pathophysiology

ANCA is frequently associated with diseases characterized by the presence of vasculitis, affecting small and medium size vessels (e.g., arterioles, capillaries, and venules). These diseases are associated with circulating autoantibodies directed against the neutrophil granule components, myeloperoxidase (MPO) and proteinase 3 (PR3). In the correct clinical context, the specificity of these autoantibodies for ANCA-associated vasculitides is as high as 98%. This group of disorders includes Wegener's granulomatosis, microscopic polyangiitis and Churg-Strauss syndrome. Despite some overlap, PR3-ANCA is particularly associated with Wegener's granulomatosis, and MPO-ANCA, with microscopic angiitis.[25,26]

BOX 58-1 CAUSES OF PULMONARY HEMORRHAGE IN CHILDREN

Infection
Bronchitis
Bronchiectasis
  Cystic fibrosis
  Primary ciliary dyskinesia
  Immunodeficiency
Lung abscess
Pneumonia

Trauma
Airway laceration
Lung contusion
Artificial airway
Suction catheters
Foreign body
Inhalation injury

Vascular Disorders
Pulmonary embolism/thrombosis
Pulmonary arteriovenous malformation
Pulmonary hemangioma

Coagulopathy
Von Willebrand's disease
Thrombocytopenia
Anticoagulants

Congenital Lung Malformations
Sequestration
Congenital pulmonary airway malformations
Bronchogenic cyst

Miscellaneous
Catamenial
Factitious
Neoplasm

Diffuse Alveolar Hemorrhage Syndromes

BOX 58-2 CAUSES OF DIFFUSE ALVEOLAR HEMORRHAGE

Immune Mediated
Idiopathic pulmonary capillaritis
Wegener's granulomatosis
Microscopic polyangiitis
Goodpasture's syndrome
Systemic lupus erythematosus
Henoch-Schönlein purpura
Behçet's disease
Cryoglobulinemic vasculitis
Juvenile idiopathic arthritis

Nonimmune Mediated
Idiopathic pulmonary hemosiderosis
Acute idiopathic pulmonary hemorrhage of infancy
Heiner's syndrome
Asphyxiation/abuse
Cardiovascular causes
  Pulmonary vein atresia/stenosis
  Total anomalous pulmonary venous return
  Pulmonary veno-occlusive disease
  Mitral stenosis
  Left-sided heart failure
  Pulmonary capillary hemangiomatosis
  Pulmonary telangiectasia

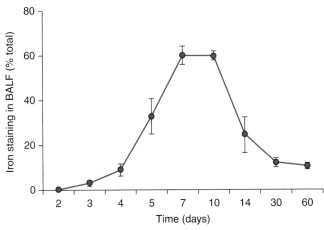

FIGURE 58-1. Time course of hemosiderin-laden macrophage production following a single episode of simulated alveolar hemorrhage in mice. (From Epstein CE, et al. *Chest.* 2001;120:2013-2020, with permission.)

The primary events leading to the onset of these necrotizing vasculitides are not known. Several hypotheses have been proposed that infectious agents can trigger and perhaps perpetuate such events.[27–30] The presence of these autoantibodies most likely reflects a pathobiological series of events involving the neutrophils and monocytes attacking the vascular endothelium of small vessels,

causing the release of autoantigens from these cells with eventual presentation to the immune system. In ANCA-associated vasculitis, it has been shown that with activation and damage of the endothelial cells, autoantibodies to endothelial cell constituents (antiendothelial cell antibodies [AECA]) are commonly produced. During this inflammatory attack on the vessel walls, the basal membrane of some vessels also can be damaged and autoantibodies to the basement membrane α3 domain of type IV collagen of the pulmonary vessels and glomeruli are produced.[26]

Other autoantibodies have been described in ANCA-associated vasculitis. These autoantibodies are likely to reflect mechanisms operating in the inflammatory cascade and may even be part of an orchestrated attack on the endothelium and basement membrane. The autoantibodies include AECA, antiglomerular basement (GBM) antibodies, antibasal membrane laminin antibodies, and antiphospholipid antibodies (APLA). With the exception of the antibasal membrane laminin antibodies, these autoantibodies are considered to be of clinical significance.

Antibodies to constituents of the endothelium have been described to be generally directed to small vessel endothelial cells, thus reflecting the typical distribution of such cells in the lungs, nose, and kidneys.[31] An increase in AECA levels has been described in patients with increasing vasculitic activity in idiopathic ANCA-associated and drug-induced vasculitis. An increase of these autoantibodies has been observed in both ANCA-negative and ANCA-positive patients during relapse of their disease. Levels of ANCA and AECA fluctuate independently, and these autoantibodies do not cross-react with the target antigens.[32]

Among patients with anti-GBM disease (also known as Goodpasture's syndrome), antibodies to the alpha domain of type IV collagen have been well described. Several groups have found anti-GBM antibodies co-occurring with ANCAs in patients with idiopathic ANCA-associated vasculitis.[33] In these patients, anti-MPO antibodies are the most specific. Some have proposed that it is essential to test for both types of autoantibodies because the co-occurrence of anti-GBM antibodies and ANCAs may be associated with more severe renal involvement leading to end-stage renal disease and poorer survival.[34]

The presence of APLA, which include anti-beta2 glyco-protein1 antibodies, anticardiolipin antibodies, and the lupus anticoagulant, is considered important in idiopathic ANCA-associated vasculitis.[35] Several reports have indicated that patients with both ANCA and APLA get more extensive and more severe disease. In drug-induced vasculitis, APLA of the IgM class are more frequently seen. If antihistone antibodies and ANCAs directed to more than one ANCA antigen are found together, a drug-induced condition should be suspected.[36]

Pulmonary-Renal Syndromes
Wegener's Granulomatosis
Wegener's granulomatosis is a necrotizing vasculitis of the small and medium-sized blood vessels associated with granulomatous inflammation that usually affects the respiratory system first and then the kidneys. Upper and lower respiratory manifestations include chronic rhinitis; sinusitis; serous otitis media; nasal cartilage destruction leading to saddle nose deformity; salivary gland swelling, subglottic stenosis, and tracheobronchial ulceration; parenchymal lung nodules or masses that tend to cavitate; and

DAH from PC.[22] Clinically, patients have dyspnea, cough with or without hemoptysis, and hypoxemia. Patients with renal involvement have hematuria with red cells and red cell casts. Other organs can be affected including the eye, heart, gastrointestinal tract, spleen, joints, skin, central nervous system, and pituitary gland.[37–56]

Laboratory evaluation should include a complete blood count (CBC) to identify anemia, erythrocyte sedimentation rate (ESR) and C-reactive protein (CRP) as nonspecific markers of inflammation, and blood chemistries and urinalysis to look for renal disease. Finally, testing for ANCA is essential because the majority of patients will have serum anti-PR3 antibodies (c-ANCA pattern).

Chest radiographs may show impressive nodules or masses with or without cavitation that are disproportionate to respiratory symptoms or pulmonary function studies. Computed tomography (CT) scans of the chest better characterizes these nodules or cavitary lesions but also may show diffuse ground glass or densities or consolidation related to DAH or airway abnormalities (Fig. 58-2). Sinus CT also may be useful in identifying sinus opacification and bony destruction.

Bronchoscopy may be indicated to define upper and lower airway lesions that include ulceration, granulomata, stenosis, and malacia. In patients with diffuse infiltrates, bronchoalveolar lavage may be bloody and reveal red blood cells and hemosiderin-laden macrophages consistent with DAH.

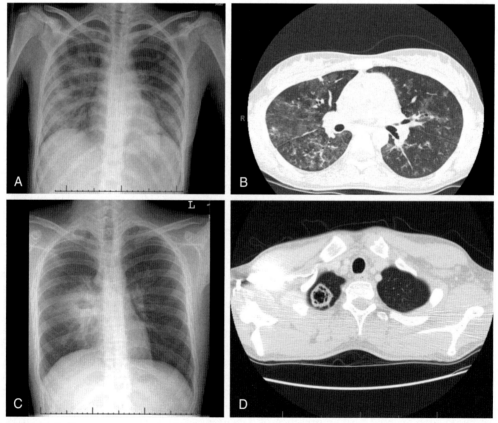

FIGURE 58-2. Radiographic findings in Wegener's granulomatosis. Radiographic findings in Wegener's granulomatosis can be variable. Chest x-rays can show diffuse alveolar infiltrates consistent with alveolar hemorrhage **(A)** with a corresponding chest CT with diffuse ground glass opacities and septal thickening **(B)**. Alternatively the chest x-ray can show no evidence of alveolar hemorrhage with cavitary lesions **(C)**. A CT scan in this case will have an absence of ground glass opacities with large cavitary lesions **(D)**.

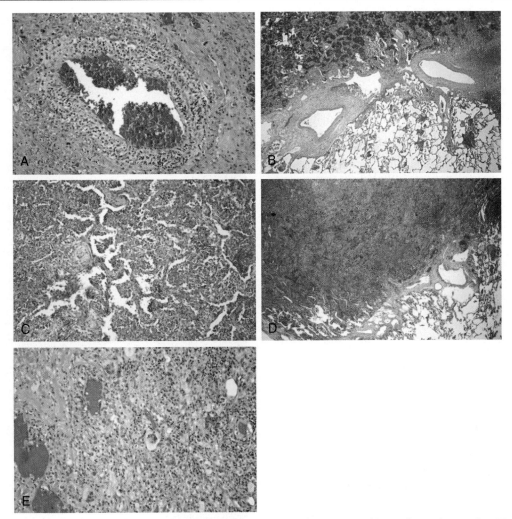

FIGURE 58-3. In Wegener's granulomatosis, there is vasculitis with parenchymal inflammation and hemorrhage. The vasculitis **(A)** involves medium-sized and smaller vessels and may be transmural and involve the complete circumference of the vessel as here, or it may involve only a portion of the vessel wall. There may be capillaritis **(B)** with hemorrhage **(C)**. Necrosis is basophilic because of its neutrophil content and is geographic **(D)**. There is abundant inflammation with lymphocytes, plasma cells, macrophages, neutrophils, and occasional multinucleate giant cells **(E)**.

Histopathologic confirmation is still considered the gold standard for the diagnosis of Wegener's granulomatosis in children. Characteristic features include a vasculitis of the medium and small vessels and capillaritis associated with necrotizing granulomata (Fig. 58-3). Biopsies from the lung or upper respiratory tract are preferred because of their high sensitivity and specificity. Kidney biopsies typically show segmental necrotizing glomerulonephritis with or without crescent formation, which is nonspecific and can be seen in other immune-mediated renal disorders.

In 1992, the Chapel Hill Consensus Conference declared that the histopathologic documentation of granulomatous involvement of the respiratory tract was not explicitly required and that the radiographic or clinical evidence highly predictive of such granulomatous pathology might be sufficient to diagnose Wegener's granulomatosis. Thus, the diagnosis of Wegener's granulomatosis now rests on clinical, serologic, radiographic, and pathologic correlations.

Treatment for pediatric Wegener's granulomatosis is broadly similar to the approach used in adults, with the goals of inducing and then maintaining remission.

Induction therapy has traditionally included glucocorticoids and cyclophosphamide. In children, we use both pulse intravenous methylprednisolone (30 mg/kg, maximum 1 g, infused once, weekly) and oral prednisone (1 to 2 mg/kg, daily). Several regimens involving oral or intravenous cyclophosphamide therapy, given over a period of 3 to 6 months, have demonstrated efficacy in inducing remission, lengthening time to relapse, and reducing adverse events.[57,58] Despite the efficacy of glucocorticoids and cyclophosphamide in inducing remission, disease relapses occur in as many as 50% of patients, and 20% to 53% may develop a relapse within the first 1 to 2 years following treatment. Disease relapses occur when the drugs are reduced or withdrawn. Given the adverse effects of cyclophosphamide, newer treatment strategies directed at B cell depletion have been tried. Rituximab appears to be as effective as cyclophosphamide and somewhat safer.[59]

Other important components of induction therapy in children include intravenous immunoglobulin (IVIG) and plasmapheresis. In addition to three open studies demonstrating beneficial effect on ANCA-associated vasculitis, a small randomized placebo-controlled trial of 34 patients showed a significantly higher rate of remission in the IVIG-treated group compared with placebo (15 vs. 6 remissions, P = 0.015).[60] In our center, IVIG is administered as part of the acute therapy and continued for at least 6 months.

Plasmapheresis has been shown to decrease morbidity in patients with primarily renal disease as part of the induction therapy.[61,62] No controlled trials are available with respect to alveolar hemorrhage and plasmapheresis; however, a retrospective analysis of 20 patients with alveolar hemorrhage who received plasmapheresis reported resolution of hemorrhage in all patients.[61] We believe that plasmapheresis should be considered in the early management of DAH due to Wegener's granulomatosis, microscopic polyangiitis, macrophage activation syndrome, anti-glomerular basement membrane antibody disease, antiphospholipid antibody syndrome, and systemic lupus erythematosus.

Following successful induction therapy, maintenance therapy traditionally has included low-dose prednisone and methotrexate or azathioprine.[63] Mycophenolate mofetil and leflunomide have been used as well.[64,65] For refractory disease, treatment options include rituximab, infliximab, and IVIG. Deoxyspergualin and antithymocyte globulin have been used in adults with ANCA-associated vasculitis, but there are no data in children.[58] Chapter 57 provides further discussion of Wegener's granulomatosis in pulmonary disease.

Microscopic Polyangiitis

Microscopic polyangiitis is a small-vessel vasculitis that, in children, appears to be more common than Wegener's granulomatosis. The presentation is similar to the other pulmonary-renal syndromes with hemoptysis, anemia, and new chest x-ray infiltrates in adults. However, hemoptysis is not always present in young children.[4,66] Patients can present with an acute, life-threatening event or with a more indolent course. Hypoxemia, often found at presentation, can be profound and requires intubation and mechanical ventilation. Although renal disease is found in some patients at presentation, a lack of renal disease does not exclude the diagnosis. Physical exam often reveals diffuse crackles, and imaging studies show characteristic but nonspecific changes of diffuse alveolar infiltrates, sometimes with a tree-in-bud pattern and septal thickening on chest CT (Fig. 58-4). Bronchoscopy and bronchoalveolar lavage reveal evidence of alveolar hemorrhage with blood-tinged fluid grossly and hemosiderin-laden macrophages on microscopic examination. In the absence of renal disease, all of the findings described above are nonspecific and cannot distinguish microscopic polyangiitis from idiopathic pulmonary hemosiderosis (IPH) or any other alveolar hemorrhage syndrome.

A diagnosis of microscopic polyangiitis is suggested by the presence of serum anti-MPO antibodies (p-ANCA pattern). In contrast, most patients with Wegener's have serum anti-PR3 antibodies (c-ANCA pattern). Lung histopathology in microscopic polyangiitis shows pulmonary capillaritis with a neutrophilic infiltration of the small arterioles, venules, and capillaries associated with fibrinoid necrosis (Fig 58-5.). The granulomatous vasculitis, characteristic of Wegener's, is not seen. As in Wegener's and other immune-mediated renal disorders,

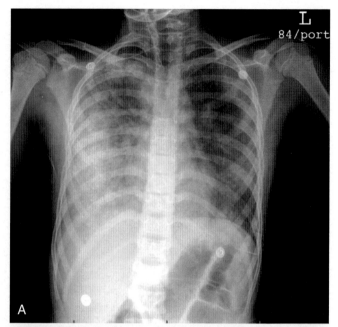

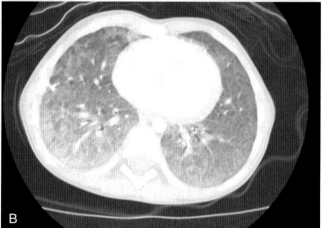

FIGURE 58-4. Radiographic findings in microscopic polyangiitis. Chest x-rays in microscopic polyangiitis shows diffuse alveolar infiltrates consistent with alveolar hemorrhage **(A)**. Chest CT also will show diffuse ground glass opacities with septal thickening that can be subtle **(B)**. These findings are nonspecific and are seen in many causes of alveolar hemorrhage.

patients with microscopic polyangiitis and renal involvement demonstrate segmental necrotizing glomerulonephritis on biopsy.

Treatment of microscopic polyangiitis is similar to that of Wegener's granulomatosis with the exception that cyclophosphamide is not always required for milder cases. In life-threatening cases, treatment should include corticosteroids, cyclophosphamide, plasmapheresis, and IVIG. After patients are disease-free for 6 months, they can be converted to maintenance therapy with low-dose prednisone and either methotrexate or azathioprine for at least 1 to 2 years. Because patients can relapse, sometimes with life-threatening consequences, we recommend that the patient be completely disease-free for a prolonged period of time before considering stopping therapy completely. Laboratory data, including CRP, ESR, and ANCAs, can be used to monitor a patient's response to therapy and to detect early relapse after treatment has been stopped.

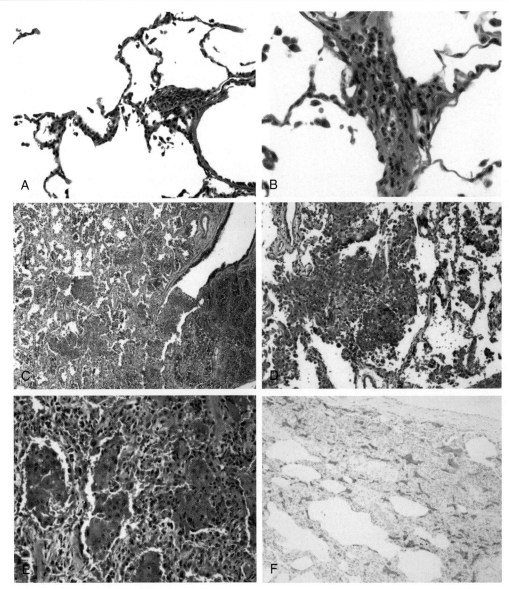

FIGURE 58-5. Small vessel vasculitis may be a feature of a number of immune-mediated vasculitic disorders that involve the lung, although in childhood, it is most often related to microscopic polyangiitis and is often associated with glomerulonephritis (pulmonary-renal syndrome). It is characterized by multiple foci of acute inflammation with clusters of neutrophils widening alveolar walls **(A)** and infiltrating the walls of small blood vessels within alveolar walls **(B).** There is often extravasation of erythrocytes with a background of diffuse hemorrhage filling airspaces **(C),** and there may be evidence of alveolar wall necrosis with fibrinous exudates and neutrophils spilling into airspaces **(D),** alveolar epithelial hyperplasia, focal organization and more diffuse alveolar wall widening **(E),** and hemosiderin deposition **(F,** iron stain).

Goodpasture's Syndrome

Similar to Wegener's and microscopic polyangiitis, Goodpasture's syndrome presents with the characteristic alveolar hemorrhage and renal disease. However, in contrast to these other pulmonary-renal syndromes that may have more systemic involvement, the disease in Goodpasture's is almost exclusively limited to the lung and kidneys.

Diagnostic imaging and bronchoalveolar lavage will yield findings consistent with nonspecific DAH. However, the classic distinguishing feature includes the detection of serum anti-GBM antibodies in serum and along the basement membrane in lung and renal tissue identified by immunofluorescent staining (Fig. 58-6). Biopsy material must be processed quickly and immunofluorescent staining applied promptly to optimize the detection of the anti-GBM antibodies.

Treatment of Goodpasture's syndrome is similar to that of the other pulmonary-renal syndromes, with corticosteroids used as primary treatment and cyclophosphamide added in severe cases. One important difference is that plasmapheresis is used in all cases of Goodpasture's syndrome to remove the circulating anti-GBM antibodies and to limit the amount of damage to the lungs and kidneys.[67–69]

Isolated Pulmonary Capillaritis

In children, isolated PC can present with classic signs and symptoms of alveolar hemorrhage without renal or other systemic manifestations.[66] Patients will have diffuse alveolar opacities on diagnostic imaging studies; low hemoglobin; hemosiderin-laden macrophages on bronchoalveolar lavage; and a normal BUN, creatinine, and urinalysis.

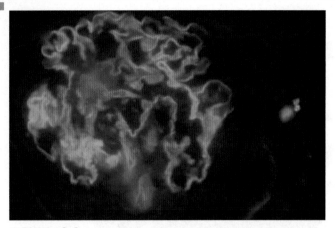

FIGURE 58-6. In Goodpasture's syndrome, diagnosis depends on the detection of antibodies with specificity for the glomerular basement membrane (anti-GBM antibodies) either in lung or kidney biopsy tissue. In this case, the kidney shows immunofluorescent staining of the glomerular basement membrane with anti-GBM antibody.

ESR and CRP are often quite elevated. Compared with IPH, PC is associated with a lower hemoglobin and higher ESR.[66] The presence of ANCA, usually of the MPO type but occasionally of the PR3 type, is often, but not always, found. In the absence of ANCA, lung biopsy is required for diagnosis. Because the neutrophilic capillaritis can be patchy and subtle, an inexperienced pathologist can easily miss the diagnosis. It is important, therefore, that an experienced pediatric lung pathologist review the slides.

As with other immune-mediated alveolar hemorrhage, isolated PC can have a fulminate presentation, and aggressive therapy, already discussed, should be instituted early.

Non-Immune-Mediated Alveolar Hemorrhage

Examples of non-immune-mediated alveolar hemorrhage include IPH, acute idiopathic pulmonary hemorrhage of infancy (AIPH), Heiner's syndrome, child abuse, and primary cardiovascular disease. Much controversy remains as to whether Heiner's syndrome, alveolar hemorrhage caused by milk allergy, actually exists.[70–72] A diverse group of cardiovascular disorders, including mitral stenosis, veno-occlusive disease, pulmonary capillary hemangiomatosis, and pulmonary telangiectasia, can result in a congestive vasculopathy with resultant hemosiderin-laden macrophages from DAH (Fig. 58-7). In a recent report of 30 cases of veno-occlusive disease and 5 cases of pulmonary hemangiomatosis, Lantuejoul and colleagues[73] found histopathologic evidence of pulmonary hemosiderosis in 80%. Pulmonary hypertension and pulmonary embolism can both cause hemosiderin-laden macrophages and should be in the differential diagnosis of pulmonary hemosiderosis.

Idiopathic Pulmonary Hemosiderosis
Previously considered the most common form of DAH, IPH is now a diagnosis of exclusion. Although IPH was reported to have a high mortality in the older literature, more recent studies have suggested a better prognosis.[74–76]

As in any alveolar hemorrhage syndrome, the clinical presentation of IPH is nonspecific with symptoms of malaise, cough, dyspnea, and tachypnea. Hemoptysis may not be present, especially in young children, who swallow their sputum. On physical examination, pallor, crackles, and clubbing, especially in long-standing disease, are present. Previously, the findings of iron-deficiency anemia; diffuse alveolar infiltrates on imaging studies; and hemosiderin-laden macrophages in sputum, gastric aspirate, or bronchoalveolar lavage were considered sufficient for diagnosis, especially when there was no evidence of systemic disease and negative autoimmune serology. Lung biopsy was not deemed necessary in such cases.[3,77]

Recent articles have shown a much higher rate of capillaritis in children than IPH, and many of the patients with capillaritis have negative serology for autoantibodies.[66] Therefore, we recommend that patients with DAH without a cardiovascular cause and negative serology undergo a lung biopsy. In IPH, the biopsy characteristically shows evidence of bland alveolar hemorrhage with multiple hemosiderin-laden macrophages in the airspaces, in the absence of significant inflammation or any evidence of capillaritis or vasculitis (Fig. 58-8). However, we emphasize that the pathologic features of capillaritis can be quite subtle, and many cases that we have reviewed where IPH was the initial diagnosis actually had PC.

It is important to distinguish between IPH and PC because the treatments are different. In general, PC is much more difficult to treat and often requires cytotoxic therapy to induce remission and prevent recurrence. In contrast, IPH can be successfully treated with corticosteroids alone in many cases, with hydroxychloroquine or azathioprine used as steroid-sparing agents when additional therapy is required. However, severe cases may warrant therapy similar to that used for life-threatening immune-mediated DAH and even extracorporeal membrane oxygenation.[78] In a recent series, 6-mercaptopurine was used successfully as long-term maintenance therapy.[79]

Acute Idiopathic Pulmonary Hemorrhage of Infancy
AIPH is a unique form of DAH that occurs in previously well infants who present with acute respiratory failure, diffuse infiltrates, and pulmonary hemorrhage. This disorder was initially reported in a cluster of 10 infants who lived in a geographically defined area of innercity Cleveland.[80] This study implicated exposure to water damage, and further investigation suggested that increased concentrations of *Stachybotrys chartarum*, a mycotoxin-producing mold, were found in the patients' homes.[81] However, the Centers for Disease Control and Prevention (CDC) critically reviewed this study, found major methodologic shortcomings, and concluded that the association between AIPH and *Stachybotrys* had not been proven.[82] More recently, in a report of four infants with AIPH in Massachusetts, two were found to have von Willebrand's disease and one other had a borderline test for von Willebrand's disease.[83]

Therefore, a coagulation evaluation needs to be performed in every child with AIPH. In addition, an

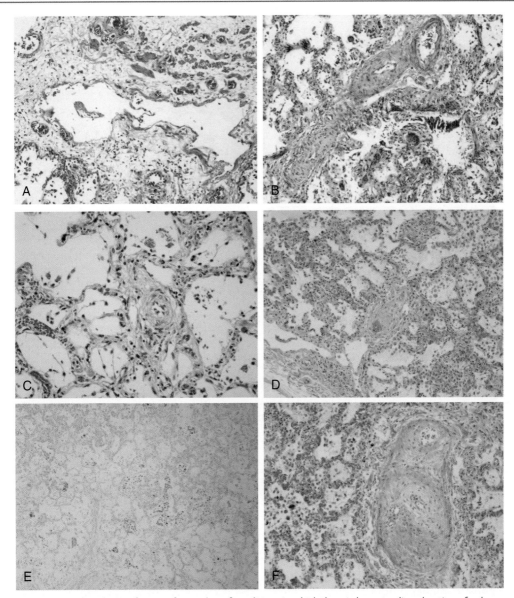

FIGURE 58-7. Congestive vasculopathy is a feature of a number of conditions in which there is long-standing elevation of pulmonary venous pressure from a variety of etiologies, including elevated left atrial pressure and pulmonary venous obstruction that includes pulmonary veno-occlusive disease. Pathologically congestive vasculopathy shows vascular remodeling affecting pulmonary veins with medial hypertrophy, arterialization, and perivenous fibrosis; lymphatics with dilatation and often lymphatic smooth muscle hyperplasia (**A**); arteries with mild medial hypertrophy and often eccentric intimal fibrosis (**B**, Movat pentachrome stain); and arterioles with more prominent muscularization (**C**). There are also parenchymal changes with edema, alveolar wall widening (**D**), and hemosiderin deposition (**E**, iron stain). In pulmonary veno-occlusive disease there is also venous intimal fibrosis that may be occlusive (**F**), and there may be arterial thrombosis and focally prominent alveolar capillary dilatation and congestion resembling foci of pulmonary capillary hemangiomatosis.

echocardiogram is indicated to screen for cardiovascular disease, and a skeletal survey and retinal exam should be performed to look for evidence of child abuse. As the cause of AIPH remains elusive, the CDC has recommended ongoing investigation and surveillance.[84]

■ APPROACH TO THE CHILD WITH PULMONARY HEMORRHAGE

Diagnosis

A systematic approach to the child with suspected pulmonary hemorrhage is required to determine the specific etiology and institute timely and appropriate therapy.

In patients with unexplained hemoptysis, diagnostic studies to consider include spiral CT with contrast to investigate for pulmonary embolism and arteriovenous malformations; tests for coagulation; and bronchoscopy to detect foreign bodies, airway hemangiomata, or tumors. Children with hemoptysis and bronchiectasis related to cystic fibrosis or other disorders rarely need additional diagnostic evaluation, but they may require intervention with bronchial artery embolization if hemoptysis is severe. In those with possible infectious pneumonia, blood and sputum cultures and a PPD should be considered with bronchoscopy, and bronchoalveolar lavage should be reserved for patients who do not respond to conventional therapy.

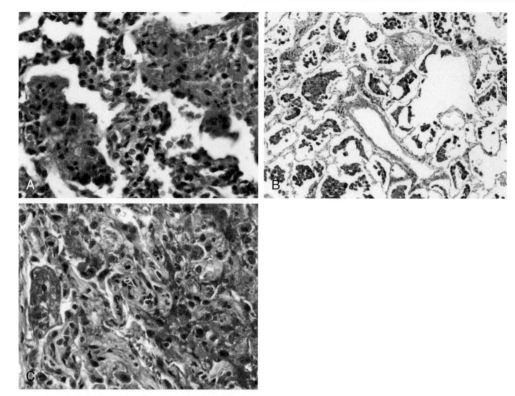

FIGURE 58-8. In idiopathic pulmonary hemosiderosis, diffuse alveolar hemorrhage **(A)** and hemosiderin-laden macrophages **(B,** iron stain) are present. Although there is mild alveolar wall fibrosis **(C,** Movat pentachrome stain) and mild alveolar epithelial hyperplasia, there is no alveolar wall or vascular inflammation.

In any child with diffuse alveolar opacities, cardiovascular causes should be ruled out by echocardiogram, CT with contrast, magnetic resonance imaging, or cardiac catheterization in selected cases. In patients with suspected or documented DAH and renal involvement, rash, joint disease, and other systemic manifestations, an immune-mediated vasculitis should be considered, and a pediatric rheumatologist should be consulted. Appropriate diagnostic studies would include an ANA profile, ANCA, CBC, ESR, CRP, urinalysis, metabolic panel, d-dimers, von Willebrand's factor, antiphospholipid antibody, lupus anticoagulant, and other tests as indicated. The identification of hemosiderin-laden macrophages in sputum, gastric aspirate, or bronchoalveolar lavage may confirm alveolar hemorrhage, but it is not specific as to the cause. Table 58-1 summarizes the distinguishing features of the alveolar hemorrhage syndromes.

In patients with DAH who have no cardiac, renal, or other systemic disease and negative ANA, ANCA, and anti-GBM antibodies, we strongly recommend that a transthoracic biopsy be done either through a mini-thoracostomy ("open") or with video-assisted thoracoscopic surgery. Lung tissue should be processed according to the guidelines set forth by the Children's Interstitial Lung Pathology Cooperative Group.[85] As discussed, histopathology of PC shows intraalveolar and interstitial red blood cells; pauci-immune hemorrhagic, necrotizing alveolar capillaritis with neutrophilic infiltration resulting in fibrinoid necrosis and dissolution of the arteriolar and venular walls; and intra-alveolar hemosiderosis. The presence of granulomatous inflammation is consistent with a diagnosis of Wegener's granulomatosis. Anti-GBM antibodies along the capillary basement membranes in the lung demonstrated by immunofluorescence are diagnostic of Goodpasture's syndrome. If only bland alveolar hemorrhage with hemosiderin-laden macrophages is found, and capillaritis is excluded, then a diagnosis of IPH can be made. It is highly recommended that the biopsy be performed early and before treatment is initiated because treatment may obscure the histologic picture.

Treatment

Treatment of pulmonary hemorrhage is based on the presentation and cause. In cases of massive hemoptysis, intubation and mechanical ventilation with high positive end-expiratory pressures may be necessary. If massive hemorrhage is unilateral, use of a double-lumen endotracheal tube allowing for airway occlusion of the affected side and ventilation of the unaffected side should be considered. Bronchial artery embolization is the treatment of choice to control bleeding. Underlying etiologies such as coagulopathy, cystic fibrosis exacerbations, pneumonia, arteriovenous malformations, or foreign bodies should be treated appropriately.

For patients with immune-mediated alveolar hemorrhage and life-threatening presentation, in addition

TABLE 58-1 CLINICAL MANIFESTATIONS OF DIFFUSE ALVEOLAR HEMORRHAGE SYNDROMES

	WG	MPA	GS	PC	SLE	IPH
Alveolar hemorrhage	++	++++	++++	++++	+	++++
Glomerulonephritis	++++	++++	++++	−	++++	−
Elevated ESR/CRP	++++	++++	+	++++	++++	+
Serologies	PR3	MPO	GBM	PR3, MPO	ANA	−
Extra-renal findings	+++	+++	−	−	++++	−

ANA, Antinuclear antibody; *CRP*, C-reactive protein; *ESR*, erythrocyte sedimentation rate; *GBM*, glomerular basement; *GS*, Goodpasture's syndrome; *IPH*, idiopathic pulmonary hemorrhage; *MPA*, microscopic polyangiitis; *MPO*, myeloperoxidase; *PC*, isolated pulmonary capillaritis; *PR3*, proteinase 3; *SLE*, systemic lupus erythematosus; *WG*, Wegener's granulomatosis.

to airway and ventilatory support, aggressive pharmacologic treatment with pulse and oral corticosteroids, cyclophosphamide, plasmapheresis, and IVIG should be given, as discussed previously. Those with less severe presentation may require corticosteroids and cyclophosphamide or another steroid-sparing agent. Following successful induction, treatment with low-dose prednisone and either methotrexate or azathioprine would be appropriate. For patients with IPH, corticosteroids and hydroxychloroquine or another steroid-sparing agent will control DAH in most cases. Newer therapies to consider include intrapulmonary instillation of activated recombinant factor VII (rFVIIa).[86]

◾SUMMARY

Because of the unique blood supply to the lungs, pulmonary hemorrhage can arise from either the bronchial or pulmonary circulation. The diagnostic considerations and management are different for each system. In patients with DAH, disorders associated with PC must be ruled out before a diagnosis of IPH can be entertained. This requires lung biopsy when serologic markers of immune-mediated disease are negative. Aggressive intervention is required for life-threatening DAH because morbidity and mortality are high.

Suggested Reading

Collins CE, Quismorio Jr FP. Pulmonary involvement in microscopic polyangiitis. *Curr Opin Pulm Med.* 2005;11(5):447–451.

Fullmer JJ, Langston C, Dishop MK, et al. Pulmonary capillaritis in children: A review of eight cases with comparison to other alveolar hemorrhage syndromes. *J Pediatr.* 2005;146(3):376–381.

Godfrey S. Pulmonary hemorrhage/hemoptysis in children. *Pediatr Pulmonol.* 2004;37(6):476–484.

Holle JU, Laudien M, Gross WL. Clinical manifestations and treatment of Wegener's granulomatosis. *Rheum Dis Clin North Am.* 36(3):507–526.

Kiper N, Gocmen A, Ozcelik U, et al. Long-term clinical course of patients with idiopathic pulmonary hemosiderosis (1979-1994): Prolonged survival with low-dose corticosteroid therapy. *Pediatr Pulmonol.* 1999;(3):180–184.

Pagnoux C, Mahr A, Hamidou MA, et al. Azathioprine or methotrexate maintenance for ANCA-associated vasculitis. *N Engl J Med.* 2008;359(26):2790–2803.

Pendergraft III WF, Preston GA, Shah RR, et al. Autoimmunity is triggered by cPR-3(105-201), a protein complementary to human autoantigen proteinase-3. *Nat Med.* 2004;10(1):72–79.

Susarla SC, Fan LL. Diffuse alveolar hemorrhage syndromes in children. *Curr Opin Pediatr.* 2007;19(3):314–320.

Update: Pulmonary hemorrhage/hemosiderosis among infants—Cleveland, 1993-1996. *MMWR Morb Mortal Wkly Rep.* 2000;49(9):180–184.

Wiik AS. Autoantibodies in ANCA-associated vasculitis. *Rheum Dis Clin North Am.* 36(3):479–489.

References

The complete reference list is available online at www.expertconsult.com

59 ENVIRONMENTAL EXPOSURES IN THE NORMAL HOST

Alan P. Knutsen, MD, James Temprano, MD, MHA, Jamie L. Wooldridge, MD, Deepika Bhatla, MD, and Raymond G. Slavin, MD, MS

HYPERSENSITIVITY PNEUMONITIS Hypersensitivity pneumonitis (HP) is an immune-mediated lung disease occurring in response to repeated inhalation of an antigen. It appears to be an underdiagnosed condition often masquerading as a recurrent pneumonia, idiopathic pulmonary fibrosis, Hamman-Rich disease, or interstitial pneumonia. HP primarily affects adults and older children, and less commonly, children under the age of 2 years.[1] HP has several synonyms, including pulmonary hypersensitivity syndrome and extrinsic allergic alveolitis. The last term seems particularly appropriate because it describes the disease in graphic terms: "extrinsic," meaning it comes from an outside source; "allergic," denoting a hypersensitivity basis; and "alveolitis," referring to that part of the lung most affected by the disease. Whichever term is used, it refers to the same basic process, a hypersensitivity reaction of the lung in response to inhalation of an antigen, most often an organic dust.

A number of factors determine the response to inhalation of an organic dust. First is the basic immunologic reactivity of the host. An atopic individual will characteristically respond with production of IgE antibody. A nonatopic person will more likely produce IgG. Second is the nature and source of the antigen. Is it small enough to reach the distal part of the lung? Is it a thermophilic organism, such that it will grow in the respiratory tract? Finally, the nature and circumstances of the exposure, is it intense and intermittent, or is it low grade and chronic? An intermittent short-term extensive exposure such as that experienced by a pigeon breeder while cleaning out the coops will cause acute reversible disease. A pet-store employee, who has intermittent, lower grade but long-term exposure, will develop a subacute form that is usually reversible. Finally, a long-term, low-grade exposure experienced by a parakeet owner may result in chronic irreversible disease.[2]

Many antigens have been implicated as causes of HP, and they can come from a wide variety of sources including animal proteins, fungi, amoeba, bacteria, medications, and chemicals. Table 59-1 classifies the causes of HP. The first example of HP was farmer's lung due to a thermophilic organism. These are unicellular branching organisms that resemble true bacteria.[3] A previously common occupational form of HP was bagassosis, or Louisiana sugarcane workers' disease.[4] Mold also can be a cause of HP, with two examples being maple bark stripper's disease, which develops in loggers who strip the bark and are exposed to *Cryptostroma corticale* underneath the bark, and malt worker's lung, which develops in brewery workers exposed to *Aspergillus clavatus* present in the moldy barley on brewery floors.[5] Probably the most common cause of HP today is avian antigen. Birds are becoming an increasingly popular as pets and serve as a potent source of antigens responsible for HP.[6] Finally, an example of a chemical source is toluene diisocyanate, which may cause disease in bathtub refinishers.[7]

Pathogenesis

The pathogenesis of HP is incompletely understood. The initial event involves sensitization to an inhaled antigen in the distal airway, but the level and duration of antigen exposure that is required for sensitization is unknown (Fig. 59-1). After antigen exposure in a sensitized individual, an acute alveolitis develops with an increase in neutrophils.[8–13] This typically peaks at 48 hours and is followed by an increase in the number of macrophages and lymphocytes.[14,15] Although a low CD4+/CD8+ T cell ratio is typically seen, a predominance of CD4 + T cells also can be found.[16]

Type III and Type IV Hypersensitivity Responses
It does appear that both type III antigen-antibody complex and type IV cell-mediated delayed hypersensitivity responses are involved (see Fig. 59-1). Antigen-specific precipitating antibodies are found in patients with HP in response to the offending antigen supporting a type III reaction[17]; however, precipitating antibodies also can be found in exposed subjects without evidence of clinical disease.[18] Inhaled soluble antigens can bind to immunoglobulin and cause complement activation, leading to increased vascular permeability and an influx of neutrophils and macrophages.[19,20] This leads to the production of interleukin (IL)-1 and IL-8, tumor necrosis factor (TNF)-α, monocyte chemoattractant protein (MCP)-1, macrophage inflammatory protein (MIP)-1α, RANTES (regulated on activation, normal T cell expressed and secreted) and CCL18, with resultant migration of leukocytes into the alveolar interstitium.[21,22] Several studies illustrate the role of cell-mediated immunity in the pathogenesis of HP.[24–30] A variety of factors, such as MIP-1α, MCP-1, CCL18, and IL-2, leads to an influx and proliferation of lymphocytes in the lung of patients with HP.[24–27] Secretion of IL-12 and MIP-1α by alveolar macrophages promotes the polarization of CD4+ Th0 lymphocytes to Th1 cells (T helper type 1), which produce interferon (IFN)-γ and are essential for granulomatous inflammation and the development of HP.[28,29]

TABLE 59-1 COMMON ETIOLOGIC ANTIGENS AND SOURCES IN HYPERSENSITIVITY PNEUMONITIS

DISEASE	ANTIGENIC SOURCE	ANTIGEN
Mold and Bacteria		
Farmer's lung bagassosis	Moldy hay and moldy plant materials	*Saccharopolyspora rectivirgula (Micropolyspora faeni) Thermophilic actinomycetes Thermoactinomyces vulgaris*
Humidifier lung	Ultrasonic cool mist humidifiers	*Bacillus subtilis Klebsiella oxytoca*
Ventilation pneumonitis	Contaminated air conditioners, humidifiers, or ventilation systems	*Amebas Thermophilic actinomycetes Thermoactinomyces saccharii*
Air conditioner lung	Moldy water in HVAC system	*Aureobasidium pullulans*
Maple bark stripper's disease	Contaminated maple logs	*Cryptostroma corticale*
Cephalosporium HP	Contaminated basement (sewage)	*Cephalosporium spp.*
Malt worker's lung disease	Contaminated brewery	*Aspergillus clavatus*
Basement shower HP	Moldy basement shower	*Epicoccum nigrum*
Summer-type HP	Japanese house dust	*Trichosporon cutaneum*
Animal Protein		
Pigeon- or bird-breeder's disease; bird fancier's lung; bird handler's lung	Pigeons, parakeets, parrots, doves and cockatiels	Avian proteins from bird excreta, feathers, or bloom
Laboratory worker's lung	Rat or gerbil urine	Rodent urinary protein
Wheat weevil disease	Infested wheat flour	*Sitophilus granaries*
Oyster shell lung	Oyster/mollusk shell protein	Shell dust
Chemicals and Drugs		
Paint refinisher's disease, bathtub refinisher's lung	Toluene diisocyanate	Varnishes, lacquer, foundry casting, polyurethane foam
Pyrethrum lung	Insecticide	Pyrethrum
Drug-induced HP	Medications	Amiodarone, cyclosporine, gold, minocycline, chlorambucil, sulafasalazine, nitrofurantoin, methotrexate, beta blockers, mesalamine

Cells, Cytokines, and Other Pulmonary Factors

Several other factors may play a role in the pathogenesis of HP. Natural killer cells (NK) are increased in the bronchoalveolar lavage (BAL) fluid and lung tissue of patients with HP and appear to provide a protective effect.[23,24] Aberrant regulatory T cell and Th17 cell function also may play a pathologic role.[25–30] Up-regulation of co-stimulatory molecules on alveolar macrophages and increased expression of L-, E-, and P-selectins may lead to the influx of various leukocytes into the lung.[31–34] MyD88, an adapter protein that interacts with several toll-like receptors (TLRs), has been found to play an important role in the inflammatory response seen in HP.[35,36] Surfactant protein A, which stimulates inflammatory cytokine release, is increased in BAL fluid from patients with HP.[37] Increased formation of free radicals, through a variety of mechanisms, also contributes to lung inflammation.[17,38–40]

Excessive accumulation of extracellular matrix components through increased levels of fibrinolysis inhibitors, such as thrombin-activatable fibrinolysis inhibitor and protein C inhibitor, or decreased activity of matrix metalloproteinases, contributes to the fibrotic process seen in chronic HP.[41,42]

Susceptibility Factors

Multiple susceptibility factors have been implicated in the pathogenesis of HP, such as cigarette smoking, viral infections, endotoxin, and genetic predisposition. Several studies have observed a negative relationship between cigarette smoking and the development of HP in similarly exposed individuals.[43–48] Many patients with HP report a viral type illness or flulike symptoms during the initial stage of disease. An acute viral infection could enhance the antigenic response in HP by increasing the

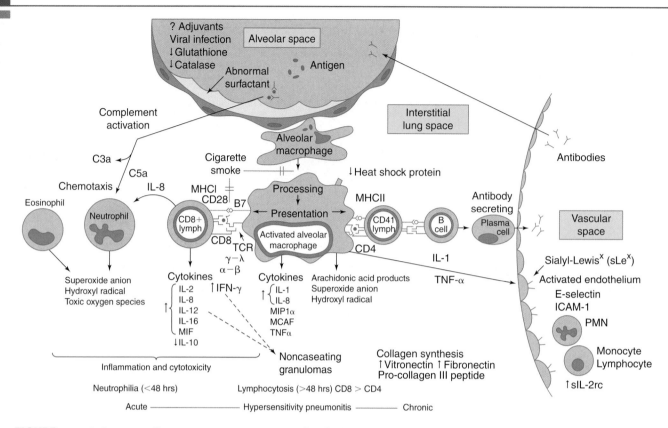

FIGURE 59-1. Pathogenesis of hypersensitivity pneumonitis. Small molecular weight antigen that enters the alveoli is engulfed by alveolar macrophages, which become activated and interact with both CD4 + and CD8 + T cells. Other cell types are attracted through chemokines and release a variety of inflammatory mediators typical of T helper cell type 1 (Th1) profile. Many factors, including adjuvants, environmental influences, surfactant composition, and balance of cytokines, influence the inflammatory responses. This response eventually leads to a lymphocytic infiltration and granuloma formation in the interstitial lung spaces and alveoli. (Used with permission from Dr. Jordan Fink and Elsevier Publishing.)

antigen presentation ability of alveolar macrophages, decreasing the clearance of antigens, and inducing the release of proinflammatory cytokines.[49] Endotoxin coexposure with antigen has been shown to augment lung pathology in a murine model of HP and may act through TLRs on macrophages, leading to a Th1 T cell response or play an indirect role in the pathogenesis of HP as an adjuvant.[24,50] Finally, various HLA haplotypes and genetic polymorphisms, such as those of the TNF-α gene promoter and IL-6 gene, have been associated with susceptibility to HP.[51–61]

Clinical Manifestations

The clinical manifestations of HP depend on the nature and circumstances of exposure; HP is divided into three stages, acute, subacute, and chronic.

Acute Stage

In the acute form of HP, such as that seen in pigeon breeders, chills, fever up to 40° C, cough, and shortness of breath are seen 4 to 6 hours after exposure. Symptoms may persist for up to 18 hours. Patients usually recover in 2 to 5 days, with episodes occurring after each subsequent exposure. Physical examination reveals only crackling and rales in the lower lung fields. HP is an example of an interstitial pneumonia in which there is a disparity between the symptoms of the patient and

the physical findings. Wheezing is uncommon because most patients exposed to organic dusts do not develop HP and asthma.

Subacute Stage

The subacute form occurs as a result of an intermittent low grade but continuous long-term exposure such as seen is in a pet-store employee. The symptoms are milder and include malaise, low-grade fever, cough, chills and progressive dyspnea often associated with anorexia and weight loss. This form is usually reversible.[62]

Chronic Stage

A long-term low-grade exposure experienced by a parakeet owner or from a contaminated home humidifier may result in chronic irreversible disease. These patients present with dyspnea, chronic cough, fatigue, anorexia and weight loss.[63]

Immunologic Studies

Laboratory evaluation generally reveals a marked leukocytosis with prominent neutrophilia during the acute phase of HP.[64] An elevation of markers of inflammation, such as erythrocyte sedimentation rate and C-reactive protein, may be seen. An elevated rheumatoid factor is found in 50% of patients along with elevation in serum IgG, IgA, and IgM.[64] Skin testing has limited value in the workup of HP. Results of a number of studies are conflicting. A high

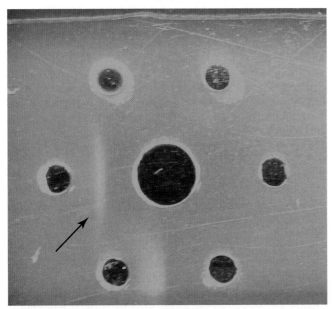

FIGURE 59-2. Ouchterlony double immunodiffusion (agar gel immunodiffusion). The center well contains patient serum and the outer wells contain different antigens. Note the strong line of precipitation between the patient's serum and the antigen *(arrow)*.

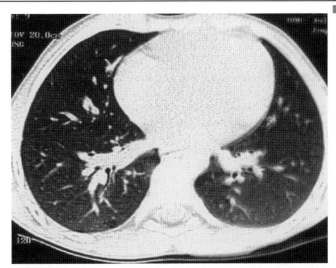

FIGURE 59-3. HRCT scan of the chest in a child with HP, demonstrating ground-glass opacities.

percentage of patients without the disease have positive skin tests reactions, and there is a lack of commercially available standardized extracts. A diagnostic hallmark of HP is an IgG precipitating antibody seen on a double gel diffusion plate (Fig. 59-2). However, the presence of precipitating antibody is only a marker of exposure, and sensitization and does not correlate with disease activity. Approximately 40% to 50% of asymptomatic exposed individuals will have precipitating antibody to the offending antigen.[65] Reports from commercial laboratories are sometimes inaccurate, and selection of a laboratory experienced in assays for the diagnosis of HP is important. Methods more sensitive than gel diffusion are available, including counterimmunoelectrophoresis (CIE), enzyme linked immunosorbent assays (ELISA), and radioimmunoassay (RIA). Lymphocyte proliferation assays to the offending antigen are usually positive in patients with HP.[66] In one study, alveolar macrophages from patients with HP enhanced the lymphoproliferative response while the response was inhibited in normal patients. This suggests that a defect in the ability of alveolar macrophages to suppress the lymphoproliferative response leads to the development of the observed lymphocytic alveolitis seen in patients with HP.[66] It should be emphasized that these studies are available only in research laboratories.

Radiologic Findings

Radiologic findings in HP correlate with the stage of disease. In acute HP, chest radiography usually demonstrates poorly defined, nodular infiltrates, but patchy ground-glass opacities or diffuse infiltrates also may occur.[24,64,67,68] It is important to note that patients with acute HP may have a normal chest radiograph after cessation of exposure and resolution of the acute episode. High-resolution computed tomography (HRCT) of the chest typically demonstrates ground-glass opacities in acute HP, but the presence of ground-glass opacities is generally a nonspecific finding (Fig. 59-3).[69,70] Ground-glass opacification represents cellular interstitial infiltration, small granulomata within the alveolar septa, or both.[70] These opacities may be found either centrally or peripherally, but are predominantly in the lower lung zones with sparing of the apices in acute HP.[20,71]

In subacute HP, a reticulonodular appearance with fine linear shadows and small nodules is typically present on chest radiograph, although the chest radiograph also may be normal as seen in acute HP.[20,71] The infiltrates in subacute HP usually predominate in the mid to upper lung zones.[20,71] HRCT of the chest in subacute HP typically demonstrates centrilobular nodules associated with larger areas of ground-glass opacity, as well as air trapping and mosaic perfusion (see Fig. 59-2).[70] Centrilobular nodules correspond to the presence of poorly marginated granulomata and active alveolitis, while mosaic perfusion indicates the redistribution of blood flow, and air trapping denotes obstructive bronchiolitis.[70] The presence of ground glass opacities, air trapping, mosaic perfusion, and areas of normal lung attenuation on the same film yields an appearance on HRCT known as the headcheese sign.[70] This is characteristic for subacute HP.

Chronic HP is characterized by diffuse reticulonodular infiltrates, volume loss, and coarse linear opacities on chest radiography.[20,67,71] The findings in chronic HP appear to be more severe in the mid to upper zones of the lung.[20,71] HRCT often demonstrates fibrotic changes that include irregular linear opacities, honeycombing, and traction bronchiectasis.[70] These changes also can be found in several other disorders such as sarcoidosis, interstitial pulmonary fibrosis, and collagen vascular diseases.[70] Centrilobular nodules are often found in chronic HP when ongoing antigen exposure is occurring. The radiographic findings in chronic HP, unlike acute HP, are unlikely to resolve when antigen exposure ceases. Several findings are not characteristically found and may be helpful in differentiating HP from other disorders. Pleural effusions or pleural thickening, as well as cavitation, calcification, or atelectasis, are usually absent in HP.[68] Hilar adenopathy, commonly seen in sarcoidosis, is rarely seen in HP.[64]

Pulmonary Function Testing and Bronchial Challenge

Pulmonary function testing typically reveals restriction with a reduction in lung volumes and a decrease in diffusion capacity for carbon monoxide (DLCO); however, obstructive, mixed obstructive and restrictive, or normal pulmonary function tests can be seen.* A decrease in airway compliance is often seen with a shift in the pressure-volume curve down and to the right.[64,71] A decrease in arterial oxygen tension (PaO_2) on arterial blood gas analysis is most commonly seen in chronic HP, but can be found in both acute and subacute forms of the disease.[16] The hypoxemia and decreased diffusion capacity may be accounted for by filling of the alveolar space with fluid and inflammatory cells. Oxygen desaturation with exercise or with sleep is not an uncommon finding.[71] Twenty percent to 40% display nonspecific airway reactivity and 5% to 10% have asthma.[68,73,74] Additionally, in patients with farmer's lung, Karjalainen and colleagues[75] showed an increased risk in developing asthma after their diagnosis of HP. The concomitant or future development of asthma after HP also has been shown in HP caused by diisocyanates, after summer-type HP and after residential mold exposure.[74,76-79]

Bronchial challenge has been studied in adults but is infrequently used in children.[71,80] These challenges can be performed either through re-exposure to the suspected setting or through a controlled challenge in an experienced laboratory. In a review by Fan,[71] 20 of 86 children with HP underwent bronchial challenge, and only 55% of these patients had positive challenges. In a large cohort of patients with bird fancier's lung, Morell and colleagues[16] reported a sensitivity of 92% and specificity of 100% using bronchial challenge to avian extracts. As the authors note in their study, bronchial challenge testing should be performed in a hospital setting with experienced staff and high-quality antigenic extracts.[16] Some difficulties that may be encountered in bronchial provocation are poor standardization of the antigen dose used for the challenge, difficulties in objectively defining a positive test, and the difficulty that many young children have in performing routine pulmonary function testing.[81]

Bronchoalveolar Lavage and Lung Biopsy

The BAL from normal individuals typically reveals a preponderance of alveolar macrophages with approximately 10% lymphocytes that have a CD4+/CD8+ ratio of 1.8.[110] After acute antigen exposure, the BAL in patients with HP reveals a predominance of neutrophils that is then followed by a lymphocytic alveolitis, which usually comprises 60% or greater of the white blood cell differential.† Historically, a low CD4+/CD8+ ratio has been associated with HP, while a CD4+/CD8+ ratio of over 3.5:1 has been associated with sarcoidosis.‡ More recent studies, however, have disputed this finding with the demonstration

of HP cases with higher CD4+/CD8+ ratios.[16,61,86] A study by Ando and colleagues[86] also suggested that the CD4+/CD8+ ratio may differ by the causative antigen and the smoking status of the patient. The BAL findings in HP also may differ based on the age of the patient. Ratjen and colleagues[23] evaluated BAL findings in children with HP. Nine subjects, 6 to 15 years of age, with acute HP were included in this study. The BAL uniformly revealed an increase in the percentage of lymphocytes and foamy macrophages in children with HP. All patients were found to either have an increased expression of HLA-DR (7 of 8 children) on BAL lymphocytes or an increase in NK cells (5 of 8 children) in BAL fluid. Importantly, there were no significant differences between normal controls and patients with HP with respect to the CD4+/CD8+ T cell ratio.

Histologic findings in HP vary based on the stage of disease.[19,21,87] Reports on the pathology associated with acute HP are few, but most note the presence of interstitial mononuclear cell infiltrates.[18,87] Granulomata and macrophages with foamy cytoplasm also have been reported.[88] The classic triad of subacute HP includes an interstitial lymphocytic-histiocytic cell infiltrate; bronchiolitis obliterans; and scattered, poorly formed, non-necrotizing granulomata.[16,19] In a large series of patients with bird fancier's lung, however, this triad was only seen in 9% of cases that underwent transbronchial lung biopsy, but at least one of the findings was present in 69% of cases.[16] Other findings commonly seen in HP include interstitial giant cells, interstitial granulomata, or Schaumann bodies.[89] In a pathologic review of 25 cases with chronic HP, giant cells, granulomata or Schaumann bodies were seen in 88% of cases, and 72% of cases exhibited a usual interstitial pneumonia (UIP)–like pattern.[89] A nonspecific interstitial pneumonia (NSIP)–like pattern or a bronchiolitis obliterans organizing pneumonia–like disease also can be seen in chronic HP.[90,91] Multiple studies have demonstrated decreased survival rates in patients with UIP-like or NSIP-like patterns of fibrosis.[89,92,93]

The usefulness of biopsy for the diagnosis of HP has been questioned.[21,94] Although the aforementioned findings are commonly seen in various stages of HP, none of the findings are pathognomonic for the disease because they can be found in other lung disorders. Most patients with HP can be diagnosed based on signs, symptoms, exposure history, radiographic, laboratory and BAL findings, obviating the need for lung biopsy. When a biopsy is performed, a surgical lung biopsy is the preferred method because it has greater diagnostic yield.[21] A study in patients with farmer's lung found limited usefulness of transbronchial biopsies as a diagnostic tool in HP.[95] Because the utility of transbronchial biopsies in HP is questioned and the majority of cases can be diagnosed without biopsy, surgical lung biopsy is usually reserved for cases when other studies do not yield a definitive diagnosis.

Etiology

There are over 200 antigens known to cause HP. The etiology of HP differs between adults and children and is due to differences in exposure. The majority of adult cases of HP are due to various occupational exposures. In children, most cases are due to household exposures, with

---

*References 20, 24, 64, 67, 68, 71, and 72.
†References 8, 9, 12, 20, 63, and 82.
‡References 20, 24, 63, 64, and 82–85.

avian antigens being the most common etiology, followed by molds.[71] A classification of the types of HP with the respective causative antigens is given in Table 59-1.

Bird Fancier's Lung

Avian antigens are the most commonly reported cause of HP in children.[71,96] Proteins derived from the bloom, serum, or excrement of several avian species have been demonstrated to cause HP. Bloom, a dust coating the feathers composed of keratin covered with IgA, is produced in large quantities by flying birds. While pigeons are the principal source of avian antigen in HP, several other birds have been implicated, such as parakeets, parrots, doves, and cockatiels.[97–103] Although bird fancier's lung is the commonest form of HP seen in children, it is still a rare disease.[96] Most pediatric reports note that children were initially treated for pulmonary infections or had multiple health care encounters before a diagnosis was made.[96,104–106] The diagnosis should be considered in any child with persistent, unexplained respiratory symptoms. The mainstay of therapy is bird avoidance, and therapy with corticosteroids is frequently required. Importantly, bird antigens have been found to persist at high levels as long as 18 months after bird elimination from the home.[107] As is the case with other forms of HP, patients with acute forms of the disease have the best prognosis, while those with chronic disease have higher morbidity.[108]

Other Environmental Exposures

HP also may result from exposure to various fungal or bacterial antigens. *Thermophilic actinomycetes*, *Neurospora*, and *Candida albicans* have been reported as causes of HP in patients that used covered swimming pools.[109,110] Residential mold contamination with *Auerobasidium pullulans* has been reported to cause HP in an adult and in child siblings.[74,111] This same species has been implicated as the etiologic agent causing HP in a child exposed to indoor hydroponics.[112] Household exposure to a fungus, *Trichosporon cutaneum*, causes summer-type HP, a common form of HP in Japan.[113] Contamination of the home with the fungus *Bjerkandera adusta* was found to cause HP in an elderly male.[77] A report of two children with HP secondary to exposure from an unventilated basement shower identified *Epicoccum nigrum* as the causative mold.[114] *Fusarium napiforme* also was found to be the etiologic agent in a 17 year old with HP due to residential mold exposure.[115] Exposure to mold or various bacteria through ultrasonic humidifiers and saunas also has been demonstrated to cause HP.[116–118] *Aspergillus fumigatus* was found to be the causative agent in a child with HP who had repeated exposure to organic compost on a playground.[119] There are also numerous reports of "hot-tub lung," caused by *Mycobacterium avium* complex, a non-tuberculous mycobacteria.[120–125] This disease typically occurs after exposure to hot water aerosols from hot tubs, showers, and swimming pools.[123] Most reports note that poor hot tub maintenance or poor personal hygiene practices contribute to the development of the disease. Some controversy does exist on whether this disease is a true representation of HP or has an infectious etiology. Patients with hot tub lung have well-formed, sometimes necrotic, granulomata, obstructive lung disease, and usually lack serum precipitating antibodies to the offending antigen, all supporting an infectious nature of the illness.[122,123] However, the clinical presentation, BAL lymphocytosis, HRCT findings, and therapeutic response to cessation of exposure and treatment with corticosteroids are consistent with HP.[121–125] *Cladosporium* also has been implicated as a cause of HP in an enclosed hot tub area.[126] Finally, "lifeguard lung," a granulomatous pneumonitis from indoor swimming pool exposure, was reported in several lifeguards exposed to water spray features at an indoor pool.[127]

Therapeutic Considerations and Prognosis

In the acute form, simple removal from the offending environment generally suffices. If symptoms are severe, the patient should be started on a tapering dose of prednisone beginning with 60 mg per day. Supportive measures might include O_2, antitussives, and antipyretics as indicated. For the repeated, acute, or subacute form, exposures should be decreased as much as possible with administration of long-term corticosteroids emphasizing alternate day therapy. The chronic form can be treated with long-term corticosteroids but only if radiographic findings and physiologic changes indicate a response.[128] Clinical follow-up should include spirometry with lung volume and diffusion capacity and chest radiograph. It is vital that the antigen responsible for HP be determined so that appropriate environmental control measures can be carried out. Several initiatives can decrease the antigenic burden. Chemicals can be added to prevent growth of an agent. A good example is propionic acid, which when added to sugarcane, eliminates the growth of the thermophilic organism responsible for bagassosis. Water should be changed frequently in humidification or air conditioning units. Storage dryers decrease the growth of mold and thermophilic organism in hay and straw. Finally, crops should be harvested when the moisture content is low. There are many ways to decrease exposure to organic dust. Dusty materials within closed spaces should be mechanically handled. Effective ventilation will remove dust from the ambient air. In some instances, personal respirators or masks may be used. Finally, when these measures have failed, the worker should be removed from the disease-producing environment.

The prognosis for patients with HP is generally good if the offending antigen is detected and avoidance measures are enforced during the acute and subacute stages. In a review of HP in children by Fan,[71] 97% of reported pediatric cases of HP had a favorable outcome when exposure was eliminated. A study in patients with farmer's lung demonstrated a recovery in DLCO up to 2 years from initial diagnosis.[129] In chronic HP, the prognosis is not as good, especially in patients with continued antigen exposure.[108] The presence of fibrosis seems to be the most important factor in prognosis because antigen class, symptom duration, and pulmonary function did not appear to be significant predictors for survival in patients with HP.[130] Fortunately, with early identification and treatment, progression to the chronic stage of HP can be avoided.

■ EOSINOPHILIC PULMONARY DISEASES

The eosinophilic lung diseases include a group of disorders that are characterized by increased peripheral blood and/or pulmonary eosinophilia (Box 59-1).[131-133] The clinical presentation of pulmonary eosinophilia consists of pulmonary symptoms, abnormal chest radiographs, and blood/sputum eosinophilia.

Biology of Eosinophils

Eosinophils are inflammatory granulocytes important in host defense principally against helminth parasites. They also play an important inflammatory role in a variety of diseases, including asthma, allergic diseases, eosinophilic esophagitis, and hypereosinophilic syndrome. Eosinophils are bone-marrow derived granulocytes.[134] The key cytokines that are critical for bone production of eosinophils are interleukin (IL)-3, IL-5, and granulocyte-monocyte-colony stimulating factor (GM-CSF), produced by CD4+ T cells. Activation of eosinophils is principally by IL-5 stimulation, which also increases tissue eosinophil survival. Tissue recruitment of eosinophils from the vascular system is stimulated by the chemokines platelet activating factor (PAF), leukotriene (LT)-D4, C5a, CCL11/eotaxin, and CCL5/RANTES. Stimulation by eotaxin is selective for only eosinophils.

Eosinophils possess a number of preformed granule-derived proteins (major basic protein, eosinophil peroxidase, eosinophil cationic protein, eosinophil-derived neurotoxin, and Charcot-Leyden crystal protein), de novo synthesized lipid mediators (LTC4, PGE1, PGE2, TXB2, 15-HETE, and PAF), and reactive oxygen species that are released upon stimulation and result in inflammation. Eosinophils synthesize a number of Th2 cytokines (IL-4 and IL-5), Th1 cytokines (IFN-γ), and chemokines (eotaxin, RANTES). Eosinophils also have Fc receptors, principally for IgA, which may regulate antibody dependent cellular cytotoxicity (ADCC) eosinophil degranulation. Thus, eosinophils are principally Th2-driven granulocytes that have potent inflammatory and tissue destructive properties.

Drug-Induced Eosinophilia

Many different drugs have been associated with the development of pulmonary eosinophilia (Box 59-2).[135-142] In fact, drug reactions are one of the most commonly reported causes of pulmonary infiltrates with blood or pulmonary eosinophilia. Sulfonamides, including sulfasalazine, were the first recognized cause of this reaction; however, more recently, it has been described with the structurally similar

drugs, sulfonylurea and chlorpropamide, and the antituberculous drug, p-aminosalicylic acid. The tricyclic compounds imipramine and carbamazepine also may cause pulmonary eosinophilia. Of the hydantoins (nitrofurantoin, dantrolene, and phenytoin), nitrofurantoin is most likely to cause an adverse pulmonary reaction. The reaction may be seen within days of starting treatment. Other drugs that have been implicated in pulmonary eosinophilia are listed in Box 59-2.

In addition to drugs, toxins from occupational exposures, such as rubber workers exposed to aluminum silicate and particulate metals, sulfite-exposed grape workers, and workers affected by Scotchguard inhalation are also linked to pulmonary eosinophilia.

A Löffler's-like syndrome has been seen in crack cocaine users. Drug reactions may be associated with the simple form of pulmonary eosinophilia-like syndrome, fulminant acute eosinophilic pneumonia-like syndrome, or they may follow a more chronic source. Symptoms normally start within a month of starting the drug and include cough, dyspnea, and fever. Histologically, there is pulmonary interstitial edema with a lymphocytic and eosinophilic infiltrate, and the alveoli contain eosinophils and histiocytes. Peripheral eosinophilia, though common, is not an invariable finding. Chest radiographs show interstitial or alveolar infiltrates and often demonstrate Kerley B lines. HRCT chest scans demonstrate areas of ground-glass attenuation; airspace consolidation; nodules; irregular lines, and sometimes, hilar adenopathy or pleural effusion.[143,144]

Drug-induced eosinophilic lung disease resembles other eosinophilic lung diseases, such as Löffler's syndrome. Thus, other causes need to be evaluated. Confirmation of the adverse reactions may be carried out by challenging the patient with a single dose of the drug. Skin testing with

---

BOX 59-1   PULMONARY DISEASES WITH EOSINOPHILIA

1. Drug- and toxin-induced eosinophilic disease
2. Helminth-associated eosinophilic lung disease
3. Fungal-associated eosinophilic lung disease
4. Acute eosinophilic pneumonia
5. Chronic eosinophilic pneumonia
6. Eosinophilic granuloma (formerly Histiocytosis X)
7. Churg-Strauss syndrome (Allergic angiitis and granulomatosis)
8. Hypereosinophilic syndrome

BOX 59-2   DRUGS THAT CAUSE EOSINOPHILIC LUNG DISEASE

Ampicillin	L-Tryptophan
Aspirin	Mephenesin carbamate
Beclomethasone dipropionate (inhaled)	Methotrexate
Bleomycin	Minocycline
Captopril	Naproxen
Carbamazepine	Nickel
Chlorpromazine	Nitrofurantoin
Clarithromycin	p-Aminosalicyclic acid
Chlorpropamide	Penicillamine
Clofibrate	Penicillin
Cocaine (inhaled)	Pentamidine (inhaled)
Cromolyn (inhaled)	Phenytoin
Desipramine	Pyrimethamine
Diclofenac	Rapeseed oil
Febarbamate	Sulfadimethoxine
Fenbufen	Sulfadoxine
Glafenine	Sulfasalazine
GM-CSF	Sulindac
Gold	Tamoxifen
Ibuprofen	Tetracycline
Imipramine	Tolazamide
IL-2	Tolfenamic acid
IL-3	Vaginal sulfonamide cream
Iodinated contrast dye	

either patch or prick tests is usually negative. *In vitro* lymphocyte transformation tests have been positive with some drugs, such as nitrofurantoin and carbamazepine. When the offending drug is discontinued, there is usually resolution of the symptoms and the eosinophilia, together with clearing of the chest radiograph. When resolution is slow, corticosteroid drugs may hasten the recover, though not invariably.

Helminth-Associated Eosinophilic Lung Diseases

Helminth-associated eosinophilic lung diseases can be characterized based on the natural life-cycle or history of the parasites[145-151] (Box 59-3). Infection in humans may occur by ingestion of eggs or larvae, penetration of skin by larvae, or inoculation of larvae by biting insects. Eosinophilic inflammation is a host response mechanism to resist these infections. Helminth infections also may lead to elevated serum IgE levels and a dominant Th2 cytokine profile. In developing countries, this Th2 response to parasites appears to decrease expression of asthma and allergic diseases.

BOX 59-3 HELMINTH-ASSOCIATED EOSINOPHILIC LUNG DISEASES

1. Transpulmonary passage of helminth larvae (Löffler 's syndrome)
   - *Ascaris lumbricoides, Ancylostoma duodenale, Necator americanus, Strongyloides stercoralis*
2. Hematogenous seeding with helminth larvae
   - Cutaneous larva migrans—nonhuman ascarids and hookworms, *Trichinella spiralis, Schistosoma*
   - Visceral larva migrans—aberrant infection—*Toxocara canis*
   - Disseminated *Strongyloides*
3. Pulmonary parenchymal invasion with helminths
   - *Paragonimus westermani* lung flukes
4. Tropical pulmonary eosinophilia—Filaria
   - *Wucheria bancrofti, Brugia malayi*

Transpulmonary Passage of Helminth Larvae

In 1932, Löffler described transient or migratory pulmonary infiltrates and peripheral blood eosinophilia in Swiss patients (132 with *Ascaris* infection acquired from soil containing human feces used as fertilizer. The nematodes that cause Löffler's syndrome are *Ascaris lumbricoides*, the hookworms *Ancylostoma duodenale* and *Necator americanus*, and *Strongyloides stercoralis*.[146,147] These organisms have infecting larvae that pass through the lungs as part of their life cycle. The larvae penetrate into the alveoli from the circulation and then ascend the airway to transit down the esophagus into the small intestines. In the intestines, the larvae mature and become adult worms.

Ascaris lumbricoides is the principal cause of Löffler's syndrome.[146,147] *Ascaris* is a ubiquitous parasite present in the soil of temperate and tropical zones. Infection is acquired by ingestion of the eggs, which hatch in the upper small intestine and free the larvae. The pulmonary symptoms develop 9 to 12 days after ingestion of the *Ascaris* eggs. Common symptoms include a nonproductive cough and substernal pain. Rales and wheezing occur in 50% of patients. Chest radiographs show nonsegmental infiltrates ranging in size from several millimeters to centimeters. The infiltrates are transitory and migratory and usually resolve over several weeks. Histopathology of the pulmonary infiltrates shows an eosinophilic inflammatory reaction to the *Ascaris* larvae. Peripheral blood eosinophilia peaks during pneumonic involvement and resolves over many weeks. Diagnosis of *Ascaris* infection is difficult at the time of pneumonitis because this would require identification of the larvae either from pulmonary secretions or gastric aspirates. Typically, the diagnosis is established by identification of *Ascaris* eggs in stool specimens, but this may not occur until 2 to 3 months after the pulmonary infiltrates (Table 59-2). IgG and IgE antibodies to the ABA-1 allergen of *Ascaris* develop earlier and may be protective. The treatment of *Ascaris* infection is albendazole or mebendazole.

TABLE 59-2 DIAGNOSIS OF HELMINTH INFECTIONS

PARASITE	MICROSCOPIC DIAGNOSIS		SEROLOGIC
	Stage	**Specimen**	
Intestinal Nematodes			
Ascaris lumbricoides	Eggs	Feces	IgE and IgG antibodies (I, Q, S)
Ancylostoma duodenale	Eggs, larvae	Feces	
Necator americanus	Eggs, larvae	Feces	
Strongyloides stercoralis	Larvae	Feces, sputum, duodenal fluid	IgG antibodies (Q, S)
Tissue Nematodes			
Trichinella spiralis	Larvae	Muscle biopsy	IgG antibodies (Q, S)
Toxocara canis	Larvae	Liver biopsy, other tissues	IgG antibodies (Q, S) (preferred)
Wuchereria bancrofti	Microfilariae	Blood, urine	IgG (CDC), antigen (blood)
Brugia malayi	Microfilariae	Blood, urine	IgG (CDC), antigen (blood)
Flukes—Trematodes			
Schistosoma spp.	Eggs	Feces, rectal snips	IgG antibodies (Q, S, CDC) Antigens (serum, urine)
Paragonimus westermani	Eggs	Sputum, feces	IgG (CDC)

CDC, Division of Parasitic Diseases, Centers for Disease Control and Prevention; *I*, IBT Laboratories; *Q*, Quest Laboratories; *S*, Speciality Laboratories..

Hookworms

Infection with hookworms also may cause Löffler's syndrome, but more rarely. Hookworms are prevalent in tropical and subtropical zones. Infection is acquired from larvae contaminated soil via ingestion or exposure to skin by *A. duodenale* and *N. americanus*.[146,147] The larvae that enter the skin cause a pruritic skin rash characterized by papules and papulovesicles, especially on the feet. The larvae are then carried by the venous circulation to the right side of the heart and to the lungs. From here, the larvae follow the route described for *Ascaris*. Larvae that are ingested develop entirely within the gastrointestinal tract, similar to *Ascaris*. Clinical symptoms, besides eosinophilic pneumonitis and eosinophilia, or include anemia caused by blood loss, abdominal pain, diarrhea, nausea, and anorexia. The diagnosis is established by identification of hookworm eggs and worms in stool specimens (see Table 59-2).

S. stercoralis has a worldwide distribution but is most prevalent in tropical and subtropical regions.[146,147] Similar to hookworm infection, *S. stercoralis* infection is acquired by exposure of the skin to larvae in the soil. Larval migration through the skin results in erythematous maculopapular lesions, especially on the feet, and creeping eruptions, "larva currens." The migration of larvae from skin to heart and lungs and then gastrointestinal tract is similar to hookworms; it takes approximately 1 month for mature eggs to develop in the intestines. The clinical manifestations include an eosinophilic pneumonitis, eosinophilia, and gastrointestinal symptoms of watery mucous diarrhea. The diagnosis is established by identification of the larvae in stool, sputum, or duodenal fluid specimens (see Table 59-2). IgG antibodies for *Strongyloides* also may be detected.

Hematogenous Seeding with Helminth Larvae

In this category, there is heavy hematogenous infection by helminth larvae or eggs causing eosinophilic pneumonitis. The etiologic helminths include nonhuman *Ascaris* and hookworms, which cause cutaneous larva migrans, and *Toxocara canis*, which causes visceral larva migrans, *Trichinella spiralis*, *Schistosoma*, and disseminated *Strongyloides*.[148–150]

Toxocara canis infection is characterized by visceral larva migrans, eosinophilia, fever, hepatomegaly, and eosinophilic pneumonitis in 32% to 44% of patients.[148–150] *Toxocara* eggs are prevalent wherever dogs are found. Infection occurs through ingestion of contaminated soil, most commonly by young children. Because the larvae do not mature, they migrate throughout the body causing visceral larva migrans.[149] A pronounced eosinophilia develops and eosinophilic granuloma formation occurs in the target organs that include the liver, lungs, brain, and eye. Serologic diagnosis is available through the Division of Parasitic Diseases, Centers for Disease Control and Prevention, Atlanta, GA (see Table 59-2).

Trichinella spiralis causing trichinellosis is acquired by ingestion of undercooked meat, primarily domestic pigs.[149] *T. spiralis* has a worldwide distribution. Two to 3 weeks after ingestion, adult worms mature in the small intestine. Larvae migrate from the gastrointestinal tract throughout the body via blood and lymphatics to principally striated muscle. The worms and larvae evoke an eosinophilic and lymphocytic inflammatory response. Clinical symptoms include myositis and, with high infectious burden, eosinophilic pneumonia, myocarditis, and encephalitis may develop. Diagnosis can be established by detection of antibodies to *Trichinella* (see Table 59-2). Treatment is with mebendazole or albendazole.

Schistosomiasis is caused by helminth parasites of the class Trematoda, which includes flukes.[148,150] Each species of *Schistosoma* uses fresh-water snails as its intermediate host. Its geographic distribution is limited to certain snail habitats, such as China, Indonesia, sub-Saharan Africa, Egypt, the Middle East, and Brazil. Humans are infected in fresh water contaminated by the fork-tailed cercariae, which penetrate the skin. Within hours of penetration, erythematous or vesicular lesions develop caused by eosinophilic and monocytic inflammatory reactions, termed "*swimmer's itch*." The *Schistosoma* larvae then migrate through the lungs causing fever and eosinophilic pneumonitis. These reactions typically resolve spontaneously. Acute schistosomiasis begins 1 to 2 months later when mature worms begin to produce eggs. At this time, there is characteristically marked eosinophilia, elevated IgE levels, elevated specific IgE and IgG antibodies to *Schistosoma*, and a Th2 cytokine response. The eosinophilic pneumonitis, which occurs during larval migrations, occurs early in infection and is manifested by fever, cough, and basilar rales, and wheezing. Chest x-rays may show basilar mottling. There is peripheral blood and pulmonary eosinophilia. Symptoms typically resolve spontaneously over a 1-month period. In patients with a heavy parasite load, a reactive pneumonitis may be seen. Diagnosis is established serologically or by identification of eggs in stool specimens (see Table 59-2). Praziquantel is the treatment of choice.

Paragonimus westermani is a helminth in the Trematodes class.[150] *P. westermani* is a lung fluke. Human infection is acquired by eating fresh-water crab or crawfish. The larvae penetrate the wall of the intestine and migrate through the diaphragm to reach the lungs. Pulmonary infection may be asymptomatic or cause a chronic cough productive of blood-streaked sputum. Eosinophilia is common. Pulmonary paragonimiasis is diagnosed by identification of eggs in stool or sputum specimens (see Table 59-2). In addition, serologic studies are useful. Treatment is with praziquantel.

Tropical pulmonary eosinophilia is caused by *Wuchereria bancrofti* and *Brugia malayi*.[146,147] *Wuchereria* and *Brugia* are classified as filarial parasites in the helminth family. These parasites are prevalent primarily in the tropics. Infection is acquired through insect bites, during which larvae are transmitted. Migration of microfilariae to the lungs causes eosinophilic pneumonitis manifested by wheezing, cough, chest pain, pulmonary infiltrates, and eosinophilia. Diagnosis is established by identification of microfilaria in blood or urine specimens (see Table 59-2). Serologic studies of IgG antibodies and filarial antigens are helpful. Diethylcarbamazine is the treatment of choice.

Disseminated strongyloidiasis may occur as a result of a hyperinfective cycle in which larvae invade all tissues.[152]

Allergic Bronchopulmonary Aspergillosis (ABPA)

Allergic bronchopulmonary aspergillosis (ABPA) is a Th2 hypersensitivity lung disease caused by bronchial colonization with *Aspergillus fumigatus* that affects approximately 1% to 2% of patients with asthma and 7% to 9% of cystic fibrosis (CF) subjects.[153–157] It is relatively uncommon in childhood, although it has been reported in children with CF from England and the United States. It was first described in adults in 1952 in England. The disease is most commonly caused by *A. fumigatus*. This is a ubiquitous mold that is commonly encountered around farm buildings, barns, stables, silos, and compost heaps. Human disease has been reported from most countries of the world. ABPA should be distinguished from other lung diseases caused by *A. fumigatus*, such as invasive aspergillosis, aspergilloma, IgE-mediated asthma from *A. fumigatus* sensitivity, and HP due to *A. fumigatus* or *A. clavus* (malt worker's disease). ABPA is characterized by exacerbations of asthma, recurrent transient chest radiographic infiltrates, and peripheral and sputum eosinophilia. *A. fumigatus* hyphae are generally found in the sputum at the time of acute exacerbations of ABPA. ABPA may lead to corticosteroid-dependent asthma, bronchiectasis, or pulmonary fibrosis. The diagnostic features of ABPA are (1) asthma or CF, (2) pulmonary infiltrates, (3) elevated total serum IgE >1000 U/mL, (4) IgE anti-*Aspergillus* antibody, (5) IgG anti-*Aspergillus* antibody, (6) peripheral blood and pulmonary eosinophilia, and (7) proximal bronchiectasis.

Pathology

The gross pathology of ABPA demonstrates cylindrical bronchiectasis of the central airways, particularly those to the upper lobes.[153–157] These airways may be occluded by "mucoid impaction," a condition in which large airways are occluded by impacted mucus and hyphae. Airway occlusion may lead to atelectasis of a segment or lobe, and if the atelectasis is long-standing, saccular bronchiectasis may result. Typically, ABPA is worse in the upper lobes than in the lower lobes. Microscopic examination of the airways shows infiltration of the airway wall with eosinophils, lymphocytes, and plasma cells. The airway lumen may be occluded by mucus-containing hyphal elements and inflammatory cells, especially eosinophils. Squamous metaplasia of the bronchial mucosa commonly develops, and sometimes granulomata form. Rarely, bronchiolitis obliterans or bronchocentric granulomatosis develops.

Pathogenesis

In the pathogenesis of ABPA, *A. fumigatus* spores 3 to 5 μm in size are inhaled and germinate deep within the bronchi into hyphae.[153–157] In addition, fragments of the hyphae can be identified within the pulmonary parenchyma. The implication of this is that there is the potential for high concentrations of *A. fumigatus* allergens to be exposed to the respiratory epithelium and immune system. *A. fumigatus* releases a variety of proteins, including superoxide dismutases, catalases, proteases, ribotoxin, phospholipases, hemolysin, gliotoxin, phthioic acid, and other toxins. The first line of defense against *Aspergillus* colonization in the lungs is macrophage and neutrophil killing of the conidia and the hyphae. In the development of ABPA, Kauffman's group proposed that *Aspergillus* proteins have a direct effect on the pulmonary epithelium and macrophage inflammation.[158,159] They demonstrated that *Aspergillus* proteases induce epithelial cell detachment. In addition, protease-containing culture filtrates of *Aspergillus* induce human bronchial cell lines to produce proinflammatory chemokines and cytokines, such as IL-8, IL-6, and MCP-1. Thus, various *Aspergillus* proteins have significant biological activity that disrupts the epithelial integrity and induces a monokine inflammatory response. This protease activity allows for enhanced allergen exposure to the bronchoalveolar lymphoid tissue immune system. This is evident by the bronchoalveolar lymphoid tissue synthesis of *Aspergillus*-specific IgE and IgA antibodies.

Recently, two genetic susceptibility factors have been proposed in the development of ABPA. Chauhan and colleagues[160–162] observed that asthmatic and CF patients who expressed *HLA-DR2* and/or *DR5* and lacked *HLA-DQ2* were at increased risk to develop ABPA after exposure to *A. fumigatus*. Furthermore, within *HLA-DR2* and *HLA-DR5*, there are restricted genotypes. In particular, *HLA-DRB1*1501* and *HLA-DRB1*1503* were reported to produce high relative risk. On the other hand, 40% to 44% of non-ABPA atopic *Aspergillus*-sensitive individuals have the *HLA-DR2* and/or *HLA-DR5* genotype. Additional studies indicated that the presence of *HLA-DQ2* (especially *HLA-DQB1*0201*) provided protection from the development of ABPA. Recently, increased sensitivity to *in vitro* IL-4 stimulation as measured by enhanced expression of the low-affinity IgE receptor (CD23) on B cells was observed in ABPA patients. This was associated with single-nucleotide polymorphisms of the IL-4 receptor alpha chain (IL-4Rα) in 92% of ABPA subjects, principally the IL-4-binding single-nucleotide polymorphism ile75val.[153,155,157]

This increased sensitivity to IL-4 is demonstrated by increased expression of CD23 and CD86 on B cells of ABPA subjects and increased CD23 expression during flares of ABPA.[153,157] CD23 is expressed on a variety of cells, including B cells, natural killer cells, subpopulations of T cells, and a subpopulation of dendritic cells. T-cell CD23 and B cell CD21 form a costimulatory pathway. T-cell CD28 and B cells CD80 and CD86 costimulatory pathways activate both T and B cells, and CD28:CD86 is important in IgE synthesis. CD86 also is found on dendritic cells that have the histamine receptor 2, which skews antigen-specific T cells to a Th2 response. In a murine model of ABPA, Kurup and colleagues have found that CD86 expression is up-regulated in the lung tissue (V.P. Kurup, Medical College of Wisconsin, personal communication). Recently, we also have observed increased CD86 expression on monocyte-derived dendritic cells of ABPA subjects. Thus, antigen-presenting cells such as monocytes and dendritic cells bearing *HLA-DR2* and/or *HLA-DR5* and increased sensitivity to IL-4 stimulation probably play a critical role in skewing *A. fumigatus*-specific Th2 responses in ABPA.

Brouard and co-workers[163] recently reported a third genetic risk, the association of the *-1082GG* genotype of the IL-10 promoter with colonization by *A. fumigatus* and the development of ABPA in CF. The *-1082GG* polymorphism has been associated with increased IL-10 synthesis; whereas the *-1082A* allele has lower IL-10 synthesis. Thus, dendritic cells expressing HLA-DR2/DR5 that have an HR2 phenotype, increased IL-10 synthesis, and increased sensitivity to IL-4 stimulation due to *IL-4RA* polymorphisms, may be responsible for skewing *Aspergillus*-specific Th2 responses in ABPA.

Recent studies in asthma have implicated the role of bronchial epithelia and mesenchymal cells forming the epithelial-mesenchymal trophic unit (EMTU) with a profibrotic response when stimulated with proteases such as Der p1 and with IL-4 and IL-13.[164] In ABPA subjects, *Aspergillus* proteases and allergen stimulation of the EMTU in conjunction with increased sensitivity to IL-4 due *IL-4RA* SNPs may result in increased bronchial epithelial secretion of IL-8, GM-CSF, and transforming growth factor (TGF-α), the ligand for epidermal growth factor leading to bronchial destruction and fibrosis.

Clinical Manifestations

Clinical symptoms of ABPA include increased coughing, episodes of wheezing, anorexia, malaise, fever, and expectoration of brown plugs. ABPA can present acutely with acute symptoms and signs associated with transient pulmonary infiltrates and eosinophilia or with mucoid impaction; it also may present an exacerbation of a chronic disease characterized by proximal bronchiectasis. It is thought that the chronic form of the disease develops following the acute process and that it can be prevented by effective therapy. In chronic ABPA, the acute episodes are superimposed on a background of chronic cough and sputum production. In adults, ABPA usually affects the younger age group of adult asthmatics, and most cases occur before 40 years of age. In pediatrics, ABPA rarely affects children with asthma, and it is usually seen in children with CF, who may simply appear to have a worsening of their pulmonary status or an acute pulmonary exacerbation of CF. ABPA does sometimes affect children with asthma, and there is a report of 3 children who developed it before 2 years of age. Physical examination shows the signs of chronic lung disease from CF or asthma, such as hyperaeration of the lungs, expiratory wheezing, a chronic productive cough, and crackles or wheezes. The chronically ill patient with bronchiectasis may have coarse crackles, weight loss, and digital clubbing.

The clinical criteria for the diagnosis of ABPA developed at a recent Cystic Fibrosis Foundation consensus conference are shown in Box 59-4. It has been suggested that a certain numbers of these criteria should be present to make the diagnosis of ABPA, although this approach has not been validated in childhood. A problem with applying the criteria in children is that usually ABPA occurs in children with CF in whom many of the criteria

---

BOX 59-4 CRITERIA FOR DIAGNOSIS OF ALLERGIC BRONCHOPULMONARY ASPERGILLOSIS IN CYSTIC FIBROSIS

Classic Case
- Acute or subacute clinical deterioration not attributable to another etiology
- Total serum IgE concentration greater than 1000 IU/mL unless patient is receiving corticosteroid therapy
- Immediate cutaneous reactivity to *Aspergillus fumigatus* while the patient is not being treated with antihistamines or *in vitro* presence of serum IgE antibody to *A. fumigatus*
- Precipitating antibodies or serum IgG antibody to *A. fumigatus*
- New or recent abnormalities on chest radiography or chest CT that have not cleared with antibiotics and standard physiotherapy

Minimal Diagnostic Criteria
- Acute or subacute clinical deterioration not attributable to another etiology
- Total serum IgE concentration greater than 500 IU/mL unless patient is receiving corticosteroid therapy. If ABPA is suspected and the total level of 200 to 500 IU/mL, repeat testing in 1 to 3 months is recommended. If patient is taking steroids, repeat when steroid treatment is discontinued.
- Immediate cutaneous reactivity to *Aspergillus fumigatus* while the patient is not being treated with antihistamines or *in vitro* presence of serum IgE antibody to *A. fumigatus*
- One of the following: (1) precipitins to *A. fumigatus* or in vitro documentation of IgG antibody to *A. fumigatus* or (2) new or recent abnormalities on chest radiography or chest CT that have not cleared with antibiotics and standard physiotherapy

---

could be due to the underlying disease. Some children with CF appear to have a clinical variant of ABPA without having all the typical criteria, and they may respond clinically to corticosteroids. Patients being considered for this diagnosis should have skin testing with *A. fumigatus* antigen.

Differential Diagnosis

Several diseases cause pulmonary infiltrates in children with asthma or CF. The differential diagnosis of ABPA should include the following: viral or bacterial pneumonia, poorly controlled asthma with mucoid impaction or atelectasis, inhaled foreign body, CF (with or without ABPA), immotile cilia syndrome, tuberculosis with eosinophilia, sarcoidosis, pulmonary infiltrates with eosinophilia, HP, and pulmonary neoplasm.

Clinical Staging

The spectrum of ABPA varies widely, from individuals with mild asthma and occasional episodes of pulmonary eosinophilia (with no long-term sequelae), to patients with fibrosis, honey-comb lung, and respiratory failure. Patterson and colleagues[165] have suggested a clinical classification with five clinical stages. Stage I is the acute stage of ABPA with many of the typical features of the disease. If this stage goes into remission, the infiltrates clear, symptoms reduce, and the serum IgE value will decline by up to 35% within 6 weeks. Stage II is remission. Stage III is an exacerbation associated with the recurrence of the initial symptoms and a twofold increase in serum IgE level. Stage IV is reached when patients need continuous corticosteroids either to control their asthma or to prevent a recurrence of ABPA. Stage V is the fibrotic stage, which is present when there is severe upper lobe fibrosis present on the chest radiograph, and it may be associated with honeycombing. The stage V lesions may not respond to corticosteroids although steroids are often necessary to maintain a bronchodilator response, and severe wheezing may develop if steroids are discontinued. Pulmonary fibrosis is an advanced complication that can lead to pulmonary hypertension and cor pulmonale.

Radiographic Findings
There are several characteristic radiographic abnormalities associated with ABPA.[154,165] The most common lesion is a large, homogeneous shadow in one of the upper lobes with no change in volume. The shadow may be triangular, lobar, or patchy, and it frequently moves to another site. "Tram line" shadows are fine parallel lines radiating from the hila that represent inflammation of airway walls. Mucoid impaction causes toothpaste shadows or gloved-finger shadows. Several adult patients have been reported with normal chest radiographs, so radiographic abnormalities are not invariably present. In these individuals, cylindrical bronchiectasis was demonstrated by tomography or CT scan.

Laboratory Investigations
Laboratory tests that support the diagnosis of ABPA are those that demonstrate allergy to the mold, such as a positive specific IgE test and positive Aspergillus precipitins.[153–157] The precipitins are only weakly positive compared with the strong reactions seen in patients with mycetomas. Culture of A. fumigatus from the sputum is only a secondary criterion for the diagnosis of ABPA because a large proportion of individuals with CF without ABPA have Aspergillus on sputum cultures. Some normal individuals and many individuals with lung diseases have small numbers of spores in their sputum; these are probably present because of passive inhalation. The presence of hyphae is more specific, and the presence of eosinophils in association with hyphal elements is suggestive of the diagnosis. The presence of eosinophilia in sputum or blood is suggestive of ABPA and is a primary diagnostic criterion. The PB eosinophil count is usually greater than 1000/mm^3, and values greater than 3000/mm^3 are common.

An increased serum IgE value is very characteristic of ABPA, and values may reach as high as 30,000 IU/mL. Usually, the value is greater than 1000 IU/mL. Much of the IgE is not specific to Aspergillus but is the result of polyclonal B cell activation. The IgE level is a very useful marker of disease activity, and it can be used to follow outpatients for "flares." The simple skin-prick test is a useful screening test because ABPA is very unlikely in patients with a negative reaction. A dual-reaction skin test with an immediate (10 to 15 minutes) and a late (4 to 8 hours) reaction occurs in one third of patients with ABPA. Alternatively, serum may be measured for the presence of specific IgE and IgG antibodies. Patients with ABPA and Aspergillus-sensitive asthma will have elevated Aspergillus specific IgE antibody, but patients with ABPA will have quantitatively increased Aspergillus-specific IgE levels. Crameri's group[168] has reported that ABPA and Aspergillus-sensitive patients have elevated

IgE antibodies to recombinant Aspergillus Asp f1, Asp f3, Asp f4, and Asp f6 allergens, and that IgE levels to Asp f4 and Asp f6 are highly specific for ABPA.

The usual pattern of serum precipitins is that immunoelectrophoresis shows one to three precipitin lines, often to only one extract.[158,165] Patients with aspergilloma will have multiple precipitin lines to all antigen extracts. Extracts of A. fumigatus contain a complex mixture of proteins that are mainly derived from the hyphae. Antigenic composition varies between batches according to the culture conditions, even within the same laboratory. There is, therefore, a lack of standardization that makes it difficult to compare results among laboratories. However, there has been some success with purification of the major antigenic components that may lead eventually to improved diagnosis. We find it best to send all our testing to one central laboratory that has well-established methods for the characterization of the serologic responses to A. fumigatus.

Therapy
Treatment is designed first to control the acute episodes and then to limit the development of chronic lung disease.[158,165] Most cases of ABPA require treatment with systemic corticosteroids, and the treatment of choice is prednisone. Steroid therapy rapidly clears the eosinophilic infiltrates and the associated symptoms; however, it is less effective at treating mucous impaction. The usual starting dose is 0.5 mg/kg/day, taken each morning, and this dose is maintained for 2 to 4 weeks while following the patient clinically and checking the chest radiograph for resolution of the acute process. After this induction treatment, the dose of prednisone should be reduced to 0.5 mg/kg given on alternate days. If mucous impaction persists and is associated with atelectasis, bronchoscopy should be performed to confirm the diagnosis and to attempt to remove the mucous plugs.

Following resolution of the acute process, the dose of prednisone should be reduced over 1 to 3 months. Chronic treatment with corticosteroids is controversial, especially in adults, because only a minority of patients with ABPA is at risk of chronic lung disease. The relationship between acute episodes and lung damage is unclear, and the precise dose of prednisone is not certain because acute exacerbations may continue while the patients are on low doses of steroids. However, children with ABPA usually have CF and may need treatment with long-term corticosteroids to prevent progressive lung damage. Therefore, we usually maintain therapy with a dose of 0.5 mg/kg on alternate days for 3 months and then, after 3 months, the dose of prednisone is tapered over a further 3 months while checking the chest radiograph and the serum IgE level for evidence of relapse. Initially, the serum IgE level should be checked at every visit, and if the level increases by twofold or more, the steroid dose should be increased. We recommend that patients are followed with serum IgE levels and chest radiographs every 6 months for the first 1 to 2 years, and then, if the child remains in remission, it should be possible to reduce the frequency of these studies.

The antifungal agent itraconazole has been used to reduce the doses of steroids that are required.[166,167]

Initially, there were only open nonrandomized studies that indicated that itraconazole is a useful adjunct to systemic corticosteroid therapy. Two recent randomized controlled trials also have favored itraconazole use. A double-blind, randomized, placebo-controlled trial of itraconazole 200 mg twice daily dose resulted in decreased IgE level and an increase in pulmonary function and exercise tolerance. Another randomized, controlled trial showed that treatment of stable ABPA in adults with 400 mg/day itraconazole resulted in a significant reduction in sputum eosinophil count, sputum eosinophilic cationic protein levels, serum IgE concentrations, and *Aspergillus*-specific IgG. There also was a reduction in episodes of exacerbation requiring treatment with systemic steroids. In the treatment of children with ABPA, we have used a dose of 10 mg/kg/day of itraconazole. Omalizumab, an anti-IgE monoclonal antibody, has been used in uncontrolled reports. Anecdotally, it has been effective, but a randomized controlled trial is necessary.

There is no place for immunotherapy in children with ABPA because it is ineffective and potentially dangerous. Inhaled anti-inflammatory agents, such as cromoglycate and beclomethasone are not generally thought to be effective. The role of inhaled spores in the pathogenesis of ABPA is unclear, but there is a seasonal incidence of ABPA that is probably related to seasonal changes in mold spore counts. Therefore, it is reasonable to advise patients with ABPA to avoid exposure to places with high spore counts, such as damp basements, barns, and compost heaps.

Prognosis

The prognosis for children with ABPA is good if the disease is detected early and treatment is started promptly. It is important that the diagnosis is made and treatment commenced before there is permanent lung damage from bronchiectasis. In such patients, there should be no progression of the disease, although relapses can occur many years later, and long-term follow-up is recommended. In children with CF, the relapses seem to be more frequent than they are in people with asthma, and careful surveillance is necessary to ensure resolution of the disease process. In some CF patients, it is difficult to wean the steroids without an increase in symptoms, such as dyspnea and wheezing; whether this is due to the underlying CF lung disease or due to patients going from stage I to stage III ABPA on withdrawal of steroids is unclear. Symptoms are not a reliable guide to therapy; therefore, it is important to reevaluate the chest radiograph and the serum IgE at regular intervals until a long-term remission is established.

Acute Eosinophilic Pneumonia

Acute eosinophilic pneumonia is a distinct clinical entity that occurs in both adults and children, with a male preponderance[169-176] (Table 59-3). Other causes of eosinophilic lung diseases, such as parasitic, drug-induced, fungal hypersensitivities, need to be excluded. The clinical manifestations include acute onset of fever, cough, and dyspnea for 1 to 5 days. There may be associated

TABLE 59-3 CHARACTERISTICS OF ACUTE AND CHRONIC EOSINOPHILIC PNEUMONITIS

CHARACTERISTIC	ACUTE	CHRONIC
Ages	Children and adults	Adults 40–50 years of age peak
Sex	Male preponderance	Female preponderance 2:1
Underlying asthma	None	50%
Symptoms	Acute febrile illness 1–5 days Fever, dyspnea, cough, myalgias, pleuritic chest pain, hypoxemia	Insidious over 7–8 months Fever, night sweats, weight loss, cough, wheezing, anorexia
PE	High fever, basilar rales, wheezing	Fever, wheezing, lymphadenopathy, hepatomegaly
Chest radiograph And CT scan	Diffuse alveolar or mixed alveolar interstitial infiltrates, pleural effusions	Dense peripheral infiltrates (negative image of pulmonary edema)
PFT	Restrictive pattern	Restrictive pattern
Lung biopsy	Diffuse acute organizing alveolar damage, eosinophilic infiltration of alveoli, interstitium, bronchial epithelium	Eosinophils and lymphocytes in alveoli and interstitium, thickened alveolar walls. Interstitial fibrosis in 50%; BO in 25%
BAL	45±11% eosinophils, 20±11% lymphocytes	>25% eosinophils, lymphocytes
Blood eosinophilia	Absent	Present
IgE level	Elevated in some	Elevated in most
Corticosteroids	Prompt response. No relapse if corticosteroids tapered over 8 weeks	Prompt response; relapse if corticosteroids discontinued within 6 months

BAL, bronchoalveolar lavage; *BO*, bronchiolitis obliterans; *CT*, computed tomography; *PE*, physical examination; *PFT*, pulmonary function testing.

pleuritic chest pain and myalgias. Patients then develop hypoxemia and respiratory failure often requiring a mechanical ventilator. Physical examination reveals high fever, respiratory distress, and basilar rales, sometimes with fever. Initial chest radiographs reveal interstitial infiltrates[171,172] that progress to diffuse alveolar infiltrates. Chest CT scans demonstrate diffuse alveolar infiltrates, pleural effusions, pronounced septal markings, and normal lymph nodes.

Pulmonary function studies demonstrate a restrictive pattern with decreased diffusing capacity. Bronchoalveolar lavage fluid reveals eosinophilia (45±11%) and lymphocytosis (20±11%). Pleural effusions are common with up to 42% eosinophils on cell count. There is evidence of eosinophil degranulation in the pleural fluid with an elevated pH. Lung biopsy specimens demonstrate eosinophil infiltration of the interstitium, alveoli and epithelium. Peripheral blood eosinophilia is typically absent; however, serum IgE levels may be elevated in some patients. The etiology of acute eosinophilic pneumonia is unknown. However, there is a dramatic response to high-dose corticosteroids, typically within 24 to 48 hours. Steroids are then tapered over an 8-week course. Relapses or recurrences are unusual.

Chronic Eosinophilic Pneumonia

Chronic eosinophilic pneumonitis is a disorder that affects primarily middle-age adults with a 2:1 female preponderance[177–181] (see Table 59-3). The etiology is unknown, and other conditions that cause eosinophilic lung diseases need to be excluded. A risk factor may be asthma, which occurs in 50% of patients. The symptoms are insidious, developing over a 7 to 8 month period. They include fever, night sweats, weight loss, cough, and wheezing. The cough is typically nonproductive. Some patients also experience lymphadenopathy or hepatomegaly.

Chest radiographs reveal extensive, bilateral, peripheral infiltrates, the so-called "negative image of pulmonary edema," which is diagnostic of chronic eosinophilic pneumonia. Chest CT scans show peripheral airspace disease and may show hilar adenopathy. Peripheral blood eosinophilia is prominent. BALF examination reveals increased eosinophils >25% and increased lymphocytes. IgE levels are also frequently elevated.

Lung biopsy specimens display moderate to extensive accumulation of eosinophils and lymphocytes in the alveoli and the interstitium with thickened alveolar walls. Sometimes multinucleated histiocytic giant cells, lymphocytes, and plasma cells are found in the alveoli, a noncaseating granuloma reaction. There is also a mild perivascular cuffing of venules with eosinophils and lymphocytes. Interstitial fibrosis has been reported in 50% of patients and bronchiolitis obliterans in 25% of patients.

Response to high-dose corticosteroids is dramatic, with resolution of symptoms within 24 to 48 hours. Radiographically, pulmonary infiltrates resolve over 10 to 21 days. Taper of corticosteroids needs to be prolonged typically more than 6 months to prevent relapse. The mean duration of corticosteroid treatment is approximately 19 months. Recurrent attacks have occurred in about one third of the patients, especially in those with asthma. Some patients have subsequently developed Churg-Strauss syndrome, raising the possibility of overlap of the two diseases. Nonetheless, long-term prognosis is excellent for most patients.

Eosinophilic Granuloma

Eosinophilic granuloma, formerly called histiocytosis X, is the benign form of the three forms of Langerhans cell histiocytosis: Letterer-Siwe disease, Hand-Schuller-Christian disease, and eosinophilic granuloma.[182] Eosinophilic granuloma affects children and young adults, particularly males. Typically, there is only a solitary lesion, but there may be multiple lesions that may be asymptomatic or may cause pain. Any bone may be involved, with the calvarium, ribs, and femur being the most common sites. Histologically, the lesions are comprised of foamy vacuolated histiocytes with variable numbers of eosinophils, neutrophils, lymphocytes, and plasma cells. The histiocytosis X cells are derived from Langerhans cell origin and are positive for CD1a and HLA-DR.

Pulmonary interstitial lung disease occurs in approximately 20% of patients with eosinophilic granuloma. Chest radiographs demonstrate an alveolar pattern in an early state. This may be followed by 3 to 10 mm nodular shadows or a reticulonodular pattern with a predilection for the apices. Fibrosis and honeycombing also may ensue. Histologically, eosinophils are present in the lesions; however, they are not present in BALF specimens.

Churg-Strauss Syndrome—Allergic Angiitis and Granulomatosis

Churg-Strauss syndrome (CSS) is also named allergic angiitis and granulomatosis because of its association in patients with asthma, allergic rhinitis, and sinusitis and with its findings of eosinophilic vasculitis and granulomatous lesions[183–196] (Box 59-5). Nearly all patients have allergic rhinitis and pansinusitis. Three phases have been described in CSS. The first phase involved development of asthma with variable severity, typically in adults. Tapering of systemic corticosteroid treatment of asthma may unmask CSS.[188] This has been reported as a risk in asthmatic patients treated with omalizumab and when the prednisone is decreased or discontinued. The second phase is characterized by the development of peripheral blood eosinophilia and eosinophilic tissue infiltrates. The third phase involves eosinophilic vasculitis of extrapulmonary organs, typically the skin, gastrointestinal tract, heart, and nervous system.

Cutaneous lesions are common, occurring in 70% of patients, variably manifesting as maculopapular rashes; petechiae; purpura or ecchymoses; and cutaneous and subcutaneous nodules, commonly on the scalp or extremities.[191] Peripheral neuropathies are common including mononeuritis multiplex and polyneuropathies.[190] Cerebral infarctions may occur and can be a cause of death. Cardiac involvement is a common cause of death and occurs in a third of patients. Gastrointestinal problems include abdominal pain, diarrhea, bleeding, and obstruction.[183–187] Pulmonary symptoms are present

BOX 59-5 FINDINGS IN CHURG-STRAUSS SYNDROME

- History of asthma
- Pulmonary
  - Patchy, transient infiltrates
  - Eosinophilic infiltration of alveoli, interstitium, blood vessels
  - Necrotizing and non-necrotizing granulomata
  - Eosinophilic angiitis
- Systemic vasculitis involving ≥2 extrapulmonary organs
  - Small and medium size arteries and veins, eosinophilic vasculitis
  - Eosinophilic granulomata
- Nasal symptoms
  - Allergic rhinitis
  - Pansinusitis
- Cutaneous
  - Maculopapular rash
  - Petechiae, purpura, ecchymoses
  - Cutaneous and subcutaneous nodules on scalp and extremities
- Cardiac
  - Hypertension
  - Pericarditis
  - Heart failure
- Gastrointestinal
  - Abdominal pain
  - Diarrhea
  - Bleeding
  - Obstruction
- Peripheral neuropathy
  - Mononeuritis multiplex
  - Polyneuropathy
- Central nervous system
- Cerebral infarction
- Hematologic
  - >1500 eosinophils/µL
- Radiologic
  - Chest x-ray: Transient pulmonary infiltrates
  - CT scan: airspace consolidation or ground-glass appearance, septal lines, bronchial wall thickening

in nearly all patients.[183–187] This is seen as patchy and transient pulmonary infiltrates demonstrated on chest radiographs.[192] Chest HRCT scans reveal a variety of findings that include airspace consolidation or interstitial ground-glass opacities, septal lines, and bronchial wall thickenings.[193]

Eosinophilia ≥1500 cells/mm³ is uniformly present.[183–187] Lung biopsy specimens demonstrate extensive eosinophil infiltration present in the interstitium, air spaces, and perivascularly.[183,184,193,194] In addition, both necrotizing and non-necrotizing granulomata may be present, involving blood vessels. The angiitis varies from eosinophilic infiltration of blood vessels to necrotizing vasculitis of small and medium-sized vessels. Biopsies of the cutaneous nodules reveal eosinophilic infiltration.

The treatment of CSS is principally with prolonged systemic corticosteroids.[183–187] If untreated, the mortality is significant, as high as 50% in the first 3 months of the onset of vasculitis. In treated patients, the mean survival is 9 years.

Hypereosinophilic Syndrome

Hypereosinophilic syndrome (HES) was first defined by Chusid and colleagues[196] in 1975, who specified the following three criteria for diagnosis: (1) absolute eosinophil count ≥1500/mm³ in peripheral blood for more than 6 months; (2) lack of evidence for parasitic, allergic, and other recognized causes of eosinophilia; and (3) end-organ dysfunction due to eosinophilic infiltration. It is now recognized that HES represents a spectrum of disorders that includes not only the previously described idiopathic HES (IHES) but also disorders characterized with eosinophilic organ infiltration that may or may not be accompanied by peripheral blood eosinophilia (i.e., eosinophilic pneumonia, eosinophil-associated gastrointestinal disorders [EGID], CSS, and eosinophilic dermatitis [Wells syndrome]).[197–199] A revised classification of HES was presented in 2006 by Klion and colleagues.[200] This classification system was the culmination of a workshop conducted by the Hypereosinophilic Diseases Working Group of the International Eosinophil Society with the intent of allowing accurate identification of the cause of hypereosinophilia, which in turn guides the clinical management of these patients. HES was classified into the following categories: myeloproliferative, lymphocytic, familial, idiopathic, overlap (blood eosinophilia ≥ 1500/mm³ with single organ involvement) and associated (blood eosinophilia ≥1500/mm³ in association with a distinct second diagnosis, such as inflammatory bowel disease etc). This classification has been subsequently revised by the same group based on disease pathophysiology (myeloproliferative vs. lymphocytic) (Box 59-6), as it is recognized that this defines not only the clinical features but also the prognosis and management of HES.[201]

BOX 59-6 HYPEREOSINOPHILIA SYNDROMES

1. Myeloproliferative variant
   a. Clonal eosinophilia
   - FIP1L1/PDGFRA-associated HES
   - Chronic eosinophilic leukemia with cytogenetic abnormalities and/or blasts on peripheral smear
   b. Features of myeloproliferative disease without proof of clonality
2. Lymphocytic variant
   c. Clonal lymphocyte population
   d. No demonstrable T cell clone but may have evidence of marked T cell activation
3. Familial
   e. Family history documented persistent eosinophilia of unknown cause
4. Undefined
   f. Benign
   - Asymptomatic with no evidence of organ involvement
   g. Complex
   - Organ dysfunction, but does not meet criteria for myeloproliferative or lymphocytic variants
   h. Episodic
   - Cyclical angioedema and eosinophilia
5. Overlap
   i. Eosinophil-associated gastrointestinal disease
   j. Eosinophilic pneumonia
   k. Eosinophilia myalgia syndrome
   l. Other organ-restricted eosinophilic disorders
6. Associated
   m. Churg-Strauss syndrome
   n. Systemic mastocytosis
   o. Inflammatory bowel disease
   p. Sarcoidosis
   q. HIV
   r. Other disorders

Adapted from Simon et al (2010).[201]

HES is more common in males and in patients 20 to 50 years old, but it also affects children. The onset of symptoms of HES are often insidious. The common presenting symptoms include fatigue, cough, dyspnea, myalgias, rash, and retinal lesions. HES may affect and damage many organs, including cardiac, cutaneous, neurologic, pulmonary, splenic, hepatic, ocular, and gastrointestinal organs. Cardiac involvement is the major cause of mortality in patients with HES. Eosinophilic endomyocardial disease and mucosal ulcers are common. Eosinophilic granules and mediators are deposited on the endocardium, resulting in myocardial degeneration and fibrosis.[197,202–208] Cardiac disease is characterized by eosinophilic endocardial myelofibrosis, cardiomyopathy, valvular disease, and mural thrombus formation. Serum tryptase levels are often elevated, and splenomegaly is present. Pulmonary disease affects up to 49% of patients with HES, and symptoms consist of chronic nonproductive cough. Asthma is not typically present. Pulmonary infiltrates may develop and may be focal or diffuse. Pulmonary fibrosis may develop. CSS may occur as an associated variant of HES.

The myeloproliferative or "classic" HES presents with features of myeloproliferative disease (i.e., hepatosplenomegaly, cytopenias, circulating myeloid precursors and increased bone marrow cellularity). Elevated serum vitamin B_{12} levels or tryptase levels may be seen.

This form of HES is thought to arise from a mutation in the hematopoietic stem cell that results in clonal expansion, predominantly of eosinophils. The majority of these patients have a cryptic interstitial deletion on chromosome 4 q12 that results in the formation of a fusion protein FIP1L1-PDGFRA that brings together the FIP1L1 and the gene for the cytoplasmic domains of the PDGFRα receptor. This gene fusion results in the formation of a constitutively active tyrosine kinase that is responsible for clonal expansion of eosinophils.[209–211] Other cytogenetic abnormalities that involve PDGFRB and fibroblast growth factor receptor have been reported in patients presenting with the myeloproliferative form of HES. This category also includes HES with features of myeloproliferative disease without proof of clonality, as well as chronic eosinophilic leukemia as defined in the World Health Organization (WHO) classification.[197]

The lymphoproliferative subtype of HES is characterized by polyclonal expansion of eosinophils, usually in response to chemokines like IL-5 produced by dysregulated T-cells. These cells have a characteristic immunophenotype (CD4+CD3- or CD3+CD4-CD8-) and may show monoclonal or polyclonal expansion. Cutaneous manifestations are common in this group of patients. Some may progress to an overt T-cell lymphoma.[200–202] The undefined subtype comprises asymptomatic eosinophilia, necrotizing eosinophilic vasculitis, episodic angioedema with eosinophilia, and other symptomatic forms of eosinophilia that do not have features of the myeloproliferative or lymphocytic forms.[200–201] It is possible that patients with these forms of HES, as well as those with the overlapping or associated HES, also have dysregulated IL-5 producing T lymphocytes.

The evaluation of patients with hypereosinophilia should begin with a meticulous search for triggering factors—drug history, travel history and habitat, and history of allergies with exclusion of underlying malignancy or collagen vascular disease. Careful assessment of organ function to evaluate eosinophil-mediated organ damage is critical.[202] In the absence of underlying disease, or if features of myeloproliferative disease are present, patients with HES should be referred to hematology/oncology for complete evaluation to exclude malignancies, which includes bone marrow examination and radiologic imaging to exclude lymphoma. The evaluation also should include exclusion of a cytogenetic abnormality by TCR gene rearrangement, and RT-PCR or FISH for FIP1L1-PDGFRA. Plasma cytokine levels, especially IL-5, should be measured, as should serum tryptase; however, these may be elevated in both the myeloproliferative and lymphocytic forms of HES.[202]

Control of the eosinophilia is important to prevent organ damage from deposition of eosinophilic mediators. Corticosteroids have been the mainstay of treatment and remain the first-line treatment for FIP1L1-PDGFRA–negative HES. Imatinib mesylate (Gleevec 100 to 400 mg per day) is a tyrosine kinase inhibitor that targets the fusion protein FIP1L1-PDGFRA[209–211]; it now constitutes the treatment of choice for the FIP1L1-PDGFRA–positive myeloproliferative variant of HES. Dramatic clinical responses to imatinib are described in FIP1L1-PDGFRA–positive HES with eosinophilia resolving within a 1-week period and reversal of organ dysfunction as early as 1 month. Other myeloproliferative variants that are negative for the FIP1L1-PDGFRA fusion protein also may respond to imatinib.[211] Other drugs including azathioprine, cyclosporine A, and hydroxyurea have been used in conjunction with corticosteroids or as steroid-sparing agents, particularly for the lymphocytic variant of HES.[202] These patients need careful monitoring for development of a lymphoid malignancy. Immunomodulatory therapy with IFN-α and monoclonal antibody to IL-5 (mepolizumab) also has been described. In two recent reports, patients with HES were treated with three doses of antibody to IL-5.[212,213] Blood eosinophils declined by tenfold and were sustained for 12 weeks after the last dose of antibody. The anti-CD52 monoclonal antibody alemtuzumab has been used to successfully treat two patients with HES.[200] Allogeneic stem cell transplant can be curative for HES.[214,215]

BRONCHIOLITIS OBLITERANS

Bronchiolitis obliterans (BO) is a rare disease of the small airways caused by severe injury leading to fibrosing and narrowing or complete obliteration.[216] It has been described in all age groups. Causes of BO include inhalation of toxic chemicals such as hydrochloric acids or nitric acids. Other associated cases include lupus erythematosus, rheumatoid arthritis, Stevens-Johnson syndrome, lung transplantation, and bone marrow transplant. The focus of this section is BO as a sequel to respiratory infection.

Postinfectious BO occurs following a lower respiratory tract infection usually of viral etiology. Adenovirus is the leading cause of postinfectious BO worldwide. Adenoviral serotypes 3, 7, and 21 demonstrate the highest virulence. A retrospective analysis of 415 pediatric patients in Argentina with acute adenoviral lower respiratory tract infections found serotype Ad7h in 76.3% of the cases.[217] Of those cases, 34% developed respiratory sequelae, and 61% died either during the acute phase of the illness or due to long-term progressive respiratory failure. A case-control study of 109 pediatric postinfectious BO cases found adenoviral infection to be strongly and independently associated with an increased risk for BO.[218] Other viruses associated with postinfectious BO include influenza, parainfluenza, measles, respiratory syncytial virus (RSV), varicella, and metapneumovirus. *Mycoplasma pneumoniae* also has been associated with postinfectious BO. Case reports of patients developing BO following acute bronchiolitis due to co-infection of RSV and adenovirus suggests that adenovirus remains the primary etiology of postinfectious bronchiolitis obliterans.[219,220]

Postinfectious BO is more prevalent in the southern hemisphere including Argentina, Brazil, Chile, Uruguay, New Zealand, and Australia.[221] However, postinfectious bronchiolitis also is diagnosed in the United States, Canada, Turkey, South Korea, and Taiwan.[216] A recent study reported an increased frequency of HLA haplotype DR8-DQB1*0302 in children with postinfectious bronchiolitis obliterans.[222] This allele has a high frequency in the Amerindian population and may explain the high frequency in South American countries.

The initial presentation of infants and children with postinfectious BO does not differ from that of acute bronchiolitis caused by RSV or other viruses. The infant becomes ill with cough and fever and then develops dyspnea and wheezing. On auscultation of the chest, wheezes and crackles are heard. The chest radiographic features consist of peribronchial thickening, increased interstitial markings, and areas of patchy bronchopneumonia. Collapse and consolidation of segments or lobes are common. Castro-Rodriguez found that in children with acute adenoviral infection, those with atelectasis on chest radiograph were more likely to develop than those without atelectasis.[223] Risk factors associated with the initial illness and subsequent development of BO includes hospitalization for more than 30 days, multifocal pneumonia, hypoxia, hypercapnia, need for intensive care, and need for mechanical ventilation.[217] The use of corticosteroids and beta-agonists during the acute illness is reported more frequently in children who developed BO than in those who do not.[223] These studies suggest that infants and children presenting with severe acute bronchiolitis should undergo testing to identify the viral etiology and assess risk factors associated with BO.

In children who develop BO, the clinical and radiographic features of the acute presentation wax and wane for weeks to months, with incomplete recovery. They demonstrate persistent tachypnea, crackles, wheezing, and hypoxemia for at least 60 days after the initial illness. There are recurrent episodes of atelectasis, pneumonia, and wheezing. A high proportion of patients with documented adenoviral pneumonia eventually develop chronic lung disease including persistent atelectasis, bronchiectasis, recurrent pneumonia, hyperinflation, and increased pulmonary markings on chest radiographs. The development of unilateral hyperlucent lung (Swyer-James syndrome) is a long-term complication of adenoviral infection.

Pulmonary function testing in infants with BO show severe fixed airflow obstruction, decreased compliance, and increased resistance, with only a small number of patients responding to bronchodilators.[218] Spirometry in older children demonstrates airflow obstruction with decreased forced expiratory volume in 1 second, decreased ratio of forced expiratory volume in 1 second to forced vital capacity, and markedly decreased forced midexpiratory flow rates. The flow-volume curve shows a severely concave expiratory loop consistent with small airway disease. Lung volumes reveal a marked increase in residual volume and total lung capacity with increase in residual volume/total lung capacity ratio. These pulmonary function test findings are typical for air trapping and hyperinflation. However, one study that used CT to diagnose BO in children found normal impulse oscillometry in one third and mild abnormalities in another third of the cases.[223] This study suggests that BO may have a wider spectrum of severity then previously recognized.

Bronchoscopy, with collection of BAL fluid, can be useful in identifying the infectious agent causing the acute illness. In the chronic phase of the disease, negative viral studies are common. Cytology from BAL shows a high white cell count with markedly increased neutrophils and increased lymphocytes. Lymphocyte subsets show an increase in activated T lymphocytes, and a decreased CD4+/CD8+ ratio suggesting that the pathogenesis of the disease involves B and T lymphocytes.[224]

HRCT of the chest has become an important tool in the diagnosis of BO.[216] Mosaic perfusion, vascular attenuation, and expiratory air trapping are diagnostic features of BO (Fig. 59-4). These findings occur in up to 100% of cases.[224,225] Bronchial wall thickening, bronchiectasis, and atelectasis also are frequent findings. The Bhalla CT scoring system was initially developed to quantify lung disease in cystic fibrosis patients.[226] However, one study suggests that the use of this scoring system in pediatric BO patients may be useful to predict the severity of lung impairment later in life.[227] It has been suggested that chest HRCT findings can have high specificity but incomplete sensitivity for the diagnosis of BO.[216]

To further aid in the diagnosis in young children, a BO score has been proposed.[228] Zero to 4 points were assigned for typical clinical history, 0 to 3 points were assigned for documented adenoviral infection, and 0 to 4 points were assigned for HRCT of the chest showing mosaic perfusion. A score ≥7 predicted the diagnosis of BO with a specificity of 100% and a sensitivity of 67%. However, a score <7 does not accurately rule out the diagnosis.

Lung biopsy has been considered the gold standard for diagnosis of BO. Because of the heterogeneous distribution of airway involvement through the lung, sampling error can occur.[216] In 30 children undergoing lung biopsy, histologic changes consistent with BO were found in 97% of the cases, but many of the lesions were mild and did

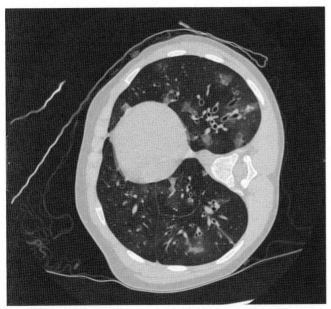

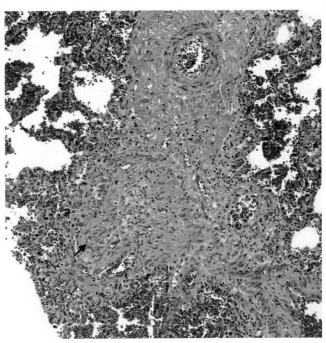

FIGURE 59-4. HRCT scan of the chest of a child with bronchiolitis obliterans demonstrating mosaic perfusion and vascular attenuation. Air-trapping is demonstrated by lack of increase in attention or decrease in lung volume in dependent lung. (Image courtesy of Alan Brody, MD, at Cincinnati Children's Hospital Medical Center, Ohio.)

FIGURE 59-5. Residual peribronchial smooth muscle *(arrow)* with adjacent maturing fibroblastic plug occluding the lumen of a bronchiole (10 × magnification). (Image courtesy of Todd Boyd, MD, at Cincinnati Children's Hospital Medical Center, Ohio.)

not correlate with the clinical severity of the disease.[221] In addition, totally obliterated airways were found in only 23% of lung biopsies versus 100% with lobectomy or autopsy. Lung biopsies have been reported as normal or nondiagnostic in up to one third of patients.[216] Thus, it is important to recognize the potential diagnostic and prognostic limitations of lung biopsy, and increasingly, the diagnosis of BO is one best considered in the context of clinical-radiographic-pathologic correlation.

When a biopsy is indicated, morphometric evaluation of the lung architecture reveals areas of hyperinflation predominating over areas of collapse.[221] On histologic examination, postinfectious BO is characterized by inflammation and fibrosis in the small airways. Chronic inflammatory cells fill the lumen of the small airways in the lung. These inflammatory cells can extend into the peribronchiolar region and less frequently into the alveoli. Small lymphoid aggregates without exuberant reactive germinal centers also have been described.[221] The inflammatory infiltrate is composed of T lymphocytes with a predominance of the CD8+ subset.[229] These findings suggest T lymphocyte-mediated airway injury as the cause of bronchiolitis obliterans.

The second histologic feature of BO is fibrous tissue creating varying degrees of luminal occlusion in the small airway. Total obliteration of the lumen by fibrotic tissue is frequently seen[221] (Fig. 59-5). An elastic stain is useful in identifying the elastic layer remnants of bronchiolar walls within the fibrotic tissue. Foamy macrophages, mucostasis, and bronchiectasis are other frequent findings. Viral inclusion bodies are usually not present.

Previously, BO was histologically classified into two subgroups—constrictive, described above, or proliferative. The proliferative type is characterized by the presence of granulation tissue plugs (Masson bodies) within the lumens of the small airways, alveolar ducts, and alveoli. Another term for the proliferative type is bronchiolitis obliterans organizing pneumonia (BOOP). More recent literature uses the term cryptogenic organizing pneumonia (COP). This disease has similar etiologies to constrictive bronchiolitis obliterans including viral infection, inhalation injuries, connective tissue disorders, and immunosuppression. The clinical features include flulike illness, dry cough, and dyspnea. Radiographic imaging reveals patchy consolidation and ground-glass opacities. Pulmonary function testing frequently shows a restrictive abnormality.[230] The connection, if any, between the two classifications of BO is unknown. The proliferative type is rarely found in the pediatric population.[221]

Treatment options for BO are limited, with most therapies having limited evidence supporting their use. Supportive care includes oxygen therapy, adequate nutritional intake, avoidance of smoke and other irritants, influenza vaccinations, and pulmonary rehabilitation. Aggressive treatment of gastroesophageal reflux may be necessary to prevent ongoing lung injury from gastric acid. A small number of patients demonstrate improvement with bronchodilators and inhaled corticosteroids.

Systemic corticosteroids are frequently used in BO, regardless of the etiology. However, the effectiveness of systemic corticosteroids remains unproven. The degree of reversible inflammation versus fibrosis in the airway most likely affects individual patient responsiveness. If beneficial, a response to systemic corticosteroids probably occurs in the earlier stages of disease before complete airway fibrosis. While there are no controlled studies, pulse therapy consisting of intravenous methylprednisolone, 30 mg/kg (maximum 1 g) infused over 1 hour daily for 3 consecutive days has been proposed.[216] If the patient demonstrates benefit, the therapy is repeated monthly for 3 to 6 months, depending on the patient's ongoing responsiveness. Other therapies reported (anecdotally) include immunomodulatory doses of intravenous immunoglobulin as a steroid-sparing agent[216] and selective TNF-α blockade for BO following lung transplantation.[231] Small studies support the use of azithromycin as a chronic immunomodulatory agent to prevent further decline in lung function.[232,233]

The outcome of patients with postinfectious BO is unclear. Multiple studies of postadenoviral BO report improvement or resolution of chronic hypoxia and wheezing episodes.[223,218] Other studies show a progressive decline in pulmonary function suggesting lifelong pulmonary impairment.[224] Death has been reported secondary to postinfectious BO.[234]

Postinfectious BO remains a rare disease of the small airways, with adenovirus as the leading cause. Although the disease is well described from a clinical, radiographic, and histologic standpoint, ongoing research is needed to identify treatment options and long-term outcomes.

References

The complete reference list is available online at www.expertconsult.com

60 RARE CHILDHOOD LUNG DISORDERS

Daniel J. Lesser, MD, Lisa R. Young, MD, and James S. Hagood, MD

■ INTRODUCTION

Although some respiratory diseases occur only rarely in the pediatric population, knowledge of these disorders is valuable from a number of perspectives. Timely diagnosis and treatment of rare disorders can only be made if the practitioner is familiar with the entity in question. Furthermore, elucidation of the pathophysiology underlying rare disorders can be applied to understanding both normal respiratory physiology and related but more prevalent disorders. Many rare lung disorders are covered in other chapters. This chapter characterizes both selected disorders with a primary respiratory component and respiratory disease occurring secondary to systemic disorders, with emphasis on interstitial lung disease. The diseases covered may present predominantly during childhood, (e.g., respiratory disorders of the lymphatic system) or adulthood, but with implications for or rare occurrence in pediatric patients (e.g., pulmonary alveolar microlithiasis [PAM] and α_1-antitrypsin [AAT] deficiency. Foundations provide invaluable information, support, and advocacy to families and patients affected by rare diseases and also function as important resources for practitioners. This chapter therefore directs the reader to selected disease—specific groups that may significantly impact care.

Respiratory Disorders of the Lymphatic System

A number of rare disorders related to dysregulation of lymphatic development occur in pediatric patients from infancy to adolescence. The normal pulmonary lymphatic system is composed of two interconnected pathways: one drains the subpleural space and outer surface of the lung, while the other follows bronchovascular bundles to drain the deeper portions of the lung (see Chapter 5).[1] In humans, the pulmonary lymphatic system begins to form approximately 6 weeks into embryonic growth with sprouting of distinct endothelial cells directly from the developing venous system.[2] A number of growth factors have been identified that direct development of the lymphatic vasculature.[3] The pathophysiology leading to lymphatic dysfunction varies among the disorders described in this section. For example, it has been hypothesized that disordered embryonic development plays a role in pulmonary lymphangiectasia (PL), a disorder that often presents in the neonatal period. In disorders that present outside of the neonatal period (e.g., lymphangiomatosis), disease is associated with abnormalities of lymphatic growth. Furthermore, a significant number of children with pulmonary lymphatic disorders also manifest lymphatic involvement of other organ systems, congenital cardiac disease, and chromosomal disorders. This section describes disorders associated with lymphatic dysfunction that have a significant component of respiratory disease. (See Chapter 21 for a further discussion of congenital lung diseases.)

Pulmonary Lymphangiectasia

Pulmonary lymphangiectasia (PL) is characterized by dilatation of pulmonary lymphatic vessels and disordered drainage, leading to accumulation of lymph within the lungs and a spectrum of respiratory disease. Although its exact incidence is not known, it has been estimated that 0.5% to 1% of neonates who die in the neonatal period have PL.[1] The majority of reported cases occur sporadically, and most present in the neonatal period or during infancy. However, cases of PL have also been described to occur during childhood and into adulthood.[4]

One commonly used classification system for PL distinguishes between disease caused by a primary developmental defect and that occurring secondary to an obstructive process impeding normal lymph drainage.[3] It has been hypothesized that primary PL occurs secondary to failure of normal regression of the large lymphatic vessels observed in the embryo at 9 to 16 weeks of gestation.[3] Some infants with primary PL present with disease that seems confined to the respiratory system, while others display more generalized symptoms characterized by lymphedema and extrathoracic involvement.[3] Secondary causes of PL usually involve congenital cardiac diseases associated with obstructed pulmonary venous flow. Thus, hypoplastic left heart syndrome, congenital mitral stenosis, and pulmonary vein atresia have all been associated with PL.[3,5] In addition to cardiac disease, thoracic duct agenesis and infection may also block lymphatic drainage and cause PL.

A number of chromosomal disorders are associated with PL, including Noonan syndrome, Hennekam syndrome, Yellow Nail syndrome, and Down syndrome.[1,3] Children with PL that is associated with chromosomal disorders are more likely to present with generalized lymphangiectasia. These patients may display a less severe pulmonary component and often have a better outcome when compared with those who present with primarily pulmonary disease during the neonatal period.[1]

Pediatric patients presenting at birth often develop respiratory distress that progresses rapidly to respiratory failure.[1] Chylous pleural effusions may be prominent, but a significant number of children with PL do not present with effusions.[1] Individuals who first develop symptoms later in infancy or during childhood usually display less severe disease when compared to those with neonatal onset. In later-presenting forms, initial symptoms include chronic tachypnea, recurrent cough, and wheezing.[4] PL in these individuals has been associated with chylothorax, chylopericardium, and chylous ascites.[3] Frequent respiratory exacerbations, possibly related to lower respiratory tract infections, can occur.[1,4]

The diagnostic workup of the child with suspected PL includes plain chest radiography, chest high-resolution computed tomography (c-HRCT), and lung biopsy. Chest radiography often reveals interstitial infiltrates and hyperinflation, with or without pleural effusion.[1] HRCT shows thickening of peribronchovascular septa and septa surrounding lobules (Fig. 60-1).[3] Lung biopsy, the gold standard for diagnosing PL, is characterized by the appearance of dilated lymphatic vessels located in the interlobular septa, near bronchovascular bundles, and/or within the pleura (see Fig. 60-1).[5] Dilated lymphatic vessels may occasionally appear cystic.[2] In addition to lymphatic findings, lung biopsy may also show thickening and widening of interlobular septa.[2] Because lymphangiectasia may be part of a systemic dysplasia, consideration should also be given to careful evaluation for extrapulmonary disease manifestations such as gastrointestinal involvement, bony disease, or skin lesions from draining lymphatic glands.

There is no known cure for PL, and treatment is primarily supportive. Respiratory failure in a significant number of neonates with PL is refractory to conventional positive pressure ventilation and high-frequency oscillation. In these cases, inhaled nitric oxide and extracorporeal membranous oxygenation (ECMO) have been used with variable success.[5] Treatment of children who present outside the neonatal period can be relatively less complex, as this form of the disease tends to be less severe. Therapy for older children with PL includes supplemental oxygen, antimicrobials, and treatment for recurrent wheezing or cough.[4]

Although the natural course of PL is variable, the disease has historically carried a high mortality rate when diagnosed in the neonatal period. More recent reports suggested improved survival with aggressive intervention and modern neonatal intensive care.[4] Subsequent to these reports, however, Mettauer and coworkers reported survival in only 1 of 7 children referred to their tertiary center.[5] The authors concluded that although the prognosis for PL is poor, the condition is survivable with aggressive intervention.[5] Furthermore, those who survive the neonatal period seem to eventually experience improvement of their disease.[4,5] Clearly, a spectrum of severity exists. With further delineation of the molecular mechanisms controlling development of the lymphatic system, it is likely that new methods of classifying and ultimately treating PL will become available. The Lymphatic Research Foundation (www.lymphaticresearch.org) aims to facilitate research regarding the lymphatic system and related disorders.

Lymphangiomatosis and Gorham-Stout Disease

Abnormal proliferation of lymphatic vessels distinguishes lymphangioma, lymphangiomatosis, and Gorham-Stout disease from other lymphatic disorders of the lung. While lymphangioma refers to a solitary malformation, lymphangiomatosis refers to the presence of multiple lymphangiomas and is less common than the occurrence of a single lymphangioma. Gorham-Stout disease is a related syndrome characterized by chylothorax and bone

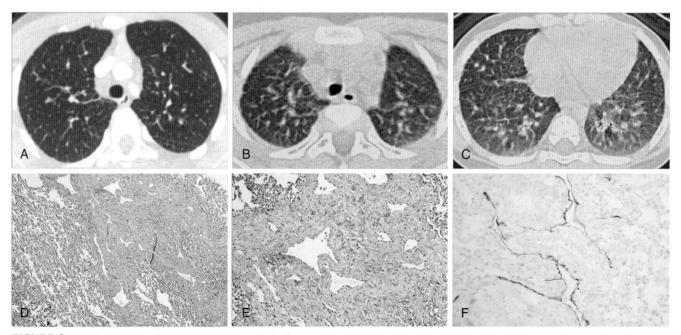

FIGURE 60-1. Chest high-resolution computed tomography from an 8-year-old (**A**) and a 2-year-old (**B** and **C**) with lymphangiectasia. Imaging shows variable intensity of interlobular septal thickening. Both children presented with nonspecific respiratory symptoms and recurrent pneumonia without identification of pathogens; neither had overt extrapulmonary manifestations of lymphatic dysplasia. Lung biopsy shows septal widening with prominent and muscularized lymphatics (**D** and **E**, hematoxylin and eosin) as illustrated by D240 immunostaining highlighting the lymphatic endothelium (**F**). (Cases provided by Lisa R. Young, MD, Cincinnati Children's Hospital Medical Center, Susie Millard, MD, Helen DeVos Children's Hospital and Michigan State University, and Gail Deutsch, MD, Seattle Children's Hospital.)

cysts, with lymphangioma seen on biopsy. Gorham-Stout disease and lymphangiomatosis both occur sporadically without a known inheritance pattern.

Lymphangiomatosis is a severe disease characterized by the occurrence of numerous lymphangiomas, often affecting multiple organs. Involvement of the liver, soft tissue, spleen, bones, mediastinum, and lungs may occur.[2,6] The disease is reported more frequently in children than in adults, and a significant number of infants are reported.[6] Lymphangiomatosis involving the thorax can manifest in the mediastinum, pleural space, chest wall, lungs, or pericardium.[7] Individuals with thoracic involvement may present with cough, chest pain, dyspnea, or wheezing.[6] Chylous effusions are often a prominent component of the clinical disease pattern of lymphangiomatosis.[2,6] Chest radiography reveals interstitial infiltrates, chest mass, effusions, or bony lesions.[2,7] In addition to multiple lymphangiomas, c-HRCT may exhibit smooth thickening of interlobular septa and bronchovascular bundles, ground-glass attenuation, or effusions.[6] Biopsies of lymphatic lesions are characterized by increased numbers of dilated lymphatic channels lined by endothelium.[2]

The natural history of lymphangiomatosis entails progressive growth of lymphangiomas that eventually compress vital structures.[7] Both young age and respiratory involvement predict a particularly poor outcome.[6] However, successfully treated cases of lymphangiomatosis with thoracic involvement have been reported.[8] Therapy for severely symptomatic pleural effusions may include thoracentesis or pleurodesis. When lymphangiomas are diffuse, complete surgical resection often is not possible.[7] Medical therapy for lymphangiomatosis using interferon-alpha 2b has been reported, with the aim of halting the lymphatic proliferation that is the hallmark of the disease.[8]

Gorham-Stout disease is characterized by proliferation of vascular structures within bones, leading to osteolytic lesions evident on radiography.[9] Chylothorax is associated with the disease, possibly related to dysplasia of lymphatic vessels at the pleura.[9] Children are more commonly affected than adults, and presenting symptoms may include cough, dyspnea, and pain.[10] The presence of chylothorax is associated with worsened prognosis in this severe disease.[9] Similar to lymphangiomatosis, anecdotal reports suggest that interferon-alpha 2b may

be trialed in the treatment of Gorham-Stout disease.[9,10] The Lymphangiomatosis & Gorham's Disease Alliance (http://lgdalliance.org) and the Lymphangiomatosis Foundation (www.lymphangiomatosis.org) are dedicated to care for those affected by these disorders. Ongoing efforts to improve the classification and phenotyping of lymphatic dysplasias, including PL and lymphangiomatosis, may lead to improved diagnostic strategies, molecular understanding, and targeted therapeutic considerations.

Lymphangioleiomyomatosis

Lymphangioleiomyomatosis (LAM) is characterized by abnormal smooth muscle proliferation and cystic destruction in the lung. This disorder presents in women of childbearing age with recurrent pneumothoraces, progressive dyspnea, and multiple lung cysts evident on c-HRCT.[11] Although lymphatic involvement is not always a prominent feature, some patients develop chylous effusions.[11] LAM is distinct from lymphangiomatosis and is differentiated based on the presence of lung cysts and distinct immunohistochemistry.[11] The disease may occur sporadically, without known inheritance pattern, or it may be associated with tuberous sclerosis complex (TSC), an autosomal dominant disease with variable penetrance.[11] Rarely, cystic pulmonary disease can occur in children with TSC (Fig. 60-2).[12] Although at least 40% of adult women with TSC have lung cysts compatible with LAM, symptomatic pulmonary disease is quite rare in girls with TSC. Furthermore, only a few pediatric cases of LAM have been reported.[13–15] The LAM Foundation (www.thelamfoundation.org) offers information, resources, and a worldwide network to those affected.

Pulmonary Alveolar Microlithiasis

PAM is an autosomal recessive disease characterized by the deposition of calcium phosphate calculi within alveoli. A gene linked to PAM has been identified, and the cause of the disease is thought to be related to disordered phosphate transport.[16] Chest radiography of affected individuals reveals sandlike micronodules indicative of calcium phosphate microliths and is one of the most striking features of the disorder (Fig. 60-3). Most pediatric patients are asymptomatic and may come to medical

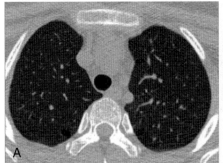
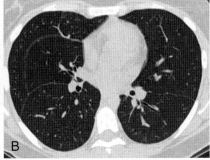
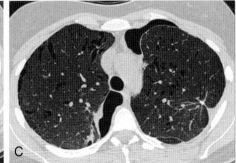

FIGURE 60-2. **A,** Chest high-resolution computed tomography from a 16-year-old female with tuberous sclerosis complex shows a few radiolucent thin-walled cysts bilaterally. These findings are consistent with very mild early lymphangioleiomyomatosis were detected on screening c-HRCT in this asymptomatic teenager. **B,** c-HRCT demonstrates only a few tiny cysts in this 17-year-old female with TSC, however, she subsequently experienced unusually rapid progression including bilateral pneumothoraces. **C,** Subsequent c-HRCT (age 18.5 years) shows diffuse cystic lung disease and residual bilateral pneumothoraces. (Case provided by Lisa R. Young, MD, Cincinnati Children's Hospital Medical Center.)

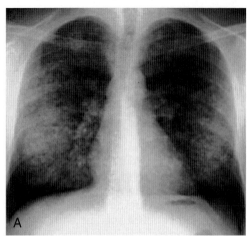
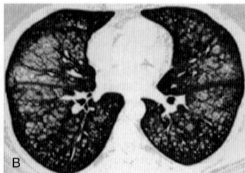

FIGURE 60-3. Radiographic features of pulmonary alveolar microlithiasis. **A,** Posteroanterior chest radiograph showing the classic "sandstorm" appearance of pulmonary alveolar microlithiasis, including diffuse, patchy, bilateral sharp micronodular disease. **B,** High-resolution computed tomographic scan of the chest showing micronodular densities. (From Brandenburg VM, Schubert H. Images in clinical medicine. Pulmonary alveolar microlithiasis. N Engl J Med. 2003;348:1555.)

attention only after a relative has been identified, or when radiography obtained for a nonrelated indication is suggestive of PAM.

In 2007, Huqun and colleagues used genome-wide single-nucleotide polymorphism (SNP) analysis to associate mutations in the *SLC34A2* gene with this disorder.[17] In addition, the *SLC34A2* gene was independently associated with PAM by applying linkage analysis to a large, consanguineous family in Turkey with multiple affected family members.[18] *SLC34A2* encodes a type IIb sodium-dependent phosphate transporter that is expressed in type II alveolar cells.[17] One of the functions of type II alveolar cells involves degradation of surfactant. Phosphate is a waste product of this degradation and may build up in cells unless properly removed. It has thus been hypothesized that failure of phosphate reuptake secondary to dysfunction of the *SLC34A2* gene product causes formation of calcium phosphate microliths, the hallmark of PAM.[16]

A significant proportion of reported cases of PAM occur in Italy, Japan, and Turkey. It is not known whether this reflects true clustering of the disease or increased awareness and reporting in these countries. Although historically the majority of reported cases of PAM describe adults, increased numbers of children with the disorder have been identified more recently. For instance, Tachibana and coworkers report 52% of a series of 111 patients identified in Japan before 15 years of age.[16] In Turkey and Italy, however, the mean age of diagnosis is 27 and 30 years, respectively.[16] This difference in age of diagnosis may reflect different rates of screening family members of affected individuals.

Diagnosis often occurs when a chest radiograph is performed for other diagnostic purposes.[19] Others are diagnosed upon presentation for screening based on the diagnosis of a family member. Individuals with PAM, especially in the pediatric population, are usually asymptomatic at the time of diagnosis.[16] Remarkably, this absence of symptoms occurs despite impressive radiologic changes evident on plain chest radiography as well as CT scan of the chest. Mariotta and colleagues reviewed the literature to describe 576 cases of the disorder and

reported the presence of symptoms (including dyspnea, cough, and chest pain) in only about half of those affected.[20] At diagnosis, pulmonary function testing is often normal or, in some cases, shows slightly decreased vital capacity or diffusing capacity.[16] Decline of pulmonary function and occurrence of respiratory insufficiency occur over decades.[16,20]

PAM is distinguished from other pulmonary diseases by its "sandstorm" appearance on plain chest film, representative of calcium-phosphate micronodules. This finding is considered by some to be pathognomonic for the disease. The micronodules evident on chest radiography often appear denser at the lung bases and can obscure the borders of the cardiac silhouette and diaphragm.[16] Sarcoidosis, tuberculosis, histoplasmosis, and idiopathic pulmonary hemosiderosis may be considered in the differential diagnosis of a patient presenting with the radiologic findings of PAM. HRCT may reveal micronodules, ground-glass opacities, subpleural interstitial thickening, and interlobular septal thickening.[21] Children with PAM may not display all of the classic radiographic features seen on plain chest radiography or CT scan. In pediatric patients, ground-glass opacification can predominate over the nodular calcific densities classically ascribed to the disease.[22]

Lack of consensus exists regarding the natural course of the disease because of the paucity of reports that describe long-term outcome. Some reports suggest that for some individuals, the symptoms of the disease are static.[19] However, a significant number of reports describe the development of pulmonary fibrosis followed by respiratory insufficiency, pulmonary hypertension, and death secondary to respiratory failure over several decades following diagnosis.[19] Although various therapies have been tried, there is presently no cure for PAM. Corticosteroids and whole lung lavage have not shown efficacy.[19] Lung transplantation has been performed successfully.[23] Disodium etidronate has been used with the aim of inhibiting precipitation of calculi and has been suggested to improve clinical and radiographic disease over the long term in two patients who were diagnosed during childhood.[23] As our understanding of the link between the mutated *SLC34A2* gene product and the presumed buildup of phosphate develops, it is hoped that new therapies to halt or slow the formation of microliths and interstitial lung disease will become available.

Gaucher Disease

The most common lysosomal storage disease, Gaucher disease (GD) is an autosomal recessive disorder caused by a mutation in the *glucocerebrosidase* gene that results in abnormal buildup of glucocerebroside. Glucocerebroside accumulates within macrophages, identified pathologically as Gaucher or foam cells. In the lung, infiltration of Gaucher cells may occur within alveoli, within interstitial spaces, around airways, or within pulmonary vasculature and may cause a form of infiltrative lung disease.[24,25] In addition to primary lung disease caused by GD, hepatopulmonary syndrome may also occur secondary to the liver disease associated with the disorder. Although clinical pulmonary disease is uncommon in GD, a significant number of patients have abnormal pulmonary function testing.[26] Chest radiography may display reticulonodular changes, and c-HRCT shows ground-glass consolidation, interstitial involvement, alveolar opacities, and bronchial wall thickening (Fig. 60-4).[27] While enzyme replacement therapy for GD decreases organomegaly and improves hematologic parameters, it has been less successful in reversing existing pulmonary disease.[24] However, this therapy may in some cases slow or prevent progressive decline in lung function.[25] Currently, the role of enzyme replacement therapy in preventing lung disease is not known. The National Gaucher Foundation (www.gaucherdisease.org) seeks treatments and a cure for Gaucher Disease.

Niemann-Pick Disease Type B

Niemann-Pick disease (NPD) is an autosomal recessive disorder characterized by deficiency of acid sphingomyelinase, leading to the accumulation of sphingomyelin within cells and tissues.[28] While type A NPD manifests as a severe neurodegenerative disorder that can often lead to death in the first 3 to 4 years of life, individuals with type B NPD usually do not have neurologic involvement and often survive into adulthood.[28] Pediatric patients with type B NPD present with hepatomegaly, splenomegaly, thrombocytopenia, and dyslipidemia.[28] A significant number of individuals with type B NPD also exhibit interstitial lung disease (ILD).[28,29] In the lung, buildup of foam cells containing sphingomyelin occurs within alveoli, alveolar walls, lymphatic spaces, and the pleural space.[30,31] Rarely, a severe form of ILD caused by NPD may present in infancy or early childhood.[31] In many cases, ILD appears more indolent, and survival well into adulthood occurs frequently.[28,30] Pulmonary function abnormalities are common and are characterized by decreased FVC, FEV_1, and diffusing capacity.[29] However, the degree to which hepatosplenomegaly and abdominal distension contribute to the reported spirometry findings is unclear. Radiographic abnormalities of c-HRCT observed in NPD include ground-glass appearance, reticulonodular densities, thickening of interlobular septa, and thickening of intralobular lines.[29] However, the severity of radiologic findings has not been found to correlate with pulmonary function testing.[29] Although no specific treatment for NPD exists, whole lung lavage has been tried with varying success for the most severe cases.[31] It is hoped that enzyme replacement therapy will eventually contribute to stabilization or improvement of lung disease associated with NPD. The National Niemann-Pick Disease Foundation (www.nnpdf.org) provides support services for individuals and families affected by the disorder.

Neurofibromatosis

Neurofibromatosis type 1 (NF-1) is an autosomal dominant disorder characterized by neurofibroma, café au lait spots, pigmented hamartomas of the iris, skeletal dysplasia, and optic glioma. Thoracic involvement

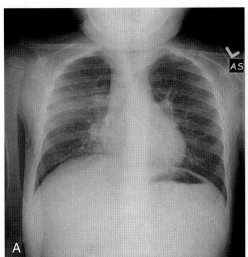
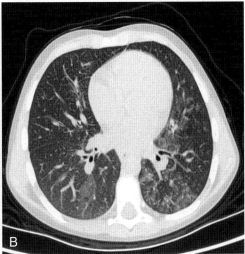

FIGURE 60-4. **A,** Chest radiograph of a 3-year-old female with Gaucher disease who had received enzyme replacement therapy since infancy reveals reticulonodular changes and areas of consolidation. **B,** Computed tomography (CT) of the chest with mosaic pattern and areas of septal thickening. Bronchoalveolar lavage revealed numerous foam cells *(not pictured)*. (Images provided by Roberta Kato, MD, Children's Hospital, Los Angeles.)

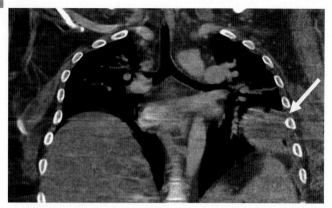

FIGURE 60-5. CT sagittal section of a 21-year-old with neurofibromatosis type I demonstrating a soft tissue mass abutting the left chest wall with adjacent atelectasis. Biopsy of the mass was consistent with neurofibroma.

in NF-1 mainly entails the presence of neurofibromas, often plexiform, that may arise from the chest wall or posterior mediastinum (Fig. 60-5).[32] Plexiform neurofibromas have multiple nerve roots and can surround vital structures, making resection complex.[32] As malignant transformation may occur, biopsy of these masses should be considered.[32] In addition to tumors and bony abnormalities affecting the thorax, NF-1 is also associated with ILD.[33] The ILD associated with NF-1 appears radiographically as large, apical thin-walled bullae and basilar fibrosis.[33] Diffuse lung disease associated with neurofibromatosis mainly occurs in adult patients and has not yet been reported in children.[33] The Children's Tumor Foundation (www.ctf.org) is dedicated to improving the health and well being of individuals and families affected by NF.

Dyskeratosis Congenita

Dyskeratosis congenita (DC) is a form of ectodermal dysplasia characterized by skin hyperpigmentation, nail dystrophy, oral leukoplakia, and bone marrow failure.[34,35] Although the most common form is inherited as X-linked recessive, the disorder may also be inherited in an autosomal dominant or autosomal recessive pattern.

A number of mutations in genes coding for proteins that function to maintain telomeres have been identified in patients with DC.[34] Approximately 20% of those with DC manifest some form of pulmonary involvement, with pulmonary fibrosis frequently described (Fig. 60-6).[35] Because of the significant number of children with DC requiring bone marrow transplant, characterization of the etiology of lung can be difficult disease when it occurs after transplant. However, a number of significant pulmonary complications, including pulmonary fibrosis and hepatopulmonary syndrome, have been described after bone marrow transplant for DC.[36,37] Therefore, it is likely that at least in some cases, development of pulmonary fibrosis is either caused by or exacerbated by the telomerase dysfunction known to occur in DC.[37] The Dyskeratosis Congenita Outreach (www.dcoutreach.com) provides information and support services to affected families.

Hermansky-Pudlak Syndrome

Hermansky-Pudlak syndrome (HPS) is an autosomal recessive disorder characterized by oculocutaneous albinism, bleeding diathesis, and pulmonary fibrosis. Notably, the disease has an especially high prevalence in a section of Puerto Rico. The underlying disorder in HPS involves disturbed formation or trafficking of intracellular vesicles. This perturbation results in dysfunction of lysosome-related organelles within a number of cell types, including macrophages and type II pneumocytes.[38,39] Clinically, lung disease usually manifests in the third or fourth decades of life.[39,40] Pulmonary function testing reveals restrictive lung disease, and HRCT indicates pulmonary fibrosis.[40] The disease may progress to death in the fourth or fifth decade of life.[40] Although a number of anti-inflammatory and immunomodulatory medications have been used to treat patients with HPS, there is currently no cure. The Hermansky-Pudlak Syndrome Network (www.hpsnetwork.org) is a support group for people and families dealing with the disorder. Ongoing investigation of the cellular mechanisms responsible for disease as well as medications targeted against pulmonary fibrosis will contribute significantly to the care of patients with HPS.

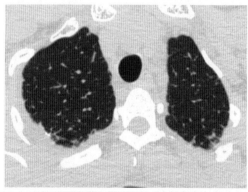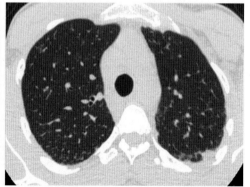

FIGURE 60-6. Chest high-resolution computed tomography images demonstrate subpleural predominant thickening of the secondary interlobular septa consistent with early pulmonary fibrosis in this 18-year-old patient with dyskeratosis congenita. (Case provided by Lisa R. Young, MD, and Ronald Bokulic, DO, Cincinnati Children's Hospital Medical Center.)

Alpha-1 Antitrypsin Deficiency

In 1963, Laurell and Erickson first discovered an association between deficiency of alpha$_1$ antitrypsin (AAT) and emphysema.[41] AAT inhibits the enzymatic breakdown of lung tissue, and its dysfunction can lead to severe obstructive lung disease. In addition, AAT deficiency causes a spectrum of liver disease ranging from mild elevation of liver function tests to cirrhosis and hepatic failure. Although AAT deficiency is not a rare disorder *per se,* pulmonary manifestations of AAT deficiency occur very rarely in children. However, familiarity with the disorder is of value to pediatric pulmonologists. AAT deficiency is one of the most common inherited diseases worldwide, and its diagnosis often goes delayed or unrecognized. Pediatric practitioners are responsible for educating patients and families regarding genetic testing for the disorder. Furthermore, AAT deficiency models how understanding of the molecular mechanisms leading to respiratory disorders contributes to clinical care.

Genetics and Pathophysiology

SERPINA1, the gene that encodes AAT, spans 12.2 kb on human chromosome 14q31-32.3.[42] AAT deficiency is inherited in a co-dominant manner, and over 100 variants of the protein have been identified. Co-dominant expression of both alleles determines the serum level of AAT. Classification occurs via the protease inhibitor (Pi) system and is based on the banding pattern of the protein on isoelectric focusing gel electrophoresis.[43] The naming of variants is based on the rate at which they migrate on the gel. For instance, "F" stands for fast, "M" for medium, "S" for slow, and "Z" for very slow. Furthermore, when multiple subtypes exist in a given class, some variants are also assigned a number or name subscript.

Various AAT phenotypes are associated with different levels of the protein, and the serum level of AAT determines the risk of emphysema. An increased risk for development of emphysema is associated with AAT levels <11 μM.[42] Serum levels of 2.5 to 7 μM are associated with PiZZ, the most prevalent disease, causing a phenotype in populations of Northern European descent.[42,43] Thus, PiZZ individuals are at increased risk of developing emphysema. In addition to categorization based on serum level of AAT, the functional activity of the gene product must also be taken into account.

AAT is a 52-kDa secreted glycoprotein that is primarily synthesized within hepatocytes as well as bronchial epithelial cells, type II pneumocytes, neutrophils, and alveolar macrophages.[43] As part of the <u>se</u>rine <u>p</u>roteinase <u>in</u>hibitor (SERPIN) family, AAT inhibits the activity of a number of proteolytic enzymes, including trypsin, neutrophil elastase, collegenase, and macrophage cathepsin.[44] The active site of AAT includes a serine residue centered on an external loop located outside of the globular protein that serves to irreversibly bind neutrophil elastase through a "mousetrap" motion (Fig. 60-7).[42,43] Once the active site of AAT has bound neutrophil elastase, the external loop swings to the opposite end of the protein and effectively inactivates the protease. Lung disease in AAT deficiency occurs primarily secondary to loss of function resulting in imbalance between levels of AAT relative to the amount of neutrophil elastase. Neutrophil elastase degrades elastin and extracellular matrix elements located within the lower respiratory tract that normally function to maintain the structural integrity of the lung.[42] As the level of AAT decreases, the risk of disease increases.

Many of the extrapulmonary (e.g., hepatic) manifestations of AAT deficiency are thought to result from accumulation of misfolded protein (toxic gain of function). Interestingly, misfolded AAT does not usually result in the typical unfolded protein response (UPR), but rather triggers an "ER overload" response characterized by chronic

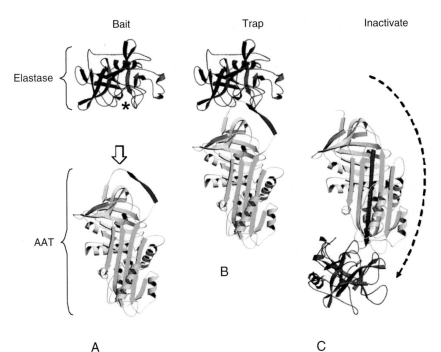

FIGURE 60-7. Alpha-1 antitrypsin "baits," traps, and irreversibly inactivates neutrophil elastase using a mousetrap-like action. AAT is a globular protein with a reactive external loop *(open arrow)* that acts as bait for neutrophil elastase by virtue of its ability to bind the active site of the protease *(asterisk)* **A,** Docking of neutrophil elastase on the reactive external loop of AAT **(B)** is associated with movement of the reactive external loop from the upper pole to the lower pole of AAT, its insertion into β-sheet A of AAT, and inactivation of the protease **(C).** (From Lomas DA, Parfrey H. Alpha1-antitrypsin deficiency. 4: Molecular pathophysiology. *Thorax* 2004;59:529-535.)

activation of the transcription factor nuclear factor-κB (NF-κB).[43] Furthermore, some of the pulmonary manifestations may result in part from extracellular (interstitial) polymerization of AAT.

Considering that not all at-risk individuals develop disease, other environmental and genetic components modulate the development of emphysema. For instance, a relationship between smoking, AAT deficiency, and development of emphysema has been well established. Thus, individuals with AAT deficiency who also smoke have an accelerated rate of developing disease. In addition to cigarette smoking, exposure to kerosene heaters, employment in agriculture, and exposure to other pollutants from biomass fuel sources have all been implicated in the development of emphysema.[42,45] Further investigation of the mechanisms by which environmental and genetic factors modify disease will help identify those at highest risk for developing emphysema.

Epidemiology and Clinical Presentation

AAT deficiency is one of the most prevalent genetic disorders worldwide. In Europe, the highest frequency of the *PiZ* allele occurs along the northwestern seaboard of the continent.[42,46] Due to the frequency of the allele, Pi ZZ is the phenotype most commonly identified in individuals who develop emphysema secondary to AAT deficiency. Furthermore, AAT deficiency is the most common genetic cause of neonatal liver disease.[45] Although prevalent, AAT deficiency remains a severely underrecognized disorder. It is estimated that only about 5% of individuals in the United States with the disorder are actually diagnosed.[45]

It should be emphasized that AAT deficiency has not been shown to typically cause severe obstructive lung disease in the pediatric population. The vast majority of children with AAT deficiency present with liver disease, often beginning with jaundice and cholestasis in the neonatal period. Liver disease associated with AAT may be sufficiently severe to cause liver failure and is one of the most common indications for liver transplantation in young children.

The mean age of presentation of lung disease in AAT deficiency is 32 to 41 years, and presentation before 25 years is rare.[42] Symptoms usually occur in smokers or those with a history of smoking. However, as detailed above, a number nonsmokers and even smokers with AAT deficiency remain asymptomatic. In addition to liver disease, AAT deficiency has also been associated with bronchiectasis, necrotizing panniculitis, and multisystemic vasculitis.[42]

Much of the available knowledge regarding AAT deficiency in children stems from a birth cohort that identified 184 individuals in Sweden, where AAT screening of 200,000 newborns occurred from 1972 to 1974.[47] These studies found lung function testing to be normal in adolescents up to 18 years of age with PiZZ.[47] In addition, the pulmonary function tests examined at this age did not differ significantly from normal controls or subjects with PiSZ.[46] However, when compared to those who do not smoke, Piitulainen and colleagues (1998) found 18-year-olds with either PiZZ or PiSZ who smoked to have lower FEV_1 and FEV_1/VC.[47] Thus, the authors concluded that the first signs of lung disease in AAT-deficient

smokers occur in adolescence.[47] At 22 years of age, pulmonary function testing, although still within normal range (mean FEV_1 98% predicted), was found to have significantly declined (mean 1.2% annual decline) when compared with testing done at 16 and 18 years.[48] Furthermore, 29% of individuals reported wheezing, and 15% had been diagnosed with asthma.[48] Thus, the authors speculated that respiratory symptoms in young adults with PiZZ may be misidentified as asthma, contributing to a delay in diagnosis for those with symptoms of AAT deficiency.[48]

Diagnosis

Decreased serum levels of AAT indicate disease and necessitate further workup. As inflammatory conditions (e.g., acute respiratory illness) can increase AAT levels above baseline, individuals with borderline ATT serum levels should be closely monitored and considered for further genetic testing.[42] Isoelectric focusing (phenotyping) identifies AAT variants and has historically been the most widely used method for diagnosis. More recently, genotyping by PCR has become the diagnostic test of choice, with phenotyping being reserved for confirmatory testing.[49]

Predispositional testing, or the testing of asymptomatic individuals at risk for developing disease, has relevance to the pediatric population. Hypothetical concerns exist regarding the psychological ramifications of being diagnosed during childhood with a disease that may not manifest for decades, if at all.[42,45] It has been speculated that knowledge of the illness may negatively impact a child's self-image or relationship with family members and peers.[42] Furthermore, concerns exist regarding the ability to secure health insurance and employment.[45] Alternatively, individuals who test negative for the disorder most likely will incur a positive emotional benefit.[42] Pediatric patients diagnosed with AAT deficiency must be counseled against tobacco use and the dangers of other relevant environmental exposures, and such counseling may be more effective when initiated at a younger age.[42,45]

Guidelines recommend testing of siblings of an individual with AAT deficiency, and genetic testing should be discussed for siblings of an individual who is heterozygous.[42] In addition, genetic testing is recommended for pediatric patients with unexplained liver disease and may be discussed with adolescents who present with persistent unexplained airflow obstruction.[42] Finally, it is recommended that genetic testing of adolescents proceed only if the adolescent is mature enough to understand the issues involved in testing, and that both assent and parental permission have been obtained.[42]

Natural Course and Treatment

Emphysema in AAT deficiency usually begins in the third or fourth decade of life, but timing of the onset of symptoms is highly variable. Treatment of respiratory manifestations of AAT deficiency centers on therapy for airways obstruction and hypoxemia, antimicrobials for secondary infection, and replacement enzyme (augmentation) therapy.[42] Augmentation therapy comprises regular administration of purified AAT and is recommended for individuals with

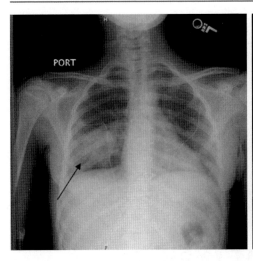
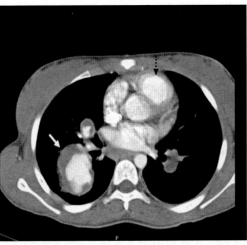

FIGURE 60-8. Chest radiography and CT angiogram of a 13-year-old female with Behçet disease with pulmonary artery aneurysms *(solid arrow)* and intracardiac thrombi *(dashed arrow)*. (From Endo LM, Rowe SM, Romp RL, et al. Pulmonary aneurysms and intracardiac thrombi due to Behçet's disease in an African-American adolescent with oculocutaneous albinism. *Clin Rheumatol* 2007;26:1537-1539.)

evidence of airflow obstruction.[42] However, replacement therapy cannot address the effects of polymerization of abnormal AAT. Future therapies may address the misfolding of AAT or use small fragment homologous replacement to correct the gene defect of Z AAT deficiency.[43]

The Alpha-1 Association (www.alpha1.org) and Alpha-1 Foundation (www.alpha1foundation.org) provide resources, support, education, and advocacy.

Behçet Disease

Behçet disease is a vasculitic disorder defined by the presence of recurrent oral ulcers, genital ulcers, eye disease (characteristically uveitis), and skin lesions.[50,51] Risk of developing the disease is associated with being a carrier of the *HLA-B51* allele.[52] Pulmonary vasculitis in Behçet disease is a severe complication and may lead to hemorrhage, infarction, and death.[51] Although most pulmonary disease observed in Behçet disease occurs in adults, pediatric patients have also been reported.[50,53] Pulmonary artery aneurysm is the most common respiratory presentation of Behçet disease and may be single or multifocal (Fig. 60-8).[51] These aneurysms occur with increased frequency in men with the disease and often present with hemoptysis.[51,52] Helical CT of the chest is the first-line imaging modality recommended if pulmonary artery aneurysm is suspected.[51,52] In addition to pulmonary artery aneurysm, pulmonary parenchymal disease is also reported. Behçet disease has been associated with pleuritis, reticulonodular or focal opacities, mass lesions, and hilar enlargement.[50-53] The majority of these findings most likely occur secondary to hemorrhage or infarction related to pulmonary vasculitis.[52] In addition, diffuse lung diseases such as organizing pneumonia, eosinophilic pneumonia, and pulmonary fibrosis have also been reported as very rare occurrences.[51,52] Treatment for Behçet disease centers on immunosuppressive and anti-inflammatory therapies. Anticoagulation is usually not recommended, because it may lead to worsening hemorrhage.[51] In summary, pulmonary problems in Behçet disease most often involve complications of vasculitis. Although rarely seen in children, the potential for life-threatening hemorrhage lends relevance to the disorder for pediatric practitioners.

■ SUMMARY

Rare lung disorders influence the care of children with respiratory diseases in a number of fundamental ways. Understanding of normal biologic function often occurs via characterization of the disrupted pathways occurring in rare diseases. This knowledge can then be applied to related diseases that occur with higher prevalence. Most importantly, the respiratory practitioner's ability to identify and care for pediatric patients with diseases that occur uncommonly will significantly impact the lives of those affected.

Suggested Reading

American Thoracic Society, European Respiratory Society. American Thoracic Society/European Respiratory Society statement: standards for the diagnosis and management of individuals with alpha-1 antitrypsin deficiency. *Am J Respir Crit Care Med.* 2003;168:818–900.

Esther Jr CR, Barker PM. Pulmonary lymphangiectasia: diagnosis and clinical course. *Pediatr Pulmonol.* 2004;38:308–313.

Faul JL, Berry GJ, Colby TV, et al. Thoracic lymphangiomas, lymphangiectasis, lymphangiomatosis, and lymphatic dysplasia syndrome. *Am J Respir Crit Care Med.* 2000;161(3 Pt 1):1037–1046.

Goitein O, Elstein D, Abrahamov A, et al. Lung involvement and enzyme replacement therapy in Gaucher's disease. *QJM.* 2001;94:407–415.

Mendelson DS, Wasserstein MP, Desnick RJ, et al. Type B Niemann-Pick disease: findings at chest radiography, thin-section CT, and pulmonary function testing. *Radiology.* 2006;238:339–345.

Tachibana T, Hagiwara K, Johkoh T. Pulmonary alveolar microlithiasis: review and management. *Curr Opin Pulm Med.* 2009;15:486–490.

Uzun O, Akpolat T, Erkan L. Pulmonary vasculitis in Behçet disease: a cumulative analysis. *Chest.* 2005;127:2243–2253.

Selected Foundations

Alpha-1 Association. www.alpha1.org.
Alpha-1 Foundation. www.alpha-1foundation.org.
Children's Tumor Foundation (Neurofibromatosis). www.ctf.org.
Dyskeratosis Congenita Outreach. www.dcoutreach.com.
Hermansky-Pudlak Syndrome Network. www.hpsnetwork.org.
LAM (lymphangioleiomyomatosis) Foundation. www.thelamfoundation.org.
Lymphangiomatosis & Gorham's Disease Alliance. http://lgdalliance.org.
Lymphangiomatosis Foundation. www.lymphangiomatosis.org.
Lymphatic Research Foundation. www.lymphaticresearch.org.
National Gaucher Foundation. www.gaucherdisease.org.
National Niemann-Pick Disease Foundation. www.nnpdf.org.

References

The complete reference list is available online at www.expertconsult.com

X

Disorders of the Immunocompromised Child

61 PRIMARY IMMUNODEFICIENCY: CHRONIC GRANULOMATOUS DISEASE AND COMMON VARIABLE IMMUNODEFICIENCY DISORDERS

Daniel R. Ambruso, MD, and Richard B. Johnston, Jr., MD

CHRONIC GRANULOMATOUS DISEASE

Chronic granulomatous disease of childhood was first described by Berendes and colleagues[1] and by Landing and Shirkey[2] as a distinct clinical entity of unknown cause.[3] The disease is characterized by recurrent infections, usually with low-grade pathogens; formation of abscesses and suppurative granulomas; and normal humoral and cellular immunity. The usual onset of symptoms is early in life (most in the first 2 years of life). The disease is generally chronic, and unless diagnosed and treated, the common outcome is death from overwhelming infection.

After the original patients, similar cases were reported using various names.[4–7] *Chronic granulomatous disease (CGD)* is now the generally accepted term for this syndrome. In 1967, Quie and colleagues[8] defined the basic step in pathophysiology as an inability of phagocytic cells to kill ingested bacteria. Baehner and Nathan[6] reported that CGD neutrophils did not undergo the phagocytosis-associated "respiratory burst" of oxygen consumption and hydrogen peroxide (H_2O_2) production that characterizes phagocytic cells.

Although all of the cases initially documented were in males, later reports described females, suggesting the possibility of autosomal-recessive variants.[9,10] In the 1970s, progress was made in elucidating the nature of the basic biochemical defect, decreased oxidase activity, a process by which oxygen (O_2) is reduced to superoxide anion (O_2^-) using NADPH as the electron source.[11–13] In 1978, Segal and Jones[13] reported the association of a b-type cytochrome and the NADPH oxidase, as well as its deficiency in CGD. Continued studies firmly defined

the relationship between X-linked CGD and deficiency of cytochrome b558.[14] In the late 1980s, the gene that is abnormal in X-linked CGD was cloned and subsequently shown to produce the heavy-chain component of the cytochrome b558 heterodimer (gp91phox).[15–17] Subsequently, the light chain (p22phox) was described and found to be the basis for the autosomal-recessive form of cytochrome b–deficient CGD.[18]

In the late 1980s and early 1990s, the molecular basis for other forms of autosomal-recessive CGD were defined. Cytosolic components p47phox and p67phox were identified, linked to distinct variants of CGD, and sequenced; and their genes were cloned.[19–22] Deficiency of p40phox has been more recently described.[23]

Thus, 84 years after Metchnikoff first posited that phagocytosis is essential in fighting infection (in 1883), studies in patients with CGD demonstrated for the first time clearly that a defect in phagocyte function is a major breach in host defense against severe infections. Since 1967, the biochemistry of the oxidase enzyme system has been elucidated, the major components defined, and the molecular basis for the most common variants of CGD described. Taking advantage of this syndrome as an "experiment of nature" has greatly expanded our knowledge of the role of the phagocyte in host defense.

CLINICAL FEATURES

The hallmark of this disease is the occurrence of purulent inflammation due to catalase-positive, low-grade pyogenic bacteria. This syndrome should be considered in any individual with recurrent catalase-positive bacterial or fungal infections. Table 61-1 summarizes the relative frequencies of the most common clinical findings in patients with CGD in the earliest reported cases—before the general use of prophylactic antimicrobial therapy.[24] A more recent analysis of infections in 368 patients enrolled in a registry for CGD[25,26] shows a general decline in most types of infection, with the notable exception of pneumonia (Table 61-2).

Of the 368 registry patients, 76% had the X-linked recessive form of CGD. The mean age at diagnosis in the registry patients was 3 years with the X-linked form and 7.8 years with an autosomal-recessive form.[25] These ages are much higher than they should be for the sake of the patient. In rare instances, the initial diagnosis has been made in adulthood. Reviews have suggested that autosomal-recessive variants generally have clinically milder disease.[26,27]

Although any organ may be involved with infections, two patterns have been evident in CGD populations across the world.[25-35] Tables 61-1 and 61-2 exemplify data from the United States. First, the inability of

TABLE 61-1 CLINICAL FINDINGS IN THE 168 EARLIEST REPORTED PATIENTS WITH CHRONIC GRANULOMATOUS DISEASE

FINDING	PERCENTAGE OF PATIENTS INVOLVED
Marked lymphadenopathy	82
Pneumonitis	80
Dermatitis	71
Hepatosplenomegaly	68
Onset by 1 year of age	65
Suppuration of nodes	62
Splenomegaly	57
Hepatic-perihepatic abscesses	41
Osteomyelitis	32
Onset with dermatitis	25
Onset with lymphadenitis	23
Facial periorificial dermatitis	21
Persistent diarrhea	20
Septicemia or meningitis	17
Perianal abscess	17
Conjunctivitis	16
Death from pneumonitis	15
Persistent rhinitis	15
Ulcerative stomatitis	15

Adapted from Johnston RB Jr, Newman SL. Chronic granulomatous disease. *Pediatr Clin North Am.* 1977;24:365-376.

TABLE 61-2 MOST COMMON INFECTIONS IN 368 PATIENTS ENROLLED IN A REGISTRY FOR CHRONIC GRANULOMATOUS DISEASE

INFECTION	PERCENTAGE OF PATIENTS
Pneumonia	79
Abscess (any)	68
Subcutaneous	42
Liver	27
Lung	16
Perirectal	15
Brain	3
Suppurative adenitis	53
Osteomyelitis	25
Bacteremia/fungemia	18
Cellulitis or impetigo	10

Data from Winkelstein JA, Marino MC, Johnston RB Jr, et al. Chronic granulomatous disease: Report on a national registry of 368 patients. *Medicine.* 2000;79:155-169.

phagocytic cells to effect microbicidal activity at the interface between the host and the environment leads to infections such as pneumonitis, infectious dermatitis, and perianal abscesses. With the involvement of the mononuclear phagocyte system, deep-seated infections result in purulent lymphadenitis, hepatomegaly, splenomegaly, and hepatic and perihepatic abscesses. At all sites of infection, microbes may be sequestered and protected from intracellular killing mechanisms and antimicrobials. Unable to destroy the microbes, the phagocytes die and release the organisms. Further microbial proliferation and leukocyte accumulation lead to the abscesses and granulomas that characterize the disorder. Septicemia may also occur because of the inability of phagocytes to localize microbial invasion.

Purulent rhinitis and otitis are common clinical features of this disease. With adequate antibiotic therapy, rhinitis clears slowly, only to recur within a few days after the treatment is discontinued. The oropharynx and gastrointestinal tract are frequently infected, with ulcerative stomatitis, gingivitis, esophagitis, rectal abscesses, perianal abscesses, and fissures being common. Urinary tract infections and glomerulonephritis, renal abscesses, and cystitis have all been reported. Gonadal infections are rare but have been described. Osteomyelitis is common: the most frequent sites include metacarpals, metatarsals, spine, and ribs.

Lymphadenitis, a characteristic clinical feature, occurs in the majority of patients during the course of the disease. It is typically chronic, suppurative, and granulomatous and very often requires surgical drainage. Cervical, axillary, and inguinal nodes are usually involved, but hilar and mesenteric lymph nodes are also commonly enlarged.

Skin lesions include impetiginous eruptions that progress slowly to suppuration. The healing process can be slow, resulting in granulomatous nodules that persist for months. These lesions may be found in any part of the body, the face and neck being the most frequent sites. Sweet's syndrome (acute febrile neutrophilic dermatosis)[36] has been associated with CGD. Furunculosis and subcutaneous abscesses may be chronic problems. Eczematoid dermatitis can be seen early in the diagnosis.

Carriers of X-linked CGD can have discoid lupus, aphthous ulcers, and systemic lupus-like symptoms.[37,38] If X-linked inactivation is skewed so that <10% of neutrophils express the normal NADPH oxidase, carrier females can have clinical CGD.[39–42] The progressive skewing of the X chromosome that occurs with age can result in adult-onset CGD in these carriers.[42]

While the major problems of patients with CGD are related to infections, these individuals can also be afflicted with a number of conditions reflecting a vigorous inflammatory response without a clear infectious cause.[27,28] Pyloric stenosis, with associated decrease in gastric emptying, is common, and sterile granulomas can be found in the pyloric antrum. Similar lesions in the small and large bowel may be associated with persistent abdominal pain, diarrhea, malabsorption, or obstruction.[43] Some of the gut lesions have been described as eosinophilic gastroenteritis, gastrointestinal dysmotility, or inflammatory bowel disease. Granulomas in the urinary bladder can result in obstructive uropathy. Pericarditis and pleuritis have been noted. Chorioretinitis was detected in 9 of 30 boys with X-linked CGD and in 3 of 15 related carriers in one clinic.[44]

The single patient reported with p40phox deficiency had a partial deficiency in the respiratory burst, no severe infections, but severe and chronic granulomatous colitis.[23] Patients with CGD can also have a typical autoimmune disease, including systemic and discoid lupus, idiopathic thrombocytopenic purpura, juvenile rheumatoid arthritis, IgA nephropathy, or antiphospholipid syndrome.[45] It seems likely that there is a common mechanism for this spectrum of inflammatory conditions, perhaps related to the fact that CGD neutrophils do not undergo normal cell death by apoptosis, are not cleared efficiently by macrophages, and therefore release toxic constituents into the tissues.[46,47] Whatever the mechanism, the response of pyloric and bladder granulomas to steroids is well documented.

■ PULMONARY COMPLICATIONS

Patient surveys, as exemplified in Tables 61-1 and 61-2, show that pneumonia continues to be one of the most common types of infection, occurring in about 80% of patients with CGD.[25–35] Pulmonary disease has also become a major cause of mortality in CGD.[25] The onset of lower respiratory tract infection may be heralded by the usual clinical presentation of fever, cough, tachypnea, pleuritic pain, and abnormal auscultatory findings. However, in some patients, particularly those with a fungal infection, few if any signs or symptoms have been noted in the presence of marked infiltration on

TABLE 61-3 MOST COMMON INFECTING ORGANISMS IN THE 368 PATIENTS IN THE CHRONIC GRANULOMATOUS REGISTRY

TYPE OF INFECTION	ORGANISM	PERCENTAGE OF PATIENTS*
Pneumonia	*Aspergillus* species	33
	Staphylococcus species	9
	Burkholderia cepacia	7
	Nocardia species	6
	Serratia species	4
Abscess— subcutaneous, liver, and/or perirectal	*Staphylococcus* species	26
	Serratia species	3
	Aspergillus species	3
Abscess—lung	*Aspergillus* species	4
Abscess—brain	*Aspergillus* species	2
Suppurative adenitis	*Staphylococcus* species	14
	Serratia species	5
Osteomyelitis	*Serratia* species	7
	Aspergillus species	5
Bacteremia/fungemia	*Salmonella* species	3
	Burkholderia cepacia	2
	Candida species	2

*Percentage of the 368 patients who had this organism isolated at least once from the infection shown.
Data from Winkelstein JA, Marino MC, Johnston RB Jr, et al. Chronic granulomatous disease: Report on a national registry of 368 patients. *Medicine*. 2000; 79:155-169.

radiography. Chronic granulomatous infiltrations, bronchiolitis obliterans, pulmonary fibrosis, bronchiectasis, interstitial lung disease, and sarcoidosis have been noted in both pediatric and adult patients.[29,48–50]

The range of microbial agents causing pulmonary infections is shown in Table 61-3. Since the 1970s, the use of daily antimicrobial therapy in CGD has reduced the rate of infections caused by *Staphylococcus aureus* and enteric bacteria,[51,52] but *Aspergillus* spp. has become a particularly troublesome offender.[25,53] Fungal infection of the lung can present as discreet nodular, miliary, or pan-lobular involvement. Fungi now cause a large percentage of infections in CGD; these typically cause less fever and can be hard to diagnose in early stages. Fungal lung involvement may spread to the pleura and adjacent bone and soft tissues of the chest wall.[54,55] Although *Aspergillus* accounts for most of the fungal agents (>80%), other agents such as *Acremonium striatum*, *Candida albicans*, *Pneumocystis carinii*, and *Paecilomyces* spp. may be isolated from infected lungs.[25,28,53] *Aspergillus* pneumonia, with or without dissemination, was the leading cause of death in the 368 registry patients (23 of 65 total deaths). *Nocardia*, atypical mycobacteria, and the bacillus Calmette-Guérin vaccine strain of mycobacteria can also cause pulmonary disease.[35]

Pulmonary lesions on radiograph include extensive infiltration of the lung parenchyma and prominent hilar adenopathy (Fig. 61-1). Bronchopneumonia, lobar

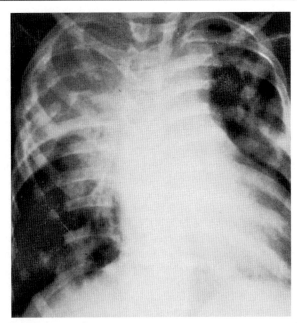

FIGURE 61-1. A chest roentgenogram from a patient with chronic granulomatous disease, showing extensive involvement of the right lung. This patient died of the overwhelming infection.

pneumonia, extensive reticulonodular infiltration, pleural effusion, pleural thickening, pulmonary abscess, and atelectasis (especially of the right middle lobe) have been described.

In spite of extensive antimicrobial treatment, the various expressions of CGD pulmonary disease often regress slowly over a period of weeks to months, or they can progress to involve an entire lobe. An unusual manifestation of pulmonary involvement observed in these patients is so-called *encapsulated pneumonia.*[56] This pneumonia is characteristically seen on roentgenography as a homogeneous, discrete, relatively round lesion; it may occur singly or in groups of two to three infiltrates (Fig. 61-2). The size and contour of the lesions may change over days or weeks or remain unchanged. Histologically, they take the form of caseating granulomas (Fig. 61-3). A homogeneous "shotgun" distribution of small granulomatous lesions can occur, which gives the radiographic appearance of miliary tuberculosis. Discoid atelectasis, thickening of the bronchi, air bronchograms, "honeycombing," loss of lobar volume, and bronchiectasis associated with hemoptysis are occasionally observed.

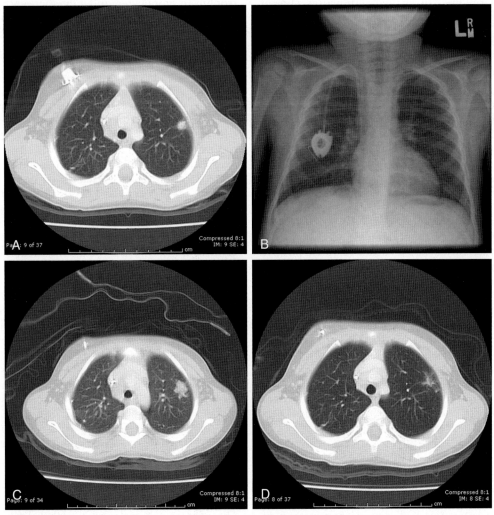

FIGURE 61-2. **A,** Encapsulated pneumonia in a patient with chronic granulomatous disease. A CT scan with nodular lesion in left upper lobe. **B,** PA chest roentgenogram for comparison at the same time as **(A)** does not demonstrate lesion. **C,** Progression of lesion. **D,** Lesion resolving in response to appropriate antifungal therapy. (Images courtesy of Thomas Hay, MD.)

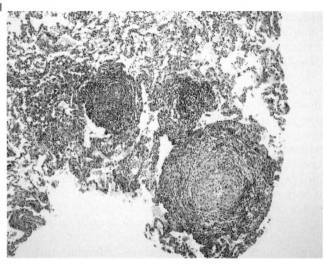

FIGURE 61-3. Typical granuloma of lung tissue removed from the patient in Figure 61-2. (Image courtesy of Kelley Capocelli, MD.)

LABORATORY FINDINGS AND DIAGNOSIS

Except for abnormalities of phagocyte function, clinical laboratory findings reflect acute or chronic infection and inflammation. Leukocytosis with neutrophilia, elevated erythrocyte sedimentation rate and C-reactive protein, and the anemia of chronic inflammation are common. The anemia is usually not caused by a deficiency of iron stores but to a decrease in iron release from the mononuclear phagocyte system and diminished utilization by the marrow.[57] It typically does not respond to iron administration but improves with resolution of infection. Evidence of hemolytic anemia with acanthocytosis suggests absence of the K_x antigen in red blood cells, a trait encoded close to the *gp91phox* gene on the X chromosome.

Screening evaluations of various aspects of immune function are usually normal, including complement, cellular immunity, and antibody production in response to immunization.[28] Polyclonal hypergammaglobulinemia is common. A deficiency of microbicidal activity against catalase-positive bacteria (e.g., staphylococci and *E. coli*) and a diminished or absent respiratory burst by neutrophils and monocytes are the essential functional and biochemical findings of CGD.

Patients with CGD have a predisposition to infections with a broad variety of bacteria and fungi (see Table 61-3). The most common organisms are *S. aureus*, enteric bacteria, and *Aspergillus*,[24,25,35,52] but unusual and rarely pathogenic organisms may cause disease in patients with CGD. Recent studies have focused on *Burkholderia cepacia* as a significant pathogen, particularly in the lung.[27,58–60] Infection by this organism was the second leading cause of death in patients in the CGD registry. Its propensity to infect patients with either CGD or cystic fibrosis is not understood.

Microbial agents associated with pulmonary infections are the same as those that cause infections in other parts of the body. Fungal pneumonitis is frequent, especially caused by *Aspergillus*. Other pulmonary pathogens include *Nocardia* spp., *P. carinii*, *Actinomyces*, and mycobacteria. Infections due to pneumococci, streptococci, and

Haemophilus spp. are no more common in children with CGD than in normal children, presumably because these catalase-negative organisms cannot protect against their own H_2O_2 production within the phagocytic vacuole.

Tissue from infected sites shows granulomas like those typically seen with intracellular parasites such as mycobacteria. Granulomas in CGD patients include mononuclear phagocytes that can contain a tan or yellow pigmented material.[2,61] Granulomas in the presence of the pathogens noted above strongly suggests the diagnosis of CGD.

Simple screening tests for CGD are currently available. The histochemical nitroblue tetrazolium (NBT) test[62] remains a reliable screening measure. Stimulation of microbicidal activity and the respiratory burst results in the reduction of O_2 to O_2^-; NBT dye is reduced by the extra electron in O_2^- and converted from a yellow, water-soluble dye to a purple insoluble substance. In normal individuals, 95% or more of phagocytic cells reduce NBT; the phagocytes from patients with the common variants of CGD do not reduce NBT. Carriers of X-linked CGD exhibit two populations of cells: normal and NBT-negative.

Fluorescence-based screening assays using flow cytometry avoid the subjective element of the NBT test. Dihydrorhodamine-123 can be readily preloaded into neutrophils or monocytes, and it interacts with oxygen metabolites produced during the respiratory burst to generate products with increased fluorescence.[63] Patients' phagocytes do not shift fluorescence after stimulation. X-linked carriers have two populations. Additionally, some CGD variants (e.g., p47phox deficiency and milder variants of X-linked CGD) have very low oxidase activity in all cells, and this technique can detect this activity. This assay is more quantitative than the NBT test because it measures oxidase activity of the entire phagocyte population and can quantify partial reduction in the respiratory burst.

A positive screening test should be confirmed with one or more quantitative tests. Bactericidal assays with *Eschericia coli* or *S. aureus* may be diagnostic.[8,64] Quantitative assays of O_2 consumption, O_2^- production, or generation of H_2O_2 can be helpful.[6,32,64,65] Finally, an analysis of the various oxidase components will define the molecular variant of CGD. Cytochrome b558 can be quantitated spectroscopically, and the individual oxidase components can be analyzed by Western blot. Several cell-free systems that can reproduce the assembly and activation of the oxidase in intact cells with the use of plasma membrane and cytosol from neutrophils may be helpful in defining the molecular variants of CGD. Identification of the genetic mutation responsible for the protein defect may be helpful for genetic counseling, prenatal studies, and judging prognosis.[66,67]

Prenatal diagnosis may be achieved with screening tests on fetal neutrophils obtained by percutaneous umbilical blood sampling. The diagnosis for some CGD variants can be made from chorionic villus or amniocyte samples using restriction fragment length polymorphism or gene analysis without the risk of fetal blood sampling.[68,69]

NADPH OXIDASE

The oxidase enzyme resides in the plasma membrane of stimulated cells, and through the oxidation of NADPH catalyzes the reduction of O_2 to O_2^-, the first step in

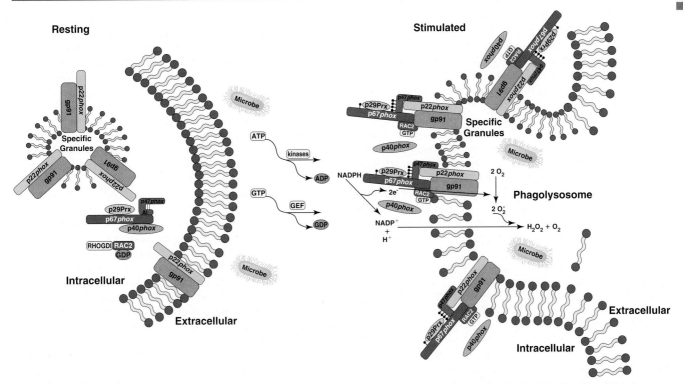

FIGURE 61-4. Schematic diagram of the NADPH oxidase enzyme system, its components, and its activation. In resting neutrophils, membrane components (gp91phox and p22phox) reside in plasma membrane and specific granules. With stimulation, degranulation of specific granules expands the amount of cytochrome b_{558} in plasma membrane and translocation of cytosolic components (rac2, p47phox, p67phox, and p40phox) and p29 peroxiredoxin 6 (p29Prx) to the plasma membrane results in assembly of an active oxidase enzyme system that uses electrons from NADPH to reduce O_2 to form O_2^-.

production of antimicrobial oxygen metabolites. Phagocyte oxidase (phox) activity results from the interaction of several components that form an enzyme complex. In resting cells, these components reside in different compartments. With stimulation of the cell, they assemble in the plasma membrane to express oxidase activity [28,70–72] (Fig. 61-4).

The main catalytic component of the oxidase is the cytochrome b558. In resting cells, 10% to 20% of total cellular cytochrome b558 appears to be located in plasma membrane, and 80% to 90% is in the membranes of specific granules. This protein is a heterodimer composed of α (p22phox) and β (gp91phox) subunits. Cytochrome b558 binds NADPH; its flavin binding site and a heme moiety are critical to shuttling electrons between NADPH and O_2.[73] With stimulation, specific granule membranes fuse with plasma membrane, increasing the amount of cytochrome b558 associated with the plasma membrane. The cytosolic oxidase components translocate to the plasma membrane and specific granules, providing an active oxidase complex that is increased in the plasma membrane.[70,71] A low–molecular weight G protein, Rap1a, is associated with cytochrome b558 and may be important in assembly and activation of the oxidase complex.[28,74]

The cytosolic oxidase components include p47phox, p67phox, and p40phox.[21,22,73] A cytosolic low–molecular weight guanosine triphosphate (GTP)–binding protein, p21rac2, is also involved, and there may be other proteins that control GTP binding to the rac2 protein.[75,76] These latter elements link with receptors on the plasma membrane and help transmit and/or amplify biochemical signals (e.g., from opsonized microbes) that regulate assembly and activation of the oxidase.

p47phox and p67phox appear to exist as a complex in the cytosol of resting cells.[73,77] Interactions between this complex, plasma membrane, and the cytoskeletal elements are critical for activation of the oxidase.[72] Precise details of the relevant domains for interactions of phox proteins, changes that occur during cell activation, and the relationship with signaling pathways has been under intense investigation in recent years and is summarized in a recent review.[78] The gene for p40phox (NCF4) has been cloned, and p40phox was identified as binding strongly to p67phox. More recent work suggests that p40phox function within the NADPH oxidase complex depends on its binding to phosphatidylinositol 3-phosphate.[23] An additional protein closely associated with p67phox has been described.[79] This 29-kd protein (termed *p29*) is categorized as a peroxiredoxin 6 by its sequence and activity. Peroxiredoxins are a class of peroxidases that oxidize H_2O_2 with sulfur groups on cysteine residues.[80] Neutrophil p29 peroxiredoxin 6 enhances O_2^- production in subcellular systems of oxidase activity and in intact cells and translocates to plasma membrane after stimulation of the respiratory burst.[81] The p29 peroxiredoxin 6 may protect the oxidase from its own toxic products or may play a role in signaling.

MOLECULAR DEFECTS AND INHERITANCE

Genetic testing documenting a patient/family mutation is currently available through commercial or research laboratories. In addition to confirming the correct classification of the patient and his or her prognosis, the specific defect will be important if more aggressive management strategies (e.g., gene therapy and/or hematopoietic stem cell transplantation) are considered. With the discovery of the various oxidase components over the past 15 years, the molecular basis of CGD has come into focus. Most patients express genetic or molecular abnormalities in one of the four major components of the oxidase: gp91phox, p22phox, p47phox, or p67phox (Table 61-4).[25,28,66,67] One patient has been reported with a mutation in *rac*2,[82] but no patients have been described with a rap-1 abnormality. p40phox, which is encoded by the *NCF4* gene on chromosome 22 (22a13.1), is reported to be diminished in individuals with p67phox deficiency, and a single patient has been described with an autosomal recessive deficiency in this component, deficiency of the phagocytosis-stimulated respiratory burst, and granulomatous colitis.[23]

The most common molecular defects in CGD are related to gp91phox and account for about 70% of all cases of this syndrome.[26,28–35,66] Located on the short arm of the X chromosome (Xp21.1), defects in the *gp91phox* gene are inherited as X-linked recessive. In the most common variety, mutations in the gene result in the lack of gp91phox protein due to mRNA or protein instability. NADPH oxidase activity is totally absent, no cytochrome b558 is seen spectrophotometrically, and no gp91phox is detected on Western blot. A defect in the membrane contribution to oxidase activity is documented with analysis in cell-free systems. Cytosol and its components are normal. Deletions; insertions; and splice site, missense, and nonsense mutations have all been described and reviewed in detail.[66]

Other variants of gp91phox deficiency have been described. Some mutations have resulted in partial loss of protein expression and diminished oxidase activity in proportion to the decrease in protein content. In some, a truncated protein is expressed. Defects are found in exons, introns, intron/exon junctions, and promotors. A few cases have been described with normal gp91phox protein expression but nearly complete absence of oxidase activity. Additional variants have been reported with the inability to interact with NADPH or with p47phox and p67phox or to bind flavin adenine dinucleotide (FAD). Severity of disease in these less common genetic variants correlates with the level of cytochrome b expression and superoxide production.

Patients who lack both the respiratory burst and cytochrome b558 and exhibit an autosomal-recessive mode of inheritance have a deficiency in p22phox, the gene for which is found on chromosome 16 (16q24). These patients account for 5% to 6% of all cases. In the usual form, the deficiency in membrane contribution of oxidase activity is accompanied by absence of the cytochrome b558 spectrum and both gp91phox and p22phox by Western blot. Analysis of cytosolic components is normal. Although fewer genetic analyses have been completed, deletion; insertion; and missense, nonsense, and splice site mutations have been described.[67] In one variant, a homozygous missense mutation affects the area of interaction between p22phox and p47phox, resulting in a normal cytochrome b558 that cannot form an oxidase complex.

Patients who exhibit an autosomal-recessive mode of inheritance but whose neutrophils contain normal amounts of cytochrome b558 may have a deficiency of either p47phox or p67phox. The gene for p47phox falls on chromosome 7 (7q11.23), and that for p67phox is on chromosome 1 (1q25). Defects in these genes account for approximately 20% and for 5% to 6% of CGD cases, respectively. Absent or nearly absent oxidase in whole cells is coupled with deficient cytosol contribution in the cell-free system and deficiency of the protein on Western blot. There appears to be much less heterogeneity in genetic mutations causing deficiency of p47phox than of p67phox.[67] Patients studied to date are either homozygous for a GT dinucleotide (ΔGT) deletion at the start of exon 2 of the *NCF-1* gene or are compound heterozygotes with GT deletion on one allele and a point mutation on the second allele. The reason for the homogeneity is that most normal individuals have *p47phox* pseudogenes, each of which colocalize with the functional gene at 7q11.23. Recombination events between the functional genes and pseudogenes lead to incorporation of ΔGT into the *NCF-1* gene. In addition to heterozygous GT changes, missense and splice junction changes have been described. In many patients studied, normal amounts of mRNA and complete absence of p47phox are found in neutrophils, suggesting translation of an unstable protein.

Relatively few molecular defects have been characterized in patients with p67phox deficiency. As with p47phox deficiency, mRNA for p67phox is usually present; but in most cases no protein is detected. Nonsense, missense, homozygous point, splice site, insertion, and deletion mutations as well as one duplication have been documented, suggesting a heterogeneity of genetic abnormalities for p67phox.[28,67]

The patient with *rac*2 deficiency presented with severe, recurrent perirectal abscesses and pyoderma, omphalitis, and poor wound healing.[82,83] His neutrophils exhibited a unique pattern of functional abnormalities, including markedly diminished random and directed migration, decreased ingestion and bactericidal activity, and absent degranulation of azurophilic granules. Expression of CD11b and degranulation of specific granules were normal. O_2^- production in response to N-formyl-methionyl-leucyl-phenylalanine and platelet-activating factor was absent, to opsonized zymosan was decreased, but to phorbol myristate acetate was normal. *Rac*2 was 30% of control, and all other oxidase components were normal. A mutation in one nucleotide of codon 57 for one *rac*2 allele resulted in a substitution of asparagine for aspartic acid. Although both the wild-type and mutant alleles were expressed, the mutant protein had a defect in the GTP binding site, could only bind guanosine diphosphate, and had a dominant-negative effect on the wild-type *rac*2 as well as other low–molecular weight GTPases.[82,83] Because of this, the oxidase and the other neutrophil functions were affected. The patient was cured by a bone marrow transplant from his human leukocyte antigen (HLA)–identical sibling.[84]

Deficiency of glucose-6-phosphate dehydrogenase (G6PD) in leukocytes, which occurs in a small number of patients with erythrocytes deficient in this enzyme, has been considered a variant of CGD.[26,85–87] Patients whose neutrophils contain less than 5% of normal activity suffer

TABLE 61-4 MOLECULAR AND GENETIC CLASSIFICATION OF CHRONIC GRANULOMATOUS DISEASE

AFFECTED COMPONENT*	CHROMOSOME LOCATION	GENE*	INHERITANCE*	SUBTYPE CLASS*	NBT/DHR (% POSITIVE)/ O₂⁻ PRODUCTION	CYTOCHROME B₅₅₈ SPECTRUM	WESTERN BLOT ANALYSIS†	FREQUENCY
gp91phox	Xp21.1	CYBB	XL	X91^0	0/0	0	Absent gp91phox Markedly decreased or absent p22phox	70%
				X91$^-$	80%-100%/3%-30% (weak)	3%-30%	Decreased gp91 and p22phox	
				X91$^-$	5%-10%/5%-10%	5%-10%	Decreased gp91 and p22phox	
				X91$^+$	0/0	100%	Normal gp91 and p22phox	
p22phox	16p24	CYBA	AR	A22^0 A22$^+$	0/0 0/0	0 100%	Absent p22 and gp91phox Normal p22 and gp91phox	5%-6%
p47phox	7q11.23	NCF-1	AR	A47^0	0/0-1%	100%	Absent p47phox	20%
p67phox	1q25	NCF-2	AR	A67^0	0/1-1%	100%	Absent p67phox	5%-6%

*Oxidase components expressed as gp91phox, p22phox, p47phox, p67phox, and their genes as *CYBB*, *CYBA*, *NCF-1*, and *NCF-2*, respectively. The superscript designates detection of protein in patient samples. A, autosomal; AR, autosomal-recessive; XL, X-linked; O, absent; –, diminished; +, present. Subtypes represented by letter designating type of inheritance. The superscript

†For Western blot analysis, abnormalities in specific phox proteins are noted. Other components not described are normal with this technique. Deficiencies in gp91phox and p22phox exhibit dimin-Activity measurements may be made in the cell-free system of activation.[70-71] In this system, activity is defined by both cytosol (and associated components) and membrane. Deficiencies in gp91phox and p22phox exhibit dimin-ished or absent membrane contribution, and deficiencies of p47phox and p67phox exhibit diminished or absent cytosol contribution.

Data from Roos D, Kuhns DB, Roesler J, et al. Hematologically important mutations: X-linked chronic granulomatous disease (third update). *Blood Cells Mol Dis.* 2010;45:246-265; Roos D, Kuhns DB, Maddalena A, et al. Hematologically important mutations: The autosomal recessive forms of chronic granulomatous disease (second update). *Blood Cells Mol Dis.* 2010;44:291-299.

from recurrent, sometimes fatal, infections. Their neutrophils do not exhibit a respiratory burst and exhibit a microbicidal defect against catalase-positive organisms. Deficiency of NADPH as the efficient electron donor to the oxidase may explain this disorder.[85]

MANAGEMENT

The key to the successful management of CGD remains early diagnosis, prophylactic antimicrobial therapy, and rapid and vigorous treatment of infections.[28,51,52,88–94] This approach begins with prophylactic daily doses of trimethoprim-sulfamethoxazole (4 to 6 mg/kg trimethoprim, 20 to 30 mg/kg sulfamethoxazole, once or divided into two doses daily), which has reduced the incidence of severe bacterial infections by 70%. Ciprofloxacin may be used as an alternative. Interferon-γ given at a dose of 1.5 mcg/kg (surface area <0.5 m²) or 50 mcg/m² (surface area ≥0.5 m²) three times weekly by subcutaneous injection also reduces the incidence and severity of infections.[89,92] Administration before bedtime along with acetaminophen reduces fever and myalgias. Daily itraconazole at 100 to 200 mg/day (4 to 5 mg/kg in two doses) taken with food has been advocated as fungal prophylaxis.[51,88] Care should be taken to avoid environmental conditions that present a high risk for exposure to *Nocardia* and fungi, especially *Aspergillus* (e.g., garden mulch, construction sites, leaves, and marijuana).

When infections develop, aggressive attempts should be made to obtain culture and antimicrobial sensitivity of organisms from localized areas. Surgical drainage, including of pulmonary abscesses or empyema, is also critical to treatment because the antimicrobials required to resolve infection do not penetrate well into abscesses.[93,94] The infected site should be aggressively débrided with prolonged drainage to prevent loculation and sequestration of infected areas.

In patients with fever and elevated C-reactive protein and sedimentation rate but no definite locus for an infection, an empiric trial of parenteral antimicrobials may be necessary. During the initiation of this therapy, definition of the infected area should be sought with routine radiographs, computed tomography or magnetic resonance imaging studies, or radionucleotide scans.

Identification of the infected site may provide clues to initial antimicrobial coverage. For example, the vast majority of liver abscesses are caused by staphylococci (see Table 61-3), and vancomycin and levofloxacin might be used initially. *Burkholderia cepacia* is found in a higher incidence in the lung, and *Serratia* is found in soft tissue and bones. For these infections, increasing the trimethoprim-sulfamethoxazole to a full therapeutic dose and adding a cephalosporin, meropenem, or levofloxacin should be considered until antimicrobial sensitivities are available. Antimicrobial coverage may be reorganized in response to antimicrobial sensitivities of recovered organisms. Initial parenteral treatment and oral antimicrobials for weeks or months may be required to resolve the infection.

If fungus is suspected or defined, vigorous antifungal therapy should be instituted. Although amphotericin has been advocated in the past, other agents may be required, such as itraconazole, voriconazole (6 mg/kg every 12 hours on day 1, and then 4 mg/kg every 12 hours), or posaconazole (200 mg, three times daily; currently approved only for children over 12 years of age and adults).[88,95–97] Prednisone may be considered for miliary involvement. Although not proved efficacious, daily granulocyte transfusions (at least 10¹⁰ granulocytes per transfusion) have been used as a supplement to aggressive surgical and antimicrobial therapy,[27,28,98] but these can cause alloimmunization, which could hamper later bone marrow transplantation.

Some patients with CGD inherit, as a closely associated X-linked allele, a deficiency in the K_x antigen affecting both erythrocytes and leukocytes.[28] This results in the lack of Kell antigens on the surface of the red blood cells, which can be associated with a chronic hemolytic anemia. In addition, transfusion of these patients can result in true isoimmunization for Kell antigens and the risk for immediate or delayed transfusion reactions.

Inflammatory conditions or obstructive lesions of the gastrointestinal tract (seen in up to 50% of patients) or genitourinary tract (in up to 70% of patients) usually respond to treatment with steroids.[43,99,100] The response may be prompt, but relapses are common.

HEMATOPOIETIC CELL TRANSPLANTATION AND GENE THERAPY

Hematopoietic cell transplantation has been attempted with mixed results.[101–105] Long-term engraftment and reversal of the defect has been documented. Sources of stem cells include bone marrow, mobilized peripheral blood, and umbilical cord blood. Although unrelated donors have been used, the majority of successful transplants have been completed with HLA-identical siblings.[101,103] In a series from the United Kingdom, transplantation led to resolution of colitis and catch-up growth in children with growth failure.[104] The best predictors of success have been absence of overt preexisting infection at the time of transplantation and transplantation at a relatively early age, before numerous infections and end-organ damage have occurred.

Many of the centers transplanting CGD patients have used a myeloablative preparative regimen. While engraftment has occurred in a high percentage of patients, the presence of concurrent infection has presented a significant risk for severe complications, and death has been common. The National Institutes of Health published its experience using a non-myeloablative preparative regimen with T cell–depleted peripheral blood stem cells from HLA-identical siblings.[103] After a median follow-up of 17 months, 8 of 10 patients had sufficient neutrophils to provide normal host defense and resolution of granulomatous lesions. Another center used marrow from matched unrelated donors; 7 of 9 patients were alive and well 20 to 79 months after transplantation.[105] Restrictive lung disease was cleared in two of these individuals. Although CGD can be cured by successful hematopoietic cell transplantation, the possibility of infections, graft rejection, and graft-versus-host disease remain major impediments, and the risks and benefits must be weighed carefully with each individual patient.

Since CGD arises from gene defects in a finite group of proteins expressed in myeloid cells, transfer of a normally functioning gene into the pluripotent stem cell would, theoretically, constitute definitive treatment. The groundwork for this approach was laid with experiments in which Epstein-Barr virus–transformed B-lymphocyte or myelomonoblastic cell lines from CGD patients with various molecular defects were transfected with complementary DNA (cDNA) for the missing oxidase component. Partial correction of protein expression and oxidase activity was obtained.[21,106,107] Reconstitution *in vivo*, however, would require transfection of normal genes into pluripotent stem cells. To this end, CD34+ peripheral blood hematopoietic progenitor cells were transduced with cDNA for p47phox, p22phox, or gp91phox.[108,109] Murine models of CGD have also provided useful information for successful application of human gene therapy trials.[110,111]

Malech and colleagues developed a model process for CGD gene therapy and employed it in a clinical trial of five patients with p47phox-deficient CGD.[112] CD34+ progenitor cells were mobilized by granulocyte colony-stimulating factor infusion, harvested by apheresis, purified, then expanded *ex vivo* in the presence of growth factors. These expanded CD34+ cells were transfected with cDNA for normal p47phox in a retroviral vector. The patients received 0.1 to 4.7×10^6 transfected cells/kg. After 3 to 5 weeks, low levels of blood neutrophils with normal ability to oxidize dihydrorhodamine were detected; but these cells declined to undetectable numbers over 3 to 6 months. Although the numbers of normal cells were too small to reconstitute the defect and the effect was not long-lasting, the general principles of this approach were demonstrated.

This experience was extended by Ott and colleagues.[113] After non-myeloablative marrow conditioning with busulfan, two young adults with X-linked CGD were treated with autologous CD34+ stem cells that had been transfected with a retrovirus vector expressing gp91phox.

Substantial gene transfer occurred in both individuals, and life-threatening infections resolved within the first few months. However, the level of gene-positive neutrophils subsequently increased as a result of oligoclonal outgrowth of cells in which the vector had inserted at the site of a proto-oncogene.[114] Bone marrow exam showed myelodysplasia with monosomy 7 in both men; one died of sepsis, and the other received an allogeneic hematopoietic stem-cell transplantation.[114,115]

Based on the clearance of severe infections achieved in the otherwise failed trial of Ott and coworkers, Kang, Malech, and colleagues treated three adult X-linked CGD patients suffering severe, unresolving infections with a different retroviral vector encoding gp91phox after busulfan marrow conditioning.[116] The three patients had 26%, 5%, and 4% oxidase-normal neutrophils initially, but these normal cells declined over time. One of the patients with a sustained level of 1.1% normal cells cleared treatment-intractable liver abscesses and has been free of infection for 3 years; a second patient with 0.03% sustained normal-cell levels resolved his *Aspergillus* lung infection that had extended to ribs and vertebrae. The patient with no detectable normal cells by 4 weeks died of

his *Paecilomyces* lung infection.[116] Thus, gene therapy has not yet cured a patient with CGD; but the field has made definite progress, and gene therapy clearly holds out hope for the future.

COMMON VARIABLE IMMUNODEFICIENCY DISORDERS

Common variable immunodeficiency disorders is now the standard term[117] for a group of disorders that are almost always associated with pulmonary complications. The group is characterized clinically by onset in the first 5 to 10 years of life or in mid-adolescence to young adulthood with recurrent bacterial infections, especially sinusitis, pneumonia, and chronic pulmonary disease. Although not common, the disorder can begin in infancy. Autoimmune disease, gastrointestinal disorders, and a predisposition to lymphoma are less commonly associated conditions. The group is characterized immunologically by decreased production of IgG in combination with low levels of IgA and/or IgM, weak or absent antibody response to immunizations, and absence of any other immunodeficiency state.

The condition was earlier thought of as a single entity and was initially referred to as *late-appearing* (or *acquired*) *hypogammaglobulinemia*. It was diagnosed in males and females and after infancy, and this term differentiated it from the earlier-described *congenital X-linked agammaglobulinemia*. As more cases were described, it was given the name *common variable immunodeficiency* (OMIM 240500). The condition is aptly named—it is common, at least among primary immunodeficiency diseases, with an estimated rate in the population of 1 in 25,000 to 30,000[118–121]—and its clinical presentation and underlying immune cellular defects vary widely. It is apparently the expression of several different conditions with multiple underlying single-gene or polygenic defects. Although it is not clear what most of these may be, it is nevertheless appropriate that the new term for the group (used in our title) emphasizes a family of disorders. In describing the *diagnosis* applied to patients within the group, we will use the abbreviation *CVID* to mean a common variable immunodeficiency disorder.

CLINICAL FEATURES

Major reviews of 248 CVID patients from the U.S.,[120] 252 patients from France,[122] and 334 patients from the European Common Variable Immunodeficiency Disorders Registry,[121] a collaborative analysis by two of the principal authors of these reviews,[123] and a review of CVID in children[124] have greatly expanded current understanding of these disorders.

The fundamental feature of CVID is insufficient production of antibodies to pathogens. Thus, almost all patients have a history of serious or recurrent infections (e.g., all but 5 of 248 patients in the U.S. cohort[120]). Table 61-5 summarizes the most common infections that occurred in the American and French cohorts, and the list reflects the experience at other centers (in particular that in references 121 and 123 and citations contained therein).

TABLE 61-5 SUMMARY OF MOST COMMON INFECTIONS IN TWO LARGE COHORTS OF PATIENTS WITH CVID

	NO. OF PATIENTS OF TOTAL 248[120] (%)*	NO. OF PATIENTS OF TOTAL 252[122] (%)*
Recurrent bronchitis, sinusitis, and/or otitis	243 (98)	
Respiratory and lung infections (total)		240 (95)
Pneumonia	190 (77)	147 (58)
Chronic lung disease, including bronchiectasis	68 (27)	92 (37)
Viral hepatitis	16 (7)	
Severe or recurrent herpes zoster infection	9 (4)	27 (11)
Severe varicella infection		10 (4)
Giardia enteritis	8 (3)	35 (14)
Pneumocystis infection	7 (3)	2 (1)
Mycoplasma pneumonia	6 (2)	
Salmonella or *Campylobacter* enteritis	6 (2)	38 (15)
Osteomyelitis or septic arthritis (2 each)	4 (2)	
Chronic mucocutaneous candidiasis	3 (1)	
Bacteremic sepsis	3 (1)	33 (13)
Bacterial meningitis	2 (<1)	20 (8)

*Number of patients (%) with the infection among the total studied.
Adapted from Cunningham-Rundles C, Bodian C. Common variable immunodeficiency: clinical and immunological features of 248 patients. *Clin Immunol.* 1999;92: 34-48; Oksenhendler E, Gerard L, Fieschi C, et al, for the DEFI Study Group. Infections in 252 patients with common variable immunodeficiency. *Clin Infect Dis.* 2008;46:1547-1554 and their accompanying texts. Cunningham-Rundles and Bodian report the experience of an academic medical center in New York City. Fifteen percent of the 248 patients developed symptoms between 2 and 10 years of age (mean age 23 years for males, 28 years for females). Oksenhendler and colleagues report the experience of DEFI, a French national study of adults with primary hypogammaglobulinemia. Fifty-nine percent of the 252 patients developed symptoms between 4 and 10 years of age (median age at onset 19 years).

Recurrent or chronic bronchitis, sinusitis, and/or otitis media occur in almost all patients and are the most common infections at onset of symptoms.[120-124] The microorganisms most commonly cultured before the diagnosis is made and treatment started are those that require antibody for optimal opsonization and phagocytosis, particularly pneumococci, *H. influenzae,* and streptococci. After treatment is started with intravenous immunoglobulin (IVIG), infections are more likely to be caused by staphylococci or an enteric pathogen, fungi (e.g., *Candida, Pneumocystis, Nocardia*), a virus (varicella-zoster virus, enteroviruses, hepatitis viruses), protozoa (especially *Giardia*), or *Mycoplasma.*[119-127] In a review of 20 patients diagnosed with CVID and an enteroviral infection, 14 had ECHO or Coxsackievirus infection and 6 had poliomyelitis, particularly caused by live polio vaccine.[126]

The clinical findings in 32 children with CVID[124] were very similar to those described in the large reviews of patients of all ages (see Table 61-5). Recurrent or chronic respiratory tract infections (88% of the children), sinusitis (78%), otitis media (78%), pneumonia (78%), bronchiectasis (34%), and intestinal tract infections (34%) were the most common infections. Two children had polio after live poliovirus immunization. An allergic disorder was present in 38% of the children and an autoimmune condition in 31%. The mean time between onset of symptoms and institution of immunoglobulin substitution therapy was 5.8 years.

On physical examination, evidence of complications may include growth retardation (9 of the 32 children)[124] or weight loss (adults), changes associated with chronic otitis or sinusitis, lymphadenopathy, splenomegaly, gingivitis, poor dentition, and signs of chronic pulmonary disease.[119-124]

Gastrointestinal disease occurs in roughly a quarter to a third of patients (15% to 47%, depending on what conditions are included),[120,122,128,129] perhaps in those who have an accompanying defect in cell-mediated immunity.[128] These disorders may be caused by infection, cancer, or autoimmune or inflammatory disease. Chronic diarrhea is the most common symptom. The etiology is not always known, but infections with *Giardia, Salmonella, Campylobacter* (see Table 61-5), CMV, or *Cryptosporidium* have been reported.[120,122,129]

Autoimmune disease develops in 20% to 25% of individuals with CVID, most often expressed as autoimmune hemolytic anemia or thrombocytopenic purpura, but also as rheumatoid arthritis, pernicious anemia, immune neutropenia, inflammatory bowel disease, or almost any known autoimmune condition.[120,122,130,131] Patients with CVID are at increased risk for malignancies, with particular susceptibility to non-Hodgkins lymphoma and gastric cancers.[119-121,132,133] Polyclonal lymphocytic infiltration expressed as enteropathy, persistent lymphadenopathy, splenomegaly, organ granulomas, or granulomatous/lymphocytic pulmonary disease, in various combinations, is one of the major phenotypes of CVID.[121]

PULMONARY COMPLICATIONS

Lung disease is the most common serious problem in patients with CVID,[120,134-137] accounting for disabling morbidity and early mortality. In large clinical studies, a quarter to about half of the patients had chronic lung disease including bronchiectasis, or restrictive or obstructive lung disease.[120,133,135,136] Bronchiectasis can be seen in children younger than 3 years of age as a result of infection and the inflammation it elicits; and it can be the presenting symptom of CVID at almost any age. Patients have been identified by being tested for immunoglobulin levels as an afterthought on their way to resection of a bronchiectatic segment of lung. In children who carry a diagnosis of CVID, the almost universal presence of chronic bronchitis may delay diagnosis of a more serious pulmonary disease.

In one study of B cell immunodeficiency in subjects older than 18 years of age, 75% of whom had CVID, bronchiectasis was detected by chest CT exam but not by chest radiograph in 8 of 19 patients; and the presence of bronchiectasis by CT did not correlate with either the presence of clinical symptoms (cough, sputum, fever) or abnormalities on pulmonary function tests.[138]

Noninfectious pulmonary disease becomes common beginning in adolescence and early adulthood.[136] Granulomatous lung disease, lymphocytic interstitial pneumonia, follicular bronchiolitis, and lymphoid hyperplasia have been grouped in patients with CVID under the term *granulomatous-lymphocytic interstitial lung disease (GLILD)*.[136,137,139,140] An example of radiographic findings from a patient with GLILD is included in Figure 61-5. This CVID subgroup is at high risk for early mortality

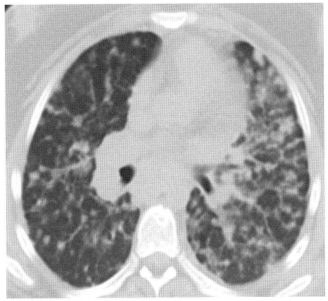

FIGURE 61-5. CT scan of a 16-year-old with biopsy-proven GLILD. Note the extensive nodular infiltrates throughout both lung fields and interstitial thickening with associated mediastinal and subcarinal adenopathy. (Image courtesy of Robin Deterding, MD.)

and B-cell lymphomas (median survival 14 years versus 29 years in other CVID groups in one careful study[136]). Human herpesvirus 8, a B-cell lymphotrophic virus, was isolated from 6 of 9 CVID patients with GLILD, 1 of 21 CVID patients without GLILD, and no controls; one CVID-GLILD patient later developed a B-cell lymphoma.[140] Granulomatous lung disease in CVID patients has been diagnosed as sarcoidosis.[120,139,141,142]

LABORATORY FINDINGS AND DIAGNOSIS

The characteristic findings in CVID are levels of IgG that are two standard deviations or more below age-adjusted means[120] and decreases in IgM and/or IgA meeting the same criteria. If first-drawn immunoglobulin levels are low, these should be confirmed to exclude the possibilities of lab error, and the patient's response to both protein and polysaccharide vaccines should be tested. A normal response should be greater than a two-fold rise from baseline.

Most patients with CVID have normal numbers of circulating B and T lymphocytes, but some patients have decreased levels of circulating phenotypic memory (CD27+) B cells or isotype-switched memory B cells (CD27+ IgD– IgM–).[143-145] Some have mildly abnormal T-lymphocyte function or phenotypic T cell markers, including T-lymphocyte proliferation in response to standard mitogens and antigens, decreased CD4+ cells and thus CD4/CD8 ratio, reduced numbers of T-regulatory cells, reduced CD19+ B cells, altered expression of IL-2 and other cytokines, defective T cell receptor signal transduction, and defective Toll-like receptor (TLR) 7 and 9 function in lymphocytes and dendritic cells.[120,121,143-152]

These phenotypic and functional lymphocyte abnormalities are rarely needed to make the diagnosis of CVID, but they are becoming increasingly important in understanding clinical phenotype and prognosis,[144-148] and they will become even more important as genetic defects are matched with these abnormalities. For example, 9% of 313 CVID patients in the French national registry presented with late-onset combined immunodeficiency associated with opportunistic infections, marked decrease in CD4+ T cells, and increased risk of granulomatous disease, gastrointestinal disease, and lymphoma.[153]

Because CVID is a diagnosis of exclusion, other conditions that may have an almost identical phenotype in some cases must be considered. These include X-linked agammaglobulinemia, hyper-IgM syndromes, and transient hypogammaglobulinemia of infancy. In the last case, cellular immunity (abnormal in about 40% of CVID patients) and response to immunization (abnormal by definition in CVID) are typically normal, and the condition is usually gone by 24 months. X-linked agammaglobulinemia results from any of several hundred mutations in the *Btk* gene, and the condition typically presents with absence of B cells and infections within the first 2 years of life. However, hypomorphic *Btk* mutations can allow some B cell formation and IgG levels that are only moderately depressed or even normal.[42,154,155] As many as 10% of CVID patients may have decreased numbers of B cells, but these are usually well above levels in Btk deficiency.

MOLECULAR DEFECTS AND INHERITANCE

It is likely that CVID results from a variety of genetic defects. Most of these probably arise from sporadic mutations, but approximately 10% of patients have family members with CVID or another humoral immune abnormality.[156] Gene defects associated with CVID are beginning to be identified. One of these is the recessive gene for inducible co-stimulator of activated T cells (ICOS) on chromosome 2q, which is thought to be important in signaling T cells for T and B cell cooperation.[157–159] One patient with ICOS deficiency presented at 18 months of age, but most developed recurrent sinopulmonary infections in adolescence or young adulthood.[157] Another CVID-associated gene encodes transmembrane activator and calcium-modulator and cyclophilin ligand (TACI) found on chromosome 17p. TACI is expressed on B cells and CD4+ T cells and is involved in isotype switching.[160,161] Mutations in this gene are found in 8% to 10% of CVID patients and are associated with susceptibility to CVID rather than directly causing it.[161,162] A defect of B-cell activating factor of the tumor necrosis factor family receptor (BAFF-R) encoded on chromosome 22q was described in siblings from one family.[163] Homozygous or compound heterozygous mutations in the gene for CD19 on chromosome 16p can be associated with a CVID phenotype.[164,165]

MANAGEMENT

As with other immunodeficiency states, prompt identification of the site of infection and infecting organism and prompt administration of antimicrobial therapy will expedite resolution and reduce the chronic complications. Treatment for an extended period may be required. Administration of prophylactic antimicrobials has not been studied and remains controversial. Immunizations may not be useful because these patients have poor antibody responses, but they are still recommended.[166] No adverse events have been reported with live vaccines, except for two cases of polio after live virus immunization, and caution should be used when considering these.

Treatment for infections should be guided by results of cultures. For acute exacerbations of bronchiectasis or sinusitis (both driven by cycles of infection and scarring), options include amoxicillin-clavulanate, cephalosporins, or fluoroquinalones (except ciprofloxacin) for 2 to 4 weeks. Inhaled glucocorticoids may reduce the cough and dyspnea with bronchiectasis but should be used sparingly, and the patient's condition should be monitored with pulmonary function testing and CT scans.

Immunoglobulin replacement has led to major improvement in the management of infections in CVID, preventing acute infections and slowing progression of chronic infections.[167] It may be given intravenously every 3 to 4 weeks or subcutaneously if venous access is poor or to circumvent severe reactions to intravenous administration. The usual starting dose is 300 to 400 mg/kg to keep trough IgG levels (drawn just before administering the next dose) in the middle of the reference range. Higher doses, up to 1 g/kg, may be required,[168] for example, to treat development of central nervous system or systemic

(muscle and liver) enteroviral infection, to which CVID patients are predisposed.[126] Immunoglobulin replacement therapy will be needed for the lifetime of the patient, monitored as IgG trough levels and adjusted as indicated. Patients with non-infectious, autoimmune disorders may require immunosuppressive therapy, but this should be undertaken cautiously. Glucocorticoids are the first-line treatment for autoimmune cytopenias; higher doses of IVIG may also be considered.[169,170] Splenectomy should be considered as a last resort as it may increase the risk for subsequent severe infections.[171] Rituximab has been used successfully in CVID patients with cytopenia.[171,172] CVID patients should be monitored for signs and symptoms of lymphoid malignancy and gastric cancer and have age-appropriate cancer screening.[120]

We are unaware of established treatment guidelines or controlled trials to inform optimal management of GLILD in patients with CVID. Anecdotal experience has shown general improvement in symptoms with corticosteroid treatment.[137] Exercise testing and full pulmonary function testing can be used to monitor the effects of therapy. CT radiographic abnormalities may not resolve though symptoms improve with corticosteroids. Cyclosporin and monoclonal antibody therapy against TNF-α or CD 20 expressed on B cells have been tried, but the experience is limited.[137]

With the advent of immunoglobulin replacement and aggressive management of infections, the risk of death from infection has been reduced dramatically. Nearly two-thirds of patients survive 20 years beyond the diagnosis.[120] The highest mortality rates currently are seen in patients with bronchiectasis, GLILD, and non-infectious complications.[121,136]

Suggested Reading

Cale CM, Jones AM, Goldblatt D. Follow up of patients with chronic granulomatous disease diagnosed since 1990. *Clin Exp Immunol*. 2000; 120:351–355.

Chapel H, Cunningham-Rundles C. Update in understanding common variable immunodeficiency disorders (CVIDs) and the management of patients with these conditions. *Br J Haematol*. 2009;145:709–727.

Cunningham-Rundles C, Bodian C. Common variable immunodeficiency: clinical and immunological features of 248 patients. *Clin Immunol*. 1999;92:34–48.

Kang EM, Choi U, Theobald N, et al. Retrovirus gene therapy for X-linked chronic granulomatous disease can achieve stable long-term correction of oxidase activity in peripheral blood neutrophils. *Blood*. 2010;115:783–791.

Nelson KS, Lewis DB. Adult-onset presentations of genetic immunodeficiencies: Genes can throw slow curves. *Curr Opin Infect Dis*. 2010; 23:359–364.

Pogrebniak HW, Gallin JI, Malech HL, et al. Surgical management of pulmonary infections in chronic granulomatous disease of childhood. *Ann Thorac Surg*. 1993;55:844–849.

Seger RA. Modern management of chronic granulomatous disease. *Br J Haematol*. 2008;140:255–266.

Urschel S, Kayikci L, Wintergerst U, et al. Common variable immunodeficiency disorders in children: Delayed diagnosis despite typical clinical presentation. *J Pediatr*. 2009;154:888–894.

van den Berg JM, van Koppen E, Ahlin A, et al. Chronic granulomatous disease: The European experience. *PLoS One*. 2009;4:e5234.

Winkelstein JA, Marino MC, Johnston Jr RB, et al. Chronic granulomatous disease: Report on a national registry of 368 patients. *Medicine*. 2000;79:155–169.

References

The complete reference list is available online at www.expertconsult.com

62 PULMONARY DISEASE IN THE PEDIATRIC PATIENT WITH ACQUIRED IMMUNODEFICIENCY STATES

Jonathan Spahr, MD, Daniel J. Weiner, MD, Dennis C. Stokes, MD, MPH, and Geoffrey Kurland, MD

INTRODUCTION

Aggressive pharmacologic, surgical, and radiotherapeutic strategies for treatment of children with oncologic diagnoses as well as transplantation of solid organs for children with end-stage organ failure (e.g., lung, heart, kidney, liver, and intestine) leave the recipients of such treatments in an immunosuppressed state. Cytotoxic medications for treatment of childhood cancers often cause bone marrow suppression and direct pulmonary toxicity; irradiation of tumors may damage organs including the lung. Ablation chemotherapy combined with radiation used to prepare patients for hematopoietic stem cell transplantation (HSCT) renders them pancytopenic during marrow engraftment and carries direct pulmonary toxicity. Immunosuppressive agents to prevent rejection of transplanted organs commonly increase the risk of opportunistic infections, many of which affect the lung. As a result, pulmonary disease in these patients is relatively common and often results in significant morbidity and mortality.

In this chapter, we will discuss pulmonary complications of solid-organ transplantation, HSCT, and treatment of childhood oncologic disease. Included in these potential complications are pulmonary infections, which will be the focus of the initial portion of this chapter. In addition, we will address important noninfectious complications; some of these are specific to underlying conditions and their treatments.

Congenital immunodeficiencies, human immunodeficiency virus (HIV)–associated acquired immunodeficiency syndrome (AIDS), and pulmonary complications of lung transplantation are discussed in Chapters 61, 63, and 64, respectively). See Chapter 74 for a further discussion of lung injury caused by pharmacologic agents including chemotherapeutics.

PULMONARY INFECTIONS IN THE IMMUNOCOMPROMISED PEDIATRIC HOST

Immunocompromised pediatric patients include the rare patients with congenital defects of innate host defenses including neutrophil abnormalities, defects affecting lymphocyte function, and defects of humoral immunity. The major expansion of the population of immunocompromised children, however, has occurred with increased HSCT and solid-organ transplantation, successful treatment of childhood malignancy, and the AIDS epidemic. In addition to increasing the at-risk population, these

developments have also led to a continuing increase in the number of identifiable pathogens. The term *opportunistic pathogen* is usually reserved for an organism typically infecting a patient with abnormal host defenses. The terms *immunodeficiency* and *compromised host* were first used in the 1960s and 1970s for patients with primary immunodeficiencies and for those who survived childhood malignancies.[1] In the following section, we will review some of the more common pulmonary infections in this patient population.

CLINICAL PRESENTATION OF PULMONARY INFECTION IN THE IMMUNOCOMPROMISED CHILD

The clinical presentations of pneumonia in the immunocompromised child are often nonspecific, and a high index of suspicion for atypical or opportunistic pathogens is required. Childhood cancer therapy, HSCT, solid-organ transplantation, primary immunodeficiencies, and AIDS are each associated with specific pulmonary pathogens.

In addition, these patients often have an atypical or more severe course even when infected with a "usual" childhood respiratory pathogen.[2] For example, viruses such as Varicella-zoster, influenza, and measles are all capable of leading to devastating pulmonary infections in the immunocompromised host. Although adenovirus can cause diffuse pneumonia in any child, it can be particularly common and catastrophic in immunocompromised hosts.[3-5]

The clinical course of opportunistic infections may be quite variable and further affected by the type and degree of remaining host defenses. For example, fungal pulmonary infections in patients with chemotherapy-induced neutropenia and defective cell-mediated immunity are often associated with mild clinical symptoms and radiographic findings until normalization of peripheral blood neutrophil counts leads to significant inflammation, lung destruction, pulmonary cavitation, and clinical deterioration. The interplay of fungal pathogens with the innate and adaptive immune systems is still under investigation. It is becoming increasingly clear that fungi can both subvert and exploit the host immune response, allowing for chronic carriage or pathogenicity. This complex response is likely mediated by various molecular interactions involving cytokines as well as cellular elements.[6-9]

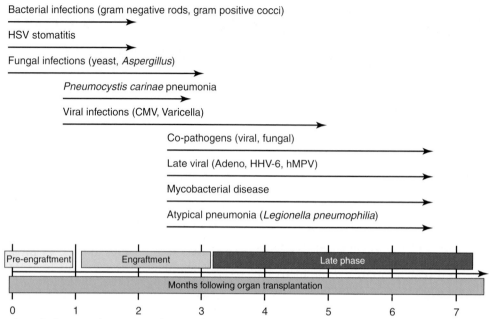

TIMELINE OF INFECTIOUS PULMONARY COMPLICATIONS

Bacterial infections (gram negative rods, gram positive cocci)

HSV stomatitis

Fungal infections (yeast, *Aspergillus*)

Pneumocystis carinae pneumonia

Viral infections (CMV, Varicella)

Co-pathogens (viral, fungal)

Late viral (Adeno, HHV-6, hMPV)

Mycobacterial disease

Atypical pneumonia (*Legionella pneumophilia*)

| Pre-engraftment | Engraftment | Late phase |

Months following organ transplantation

0   1   2   3   4   5   6   7

FIGURE 62-1. Timeline of infectious pulmonary complications following solid-organ transplantation.

INFECTIOUS RISKS SHARED BY MALIGNANCY, SOLID-ORGAN TRANSPLANTATION, AND HEMATOPOIETIC STEM CELL TRANSPLANTATION

The immune system has multiple components. Disorders of the immune system can be divided into those involving *innate* and *adaptive* components. There are physical barriers to infectious agents, including skin and mucosal cells. Humoral components of the immune system include immunoglobulins, complement, and other nonspecific antibacterial molecular species (e.g. defensins) important to innate pulmonary defenses.[10] Cellular components include phagocytic cells, particularly neutrophils, and lymphocytes. See Chapters 7 and 61 for a more complete description of the development, interactions, and defects of each of these components.

Patients undergoing treatment for malignancy, HSCT, or solid-organ transplant have periods of immunosuppression that vary in length and severity. The recovery of the immune system after myeloablative conditioning followed by HSCT, for example, can be divided into three phases. The *pre-engraftment* or *early phase*, from day 0 to day 30 or sooner, encompasses the time of marrow recovery leading to normalization of the peripheral neutrophil count; the *post-engraftment phase* is considered day 30 to day 100 after HSCT; and the *late phase* follows day 100 post-HSCT. For patients with HSCT, each phase is characterized by a susceptibility to certain types of infections correlating with the status of the immune system at that time point.[11] Following solid-organ transplantation, patients tend to be more immunosuppressed early in the posttransplant period. Patients with malignancies often receive chemotherapy in a cyclic pattern, leading to periods of severe marrow suppression followed by periods of recovery.

Figure 62-1 demonstrates the different phases of immunodeficiency in which certain infectious organisms may predominate. As occurs with individuals who are not immunosuppressed, respiratory viruses and community-acquired bacteria are quite common in individuals who are immunosuppressed. Those who are immunosuppressed, however, have a greater propensity for infection with a wider variety of organisms (opportunistic infections, Table 62-1).

COMMON PULMONARY INFECTIOUS AGENTS IN THE IMMUNOCOMPROMISED PEDIATRIC HOST

Viral Pathogens (See also Chapter 28)

Cytomegalovirus

Cytomegalovirus (CMV) is a common herpesvirus infection of both neonates and older immunocompromised children.[12-13] Viral carriage does not always lead to disease, however, and the progression from carriage to disease depends on many factors including the age and the immune status of the infected individual. The organism can be acquired *intrapartum* or from breast milk, saliva, or blood (via infected white blood cells). Both humoral and cellular immune mechanisms are important in establishing protection against CMV. Individuals who are CMV-seronegative prior to immunosuppression because of transplantation or chemotherapy are at increased risk of CMV disease by acquisition of virus from *de novo* infection, from blood products that contain virions, or from transplanted organs from CMV-seropositive individuals. CMV-seropositive individuals who require immunosuppression also run a significant risk for "reactivation" disease, including CMV pneumonia.

TABLE 62-1 TYPICAL PULMONARY PATHOGENS ASSOCIATED WITH ACQUIRED IMMUNODEFICIENCY STATES

	BACTERIAL	FUNGAL	VIRAL/PROTOZOAL/OTHER
Neutropenia			
Chronic	*Haemophilus influenzae, Streptococcus pneumoniae, Staphylococcus aureus, Klebsiella* spp.	—	—
Acute	*S. aureus*	—	—
Immunosuppressive Therapy	*S. aureus, Listeria* spp., *Mycobacterium tuberculosis*	*Aspergillus* spp., *Mucor* spp., *Histoplasma* spp.	Cytomegalovirus (CMV), *Pneumocystis jirovecii,* Varicella-zoster virus (VZV), *Toxoplasma* spp., Herpes simplex virus, *Cryptococcus* spp.
Bone Marrow Transplant			
Early (<30 days)	*Pseudomonas* spp., other Gram-negative and Gram-positive spp.	*Candida* spp.	—
Late (>30 days)	*S. aureus*	*Aspergillus* spp.	CMV, *Toxoplasma* spp., VZV, *P. jirovecii,* Epstein-Barr virus, adenovirus
Late (>100 days)	Encapsulated Gram-positive (*H. influenzae, S. pneumoniae*)	—	VZV

CMV-infected cells typically contain basophilic nuclear inclusions surrounded by a clear halo, giving them an "owl eye" appearance; such inclusions are typically seen in alveolar cells. The pathology of CMV pneumonitis varies from diffuse, discrete parenchymal hemorrhagic nodules to diffuse alveolar damage or chronic interstitial pneumonitis. The radiographic pattern of CMV pneumonia is usually a diffuse reticulonodular pattern that is less "alveolar" than is seen in pneumonia caused by *Pneumocystis jirovecii* (described later in the chapter). Chest high-resolution computed tomography (c-HRCT) most commonly reveals patchy or diffuse ground-glass attenuation, and more diffuse pulmonary involvement may be predictive of disease progression.[14]

Prior to the availability of effective antiviral therapy, approximately 50% of patients with aplastic anemia or hematologic malignancy treated by allogeneic HSCT developed CMV infection and CMV pneumonia,[15] with up to 90% mortality. CMV may also be a co-pathogen with other opportunistic organisms, including *P. jirovecii,* Epstein-Barr virus (EBV) and *Aspergillus.*

The diagnosis of CMV pneumonia is usually made by demonstration of typical inclusions in lung tissue. Urinary excretion of CMV can be coincident but not necessarily causally related to disease. The most important method for CMV detection in blood and other fluids (e.g., BAL) are those that estimate the quantity of virus or viral DNA. Of these, determination of CMV DNA using polymerase chain reaction (PCR) is quite sensitive and widely available.[16] Determination of the presence of the CMV protein pp65 within peripheral white blood cells is also useful to identify patients harboring the organism. PCR for CMV detection in the blood has become a more commonly used noninvasive test to follow at-risk patients following HSCT or solid-organ transplant recipients in order to more accurately predict the development of CMV disease. PCR detection of CMV precedes culture isolation of CMV and persists longer than culture-positivity.

Techniques for identifying CMV in BAL include immunofluorescence, DNA hybridization, or microplate culture combined with CMV antigen detection using monoclonal antibodies. Though highly sensitive, these techniques must be interpreted cautiously because CMV can be a commensal and may be coincidentally present without being the cause of disease.

The use of CMV-negative blood products has reduced the incidence of CMV pneumonia in seronegative transplant patients. Prophylactic and pre-emptive strategies for patients at risk have utilized ganciclovir, foscarnet, and high-titer anti-CMV IgG and have led to a substantial reduction in the incidence and mortality of CMV disease.[11,17] Valganciclovir (the L-valyl ester and pro-drug of ganciclovir) has improved oral bioavailability compared with ganciclovir and is now the preferred drug for the prevention and treatment of CMV disease.[18]

"Late" CMV has been observed in HSCT recipients with active graft-versus-host disease (GVHD); with low CD4 counts; and with a history of prior CMV reactivation or extended use of anti-CMV treatment or prophylaxis.[19] Reduced-intensity conditioning regimens for HSCT (so-called "mini-transplants") with fludarabine, single-dose radiation, and posttransplant cyclosporine and mycophenolate mofetil is an emerging treatment for patients who are not candidates for standard myeloablative conditioning.[20] These patients have a shorter period of neutropenia and a lower risk for CMV disease and viremia during the first 100 days, but they subsequently may have a delayed onset of CMV disease. Unlike early-onset disease, which is characterized mainly by interstitial pneumonitis,[21] late-onset CMV manifestations include retinitis, marrow failure, and encephalitis.[19,22]

Respiratory Syncytial Virus and Other Common Respiratory Viruses

Respiratory syncytial virus (RSV) and other common respiratory viruses (e.g., parainfluenza, influenza, bocavirus, and rhinovirus) have long been recognized as important pathogens in adult recipients of HSCT as well as pediatric leukemia patients.[23] Although they usually cause upper respiratory tract infections, they commonly progress to involve the lower respiratory tract, carrying significant morbidity and mortality.[24] Chest radiographs may have diffuse but nonspecific densities. Nasopharyngeal swabs or washings with culture or enzyme immunoassay (EIA) are the most commonly used diagnostic tools for most viral pathogens including RSV. Newer technologies, including reverse-transcriptase polymerase chain reaction (RT-PCR) and direct immunofluorescence assays, may prove to be specific, sensitive, and more rapid for detection,[25] although further clinical studies are required. Studies of the use of the antiviral agent Ribavirin in treating adult recipients with RSV have suggested that early administration of aerosolized Ribavirin before significant lower respiratory disease develops is superior to intravenous Ribavirin treatment.[24] There is also support for the use of the monoclonal anti-RSV antibody known as Palivizumab in patients who develop RSV following HSCT; however the largest study was in adults, and all patients also received inhaled Ribavirin.[26] While there is less published data concerning these pathogens in pediatric HSCT recipients, the increased likelihood of childhood exposure in schools and other environments should lead the clinician to consider such pathogens when evaluating an immunosuppressed child with upper or lower respiratory illness of uncertain etiology.

Varicella-Zoster Virus and Herpes Simplex Virus

Varicella-zoster virus (VZV) and herpes simples virus (HSV) are DNA viruses that typically cause benign infections of the skin and mucous membranes. However, VZV and HSV can lead to visceral dissemination and pneumonia in certain high-risk groups, including neonates, cancer patients, AIDS patients, those with congenital defects of cell-mediated immunity, and recipients of solid-organ transplants or HSCT).[27] Before the availability of specific antiviral therapy, VZV pneumonitis occurred in approximately 85% of cancer patients with visceral dissemination, with a resultant mortality of 85%. Pneumonitis is much less common with reactivation of herpes zoster and HSV, but it is a potentially serious infection following HSCT and in oncology patients.

The clinical presentation of VZV or HSV pneumonitis is nonspecific and includes fever, cough, dyspnea, and chest pain. Patients with VZV who have an increasing number of skin lesions, abdominal or back pain, or persistent fevers should be considered at high risk for dissemination. HSV pneumonitis may be more subtle in its presentation, and pneumonitis can occur in the absence of mucocutaneous lesions in newborns and HSCT recipients. Chest radiographs of herpesvirus pneumonias typically show ill-defined, bilateral, scattered nodular densities, first seen in the peripheral lung fields with subsequent coalescence into more extensive infiltrates. Microscopically, the infection involves alveolar walls, blood vessels, and small bronchioles. Electron microscopy shows intranuclear viral inclusions. Hemorrhage, necrosis, and extensive alveolar edema are seen in severely affected areas of lung; hemorrhagic tracheitis and bronchitis can also be seen. Secondary infections with bacterial pathogens were more commonly seen in the preantibiotic era, but with the emergence of resistant organisms such as Methicillin-resistant *Staphylococcus aureus*, this remains a worrisome complication.

Interstitial lung disease secondary to HSV infection has been reported following HSCT, but this is relatively rare[28] and far less common than CMV-related interstitial lung disease in this population.

Varicella-zoster immune globulin can modify or prevent VZV infection in high-risk hosts exposed to the virus if given within 48 to 72 hours of exposure. VZV immune globulin, antiviral therapy with acyclovir and related drugs, and routine varicella vaccinations have been effective in reducing the incidence of serious VZV pneumonias in immunocompromised hosts. In the case of HSV pneumonitis, acyclovir may not always be protective against respiratory complications. *In vitro* testing for antiviral sensitivity and the administration of alternative antiviral treatment may be warranted when proven *HSV* pneumonitis occurs.[29]

Herpesvirus Type 6

Human herpesvirus 6 (HHV-6) is a DNA virus and is the etiologic agent of roseola. It can persist in normal hosts following infection and has been shown to integrate into the host genome in 0.2% to 2% of the population.[30–31] Immunosuppression can lead to reactivation of HHV-6, resulting in fever, hepatitis, bone marrow suppression, encephalitis, and interstitial pneumonia.[32–33] Human herpesvirus 6 may also be associated with co-infection by CMV and other pathogens. Antiviral compounds with activity against CMV (e.g., ganciclovir, foscarnet, and cidofovir) are also active against HHV-6.[34]

Human Metapneumovirus

Human metapneumovirus (hMPV) accounts for large proportion of cases previously relegated to "undiagnosed" respiratory infections, particularly in young children.[35–36] Its epidemiology is similar to that of RSV (i.e., winter epidemics, with variation in severity from year to year). Martino and colleagues[37] recently described isolation of hMPV as a primary pathogen in 11 of 177 (6.2%) of nasopharyngeal aspirates from symptomatic adult HSCT recipients. An additional 5 patients had hMPV as a copathogen—1 with Aspergillus, 1 with Aspergillus and CMV, and 3 with other respiratory viruses (Adenovirus, RSV, or influenza). Fifty percent of the infections were considered nosocomial; pneumonia complicated hMPV-upper respiratory tract infections in 4 of 9 (44%) and 1 of 7 (14%) allo-HSCT and auto-HSCT recipients, respectively. More worrisome, Englund and coworkers[38] reported real-time PCR evidence of metapneumovirus in 5 of 163 (3%) of BAL samples obtained in HSCT recipients experiencing respiratory disease. Of these 5 patients, 4 died of respiratory failure, and most carried a diagnosis of "idiopathic pneumonia syndrome" (discussed further later in the chapter). More recently, Evashuk and colleagues reported metapneumovirus infection leading to severe respiratory failure in an infant recovering from liver transplantation.[39] It is likely that further investigations will reveal that hMPV is an important new viral pathogen in immunocompromised adults and children.[40]

Adenovirus

Adenovirus is a DNA virus that is a common cause of community-acquired lower respiratory tract disease. Serotypes 3 and 7 are associated with epidemics of bronchiolitis and pneumonia in the general population. In immunocompromised patients (e.g., HSCT recipients), adenovirus infections can lead to gastrointestinal, urologic, and pulmonary morbidity with disseminated disease that is associated with a high mortality.[5] Adenovirus typically causes fever, pharyngitis, cough, and conjunctivitis. Pneumonia is usually mild in normal hosts, but rapid progression, with necrotizing bronchitis and bronchiolitis, can occur in immunocompromised patients. The radiographic picture is nonspecific and resembles other causes of diffuse pneumonia. Failure of pneumonia to respond to standard therapy, particularly in the setting of epidemic acute respiratory disease in the community or hospital staff, should raise suspicion of adenovirus involvement.

The diagnosis is usually made by lung biopsy or brushings demonstrating typical adenoviral inclusions, or by culture, but the diagnosis may be delayed by institution of empiric antimicrobial and antifungal therapy and delay in invasive procedures. PCR to quantify adenoviral DNA in blood or other fluids is now available[41–42] and in some circumstances may be useful as a screening tool. The antiviral agent Cidofovir has been shown to have activity against adenovirus, but more study is needed before it can be universally recommended.[43] Because very low T cell counts in HSCT recipients are a major risk factor for disseminated disease in patients found to harbor adenovirus and because PCR is quite sensitive, algorithms have been proposed for determining which patients might benefit from antiviral treatment with agents such as Cidofovir.[44–45] Meanwhile, supportive therapy for affected patients includes oxygen, treatment of bacterial superinfections, intravenous (IV) immunoglobulin, and assisted ventilation.

Fungal Pathogens (See also Chapter 34)

Pneumocystis Jirovecii (Formerly P. Carinii)

Pneumocystis has been an organism of uncertain taxonomy and was regarded as a parasite because of its resemblance to cystic spore-forming protozoa. DNA sequencing of 16 S-like ribosomal RNA of *P. carinii* with phylogenetic analysis demonstrates that it is much more closely related to fungi than to protozoal organisms.[46] There are several animal models for infection with *Pneumocystis*, with no evidence of cross-infection across species. The nomenclature *P. carinii* is now reserved for the organism that infects rats, while *P. jirovecii* is the organism isolated in humans[47] The term *PCP*, initially an acronym for *Pneumocystis carinii* pneumonia, is retained with *P. jirovecii* pneumonia, now indicating *Pneumocystis* pneumonia.

The organism exists in two forms in tissues: the more common trophic, or trophozoite, and the cystic form containing sporozoites.[48] The trophozoites measure 2 to 5 μm and stain best with Giemsa stains, but they are not visible with Grocot-Gomori methenamine–silver nitrate or toluidine blue O stains, which stain the 5- to 8-μm cyst forms. The cysts are spherical or cup-shaped and often appear to contain up to eight 1- to 2-μm sporozoites within the cyst wall. The organism cannot be cultured from routine clinical specimens and must be identified in tissue, sputum, or bronchoalveolar lavage (BAL). The trophozoites appear to attach to type I cells through surface glycoproteins related to lectins and there undergo encystation. This interaction leads to cell injury directly or through soluble factors. The alveoli of lungs infected with *P. jirovecii* are filled with trophozoites and protein-rich debris, and the altered permeability produced by the organism contributes to the development of pulmonary edema and surfactant abnormalities, which lead to decreased pulmonary compliance and altered gas exchange. Latent infection with *P. jirovecii* was thought to be common, since serologic studies indicated that 40% of children had antibodies to the organism, and more recent studies using sensitive polymerase chain reaction assays have found evidence of *P. jirovecii* in the nasopharynx and lungs of normal infants. Colonization appears to be common in immunocompromised patients but less common in normal hosts, and there is some evidence of patient-to-patient transmission. Reactivation of latent infection in the immunocompromised host, previously felt to be the most likely explanation for disease, has been called into question by epidemiologic data suggesting new acquisition of airborne organisms.[48]

In patients with congenital or acquired immunodeficiency, the clinical features of PCP are nonspecific and include dyspnea, tachypnea, fever, and cough. Cyanosis occurs later, but early hypoxemia with a mild respiratory alkalosis is common. The most common chest radiographic finding is diffuse bilateral infiltrates.

P. jirovecii pneumonia can be treated by several medications, although trimethoprim-sulfamethoxazole (TMP-SMZ) is the preferred agent for both prophylaxis and treatment in children as well as adults.[48] The earliest drug available for PCP was the dihydrofolate reductase inhibitor pentamidine, which was associated with a high rate of immediate adverse reactions including hypotension, tachycardia, and nausea as well as hypoglycemia and nephrotoxicity. Pentamidine may be administered by the aerosol route for treatment of or prophylaxis to prevent PCP in at-risk patients, but its effectiveness is highly dependent on the delivery system used. Other "second-line" medications that have activity against *P. jirovecii* include combination therapy of clindamycin and primaquine, dapsone (sometimes combined with trimethoprim), and atovaquone.[48–50] Limited studies and case reports of the use of the antifungal agent caspofungin have shown some promise, but more studies are necessary.[51–52] A newer form of combination therapy, reported for patients with AIDS, is trimetrexate-folinic acid,[53] but this too will require further evaluation. For proven PCP infection with moderate to severe hypoxemia, high-dose TMP-SMZ with adjuvant glucocorticoid therapy remains the treatment of choice.[48,54]

Patients at known risk for *P. jirovecii* generally receive prophylaxis. For pediatric oncology and immunocompromised patients, oral TMP-SMZ given 3 days per week is effective. However, if patients or parents are noncompliant, there is a risk of breakthrough pneumonias on this schedule. For most patients TMP-SMZ remains the drug of choice, but other prophylactic regimens have been used.[48]

Aspergillus Species

Aspergillus is a group of ubiquitous fungal organisms found in soil and other settings, including the hospital environment. *Aspergillus fumigatus* is the most common species to cause pneumonia in immunocompromised hosts, but other pathogenic species include *Aspergillus niger* and *Aspergillus flavus*.[55] Invasive *Aspergillus* is most commonly seen in pediatric patients with malignancy (especially acute myelocytic leukemia) and HSCT.[56]

In tissue, the organisms are seen as septate hyphae with regular 45-degree dichotomous branching and are best observed with methenamine silver staining (Fig. 62-2). *Aspergillus* causes both acute invasive pulmonary aspergillosis and a more chronic necrotizing form. The former occurs most commonly in patients undergoing cancer therapy as well as other immunocompromised patients (e.g., those with aplastic anemia). Aspergillosis of the lung is often preceded by or accompanied by invasion of the nose and paranasal sinuses in susceptible hosts. Confirmed risk factors for aspergillosis include prolonged neutropenia, concurrent chemotherapy and steroid therapy, and

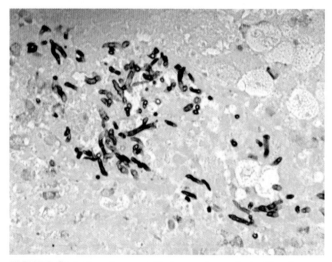

FIGURE 62-2. Invasive aspergillosis seen in a patient with pulmonary complications post-HSCT. Methenamine silver stain, 400×.

broad-spectrum antimicrobial therapy. Cutaneous aspergillosis is often observed in patients with disseminated disease.

In the lungs, *Aspergillus* can cause tracheobronchitis, pneumonia, abscesses and cavity formation, and diffuse interstitial pneumonia. The organisms often extend along blood vessels, and nodular lesions of necrosis surrounded by air often develop within an area of pneumonia, leading to the typical air crescent sign seen on c-HRCT. While strongly suggestive of *Aspergillus* infection, this finding usually is seen early in the disease process and later is replaced by the more common findings of nodular infiltrates with or without cavitation. c-HRCT is much more sensitive than plain radiographs and can reveal early evidence of cavitation.

The diagnosis of *Aspergillus* pneumonia is generally made by tissue examination. *Aspergillus* can be isolated from BAL in approximately 50% of cases, and needle aspiration biopsy of peripheral lung lesions can also demonstrate typical fungal lesions.[57] Although direct tissue sampling by needle biopsy or transbronchial biopsy is recommended for diagnosis, the angioinvasive nature of *Aspergillus* increases the risk of bleeding or secondary infection following such procedures.[58] Isolation of *Aspergillus* from a nasal culture in a patient with typical clinical risk features (i.e., prolonged neutropenia, progressive nodular infiltrates, cavitary lesion) may be helpful, but negative cultures do not exclude *Aspergillus*. *Aspergillus* galactomanan antigen detection in blood and BAL fluid as well as other noninvasive tests under development offer the promise for accurate diagnosis without more invasive procedures (e.g., needle biopsy or transthoracic lung biopsy),[59–60] although more studies are necessary to demonstrate their utility in clinical practice.[60–61]

Although Amphotericin B was initially the sole antifungal agent with activity against *Aspergillus*, newer agents are available and include the orally-available itraconazole and voriconazole, which have excellent activity against *Aspergillus;* of these, voriconazole may become the treatment of choice for invasive aspergillosis.[62–64] Alternative therapies for aspergillosis include lipid formulations of amphotericin B, caspofungin, or intravenous itraconazole. The utility of surgical excision of *Aspergillus* lesions is somewhat controversial. Invasive pulmonary aspergillosis during treatment of hematologic malignancy is generally considered a contraindication to subsequent bone marrow transplant, but adult patients treated with amphotericin B and surgery have survived free of disease and without reactivation of *Aspergillus* following transplantation. The outcome of *Aspergillus* pneumonia depends primarily on such host factors as degree of immunosuppression and recovery of neutrophil counts as well as early diagnosis and treatment.[65]

Mucor and Rhizopus

Mucormycosis includes fungal disease caused by organisms in the order Mucorales, including a variety of species in the genera *Rhizopus, Mucor,* and *Cunninghamella.*[66] In tissues they are differentiated from *Aspergillus* by their broad, nonseptate hyphae that branch at angles up to 90 degrees and have an appearance of "twisted ribbons." *Rhizopus* organisms cause disease only in patients with underlying disease. In adults, they are associated with chronic acidosis states, such as diabetes mellitus with ketoacidosis. Most pediatric cases of pneumonia occur in the oncology population, where *Rhizopus* is found in the same risk groups as *Aspergillus*.

Pneumonia due to *Rhizopus* is usually an insidious segmental pneumonia that is slowly progressive despite antifungal therapy. Persistent fever, chest pain, hemoptysis, and weight loss are typical. Cavitation may occur, and dissemination to brain and other sites occurs as a result of the propensity of the organism to invade blood vessels. Death may occur suddenly with massive pulmonary hemorrhage, mediastinitis, or airway obstruction. The specific diagnosis usually depends on demonstration of the organism in open, transbronchial, or needle aspiration lung biopsy specimens. As with *Aspergillus*, treatment with amphotericin B and possible surgical resection as early as possible is critical to achieving a cure. Posaconazole has good activity against mucormycosis, which can be aggressive and relatively resistant to voriconazole.[67-68] If present, correction of chronic acidosis also appears to be important in some forms of *Rhizopus* disease.

Candida Species

Though important as a cause of fungal sepsis and secondary hematogenous pulmonary involvement, primary *Candida* pneumonia is unusual. *Candida albicans* and *Candida tropicalis* are the most important causes of fungal sepsis and secondary pulmonary involvement. Neutropenic children colonized with *C. tropicalis* are at a 10-fold higher risk for dissemination than are children colonized with *C. albicans*. Patients with HIV infection, primary immunodeficiencies, or prolonged neutropenia are at greatest risk, but other predisposing conditions include diabetes, corticosteroid administration, broad-spectrum antimicrobial treatment, intravenous hyperalimentation, and presence of deep venous access devices (conditions common to the patient with solid-organ transplantation or HSCT).

In tissue, silver stains show oval budding yeasts 2 to 6 μm in diameter with pseudohyphae. The prominent clinical features of primary *Candida* pneumonia include bronchopneumonia, intra-alveolar exudates, and hemorrhage. Amphotericin B is usually the treatment of choice for invasive *Candida* infections, along with flucytosine if synergism is desired. The imidazole antifungal agents, including ketoconazole, fluconazole, and itraconazole, have activity against *C. albicans* and have been used successfully. Although fluconazole prophylaxis and the use of hematopoietic growth factors have led to a reduction in the frequency of early *Candida* infections in patients at risk, many institutions have experienced an increase in azole-resistant non-*albicans Candida* infections.[69,75] In response to this, caspofungin appears to be an excellent alternative with less toxicity than amphotericin B and improved coverage against systemic *Candida* infections when compared with fluconazole.[64,76-77] A recent Cochrane review of various antifungal treatments points out the relative benefits of liposomal Amphotericin as well as the need for further controlled clinical trials to determine the optimal treatment for deep fungal infections in the pediatric host.[78]

Histoplasmosis and Blastomycosis

Histoplasma capsulatum and *Blastomyces dermatitidis* are ubiquitous soil fungi endemic to the eastern and southeastern United States. Histoplasmosis is especially associated with exposure to bird or bat fecal material[79]; as a result, it is a fairly common infection in immunocompetent children and may be asymptomatic or lead to an acute pneumonia with fever, hilar adenopathy, and pulmonary infiltrates. Blastomycosis is a less common but more serious infection. Both can cause chronic granulomatous pulmonary disease and lead to extrapulmonary dissemination.

In the immunocompromised patient, particularly pediatric oncology patients, histoplasmosis may be seen as an acute illness with fever, cough, and diarrhea, or in a disseminated form with additional features of hepatosplenomegaly, fever, and adenopathy.[80] Interestingly, neutropenia is not always associated with *H. capsulatum* infections. Chest radiographs or c-HRCT scans usually demonstrate hilar adenopathy and nodular parenchymal disease in both forms of the disease. Blastomycosis is much less common in adult or pediatric oncology patients, and may be associated with dermatologic manifestations such as skin ulcers in addition to diffuse chronic pulmonary infiltrates.[81]

Amphotericin B is indicated for both histoplasmosis and blastomycosis in immunocompromised hosts. Itraconazole is also effective for histoplasmosis and moderate blastomycosis without central nervous system involvement.

Cryptococcus Neoformans

Cryptococcus neoformans is a yeast that causes protean clinical manifestations in immunocompromised patients, often involving the meninges, endocardium, skin, and lymph nodes.[82] The lungs are the portal of entry for *C. neoformans*, and pulmonary involvement may be minimal if dissemination occurs quickly. Pneumonia is typically accompanied by chest pain, fever, and cough. The diagnosis of cryptococcosis relies on demonstration of the organism histologically, in biopsy tissue or pleural fluid[83] or by culture methods.[84] Although controlled trials are lacking, the recommended treatment in immunosuppressed patients is IV amphotericin B and oral flucytosine followed by fluconozole.[84-85]

Rarer Fungal Pneumonias

Several recent trends have been noted in fungal infections. Among them is the increased identification of rarer fungal pathogens including saprophytic fungi (e.g., *Trichosporon beigelii* and *Fusarium* spp.). These fungi cause skin and soft-tissue infections and occasionally invade the lungs and sinuses. For example, *Scedosporium apiospermum* (formerly *Pseudallescheria boydii*) causes invasive disease in solid-organ transplant patients, with lung involvement in 50%[86]; it is difficult to distinguish histologically from *Aspergillus*.[87-88] These fungi are thus often difficult to diagnose, and, unlike *Aspergillus*, their response to therapy with amphotericin B may be very poor. Newer azole agents such as posaconazole and voriconazole have activity against *Fusarium* spp. and *Scedosporium* spp. and should be considered if these species are isolated from immunosuppressed patients.

Bacterial Pathogens

The bacterial pathogens (see also Chapter 29) associated with pneumonia in immunocompromised hosts include the pathogens typically associated with pneumonia in children, such as S. *aureus* (particularly methicillin-resistant strains), *H. influenzae*, and *S. pneumoniae*. *Pseudomonas aeruginosa* is an additional important cause of pneumonia and sepsis in hospitalized immunocompromised children. Significant risk factors for bacterial infections include neutropenia, the presence of indwelling venous catheters, and perineal skin lesions. More unusual bacterial causes of pneumonia include *Listeria monocytogenes,* a Gram-positive rod that causes primarily septicemia with subsequent pulmonary involvement in immunocompromised patients. Corynebacteria (commonly called *diphtheroids*) are Gram-positive bacilli or coccobacilli that exist as saprophytes on mucous membranes and skin. *Corynebacterium jeikeium* is a strain from this group that may lead to sepsis and pneumonia in oncology and HSCT patients.[89] *Listeria* can be successfully treated with ampicillin plus an aminoglycoside, but newer cephalosporins are not active against *Listeria*. C. *jeikeium* is resistant to most antimicrobials except vancomycin. Other rare Gram-negative organisms that cause pneumonia in the immunocompromised host include *Legionella pneumophila* and *Capnocytophaga* sp. It is important to realize that factors such as geographic location, changes in infection control, prophylactic antimicrobial protocols, and technological advances all have an effect on microbial predominance.[90–91]

Mycobacteria

With the onset of the AIDS epidemic, disease caused by both *Mycobacterium tuberculosis* and atypical strains such as *Mycobacterium avium-intracellulare* have been increasingly recognized in both AIDS and non-AIDS immunodeficient populations.[92] (See also Chapter 33.)

The development of disseminated *M. tuberculosis* following HSCT is a serious and often fatal complication[93] (Fig. 62-3). Based on data from developed countries, *Mycobacterium tuberculosis* infections are rare in HSCT recipients.[94–96] However, the incidence of tuberculosis in the HSCT population directly reflects its incidence in the general population. In Turkey, where tuberculosis is endemic (35 per 100,000 population versus 7 per 100,000 in the United States), tuberculosis was 40 times more common in allo-HSCT patients than in the general population.[97] The presence of multidrug-resistant strains of *M. tuberculosis* (indirectly related to treatment of HIV disease) is of great concern[98] and has led some programs to maintain a high index of suspicion for tuberculosis and to treat HSCT recipients with this complication for longer periods of time, often with multidrug regimens.[95]

Nontuberculous mycobacterial (NTM) infections can be either catheter-related or respiratory infections.[99] Mere isolation of NTM on BAL may not be of pathogenic significance unless there is evidence of tissue invasion or

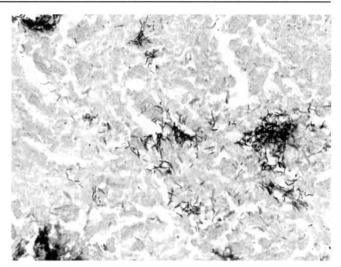

FIGURE 62-3. Acid-fast organisms in a patient with end-stage lung disease following HSCT. Acid-fast stain, 1000×.

concomitant bacteremia is present. Treatment requires two to four antimicrobials guided by *in vitro* susceptibility testing, and removal of indwelling catheters (if contaminated) as well as surgical debridement of subcutaneous tunnel infection sites.[99]

Legionella pneumophila

Patients undergoing bone marrow and solid-organ transplantation are particularly susceptible to *Legionella* infections caused by prolonged neutropenia and abnormalities in cell-mediated immunity. Legionnaires' disease (LD) can be acquired by inhalation of aerosols containing *Legionella pneumophila* or by microaspiration of contaminated drinking water.[100] LD should always be in the differential diagnosis of pneumonia among HSCT recipients. Appropriate tests to confirm LD include culturing sputum, BAL, and tissue specimens; testing BAL specimens for *Legionellae* by direct fluorescent antibody; examining for *Legionella pneumophila* serogroup one antigen in urine; and performing testing for five S rRNA PCR of either BAL, urine, or serum samples.[101–102]

Parasitic Agents (See also Chapter 36)

Toxoplasma Gondii and *Cryptosporidium Parvum*

Toxoplasma gondii infects cats and other animals and secondarily infects humans, causing congenital toxoplasmosis during intrauterine infection. Primary infection later in life usually causes only lymphadenopathy and mild systemic symptoms.[103] *Cryptosporidium parvum* infects a variety of hosts, including immunosuppressed individuals. Its usual routes of transmission are water- or food-borne, but person-to-person transmission is possible.[104] *Toxoplasma* primarily causes central nervous system disease, but disseminated disease with secondary pulmonary involvement can occur, presenting with shortness of breath, cough, fever, and bilateral interstitial infiltrates.[105] *Cryptosporidium parvum* causes severe diarrhea, but disseminated disease with pulmonary involvement can occur. Treatment of *T. gondii* is with pyrimethamine-sulfadiazine, while treatment of C. parvum is rapidly evolving, with combination therapy of azithromycin-paramomycin[106] being supplanted by the more effective nitazoxanide in many parts of the developing world.[107]

Pulmonary Co-Infections

Late after solid-organ transplantation or in the late-phase infections following HSCT, it is not unusual to find co-pathogens, that is, isolation of more than one pathogenic species of bacteria, fungus, or opportunistic virus from BAL or lung biopsy specimens. For example, pulmonary co-pathogens may be isolated in as many as 53% of patients with parainfluenza pneumonia.[108] HSCT recipients with CMV disease or respiratory viral infections are more susceptible to invasive fungal infections, especially Aspergillus.[109] Alangaden and colleagues described occurrence of Gram-negative bacilli and Aspergillus infections among allogeneic bone marrow transplant recipients with chronic GVHD requiring long-term steroid use.[110] In our own series of patients, we have seen a variety of microorganisms, including E. coli, Aspergillus fumigatus, Enterococcus, and Nontuberculous mycobacterial species (NTM) either as pulmonary colonizers or co-pathogens. Chronic colonization of the airways of patients with GVHD may be analogous to colonization of the respiratory tract with Pseudomonas and Aspergillus species in patients with cystic fibrosis, possibly suggesting an alteration in the homeostasis of the respiratory mucosa, mucociliary clearance, and airway surface liquid. Recovery of bacteria from respiratory secretions in this scenario may represent airway colonization rather than invasive parenchymal disease.

■ NON-INFECTIOUS PULMONARY COMPLICATIONS IN THE IMMUNOCOMPROMISED PEDIATRIC HOST

Immunocompromised patients are at risk for a variety of non-infectious complications that simulate infection and complicate the diagnostic evaluation. The following section will discuss the non-infectious complications seen in patients who are immunocompromised followed by a brief discussion regarding common diagnostic testing employed when evaluating such patients.

■ PULMONARY COMPLICATIONS OF CHILDHOOD TUMORS AND THEIR TREATMENT

Childhood cancers are treated with a combination of surgery (primarily for solid tumors), chemotherapy, and radiotherapy. Pulmonary toxicity in pediatric cancer survivors has been the subject of a recent review.[110a] See Chapter 74 for a further discussion of pulmonary toxicity from chemotherapy. Radiation therapy is an integral component of curative treatment for a variety of oncologic malignancies, both for the treatment of primary tumors and for those patients with distant metastases. A common site for metastases is the lung, particularly in diseases such as Wilms' tumor, sarcomas, and hepatoblastoma. Whole lung irradiation (WLI) is often used as adjuvant therapy for patients with distant lung metastases. Unfortunately, lung tissue is particularly sensitive to the effects of radiation, and the untoward effects of WLI are a concern, both during and well beyond the end of therapy. Additionally, total body irradiation (TBI) is commonly used as part of pretransplant conditioning regimens.

Therapeutic doses of radiation can cause acute (radiation pneumonitis) and chronic (radiation fibrosis) lung injury. The incidence of acute radiation pneumonitis is up to 15% of adults treated for breast and lung cancers and Hodgkin's disease, but the incidence in pediatric patients is less well described.[111] The incidence may be dependent on the radiation dose, fractionation, and volume of lung exposed,[112] as well as concurrent chemotherapy.[113] At thoracic radiation doses approximating 1000 cGy or more, total lung capacity and diffusing capacity may be significantly impaired.[114–116] Some chemotherapeutic agents (bleomycin, dactinomycin) have additive toxicity with radiation, and others (actinomycin D and adriamycin) can result in a "radiation recall" effect, with delayed presentation of toxicity, up to 6 weeks later.[117]

Acutely, radiation injury results in release of a number of pro-inflammatory cytokines that can cause subendothelial and perivascular damage. Over time, this causes type II pneumocyte hypertrophy and infiltration of inflammatory cells.[118] Radiation pneumonitis typically presents 30 to 90 days after radiation therapy with symptoms of cough, dyspnea, hypoxemia, and pleuritic pain. Examination may reveal crackles or a pleural friction rub, and chest radiography may show diffuse haziness or ground-glass densities. Early injury may be detected by decreases in diffusing capacity for carbon monoxide. The differential diagnosis for this presentation clearly includes infections and other etiologies that must be excluded. Treatment of radiation pneumonitis usually involves systemic corticosteroids, based on a murine model of radiation toxicity.[119]

Radiation fibrosis may appear 6 to 24 months after radiation therapy. It is usually but not always proceeded by symptoms of radiation pneumonitis, and itself most commonly presents with progressive dyspnea. Radiographically, there may be streaky densities, decreased lung volume or atelectasis, or pleural thickening. Pulmonary function findings include hypoxemia, a restrictive defect, and decreased diffusing capacity. Histologic findings include pleural and subpleural fibroses, interstitial fibrosis, interstitial pneumonitis, interlobular septal fibrosis, and obliteration of pulmonary vessels (Fig. 62-4). Unfortunately, there is no useful treatment for radiation fibrosis. Some patients with severe lung disease as a result of radiation fibrosis have undergone lung transplantation. As such, efforts should be focused on prevention (with considerations of shielding, dose, and effects of other agents) and close monitoring for patients at high risk.

Analysis of self-report data from the Childhood Cancer Survivor Study[120] cohort showed that, in survivors who were more than 5 years from diagnosis and received radiation to the chest or total body irradiation,

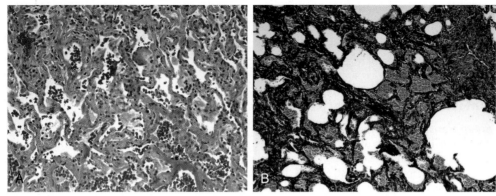

FIGURE 62-4. Radiation fibrosis. **A,** H&E stain, 20×, showing pleural, subpleural, and interstitial fibrosis; foci of chronic interstitial pneumonitis; and irregular scars within the parenchyma. The interlobular septa are fibrotic and thickened with obliteration of some of the pulmonary vasculature. **B,** Trichrome stain showing significant collagen deposition.

there was a statistically significant increase in the relative risk of developing late pulmonary complications including lung fibrosis, emphysema, recurrent pneumonia, chronic cough, persistent shortness of breath, and abnormal chest wall development. As more children survive cancer and live well into adulthood, it is important to consider the late effects associated with WLI.[113] Beyond the lung parenchyma itself, radiation can also impair the growth of the muscle, cartilage, and bone of the thorax. Studies in adults receiving WLI suggest that mild restrictive disease usually resolves over a period of 2 to 4 years. However, the ongoing development of the chest wall and the lung in children makes the impact of such toxic therapy quite different. Continued alveolar multiplication occurs until 2 to 4 years of age, and alveolar enlargement continues for some time after that.[121] The growing chest wall may also be impacted by radiation treatment. These important differences suggest that findings from adult studies may not be able to be extrapolated to pediatric patients. There is a paucity of contemporary data on the long-term sequelae of whole lung irradiation in pediatric patients.

Weiner and colleagues reported a retrospective review of pulmonary function in 30 children who had received WLI[122] for treatment of malignancy. At a median of almost 3 years postradiation, 20% of subjects had moderate or severe reduction in FEV_1, 43% had moderate or severe reduction in TLC, and 43% had moderate or severe reduction in diffusing capacity. At least two patients demonstrated a clear progressive decline over time. These authors suggested that recognition of early abnormalities might allow for earlier intervention for radiation pneumonitis (e.g., corticosteroid therapy) and that it cannot be presumed (as in adults) that loss of lung function after radiation is transient.

Benoist and coworkers[115] followed 48 children treated with WLI for Wilms' tumor for 2 to 17 years following treatment. Two subjects had clinical evidence of radiation pneumonitis shortly after treatment, which resolved within 3 to 8 weeks. In this study, the percentage of patients with abnormal TLC or lung compliance increased over time, with reduced TLC observed in 50% at 6 months and >90% at 6 years. These authors posit that early lung function abnormalities are caused by

parenchymal lung injury, while later effects result from impaired chest wall growth. These findings argue for continued pulmonary follow-up of children treated with thoracic irradiation.

PULMONARY COMPLICATIONS FOLLOWING SOLID-ORGAN TRANSPLANTATION

Pulmonary Edema, Pleural Effusions, and ARDS

Pulmonary edema can occur posttransplant as a result of increased hydrostatic pressure (e.g., caused by fluid and blood product administration or poor left ventricular function) or decreased oncotic pressure (e.g., caused by hypoalbuminemia), or as a result of increased vascular permeability (e.g., caused by immune-mediated transfusion-related acute lung injury [TRALI]).

Pleural effusions may also occur as a result of increased hydrostatic or decreased oncotic pressure. Lymphatic vessels that drain the lungs can be overwhelmed or disrupted in transplantation. Infection or injury in the thoracic, mediastinal, or abdominal cavity can lead to sympathetic effusions or empyema. Finally, abdominal ascites fluid (i.e., in patients with liver or kidney disease) can translocate through pores in the diaphragm and enter the pleural space.

Pleural effusions can occur in up to 40% of children who undergo liver transplantation,[123] are predominantly right-sided, and are thought to occur as a result of disruption of diaphragmatic lymphatic channels.[124] Effusions exclusively in the left pleural space following liver transplantation should prompt evaluation for other causes. Generally, pleural effusions following liver transplantation will enlarge over the first week following transplantation and then resolve over the ensuing 3 to 4 weeks. Between 14% and 25% of pediatric patients require pleural drainage because of significant respiratory compromise.[125-126] Not surprisingly, pleural effusions significantly increase the duration of mechanical ventilation and ICU days.[126] Persistent pleural effusions may be a sign that acute rejection of the liver allograft is occurring.[127]

Acute respiratory distress syndrome (ARDS) is a devastating complication in up to 15% of liver transplant recipients in the immediate postoperative period. This is primarily caused by sepsis, but in the case of liver and small bowel transplantation, other risk factors should be considered as potential causes (e.g., severe malnutrition of the recipient, the extensive and prolonged abdominal surgery, massive intraoperative blood transfusion, and aspiration in the early post-transplant period).[128]

Impairment of Respiratory Mechanics

The extensive surgery in the upper abdomen that occurs during orthotopic liver transplantation can have significant effects upon diaphragmatic excursion, especially on the right side. Diaphragmatic dysfunction can also occur in heart, kidney, and small bowel transplantation, but to a lesser degree than after liver transplantation. Poor excursion of the diaphragm can lead to impaired cough and airway clearance, resulting in atelectasis and pneumonia. Diaphragmatic function can be impaired by swelling in the subdiaphragmatic area, as well as phrenic nerve injury when the suprahepatic vena cava is clamped during liver transplantation. Diaphragmatic dysfunction or paralysis was found in 8% to 11% of pediatric liver transplant recipients,[126-127] and with more sensitive techniques phrenic nerve conduction abnormalities were seen in up to 80% of adult liver transplant recipients.[129] For adults, the injury to the right phrenic nerve does not seem to have significant impact on recovery as determined by duration of mechanical ventilation or hospital stay. In infants and small children, compromise of one diaphragm can lead to more respiratory distress, atelectasis, and pneumonia, as well as longer duration of mechanical ventilation and ICU stays.[126]

Recruiting atelectatic lung and performing adequate airway clearance in the post–liver transplant period can be challenging because of pain and the "fresh" surgical sites. This is especially true for patients in whom the abdomen is not completely closed in the immediate postoperative period. In this situation, the important abdominal muscles that are needed for cough are impaired. Patients may require noninvasive positive pressure ventilation (NIPPV) after extubation. Airway clearance and the use of a mechanical in-exsufflator (Cough Assist device) can help to clear secretions and prevent atelectasis in the immediate postoperative period. Since physiotherapy to the chest wall may be painful after sternotomy, oscillating positive expiratory pressure devices (e.g., Flutter, Acapella, Quake) and incentive spirometry (in patients who can cooperate) and intrapulmonary percussive ventilation (in those that cannot cooperate) can be invaluable in the postoperative period. When diaphragmatic dysfunction or paralysis is present, plication of the diaphragm can be considered (and was utilized in 25% of patients with diaphragm paralysis).[127] However, plication should only be considered if phrenic nerve function has not returned after a period of observation with noninvasive management of at least 90 days, or if the patient develops clinical respiratory deterioration.

Medication Toxicity

Early infusion of cyclosporine has been reported to cause ARDS in patients receiving liver transplantation.[128] Fortunately, most medications used for immunosuppression in the post–organ transplantation period do not have direct toxicity to the lung. Two exceptions are the mammalian targets of rapamycin (mTOR) inhibitors, sirolimus (rapamycin), and everolimus. Both are potent immunosuppressants that confer less nephrotoxicity than calcineurin inhibitors. They have been increasingly popular because of their overall favorable side-effect profile. However, sirolimus and everolimus have been shown to cause interstitial pneumonitis at both therapeutic and supratherapeutic drug levels.[130-134] One transplant center has reported a 2.9% incidence of sirolimus- and everolimus-related pneumonitis in renal transplant patients.[133]

Sirolimus-induced interstitial pneumonitis can occur acutely, but the onset is usually slow and may escape early detection. Patients usually present with dyspnea on exertion (66% to 90%), dry cough (75% to 100%), and fever (60% to 87%). Lung function testing may reveal a restrictive defect. Plain films and CT scans of the chest might reveal an interstitial pattern with interstitial infiltrates, consolidation, or ground-glass opacification with lower lobe predominance. BAL and biopsy specimens can show patterns of lymphocytic alveolitis, pulmonary hemorrhage, or organizing pneumonia.[132-133] Treatment requires discontinuation of the causative medication, and resolution is generally prompt, although radiographic abnormalities may persist. Corticosteroid use should be considered and may be effective, although supportive data are limited.[133]

Posttransplant Lymphoproliferative Disease (PTLD)

Immunosuppression required for solid-organ transplant recipients place them at increased risk for developing posttransplant lymphoproliferative disease (PTLD).[135] PTLD typically stems from an immunosuppressive regimen that causes T lymphocyte depletion, which then leads to uncontrolled EBV-driven B cell proliferation. This unregulated growth of B cells can range from benign polyclonal B lymphocyte expansion to aggressive immunoblastic B cell lymphomas.[136] Less frequently, PTLD also can result from T cell or natural killer (NK) cell proliferation.[137-138] Analysis of EBV viral load in the peripheral blood is an integral component of post-transplant monitoring. Screening of the at-risk patient population may be the earliest means of detecting the presence of EBV as a marker for PTLD prior to the onset of clinical symptoms. PTLD can present without symptoms, but shortness of breath, cough, and upper airway obstruction were the most common symptoms in those with pulmonary PTLD. Increasing EBV load may signify a need to adjust the patient's immunosuppressive regimen. Because CMV may be a co-infecting agent in these patients, prophylactic antiviral therapy and CMV PCR monitoring are also recommended.[139] In patients who present with pulmonary disease, nodular abnormalities are the most common finding (Fig. 62-5A, B), although

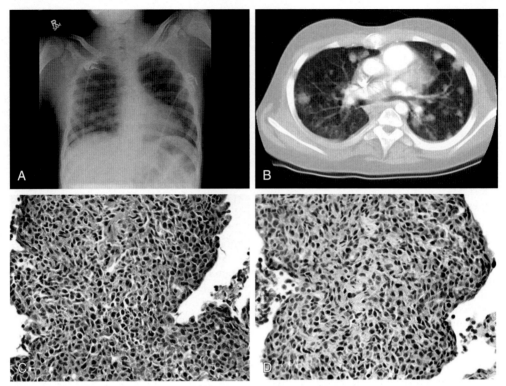

FIGURE 62-5. Posttransplant lymphoproliferative disease. **A,** Anteroposterior chest radiograph. **B,** Computed tomography scan. **C,** Histopathology showing monomorphic clonal expansion of lymphocytes that express Epstein Barr early RNA **(D).**

lymphadenopathy, consolidations, or effusions may be seen on chest imaging.[140] Even when PTLD is strongly suggested by the combination of increasing EBV load and typical radiographic findings, biopsy material should be obtained to confirm the diagnosis histologically (see Fig. 62-5C) and assess for the presence or absence of EBV–early RNA (EBER)-staining cells (see Fig. 62-5D). In addition, it is useful to characterize cell surface markers such as CD20, which may guide therapy.

PTLD occurs in approximately 3% to 9% of heart transplant recipients[139,141-142] and up to 20% of intestinal transplant recipients.[143] PTLD can occur following kidney and liver transplantation as well, but less frequently. PTLD arising in the lung is much more common following heart, lung, and heart-lung transplantation than following transplantation of abdominal organs. The median onset of PTLD is typically within 24 months following solid-organ transplantation.

A significant risk factor for PTLD is seroconversion of an EBV-naïve recipient, either by primary infection in a previously uninfected recipient or by transplantation of a graft from an EBV-seropositive donor. Other risk factors include a high degree of immunosuppression, Rh factor negativity, Rh mismatch, and recipient CMV seronegativity.[141-142,144] In a multicenter study of PTLD following pediatric heart transplantation, the respiratory system was the second most common site of involvement occurring in 25% of those with PTLD.[139] In the study population, 87% were EBV-positive, and there was 25% 1-year mortality after diagnosis of PTLD. Most case series of PTLD following solid-organ transplantation report that there is an increase in

mortality reflecting the severity of the disease itself or its treatment, specifically the treatment effects upon the transplanted organ.

Isolated pulmonary PTLD is uncommon in patients with transplanted abdominal organs, and imaging of the abdomen should accompany pulmonary imaging if PTLD is suspected. All transplant patients with systemic symptoms (i.e., fever, night sweats, and weight loss) should be suspected of having PTLD. Nonetheless, infection and other malignancies can present with similar symptoms, and therefore these entities should be considered when confronted by solid-organ transplant recipients with systemic symptoms. Kaposi's sarcoma (KS) is one such malignancy that can affect immunosuppressed individuals and can have similar radiographic findings (nodular densities with lymph node enlargement). Fortunately, lung involvement of KS is rare.

Initial therapy for PTLD is the reduction of immunosuppression to reduce the degree of T lymphocyte depletion. This reduction can be associated with further complications (e.g., graft rejection) and still may be insufficient.[145-146] Thus, some have employed novel assays of immune function to monitor the degree of immunosuppression while at the same time monitoring EBV viral load.[147] Antiviral agents, intravenous immunoglobulin including anti–B cell immunotherapy with the monoclonal anti-CD-20 antibody (rituximab) have been attempted with varying degrees of success.[148] Recognition and reduction of risk factors and serial monitoring of EBV DNA in blood of high-risk HSCT recipients are important.[149] The main complication of rituximab therapy is prolonged B cell depletion and hypoimmunoglobulinemia.[150]

Anti-CMV therapy should be continued in patients at risk for this co-infection, but it may not decrease the cellular proliferation of PTLD because there is very little active EBV replication in these lesions.

Other Noninfectious Pulmonary Complications of Solid-Organ Transplantation

Many pulmonary complications that arise pretransplantation may not completely or immediately resolve posttransplantation. Metastatic pulmonary calcifications can occur in patients with kidney or hepatic failure, and, while usually benign, can lead to restrictive lung disease. Furthermore, their nodular appearance on chest radiographs can mimic nodules from infection or malignancy (see previous section).

Pulmonary conditions such as alveolar simplification[151] and Primary Ciliary Dyskinesia (PCD)[152] can be associated with congenital heart disease, including those associated with heterotaxy, and they may not have been recognized before heart transplantation. These conditions should be considered if unexpected pulmonary complications including prolonged hypoxemia and recurrent atelectasis develop in the posttransplant period.

Hepatopulmonary syndrome (HPS) and porto-pulmonary hypertension (PPHTN) are two entities that occur in end-stage liver disease and can significantly improve with liver transplantation. However, improvement is not universal or even expedient. In the case of HPS, significant hypoxemia can occur as a result of dilation of pulmonary capillaries, and this may persist in the postoperative period, leading to prolonged mechanical ventilation and use of supplemental oxygen. Typically, resolution of hypoxemia from HPS occurs over the initial 8 months.[153]

Severe cases of PPHTN may preclude liver transplantation as the operative mortality increases as the severity of pulmonary hypertension increases. Additionally, PPHTN can recur or occur de novo after liver transplantation. Posttransplant pulmonary hypertension (PHTN) can occur in those with pretransplant HPS, those with recurrent liver disease, and those with no apparent liver disease and isolated PHTN. Severe PHTN in either the pretransplant or posttransplant period increases the risk of mortality.[154–155] Continuous infusion of prostaglandins can serve to lower pulmonary pressures, acting as a bridge to transplant and attenuating surgical risk.

Venous thromboemboli (VTE) can occur in the posttransplant period, thus leading to respiratory distress and hypoxemia, but they are uncommon in pediatric patients. Renal transplant patients may be at higher risk because of manipulation of pelvic veins, although this has mainly been reported in adult patients.[156]

▰ PULMONARY COMPLICATIONS OF HEMATOPOIETIC STEM CELL TRANSPLANTATION

Significant advances in transplantation immunology as well as innovations in chemotherapy and irradiation have allowed HSCT to become a more viable therapy for the treatment of hematologic diseases. The science of bone marrow transplantation, which began as the allogeneic transplantation of whole bone marrow, has progressed to include allogeneic altered marrow (e.g., T cell depleted), autologous marrow, and HSCT. Despite many advances, even the most experienced transplant centers encounter significant posttransplantation morbidity and mortality. Infectious and noninfectious pulmonary complications remain common following marrow transplantation both in adults[157–159] and children.[160–163] While most of the studies of HSCT recipients deal with adults rather than children, many important principles apply across age barriers. Although different sources of stem cells for transplantation (e.g., allogeneic or autologous) portend different risks of particular complications, we will describe potential complications in a more general fashion and will refer to relative incidences when appropriate. In addition, we will refer to these procedures collectively as HSCT.

Pretransplant Factors

Some pre-existing diseases that themselves are treated with HSCT may have significant pretransplant pulmonary complications. An example is sickle cell disease (SCD), which can be complicated by acute chest syndrome and pulmonary infarction[164] as well as pulmonary hypertension.[165] Either of these complications is likely to have a negative effect on pulmonary function following HSCT.

Patients with underlying malignancies may have been treated with cytoreductive agents or irradiation targeting the lung. Several chemotherapeutics, including bleomycin, busulfan, and cyclophosphamide, are known pulmonary toxins, leading to a range of pulmonary complications including fibrosis and pneumonia.[166] These pulmonary toxins are discussed in more detail in Chapter 74. Lung irradiation, either as treatment of a primary malignancy, pulmonary metastatic disease, or as part of a conditioning regimen in preparation for HSCT can also result in pulmonary disease, manifesting mainly as either pneumonitis or pulmonary fibrosis.[167]

It is critical that patients previously exposed to treatments that are potentially "pneumotoxic" have pre-HSCT pulmonary screening (Table 62-2). In patients who are capable of cooperating, pulmonary function testing (PFT), including the determination of lung volumes,

TABLE 62-2 RECOMMENDATIONS FOR PULMONOLOGY EVALUATION PRIOR TO HEMATOPOIETIC CELL TRANSPLANTATION

History/physical examination
Chest radiograph
High-resolution, thin cut, computed tomography (CT) scan of chest
Pulmonary function testing*:
   Spirometry
   Lung volumes
   Transfer factor (diffusing capacity)
   Maximal inspiratory/expiratory pressure
6-minute walk test

*Pulmonary function testing will depend on patient age and cooperativity.

flows, diffusing capacity, and respiratory muscle strength, can document the presence of lung disease prior to immunosuppressive chemotherapy or transplantation. Abnormalities in PFTs may represent a manifestation of the underlying illness (e.g., neoplasm with pulmonary metastatic disease), complications of the underlying illness (e.g., pulmonary infarction secondary to sickle cell anemia), or other pre-existing pulmonary conditions (e.g., asthma).[168] PFTs remain useful during oncologic treatment or posttransplantation and can be especially important as adjuncts to radiographic evaluation of intercurrent illness affecting the lung. A recent report suggests that pre-HSCT pulmonary function can predict post-HSCT survival,[169] but further studies are needed to determine if there are PFT parameters that are both specific and sensitive to determine patients who should not undergo HSCT. Musculoskeletal weakness is both a common pre-existing condition and a known complication of HSCT[170]; several relatively simple tests (6-minute walk test and respiratory muscle strength test) are useful in identifying patients at risk,[171] allowing for musculoskeletal rehabilitation and nutritional support in both the pre- and post-HSCT period.

Spirometry and plethysmography can also be accomplished in infants and toddlers who are unable to cooperate with traditional testing. See Chapter 11 for a further discussion of these techniques. The information from infant lung function testing can be used in a very similar way to that from standard lung function testing, although there are, as yet, no data looking at outcomes and infant lung function in pediatric oncology patients. Additionally, the diffusing capacity measurement may be the most sensitive test for detecting early lung injury from chemotherapy or radiation. Unfortunately, there is no system commercially available at the present time to perform these measurements in infants/toddlers. It is possible that iatrogenic pulmonary disease from chemotherapy or radiotherapy may be common in the developing lung, and further studies in this population are of great importance.

As might be expected, the impact of some conditioning regimens on post-HSCT pulmonary complications has led to alterations in the intensity of these regimens. A recent report demonstrated that this approach may lead to improved survival with diminished toxicity in selected circumstances such as in recipients with primary immunodeficiency who are to receive HSCT from an HLA-matched unrelated donor[172] or in patients with SCD.[172–173]

There are a variety of other pre-HSCT factors that may adversely affect post-HSCT pulmonary status and complications. These consist of pulmonary infections, including viral illnesses, thoracic surgical procedures, chronic aspiration, and gastroesophageal reflux. Severe lower respiratory infections, particularly invasive fungal disease, can increase the risk of both recurrent infection and pulmonary debilitation post-HSCT. The increased risk of recurrent fungal infection in patients undergoing intensive chemotherapy[174] led to more widespread use of antifungal prophylaxis to prevent recurrence following HSCT.[175] This practice has allowed consideration of HSCT in these high-risk patients.[176–177]

Thoracic surgical procedures prior to HSCT may include lobectomy or wedge resection of pulmonary metastatic disease or for surgical diagnosis of localized fungal infections. The risk of HSCT closely following thoracic surgery is probably increased, but this may depend upon the type of surgical approach taken, the amount of lung tissue removed, the patient's underlying nutritional status, and other factors such as neutropenia. Such procedures also carry the risk of postoperative pain and splinting, decreased cough, and resultant atelectasis; in addition, chest tube placement is common following open thoracotomy, which may prolong the postoperative recovery, although tube thoracostomy is not an absolute contraindication to HSCT.[178]

Cytoreductive therapy and irradiation alter host defenses and disturb mucosal integrity, potentially leading to colonization with potential pathogens. Potential HSCT recipients with dysphagia or odynophagia should be evaluated for esophagitis, as the damaged esophageal mucosa, aided by neutropenia, increases the risk of esophageal colonization with organisms including *Candida* and *Herpes simplex*. Esophagoscopy may help direct therapy for such patients.[179] In addition, gastroparesis and delayed gastric emptying resulting in nausea, gastroesophageal reflux, or decreased oral intake may be seen following HSCT.[180–181]

Malnutrition is common in pediatric patients being considered for HSCT, and accurate determination of the degree of malnutrition is important.[182] Because myeloablative and irradiative conditioning regimens can lead to mucositis affecting oral intake and because malnutrition is felt to be an independent risk factor for mortality following HSCT,[183] the use of enteral or parenteral feeding is common following HSCT.[184–185] Newer strategies, designed to decrease regimen-related toxicity such as mucositis by a combination of vitamins, ursodeoxycholic acid, and parenteral nutrition, suggest that improved nutritional support may itself promote earlier engraftment and a decrease in toxicity.[186]

Early Noninfectious Posttransplant Complications (See also Figure 62-6)

Oral and Perioral Complications

Oral mucositis affects the majority of patients undergoing HSCT[187] and can lead to dysphagia as well as laryngeal or epiglottic edema resulting in upper airway obstruction. It is recognized to increase the risk of infection, lengthen hospital stay, and increase the cost of care.[188] Although oral mucositis likely represents the sequelae of intensive chemotherapy and irradiation,[189] other important factors (e.g., bacterial colonization of the mucosal surface, upregulation of proinflammatory cytokines, and oxidative radical production) play an important role.[187,190–191] It is usually seen within the first week of irradiation and reaches its peak 1 to 2 weeks following HSCT.[192] Impaired mucociliary clearance in the nasopharynx, along with oropharyngeal mucositis, can lead to both upper and lower airway complications including sinusitis, oropharyngeal bleeding, upper airway obstruction, stridor, and aspiration pneumonia. Advances in the understanding of the pathophysiology of oral mucositis have led to newer treatments

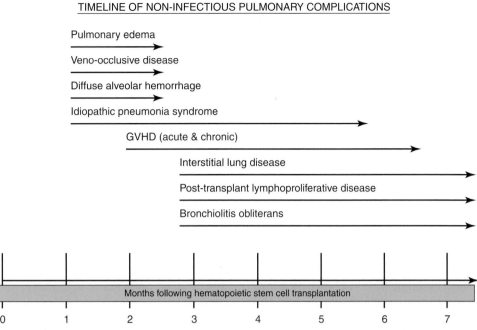

TIMELINE OF NON-INFECTIOUS PULMONARY COMPLICATIONS

Pulmonary edema

Veno-occlusive disease

Diffuse alveolar hemorrhage

Idiopathic pneumonia syndrome

GVHD (acute & chronic)

Interstitial lung disease

Post-transplant lymphoproliferative disease

Bronchiolitis obliterans

Months following hematopoietic stem cell transplantation

0   1   2   3   4   5   6   7

FIGURE 62-6. Timeline of noninfectious pulmonary complications following hematopoietic stem cell transplantation.

including dietary manipulation, mucosal administration of monochromatic light, and the administration of cytokines such as keratinocyte growth factor.[186-187,193]

Pulmonary Edema and Capillary Leak Syndrome

Pulmonary edema in the posttransplant period is relatively common[162,194-195] and is characterized by a rapid onset usually within the 2 to 3 weeks following HSCT. Potential etiologies include increased hydrostatic pressure from either overvigorous rehydration or fluid overload via parenteral nutrition, cardiac dysfunction following the use of anthracyclines, and renal toxicity following cyclophosphamide. Other causes of increased pulmonary capillary permeability may include sepsis and direct pulmonary toxicity secondary to irradiation and chemotherapy. Clinical features may include dyspnea, tachypnea, weight gain, hypoxemia, and basilar crackles on chest auscultation. Chest radiographs often show bilateral infiltrates, and pleural effusions may also be present. Treatment usually involves vigorous diuresis. A recent single case report suggests that blocking vascular endothelial growth factor-A (VEGF-A) with the monoclonal antibody Bevacizumab may improve capillary leak syndrome,[196] but further studies are needed before this can be considered standard therapy.

Peri-Engraftment Respiratory Distress Syndrome

This entity has a low incidence (~5%) and occurs within the first 14 days following HSCT, at a time coinciding with neutrophil engraftment.[197-199] The characteristic clinical and radiographic features include hypoxemia and respiratory distress. Chest radiographic findings include diffuse edema and pulmonary infiltrates and in some cases pleural effusion.[200] BAL and other invasive studies are consistently negative for pathogens. While its name and timing might suggest a specific pathology, there are no biochemical markers or pathognomonic histopathologic

findings to distinguish it from other forms of respiratory distress in the period closely following HSCT. Therapy is supportive, and although steroids have often been utilized for treatment, their efficacy is unproven.

Idiopathic Pneumonia Syndrome

Idiopathic pneumonia syndrome (IPS; also known as *idiopathic interstitial pneumonitis*) has a reported incidence of 5% to 10% in adult HSCT recipients,[201-202] although the incidence in pediatric recipients is more difficult to assess. A National Heart, Lung, and Blood Institute Workshop[203] refined the definition of IPS and established clinical and diagnostic criteria for it. Accordingly, the clinical manifestations of IPS include dyspnea, nonproductive cough, hypoxemia, and crackles on auscultation; pulmonary function testing reveals a restrictive pulmonary physiology, and diffuse or nonlobar infiltrates are seen on chest radiograph. In order to confirm this diagnosis, BAL cultures must be negative for bacterial, viral, and fungal pathogens; a second negative BAL is recommended 2 to 14 days following the initial BAL. Open lung biopsy is not specifically suggested, although transbronchial biopsy may be considered if the patient's condition will allow it. Pathologically, IPS can have two distinct histopathologic types: interstitial pneumonia and diffuse alveolar damage. IPS is typically an early complication of HSCT. Previous reports of IPS incidence described a bimodal pattern, with an initial peak approximately 2 weeks and a later peak 6 to 7 weeks post-HSCT.[203] While an entity essentially identical to IPS can be seen >100 days following HSCT, the incidence of this much later complication is unknown.

Of special interest is a review of more than 1,000 HSCT recipients[202] in which the overall incidence of IPS was 7.3%, with no significant difference in incidence between recipients of autologous and allogeneic HSCT. Pediatric patients (<20 years of age) had a slightly lower incidence of IPS. The median time between HSCT and onset of symptoms of IPS was 21 days; the hospital mortality was 74% and multi-organ failure rather than isolated respiratory failure was associated with mortality. Potential causes for IPS have included direct pulmonary toxicity resulting from pre-HSCT conditioning, as well as immunologically-mediated factors resulting from alloreactivity,[204–207] although the previously-described report of Englund[38] raises the possibility of metapneumovirus as a contributor to the pathogenesis of IPS.

Treatment for IPS remains supportive; steroids, although often used, have not been shown to have a beneficial effect. The need for mechanical ventilation in these patients is associated with a poor prognosis, and most patients requiring this degree of support do not survive.

Diffuse Alveolar Hemorrhage (DAH)

Although pulmonary hemorrhage diagnosed by BAL was first reported in immunocompromised patients older than 30 years ago,[208] Robbins and colleagues are generally credited with the description of what is known as diffuse alveolar hemorrhage (DAH) in recipients of HSCT.[209] This entity appears to be much more common in adult than in pediatric recipients of HSCT.[209–210] It usually appears within 30 days post-HSCT and coincides with marrow recovery. Of interest is the finding of relative BAL neutrophilia, despite peripheral leucopenia.[209]

A recent retrospective analysis of pediatric HSCT recipients suggests that the incidence of DAH is approximately 5%, with allogeneic recipients being at higher risk.[211] The clinical onset is often relatively sudden and rapidly progressive, with dyspnea, hypoxemia, and crackles on auscultation. On BAL, the characteristic feature is that with each successive aliquot instilled, the effluent becomes more hemorrhagic[209]; however, the specificity and sensitivity of the findings are not completely clear. Agusti and coworkers reported on 4 of 8 HSCT recipients who had DAH on postmortem and nonhemorrhagic BALs, while 7 of 13 patients without pathologically proven DAH had hemorrhagic BALs.[212] Thus, clinical correlation, timely performance of BAL, and sampling of multiple sites may be important in establishing the presence or absence of DAH.

Pulmonary and Hepatic Veno-Occlusive Disease (VOD)

First reported by Troussard and colleagues, this entity presents as a form of pulmonary hypertension, with dyspnea, signs of right-sided heart failure, and pulmonary infiltrates on chest radiograph.[213] Children compose the most significant proportion of HSCT recipients affected by VOD.[214–215] Hepatic VOD, another vascular complication of HSCT, is often associated with pulmonary VOD and interstitial pneumonitis.[216] In both, small veins and venules are partially or completely occluded by intimal fibrosis. The explanation of the relatively common coexistence of hepatic and pulmonary VOD is unknown. Possibilities include coexistent underlying toxicities or genetic factors.[217]

The diagnosis of pulmonary VOD requires a high index of clinical suspicion, as many cases reported in the literature are diagnosed postmortem.[215] Some recent reports suggest that serum levels of vascular endothelial growth factor or plasma protein C activity may be useful surrogate markers for the development of VOD,[218–219] but larger controlled studies will be needed before their routine use can be recommended. Echocardiography, cardiac catheterization, BAL to rule out intercurrent infection, and transbronchial or transthoracic lung biopsy are potential clinical investigations that should be tailored to the patient's condition and the clinical circumstances. Treatment options for pulmonary VOD are few, although recent reports demonstrate that defibrotide, a polydisperse oligonucleotide with fibrinolytic and antithrombotic properties,[220–221] may be effective therapy for hepatic VOD.[217,222] There are also recent reports of its utility in preventing VOD in HSCT recipients at increased risk for this complication.[223]

Pulmonary Function Following HSCT

A significant proportion of children who undergo HSCT have abnormalities in pulmonary function testing both soon after HSCT and later after engraftment has taken place.[163,169,224] As described earlier in the chapter, determination of pulmonary function prior to immunosuppressive chemotherapy or transplantation will serve as a reference point for studies obtained later in the patient's course.

Ginsberg and coworkers[169] reported a retrospective analysis of serial pulmonary function tests (PFTs) in 457 patients undergoing HSCT at two large tertiary pediatric hospitals. Of these subjects, 273 had at least one pretransplant PFT. The majority of patients had normal or mildly reduced spirometry (FVC and FEV_1) and lung volumes prior to transplant. In addition, the majority had a decreased diffusing capacity, with 25% having moderately or severely reduced diffusion. Following HSCT, FVC and FEV_1 decreased significantly over the first 6 months, improved slightly between 6 and 12 months, and remained stable at 1 to 2, 2 to 5 and more than 5 years. Diffusing capacity also decreased 6 months post-HSCT, with gradual but incomplete improvement by 5 years posttransplant. In a multivariate analysis, patient age, underlying diagnosis, and transplant type (autologous versus allogeneic) all had independent predictive value for decline in DLCO following HSCT. Similar reports describe pulmonary function abnormalities in those who have received HSCT with total body irradiation (TBI) conditioning.[225–227] Again, regular pulmonary function testing is recommended after transplantation, in particular in subjects at higher risk of lung injuries, such as those receiving transplants after more than one relapse of an underlying malignancy, those receiving allogeneic transplants, those receiving cytotoxic medication, and those having suffered from pre-transplant pulmonary infections.

Late Noninfectious Posttransplant Complications

The differential diagnosis of late-onset pulmonary complications extends from the complications listed in the early noninfectious group to include bronchiolitis obliterans (BO), possibly associated with underlying chronic GVHD, cryptogenic organizing pneumonia (formerly *bronchiolitis obliterans organizing pneumonia,* or BOOP) and posttransplant lymphoproliferative disorder (PTLD).[105]

Additionally, persistent post-HSCT pulmonary findings of VOD and IPS continue to occasionally complicate the late posttransplant course.

Bronchiolitis Obliterans

Chronic lower airways obstruction is the most common late pulmonary complication following HSCT.[159,228] BO is most commonly associated with evidence of chronic GVHD and is much more common following allogeneic, as opposed to autologous, marrow transplantation. Additional risk factors include early posttransplant viral infection and advanced age of the recipient.[105,229] Symptoms are generally seen 12 to 24 months after HSCT but have been described as early as 90 days after transplantation. The primary symptoms reported at clinical presentation include dyspnea, wheezing, and nonproductive cough; fever is not common.

The chest radiograph is often normal, although high-resolution lung CT scans may demonstrate some characteristic abnormalities. The most common chest CT findings in BO is a heterogeneous pattern with areas of patchy hyperaeration, areas with bronchial dilatation, and other areas characterized by hypoattenuation or increased density.[230-231] This combination of findings is often referred to as *mosaic perfusion;* although not pathognomonic, this pattern is highly suggestive for BO (Fig. 62-7A).

Pulmonary function testing is illuminating, with evidence of air flow obstruction as shown by a decrease in FEV_1 and a reduction of the FEV_1/FVC ratio.[201] The degree of air trapping seen on CT images may correlate with the pulmonary function abnormality. Confirmatory biopsy to make the diagnosis of BO is rarely indicated based on the sensitivity of these studies.[159,232]

The diagnosis of post-HSCT BO is often made based on the clinical presentation of cough, dyspnea, and the insidious nature of the presentation. Additionally, there may be changes in lung function testing when screening asymptomatic patients.[233] Overall, up to 10% of allogeneic transplant recipients will have some degree of BO and chronic air flow obstruction.[234] Lung biopsy may be performed for confirmation of the diagnosis and to exclude other causes; this may demonstrate subepithelial fibrotic changes in the airways, a common pathologic finding in BO (Fig. 62-7B). The insidious nature of this process, together with continuing inflammatory changes involving the airways and parenchyma, can result in end-stage lung disease with diffuse areas of bronchiectasis and fibrosis[235] (Fig. 62-7C).

Chronic GVHD has been associated with BO, but no definitive link has been determined. The incidence is variable, with reports ranging from 2% to 20%.[229] The lack of direct evidence of small airway inflammation resulting in BO leads to the implication that donor T helper cell alloreactivity causes distal airway epithelial cell injury, which, in turn, leads to the pathologic changes seen.[231] Patients undergoing aggressive treatment for chronic GVHD, as well as those who had specific conditioning regimens utilizing busulfan and irradiation,[234] are at most risk for BO; however, these simply remain recognized associations resulting in an increased incidence of airways obstruction without a defined mechanism.

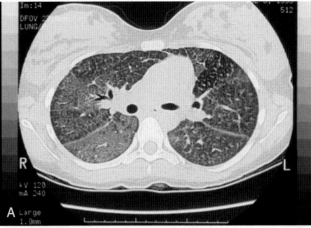

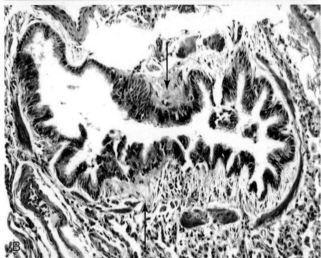

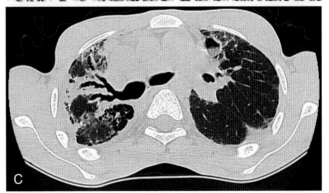

FIGURE 62-7. Bronchiolitis obliterans. **A,** Early changes of bronchiolitis obliterans as seen on this chest high-resolution CT scan. Note the changes consistent with mosaic perfusion *(arrows),* characterized by areas of varying attenuation. **B,** This photomicrograph of an airway demonstrates subepithelial fibrosis *(arrows).* Trichrome stain, 100×. **C,** Severe lung disease following HSCT as seen on chest high-resolution CT scan. Note bronchomegaly and bronchiectasis, seen best in the right upper lobe. Additional findings included widespread fibrosis of the right upper lobe and lingula, with relative sparing of the left lower lobe, and bilateral pleural thickening.

Therapy for post-HSCT BO remains centered on augmenting immunosuppression. Calcineurin-inhibitors and azathioprine, as well as steroids have reduced the decline in lung function and have shown improvement in a small proportion of subjects.[236] Recent data suggests azithromycin, a macrolide antimicrobial, may improve lung function in patients suffering from BO post-HSCT.[237] Additionally, cycled high-dose corticosteroids have been shown to reduce oxyhemoglobin desaturation and improve FEV_1 in a small cohort of pediatric patients following transplant.[238]

The benefit provided by these novel therapies may help clarify the mechanism of injury leading to BO following HSCT. Because alloreactivity and inflammation have been implicated as contributing causes of BO, the clinical approach to treatment has included both anti-inflammatory and immunomodulatory medications. There is evidence that infliximab, a monoclonal anti-tumor necrosis factor-alpha (TNF-α) antibody, may be a useful treatment of acute GVHD (especially involving skin and GI tract).[239–240] An isolated case report suggested that infliximab may be a useful treatment of BO.[241] Whether this will be an effective modality for all HSCT recipients awaits prospective multicenter randomized controlled trials.

Interstitial Lung Diseases

Interstitial lung disease, which presents with a restrictive pattern and diffusion impairment on pulmonary function testing, has also been reported as a late posttransplant complication. Here, the typical presentation is that of an asymptomatic subject, who on posttransplant monitoring is found to have a progressive decline in the vital capacity and/or diffusion capacity for carbon monoxide.[233] Whereas IPS may be the etiology for these changes, irradiation, chemotherapy, infectious pneumonitis, and BOOP could all contribute to these PFT alterations. Despite efforts to develop a good predictive model, these authors were unable to demonstrate any specific covariates that might predict the PFT. This may be similar to an entity seen in adult HSCT recipients and termed *delayed pulmonary toxicity syndrome*.[242]

Although the diagnosis is often delayed if based on lung function testing alone, certain predisposing conditions should raise awareness of the potential for developing this restrictive pattern. Some of these may extend from the early posttransplant period and include infection and veno-occlusive disease. However, the most common cause remains pre-HSCT exposure to cytotoxic drugs or irradiation. Alkylating agents, such as Lomustine (CCNU) or Carmustine (BCNU); cyclophosphamide; methotrexate; and busulfan have all been implicated in causing late pulmonary toxicity including pulmonary fibrosis.[243] Although steroids may result in clinical improvement,[242] full diagnostic studies should be undertaken to rule out deterioration related to known pretransplant pulmonary causes as well as to rule out infectious etiologies.

Cryptogenic organizing pneumonia (COP), formerly known as *bronchiolitis obliterans with organizing pneumonia* or *BOOP*, differs from BO histologically, physiologically, and, most significantly, in its response to treatment. It is histologically distinguished by patchy areas of consolidation with polypoid plugs of loose organizing connective tissue in the respiratory bronchioles and alveolar ducts.[230,244–245] Associated inflammation may be mild to moderate, but the proliferative bronchiolitis is manifest by patchy infiltrates on chest radiograph and by restriction on pulmonary function testing.[159,245] Unlike many other post-HSCT complications, BOOP/COP often improves with corticosteroid therapy. However, it is critical to rule out other post-HSCT complications, particularly infections that may cause similar symptoms and pulmonary radiographic changes. For this reason, bronchoscopies with BAL as well as open lung biopsy are often required to seek potential infectious causes as well as to document the histopathology of the lung.[232] Additionally, a response to steroids will help to differentiate between BO and BOOP/COP if the diagnosis is obscure despite studies such as bronchoscopy and open lung biopsy.[246]

Posttransplant Lymphoproliferative Disorder

Posttransplant lymphoproliferative disorder (PTLD) can occur after HSCT, as it does after solid-organ transplantation (described earlier in the chapter). In this population, allogeneic transplants, human leukocyte antigen (HLA) mismatched transplants, T cell–depleted grafts, and Epstein-Barr virus (EBV) seronegative recipients who receive transplants from EBV seropositive donors are at increased risk.[247] The pathogenesis, monitoring, and treatment of PTLD in the HSCT recipient are similar to those described previously for the solid-organ transplant recipient. The presentation is usually within the first year following HSCT, with the peak incidence 1 to 5 months after transplant.

Pulmonary Alveolar Proteinosis

Pulmonary alveolar proteinosis (PAP) has rarely been described in conditions associated with immune impairment including post-HSCT.[159,248] This condition is associated with the excessive accumulation of surfactant lipoprotein in the alveolar space and results in defective air exchange and hypoxemia. The diagnosis can be suggested on CT and is easily made on BAL, where the distinctive finding is the lipoproteinaceous milky white fluid recovered from the lower airway. This finding can be subsequently confirmed via laboratory analysis.[159] The treatment for PAP requires the physical removal of this excessive surfactant material, usually by sequential lavage.[249]

Respiratory Failure

Chronic respiratory complications following HSCT, particularly BO and interstitial lung disease, can lead to respiratory insufficiency and, ultimately, respiratory failure. Because of this, monitoring the pulmonary and cardiac status of HSCT recipients who have these complications will allow the clinician to intervene appropriately with treatment when possible. Unfortunately, the treatments for BO and interstitial lung disease are unsuccessful too often. For such conditions with end-stage lung disease, lung transplantation may be a treatment option,[250] but many lung transplant programs prefer to replace lungs before respiratory failure leads to the need for chronic intubation or tracheostomy tube placement with mechanical ventilation. As in the case of other chronic lung diseases such as cystic fibrosis,[251–252] the use of noninvasive ventilatory support will likely play an increasingly important role in allowing patients to be "bridged" to lung transplantation while remaining awake and, to some extent, ambulatory or at least more active. In addition, noninvasive ventilation can be used in immunosuppressed patients[253] as well as solid-organ recipients[254] who have acute respiratory insufficiency secondary to pulmonary infections. Such patients may thereby avoid intubation while the acute pulmonary infection leading to respiratory insufficiency is treated.

DIAGNOSTIC APPROACH TO PULMONARY DISEASE IN THE IMMUNOCOMPROMISED PEDIATRIC HOST

Radiographic Findings

In pediatric patients with either oncologic disease or other circumstances that will necessitate significant immunosuppression, radiographic evaluation including chest radiographs or, in selected cases, CT scans will help define pulmonary abnormalities before proceeding to further treatment such as ablative chemotherapy and HSCT. These preliminary studies will be useful should post-HSCT pulmonary complications such as pulmonary edema, pulmonary hemorrhage, pneumonia, or BO develop.[105]

In the immunocompromised patient, the common causes of general radiographic patterns are shown in Table 62-3, but it must be emphasized that appearances on plain chest radiograph are often deceptive and are usually not helpful in making a specific diagnosis. CT scans are much more sensitive in revealing the extent of pulmonary disease and can demonstrate other findings such as early cavitation or visceral fungal lesions. In addition, CT can better demonstrate pulmonary anatomy, directing approaches to bronchoscopy or biopsy.

Common radiographic findings include air-space consolidation, ground-glass opacities, nodules, and air trapping. Nodular opacities are common radiographic manifestations, ranging from relatively large and discrete, to smaller that appear to run along bronchovascular bundles (tree-in-bud pattern). Factors such as a patient's medications, the duration of patient symptoms, and the underlying patient immune status can help narrow the clinician's focus, improving decisions related to the choices of treatment or diagnostic testing.

NONINVASIVE DIAGNOSTIC STUDIES

Pulmonary function testing (PFT) can be a useful adjunct to other noninvasive studies when evaluating a patient with acute pulmonary complications. PFTs alone will rarely provide strong evidence of a specific diagnosis, but there are important exceptions to this. The first is the chronic and progressive decrease in diffusing capacity coupled with a decrease in TLC, which commonly is seen secondary to interstitial disease from radiation pneumonitis. The second is the progressive development of air flow obstruction and air trapping as is seen with BO. PFTs otherwise, however, must be viewed in the context of other factors including the patient's degree of immunodeficiency, the type of pulmonary symptoms and signs, and the timing of symptoms relative to previous therapy. More important is the utility of following PFTs longitudinally in patients with acquired immunosuppression, as this may alert the

TABLE 62-3	DIFFERENTIAL DIAGNOSIS OF RADIOGRAPHIC ABNORMALITIES
Airspace Consolidation	Hospital/community acquired pneumonia Fungal pneumonia Aspiration pneumonitis/pneumonia Idiopathic pneumonia syndrome Tuberculosis/nontuberculous mycobacteria DAH ARDS Pulmonary edema TRALI
Nodule	Discrete Fungal infection Nocardia infection Metastatic calcification PTLD Malignancy Septic emboli Tree-in-bud pattern Viral pneumonia Bacterial pneumonia BOS
Ground-Glass Opacities	Pulmonary edema TRALI ARDS DAH Cytomegalovirus *Pneumocystis jirovecii* Common viruses (e.g., influenza, RSV, parainfluenza) Drug toxicity
Mosaic Attenuation	Air trapping BOS Viral infection Vascular disease Pulmonary hypertension/porto-pulmonary hypertension Venous thromboembolism

ARDS, Acute respiratory distress syndrome; *BOS,* bronchiolitis obliterans syndrome; *DAH,* diffuse alveolar hemorrhage; *PTLD,* posttransplant lymphoproliferative disease; *RSV,* respiratory syncytial virus; *TRALI,* transfusion-related acute lung injury.

clinician to the development of more chronic complications, most importantly BO.

The majority of the data on post-HSCT pulmonary function is from adults, although several pediatric case series have been described.[163,169,224,255–257] Pre-HSCT therapy, including chemotherapy directed at underlying malignancies and marrow ablation therapy, is an important risk factor for the development of pulmonary sequelae. In addition, patient age is important, as the continuing lung development of pediatric patients may alter the risk of pulmonary toxicity from chemotherapeutic or marrow ablation regimens, lung irradiation, or immunosuppressive medications posttransplantation. Specific agents that may cause pulmonary injury include busulfan, cyclophosphamide, methotrexate, BCNU, and radiation.[258] See Chapter 74 for a further discussion of these agents.

Sputum produced by cough induced with inhalation of hypertonic saline aerosols has been useful in older children with immunocompromise and PCP. Gastric aspirates can be used in the younger child and are particularly helpful when the pathogen being considered is not a usual colonizing organism of the upper airway (e.g., tuberculosis). If the child requires endotracheal intubation for respiratory distress, endotracheal aspirates are easy to obtain.

The ability to detect capsular polysaccharide antigens of bacterial pathogens even after antimicrobials have been administered is occasionally helpful in hospitalized patients. A number of tests for direct detection of fungal antigens have been described (e.g., the serum galactomannan assay for *Aspergillus*), although its sensitivity and specificity in children may be less than in adult patients.[56] Direct immunofluorescence can be used to detect *Legionella* sp. with high sensitivity and specificity.[102] Enzyme-linked immunosorbent assays or direct immunofluorescence tests of blood or BAL are now available for the rapid diagnosis of respiratory syncytial virus, influenza A virus, parainfluenza viruses, *Chlamydia*, and mycobacterial infections.[259] Viral cultures are generally available, and the shell vial technique for rapid identification of CMV is very useful.

Genetic probes for detecting respiratory viruses *P. jirovecii*, *Legionella*, *Mycobacterium*, and *Mycoplasma pneumoniae* are now commercially available, and the ability of the polymerase chain reaction to amplify specific regions of genomic DNA or RNA should allow a broader application of these sensitive diagnostic approaches in the immunocompromised patient, particularly when combined with BAL to obtain specimens. Diagnostic tests for the rapid detection of potential respiratory pathogens is an area of expanding importance, and a recent review summarizes several technologies including nucleic acid amplification tests (NAATs).[260]

▪▪▪ INVASIVE DIAGNOSTIC STUDIES

Unfortunately, radiography and other noninvasive diagnostic studies rarely result in a specific diagnosis in the immunocompromised child with pulmonary disease. In that circumstance, one is often faced with either continuing empiric antimicrobial therapy or performing a more invasive diagnostic study to make a specific diagnosis. Fortunately, the safety and availability of these studies have improved significantly over last decade.

Flexible Bronchoscopy and Bronchoalveolar Lavage

Flexible bronchoscopy is safe in experienced hands and provides excellent diagnostic material in the immunocompromised child with pneumonia.[261–262] See Chapter 9 for a detailed discussion. Indications for bronchoscopy in children with pneumonia generally include (1) failure of pneumonia or fever to clear with appropriate antimicrobial therapy, (2) suspicion of endobronchial obstruction by infection or tumor, (3) recurrent pneumonia in a lobe or segment, and (4) suspicion of unusual organisms. Although the yield of gastric aspiration or BAL is probably superior to bronchoscopy for suspected tuberculosis,[263] bronchoscopy has the added value of allowing evaluation for endobronchial disease or bronchial compression.[264] Simple cytology brushing obtained through the pediatric bronchoscope can be used for cytologic examination and viral cultures, but the yield is usually low.

The bronchoscope suction channel may become contaminated by upper airway organisms during the procedure, and simple washings obtained through the bronchoscope channel are generally less useful than quantitative cultures of BAL. Nonetheless, BAL is the most useful bronchoscopic technique in the immunocompromised host, and a variety of infectious and noninfectious diagnoses can be made by BAL. Further, BAL is generally safe, even in patients with thrombocytopenia.

Although bronchoscopy with BAL is important and well tolerated, its limitations should also be appreciated. In immunocompromised patients who have received empiric broad-spectrum antimicrobial therapy for some period of time, the yield of BAL in isolating a new bacterial pathogen is likely to be low.[265] In oncology patients and other non-AIDS immunocompromised patients, the number of *P. jirovecii* organisms is usually low compared with AIDS patients, and BAL may be falsely negative.[266] In populations receiving prophylaxis for this infection, the yield for PCP will also probably be low. CMV can also be diagnosed rapidly by bronchoscopy, but CMV may be a commensal rather than an infecting organism. As discussed earlier, patients may have co-pathogens that are the predominating organism, rather than CMV. *Aspergillus* and other fungi are often difficult to diagnose by bronchoscopy, particularly early in the infection when therapy is most likely to be effective. In pediatric HSCT recipients, fungal infections were the most common infection diagnosed by BAL, but the yield was only 17% in the early conditioning (pre-HSCT) period (where broad-spectrum antimicrobial coverage was common) compared with 82% following transplant.

Transbronchial biopsies can also be taken via the flexible bronchoscope. Though safe in older patients, transbronchial lung biopsies may yield an unacceptable number of false-negative results in immunosuppressed patients and are most useful when organisms such as *P. jirovecii* or granulomatous lesions are probable. The standard pediatric bronchoscopes, 2.8 or 3.6 mm in diameter, have suction/biopsy channels of only 1.2 mm diameter, accommodating biopsy forceps of only 1 mm diameter. The resultant biopsies from such forceps are quite small, leading to the risk of false-negative biopsies in infants. Older children are more likely to tolerate larger bronchoscopes with 2 mm (or larger) channels, allowing for the passage of 1.8-mm forceps and larger biopsy samples. Reported experience with transbronchial biopsies in pediatric patients is limited, but transbronchial biopsy has a significant role in monitoring acute rejection and infections in the pediatric lung transplant patient and in skilled hands can be done with conscious sedation and a transnasal approach in the older child.[267] Transbronchial biopsy for the diagnosis of BO complicating HSCT is not recommended, as it is difficult to obtain adequate tissue using this technique.

Transthoracic Needle Aspiration Biopsy

Needle aspiration of the lung has been used for the diagnosis of PCP in pediatric cancer patients and for the diagnosis of localized infections in other immunosuppressed patients. Pneumothorax has been reported as a relatively frequent complication of the needle aspirates done for PCP,[268] and this risk must be considered even with more modern "thin"-needle techniques. The use of CT guidance greatly improves the yield and safety of transthoracic needle aspiration biopsy, particularly in the presence of peripheral nodular disease. As a result, it is the procedure of choice for children with peripheral lesions that are difficult to reach with a flexible bronchoscope, as they can safely be sampled, avoiding an open biopsy.[269]

Open-Lung Biopsy

Open-lung biopsy (OLB) is the gold standard by which other pulmonary diagnostic modalities are judged. Its advantages include the larger amount of lung tissue sampled and the ability to sample different lobes. Using current surgical techniques, OLB is generally a procedure with a low morbidity[270] that can be done rapidly and allows the surgeon to select optimal tissue for culture and microscopic examination. "Mini-thoracotomy" and lingular biopsy may be all that is necessary in patients with diffuse pulmonary processes, significantly reducing the morbidity of the procedure.

Biopsy using video-assisted thoracoscopy (VATS) is now supplanting OLB in many centers, as it can be performed safely in very small infants[271] and does not require chest tube placement following biopsy.[272] Mechanical ventilation is no longer considered a contraindication to VATS.[273] Complications such as respiratory failure, thrombocytopenia, or coagulopathies, and prior antimicrobial /antifungal therapy increase the risk of VATS as well as OLB and may also reduce the diagnostic yield.

Some studies have questioned how often lung biopsy results will lead to a change in therapy, if one excludes patients with organisms covered by empiric therapy such as *P. jirovecii* and nonspecific histologic findings without specific therapies such as fibrosis or nonspecific lung injury. Published results on OLB and VATS in immunocompromised pediatric patients have indicated yields that range from 36% to 94% for a specific diagnosis and generally support the utility of either procedure.[232,270,274-276]

Although OLB or VATS is the procedure of choice for obtaining definitive diagnostic information in immunosuppressed patients with pulmonary infiltrates, other invasive procedures (e.g., bronchoscopy with BAL as well as CT-guided needle biopsy) may be more appropriate. In addition, timing of procedures in immunocompromised patients is often difficult, requiring an understanding of each patient's history and response to therapy. If the patient is improving with empiric therapy, any invasive procedure may not be warranted. On the other hand, if a patient is deteriorating despite therapy, then moving expeditiously to a more definitive diagnostic procedure is advised. Early bronchoscopy is relatively safe and may provide a diagnosis without the need for a more invasive procedure. Limitations of bronchoscopy with BAL, however, must be acknowledged. For example, CT-guided needle biopsy has a higher diagnostic yield for isolated peripheral nodular disease. If a more extensive biopsy is deemed necessary, the choice of OLB or VATS will depend on the condition of the patient and the available expertise, both surgical and anesthetic. In most centers with experienced surgical and anesthetic staff, either procedure is relatively safe, especially when performed before respiratory failure ensues. Even in this situation, OLB or VATS may be indicated in order to establish a specific diagnosis.

Suggested Reading

Catherinot E, Lanternier F, Bougnoux M-E, et al. *Pneumocystis jirovecii* Pneumonia. *Infect Dis Clin North Am.* 2010;24:107–138.

Centers for Disease Control and Prevention, Infectious Disease Society of America, American Society of Blood and Marrow Transplantation. Guidelines for preventing opportunistic infections among hematopoietic stem cell transplant recipients. *MMWR Recomm Rep.* 2000;49(RR-10): 1–125 CE1–7.

Collin BA, Leather HL, Wingard JR, et al. Evolution, incidence, and susceptibility of bacterial bloodstream isolates from 519 bone marrow transplant patients. *Clin Infect Dis.* 2001;33:947–953.

Frey NV, Tsai DE. The management of posttransplant lymphoproliferative disorder. *Med Oncol.* 2007;24:125–136.

Gamba P, Midrio P, Betalli P, et al. Video-assisted thoracoscopy in compromised pediatric patients. *J Laparoendoscop Adv Surg Tech A.* 2010;20:69–71.

Ginsberg JP, Aplenc R, McDonough J, et al. Pre-transplant lung function is predictive of survival following pediatric bone marrow transplantation. *Pediatr Blood Cancer.* 2010;54:454–460.

Gower WA, Collaco JM, Mogayzel Jr PJ. Lung function and late pulmonary complications among survivors of hematopoietic stem cell transplantation during childhood. *Paediatr Respir Rev.* 2010;11:115–122.

Gower WA, Collaco JM, Mogayzel Jr PJ. Pulmonary dysfunction in pediatric hematopoietic stem cell transplant patients: non-infectious and long-term complications. *Pediatr Blood Cancer.* 2007;49:225–233.

Kotloff RM, Ahya VN, Crawford SW. Pulmonary complications of solid organ and hematopoietic stem cell transplantation. *Am J Respir Crit Care Med.* 2004;170:22–48.

Kumar D. Emerging viruses in transplantation. *Curr Opin Infect Dis.* 2010;23:374–378.

Kurland G, Michelson P. Bronchiolitis obliterans in children. *Pediatr Pulmonol.* 2005;39:193–208.

Mertens AC, Yasui Y, Liu Y, et al. Pulmonary complications in survivors of childhood and adolescent cancer. A report from the Childhood Cancer Survivor Study. *Cancer* 2002;95:2431–2441.

Steinbach WJ. Invasive aspergillosis in pediatric patients. *Curr Med Res Opin.* 2010;26:1779–1787.

Yang F, Li Y, Braylan R, et al. Pediatric T-cell post-transplant lymphoproliferative disorder after solid organ transplantation. *Pediatr Blood Cancer.* 2008;50:415–418.

Yen KT, Lee AS, Krowka MJ, et al. Pulmonary complications in bone marrow transplantation: a practical approach to diagnosis and treatment. *Clin Chest Med.* 2004;25:189–201.

Yoshihara S, Yanik G, Cooke KR, et al. Bronchiolitis obliterans syndrome (BOS), bronchiolitis obliterans organizing pneumonia (BOOP), and other late-onset noninfectious pulmonary complications following allogeneic hematopoietic stem cell transplantation. *Biol Blood Marrow Transplant.* 2007;13:749–759.

References

The complete reference list is available online at www.expertconsult.com

63 RESPIRATORY DISORDERS IN PEDIATRIC HIV INFECTION

MEYER KATTAN, MD, AND HEATHER J. ZAR, MD, PhD

Respiratory diseases are the most common complications occurring in children infected with the human immunodeficiency virus (HIV). Before the availability of antiretroviral therapy and establishment of programs to prevent vertical HIV transmission to infants, acute respiratory infections were a major cause of morbidity and mortality globally. Since then, we have made significant strides in understanding the virus and developing strategies to prevent transmission and slow disease progression. In high-income countries (where early identification of HIV-1–infected infants is possible and medications are readily available for both treatment of HIV-1 infection and prophylaxis of opportunistic infections), there has been a marked reduction in the rates of opportunistic infections and the rates of acute pulmonary disease.[1] Nevertheless, respiratory illness remains the most common cause of morbidity in HIV-infected children on highly active antiretroviral therapy (HAART).

Countries in sub-Saharan Africa and Asia currently have the major burden of HIV-1–infected children. Prevention of vertical transmission and early identification and treatment of HIV-1 infection and its complications remain unavailable to large segments of the population in these areas. The spectrum of respiratory illness in these countries is similar to the early reports from high-income countries but is exacerbated by high rates of infectious diseases (e.g., tuberculosis [TB]) and coexisting poverty-related factors (e.g., malnutrition and biomass fuel exposure). In addition, an increased vulnerability to respiratory infectious diseases has been reported in HIV-exposed but uninfected children compared to unexposed children in these regions.[2] As prevention and treatment programs in poorly resourced areas are strengthened and more available, this group of children will be increasingly important in considering the burden of respiratory disease.

ETIOLOGY AND PATHOGENESIS

HIV-1 is a retrovirus, which is a heterogeneous group of lipid-enveloped RNA viruses. HIV-1 comprises several subtypes designated as A to K with different geographic distributions. Through the action of its enzyme, reverse transcriptase, DNA is synthesized from RNA, which is then integrated into the host DNA genome. Most retroviruses contain only three gene regions. The *gag* (group antigen gene) encodes the core nucleocapsid proteins. The viral core contains four nucleocapsid proteins, p24, p17, p9, and p7. The *env* (envelope) genes encode the surface core proteins of the virus. HIV-1 has two major viral envelope proteins: the external gp120 and the transmembrane gp41 (Fig. 63-1). The *pol* (polymerase) gene gives rise to viral enzymes (e.g., reverse transcriptase, protease, and endonuclease). In addition to the *gag*, *pol*, and *env* genes, the 9-kilobase RNA genome of HIV-1 contains at least six additional genes (*vif*, *vpu*, *vpr*, *tat*, *rev*, and *nef*) that code for proteins involved in the regulation of gene expression.

The human CD4+ T lymphocyte is the major cellular target for HIV-1. The HIV-1 gp120 envelope protein binds to the CD4 molecule on the host cell membrane with strikingly high affinity. This leads to entry of the virus into the T cell and integration of the viral genome into the host DNA. Infection with HIV results in profound changes in T lymphocyte function. There is progressive depletion of CD4+ helper lymphocytes. In the first 9 months of life, the rate of decline of CD4+ cells in HIV-1–infected infants is double that of noninfected infants.[4] CD4+ depletion is an indicator of severity of HIV-1 infection because the incidence of opportunistic infections and other complications correlates with the number and percentage of CD4+ lymphocytes.

HIV-1 also infects monocytes, macrophages, and dendritic cells, but it has much less pronounced cytopathic effects in these cells. Therefore, infected monocytes serve as a reservoir for HIV-1, thus allowing further dissemination of the virus throughout the body.

B cell dysfunction also occurs with hyperimmunoglobulinemia commonly present in untreated infants.[5] If there is defective B cell function early in life, before the development of specific memory cells, severe infection with otherwise common organisms may result. Studies indicate that HIV-1–infected children have an impaired ability to produce and maintain antibodies to pediatric vaccines, and this inability appears early in life.[6,7]

DEFINITION

HIV-1 infection results in a disease spectrum ranging from asymptomatic infection to severely symptomatic cases. Infected patients who are asymptomatic are classified as CDC Class N. Asymptomatic patients may have abnormal immune function. Symptomatic patients are classified as CDC Category A, B, or C depending on the severity of the signs and symptoms. The CDC surveillance definition for AIDS is an illness characterized by the presence of an indicator disease (e.g., encephalopathy, *Pneumocystis jirovecii* pneumonia [PCP], lymphoid interstitial pneumonia) and documentation of HIV-1 infection. Any condition listed in the surveillance case definition

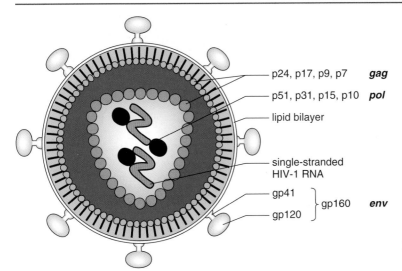

p24, p17, p9, p7   *gag*

p51, p31, p15, p10   *pol*

lipid bilayer

single-stranded
HIV-1 RNA

gp41 }
gp120 } gp160   *env*

FIGURE 63-1. Schematic representation of the human immunodeficiency virus (HIV-1). Two single-stranded RNA chains are surrounded by a nucleocapsid polypeptide. A lipid envelope surrounding the viral core contains the viral envelope proteins gp 41 and gp 120. *Gag, env,* and *pol* are the gene regions coding for the respective proteins. (Adapted from Graham BS, Wright PF: Candidate AIDS vaccines. *N Engl J Med* 1995; 333:1332.)

for AIDS (except for lymphoid interstitial pneumonitis or pulmonary lymphoid hyperplasia) places the child in Category C. An alternative clinical staging system is that used by the World Health Organization (WHO), which grades infants and children from stage 1 (asymptomatic) to stage 4. In this grading system, pulmonary diseases such as pulmonary TB or HIV-associated lung disease (including bronchiectasis) fulfill the criteria for stage 3 disease. AIDS-defining conditions such as recurrent severe bacterial infections, PCP, or extrapulmonary TB are criteria for stage 4 disease. Immunologic staging, based on the CD4 percentage and absolute CD4 count, is useful as a prognostic tool for disease severity. The CDC immunologic classification ranges from no immunosuppression to severe immunosuppression (Table 63-1).

EPIDEMIOLOGY

An estimated 2.5 million children younger than 15 years of age live with HIV-1 infection, 90% of whom reside in low- or middle-income countries, predominantly sub-Saharan Africa.

Since the initiation of screening of blood products, perinatal transmission accounts for most new cases of HIV-1 infection in children younger than 13 years of age. Perinatal transmission can occur *in utero,* intrapartum, and through breast feeding. Breast feeding is an important modality of transmission of HIV-1 infection. Avoidance of breast feeding is recommended in resource-rich countries.

The WHO recommends exclusive breast feeding for infants of HIV-1–positive women for the first 6 months of life in resource-limited settings accompanied by maternal antiretroviral therapy. Antiretroviral therapy during and after pregnancy reduces mother-to-child transmission and is recommended for women in resource-poor countries who breast feed.[8] Sexual abuse is another mode of infection in young children.[9] Adolescents, like adults, acquire HIV-1 infection primarily through sexual transmission or intravenous drug abuse.[10]

The maternal viral load is the major risk factor for perinatal transmission. The use of zidovudine administered during pregnancy after the first trimester and during labor, and administered to the newborn for 6 weeks reduced the transmission rate from 26% to 8%.[11] Subsequent cohort studies have reported lower transmission rates when zidovudine is combined with elective Caesarian section or use of highly active antiretroviral regimens that reduce maternal viral load to very low levels. The risk for transmission is less than 2% with perinatal antiretroviral regimens and maternal viral load levels below 1000 copies/mL.[12–14]

DIAGNOSIS

For children younger than 18 months of age, the preferred test for diagnosis is the HIV DNA or RNA polymerase chain reaction (PCR) assay. Approximately 30% to 40% of HIV-infected newborn infants will have a positive PCR

TABLE 63-1 IMMUNOLOGIC CATEGORIES BY AGE AND CD4+ MEASUREMENTS IN HIV-INFECTED CHILDREN

IMMUNE STATUS	AGE UP TO 12 MONTHS	AGE> 12 MONTHS TO 6 YEARS	6 YEARS OR OVER
No significant immunosuppression	>35%*	>25%	>500 cells/µl
Mild immunosuppression	25%-34%	20%-24%	350-499 cells/µl
Advanced immunosuppression	<20%-24%	<15%-19%	<200-349 cells/µl
Severe immunosuppression	<20%	<15%	<200 cells/µl

*CD4 percentage of total lymphocytes

at 48 hours of age, indicative of *in utero* transmission. By 2 weeks of age, more than 90% of infected infants will have detectable HIV-DNA, with 95% testing positive at 1 month of age. In areas with high HIV prevalence, the PCR should be repeated every 6 months during breast feeding and at least 6 weeks after discontinuing breast feeding if the initial PCR was negative.

For children older than 18 months of age, testing for HIV-1 antibody is adequate for diagnosis, as a positive test almost always indicates infection. An enzyme-linked immunosorbent assay (ELISA) detects specific antibody to the virus. The test may be confirmed using an immunoblot analysis (Western Blot). Maternal HIV antibodies usually become undetectable in infants by 15 months of age but may be present until 18 months of age. Therefore, standard HIV-IgG serologic assays cannot be used in the first 18 months of life to distinguish infection in the child from maternal antibodies.

An HIV-exposed but uninfected child younger than 18 months of age may have a positive HIV-1 antibody test, but a negative HIV DNA PCR assay.

NATURAL HISTORY OF HIV-1 INFECTION IN CHILDREN

In perinatally infected children who are untreated, there is a rapid increase in HIV RNA levels to several hundred thousand per milliliter within 1 month of birth that then decrease very slowly in the first 2 years of life.[15] Immunologic dysfunction occurs early in untreated infants, and symptoms and opportunistic infections occur in the first year of life. Earlier diagnosis, antiviral therapy, and prophylactic strategies for opportunistic infections have altered the course and character of the disease and its complications. The introduction of protease inhibitors and non-nucleoside reverse transcriptase inhibitors for treatment of HIV-1 infections made possible the use of HAART. In infants, HAART should be initiated as soon as the diagnosis of HIV infection is made irrespective of CD4 measures, as early use is associated with a substantial reduction in infant mortality and opportunistic infections.[16] For children older than 1 year of age, HAART should be initiated based on CD4 counts or clinical staging.

HIV AND LUNG DEFENSE

The profound immunologic alterations caused by HIV result in a spectrum of infectious and non-infectious lung diseases (Table 63-2). In the lung, as in peripheral blood, HIV infects pulmonary lymphocytes, and infection can be identified in lymphocytes obtained from bronchoalveolar lavage fluid (BAL).[17] The virus decreases the number of CD4+ cells and also causes infiltration of CD8+ lymphocytes in the interstitial and alveolar spaces. This is mediated by cytokines, including IL-15 from alveolar macrophages, which induce T cell proliferation and stimulate T cell migration.[18] The number of natural killer cells is increased in BAL fluid of HIV-1–infected individuals, but they lose their functional capabilities with

TABLE 63-2 PULMONARY COMPLICATIONS OF HIV INFECTION

Infections
Viruses
Cytomegalovirus
Respiratory syncytial virus
Herpes simplex virus
Parainfluenza virus
Influenza virus
Adenovirus
Bacteria
Encapsulated organisms (e.g., *Streptococcus pneumoniae,
    Haemophilus influenzae, Staphylococcus aureus*)
Gram-negative organisms (e.g., *Escherichia coli, Klebsiella,
    Pseudomonas aeruginosa*)
Mycobacterium tuberculosis
Mycobacterium avium-intracellulare
Fungi
Pneumocystis jirovecii
Candida albicans
Histoplasma capsulatum
Cryptococcus neoformans
Aspergillus species
Coccidioides immitis
Interstitial pneumonia
Lymphoid interstitial pneumonia
Pulmonary lymphoid hyperplasia
Desquamative interstitial pneumonia
Malignancies
Kaposi's sarcoma
Lymphoma

progression of disease.[19] Alveolar macrophages obtained by BAL can also be infected with HIV.[20] Although some components of macrophage defense are preserved during HIV-1 infection, lack of activation signals from T lymphocytes impairs effective defense by macrophages.

PULMONARY DISORDERS

Infants who are infected by vertical transmission have no recognizable pulmonary disease at birth attributable to HIV.[21] The incidence of respiratory distress syndrome and bronchopulmonary dysplasia is similar in infected and uninfected children born to HIV infected mothers.[22] In untreated infants, the initial symptoms and signs of HIV-1 infection include hepatosplenomegaly, lymphadenopathy, pulmonary disease, and sepsis.[23,24] A pulmonary problem may often be the presenting manifestation of HIV-1 infection.

In a prospective birth-cohort study in the United States, the rate of lower respiratory tract infections in HIV-1–infected children in the first year of life was 2.8 times greater than the rate of uninfected children born to HIV-1–infected mothers.[25] In a prospective study from Rwanda, the risk of developing severe pneumonia among infected children was three times greater than among uninfected children.[26] The highest incidence of pneumonia occurred in the first 12 months of life. The incidence rate for pneumonia excluding PCP in the pre-HAART era was between 20 and 25 per 1000 child-years in the first 12 months.[25,27] In a prospective cohort enrolled at a mean age of 40 months, 25% of children developed an acute pneumonia over 3 years, and 34% had multiple episodes.[27]

The introduction of HAART has reduced the incidence rates of opportunistic infections and improved survival. PCP, lymphocytic interstitial pneumonia (LIP), and bacterial pneumonia were the pulmonary complications most frequently encountered in the pre-HAART era. Pulmonary infections have declined in the HAART era in regions where these medications are readily accessible. For example, in HIV-1–infected children in the United States, the incidence rates of bacterial pneumonia decreased from 11.1 per hundred person-years in the pre-HAART era to 2.2 during the HAART era and of *P. jirovecii* from 1.3 per hundred person-years to 0.09.[1]

A prior history of an AIDS defining recurrent bacterial infection and a low CD4+ count are risk factors for the development of acute pneumonia.[27] Higher levels of baseline HIV RNA (especially with HIV RNA >1 million copies/mL) are associated with a higher rate of acute pneumonia. In children younger than 12 months of age, a low CD4+ cell count in the infant and a low maternal CD4+ count appear to be risk factors for pneumonia.[25] The rate of decline of CD4+ cells during the first year of life is also associated with development of lower respiratory tract infection (Table 63-3).

Pulmonary disease is an important cause of HIV-related death. Infections are the most prevalent underlying cause of death for children younger than 5 years of age, two-thirds of which are pulmonary infections. The frequency of pulmonary disease as a cause of death decreases with age. In the prospective Pediatric Pulmonary and Cardiovascular Complications of Vertically Transmitted HIV Study, chronic lung disease was present in 58% of children who died but was rarely a direct cause of death.[28]

The etiology of pulmonary infections is varied. Bacterial pneumonias with both Gram-negative and Gram-positive organisms and viral pneumonias occur more frequently in HIV-1–infected children. Mixed infections with combinations of bacterial, viral, mycobacterial, and fungal isolates are common. In many cases, no organisms are isolated. This is partly a result of the difficulty in obtaining diagnostic specimens in children and the poor sensitivity of the available diagnostic tests.

With the successful prevention of mother-to-infant transmission with antiretroviral regimens, there is a growing population of uninfected infants born to HIV-1–infected mothers. A prospective study in the United States indicated that uninfected children born to HIV-1–infected mothers were not more susceptible to pulmonary disease than those born to uninfected mothers.[25] In resource-poor countries, there are higher rates of infections including pneumonia related to factors such as poor sanitation, household crowding, and poor placental transfer of maternal antibodies. In these areas, HIV-1–exposed uninfected children have an increased risk of severe pneumonia and treatment failure compared to HIV-1–unexposed children.[2]

Bacterial Pneumonia

Bacterial pneumonia occurs more frequently in HIV-1–infected children than uninfected children because of defects in both cellular and humoral immunity. HIV-1–infected children are at risk for more severe pneumonia including bacteremic disease.[2] During the pre-HAART era, serious bacterial infections, particularly pneumonia, followed by bacteremia were the most commonly reported opportunistic infections in children, with an event rate of 15 per 100 child-years.[29] In addition, minor bacterial respiratory infections such as sinusitis and otitis media were even more common (17 to 85 per 100 child-years).[30] The incidence of pneumonia has reduced substantially with the use of HAART, declining to a rate of 2.2 to 3.1 per 100 child-years, which is similar to that in HIV-1–uninfected children.[1,31] However in low- or middle-income countries, pneumonia remains a major cause of hospitalization and mortality.[32]

HIV-1–infected children are susceptible to developing pneumonia from a broader range of pathogens than HIV-1–negative children. *Streptococcus pneumoniae* is the most commonly reported bacterial pathogen causing pneumonia and bacteremic illness. The incidence of pneumococcal bacteremia or invasive disease is 9 to 43-fold greater in HIV-infected children compared to uninfected children.[33] *Staphylococcus aureus* has been increasingly reported in HIV-1–infected children, with a higher incidence in HIV-1–infected children compared to uninfected children.[34,35] In low- and middle-income countries, *Haemophilus influenzae*, *Escherchia coli*, and *Salmonella* spp. were the most common Gram-negative organisms.[36] Using postmortem percutaneous lung aspirates from children in Zimbabwe, Ikeogu found *Klebsiella* and *Pseudomonas* spp. to be the most common Gram-negative organisms.[37] Polymicrobial disease (e.g., bacterial-viral, bacterial-pneumocystis, and bacterial-mycobacterial infections) are frequent and are associated with a worse prognosis, with mortality increasing exponentially with increased number of pathogens.[2] *Bordetella pertussis* has been reported in children with respiratory distress and cough.[38] The increasing incidence of antimicrobial-resistant bacteria that colonize the nasopharynx and that cause disease among HIV-1–infected children is of concern.[35,39]

TABLE 63-3	MEAN RATE OF DECLINE OF CD4+ LYMPHOCYTE COUNT IN FIRST YEAR OF LIFE BEFORE DEVELOPING LOWER RESPIRATORY TRACT INFECTION (LRI) OR PNEUMOCYSTIS PNEUMONIA (PCP)
	CELLS/MM³/MONTH
HIV-uninfected	55 ± 9
HIV-infected, no LRI	134 ± 20
HIV-infected, with LRI	266 ± 61
HIV-infected, with PCP	375 ± 112

HIV, Human immunodeficiency virus.
From Kattan M, Platzker A, Mellins RB, et al. Respiratory diseases in the first year of life in children born to HIV-1-infected women. *Pediatr Pulmonol.* 2001;31:267-276.

Bacterial pneumonia is usually a presumptive diagnosis in a child with respiratory signs or symptoms and an abnormal chest radiograph, as identification of a bacterial pathogen is frequently not possible because of difficulty in obtaining an appropriate specimen and poor diagnostic sensitivity of tests. Isolation of an organism from a normally sterile site such as blood is useful, but bacteremic illness occurs in a minority of pneumonia cases. Identification of an organism from respiratory secretions may not distinguish a colonizing organism from those causing disease. However, sputum induction using hypertonic saline was useful for identifying a cause of pneumonia in young South African children (median age 6 months) in whom M. tuberculosis, PCP, or bacteria were identified.[40] An organism other than common oral flora obtained from BAL accompanied by neutrophils strongly suggests a bacterial cause of pneumonia.

Treatment of bacterial pneumonia should be with broad-spectrum antimicrobials and supportive measures (e.g., oxygen) as required. The principles of treatment of bacterial pneumonia in HIV-1–infected children are similar to those in immunocompetent patients. Revised WHO guidelines for management of pneumonia in HIV-1–infected children now advise ampicillin and gentamicin or ceftriaxone as first-line therapy for bacterial pneumonia (www.who.int). The use of case management guidelines for treatment of pneumonia, as contained in the WHO Integrated Management of Childhood Illness (IMCI) program, are effective for reducing pneumonia and all-cause mortality,[41] but they require adaptation for use in high HIV prevalence areas.[2]

Immunization with conjugate vaccines provides protection against specific bacterial infections. Although the efficacy of pneumococcal vaccine (PCV) for prevention of invasive pneumococcal disease and pneumonia is lower in HIV-1–infected children compared to uninfected children, the overall burden of disease prevented is much greater among HIV-1–infected children because of the higher burden of pneumococcal disease.[33,42] Thus the overall vaccine-attributable reduction in invasive pneumococcal disease was almost 60 times higher in HIV-1–infected children compared to uninfected children, while the reduction in pneumonia was 15-fold greater.[43] As most of the pneumococcal serotypes traditionally associated with antimicrobial resistance are included in PCV, vaccination has also been associated with a reduction in infections with antimicrobial-resistant pneumococci.[42] Pneumococcal vaccination is indicated for HIV-1–infected children according to the regular immunization schedule.[44] The long-term efficacy of PCV wanes in HIV-infected children who are not on HAART. Vaccine efficacy against invasive disease declined from 65% 2.3 years postvaccination to 39% by 6 years of age in HIV-1–infected children in the absence of a booster dose, while efficacy was maintained in HIV-1–uninfected individuals. Re-immunization after 3 to 5 years is therefore recommended in children not on HAART.[45]

The Haemophilus influenzae type b (Hib) conjugate vaccine also has reduced efficacy in HIV-1–infected children compared to HIV-1–uninfected children who are not on HAART.[46] However, similar to PCV, a substantial proportion of immunized HIV-infected children will be protected from Hib-related pneumonia and invasive disease because of the increased disease burden in HIV-infected children. HIV-1–infected children should therefore be immunized with Hib vaccine according to the routine childhood immunization schedule. In resource-poor countries, where nutritional deficiencies are common, supplementation with vitamin A and zinc conferred additional protection against pneumonia in HIV-1–infected children.[47,48]

In the pre-HAART era, intravenous immune globulin (IVIG) was effective in reducing serious bacterial infections in children with symptomatic HIV-1 infection, but this occurred only in those children not receiving trimethoprim-sulfamethoxazole (TMP-SMX) prophylaxis.[49] IVIG is therefore currently recommended only in HIV-1–infected children in combination with antiretroviral agents only for those with hypogammaglobinemia (IgG <400 mg/dL), or those who fail to form antibodies to common antigens.[44]

Tuberculosis

The incidence of tuberculosis (TB) has increased in parallel with the HIV epidemic. The two diseases are strongly related; HIV predisposes to TB disease while infection with Mycobacterium tuberculosis worsens HIV-associated immunosuppression and hastens progression to AIDS. In one report from Zambia, the HIV seroprevalence rate in children with TB disease was 55.8% compared to 9.6% in a control population at the same hospital.[50] Children with HIV-1 infection are likely to be in contact with HIV-1–infected adults with TB and therefore are more susceptible to TB infection and disease. Moreover, HIV-infected children progress more rapidly to disease and disseminated illness following mycobacterial infection. Mortality from TB is higher in HIV-1–infected children than uninfected children, with co-infected children having a poorer clinical and radiologic response to treatment.[51] Because of the association of TB and HIV-1 infection, children presenting with TB disease should be tested for HIV infection.

The clinical manifestations of TB in HIV-1-infected children are similar to those in uninfected children, with pulmonary TB (PTB) occurring predominantly. However, disease in HIV-1–infected children may be more severe, and extrapulmonary disease (e.g., military disease or TB meningitis) may occur more commonly than in HIV-1–uninfected children.[52] Clinical presentation of PTB includes chronic cough and failure to thrive, but PTB frequently may present as an acute pneumonia. Chest radiographic changes are nonspecific for TB, and interpretation is subject to wide interobserver variation; however the presence of lymphadenopathy, cavitary disease, or a miliary pattern may suggest Mycobacterium tuberculosis disease (Fig. 63-2).[53] The use of scoring systems for diagnosis of PTB perform poorly with wide variability especially in HIV-1–infected children.[54]

Annual screening of HIV-infected children for M. tuberculosis infection is recommended using the tuberculin skin test in children who have a negative test. A reaction greater than 5 mm is considered positive.[55] However, the sensitivity

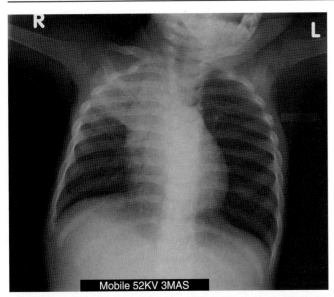

FIGURE 63-2. Chest radiograph of an HIV-infected child with culture confirmed tuberculosis. Note the marked tracheal and right bronchial compression by lymphadenopathy and the right upper lobe consolidation.

Mobile 52KV 3MAS

of skin testing is much reduced in HIV-1–infected children compared to uninfected children because of anergy; a blood interferon (IFN) gamma assay has a higher sensitivity and specificity for diagnosis of *M. tuberculosis* infection in HIV-1–infected children.[56] These measure IFN-gamma release from lymphocytes after stimulation with *M. tuberculosis*–specific antigens. Two commercially produced FDA-approved assays have been developed: T-Spot and Quantiferon Gold. However, discordance between skin test and IF results has been reported, and neither can distinguish infection from disease.[57]

If PTB is suspected in an HIV-1–infected child with a pulmonary infiltrate, specimens for microbiologic confirmation should be obtained. Bacteriologic confirmation of PTB in infants and children is underutilized, especially in hospitalized children. Examination of expectorated sputum is the recommended initial test performed to diagnose TB in the older child who can produce sputum. In children who cannot expectorate, sputum induction using 3% to 5% hypertonic saline has been shown to be effective and safe, even in infants, with a yield that is higher than gastric lavage for culture confirmation.[58] In addition, use of induced sputum has been shown to be useful and effective for microbiologic confirmation of TB in young children in community-based studies.[59,60] At least two specimens should be obtained, as a second specimen increases the microbiologic yield by approximately 20%.[58] The availability of rapid PCR-based molecular methods (Xpert MTB/RIF [Xpert]) for detection of *M. tuberculosis* enables rapid diagnosis of TB and detection of drug resistance on a sputum specimen. Xpert has a reported sensitivity of approximately 75% in children, with a specificity of approximately 99%. The WHO has endorsed Xpert as the first-line investigation to replace smear microscopy as the initial diagnostic test for suspected HIV-associated TB or multidrug-resistant (MDR) PTB in children and adults (www.who.int). The potential to rapidly make a microbiologic diagnosis at the point

of care including rapid identification of drug resistance makes the use of sputum induction in children even more imperative. The organism can be isolated from BAL or from lung tissue obtained by biopsy; however, the evidence suggests that the yield for *M. tuberculosis* is higher from gastric lavage compared to BAL.[61,62]

Empiric therapy for pulmonary TB in HIV-1–infected children should include 4 drugs (INH, rifampicin, pyrazinamide, and either ethambutol or streptomycin) daily for a 2-month induction period followed by 4 months of daily isoniazid and rifampin. Modification of therapy should be made based on susceptibility testing. Higher drug doses than have been previously used are now recommended. The minimum duration of treatment is 6 months, with some experts recommending up to 9 months, especially in severely immunocompromised children who are at increased risk of TB relapse.[44,63] Adjunctive corticosteroids are recommended for endobronchial disease with bronchial obstruction at a dose of 1 to 2 mg/kg/day tapered over 6 to 8 weeks.

For children on HAART, the antiretroviral regimen should provide optimal TB and HIV therapy and minimize potential toxicity and drug interactions. Rifampicin is compatible with all nucleoside reverse transcriptase inhibitors (NRTIs), therefore two NRTIs should be used as the backbone of antiretroviral therapy. However, rifampicin induces hepatic Cytochrome P450 enzymes and reduces the levels of some antiretroviral agents, particularly the protease inhibitors (PIs) and, to a lesser extent, the nonnucleoside reverse transcriptase inhibitors (NNRTIs). Therefore, rifampicin should preferably be used with an NRTI-based regimen rather than with a PI-based regimen. For children older than 3 years of age, two NRTIs with the NNRTI efavirenz is recommended. For children younger than 3 years of age, two NRTIs with the NNRTI nevirapine may be used. Alternatively, if a PI is used, a boosted regimen (e.g., additional ritonavir boosting with lopinavir/ritonavir) is recommended.[64] Adding additional ritonavir to lopinavir/ritonavir sufficient to achieve milligram-for-milligram parity may achieve adequate lopinavir levels, but doubling the dose of lopinavir/ritonovir is ineffective.[64,65] Rifabutin is a less potent inducer of the P450 enzymes and is therefore a suitable alternative to rifampicin, but there is limited experience with its use in children. For a child who is not yet on HAART, the decision when to initiate antiretroviral therapy depends on the child's clinical and immunologic condition. HAART may be deferred for children with mild immunosuppression. Deferred HAART initiated after 2 to 4 weeks of TB therapy reduces the risk of immune reconstitution inflammatory syndrome (IRIS). IRIS is discussed in detail later in the chapter.

For MDR PTB, a minimum of three drugs to which the organism is susceptible should be given. Streptomycin, cycloserine, or ethionamide may be substituted for ethambutol (see Chapter 33). In children with MDR TB (isoniazid- and rifampin-resistant), regimens should be individualized based on the resistance pattern of the organism from the child or source case. Daily therapy should be given for at least 12 months. Second-line drugs include clarithromycin, azithromycin, and ciprofloxacin. Directly observed therapy should be used when possible to ensure adherence to medication.

Primary INH prophylaxis for HIV-1–infected children living in a high TB prevalence area has been reported to reduce mortality by approximately 50% and TB incidence by approximately 70% in the setting of limited access to HAART.[66] The impact in children established on HAART is less clear, but further study suggests that INH prophylaxis may reduce TB incidence in such children, even when they are taking HAART.[67] The WHO has recently issued a revised policy for INH prophylaxis in HIV-1–infected children, advising use in high TB prevalence areas in children who are older than 1 year. The optimal duration of prophylaxis is unknown, but extended use appears safe and effective; WHO policy now recommends prophylaxis for up to 3 years in high TB prevalence areas.

Secondary prophylaxis should be given to all HIV-1–infected children (irrespective of the tuberculin skin test or interferon gamma test) following exposure to a close contact with TB, once TB disease has been excluded in the child. INH prophylaxis is given for 6 to 9 months. If the source case has an INH-resistant strain, rifampicin should be used for prophylaxis. If the strain is MDR, then two drugs to which the strain is susceptible should be used.[44]

BCG vaccine is contraindicated in HIV-1–infected children because of the high risk of developing disseminated disease and of death.[68] Key to TB control in HIV-1–infected children is adequate public health measures with good contact and source tracing and adherence to medication regimens. In addition, integrating TB and HIV services and the use of HAART are essential to reducing the TB caseload.

Mycobacterium Avium Complex

Mycobacterium avium complex (MAC) is ubiquitous in the environment and is found in water, soil, and dairy products. Before the HIV epidemic, MAC infrequently caused disease. In contrast, MAC was a common opportunistic infection in HIV-1–infected children in the pre-HAART era. Clinically, disease results either from localized infection or from disseminated disease. Localized disease includes cervical adenitis, pneumonitis, hepatic dysfunction, and abscesses. In HIV-1–infected patients, respiratory symptoms are not a prominent feature, but tachypnea and chronic lung infiltrates may be present. The importance of the organism in the bronchial secretions is unclear, but it most likely reflects disseminated disease rather than pulmonary infection. Symptoms caused by disseminated MAC infection are nonspecific including fever, weight loss, night sweats, cachexia, and diarrhea. None of 22 children with MAC in one series of children with AIDS had respiratory symptoms.[69] Children with MAC were older and had lower CD4+ cell counts than non-MAC children. Patients with disseminated MAC have a poor prognosis.[70] Of children who died in one report, 42% had disseminated MAC, and in 24% it was the underlying cause of death.[28]

Recommendations for prophylaxis and therapy for disseminated MAC in patients with HIV have been published.[44] A minimum of two agents is recommended to minimize the development of resistant strains. Treatment should include either azithromycin or clarithromycin with ethambutol as a second drug. For disseminated disease, a third or fourth drug (clofazimine, rifabutin, rifampin, ciprofloxacin, or amikacin) may be added. Improved immunologic status is essential to controlling MAC infection; HAART should be initiated in children who are not on antiretroviral therapy. The optimal timing of HAART is unclear; at least 2 weeks of antimycobacterial therapy is recommended prior to starting HAART to minimize the potential for IRIS.[44]

Primary prophylaxis with clarithromycin or azithromycin is recommended for severely immunosuppressed children with CD4+ cell counts <50/μL if older than 6 years of age, <75/μL if 2 to 6 years of age, CD4+ <500/μL if 1 to 2 years of age, and <750/μL if younger than 1 year of age.[44] Prophylaxis may be discontinued in children older than 2 years of age who are stable on HAART for 6 months or longer and who have sustained immune recovery as indicated by CD4+ measurements.

◼ VIRAL INFECTION

Pneumonia associated with common viral pathogens (e.g., respiratory syncytial virus [RSV], influenza, parainfluenza, herpes simplex, human metapneumovirus, and adenovirus) occurs in HIV-1–infected children.[24,71-74] HIV–1-infected children with viral lower respiratory tract infection have more severe disease compared to uninfected children and are likely to develop pneumonia rather than bronchiolitis.[35] Prolonged duration of RSV antigen shedding for up to 90 days has been observed in HIV-1–infected children.[75] Concomitant bacterial or other opportunistic infections may occur. Measles virus and Varicella-zoster virus can cause severe pulmonary disease.[76] In a report from Cote d'Ivoire, Africa, measles giant cell pneumonia was more common in HIV-1-infected children older than 15 months of age compared with HIV-negative children.[77] Acyclovir or valacyclovir are the agents of choice for Varicella infection. HIV-1–infected children with influenza should be treated with a neuraminidase inhibitor such as oseltamivir for 5 days (ideally within 72 hours) of symptom onset, as this may reduce severity of disease and complications. High-dose vitamin A should be given to children with measles.

Cytomegalovirus (CMV) is a herpesvirus that can cause retinitis, encephalitis, colitis, and pneumonitis in HIV-1–infected patients. HIV-infected infants have higher rates of CMV acquired during the first 4 years of life compared with uninfected infants born to HIV-positive mothers.[78] CMV infection is more likely to occur in children with low CD4+ counts. Coinfection of HIV and CMV stimulates HIV replication and more rapid HIV disease progression.[79] CMV disease has been reduced through use of HAART. CMV is the second most commonly identified pathogen in postmortem studies of HIV-infected children dying from pneumonia, identified in around 20% of cases in contrast to HIV-uninfected children where the virus is uncommon.[80] However, CMV-pneumocystis coinfection was common, making it difficult to define the contribution of CMV to severity of disease. Antemortem diagnosis of CMV pneumonitis is difficult as isolation of CMV from respiratory secretions may represent infection but not disease; definitive diagnosis requires a lung biopsy. A study of HIV-1–infected South African infants hospitalized with severe pneumonia reported that approximately 70% of children had CMV viremia as detected by PCR, while 36% also had CMV identified in BAL fluid or induced sputum.[81] Children with CMV-associated pneumonia had a 2.5-fold higher mortality than those without CMV pneumonia, despite treatment with ganciclovir in most. However, this association was not evident when adjusting for severe immunosuppression, indicating that CMV pneumonia may be a marker of severe immunosuppression. The presence or absence of CMV with PCP made no difference in the short-term outcome or long-term survival in adults and children in a retrospective review of cases.[82,83]

Histologically, alveolar macrophages, type II pneumocytes, bronchial and bronchiolar epithelial cells, and capillary endothelial cells may manifest cytomegaly and nuclear and cytoplasmic inclusions. The degree of interstitial pneumonitis varies because of concomitant infections. Ganciclovir should be used for treatment of CMV pneumonia and oral valganciclovir may be substituted once clinical improvement has occurred for a total of 6 to 8 weeks of therapy. To prevent recurrence, prophylactic valganciclovir should be given to children with severe immunsuppression. Initiation of HAART is crucial to contain CMV infection and prevent recurrence of disease; prophylaxis may be discontinued once sustained immune reconstitution has been achieved with HAART.

Strategies to prevent other viral infections are available. Yearly inactivated influenza vaccine should be given to children 6 months of age and older. HIV-1–infected children mount antibody responses to influenza vaccination, but antibody titers are lower than in HIV-negative controls.[84] Varicella and measles vaccines are recommended for children who are not severely immunocompromised. Passive immunization should be given to children who are exposed to measles with intramuscular immunoglobulin within 6 days of exposure. Postexposure prophylaxis with human Varicella immune globulin (VariZIG) or Varicella-zoster immune globulin (VZIG) should be given to unvaccinated children or those who are moderate or severely immunosuppressed within 96 hours of a close contact with a person who has chickenpox.

PNEUMOCYSTIS JIROVECII PNEUMONIA

Pneumocystis jirovecii (previously Pneumocystis carinii) was originally classified as a protozoan but is now regarded as a fungus. Two morphological forms of the organism are found in infected lungs: thin-walled single-nucleated trophozoites adherent to type I pneumocytes and thick-walled cysts containing four to eight single-nucleated sporozoites. The organism attaches to the alveolar epithelium, resulting in desquamation of alveolar cells. As the infection progresses, a diffuse desquamative alveolitis ensues, and the alveoli become filled with a foamy exudate consisting of alveolar macrophages and cysts containing sporozoites. Interstitial inflammation becomes evident.

P. jirovecii is the most common pathogen identified in HIV-1–infected infants with pneumonia who are not on prophylaxis or HAART.[85,86] The incidence is highest in the first year of life, peaking at 3 to 6 months of age. The incidence during the first year of life in the pre-HAART era was estimated to range from 10% to 42% in antemortem studies[85-87] and up to 52% in postmortem studies.[51,77,80,88-91] Clinical features include acute onset of cough, fever, tachypnea, and hypoxia. Normal, decreased breath sounds or crackles may be present on auscultation; hypoxia may be severe. A high plasma HIV RNA load strongly predicts PCP; CD4+ measures may be less useful, especially in young children. Approximately one quarter of children younger than 12 months of age had CD4+ counts >1500 cells/mm[3] at the time of PCP diagnosis.[92,93] However, a rapid rate of decline in CD4+ is associated with the development of PCP in children, and low CD4+ counts in older children are associated with PCP.[25]

There is a high rate of respiratory failure and need for mechanical ventilation among children with PCP. Early reported experience indicated a mortality rate exceeding 40% with the initial episode and the majority surviving less than a year subsequent to the episode.[86,94,95] The survival rate in HIV-infected children not on HAART following PCP is lower than with other disease manifestations.[92] A possible explanation for decreased survival after PCP is that the presence of P. jirovecii can increase HIV replication. It has been demonstrated that HIV production by alveolar lymphocytes obtained from BAL fluid is increased during PCP.[96] Alternatively, acquiring PCP may simply be a marker for poorer immunity and progression of disease.

The usual laboratory findings with PCP include a normal white blood cell count, an elevated lactic dehydrogenase (LDH), and normal immunoglobulin G (IgG). LDH levels >1000 IU/L are associated with PCP but are not specific.[24] The most common changes on chest radiographs are increased lung volumes, diffuse bilateral opacification, or reticulonodular infiltrates most prominent in the perihilar region and extending peripherally (Fig. 63-3).[97] Air bronchograms, focal infiltrates, a normal radiograph, pneumothorax, pulmonary interstitial emphysema, and pneumatoceles have also been described.

Diagnosis of PCP relies on the identification of the organism from bronchial washings, sputum, or lung tissue. BAL with fiberoptic bronchoscopy is a reliable method for establishing the diagnosis.[71] In intubated patients, instillation of 2 to 3 aliquots of 5 to 10 mL saline into the endotracheal tube followed by suctioning also provides a high yield. Sputum induction with 3% saline generated by an ultrasonic nebulizer can be useful for diagnosis.[40,98] The diagnostic yield using this technique is variable and is dependent upon the experience of those collecting and interpreting the specimen as well as the diagnostic test. Nasopharyngeal aspirates have been used to identify P. jirovecii, but the yield is lower than with induced sputum using staining methods.[40,86] Upper respiratory tract secretions (nasopharyngeal aspirate) provide a similar yield to lower respiratory secretions (BAL or induced sputum) when PCR based diagnosis is used.[99]

Methenamine silver, toluidine blue O, and fluorescein-conjugated monoclonal antibody are stains that identify the thick-walled cysts of P. jirovecii. Fluorescein

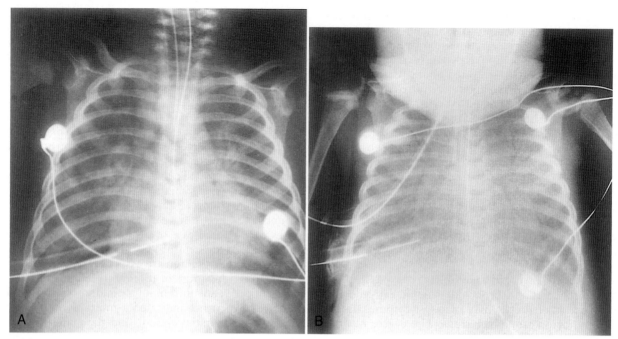

FIGURE 63-3. Chest radiograph of a 3-month-old infant presenting with *Pneumocystis jirovecii* pneumonia. **A,** The initial radiograph shows a bilateral infiltrate most prominent in the perihilar region. **B,** A chest radiograph taken 1 week later shows progression of disease with opacification of both lung fields.

staining is more sensitive than other staining methods. Trophozoite forms are identified with Giemsa stain or modified Wright-Giemsa stain. Much higher sensitivity is reported for PCR-based diagnosis compared to immunofluorescence.[99,100,101]

High-dose intravenous TMP-SMX is the treatment of choice for PCP. The conventional dose is trimethoprim 15-20 mg/kg/day and sulfamethoxazole 75-100 mg/kg/day for 21 days. Oral treatment can be given to complete the 21-day course when there is clinical improvement or if disease is mild. Revised WHO management guidelines recommend empiric therapy with TMP-SMX in HIV-infected or exposed infants with pneumonia (http://whqlibdoc.who.int/publications/2010/9789241548083_eng.pdf).

A clinical response is usually observed in 5 to 7 days, although deterioration in the patient's condition may occur in the first few days of therapy. Side effects to TMP-SMX include rashes and thrombocytopenia. An alternative treatment for PCP is pentamidine administered intravenously or intramuscularly (4 mg/kg/dose once daily) if the TMP-SMX is not well tolerated or there does not appear to be a response after 1 week of treatment with TMP-SMX. The intramuscular route is painful and can cause sterile abscesses, so it should be avoided if possible. Side effects from pentamidine include pancreatitis, renal dysfunction, and both hyperglycemia and hypoglycemia. Other alternatives include atovaquone, dapsone with trimethoprim, trimetrexate glucuronate with leucovorin, and clindamycin with primaquine.[44]

A National Institutes of Health consensus panel has recommended that corticosteroids be used as an adjunct to therapy in hypoxic adults with PCP based on studies showing improved survival and decreased incidence of respiratory failure.[102] Moderate to severe infection has been defined for this purpose as partial pressure of oxygen in arterial blood (PaO_2) <70 mm Hg in room air or an alveolar-arterial oxygen gradient more than 35 mm Hg. Good controlled clinical trials using corticosteroids in children with PCP have not been conducted, but uncontrolled data suggest that corticosteroids are beneficial[103] at a dose of 1 mg/kg/dose twice daily for 5 to 7 days, followed by a tapering dose over the next 7 to 12 days.[104] The reliability of extrapolation from adult studies is limited because of the immaturity of the child's immune system. In addition, PCP usually is a primary infection in infants, whereas PCP may represent reactivation in adults.

Early treatment with HAART and use of PCP prophylaxis has had a dramatic effect on reducing the incidence of the disease. Because of the high mortality and morbidity associated with PCP, prevention should be the primary objective. Prophylaxis is highly effective in preventing PCP. Guidelines for prophylaxis for PCP prophylaxis for children infected with or prenatally exposed to HIV are shown in Table 63-4. Prophylaxis for PCP is recommended in all infants born to HIV-1–infected mothers beginning at 4 to 6 weeks of age. Prophylaxis can be stopped once HIV-1 infection in the infant has been excluded if breast feeding is not occurring. For HIV-1–infected children, prophylaxis should continue throughout the first year of life. Discontinuation of PCP prophylaxis should be considered for HIV-1–infected children when, after receiving HAART for at least 6 months, the CD4+ percentage is ≥15% or the CD4+ count is ≥200 cells/μL for those older than 6 years of age and the CD4+ percentage is ≥15% or the CD4+ percentage is ≥500 cells/μL for children 1 to 5 years of age for more than 3 consecutive months. The same criteria can be used in patients who have experienced an episode of PCP if older than 1 year of age.

TMP-SMX is the drug of choice for prophylaxis. The recommended regimen is 150 mg TMP/m²/day with 750 mg SMZ/m²/day administered orally in divided doses twice a day three times per week on consecutive days.

TABLE 63-4 CDC GUIDELINES FOR PCP PROPHYLAXIS FOR HIV-EXPOSED AND HIV-INFECTED CHILDREN

AGE	PCP PROPHYLAXIS
Birth to 4-6 weeks, HIV exposed	No
4-6 weeks to 4 months, HIV exposed	Yes
4-12 months	
HIV infected or indeterminate	Yes
HIV exposed, not infected	No
1-5 years, HIV infected	CD4+ count <500 cells/μL or CD4+ % <15%
≥5 years, HIV infected	CD4+ count <200 cell/μL or CD4% <15%

CDC, Centers for Disease Control and Prevention; *HIV,* human immunodeficiency virus; *PCP,* pneumocystis pneumonia.

Alternatively, prophylaxis can be given 7 days a week. TMP-SMX prophylaxis may also be effective for reducing bacterial infections; daily therapy is associated with a lower incidence of bacteremia than thrice-weekly therapy.[105] If TMP-SMX is not tolerated, alternative prophylactic regimens include dapsone 2 mg/kg (not to exceed 100 mg) administered orally once daily or atovaquone 30 mg/kg once daily for children 1 to 3 months of age and older than 24 months of age and 45 mg/kg for infants 4 to 24 months of age. In children older than 5 years of age who cannot take TMP-SMX, dapsone, or atovaquone, aerosolized pentamidine 300 mg administered via inhaler once monthly is recommended.

FUNGAL INFECTIONS

Opportunistic fungal infections can cause severe pulmonary disease in children with HIV-1 infection, but the number of reported cases is small. The most common infections are with *Candida* spp., *Cryptococcus neoformans, Histoplasma capsulatum, Coccidiodes immitis,* and *Penicillium marneffei.* Dissemination of infection is common, and treatment is difficult. Constitutional symptoms (e.g., weight loss and fever) may reflect extrapulmonary involvement.

Cryptococcus usually presents as meningitis, but it can involve the lungs and cause interstitial pneumonia.[106] *Histoplasma capsulatum* most commonly affects the lungs but is likely to become disseminated in HIV-1–infected patients.[107,108] Standard serologic tests can be positive for both coccidiomycosis and histoplasmosis, but false-negative results occur in the most profoundly immunocompromised patients.[109] Skin testing is not useful because of problems with anergy and lack of standardization of most fungal skin test preparations. Cultures of bone marrow, cerebrospinal fluid, and lymph node or lung biopsy

can make the diagnosis. *Candida* spp. are often found in the oropharynx and esophagus in HIV-1–infected children. Tracheobronchial candidiasis and pulmonary infection are less common. Isolation of *Candida* from BAL fluid most likely represents an oropharyngeal contaminant because pulmonary infection is rarely confirmed on lung biopsy. Tissue invasion should be demonstrated on bronchial or lung biopsy to confirm the diagnosis.

Aspergillus infection has been reported in patients with HIV-1 infection. It occurs late in the course of HIV-1 infection and usually follows corticosteroid use or neutropenia.[110] Aspergilloma and invasive cavitary aspergillosis have been described.[111,112] *Aspergillus* infection can cause formation of a fungal pseudomembrane resulting in severe airway obstruction.[113] Transmural and peribronchial extension of the infection occurs (Fig. 63-4). The most prominent symptoms are cough and fever. In the obstructive form, dyspnea is noted.

Amphotericin-B is the drug of choice for most life-threatening fungal infections. Alternative regimens include fluconazole and itraconazole. However, even with treatment, relapse and mortality is high. Some form of chronic suppressive therapy is often given following infection.

CHRONIC LUNG DISEASE

Chronic lung disease is common in HIV-infected children with increasing age, particularly in the absence of HAART.[114] A longitudinal birth cohort study reported a cumulative incidence of chronic radiographic lung changes in HIV-infected children of 33% by 4 years of age. The most common chronic radiologic changes were increased bronchovascular markings, reticular densities, and bronchiectasis. Chronic changes were associated with lower CD4+ cell counts and higher viral loads; radiologic resolution of these may reflect declining immunity. Parenchymal consolidation persisting for 3 or more months was present in 8% of HIV-1–infected children, nodular changes persisting 3 or more months in 8%, and reticular changes or increased bronchovascular markings persisting for 6 or more months in 14%. These radiographic changes were associated with an increased frequency of clubbing, crackles, tachypnea, and decreased oxygen saturation. Mortality in the HIV-1–infected children with chronic radiographic changes was not different from mortality in HIV-1–infected children without these changes.

The spectrum of chronic HIV-associated lung disease includes LIP, chronic infections, immune reconstitution inflammatory syndrome (IRIS), bronchiectasis, malignancies, and interstitial pneumonitis.

Lymphoid Interstitial Pneumonitis/ Pulmonary Lymphoid Hyperplasia

The most commonly reported chronic lung disease is LIP/PLH complex. The presence of this condition places an HIV-infected child in the moderately symptomatic category (Category B) of the CDC classification. A report from a prospective birth cohort pre-HAART indicated that chronic nodular densities were observed in 8% of

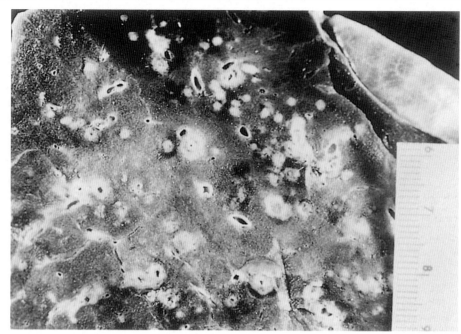

FIGURE 63-4. Cut section of lung from a 15-year-old with hemophilia and human immunodeficiency virus infection who developed airway obstruction from *Aspergillus* infection. Note the diffuse peribronchial and peribronchiolar cuffing. (From Pervez NK, Kleinerman J, Kattan M, et al. Pseudomembranous necrotizing bronchial aspergillosis. A variant of invasive aspergillosis in a patient with hemophilia and acquired immune deficiency syndrome. *Am Rev Respir Dis.* 1985;131:962.)

patients by 5 years of age.[114] In HIV-1–infected children 5 years of age or younger who died at home in Zimbabwe, 9% had LIP on autopsy.[37]

The pathology consists of a diffuse infiltration of lymphocytes in the interstitium and scattered nodules of mononuclear cells 0.5 mm in diameter. The mononuclear cells consist of lymphocytes, plasma cells, immunoblasts, and histiocytes. In LIP, the infiltration is diffuse throughout the parenchyma. In PLH, the infiltration is primarily adjacent to the bronchial and bronchiolar walls and consists of bronchial-associated lymphoid tissue hyperplasia (Fig. 63-5). The etiology of the abnormal lymphoproliferative response is unclear. The principal hypotheses are that lymphoproliferation is a response to the HIV alone or coinfection with another virus. Epstein-Barr viral DNA has been found in lung biopsies of children with LIP, and HIV RNA has been identified in the lungs of infants with LIP.[115-117] However, a causal relationship between EBV and LIP/PLH has not been confirmed.

The onset of LIP/PLH is insidious and the course slowly progressive. It usually becomes evident after the first year of life with a median age of onset of 2.5 to 3 years of age.[92] However, reticulonodular changes on chest radiographs may be observed before 12 months of age.[114] Cough or tachypnea may be present. Auscultation of the chest may be normal or reveal crackles and wheezes. Generalized lymphadenopathy, hepatosplenomegaly, clubbing, and parotid gland enlargement are commonly associated physical findings. Admission rates for lower respiratory tract illness are higher for children with LIP/PLH compared to HIV-1–infected children without LIP/PLH.[118]

The chest radiograph typically shows a bilateral diffuse interstitial reticulonodular pattern with or without hilar adenopathy.[114,119] Elevated serum immunoglobulin levels are associated with LIP/PLH.[24] Serum IgG levels >2500 mg/dL are strongly associated with LIP/PLH. Lung biopsy establishes the diagnosis. However a presumptive diagnosis of LIP/PLH can be made based on the clinical findings and the typical reticulonodular radiographic pattern lasting more than 2 months without another documented cause. In a longitudinal study, resolution of the chronic nodular radiographic findings occurred in 61% of children.[114] The radiographic resolution was not associated with any clinical improvement. Thus radiographic resolution of nodular changes may be an indicator of immunologic deterioration.

Treatment of LIP/PLH is nonspecific. Inhaled bronchodilators may provide symptomatic relief. Oxygen is administered for hypoxemia. Although treatment of LIP/PLH with corticosteroids has been reported to improve hypoxemia in a small number of patients, controlled clinical trials have not been carried out.[120]

Some cases of LIP/PLH progress to a lymphoproliferative disorder characterized by polyclonal, polymorphic B-cell content without evidence of cellular atypia, necrosis, or prominent mitotic activity but with extranodal systemic and prominent pulmonary involvement (Fig. 63-6).[121] Some cases have progressed to malignant lymphoma.

CHRONIC INFECTION

Chronic lung disease may result from recurrent or persistent pneumonia caused by bacterial, mycobacterial, viral, fungal, or mixed infections. In reports from Africa, TB is one of the most common causes of chronic lung disease.[122] Localized or disseminated disease from *M. bovis* or the nontuberculous mycobacteria (NTM) (particularly *M. avium-intracellulare* complex) may also result in chronic disease. Chronic PCP infection can result in chronic interstitial disease or cysts.[123,124]

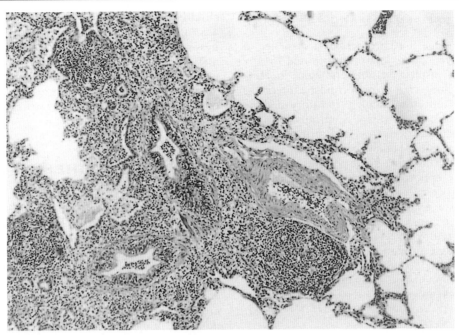

FIGURE 63-5. Lung biopsy from a child with pulmonary lymphoid hyperplasia. Note the interstitial and peribronchiolar lymphoid infiltration.

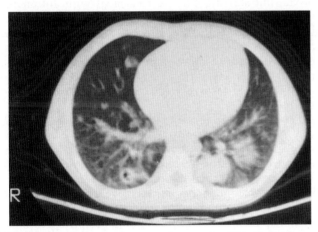

FIGURE 63-6. Computed tomography scan of a child with a polyclonal lymphoproliferative disorder. Nodular infiltrates are present bilaterally with large nodules evident in the left lower lobe.

BRONCHIECTASIS

Bronchiectasis is an important cause of chronic infiltrates and atelectasis on chest radiographs. This should be suspected when radiographs show persistent abnormalities in the same lobe for more than 6 months. The diagnosis can be confirmed with chest high-resolution computed tomography scan (c-HRCT) demonstrating dilated tubular structures. Bronchiectasis with HIV-1 infection has been associated with LIP.[125] It is possible that the lymphocytic infiltration into the mucosa and submucosa of the bronchiole leads to destruction, fibrosis, atelectasis, and subsequently, bronchiectasis. Other mechanisms of development of bronchiectasis include acute or chronic infection, a direct effect of HIV on the lung, and persistent atelectasis. Development of bronchiectasis is associated with the severity of immunosuppression. A retrospective review of 749 HIV-infected children (mostly before the availability of HAART) found that all 19 who developed bronchiectasis were CDC immunological category stage 3.[126] Therapy includes physiotherapy and aggressive treatment of intercurrent infections.

IMMUNE RECONSTITUTION INFLAMMATORY SYNDROME

With increasing use of HAART, an immune reconstitution inflammatory syndrome (IRIS) associated with mycobacterial infection and with other opportunistic infections (e.g., CMV) has been reported.[127] IRIS may occur weeks to months after initiation of HAART therapy and may result either from unrecognized mycobacterial infection or from a florid immune response directed against a mycobacterial antigen in those already on therapy.[127] IRIS has been described with different mycobacterial species including *M. tuberculosis, M. bovis,* or MAC infection.[128–131] IRIS is increasingly being recognized in HIV-infected children from high TB prevalence areas.[128,129,131] Clinically, IRIS is characterized by a paradoxical worsening in signs with increasing lymphadenopathy and new clinical and radiological respiratory signs.[128,129,131] The tuberculin skin test may become positive, and chest radiographs may show development of lymphadenopathy or new infiltrates. IRIS must be distinguished from other infections, MDR TB, or nonresponse to TB therapy caused by nonadherence. To minimize the risk of IRIS, HIV-infected children with confirmed or probable TB should be treated with anti-tuberculosis drugs for a few weeks before commencing HAART, where possible.[128] When IRIS develops in a child who was unknown to have TB, therapy for TB should be initiated. If lymphadenopathy or respiratory signs are particularly severe, oral corticosteroids may be beneficial, although there are no controlled trials in children.[128]

DIFFUSE ALVEOLAR DAMAGE

Diffuse alveolar damage (DAD) describes a sequence of events following severe acute lung injury caused by any one of a variety of insults. Possible etiologies in HIV-infected patients include viral or opportunistic infections such as *P. jirovecii* infection, adult respiratory distress syndrome, and oxygen toxicity.[132,133] Clinically, DAD is characterized by respiratory distress and diffuse pulmonary infiltrates. This entity should be suspected if there is persistent hypoxia following acute respiratory failure from PCP or other opportunistic infections. Recurrent episodes of respiratory failure may represent viral infections superimposed on a lung with DAD.

The early exudative stage of DAD occurring over 2 or 3 days is characterized by alveolar and interstitial edema and hyaline membrane formation. This progresses to a proliferative stage after one week in which there is hyperplasia of type II pneumocytes, desquamation of alveolar lining cells, and thickening of the interstitium with fibroblast proliferation.

PULMONARY TUMORS

Children with HIV have an increased risk of malignancy, occurring in 2.5% of children with AIDS in the United States[64] Non-Hodgkins lymphoma (NHL) is most common, followed by Kaposi's sarcoma (KS), leiomyosarcoma, and Hodgkin's lymphoma.[64] Primary NHL may arise in a lymph node or be extranodal. AIDS-related NHL may occur in almost any extranodal site including the lungs. In addition, pulmonary disease may result from dissemination from a primary focus.

In African HIV-infected children, KS is the most common AIDS-defining malignancy, probably due to the prevalence of human herpesvirus 8 infection (HHV-8).[134,135] In high-income settings, most cases of KS in the pediatric age group have occurred in adolescents.[136] KS lesions may produce upper airway obstruction. Pulmonary dissemination may result in chronic progressive dyspnea, cough, and fever; hemoptysis may occur with endobronchial lesions. Chest radiograph abnormalities include bilateral adenopathy, perihilar infiltrates, pleural effusion, or combinations of interstitial, alveolar, or nodular patterns.

Pulmonary tumors of smooth muscle origin in children have been reported. The airways, lungs, and pulmonary veins have been found to have nodular masses, which on biopsy have been leiomyoma and leiomyosarcoma.[137] Pseudolymphomas and lymphomas have also been reported.

UPPER AIRWAY DISEASE

Lymphoid proliferation occurs with HIV-1 infection, and it is therefore not surprising that tonsillar and adenoidal hypertrophy and pharyngeal infiltration is observed. This has resulted in upper airway obstruction in children with HIV-1 infection. It is unclear if upper airway obstruction occurs with greater frequency in HIV-1–infected children compared to uninfected children. Lymphoid infiltration of the epiglottis has also been described with gradual onset of drooling and dysphagia. Biopsy showed acute and chronic inflammation, with granulation tissue and lymphoid follicles in the submucosa.[138] *Candida* supraglottitis has been described with a slowly progressive course and lesions on the epiglottis, arytenoid cartilages, and aryepiglottic folds.[139]

APPROACH TO THE HIV-1–INFECTED PATIENT WITH RESPIRATORY SYMPTOMS

Fever and tachypnea are common presenting features in a child with HIV-1 infection. The likelihood of severe respiratory complications increases with decreasing CD4+ cell count. A chest radiograph, arterial blood gas or oxygen saturation, complete blood count, and respiratory and blood culture should be obtained in the HIV-infected child with acute respiratory symptoms. Mixed infections are common, and investigations for bacterial, viral, pneumocystis, fungal, or mycobacterial pathogens may be indicated.

A self-limited viral illness is likely if the child is normoxic, but starting empiric treatment with antimicrobials is warranted pending the results of cultures. A diffuse nodular infiltrate with hilar adenopathy in the absence of hypoxemia suggests LIP/PLH. Persistent lobar infiltrates of more than 6 months duration with normal oxygen saturation may be indicative of bronchiectasis. In such cases, c-HRCT is helpful in establishing the diagnosis.

If hypoxemia is present, PCP is more likely, particularly if the child has not received PCP prophylaxis. If there are barriers to obtaining a microbiologic diagnosis, treatment for presumptive PCP with TMP-SMX should be started. In addition, empiric treatment with a β-lactam is recommended for less severe pneumonia, and ampicillin and an aminoglycoside or a third-generation cephalosporin for severe pneumonia. Empiric treatment for CMV pneumonitis should be considered in children with severe pneumonia or when CMV is recovered from respiratory secretions and from a blood specimen. In areas of high TB prevalence, investigations for TB should be done including a tuberculin skin test; interferon gamma assay; and two induced sputum specimens for rapid molecular detection (if available), smear, and culture.

Ventricular dysfunction and cardiomyopathy have been observed in pediatric HIV-1 infection.[140] Therefore, it is important to exclude cardiac disease with congestive heart failure as a cause of respiratory symptoms.

SUMMARY

Respiratory diseases cause major morbidity and mortality in HIV-1–infected children, particularly in low- and middle-income countries. The spectrum of pulmonary diseases in industrialized and low- or middle-income countries is similar, but infectious complications (e.g., PCP, tuberculosis, and measles pneumonia) are more common in the latter. In low- or middle-income countries, underlying malnutrition may complicate the clinical outcome. General and specific preventive strategies are effective for reducing respiratory morbidity. Early use of HAART is highly effective for reducing the incidence of opportunistic infections, pulmonary morbidity, and mortality. Exposure to environmental tobacco smoke and indoor air pollution should be minimized. Attention to nutritional deficiencies can further decrease morbidity and mortality in HIV-1–infected children. Preventive interventions including immunization, and use of co-trimoxazole prophylaxis reduces the incidence of specific respiratory infections.

Suggested Reading

Bliss SJ, O'Brien KL, Janoff EN, et al. The evidence for using conjugate vaccines to protect HIV-infected children against pneumococcal disease. *Lancet Infect Dis.* 2008;8:67–80.

Calder D, Qazi S. Evidence behind the WHO guidelines: hospital care for children: What is the aetiology of pneumonia in HIV-infected children in developing countries? *J Trop Pediatr.* 2009;55:219–224.

Cotton MF, Wasserman E, Smit J, et al. High incidence of antimicrobial resistant organisms including extended spectrum beta-lactamase producing *Enterobacteriaceae* and methicillin-resistant *Staphylococcus aureus* in nasopharyngeal and blood isolates of HIV-infected children from Cape Town, South Africa. *BMC Infect Dis.* 2008;8:40.

Frigati LJ, Kranzer K, Cotton MF, et al. The impact of isoniazid preventive therapy and antiretroviral therapy on tuberculosis in children infected with HIV in a high tuberculosis incidence setting. *Thorax.* 2011;66:496–501.

Gona P, Van Dyke RB, Williams PL, et al. Incidence of opportunistic and other infections in HIV-infected children in the HAART era. *JAMA.* 2006;296:292–300.

Gray D, Zar HJ. Community acquired pneumonia in HIV-infected children: a global perspective. *Curr Opin Pulm Med.* 2010;16(3):208–216.

Kattan M, Platzker A, Mellins RB, et al. Respiratory diseases in the first year of life in children born to HIV-1-infected women. *Pediatr Pulmonol.* 2001;31:267–276.

Kovacs A, Schluchter M, Easley K, et al. Cytomegalovirus infection and HIV-1 disease progression in infants born to HIV-1-infected women. Pediatric Pulmonary and Cardiovascular Complications of Vertically Transmitted HIV Infection Study Group. *N Engl J Med.* 1999;341:77–84.

McNally LM, Jeena PM, Gajee K, et al. Effect of age, polymicrobial disease, and maternal HIV status on treatment response and cause of severe pneumonia in South African children: a prospective descriptive study. *Lancet.* 2007;369:1440–1451.

Mofenson LM, Brady MT, Danner SP, et al. Guidelines for the Prevention and Treatment of Opportunistic Infections among HIV-exposed and HIV-infected children: recommendations from CDC, the National Institutes of Health, the HIV Medicine Association of the Infectious Diseases Society of America, the Pediatric Infectious Diseases Society, and the American Academy of Pediatrics. *MMWR Recomm Rep.* 2009;58:1–166.

Morrow BM, Hsaio NY, Zampoli M, et al. Pneumocystis pneumonia in South African children with and without human immunodeficiency virus infection in the era of highly active antiretroviral therapy. *Pediatr Infect Dis J.* 2010;29:535–539.

Norton KI, Kattan M, Rao JS, et al. Chronic radiographic lung changes in children with vertically transmitted HIV-1 infection. *AJR.* 2001;176:1553–1558.

Shearer WT, Quinn TC, LaRussa P, et al. Viral load and disease progression in infants infected with human immunodeficiency virus type 1. Women and Infants Transmission Study Group. *N Engl J Med* 1997;336:1337–1342.

Shearer WT, Rosenblatt HM, Schluchter MD, et al. Immunologic targets of HIV infection: T cells. NICHD IVIG Clinical Trial Group, and the NHLBI P2C2 Pediatric Pulmonary and Cardiac Complications of HIV Infection Study Group. *Ann N Y Acad Sci* 1993;693:35–51.

Simonds RJ, Oxtoby MJ, Caldwell MB, et al. *Pneumocystis carinii* pneumonia among US children with perinatally acquired HIV infection. *JAMA.* 1993;270:470–473.

Zar HJ, Apolles P, Argent A, et al. The etiology and outcome of pneumonia in human immunodeficiency virus-infected children admitted to intensive care in a developing country. *Pediatr Crit Care Med.* 2001;2:108–112.

References

The complete reference list is available online at www.expertconsult.com

64 PEDIATRIC LUNG TRANSPLANTATION

Stuart Sweet, MD, PhD, and Blakeslee Noyes, MD

With reports of successful heart-lung and lung transplantation in adults in the early 1980s,[1,2] the application of lung transplantation to the pediatric population became an appealing prospect. Early reports of success in children undergoing lung transplantation[3-5] led to a marked increase in such procedures beginning in the early 1990s. Between 1986 and mid-2007, nearly 1100 lung transplantations and more than 500 heart-lung transplantations in patients younger than 17 years of age were reported to the Registry for the International Society for Heart and Lung Transplantation.[6] In these children, the number of lung transplant procedures performed annually over the past decade has varied between 60 and 80, though recent data suggest a plateau of approximately 70 performed per year. Historically, heart-lung transplantation was considered for patients with end-stage lung disease, with the relatively healthy native recipient heart considered for use in a "domino" transplant. Heart-lung transplant was also considered in patients with right ventricular failure associated with severe pulmonary hypertension. However, in the current era, heart-lung transplant is typically reserved for cases associated with left ventricular failure or congenital heart disease not amenable to surgical repair. Thus, the number of heart-lung transplants performed has dropped below 20 per year worldwide. Typically 30 to 35 centers report pediatric lung transplants, yielding a statistical average of two to three transplants per center annually. In reality, a few centers perform the majority of these procedures, while most centers perform very few.[6] The number of lung transplants performed yearly is far below the number of other solid-organ transplants such as heart, liver, and kidney transplantation. This relative paucity is likely due to multiple factors, including lower prevalence of end-stage pulmonary diseases in children, improved therapies for cystic fibrosis (CF) and pulmonary hypertension, significantly lower procurement rate of donor lungs, and the small number of pediatric lung transplant centers in the United States and worldwide.[7] Notwithstanding changes in the allocation of lung allografts (discussed later in the chapter), the mortality rate for pediatric candidates 1 to 11 years of age awaiting lung transplantation remains higher than that in adults, underscoring the need to expand the potential donor pool and perhaps the number of centers performing this procedure.[8]

INDICATIONS AND TIMING

Indications for lung transplantation in children have undergone considerable change in the last two decades as experience with this procedure has grown. Lung transplantation has been performed successfully, even in young infants with distinctly uncommon problems such as surfactant protein B deficiency or alveolar capillary dysplasia.[9,10] The most common diagnoses for which children are transplanted are shown in Figure 64-1 according to the age in years at time of transplantation. In children younger than 1 year of age, the most common indications are pulmonary hypertension, usually associated with congenital heart disease, other pulmonary vascular diseases, primarily pulmonary vein stenosis, and, rarely, alveolar capillary dysplasia. Disorders of surfactant metabolism include surfactant protein B and C deficiencies, and *ABCA3* transporter mutations. Less common indications include interstitial lung disease, bronchopulmonary dysplasia,[4] and pulmonary hypoplasia. In children 1 to 11 years of age, CF becomes the most common indication. In patients 12 to 17 years of age, nearly 70% of pediatric lung transplants are performed for CF patients. In children 1 to 11 years of age, disorders leading to pulmonary hypertension remain a common indication. The relative percentage of children with primary pulmonary hypertension coming to lung transplant has diminished significantly during the past decade, largely because of the introduction of effective medical therapies including prostaglandins (epoprostenol), PDE inhibitors (bosentan) and sildenafil.[6] Surprisingly, in spite of a steady increase in the median survival for CF, the relative percentage of children with CF receiving lung transplants has not changed appreciably in recent years.

Historically, timing of referral for lung transplant has been predicated on matching predictions of mortality with the anticipated waiting time for donor lungs. For example, studies in CF led to recommendations for referral for lung transplantation once the forced expired volume in 1 second (FEV$_1$) declined below 30% predicted.[11] Although more recent studies have attempted to add to these criteria,[12,13] none have improved significantly on the ability to predict waiting list mortality. Even in the best model, the positive predictive value is less than 50%.[12] In other diseases leading to lung transplant, criteria are less clear. Before committing a child to lung transplant, given absent or imperfect disease-specific criteria, most pediatric centers carefully consider multiple factors beyond lung function including growth and nutrition status, frequency of hospitalizations, and potential for improvement in overall quality of life.

During the past 5 years, listing practices for children older than 12 years of age and adults have been affected in the United States by the adoption in 2005 of the "Lung Allocation System" (LAS) by the Organ Procurement and Transplantation Network (OPTN).[14] Based on models of waiting list mortality and posttransplant survival, the new system attempts to allocate donor lungs to maximize the 1-year transplant survival benefit. The survival models

INDICATIONS FOR PEDIATRIC LUNG TRANSPLANTATION

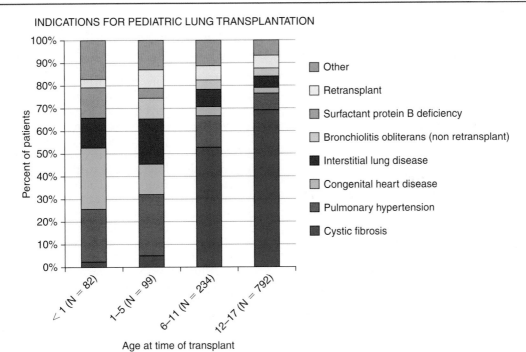

FIGURE 64-1. Indications for pediatric lung transplant. (Data adapted from Aurora P, Edwards LB, Christie JD, et al. Registry of the International Society for Heart and Lung Transplantation: Twelfth Official Pediatric Lung and Heart/Lung Transplantation Report—2009. *J Heart Lung Transplant*. 2009;28:1023-1030.)

are based on diagnosis, and other factors including age; height and weight; need for supplemental oxygen; pulmonary arterial pressures; 6-minute walk distance; and lung function. Since adoption of the LAS, waiting time and waiting list mortality have decreased in the United States.[8] However, it is not surprising that an increased number of sicker patients are receiving transplants and a significant proportion of those patients (primarily those requiring mechanical ventilation) have had poorer overall survival than historical lung transplant cohorts because the contribution of the waiting list mortality to the LAS is twice that of posttransplant survival.[15]

$$LAS = \text{posttransplant survival} - 2 \times \text{waiting list}$$
$$\text{survival, normalized to a 0-to-100 scale}$$

An important aspect of the LAS is the potential for serially collected data from patients listed for lung transplant to be used for refinement of the underlying models that generate the priority score. At the time of this writing, the OPTN Thoracic Committee is considering updates to the models based on more recent transplant cohorts and the addition of other data elements. For children younger than 12 years of age, in an effort to reduce waiting list mortality for younger children, lung allocation was modified in fall 2010 to create two urgency tiers, similar to the status one and two in heart transplant allocation. It is difficult to predict the long-term benefit of this change.

CONTRAINDICATIONS

As experience with pediatric lung transplant has grown, the number of absolute contraindications has declined, with most considered *relative* contraindications based

on each transplant center's experience and expertise (Table 64-1).[16] Absolute contraindications to pediatric lung transplantation include systemic disease affecting other organ systems, such as malignancy; HIV; hepatitis B or C; tuberculosis; or liver, renal, or left ventricular failure. In some transplant centers however, multiorgan transplantation (e.g., liver-lung transplantation) may be an option in selected patients with failure of an organ other than the lung. In CF patients, *B. cepacia* complex (BCC) organisms are often a concern. Initially, all BCC organisms were thought to lead to poor outcome after lung transplantation, but more recent analyses have suggested that only colonization with *B. cenocepacia* (formerly BCC, Genomovar III) and a related organism, *B. gladioli*, carries significant risk.[17-19] *B. cenocepacia* colonization remains an absolute contraindication to lung transplant at a significant percentage of pediatric centers. Infection or colonization with *Aspergillus*, atypical mycobacteria, or multiresistant organisms are relative contraindications in patients with CF. It is not uncommon for lung transplant candidates to present unique and complex challenges to the transplant center including malnutrition, diabetes, osteoporosis or osteopenia, vertebral compression fractures, and the use of systemic corticosteroids. These are considered relative, but not absolute, contraindications.

Prior pleurodesis—either chemical or surgical—is not a contraindication to transplant but may prolong the ischemic time because of excessive bleeding from the parietal pleura, particularly when cardiopulmonary bypass and attendant heparinization is employed.

Finally, psychosocial concerns for children, particularly nonadherence, can be particularly challenging, especially when the responsibility for adherence is shared with

Section X

TABLE 64-1 **CONTRAINDICATIONS TO PEDIATRIC LUNG TRANSPLANTATION**

ABSOLUTE	RELATIVE
Active malignancy within 2 years*	Pleurodesis
Sepsis	Renal insufficiency
Active tuberculosis	Markedly abnormal body mass index
Severe neuromuscular disease	Mechanical ventilation
Documented, refractory nonadherence	Scoliosis
Multiple organ dysfunction[†]	Poorly controlled diabetes mellitus
Acquired immunodeficiency syndrome	Osteoporosis
Hepatitis C with histologic liver disease	Chronic airway infection with multiply resistant organisms[‡] Fungal infection/colonization Hepatitis B surface antigen positive

*Some centers prefer a disease-free interval of 5 years.
[†]Consider heart-lung transplant with concomitant left ventricular insufficiency or irreparable congenital heart disease, liver-lung transplant with concomitant hepatic failure.
[‡]For some transplant centers, infection with *B. Cepacia* complex organisms, particularly genomovar III (*B. cenocepacia*), is an absolute contraindication.
Adapted from Faro A, Mallory GB, Visner GA, et al. American Society of Transplantation executive summary on pediatric lung transplantation. *Am J Transplant.* 2007;7:285-292.

the child's parents. Decisions about how to handle such cases—without creating the perception that the parent's misbehavior led to the child being denied the opportunity for transplant—must be an individualized, shared responsibility of both the referring center and the transplant center. For families in which nonadherence to a recommended treatment regimen is recognized, some centers recommend formulation of a contract between the referring physician and family that outlines the need for strict adherence to a treatment program over a 3- to 6-month period prior to evaluation/listing for lung transplant. In general, adherence concerns only become an absolute contraindication when they occur in combination with other medical risk factors, or after failure over time on the part of the child and family to meet a set of agreed-upon expectations for care and follow-up. In contrast, a significant psychiatric or mental health disorder in either the primary caregiver or the patient is considered an absolute contraindication to transplant.

SURGICAL TECHNIQUE

Potential donor lungs are evaluated using arterial blood gases, chest radiographs, airway cultures, and airway examination by bronchoscopy. The donor history is reviewed for signs and symptoms of acute viral infection. In addition, the donor is routinely screened for hepatitis A, B, and C; HIV; Varicella-zoster; cytomegalovirus (CMV); Epstein-Barr virus (EBV); and herpesvirus.[20]

In virtually all pediatric transplant procedures, cardiopulmonary bypass with heparinization is used for the implantation procedure. The surgical approach is via a bilateral anterolateral transsternal incision (i.e., the "clamshell" incision), which optimizes visualization and access to both pleural spaces. The great majority of children undergo bilateral sequential lung transplantation with telescoped bronchial-to-bronchial anastomoses. Pericardial or peribronchial lymphatic tissue from the donor and recipient is used to cover the anastomosis. This improves the blood supply to the anastomosis and may reduce the exposure of adjacent vascular structures to infection in the event of airway infection and subsequent dehiscence.[21,22] In patients with CF, careful attention to maintaining sterility of the donor allograft requires vigorous washing of the recipient trachea and bronchial stumps with an antimicrobial solution prior to implantation.

Heart-lung transplantation is rarely used in children in the United States at this time.[6] Even in the presence of marked right ventricular hypertrophy associated with pulmonary hypertension, successful bilateral lung transplantation is generally associated with resolution of right ventricular dysfunction.[23,24] In patients with pulmonary hypertension caused by a congenital heart defect, intracardiac repair of the anatomic defect may take place at the time of bilateral lung transplant, obviating the need for heart-lung transplantation.[25] Single-lung transplantation is used infrequently among children, and much less than in adults.[6]

Success with living-donor lobar lung transplantation was first reported by Starnes in 1994.[26] In this procedure, a right lower lobe from one healthy donor and a left lower lobe from another (generally a family member) are implanted in the recipient. Typically, this technique has been used in both adults and children in the setting of rapidly progressive respiratory failure when cadaveric lung allografts were judged unlikely to be available, or when further deterioration in clinical status would make the patient ineligible for deceased donor transplantation. Although living donor lung transplant has virtually disappeared in the United States since the introduction of the LAS, it is still used in Japan where access to donor organs suitable for children has been restricted.

Other strategies for increased availability of organs for children and other smaller recipients include donor downsizing using linear stapling devices or lobectomy and lobar transplant.[27]

POSTTRANSPLANT MANAGEMENT

Immunosuppressive Regimen

In the immediate preoperative period, triple-drug immunosuppression and directed antimicrobial therapy is begun. In virtually all circumstances, immunosuppression consists of a calcineurin inhibitor (either tacrolimus or cyclosporine [CSA]), a cell cycle inhibitor (azathioprine or mycophenolate mofetil [MMF]), and corticosteroids. There has been a trend in recent years toward the use of tacrolimus and MMF over cyclosporine and azathioprine. At the end of the first year, 70% of pediatric lung transplant recipients are on tacrolimus, and 55 percent are on

MMF.[6] Because lung transplant recipients have a higher risk for rejection episodes than other solid-organ transplant recipients, more intense immunosuppression regimens have been developed.[28] For example, the initial targets for trough levels for tacrolimus and cyclosporine are typically in a range of 10 to 20 ng/mL and 300 to 500 ng/mL, respectively. Initial dosing for prednisone is typically 0.5 to 1 mg/kg per day with the goal of 0.25 to 0.5 mg/kg per day by 3 to 4 months after transplant, depending on the clinical course. Nearly all patients remain on prednisone at 1 and 5 years posttransplant.[6] In addition, the use of induction immunotherapy at the time of transplant remains widely used in pediatric lung transplantation; recent data indicate that over 40% of patients receive either a polyclonal agent (anti-lymphocyte or antithymocyte globulin) or, more commonly, an IL-2 receptor antagonist (daclizumab or basiliximab).[6]

Antimicrobial Regimen

Most patients receive intravenous antibiotics before and after lung transplantation based on the most likely potential infecting organisms. Cultures from the donor may allow precise choices of antibiotics. In patients without CF, a single antibiotic with broad Gram-positive and Gram-negative coverage is typically used for 7 to 10 days posttransplant. In recipients with CF, their pretransplant sputum flora cultures help guide therapy; typically, such antimicrobial therapy is directed against Gram-negative organisms, commonly *Pseudomonas aeruginosa* and occasionally *Achromobacter* spp. More recently, vancomycin is included to cover methicillin-resistant *Staphylococcus aureus* (MRSA), which is often isolated from children with CF and advanced lung disease. In CF patients in whom *Aspergillus fumigatus* has been found, many transplant centers use voriconazole or anidulofungin postoperatively and, in some circumstances, aerosolized amphotericin, oral itraconazole, or oral voriconazole.[7] Prophylaxis against *Pneumocystis carinii* is begun shortly after transplant with trimethoprim/sulfamethoxazole (TMP/SMX) and is administered three times weekly. In patients unable to tolerate TMP/SMX, nebulized pentamidine, oral atovaquone, or dapsone are alternatives. Oral nystatin is begun in the early posttransplant period to reduce the likelihood of candidal disease.

Although the availability of ganciclovir has reduced the significance of CMV in lung transplant recipients, CMV remains a serious potential complication associated with an increased risk of mortality.[29,30] The approach to CMV prophylaxis in the pediatric lung transplant recipient is controversial, varying considerably among transplant centers. In most instances, CMV prophylaxis is not administered when both recipient and donor are CMV seronegative.[31] If either the donor or recipient is seropositive for CMV, ganciclovir or valganciclovir are administered for 4 to 12 weeks posttransplant. More recent studies have suggested a potential benefit to extending the duration of prophylaxis (with IV ganciclovir or oral valganciclovir) to 6 months or longer.[32,33] Some pediatric centers administer CMV hyperimmune globulin (CMVIg) in conjunction with ganciclovir based on reports of improved outcomes with CMV disease in adult patients.[34] However, the long-term benefit of CMVIg remains unclear.[35]

Management Issues Unique to Pediatrics

Although guided by the strategies used in adult lung transplant recipients, several important differences exist in therapy and monitoring for pediatric lung transplant recipients, most importantly related to the ability to diagnose chronic allograft dysfunction or bronchiolitis obliterans syndrome (BOS) (defined later in the chapter).

Although spirometry is essential for the clinical diagnosis of BOS, spirometry is generally not available or reliable until children reach 6 years of age. Using thoracoabdominal compression techniques, infant pulmonary function testing can identify the presence of airflow obstruction, but it requires specialized equipment and experience.[36,37] In addition, such tests cannot be performed as frequently as conventional spirometry because they require anesthesia, and infant pulmonary function testing is not addressed in the most recent BOS criteria.[38]

An additional limitation in infants and toddlers relates to transbronchial biopsies. Although transbronchial biopsy forceps small enough to fit in the suction channels of endoscopes used for bronchoscopy in young children became available in the 1990s, the smaller forceps typically yield much smaller pieces of tissue; obtaining tissue for the diagnosis of rejection in infants may therefore be somewhat challenging.

Therapeutic challenges also exist. For example, newer immunosuppressant and anti-infective agents are often not provided in the liquid forms required for young children. Management of liquid forms can be difficult for patients and families as they usually must be compounded by local pharmacies and may have a short shelf life. Managing the use of liquid forms may also be challenging for transplant centers because dosing decisions must often be made in the absence of absorption and pharmacokinetic data for infants and children.

COMPLICATIONS

Complications following lung transplantation occur in predictable timelines: in the first weeks after transplant, the most common complications are related to the condition of the donor organs and the surgical procedure; an early phase, 1 to 6 months following transplant is when infectious and acute immunologic complications become more prevalent; and a late phase, after 6 months following transplant, when chronic immunologic complications such as bronchiolitis obliterans and malignancies are observed more frequently (Table 64-2).

Immediate Posttransplant Phase

Since virtually all pediatric lung transplant procedures are performed with cardiopulmonary bypass, postoperative bleeding, particularly in the pleural space or at the site of the vascular anastomoses, is a common concern.[4] Other complications of the surgical procedure

TABLE 64-2 TIMING OF COMPLICATIONS AFTER LUNG TRANSPLANTATION

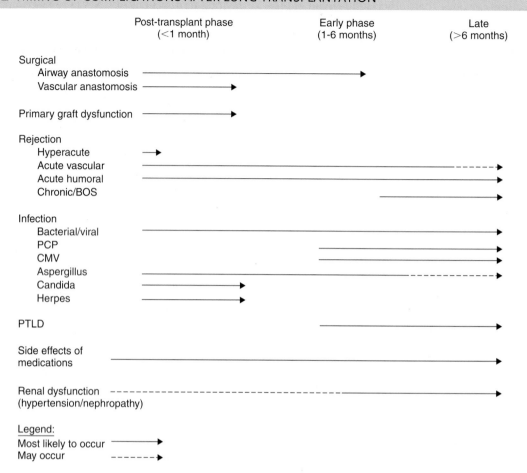

include injury of the phrenic or recurrent laryngeal nerve, causing diaphragmatic or vocal cord dysfunction. Dehiscence at either the vascular or bronchial anastomoses may require prompt surgical attention and an early return to the operating room. Most transplant centers perform flexible bronchoscopy within 24 to 48 hours of transplantation to obtain cultures from the lower airways and to assess the integrity of the airway anastomosis. Fortunately, dehiscence of the airway anastomosis has become rare since the development of techniques to cover the anastomosis with vascularized tissue.[21,22,39] However, other airway complications occur at a frequency comparable to that seen in adult lung transplant recipients including fibrotic strictures, excessive granulation tissue, or airway collapse at the site of the anastomosis.[40,41] In the event of the development of stenosis of the airway lumen, balloon dilatation or stent placement by bronchoscopy may be necessary. Mechanisms invoked to explain the development of anastomotic narrowing include donor airway ischemia, impaired airway healing, and barotrauma if prolonged ventilation is needed after transplantation.[40]

Lung allograft rejection remains problematic, representing an important obstacle to long-term success of transplantation, particularly in comparison to other solid-organ transplant procedures. A variety of mechanisms have been proposed to explain this discrepancy, including

the richness of immune effector cells resident in the pulmonary vasculature and lymphatic system; the ongoing daily exposure of the vast epithelial surface of the lung allograft to potential environmental irritants, toxins, and pathogens; and the fact that the lungs are exposed to the entire cardiac output.[42]

Hyperacute rejection within hours of transplant is a rare, potentially catastrophic complication in the immediate posttransplant period that is associated with circulating recipient antibodies that bind to donor human leukocyte antigen (HLA) molecules on vascular endothelium, leading to significant graft ischemia.[4] It can be prevented by screening the recipient for anti-HLA antibodies and avoiding donors with related antigens. However, because the logistics of organ allocation often preclude HLA information being available at the time of organ offer, this approach is typically reserved for patients with antibodies to a significant percentage of HLA types. Alternatively, patients with a low percentage of antibodies reactive to the spectrum of HLA antigens undergo cross-matching at the time of transplant. Patients with positive cross-matches are usually treated with plasmapheresis to prevent hyperacute rejection.

The most common problem that occurs in the first posttransplant week is primary graft dysfunction (PGD) related to re-implantation lung injury.[43,44] PGD is associated with the procurement procedure and duration of ischemia prior to implantation; the generation of hydroxyl radicals and pro-inflammatory cytokines during ischemia may be causative factors.[45–47] Complications related to graft dysfunction vary from mild, noncardiogenic pulmonary edema to a picture of acute respiratory distress syndrome histologically characterized as diffuse alveolar damage. Patients generally have marked hypoxemia and diffuse infiltrates. Treatment is supportive, with careful fluid management and ventilatory support;[48] extracorporeal membrane circulatory support has also been used in selected cases.[49,50] Although early retransplantation may be considered, outcomes in this setting are generally poor.[51]

Acute rejection is much more common than hyperacute rejection; a majority of patients undergo at least one episode. Acute rejection can occur as early as 1 week after transplantation or as long as 2 to 3 years later. Most commonly, episodes of acute rejection occur 2 to 12 weeks after transplantation.[42] Nonspecific signs and symptoms of acute rejection include cough, fever, dyspnea, hypoxemia, and radiographic changes. Lung function studies, if available, tend to show an obstructive pattern. Chest examination may show tachypnea and crackles. Since these symptoms are not specific for rejection and are difficult to differentiate from infection, evaluation by bronchoscopy with bronchoalveolar lavage and transbronchial biopsy (TBBx) is generally indicated, particularly for patients presenting in the first 3 months after transplant. Histologically, biopsy specimens show perivascular lymphocytic infiltrates with or without airway inflammation. They are classified according to a standardized scoring system.[52,53] Because patients with acute rejection may be asymptomatic, many transplant centers advocate surveillance bronchoscopy with transbronchial biopsy on a scheduled basis (e.g., at 2 weeks, 1, 2, and 3 months after transplant, at quarterly intervals for the first year, and semi-annually thereafter).[16] Smaller numbers of transplant centers perform bronchoscopy and biopsies only when symptoms of lower respiratory tract disease become manifest, arguing that long-term outcomes are unaffected with this approach.[54] Support for screening biopsies during the first posttransplant year has been increased by publication of data suggesting that a single episode of minimal acute rejection is an independent risk factor for chronic rejection.[55,56] However, this finding was not confirmed in a multicenter analysis of pediatric lung transplant recipients.[57]

Treatment of acute rejection consists of 10 mg/kg of intravenous methylprednisolone daily for three days. For persistent or recurrent acute rejection, lympholytic therapy (e.g., with antithymocyte globulin) may be administered, or the daily immunosuppressive regimen may be altered or enhanced. Although episodes of acute rejection are common after lung transplantation (perhaps even expected), data suggest that transplant recipients younger than 3 years of age may have fewer episodes of acute rejection than older children or adults.[58–60]

Sources of increased risk of infection in the immediate posttransplant period (and beyond) are multifactorial and include organisms present in the donor at the time of procurement, the intensity of immunosuppression, the loss of a normal cough reflex owing to both postoperative pain and the disruption of afferent and efferent nerves responsible for coordinating the cough response, impairment of mucociliary transport, and alteration in trafficking of immune effector cells to regional lymph nodes.[61] Despite the use of prophylactic antimicrobials in the perioperative period (discussed earlier in the chapter), recipient factors (particularly in patients with CF) and donor factors (e.g., active viral infection) may lead to significant infectious complications early in the postoperative period. Younger children appear to be at greatest risk for early viral infections, perhaps because they are less likely to have developed immunity.[9] In CF transplant recipients, the chronically infected lungs may cause seeding of the blood or mediastinum with recipient airway flora during explantation. Further, chronic sinus disease typical of CF is a potential source of infection to the allograft and has led some transplant centers to advocate pretransplant sinus surgery coupled with antimicrobial washing of the sinuses.[62,63] A recent retrospective analysis of sinus surgery in patients with CF undergoing transplant at a major transplant center showed no survival benefit associated with pretransplant sinus surgery.[64]

Early Phase (1 to 6 Months)

Infection

During this period, the risk of infectious complications is typically highest, especially in patients who have received an induction agent. Initially, concern is for organisms carried with the donor organs during implantation or (primarily in the case of CF) harbored in the upper and lower airways of the recipient. Subsequently, community and nosocomial organisms may cause infection as may opportunistic pathogens (e.g., pneumocystis, *Candida*). Patients who are seropositive for CMV or who are seronegative and receive lungs from a CMV-positive donor are at particular risk for CMV disease during this early phase because most prophylactic regimens against CMV are completed during this period.

Clinical manifestations of CMV infection vary from a febrile, viral syndrome associated with leukopenia to invasive disease with viremia affecting, most commonly, the lung but also other organs, particularly the GI tract. In CMV pneumonitis, patients may develop a constellation of signs and symptoms including cough, fever, chills, respiratory distress, crackles, and diffuse interstitial infiltrates. Isolation of CMV by bronchoalveolar lavage (BAL) or TBBx in the setting of a typical clinical picture is strongly suggestive of CMV pneumonia, although it is worth noting that asymptomatic shedding of CMV occurs. Treatment for CMV includes IV ganciclovir for 2 to 6 weeks and, in some centers, adjunctive therapy with CMV hyperimmune globulin. Oral valganciclovir may be administered for 2 to 3 months after completion of the IV ganciclovir course.

In the pre-ganciclovir era, the incidence of CMV disease in mismatched recipients reached 75% or higher in the first 6 months after transplant,[65] and CMV pneumonitis was a risk factor for the subsequent development of BO.[66] With the availability of ganciclovir for prophylaxis and treatment, the frequency of

CMV pneumonitis has decreased and the significance of CMV disease in the lung transplant population is less clear.[67,68]

Pneumocystis carinii was a common problem in lung transplant recipients in the early phase after transplant before routine administration of TMP/SMX began in the late 1980s. As with other solid-organ recipients, TMP/SMX prophylaxis has resulted in a marked decline in disease attributable to this fungus in lung transplant recipients. Patients ill with *Pneumocystis* present with acute onset of fever, respiratory distress, hypoxemia, and interstitial infiltrates. Silver or fluorescent staining of BAL specimens demonstrate organisms with a typical morphology and is diagnostic of disease. Intravenous TMP/SMX is the treatment of choice.

Viral infections can be particularly problematic during this period. Adenovirus[69] and paramyxoviruses including parainfluenza and respiratory syncytial virus (RSV) can cause significant lung injury or mortality.[70,71] Many centers treat these viruses aggressively with cidofovir and ribavirin, respectively.[71–73] Fungal infections also pose significant risk.[74]

Rejection

In addition to acute rejection, which has its peak incidence during this period, it has recently become clear that the posttransplant development of donor-specific anti-HLA antibodies can lead to antibody-mediated lung allograft injury.[75] The clinical manifestations of humoral lung allograft rejection are difficult to differentiate from infection or acute cellular rejection. Patients present with dyspnea, pulmonary infiltrates, and decreased lung function. Although there is no clear consensus on criteria for diagnosis, the presence of circulating donor-specific antibodies (identified using solid-phase flow cytometry techniques), alveolar capillary complement (C4d) deposition, and capillaritis in the setting of allograft dysfunction is usually considered sufficient evidence.[76] Treatment of humoral rejection is also controversial. Most centers use some combination of steroids, plasmapheresis, intravenous immunoglobulin, and B-cell reduction (cytoxan or rituximab).[77] The role of newer agents such as bortezomib (a proteosome inhibitor targeted at plasma cells) or complement inhibitors such as eculizumab remains to be elucidated.[78,79]

Medication Side Effects

Triple-drug immunosuppressive therapy has offered a therapeutic approach that allows long-term success in solid-organ transplantation. However, the side effects of these medications can be troublesome enough in some patients to ultimately affect functional outcome and quality of life. The degree of immunosuppression is a delicate balance between too much, with risks for the development of opportunistic infections, and too little, with its attendant risks of allograft rejection.

CSA and tacrolimus are both associated with hypertension and nephropathy, though these may be less severe with tacrolimus.[80] The risks of renal dysfunction with cyclosporine or tacrolimus are compounded by the frequent use of other nephrotoxic drugs such as aminoglycosides, ganciclovir, or amphotericin. One year after lung transplantation, 42% of patients have hypertension and 10.5% have renal dysfunction; this rises to 69% and 22%, respectively, 5 years after transplant.[6] Hirsutism and gingival hyperplasia appear to occur more frequently in cyclosporine-based immunosuppression.[80] Calcineurin inhibitors (CNI) also cause neurologic toxicity, and seizures, headache, and sleep disturbance are common problems in the first months following transplant.[81] In patients with CF, inconsistent and erratic metabolism and absorption of CNI can occur and underscores the need for close monitoring of blood levels. Routine blood counts are necessary for patients receiving azathioprine or MMF because of their effects on white blood cell counts. Systemic and oral corticosteroids have the potential to cause a host of well-known side effects. For example, daily use of oral corticosteroids may lead to glucose intolerance and diabetes, particularly in patients with CF, with prevalence rates of more than 30% in long-term survivors of lung transplantation.[6] Patients receiving tacrolimus have a higher risk of developing diabetes than those receiving CSA.[82]

Late Phase (More than 6 Months)

Ongoing complications in the late phase include those related to infection, drug toxicity, acute cellular and humoral rejection, and airway anastomotic narrowing. Posttransplant lymphoproliferative disease (PTLD) and BO, two very serious complications, also become apparent.

Posttransplant Lymphoproliferative Disease

The incidence of malignancy after lung transplantation in children is 5.9% 1 year after transplant and increases to 13.1% at 5 years; PTLD is by far the most common malignancy.[6] PTLD is generally an EBV-driven lymphoma in an immunosuppressed patient[83,84] and appears to occur more commonly in lung transplant recipients (as compared with other solid-organ transplant recipients), in patients with CF, and in children as compared to adults.[85] These findings are probably explained by the intensity of immunosuppression in lung transplant recipients and the fact that many pediatric patients are EBV-seronegative at the time of transplantation.[84]

Manifestations of PTLD are protean, often vague, and often confusing. A high index of suspicion is required because early diagnosis and treatment improves the likelihood of resolution of disease. In the first posttransplant year, the most common site of PTLD involvement in lung transplant patients is the allograft.[86] Although PTLD can be asymptomatic, symptoms of cough, fever, and dyspnea are not uncommon. The typical radiographic finding is single or multiple round or ovoid pulmonary nodules.[87] Involvement of lymph nodes draining the chest is not uncommon. After the first year, the incidence of extrapulmonary PTLD increases. Other sites of involvement in PTLD include the GI tract, the skin, and other lymphatic tissue including lymph nodes and the nasopharynx.[88,89] Elevated quantitative measurement of EBV by polymerase chain reaction (PCR) has been shown to be a sensitive and somewhat specific marker for PTLD; most centers monitor this test on a regular basis.[90] In addition, positron emission tomography can be a sensitive and specific test that is often performed when EBV PCR or other clinical indicators raise suspicion for PTLD.[91] Once a suspicious lesion is identified, histologic diagnosis is important for prognostic purposes. CD20-positive tumors may be more amenable to antibody therapy. A monomorphous histologic pattern has a worse prognosis.[92]

If PTLD is identified early, the mainstay of treatment is reduction in immunosuppression alone. Although some adult centers reduce immunosuppression based only on the presence of elevated EBV PCR,[93] a recent study suggests caution with this approach in children.[94] Although reduced immunosuppression can be successful in some patients, in many cases additional therapy is needed. Most centers now use therapy modeled after the Children's Oncology Group protocol ANHL 0221, which includes Ritixumab, an anti-CD20 monoclonal antibody shown to be effective in non-Hodgkin's lymphoma, low-dose cytoxan, and prednisone. This approach has been promising in pediatric solid-organ transplant recipients with PTLD.[95]

Bronchiolitis Obliterans and Bronchiolitis Obliterans Syndrome

BO is the greatest obstacle to long-term success of adult and pediatric lung transplantation. By 6 years after lung transplantation in children, only 40% of survivors are free of BO, a worrisome figure since BO is the leading cause of death after the first year posttransplant.[6] Histologic analyses of lesions of BO show progressive and irreversible stenosis of the bronchiolar lumen, eventually resulting in fibrosis and near-occlusion of the airway lumen with collagen.[68]

BO is generally equated with chronic lung allograft rejection, although the immunologic basis of BO remains poorly understood. Diagnosis of BO from tissue obtained by TBBx may be difficult because of the patchy and uneven distribution of the disease. As a result, the term *bronchiolitis obliterans syndrome (BOS)* has evolved as the physiologic surrogate for BO.[38] Among the criteria used to establish a diagnosis of BOS is an otherwise unexplained fall in FEV_1 of greater than 20% from the best previous baseline studies.

A variety of risk factors for the development of BOS have been proposed, most based on single-center studies. A comprehensive review of these reports identified acute rejection as the only consistent risk factor, with acute rejection episodes occurring more than 3 months posttransplant carrying the greatest significance.[66] The presence of lymphocytic bronchitis/bronchiolitis (the so called "B" grade) was also significant, particularly when observed beyond 6 months following transplant. The role of CMV (on the basis of donor/recipient serology, CMV "infection," or CMV pneumonitis) as a risk factor was deemed inconclusive, likely due in part to the use of ganciclovir prophylaxis and treatment.[67,68] More recently, the presence of anti-HLA antibodies[96,97] as well as autoantibodies to structural proteins (e.g., alpha tubulin and collagen V) have been identified as risk factors.[98,99] In addition, gastroesophageal reflux has been identified as a risk factor, with some evidence that fundoplication can reduce the incidence of BO.[100,101] An association between community-acquired respiratory

viruses (i.e., paramyxoviruses, influenza, adenovirus) has been suggested.[102,103] Finally, nonadherence with the immunosuppressive regimen can also result in BO.[104] In contrast, there are center-specific data showing that younger children[60] and patients receiving living-related lobar transplantation[105,106] are at *lower* risk for developing BOS. Currently, the most prevalent hypothesis is that BO represents a final common pathway resulting from the immune response to an airway injury induced by one or more of these risk factors, leading to chronic epithelial airway damage and eventually severe airway obstruction.[107] The consistent identification of acute rejection as a risk factor for BO reinforces the importance of routine surveillance bronchoscopy to detect and treat subclinical acute rejection. As noted earlier in the chapter, this issue is further complicated by reports that episodes of minimal acute rejection (Grade A1) were a risk factor for early-onset BO.[55,56] Although the consensus approach to Grade A1 rejection in *asymptomatic* patients has been observation, to reduce the risk for early development of BO, the possibility of altering or enhancing immunosuppression in this setting has been entertained.

Treatment of BO is problematic at best, with augmented immunosuppression the general recommendation. Some transplant centers endorse changing the immunosuppressive regimen from CSA to tacrolimus, with anecdotal reports of success (though most pediatric centers no longer use CSA as the primary CNI).[108] The use of azithromycin three times weekly as an anti-inflammatory agent appears to benefit a subset of patients, typically those with airway neutrophilia, leading to the suggestion that BO has two phenotypes based on azithromycin responsiveness.[109] Antilymphocyte agents such as antithymocyte globulin or OKT3 may be effective adjunctive therapy in some patients.[110] Recently, treatment with photopheresis has shown some benefit.[111,112] As with PTLD, early identification and treatment are most likely to be effective. In many patients however, progression of disease is inexorable and often complicated by infection with bacterial or viral pathogens. The goal of therapy is to ameliorate the chronic rejection, reduce the risk of infectious complications, and prevent further deterioration in lung function. Many centers consider retransplantation as an option in patients with progressive decline in lung function.

OUTCOMES

Survival

Survival after pediatric lung transplantation for patients transplanted between January 1990 and June 2007 is depicted in Figure 64-2A. There is no statistical difference in survival rates among the different age groups shown, with a 50% survival rate of 4.5 years collectively. When analyzed by era (Fig. 64-2B), 1- and 5-year survival rates improved significantly from 67% and 43%, respectively, in the era between 1988 and 1994 to 83% and 50%, respectively, in the recent era (2002 to 2007). This improvement mostly reflects better early outcomes, however.[6] This does not compare favorably

Section X

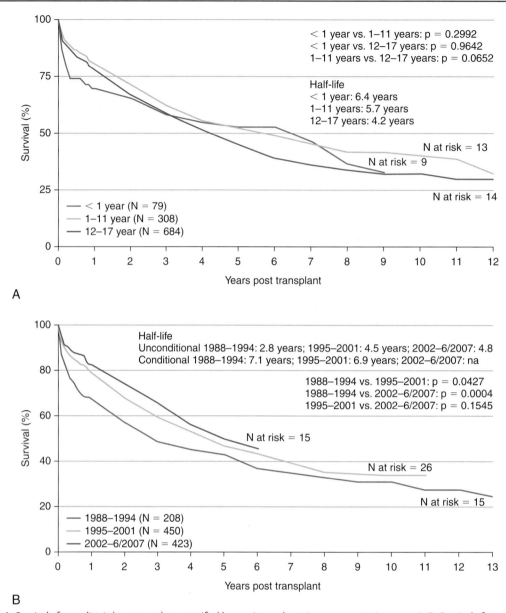

FIGURE 64-2. A, Survival after pediatric lung transplant, stratified by age (transplants January 1990 to June 2007). **B,** Survival after pediatric lung transplant, stratified by era of transplant. (Reprinted with permission from Aurora P, Edwards LB, Christie JD, et al. Registry of the International Society for Heart and Lung Transplantation: Twelfth Official Pediatric Lung and Heart/Lung Transplantation Report—2009. *J Heart Lung Transplant.* 2009;28:1023-1030.)

with pediatric patients undergoing heart transplantation where the half-life is closer to 12 to 13 years.[113] In the most recent ISHLT report, analyses of risk factors for 1-year mortality demonstrated, in addition to the era effect noted above, increased mortality in patients on the ventilator at the time of transplant (RR 3.62) and lower mortality in patients receiving transplants in centers performing more than 5 transplants per year (RR 0.71). Risk factors for 5-year mortality again include an era effect as well as being on a ventilator prior to transplant (RR 2.46). Data from a large pediatric center suggests that the mortality risk associated with ventilator use is not seen in infants.[60] Younger children had lower 5-year mortality than adolescents (RR 0.76 for 1 to 11 years of age and RR 0.55 for younger than 1 year of age), typically ascribed to poor adherence in adolescence.[6]

Transplant Benefit, Functional Outcome, and Quality of Life

Although generally viewed as a means for prolonging life, a recent provocative paper by Liou and colleagues[114] challenged the concept that pediatric lung transplant in the United States has achieved that goal. In contrast to an earlier report indicating a survival benefit from a group in the United Kingdom,[115] the validity of the recent study was challenged based on the fact that the dataset was biased against transplantation because covariates were obtained well before the time of transplant and estimates of benefit were based on factors that could change between listing and transplant.[116] Nonetheless, an important finding in the study was that 57% of the children listed for lung transplant in the United States had a predicted survival of 5 years or greater,[114] suggesting that the waiting time–based system in the United States may have led to patients being listed well before transplant would have provided a survival benefit. Though the new lung allocation system may have mitigated this concern, better predictors of waiting list mortality for pediatric lung transplant candidates are needed to ensure transplant has a reasonable chance of conferring survival benefit.

The Liou study[114] also reinforced the need for inclusion of objective evaluation of quality of life in assessments of transplant benefit. Perhaps not surprisingly, the quality of life and survival in adult lung transplant recipients was better than candidates who remained on the waiting list.[117–119] Nonetheless, extrapolation to children and adolescents must be approached cautiously. Although 80% of lung transplant survivors report no activity limitations at 1, 3, and 5 years posttransplant, there are few well-controlled studies regarding quality of life in children undergoing lung transplantation. Nixon found a 24% improvement in quality of well being in a small number of recipients after transplantation.[120] More recently, a group of 47 thoracic organ recipients (of whom 6 were lung transplant recipients) scored lower on a health status questionnaire administered to the parent or caregiver compared to a normal population but were similar to children with asthma, juvenile rheumatoid arthritis, and intractable epilepsy.[121] It is worth emphasizing that assessments of quality of life are difficult and affected by the child's baseline capabilities prior to transplant and their expectations after transplant.[120] In addition, measures of childhood development must also be included. Systematic assessment of quality of life and developmental impact of transplant on pediatric recipients remains an underexplored area of pediatric lung transplantation.

Growth

Somatic growth after lung transplant is an ongoing problem for most transplant recipients, partly because of substandard pretransplant nutritional status and the continued use of systemic corticosteroids after the transplant procedure. Improving nutritional status and maximizing growth is an important goal after transplant.

Since the early reports of successful lung transplantation in young children, concerns have been raised about the potential for lung allograft growth.[3] Animal data indicate that allogeneic lung transplantation is associated with an increase in lung volumes and airway size with age.[122] Although spirometry and lung volume measurements following lung transplant have been reported to be normal in infants[123] and older children,[58] these measurements may reflect increased volume of each alveolar unit rather than alveolar tissue growth or increased surface area for gas exchange. Serial CT scan data to support growth of intrathoracic airways over time was reported by Ro and coworkers.[124] However, the diffusing capacity of carbon monoxide (DLCO) did not show an appreciable increase in a single-center study of pediatric recipients of cadaveric and living-donor transplants.[125] Although DLCO provides a better estimate of gas exchange surface area, it is not easily measurable in infants. Thus, further study is required to determine whether surface area for gas exchange increases as lung volumes increase in pediatric lung transplant recipients.

Causes of Death

Causes of death after pediatric lung transplantation are depicted in Figure 64-3. Graft failure and infection are important causes of death in the first year after transplant. In the first 30 days after transplant, surgical complications are an important cause of death. After the first 30 days and before 1 year posttransplant, infection from any cause accounts for roughly 40% of deaths. By 1 to 3 years following transplant, BO becomes the leading cause of death, accounting for nearly 40% of the mortality. Infection remains an important cause of death throughout the follow-up period. Although these represent the most recent data available from the International Society of Heart and Lung Transplantation, there has been little shift in the distribution of causes of death compared to previous registry data.[6]

Future Directions

In summary, although presenting unique challenges related to pediatrics, lung transplant is a lifesaving option for infants, children, and adolescents with end-stage pulmonary parenchymal and vascular disease. In spite of improvements in survival during the past decade,[6] long-term survival rates remain poor compared to heart and other solid-organ transplants.

Moreover, the shortage of organ donors and of lung transplant centers coupled with increased numbers of adults receiving lung transplants will likely limit access to this procedure to fewer than 100 children annually. Efforts to increase awareness about organ donation will likely remain the cornerstone of efforts to increase the number of transplants performed in the United States and worldwide.

With improved survival will come increased focus on growth and development as well as increased need to minimize the deleterious effects of immunosuppression on these critical processes. Improving poor outcomes in the adolescent population will remain an important priority.

Removing BO as the key obstacle limiting long-term survival will continue to be a priority in lung transplant research. Uniform treatment strategies and multicenter collaborations will be needed to identify strategies for earlier diagnosis and determine treatment efficacy as few centers perform enough transplants each year to adequately power such studies. A key research opportunity may be exploring the reduced incidence of rejection and BO in the naïve but developing immune system of infants.[59,60]

In spite of these obstacles, over 1600 children in the last 3 decades have been given a chance for long-term survival because of the success of lung and heart-lung transplantation. Although recent improvements in outcome for children with CF and pulmonary hypertension will hopefully reduce the number children needing lung transplants, those who do should continue to benefit.

Section X

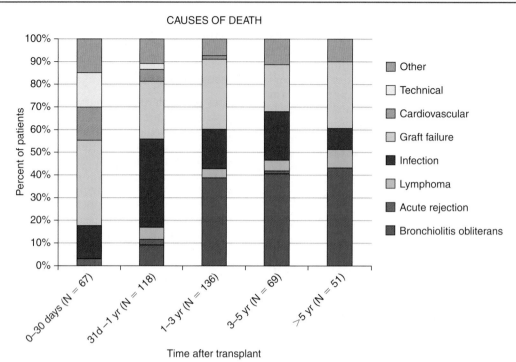

FIGURE 64-3. Causes of death after pediatric lung transplant. (Data adapted from Aurora P, Edwards LB, Christie JD, et al. Registry of the International Society for Heart and Lung Transplantation: Twelfth Official Pediatric Lung and Heart/Lung Transplantation Report—2009. *J Heart Lung Transplant.* 2009;28:1023-1030.)

Suggested Reading

Arcasoy SM, Fisher A, Hachem RR, et al. ISHLT Working Group on Primary Lung Graft Dysfunction. Report of the ISHLT Working Group on Primary Lung Graft Dysfunction part V: predictors and outcomes. *J Heart Lung Transplant.* 2005;24:1483–1488.

Aurora P, Edwards LB, Christie JD, et al. Registry of the International Society for Heart and Lung Transplantation: Twelfth Official Pediatric Lung and Heart/Lung Transplantation Report—2009. *J Heart Lung Transplant.* 2009;28:1023–1030.

D'Ovidio F, Keshavjee S. Gastroesophageal reflux and lung transplantation. [Review]. *Dis Esophagus.* 2006;19:315–320.

Egan TM, Murray S, Bustami RT, et al. Development of the new lung allocation system in the United States. *Am J Transplant.* 2006;6(5 Pt 2):1212–1227.

Estenne M, Maurer JR, Boehler A, et al. Bronchiolitis obliterans syndrome 2001: an update of the diagnostic criteria. [Review]. *J Heart Lung Transplant* 2002;21:297–310.

Glanville AR. Antibody-mediated rejection in lung transplantation: myth or reality? *J Heart Lung Transplant.* 2010;29:395–400.

Orens JB, Boehler A, de Perrot M, et al. A review of lung transplant donor acceptability criteria. [Review] *J Heart Lung Transplant* 2003;22:1183–1200.

Sandrini A, Glanville AR. The controversial role of surveillance bronchoscopy after lung transplantation. [Review] *Curr Opin Organ Transplant* 2009;14:494–498.

Stewart S, Fishbein MC, Snell GI, et al. Revision of the 1996 working formulation for the standardization of nomenclature in the diagnosis of lung rejection. *J Heart Lung Transplant.* 2007;26:1229–1242.

Sweet SC, Aurora P, Benden C, et al. Lung transplantation and survival in children with cystic fibrosis: solid statistics—flawed interpretation. *Pediatr Transplant.* 2008;12:129–136.

References

The complete reference list is available online at www.expertconsult.com

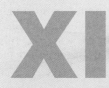

XI
Aerodigestive Disease

65 THE AERODIGESTIVE MODEL

Robin T. Cotton, MD, FACS, FRCS(C)

The development of our aerodigestive model was an outgrowth of advances made in the care of critically ill neonates. Although these advances resulted in significantly increased survival rates, infants were frequently left with multiple problems arising from their underlying condition or its subsequent management. Many were tracheotomy dependent and in need of airway reconstruction. Others required the care of subspecialists in otolaryngology, pulmonary medicine, gastroenterology, and surgery. Given the complexity of these patients and the enormous burden on families who came to Cincinnati Children's Hospital Medical Center (primarily for airway reconstruction), it was crucial for our involved pediatric subspecialists to develop a model for the delivery of efficient, unfragmented care.

In view of the success we have achieved, the objective of this section is to provide the reader with more in-depth information regarding key aspects of our model and the children who benefit tremendously from the horizontally integrated approach that we have implemented.

◼ PATIENT OVERVIEW

Our interdisciplinary model was developed to address the needs of a wide spectrum of patients with interrelated pathologies that fall into the following classifications:
• Patients with airway issues stemming from congenital, acquired, structural, or physiologic etiologies

• Patients with pulmonary issues, including bronchopulmonary dysplasia, aspiration bronchiectasis, oxygen and/or ventilator dependence, and chest wall abnormalities
• Patients with gastrointestinal issues, including gastroesophageal reflux disease, eosinophilic esophagitis, and esophageal dysmotility
• Patients with feeding issues such as oral aversion, choking, aspiration, or dysphagia
• Patients with central or obstructive sleep apnea who have associated genetic or neurologic issues

The Interdisciplinary Team

Ideally, the interdisciplinary team should comprise physicians and other professionals with expertise in the evaluation and treatment of these challenging patients. Subspecialists play the major role in patient care in otolaryngology, pulmonary medicine, gastroenterology, surgery, and anesthesia; the care they provide is coordinated by nurse practitioners and nurses. Intensivists, radiologists, geneticists, pediatricians with expertise in developmental and behavioral issues, and speech and language pathologists are also key players. Other interdisciplinary programs (e.g., the feeding team and sleep center) provide care for selected patients, and a wide array of other health professionals become involved as needed (Fig. 65-1).

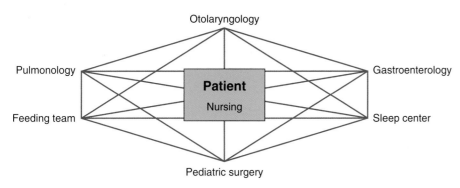

FIGURE 65-1. The interdisciplinary model.

Screening and Evaluating Potential Patients

Potential patients from either within or outside the institution are initially screened via a telephone interview by a nurse practitioner. This initial step provides information that leads to a preliminary evaluation and management plan. After a thorough review of the patient's medical history, a lead physician is chosen based on the patient's primary presenting problem. At weekly interdisciplinary team meetings, physicians discuss pertinent and pressing clinical issues with other team members and decide on appropriate diagnostic tests that the patient should undergo. These tests are then scheduled in a coordinated fashion so as to minimize the burden on patients and their families, eliminate unnecessary visits to the hospital, and avoid repeated use of anesthetics. After the initial assessment, team members conduct a thorough review of diagnostic test results and develop a detailed interdisciplinary management plan. In carrying out this plan, close collaboration is maintained among all team participants.

SUMMARY

The evolution in medicine over the past 4 decades has created a pediatric patient population that suffers from complex disorders involving the airway and digestive tract. In our experience, optimal patient-centered care is best provided by using a well-coordinated interdisciplinary team approach.

66 ASPIRATION

R. Paul Boesch, DO, MS, and Robert E. Wood, MD, PhD

Aspiration refers to the penetration of material below the subglottic area and into the lower airways. There are two main aspiration syndromes: 1) an acute aspiration event quickly progressing to acute pneumonitis and possibly respiratory failure and 2) chronic repeated aspiration of very small volumes that leads to a persistent smoldering inflammatory state and eventually results in chronic lung injury. Acute aspiration of a large volume of gastric contents or even small volumes of hydrocarbon-containing liquids induces a severe toxic injury to airway mucosa with mucosal edema, bronchorrhea, and airway obstruction. Injury to terminal respiratory units causes pulmonary edema and an ARDS-like syndrome that may be life-threatening.[1,2] Injury to terminal respiratory units is more common with hydrocarbon aspiration as the volatile liquid produces a vapor that is subsequently inhaled deeper into the lungs. Long-term pulmonary fibrosis may follow hydrocarbon aspiration. Nonvolatile lipid-containing liquids (e.g., mineral oil) are not absorbable, and aspiration results in persistent lipoid pneumonia, bronchiolar obstruction, and chronic lung injury. For lipoid pneumonia, repeated bronchoalveolar lavage (BAL) may be both diagnostic and therapeutic.[3] Chronic pulmonary aspiration is a common problem in pediatrics and remains a diagnostic and therapeutic challenge. Chronic aspiration is almost always a consideration in the evaluation of the "aerodigestive" patient and will therefore be the focus of the remainder of this chapter.

Chronic pulmonary aspiration represents the repeated passage of food material, gastric refluxate, or saliva into the subglottic airways in sufficient quantities to cause chronic or recurrent respiratory symptoms.[4,5] Aspiration is an intermittent occurrence resulting from failure of airway protection that occurs in the setting of repeated opportunities for aspiration to occur. These opportunities may be nearly continuous, such as with severe hypopharyngeal pooling of oral secretions, or intermittent such as with reflux of gastric contents above the upper esophageal sphincter or swallowing dysfunction. Opportunities to aspirate may be limited to specific consistencies, such as during swallowing of thin liquids. Safe swallowing and airway protection from aspiration requires effective integration and coordination of deglutition and respiration as both share the same aerodigestive tract. Failures in this coordination may be caused by anatomic abnormalities within the aerodigestive tract, disruptions of the complex neurologic sensorimotor networks of swallowing and respiration, or functional disorders of the esophagus or muscles of deglutition (Fig. 66-1).

Chronic aspiration is very common in aerodigestive patients as they generally present with complicated underlying medical conditions, including feeding failure, gastroesophageal reflux (GER), neurologic injury, chronic respiratory disease, tracheostomy, impaired laryngeal function, and airway lesions resulting in obstructed breathing, or abnormal connections between the airway and gastrointestinal tract. Such patients commonly have congenital syndromes predisposing to aspiration or were born very prematurely. Because of their complex multisystem disorders, it may be difficult to distinguish between the symptoms of other underlying conditions (e.g., bronchopulmonary dysplasia or tracheobronchomalacia) and chronic aspiration. The symptoms of chronic aspiration are common to many respiratory conditions, and a reliance on symptoms of dysphagia and recurrent pneumonias will fail to identify many children with significant chronic lung injury from aspiration. The most common symptoms of chronic aspiration include: chronic cough, wheezing, congestion, choking or gagging with feeds, failure to thrive, apnea, intermittent fever spikes, and recurrent chest infections. The parental report of "wet vocal quality" or "wet breathing" may be the most predictive symptoms of aspiration.[6]

Chronic pulmonary aspiration results in significant morbidity. Children may be hospitalized for recurrent pneumonias and commonly develop progressive lung injury and bronchiectasis. Significant bronchiectasis may persist into adulthood and result in respiratory failure. Chronic pulmonary aspiration is the leading cause of death in neurologically impaired patients and those with congenital syndromes such as Cornelia de Lange and Cri du Chat.[7,8] Some children, particularly those without neurologic injury, are diagnosed inappropriately as having asthma and may develop irreversible lung injury before chronic aspiration is suspected, identified, and treated. The histopathology of chronic aspiration is that of bronchiolocentric organizing pneumonia with [9-12] (Fig. 66-2). This correlates with findings of bronchiolar obstruction and injury seen on chest high-resolution computed tomography (c-HRCT): centrilobular ("tree-in-bud") opacities and bronchiectasis.[10,13,14] In animal models of chronic aspiration, repeated aspiration of small food particles results in the greatest injury as a chronic foreign body reaction causes damage to the architecture of the lung parenchyma. In animal models of a single small aspiration event, the effect the inflammatory response to small food particles is amplified by acidification of the aspirated material.[15]

ASPIRATION CAUSED BY SWALLOWING DYSFUNCTION

Normal swallowing is a complex process that is dependent upon intact anatomy and well-organized sensory and motor function of specific cranial and cervical nerves. The oral phase is voluntary and includes acceptance and preparation of the food bolus, which includes sucking or chewing and manipulating a bolus on the tongue. The bolus is usually delivered to the pharynx in

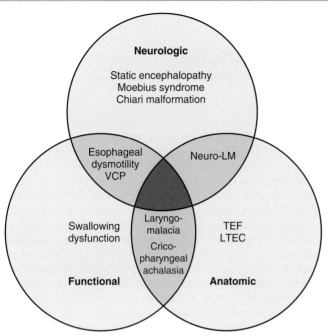

FIGURE 66-1. Interrelationship of neurologic, anatomic, and functional causes of chronic aspiration. *VCP*, vocal cord paralysis; *Neuro-LM*, neurologic-variant laryngomalacia; *TEF*, tracheoesophageal fistula; *LTEC*, laryngotracheoesophageal cleft.

voluntary fashion, but premature spillage of material into the hypopharynx can occur if oral movements are not coordinated. Once bolus delivery occurs, the involuntary pharyngeal phase is triggered and airway protection takes place. This is a sequential event involving cessation of respiration, adduction of the true vocal folds in association with horizontal approximation of the arytenoid cartilages, closure of the false vocal folds, and retroversion of the epiglottis. The combination of elevation of the larynx and contraction of intrinsic laryngeal muscles allows the epiglottis to serve as a gutter, diverting food and liquids laterally into the pyriform sinus region. The larynx is elevated under the base of the tongue, facilitating the stretching and opening of the cricopharyngeus, as the pharyngeal constrictors shorten the pharynx and propel the bolus through the upper esophageal sphincter. Once passage of the bolus occurs, the larynx returns to its resting position and the airway reopens. The bolus is subsequently transported to the stomach by peristalsis, aided by gravity.

Development of Swallowing

Development of swallowing begins early in fetal development, and development of the aerodigestive tract develops integrated with the development of the respiratory centers of the brainstem. Central pattern generation in the brainstem controls and coordinates movements of mastication, respiration, and deglutition through adaptive networks of interneurons densely bundled within the nucleus ambiguus and nucleus tractus solitarius.[16,17] These central pattern generators respond to suprabulbar signals as well as sensory feedback. Cortical input facilitates the oral phase and the initiation of the pharyngeal phase of swallowing, while sensory afferent feedback is transmitted via cranial nerves (CN) V, VII, IX, and X. Primary motor efferent activity for swallowing is provided by CN V, VII, IX, XII, and cervical nerves C1 to C3. Ultrasound studies have demonstrated pharyngeal swallowing as early as 10 to 14 weeks gestation, nonnutritive sucking and swallowing at 15 weeks, and suckling with anterior to posterior tongue movements between 18 and 24 weeks gestation. At 26 to 29 weeks gestation, reflexes between taste buds and facial muscles can be demonstrated, and nonnutritive sucking on a pacifier may be observed. Some infants can feed by mouth at 32 to 33 weeks, although 34 weeks is the earliest that infants may sustain full nutrition and hydration orally. Beyond term, swallowing matures, characterized by increased sucking and swallowing rates, longer sucking bursts, and larger volumes per suck.

Mechanisms of Aspiration During Swallowing

Protection against aspiration is provided by the functional anatomy of swallowing and by protective reflexes; any breakdown in the structure, effectiveness, or coordination of these components may result in failure of safe swallowing. As mentioned earlier in the chapter, a food bolus should be adequately prepared in the mouth and delivered to the pharynx at an appropriate time, coordinated with breathing. Delayed initiation of swallowing will allow the bolus to enter the pharynx before the protective actions of the pharyngeal phase occur, leaving the laryngeal inlet susceptible to penetration and aspiration. Inadequate laryngeal elevation will result in impaired epiglottic function and leaves the posterior larynx in

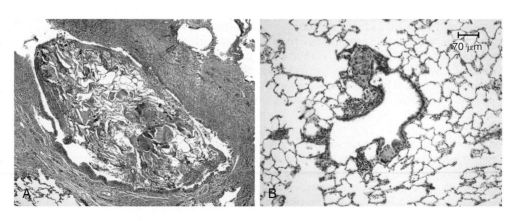

FIGURE 66-2. Histopathology of chronic aspiration. **A,** Lung biopsy from a 6-year-old suspected of interstitial lung disease but found to have bronchiolocentric inflammation filling of the airway lumen with inflammatory cells, giant cells, and vegetable matter. **B,** Early development of peribronchiolar inflammation with giant cells in a 10-week-old rat following tracheal instillation of 0.4 mL/kg of soy infant formula and ground rat chow 3 times a week for 6 weeks.

closer approximation to the bolus as it passes through the hypopharynx. At this point, weakness in the pharyngeal squeeze or impaired opening of the upper esophageal sphincter will allow the bolus to persist for a greater duration in the hypopharynx, creating the potential for overflow into the open airway. Regurgitation of food from either the esophagus or stomach also creates this problem. If there is an inadequate dam protecting the posterior larynx (such as occurs with a laryngeal cleft or deep interarytenoid notch), the bolus may then more easily penetrate the laryngeal inlet.

The actions of the intrinsic laryngeal muscles, innervated by the superior laryngeal nerve and recurrent laryngeal nerve, are of major importance to airway closure during swallowing. The intrinsic muscles (i.e., the cricothyroid, posterior cricoarytenoid, lateral cricoarytenoid, thyroarytenoid, transverse and oblique arytenoids, and vocalis) serve as sphincters, adductors, abductors, tensors, and relaxers of the structures critical to the opening and closing of the airway. The supraglottic larynx is densely populated with various types of sensory receptors, including mechanical, chemical, and thermal receptors. The sensitivity and response of each of these receptor types varies with age. In infants, mechanical stimulation of the larynx invokes reflex swallowing and apnea, whereas in older children laryngeal closure and cough are predominant reflexes. Diminished laryngeal sensation is a tremendous challenge to safe swallowing such that swallowing of even normal oral secretions may not be triggered, and frank aspiration results when any penetration occurs. Decreased laryngeal sensation correlates very highly with aspiration.[18–20]

Swallowing Dysfunction in Specific Populations

Chronic pulmonary aspiration secondary to swallowing dysfunction most often occurs secondary to central or peripheral neurologic disease, functional immaturity, or anatomic limitations (Table 66-1). While most children who aspirate have some combination of these factors, there exist children who have swallowing dysfunction (usually delayed initiation of swallowing) with aspiration sufficient to cause chronic respiratory symptoms and lung injury without any identifiable anatomic, neurologic, or developmental limitations.[21–23] These children may require gastrostomy tube placement, but generally the swallowing dysfunction resolves between 2 and 3 years of age.

The newborn infant, and particularly the preterm infant, are particularly susceptible to aspiration caused by tenuous coordination between sucking, swallowing, and breathing. Children and adults typically initiate swallowing during the mid-expiratory phase, with an obligatory deglutition apnea, followed by further expiration to help prevent aspiration of residual liquid.[24,25] Term infants younger than 6 months of age will most often swallow at the very end of inspiration and the onset of expiration.[25] Premature infants have more varied phase relationships due to variable rates of development of coordination between central deglutition and respiration.[26,27] Swallowing may occur at the cusp of inspiration at times, and respiration may intrude on the deglutition apnea.

TABLE 66-1 CONDITIONS ASSOCIATED WITH CHRONIC PULMONARY ASPIRATION

Prematurity

Congenital Anatomic Abnormalities

Esophageal atresia
Tracheoesophageal fistula
Laryngotracheoesophageal cleft
Choanal stenosis or atresia
Cleft palate
Macroglossia
Laryngomalacia
Microgastria
Vascular ring
Tracheal stenosis
Cystic hygroma
Laryngeal/pharyngeal vascular malformation
Tracheostomy

Acquired Anatomic Abnormalities

Laryngeal/pharyngeal tumors
Laryngeal/pharyngeal trauma

Congenital Syndromes

CHARGE Association
Möbius
Pfeiffer
Cornelia de Lange
Cri du chat

Gastrointestinal

Esophageal dysmotility
Esophageal foreign body
Cricopharyngeal achalasia
Gastroesophageal reflux

Central Nervous System

Depressed consciousness
Static or progressive encephalopathy
Traumatic brain injury
Cerebrovascular accident
Hydrocephalus

Peripheral Neurologic

Arnold Chiari malformation
Vocal cord paralysis
Neurologic-variant laryngomalacia

Neuromuscular

Muscular dystrophy
Myotonic dystrophy
Spinal muscle atrophy
Myasthenia gravis
Guillain-Barré syndrome

Otherwise Normal Child with Isolated Aspiration

Fatigue of the swallowing mechanism can also develop toward the end of a prolonged feeding session, especially in infants with respiratory disease and increased work of breathing.

Chronic aspiration is highly prevalent in children with neurologic impairment such as static encephalopathy and neuromuscular disorders. Children with neurologic impairment frequently require prolonged feeding times. Choking with feeding, chest infections, and dysphagia may be present in nearly all children with severe cerebral palsy.[28–30] Aspiration may occur before, during, or after a swallow and often does not provoke cough clearance. Common mechanisms include poor oral preparation, neck extension impairing laryngeal elevation, premature spillage of liquids, poor pharyngeal clearance with excessive residual, and poor esophageal opening.[31] Aspiration is the most common cause of death in these patients.[32] The prevalence of feeding disorders is very high in children and adolescents with neuromuscular disorders such as spinal muscle atrophy, Duchenne muscular dystrophy, and myotonic muscular dystrophy.[33–36] While some diseases have specific contributing characteristics (e.g., macroglossia in Duchenne muscular dystrophy), nearly all are associated with prolonged transit time, poor laryngeal elevation, decreased pharyngeal squeeze, and persistent pharyngeal residual related to neuromuscular weakness. These patients are particularly subject to fatigue with prolonged oral feeding.

Peripheral neurologic diseases and injury can result in chronic pulmonary aspiration. Vocal cord paralysis (bilateral more than unilateral) as may result from a difficult delivery or surgery within the mediastinum may both interfere with coordination of respiration and swallowing and impair protective posterior glottic closure. Congenital syndromes that result in lower cranial nerve dysfunction such as Möbius syndrome or CHARGE association (coloboma, heart defect, atresia choanae, retarded growth and development, genital hypoplasia, ear anomalies) are very frequently complicated by chronic aspiration. Among children with CHARGE association, dysphagia and aspiration is as common as most of the major associations.[37,38] Similarly, dysphagia with vocal cord dysfunction, pharyngoesophageal dysmotility, and aspiration can be a presenting feature of Arnold-Chiari malformations due to compression of the brainstem and the subsequent effect on lower cranial nerve function.[39,40] Cricopharyngeal achalasia may be associated with Arnold-Chiari malformations but may also be a congenital cause for aspiration.[41–43] Cricopharyngeal achalasia creates opportunities for aspiration due to delayed passage of food bolus into the esophagus and increased pooling of food and oral secretions in the hypopharynx.

Anatomic abnormalities anywhere along the aerodigestive tract may impact deglutition and result in increased risk for chronic aspiration. Children with craniofacial malformations (e.g., choanal stenosis and cleft palate) are susceptible to chronic aspiration caused by decreased coordination of swallowing and breathing. Crowding of the pharyngeal airway caused by macroglossia or retrognathia creates risks for aspiration. Neck cysts and tumors may narrow and distort the upper aerodigestive tract as well as impair the movements of laryngeal and pharyngeal structures of deglutition. These include cystic hygromas, lymphatic malformations, neuroblastomas, and hemangiomata. The upper airway anatomy can also be distorted by caustic ingestion, thermal inhalational injury, or trauma. Lingual and palatine tonsil hypertrophy may also be associated with aspiration, particularly in neurologically impaired patients, and treatment may improve dysphagia.[44,45] Any lesion resulting in persistent or intermittent upper airway obstruction can disrupt the timing of the swallow. Laryngomalacia is the best recognized of these causes, as feeding problems are the second-most common presenting symptom behind stridor.[46–48] Surgical treatment can effectively improve both stridor and aspiration caused by laryngomalacia with tight aryepiglottic folds or tall prolapsing arytenoids.[49] Supraglottoplasty should be considered cautiously in patients with apparent laryngomalacia caused by poor upper airway tone (i.e. "neurologic-variant laryngomalacia"), as aspiration may be worsened following surgery.

Anatomic abnormalities such as tracheoesophageal fistula (TEF) and laryngotracheoesophageal cleft (LTEC) also result in aspiration during swallowing, though not due to abnormalities in deglutition. These cause a direct connection between the esophagus and the airway, and most TEFs are detected at birth. Aspiration of thin liquids drunk quickly is the typical history for a LTEC. H-type TEF and LTEC are difficult to detect, and diligent investigation by a skilled rigid bronchoscopist is generally required. Even mild LTEC (types 1 and 2) may be associated with significant symptoms (e.g., stridor, feeding problems, recurrent respiratory infections), even when radiographic swallowing studies do not demonstrate frank aspiration.[50,51]

Children with chronic pulmonary aspiration frequently have tracheostomy tubes because of their underlying medical conditions and for pulmonary toilet. The presence of a tracheostomy tube affects many important components of swallowing, causing impaired laryngeal elevation, alterations in timing, and prevention of the rise in intratracheal pressure. While an association between impaired swallowing and the presence of a tracheostomy tube has been documented, there is no study that demonstrates the development of de novo aspiration following tracheostomy placement in children.[52–54] Children with tracheostomies who chronically aspirate may benefit from use of a one-way speaking valve when anatomically appropriate. This restores physiologic PEEP and allows subglottic pressure to elevate with swallowing. This can also be achieved with positive pressure applied to the tracheostomy tube by CPAP or a ventilator.

EVALUATION OF SWALLOWING

Swallowing function can be evaluated by clinical examination by a trained speech and language pathologist, by radiographic investigation, or endoscopically. Each method has strengths and weaknesses. Clinical evaluations by trained providers provide excellent evaluation of the feeding behaviors, aversions, and oral motor skills. They also provide good screening for possible aspiration. One study reported a negative predictive value of 89% for aspiration of liquids, yet the reported positive predictive value was worse: 54% for liquids and 18% for solids.[55] When the clinical exam suggests aspiration, a swallowing study should be performed to confirm it.

Radiographic Evaluation of Swallowing

Radiographic tests are the most commonly utilized method for evaluation of deglutition. Videofluoroscopic swallow studies (also known as *modified barium swallows*) have the ability to directly evaluate the oral, pharyngeal, and esophageal phases of swallowing.[55–58] This assessment can be made utilizing consistencies similar to what the child is accustomed to eating. Any abnormality in bolus formation, timing of swallow, and competence of velopharyngeal valve can be observed. Aspiration and penetration of food material caused by premature spillage, delayed initiation of swallow, ineffective swallow, pooling of residual material in the hypopharynx, cricopharyngeal achalasia, or aspiration of refluxed material can be seen. Passage of the bolus through the esophagus can be evaluated, and aspiration through a laryngeal cleft or H-type tracheoesophageal fistula can be seen (although with poor sensitivity). Compensatory interventions and feeding recommendations can be made and evaluated at the time of the study.

Videofluoroscopic swallow studies have limitations. It must be kept in mind that they represent a snapshot and that the accuracy can be affected by patient cooperation, position, current state of health, volume of food taken, the number of swallows evaluated, and being "rushed" by the evaluator. Every attempt should be made to replicate feeding as it is done in the home and during a period of baseline health. Owing to the episodic nature of aspiration, a normal swallow study cannot entirely rule out aspiration of feeds. Generally, a videofluoroscopic swallow study is a standard evaluation for direct aspiration ("from above") for children in whom clinical evaluation has suggested abnormal swallowing.

Endoscopic Evaluation of Swallowing

Swallowing function can also be evaluated via a fiberoptic endoscopic evaluation of swallowing (FEES). This evaluation may be performed by a trained otolaryngologist, a speech and language pathologist (SLP), or both working together. FEES requires no sedation or radiation exposure and, in contrast to radiographic swallow studies, is completely portable. This allows FEES to be performed at the bedside and in whatever type of seat or wheelchair the child is accustomed to feeding. A small flexible nasopharyngoscope is passed transnasally and positioned between the soft palate and epiglottis. Multiple swallows are visualized directly by the otolaryngologist, the SLP, and the child's home caregivers via a video monitor. The oral and pharyngeal phases can be assessed, but the scope is blind to events occurring during pharyngeal contraction. Children can be fed the same food they are accustomed to eating at home, the consistencies can be varied, and the effectiveness of implemented compensatory and therapeutic swallowing techniques can be assessed. The ability of the caregiver to observe the aspiration event and the effectiveness of feeding techniques provides direct feedback.

Role of Radiographic and Endoscopic Tests in the Evaluation of Aspiration

Radiographic swallow studies and FEES are both valuable tools for the evaluation of deglutition, but they have unique strengths and weaknesses (Table 66-2). They are

TABLE 66-2 COMPARISON OF VSS AND FEES

VIDEOFLUOROSCOPIC SWALLOW STUDY	FIBEROPTIC ENDOSCOPIC EVALUATION OF SWALLOWING
Improves clinical examination of swallowing	Improves clinical examination of swallowing
Evaluates oral, pharyngeal, AND esophageal phases of deglutition	Blind to actual moment of swallow
Limited evaluation of anatomy	Does not evaluate esophageal phase
Evaluates multiple consistencies	Evaluates functional anatomy of swallow
May lack sensitivity: Less eaten→ less sensitive	Evaluates multiple consistencies
Feeding recommendations made at time of study	Evaluates airway protective ability and sensation (even if does not eat)
Widely available	Feeding recommendations made at time of study
Radiation exposure	Not widely available
Not portable, non-invasive	No radiation
	Portable but invasive
	Good caregiver feedback

equally sensitive in their abilities to detect delayed initiation of swallow, penetration, aspiration, and postswallow residue.[59–61] A prospective, randomized trial in dysphagic adults found no differences in pneumonia outcomes whether feeding recommendations were made based on FEES or videofluoroscopic swallow study results.[62] Radiographic swallow studies can improve their sensitivity when many swallows can be observed, especially as the effects of fatigue may become evident. However, radiographic assessment of the child who has not been orally feeding (because of prolonged illness or oral aversions) is very limited. FEES is useful in these situations as aspiration risk can be evaluated by assessing vocal cord function, excessive pooling of oral secretions, or by placing a few drops of colored food dye on the tongue and observing for aspiration or penetration.[63] Laryngeal sensation and protective reflexes can be further assessed by the addition of sensory testing (FEES-ST) in which graded bursts of air are applied to an aryepiglottic fold while observing for a laryngeal adductor response.[63,64] This allows FEES to evaluate children who may aspirate oral secretions or to assess a non-orally feeding child's safety to begin eating by mouth. Detection of aspiration through a laryngeal cleft can be improved due to the superior visualization of laryngeal anatomy. FEES is particularly useful in the assessment of postoperative aspiration risk for a child with a high-grade subglottic stenosis in whom airway reconstructive surgery is being planned. Both radiographic swallow studies and FEES are useful and complementary because of the different types of information they provide.

ASPIRATION OF GASTROESOPHAGEAL REFLUX

Not all aspiration occurs directly via dysfunctional swallowing. There is a well-documented relationship between GER and chronic respiratory symptoms such as: wheezing, chronic cough, nocturnal cough, apnea, and recurrent chest infections.[65–68] While there may be multiple possible mechanisms for GER-related respiratory symptoms, it is clear that chronic aspiration of gastric contents does occur.[69–71] The effect of chronic microaspiration of acidic material on the development of *chronic* lung injury is not entirely clear. With reflux aspiration, there are other factors besides pH; pepsin, bile acids, and food particulates are all present in gastric fluid and may play a role in the pathophysiology of lung injury. Experimental instillation of weakly acidic liquid (pH >2.5) into the lungs of animals results in an immediate inflammatory response and pneumonitis.[72] The acute effects of a single small-volume instillation subsequently resolve. In an animal model of chronic aspiration, histopathologic changes were completely independent of acidity and were more related to the presence of the food particulates.[12,15] If it is the gastric contents themselves, independent of acidity that results in lung injury, then acid suppression may not prevent the chronic lung injury from aspiration. In addition, the use of acid-suppressing medications increases gastric colonization by bacteria and may result in aspiration of material with greater bacterial density.[73,74] This potential has been demonstrated in multiple adult studies of ventilator-associated pneumonia but not in the single prospective trial in a pediatric intensive care unit.[73,75–78]

GER is quite common in children with chronic respiratory diseases.[68,79–81] The risk of aspiration from reflux is increased when there is coexisting swallowing dysfunction, decreased laryngeal sensation, tachypnea, or upper airway obstruction. GER and aspiration may also occur in cases of esophageal dysmotility, compression, or stenosis, and it is particularly difficult to manage.

Evaluation of Reflux Aspiration

There are several diagnostic modalities available for the diagnosis of GER, yet none are sufficiently sensitive and specific to reliably prove aspiration. While a certain amount of acid exposure may be expected to cause esophagitis, establishment of norms for reflux aspiration is not possible. Certainly some individuals may have a moderate amount of reflux and not aspirate, while others may protect their airways so poorly that any amount of reflux results in aspiration and lung injury. Therefore, episodes of reflux to or above the upper esophageal sphincter should be thought of as opportunities to aspirate, rather than proof of aspiration itself.

Lipid-Laden Macrophage Index

Biomarkers obtained from the lungs have been sought and evaluated in order to identify children with significant aspiration, especially those who are suspected of aspirating refluxate. The most extensively studied biomarker is the calculation of a quantitative index of lipid-containing macrophages in BAL fluid. Theoretically, an increased prevalence of lipid-filled macrophages in the lower airway suggests aspiration of food during swallowing or following reflux from the stomach. While several studies have found higher levels of lipid in the BAL of children with chronic aspiration than those without, many others have not.[68,82–87] This inconsistency is even more striking viewed across studies, even when the methodology for lipid-laden macrophage index (LLMI) is the same (Fig. 66-3). This variability may represent an inherent limitation in the LLMI itself, reflect differences in groups characterized as aspirators due to lack of a gold standard, or demonstrate that the presence of GER and respiratory symptoms only presumes aspiration as the mechanism. This last point is highlighted by two studies evaluating the correlation of proximal reflux events, detected by esophageal impedance and pH monitoring, to LLMI. Borrelli and colleagues found correlation between reflux episodes to the proximal esophagus (total and non-acid) in children with recurrent consolidations, asthma, and laryngotracheitis, though only two subjects had LLMI greater than the commonly cited threshold of 100.[88] Rosen and coworkers also evaluated children with possible GER and respiratory symptoms.[89] The authors compared proximal reflux events between those that had LLMI greater than and less than 100 and found a trend toward fewer events in those with LLMI greater than 100. This lack of correlation between proximal reflux events and LLMI is consistent with data from our own center.

Other Biomarkers of Reflux Aspiration

As elevated lipid-containing macrophages would not be expected to be specific for aspiration caused by reflux, recent efforts have sought to evaluate biomarkers of gastric origin. Gastric pepsin is the most extensively evaluated of these biomarkers. Krishnan and colleagues found pepsin in the tracheal aspirates of those children undergoing endoscopy who had both respiratory symptoms and esophagitis, but not in those without.[90] Since then, pepsin has been evaluated as a biomarker of aspiration in intubated premature infants, pediatric critical care patients, and lung transplant recipients.[91–96] In intubated premature infants, pepsin is almost invariably found in endotracheal aspirates, with concentrations increasing over time; higher concentrations are associated with development of severe bronchopulmonary dysplasia.[91,92] In these studies, pepsin did not appear to arrive in the airway via production by airway epithelium or hematogenous spread, yet the almost ubiquitous presence of pepsin (even in infants not enterally fed) would seem to limit its utility as a biomarker of significant reflux aspiration. Similarly, the finding of pepsin in tracheal aspirates of older intubated children (whether fed by nasogastric or nasojejunal tube) may signify that pepsin may not be a clinically useful biomarker of aspiration, or that reflux aspiration is omnipresent in most intubated infants and children, regardless of feeding status, after a few days. It is important to remember that most of these studies have evaluated the presence of pepsin in tracheal aspirates obtained repeatedly, and therefore results obtained on a single BAL may be different.

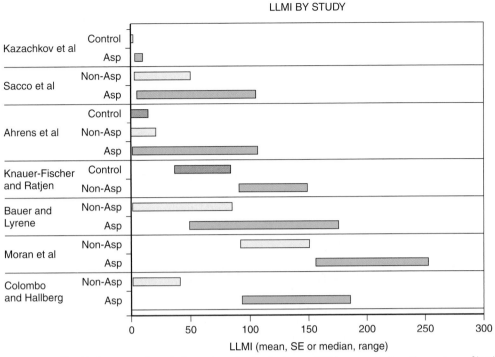

FIGURE 66-3. Comparison of lipid-laden macrophage index on bronchoalveolar lavage (BAL) across studies. Comparison of lipid-laden macrophage indices *(LLMIs)* across studies to demonstrate overlapping ranges between controls, children with aspiration (Asp), and children without aspiration *(Non-Asp)*. Despite a similar grading system, nonaspirating children in some studies have a higher LLMI than aspirating children in others.

Treatment Considerations for Reflux Aspiration

There are various treatment options for GER, and a full discussion is beyond the scope of this chapter. When considering therapeutic options for reflux aspiration (as opposed to reflux esophagitis), it is essential to recognize that acid suppression does not reduce the number of reflux events, only the pH of such events. Acid suppression in the context of reflux aspiration may result in the aspiration of material with a higher bacterial density caused by colonization of the proximal GI tract.[73,77,97] Perturbations in local lung defense (e.g., chronic inflammation and degradation of surfactant proteins) combined with the increased bacterial density of aspirated material may result in increased infection and lung injury.[98] Therefore, children who are unable to adequately protect their airways from aspiration caused by reflux require an intervention, generally surgical, that will decrease the number of reflux events to their proximal esophagus. Surgical options generally include transpyloric feeding (i.e., gastrostomy-jejunostomy or jejunostomy tubes) or fundoplication. Fundoplication is the most commonly utilized surgical procedure and is often successful in resolving reflux, and in some studies demonstrates efficacy in reducing respiratory symptoms attributed to reflux.[99-102] Unfortunately, in neurologically impaired children there is a greater incidence of both chronic aspiration and GER, and a greater likelihood of failure of fundoplication, increased incidence of post-fundoplication retching, and decreased efficacy in reduction of respiratory symptoms.[99,102-107] In children with esophageal dysmotility, a fundoplication must be created carefully so as not to impede forward transit of food or oral secretions through the esophagogastric junction because this may worsen aspiration. Jejunostomy feedings may allow adequate feeding and decrease respiratory symptoms caused by aspiration without the concerns for gas bloat or retching, however there are other issues.[108,109] Jejunostomies do not prevent reflux of gastric secretions, do not allow the convenience of bolus feeding, and carry the risk of intussusception and repeated displacement. Another use for gastrojejunostomy is diagnostic. In a child with an existing gastrostomy, a trial of conversion to a gastrostomy-jejunostomy tube may test the potential impact of an antireflux procedure on respiratory symptoms that are suspected to be caused by reflux aspiration.

ASPIRATION OF ORAL SECRETIONS

Chronic aspiration of saliva is the least-commonly recognized form of aspiration and may not be diagnosed until significant lung injury has developed. The oral cavity contains a high density of bacteria and yeast that can cause lung infections if aspirated in sufficient quantity.[110] Most neurologically impaired children who aspirate oral secretions do so because of severe swallowing incoordination and absent laryngeal sensation rather than excessive production of saliva.[111] Other conditions commonly associated with both swallowing dysfunction and aspiration of saliva include CHARGE association, Möbius syndrome, congenital high airway obstruction syndrome (CHAOS), and vocal cord paralysis. It is unusual for a child without severe swallowing dysfunction to aspirate oral secretions. Children with cricopharyngeal achalasia, severe esophageal dysmotility, stricture, or diverticulum are exceptions. These children may pool saliva excessively in their hypopharynx and aspirate at night because of a combination of depressed protective reflexes during sleep and the absence of gravity assistance in the drainage of secretions from the esophagus into the stomach.

Evaluation of Salivary Aspiration

Aspiration of saliva is best evaluated by FEES or FEES-ST, as pooling and aspiration of oral secretions can be visualized directly. The lack of a compensatory cough or laryngeal adductor reflex further supports the likelihood that significant pathologic aspiration of saliva is occurring. Radionuclide salivagrams are performed by placing a small quantity of radiotracer in the buccal space and recording serial images until there is clearance from the mouth. The presence of activity in the trachea or bronchi indicates aspiration of saliva. While these tests are likely very specific, they are infrequently positive in children highly suspected of aspiration and correlate poorly with other tests for aspiration.[112–115] In children with a tracheostomy, aspiration of saliva can be evaluated by placement of 1 to 2 drops of green food dye in the buccal space, a few times a day, for several days and having a caregiver keep a diary of suctioning of colored secretions from the tube. While the basis of the test is the same as the radionuclide salivagram, repeated administration captures a longer window of time and may improve sensitivity.

Treatment of Salivary Aspiration

Treatment of salivary aspiration may be medical or surgical. Oral anticholinergic medications decrease salivation and therefore may decrease the amount of saliva available to aspirate. These medications do not specifically affect saliva production, however, and adverse effects are common. These include behavioral changes, constipation, dry mouth, urinary retention, flushing, nasal congestion, vomiting, and diarrhea.[116–118] Of greater concern is the potential for thickening of tracheal and bronchial secretions that could result in life-threatening mucus plugging of airways or tracheostomy tubes. For this reason, they should be used with great caution in infants, children with neuromuscular diseases, and those with small tracheostomy tubes. Production of saliva can be specifically reduced either by injection of glands with botulinum toxin, ligation of salivary ducts, or removal of salivary glands. The submandibular glands are most frequently treated by injection, excision, or duct ligation as they are responsible for the majority of baseline saliva production. Parotid glands are the major secretors of saliva in anticipation of eating and are therefore commonly treated, by injection or duct ligation, at the same time as the submandibular glands. Botulinum toxin injection, duct ligation, and gland excision have all demonstrated efficacy in reduction of drooling and decreasing respiratory infections.[119–123] Botulinum toxin injection results in a limited duration of effect (which may be desirable or undesirable), while the effects of salivary gland excision or duct ligation are generally long-lasting.

■ EVALUATION OF LUNG INJURY CAUSED BY ASPIRATION

As the lung is the end organ of damage from chronic aspiration, it makes sense to confirm the presence and extent of lung injury from aspiration. As mentioned, evaluations of swallowing dysfunction and GER are imperfect, and many interventions to prevent aspiration require major surgery or lifestyle modifications. Therefore, one should confirm that identified abnormalities in swallowing function are sufficient to cause lung injury. This will inform the "urgency" to intervene. Chest radiographs are readily available and are usually abnormal in children with chronic aspiration. Hyperaeration, segmental or subsegmental infiltrates, and peribronchial thickening may be seen; usually in multiple lobes and in a dependent distribution. The findings on plain chest radiograph, however, are very nonspecific and are of little use in differentiating chronic aspiration from other diffuse lung diseases. Furthermore, chest radiographs are not very sensitive with regard to detecting bronchiectasis from chronic aspiration.

C-HRCT is more sensitive than plain radiographs in the detection and definition of early airways and parenchymal disease in pediatric patients.[124,125] Ideally suited to evaluate diffuse lung diseases, c-HRCT is capable of identifying signs of small airway disease such as centrilobular ("tree-in-bud") opacities, bronchial thickening, and subsegmental atelectasis, and it is the current gold standard for diagnosis of bronchiectasis. These findings on c-HRCT are representative of those found on lung histopathology.[10,13,14] While these findings are not specific for chronic pulmonary aspiration, the presence of these findings in a multilobe-dependent distribution in a child with known dysphagia or GER provides strong evidence for aspiration lung injury (Fig. 66-4). Though specific protocols may vary, commonly thin (1-mm) images are obtained at intervals of 10 mm during a controlled inspiratory breath hold. Although there is appropriate concern over excessive exposure to ionizing radiation,

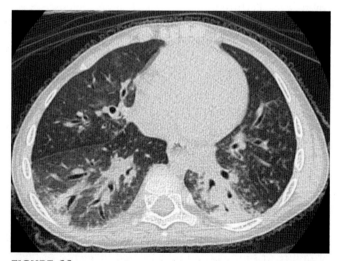

FIGURE 66-4. Lung injury caused by chronic aspiration. Chest high-resolution computed tomography (c-HRCT) shows dependent bronchiectasis, consolidations, and centrilobular opacities in a child with chronic aspiration caused by recurrent tracheoesophageal fistula.

HRCT uses limited sampling that allows radiation doses to be minimized; current protocols can deliver doses equivalent to 6 weeks of ambient radiation exposure.[126] It is necessary to be aware of the protocols used in one's own institution.

MULTIDISCIPLINARY APPROACH TO CHRONIC ASPIRATION

The evaluation and treatment of a child suspected of chronic pulmonary aspiration is best performed by a multidisciplinary team. By way of example, how else might we sort out the causes for respiratory symptoms in the following child: 2 years old, 25-week premature birth with chronic lung disease, tachypnea, wheezing with chest congestion, hypoxemia with sleep and illness, snoring with sleep, moderate tracheobronchomalacia, and a deep interarytenoid notch? In addition, the child has mild oral aversion and premature spillage and penetration with liquids. He is status post-fundoplication with a small paraesophageal hernia and takes some feeds orally and some by gastrostomy. Clearly a child such as this has a complex interaction of pulmonary, airway, and gastrointestinal pathology. Chronic aspiration may be a component of the symptoms and if left untreated would lead to progressive lung injury and associated morbidity. A broad evaluation of all the contributing factors is required, with the development of a coordinated approach to systematically address the most significant contributors to disease, but without disrupting successful compensatory mechanisms the child may have developed. With advancements in perinatal medicine, children such as these are increasingly common.

The key components of such a multidisciplinary team include a pulmonologist, otolaryngologist, gastroenterologist, and speech and language pathologist. Given the frequency with which certain inherited diseases result in aerodigestive disorders, a geneticist can be a very useful person on the team. Other supporting team members include a cardiothoracic surgeon, general surgeon, neurosurgeon, radiologist, cardiologist, neurologist, and occasionally an orthopedist. With so many services potentially involved, coordination of care is of paramount importance.

Ideally, each service involved would have an opportunity to obtain a primary history and examine the child, and then the providers would meet as a group and plan a coordinated evaluation. It is beneficial to have one individual identified as the primary provider to discuss the plan with the caregivers and answer their questions. This prevents the family from having to seek out different providers with different questions and then interpret various recommendations. All children suspected of chronic pulmonary aspiration should have their swallowing evaluated by videofluoroscopic swallowing study, FEES, or both. The method for evaluation of swallowing should be determined based on available expertise, the child's clinical situation, and the relative strengths and weaknesses of each test. Evaluation for GER may also be considered. For children with impaired swallowing or GER, c-HRCT can identify when there has been lung injury attributable to

chronic aspiration. If dependent bronchiectasis is present, it may be difficult to determine if this is a result of prior or ongoing aspiration. This is especially true when children are referred for evaluation after having had their feeding altered or having received a fundoplication.

Evaluation of the Aerodigestive Tract

Once we are convinced that there is chronic aspiration sufficient to cause lung injury, a search for underlying causes should be undertaken. This always includes a thorough assessment of the anatomy of the aerodigestive tract. A fundamental component of this is bronchoscopy. Bronchoscopy may be undertaken using rigid or flexible instruments, and there are relative strengths and weaknesses to each. Flexible bronchoscopy provides assessment of the entire upper and lower airways and can identify pathology from the nose to the distal bronchi. Flexible bronchoscopy is particularly well-suited to identifying dynamic airway lesions such as laryngomalacia, pharyngomalacia, tracheomalacia, and bronchomalacia, which a rigid bronchoscopy approach may obscure. In addition, flexible bronchoscopy allows for the performance of BAL. Paired with c-HRCT, BAL can help determine if lung injury is caused by prior or ongoing aspiration. The presence of increased secretions with an inflammatory profile on BAL (with or without elevated lipid-laden macrophages) would provide supporting evidence for ongoing aspiration, even though it lacks the specificity to prove it outright.

Rigid bronchoscopy should be considered an essential evaluation in a child with chronic aspiration. While evaluation of upper airway dynamics and ability to obtain diagnostic BAL may be limited, rigid instruments are far superior to flexible for the identification of laryngeal clefts, H-type tracheoesophageal fistula, and cricopharyngeal achalasia (Fig. 66-5). Even in a patient with a known laryngeal cleft, flexible bronchoscopes fail to detect or evaluate the extent of them most of the time. The direct approach to the posterior larynx, cricoid, and proximal trachea with instruments capable of manipulating tissue makes this possible. Even rigid bronchoscopists can easily miss laryngeal clefts (especially types 1 and 2) unless a specific effort is made to look for them. In reality, the practice of combined bronchoscopy, rigid and flexible, performed concurrently, offers certain distinct advantages. With this approach, both the pulmonologist and the otolaryngologist have the opportunity to see the static and dynamic airway anatomy firsthand in its entirety, can observe the status of the lower airways, and have a dialog regarding an integrated care plan. The addition of evaluation by a gastroenterologist, as part of a "triple endoscopy," adds an evaluation for potential reflux aspiration, acid esophagitis, eosinophilic esophagitis, and anatomic abnormalities of the upper gastrointestinal tract. This is especially important if the child is being evaluated in preparation for airway reconstruction. Given that these children often require both medical and surgical intervention, this combined approach makes logical sense, and the multidisciplinary evaluation leads to a consistent, cohesive assessment and plan to be delivered to the family.

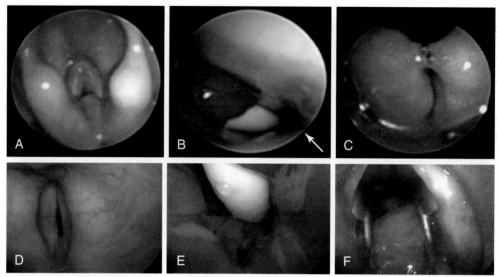

FIGURE 66-5. Evaluation of laryngoesophagotracheal cleft (LTEC) by rigid and flexible bronchoscopes. **A, B,** and **C,** Evaluation of LTEC (type 3) with flexible bronchoscope: **A,** Redundant tissue in the interarytenoid space or posterior commissure is very suspicious for LTEC. **B,** Note that the distal extent of cleft cannot be seen clearly *(arrow)*, though the scope can slide posteriorly and into the esophagus. **C,** A post-cricoid "seam" is also suspicious for LTEC. Note that it is very unusual to be able to see even such a large cleft this well with a flexible bronchoscope. **D, E,** and **F,** Evaluation of the same patient with a rigid bronchoscope: **D,** similar view of redundant tissue in interarytenoid space. **E,** Direct approach to posterior glottis and upper trachea, as well as laryngeal suspension, aids in clear definition of distal extent of cleft. **F,** Various instruments can be utilized by the otolaryngologist to further define the extent of the cleft.

Suggested Reading

Boesch RP, Daines C, Willging JP, et al. Advances in the diagnosis and management of chronic pulmonary aspiration in children. *Eur Respir J.* 2006;28:847–861.

Delaney AL, Arvedson JC. Development of swallowing and feeding: prenatal through the first year of life. *Dev Disabil Res Rev.* 2008;14:105–117.

Pasteur MC, Bilton D, Hill AT. British Thoracic Society Bronchiectasis non-CF Guideline Group. British Thoracic Society guideline for non-CF bronchiectasis. *Thorax.* 2010;65(suppl 1):i1–i58.

References

The complete reference list is available online at www.expertconsult.com

67 FEEDING, SWALLOWING, AND VOICE DISORDERS

J. Paul Willging, MD, Alessandro de Alarcon, MD, Claire Kane Miller, PhD, Lisa N. Kelchner, PhD, CCC-SLP, BRS-S, and Scott Pentiuk, MD, MeD

The upper aerodigestive tract is the confluence of the respiratory, digestive, and phonation systems. Precise integration of functions is required for protection of the lower airway from aspiration during swallowing and for adequate production of voice. There are a variety of anatomic and neurologic etiologies that may affect the structural integrity and interrelated physiology of feeding, swallowing, and phonation. In particular, congenital or acquired conditions involving the supraglottic, glottis, or subglottic airway require airway surgical interventions that may have an effect on laryngeal function for airway protection, swallowing, and voicing.[1-5] Any necessary reconstruction procedures involve anatomic alteration of the laryngeal anatomy; therefore, careful preoperative assessment of laryngeal anatomy and function pertinent to swallowing and phonation is required. Many children with complex airway conditions also have concomitant neurodevelopmental delays that place them at even higher risk for communication, feeding, and swallowing disorders.[6] The multifactorial nature of feeding, swallowing, and voice disorders involves multiple disciplines in the evaluation and management process, and therefore, a team approach is best. This chapter will review the multidisciplinary perspectives on clinical and instrumental evaluation and management of infants and children with feeding, swallowing, and voice disorders.

ANATOMY, PHYSIOLOGY, AND NEURAL CONTROL PERTINENT TO FEEDING, SWALLOWING, AND PHONATION

The larynx serves three functions: connection of the upper and lower respiratory airway, closure for protection of the lower airway during swallowing, and generation of sound for voice. Identification of the maturational changes that occur in the anatomy of the aerodigestive tract and in the ontogeny of feeding, swallowing, and voice production is fundamental in delineating physiologic abnormalities and in defining the effect of compensatory strategies for improvement of laryngeal function.

In terms of anatomy, there are differences in the size and location of the structures associated with the key laryngeal functions in the infant as compared to the child or adult. At birth, the larynx is positioned relatively high in the neck, located adjacent to cervical vertebrae C1 to C3, and later descending to levels C6 to C7. The overall size of the infant larynx is approximately one third that of the adult, with the membranous portion of the true vocal folds (TVFs) measuring approximately 2 to 3 mm and the bulkier cartilaginous portion measuring approximately 3 to 4 mm.

There is a slight downward slant of the TVFs (posterior to anterior). The thyroid cartilage of the pediatric larynx is rounded, the epiglottis may have an omega shape, and the cricoarytenoid joints and vocal processes are proportionately larger than in the adult larynx.[7] The delicate respiratory epithelium that lines the infant airway is particularly prone to injury from prolonged or traumatic intubation, and the subglottic region is often the site for reactive stenosis.[8] The length of the membranous portion of the vocal folds increases and the arytenoid cartilages debulk as the child grows. Puberty is a time of rapid laryngeal growth, especially in males, and it is the developmental period when the length of the folds reach adult size (e.g., 17 to 21 mm for males; 11 to 15 mm for females).[9] Histologic differentiation of the pediatric vocal fold cover is not fully understood, but the process is thought to continue from infancy into the early teens. The TVFs of infants and young children are thinner, and the lamina propria is composed of a uniform single layer versus the three discreet layers known to be present in adults (i.e., superficial, intermediate, and deep layers). The vocal fold ligament is not fully formed until after puberty, and during childhood the thyroarytenoid muscle has a greater percentage of collagen.[7,10,11]

The small size and shape of the oral cavity relative to the tongue facilitates early sucking as the buccal fat pads provide lateral stability for efficient tongue motion. As the infant grows, the prominent buccal pads decrease, the oral cavity increases in size, and the relative size of the tongue decreases. More space is available for differentiated tongue movements during both feeding and vocalization. Elongation of the pharynx occurs as does the maturational descent of the larynx from C3 to C6 by approximately 3 years of age. As the larynx descends, increased neuromuscular control of the structural elements of the pharynx is critical for maintenance of airway protection during swallowing.[12]

In addition to the anatomic interrelation of the structures involved in feeding, swallowing, and voicing, there is common neural control that is composed of cortical influences, peripheral afferent signals, nerve networks, and efferent responses driven by motor neurons The oral, nasal, pharyngeal, and laryngeal structures are primarily innervated by branches of cranial nerves I, V, VII, IX, X, XI (vagal branch), XII, and branches of the upper cervical nerves. There are further structural and regulatory interrelationships within the brainstem, specifically the medulla (e.g., central pattern generator). Afferent input for swallowing is primarily located in the nucleus tractus solitarius (NTS); efferent control is localized in the nucleus ambiguus (NA) and the dorsal motor nucleus of CN X. Likewise, afferent input is received by the NTS for respiration, with efferent respiratory control via premotor neurons in the NTS and NA that project to the spinal cord motor neurons and innervate the respiratory skeletal musculature. Central control of vocalization becomes highly differentiated during the first few months of life as laryngeal functions develop and transition from primarily protective reflexes to intentional vocal use for communication occurs.

Feeding Skill Development

Feeding gradually evolves from a reflexive behavior in infants to a cortically regulated behavior during the first 2 years of life (Table 67-1). Anatomic changes in oral and pharyngeal structural relationships as well as maturation of the central nervous system during the first 2 years of life are reflected in the transition to mature oral motor/feeding and swallowing skills. Sucking occurs early *in utero* and continues as the primary means of obtaining nutrition for the first 3 to 4 months of life.[13] As the motor and digestive systems mature, smooth solids such as strained or pureed foods are introduced at approximately 4 to 6 months of age. Head control and stability improve with differentiation of tongue movements at 7 to 9 months of age, at which time increased food textures are presented. Continued emergence of active oral motor movements such as tongue lateralization and rotary chewing facilitate the transition to table foods at around 1 year of age. By 2 years of age, oral motor/feeding and swallowing skills are in place, with refinements in oral motor movements as the child continues to mature.[14]

Phases of Swallowing

The swallowing process is composed of the oral preparatory, oral, pharyngeal, and esophageal phases. For an efficient oral phase of swallowing to occur, it is crucial to have normal anatomy and intact gross discriminative and special sensory input from olfaction via CN I and the oral cavity via CN V (V2 and V3), VII, IX, and X. It is also crucial to have intact muscular strength and coordination of the buccal and oral musculature. Adequate oral preparation of the bolus, followed by posterior transfer of the bolus to the hypopharynx via tongue base retraction and simultaneous closure of the soft palate against the posterior pharynx occurs. Once the oral bolus is transferred to the hypopharynx, airway protection must occur during the pharyngeal swallowing phase to prevent aspiration. Tactile receptors in the pharynx provide sensory stimulation to the medullary swallow center, and swallowing is initiated via the nucleus ambiguus and the dorsomedial vagal nucleus.[15]

Airway protection during the pharyngeal phase of the swallow occurs as a sequence involving the cessation of respiration (swallowing apnea), adduction of the TVFs in association with the medial approximation of the arytenoid cartilages, compression of the ventricular vocal folds, and retroversion of the epiglottis.[16] At the instant of swallow, the larynx is elevated under the base of the tongue, facilitating the stretching and opening of the cricopharyngeus, as the pharyngeal constrictors shorten the pharynx and propel the bolus into the upper esophageal sphincter. Once passage of the bolus has occurred, the

TABLE 67-1 ORAL MOTOR/FEEDING SKILL DEVELOPMENT

AGE RANGE	SKILL	FOOD TYPES
Birth to 4 months	Sucking predominates	Liquid (breast milk, formula)
4-6 months	Anterior-posterior tongue movements for efficient transfer of smooth solids	Pureed, smooth, semi-solid foods
7-9 months	Efficient sucking, emergent skills for cup drinking Emergence of tongue lateralization Vertical chewing motion in response to solids	Semi-solids with increased textures (e.g., cottage cheese, regular applesauce, fruited yogurt) Solid items (e.g., very easily dissolvable cereal pieces, soft cookies, shredded cheese)
9-12 months	Increasing lateral tongue movements for mastication of foods Vertical chewing pattern with emergence of lateral tongue movements Transition to cup drinking Trend toward less formula intake as solid intake increases	Fork-mashed or slightly blended table foods Transitioning toward easy to manage solid foods (e.g., scrambled eggs, toast strips, pasta pieces, crunchy but dissolvable cookies, and crackers)
12-18 months	Consistent tongue lateralization Emergence of mature rotary chewing pattern	Easy to manage solid foods (e.g., crackers, breads, casseroles, soft fruit pieces, and tender meat such as flaked fish or chicken)
19-24 months	Chewing efficiency increases Cup drinking	Table foods requiring greater mastication (e.g., tender meats, steamed vegetables, and fruits)
24 months	Oral motor/feeding skills have emerged, with refinement in skills to continue	Wide range of textures

larynx returns to its resting position, the airway reopens, and respiration resumes. Swallowing apnea and glottic closure are linked events, though swallowing apnea has been described to occur as a result of a dedicated neural command.[17] The exact neural control mechanisms are unknown, though past and recent investigations suggest that a designated neural command from the central pattern generator within the medullary brainstem occurs.[15,17,18] The specific respiratory phase patterns and duration of apneic pause in relation to normal and abnormal swallowing parameters in the pediatric population is presently unknown; however, there is emerging data regarding respiration and nutritive swallowing parameters in the infant population.[19]

The neurologic arch that allows for airway protection is described as the laryngeal adductor reflex (LAR).[20] The supraglottic area contains chemoreceptors, mechanoreceptors, thermal receptors, and baroreceptors (i.e., stretch/pressure receptors) that are highly sensitive to specific kinds of sensory input. The LAR is activated by mechanical or chemical stimulation of the supraglottic mucosa in the region of the aryepiglottic fold.[20] The internal branch of the superior laryngeal nerve transmits sensory information via the special visceral afferent fibers to the inferior nodose ganglion. The information passes to the nucleus solitarius, which is responsible for the regulation of swallowing and respiration. The efferent response initiated at the nucleus ambiguus and dorsal motor nucleus of CN X results in glottic closure and inhibition of respiration with or without a swallow.[21–24]

The actions of the intrinsic laryngeal musculature are of major importance to phonation and to airway closure during swallowing. The intrinsic muscles (i.e., cricothyroid, posterior cricoarytenoid, lateral cricoarytenoid, thyroarytenoid [vocalis], and the transverse and oblique arytenoids) serve to adduct, abduct, and tense the vocal folds as well as open and close the laryngeal valve. The cricothyroid stretches and tenses the vocal fold and is innervated by the external branch of the superior laryngeal nerve. The posterior cricoarytenoid is the sole abductor of the vocal folds and is innervated by the recurrent laryngeal nerve. The lateral cricoarytenoid adducts the interligamentous portion of the vocal fold and is supplied by the recurrent laryngeal nerve. The thyroarytenoid and the transverse and oblique arytenoids are likewise innervated by the recurrent laryngeal nerve. The thyroarytenoid works to relax the vocal folds. Its medial portion, the vocalis, relaxes the posterior vocal ligament while maintaining and increasing tension of the anterior portion. The transverse and oblique arytenoids close the intercartilaginous portion of the glottis.

During the pharyngeal phase of the swallow, the upper esophageal sphincter relaxes and allows the bolus to enter the esophagus, initiating the esophageal phase of the swallow. Peristaltic contractions propel the bolus through the esophagus, and the lower esophageal sphincter subsequently relaxes to allow the bolus to pass into the stomach. Propagation of the peristaltic wave is reliant upon the intrinsic myenteric plexus and on vagal afferents.[15]

CONDITIONS ASSOCIATED WITH FEEDING, SWALLOWING, AND AIRWAY PROTECTION PROBLEMS

Difficulty with the oral, pharyngeal, or esophageal phases of swallowing may occur as a result of structural, neurologic, cardiorespiratory, metabolic, or inflammatory disorders (Table 67-2). The etiologies may be congenital or acquired, and the interactions of the developing respiratory, neurologic, and gastrointestinal systems create numerous variables to consider.

Anatomic abnormality in any of the structures from the nasal cavity to the gastrointestinal tract has the potential to disrupt the processes of feeding, swallowing, and ability to achieve and maintain airway closure and protection. Anatomic defects in the oral cavity or

TABLE 67-2 CONDITIONS ASSOCIATED WITH DYSFUNCTION IN THE ORAL, PHARYNGEAL, AND ESOPHAGEAL PHASES OF SWALLOWING

ORAL/ PREPARATORY	PHARYNGEAL	ESOPHAGEAL
Cleft lip/cleft palate	Cricopharyngeal achalasia	Tracheoesophageal fistula
Choanal atresia	Arytenoid prolapse	Eosinophilic esophagitis
Macroglossia	Laryngeal cleft	Vascular ring
Micrognathia	Vocal cord paralysis	Gastroesophageal reflux disease
Oral hypotonia	Laryngo-pharyngitis	Esophageal dysmotility
Oral sensory-motor dysfunction		Achalasia
Cranial nerve paralysis		Esophageal stricture

oropharynx create difficulty in the oral phase of swallowing and include craniofacial syndromes, cleft lip and cleft palate, and macroglossia.[25,26] Congenital defects of the larynx, trachea, or esophagus (e.g., laryngomalacia, laryngeal cleft, or tracheoesophageal fistula) are associated with airway compromise as well as esophageal phase abnormalities.[27] Surgical reconstruction may alleviate the obstructive structural defects, though problems may persist with phonation and laryngeal function during swallowing.[2,3] Tracheoesophageal fistula repair can alter nerve function and esophageal motility leading to prolonged bolus clearance and increased risk for gastroesophageal reflux (GER).[28] There is also the risk of stricture formation at the repair site as well as possible recurrence of the fistula, leading to aspiration.

Neurologic conditions are by far the most common etiology of potential feeding, swallowing, and airway protection problems. Neuromotor impairment as a result of cortical dysfunction, abnormality in the brainstem, or cervical cord injury may affect laryngeal functions that are critical for adequate feeding/swallowing, phonation, and airway protection. Such problems include cerebral palsy, vocal fold paralysis, Arnold-Chiari malformation, cricopharyngeal achalasia, and cranial nerve abnormalities associated with syndromes such as CHARGE association (coloboma, heart defect, atresia choanae, retarded growth and development, genital hypoplasia, ear anomalies), and Moebius syndrome.

Cardiorespiratory compromise secondary to airway abnormalities (e.g., subglottic stenosis, airway edema, and other structural issues) may be reflected in an infant's inability to coordinate respiration and swallowing, and it is often apparent during initial attempts at oral feeding. Feeding-related apnea or episodes of bradycardia may occur. In older infants and children, problems with respiratory compromise are reflected in poor respiratory support during phonation and poor coordination or inappropriate timing of airway protection during swallowing, resulting in coughing, choking, noisy breathing, or recurrent episodes of pneumonia, bronchitis, or atelectasis.[29]

Inflammatory processes such as esophagitis from chronic GER or chronic inflammation/irritation secondary to eosinophilic esophagitis may result in airway manifestations that can interfere with the development of oral motor and feeding skills as well as with swallowing.[30-32] These diseases are increasingly being recognized in children with complex airway disease and are discussed in more detail in Chapters 66 and 68. Chronic reflux or irritation to the laryngeal area has been associated with airway reconstruction failure.[8] Hyposensitivity in the pharyngeal and laryngeal area from chronic reflux irritation may result in poor sensory awareness and a higher risk for aspiration.[23]

Specific Airway Conditions and the Effect on Feeding, Swallowing, and Voice

Pathologic airway conditions in pediatric patients include congenital or acquired subglottic stenosis, glottic stenosis, laryngotracheal stenosis, laryngeal webs or atresia, and tracheal lesions. Congenital subglottic stenosis is relatively rare and typically occurs in conjunction with genetic syndromes or laryngeal malformations. Acquired laryngotracheal stenosis is more common, occurring after manipulation or insult to the airway. Such conditions include subglottic stenosis as a result of prolonged or traumatic intubation, hypopharyngeal stenosis secondary to trauma or caustic agent inhalation or ingestion, vocal fold paralysis as a result of surgical intervention, and tracheal stenosis following intubation. Tracheotomy with later surgical intervention for reconstruction and expansion of the airway is often necessary. The surgical reconstruction techniques are selected based upon the extent and location of the airway lesion and are designed to expand or resect the airway. Avoidance of damage to the recurrent laryngeal nerve as well as to intact laryngeal structures is a primary goal. As discussed previously, an important consideration is the effect that the necessary surgical interventions may have upon the laryngeal functions of phonation and airway protection during swallowing. As children with complex airway conditions may have persistent aspiration or severe reflux, they may be candidates for fundoplication prior to airway reconstruction. It should be noted that these procedures can worsen unrecognized esophageal dysmotility, leading to symptoms of gagging and retching.[33]

Postsurgical issues have been described in regard to voice and swallowing.[1-5] Airway expansion procedures may involve the placement of anterior and/or posterior grafts that are stabilized via an in-dwelling airway stent during the postoperative period. Swallowing and voice production are possible during the period that the stent is in place, however difficulties may arise, depending upon the necessary location of the stent. If placement of the stent is necessary at the glottic level, both phonatory and swallowing dynamics are affected. If the stent location extends to the level of the arytenoids, or to the base of the epiglottis, swallowing function, in particular, is significantly compromised. Patients who undergo placement of posterior grafts may be at risk for destabilization of the cricoarytenoid joint and lateral cricoarytenoid muscles, and are therefore at particular risk for difficulty with airway protection during swallowing and significant degrees of dysphagia.[5] The presence or extent of any postoperative dysphonia will depend on

the integrity of the vibratory surface of the vocal fold mucosa and function of the intrinsic laryngeal muscles and cricoarytenoid joint motion.

■ EVALUATION AND MANAGEMENT

Identification and management of feeding, swallowing, and voice disorders is best done by a multidisciplinary team. The issues span the scope of multiple disciplines, so ideally members of a team include otolaryngologists, gastroenterologists, pulmonary medicine specialists, speech pathologists, occupational therapists, dietitians, behavioral psychologists, and social workers.[34]

In regard to feeding and swallowing assessment, obtaining a detailed history of the child's medical history, development, diet, and feeding patterns is essential. Clinical interview questions include the types of foods and liquids typically ingested, tolerance of different textures and volume, and the child's typical behavior during meals. Specific inquiries should be made regarding respiratory status, history of recurrent respiratory infections or pneumonia, upper airway noise, stridor associated with feeding, or any interventions or operations involving the aerodigestive tract. A thorough clinical assessment of nonnutritive and nutritive oral motor skills is conducted. Clinical assessment of oral motor/feeding skills should include assessment of parent-child interaction during feeding, as disordered interactions may exacerbate feeding difficulties. Clinical signs and symptoms of possible swallowing dysfunction have been noted, including gagging, coughing, choking, color changes, increased noisiness during or after feedings, periods of apnea or bradycardia associated with feeding, increased difficulty with secretion management, frequent suctioning needs, or evidence of food or liquid in the tracheostomy tube.

Instrumental Assessment of Swallowing Function and Airway Protection

If clinical signs or symptoms of possible difficulty with airway protection during swallowing are noted during the clinical feeding evaluation, objective studies to assess airway protection during swallowing are indicated. The most common instrumental examinations include the video swallow study (VSS) and fiberoptic endoscope evaluation of swallowing (FEES). A joint FEES and voice assessment may be efficacious when there are indications for both voice and endoscopic swallowing assessment. Indications for the pediatric FEES study and the video swallow study are listed in Table 67-3. The relative advantages and disadvantages of each examination are summarized in Table 67-4.

The pediatric VSS is beneficial as it provides clear visualization of all phases of the swallow under fluoroscopy.[35] Delineation of tongue motion during bolus preparation, and adequacy of tongue base retraction for swallowing initiation is analyzed. Bolus transfer through the pharynx and upper esophageal sphincter is clearly visualized. Abnormalities in the swallowing process such premature bolus transfer, delayed initiation of swallowing response, inadequate pharyngeal clearance following swallowing, penetration of the bolus into the larynx, and aspiration

TABLE 67-3 INDICATIONS FOR VIDEOFLUOROSCOPY AND/OR FIBEROPTIC ENDOSCOPIC EVALUATION OF SWALLOWING

VIDEOFLUOROSOPIC SWALLOWING STUDY	FIBEROPTIC ENDOSCOPIC EVALUATION OF SWALLOWING (FEES)
Baseline assessment of swallowing function: Need overall view of oral, pharyngeal, and esophageal phases of swallowing	Known or suspected structural abnormality with implications for airway protection during swallowing
Need to view sequential swallow sequences	Questionable secretion management ability
Need to exclude structural problem in the esophagus, stomach, or duodenum as a source of dysphagia	Patient accepts minimal amounts of food/liquid orally

TABLE 67-4 ADVANTAGES AND DISADVANTAGES OF PEDIATRIC FEES

ADVANTAGES	DISADVANTAGES
Specific focus on airway protection during swallowing	Possible discomfort with scope passage
Provides assessment of patient ability to manage secretions	Presence of scope may induce gagging and vomiting in patients with hypersensitive responses
Does not require alteration of food or liquid with contrast	View is obscured during swallowing contraction; can only view events before and after "white-out"
No radiation exposure	Focus of exam is limited to primarily the pharyngeal phase
Can determine readiness to transition to oral feeding in regard to airway protection ability	Lack of view during rapid sequential swallowing (bottle feeding)
Effect of compensatory strategies on improvement of swallowing function/safety can be determined during exam	Contraindicated for patients with choanal atresia, nasal stenosis, nasal obstruction, pharyngeal stenosis
Visual picture of swallowing may provide beneficial feedback to family	Requires special training

of the bolus are readily identified. Patient reaction or response to abnormalities in the swallowing process can be assessed. For example, protective reaction or adequacy of clearing response to episodes of aspiration can be ascertained. Compensatory strategies can be implemented to assist with maintenance of airway protection during swallowing or to improve swallowing efficiency. Positioning adjustments, increasing liquid viscosity/texture alteration, or postural strategies (e.g., chin flexion or head tilting)

may be implemented to assess effect on improving swallowing dynamics and improving airway protection during swallowing.

Disadvantages to the pediatric VSS include radiation exposure to the patient and to the feeder. The necessary addition of barium to the food and liquid potentially decreases the child's willingness to eat or drink during the examination. Implementing compensatory strategies adds to the overall radiation exposure time, limiting the extent to which options can be tested. Infants or children who have only negligible amounts of oral intake are not appropriate candidates for a VSS as a sufficient amount of contrast must be ingested to obtain adequate imaging.

A FEES study to assess airway protection ability as well as adequacy of airway protection during swallowing is indicated for patients who have never fed orally or who have minimal oral intake. FEES is accomplished via transnasal passage of a pediatric endoscope, and it permits direct visualization of pharyngeal and laryngeal structures, function, management of secretions, intactness of sensation, and spontaneous swallows.[36] The swallowing assessment is performed using the patient's normal foods and liquids and customary mode of intake. However, information regarding secretion management and ability to generate spontaneous swallows can be achieved without requiring the patient to ingest food or liquid. The focus of the pediatric FEES study is on airway protection ability and sensation, and it is exceptionally helpful if there is a known or suspected structural abnormality of the pharynx or larynx. Compensatory strategies to assist with achieving airway protection during swallowing (e.g., those used during the VSS) can be implemented without concern for prolonged radiation exposure. Patients who are being evaluated for possible airway reconstruction procedures are particularly appropriate candidates for FEES as information regarding integrity of structures and function is made available.[37] Assessment of current swallowing ability and laryngeal function provides the information necessary to proceed with surgical intervention designed to rebuild and preserve total laryngeal function. A clinical swallowing assessment in conjunction with the pediatric FEES examination has been shown to identify patients with difficulty achieving airway protection preoperatively, and to identify patients likely to require short-term swallowing treatment postoperatively.[38]

One distinct advantage of the pediatric FEES exam is the ability to obtain information regarding the patient's laryngopharyngeal sensory threshold, fundamental to airway protection integrity. The adequacy of the LAR for protection from aspiration can be assessed by gently tapping the endoscope in the region of the aryepiglottic fold, for observation of reflexive glottic closure. In addition, more precise laryngopharyngeal sensory discrimination testing is possible using a calibrated duration and intensity controlled air pulse to the aryepiglottic fold region through an endoscope specifically designed for this purpose.[21]

Disadvantages to the pediatric FEES examination include possible discomfort with endoscope passage, though topical anesthesia (1:1 mixture of oxymetazoline and 2% pontocaine) can be administered nasally prior to the exam to increase patient comfort. In addition, use of lidocaine gel on the scope facilitates numbing of the nasal passageway and may also increase patient comfort with the procedure. Patients with oral hypersensitivity or oral aversion may have a gagging reaction in response to the tactile stimulation of the instrument. The specific focus of the FEES exam is limited to the pharyngeal phase of the swallow. There is a loss of view or "white-out" during the swallow caused by pharyngeal contraction and subsequent light deflection. The loss of view during sequential swallowing such as during bottle-feeding is not advantageous. FEES is contraindicated in patients who present with choanal atresia, nasal stenosis, nasal obstruction, or pharyngeal stenosis.

Additional Evaluations

Additional testing may be performed as indicated by the patient's history and exam. Further imaging studies include an upper GI or esophagram to define the upper gastrointestinal anatomy. Endoscopy is important for detecting mucosal abnormalities such as laryngitis or esophagitis as well as structural abnormalities. This can include assessment with microlaryngoscopy, bronchoscopy, and upper endoscopy. At our institution, these procedures are often coordinated and performed sequentially in order to limit exposure to anesthesia as well as to maximize shared communication and planning between subspecialties and families.

Impedance probe monitoring is another useful test for GER and provides information regarding esophageal clearance. Though impedance is gaining popularity in the evaluation of children, esophageal manometry remains the gold standard for motility. Children with frequent vomiting or evidence of severe GER may also benefit from a gastric emptying scan. An MRI of the brain may be needed to evaluate for possible neurologic causes of dysphagia such as Arnold-Chiari malformation.

Management Strategies

The approach to intervention for feeding, swallowing, and phonation issues is individualized for each patient as they tend to be multifactorial in nature. Treatment strategies for feeding and swallowing dysfunction are summarized in the following section. Assessment and management of voice issues will be discussed later in the chapter.

Treatment approaches to feeding and swallowing issues (dysphagia) are composed of direct rehabilitative maneuvers/exercises and the use of compensatory strategies such as sensory stimulation, alterations in positioning for feeding, the use of specialized feeding equipment, and the implementation of specific behavioral approaches to facilitate positive and productive feeder/child interactions. The specific approach is determined by the medical issues present, the child's developmental level, and the types of sensory and motor issues that are contributing to the feeding and swallowing dysfunction.

In regard to ensuring optimum nutrition, supplemental feeding access via nasogastric tubes or gastrostomy placement may be helpful during the oral feeding treatment period. The supplemental feeding allows the child to receive calories needed for adequate growth as they develop more functional swallowing skills and progress with feeding therapy. Treatment techniques focus on improving the child's oral motor skills to assist with feeding efficiency and ability to progress with food of increased texture. Treatment may also include methods to assist with overcoming sensory processing and oral sensory discrimination issues that may be contributing to the overall oral feeding difficulty. In cases of severe dysphagia, supplemental feeding methods may provide total nutrition; however, allowing the child to have some degree of oral stimulation, even if this consists only of tastes without appreciable volume, promotes social interaction at mealtime and may assist in preventing the development of oral aversion or resistance to oral feeding.

It is important to recognize behavioral overlays that may occur in this population. In general, oral aversion and resultant poor oral intake may have a strong underlying behavioral component in some children.[39] Parents or caretakers may be afraid to present oral feedings because of their child's medical complexity, or they may view the child as "vulnerable" and not provide mealtime structure or organization. Children with complex airways and multiple medical issues who undergo periods of time without oral intake can develop aversions that persist even after their underlying condition is corrected.

In a select group of children, innovative feeding practices are needed. For example, our center has trialed giving pureed foods into the gastrostomy for children with gagging and retching behaviors following fundoplication surgery. This method of feeding can decrease symptoms and allow children to be more receptive to taking food orally.[40]

Empiric data are limited regarding the efficacy of therapeutic strategies to assist with development of compensatory swallowing techniques postoperatively in airway reconstruction patients. Introduction of a modified supraglottic swallowing sequence to assist with achieving compensatory airway closure during swallowing has been described as effective in small patient samples.[5] Indirect treatment strategies include the alteration of textures and liquids (i.e. thickening liquids) to slow liquid flow and provide an increased time interval for use of supraglottic strategies to assist with airway closure. Alternating solid intake with liquid intake to assist with pharyngeal clearance has also been described as an effective strategy in the postoperative airway reconstruction period.

▬ VOICE

Normal voicing depends on the general health of the individual as well as the integrity of the structures and physiology of the central and peripheral nervous systems, pulmonary system, larynx, and upper aerodigestive tract. Vocal fold vibration requires the buildup of subglottal air pressure (P_{sub}) that overcomes the resistance of the partially adducted vocal folds. The pressure of the the airstream causes separation or lateral motion of the vocal fold edges, which occurs in an inferior to superior sequence. As the pulmonary airstream flows through the narrow, constricted transglottal space, its velocity increases, creating suction forces (attributed to the Bernoulli effect), that, along with myoelastic recoil forces, draw the lower lip (and then upper lip) of the folds back together. Return of the vocal fold edges to a near midline position results again in an increase in P_{sub}, and a subsequent cycle starts. This simplified version of the classic description of phonation is based largely on van den Berg's description of the myoelastic aerodynamic theory of vibration (re)introduced in 1958.[7] Titze expanded on this theory in 1994 by describing how the behavior of supraglottic airstream contributes to sustaining phonation.[41] More recent work in computer and biobehavioral modeling of air flow through the larynx continues to advance our understanding of air flow vortices and phonation,[42] but most of these models are based on the adult phonatory system.

Acquired and congenital voice disorders are reported to occur in 6% to 23% of all children at some point during childhood, making communication difficult and creating potential obstacles for learning.[43] Moreover, a weak or dysphonic cry may be one of the first indicators of a health concern in a newborn.[44] Medically fragile children who experience long periods of aphonia during critical periods of language development (birth to 3 years) are known to be at risk for delayed communication skills.[45–47] The range of etiologies associated with pediatric voice disorders can include those related to use (e.g., nodules, puberphonia, paradoxical vocal fold dysfunction), structure dysfunction (e.g., anterior webs, glottic and subglottic stenosis), disease (e.g., recurrent respiratory papillomatosis), neuromotor dysfunction (e.g., unilateral or bilateral vocal fold paralysis), reflux (e.g., edema and erythema), and those related to congenital causes or iatrogenic injuries (e.g., scarring). In children who have complex airway conditions requiring numerous reconstruction surgeries, anatomic changes may include off-level and scarred vocal folds, cricoarytenoid joint immobility, and arytenoid prolapse. These types of changes can result in variable voice outcomes, causing the child to compensate by compressing supraglottic structures in order to produce a voice.[48]

Pediatric Voice Assessment

Assessment of a child who presents with a voice disorder should include collaboration between a physician and a voice specialist (i.e., a speech language pathologist [SLP]) for evaluation of the patient's health and voice use history; acoustic, aerodynamic, endoscopic, perceptual parameters; and handicapping or quality of life effects. Under ideal circumstances, the medical evaluation of the patient is in close proximity, both in time and location, to that of the SLP. The physician exam typically includes the physical examination of the head and neck, a related medical workup, and an indirect examination of the larynx using a mirror, flexible endoscopy, or digital endoscopy. When either anatomic or cooperation issues preclude an optimal view of the patient's larynx, examination of the child under anesthesia may be indicated. Referral for more extensive assessment of the patient's voice may be made to an SLP who specializes in voice disorders.

Current clinical voice instrumentation technology permits the trained SLP to describe and quantify parameters of laryngeal and vocal function for clinical and research purposes.[49,50] Data collection requires access to a soundproof or quiet area, specialized computer-based software for recording and acoustic analyses, a high-quality microphone, and calibration protocols. Measures such as average fundamental frequency (F_0) and intensity (I_0), frequency range, harmonics-to-noise ratio (HNR), average air flow rate (mL/sec), and estimated subglottic pressure (cm/H_2O) allow the clinician to determine if structural abnormalities (e.g., lesions, scarring, or paralysis) are limiting vocal fold tension changes or altering frequencies and intensity during connected speech. Specialized instrumentation (e.g., Phonatory Assessment System, KayPentax) can be used for the collection of the acoustic and aerodynamic measures.[50,51] Normative data for each of these measures are available that allow the clinician to compare values obtained from an evaluation to children of similar age and gender.[52] These values reveal the efficiency of laryngeal valving during voicing and can reflect normal, hyperfunctional, or hypofunctional conditions. For example, hyperfunctional voice disturbances (e.g., excessive vocal fold/laryngeal compression) are evident in elevated P_{sub} and lower air flow rates. These measures suggest that increased pressures are needed to initiate vocal fold vibration, and that air flow is through a more constricted larynx. Conversely, hypofunctional voice disturbances are reflected in lower P_{sub} and higher air flow rates, indicating incomplete or weak approximation of the vocal folds (e.g., unilateral vocal fold paralysis).

Perceptual ratings of vocal quality in the voice-disordered individual are considered a standard outcome measure, despite their subjective nature. Expert and consumer perceptions of voice quality drive satisfaction with medical, surgical, and behavioral treatments.[53] Perceptual instruments are typically scaled and categorized as being equal appearing/ordinal (descriptor-based numeric ratings) or visual analog indicating severity levels for the described attributes. The Consensus Auditory Perceptual Evaluation of Voice (CAPE-V), now widely used in clinical settings, was introduced in 2003[54] and uses a 100-mm visual analog scale for experts to rate overall severity of the voice disorder as well as perceived degrees of breathiness, raspiness, strain, and changes in pitch and intensity.[55]

Laryngeal digital endoscopy is the imaging technique used to assist in the diagnosis of all voice disorders across the lifespan. Accomplished using transoral rigid or transnasal flexible endoscopes, this method permits a dynamic image that provides information regarding the nature of gross laryngeal function (e.g., arytenoid mobility, TVF level, glottic closure) and, if stroboscopy is employed, vocal fold vibration. Documentation of the presence or absence of laryngeal pathology and a permanent record of the exam is obtained.[56] The advantages of the rigid scope include higher magnification and brighter light source. The feasibility of using transoral rigid endoscopy in clinical pediatric voice practice has been documented.[57] However, for practical and some preferred reasons, nasendoscopy remains the typical clinical method of laryngeal examination for younger children.[58] The ability of any individual child to cooperate with either type of exam depends on his or her understanding, maturity, anatomy, and adequate preparation (along with their parents) for the examination process.

Stroboscopy permits the observation of discreet vibratory behaviors during production of sustained vowels. It uses a light pulsed at a frequency slightly slower than the average fundamental frequency of the patient's voice signal, resulting in an image that is actually created from points of successive (vibratory) cycles, visually fused. As such, stroboscopy requires a relatively stable acoustic signal in order for the vibration of the vocal folds to be adequately tracked and interpreted. Specific parameters of vocal fold vibration assessment include configuration of glottic closure, mucosal wave, amplitude of vibration, phase symmetry, and phase closure. Characterization of vibratory parameters as examined by stroboscopy are not yet fully described for the pediatric population. However, the ability to endoscopically assess parameters of general laryngeal function is well established and has continued to improve with advancements in technology.[59,60] High-speed digital endoscopy, conducted in a similar fashion, overcomes the limitations of stroboscopy because it records the vibration of the vocal folds in real time and does not rely on the quality of the voice signal.[61] It permits the visualization and quantification of cycle-to-cycle vibratory parameters as well as issues related to voice onset/offset and vocal fold edge asymmetries. At the present time however, in most modern pediatric voice clinics, the use of high-speed endoscopy for clinical purposes is limited.

Treatment of Pediatric Voice Disorders

Medical-Surgical Treatment

The goal of medical-surgical interventions for the child with voice and/or airway disease is to eliminate or control disease and restore the integrity of the laryngeal airway while preserving laryngeal function related to airway protection and voicing. Immediate surgical intervention is required for airway conditions such as bilateral TVF paralysis, congenital web, congenital or acquired subglottic stenosis, laryngeal injury, and severe obstructive airway disease (e.g., recurrent respiratory papillomatosis [RRP]). Restorative surgeries aimed at successful decannulation and reconnection of a functional upper and lower airway involve expansion or resection techniques that can be single- or double-staged. Related techniques (e.g., cordotomy, arytenoidectomy, or lateralization) may also be used alone or in conjunction with larger reconstructions to expand the airway.[62] Postoperative voice outcome is variable and is affected by both the underlying laryngeal pathology and the surgical intervention (i.e., resection or augmentation). Adequate expansion of the airway may preclude complete midline approximation of the TVFs, which, in turn, affects voicing ability. Reconstruction of the voice following airway reconstruction may involve procedures to realign the glottis or procedures to minimize operative glottic gaps. The process is often painstaking and should be carried out with the outmost care to avoid potential airway compromise. Techniques to *minimize* glottic incompetence caused by unilateral vocal fold paralysis include temporary medialization options such as injection of gel-foam, Radiesse Voice gel, Restalayne, or other similar products into the lateral aspect of the TVF. Options for long-term management of unilateral vocal fold paralysis include longer-term injections (Radiesse Voice or autologous fat), ansa-cervicalis to recurrent laryngeal nerve reinnervation, or

medialization laryngoplasty with a Gortex or silastic implant. Medialization laryngoplasty should be considered only after a child has gone through puberty and the larynx is at its adult size.

The most common cause of hoarseness in children is vocal fold nodules.[63] The initial treatment approach tends to be conservative, although clear guidelines for management do not exist. Most treatment approaches involve changing traumatic phonatory behaviors (e.g., screaming and shouting) and encouraging compliance with recommended behavioral treatments. Additional medical management may include treatment of reflux or looking for other causes of inflammation (e.g., eosinophilic esophagitis, allergy, asthma). Surgical intervention tends to be reserved for select cases when other therapies have failed after sincere efforts to comply with behavioral changes. Unilateral vocal fold cysts are almost always removed surgically but pre and post speech therapy is recommended to facilitate vocal health.

RRP is the second most common reason for hoarseness in children.[64] The goal of any treatment for RRP is to manage the tumor burden, contain the disease, and improve or maintain voice quality. Typically surgical management involves laser ablation (e.g., CO_2, Potassium-titanyl-phosphate [KTP], or pulsed dye), microdebridement, sharp resection, or cautery ablation. Severe cases may require tracheotomy. Adjunctive treatment for RRP is not standardized and is usually considered for severe cases (more than four trips to the operating room per year or frequent need for debridement secondary to airway obstruction).

Medical management of reflux is an important component as either a single or multimodal approach to treating any condition that results in a voice disorder. In some instances, medical management of reflux is considered prophylactic, particularly when used to control laryngeal irritation and promote healing during the perioperative time period. In other instances, reflux may be the primary cause of the voice disorder, necessitating aggressive, prolonged medical treatment.

Behavioral Treatment

Recommended components of any voice therapy approach include increasing the general and specific awareness of vocal behaviors to be changed; education; and emphasis on vocal hygiene, age-appropriate direct voice therapy techniques, and generalization exercises.[65,66] Pediatric voice therapy programs are eclectic but individualized, using a variety of techniques that are based on treatment goals and the child's ability. Behavioral modifications of phonotraumatic behaviors as well as modification of adult tested techniques such as resonant voice therapy[67] are designed to reduce laryngeal tension and strain. Resonant voice therapy can be adapted for use with children as can vocal function exercises,[68] a technique designed to increase sustained phonation times and focus of acoustic energy. Such approaches are easily understood and use a systematic daily practice regimen intended to reinforce positive changes in the sensory motor components of voice production. Newer treatment approaches that take advantage of digital interactive gaming technology may prove beneficial in both motivating and reinforcing treatment objectives as well as improving compliance. Yet, few studies have investigated the direct effect of pediatric voice therapy, and exact outcomes in response to specific techniques are unclear.[66] In part, this can be attributed to the difficulty of conducting such trials in pediatric populations within the venues of education and medicine. All voice therapy programs require participation and involvement of parent and family members.

Behavioral treatments aimed at improving voice quality in the child with a complex airway condition (e.g., post–airway reconstruction) use standard strategies and techniques that must be adapted for the specific needs of the child. For example, it is not uncommon for a child post–airway reconstruction to use alternate laryngeal tissue (e.g., ventricular folds) to produce voice. Changes and improvements in (ventricular) vocal quality can be accomplished, resulting in a more perceptually appealing outcome that requires less effort from the child.

■ SUMMARY

Analysis of specific laryngeal functions associated with voice and swallowing in the pediatric population is best accomplished through clinical and instrumental examinations. Identification of current laryngeal function and awareness of changes that may occur in association with specific reconstruction procedures assist clinicians in designing appropriate and effective treatment plans. Based on the number of interacting variables and possible comorbidities, a team approach to airway, swallowing, and voice assessment and management is key to the child's ultimate health outcome and quality of life.

References

The complete reference list is available online at www.expertconsult.com

68 GASTROESOPHAGEAL REFLUX DISEASE AND EOSINOPHILIC ESOPHAGITIS IN CHILDREN WITH COMPLEX AIRWAY DISEASE

Scott Pentiuk, MD, MeD, Phil E. Putnam, MD, and Marc Rothenberg, MD, PhD

Children who have complex airway conditions often have concomitant gastrointestinal (GI) disease, most notably gastroesophageal reflux disease (GERD), eosinophilic esophagitis (EoE), dysphagia, or disordered motility. These children often have a history of prematurity and neurodevelopmental delay along with other attendant comorbidities associated with prolonged NICU admissions. They also may have syndromes that lead to structural abnormalities such as esophageal atresia with or without tracheoesophageal fistula (TEF). These GI conditions may contribute to the disordered breathing that is commonly caused by lung disease of prematurity complicated by structural anomalies (congenital or acquired). Simultaneous management of the airway and the GI disease is required for optimal outcome.

GASTROESOPHAGEAL REFLUX DISEASE

Children who have complex airway anomalies may be at higher risk for GERD. The exact prevalence of GERD in this population is unknown, though it is generally believed to be up to 70% in children who have complex medical conditions such as developmental delay and post-TEF repair.[1,2]

It is important to distinguish gastroesophageal reflux (GER) from GERD. Reflux occurs in normal individuals and is the inconsequential transient return of gastric contents into the esophagus, whereas GERD is defined as symptoms and/or mucosal changes related to excessive stomach acid regurgitation into the esophagus and oropharynx.[3] Normal children demonstrate reflux into their esophagus multiple times per day, half of which are generally nonacid in nature.[4] In patients who have a history of swallowing dysfunction, there is evidence that episodes of reflux reaching the level of the proximal esophagus can cause airway damage and lead to pneumonia and respiratory tract infections.[5] GERD may be caused by the altered thoracoabdominal pressure relationships that exist in children who have obstructive airway disease. Thus GERD is frequently a consequence rather than a primary cause of asthma symptoms or pulmonary exacerbations in cystic fibrosis. Nevertheless, GERD may contribute to symptoms in these conditions.

GERD is also associated with weight gain and obesity in adult women.[6] Evidence for this association in pediatric age patients is less compelling. Nevertheless, clinical consideration of GERD in children should recognize the potential for interactions between excess weight, sleep-disordered breathing, asthma, and GERD.[7]

The symptoms of GERD affecting the airway are wide-ranging and include reactive airways disease, chronic cough, voice hoarseness, and difficulty swallowing.[3,8] Mucosal abnormalities including laryngeal edema, cobblestoning, and mucosal erythema, are nonspecific and do not prove reflux disease. Likewise, the absence of these findings does not exclude the presence of reflux.[3]

True acidic GER can lead to mucosal injury in the larynx, conducting airways and lung tissue. Acidic aspiration has been long known to cause mucosal sloughing and neutrophilic inflammation in alveolar tissue.[9] There is evidence that acid reflux decreases laryngeal sensitivity, which could increase the risk for aspiration.[10] Even nonacid reflux has been linked with a higher frequency of chronic lung disease in adults.[11] On the other hand, poorly controlled asthma did not benefit from treatment with esomeprazole in patients who also had asymptomatic GERD in a 24-week placebo-controlled blinded study, which demonstrates the difficulty in establishing the cause-effect relationship between reflux disease and laryngeal or airway symptoms.[12] GERD may be present as a comorbidity that has no impact on the airway, or it may cause or exacerbate airway symptoms.

Data regarding the relationship between GERD and reconstructive airway surgery are sparse. Carron and colleagues demonstrated that simulated GER caused increased inflammation in cartilage grafts in a rabbit model after laryngotracheoplasty compared to controls.[13] However, they were unable to show that reflux led to increased failure in the rabbit cartilage grafts. Several authors note that treatment of children with proton pump inhibitor therapy to prevent GER improves outcome in children after airway reconstruction, but these studies are all retrospective or represent just expert opinion.[14–16] Zalzal and coworkers showed that children who had documented GERD had similar outcomes to those who did not have GERD after laryngotracheal reconstruction for laryngeal stenosis, irrespective of treatment.[17] Regardless, there is sufficient concern that GER might negatively impact the results of airway reconstruction surgery that empiric antireflux therapy is often prescribed.

Diagnosis

The diagnosis of GERD depends on the demonstration that there are untoward consequences from reflux events. There is no single gold standard test. The diagnosis may be made presumptively based on clinical history alone when there is effortless regurgitation or heartburn. When regurgitation is not present in a child who has non-GI symptoms that could be caused by GERD, additional testing to detect reflux events or to document esophageal mucosal injury is possible. There is no single test that proves that reflux is responsible for a particular airway symptom, but a successful empiric trial of a proton pump inhibitor or H_2 blocker is suggestive.

Children with persistent symptoms or who need diagnostic studies prior to therapy may undergo endoscopic evaluation or multichannel intraluminal impedance plus pH-metry (MII-pH). The latter is a 24-hour study that measures the frequency, duration/clearance, height of reflux, and duration of acid exposure in the esophagus by means of a catheter placed via the nose. Upper GI endoscopy permits visual inspection and biopsy of the esophageal mucosa to detect acid injury ranging from microscopic abnormalities on histology to gross mucosal ulceration. However, there is controversy as to how to interpret the biopsy findings as due to acid reflux disease.[3] Children who aspirate refluxed gastric contents may have pepsin identified in their broncheoalveolar lavage, though the absolute sensitivity and application of this test remains to be determined.[18] Upper GI series with barium is not adequate for the diagnosis of GERD as the ingested contrast media commonly refluxes back into the esophagus, even in normal individuals. However, the test is commonly performed to evaluate the upper GI anatomy in patients who vomit or have dysphagia.

Treatment

Standard medical therapy for GERD is acid suppression with either a proton pump inhibitor or H_2 blocker. It is important to remember that nonacid reflux will still occur even with adequate doses of medication. Children who do not seem to respond to acid suppression may require additional evaluation for eosinophilic esophagitis or gastroparesis as discussed later in the chapter.

Medical therapy to limit the number of reflux episodes, irrespective of acidity, is quite limited. Metoclopramide has been used for GERD but has limited effectiveness and a high risk of side effects, including tardive dyskinesia.[19]

Children with recalcitrant GERD may benefit from antireflux surgery as it effectively abolishes reflux and the attendant symptoms. Aspiration of refluxed gastric contents is controlled by fundoplication, but aspiration during swallowing is not affected. Fundoplication is associated with a number of complications, such as gagging/retching, gas bloat, or dumping syndrome, so it should be reserved for those patients who cannot be managed medically.[20]

DISORDERS OF MOTILITY

It is also important to consider that children with complex airway conditions may also have gastric or esophageal motility disorders. Esophageal dysmotility can be idiopathic but may also relate to nerve disruption following surgery, such as tracheoesophageal fistula repair or Nissen fundoplication. Children may present with inability to swallow, regurgitation, or intractable GER symptoms. Upper GI may show poor clearance of contrast in the absence of a stricture. MII-pH testing is normally employed to detect reflux and associated symptoms with retrograde fluid movement in the esophagus, but the analytical software may also be used to evaluate antegrade esophageal emptying of swallowed (and refluxed) material. Esophageal peristalsis may be diminished, absent, or even retrograde on manometric testing.

Disorders of gastric emptying present with symptoms such as nausea, early satiety, and vomiting, often from meals ingested many hours prior.[21] In children for whom there is concern for poor stomach emptying, a nuclear gastric emptying scan can provide a quantitative assessment, but does not establish the underlying cause of delay.

Treatment for motility disorders of the esophagus is often supportive as there are no commonly employed medications that improve esophageal peristalsis. Children may need to restrict bolus size and often require a significant proportion of their calories by liquid formulas. Because of the risk of worsening gagging and retching after surgery, we typically do not recommend fundoplication in children with esophageal or gastric dysmotility, though there are few data in the literature.

Erythromycin is an antimicrobial with a prokinetic side effect that is employed to improve gastric emptying. It does not have significant impact on GER, but it can improve symptoms of impaired gastric emptying. Other possible therapies include endoscopic administration of Botox to the pylorus (with or without concomitant pyloric dilatation (temporary relief) and surgical pyloroplasty (for long-term relief). Gastric pacemakers are under development.[22]

EOSINOPHILIC ESOPHAGITIS

An increasingly recognized cause of inflammation of the esophagus is eosinophilic esophagitis (EoE). This clinicopathologic entity is defined by the presence of >15 eosinophils/HPF on microscopic biopsy of the esophagus in the absence of GERD or any other condition that could promote eosinophilic inflammation.[23] Eosinophils are not found in the normal esophagus but can be increased in a variety of diseases including GERD, celiac disease, Crohn's disease, hypereosinophilic syndrome, and eosinophilic gastroenteritis.[24] Proof that children have EoE rather than GERD is established by their failure to respond fully to acid suppression or by a negative MII-pH study.

EoE is a spectrum of conditions, most commonly a manifestation of allergic disease, as it resolves with elimination of food antigens. It has features of IgE-mediated processes (e.g., positive skin tests to common food allergens) but is mainly associated with chronic Th2-associated hypersensitivity immune responses. There is a 3 to 1 male-to-female predominance, and two thirds of patients have an atopic phenotype (i.e., asthma, eczema, or food allergy). There is a genetic predisposition for EoE, so several family members may carry the diagnosis.[25]

Symptoms of EoE can be similar to those of GERD. Notably, younger children seem to present with symptoms such as vomiting, reflux-like symptoms, and a feeding disorder. Older children may present with abdominal pain, whereas adolescents more commonly present with symptoms of dysphagia or food impactions.[26–28]

EoE has been diagnosed in children who presented with recurrent croup, chronic cough, sinusitis, congestion, or choking episodes.[29,30] At our institution, undiagnosed EoE has been discovered in children who previously failed airway reconstruction, although its precise role in that failure remains uncertain. Nevertheless, because there is sufficient concern that EoE might pose difficulties after airway reconstruction, we treat EoE and confirm histologic recovery prior to reconstructive airway surgery.

Diagnosis

Because the symptoms of EoE are otherwise nonspecific, a high degree of suspicion is needed to proceed with endoscopy to make the diagnosis, which is established when there are >15 eosinophils/HPF in a patient who does not have reflux or another condition. As EoE can be a patchy disease, it is recommended that a minimum of five biopsies of the esophagus be examined pathologically.[31]

The endoscopic features of EoE are characteristic but nondiagnostic, and they include thickening, furrowing of the esophageal mucosa, and white plaques that are eosinophilic microabscesses on the surface. However, an estimated 25% of cases with EoE present with normal endoscopic appearance.[32]

Treatment

Treatment for EoE includes dietary antigen elimination or topical steroids. Food allergy testing may identify the potential offending antigen, and patients may start a directed elimination diet. Another diet empirically eliminates six common food antigens (milk, soy, egg, fish, nuts, and wheat) and has been effective in up to 80% of patients.[33] Elemental formula diets are extremely effective but so unpalatable in older children that they often require NG- or G-tube access.[34] Topical steroids, including swallowed fluticasone or budesonide, directly reduce the mucosal inflammation in up to 80% of patients.[35,36]

Unfortunately, symptom resolution does not imply resolution of the histologic inflammation.[37] Because chronic persistent eosinophilic inflammation is associated with lamina propria fibrosis and stricture development, repeat endoscopy is recommended to confirm histologic remission of the disease, even if symptoms have diminished.[23]

Suggested Reading

GERD

Orenstein SR. An overview of reflux-associated disorders in infants: apnea, laryngospasm, and aspiration. *Am J Med* 2001;111(suppl 8A):60S–63S.
Tighe MP, Afzal NA, Bevan A, et al. Current pharmacological management of gastro-esophageal reflux in children. *Paediatr Drugs.* 2009;11:185–202.
Vandenplas Y, Rudolph CD, DiLorenzo C, et al. Pediatric gastroesophageal reflux clinical practice guidelines: Joint recommendations of the North American Society for Pediatric Gastroenterology, Hepatology, and Nutrition (NASPGHAN) and the European Society for Pediatric Gastroenterology, Hepatology, and Nutrition (ESPGHAN). *J Pediatr Gastroenterol Nutr.* 2009;49:498–547.

Eosinophilic Esophagitis

Dauer EH, Ponikau JU, Smyrk TC, et al. Airway manifestations of pediatric eosinophilic esophagitis: a clinical and histopathologic report of an emerging association. *Ann Otol Rhinol Laryngol.* 2006;115:507–517.
Furuta G, Liacouras C, Collins M, et al. Eosinophilic esophagitis in children and adults: A systematic review and consensus recommendations for diagnosis and treatment. *Gastroenterology.* 2007;133:1342–1363.
Rothenberg ME, Mishra A, Collins MH, et al. Pathogenesis and clinical features of eosinophilic esophagitis. *J Allergy Clin Immunol.* 2001;108:891–894.

References

The complete reference list is available online at www.expertconsult.com

69 LARYNGEAL AND TRACHEAL AIRWAY DISORDERS

Alessandro de Alarcon, MD, Robin T. Cotton, MD, and Michael J. Rutter, MD

Advances in the management of critically ill infants with extreme prematurity, complex congenital anomalies, airway trauma, and infectious diseases concomitantly created a new subset of patients with complex airway problems. The overall management of these patients often includes surgical airway intervention. Evaluation requires a global perspective, with assessments of both the airway and the child's overall health status. This broad-based approach provides information that is crucial to the success of airway reconstruction.

We have found that minimizing the risk of operative failure can best be achieved through the collaborative efforts of a well-coordinated interdisciplinary team. Thorough clinical and operative examinations should be performed, with involved health professionals being aware of conditions and risk factors that can significantly impact clinical outcomes.

This chapter presents an overview of the critical aspects of otolaryngologic management of this complex patient population in the context of the collaborative model used at our institution. We briefly discuss the initial assessment, mitigating factors that can affect airway reconstruction, and perioperative management of specific airway pathology.

OPERATIVE ASSESSMENT

The operative evaluation is performed by the interdisciplinary team, with input from each physician being crucial. This evaluation comprises three endoscopic procedures performed consecutively with the patient under a single anesthesia: (1) flexible bronchoscopy with bronchoalveolar lavage (BAL); (2) microlaryngoscopy and rigid bronchoscopy; and (3) esophagoduodenoscopy (EGD) with biopsy. For patients in whom gastroesophageal reflux (GER) is suspected or in whom GER would have negative consequences on subsequent management, objective evaluation of GER is recommended. Each component of this endoscopic evaluation is aimed at identifying possible pathology and risk factors that can affect the success of airway reconstruction.

Flexible Bronchoscopy

Flexible bronchoscopy offers several advantages over rigid bronchoscopy. It can identify particular areas that can cause airway obstruction and that may be underappreciated or missed with a rigid bronchoscope. More specifically, flexible bronchoscopy provides better assessment of disorders such as glossoptosis, laryngomalacia, tracheomalacia, and bronchomalacia. Evaluation of the distal airway may provide additional information on vascular compression, bronchiectasis, and assessment of aspiration by BAL. (See Chapter 66 for a more detailed discussion.)

Microlaryngoscopy and Rigid Bronchoscopy

Microlaryngoscopy and rigid bronchoscopy are performed with the primary goal of identifying anatomic levels of airway obstruction from the larynx to the carina. The supraglottis is evaluated with attention given to the possibility of supraglottic obstruction such as laryngomalacia and supraglottic stenosis. The vocal fold level is then evaluated for posterior glottic stenosis, anterior glottic web, and laryngeal cleft. If vocal fold immobility is suspected or seen on the fiberoptic endoscopic evaluation of swallowing (FEES) or on voice evaluation, the cricoarytenoid joints should be palpated to determine if there is any fixation of the joint.

Rigid bronchoscopy is performed using a combination of Hopkins rod telescopes and rigid bronchoscopes. The subglottis is evaluated initially. If subglottic stenosis is present, it is classified by the Cotton-Myer scale[1] and sized using appropriate endotracheal tubes (Table 69-1). Additionally, the length of stenosis and the proximity to the vocal folds is assessed and documented. If a tracheotomy is in place, attention is paid to the evaluation of the suprastomal area, considering the possibility of suprastomal collapse, granuloma, intratracheal skin tract, and high tracheotomy. The trachea is evaluated to the level of the carina, looking for additional pathology, including tracheal stenosis, complete tracheal rings, tracheoesophageal fistula (TEF), TEF pouches, vascular compression, and tracheomalacia.

Esophagoduodenoscopy

Evaluation of the upper gastrointestinal tract can provide information that is crucial in decision making as to future surgery. Inflammation in the laryngotracheal complex can be caused by conditions of the upper gastrointestinal tract, resulting in an "active" (i.e., inflamed) larynx. Poor wound healing and scarring is more likely to occur in this setting. The two gastrointestinal conditions associated with laryngeal inflammation are eosinophilic esophagitis (EE) and gastroesophageal reflux disease (GERD). The diagnosis of EE is made by esophageal biopsy. Laryngeal inflammation may resolve with appropriate treatment of the underlying condition, permitting surgical reconstruction with a lower risk of complication.

TABLE 69-1 COTTON-MYER GRADING SCALE

PERCENTAGE OF OBSTRUCTION BY ACTUAL ENDOTRACHEAL TUBE SIZE

Patient age	Normal ID (mm)	Normal OD (mm)	Percentage of obstruction with actual endotracheal tube size								
			ID = 2.0	ID = 2.5	ID = 3.0	ID = 3.5	ID = 4.0	ID = 4.5	ID = 5.0	ID = 5.5	ID = 6.0
Premature	2.0	2.8	0%								
	2.5	3.6	40%	0%							
	3.0	4.3	58%	30%	0%						
0–3 mo	3.5	5.0	68%	48%	26%	0%					
3–9 mo	4.0	5.6	75%	59%	41%	22%	0%				
9 mo to 2y	4.5	6.2	80%	67%	53%	38%	20%	0%			
2y	5.0	7.0	84%	74%	62%	50%	35%	19%	0%		
4y	5.5	7.6	86%	78%	68%	57%	45%	32%	17%	0%	
6y	6.0	8.2	89%	81%	73%	64%	54%	43%	30%	16%	0%

ID – Inside diameter, OD – Outside diameter

Grade I	Grade II	Grade III	Grade IV
No obstruction — 50% obstruction	51% obstruction — 70% obstruction	71% obstruction — 99% obstruction	No detectable lumen

Swallowing and Voice Evaluations

Preoperative swallowing and voice evaluations can be crucial, as both assessments may alter an otherwise sound surgical plan.

If there is a suspicion of ongoing aspiration, if surgery will involve the glottis, or if surgery will repair a stenosis that may be preventing aspiration, then a swallowing evaluation should be pursued. The two most commonly used evaluations of swallowing are videofluoroscopic swallow study (VSS) and FEES. These complementary evaluations can assess ongoing aspiration with swallowing as well as the likelihood of future aspiration.[2,3] The advantages of FEES are that the laryngeal protective mechanisms can be visualized by the surgeon, vocal fold motion can be documented, and the potential risk of aspiration can be assessed prior to airway surgery.

Another evaluation that may be useful in children who have a tracheotomy is dye testing. Through the use of green food coloring, aspiration in general as well as specific causes of aspiration can be assessed as follows: dye can be placed on the tongue to evaluate aspiration of saliva or secretions; a particular consistency of food can be dyed to assess for consistency-specific aspiration; and gastrostomy tube feeds can be dyed to assess aspiration of refluxed feeds. Aspiration is suspected if stained secretions or feeds are noted from the tracheotomy during feeding or at any time after feeding. Dye testing provides no value in the evaluation of aspiration in children with a grade IV (complete) stenosis. Information obtained from a swallowing evaluation becomes crucial in planning the operative procedure and in counseling the family about the potential risk of aspiration.

Because many airway reconstructive procedures involve a compromise between voice quality and airway improvement, preoperative voice evaluation has become increasingly important.[4–6] This evaluation provides key information regarding the impact of the initial surgery on voice, the potential impact of further surgery on voice, and

the status of vocal cord mobility. In some cases, operative planning can be modified to offer a better balance between long-term voice and airway concerns. When vocal fold immobility is noted on the voice evaluation, the surgeon should search for the specific etiology of the immobility, as various conditions may appear similar on voice evaluation but may be treated differently (e.g., posterior glottic stenosis, vocal cord paralysis, and fixation of the cricoarytenoid joints). This assessment is best done during microlaryngoscopy and bronchoscopy. Counseling families about the impact of airway surgery on future voice quality and the options of voice therapy is also an important part of the overall process.

■ MITIGATING FACTORS

Bacterial Colonization

Because of the prevalence of colonization by methicillin-resistant *Staphylococcus aureus* (MRSA) and *Pseudomonas aeruginosa* in our patients with complex aerodigestive problems (approximately 30%), we recommend screening for these bacteria by culture of the nares and tracheal aspirate. Both MRSA and *Pseudomonas aeruginosa* have a predilection for infecting cartilage and can lead to operative failure. Patients who are found to be positive are treated with perioperative and postoperative antimicrobial therapy (Table 69-2). In our experience, this protocol decreases the risk of infection-related morbidity (authors' unpublished data).

Eosinophilic Esophagitis

EE is an uncommon disorder that, if left untreated, may have a significant effect on the aerodigestive tract. Many patients who have EE also have esophageal, laryngotracheal, and sinonasal complaints; however, some patients are asymptomatic.[7] The diagnosis of EE is

TABLE 69-2 PERIOPERATIVE AND OPERATIVE ANTIBIOTIC PROTOCOL FOR BACTERIAL COLONIZATION

ORGANISM	PERIOPERATIVE	INTRAOPERATIVE	POSTOPERATIVE
Methicillin-resistant *Staphylococcus aureus*	Bactrim DS: 6-12 mg/kg/day, 72 h before; Bactroban intranasal 72 h before	Vancomycin: 15 mg/kg 1 h before incision followed by q6h × 2 doses (maximum)	Bactrim DS: 6-12 mg/kg/day for 2 weeks; Vancomycin 15mg/kg/24 hr × 48 h
Pseudomonas aeruginosa	Ciprodex: intratracheal 72 h before	Piperacillin/Tazobactam: 100 mg/kg 1 h before incision followed by q6h dosing	Ciprodex: Begin 1 week after surgery through tracheal tube; Piperacillin/Tazobactam 100 mg/kg q6h for 1 week after surgery

made by histologic examination of biopsies taken from the esophagus at the time of esophageal endoscopy. In patients who have active EE, the laryngotracheal complex is often inflamed. Surgery in the presence of active EE often elicits a brisk inflammatory response that can lead to graft failure or re-stenosis. If EE is present, the authors recommend medical management followed by repeat endoscopy with biopsies. Once biopsies demonstrate no active EE, surgery may be performed. (See Chapter 68 for a more detailed discussion on EE and its treatment.)

Gastroesophageal Reflux Disease

The evaluation for GERD can include esophagoscopy with biopsies, esophagram, impedance probe, and dual pH probe testing. Because of the potential impact of this condition on postoperative healing, the authors routinely administer prophylactic preoperative and postoperative therapy to patients undergoing airway reconstruction. Most patients are managed with a daily proton pump inhibitor and nighttime H_2 blocker therapy. Patients continue the antireflux regimen for up to 1 year following successful reconstruction. Nonacidic reflux also can play a role. The authors believe that in some cases non-acidic reflux can cause damage in the reconstructed airway and potentially lead to operative failure. When medical treatment fails or nonacidic reflux is suspected, a Nissen fundoplication should be considered before airway reconstruction.[8–10]

Obstructive Sleep Apnea

Obstructive sleep apnea (OSA) can be difficult to diagnose and treat, and it can cause failure in an otherwise well-executed operative plan. In children who have multilevel airway obstruction, including a known fixed airway lesion above a tracheotomy, OSA may be difficult to identify because the tracheotomy cannot be capped during a sleep study. In these cases, a two-stage airway reconstruction is often performed, leaving the tracheotomy in place, which allows for later assessment of OSA.

Pulmonary Disease

Unrecognized or untreated pulmonary disease can increase the risk of operative failure. This broad classification of pathology encompasses numerous diseases that affect the upper and lower respiratory systems, including unrecognized but significant aspiration, bronchopulmonary dysplasia, tracheomalacia, bronchomalacia, cystic fibrosis, and reactive airway disease. Failure to identify any of these disease processes, even when the commonly found subglottic stenosis is identified and treated, can result in significant airway obstruction and operative failure. Collaboration with a pediatric pulmonologist is important, not only in the diagnosis, but also in both the short- and long-term management of these patients. When significant pulmonary disease is identified, it is crucial that surgery be delayed until this pathology is treated.

Inappropriate Patient Selection

Patient selection can significantly affect overall clinical outcome. Although the goal of creating an anatomically normal airway at the site of reconstruction may be achieved from a technical perspective, if a child remains dependent on a tracheotomy because of oxygen or ventilation requirements, or suffers from chronic aspiration, then in a more global sense the operation has failed.

▬ OPTIMIZATION

Optimizing patient status before surgery plays a central role in airway management and is crucial to the success of surgery. This point cannot be overemphasized. Many of our patients have multiple comorbidities that complicate treatment. Inadequate management of the aforementioned mitigating factors can have a negative impact on an otherwise well-conceived and well-executed surgical plan.

▬ MANAGEMENT OF AIRWAY PATHOLOGY

Laryngomalacia

Laryngomalacia is the most common cause of stridor in newborns.[11] Symptoms are usually observed at birth or within the first few days of life. Stridor is generally mild, but it typically worsens with feeding, crying, and lying in a supine position. In 50% of patients, stridor worsens during the first 6 months of life. A subset of children with severe laryngomalacia (5%) may present with a spectrum of symptoms, including apnea, cyanosis, severe retractions, and failure to thrive. Also, many patients suffer from clinically significant reflux. In extremely severe cases, cor pulmonale is seen. Although laryngomalacia usually resolves spontaneously by 1 year of age, severe disease necessitates surgical intervention.

Diagnosis is confirmed by flexible transnasal fiberoptic laryngoscopy. Characteristic findings include short aryepiglottic folds, with prolapse of the cuneiform cartilages. In some patients, a tightly curled (Ω shaped) epiglottis is observed. Because of the Bernoulli effect, characteristic collapse of the supraglottic structures is seen on inspiration. Inflammation indicative of reflux laryngitis may also be seen.

Determining whether or not to intervene surgically is based more on the severity of symptoms than on the endoscopic appearance of the larynx. Patients with laryngomalacia rarely present with acute airway compromise. In the 5% who require surgical intervention, this may be planned within 1 to 2 weeks of presentation. Preoperative management of GER is recommended.

Supraglottoplasty (also referred to as *epiglottoplasty*) is currently the operative procedure of choice. This procedure is quick and effective and can be adapted to the infant's specific laryngeal pathology. Both aryepiglottic folds are divided, and one or both cuneiform cartilages may also be removed. If the aryepiglottic folds alone are divided, postoperative intubation is generally not required. However, if more extensive surgery is performed, overnight intubation is prudent.

Following supraglottoplasty, patients should be observed overnight in the intensive care unit. In some children, obstruction persists postoperatively. Repeat fiberoptic laryngoscopy at the bedside is valuable in determining whether this can be attributed to laryngeal edema or persistent laryngomalacia that necessitates further surgery. Reflux management is helpful in minimizing laryngeal edema. Occasionally, although the postoperative appearance of the larynx is adequate, obstructive symptoms are ongoing. Such cases may have an underlying neurologic component, which becomes more evident with time. Supraglottoplasty in these children often fails, thus requiring tracheotomy placement.

Vocal Cord Paralysis

Vocal cord paralysis is the second most common cause of stridor in newborns, and it may be either congenital or acquired.[12] Congenital vocal cord paralysis generally manifests bilaterally. Although it is usually idiopathic, it is sometimes seen in children with central nervous system pathology (e.g., hydrocephalus and Arnold-Chiari malformation of the brainstem). Most children with bilateral paralysis present with significant airway compromise, though with an excellent voice. They usually do not aspirate. Acquired disease is generally, though not always, a unilateral condition arising from iatrogenic injury to the recurrent laryngeal nerve. Because of the length and course of the left recurrent nerve, this is far more likely to be damaged than the right recurrent laryngeal nerve. As such, acquired disease usually affects the left vocal cord. Risk factors for acquired paralysis include patent ductus arteriosus repair, the Norwood cardiac repair, and esophageal surgery, particularly TEF repair. In older children, thyroid surgery is an additional risk factor. Unlike children with bilateral vocal cord paralysis, most children with unilateral disease have an acceptable airway, but a breathy voice. These children are at a slightly higher risk of aspiration.

The diagnosis of vocal cord paralysis is established with awake flexible transnasal fiberoptic laryngoscopy or stroboscopy. Once paralysis has been confirmed, management depends on a number of factors. Children with acquired vocal cord paralysis (whether unilateral or bilateral) may experience spontaneous recovery several months after nerve injury; however, this occurs only if the nerve is stretched or crushed but is otherwise intact.

Children with unilateral paralysis can be initially managed with observation, temporary injection medialization, or speech and voice therapy. Determining the appropriate option is based on a discussion with the patient's family, taking into account the need for restoration of normal voice and improvement of aspiration. Regardless of which option is chosen, these children should be observed for at least 1 year prior to any permanent intervention. If paralysis persists after this period of time and there is a functional deficit, long-term interventions such as ansa-cervicalis re-innervation, permanent medialization laryngoplasty, or long-term injection medialization (fat or Radiesse) are considered. These options are discussed with the family and are often influenced by the age of the child and the presence of comorbidities. Medialization laryngoplasty is best performed after puberty.

For patients with bilateral paralysis associated with an underlying disease process, successful treatment of that disease may reverse the paralysis; however, up to 90% of these infants ultimately require tracheotomy placement. Given that up to 50% of children with congenital idiopathic bilateral vocal cord paralysis have spontaneous resolution of their paralysis by 1 year of age, surgical intervention to achieve decannulation is almost always delayed until patients are older than 1 year of age.

Several surgical options have been used for patients with bilateral paralysis, and no particular option offers a universally acceptable outcome. The aim of surgery is twofold: (1) to achieve an adequate decannulated airway while maintaining voice and (2) to prevent aspiration. Surgical options include laser cordotomy, partial or complete arytenoidectomy (endoscopic or open), vocal process lateralization (open or endoscopically guided), and posterior cricoid cartilage grafting. In a child with a tracheotomy, it is often prudent to maintain the tracheotomy to ensure an adequate airway prior to decannulation. In a nontracheotomized child, a single-stage surgical procedure can be carried out. Acquired bilateral vocal cord paralysis that does not resolve spontaneously is usually less responsive to treatment than idiopathic vocal cord paralysis. In these cases, more than one operative intervention may be required to achieve decannulation. In patients who have undergone such interventions, postextubation stridor may respond to continuous positive airway pressure (CPAP) or high-flow nasal cannula. The postoperative risk of aspiration should be evaluated by a VSS before the child returns to a normal diet. During the initial postoperative weeks, some children have an increased risk of aspirating with certain textures, especially thin fluids.

Laryngeal Webs

Laryngeal webs result from a failure of recanalization of the glottic airway in the early weeks of embryogenesis. In severe cases, as recanalization commences posteriorly and progresses anteriorly, complete laryngeal atresia may occur. In less severe cases, a thin anterior glottic web may be the only remnant of the recanalization process. The web is typically thickened anteriorly and thins out toward the posterior edge.

Although some anterior glottic webs are gossamer thin, most are thick and generally associated with a subglottic "sail" that compromises the subglottic lumen. Patients have varying degrees of glottic airway compromise, which usually manifests in an abnormal cry or respiratory distress. Thin webs may elude detection, as neonatal intubation for airway distress may lyse the web.

Thick webs require open reconstruction with either reconstruction of the anterior commissure or placement of a laryngeal keel.[13] The presence of thick membranous webs requires placement of a tracheotomy in approximately 40% of patients.

Subglottic Stenosis

Subglottic stenosis (SGS) can be either congenital or acquired. Congenital SGS in the neonate is defined as a lumen 4.0 mm in diameter or less at the level of the cricoid cartilage. SGS is thought to result from a failure of the laryngeal lumen to recanalize, and it is one of a continuum of embryologic failures that include laryngeal atresia, stenosis, and webs. Congenital SGS is often associated with other congenital head and neck lesions and syndromes (e.g., a small larynx in a patient with Down syndrome). Acquired SGS is far more common and is typically a sequel of prolonged neonatal intubation, often with an inappropriately large endotracheal tube. Other cofactors for the development of acquired SGS include reflux and EE.

Levels of SGS severity are graded according to the Myer-Cotton grading system (see Table 69-1). In its mildest form (no obstruction to 50% obstruction), congenital SGS appears as a normal cricoid cartilage with a smaller than average diameter, usually elliptical in shape. Mild SGS may manifest in recurrent upper respiratory infections (often diagnosed as croup) in which minimal subglottic swelling precipitates airway obstruction. In a young child, the greatest obstruction is usually 2 to 3 mm below the true vocal folds. More severe cases may present with acute airway compromise at delivery. If endotracheal intubation is successful, the patient may require intervention before extubation. When intubation cannot be achieved, tracheotomy placement at the time of delivery may be life-saving. It is important to note that infants typically have surprisingly few symptoms. Even those with grade III SGS (71% to 99% obstruction) may not be symptomatic for weeks or months.

Children with mild acquired SGS may be asymptomatic or minimally symptomatic. Observation rather than intervention may therefore be appropriate. This is often the case for children with grades I or II SGS. Those with more severe SGS (grades III and IV), however, are often symptomatic, with either tracheal dependency or stridor and exercise intolerance.

Radiologic evaluation of an airway that is not intubated may provide the clinician clues about the site and length of the stenosis. Useful imaging modalities include inspiratory and expiratory lateral soft-tissue neck films, fluoroscopy to demonstrate the dynamics of the trachea and larynx, and chest radiograph. However, the single most important investigation is high-kilovoltage airway films. These films are taken not only to identify the classic "steepling" observed in patients with SGS, but also to identify possible tracheal stenosis. The latter condition is generally caused by complete tracheal rings, which may predispose the patient to a life-threatening situation during rigid endoscopy.

Whether SGS is congenital or acquired, evaluation requires endoscopic assessment, which is considered the gold standard. Endoscopy is necessary for the diagnosis of laryngeal stenosis. Precise evaluation of the endolarynx should be carried out, including grading of the subglottic stenosis. Stenosis caused by scarring, granulation tissue, submucosal thickening, or a congenitally abnormal cricoid cartilage can be differentiated from SGS with a normal cricoid, but endoscopic measurement with endotracheal tubes or bronchoscopes is required for an accurate evaluation.

In a patient with congenital SGS, the larynx will grow as the patient grows. As such, after initial management of SGS, the patient may not require further surgical intervention. However, if initial management requires intubation, the risk of developing an acquired SGS in addition to the underlying congenital SGS is considerable.

Unlike congenital SGS, acquired SGS is unlikely to resolve spontaneously and thus requires intervention. Reconstruction of the subglottic airway is a challenging procedure, and the patient's condition should be optimized before undergoing surgery. In children with mild symptoms and a minor degree of SGS, endoscopic intervention may be effective. Endoscopic options include radial incisions (cold steel or laser) through the stenosis, laryngeal dilatation, the application of topical or injected steroids, and topical mitomycin. More severe forms of SGS are better managed with open airway reconstruction. Laryngotracheal reconstruction using costal cartilage grafts placed through the split lamina of the cricoid cartilage is reliable and has withstood the test of time.[14,15] Costal cartilage grafts may be placed through the anterior lamina of the cricoid cartilage, the posterior lamina of the cricoid cartilage, or both. These procedures may be performed as a two-stage procedure, maintaining the tracheal tube and temporarily placing a suprastomal laryngeal stent above the tracheal tube. Alternatively, in selective cases, a single-stage procedure may be performed, with removal of the tracheal tube on the day of surgery and with the child requiring intubation for 1 to 14 days.[16,17] Higher decannulation rates have reportedly been achieved with cricotracheal resection than with laryngotracheal reconstruction in the management of severe SGS.[18,19] Cricotracheal resection is, however, a technically demanding procedure that carries a significant risk of complications.

Vascular Compression

Although vascular compression of the airway is not uncommon, most affected children are either asymptomatic or only minimally symptomatic. Forms of vascular compression affecting the trachea include innominate artery compression (most common), double aortic arch, and pulmonary artery sling. While symptomatic vascular compression of the trachea or bronchi is rare, it is associated with marked symptoms, including biphasic stridor, retractions, a brassy cough, and "dying spells." Symptoms tend to exacerbate when the child is distressed. Vascular rings that result from a retroesophageal subclavian artery and a ligamentum arteriosum are less likely to be associated with airway compromise. Bronchial compression by either the pulmonary arteries or aorta may be significant, but in the absence of associated major cardiac anomalies, it is typically a unilateral problem.

The diagnosis of airway compression is best established with rigid and/or flexible bronchoscopy. Thoracic imaging is then useful in assessing the intrathoracic vasculature. Imaging modalities generally include high-resolution computed tomography (HRCT) with contrast enhancement and 3-D reconstruction, magnetic resonance imaging (MRI), magnetic resonance angiography (MRA), and echocardiography. In some cases, angiography is required.

In a neonate with acute airway compromise, intubation may be required to stabilize the airway prior to definitive treatment. In some cases, CPAP offers a degree of temporary improvement, as segmental tracheomalacia may be present in the region of the vascular compression. Prolonged intubation should be avoided because of the risk of forming an arterial fistula from erosion of an endotracheal tube into the area of compression. Similarly, while tracheotomy will establish an unobstructed airway, there is also an increased risk of an arterial fistula into the airway.

The surgical management of symptomatic vascular compression varies, depending on individual pathology. Strategies for managing innominate artery compression include thymectomy and aortopexy; however, if little thymus is present, an alternative procedure is re-implantation of the innominate artery more proximally on the aortic arch. A double aortic arch requires ligation of the smaller of the two arches, which is usually the left. A pulmonary artery sling is transected at its origin, dissected free, and re-implanted into the pulmonary trunk anterior to the trachea. There is a high incidence of complete tracheal rings in children with a pulmonary artery sling, and these should be repaired at the time of vascular repair.

Although alleviating vascular compression improves the airway, it takes time for the airway to completely normalize. This is a consequence of long-standing vascular compression having adversely affected the normal cartilaginous development of the compressed segment of trachea, with resultant cartilaginous malacia or stenosis.

Until the airway normalizes, children who are persistently symptomatic may require stabilization with a tracheotomy. Tracheal stabilization with the use of intratracheal stents is alluring, but the incidence of complications under such circumstances is nevertheless high. Placement of a temporary tracheotomy is thus a more desirable alternative.[20]

Posterior Laryngeal Clefts

Posterior laryngeal clefts result from a failure of the laryngotracheal groove to fuse during embryogenesis. In a widely used anatomic classification system, these clefts are divided into four subtypes associated with varying levels of severity; type 1 cleft is the least severe and type 4 cleft is the most severe.[21] Other associated anomalies are common and may be divided into those that affect the airway and those that do not. Associated airway anomalies include tracheomalacia (>80%) and TEF formation (20%). Non-airway associations include anogenital anomalies and GER. The most common syndrome associated with posterior laryngeal clefting is Opitz-Frias syndrome, which is characterized by hypertelorism, anogenital anomalies, and posterior laryngeal clefting.

Although aspiration is the hallmark clinical feature of this disorder, signs and symptoms may be nonspecific, making the diagnosis elusive. Symptoms may also include apnea, recurrent pneumonia, feeding difficulties, and airway obstruction.

VSS and FEES may suggest the risk of aspiration for children with clefts, however a definitive diagnosis requires rigid laryngoscopy and bronchoscopy, with the interarytenoid area being specifically probed to determine if a posterior laryngeal cleft is present.

Initial management decisions should consider whether the infant requires tracheotomy placement, gastrostomy tube placement, or Nissen fundoplication. Although none of these procedures is essential, each increases the likelihood of successful cleft repair. Protection against aspiration is also crucial, and nasojejunal feeding may be a useful way of stabilizing an infant. Surgical repair may be performed endoscopically for most type 1 and some type II clefts; however, longer clefts that extend into the cervical or thoracic trachea require open repair. The transtracheal approach is advocated in that it provides unparalleled exposure of the cleft while protecting the recurrent laryngeal nerves. A two-layer closure is recommended, with the option of performing an interposition graft if warranted; a useful interposition graft is a free transfer of clavicular or tibial periosteum, or costal cartilage. Because all clefts are prone to anastomotic breakdown, repeat endoscopy and postoperative swallow studies should be performed to evaluate persistent aspiration and confirm a successful functional repair.[22]

Tracheomalacia

Tracheomalacia is the most common congenital tracheal anomaly. Most children are either asymptomatic or minimally symptomatic, and most cases involve posterior malacia of the trachealis, with associated broad tracheal rings. Commonly associated abnormalities include laryngeal clefts, TEF, and bronchomalacia. Presenting symptoms include a brassy cough, wheezing, respiratory distress when agitated, and dying spells. Diagnosis is established with rigid or flexible bronchoscopy while maintaining spontaneous respiration. The key elements of diagnosis include: (1) ascertaining the severity of the malacia; (2) ascertaining the location of the malacia, particularly the possible presence of associated bronchomalacia; and (3) determining whether positive pressure support improves the malacia.

Although mild tracheomalacia is watched expectantly and anticipated to improve with time, more severe symptoms warrant intervention.[23] The most common intervention is tracheotomy placement, with the tip of the tracheotomy tube bypassing the malacic segment. Positive pressure support delivered through the tracheotomy tube assists with the management of associated bronchomalacia. While there is currently no definitive surgical approach to repair tracheomalacia, this is an area of active research.

Complete Tracheal Rings

Complete tracheal rings are a rare, though life-threatening anomaly that presents with progressive worsening of respiratory function over the first few months of life, stridor, retractions, and marked exacerbation of symptoms during intercurrent upper respiratory tract infections. Children with distal tracheal stenosis usually have a characteristic biphasic wet-sounding breathing pattern that transiently clears with coughing; this pattern is referred to as "washing machine breathing." The risk of respiratory failure increases with age.

An initial high-kilovolt airway radiograph may indicate tracheal narrowing; however, the diagnosis is established with rigid bronchoscopy. This should be performed with utmost caution, using the smallest possible telescopes, as any airway edema in the region of the stenosis may turn a narrow airway into an extremely critical airway. If the stenosis is severe, the stenotic airway should not be instrumented, even with the smallest telescope. The initial bronchoscopic view is often sufficient to establish the diagnosis, thereby avoiding the risk of airway edema. Because 50% of children have a tracheal inner diameter of approximately 2 mm at the time of diagnosis, the standard interventions for managing a compromised airway are not applicable. More specifically, the smallest endotracheal tube has an outer diameter of 2.9 mm, and the smallest tracheotomy tube has an outer diameter of 3.9 mm; hence, the stenotic segment cannot be intubated. This may leave extracorporeal membrane oxygenation (ECMO) as the only viable alternative for stabilizing the child. This situation is best avoided by performing bronchoscopy with the highest level of care. Over 80% of children with complete tracheal rings have other congenital anomalies, which are generally cardiovascular in origin. As such, investigation should include a contrast-enhanced chest HRCT scan and an echocardiogram. Specifically, a pulmonary artery sling should be excluded, as this is a common association, and if present, should be repaired concurrent with the tracheal repair. Most children with complete tracheal rings require tracheal reconstruction.[24] The recommended surgical technique is the slide tracheoplasty.[25] This approach yields significantly better results than any other form of tracheal reconstruction and is applicable to all anatomic variants of complete tracheal rings.

References

The complete reference list is available online at www.expertconsult.com

XII

Other Diseases with a Prominent Respiratory Component

70 AIR AND LIQUID IN THE PLEURAL SPACE

MARK MONTGOMERY, MD, FRCP(C)

The pleura plays an integral role in respiration. The potential pleural space couples the lung with the chest wall and provides an integrated respiratory system. Consequently, disorders of the pleura constitute an important cause of morbidity and mortality in infants and children. Prompt recognition and appropriate management of these disorders can avert a more serious cardiorespiratory catastrophe. This chapter discusses the anatomic features of the pleural membranes and fluid, the physiology of liquid transport in the potential space, and the various disorders of liquid and air accumulation and their management.

◼◼◼ANATOMY OF THE PLEURAL SPACE

Anatomic Features

The pleural space is a potential space, 10 to 24 μm wide, defined by the parietal and visceral pleurae.[1,2] The parietal pleura covers the inner aspect of the chest wall and diaphragm. The visceral pleura is tightly adherent to the surface of the lungs and to interlobar fissures. A thin film of liquid separates the two surfaces. An understanding of pleural function requires an appreciation of the structure of these membranes.

Parietal Pleura

The parietal pleura consists of a single layer of flat, cuboidal mesothelial cells, 1 to 4 μm thick, supported by loose connective tissue.[3] Blood vessels, nerves, and lymphatic vessels invest the connective tissue. The arterial supply is derived from the intercostal and internal mammary arteries. Venous blood drains to the systemic circulation. The parietal pleura possesses nervous innervation from the

sensory branches of the intercostal and phrenic nerves. The parietal pleura has direct connection to the lymphatic vessels. The surface of the parietal pleura contains stomas that are 2 to 12 μm in diameter and exhibit preferential caudal distribution.[4] The stomas may exhibit as much as a 10-fold increase in size with inspiratory maneuvers. Stomas are instrumental in clearing fluid and particle accumulations via the lymphatic glands. Lymphatic vessels are located in the submesothelial layer of the parietal pleura. The anterior parietal pleura drains to the internal intercostal lymph nodes, and the posterior parietal pleura drains to the lymph nodes located along the internal thoracic artery. The presence of sensory innervation and stomas distinguishes the parietal pleura from the visceral pleura.[5]

Visceral Pleura

The visceral pleura is a complex and delicate membranous structure. There is a single mesothelial layer of cuboidal cells overlying the basement membrane, and there are multiple submesothelial layers of connective tissue. Microvilli, which are 0.1 μm wide and 3 to 6 μm long, are evident on the apical surfaces of the visceral mesothelial cells. The microvilli participate in the homeostasis of the pleural fluid and contribute to transmembrane solute and fluid movement. Further, vesicles contained within the microvilli trap particles and glycoproteins, thereby reducing friction between the visceral and parietal pleurae.[6] Blood supply to the visceral pleura is via the bronchial arteries, with a minor contribution from the pulmonary circulation. The connective tissue underlying the mesothelial layer is richly endowed with type 1 collagen and provides much of the tensile strength of the pleura. The lymphatic glands drain to the mediastinal nodes, following the course set by the pulmonary veins and arteries. The visceral pleura has no sensory innervation, but it is supplied by branches of the vagus and sympathetic trunks.

PHYSIOLOGY OF THE PLEURAL SPACE

Formation and Absorption of Pleural Fluid

The pleural membranes are permeable to liquid. Normally, the influx and outflow of pleural fluid is in steady state and results in a small, but measurable, amount (0.1 to 0.2 mL/kg) of sterile, colorless liquid.[7, 10] The pleural liquid is thickest over dependent areas of the thorax. The fluid provides union and prevents friction between the visceral and parietal pleurae. Normal pleural fluid contains 15 gm/L protein and is alkaline (pH 7.60). There are approximately 1700 cells/mm³, consisting of 75% macrophages, 23% lymphocytes, and 2% mesothelial cells.[8] Pleural fluid homeostasis is a balance among production of pleural fluid, competence of the pleural membrane, and absorption of pleural fluid via microvilli, capillary membranes, and lymphatic stomas.

A rational understanding of the accumulation of excess pleural liquid requires knowledge of normal liquid transport into and out of the pleural cavity. Fluid influx and outflow are described by Starling forces and also are determined by clearance via lymphatic stomas.[9] Nearly 90% of the original amount of pleural liquid filtered out of the arterial end of the capillaries is re-absorbed at the venous end. The remainder of the filtrate (10%) is returned via the lymphatic glands. The balance between filtration and re-absorption forces determines the direction of liquid movement. Starling described a classic approach to convective (bulk) liquid movement between vascular and extravascular compartments, which is described in Chapter 43.

There is a net pressure of 9 cm H_2O (filtration pressure) at the parietal pleural capillary level, tending to drive liquid into the pleural space. In contrast, a net driving pressure of −10 cm H_2O (absorption pressure) is acting on the visceral pleural capillaries, driving liquid from the pleural space into the capillaries (Table 70-1). Net liquid absorption from the pleural space occurs because absorption pressure is slightly greater than filtration pressure. Increased negative pressure develops in the liquid between the contact points of the visceral and parietal pleurae because of increased stretching and deformation at these sites. Ultimately, the negative pleural liquid pressure equilibrates with the absorption pressure. Thus, the pleural space is kept virtually liquid-free, a state that represents equilibrium between filtration and absorption.

Pleural absorption of liquid is augmented by intercostal and diaphragmatic activity (e.g., deep breathing exercises), which results in increased vascular and lymphatic uptake owing to dilation of the lymphatic stomas and the dehiscences formed between mesothelial cells of the visceral pleura. Predictably, hypoventilation decreases absorption of particulate matter from the pleural space. Moreover, markedly negative intrapleural pressures throughout the respiratory cycle (e.g., those occurring with atelectasis or with continuous suction on closed thoracostomy tubes) will contribute to the generation of pleural fluid.

The parietal pleura plays a vital role in the clearance of excess pleural fluid. The capacity of the lymphatic system to drain the pleural space is tremendous via stomas in the parietal pleura. The rate of fluid transport from the pleural space through the lymphatic glands increases in a linear fashion to exceed the usual rate of fluid production by almost 30-fold. The ability of the parietal pleura to markedly enhance fluid absorption via the stomas is crucial to preventing and clearing fluid accumulation.

Maintenance of an Air-Free Pleural Space

The pleural membranes are permeable to gas, yet the pleural space is free of air. The difference between total gas pressure in the venous system and that in the pleural space accounts for this fact. Partial pressures of gases in the venous blood at sea level are: partial pressure of oxygen (Po_2) = 40 mm Hg, partial pressure of carbon dioxide (Pco_2) = 46 mm Hg, partial pressure of nitrogen (PN_2) = 573 mm Hg, and partial pressure of water (PH_2O) = 47 mm Hg. The sum of these is 706 mm Hg, which is 54 mm Hg (73 cm H_2O) less than atmospheric pressure (at sea level). Because total gas pressure in venous blood is approximately 73 cm H_2O subatmospheric, and intrapleural pressure at resting lung volume is approximately 5 cm H_2O subatmospheric, there is a pressure gradient of approximately 68 cm H_2O, favoring continuing absorption of gas from the pleural space into the circulation. Thus, provided there is no continuing air leak to the pleural space from the

TABLE 70-1 STARLING RELATIONSHIP IN THE PARIETAL AND VISCERAL PLEURA	PARIETAL PLEURA	VISCERAL PLEURA
Force Moving Liquid into the Pleural Space (cm H_2O)		
Capillary hydrostatic pressure	30	11
Interstitial hydrostatic pressure (pleural pressure)	−5	−5
Oncotic pressure of the pleural liquid	−6	−6
Total (cm H_2O)	41	22
Force Moving Liquid into the Pleural Capillaries (cm H_2O)		
Plasma oncotic pressure	32	32
Net Force (cm H_2O)	−9 (out)	10 (in)

atmosphere, gas volume within the pleural space diffuses out until all of the gas disappears, at a rate of 100 mL/wk, so normally the pleural space is kept totally gas-free. Furthermore, the partial pressure of nitrogen in the capillary and venous blood is the major contributor to the total partial pressure of gas in the pleural space. The clinical practice of using supplemental oxygen therapy to reduce the P_{N_2} and speed resorption of a small pneumothorax is based on this principle.[11] It has been demonstrated that 100% oxygen breathing can increase the rate of absorption of loculated pleural air by six-fold.[12]

ACCUMULATION OF EXCESS PLEURAL LIQUID

Pathogenesis

The normal state of a nearly liquid-free pleural cavity represents equilibrium between pleural liquid formation (filtration) and removal (absorption). Fundamentally, excess liquid accumulates in the pleural cavity (effusion) whenever filtration exceeds removal as a result of: (1) increased filtration associated with normal or impaired absorption, (2) normal filtration associated with inadequate removal, or (3) addition of exogenous fluid (peritoneal cavity or intravenous fluid extravasation).[13,14] Thus, disequilibrium

may be caused by disturbances in the Starling forces that govern filtration and absorption, alterations in lymphatic drainage, or both.

Various clinical disorders can alter vascular filtration and absorption in the pleural capillaries as well as lymphatic flow (Table 70-2).[6] Inflammation (e.g., pleural infection, rheumatoid arthritis, systemic lupus erythematosus, pulmonary infarction) or direct toxic damage to the endothelium may increase the filtration coefficient. The increase in the filtration coefficient allows protein loss from the capillaries and accumulation in the pleural cavity, thereby increasing oncotic pressure in the interstitial space. Local blood flow may increase in response to inflammation, resulting in an increase in capillary hydrostatic pressure. The net consequence of these changes is increased liquid and protein transudation into the pleural cavity that exceeds the normal capacity of lymphatic drainage. In all conditions that result in pleural effusion caused by abnormality in the pleural membrane, there will be an excess of protein or other large molecules in the pleural fluid.

Pleural fluid formation is enhanced in the face of increased capillary hydrostatic pressure or more negative hydrostatic pressure in the interstitial space.[13] Hydrostatic pressure increases with systemic venous hypertension (e.g., pericarditis, right-sided heart failure caused by overinfusion of blood or fluid, superior vena cava syndrome)

TABLE 70-2 PATHOPHYSIOLOGY OF PLEURAL LIQUID ACCUMULATION

PRIMARY MECHANISM	CLINICAL DISORDERS	PLEURAL EFFUSION
Altered Starling Forces		
Increased capillary permeability (K_f)	Pleuropulmonary infection; circulating toxins; systemic lupus erythematosus; rheumatoid arthritis; sarcoidosis; tumor; pulmonary infarction; viral hepatitis	Exudate
Increased capillary hydrostatic pressure (P_c)	Overhydration; congestive heart failure; venous hypertension; pericarditis	Transudate
Decreased hydrostatic pressure of the interstitial space (P_{is})	Trapped lung with chronic pleural space; post-thoracentesis	Transudate
Decreased plasma oncotic pressure (π_{pl})	Hypoalbuminemia; nephrosis; hepatic cirrhosis	Transudate
Increased oncotic pressure in the interstitial space (π_{is})	Pulmonary infarction	Exudate
Inappropriate Lymphatic Flow		
Inadequate outflow	Hypoalbuminemia; nephrosis	Transudate
Excessive inflow	Hepatic cirrhosis with ascites; peritoneal dialysis Mediastinal radiation, superior vena caval syndrome, fibrosis; pericarditis; tuberculosis; lymphoma, mediastinal hygroma; hereditary lymphedema, congenital chylothorax	Transudate or exudate
Impaired flow	Mediastinal lymphadenopathy and thickening of the parietal pleura; obstruction or chyle of the thoracic duct; developmental hydroplasia or defect	Exudate, transudate
Disruption of the diaphragmatic lymphatic glands	Pancreatitis; subphrenic abscess	Exudate
Vascular leak	Trauma; spontaneous rupture; vascular erosion by a neoplasm; hemorrhagic disease	

or because of pulmonary venous hypertension (e.g., congestive heart failure). The resulting increased accumulation of pleural liquid (hydrothorax) is caused by increased driving pressure in the systemic capillaries. The creation of a markedly subatmospheric pleural pressure (e.g., persistent high negative pressures occasionally used during tube thoracostomy drainage), even in the presence of normal hydrostatic pressure in the pleural capillaries, may also result in increased fluid filtration from the pleural capillaries. This mechanism also explains effusions that occur after pneumonectomy, recurrence of effusion after repeated thoracenteses, and the increasing effusion that occurs in tuberculosis, consequent to visceral pleural thickening, fibrosis, and permanently atelectatic lungs. Oncotic pressure (π) determines how effectively fluid is re-absorbed. Net absorption by the visceral pleura is reduced to zero by an increase in the pleural liquid protein concentration of more than 40 g/L (an exudative pleural effusion) in the presence of a normal plasma protein concentration. When plasma oncotic pressure is significantly reduced (e.g., hypoalbuminemia caused by nephrosis), parietal pleural filtration is increased and visceral pleural absorption is reduced. In all of these conditions, excess pleural fluid remains an ultrafiltrate, with normal concentrations of pleural fluid protein.

Proper functioning of the lymphatic stomas and system are essential in clearing the pleural space of excess fluid. If lymphatic channels are unable to provide adequate drainage, pleural effusion ensues. Lymphatic drainage may be impeded as a result of: (1) systemic venous hypertension; (2) mediastinal lymphadenopathy (e.g., lymphoma or fibrosis); (3) fibrosis of the parietal pleura (e.g., tuberculosis); (4) obstruction of the thoracic duct (e.g., chylothorax); and (5) developmental hypoplasia of the lymphatic channels (e.g., hereditary lymphedema). On occasion, the lymphatic system is overloaded by absorption of peritoneal fluid (e.g., liver cirrhosis with ascites, peritoneal dialysis) via the diaphragmatic lymphatic glands.[14] The result is escape of excess lymphatic fluid under increased pressure into the pleural cavity, where pressure is normally subatmospheric, and development of a hydrothorax. The contribution of an abnormality in the lymphatic system must be considered in the evaluation of ongoing development of a pleural effusion.

In summary, a single clinical disorder may cause pleural effusion through one or several mechanisms. Moreover, clinical disorders may coexist. The characteristics of abnormal collections of pleural fluid reflect these mechanisms and greatly assist in establishing the etiology of pleural effusions.

Functional Pathology

The degree of dysfunction is determined by the rapidity of development of pleural effusion and the quantity of pleural fluid, as well as by the nature of the underlying disorder and the status of cardiopulmonary reserve. The usual result of pleural effusion is limited lung inflation, with a resultant decrease in vital capacity. Pleural inflammation is associated with pain that worsens with deep breathing, limiting full lung expansion. Pleuritic pain may resolve as pleural fluid increases because contact between the irritated pleural membranes is reduced. In all cases of pleural fluid accumulation, the underlying lung and corresponding chest wall are uncoupled, and function may not be coordinated. Further, elastic resistance to lung distention increases, thereby limiting lung expansion. Compressive atelectasis may contribute to decreased lung expansion, ventilation-perfusion mismatch, and hypoxemia. Pleural fluid may also distort the chest wall. The chest wall may bulge outward, with downward displacement of the ipsilateral hemidiaphragm. Inspiratory muscles are then placed at a mechanical disadvantage, compromising inspiratory efforts. Rarely, a large pleural effusion will produce mediastinal shift, decreasing venous return and compromising cardiac output. Therapy may also contribute to ongoing pulmonary compromise. Pain caused by thoracentesis or indwelling chest tubes may limit full inspiration. Ongoing use of suction for chest tube drainage may promote continued development and removal of pleural fluid. Chronic loss of protein or lipids as a result of chest tube drainage may result in malnutrition.

History and Physical Examination

Pleural effusion is usually secondary to an underlying disorder. The underlying disease determines the predominant systemic symptoms. Until accumulation of pleural liquid increases enough to cause cardiorespiratory difficulties (e.g., dyspnea, orthopnea), pleural effusion may be asymptomatic.[15] Symptoms of direct pleural involvement include chest pain, chest tightness, and dyspnea. Older children may have sharp pleuritic pain on inspiration or a cough that is caused by stretching of the parietal pleura. The locus of pleurisy determines the site of pain, which may be felt in the chest overlying the site of inflammation or may be referred to the ipsilateral shoulder if the central diaphragm is involved or to the abdomen if the peripheral diaphragm is involved. Severe chest pain inhibits respiratory movement and causes dyspnea. As effusion increases and separates the pleural membranes, pleuritic pain becomes a dull ache and may disappear.

Attention to chest findings on physical examination is important, particularly if only a small amount of pleural fluid is present. Pleural rub caused by roughened pleural surfaces may be the only finding early in the course of disease, and it may be heard during inspiration and expiration. As pleural effusion increases, pleural rub is lost. Thus, pleural rub indicates the absence of significant pleural effusion. Diminished thoracic wall excursion, fullness of the intercostal spaces, dull or flat percussion, decreased tactile and vocal fremitus, diminished whispering pectoriloquy, and decreased breath sounds are easily demonstrated over the involved site in an older child with moderate effusion. However, breath sounds in a neonate with moderate pleural effusion may be deceptively loud and clear throughout both lung fields because of the small chest volume. Additional signs of pleural effusion include displacement of the trachea and cardiac apex toward the contralateral side and splinting of the involved hemithorax, resulting in scoliosis concave to the affected side.

Frequent reassessment must continue after the detection of pleural fluid. The underlying condition resulting in pleural disease must be determined. Knowledge of the mechanisms that resulted in pleural effusion and the expected natural history or response to therapeutic interventions is essential to monitor the progress of the child with pleural effusion.

Section XII

Chest Imaging

A standard posteroanterior chest radiograph is relatively insensitive in detecting pleural effusion. In general, a minimum of approximately 400 mL of pleural liquid is required for roentgenographic visualization in upright views of the chest.[16] An expiratory view may accentuate pleural fluid, which is seen as a straight, radiodense line.[17] Obliteration of the costophrenic angle (Fig. 70-1) is the earliest radiologic sign of pleural liquid accumulation. When effusion is moderate, chest radiographs demonstrate uniform water density and widened interspaces on the affected side, with displacement of the mediastinum to the contralateral hemithorax. In acutely ill children, when only a supine view is available, detection of

pleural fluid is problematic. Generalized haziness of the affected hemithorax or accentuated pleural reflection may be the only clue to this disorder (Fig. 70-2). Standard posteroanterior chest radiographs may be inadequate to fully evaluate pleural fluid.

Lateral decubitus radiographs provide valuable information about the quantity and quality of effusions, allow evaluation of the underlying parenchyma, and assist in planning investigations and therapy. Thin, mobile (nonloculated) pleural fluid will layer out on the dependent side (Figs. 70-3 and 70-4). Lateral decubitus views with the unaffected side inferior may enhance visualization of the underlying parenchyma on the affected hemithorax. Placing the unaffected side superior enhances the

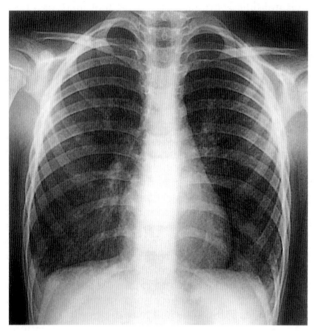

FIGURE 70-1. Posteroanterior chest radiograph demonstrating lung hyperinflation and perihilar interstitial infiltrates, consistent with *Mycoplasma* pneumonia. Blunted costophrenic angles indicate small bilateral pleural effusions.

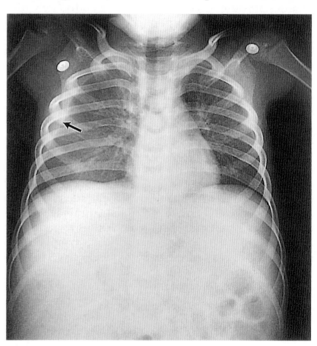

FIGURE 70-2. Anteroposterior supine chest radiograph with pleural fluid evident between the chest wall and the lung *(arrow)*. Note the generalized increased haziness of the right hemithorax caused by the accumulation of pleural fluid.

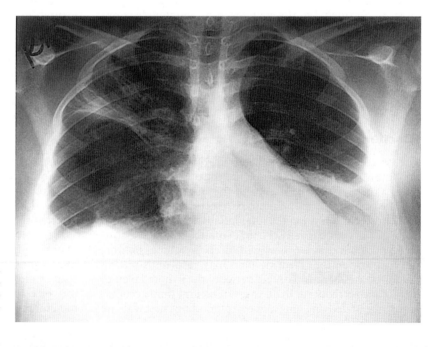

FIGURE 70-3. Posteroanterior erect chest radiograph demonstrating bilateral pleural effusions, with the effusion on the left greater than that on the right. Also evident are atelectasis in the right upper lobe and consolidation in the left lower lobe.

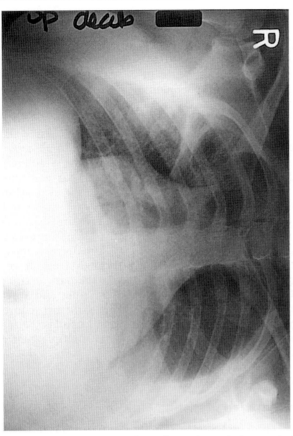

FIGURE 70-4. Left lateral decubitus chest radiograph showing the layering of a nonloculated left pleural effusion.

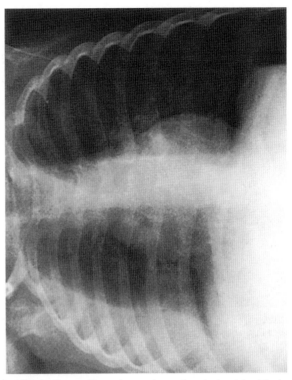

FIGURE 70-6. Decubitus chest radiograph with the right side dependent, obtained in the same patient as in Figure 70-5, confirming the presence of a free-flowing right pleural effusion.

evaluation of pleural effusion. As little as 50 mL of pleural liquid can be detected with properly exposed lateral decubitus views; this liquid is seen as a layering of liquid density in the dependent portion of the thoracic cavity. Moreover, a decubitus film demonstrating more than 10 mm of pleural fluid between the inside of the chest wall and the lung indicates an effusion of sufficient volume for thoracentesis. Decubitus films may also demonstrate infrapulmonary pleural effusion (Figs. 70-5 and 70-6). Failure

of the liquid to shift from the upright to the decubitus view indicates loculation, as commonly seen in staphylococcal empyema (Figs. 70-7 and 70-8). Evaluation of the parenchyma and differentiation of loculated effusion caused by pleural fibrosis or infiltration may require adjunctive imaging modalities.

Ultrasonography can differentiate pleural thickening from effusion, preventing fruitless attempts at diagnostic thoracentesis, and may identify the best site for

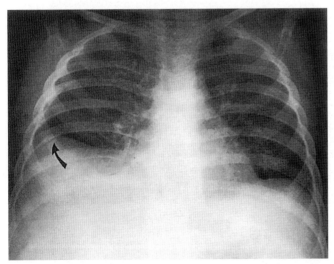

FIGURE 70-5. Upright chest radiograph of a child with nephrotic syndrome, demonstrating right infrapulmonary pleural effusion. The right hemidiaphragm shows peak elevation laterally *(arrow)* and relative lucency of the costophrenic sinus, which are signs that indicate an intrapulmonary location of the liquid.

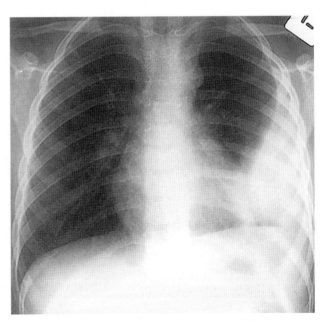

FIGURE 70-7. Posteroanterior erect chest radiograph demonstrating a large left empyema. Concomitant passive atelectasis of the adjacent lung is noted.

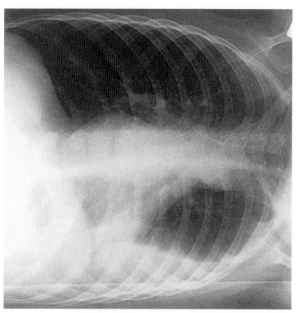

FIGURE 70-8. Left lateral decubitus chest radiograph showing no change in the configuration of the left empyema, indicating that it is loculated.

Computed tomography (CT) scans are extremely helpful in evaluating the pleura and the underlying parenchyma in large loculated effusions[18] Pleural thickening or a mass is readily apparent (Fig. 70-10). The parietal pleura readily enhances in the presence of an empyema (Fig. 70-11). A loculated parapneumonic effusion is differentiated from a lung abscess by the angle made between the fluid-filled mass and the chest wall. An empyema usually creates an obtuse angle where it meets the chest wall, in contrast to the acute angle produced by an abscess. CT scan may be extremely helpful in making a differential diagnosis. Magnetic resonance imaging has not demonstrated an advantage over CT scans in the evaluation of pleural disorders.

Further thoracic imaging techniques are required to demonstrate bronchopleural fistulas. One approach is by sinography. Radiopaque contrast material is injected into the affected pleural space through a needle or an existing chest tube (Fig. 70-12). As the patient coughs, the contrast material opacifies the fistula and spreads throughout the bronchial tree. This is the procedure of choice for peripherally situated small fistulas. Selective bronchography is used to delineate multiple centrally located fistulas.

thoracentesis, or insertion of a thoracostomy tube. Moreover, ultrasound will detect loculations and identify the quality of effusion. Anechoic pleural fluid (Fig. 70-9A) may be either a transudate or an exudate. Demonstrable multiple echogenic foci indicate an exudate or an empyema (Fig. 70-9B). With an empyema, there may be accentuation of the visceral pleura caused by thickening of the visceral pleura, compressive atelectasis, or consolidation of the adjacent parenchyma. Thus, the border between the pleural fluid and the parenchyma may be accentuated. Differentiation of a solid mass from echogenic pleural fluid is apparent by variations in the latter with breaths. A wealth of information is available from sonographic evaluation of a pleural disorder.

Examination of Pleural Fluid

Evacuation of liquid by thoracentesis confirms the clinical and radiologic diagnosis of effusion. The specimen may provide the only evidence on which to make the diagnosis of certain disease states or to exclude others.[19-21]

There are multiple techniques used for obtaining pleural fluid by thoracentesis. Regardless of the procedure used, similar principles apply. An excellent resource produced by the *New England Journal of Medicine* is available online at www.youtube.com/watch?v=6-9W-Y2dbpc; for thoracoscopic views, see www.videosurf.com/video/decortication-for-pleural-empyema-60812485?vlt=kosmix

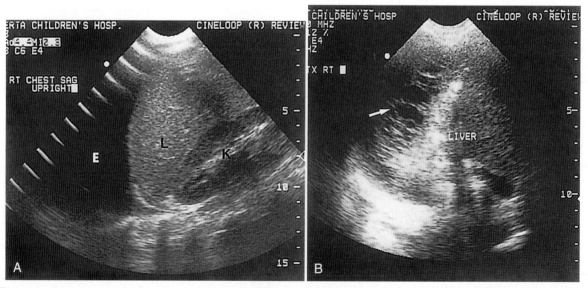

FIGURE 70-9. A, Sagittal sonogram of the lower right hemithorax and the upper quadrant. A large anechoic right pleural effusion *(E)*, the liver *(L)*, and the kidney *(K)* are identified. This is the appearance of a nonloculated uncomplicated pleural effusion. **B,** Transverse sonogram of the right upper quadrant 6 days later demonstrates a lesion of mixed echogenicity *(arrow)* posterolateral to the liver, which is consistent with an empyema.

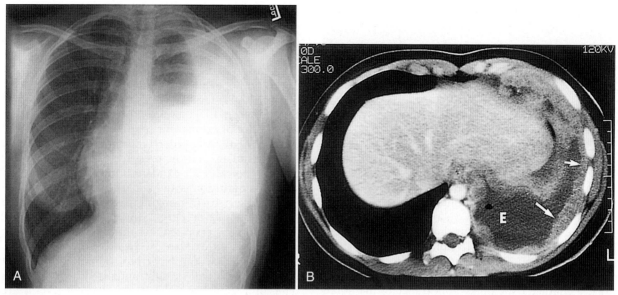

FIGURE 70-10. **A,** Posteroanterior erect chest radiograph illustrating a large left pleural effusion. The pleural fluid obscures evaluation of the underlying left lung. Mass effect, with shift of the mediastinum to the right, is noted. **B,** Axial enhanced computed tomography scan of the lower chest demonstrates a lobulated mass along the left pleural surface *(arrows),* surrounding the left hydrothorax *(E).*

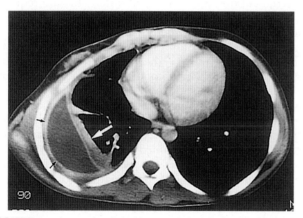

FIGURE 70-11. Axial enhanced computed tomography image of the chest. A loculated empyema with a peripheral enhancing rim *(small black arrows)* is identified within the lower right hemithorax. The rim is smooth in contour and of minimal thickness. Concomitant atelectasis of the adjacent lung is noted *(large white arrow).*

and www.kosmix.com/topic/pleural_empyema/Video.[22] The clinician must be knowledgeable about the procedure and the anatomy of the pleural space. The child and parents should be aware of the need for thoracentesis and knowledgeable about the procedure. Consideration should be given to the use of short-duration sedation, if needed. The child should have vascular access, and supplemental oxygen should be available. The site of thoracentesis should be determined clinically by percussion and confirmed with ultrasound. The site of thoracentesis should be 1 to 2 cm below the site of dullness or the superior level of the effusion as determined by ultrasound. In cases of pleural irritation, diaphragmatic splinting may occur, thus elevating the hemidiaphragm, and dullness to percussion may be caused by fluid or subdiaphragmatic organs. If ultrasound is used to locate the pleural fluid to be tapped, then thoracentesis should be performed at the time of ultrasound. Localization of the fluid may be lost if the site is only marked at the time of ultrasound because the same

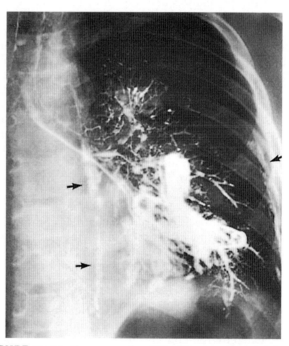

FIGURE 70-12. Pleurogram of a child with a bronchopleural fistula, demonstrating the contrast material in the pleural cavity *(arrows)* and airways. Lipiodol was injected through a chest tube.

body position may not be duplicated later. Portable ultrasound is an excellent approach. After the site of thoracentesis is determined, adequate analgesia is provided. With strict aseptic technique, a thoracentesis needle or large-bore intravascular catheter is introduced just above the rib. This placement avoids the intercostal nerve and vascular bundle. Attention must be paid to ensure that the needle is not introduced beyond the fluid and into the lung. A chest radiograph should be obtained after thoracentesis to ensure that a pneumothorax has not been created and to evaluate the underlying lung parenchyma.

BOX 70-1   PHYSICAL AND CHEMICAL CHARACTERISTICS OF CHYLE

Sterile
Ingested lipophilic dyes stain the effusion
Cells are predominantly lymphocytes
Sudan stain shows fat globules
Total fat content exceeds that of plasma (e.g., ≤660 mg/dL)
Protein content is half of or the same as that of plasma (usually ≥3.0 g/dL)
Electrolyte count is the same as that of plasma
Blood urea nitrogen level is the same as that of plasma
Glucose level is the same as that of plasma

The gross appearance of the liquid may be a clue to the cause of effusion.[23] Pale, clear, yellow liquid suggests a transudate. Aspiration of chylous liquid (Box 70-1) suggests injury to the lymphatic channels (e.g., neoplasm, tuberculosis, surgery) or spontaneous anatomic leakage of chyle (e.g., congenital chylothorax). In congenital chylothorax, a characteristic milky appearance of the liquid and the presence of chylomicrons are seen only after oral feedings have been started. Pleural liquid may assume the appearance of chyle, which is milky white and opalescent. If further analysis does not show fat globules, chylomicrons, or a turbid supernatant, the effusion is called *chyliform*. The milky appearance represents fatty degeneration of pus and endothelial cells. It may be seen in longstanding cases of purulent effusion. Bloody fluid implies vascular erosion from a malignant tumor or trauma to the intercostal or chest wall vessels. Brisk and massive bleeding is seen when the systemic circulation is involved because systemic pressure is six-fold higher than pulmonary pressure. A purulent specimen indicates bacterial infection of the pleura. Fluid with a chocolate brown or anchovy paste appearance suggests amebiasis. Anaerobic pleural infections have a characteristic putrid odor.

Laboratory evaluation of pleural fluid will allow evaluation of the integrity of the pleural membrane. The first point in clinical decision making regarding pleural effusion is to establish whether the effusion is a transudate or an exudate. If the pleural membrane is intact, then a transudate results. There is an abnormality in the Starling forces (altered hydrostatic or oncotic pressure) or fluid movement from the peritoneal cavity across the diaphragmatic pores. In clinical scenarios in which the pleural membranes are intact, the fluid is an ultrafiltrate, whereby the concentration of protein and large molecules is not increased. In contrast, exudative pleural effusion results when the integrity of the pleural membrane is impaired. There is leakage of protein or other large molecules across the membrane. Inflammation of the pleural membrane, pleural or mediastinal malignancy, and infection in the pleural space are the most likely causes of exudative effusion. The criteria used to characterize pleural effusion as an exudate (Light's criteria) include: (1) the ratio of pleural fluid to serum protein level is >0.5; (2) the ratio of pleural fluid to serum lactate dehydrogenase (LDH) level is >0.6; and (3) the ratio of pleural fluid to serum LDH level is greater than two thirds of the upper limit of normal for serum levels (Table 70-3).[21,23,24] Absence of all three criteria indicates that the pleural fluid is a transudate, and the presence of any one of the three criteria indicates an exudate. Other minor criteria that suggest an effusion is an exudate include elevated pleural liquid cholesterol (>45 mg/dL, 1.16 mmol/L) and a pleural liquid protein level >30 g/L. In clinical scenarios in which a transudate is expected, yet the pleural effusion is characterized as an exudate by Light's criteria, further biochemical analysis can be helpful. Serum and pleural fluid albumin levels will be substantially different in an exudate. In a transudate, the serum albumin level is greater than the pleural level by at least 1.2 mg/dL (12 g/L). At minimum, pleural fluid levels of total protein, LDH, and glucose should be determined on all samples. Further, bacterial culture, cell count, and differential are required on all samples. The need for cytology and further biochemical analysis is dictated by the clinical scenario.

A red blood cell count of 5000 to 10,000/μL imparts a bloody appearance to the pleural fluid. Automated determination of the red blood cell count in pleural fluid is often inaccurate, possibly because of the confusing assortment of debris in the fluid. Blood in the pleural fluid caused by thoracentesis tends to vary in intensity during the procedure. Further, platelets are present in pleural fluid obtained during a traumatic tap. Hemothorax is present if the hematocrit of the pleural fluid is more than 50% of the hematocrit of the peripheral blood. In the absence of trauma, the usual causes of bloody pleural effusion include malignancy, lung infarction, and postpericardiotomy syndrome.

Obtaining the number and type of white blood cells in the pleural fluid assists in determining the etiology of effusion.[24-26] Eighty percent of transudates have white blood cell counts of up to 1000/μL. Monocytes, lymphocytes, and macrophages are the predominant white blood cells in a transudate. Lymphoma and tuberculosis characteristically produce pleural effusions with white blood cell counts of <10,000/μL, of which approximately 85% are lymphocytes. Lymphocytes are also commonly seen in the pleural fluid of patients with sarcoidosis, chronic rheumatoid arthritis, chylothorax, and yellow nail syndrome. White blood cell counts in patients with parapneumonic

TABLE 70-3   CHEMICAL SEPARATION OF TRANSUDATES AND EXUDATES*

Type of Effusion	PLEURAL LIQUID CONCENTRATION		PLEURAL/SERUM CONCENTRATION RATIO	
	Protein	LDH	Protein	LDH
Transudate	<3 g/dL	<2/3*	<0.5	<0.6
Exudate	≥3 g/dL	>2/3	≥0.5	≥0.6

*Pleural lactate dehydrogenase levels should be less than two thirds of the upper level of serum lactate dehydrogenase. *LDH*, Lactate dehydrogenase.

effusion, empyema, acute pancreatitis, and lupus pleuritis are usually >10,000/μL. Frank pus is caused by the combination of leukocytes, fibrin, and cellular debris. Consequently, the white blood cell count of a grossly purulent effusion may be lower than expected. Eosinophilia, greater than 10% eosinophils, usually results from pleural injury and signifies recent hemothorax or pneumothorax. Pulmonary infarction, parasitic or fungal infection, and drug hypersensitivity reactions are other causes of eosinophilic pleural effusions. Basophils usually represent leukemic involvement of the pleura. Cytology of the pleural fluid is essential for an undiagnosed lymphocytic effusion, a basophilic effusion, or an exudate in the presence of malignancy at another site.

Biochemical analysis of a pleural effusion provides further information regarding its nature and etiology.[23,26] Moreover, pleural fluid pH that is >7.45 or greater than blood pH is consistent with a transudate. Samples sent for pleural fluid pH should be handled, transported, and analyzed in the same way as arterial blood samples. Pleural fluid pH <7.30 occurs in the presence of increased carbon dioxide production (e.g., infection), acid leak into the pleural space (e.g., esophageal rupture), or a decrease in normal hydrogen ion transport from the pleural space (e.g., pleuritis, pleural fibrosis). The pH of the pleural fluid supplies prognostic information. It differentiates between causes of high pleural fluid amylase: pH <7.3 indicates esophageal rupture, and pH >7.3 indicates pancreatitis. A nontuberculous parapneumonic effusion with a pH of less than 7.20 indicates a high probability of loculation. Pleural effusions with pH <7.10, an LDH level >1000 IU/L, and a glucose level <50% of blood glucose should be considered parapneumonic effusions. LDH levels provide additional information beyond the characterization of transudates or exudates. A high LDH level in the face of normal or near-normal levels of pleural fluid protein suggests malignancy or pleural infection. Pleural fluid glucose is <50% of blood values in cases of decreased transport to the pleural space or increased uptake. Empyema, tuberculosis, rheumatoid arthritis, lupus pleuritis, pancreatitis, malignancy, and esophageal rupture reduce pleural fluid glucose levels. All pleural fluid samples should be cultured appropriately, including tuberculosis and fungal cultures, in the proper clinical setting.

A chylous effusion is characterized by a normal pleural fluid/serum glucose concentration ratio (>0.5), the presence of chylomicrons, the presence of triglycerides, and an abundance of T lymphocytes. The pleural fluid pH is normal.[28]

Extravasated infusates or effusions secondary to peritoneal dialysis produce a characteristic biochemical picture. The milky appearance or color may be similar to that of the infusate. The pleural liquid glucose level is greater than the blood glucose level. Nevertheless, the pleural glucose level is less than that of the infusate due to active transport. Pleural liquid LDH levels are low. The fluid may have a neutrophilic predominance or may be hemorrhagic, as shown by cell counts.

Pleuritis caused by collagen vascular disease can be further evaluated by assays of the pleural fluid. Pleural fluid rheumatoid factor levels exceeding blood levels and pleural fluid titers >1:320 are positive for rheumatoid arthritis. Similarly, pleural fluid antinuclear antibody titers >1:160, or greater than serum levels, are positive for lupus pleuritis.

Pleural Biopsy

Parietal pleural biopsy is indicated in patients with unexplained inflammatory pleural effusion. This typically occurs in the context of malignancy—either as a primary cause or as a precursor for infection during periods of immunosuppression.[29] The procedure may be performed either percutaneously at the bedside with a specially designed needle, during thoracoscopy, or by open thoracotomy under general anesthesia. Although a variety of special cutting needles have been developed for bedside use, the majority of these procedures are now done in the operating room with thoracoscopy.

The specific needles used for percutaneous sampling, namely, the Cope, Abrams Ballestero, Vim-Silverman, and Harefield needles, vary slightly, but in general they obtain a sample of pleural tissue via a side-biting mechanism. The Harefield needle allows aspiration of liquid at the time of pleural biopsy. The tissue specimen includes portions of intercostal muscle and the adjoining parietal pleura. It is approximately 4 mm in diameter and is sent for histologic and culture studies. The liquid in the pleural space prevents the needle from puncturing the lung. Thus, biopsy is most easily accomplished at the time of initial thoracentesis, when there is the least chance of lacerating the underlying lung. The greatest value of percutaneous parietal biopsy is in clinical disorders that cause lymphocytic pleural effusions and widespread involvement of the pleural surface (e.g., tuberculosis, tumors).

Management of Noninflammatory Pleural Effusions and Transudates

Treatment of transudates and hemorrhagic and chylous pleural effusions is directed at supportive therapy of the functional disturbances and at specific management of the underlying disorder. Evacuation of a transudate after the initial diagnostic thoracentesis is indicated only for relief of dyspnea and other cardiorespiratory disturbances caused by mediastinal displacement. Intercostal tube drainage may be provided in lieu of repeated thoracenteses, depending on the child's tolerance of the procedures and the progression of the underlying disorder. Diuretics administered to some patients may slow re-accumulation of the transudate and may decrease or eliminate the need for frequent thoracentesis. Specific treatment of the underlying disorder emphasizes the need for thorough history taking and meticulous physical examination to arrive promptly at an accurate clinical diagnosis. Cardiovascular and renal causes (e.g., congestive heart failure, nephrosis) and lymphatic disorders that cause inappropriate lymphatic flow are managed accordingly. Pleural transudates caused by fluid overload (e.g., from intravenous infusion) or overload of lymphatic drainage (e.g., ascites, peritoneal dialysis) may require only diuresis or may resolve spontaneously.

HEMOTHORAX

The treatment of hemothorax associated with shock requires immediate expansion of the vascular volume and direct surgical repair of bleeding vessels. In general, a requirement for blood transfusion of more than 20 mL/kg or ongoing blood loss of >3 mL/kg/hr is an indication for immediate thoracotomy. Smaller bleeds should be evacuated because healing may be associated with pleural adhesions. Cautious use of fibrinolytic enzymes instilled into the pleural cavity may help if clots have formed. Chest pain is relieved by analgesics.

CHYLOTHORAX

Chylothorax poses unique problems in management.[30,31] Immediate thoracentesis is required for life-threatening cardiorespiratory embarrassment. In the absence of a life-threatening situation, the initial treatment of neonatal and most cases of postsurgical or traumatic chylothorax includes: (1) single thoracentesis, with complete drainage of chyle; (2) nutritional support; and (3) close surveillance of the patient's nutritional status and immune competency. Flow through the thoracic duct must be reduced enough to allow the defect to heal. The use of a medium-chain triglyceride diet, with avoidance of fatty meals containing long-chain fatty acids, significantly reduces lymph flow (up to 10-fold) because medium-chain triglycerides are absorbed directly into the portal venous blood and contribute little to chylomicron formation. Cessation of chylous effusion should occur by the end of the second week of treatment. However, even with the use of medium-chain triglycerides and avoidance of long-chain fatty acids, there may still be substantial flow through the thoracic duct and continued development of the chylothorax. Discontinuation of oral feeding and the use of total parenteral nutrition are often required. Vitamin supplements are added to avoid deficiency states. No surgical treatment is considered for 4 to 5 weeks to allow sufficient time for closure of lymphatic channel fistulas. With the foregoing therapeutic program, most patients respond favorably, with progressive weight gain and cessation of the chylothorax.[31,32] The use of intravenous somatostatin or octreotide assists in the control of chylothorax. In the few treatment-resistant cases, thoracotomy is required. Giving the patient a small amount of a high-fat substance (e.g., cream) preoperatively assists in the detection of the thoracic duct defect at thoracotomy. Rarely, chylothorax is caused by lymphangiomatosis involving the ribs. In these cases, abnormalities are detected on chest radiograph, and there is little response to the dietary manipulations discussed earlier in the chapter.

Management of Exudates and Empyema

Inflammation of the pleural membranes (e.g., pleurisy, pleuritis) is usually a consequence of diseases elsewhere in the body and rarely of disturbances residing primarily in the pleura. The inciting process may be infection, neoplasm, trauma, pulmonary vascular obstruction, systemic granulomatous disease, or a generalized inflammatory disorder affecting the serous membranes.

TABLE 70-4 ETIOLOGIC SPECTRUM OF PLEURISY AND EMPYEMA

ORIGIN AND NATURE OF INFLAMMATION	CLINICAL EXAMPLES
Primary in the Pleura	
Neoplasm	Primary pleural mesothelioma
Trauma	After cardiothoracic surgery, lung aspiration and percutaneous pleural biopsy, thoracic irradiation therapy
Contiguous Structures	
Lung infection	Pneumonia (aerobic and anaerobic bacterial, tuberculous, fungal, viral, mycoplasmal, echinococcal), bronchopleural fistula
Chest wall and infection	Chest wall contusion and abscess, intraabdominal abscess (subphrenic and subdiaphragmatic hepatic), acute hemorrhagic pancreatitis, pancreaticopleural fistula
Mediastinal infection and neoplasm	Acute mediastinitis (secondary to esophageal rupture), mediastinal tumors
Systemic Diseases	
Septicemia	Distant sites of suppuration
Malignancy	Lymphoma, leukemia, neuroblastoma, hepatoma, multiple myeloma
Vascular obstruction	Pulmonary infarction
Connective tissue or collagen disorder	Systemic lupus erythematosus, polyarteritis, Wegener's granulomatosis, rheumatoid arthritis, scleroderma, rheumatic fever
Granulomatous disease	Sarcoidosis

Table 70-4 classifies clinical disorders that may cause pleurisy and empyema according to the original site and nature of the inciting process. Infection from adjacent pulmonary and subdiaphragmatic foci reaches the pleura by contiguous spread. Bacteria occasionally reach the pleural cavity via a bronchopleural fistula, through a traumatic breach of the chest wall, or by way of the circulation from distant sites of suppuration. Trauma after certain diagnostic and therapeutic cardiothoracic procedures irritates the pleura, which may become secondarily infected. Pulmonary embolism (thrombus, fat, or gas) results in focal parenchymal necrosis that spreads to involve the pleural surface, causing pleurisy, with or without effusion. Connective tissue disorders, such as systemic lupus erythematosus and rheumatoid arthritis, may involve the pleura as part of the more widespread inflammatory process.

Primary neoplasms of the pleura, including benign and malignant mesothelioma, are rare causes of exudative pleural effusions in children. Metastatic involvement of the pleura may arise directly from pulmonary parenchymal lesions or through contiguous spread of a metastatic lung lesion. Neoplastic masses may obstruct the lymphatic channels, decreasing the removal of proteins from the pleural space. Pleural irritation may occur after certain diagnostic procedures (e.g., needle aspiration of the lung, percutaneous pleural biopsy) or therapeutic interventions (e.g., radiation therapy for mediastinal malignancy, cardiothoracic surgery). Fortunately, the risk of secondary purulent pleurisy caused by medical intervention is low.

Thoracoabdominal infections are the major origin of pleurisy with effusion.[32,33] Up to 20% of children with viral and Mycoplasma pneumonia have effusions. These are usually transient and of minor importance.[34,35] On occasion, however, the effusions may be massive and cause respiratory distress, necessitating prompt drainage, or they may be recalcitrant and cause prolonged morbidity in infants, with concurrent malnutrition. Nonetheless, the effusions rarely become loculated.

Pulmonary tuberculosis usually causes fibrinous, or "dry," pleurisy until the caseous materials containing the tuberculous antigen leak into the pleura via the pleural circulation.[36] Considerable effusion then results from the specific allergic reaction of the pleural membranes. The onset of effusion is within 6 months of the primary infection, coincident with the development of cell-mediated immunity.[37] The cellular character of the exudate is lymphocytic. Effusion is usually on the side of the primary parenchymal focus. Bilateral effusions indicate hematogenous dissemination from a remote focus. Frank tuberculous empyema is rare, occurring in only approximately 2% of cases of tuberculous pleurisy, particularly those complicated by bronchopleural fistula.

Nontuberculous bacterial pneumonias are the most frequent cause of inflammatory pleural effusions, or parapneumonic effusions.[38-40] Such an effusion may loculate owing to pleural adhesions, or may be purulent. Box 70-2 lists, in order of descending prevalence, the predominant aerobic and anaerobic isolates of empyema. The opportunity to establish a specific etiologic agent depends on the patient's age, the nature of the underlying disease, the laboratory culture methods used, and the timing of the initiation of antimicrobial therapy. *Staphylococcus aureus*

BOX 70-2 BACTERIOLOGY OF NONTUBERCULOUS EMPYEMA

Aerobic Bacteria
Streptococcus pneumoniae
Staphylococcus aureus
Streptococcus pyogenes
Haemophilus influenzae type b
Escherichia coli
Klebsiella species
Pseudomonas aeruginosa

Anaerobic Bacteria
Microaerophilic streptococci
Fusobacterium nucleatum
Bacteroides melaninogenicus
Bacteroides fragilis
Peptococcus
Peptostreptococcus
Catalase-negative, non–spore-forming, Gram-positive bacilli

---

is the single most common pathogen causing empyema in infants younger than 2 years of age. Superficial skin lesions, osteomyelitis, and cystic fibrosis are conditions associated with staphylococcal empyema. *Haemophilus influenzae* type b is now an infrequent causative agent for empyema because of the widespread use of immunization. *Streptococcus pneumoniae* is commonly responsible for empyema. Group A streptococcus has reemerged as a significant agent that causes empyema in later childhood and adolescence. Antimicrobial therapy for community-acquired loculated parapneumonic effusion must provide coverage for these agents.[41] Additional coverage for Gram-negative infections should be considered in children with nosocomial pneumonia, particularly that caused by *Pseudomonas aeruginosa*.

Anaerobic pleuropulmonary infections, which are uncommon in children, have distinctive clinical characteristics. More than 90% of patients have periodontal infections, altered consciousness, and dysphagia.[42] Aspiration of a large volume of oropharyngeal secretions occurs in the presence of disturbed clearing mechanisms. It is therefore not surprising that the three predominant pleural anaerobic isolates—microaerophilic streptococci, *Fusobacterium nucleatum*, and *Bacteroides melaninogenicus*—compose the normal flora of the upper respiratory tract and that the primary pulmonary disease (e.g., lung abscess, necrotizing pneumonia) is usually located in gravity-dependent lung segments. The clinical course is generally insidious and indolent. Mediastinal and subdiaphragmatic foci of infection are also common sites of origin for anaerobic empyema.

Except for septicemia from contiguous or distant sites of suppuration, the systemic origins of pleurisy generally produce nonpurulent effusion. Effusion secondary to pulmonary embolism of venous thrombi, fat, or gas is rare in childhood, although it may be a serious consequence of malignancy. Pleurisy may be associated with connective tissue disorders, such as lupus erythematosus and rheumatoid arthritis, and, in this case, it is part of a more widespread inflammatory process.

In summary, various clinical disorders resulting from a myriad of inflammatory origins can induce pleurisy and empyema. Certain clinical settings are distinctive for specific bacterial isolates. Treatment of inflammatory pleural disorders is aimed at specific management of the underlying cause as well as relief of functional disturbances caused by the inciting clinical disorder, associated pleural involvement, and concurrent complications. Therapy is both medical and surgical. A prompt, specific etiologic diagnosis is optimal for management.

General supportive measures include bed rest for the acutely ill child and appropriate analgesia. Fluid management must be sufficient to replace increased losses caused by fever and tachypnea. Supplemental oxygen should be administered to the child with hypoxia or increased work of breathing. It is imperative to recognize that irritability may be caused by pain, high fever, distressing cough, or hypoxia. Lying on the affected side may provide temporary relief by splinting the involved thorax.

The development of effusion after "dry" pleurisy usually provides relief from pain. However, accumulation of an excessive amount of pleural liquid necessitates thoracentesis to relieve dyspnea. Repeated thoracentesis and, eventually, continuous chest tube drainage are indicated if rapid re-accumulation of effusion induces dyspnea and dominates the clinical picture, as commonly occurs in neoplasm. Although most effusions caused by a noninfectious inflammatory process require only drainage to relieve dyspnea, additional specific measures may be indicated in the presence of certain underlying systemic diseases. Systemic and intrapleural instillation of chemotherapeutic agents and mediastinal irradiation of the involved nodes or primary tumor sites are used to control pleural effusion in lymphoma. Prednisone ameliorates dyspnea as well as cough, anorexia, and weight loss in sarcoidosis. Corticosteroids increase the rate at which tuberculous effusion resolves and fever returns to normal, but definitive proof of their value on eventual ventilatory function has not been shown. If steroids are to be used to help alleviate dyspnea, concomitant antituberculous chemotherapy is essential. Tuberculous effusions usually clear within 6 months of treatment with isoniazid, rifampin, and pyrazinamide. Asymptomatic noninfectious pleural exudates require only management of the underlying disorder. Improvement in the underlying systemic disease is paralleled by resolution of the accompanying pleural exudate.

Pleural effusions caused by infection require specific antimicrobial treatment and certain surgical considerations. Significant early morbidity and mortality rates are associated with uncontrolled infection of the pleural space. The management of loculated parapneumonic effusions is variable and evolving with the development of new surgical modalities.[43–47] The principal underlying treatment is to control and evacuate infection and balance the benefits of treatment with the risks and complications. Hence, treatment approaches must be individualized based on the child's current condition and preexisting health status and the characteristics of the pleural fluid. Parenteral antimicrobial therapy is required. The initial choice of antimicrobial agents is based on the clinical data, the bacterial epidemiology in the community, and the known pharmacologic properties of the drugs. Dosage must be adequate, and initial administration should be by the intravenous route. Infection may be polymicrobial, so more than one antimicrobial drug must be given initially. Subsequent changes in antimicrobial coverage are guided by the results of culture and sensitivity tests. A guide to antimicrobial therapy for nontuberculous bacterial pleurisy and empyema is presented in Table 70-5. Physicians always must be aware of the potential side effects of the drugs on various target organs and must be prepared to use alternative drugs, if necessary. Unlike adults, children with empyema usually do not have the long-term sequelae of fibrothorax or trapped lung.[48–51] Regardless of the interventions used or avoided, children are not at the same risk of long-term sequelae from empyema. Management decisions revolve around strategies to promote prompt control of infection and resolution of respiratory compromise.

Recent studies suggest that early introduction of video-assisted thoracoscopy (within 4 days of admission and therapy) is beneficial to reduce hospital stay and enhance resolution of the empyema.[52–54]

TABLE 70-5 A GUIDE TO ANTIMICROBIAL THERAPY FOR BACTERIAL PLEURISY AND EMPYEMA

INFECTING AGENT	DRUG AND DOSAGE (PER KILOGRAM PER DAY) ROUTE AND DURATION*
Aerobic Bacteria	
Staphylococci	Cloxacillin, 100-200 mg, divided in 3-6 doses, IV initially, for 3-4 weeks Clindamycin, 24-40 mg/kg, divided in 3-4 doses
Haemophilus influenzae	Cefotaxime, 200 mg/kg, maximum of 8 g/day, divided in 4 doses or Ceftriaxone, 80-100 mg/kg, divided in 1-2 doses
Pneumococcus and streptococci	Penicillin G, 250,000-400,000 units/kg, divided in 4-6 doses
Escherichia coli and Klebsiella	Cefotaxime, 200 mg/kg, maximum of 8 g/day, divided in 4 doses
Pseudomonas aeruginosa	Ticarcillin, 200-300 mg/kg, divided in 4-6 doses or Ceftazidime, 30-50 mg/kg, maximum of 6 g/day, divided in 3 doses with Tobramycin, 5-7 mg/kg, divided in 3 doses
Anaerobic bacteria†	
Bacteroides fragilis	Clindamycin, 24-40 mg/kg, divided in 3-4 doses
All except *B. fragilis*	Clindamycin, 24-40 mg/kg, divided in 3-4 doses or Penicillin G, 250,000-400,000 units/kg, divided in 4-6 doses

*The lower dose in the dosage range and less frequent intervals of administration are recommended for neonates.
†The duration of therapy for anaerobic pneumonitis requires an adjustment if the lung lesions go on to cavitate. Often 6 to 12 weeks of therapy is required before the lung lesions clear or only a small, stable residual lesion is left.
IV, Intravenously; *kg*, kilogram body weight.

Removal of infected pleural fluids should be considered in all cases. If there is a mobile pleural effusion, then diagnostic thoracentesis is worthwhile. Thoracentesis is performed to relieve dyspnea during the acute stage and is repeated as required; it may be all that is necessary for free-moving effusions with pH >7.20. When the fluid is still mobile and is not loculated, diagnostic thoracentesis can also be therapeutic. An attempt should be made to remove as much fluid as possible. The use of repeated thoracentesis has been supplanted by insertion of a chest drain to provide ongoing drainage of pleural effusion. The technique for thoracentesis is as previously described, with important modifications. The initial thoracentesis should be performed with a large-bore intravenous catheter. A large-bore needle is required for drainage of thick secretions. However, a large-bore needle increases the risk of trauma to the chest wall and lung. The provision of appropriate sedation and analgesia is paramount to successful initial drainage of infected fluid. Consultation with anesthesia colleagues is important to ensure that appropriate analgesia, sedation, and patient monitoring are provided for the procedure. Immediate closed-tube thoracostomy is indicated when examination shows frank pus in the pleural fluid, a positive Gram stain, pH <7.20 or >0.05 units below arterial pH, or massive effusion associated with overwhelming sepsis. Application of negative pressure to the tube enhances obliteration of the empyema space and reexpansion of the lung. A thoracostomy tube has a larger bore than an intravenous catheter and, theoretically, improves drainage from the pleural space. The vast majority of pleural drainage occurs in the first 12 to 24 hours. An empyema or a parapneumonic effusion can loculate within 24 to 48 hours of the initiation of appropriate antimicrobials. Once the pleural fluid is loculated, further attempts at thoracentesis or chest tube drainage are fruitless, and the benefits of instrumenting the pleural space must be weighed carefully against the risks. If the child is responding to antimicrobial therapy, with improved appetite, increased energy level, and defervescence, then surgical intervention is not required. If there is slow resolution of symptoms, an option to enhance clearance of an empyema is the use of streptokinase or urokinase to lyse pleural adhesions and promote tube thoracostomy drainage.[55] The method used to instill urokinase is age dependent. For children under 10 kg, 10,000 units in 10 mL of normal saline is instilled through the chest tube, and for children weighing over 10 kg, 40,000 units in 40 mL of normal saline is used. The drug is administered twice daily with a 4-hour dwell time for 3 days.[55] The child with ongoing respiratory compromise and constitutional symptoms should be considered for video-assisted thoracoscopic surgery. In some centers, the safety and tolerability of video-assisted thoracoscopic surgery has led to earlier introduction of surgery to evacuate the pleural space. With specific parenteral antimicrobial therapy and timely provision of appropriate pleural drainage, patients should recover completely from an episode of bacterial pleurisy and empyema. Symptoms usually resolve in stages, with improved energy and appetite preceding the resolution of fever. Once chest drainage is <30 mL/day and the patient's constitutional symptoms have improved, the chest tube may be removed. Intravenous antimicrobials should be used until the constitutional symptoms have resolved for several days. The total duration of antimicrobial administration (intravenous and oral) is at least 3 to 4 weeks. Findings on chest radiograph will resolve slowly, lagging behind clinical improvement. The clinician must take care to follow radiographic improvement in a child who is asymptomatic. Obtaining occasional chest radiographs to follow the resolution of empyema is appropriate. Residual pleural thickening will be present on chest radiographs taken even 6 months after the acute event. As long as the child is asymptomatic, infrequent imaging to follow resolution of empyema is appropriate.

Prognosis

The outlook in inflammatory pleural disorders depends on the nature of the underlying clinical problem, the nature and extent of pleural disease, the age of the patient, the timing of initiation of therapy, and the occurrence of complications. Noninfectious pleurisy and effusions resolve with resolution of the underlying systemic problem. Malignant pleurisy carries an extremely grave prognosis, whereas viral and *Mycoplasma* pleural diseases generally resolve spontaneously with time. Patients with empyema have a more prolonged and complicated hospital course and may require longer follow-up after returning home than patients with non-empyemic, free-moving pleural liquid. Parapneumonic effusions and empyema still produce significant morbidity and mortality. Only 50 years ago, the mortality rate associated with empyema approximated 100%. Most recent series report case fatality rates of 6% to 12%, with the highest rates among infants younger than 1 year of age. Prompt and adequate therapy during the acute phase should result in complete recovery. Complications (e.g., bronchopleural fistula and tension pneumatoceles) are rare but may delay full recovery. Fibrothorax is extremely rare. In contrast to adults, infants and children have a remarkable ability to resolve pleural thickening, with no effect on subsequent lung growth and function.

■ AIR IN THE PLEURAL SPACE

Etiology and Pathogenesis

Intrapleural accumulation of air (pneumothorax) ensues whenever the pleural space has a free communication with the atmosphere, either from a chest wall defect through the parietal pleura or from alveolar rupture. Rarely, pneumothorax results from infection with gas-producing microorganisms. A chest wall defect can be iatrogenic or from a penetrating injury from a missile or projectile.[56] Thoracic trauma, including compressive blunt injury caused by vehicular accidents, falls, and external cardiac massage, can rupture the lung. Infants and children are prone to internal injury from blunt trauma because of the greater compressibility of the chest wall. Thus, laceration or transection of major airways may accompany chest trauma, even without fractured rib fragments or obvious external injury.

During assisted ventilation, sometimes the escaping air dissects along perivascular planes centripetally, to the hilum, where it ruptures into the mediastinum (pneumomediastinum) and then through the visceral pleura, into the pleural space (Fig. 70-13). Alternatively, when under tension in the interstitial space, air may rupture directly through the visceral pleura, into the pleural space. When the air leak is confined to the interstitium, the condition is known as *pulmonary interstitial emphysema* (Fig. 70-14). When under sufficient pressure, air may dissect out of the thorax, along subcutaneous tissue planes (subcutaneous emphysema), or into the peritoneal cavity (pneumoperitoneum) (Fig. 70-15).[57,58] Less commonly, air that ruptures into the mediastinum may

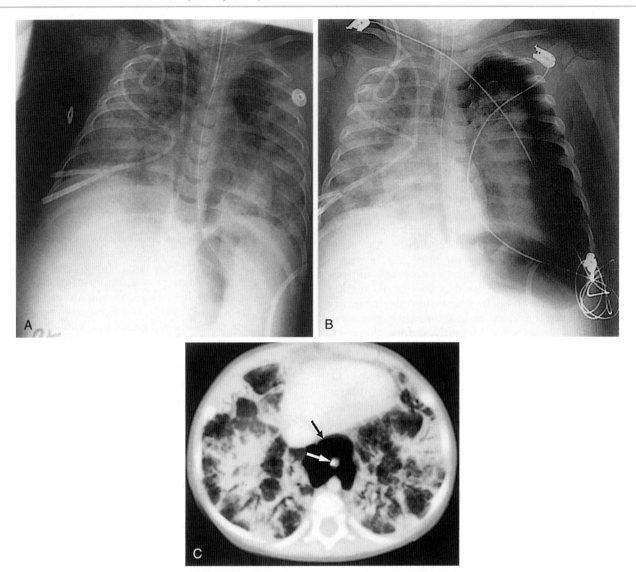

FIGURE 70-13. A, Anteroposterior chest radiograph of a patient with acute myelocytic leukemia and acute respiratory distress syndrome (ARDS). A large pneumomediastinum is evident from the hyperlucency overlying the thoracic vertebrae. **B,** Chest radiograph 1 day later demonstrates a large left tension pneumothorax and increasing pneumomediastinum, highlighting the left border of the heart. **C,** Enhanced axial chest computed tomography using lung windows demonstrates diffuse alveolar opacities throughout both lungs, consistent with ARDS, and a large pneumomediastinum, as depicted by the air *(black arrow)* encircling the esophagus *(white arrow).*

dissect into the pericardial space (pneumopericardium). Box 70-3 lists the clinical entities that result from air leak caused by lung rupture.

In the neonatal period, lung rupture can result from prolongation of the high transpulmonary pressure required during the first few breaths to inflate an airless lung, which opens sequentially. Prolonged application of high transpulmonary pressure across the normally aerated portions of the lung occurs because some of the airways may be occluded by aspirated blood, mucus, meconium, or squamous epithelium. The incidence of symptomatic spontaneous pneumothorax in the newborn period is approximately 0.5%, whereas a radiographic survey of neonates detected an incidence of approximately 3%. The newborn is particularly susceptible to uneven alveolar distention because the pores of Kohn, which normally allow interalveolar air distribution, are underdeveloped.

Outside of a complication of assisted ventilation, the most common presentation of pneumothorax is a spontaneous pneumothorax, occurring without warning in an individual with no overt underlying lung disease. Spontaneous pneumothorax is much more common in males than females.[59] Risk factors for a spontaneous pneumothorax include a tall lean body habitus (e.g. Marfan's syndrome)(Fig. 70-16) and cigarette smoking.[60] Air leak usually occurs from rupture of apical blebs, as opposed to dissection along the intrapulmonary vascular bundle.

The pathogenesis of pneumothorax in the older child can be disease-specific.[60a] Pneumothorax may be spontaneous, with no apparent underlying lung disease. Conversely, pneumothorax may complicate parenchymal infections and necrosis, pulmonary parenchymal tumors (e.g., pulmonary sarcomas that outgrow the blood supply and become necrotic), or lung infarction secondary

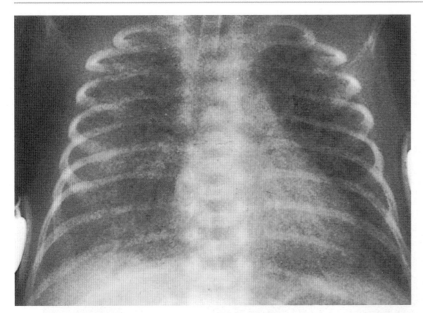

FIGURE 70-14. Chest radiograph of a neonate with hyaline membrane disease, demonstrating interstitial emphysema of the right lung.

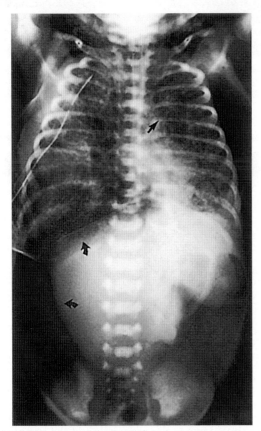

FIGURE 70-15. Chest radiograph of a neonate with hyaline membrane disease, demonstrating pneumomediastinum *(straight arrow)*, massive subcutaneous emphysema, and pneumoperitoneum that is pushing the liver down *(curved arrows)*.

BOX 70-3 CLINICAL SPECTRUM OF AIR LEAK PHENOMENA SECONDARY TO RUPTURE OF ALVEOLI
Interstitial emphysema
Pneumomediastinum
Pneumothorax
Subcutaneous emphysema
Pneumoperitoneum
Pneumopericardium
Pulmonary pseudocyst
Pulmonary venous gas embolism

Functional Pathology

Pneumothorax uncouples the lung from the chest wall. Regardless of the age of the patient and the underlying cause of pneumothorax, massive or continued air leak elevates the intrapleural pressure to above atmospheric pressure, a condition known as *tension pneumothorax.* The ipsilateral lung collapses because its elastic recoil can no longer be counteracted by the outward pull of a previously subatmospheric pleural pressure. The contralateral lung is overexpanded during inspiration, and, as a result, greater retractive force develops, pulling the mediastinum toward it during expiration and impeding venous return to the heart. Because ventilation is impaired, greater inspiratory efforts develop in an attempt to generate sufficient negative pleural pressure to ventilate the normal lung, aggravating the tension pneumothorax, shifting the mediastinum further, and severely impeding systemic venous return to the heart. Hypoxemia and hypercapnia result. Compensatory tachycardia occurs and further decreases diastolic filling and ventricular output, with cardiac standstill imminent unless the pulmonary tamponade is decompressed. Lung collapse per se does not contribute in a major way to poor gas exchange because there is redistribution of pulmonary blood flow to the normal lung, which will have lower vascular resistance.

In addition to the intrapleural pressure that develops and the inherent elastic recoil of the lung, the degree of

to vascular emboli. Furthermore, abnormality of the pulmonary parenchyma, as with sarcoidosis, histiocytosis, or interstitial lung disease predisposes to secondary pneumothorax. Airway abnormalities with resultant overdistension of peripheral pulmonary parenchyma, as with asthma, cystic fibrosis, emphysema, or mucoid impaction of the airway may result in lung rupture.

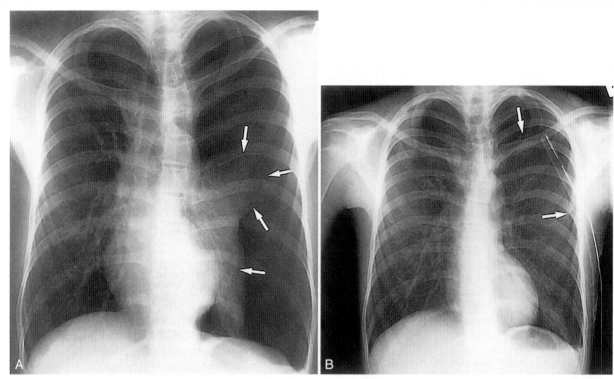

FIGURE 70-16. **A,** Posteroanterior chest radiograph demonstrating a spontaneous left tension pneumothorax, with a shift of the cardiac silhouette and the mediastinum to the right. The left hemidiaphragm is flattened. The left lung is completely collapsed. **B,** Posteroanterior chest radiograph after insertion of a chest tube on the left shows a residual moderately sized pneumothorax. A small bleb is identified along the superior aspect of the left upper lobe. This patient has Marfan's syndrome. Arrows on each radiograph indicate lung margins.

lung collapse also varies with the cause of pneumothorax and the presence of visceroparietal adhesions. Chronic lung disease that decreases lung elastic recoil and concomitant pleural adhesions prevents total collapse.

History and Physical Examination

Symptoms of pneumothorax vary according to the extent of lung collapse, the degree of intrapleural pressure, the rapidity of onset, and the age and respiratory reserve of the patient. A patient may have sudden cardiorespiratory collapse without clinical warning or antecedent roentgenographic changes, or he or she may be asymptomatic, with the diagnosis made initially on the basis of chest roentgenogram. Early recognition of lung rupture requires keen awareness of its possibility, particularly in patients with conditions known to be associated with this complication (Box 70-4). Pneumothorax may also be a spontaneous event, unrelated to any known cause, particularly in newborn infants and tall, lean adolescents and young adults.

In an otherwise normal neonate, symptoms of spontaneous pneumothorax are often subtle, and physical findings are misleading because abnormalities may not be immediately discernible. Certain clinical features, however, have been seen on close observation: (1) the infant is unusually irritable; (2) tachypnea with a respiratory rate >60 breaths/min is invariably seen; and (3) chest bulging is usually noticeable, especially with unilateral pneumothorax. A shift of the cardiac impulse away from the site of pneumothorax is a useful sign, but often it cannot be detected confidently. It is also difficult to identify diminished air entry on the ipsilateral side because of the small

BOX 70-4 Conditions Associated with Alveolar Rupture

First breath
Diagnostic and therapeutic maneuvers
Thoracentesis
Aspiration lung biopsy
Percutaneous pleural biopsy
Cardiothoracic surgery
Resuscitation
Ventilator therapy, especially with positive end-expiratory pressure
Lower respiratory tract diseases
Hyaline membrane disease
Aspiration syndrome
Asthma
Cystic fibrosis
Tuberculosis (cavitary, miliary)
Pneumonia and bronchiolitis
Malignancy (primary or metastatic)
Blunt thoracic trauma

size of the newborn chest. Grunting, retraction, and cyanosis are noted late in the progression of the complication.

In a newborn with underlying lung disease requiring mechanical respiratory assistance, certain observations are useful to note. Sudden deterioration, accompanied by decreased compliance of the respiratory system and the need for increased inspiratory pressure, suggests a diagnosis of tension pneumothorax, which necessitates prompt needle decompression. Changes in vital signs include decreases in heart rate, blood pressure, and respiratory rate, and narrowing of pulse pressure. Even when deterioration is gradual, auscultation is often unreliable because breath sounds from the remaining expansible areas of the lungs are clearly transmitted across the small newborn chest during mechanical ventilation.

Although certain limitations of physical examination of the chest have been alluded to, periodic physical reappraisal remains important and must be done whenever a patient shows clinical worsening, deterioration in arterial gas tensions, or both. Additional nonroentgenographic tools for monitoring infants for pneumothorax in high-risk situations (e.g., in hyaline membrane disease, meconium aspiration, mechanical ventilation) should be used; they include continuous electrocardiographic display on the oscilloscope[61] and monitoring of arterial oxygen saturation. In neonates, chest transillumination with a powerful fiberoptic light probe has been effectively applied to the diagnosis of pneumothorax at the bedside and has a distinct advantage. These techniques allow for more focused use of the chest radiograph in following these neonates.

Roentgenographic confirmation is essential when the physical findings are minimal and cardiorespiratory function is only modestly altered. An anteroposterior chest film supplemented by a horizontal beam cross-table lateral view, with the patient supine or in the decubitus position, can detect even relatively small amounts of intrapleural or mediastinal air. Pneumothorax must be differentiated from lung cyst and lobar emphysema. In both of these conditions, the lower border of the radiolucency is crescentic; in addition, attenuated lung markings may appear lateral to this line. A congenital diaphragmatic hernia is readily identified in the following way: a nasogastric tube with a radiopaque tip is used for decompression and left in place while a radiograph is taken; if the radiograph shows the tip in the thoracic cavity, then a diaphragmatic hernia is present.

In an older child, certain conditions (including bronchiolitis, asthma, cystic fibrosis, pertussis syndrome, hydatid cyst, progressive primary pulmonary tuberculosis, metastatic sarcoma, staphylococcal pneumonia, and blunt thoracic injury) alert the clinician to the risk of pneumothorax. The diagnosis is suspected when a patient has sudden, severe cardiorespiratory collapse, or less seriously, shallow breathing and sudden pain in the chest or referred to the shoulder. Contributory factors include frequent paroxysms of cough, severe underlying lung disease, and the use of a respirator. Pneumothorax is not as difficult to detect in older children as it is in the newborn because abnormal physical findings are more apparent. Nonetheless, in children with diffuse, obstructive lung disorders, the physical signs of the underlying disease may be similar to those of pneumothorax and may be unchanged by the development of this complication, except for shift of the trachea and the apical beat. Even the latter may be difficult to locate in light of overinflation. The scratch sign, which is a loud, harsh sound heard over the midsternum when the affected side is stroked with a dull instrument or a finger, may be elicited.

Radiologic confirmation is helpful. There is little information added by an expiratory view.[62] The size of the pneumothorax can be estimated from the following formula:[62a]

$$\text{Size of pneumothorax (\%)} = (1 - [L^3 / H^3]) \times 100 \quad [62a,64]$$

where L is the diameter of the lung and H is the diameter of the hemithorax on upright inspiratory chest radiograph. Collapse of the lung halfway to the lung border can also approximate a "medium" pneumothorax. Moreover, a distance of 2 cm from the interior border of the chest wall to the collapsed lung edge, measured at the hilum, represents the distinction of a large- from a small-sized pneumothorax. The existence of a 2-cm space from lung edge to chest wall suggests the presence of a 50% pneumothorax.[65]

The clinician should be mindful that air tends to collect anteriorly, as opposed to liquids that accumulate more in dependent areas of the thorax. In the presence of intrapleural air, consideration should be given to other air leak phenomena. Pneumomediastinum rarely results in cardiopulmonary compromise, but it may precede pneumothorax. Air may also dissect to the pericardium, producing tamponade, or to the peritoneum, where differentiation from a ruptured abdominal viscus is essential. With subcutaneous emphysema, palpable crepitations may be present over the neck and torso.

Management

In room air, the pleural space is cleared of 1.25% of the volume of the hemithorax every 24 hours.[66]

When pneumothorax is present, intrapleural gas absorption can be hastened considerably (about six- to seven-fold, to almost 10%/day), if the gas is loculated (there is no continuous air leak), by breathing 100% oxygen. Breathing 100% oxygen washes out nitrogen from the body without significantly increasing venous P_{O_2}. Under ordinary circumstances, arterial blood is almost completely saturated with oxygen during air breathing; therefore, oxygen breathing changes the arterial oxygen content by increasing only the amount of oxygen dissolved in plasma. The increase in dissolved oxygen that occurs with a change from air to oxygen breathing is approximately 1.5 volumes percent. Because the difference in arteriovenous oxygen content remains, on average, 5 volumes percent, and the steep part of the oxyhemoglobin dissociation curve is in effect, breathing 100% oxygen increases venous P_{O_2} from 40 to approximately 50 torr. This increase in venous P_{O_2} is accomplished while P_{N_2} goes to nearly zero, and therefore total venous gas pressure is approximately 143 mm Hg, or 617 mm Hg (800 cm H_2O) less than atmospheric pressure. Thus, breathing 100% oxygen will hasten the absorption of loculated gas.[66]

Individuals with small (less than 15%) pneumothorax who are asymptomatic can be observed and do not necessarily require intervention.[66a] There should be resolution of the pneumothorax within 12 days.

In the presence of underlying disease, direct mechanical evacuation of intrapleural air should be performed unless the pneumothorax is very small, the underlying disorder is mild, and the patient's clinical status is stable. Close clinical and blood gas monitoring is an integral part of management.

The appropriate use of interventions in a spontaneous primary pneumothorax is evolving. Specific clinical settings mandate decompression and evacuation of intrapleural air.[67] Evacuation of intrapleural air is essential in all patients who are breathless.[65] Furthermore, pleural air should be evacuated before air transport. The reduction in barometric pressure with ascent increases the volume of intrapleural air, possibly converting a small pneumothorax to tension pneumothorax in transit. Tube thoracostomy provides an escape for intrapleural air should the volume increase. Needle aspiration of a pneumothorax is often sufficient and has shown equivalence to immediate insertion of a chest drain.[68] Needle aspiration of a pneumothorax is successful in approximately 60% of cases, and if unsuccessful, then a chest drain should be used to evacuate the pleural air.[65] A small-bore chest tube inserted into the chest by the Seldinger technique is as effective as larger-bore chest tubes. There is no need for application of suction to speed evacuation of the pleural air; simply providing an underwater seal or Heimlich valve is usually adequate. Low-grade suction (10 to 20 cm H_2O) may be applied if there is continuing air leak after 24 hours of straight drainage.

Shortly after the procedure, a chest radiograph should be taken to assess lung expansion. The drainage tube is left in place for an average of 3 days, until there has been no air leak for 24 hours. Cessation of air leak is recognized by cessation of bubbling in the drainage collection system during the respiratory cycle. Observing the swing of the water meniscus, which normally oscillates during respiration, ensures patency of the tube. After cessation of air leak is established and complete lung expansion is confirmed by roentgenography, the tube is withdrawn. The tube should not remain in place, clamped, for an extended period before withdrawal. Narcotic analgesics are indicated to reduce pleuritic pain associated with tube removal. If possible, based on the child's age, understanding, and cooperation, the tube should be removed during an expiratory breath-hold. This maneuver maintains positive pleural pressure, reducing the incidence of recurrence of pneumothorax with chest tube removal.

Various agents have been used to produce pleurodesis and reduce recurrence rate, including talc, tetracycline, autologous blood, and fibrin glue.[69-71] Introduction of a talc slurry has been associated with adult respiratory distress syndrome and respiratory failure. Selection of the best agent to use, the timing of use, and use of video-assisted thoracoscopy remains a matter of debate and is individualized to the unique patient being treated.

Management of pneumothorax in patients with cystic fibrosis involves several considerations. With the first occurrence of a small, asymptomatic, unilateral pneumothorax, resolution is typical after expectant care in the hospital and treatment of the acute pulmonary infection. If spontaneous resolution does not occur or if the initial episode is a large pneumothorax, chest tube drainage is required. After most of the intrapleural air has been evacuated, CT scan is recommended in patients with persistent or recurrent pneumothorax. If an apical bleb is found, then thoracoscopic resection is indicated. If no bleb is found, then either thoracoscopic or sclerosing pleurodesis is indicated. Due to the advent of lung transplantation in cystic fibrosis, discussion should be held with the transplant center before any procedure that obliterates the pleural space is performed. Moreover, new forms of chest physiotherapy that involve positive expiratory therapy should be withheld for 2 to 3 months to ensure that the ruptured bleb has healed. The long-term prognosis in cystic fibrosis after pneumothorax is poor, with a median survival time of 30 months.

Prognosis

Recurrence of spontaneous pneumothorax is common, ranging in incidence from 40% to 87%. The risk of recurrence is increased if the initial episode is slow to resolve (>7 days), and if there is ongoing cigarette smoking following development of a spontaneous pneumothorax. Moreover, each recurrence increases the incidence of further recurrence. To decrease the risk of recurrence, children should avoid scuba diving. On a temporary basis, 4 weeks after resolution of pneumothorax, all air travel, contact sports, and playing brass or woodwind musical instruments is to be avoided. Both CT scans and thoracoscopy have proven useful in detecting blebs in cases of recurrent or slow-to-resolve air leak. Consideration should be given to these further investigations and to pleurodesis if the initial pneumothorax occurs in individuals whose habitus or underlying lung disease places them at increased risk for recurrence.

Suggested Reading

Balfour-Lynn IM, Abrahamson E, Cohen G, et al. BTS guidelines for the management of pleural infection in children. *Thorax*. 2005;60(suppl 1): i1–i21.

Baumann MH, Strange C, Heffner JE, et al. Management of spontaneous pneumothorax. An American College of Chest Physicians Delphi Consensus Statement. *Chest*. 2001;119:590–602.

Kalfa N, Allal H, Lopez M, et al. Thoracoscopy in pediatric pleural empyema: a prospective study of prognostic factors. *J Pediatr Surg*. 2006;41:1732–1737.

Light RW. *Pleural Diseases*. 5th ed. Baltimore: Williams & Wilkins; 2007.

Macduff A, Arnold A, Harvey J, on behalf of the BTS Pleural Disease Guideline Group. Management of spontaneous pneumothorax: British Thoracic Society Pleural Disease Guideline 2010. *Thorax*. 2010;65(suppl 2):ii18–ii31.

McLaughlin FJ, Goldmann DA, Rosenbaum DM, et al. Empyema in children. Clinical course and long-term follow-up. *Pediatrics*. 1984;73:587–593.

Müller K-M. Principles of anatomy and pathology of the pleura. *Eur Respir Mon*. 2002;22:1–27.

Noppen N, Alexander P, Driesen P, et al. Manual aspiration versus chest tube drainage in first episodes of primary spontaneous pneumothorax: a multicenter, prospective, randomized pilot study. *Am J Respir Crit Care Med*. 2002;165:1240–1244.

Redding GJ, Walund L, Walund D, et al. Lung function in children following empyema. *Am J Dis Child*. 1990;144:1337–1342.

References

The complete reference list is available online at www.expertconsult.com

71 PRIMARY CILIARY DYSKINESIA

Margaret W. Leigh, MD

Primary ciliary dyskinesia (PCD) is an inherited disorder characterized by defects of motile cilia that are associated with impaired ciliary motion. Ongoing molecular genetic studies in PCD have identified disease-causing mutations within several genes encoding structural and functional proteins within ciliated cells. In PCD, dysfunction of respiratory tract cilia results in ineffective clearance of mucous secretions and inhaled particles, including bacteria. Consequently, recurrent or persistent rhinitis, sinusitis, otitis media, and bronchitis are characteristic clinical features of PCD. Bronchiectasis is the predominant pulmonary complication. Approximately 50% of individuals with PCD have *situs inversus totalis* or other laterality defects attributed to dysfunction of nodal cilia during embryonic development. Male infertility is common in PCD because defects in sperm tail structure and function may mirror those in respiratory cilia.

HISTORICAL BACKGROUND AND NOMENCLATURE

In the 1930s, Kartagener described a clinical syndrome (previously identified by others) manifested by the triad of situs inversus, chronic sinusitis, and bronchiectasis[1] that later was defined as Kartagener's syndrome. Several decades later, Afzelius and others noted that patients with Kartagener's syndrome as well as other patients with chronic sinusitis and bronchiectasis have defects in the ultrastructural organization of cilia.[2-4] Initially, the term *immotile cilia syndrome* was used to describe this disorder. Subsequent studies demonstrated that cilia are often motile but their beat is uncoordinated and ineffective. The name was changed to *primary ciliary dyskinesia* to more appropriately describe the spectrum of ciliary dysfunction and to distinguish "primary" or genetic ciliary defects from "secondary" or acquired defects associated with epithelial injury from insults such as viral respiratory tract infections or exposure to toxic agents.

CILIA: STRUCTURE AND FUNCTION

Motile Cilia

The large airways and contiguous structures (i.e., the nares, paranasal sinuses, and middle ear) are lined by a ciliated, pseudostratified columnar epithelium that is important for mucociliary clearance. The cells on the luminal surface of this epithelium are predominantly ciliated cells with interspersed goblet cells. Other epithelia that contain motile cilia are found in the ependyma of the brain and in the fallopian tubes. Flagella (e.g., tails of spermatozoa) have a core structure similar to that of cilia with the same fundamental motility characteristics.

Mature respiratory ciliated cells contain approximately 200 cilia of uniform size with an average length of 6 µm and diameter of 0.2 µm. Each normal cilium contains an array of longitudinal microtubules consisting of nine doublets arranged in an outer circle around a central pair (Fig. 71-1). The microtubules are anchored by a basal body in the apical cytoplasm of the cell. Several different proteins contribute to ciliary structure and function. Tubulin, a dimeric molecule with distinct α- and β-subunits, is the principal protein of microtubules. A network of structural proteins provide intertubular linkages to maintain the "9+2" configuration pattern of microtubules in healthy cilia. The protein nexin links the outer microtubular doublets, creating a circumferential network, and radial spokes connect the outer microtubular doublets with a central sheath of protein that surrounds the central tubules. Dynein is attached to the microtubules as distinct inner and outer "arms," recognizable on electron micrographs of ciliary cross-sections, and is thought to participate in the provision of energy for microtubule sliding through adenosine triphosphatase (ATPase) activity. Inner and outer dynein arms are attached to each microtubule doublet at distinct intervals—approximately 25 nm for outer dynein arms and approximately 100 nm for inner dynein arms. The outer dynein arms (closer to the cell membrane) are longer and form a hook, while the inner dynein arms (closer to the central pair of microtubules) are short and straight. Each dynein arm is a multimer of two to three heavy chains (400 to 500 kd), two to four intermediate chains (45 to 110 kd), and at least eight light chains (8 to 55 kd),[5,6] with each dynein chain protein encoded by a distinct gene. The dynein heavy chains contain the ATPase that provides the energy for ciliary movement.

Ciliary bending results from the longitudinal displacement of adjacent microtubular doublets. Because nexin links maintain the axonemal relationships and the basal bodies anchor the microtubules, the sliding of the outer microtubules is converted into a bending movement of the cilia. Ciliary motion takes place within an aqueous layer of airway surface liquid and is divided into two phases: an effective stroke phase that sweeps forward and a recovery phase during which the cilia bend "backward" and extend into the starting position for the stroke phase. Typically, the tips of cilia contact the overlying mucus during the stroke phase to propel mucus forward, but during the recovery phase, cilia lose contact with the mucus. Normal human cilia bend in a rapid, rhythmic, wavelike motion within a single plane. The ciliary beat frequency is faster in the proximal airways than in the distal airways (~12 beats/second in the nose and trachea versus 8 beats/second in the bronchioles) and is faster in children than in adults (nasal ciliary beat frequency is close to 13 beats/second in young children versus 11.5 beats/second in adults).[7] In healthy epithelium,

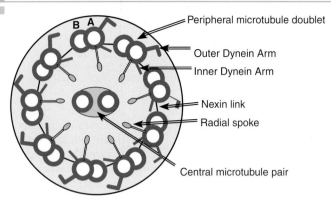

FIGURE 71-1. Diagrammatic cross-section representation of a normal cilium. The nine outer doublet microtubules and the central pair of microtubules are interconnected by radial spokes and nexin links. Outer and inner dynein arms are attached to the A subunit of the peripheral doublets.

cilia are aligned spatially with parallel orientation of the central pair of tubules in adjacent cilia; therefore, ciliary motility is maintained in the same general orientation along the length of airways. Normal mucociliary transport rates may be as rapid as 20 to 30 mm/min. Although the regulation of ciliary actions is complex and not fully understood, it is clear that several signaling mechanisms, including intracellular Ca^{2+}, cyclic adenosine monophosphate, extracellular nucleotides such as adenosine triphosphate, and airway nitric oxide (NO) play key roles in regulating ciliary beat frequency.[8–11]

Embryonic Nodal Cilia and Primary (Sensory) Cilia

At the time of gastrulation, a region on the ventral surface of the embryo designated the *ventral node* contains cells with a single cilium per cell. Recent studies have shown that these nodal cilia are motile and generate directional flow of fluid that is important for directing left-right asymmetry in the developing embryo.[12] The ultrastructure of embryonic nodal cilia has many features of epithelial motile cilia including the circular array of 9 microtubule doublets with inner and outer dynein arms; however, there is no central pair of microtubules, hence a $9+0$ array.[12] Unlike the planar power stroke with recovery phase seen in respiratory cilia, these nodal cilia beat in a rotary fashion; and, the direction of the nodal flow is determined by the tilt of the rotational axis of the cilia.[12]

Primary or sensory cilia are found in cells throughout the body.[6,13] Typically, primary cilia appear as a single cilium per cell and have a $9+0$ structure (like nodal cilia); however, these primary cilia do not have dynein arms and are not motile. Otherwise, primary cilia and motile cilia share many proteins and structures. The primary functions of primary cilia have been linked to sensory and signaling pathways.[6,13] Conceivably, motile cilia share some of these sensory and signaling functions. Defects in the assembly and function of primary cilia have been linked to a wide variety of disorders (primary ciliopathies), including polycystic kidney disease, Bardet-Biedl syndrome, Joubert syndrome, and retinitis pigmentosa.[6,13] Better

definition of the molecular basis for primary ciliopathies has raised interest in a potential overlap between primary ciliopathies and PCD.

ULTRASTRUCTURAL CILIARY DEFECTS IN PRIMARY CILIARY DYSKINESIA

By routine light microscopy, the ciliated epithelium of patients with PCD may appear normal. Examination of the ultrastructural organization of cilia by transmission electron microscopy has identified a number of distinct ciliary defects in patients with PCD, including defects in the dynein arms, radial spokes, and nexin links as well as microtubular transpositions (Box 71-1, Fig. 71-2). These distinct ultrastructural defects are generally apparent in cilia throughout the airways, middle ear, and oviduct, as well as in sperm tails, providing evidence that PCD is a generalized disorder of genetic origin.

DYNEIN ARM DEFECTS

Dynein arm defects occur in approximately 80% of PCD patients and include complete absence of both inner and outer dynein arms[2,14] as well as complete or partial absence of either the inner or the outer dynein arms.[15,16] Outer dynein arms are easy to identify because the periphery of the axoneme contains scant electron-dense material. However, inner dynein arms project into the central portion of the axoneme where there is more abundant overlying electron-dense material that can obscure margins and confound the ability to discern the inner dynein. Some investigators have used computer-assisted image analysis to improve visualization of inner dynein arms, thereby enhancing the ability to detect inner arm defects.[17] Because partial absence of inner dynein arms may be observed in normal subjects without recent respiratory infections or other identifiable insults, the diagnosis of PCD in individuals with partial absence of inner dynein arms can be challenging.[16]

BOX 71-1 ULTRASTRUCTURAL DEFECTS IN PRIMARY CILIARY DYSKINESIA

Dynein Arm Defects
Total or partial absence of inner and outer dynein arms
Total or partial absence of inner dynein arms
Total or partial absence of outer dynein arms
Shortening of dynein arms

Radial Spoke Defects
Total absence of radial spokes
Absence of radial spoke heads

Microtubular Transposition
Absence of the central pair of tubules with transposition of outer doublet to the center

Other
Ciliary disorientation
Ciliary aplasia
Absence of nexin links
Basal body anomalies
Central microtubular agenesis
Normal ultrastructure but impaired function

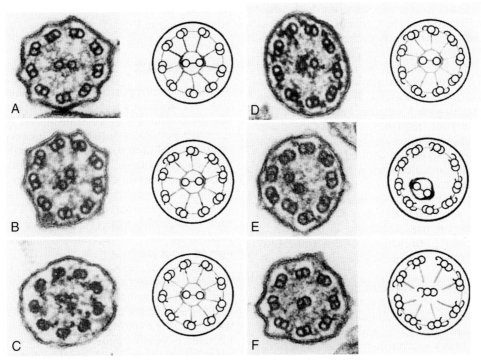

FIGURE 71-2. Specific ciliary defects that cause primary ciliary dyskinesia. Each panel shows transmission photomicrograph of ciliary cross-section *(left)* with corresponding diagrammatic representations *(right)*. **A,** Dynein arm defect: total absence of outer and inner dynein arms. **B,** Dynein arm defect: partial absence of outer and inner dynein arms (~60% of dynein arms are absent). **C,** Dynein arm defect: absence of outer dynein arms. **D,** Dynein arm defect: absence of inner dynein arms. **E,** Radial spoke defect: absence of radial spokes with eccentric central core. **F,** Microtubular transposition defect: absence of central tubules with transposition of one doublet to the central axis of the cilium. (**A, B,** and **D,** original magnification × 106,000; **C,** original magnification × 104,000; **E,** original magnification × 140,000; **F,** original magnification × 110,000.) (Photomicrographs courtesy of J.M. Sturgess and J.A.P. Turner.)

RADIAL SPOKE DEFECTS

A number of radial spoke defects have been associated with ciliary dysmotility, including total absence of radial spokes and absence of radial spoke heads.[18] These defects are recognized by an eccentric position of the central pair of microtubules that are normally stabilized in a central position by the radial spokes. Central displacement of one of the outer microtubular doublets may also occur.

MICROTUBULAR TRANSPOSITION DEFECT

A characteristic alteration in the 9 + 2 configuration of axonemal microtubules has been described in some families with PCD. Typically, the central pair of tubules is missing, and one of the outer microtubular doublets is transposed to the center in both cilia and flagellae.[19]

OTHER DEFECTS

A number of other defects have been identified in patients with ciliary dysmotility, including ciliary aplasia (absence of cilia and no apparent ciliogenesis), ciliary disorientation (misalignment of the central pairs of microtubules in adjacent cilia),[20] absence of nexin links,[21] basal body anomalies, and central microtubular agenesis.[22] All of these defects may be apparent to some degree following

insults such as viral infections; therefore, it is not clear whether these are primary or secondary defects. One approach to discern whether defects are acquired or congenital is to examine ciliary ultrastructure after a prolonged period in cell culture during which cells dedifferentiate and then reciliate. If the defect does not persist after reciliation, then the defect is more likely an acquired defect as shown for ciliary disorientation.[23] In some patients with typical clinical manifestations of PCD and ciliary dysmotility, ciliary ultrastructure appears normal, suggesting other defects that affect function but not structure. Recent genetic studies have confirmed PCD in some of the individuals with normal ultrastructure.[24] With further definition of the multiple genes and gene mutations involved in PCD, genetic confirmation of the diagnosis in individuals with normal or "nonclassic" ultrastructural defects in cilia will become more frequent (see the Genetics section later in the chapter).

FUNCTIONAL CILIARY DEFECTS IN PRIMARY CILIARY DYSKINESIA

Ciliary motion may be assessed by videomicroscopy of freshly excised ciliated epithelium obtained by scrape or brush biopsy of the inferior surface of the nasal turbinate, or by bronchial brush biopsy. Freshly excised ciliated cells maintain ciliary beating for several hours if placed in appropriate culture media. In PCD, the cilia may be immotile or dyskinetic. Recent studies using high-speed videomicroscopy have shown that certain beat patterns are associated with specific ultrastructural defects; specifically, absence of outer dynein arms is associated with immotility or a slightly flickering beat pattern; isolated inner dynein arm defects or radial spoke defects are associated with a slow, stiff motion; and ciliary transposition defects are associated with a circular beat pattern that may have a normal beat frequency but lacks the directional bend.[25] A number of other disorders including viral infections and asthma can cause acquired ciliary dysfunction.[26] By placing cells in culture for a prolonged period to allow cells to dedifferentiate and undergo ciliogenesis, acquired ciliary dysfunction can be reduced.[27] At the time of this writing, assessment of ciliary beat pattern and ciliary beat frequency is used as an aid in diagnosis at specialized PCD centers, but it has not been sufficiently standardized for widespread clinical screening or diagnosis of PCD.

Effectiveness of ciliary beat can be evaluated by measuring mucociliary clearance. As a screening assessment of mucociliary clearance, some clinicians apply saccharin particles to the anterior nares and measure the time interval until the sweet saccharin is tasted (saccharin test).[28] This procedure has limited usefulness in children because the patient must lie still with no sneezing, sniffing, or coughing for up to 1 hour. In specialized centers, nasal or lung mucociliary clearance is determined by using a gamma counter to measure the rate of removal of inhaled radiolabeled particles.[29,30] When cough is suppressed, patients with PCD have no (or little) clearance of isotope from the lung.[29-33] Unlike in cystic fibrosis, cough clearance in PCD is preserved and serves as a compensatory clearance mechanism.[33] A few centers are using mucociliary clearance as a diagnostic test for PCD.[34]

NASAL NITRIC OXIDE IN PRIMARY CILIARY DYSKINESIA

In 1994, Lundberg and colleagues reported that children with Kartagener's syndrome (situs inversus, chronic sinusitis, and bronchiectasis) produced very little nasal NO.[35] Subsequent studies have demonstrated that nasal NO is extremely low (5% to 15% of normal) in PCD patients,[36-39] and hence may be useful for screening for PCD. NO is formed by the nitric oxide synthase (NOS) enzyme system, in the presence of appropriate substrate (L-arginine and oxygen) and cofactors including tetrahydrobiopterin. In normal adults, production of NO from the nose (primarily from paranasal sinuses) is 10- to 50-fold greater than that from the lower airways. Accurate assessment of nasal NO production requires maneuvers for palate closure, breath holding, or intubation to exclude contaminating gases from the lower airway that have much lower NO concentrations. Preschool children cannot cooperate with palate closure or breath-holding maneuvers, therefore assessment of nasal NO production has limited use as a screening test in young children.[40] The mechanism for altered nasal NO production in PCD has not been defined. Interestingly, some patients with cystic fibrosis also have low nasal NO, but not as low as in PCD.[36]

GENETICS

PCD has been reported in many ethnic groups without apparent racial or gender predilection. In most families, PCD appears to be transmitted by an autosomal-recessive pattern of inheritance; however, rare instances of autosomal-dominant or X-linked inheritance patterns have been reported.[41,42] Parents of affected children are normal and have no evidence of impaired ciliary structure or function, but they may have intermediate nasal NO values.[39] The estimated incidence of PCD is 1 in 15,000 to 1 in 20,000 births. The incidence of *situs inversus* is random within affected families, suggesting that this phenotype is not genetically determined.

Genetic heterogeneity of PCD is suggested by the numerous ultrastructural phenotypes[43,44] and has been confirmed in molecular genetic studies that initially focused on genes encoding dynein arm proteins and more recently expanded to include genes encoding other proteins in ciliated cells. Through a collaborative international research effort, great progress has been made in the identification of PCD genes through targeted screening of candidate genes.[45-47] The axoneme of cilia and flagellae is conserved phylogenetically with remarkably high sequence conservation between flagellar proteins in unicellular organisms (e.g., *Chlamydomonas*, a flagellate alga) and mammalian ciliary proteins. The entire genome for *Chlamydomonas* has been sequenced, and genetic mutation analyses in dysmotile mutant strains of *Chlamydomonas* have identified numerous mutated genes.[6] The human homologues of these *Chlamydomonas* genes have been screened as candidate genes for PCD and several have been identified as PCD genes.

To date, 11 PCD genes have been identified, including genes for dyneins, radial spoke proteins, and proteins involved in axonemal assembly (Table 71-1). Mutations in five outer dynein arm genes have been identified in PCD families: two dynein heavy chain genes (*DNAH5*[48-51] and *DNAH11*[24,52,53]) and two dynein intermediate chains (*DNAI1*[54-58] and *DNAI2*[59,60]) and one light/intermediate chain (*TXNDC3*[61]). With the exception of *DNAH11*, disease-causing mutations in these outer dynein arm proteins are associated with absence or marked truncation of the outer dynein arms and abnormal ciliary beat that is slow, stiff, and dyskinetic. In PCD patients with *DNAH11* mutations, the ciliary ultrastructure is normal and a subtle ciliary beat alteration is seen with a slight stiffness to the midportion of the cilia and a hyperkinetic beat. Several other outer dynein arm genes and inner dynein arm genes have been screened, but no disease-causing mutations have been identified to date.

Mutations in two radial spoke head genes (*RSPH9*[62,63] and *RSPH4A*[63]) have been identified in PCD families. The ultrastructural defect associated with mutations in these radial spoke genes consists of intermittent loss of the central pair of microtubules and transpositions

TABLE 71-1 GENES WITH DISEASE-CAUSING MUTATIONS IN PCD PATIENTS WITH ASSOCIATED ULTRASTRUCTURAL AND FUNCTIONAL CILIARY DEFECTS

HUMAN GENE	PROTEIN ENCODED BY GENE	ULTRASTRUCTURAL CILIARY DEFECT	FUNCTIONAL DEFECT IN CILIARY MOVEMENT
DNAH5	Dynein heavy chain 5	Outer dynein arms—absent or only a short stub	Slow, stiff, dyskinetic beat
DNAI1	Dynein intermediate chain 1	Outer dynein arms—absent or only a short stub	Slow, stiff, dyskinetic beat
DNAI2	Dynein intermediate chain 2	Outer dynein arms—absent or only a short stub	Slow, stiff, dyskinetic beat
TXNDC3	Thioredoxin domain-containing protein 3, a dynein light/ intermediate chain	Outer dynein arms—some normal, some absent or short	Regions with slow, stiff, dyskinetic beat
DNAH11	Dynein heavy chain 11	Normal ultrastructure	Rapid beat with subtle limitation of cilia bending
RSPH9	Radial spoke head protein 9	Central apparatus—intermittent central pair loss and transpositions of peripheral doublet to center	Circular ciliary beat
RSPH4A	Radial spoke head protein 4A	Central apparatus—intermittent central pair loss and transpositions of peripheral doublet to center	Circular ciliary beat
C14 or f104 (previously KTU/PF13)	Kintoun, the cytoplasmic protein involved in dynein arm assembly	Outer and inner dynein arms—absent	Immotile
LRRC50	Leucine-rich repeat-containing protein, presumably involved in dynein arm assembly	Outer and inner dynein arms—absent	Immotile
CCDC39	Coiled-coil domain-containing protein 39, the axonemal protein involved in the assembly of inner dynein arms, nexin links, and radial spokes	Absent inner dynein arms, axonemal disorganization with absence or displacement of central pairs, and/or mislocalized peripheral doublets	Dyskinetic beat
CCDC40	Coiled-coil domain-containing protein 40, the axonemal protein involved in the assembly of inner dynein arms, nexin links, and radial spokes	Absent inner dynein arms, axonemal disorganization with absence or displacement of central pairs and/or mislocalized peripheral doublets	Rigid but fast flicker beat

of peripheral doublets toward the center (with the exception of one case with *RSPH9* mutations in which ultrastructure was normal). Ciliary beat is circular as seen in nodal cilia; therefore, nodal ciliary function is likely normal. Not surprisingly, situs inversus has not been observed in individuals with mutations in radial spoke genes.

Several genes for proteins involved in assembly of the axoneme have been identified as PCD genes. Disease-causing mutations in two of these genes (*Ktu/PF13*[64] and *LRRC50*[65,66]) are associated with absence of both inner and outer dynein arms and immotile cilia. Disease-causing mutations in the other two (*CCDC39*[67] and *CCDC40*[68]) are associated with loss of inner dynein arms and central apparatus defects. The wide variety of genes associated with PCD confirms genetic heterogeneity. Advances in molecular genetics technology provide opportunities to accelerate the identification of additional PCD genes through more comprehensive screening of the entire exome or entire genome.

CLINICAL FEATURES OF PRIMARY CILIARY DYSKINESIA IN CHILDREN

Patients with different ultrastructural defects and different PCD genetic defects manifest similar clinical features. To date, the only documented exception is that an isolated absence of the central pair of microtubules (central pair agenesis) and/or a genetic defect in radial spoke head proteins (*RSPH9* and *RSPH4A*) have not been associated with laterality defects (*situs inversus totalis* or heterotaxy).[62,63,69] Children present with a history of chronic, productive cough and a combination of chronic and recurrent respiratory infections, including rhinitis, sinusitis, otitis media, bronchitis, and pneumonia.[39,45,70,71] The majority of PCD patients have a history of respiratory problems in the newborn period (i.e., tachypnea, cough, hypoxemia) attributed to neonatal pneumonia, transient tachypnea of the newborn, or aspiration pneumonitis; however, the possibility of PCD is rarely considered except in patients with situs inversus, persistent atelectasis, persistent pneumonia, or a family history of PCD.[39,72,73] More typically, the diagnosis is made in children and young adults who have chronic cough, sinusitis, and otitis media. The clinical and radiographic findings in children are summarized in Boxes 71-2 and 71-3.

LOWER RESPIRATORY TRACT MANIFESTATIONS

Chronic cough is an almost universal feature of PCD. Typically, the cough is productive and most apparent in the early morning but may also occur at night or in association with exercise. Sputum may be mucoid or purulent. Most patients describe yellow or yellow-green sputum that clears with antimicrobial therapy. In many children, exercise tolerance is normal but becomes impaired with advancing obstructive airways disease in older children and young adults. Findings on chest examination are variable. Some patients have localized crackles that may or may not clear following forceful cough, and some may have hyperinflation of the chest. Wheezing is relatively uncommon. Digital clubbing may be apparent in older patients with bronchiectasis.

BOX 71-2 PRIMARY CILIARY DYSKINESIA: CLINICAL FINDINGS IN CHILDREN

Frequent (in >60% of Children)
Respiratory distress during the neonatal period
Chronic productive cough
Recurrent pneumonia
Air flow obstruction
Chronic rhinitis and rhinorrhea
Chronic otitis media
Chronic sinusitis
Male sterility

Common (in 20% to 60% of Children)
Situs inversus
Nasal polyps
Conductive hearing loss
Tympanic membrane perforation
Digital clubbing (more prevalent in adults than in children)

BOX 71-3 PRIMARY CILIARY DYSKINESIA: RADIOGRAPHIC FINDINGS IN CHILDREN

Frequent (in >60% of Children)
Hyperinflation
Bronchial wall thickening
Segmental or subsegmental atelectasis
Mucosal thickening of the paranasal sinuses

Common (in 20% to 60% of Children)
Situs inversus
Bronchiectasis
Opacification of paranasal sinuses

Bacterial cultures of bronchoscopic aspirates yield a number of organisms that may be inhaled or aspirated from the upper respiratory tract, such as nontypeable *Haemophilus influenzae, Staphylococcus aureus, Streptococcus viridans,* and *Streptococcus pneumoniae.* Older patients with long-standing disease may be chronically infected with *Pseudomonas aeruginosa,*[39,74] although young children with PCD may be infected with this organism, at least transiently. Nontuberculous Mycobacteria, particularly *Mycobacterium avium* complex and *Mycobacterium abscessus,* have been recovered in respiratory cultures from older children and adults with PCD.[39] Early studies identified chest radiographic findings in children with PCD, including (in order of frequency) hyperinflation, bronchial wall thickening, segmental atelectasis/consolidation, situs inversus, and bronchiectasis.[75] More recent studies, evaluating changes on chest CT, suggest that bronchial wall thickening and mucus plugging are more prevalent than hyperinflation and air trapping.[76-78] Bronchiectasis may occur in early childhood and becomes more prevalent with age such that close to 100% of adults with PCD have bronchiectasis.[76-79] Typically, these radiographic findings, including bronchiectasis, are most apparent in the middle lobe, lingula, and lower lobes. With the exception of situs inversus, these radiographic features may be apparent in other chronic disorders, including cystic fibrosis, immunodeficiency, and chronic aspiration.

Pulmonary function tests may be normal during early childhood but more typically demonstrate obstructive airway disease that becomes more severe in adulthood. Typical findings include decreased flow rates (forced expiratory flow between 25% and 75% of vital capacity [$FEF_{25\%-75\%}$] and forced expiratory volume in 1 second [FEV_1]), increased residual volume (RV), and increased ratio of residual volume to total lung capacity (RV/TLC). Bronchodilator responsiveness is variable. Longitudinal analyses of children with PCD suggest that lung function may remain stable over relatively long periods of time; however, there is a wide variation in the course of lung function in PCD.[80-82]

NOSE AND PARANASAL SINUSES

Nasal congestion, a common presenting feature, is often present in early infancy, with little to no seasonal variation. Most patients describe chronic mucopurulent nasal drainage. Typically, sinus radiographs or computed tomograms demonstrate mucosal thickening, cloudiness, or opacification of all paranasal sinuses, even in the absence of sinus symptoms. Anosmia, hyponasal speech, and halitosis are more apparent in severely affected patients.

MIDDLE EAR

Chronic otitis media of variable severity is present in almost all patients with PCD. At the time of diagnosis, many patients older than 2 years of age have a history of either chronic tympanic membrane perforations or have had tympanostomies with insertion of ventilation tubes into the tympanic membranes. Many have conductive hearing loss, at least intermittently, during early childhood that improves by adolescence.[83] Middle ear findings may be most helpful in distinguishing PCD from cystic fibrosis or other causes of chronic lung disease.

SITUS INVERSUS TOTALIS AND OTHER LATERALITY DEFECTS

Situs inversus totalis occurs in nearly 50% of patients with PCD. Typically, all viscera in the chest and abdomen are transposed (i.e., *situs inversus totalis*). The underlying basis for situs inversus totalis in PCD has been attributed to dysfunction of the embryonic nodal cilia that play a key role in directing normal rotation of viscera.[48,54,84] Without functional nodal cilia, thoracoabdominal laterality becomes random. This randomness of laterality in PCD has been demonstrated in genetically identical twins with PCD: one with situs solitus and one with situs inversus totalis,[85] as well as in dynein knockout mouse models.[48,54,86,87] Recent studies have demonstrated that heterotaxy (i.e., *situs ambiguus* or organ laterality defects other than *situs inversus totalis*) occurs in at least 6% of individuals with PCD.[69] Heterotaxia is often associated with complex congenital heart disease and includes a wide array of laterality defects such as abdominal *situs inversus,* polysplenia (left isomerism), and asplenia (right isomerism and Ivemark syndrome).[88] Over 100 genes have been linked to laterality defects, including PCD genes, which has led to greater focus on the overlap between PCD and the full spectrum of laterality defects between *situs solitus* and *situs inversus totalis*.[89]

GENITOURINARY SYSTEM

Male infertility is common and attributable to impaired sperm motility. The ultrastructural and functional defects in cilia are mirrored in sperm flagellae in some but not all PCD patients.[14,90] The occurrence of ultrastructural ciliary defects in ciliated cells lining fallopian tubes[91,92] has led to speculation that infertility and ectopic pregnancies could be increased in women with primary ciliary defects, but this association has not been examined systematically.

OTHER

Hydrocephalus has been reported in a few patients with PCD[93–95] and in some knockout mouse models for PCD; ultrastructural and functional defects in ventricular ependymal cilia provide a theoretical basis for this association. Defective leukocyte migration has been reported in a few PCD patients, suggesting that the cytoplasmic microtubules of leukocytes may be altered, but specific defects in neutrophil chemotaxis have not been defined.[96,97]

DIAGNOSIS OF PRIMARY CILIARY DYSKINESIA

Definitive diagnosis of PCD can be challenging and requires involvement of specialized centers with expertise in clinical features of PCD, as well as the different tests to assess ciliary motility, ciliary ultrastructure, nasal NO measurement, mucociliary clearance, and genetic defects.[45,47,98–100] Suitable samples for examination of ciliary motility and ultrastructure include nasal biopsy obtained by brushing or curettage of the inferior surface of the nasal turbinates, or bronchial brush biopsy. Identification of impaired motility and one of the specific ultrastructural defects in a patient with chronic cough, sinusitis, and otitis media provides solid evidence for the diagnosis. Airway insults such as exposure to pollutants and respiratory viral infections may be accompanied by nonspecific ultrastructural changes in cilia that impair motility. Therefore, analysis of ciliary ultrastructure should be performed by an electron microscopist who has extensive experience examining ciliated cells. Despite expert review, the ultrastructural analysis may be inconclusive in some cases because of uncertainty in distinguishing primary from secondary ciliary defects; long-term follow-up and repeat biopsies may be needed before a firm diagnosis can be made. The role of nasal NO measurement in the diagnostic evaluation has not been defined; however, recent studies suggest that this assay may be a useful screening test for PCD or may serve as an adjunctive diagnostic test in individuals with "uncertain" ciliary ultrastructural studies.[36–39] With further advances in identification of PCD genes, genetic testing may become useful for diagnostic testing.

TREATMENT

At present, no specific therapeutic modalities are available to correct ciliary dysfunction, and there has been no large randomised controlled trial of any treatment. Management should include aggressive measures to enhance clearance of mucus, prevent respiratory infections, and treat bacterial superinfections.[70]

Approaches to enhance mucus clearance in PCD are similar to those used in the management of cystic fibrosis. Chest percussion and postural drainage facilitate clearance of distal airways. Because cough is an effective clearance mechanism, patients are encouraged to cough and to engage in activities such as vigorous exercise that stimulate cough. All patients and families should be counseled about the importance of cough and instructed to avoid cough suppressants. Bronchodilators such as albuterol may aid mucus clearance in patients who are bronchodilator responsive. As in cystic fibrosis, anti-inflammatory agents, deoxyribonuclease, nebulized hypertonic saline, and other measures to facilitate airway clearance may be beneficial; however, specific indications and utility in PCD have not been defined.

A number of measures to prevent respiratory tract infection and irritation should be considered. PCD patients should receive routine immunizations that provide protection against a number of respiratory pathogens, including pertussis, measles, and *Haemophilus influenzae* type b, as well as the pneumococcal vaccine and a yearly influenza virus vaccine. Preventive counseling should include avoidance of exposure to respiratory pathogens, tobacco smoke, and other pollutants and irritants that may damage airway mucosa and stimulate mucus secretion.

Prompt institution of antimicrobial therapy for bacterial superinfections (bronchitis, sinusitis, and otitis media) is crucial for preventing irreversible damage. Sputum Gram stain and culture results may be used to direct appropriate choice of antimicrobial therapy. In some patients, symptoms recur within days to weeks after completing a course of antimicrobials. This subgroup may benefit from extended use of a broad-spectrum antimicrobial such as trimethoprim-sulfamethoxazole.

Surgical intervention may be indicated for specific complications. Tympanostomy with ventilation tube placement has been used to control chronic serous otitis media that persists despite antimicrobial therapy. Tympanostomy placement may improve hearing, but it is often complicated by offensive otorrhea; therefore, there is ongoing debate about indications and utility of this intervention in PCD.[83,101] Sinus drainage may benefit patients with severe sinusitis that does not respond to antimicrobial therapy. Lobectomy may be considered in patients with localized bronchiectasis or atelectasis that is thought to be a nidus for chronic infection. However, lobectomy should be approached cautiously, recognizing that removal of any functioning lung tissue in patients with progressive lung disease could have adverse long-term consequences. Lung transplantation (including heart-lung, bilateral lung, and living related bilateral lung transplantation) has been performed successfully in PCD patients with end-stage lung disease (with surgical modifications for patients with situs inversus).

PROGNOSIS

Chronic lung disease with bronchiectasis and some degree of pulmonary disability has been the usual outcome. Progression of lung disease is quite variable, and a number of individuals have experienced a normal or near-normal life span. Several longitudinal studies suggest that aggressive approaches to airway clearance and controlling lung infection can retard progression of lung disease.[80–82]

PCD AND POTENTIAL OVERLAP WITH PRIMARY CILIOPATHIES

Advances in our understanding of the genetics and molecular abnormalities in sensory cilia have helped define a diverse group of diseases, or primary ciliopathies. Primary cilia are found in almost all cells at some time in development and play key roles in sensation and signaling; therefore, primary ciliopathies include a wide range of disorders. Some primary ciliopathies are manifested primarily in one organ (e.g., retinitis pigmentosa, polycystic kidney disease, or nephronophthisis), while others are manifested as complex syndromes (e.g., Bardet-Biedl syndrome, Joubert syndrome, Leber's congenital amaurosis).[102] Rare case reports have demonstrated features of PCD and primary ciliopathies in the same patient, which has heightened interest in potential overlapping ciliopathies. Several individuals and families have been identified with both retinitis pigmentosa and PCD, suggesting that some ciliary defects may affect both sensory and motile cilia.[103–108] Similarly, a family with mutations in OFD1 (linked to the primary ciliopathy syndrome, oral-facial-digital type 1 syndrome) had clinical features and functional respiratory ciliary studies consistent with primary ciliary dyskinesia.[109] Several adults with autosomal dominant polycystic kidney disease (a well-defined primary ciliopathy), have bronchiectasis, suggesting dysfunction of respiratory cilia.[110] With more careful evaluation for evidence of motile cilia function within individuals with primary ciliopathies and evidence of primary ciliary dysfunction within individuals with PCD, other overlapping ciliopathy syndromes are likely to emerge.

References

The complete reference list is available online at www.expertconsult.com

72 CHILDHOOD PULMONARY ARTERIAL HYPERTENSION

Erika Berman Rosenzweig, MD, and Robyn J. Barst, MD

Pulmonary arterial hypertension (PAH) is a serious progressive condition with a poor prognosis if not identified and treated early. Until recently, the diagnosis of idiopathic pulmonary arterial hypertension (IPAH, formerly termed *primary pulmonary hypertension [PPH]*) was virtually a death sentence, particularly for children, with a median survival of less than 1 year.[1] The data in the Primary Pulmonary Hypertension NIH Registry illustrated the worse prognosis for children than adults.[1] In this registry, the median survival for all of the 194 patients was 2.8 years, whereas it was only 0.8 years for children. Fortunately, there has been promising progress in the field of PAH over the past several decades, with significant advances in treatment that can improve quality of life, exercise capacity, hemodynamics, and survival.[2-5] Nevertheless, extrapolation from adults to children is not straightforward. This chapter will review childhood PAH with an emphasis on the latest therapeutic advances.

DEFINITION AND CLASSIFICATION

The definition of PAH, which was modified in 2008, is the same for both children and adults; it is a mean pulmonary arterial pressure ≥25 mm Hg at rest, with a normal pulmonary artery wedge pressure (i.e., ≤15 mm Hg) and an elevated pulmonary vascular resistance (PVR).[6] Although a specific minimum elevation in PVR was taken out of the revised definition, one must remain cognizant that by definition, PAH requires an increased PVR. This is especially important when assessing patients with associated congenital systemic to pulmonary shunts. PAH occurs in the "pre-capillary" pulmonary vascular bed and therefore excludes causes of pulmonary venous hypertension (e.g., mitral stenosis). While exercise hemodynamic abnormalities are no longer included in the updated definition of PAH, they still may be an important measure in some children because children with PAH often have an exaggerated response of the pulmonary vascular bed to exercise. The exclusion of exercise-induced PAH was based on the difficulty in reliably obtaining complete exercise hemodynamics and the concern that some subjects could be misdiagnosed as having exercise-induced PAH. Children also have a greater vasoreactive response to hypoventilation than adults. Not uncommonly, children with a history of recurrent exertional or nocturnal syncope have a resting mean pulmonary artery pressure that markedly increases with exercise and with modest systemic arterial oxygen desaturation during sleep.

In 1998, at the Primary Pulmonary Hypertension World Symposium, clinical investigators from around the world proposed a new diagnostic classification; this classification categorized pulmonary vascular disease by similar clinical features and histopathology. The classification reflected the recent advances in the understanding of pulmonary hypertensive diseases as well as recognized the similarity between IPAH and PAH associated with other conditions (APAH). At the 2003 World Pulmonary Hypertension Symposium, the term *primary pulmonary hypertension* was changed to *idiopathic pulmonary arterial hypertension* reflecting the fact that this is a diagnosis of exclusion with exact cause(s) yet unknown. Thus, in addition to IPAH (both sporadic and familial), PAH associated with congenital heart disease (CHD); connective tissue disease (CTD); portal hypertension; HIV infection; drugs and toxins (including anorexigens); and persistent pulmonary hypertension of the newborn (PPHN) were classified along with IPAH as Group I pulmonary *arterial* hypertension. In 2008, the diagnostic classification system was updated further (Box 72-1[6]); for example, sickle cell–associated PAH was added to PH Group 1, and the term *familial PAH* was abandoned in favor of *heritable PAH (HPAH)*, defined to include all subjects with FPAH plus any patients with an identified genetic mutation regardless of whether there was a family history of PAH. In this most recent classification, IPAH only refers to a patient without a family history and without an identified genetic mutation (see Box 72-1). This classification separates PAH from pulmonary venous hypertension, pulmonary hypertension associated with disorders of the respiratory system or hypoxemia, pulmonary hypertension caused by chronic thrombotic or embolic disease, and pulmonary hypertension caused by disorders directly affecting the pulmonary vasculature. The clinical classification also provides rationale for considering many of the therapeutic modalities that have been demonstrated to be efficacious for IPAH, for PAH associated with the other PH Group 1 conditions based on similar clinical features, pathology, and pathobiology.

Pulmonary arterial hypertension may be further classified into three clinical entities by physiologic characteristics. First, there is the group of patients who have PAH from infancy in whom the PVR remains elevated, for example, PPHN. This may resolve in the neonatal period or persist well beyond infancy. Second, there is PAH associated with a large, unrestrictive, congenital systemic-to-pulmonary shunt that causes pulmonary vascular disease from increased shear stress (increased pulmonary blood flow). Ultimately, there is a reversal of shunting leading to central cyanosis for which the term the *Eisenmenger complex* was coined by Paul Wood. In these cases, right ventricular function is usually preserved, at least for a number of years, because of decompression of the right ventricle at the expense of right-to-left shunting and central cyanosis.

BOX 72-1 UPDATED CLINICAL CLASSIFICATION OF PULMONARY HYPERTENSION

1. Pulmonary Arterial Hypertension (PAH)
1.1. Idiopathic PAH
1.2. Heritable
1.2.1. BMPR2
1.2.2. ALK-1, endoglin (with or without hereditary hemorrhagic telangiectasia)
1.2.3. Unknown
1.3. Drug- and toxin-induced
1.4. Associated with
1.4.1. Connective tissue diseases
1.4.2. HIV infection
1.4.3. Portal hypertension
1.4.4. Congenital heart diseases
1.4.5. Schistosomiasis
1.4.6. Chronic hemolytic anemia
1.5. Persistent pulmonary hypertension of the newborn
1'. Pulmonary veno-occlusive disease (PVOD) and/or pulmonary capillary hemangiomatosis (PCH)

2. Pulmonary Hypertension Caused by Left Heart Disease
2.1. Systolic dysfunction
2.2. Diastolic dysfunction
2.3. Valvular disease

3. Pulmonary Hypertension Caused by Lung Diseases and/or Hypoxia
3.1. Chronic obstructive pulmonary disease
3.2. Interstitial lung disease
3.3. Other pulmonary diseases with mixed restrictive and obstructive pattern
3.4. Sleep-disordered breathing
3.5. Alveolar hypoventilation disorders
3.6. Chronic exposure to high altitude
3.7. Developmental abnormalities

4. Chronic Thromboembolic Pulmonary Hypertension

5. Pulmonary Hypertension with Unclear Multifactorial Mechanisms
5.1. Hematologic disorders: myeloproliferative disorders, splenectomy
5.2. Systemic disorders: sarcoidosis, pulmonary Langerhans cell histiocytosis: lymphangioleiomyomatosis, neurofibromatosis, vasculitis
5.3. Metabolic disorders: glycogen storage disease, Gaucher disease, thyroid disorders
5.4. Others: tumoral obstruction, fibrosing mediastinitis, chronic renal failure on dialysis

From Simonneau G, Robbins IM, Beghetti M, et al. Updated clinical classification of pulmonary hypertension. *J Am Coll Cardiol.* 2009;54(1 Suppl):S43-S54.

Lastly, there is classic "IPAH" in which a vasculopathy occurs within the pulmonary arterioles leading to right heart pressure overload. Patients with congenital systemic to pulmonary shunts who have pulmonary vascular disease from left-to-right shunting and increased shear stress and subsequently undergo closure of the defect will behave physiologically just as an IPAH patient does with an increased pressure load to the right ventricle and the absence of central cyanosis. There may be an overlap between these entities, for example, CHD and elevated PVR from birth in which there was never left-to-right shunting leading to increased shear stress, but rather right-to-left shunting and the absence of congestive heart failure symptoms and lack of failure to thrive from the beginning.

While the classification helps our understanding of the pathophysiology of PAH patients, it also has implications for the natural history, which will be discussed later in the chapter. Despite the different physiologic classifications of PAH, the histopathologic changes are virtually identical, and thus similar treatment strategies have evolved. As insight is advanced into the mechanisms responsible for the development of PAH, the introduction of novel therapeutic modalities will hopefully increase the overall efficacy of therapeutic interventions for PAH.

NEONATAL PULMONARY HYPERTENSION

Persistent Pulmonary Hypertension of the Newborn

PPHN is a unique form of PAH, which most often resolves completely with proper intervention. PPHN is a syndrome characterized by increased PVR, right-to-left shunting (at the atrial and/or ductal level), and severe hypoxemia.[7] PPHN is frequently associated with pulmonary parenchymal abnormalities (e.g., meconium aspiration, pneumonia, or sepsis) or may occur when there is pulmonary hypoplasia, maladaptation of the pulmonary vascular bed postnatally as a result of perinatal stress, or maladaptation of the pulmonary vascular bed *in utero* from unknown causes. In some instances, there is no evidence of pulmonary parenchymal disease and the "injury" that is the "trigger" of the PAH is unknown. Although some children die during the neonatal period despite maximal cardiopulmonary therapeutic interventions, PPHN is almost always transient,[8-10] with infants recovering completely without requiring long-term medical therapy. In contrast to these infants, patients with IPAH as well as PAH related to the other conditions discussed earlier in the chapter, appear to require treatment indefinitely. It is possible that in some neonates the PVR doesn't fall normally after birth and goes unrecognized during the neonatal period; the patient is then diagnosed with PAH at a later date as the pulmonary vascular disease progresses. Pathologic studies examining the elastic pattern of the main pulmonary artery[11,12] suggest that IPAH is present from birth in some patients, although it is acquired later in life in others. The histopathologic changes have also illustrated increased muscularity of the peripheral pulmonary arterioles, similar to IPAH.[13]

Misalignment of the pulmonary veins with alveolar capillary dysplasia is often diagnosed as PPHN; however, it is a separate entity, that is, a rare disorder of pulmonary vascular development that most often is diagnosed only after an infant has died from fulminant PAH[14] (see Chapter 55). Features that should raise a clinician's suspicion of the possibility of alveolar capillary dysplasia include association with other nonlethal congenital malformations, late onset of presentation (i.e., after 12 to 24 hours of age), and severe hypoxemia refractory to medical therapy. Infants most often present with severe PAH with transient responses to inhaled nitric oxide, as well as transient responses after intravenous epoprostenol is added to the inhaled nitric oxide, but then become refractory to the treatment with virtually all infants subsequently dying within the first several weeks of life. There may be a heterogeneous involvement in the pulmonary parenchyma that delays presentation in some patients. This variability in clinical severity and histopathology is consistent with the marked biologic variability that occurs in many forms of PAH. When pulmonary hypertension results from neonatal lung disease such as meconium aspiration, the pulmonary vascular changes are most severe in the regions of the lung showing the greatest parenchymal damage.

PULMONARY ARTERIAL HYPERTENSION IN CHILDHOOD

The remainder of this review will focus on PAH beyond the neonatal period. Whether the pulmonary hypertension is due to increased flow or resistance depends on its cause.

PAH/CHD: By definition, hyperkinetic pulmonary hypertension refers to PAH from congenital systemic to pulmonary communications with increased pulmonary blood flow, e.g., ventricular septal defect, or patent ductus arteriosus. Pulmonary venous hypertension is caused by disorders of left heart filling (e.g., pulmonary venous obstruction, mitral stenosis, or left ventricular failure). In the absence of left heart obstruction or dysfunction leading to pulmonary venous hypertension, the pulmonary artery wedge pressure and left ventricular end diastolic pressure are normal. Pulmonary arterial hypertension related to unrepaired congenital heart disease (i.e., Eisenmenger syndrome) is thought to develop after exposure to hyperkinetic shear stress following a period of normal PVR and increased pulmonary blood flow. Several types of congenital heart defect are associated with a greater risk for the development of pulmonary vascular disease. However, approximately one third of patients with all forms of uncorrected congenital heart disease will die from pulmonary vascular disease if not dying earlier from an unrelated cause.[15] It is not known why some children with the same underlying congenital heart defect develop irreversible pulmonary vascular obstructive disease in the first year of life and others maintain "operable" levels of pulmonary vascular resistance into the second decade and beyond. In children whose congenital heart disease is diagnosed later in life, one needs to determine whether the patient is "operable" or has "irreversible" pulmonary vascular disease. In the past, the evaluation of "operability" included anatomic criteria (Heath-Edwards classification) based on microscopic findings from lung biopsies to aid in the determination of "operability."[16] However, lung biopsies carry a significant risk of morbidity and mortality in this population. Furthermore, the pulmonary vascular disease can be quite heterogeneous and thus a biopsy from one area of the lung may not necessarily represent the overall pulmonary vascular disease in both lungs. The current approach is to use acute pulmonary vasodilator testing during cardiac catheterization to evaluate "operability." The assessment of surgical operability requires an accurate evaluation of the degree of pulmonary vasoreactivity or reversibility. It is important to determine whether the elevated PVR index (PVRi) responds favorably to acute pharmacologic vasodilatation, with a fall into the near-normal range for PVRi (to ≤ 3 Wood units $\times$ m^2). In the past decade, studies with inhaled nitric oxide and intravenous epoprostenol have been useful both in preoperative evaluations as well as in the treatment of postoperative patients with elevated PVR.[17-21] The availability of pulmonary vasodilators such as inhaled nitric oxide for perioperative management of pulmonary hypertension have allowed for surgical "correction" in select patients who present later in life with borderline elevated PVRi in the range 3 to 5 Wood units $\times$ m^2. If a patient with elevated PVR is being considered for surgery, there is an increased risk of postoperative pulmonary hypertensive crises. Thus, knowing if the pulmonary circulation will respond favorably to inhaled nitric oxide or intravenous prostacyclin can help guide the management of this potentially life-threatening postoperative complication.[16,22] For patients with an elevated PVRi (at least 3 Wood units $\times$ m^2, and particularly >6 Wood units $\times$ m^2), surgical closure of a systemic-to-pulmonary communication can be catastrophic and lead to severe right-sided heart failure since the "pop-off" valve for the right ventricle is suddenly removed.

IPAH/HPAH: Idiopathic pulmonary arterial hypertension (IPAH) and heritable pulmonary arterial hypertension (HPAH), subtypes of PH Group 1 PAH, are characterized similarly by progressive pulmonary arterial vascular obliteration and subsequent right-sided heart failure if untreated. A PAH patient is subclassified as having IPAH when the patient meets the hemodynamic criteria of PAH[5] and all other associated forms of PAH (APAH) have been ruled out. HPAH (previously referred to as *FPAH, familial pulmonary arterial hypertension*) occurs when there is a family history of PAH or identification of one of the genetic mutations associated with PAH, regardless of whether or not there is a family history. Although HPAH may represent a different clinical phenotype, both IPAH and HPAH likely represent overlapping diagnostic subgroups of PAH and are classified with other forms of PH Group 1 PAH because of similar characteristics, histopathologic changes, and treatment responses.

Epidemiology

The exact incidence and prevalence of IPAH/HPAH in children worldwide is unknown. Adult studies have reported an overall incidence of approximately one to two new IPAH cases per million in industrialized countries.[23-25] In the French and Scottish registries, the prevalence of Group I PAH was reported as 15 to 50 PAH cases per million adults and included APAH cases.[23,25] With respect to children, a national cohort study of IPAH children in the United Kingdom followed over 7 years reported a lower incidence and prevalence compared to adults.[26] The incidence of childhood IPAH was 0.48 cases per million children per year, and the prevalence was 2.1 cases per million.[26] Of these patients, 7.8% had HPAH similar to reports in adults. The difference between the prevalence in the French registry and the UK childhood registry may be attributable in part to PAH cases (including anorexigen-related and CTD) included in the adult French registry that are not seen in children. A French pediatric registry reported a 4.4 per million prevalence of pediatric IPAH/HPAH.[27] However, this prevalence does not include APAH-CHD—a subgroup of PAH that is considered to make up at least 50% of pediatric PAH. Thus the "best" estimate for prevalence of pediatric PAH is approximately 10 per million.

Although the disease is rare, with improved diagnostics and increased awareness it appears that more patients (both children and adults) have PAH than was previously recognized. On occasion, infants who have died with the presumed diagnosis of sudden infant death syndrome had IPAH diagnosed at postmortem examination. The female preponderance in adult patients with IPAH previously reported as approximately 1.7:1 females to males[28] is similar to earlier reports in children with IPAH (i.e., 1.8:1), with no significant difference in younger children compared to older children.[26,29] More recent reports from the United States have reported a higher female preponderance in adults with PAH (i.e., ~4:1), with the gender ratio in the pediatric patients more similar to previous reports (i.e., ~2:1).[30]

Natural History

Historically, untreated IPAH exhibited a course of progressive right-sided heart failure and early death. In contrast, children with unrepaired congenital to systemic shunts often lived for at least several decades without targeted treatment. Several large survival studies of primarily adult patients with IPAH were conducted in the 1980s prior to the current treatment era. These retrospective and prospective studies yielded quite uniform results: adult patients with IPAH who did not have lung or heart-lung transplantation had actuarial survival rates at 1, 3, and 5 years of 68% to 77%, 40% to 56%, and 22% to 38%, respectively.[1,31,32] During the era before the use of continuous intravenous epoprostenol (approved in 1995), in children who were nonresponders to acute vasodilator testing and therefore not candidates for oral calcium channel blockade, the 1-, 3-, and 5-year survival rates were 66%, 52%, and 35%, respectively.[33] In a more recent treatment era using epoprostenol treatment for nonresponders and calcium channel blockade for acute responders, the 10-year survival rate for children was estimated at 78%.[34] However, there is significant biologic variability in the natural history of the disease in both adults and children, with some patients having a rapidly progressive downhill course resulting in death within several weeks after diagnosis and others surviving for at least several decades. In contrast, the long-term natural history for patients with unrepaired APAH-CHD is much more favorable with survival often into the fourth to fifth decade. However, similar to other forms of PAH, the natural history of Eisenmenger syndrome also demonstrates a wide spectrum of variability. Nevertheless, the overall natural history for Eisenmenger patients has been significantly better than for patients with IPAH.[32] For a classic Eisenmenger patient, death in childhood is unusual with most patients surviving into their mid twenties to thirties. Patients have even survived to the seventh decade, although this is rare. The better prognosis for Eisenmenger patients is likely due to the presence of a "pop-off" valve. For Eisenmenger patients or patients with a CHD and elevated PVRi (≥ 3 to 5 U × m^2), closing the heart defect can change the natural history from that of an Eisenmenger patient to the worse prognosis of an IPAH patient. Therefore, operability needs to be assessed carefully if closure is being considered. For borderline patients, one may consider closure of the CHD leaving a smaller residual defect or creating an "atrial septal defect," that is, by performing an atrial septostomy. There is also debate as to whether an atrial communication is as effective a "pop-off" as a shunt at the ventricular level because shunting at the atrial level would require significant elevation in right ventricular end diastolic pressure.

Pathobiology

Vasoconstriction

There have been many recent advances in the understanding of the pathobiology of PAH; pulmonary vascular disease is a multifactorial disease with several causes that lead to a final common histopathologic vasculopathy. Recent investigations in the basic science arena have uncovered several different biochemical/mechanistic features of pulmonary vascular obstructive disease that have lead to novel treatments. These include abnormalities of the prostacyclin pathway, the endothelin system, and nitric oxide production/availability. In 1977, Wagenvoort and Wagenvoort hypothesized that "primary pulmonary hypertension" (IPAH) is a disease of individuals with hyperreactive pulmonary arterioles in whom various stimuli initiate vasoconstriction, with subsequent development of the characteristic vascular lesions."[35] While the early focus for treatment of this disease stemmed from this hypothesis, that is, finding the ideal pulmonary vasodilator, evidence over the past 2 decades has pointed to other vasoproliferative abnormalities. In infants, the pathobiology suggests failure of the neonatal vasculature to relax, in addition to a striking reduction in arterial number/surface area. However, with time, the changes become fixed with a vasodilator-unresponsive component that appears temporally related to the development of thickened vascular media and adventitia with dramatic increases in the deposition of structural matrix proteins such as collagen and elastin in the pulmonary arterial wall.[36] In older children, intimal hyperplasia, occlusive changes, and plexiform lesions are found in the pulmonary arterioles. Despite significant advances in the understanding of the pathobiology of IPAH, the mechanisms that initiate and perpetuate this disease remain speculative. Adults with IPAH often have severe plexiform lesions and what appear to be "fixed" pulmonary vascular changes. In contrast, children with IPAH have more pulmonary vascular medial hypertrophy with less intimal fibrosis and fewer plexiform lesions. In the classic autopsy studies by Wagenvoort and

Wagenvoort in 1970,[37] medial hypertrophy was severe in patients younger than 15 years of age, and it was usually the only abnormality seen in infants. Among the 11 children younger than 1 year of age at the time of death, all had severe medial hypertrophy, yet only three had intimal fibrosis; two had minimal intimal fibrosis, one had moderate intimal fibrosis, and none had plexiform lesions. With increasing age, intimal fibrosis and plexiform lesions were seen more frequently. These postmortem studies suggested that pulmonary vasoconstriction, leading to medial hypertrophy, may occur early in the course of the disease and may precede the development of plexiform lesions and other fixed pulmonary vascular changes. The observations may offer clues to the observed differences in the natural history and factors influencing survival in children with IPAH compared to adult patients. In general, younger children appear to have a more reactive pulmonary vascular bed relative to both vasodilatation and vasoconstriction. Severe acute pulmonary hypertensive crises occur in response to pulmonary vasoconstrictor "triggers" more often in young children than in older children or adults. Based on these pathologic studies, the most widely proposed mechanism for IPAH until the late 1980s and early 1990s was pulmonary vasoconstriction.[36–39]

Endothelial Dysfunction

Endothelial dysfunction appears to be a key factor in mediating the structural changes that occur in the pulmonary vasculature in PAH. The integrity of the pulmonary vascular endothelium is critical for maintaining vascular tone, homeostasis, barrier function, leukocyte trafficking, transduction of luminal signals to abluminal vascular tissues, production of growth factors, and cell signaling with autocrine and paracrine effects.[40] In addition, abnormalities in vasoactive mediators appear to contribute to the pathobiology of PAH. Whether these perturbations are a cause or consequence of the disease process remains to be elucidated[41–48] (Fig. 72-1).

One theory is that there may be a "trigger" for endothelial activation in "genetically susceptible patients." Endothelial activation can then lead to apoptosis of quiescent cells, destabilization of the pulmonary vascular intima, and uncontrolled proliferation of endothelial cells with progression to the classic plexiform lesions. Once the vascular wall is damaged, proliferative mediators may cross into the matrix and lead to degradation of matrix and proliferation of smooth muscle.

The vascular endothelium is now recognized as an important source of locally active mediators that contribute to the control of vasomotor tone and structural remodeling, and it appears to play a crucial role in the pathogenesis of PAH.[49] Various studies suggest that imbalances in the production or metabolism of vasoactive mediators produced in the lungs, as well as substances involving control of pulmonary vascular growth, may be important in the pathogenesis of PAH. These may include increased thromboxane, endothelin, and serotonin, and decreased prostacyclin[41,42] and nitric oxide,[43–45,48] as well

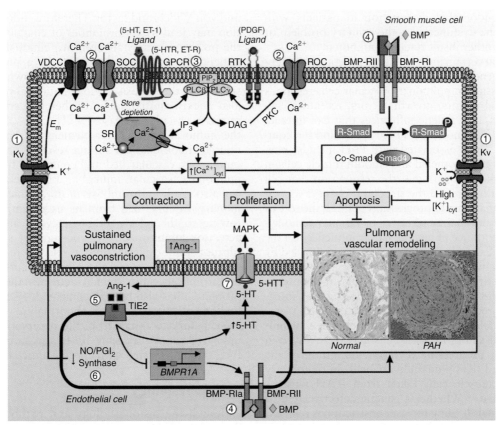

FIGURE 72-1. Possible pathobiologic mechanisms of pulmonary arterial hypertension. (From McLaughlin VV, Archer SL, Badesch DB, et al. ACCF/AHA 2009 expert consensus document on pulmonary hypertension: a report of the American College of Cardiology Foundation Task Force on Expert Consensus Documents and the American Heart Association. *J Am Coll Cardiol.* 2009;53:1573-1619.)

as changes in VEGF and xanthine oxidoreductase.[41–45,48,50] The endothelial cell dysfunction seen in association with PAH leads to the release of *vasoproliferative* substances in addition to *vasoconstrictive* agents that ultimately result in progression of the pulmonary vascular remodeling and progressive vascular obstruction and obliteration. Stewart and colleagues[44] and Giaid and coworkers[51] reported elevated circulating levels of endothelin, a potent vasoconstrictor and mitogen, in patients with various forms of PAH and PH with increased local production of endothelin by the pulmonary arterial endothelium reported in the PAH patients.[44] Endothelial dysfunction also likely results in the release of chemotactic agents, leading to the migration of smooth muscle cells into the vascular wall, which may lead to the characteristic pulmonary arteriolar medial hypertrophy and hyperplasia. This endothelial dysfunction, coupled with the excessive release of locally active thrombogenic mediators, promotes a procoagulant state, leading to further vascular obstruction. The process is characterized, therefore, by an inexorable cycle of endothelial dysfunction leading to the release of vasoconstrictive, vasoproliferative, and prothrombotic substances, ultimately progressing to vascular remodeling and progressive vascular obstruction and obliteration. Despite our lack of complete understanding of the pathogenesis of PAH, these imbalances and abnormalities have changed the focus of clinical drug development from chronic vasodilator therapy alone, to the evaluation of therapeutic agents that may reverse the vasoproliferation, and ultimately result in pulmonary vascular regression and reverse remodeling. Although various studies have demonstrated endothelial dysfunction in patients with PAH, whether the dysfunction is the primary problem or secondary to another insult remains unknown.

The theory that certain individuals are genetically susceptible has led to genetically oriented research. It is now clear that gene expression in pulmonary vascular cells responds to environmental factors, growth factors, receptors, signaling pathways, and genetic influences that can interact with each other. The molecular processes behind the complex vascular changes associated with PAH include: phenotypic changes in endothelial and smooth muscle cells in hypertensive pulmonary arteries, the recognition that cell proliferation contributes to the structural changes associated with the initiation and progression of PAH, the role of matrix proteins and matrix turnover in vascular remodeling, and the importance of hemodynamic influences on the disease process. Examples of effector systems controlled by gene expression include transmembrane transporters; ion channels; transcription factors; modulators of apoptosis; kinases; and cell-to-cell interactive factors such as integrins, membrane receptors, growth factors, and cytokines.

In addition, defects in the potassium channels of pulmonary vascular smooth muscle cells may be involved in the initiation or progression of IPAH. Inhibition of the voltage-regulated (Kv) potassium channels in pulmonary artery smooth muscle cells taken from IPAH patients has been reported.[52] Whether a genetic defect related to potassium channels leading to vasoconstriction is relevant to the development of IPAH in some patients remains unknown. These studies suggest that IPAH is a disease of "predisposed" individuals in whom various "stimuli"

may initiate the pulmonary vascular disease process. By identifying molecular mechanisms that are linked to epidemiologic risk factors, as well as developing molecular, genetic, biochemical, and physiologic tests to monitor and diagnose IPAH, novel treatment strategies will improve therapeutic interventions for IPAH. There may be different subsets of patients in whom vasoconstriction is the predominant feature, and those in whom vascular injury or endothelial dysfunction is the primary problem. Even so, these components appear closely intertwined. Whether these physiologic processes (vasoconstriction versus vascular injury) are a cause or a consequence of the disease remains unclear.

Studies during the past 15 years have suggested a genetic predisposition for developing PAH in up to 10% of individuals affected. Mutations of the bone morphogenetic protein receptor 2 *(BMPR2)* gene were first described in individuals with familial PAH,[53–56] with a decrease in the alveolar density of *BMPR* expression in patients with documented IPAH. Other candidate genes have also been identified such as *ALK-1* (which encodes TGF-β receptor) and endoglin (an inducer of angiogenesis, endothelial cell survival, and vessel stabilization). Future investigations will focus on these genetic influences on the pathogenesis of PAH as well as impact on clinical phenotype. Whether therapeutic manipulations based on genetic factors will be feasible in the future, as we focus attention on individualized therapy, is intriguing.

The endothelium also has a key role in maintaining normal coagulation through elaborating various factors such as heparin sulfates, urokinase type plasminogen activator, and von Willebrand factor. Therefore endothelial dysfunction may lead to abnormalities of coagulation leading to the prothrombotic state seen in pulmonary hypertension patients. In addition, there may be a physiologic effect from pulmonary arteriole lumen narrowing that leads to stasis and thrombosis.[57] Coagulation abnormalities may also coexist, initiating or further exacerbating the pulmonary vascular disease.[58,59] The interactions between the humoral and cellular elements of the blood on an injured endothelial cell surface result in remodeling of the pulmonary vascular bed and contribute to the process of pulmonary vascular injury.[60,61] Endothelial cell damage can also result in thrombosis *in situ,* transforming the pulmonary vascular bed from its usual anticoagulant state (owing to the release of prostacyclin and plasminogen activator inhibitors) to a procoagulant state.[62] Elevated fibrinopeptide-A levels and p-selectin in IPAH patients also suggest that *in situ* thrombosis occurs.[63] A reduction in thrombomodulin (which activates the anticoagulant protein C) has also been documented.[64,65] Further support for the role of coagulation abnormalities at the endothelial cell surface comes from the observational reports of improved survival in adult IPAH and anorexigen-induced PAH patients treated with chronic anticoagulation.[2,66,67]

Pathophysiology

Although the histopathology and pathobiology in children with IPAH is similar to that seen in adult patients, there may be differences in the pathophysiology that alter the clinical presentation, natural history, and outcome in children. For example, children appear to have differences in their hemodynamic parameters at the time of diagnosis compared with adult patients.[68] Children with IPAH most often have a normal cardiac index at the time of presentation as opposed to adults who frequently present in clinical right-sided heart failure with a low cardiac index. This may reflect earlier diagnosis and explain why children tend to have a greater response rate to acute vasodilator testing than adults.

A brief review of the normal physiology of the pulmonary circulation will enable a better understanding of the pathophysiology of the pulmonary vascular bed. The normal decrease in PVR occurs soon after birth and reaches normal adult levels by 4 to 6 weeks of life. The normal pulmonary vascular bed is a low-pressure, low-resistance, highly distensible system that can accommodate large increases in pulmonary blood flow with minimal elevations in pulmonary arterial pressure. In PAH, however, this capacity to accommodate increases in pulmonary blood flow is lost due to the increase in PVR leading to increases in pulmonary arterial pressure at rest and further elevations in pulmonary arterial pressure with exercise. The right ventricle hypertrophies in response to this increase in afterload. If there has been a gradual exposure over time, the right ventricle has the ability to remodel and adapt to the pressure overload by recruitment of sarcomeres and hypertrophy of myocytes. The adaptation of the right ventricle to increased afterload such as in IPAH or congenital heart defects with increased right ventricular afterload (e.g. pulmonic stenosis) is a double-edged sword. The right ventricular hypertrophy will assist the right ventricle in pumping against the increased afterload; however, this occurs at a cost to left ventricular integrity. Under normal conditions, the right ventricle is crescent-shaped with the right ventricular free wall and interventricular septum concave around the left ventricle at both end-diastole and end-systole. During systole, the left ventricle contracts toward a central axis, while the right ventricular free wall and septum contract in parallel. With right ventricular hypertrophy, the interventricular septal orientation flattens and ultimately commits to the right ventricle in severe cases. This may lead to a vicious cycle of left ventricular diastolic dysfunction and subsequent worsening of right-sided heart failure in severe cases.[69,70] In the early stages, the right ventricle is capable of sustaining normal cardiac output at rest, but the ability to increase cardiac output with exercise is impaired. As pulmonary vascular disease progresses, the right ventricle fails and resting cardiac output decreases. As right ventricular dysfunction progresses, right ventricular diastolic pressure increases with clinical onset of right ventricular failure, the most ominous sign of pulmonary vascular disease. Dyspnea is the most frequent presenting complaint in adults and children with IPAH; it is caused by impaired oxygen delivery during physical activity as a result of an inability to increase cardiac output in the presence of increased oxygen demands. Syncopal episodes, which occur more frequently with children than with adults, are often exertional or postexertional and imply a severely limited cardiac output, leading to a decrease in cerebral blood flow. Peripheral vasodilatation during physical exertion can exacerbate this condition.

The two most frequent mechanisms of death in PAH are progressive right ventricular failure and sudden death, with the former occurring more often, especially in adults.[1] Progressive right ventricular failure leads to dyspnea and a progressive decrease in cardiac output. Complicating illnesses such as pneumonia can be fatal as alveolar hypoxia causes hypoxic pulmonary vasoconstriction, leading to an inability to maintain adequate cardiac output and resulting in cardiogenic shock and death. When arterial hypoxemia and acidosis (respiratory and/or metabolic) occur, life-threatening arrhythmias may develop. Postulated mechanisms for sudden death include bradyarrhythmias and tachyarrhythmias, acute pulmonary emboli, acute pulmonary arterial aneurysm rupture, massive pulmonary hemorrhage, and sudden right ventricular ischemia. Hemoptysis appears to be caused by pulmonary infarcts from secondary arterial thromboses.

Diagnosis and Assessment

The diagnosis of IPAH is one of exclusion. It is critical to exclude all likely related or associated conditions that might be managed differently. A detailed history and physical examination, as well as appropriate tests, must be performed to uncover potential causative or contributing factors, many of which may not be readily apparent. A family history of pulmonary hypertension, connective tissue diseases, congenital heart disease, other congenital anomalies, and early unexplained deaths may be contributory. If the family history suggests familial PAH, careful screening of all first-degree relatives is recommended. Genetic testing is also available in select centers. Additional issues to address include obtaining a detailed birth/neonatal history, a medication history including psychotropic drugs, appetite suppressants, and over-the-counter drugs, and inquiring about exposure to high altitude or to toxic cooking oil,[71,72] travel history, and any history of frequent respiratory tract infections, or venous or arterial thrombi. The answers to these questions may offer clues to a possible "trigger" for the development of the PAH.

The diagnostic evaluation in children suspected of having PAH is similar to that of adult patients (Fig. 72-2[73]), with the exception of certain conditions that rarely occur in children (e.g., chronic thromboembolic pulmonary hypertension). Determination of WHO functional class also can be a helpful gauge of clinical stability or disease progression in children as in adults (Box 72-2).[74]

Hemodynamics/Cardiac Catheterization

Despite advances in noninvasive technology, cardiac catheterization remains the gold standard for the diagnosis of PAH, assessing disease severity and prognosis, and the selection of appropriate treatment. As shown in the diagnostic guidelines (see Fig. 72-2[73,75]), all children should undergo a diagnostic cardiac catheterization (to confirm the diagnosis of suspected PAH) with acute pulmonary vasodilator testing using a short-acting vasodilator to determine acute vascular responsiveness. The younger the child is at the time of diagnosis, the more likely that the child will respond to acute testing, but there is wide variability.[33] The presence of a robust response to acute

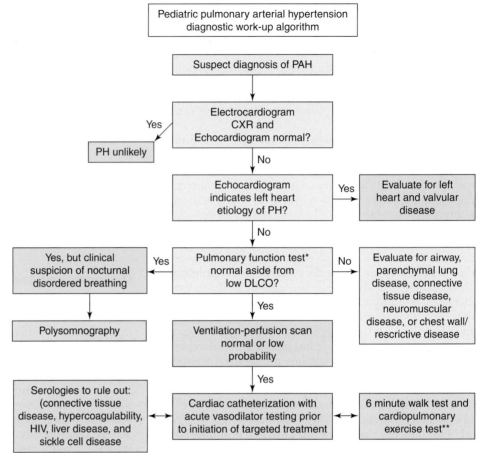

FIGURE 72-2. Diagnostic workup for patients with suspected pulmonary arterial hypertension. *If unable to obtain a reliable test in a young child and there is a high index of suspicion for underlying lung disease, the patient may require further lung imaging. **Children older than 7 years of age can usually perform reliably to assess exercise tolerance and capacity in conjunction with diagnostic workup. *PH,* pulmonary hypertension; *PAH,* pulmonary arterial hypertension; *CXR,* chest x-ray, *HIV,* human immunodeficiency virus. (From Rosenzweig EB, Feinstein J, Humpl T, et al. Pulmonary arterial hypertension in children: diagnostic work-up and challenges. *Progr Pediatr Cardiol.* 2009;27:7-11.)

BOX 72-2 WORLD HEALTH ORGANIZATION FUNCTIONAL CLASSIFICATION*

Class I: Patients with pulmonary hypertension but without resulting limitations of physical activity. Ordinary physical activity does not cause undue dyspnea or fatigue, chest pain or near syncope.

Class II: Patients with pulmonary hypertension resulting in slight limitation of physical activity. They are comfortable at rest. Ordinary physical activity causes undue dyspnea or fatigue, chest pain or near syncope.

Class III: Patients with pulmonary hypertension resulting in marked limitation of physical activity. They are comfortable at rest. Less than ordinary activity causes undue dyspnea or fatigue, chest pain or near syncope.

Class IV: Patients with pulmonary hypertension with inability to carry out any physical activity without symptoms. These patients manifest signs of right-sided heart failure. Dyspnea and/or fatigue may even be present at rest. Discomfort is increased by any physical activity.

---

*Modified for pulmonary hypertension from the New York Heart Association Functional Classification, 1998 2nd World Symposium on Pulmonary Arterial Hypertension.

---

vasodilator testing usually predicts long-term response to high-dose oral calcium channel blockade therapy. Unfortunately, there are no additional hemodynamic or demographic variables that accurately predict whether or not a child will respond to acute vasodilator testing. It appears that HPAH patients are less likely to respond to acute vasodilator testing and therefore less likely to

respond to chronic calcium channel blockade treatment.[76,77] Several studies suggest that up to 30% to 40% of children with IPAH may manifest a robust response to acute vasodilator testing and thus near-complete reversibility with chronic oral calcium channel blockade therapy, while others may have what appears to be irreversible disease; the duration of symptoms prior to diagnosis does not appear to correlate with the likelihood of an acute response or lack thereof. These observations underscore the marked biologic variability in the time course of IPAH and serve to emphasize the need to individualize the therapeutic approach. The currently recommended vasodilators for acute vasodilator drug testing are either inhaled nitric oxide or intravenous epoprostenol. Patients who are responsive to acute vasodilator testing are likely to have a favorable response with acute calcium channel blocker testing and subsequently with long-term oral calcium channel blockade treatment.[2,33] Historically, a significant response to acute pulmonary vasodilator testing has been considered a reduction in mean pulmonary arterial pressure of at least 20%, with no change or an increase in cardiac output. More recently, the definition of a significant "acute response" has been modified for adult patients to better predict long-term response to calcium channel blockade therapy.[78] However, it is unclear whether this modified definition better predicts long-term response to calcium channel blockade in children as it appears to do in adults. Patients who do not manifest a response to acute vasodilator testing are unlikely to have clinical benefit from chronic oral calcium channel blockade therapy. Furthermore, acute deterioration and decompensation may occur with empiric calcium channel blockade therapy in patients who are not acutely responsive,[79,80] particularly in children with underlying lung disease. Empiric treatment with calcium channel blockade is not recommended, and it can be detrimental (resulting in fatal cardiogenic shock) in addition to not being efficacious.

Clinical Presentation

The presenting symptoms in children with PAH are highly variable. Infants with PAH often present with signs of low cardiac output (e.g., tachypnea, tachycardia, poor appetite, failure to thrive, lethargy, diaphoresis, and irritability). Some infants have crying spells, presumably as a result of chest pain that cannot be otherwise verbalized. In addition, infants and older children may develop cyanosis with exertion, due to right-to-left shunting through a patent foramen ovale or congenital heart defect. The patent foramen ovale serves as a "pop-off" valve for the hypertensive right heart in children without other systemic to pulmonary communications. Children without adequate shunting through a patent foramen ovale or CHD may present with syncope due to the inability to achieve an adequate cardiac output with exertion. After early childhood, children present with similar symptoms to adults. In older children, the most common symptoms are exertional dyspnea, fatigue, and, occasionally, chest pain. Chest pain, or angina, results from right ventricular ischemia and is often underappreciated. Clinical right ventricular failure is rare in young children, occurring most often in children older than 10 years of age with severe longstanding PAH. Peripheral edema is generally a reflection of right ventricular failure and is more likely to be associated with advanced pulmonary vascular disease. The interval between onset of symptoms and time of diagnosis is usually shorter in children than in adults, particularly in young children who present with syncope. In addition to exertional or postexertional syncope, children may present with "hypoxic" seizures resulting from exertional syncope or exaggerated pulmonary vasoconstriction caused by systemic arterial oxygen desaturation during sleep (particularly in the early morning hours).

Physical Examination

Physical Signs

On physical examination, signs differ for children with and without an intracardiac or extracardiac shunt. In patients who have undergone "corrective" surgery for their congenital heart defects, the physical findings may be identical to patients with IPAH or other types of Group I PAH. Many of the physical findings in children with associated forms of PAH are similar to those with IPAH (see Box 72-1). Careful attention should be paid to the cardiac examination and other signs of systemic venous congestion related to right "pump" failure. The cardiac signs of elevated right ventricular systolic pressure include a loud single P2, a murmur of tricuspid

insufficiency, and a murmur of pulmonary insufficiency. A pansystolic murmur of tricuspid regurgitation is very common. The high-pitched diastolic murmur of pulmonary insufficiency may be heard at the left upper sternal border and usually relates to the high pulmonary arterial pressures and dilatation of the main pulmonary artery. In addition, there may be an S3 or S4 right ventricular gallop. An increase in the pulmonic component of the second heart sound and a right-sided fourth heart sound are early findings. When heard, a right ventricular third heart sound generally reflects advanced disease. Jugular venous distention, although rare in children, may be present with a prominent *a* wave. Hepatomegaly may also be present. Because the liver capsule is more distensible in children, the size of the liver is a good marker of the degree of right-sided heart failure and response to therapy. Ascites and peripheral edema can also occur in advanced cases. Other findings may implicate a systemic cause for the pulmonary arterial hypertension (e.g. the rash of systemic lupus erythematosus). Clubbing and central cyanosis may be present in children with underlying lung disease or Eisenmenger syndrome. Clubbing is not a typical feature of IPAH, although on rare occasions it has been observed in patients with longstanding disease who develop chronic hypoxemia secondary to right-to-left shunting via a patent foramen ovale. Clubbing of the digits is very rare following early complete surgical repair of a congenital heart defect unless there is underlying pulmonary disease, since these patients are no longer cyanotic.

TREATMENT

Although there is neither a cure for PAH nor a single therapeutic approach that is uniformly successful, therapy has dramatically improved over the past several decades, resulting in sustained clinical and hemodynamic improvement as well as increased survival in many children with various types of PAH.[33] An overview of our current approach and guidelines for treatment is shown in Fig. 72-3. Noninvasive studies obtained prior to initiating therapy, as well as periodically thereafter, are useful in guiding changes in therapeutic regimens, particularly in light of recent advances with various novel therapeutic agents.

General Measures

The pediatrician plays an invaluable role in the care of children with PAH. Because children often have a more reactive pulmonary vascular bed than adult patients, any respiratory tract infection that results in ventilation/perfusion mismatching from alveolar hypoxia can result in a serious or even catastrophic acute pulmonary hypertensive crisis if not treated aggressively. Influenza and pneumococcal vaccinations are recommended unless there are contraindications. Antipyretics should be administered for temperature elevations greater than 101° F (38° C) to minimize the consequences of increased metabolic demands on an already compromised cardiorespiratory system. Children may also require aggressive therapy (e.g., inhaled nitric oxide) for acute pulmonary

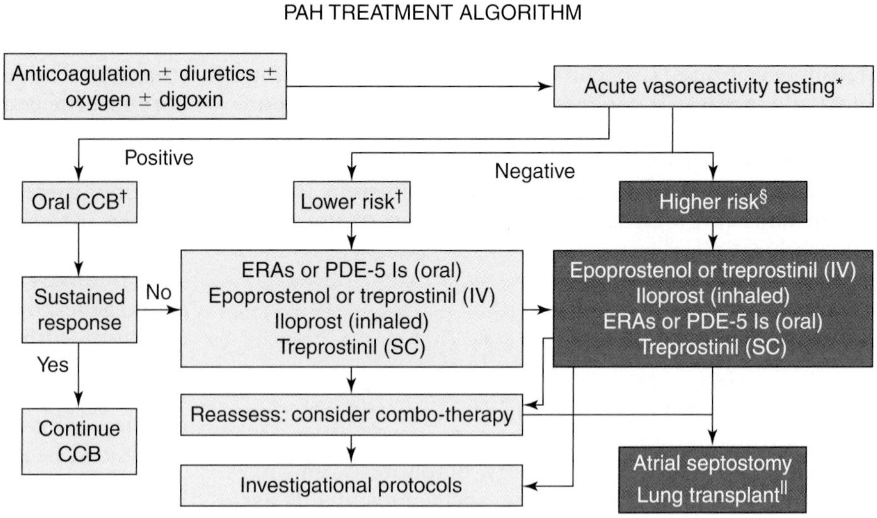

PAH TREATMENT ALGORITHM

FIGURE 72-3. Treatment algorithm for pulmonary arterial hypertension. *CCB,* Calcium channel blocker; *ERA,* endothelin receptor antagonist; *PGI2,* prostacyclin; *PDE 5,* phosphodiesterase type 5. (From McLaughlin VV, Archer SL, Badesch DB, et al. ACCF/AHA 2009 expert consensus document on pulmonary hypertension: a report of the American College of Cardiology Foundation Task Force on Expert Consensus Documents and the American Heart Association. *J Am Coll Cardiol.* 2009;53:1573-1619.)

hypertensive crises that occur during episodes of pneumonia or other infectious diseases. Patients may require antitussive medications during upper respiratory infections to prevent excessive coughing, which increases pulmonary arterial pressures and can result in acute pulmonary hypertensive crises. Decongestants with pseudoephedrine should be avoided as they may exacerbate the pulmonary hypertension. Diet and medical therapy should be used to prevent constipation, since Valsalva maneuvers transiently decrease venous return to the right side of the heart and may precipitate syncopal episodes.

Anticoagulation

Consideration of chronic anticoagulation in children with PAH is based on observational studies in adults with IPAH.[2,31,67] The lung histopathology often demonstrates thrombotic lesions in small pulmonary arterioles in both adult and pediatric patients with IPAH and other forms of APAH. Some patients have an underlying coagulopathy (e.g., antiphospholipid syndrome, or protein C/S deficiency). In patients with poor right ventricular function, thrombi can form within the ventricle, and postmortem examinations of patients with pulmonary vascular disease who have died suddenly often demonstrate fresh clot in the pulmonary vascular bed. Whether or not secondary thrombosis *in situ* is a significant exacerbating factor in patients with a normal resting cardiac output is unknown. In addition, even a small pulmonary embolus can be life-threatening in patients who cannot vasodilate or recruit additional pulmonary vessels. Clinical data supporting the chronic use of anticoagulation is limited but supportive. Warfarin has been shown to be associated with improved survival in two retrospective adult observational studies, and one prospective adult observational study (in patients who were not responsive to acute vasodilator testing); all three studies were in adult patients with IPAH/HPAH or PAH associated with anorexigen exposure.[2,31,67] The dosage of anticoagulation usually recommended is that to achieve an INR of 1.5 to 2; however, certain clinical circumstances (e.g., positive lupus anticoagulant, positive anticardiolipin antibodies, Factor

V Leiden, Factor II 20210A variant,[81-84] and documented chronic thromboembolic disease) may require dose adjustment to maintain a higher INR. For patients at a higher risk of bleeding (e.g., patients with significant thrombocytopenia), the dosage should be adjusted to maintain a lower INR. Whether or not chronic anticoagulation is efficacious as well as safe for children with pulmonary hypertension remains to be determined. Our approach has been to anticoagulate children who are hypercoagulable or in right-sided heart failure, similar to the approach for adult patients. In children who are extremely active, particularly toddlers, we recommend maintaining an INR less than 1.5 unless there is severe pulmonary vascular disease. Antiplatelet therapy with aspirin or dipyridamole does not appear to be effective in areas of low flow, where thrombosis *in situ* is known to occur. However, studies have not been done to evaluate such agents in PAH. Parents should be advised to avoid administering other medications that could interact with the warfarin unless the possible interactions are known, and the dose of the warfarin is adjusted as needed. Similar to the approach with adult pulmonary hypertension patients, if anticoagulation with warfarin is contraindicated or dose adjustments are difficult, low–molecular weight heparin at a dose of 0.75 to 1 mg/kg by subcutaneous administration once or twice daily may be a reasonable alternative. However, the long-term side effects of heparin, such as osteopenia and thrombocytopenia, are of concern. To date there are no studies comparing the safety and efficacy of anticoagulation with warfarin to heparin. There may be additional benefits of heparin on the pulmonary vascular bed. Experimental studies by Thompson and colleagues, *in vivo*[85] and Benitz and coworkers *in vitro*[86] suggest that vascular smooth muscle growth inhibitors such as heparin may be useful in preventing progression of pulmonary vascular disease.

Calcium Channel Blockade

Calcium channel blockers are a chemically heterogeneous group of compounds that inhibit calcium influx through the slow channel into cardiac and smooth muscle cells.

Their usefulness for select patients with PAH is based on their pulmonary vasodilator effects. Acute vasodilator testing during right-heart cardiac catheterization is a critical part of the initial assessment of patients with PAH to determine the appropriate initial treatment course. Chronic calcium channel blockade is efficacious for patients ("responders") who demonstrate a robust acute response to vasodilator testing (i.e., a decrease in mean pulmonary arterial pressure by $\geq 20\%$ from baseline with no clinically significant decrease in cardiac output, and a decrease or no change in the ratio of PVR to systemic vascular resistance),[87,88] although not all acute "responders" have a sustained long-term response.[33] In contrast, patients who do not respond acutely fail to respond to long-term calcium channel blockade.[2,33] In general, these patients ("nonresponders") will respond to long-term treatment with an intravenous prostacyclin, such as epoprostenol, and may respond to other novel treatments.[88] The term *nonresponder* is only used with respect to acute vasodilator testing and calcium channel blockade response.

Fewer than 10% of adult patients with IPAH will respond to chronic oral calcium channel blockade,[2] as documented by improvement in symptoms, exercise tolerance, hemodynamics, and survival. The current definition for an acute responder in adult PAH has changed from a decrease in mean PAP and PVR $\geq 20\%$ with no clinically significant decrease in cardiac index to a decrease in mean PAP by $>10\,$mm Hg to an absolute value of $<40\,$mm Hg with no clinically significant decrease in cardiac index.[87,89,90] The definition was changed based on long-term survival data in IPAH adult patients in whom calcium channel blockade had been started using the earlier definition. It remains unclear whether this change in definition will be adequately sensitive and specific for identifying long-term responders to calcium channel blockade. A significantly greater percentage of children than adults are acute responders (up to 40%) and can be effectively treated with chronic oral calcium channel blockade for at least some time; this duration of effective therapy can vary from months (which is unusual) to several decades.[33,34] For acute responders, most studies have used calcium channel blockers at relatively high doses (e.g., long-acting nifedipine 120 to 240 mg daily or amlodipine 20 to 40 mg daily); however, the optimal dosing for both children and adult patients with PAH is uncertain. Because of the frequent occurrence of significant adverse effects with calcium channel blockade therapy in nonresponders, including systemic hypotension, pulmonary edema, right ventricular failure, and death, treatment with calcium channel blockers is not recommended for patients in whom acute effectiveness has not been demonstrated. This supports the importance of an initial assessment by cardiac catheterization with acute vasodilator testing before prescribing a long-term pulmonary vasodilator.

Serial Reevaluations

Serial reevaluations, including repeat vasodilator testing to maintain an "optimal" chronic therapeutic regimen, are essential to the care of children with PAH. In our experience, acute responders who are treated with chronic

oral calcium channel blockade therapy continue to do exceedingly well as long as they remain acutely reactive to vasodilator testing on repeat cardiac catheterizations.[34] In contrast, children who are initially acute responders and are treated with chronic calcium channel blockade and who then stop demonstrating active vasoreactivity on repeat testing usually deteriorate clinically and hemodynamically despite continuation of chronic calcium channel blockade therapy. If they are then treated with continuous intravenous epoprostenol, they will probably demonstrate improvement similar to the experience with children who are nonresponders. Other novel therapeutic agents, discussed later in the chapter, also may be considered for these patients.

Targeted Therapy

Prior to 1995, there were no approved therapies for PAH. However, since then, 20 randomized controlled trials with 9 compounds as monotherapy have been completed in adult PAH patients. In addition, 6 randomized controlled trials evaluating combinations of agents have been completed (e.g., endothelin-receptor antagonists [ERAs] and phosphodiesterase [PDE]-5 inhibitors, or prostacyclin analogs and ERAs or PDE-5 inhibitors). Approximately 5000 patients, the vast majority being adults, have participated in these studies aimed at developing effective treatments for PAH. The conclusions derived from clinical trials over the past 15 years have permitted us to develop an evidence-based treatment algorithm for adult patients with PAH. This algorithm is used worldwide, subject to the availability of specific drug therapies (see Fig. 72-3[90]). However, despite there being eight drugs currently approved for adult PAH, there are no drugs currently approved for pediatric PAH. Based on similarities between pediatric and adult PAH, consensus recommendations for pediatric PAH have, to date, been extrapolated from adult data with off-label use in children. Although off-label use in pediatric patients appears to have significantly improved overall quality of life and outcomes for many children with PAH, without adequate long-term safety studies and determination of optimal dosing, we may not be treating these children optimally. Nevertheless, treatment for pediatric PAH currently uses the adult evidence-based guidelines.

Treatment of IPAH initially focused on the use of vasodilators in the hope that an increase in pulmonary vascular tone significantly contributed to the high pulmonary arterial pressures. Although the bulk of the pulmonary vascular obstruction was clearly anatomic, vasodilators offered the prospect not only of decreasing pulmonary arterial pressures somewhat, and therefore the hemodynamic burden on the right ventricle, but also of prompting reversibility of the anatomic lesions. Unfortunately, the use of vasodilators, which could affect the systemic as well as the pulmonary circulation, led to progressive disenchantment with one agent after another.

Fewer than 10% of adult IPAH patients and even fewer patients with PAH associated with other conditions such as connective tissue disease or congenital heart disease respond acutely to vasodilator testing and are candidates for whom treatment with calcium channel blockade can be considered. A landmark development for patients who failed to satisfy the criteria for a good hemodynamic response to acute vasodilator testing was the demonstration that such patients respond to continuous infusion of epoprostenol. That is, patients who fail to respond acutely to intravenous epoprostenol can respond chronically. Indeed, a substantial number of such patients have been treated this way for many years or have used continuous intravenous epoprostenol as a transition to transplantation or newer drug therapies. During this evolution, heart-lung and then lung transplantation became increasingly feasible and available, although the donor supply is still a significant limiting factor. More recently, the development of oral medications that block the receptors for endothelin or that augment the effects of endogenous nitric oxide by inhibiting phosphodiesterase type-5 (the enzyme responsible for the inactivation of cyclic guanosine monophosphate) have been shown to be effective therapies and may obviate the need for prostacyclin therapy in many PAH patients. Alternative forms of delivery of longer-acting prostacyclin analogs, including subcutaneous and aerosolization, have also been developed and may prevent (or delay) the need for parenteral prostacyclin therapy in many patients.

As a result of these advances, a PAH patient has several therapeutic options. However, none of these modalities is free of complications, and one must remember that all of these drugs were evaluated primarily in adult patients and not in children. Thus, safety concerns for a class of drugs may be more or less in children based on their metabolism being different than adults. Many affected children are still growing, with ongoing lung development, and the optimal doses are not necessarily being used (or known). Pediatric PAH patients appear to do better with higher doses on a per-kilogram basis for at least several of the PAH drugs (e.g., calcium channel blockers and prostacyclin analogs such as epoprostenol), but it remains unknown whether this will apply to other PAH drugs. Endothelin receptor antagonists can cause hepatic injury. The continuous infusion of a prostacyclin analog has the risks associated with a permanently placed intravenous catheter, such as bacteremia, sepsis, or thromboembolic events. Transplantation offers the substitution of immunosuppression and its attendant risk of infection as a "better" or alternative option to RV failure. Despite the limitations of each of these therapeutic modalities, together they provide a graduated therapeutic approach that has provided, at each stage, a better quality of life for many children with PAH.

Prostacyclin Analogs

Intravenous Prostacyclin (Epoprostenol)

Epoprostenol (prostacyclin) has been used since its approval in 1995 with great success. It improves hemodynamics, quality of life, and exercise capacity in patients with IPAH and PAH associated with other conditions such as CHD, connective tissue disease, HIV infection, and portal hypertension, and increases survival in IPAH/HPAH. By the late 1990s, epoprostenol became the gold standard for treatment of IPAH in patients who were not responsive to acute vasodilator testing and therefore would not benefit from chronic oral calcium channel blockade. Epoprostenol (prostacyclin, prostaglandin I_2), a metabolite of arachidonic acid, and its analogues continue to be a major focus for treatment for a variety of forms of PAH. The pulmonary endothelium naturally elaborates prostacyclin into the bloodstream, where it has a short biologic half-life (2 to 3 minutes). In principle, prostacyclin is attractive for the treatment of PAH on several accounts. It has been shown to: (1) be a pulmonary vasodilator, (2) inhibit platelet aggregation, (3) inhibit proliferation of vascular smooth muscle, (4) improve endothelial dysfunction, and (5) be a possible cardiac inotrope.

The use of prostacyclin or other prostacyclin analog for the treatment of IPAH is supported by the demonstration of an imbalance in the thromboxane to prostacyclin metabolites in patients with IPAH,[42] as well as the demonstration of a reduction in prostacyclin synthase in the pulmonary arteries of IPAH patients.[47] Although chronic intravenous epoprostenol improves exercise tolerance, hemodynamics, and survival in IPAH patients, its mechanism(s) of action remains unclear.[3,4,89-93] Epoprostenol lowers pulmonary arterial pressure, increases cardiac output, and increases oxygen transport. These effects occur with long-term use, even if there is no acute response to vasodilator testing supporting the premise that epoprostenol has additional properties (other than as a pulmonary vasodilator) resulting in pulmonary vascular remodeling.[33] The optimal dose of intravenous epoprostenol is unclear. The dose (ng/kg/min) is titrated incrementally, with the most rapid increases during the first several months of epoprostenol use. Although a mean dose at 1 year in adult patients is approximately 20 to 40 ng/kg/min, the mean dose at 1 year in children, particularly young children, is closer to 50 to 80 ng/kg/min, but there is significant patient variability in the "optimal" dose.

Because epoprostenol is chemically unstable at neutral pH/room temperature and has a short half-life (1 to 2 minutes), chronic epoprostenol treatment requires a continuous intravenous delivery system with cold packs to maintain stability. Permanent central venous access is required to administer the medication. Thus, serious complications are associated with its use such as line sepsis, local site infection, and catheter dislodgment. In addition, pump malfunction may lead to a sudden bolus of epoprostenol (rare), or interruption of the medication that can cause severe rebound pulmonary arterial hypertension. Therefore, a search for alternate routes of drug delivery has led to the clinical development of oral, inhaled, and subcutaneous prostacyclin analogs. Treprostinil, a longer-acting prostacyclin analog, is approved for continuous subcutaneous, continuous intravenous, or inhaled (administered 4 times daily) use. Aerosolized iloprost, another stable prostacyclin analog approved for the treatment of PAH, is administered 6 to 9 times daily.

Inhaled Prostacyclin Analogs (Iloprost, Treprostinil)

Iloprost, an inhaled prostacyclin analog, may be advantageous because of the potential benefits of inhaled delivery that may avoid some of the systemic side effects, including hypotension, which can accompany epoprostenol use. Iloprost is a more stable synthetic analog of prostacyclin.[94]

It has a similar molecular structure to prostacyclin and acts through prostacyclin receptors on vascular endothelial cells.[95,96] Iloprost has both vasodilator and platelet aggregation inhibition properties similar to prostacyclin.[94] It has a biological half-life of ~20 to 25 minutes in humans.[97] It has been shown to have more pronounced short-term hemodynamic effects than inhaled nitric oxide in patients with IPAH.[98–101]

Inhaled iloprost (6 to 9 times a day [median dose 30 mcg/day]) was approved in 2004 for the treatment of PAH.[102] The noninvasive delivery system makes it appealing, but the need for 6 to 9 treatments per day (each lasting 5 to 15 minutes) can be a burden for patients, particularly children. Further, the currently approved inhalation devices may be challenging for routine administration in young children. Randomized trials of inhaled iloprost versus intravenous epoprostenol are warranted, although the feasibility of such trials is problematic.

The acute effects of inhaled nitric oxide have also been compared with aerosolized iloprost for children with pulmonary hypertension and congenital heart defects and found to be equally efficacious.[103] Although additive effects have been suggested when the two agents are used together, in this study there were no additive or synergistic effects.

In 2009, the prostacyclin analog treprostinil was approved in its inhalation form for PAH.[104] Based on a longer half-life than iloprost, inhaled treprostinil is given 4 times per day as opposed to 6 to 9 times per day for inhaled iloprost. To date, there are no safety and efficacy data in children. However, the delivery system may be easier for younger children to administer effectively compared with inhaled iloprost. Future investigations of its safety and efficacy in the pediatric population are warranted.

Subcutaneous/Intravenous Prostacyclin Analog (Treprostinil)

Treprostinil sodium is a chemically stable prostacyclin analog that shares at least some of the pharmacologic actions of epoprostenol. Acute hemodynamic effects with treprostinil are similar to those observed with intravenous epoprostenol in patients with IPAH, however treprostinil is stable at room temperature and neutral pH and has a longer half-life (2 to 3 hours) when administered subcutaneously.[105] Similar to epoprostenol, treprostinil is infused continuously by a portable pump and can be administered either subcutaneously or intravenously. Treprostinil was approved in 2002 for subcutaneous infusion and in 2004 for intravenous infusion.[106] The risk of central venous line infection is eliminated when treprostinil is used subcutaneously. Although no serious adverse events related to treprostinil or the delivery system when used subcutaneously have been reported, discomfort at the infusion site is common and may not be well tolerated by children.[107]

Endothelin Receptor Antagonists

Endothelin (ET-1) is a potent mitogen and vasoconstrictor that is produced in excess by the hypertensive pulmonary endothelium.[108] Circulating levels of endothelin are increased in patients with PAH, and the magnitude of elevation correlates with survival.[109] There are at least two different receptor subtypes: ET_A receptors are localized on smooth muscle cells and mediate vasoconstriction and proliferation,[110] while ET_B receptors are found predominantly on endothelial cells and are associated with: (1) endothelium-dependent vasorelaxation through the release of vasodilators (i.e., prostacyclin and nitric oxide), (2) clearance of ET, and (3) vasoconstriction (on smooth muscle cells) and bronchoconstriction.[111,112] Bosentan, an orally active twice-daily dual ET_A and ET_B receptor antagonist, was approved in 2001 based on studies in adult patients.[113,114] This was a significant advance in the field of PAH in that prior to 2001 there were no oral therapies approved for PAH. In a small, two center open-label study in 19 pediatric patients with IPAH, or PAH associated with congenital heart defects, bosentan improved hemodynamics after 12 weeks of treatment[115] with uncontrolled long-term data suggesting maintenance of efficacy in children with PAH.[116,117] The drug is generally well tolerated, however liver function must be monitored monthly as bosentan can produce significant hepatic dysfunction in ~8% of adult patients and ~3% of pediatric patients.

Two selective oral ET_A receptor antagonists (sitaxsentan and ambrisentan) have also been developed.[118–120] The rationale for selective ET_A receptor blockade is that it may benefit patients by blocking the vasoconstrictor effects of the ET_A receptor while maintaining the vasodilator and clearance effects of the ET_B receptor. Due to a drug interaction between sitaxsentan and warfarin decreasing the metabolism of warfarin, significantly lower doses of warfarin are needed to maintain a therapeutic INR. Sitaxsentan is currently only approved outside the United States. Ambrisentan was approved for PAH in 2007.[120] Currently, data on the use of sitaxsentan and ambrisentan in children are lacking. Although the risk of increased hepatic transaminases appears to be less with the ET_A selective receptor antagonists than with bosentan, all ERAs to date carry a risk of hepatic injury.

The use of ERAs (both dual receptor and selective ET_A receptor antagonists) appears promising for children with PAH. For patients who do not have an acute response to vasodilator testing or have failed treatment with oral calcium channel blockade, ERAs may offer a viable treatment option. Furthermore, in the future, the addition of ERAs to chronic calcium channel blockade therapy or to epoprostenol or another prostacyclin analog therapy may increase the overall efficacy of treatment for PAH in children.

Nitric Oxide

Nitric oxide (NO) is synthesized in endothelial cells from one of the guanidine nitrogens of L-arginine by the enzyme NO synthase. It has proved to be the endothelium-derived relaxing factor that contributes to the low initial tone of the pulmonary circulation. It has the advantage over other vasodilators of selectively relaxing pulmonary vessels without affecting systemic arterial pressure. NO is currently being used as an acute test of vasoreactivity in a wide variety of pulmonary hypertensive states and is approved for PPHN.[121,122] When inhaled, the rapid combination of

NO and hemoglobin inactivates any NO diffusing into the blood, preventing systemic vasodilatation. NO is therefore a potent and selective pulmonary vasodilator when administered by inhalation. NO may also have antiproliferative effects on smooth muscle and inhibit platelet adhesion. Inhaled NO has been demonstrated to be safe and efficacious in the treatment of PPHN.[121,122] Inhaled NO has been useful for determining "operability" of patients with CHD. It has also been used for the treatment of IPAH exacerbations, perioperative pulmonary hypertension following cardiac surgery, and other forms of PAH. Clinical trials are in progress evaluating the safety and efficacy of chronic inhaled NO in patients with inadequate responses to the currently approved PAH therapies.

Phosphodiesterase Inhibitors

Phosphodiesterase type 5 (PDE 5) inhibitors prevent the breakdown of cyclic GMP, thereby raising cyclic GMP levels. This effect should potentiate the pulmonary vasodilatation with NO. Sildenafil (orally active 3 times daily) and tadalafil, (orally active once daily), both PDE 5 inhibitors, enhance NO activity by inhibiting PDE 5, the enzyme responsible for catabolism of cyclic guanosine monophosphate. They were approved for the treatment of PAH in 2005 and 2009, respectively.[123–126] Phosphodiesterase type 5 inhibitors may also be particularly beneficial in conjunction with chronic inhaled NO, where withdrawal of NO may lead to rebound pulmonary hypertension. Intravenous, long-acting oral, or aerosolized forms of PDE 5 inhibitors all have therapeutic appeal. The effects of intravenous sildenafil were compared with inhaled NO in preoperative and postoperative patients with congenital heart disease and elevated pulmonary vascular resistance.[127] In this study, intravenous sildenafil was as effective as inhaled NO in children with congenital heart disease. Carefully designed short- and long-term studies of the safety and usefulness of PDE 5 inhibitors in combination with inhaled NO are warranted.

Gene Therapy

With the identification of the *HPAH* gene, a mutation in the *BMPR2* protein at chromosomal locus 2q33 that is associated with FPAH in selected families, attention has focused on gene replacement therapy. An alternative therapeutic approach has been to induce the overexpression of vasodilator genes, notably endothelial NO synthase and prostacyclin synthase, since patients with various forms of PAH have been shown to have deficiencies in both. Given the preliminary clinical observations that exogenous administration of chronic NO or epoprostenol may have salutary effects on even advanced forms of the disease, it seems worthwhile to pursue these alternative modes of "drug delivery." Advances in our understanding of the genetic predisposition associated with at least some, if not all, patients with PAH, suggest that gene therapy may be possible in the future.

Oxygen

Some patients who remain fully saturated while awake demonstrate modest systemic arterial oxygen desaturation with sleep, which appears to be caused by mild hypoventilation.[128] During these episodes, children with pulmonary hypertension may experience severe dyspnea, as well as syncope, with or without hypoxic seizures. Desaturation during sleep usually occurs during the early morning hours and can be eliminated by using supplemental oxygen. We recommend that children have supplemental oxygen available at home for emergency use. Children with PAH should be treated with supplemental oxygen during any significant upper respiratory tract infections if systemic arterial oxygen desaturation occurs. Children with desaturation caused by right-to-left shunting through a patent foramen ovale usually do not improve their oxygen saturation with supplemental oxygen, although oxygen supplementation may reduce the degree of polycythemia in these children. A small study of children with Eisenmenger syndrome demonstrated improved long-term survival with supplemental oxygen.[129] However, in a subsequent study with 23 adult patients with Eisenmenger syndrome, there was no significant improvement in survival with nocturnal oxygen.[130] Some children experience arterial oxygen desaturation with exercise as a result of increased oxygen extraction in the face of fixed oxygen delivery and may benefit from ambulatory supplemental oxygen. In addition, children with severe right ventricular failure and resting hypoxemia, resulting from a markedly increased oxygen extraction, should also be treated with chronic supplemental oxygen therapy. Supplemental oxygen is also recommended for air travel to avoid alveolar hypoxia and exacerbation of the pulmonary hypertension.

Additional Pharmacotherapy: Cardiac Glycosides, Diuretics, Antiarrhythmic Therapy, Inotropic Agents, and Nitrates

Although controversy persists regarding the value of digitalis in IPAH,[131] children with right-sided heart failure may benefit from digitalis in addition to diuretic therapy. Diuretic therapy must be initiated cautiously because these patients are preload-dependent to maintain optimal cardiac output. Despite this, relatively high doses of diuretic therapy are often needed. Although malignant arrhythmias are rare in pulmonary hypertension, treatment is appropriate for documented cases. Atrial flutter or fibrillation often precipitates an abrupt decrease in cardiac output and clinical deterioration due to loss of the atrial component. As opposed to healthy children, in whom atrial systole accounts for approximately 25% of the cardiac output, atrial systole in children with IPAH often contributes as much as 70% of the cardiac output. Therefore, aggressive treatment of atrial flutter or fibrillation is advised.

Although, there are no studies on the usefulness of intermittent or continuous treatment with inotropic agents, dobutamine can be used for additional inotropic support in conjunction with continuous intravenous epoprostenol in children with severe right ventricular dysfunction, as a bridge to transplantation. Children have also benefited from short-term inotropic support during acute pulmonary hypertensive crises to augment cardiac output during a period of increased metabolic demand.

Oral and sublingual nitrates have been used to treat chest pain in some children with IPAH, although the experience with these agents remains limited. Children who complain of chest tightness, or pressure, or vague discomfort that is responsive to sublingual nitroglycerin should be treated with chronic oral nitrates as well as sublingual nitroglycerin.

Atrial Septostomy

Children with recurrent syncope in severe right-sided heart failure have a very poor prognosis.[1,132] Exercise-induced syncope is caused by systemic vasodilation, with an inability to augment cardiac output (through a fixed pulmonary vascular bed) to maintain adequate cerebral perfusion. If right-to-left shunting through an interatrial or interventricular communication is present, cardiac output can be maintained or increased if necessary. In addition, right-to-left shunting at the atrial level alleviates signs and symptoms of right-sided heart failure by decompression of the right atrium and right ventricle. Increased survival has been reported in patients with IPAH with a patent foramen ovale, although this remains controversial.[133] Patency of the foramen ovale may improve survival if it allows sufficient right-to-left shunting to maintain cardiac output. Successful palliation of symptoms with atrial septostomy has been reported in several series.[134–138] In our experience, PAH patients with recurrent syncope or right-sided heart failure improve clinically as well as hemodynamically following atrial septostomy; patients experience no further syncope, and signs and symptoms of right-sided heart failure improve. Although systemic arterial oxygen saturation decreases, overall cardiac output and oxygen delivery improve despite the right-to-left shunting at the atrial level. In our experience, atrial septostomy results in a survival benefit; the survival rates at 1 and 2 years are 87% and 76%, respectively, compared with conventional therapy (64% and 42% at 1 and 2 years, respectively).[139] Thus, although atrial septostomy does not alter the underlying disease process, it may improve quality of life and represent an alternative for selected patients with severe IPAH. However, this invasive procedure is not without risk; our indications for the procedure include recurrent syncope or right ventricular failure despite maximal medical therapy, and as a bridge to transplantation. Although there is a worldwide experience with more than 100 patients, the procedure of atrial septostomy should still be considered investigational. Closure of the atrial septal defect can be performed at the time of transplantation.

Transplantation

While successful heart-lung transplantation, as well as single and double lung transplantation with repair of congenital heart defect(s) has been available for more than 20 years, there are several limitations to these procedures. A limited number of centers perform the procedures in children, and the availability of suitable donors is limited. Furthermore, the high incidence of chronic allograft rejection or bronchiolitis obliterans in the transplanted organs of these patients (25% to 50%) and the potential consequences of lifelong immunosuppression are of great concern.[139] Both single and bilateral lung transplantation have been performed in pediatric patients with pulmonary vascular obstructive disease including patients with severe right ventricular failure.[140] Currently, the overall 1-year, 5-year, and 10-year survival rates following lung transplantation for PAH patients is 64%, 44%, and 20%, respectively.[139–142] There has been no significant improvement in survival in more recent years (e.g., 1998 to 2001 versus 1992 to 1998). For untreated Eisenmenger patients, the natural history is much more favorable. The 5-year and 25-year survival rate is greater than 80% and 40%, respectively, for untreated Eisenmenger patients,[142] as opposed to following lung transplantation with a 1-year and 5-year survival of 52% and 39%, respectively.[139] Thus, transplantation is most often reserved for WHO functional class III and IV patients with PAH who have progressed despite optimal medical therapy (see Box 72-2). As progress is made in the medical management of PAH, the indications for transplantation will change. The course of the disease and the waiting time must be taken into account when referring for transplantation. Ideally, children should be listed when their probability of 2-year survival without transplantation is 50% or less. While there are advantages and disadvantages to each operation, that is, lung (single or double) versus heart-lung transplantation, there is currently no consensus regarding the optimal procedure. The availability of donor organs often influences the choice of procedure. It is possible that data on long-term survival will demonstrate a survival advantage of one procedure over another. Although lung and heart-lung transplantation are imperfect therapies for PAH, when offered to appropriately selected patients, transplantation may improve survival with an improved quality of life. Early referral to a center with expertise in pediatric lung and heart-lung transplantation will decrease pretransplantation mortality and allow families to have adequate time to make an informed and thoughtful choice about this therapy. Living related donor transplantation remains controversial; although living related donor transplantation has been successful, there is limited experience.[143,144]

■ SUMMARY

Recent therapeutic advances have significantly improved the prognosis for children with PAH. Nevertheless, PAH remains a serious condition that is extremely challenging to manage. Chronic vasodilator therapy with calcium channel blockade in acute responders to vasodilator testing, and continuous intravenous epoprostenol in nonresponders appears to be effective in children, with observational studies reporting improved survival, hemodynamics, and symptoms.[2–4,93,145–148] Additionally, prostacyclin analogs administered by inhalation, continuous subcutaneous, or continuous intravenous infusion; oral ERAs; and oral PDE 5 inhibitors are available for the treatment of PAH. Although not approved for PAH, inhaled NO is frequently used in the acute setting, with chronic administration undergoing evaluation. In a carefully controlled setting, there may be a role for transitioning PAH children who have had an excellent response to long-term intravenous epoprostenol therapy to oral or inhaled agents.[149] In the future, there will undoubtedly be more treatment options for patients with PAH. However, in the early stages of use, and without controlled studies for comparison, the newer agents should be used cautiously with close monitoring for treatment failure. Based on distinct mechanism(s) of action, combination therapy may further improve the overall efficacy of treating a child's PAH. Future developments in vascular biology will improve our understanding of the etiologies of PAH and its pathobiology, as well as provide rationale for more specific medical therapies. The current treatment algorithm for pediatric patients, extrapolated from adult evidence-based guidelines, will continue to evolve as newer agents become available (see Fig. 72-3). It remains unknown whether these new agents will prove to be as effective as intravenous epoprostenol in selected children. Additionally, with increasing collaborative efforts between pharmaceutical companies, regulatory agencies, and academia, the future of clinical drug development for pediatric patients looks bright. Such studies should further the advances made to date

in treating children with PAH because, even when the disease is similar between children and adults, children are not merely "small adults." Optimal care for pediatric patients requires knowledge of the therapies assessed in pediatric patients in addition to study in adult patients.

We hope that by increasing our understanding of the pathobiology of PAH, novel treatment strategies will continue to evolve, and one day we will be able to prevent and cure this disease.

References

The complete reference list is available online at www.expertconsult.com

73 THE LUNG IN SICKLE CELL DISEASE

Robert C. Strunk, MD, and Michael R. DeBaun, MD

DEFINITIONS, EPIDEMIOLOGY

Sickle cell disease (SCD) results from the presence of sickle hemoglobin (HbS) that polymerizes in a deoxygenated state, producing rigid, sickled erythrocytes that occlude the microvasculature. Resulting vaso-occlusive episodes may occur in any organ of the body with tissue ischemia and ultimately organ infarction. SCD produces high rates of morbidity and mortality and has profound effects on quality of life for affected individuals and their families. Pulmonary physicians need to be familiar with the disease because of frequent occurrence of chronic respiratory symptoms that affect daily functioning, development of chronic lung disease that can be associated with pulmonary hypertension and death, and acute chest syndrome (ACS) that can progress suddenly and cause death. In addition, an interaction between SCD and asthma, a comorbid condition, increases both morbidity and mortality.

SCD is one of the most common genetic diseases screened for in the newborn period in the United States, occurring in 1 in 2647 infants regardless of race and 1 in 400 African-American children. Even in the entire population, SCD is more common than primary congenital hypothyroidism or cystic fibrosis (which occurs in 1 in 3000 and 1 in 3900 births, respectively). SCD occurs in several phenotypes. In the most severe form, a patient is either homozygous for the HbS allele or heterozygous for HbS and β-null thalassemia (SCD-Sβ⁰, when there is no β chain production), both of which yield the majority of hemoglobin (Hb) as HbS (SCD-SS or sickle cell anemia). Less severe disease occurs when the patient is heterozygous for HbS and for another hemoglobin mutation, such as HbC (SCD-SC) or β-plus thalassemia (SCD-Sβ⁺, when there is some β chain production), when a smaller percentage of Hb is HbS. Sickle cell trait, with only a single copy of HbS, occurs in approximately 8% of African-American individuals. It is commonly a benign condition because the normal hemoglobin (HbA) constitutes most of the hemoglobin.

PATHOPHYSIOLOGY

Sickling and Inflammation

In SCD, the primary molecular defect in the *beta globin* gene results in a cascade of cellular events that produce polymerization of HbS, most notably when it is in a deoxygenated state. These events culminate in vaso-occlusive episodes, the hallmark of the disease. HbF is noted to inhibit the process of polymerization, and disease severity is diminished in individuals who are born with high HbF levels that continue throughout adulthood (HbS hereditary persistent fetal hemoglobin) or when HbF production is increased pharmacologically, such as with regular use of hydroxyurea.

During the last several years, increasing attention has been focused on the contribution of hemolysis to the pathogenesis of SCD. Hemolysis results in the release of intracellular red blood cell arginase and free hemoglobin. As arginase degrades arginine, the substrate for nitric oxide (NO) synthase, there is an obligatory depletion in the amount of NO.[1] Additionally, free hemoglobin binds to and acts as a biologic sink for NO, further reducing NO bioavailability.[2] Decreased NO has been postulated as the key component for endothelial dysfunction, resulting in several clinical manifestations, the hallmark of which is an elevated tricuspid regurgitant jet velocity (TRJV) as assessed by Doppler echocardiography, a proxy for an elevated pulmonary artery pressure. Among adults with SCD, a TRJV ≥ 2.5 m/sec is associated with a rate ratio for death of 10.1.[3] Further evidence is evolving to support or refute the clinical relevance of and a mechanism for the association between hemolysis, NO, and elevated TRJV in children with SCD.

Inflammation is a significant component of SCD, with the airway uniquely susceptible to effects of the pro-inflammatory state associated with SCD and also effects of infection, allergens in sensitized individuals, and irritants. Evidence to support the importance of ongoing inflammation includes elevated levels during periods of apparent wellness of white blood cells,[4] TNFα,[5] and soluble vascular cell adhesion molecule-1 (sVCAM-1),[6] among many others. Much investigation of the role of inflammation has focused on vascular endothelium, as adhesion of the sickle erythrocytes, leukocytes, and platelets to the microvascular endothelium is promoted by increased levels of circulating inflammatory cytokines, which contributes to further obstruction of arterioles.

CLINICAL MANIFESTATIONS

The most common manifestations of SCD include susceptibility to life-threatening infections (particularly caused by encapsulated organisms such as *Streptococcus pneumoniae* and *Haemophilus influenzae* type B), recurrent pain episodes that often require treatment with opioids at home (or hospitalization for parenteral therapy), ACS, and cerebral infarcts, both overt and silent.

The epidemiology, natural history, and treatment of renal, CNS, and other end-organ complications that occur in SCD are extensive and beyond the scope of this chapter. In this chapter, we will focus primarily on the pulmonary complications associated with SCD.

Acute Chest Syndrome

Acute chest syndrome (ACS) has been defined by a consensus of investigators at the Comprehensive Sickle Cell Centers as an acute illness characterized by fever with or without respiratory symptoms, accompanied by a new radiodensity on chest radiograph.[7] ACS is the second most common reason for hospitalization following pain episodes,[8] occurring more often in patients with SCD-SS and SCD-Sβ[0] than in patients with SCD-SC and SCD-Sβ[+].[9] The incidence is highest in children 2 to 4 years of age.[9] At diagnosis, inspiratory crackles are the most common clinical finding (75% of young children and 81% of adults), but wheezing is also common (33% of young children and 16% of adults).[10]

ACS includes several features that can be produced by other processes, particularly in young children. The ability to distinguish ACS, an idiopathic pulmonic process specific to SCD, from other pulmonary disease is challenging. The finding of wheezing is important, as many young children can have transient wheezing with viral infection, and an accompanying new radiodensity could represent simply associated atelectasis. In addition, an acute asthma exacerbation at any age could also be mislabeled ACS, as asthma episodes are commonly accompanied by fever as a sign of an underlying viral infection initiating the exacerbation, with infiltrates due to atelectasis. Neither of these types of illnesses would represent true ACS episodes and may need to be treated differently. As in other settings, viral-induced wheezing is noted by the exposures and the timing of viral disease epidemics in the community. Asthma may be suggested by predictive factors similar to children without SCD, such as presence of eczema or a history of asthma in the mother or father, or presence of specific allergen sensitivities that would be sought when there is a high index of suspicion from the personal and family histories.

The course of ACS can be rapid and may prove fatal in both children and adults. ACS is the leading cause of premature death in SCD and affects approximately 50% of patients with SCD-SS at least once in their lifetime.[8,11] The etiology of ACS is multifactorial, and the pathogenesis is not completely understood. In a large prospective study, the cause of ACS was not identified in 46% of episodes; in patients with an identified etiology, infection (29.4%), fat embolism (8.8%), and pulmonary infarction (16.1%) are most common.[10] Infectious agents identified include viruses (6.4%), chlamydia (7.2%), mycoplasma (6.6%), bacteria (4.5), and mixed or miscellaneous (4.7%).[10]

Chronic Lung Disease

Clinical observations and published cross-sectional data have led to the speculation that lung function evolves in children and adolescents with SCD from normal to obstruction to restriction. The exact timing of onset of pulmonary function abnormalities is not known. Only one study has examined pulmonary function in infants. Koumbourlis and colleagues studied 20 young children 3 to 30 months of age and described abnormal lung function, primarily obstructive.[12] In general, children with SCD-SS had more abnormal lung function than those with SCD-SC, consistent with findings in older children. Studies in children 5 to 18 years of age have found normal spirometry in 71%, with small percentages of restrictive (13%) or obstructive (16%)

physiology.[13-19] Nickerson and coworkers used cross-sectional data from the Cooperative Study for Sickle Cell Disease (CSSCD) to study changes in pulmonary function with age and found a decline in all spirometry values with increasing age in children with SCD-SS.[20] Others have also found a prevalence of abnormal lung function greater in adolescents than in younger children. For example, MacLean and colleagues[14] found restrictive physiology in 0.9% of children at 8 years of age but in 18.7% at 17 years of age.

Longitudinal pulmonary studies from childhood to adulthood are needed to determine the exact progression of lung disease along this proposed spectrum and to identify clinical and disease course factors associated with pulmonary function changes. Several studies have been completed using pulmonary function tests obtained for clinical purposes, with individual patients followed for intervals (means) of 3.5 years to 4.2 years.[16] In all of these studies, data were spliced together to obtain information about changes in lung function over time. Each study showed lower lung function in older adolescents than in school-age children, similar to the findings of Nickerson and coworkers.[20] Field and colleagues[21] compared lung growth in children with SCD-SS to normal children in the Harvard Six Cities Study, comparing each case to an age-, gender-, and height-matched child with African-American race in the normal group. Longitudinal FEV_1 was lower for boys and girls with SCD-SS compared to normal children. Girls with SCD-SS showed lower longitudinal FVC and FEV_1/FVC, but there was no difference in these two spirometry values in boys.[21] Matching by gender in addition to age and height allowed the investigators to suggest that gender may influence the risk of developing abnormal lung function and airways obstruction. Studies are needed to define the role of gender as well as to examine other risk factors in the evolution to chronic lung disease.

Chronic lung disease is a major cause of morbidity and mortality in older adolescents and adults.[3,22] Several authors have published cross-sectional studies of lung function in patients in late adolescence and adulthood and found restriction most common (31%), but also obstruction alone (32%) or mixed with restriction (11%). A greater predominance of restriction (approximately 90%) was found by Klings and colleagues[23] using data collected in the CSSCD to study lung function in 310 adults between 20 and 67 years of age (mean 30.7 ± 10.3), with decreases in TLC and abnormalities in DLCO. Chronic lung disease most likely has its start in the pediatric population; however, little is known about the clinical course in the child or adolescent with SCD that results in chronic lung disease. Powars first postulated that ACS episodes are the most important risk factor for the development of chronic lung disease,[22] but other authors have found the role of prior ACS episodes in the evolution of restrictive lung disease unclear.[23]

Sylvester and colleagues[24] studied chest high-resolution CT scans in 33 adults, 17 to 67 years of age, 30 of whom had abnormalities, most prominently lobar volume loss, prominent central vessels, a reticular pattern, and ground-glass opacification. Lobar volume loss was negatively correlated with FEV_1, FVC, and TLC. These findings are consistent with the speculation that restrictive lung disease is caused by fibrotic interstitial abnormalities, and these abnormalities are common in adults.

ROLE OF ABNORMAL PULMONARY FUNCTION TESTS AND FUTURE MORBIDITY

An association between the abnormalities in lung function and types and frequencies of morbidity in children with SCD has also been proposed, but there have been limited studies. Boyd and coworkers[15] studied 102 children for whom morbidity data were available for a mean length of follow-up of 3.8 years after spirometry and lung volumes had been obtained. Lower airway obstruction, but not a restrictive pattern or bronchodilator reactivity, was associated with an increased rate of hospitalization for pain or ACS. The association of lower airway obstruction and pain was present, even among children without a doctor diagnosis of asthma, a known risk factor for increased morbidity (see later in the chapter). Additional studies are needed to confirm an effect of lower airway obstruction on future morbidity and to define the pathophysiology of this effect.

Low O$_2$ Saturation

Low oxygen saturation (SpO$_2$) is commonly found in children with SCD, and daytime SpO$_2$ assessments are becoming a routine practice in many sickle cell clinics. A low SpO$_2$ may be related to a history of ACS, older age, low fetal Hb levels, OSA, asthma, and hemoglobin level. The association between Hb level and SpO$_2$ is unique to SCD and is not well explained. However, it is most likely related to a combination of factors that include the fact that the pulse oximetry machines are calibrated for normal hemoglobin and not HbS, and that individuals with SCD have an increase amount of dyshemoglobins (methemoglobin and carboxy hemoglobin) that offset the SpO$_2$ measurement. Recent studies have demonstrated that the level of SpO$_2$ does not predict future morbidity.[25]

Measurement of SpO$_2$ with pulse oximetry at well visits and during illness is strongly recommended in SCD; however, caution must be exercised when interpreting the results, particularly given the observation that as many as 10% of apparently healthy children with SCD will have a pulse oximetry reading <90%,[25] and, unlike children with a normal Hb, an SpO$_2$ of <90% does not necessarily correspond to alveolar hypoxia. Further, given that the SpO$_2$ may be closer to the steepest point of the oxygen disassociation curve and is related to the fluctuations in hemoglobin levels, the SpO$_2$ is susceptible to a wider range than expected when compared to children without SCD. Mullin and colleagues[26] demonstrated that the variability in SpO$_2$ at times of wellness was related to an initial value SpO$_2$. When baseline saturation was ≤92%, SpO$_2$ varied over time approximately 5% on average with no evidence of any change in clinical status.[26]

Measurement of SpO$_2$ in children may have clinical importance when evaluating cardiac disease. In a cross-sectional study, Johnson and coworkers[27] demonstrated that left ventricular hypertrophy and diastolic dysfunction in children with SCD were related to sleeping and waking oxygen desaturation. Longitudinal studies are required to determine if there is causal relationship or simply an association of SpO$_2$ with cardiac dysfunction.

Sleep-Disordered Breathing

Obstructive sleep apnea (OSA) is a common childhood condition with a prevalence of approximately 2% to 3%. Several authors have speculated that OSA could play a causal role in vaso-occlusive and other adverse health outcomes in children with SCD. Children with SCD may be at increased risk for the development of OSA because of greater propensity for lymphoid hyperplasia and airway narrowing related to facial features associated with bone marrow hyperplasia. Limited data exist regarding the prevalence of OSA in children with SCA. One study of 50 children estimated that one-third of the children with upper airway symptoms had sleep-related upper airway obstruction based on overnight limited-channel cardiorespiratory studies.[28] To investigate a possible effect of nocturnal desaturation on morbidity, Hargrave and colleagues[29] demonstrated that the mean nocturnal SpO$_2$ was associated with the rate of pain over an average follow-up of 4.6 years; however, no threshold that conferred a higher rate of pain was identified.[29] This study, similar to most of the studies linking nocturnal respiratory dysfunction to adverse outcomes in children with SCD, recorded only nocturnal oxyhemoglobin saturation without other measures of sleep, breathing, or upper airway obstruction.

Marshall and colleagues studied auto-adjusting positive airway pressure in children with sleep-disordered breathing and found improved cognition (processing speed and attention) and a tendency to decreased pain after 6 weeks of treatment.[30] Supplemental O$_2$ was used to maintain SpO$_2$ ≥94%, with no bone marrow suppression, rebound pain, or serious adverse events observed in patients receiving supplemental O$_2$ in the 6 weeks of the trial. Currently, supplemental O$_2$ and positive airway pressure are not recommended until further studies replicate this single study, which does suggest that use of O$_2$ supplementation may not be associated with significant sequelae.

It is quite possible that early detection and treatment of OSA in this vulnerable pediatric population may improve their health outcomes. Currently no evidence supports whether application of practice guidelines intended for the general pediatric population to screen for OSA (based on ascertainment of symptoms such as snoring, observed apnea, restless sleep, or daytime sleepiness) are applicable to children with SCD. Until guidelines are developed specifically for children with SCD, we recommend following the AAP guidelines for patients with suspected SDB.

Pulmonary Hypertension

The average lifespan of individuals with SCD-SS is in the mid-forties.[8] Although there is some controversy surrounding whether an elevated TRJV measurement is associated with pulmonary arterial hypertension, there is no doubt that an elevated TRJV (i.e., >2.5 m/sec) is associated with increased mortality, with a 2-year mortality rate of nearly 15% in adults.[3] Potential etiologic factors causing elevated TRJV include hemolysis interfering with nitric oxide–mediated vasodilatation, left ventricular dysfunction, pulmonary thromboembolism, airway hyperresponsiveness (AHR), and sleep-disordered breathing, with hemolysis the predominant mechanism. The prevalence of elevated TRJV is 25% to 30% in adults and 30% in children with SCD.[31] However, no evidence exists that increased TRJV is associated with increased mortality in children. Left ventricular dilation and diastolic dysfunction has been found in adults and children with SCD, and it may have prognostic implications.

Airway Lability

Airway lability, measured either as an increased response to bronchodilators or hyperresponsiveness to cold air, exercise, or methacholine, has been demonstrated in many SCD children. Bronchodilator reactivity was found in up to 54% of children,[15,18,32] with highest percentages in those with airway obstruction.[15] The presence of AHR in SCD was initially studied with cold air and exercise challenges, with prevalence up to 78% overall and up to 83% in those with a history of wheezing that improved with the use of a bronchodilator.[33] The prevalence of positive methacholine challenges is similar to that found with challenge by the other techniques.[34-35] Initially it was thought that methacholine challenges in children with SCD were without significant increased risk, but a recent case report of the onset of significant diffuse body pain after a challenge indicates that caution must be taken in the use of this procedure.[36]

Unlike children without SCD, methacholine responsiveness in children with SCD-SS was not correlated with doctor-diagnosis of asthma, history of wheeze in the absence of a cold, FEV_1 % predicted, FEV_1/FVC % predicted, bronchodilator reactivity, exhaled nitric oxide, allergy skin tests, or eosinophil count.[37] An elevated serum IgE was the only feature of asthma that was an independent predictor of methacholine responsiveness.

Results from any of the challenge procedures have yet to yield an understanding of the pathophysiology of SCD lung disease or development of treatments to prevent morbidity, although a recent study suggests that hemolysis may be associated with increased levels of airway responsiveness to methacholine.[37] Interestingly, the presence of AHR was not associated with increased prevalence of ACS.[32] These results suggest that assessing airway responsiveness may have a limited role in the diagnostic evaluation of children with SCD.

Role of Asthma in Worsening Morbidity

Several lines of evidence indicate that the presence of a doctor diagnosis of asthma increases morbidity in individuals with SCD. This association was first observed in a retrospective case-control study of children hospitalized for pain, in which patients admitted for pain were 4-times as likely to develop ACS if a doctor-diagnosis of asthma was recorded in the chart.[38] In a subsequent study, a history of asthma was associated with increased rates of both pain and ACS in the prospective cohort study of infants followed with SCD-SS for a mean of 12 years in the CSSCD.[39] In this study, children with asthma had twice as many episodes of ACS (0.42 episodes per patient-year versus 0.20 episodes per patient-year, p<0.001) and a shorter time to first ACS episode (3.5 years versus 7.3 years, p<0.003) when compared to children without asthma. Incidence rates by age for ACS and pain were increased in patients with asthma (Fig. 73-1). Other authors have confirmed the association between physician-diagnosed asthma and increased rates of ACS[32,40] and indicated that asthma exacerbations may predispose to ACS episodes.[41] Additionally, asthma was determined to be an independent risk factor for death among individuals with sickle cell anemia.[38]

Features consistent with the presence of asthma, airway obstruction, and airway lability are common in SCD patients, suggesting that preventive treatment for asthma may help reduce the morbidity of ACS, but no randomized trials have been performed.

Atopy

Atopy, as defined by the presence of a positive skin test to an aeroallergen, is present in similar prevalence to normal controls, approximately 35%.[32] A single study provides evidence that atopy is associated with an increased frequency of recurrent ACS episodes, and that asthma

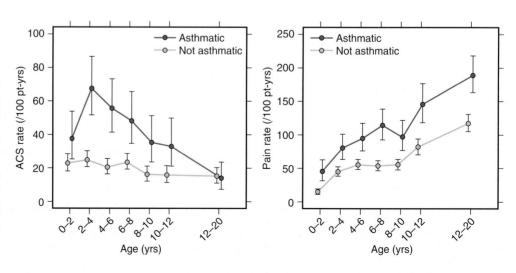

FIGURE 73-1. Age-specific incidence rates of ACS and pain events classified by clinical asthma status. The overall incidence rate of ACS events is higher in patients with asthma (0.42 events per patient-year) when compared to patients without asthma (0.20 events per patient-year, p<0.001). The overall incidence rate of painful events is higher in patients with asthma (1.11 events per patient-year) when compared to patients without asthma (0.58 events per patient-year, p<0.001). Line segments are point-wise exact 95% confidence intervals.

is much more associated with ACS when it is associated with allergic sensitization[32]; however, further studies are required for validation.

◼ CARE

Chronic

Guidelines for chronic care include, most fundamentally, regular follow-up with a hematologist at a sickle cell center. Involvement of a pulmonary physician should occur when there are symptoms suggestive of asthma and when there is even a single episode of severe ACS requiring blood transfusion therapy or intensive care unit admission. Table 73-1 presents guidelines for the care of children to recognize early pulmonary and cardiac morbidity and to reduce their impact.

In the last two decades, several well-established preventive strategies have been developed to decrease the morbidity associated with many of the complications of SCD. Use of penicillin twice daily for children up to 5 years of age and conjugated vaccines for *Streptococcus pneumoniae* and *Haemophilus influenzae* type B have dramatically decreased these infections and concomitantly the fatality rate. Supplemental folic acid is also used prophylactically after 1 year of age to maintain effective erythropoiesis. Use of hydroxyurea, an agent used primarily to increase the amount of HbF, is associated with an approximately 50% reduction in the incidence of pain episodes, ACS episodes, and the need for blood transfusions.[42] The results of a randomized trial led to FDA approval of hydroxyurea as a prophylactic agent for the prevention of pain in adults.[42] Hydroxyurea has been established as a safe agent in children and is commonly used in children with SCD.

An alternative, effective, but seldom-used strategy for the prevention of vaso-occlusive pain episodes is short-term use of regular blood transfusion therapy designed to keep the HbS levels <30%. This approach is commonly reserved for patients who have a debilitating course that severely impedes their daily functioning, such as attending school or participating in family activities. Typically it is offered for only a brief period of time, usually less than 12 months, while other options are explored. These other adjuvant therapies included re-educating the patient on how to manage pain without opioids or using nonmedicinal strategies. However, the regular blood transfusions come at a cost, including excessive iron stores that eventually require daily treatment with iron chelators, and alloimmunization.

Inherent in these recommendations is adherence with daily medications. Studies of adherence have found that

TABLE 73-1 GUIDELINES FOR THE CARE OF CHILDREN TO RECOGNIZE EARLY PULMONARY AND CARDIAC MORBIDITY AND TO REDUCE THEIR IMPACT

TEST OR THERAPY	FREQUENCY	RATIONALE
Review of systems for atopy and asthma (all children with SCD)	Annually, starting at 1 year of age. If history is positive, refer to allergy or asthma specialist.	Atopy is a risk factor for asthma. Children with asthma and SCD are at increased risk of vaso-occlusive episodes and ACS.
Assessment of lung function by spirometry (all children with SCD)	Annually in all children with SCD starting at 6 years of age. With every visit for children with SCD and asthma, maximum 4 times per year. Bronchodilator challenge should be done in children with obstruction (FEV_1/FVC <95% CI).	Children with SCD may have obstructive and restrictive defects.
Assessment of defects in lung function by lung volumes with plethysmography (all children with SCD)	Starting at 6 years of age: Every 5 years in children with no asthma or ACS episodes. Every 2 to 3 years in children with asthma or ACS episodes.	Children with SCD may have obstructive and restrictive defects.
Treatment of children with SCD and asthma per NHLBI guidelines (all children with SCD)	Indefinitely. Once diagnosed with asthma, children should be assessed at least every 6 months for persistent symptoms.	Treatment of persistent asthma in children without SCD with daily inhaled corticosteroids is effective in reducing asthma hospitalizations and symptom-days.
Review of systems for sleep-disordered breathing (sleep apnea) (all children with SCD and asthma)	Annually by history. If history is positive, refer to pulmonologist for evaluation.	Children with nocturnal hypoxemia have higher rates of vaso-occlusive pain episodes.
Appointment with pulmonologist, allergist, or asthma specialist (all children with SCD and asthma)	At least annually for children with SCD and mild asthma. At least every 6 months for children with SCD and moderate to severe asthma.	Children with asthma and SCD are at increased risk of vaso-occlusive episodes and ACS.
Assessment for elevated tricuspid regurgitant jet velocity and pulmonary hypertension by 2-D echocardiography (all children with SCD)	At least once between 16 and 18 years of age.	A tricuspid regurgitant jet velocity >2.5 m/s is associated with an increased risk of death in adults. Effective intervention is not well defined.

only about 60% of prescriptions are refilled in a timely manner over the course of a year,[43] indicating the need to focus on this facet of care at each clinic visit.

CARE FOR ACUTE EPISODES

Pain

Once a pain episode has begun, there is no established treatment to quickly control the event and opioids are usually required; thus the emphasis is on preventing the pain episodes.

Acute Chest Syndrome

Acute treatment of ACS should include the standard supportive measures offered to any child with an increased respiratory effort. These treatments include, but are not limited to, oxygen support to keep the SpO_2 >92%, close monitoring, and appropriate antimicrobial therapy to treat presumptive infection for the most common offending pathogens: *Streptococcus pneumoniae* with a third generation cephalosporin, and mycoplasma or chlamydia with a macrolide. Both these pathogens are common in ACS[44] and are believed to be more virulent in SCD. Some have suggested the use of albuterol as treatment,[45] and it is certainly worth a trial, especially in children with a past diagnosis of asthma. There have been no randomized trials of this approach.

In the only randomized intervention trial for ACS, children treated with IV dexamethasone (0.3 mg/kg every 12 hours x4 doses) recovered more quickly than those who received placebo[46] but had a higher rate of rehospitalization within 72 hours of discharge (27% in treatment versus 5% in placebo). Concern has been raised by other authors that use of systemic corticosteroids during episodes of ACS may increase length of stay in addition to the higher rate of rehospitalization. The adverse impact of systemic corticosteroids is also noted when these drugs are used chronically to treat comorbid autoimmune diseases, with initiation of therapy associated with increased frequency of painful crises, ACS, stroke, renal infarction, and avascular necrosis of the femoral head.[47]

In the setting of ACS, when there is rapid deterioration, children should be under the supervision of clinicians and facilities equipped to provide both simple and exchange blood transfusion therapy. In addition, if not present locally, such children should be transferred to a facility that has a pediatric intensive care unit so that the health care team can perform intubation or even use extracorporeal membrane oxygenation (ECMO) if necessary. ECMO has been successfully employed to prevent death, albeit in a nonrandomized clinical trial setting. The timing and approach for these more aggressive therapies are not well established but should be directed by a multidisciplinary team that includes, but is not limited to, a pediatric hematologist, pulmonologist, and critical care specialist.

There is substantial evidence that hydroxyurea is effective in preventing ACS in adults with SCD. Before using hydroxyurea in a child, individual pulmonary exacerbations should be evaluated for the possibility that they were viral-induced bronchiolitis or an asthma exacerbation, both of which are associated with atelectasis and can be confused with ACS. Before starting hydroxyurea, careful consideration should be given to the the question of whether the patient has undiagnosed or undertreated asthma.

Similar to the primary prevention of vaso-occlusive pain episodes with regular blood transfusion therapy, ACS can be prevented with regular blood transfusions with the goal of keeping the HbS level <30%. However, this therapy is typically reserved only for patients with repeated life threatening ACS episodes, which are not a direct consequence of poorly treated asthma, or are refractory to an adequate trial of hydroxyurea. Regular blood transfusion therapy should only be instituted for a defined period of time because the known consequences of excessive iron stores are not outweighed by the unknown long-term benefits of preventing ACS.

Vaso-occlusive episodes that require hospitalization and treatment with opioids are a major risk factor for ACS. In such circumstances, regular use of incentive spirometry dramatically reduces the rate of ACS. In a randomized clinical trial in which adult patients were allocated to receive incentive spirometry or observation, 10 maximal inspirations every 2 hours between 8:00 AM and 10:00 PM reduced progression to ACS by 50%.[48] Consequently, the use of incentive spirometry for all patients admitted to the hospital for pain has become standard medical care and should be an active component of supportive therapy.

Use of medications to control chronic asthma has been proposed in SCD based on the observations that ACS is more common in individuals with doctor-diagnosed asthma and that airway obstruction and airway lability are common. While both inhaled corticosteroids and leukotriene modifiers are being used in many clinical settings, there are no controlled studies to demonstate their usefulness, either to prevent ACS or to control recurrent respiratory symptoms.

SUMMARY

Pulmonary disease in children with SCD produces significant morbidity and mortality. A doctor-diagnosis of asthma has clear implications for the course of SCD, with increased rates of both pain and ACS. The mechanisms of the relationship between asthma and increased morbidity are not well understood, and there is no information about the role of treatments known to be effective for control of asthma in children without SCD. While cross-sectional studies have documented normal lung function in early childhood and restrictive disease in adulthood, little is known about the risk factors for progression rates of lung disease and how to prevent progression. The role of sleep-disordered breathing and its relationship to morbidity and mortality in SCD has only begun to be elucidated. The etiology, natural history, and optimal treatment for progressive lung disease is still unknown. Given that there is much to be learned before pulmonary disease and sleep-disordered breathing can be managed more effectively, there is a clear role for pediatric pulmonologists in studying this complex disease.

Suggested Reading

Bernini JC, Rogers ZR, Sandler ES, et al. Beneficial effect of intravenous dexamethasone in children with mild to moderately severe acute chest syndrome complicating sickle cell disease. *Blood.* 1998;92:3082–3089.

Boyd JH, Macklin EA, Strunk RC, et al. Asthma is associated with acute chest syndrome and pain in children with sickle cell anemia. *Blood.* 2006;108:2923–2927.

Castro O, Brambilla DJ, Thorington B, et al. The acute chest syndrome in sickle cell disease: incidence and risk factors. The Cooperative Study of Sickle Cell Disease. *Blood.* 1994;84:643–649.

Field JJ, DeBaun MR, Yan Y, et al. Growth of lung function in children with sickle cell anemia. *Pediatr Pulmonol.* 2008;43:1061–1066.

Gladwin MT, Sachdev V, Jison ML, et al. Pulmonary hypertension as a risk factor for death in patients with sickle cell disease. *N Engl J Med.* 2004;350:886–895.

Klings ES, Wyszynski DF, Nolan VG, et al. Abnormal pulmonary function in adults with sickle cell anemia. *Am J Respir Crit Care Med.* 2006;173:1264–1269.

MacLean JE, Atenafu E, Kirby-Allen M, et al. Longitudinal decline in lung volume in a population of children with sickle cell disease. *Am J Respir Crit Care Med.* 2008;178:1055–1059.

Platt OS, Brambilla DJ, Rosse WF, et al. Mortality in sickle cell disease. Life expectancy and risk factors for early death. *N Engl J Med.* 1994;330:1639–1644.

Powars D, Weidman JA, Odom-Maryon T, et al. Sickle cell chronic lung disease: prior morbidity and the risk of pulmonary failure. *Medicine (Baltimore).* 1988;67:66–76.

Vichinsky EP, Neumayr LD, Earles AN, et al. Causes and outcomes of the acute chest syndrome in sickle cell disease. National Acute Chest Syndrome Study Group. *N Engl J Med.* 2000;342:1855–1865.

References

The complete reference list is available online at www.expertconsult.com

74 LUNG INJURY CAUSED BY PHARMACOLOGIC AGENTS

MARIANNA M. HENRY, MD, MPH, AND TERRY L. NOAH, MD

Numerous drugs can cause pulmonary or pleural reactions in children. The most frequent offenders are chemotherapeutic agents used in the treatment of childhood neoplasms (Table 74-1), although toxic effects of other agents are increasingly recognized (Table 74-2).[1,2] Diffuse interstitial pneumonitis and fibrosis constitutes the most frequent clinical syndrome. Hypersensitivity lung disease, noncardiogenic pulmonary edema, pleural effusion, bronchiolitis obliterans, and alveolar hemorrhage are also encountered.

Although some drug-induced pulmonary damage is reversible, persistent and even fatal dysfunction may occur. Lung reactions occasionally are temporally remote from exposure to chemotherapeutic agents. Depending on the agent involved, the reaction may or may not be dose related. The mechanism of toxicity is thought to be direct injury to lung cells in most cases, but immunologic and central nervous system–mediated mechanisms seem to play a role in the toxicity of certain agents. Identified risk factors associated with cytotoxic drug therapy vary, but include cumulative dose, age of patient, prior or concurrent radiation, oxygen therapy, and use of other toxic drugs. Most reactions to noncytotoxic drugs appear to develop idiosyncratically. When patients are treated with combinations of potentially toxic drugs or with a toxic drug plus irradiation to the chest or high concentrations of oxygen (as is common in the treatment of childhood cancers), specific offenders often cannot be identified. There is little if any evidence that children are more susceptible to drug-related pulmonary injury, and in fact they may be less susceptible to some agents such as bleomycin.

The clinical presentation of drug-induced lung disease often includes fever, malaise, dyspnea, and nonproductive cough. Radiologic studies almost always demonstrate diffuse alveolar and/or interstitial involvement. Segmental or lobar disease, particularly if unilateral, should suggest another diagnosis. Abnormal pulmonary function, indicative of restrictive or obstructive disease, may be found before appearance of roentgenographic lesions. Chest CT may also provide early evidence of parenchymal abnormalities. Hypoxemia is an early and clinically important functional consequence. Pathologic features do not distinguish among most drugs and most often consist of interstitial thickening with chronic inflammatory cell infiltrate in the interstitial or alveolar compartment, fibroblast proliferation, fibrosis, and hyperplasia of type II pneumocytes, which contain enlarged hyperchromatic nuclei.[3] With hypersensitivity reactions, the interstitial infiltrate includes substantial numbers of eosinophils. Interstitial pneumonitis can be part of the multisystem syndrome known as "drug-induced hypersensitivity syndrome/drug rash with eosinophilia and systemic symptoms" (DIHS/DRESS).[4] Other diagnoses, such as infection, pulmonary hemorrhage, lung disease related to an underlying disorder, and radiation damage, must be considered in patients with suspected drug-induced lung injury. Bronchoalveolar lavage (BAL) is increasingly utilized to provide microbiologic and cytologic information essential to differential diagnosis and as a tool to begin to identify disease markers and potential pathogenetic mechanisms.[5]

Practical criteria for diagnosing drug-induced lung disease have been suggested by Allen.[6] These include (1) no other likely cause of lung disease; (2) symptoms consistent with the suspect drug; (3) time course compatible with drug-induced lung disease; (4) compatible tissue or BAL findings; and (5) improvement after the drug is discontinued.

CYTOTOXIC DRUGS USED IN CANCER THERAPY

Survivors of childhood cancers have often been exposed to multiple cytotoxic agents with potential lung toxicity, in addition to radiation, and are thus at increased risk for long-term pulmonary complications from these agents. A recent review by the Children's Oncology Group Guideline Task Force on Pulmonary Complications recommended that health care providers following such children receive a standardized cancer treatment summary from their oncologist to assess the risk for pulmonary complications; pediatric cancer survivors who received bleomycin or who are subsequently undergoing general anesthesia for procedures should have lung function monitored.[7]

ANTIBIOTICS

Bleomycin

Bleomycin is a mixture of peptide antibiotics obtained from *Streptomyces verticillus*. Its major use in children is in the treatment of Hodgkin's disease and other lymphomas. Because of the high frequency of pulmonary reactions and the utility of bleomycin for generating animal models of lung fibrosis, this agent has been studied more thoroughly than others. Pulmonary damage develops in two distinct patterns, most commonly progressive fibrosis and uncommonly an acute hypersensitivity reaction.

Pulmonary disease secondary to bleomycin occurs in as many as 40% of patients receiving the drug,[8] though frequency of reactions in children is not well documented. Multivariate analyses of follow-up data from the

TABLE 74-1 CYTOTOXIC DRUGS USED IN CANCER THERAPY

	INCIDENCE (%)	MORTALITY (%)	CLINICAL/PATHOLOGIC SYNDROMES
Bleomycin	2-40	1-10	IP/PF, H, P Eff, EP
Cyclophosphamide	≤1	40	IP/PF, PE, B
Chlorambucil	*	≤50	IP/PF
Busulfan	2-43	**	IP/PF, P Eff
Melphalan	*	≤60	IP/PF
Carmustine	10-30	15-90	IP/PF
Methotrexate	8	1	IP/PF, H, PE, P Eff
6-Mercaptopurine	*	**	IP/PF
Cytosine arabinoside	13-28	50	IP/PF, PE, BOOP, DMD
Gemcitabine	*	*	IP, B, PE
Fludaribine	9	*	IP/PF
Hydroxyurea	*	*	H
Paclitaxel	4-9	0	H
Docetaxel	73	0	Decreased DL_{CO}
Imitanib	*	*	P Eff, PE
Interleukin-2	>50	0	PE, P Eff
All-*trans* retinoic acid (ATRA)	5-27	5-29	IP, P Eff, PE, AH

*Infrequent case reports.
**Unknown.
BOOP, Bronchiolitis obliterans organizing pneumonia; *B,* bronchospasm; *DMD,* diffuse micronodular disease; *EP,* eosinophilic pneumonitis; *H,* hypersensitivity lung reaction; *IP,* interstitial pneumonitis; *PE,* pulmonary edema (noncardiogenic); *P Eff,* pleural effusion; *PF,* pulmonary fibrosis.

multicenter Childhood Cancer Survivor Study indicate that the use of bleomycin is significantly associated with lung fibrosis (RR 1.7), bronchitis (RR 1.4), and chronic cough (RR 1.9) ≥5 years postdiagnosis.[9] Bleomycin-induced pneumonitis may be diagnosed years after its use, as reported in a 15-year-old girl who had received bleomycin as an infant for yolk sac carcinoma.[10] Significant lung damage rarely occurs in adults at cumulative doses less than 150 mg. When more than 283 mg/m[2] is administered, 50% of adult patients develop severe pneumonitis.[11] Pulmonary damage is more severe in elderly than in young patients and in those with reduced glomerular filtration rate.[8] Slow intravenous administration results in less lung disease than intramuscular injection or intravenous bolus. The combination of radiotherapy or high inspired oxygen concentrations and bleomycin produces more lung injury than either alone. Pulmonary toxicity associated with relatively small quantities of bleomycin has been reported during combination drug therapy,[12] and pediatric sarcoma or Hodgkin's disease patients receiving bleomycin have increased risk for radiation pneumonitis.[13]

Pulmonary injury caused by bleomycin occurs by direct injury to cells as well as by secondary immunologic reactions. Direct toxicity may be mediated by oxidant injury, either through the production of reactive oxygen metabolites or through inactivation of antioxidants. Data supporting this mechanism include the findings that pretreatment of rodents with antioxidants or upregulation of the antioxidant gene transcription factor Nrf2 can reduce subsequent bleomycin-induced pulmonary fibrosis.[14–16] Additionally, bleomycin may directly induce senescence or apoptosis of type II epithelial cells.[17–19] Bleomycin also generates production of inflammatory mediators by lung cells.[20–25] Inflammatory cells may participate in further oxidant and proteolytic damage to lung cells.[26] Bleomycin promptly increases collagen synthesis by fibroblasts, an effect that may be mediated by transforming growth factor β.[27] Anti-inflammatory agents, antioxidants, and, specifically, nebulized heparin or urokinase can inhibit bleomycin-induced lung damage in animal models.[28,29] Gunther and colleagues[30] have reported complete abrogation of bleomycin-induced pulmonary fibrosis in rabbits using nebulized heparin or urokinase.

Bleomycin-induced lung disease can begin insidiously. Asymptomatic patients may have decreases in arterial oxygen saturation and carbon monoxide diffusing capacity (DL_{CO}). As the illness progresses, there is a decline in vital capacity and total lung capacity, characteristic of restrictive lung disease. In both interstitial pneumonitis and hypersensitivity lung reactions, patients typically present

TABLE 74-2 NONCYTOTOXIC AND OTHER DRUGS

	RECORDED CASES OR INCIDENCE	MORTALITY	CLINICAL / PATHOLOGIC SYNDROMES
Nitrofurantoin	>500 adult 8 pediatric	8%	H, IP/PF, B, AH, P Eff, BOOP, GIP
Sulfasalazine	>50 adult	2 cases	H, BOOP, FA, B
Diphenylhydantoin	7 adult 5 pediatric	0	H, B, BOOP
Carbamazepine	7 adult 7 pediatric	0	H, IP/EP, B, BOOP
Levetiracetam	1 pediatric	0	IP
Minocycline	>50 adult and adolescent	*	EP
Pencillamine	>40 adult 1 pediatric	50% (AH, BO)	H, DA, BOOP, AH
Leflunomide	>30 adult	20%	IP, DAD
Azathioprine	*	**	IP/PF, BOOP
Amiodarone	5%-15% 4 pediatric	5%-10%	H, IP/PF, BOOP, ARDS, P Eff, AH
Pegylated interferon	*	7%	IP

*Infrequent case reports.
**Unknown.
AH, Alveolar hemorrhage; *ARDS*, adult respiratory distress syndrome; *B*, bronchospasm; *BO*, bronchiolitis pneumonia; *DA*, diffuse alveolitis; *DAD*, diffuse alveolar damage; *EP*, eosinophilic pneumonia; *FA*, fibrosing alveolitis; *GIP*, giant cell interstitial pneumonia; *H*, hypersensitivity lung reaction; *IP/PF*, interstitial pneumonitis/pulmonary fibrosis; *PE*, pulmonary edema; *P Eff*, pleural effusion.

with a dry hacking cough and dyspnea; these signs occur only on exertion in mild cases, but profound respiratory distress accompanies advanced illness. Fever suggests a hypersensitivity reaction. Physical examination reveals tachypnea and fine crackles. Chest roentgenograms in symptomatic patients most commonly demonstrate diffuse linear densities. A widespread reticulonodular or alveolar pattern may also be seen. Chest CT is more sensitive for detection of early interstitial disease, and in animal models chest CT findings correlate well with pathologic changes.[31,32] Biopsy specimens usually reveal interstitial pneumonitis, fibrosis, and extensive alveolar damage with hyperplasia of type II cells, most prominently in subpleural and basilar regions.

Patients receiving bleomycin should be monitored by serial determinations of DL_{CO}. Chest CT may also be useful for monitoring disease progression, although radiation exposure from this source cannot be ignored.[32] Therapy of bleomycin-induced pneumonitis consists largely of supportive measures. Withdrawal of the drug at the onset of toxicity must be considered. Careful monitoring of oxygen therapy to avoid excessive exposure is imperative.[33] Although the inflammatory cell element resolves substantially with therapy, much of the fibrotic damage is irreversible. Treatment with bleomycin is a significant predictor of long-term respiratory symptomatology and pulmonary function decrements in survivors of Hodgkin's disease.[34] The use of steroids is controversial, but reversal of severe toxicity has been documented in some patients after use of high-dose steroids.[35] In the few patients exhibiting hypersensitivity reactions or eosinophilic pneumonitis with bleomycin,[36] corticosteroids have a definite role.

ALKYLATING AGENTS

Cyclophosphamide

Cyclophosphamide is widely used in the treatment of leukemias, lymphomas, and nonmalignant illnesses. Although pulmonary toxicity is uncommon, it does produce severe and even fatal lung damage.[37,38] Data from the Childhood Cancer Survivor Study indicate a significantly increased long-term risk for supplemental oxygen requirement, recurrent pneumonia, chronic cough, dyspnea on exertion, and bronchitis.[9] Frankovich and coworkers[39] reported a series of 34 children who underwent autologous bone marrow transplant for relapsing Hodgkin's disease and were treated with cyclophosphamide in combination with etoposide and either carmustine, chloroethylcyclohexylnitrosourea, or irradiation. Fifteen of these patients developed lung injury syndromes including interstitial pneumonitis, acute alveolitis, diffuse alveolar hemorrhage, ARDS, and bronchiolitis obliterans. Four of the patients died of pulmonary complications. In this series, a history of atopy was associated with pulmonary complications. Experiments in rodents indicate that as for bleomycin, both oxidant and inflammatory or immune mechanisms are involved in cyclophosphamide lung toxicity.[40–43] Acute IgE-mediated systemic reactions have been reported, including angioedema and bronchospasm. Cyclophosphamide also may predispose to toxicity when medications such as bleomycin, azathioprine, and carmustine are used subsequently.

Little is known about the relationship of dose, duration, and frequency of administration to the appearance of parenchymal disease in humans, though cytotoxicity appears to be dose-related in rats.[41] Pulmonary reactions have occurred following total doses between 0.15 and 50 g. Pulmonary disease may begin during cyclophosphamide therapy or weeks to years after.[44,45] A striking feature in pediatric cases has been chest wall deformity secondary to failure of lung growth during the adolescent growth spurt.[45] Subacute dry cough and dyspnea herald the onset of pulmonary toxicity; malaise, anorexia, and weight loss follow.[44,46] Physical examination reveals tachypnea and diffusely diminished breath sounds. Chest roentgenograms may show diffuse bilateral infiltrates, sometimes with pleural thickening. Pulmonary function testing reveals hypoxemia and restrictive lung disease. Biopsy and postmortem specimens show interstitial fibrosis, alveolar exudates, and atypical alveolar epithelial cells.[44,46] Withdrawal of the drug, supportive therapy, and corticosteroids are the recommended treatment.

Chlorambucil

Chlorambucil is used in the treatment of leukemias, some lymphomas, nephrosis, and inflammatory conditions such as sarcoidosis.[47] Several reports indicate that the drug produces pulmonary toxicity, albeit rarely. Little is known concerning the dose or duration of therapy necessary to produce lung damage. Patients develop cough, dyspnea, fatigue, and weight loss that appears 6 months to 3 years after initiation of therapy and progressively worsens.[48,49] Physical examination reveals tachypnea and fine bibasilar crackles. Chest roentgenograms demonstrate a diffuse interstitial infiltrate. Pulmonary function tests indicate restrictive lung disease accompanied by a defect in DL_{CO}. Histopathologic findings are similar to those associated with busulfan and cyclophosphamide therapy.[48,49] Although improvement with discontinuation of the drug and corticosteroid therapy has been reported,[50] progression of disease may occur approach.[48]

Other Alkylating Agents

Busulfan (Myleran) is used to treat chronic myelogenous leukemia, which occurs occasionally in childhood, and in some preparative regimens for bone marrow transplantation. Four percent of adult patients undergoing long-term treatment with this drug develop interstitial pneumonitis and fibrosis.[51] Mertens and colleagues[9] reported increased long-term risk for supplemental oxygen requirement and pleurisy after busulfan treatment. As with chlorambucil, pulmonary injury is usually not evident for many months after initiation of treatment. Radiation and previous cytotoxic therapy are risk factors.[52] The clinical syndrome is similar to that produced by the other alkylating agents.[51] Treatment consists of discontinuation of busulfan. Efficacy of corticosteroids is unproven, but a carefully monitored trial is indicated because of the poor prognosis.

An increase in incidence of alveolar hemorrhage has been reported when *etoposide* (VP-16) was added to a regimen of busulfan and cyclophosphamide for bone marrow transplantation; toxicity in this study was largely confined to patients who had been given prior chest radiotherapy.[53] However, Quigley and coworkers[54] found that in children, preparative regimens for bone marrow transplantation that included busulfan were associated with preservation of pulmonary function compared to regimens using other combination high-dose chemotherapeutic regimens or total body irradiation.

Melphalan is used primarily in the treatment of multiple myelomas and hence is employed infrequently in pediatrics. Although overt toxicity is unusual, the frequency of epithelial changes and fibrosis at autopsy may be as high as 50%.[55] Bronchial epithelial cell proliferation has been an unusual finding. Otherwise, the pathologic changes are typical for alkylating agents and may be reversible with discontinuation of the drug.[56]

◼ NITROSOUREAS

Carmustine

Carmustine, also called BCNU, is a synthetic antineoplastic compound. Its major use is in the therapy of lymphomas and gliomas. The incidence of BCNU pulmonary toxicity is quite variable; 20% to 30% of treated patients develop some lung disease.[57,58] The total dose administered, duration of therapy, and preexistence of lung disease are the most accurate predictors of pulmonary toxicity. Most patients with symptomatic respiratory disease have received large cumulative doses ($>777 \, mg/m^2$). Patients with toxicity also appear to have received the drug over a shorter period, irrespective of the total dose given. The onset of pulmonary symptoms has been noted between 30 and 371 days after institution of therapy, sometimes after BCNU has been discontinued. Young patients reportedly are at greater risk, but this may be the result of relatively higher doses and increased numbers of therapy cycles because of greater general tolerance. Mertens and colleagues[9] reported a significant risk for supplemental oxygen requirement among children older than 5 years of age status post-BCNU or -lomustine (CCNU) treatment. A study of 73 children with high-grade glioma treated with the combination of BCNU, cisplatin, and vincristine reported that 7 children developed interstitial pneumonitis, which was fatal in 6.[59] Radiation therapy may be synergistic. In adult patients, female gender and combination with cyclophosphamide have been identified as risk factors for pulmonary complications.[58,60]

Patients with BCNU pulmonary toxicity exhibit much the same clinical picture as that described for bleomycin.[57] Histologic findings are also similar. In a study of 8 patients who underwent lung biopsy 12 to 17 years after treatment with BCNU, there was electron microscopic evidence of ongoing endothelial and epithelial damage, suggesting long-term toxic effects of the drug.[61] One of these patients died with pulmonary hypertension due to interstitial fibrosis. The disease is fatal in approximately 15% of those affected.

Therapy is essentially supportive. Corticosteroids are often administered concomitantly with BCNU for brain tumors and afford no protection from subsequent pulmonary toxicity. However, corticosteroids may offer some benefit in the treatment of early stages of acute disease. Thymidine has been used as a biomodulator to protect from BCNU pulmonary toxicity in patients with malignant melanoma and may act via modulation of DNA repair enzymes in normal tissue.[62] In a rat model, metallothionein attenuated BCNU toxicity via antioxidant effects.[63]

ANTIMETABOLITES

Methotrexate

Methotrexate (4-aminopteroylglutamic acid) is a folic acid antagonist used in the treatment of several childhood malignancies, notably leukemias and osteogenic sarcoma as well as nonmalignant conditions such as rheumatoid arthritis and psoriasis.[64,65] The lung inflammation induced by methotrexate appears to be linked to activation of the p38 MAP kinase signaling pathway, with subsequent cytokine activation.[66] Prevalence rates of 0.3% to 11.6% have been reported for pulmonary toxicity caused by methotrexate, but ascertainment of its effects is complicated by the frequent use of combination therapy and the tendency of underlying diseases such as rheumatoid arthritis to also cause lung disease.[65] No correlation has been found between lung toxicity and dose of methotrexate, and pneumonitis may occur remotely.

The clinical features of methotrexate lung toxicity are consistent with a hypersensitivity pneumonitis.[67] Disease usually begins with a prodrome of headache and malaise, followed by dyspnea and dry cough. Pleuritic pain is rare. Fever may also occur. Physical examination reveals tachypnea, diffuse crackles, cyanosis, and occasionally skin eruptions. Hypoxemia is observed in 90% to 95% of patients, and mild eosinophilia has been reported in 41%.[65] Few reports have documented pulmonary function changes, but decreased DL_{CO} may occur.[68] Lung function testing in a series of children with juvenile rheumatoid arthritis who received methotrexate showed a similar incidence of abnormal function, including DL_{CO}, to a control population not receiving methotrexate.[69] The most common abnormalities on chest radiographs are bilateral interstitial infiltrates or mixed interstitial and alveolar infiltrates. Lung biopsy in adults reveals interstitial pneumonitis with lymphocytic and sometimes eosinophilic infiltrates, bronchiolitis, and granuloma formation consistent with a hypersensitivity reaction, although type II alveolar cell hyperplasia typical of cytotoxicity has also been found.[70,71] BAL fluids typically show lymphocytosis with variable CD4/CD8 ratios and moderate neutrophilia.[72,73]

Diagnosis of methotrexate-induced pneumonitis is difficult because this condition may mimic other diseases. Pulmonary infection must be excluded, particularly if high-dose methotrexate is used or if the underlying disease is associated with immunosuppression. Therapy consists of withdrawal of the drug and administration of corticosteroids, but the latter has not been analyzed in controlled trials. Treatment with folinic acid (leucovorin rescue) does not prevent methotrexate lung toxicity.[65] Outcome is usually favorable with clinical improvement preceding radiographic and pulmonary function improvement.[65,74] Two fatal outcomes in arthritis patients with a history of lung toxicity suggest that retreatment should be avoided after recovery from methotrexate lung injury.[75]

6-Mercaptopurine, Cytosine Arabinoside, and Gemcitabine

Scattered case reports have linked pulmonary dysfunction to 6-mercaptopurine and cytosine arabinoside. In addition, an autopsy study of patients who had leukemia and who received cytosine arabinoside within 30 days of death demonstrated significant pulmonary edema for which there was no obvious other explanation in most instances. An adult patient receiving low-dose cytosine arabinoside (20 mg/m²/day) and recombinant human granulocyte-macrophage colony-stimulating factor (GM-CSF) developed ARDS on day 12 and died 40 days after initiation of therapy.[76] In a recent report, 5 of 22 pediatric patients receiving Ara-C (1 to 1.5 g/m²/day) for treatment of acute myelogenous leukemia developed pulmonary insufficiency secondary to noncardiogenic pulmonary edema. The outcome was fatal in 3 of 5 patients.[77] Bronchiolitis obliterans organizing pneumonia (BOOP) developed in an adult patient with chronic myelogenous leukemia after treatment with Ara-C in combination with interferon-alpha; the condition resolved after discontinuation of these agents.[78] Chagnon and coworkers[79] described a series of 6 young adults with acute myelogenous leukemia who developed fever and diffuse micronodular lung disease associated with high-dose Ara-C. *Gemcitabine*, a similar drug in structure and metabolism to Ara-C, has been associated with ARDS in three patients.[80] These authors reported that corticosteroids and diuretics were helpful, but two of the three patients died. Gemcitabine has also been associated with dyspnea, bronchoconstriction, and nonspecific pneumonitis, particularly in Hodgkin's disease patients also treated with bleomycin.[81] The nucleoside analog fludaribine, used in the treatment of lymphoma and chronic lymphocytic leukemia, is associated with steroid-responsive interstitial disease in 9% of cases.[82]

Other Cytotoxic Agents

Procarbazine, VM-26, and vinca alkaloids (vinblastine and vindesine) have been associated with pulmonary injury, but in all cases other agents may have contributed. Three of 5 young adults treated with a regimen of vinblastine, doxorubicin, bleomycin, and dacarbazine for Hodgkin's disease, and granulocyte colony-stimulating factor (G-CSF) to increase neutrophil counts, developed pulmonary toxicity in one report.[12] G-CSF may thus potentiate the lung toxicity of these agents. Reactions to procarbazine have been of the hypersensitivity type. Hydroxyurea has been reported to induce severe, corticosteroid-responsive, hypersensitivity pneumonitis.[83] Paclitaxel is a plant-derived taxane agent that has been used against a broad range of tumors, including breast, ovarian, lung, head, and neck cancers. It has been associated with a high frequency of hypersensitivity pneumonitis reactions. Lung biopsy has shown interstitial pneumonitis, and BAL fluid has shown eosinophilia and lymphocytosis with a depressed CD4/CD8 ratio.[84] In a 5-year review of a series of cancer patients who received monthly paclitaxel infusions, the incidence of hypersensitivity reactions was 4%, and pretreatment with dexamethasone, diphenhydramine, and H_2 blockers was effective in preventing recurrence.[85] Interstitial pneumonitis is more common when paclitaxel is combined with radiation therapy [86] and has been reported in association with a paclitaxel-eluting coronary artery stent.[87] Docetaxel, a semisynthetic taxane, has been proposed as a safer alternative but has also occasionally been associated with severe hypersensitivity reactions.[88,89] A series of asymptomatic adult cancer patients who received docetaxel monotherapy for non-lung cancers had a small but significant drop in lung function posttreatment.[90] Oxaliplatin appeared to cause cryptogenic organizing pneumonitis in a 30-year-old patient being treated for colorectal cancer.[91]

Gefitinib is an inhibitor of the tyrosine kinase activity of the epidermal growth factor receptor (EGFR). It inhibits the growth of human cancer cell lines expressing EGFR in preclinical studies. In clinical trials in patients with non–small cell lung cancer, geftinib was associated with development of interstitial lung disease in about 1% of patients. Patients presented with acute dyspnea with or without cough or fever, at a median of 24 to 42 days after starting treatment. About one-third of cases of geftinib-associated interstitial lung disease have been fatal.[92,93] Another tyrosine kinase inhibitor, imitanib, is used in treatment of chronic myelogenous leukemia and has been associated with pleural effusion and pulmonary edema in a small number of cases.[94] Such drugs targeting specific molecular pathways are likely to be increasingly used in cancer treatment in the future.[95]

Interleukin-2 (IL-2) has been used as an antitumor factor that stimulates lymphokine-activated killer (LAK) cell and natural killer cell activity. It is sometimes given in combination with LAK cells. Although a number of systemic side effects (e.g., fever and hypotension) are seen, its major toxicity appears to be a vascular leak syndrome characterized by fluid retention, peripheral edema, ascites, pleural effusion, and pulmonary edema.[96] This syndrome has been described in children with ALL treated with IL-2.[97] Infusion of IL-2 in cancer patients has resulted in increased alveolar-arterial oxygen gradients and decreased FVC, FEV_1, and DL_{CO}.[98,99] A retrospective review of chest radiographic abnormalities in 54 patients with metastatic cancer receiving IL-2 revealed that 52% developed pleural effusion, 41% developed pulmonary edema, and 22% developed focal infiltrates. While most changes resolved by 4 weeks after therapy, residual pleural effusion was sometimes seen primarily in patients receiving IL-2 by intravenous bolus rather than by continuous infusion.[100] Lung histopathology in rodents shows widespread mononuclear and eosinophilic infiltration of parenchyma, increased lung weight, and endothelial damage.[101] Mechanisms implicated are increased generation of oxygen-free radicals, activation of complement by IL-2, and injury mediated by TNF-α.[102–104] Rapid recovery from the toxic effects of IL-2 followed withholding of treatment in most cases.[99]

All-*trans* retinoic acid (ATRA), a vitamin A derivative with multiple regulatory activities in the lung, is effective as induction and maintenance chemotherapy for acute promyelocytic leukemia (APL). Its major toxicity is a syndrome including fever, weight gain, peripheral edema, respiratory distress, interstitial infiltrates, pleural and pericardial effusions, hyperleukocytosis, intermittent hypotension, and acute renal failure. Chest CT shows small, irregular parenchymal lung nodules and pleural effusions.[105] The incidence of ATRA syndrome was 26% in a large series of APL patients followed prospectively.[106] Among patients developing ATRA syndrome, mortality was 2% including a 4-year-old child. Mean duration of therapy before the syndrome appeared was 11 days with a range of 2 to 47 days. Nicolls and colleagues[107] reported an 18-year-old patient with APL who developed diffuse alveolar hemorrhage 15 days after starting ATRA. Lung histology in patients who died of ATRA syndrome showed differentiation of APL cells, endothelial cell damage, and leukocyte infiltration.[106] ATRA may upregulate TNF receptors on lung cell lines.[108] In a murine model of APL, ATRA increased lung and heart expression of chemokines MIP-2 and KC, suggesting that pro-inflammatory cytokines play a role.[109] Treatment for ATRA syndrome consists of prompt initiation of corticosteroids. Tallman and coworkers[106] used dexamethasone 10 mg per day and found that the syndrome resolved rapidly in most patients, even if ATRA was continued. These authors suggested that ATRA may be safely restarted in most patients once the syndrome has resolved. The *cis*-retinoic acids used for the treatment of neuroblastoma have not been associated with lung toxicities.

NON-CYTOTOXIC AND OTHER DRUGS

Nitrofurantoin

Nitrofurantoin is an antimicrobial agent used for prophylaxis of urinary tract infections. Significant pulmonary reactions are relatively common; more than 500 cases have been reported, including children (see Table 74-2).[110–115] Pulmonary reactions occur in two distinct clinical patterns. In the more common acute presentation, patients report abrupt onset of fever, cough, and dyspnea within hours to 2 weeks after initiation of therapy. Rash and flulike symptoms may occur. Diffuse fine crackles and, rarely, wheezes are noted. Bilateral interstitial or alveolar infiltrates with or without pleural effusion are characteristically present, though chest radiographs may be normal. Physiologic abnormalities include hypoxemia, evidence of a restrictive ventilatory defect, and reduced DL_{CO}. Eosinophilia, leukocytosis, and an elevated sedimentation rate may accompany the reaction. Symptoms and chest radiographic abnormalities usually resolve within several days after withdrawal of the drug. Pulmonary histopathology of the acute syndrome has not been well defined as patients improve rapidly, making biopsy unnecessary. Alveolar hemorrhage has been described in two patients.[116,117]

In the less common chronic presentation, patients develop insidious onset of cough, dyspnea, and chest pain after months to years of nitrofurantoin therapy.[118] Fever may be present. A lupus-like syndrome has also been reported.[114] Crackles are heard, and diffuse interstitial infiltrates are present on chest radiographs. Pleural effusion is less common than in the acute reaction. Physiologic abnormalities are similar to those found in the acute reaction but are often more severe. Eosinophilia, elevated gamma globulin and hepatic enzymes, and positive reactions for antinuclear antibodies are often found. Pulmonary histopathology typically reveals interstitial pneumonitis with variable fibrosis. Desquamative interstitial pneumonia, BOOP, and giant cell interstitial pneumonia have also been reported in several adults on long-term nitrofurantoin therapy.[119-121] Treatment includes withdrawal of the drug and supportive measures. Corticosteroids have been used with apparent benefit; however, controlled studies to evaluate efficacy are not available. Resolution of symptoms, physiologic dysfunction, and radiographic abnormalities require weeks to months and may be incomplete. Approximately 8% of adult cases with the chronic syndrome are fatal.

The findings of eosinophilia, elevation of sedimentation rate, and positive antinuclear antibodies support a role for immunologic mechanisms of injury.[122] The drug may also damage the lungs by promoting production of toxic oxygen species.[123-125]

Sulfasalazine

Sulfasalazine, a combination of sulfapyridine and 5-aminosalicylic acid, is used primarily in the treatment of ulcerative colitis. Adverse reactions occur in approximately 20% of recipients, but pulmonary reactions are uncommon; 50 cases were identified in a recent review.[126-130] Diagnosis can be a challenge because ulcerative colitis is at times associated with lung disorders including bronchitis, BOOP, bronchiectasis, and interstitial pneumonitis.[131-133] Patients experiencing drug-related illness report acute onset of fever, cough, dyspnea, and chest pain 1 to 6 months into therapy. Fine crackles are usually present. Bilateral alveolar densities, eosinophilia, hypoxemia, and obstructive and occasionally restrictive pulmonary function patterns have been noted. Cytology from BAL fluid has no consistent pattern of cell predominance. Histopathologic lesions include interstitial pneumonitis with fibrosis, fibrosing alveolitis, and bronchiolitis obliterans with or without a component of organizing pneumonia. Discontinuation of the drug usually results in resolution of symptoms and radiographic abnormalities in several weeks to months. Corticosteroids may accelerate improvement, although effectiveness is not well established. Two fatalities have been reported.[134] The mechanism of toxicity is unknown.[130]

Diphenylhydantoin, Carbamazepine, and Levetiracetam

The anticonvulsant agents diphenylhydantoin and carbamazepine have been associated rarely with acute pulmonary disease as part of a generalized hypersensitivity reaction, including the syndrome of drug reaction with eosinophilia and systemic symptoms (DRESS syndrome).[135-140] Clinical manifestations include fever, cough, dyspnea, and rash occurring typically 2 to 8 weeks after initiation of therapy. Facial swelling and lymphadenopathy may be prominent. Crackles and, rarely, wheezes are heard; bilateral interstitial or alveolar infiltrates, sometimes with hilar adenopathy, are seen on chest radiographs. Associated findings include eosinophilia, elevated liver enzymes, hypoxemia with a restrictive pattern of lung function, and reduced DL_{CO}. Cell counts from BAL fluid reveal lymphocyte predominance, and lung biopsy typically shows interstitial pneumonitis, possibly with mild fibrosis, and rarely BOOP.[141,142] Ventilatory failure has been described.[142] Rapid improvement occurs over days to weeks following discontinuation of the drug, though manifestations may linger with multisystem involvement. Resolution may be hastened by corticosteroid administration. Interestingly, carbamazapine hypersensitivity has been implicated in the occurrence of interstitial pneumonitis/eosinophilic pneumonia in an adolescent with CF on immunosuppressive therapy following lung transplant.[143] Levetiracetam has been associated with biopsy demonstrating diffuse interstitial lung disease in a child.[144]

Minocycline

Multisystem hypersensitivity with a prominent component of skin rash has been associated with minocycline. More than 50 cases have involved the lung, often in adolescents and young adults treated for acne.[137,145-148] Eosinophilic pneumonia has been suggested by the finding of excess eosinophils in blood or BAL fluid or identified on lung biopsy. Minocycline-associated lupus has been well described. Infrequently, significant organ dysfunction with or without lung involvement has been reported including hyperthyroidism or hypothyroidism, renal failure, hepatitis (sometimes in an autoimmune pattern), and, rarely, myocarditis.[149-151] Withdrawal of the drug typically prompts improvement, though resolution may require months. Corticosteroids may accelerate improvement and have been used in combination with immunosuppression for autoimmune hepatitis. Hypersensitivity to doxycycline has been implicated in a single case involving respiratory failure.[152]

Penicillamine

Penicillamine, a chelating agent, is commonly used to treat Wilson's disease, cystinuria, and lead poisoning and, occasionally, rheumatoid arthritis and primary biliary cirrhosis. A conclusive association of this agent with lung disease is problematic because similar lung disorders occur in underlying diseases.[153,154] More than 40 cases of penicillamine-associated lung disease are reported, primarily in patients with rheumatoid arthritis.[155,156] Several patterns have been described: diffuse alveolitis; hypersensitivity pneumonitis; alveolar hemorrhage with or without associated acute glomerulonephritis, similar to Goodpasture's syndrome; and obstructive airway disease characterized pathologically as bronchiolitis obliterans. Duration of therapy before onset of symptoms tends to be short in patients with hypersensitivity reactions (<2 months), intermediate with diffuse alveolitis and bronchiolitis obliterans (3 to 19 months), and prolonged with alveolar hemorrhage (7 months to 20 years, but typically 2 to 7 years). Cough and dyspnea develop progressively over several weeks but may begin abruptly in hypersensitivity reactions with hemoptysis. Crackles and occasional wheezes are present. Elevation of sedimentation rate, increased serum IgE, and eosinophilia may be noted. Chest radiographs show diffuse alveolar or interstitial infiltrate, hyperinflation alone or no changes. Hypoxemia and severe obstructive lung disease are usually identified in patients with bronchiolitis obliterans, or restrictive disease in those with alveolitis or hypersensitivity disease. Discontinuation of the drug and corticosteroid therapy is warranted in most cases. Diffuse alveolitis and hypersensitivity pneumonitis generally improve using this approach, although some patients have residual lung disease. Response to corticosteroids alone has been disappointing in most cases of bronchiolitis obliterans and alveolar hemorrhage. Addition of azathioprine or cyclophosphamide in combination with plasmapheresis has been beneficial in several patients with Goodpasture's-like syndrome and in a single patient with bronchiolitis obliterans.[156-160]

Leflunomide

Leflunomide, an immunomodulatory drug that inhibits pyrimidine synthesis in activated lymphocytes that is used in treatment of rheumatoid arthritis and other autoimmune disorders, has been associated rarely with significant lung injury.[161-173] Injury appears to be more likely in those with underlying interstitial lung disease.[174,175] Presentation typically includes acute onset of cough and dyspnea 12 to 20 weeks after its introduction (occasionally after its discontinuation) with crackles on exam and bilateral patchy densities on chest radiograph. Ground glass and reticular/interstitial densities are identified on chest CT. The most common histologic abnormalities are diffuse alveolar injury and interstitial pneumonia. Leflunomide should be discontinued when injury related to the drug is suspected. Because of its long half-life, some have advocated treatment with cholestyramine, though benefit is uncertain.[176] Steroid therapy has been recommended; however, effectiveness is unclear. Mortality of nearly 20% has been described in early reports.

Azathioprine

Azathioprine, an immunosuppressive agent, is used in a variety of pediatric clinical conditions including renal transplantation, inflammatory bowel disease, autoimmune disorders, idiopathic pulmonary hemosiderosis, and fibrosing alveolitis.[177] A small number of cases of dose-related toxicity have been reported in adults, largely after renal transplantation.[178] Fever and hypoxemia are major presenting manifestations. Lung biopsy specimens reveal diffuse alveolar damage including hyaline membranes, interstitial pneumonitis with fibrosis, and BOOP.[178,179] A hypersensitivity-like reaction including fever and hemoptysis was reported in a 21-year old treated with azathioprine for end-stage glomerulonephritis.[180] Improvement may follow withdrawal of the drug or treatment with corticosteroids or cyclophosphamide. Progressive deterioration and death have occurred in about one half of patients.

Other Immunomodulatory Agents

Drugs targeting or modifying immune pathways are increasingly used for a variety of chronic inflammatory diseases and after transplantation. Most information on pulmonary toxicities of these agents is from adult literature. Rituximab, a monoclonal antibody against CD20 expressed on B lymphocytes, has been associated with interstitial pneumonitis.[181] Infusion of alemtuzumab (Campath), a humanized monoclonal antibody against CD52 expressed on all lymphocytes, as well as some NK cells and monocytes, was associated with severe bronchospasm responsive to steroids in an adult with chronic lymphocytic leukemia.[182] Cetuximab, an anti-EFGR monoclonal antibody, caused dyspnea with infusion in 13% of adult colorectal cancer patients.[183] Trastuzumab, a humanized monoclonal antibody against the EGFR, has become standard treatment of HER2-expressing breast cancer. Acute interstitial pneumonitis developed after its infusion in a 56-year-old.[184] Infliximab (Remicade) is a TNF-α inhibitor used in the treatment of rheumatic and inflammatory bowel disease at all ages. Villeneuve and colleagues[185] described a 70-year-old with rheumatoid arthritis who developed acute interstitial pneumonitis after his third infusion of infliximab. Standard treatment for hepatitis C in children and adults is a combination of pegylated interferon and ribavirin. Interstitial pneumonitis with a 7% mortality was reported in adult HCV patients, treated with peg interferon α-2b.[186] Chronic use of sirolimus (rapamycin), an immunosuppressive agent used as an alternative to calcineurin inhibitors, was associated with evidence of interstitial pneumonitis or BOOP in 24 adults after renal transplant.[187]

Amiodarone

Amiodarone, a benzofurane derivative with Class III antiarrhythmic activity, is used in the treatment of serious cardiac rhythm disturbances.[188] Pulmonary toxicity is the most serious complication of therapy.[189-193] Risk of lung toxicity appears to be dose related. Approximately 5% to 15% of patients who take ≥500 mg/day and 0.1% to 0.5% of those who take up to 200 mg/day develop drug-related lung disease.[192] Most affected patients have been adults; however, lung toxicity has been reported in at least four children.[194-197] Exposure to elevated concentrations of oxygen may be risk factor.

Patients with this complication insidiously develop cough, dyspnea with exertion, weight loss, weakness, and, in some instances, pleuritic chest pain and fever, usually during the first year of therapy. Approximately one-third have an acute onset of symptoms, more consistent with hypersensitivity pneumonitis. Chest examination reveals tachypnea, crackles, and, occasionally, a pleural friction rub. Diffuse or asymmetrical interstitial or alveolar infiltrates are typically present on chest radiographs. Pleural effusion is uncommon.[198] High resolution chest CT scan shows bilateral involvement with ground-glass opacities accompanied by a crazy-paving pattern with or without subpleural consolidation and bronchial wall thickening or dilation.[199] Laboratory findings include leukocytosis, elevated hepatic enzymes, and a high sedimentation rate. Physiologic abnormalities include hypoxemia, restrictive lung disease, and impaired diffusion. ARDS has been described rarely in treated adults undergoing thoracic surgery and has been associated with mortality of 50%.[200] Lung biopsy reveals infiltration of alveolar septae with lymphocytes, plasma cells, and histiocytes; patchy fibrosis; hyperplasia of type II pneumocytes; and intra-alveolar foamy macrophages representing lysosomal accumulation of phospholipids.[201,202] Foamy macrophages can also be recovered in BAL fluid. Although their presence is not pathognomonic of drug-induced injury, it has been suggested that their absence makes the diagnosis unlikely. Discontinuation of the drug results in rapid symptomatic improvement in most patients and resolution of physiologic and radiographic abnormalities over several months. Clinical evidence supports corticosteroid treatment. Recurrence of symptoms has been observed in some patients as steroid doses are tapered, potentially related to extended storage of drug in the lung. Alternative approaches are limited for patients who must remain on amiodarone because of life-threatening refractory dysrhythmias. Reinstitution of amiodarone therapy at lower doses after resolution of pulmonary disease alone or in combination with low-dose corticosteroid therapy has been successful in a few patients.[203]

The mechanism by which amiodarone causes lung injury is unknown. The most striking morphologic alterations that require explanation are the accumulation of multilamellar bodies in the cytoplasm of various cells and inflammation. Direct toxicity is supported by the finding that amiodarone injured cultured pulmonary arterial endothelial cells at concentrations equivalent to those reported in lung tissues of toxic patients.[204] Cellular accumulation of phospholipid was also observed in these drug-exposed cultured endothelial cells, an event that may cause cell injury. The mechanism of phospholipid accumulation is thought to be related in part to inhibition of phospholipid degradation secondary to reduction in activities of lysosomal phospholipases A_1 and A_2 induced by the drug.[205,206] Oxidant-mediated lung injury,[207,208] apoptosis of pulmonary epithelial cells,[209] leakage of the alveolar-capillary membrane,[210] and indirect, immune-mediated mechanisms[211–213] have been suggested. Amiodarone can alter patterns of cytokine secretion by alveolar macrophages and activate natural killer cells, but it is unclear whether these changes are initiating events or consequence of injury.[206] Regardless of mechanism, injury can lead to fibrosis.

OTHER AGENTS

Acute respiratory deterioration has been observed when the antifungal agent amphotericin B is administered to potentially septic, neutropenic patients receiving leukocyte transfusions. Patients develop the acute onset of cough, hemoptysis, dyspnea, and hypoxemia in association with the appearance of new infiltrates on chest radiographs. In one study, this syndrome developed in 64% of courses of combined therapy compared with 6% of courses of leukocyte transfusions alone.[214] Subsequent studies have questioned the role of a specific interaction between amphotericin B and granulocyte transfusions in episodes of respiratory deterioration.[215] Approximately 20 pulmonary reactions have been reported to amphotericin B or to the newer lipidic formulations, including 2 in children.[216] Symptoms tend to resolve relatively quickly when the infusion is stopped. The pathophysiology of these reactions is unclear, though development of pulmonary hypertension may be an important component. Amphotericin injures endothelial cells directly, causes neutrophil-independent injury with oxidant stress and production of eicosanoids, and releases cyclo-oxygenase products of arachadonic acid metabolism.[216] Infusion-related toxicity of amphotericin B also likely involves massive release of inflammatory cytokines such as IL-1β and TNF-α.[217]

A number of other drugs have been implicated sporadically in the development of hypersensitivity/eosinophilic lung disease. Table 74-3 shows a representative list with a focus on medications that may be given to children or adolescents.[147,218–236] An extensive compilation has been published by Allen and coworkers.[6] Churg-Strauss syndrome (i.e., asthma, eosinophilia, neuropathy, pulmonary infiltrates, and sinus disease) has been linked to leukotriene antagonists in a small number of asthma case reports, including some in children.[231–233] Aspirin and other NSAIDs induce bronchoconstriction via altered eicosanoid metabolism in patients with aspirin-induced asthma syndrome, but this condition presents almost entirely in adults.[237,238]

TABLE 74-3 ADDITIONAL DRUGS ASSOCIATED WITH HYPERSENSITIVITY/EOSINOPHILIC LUNG DISEASE

Penicillin	Para-aminosalicylic acid	Cocaine
Ampicillin	Isoniazid	Heroin
Tetracycline	Cromolyn sodium	Dantrolene
Minocycline	Zafirlukast*	Chlorpropamide
Erythromycin	Montelukast*	Hydralazine
Clarithromycin	Methylphenidate	Enalapril
Cephalosporins	Imipramine	Captopril
Sulfa-containing antimicrobials	Nonsteroidal anti-inflammatory agents†	Ranitidine
Daptomycin	Trazodone‡	Mesalamine

*Associated with Churg-Strauss syndrome.
†Includes naproxen, sulindac, piroxicam, fenbufen, diclofenac, and ibuprofen.
‡With overdose.

TABLE 74-4 NONCYTOTOXIC DRUGS ASSOCIATED WITH NONCARDIOGENIC PULMONARY EDEMA

Aspirin*	Naloxone	Haloperidol
Propoxyphene*	Nitric oxide	Phenothiazines
Calcium channel blockers*	Morphine	Ethchlorvynol*
Propranolol	Heroin*	Tricyclic antidepressants*
Epinephrine	Methadone*	Hydrochlorothiazide
Phenylephrine	Cocaine	Acetazolamide
Lidocaine	Tocolytic agents	Radiographic contrast media

*Pulmonary edema associated with overdose.

Drugs producing a clinical syndrome consistent with noncardiogenic pulmonary edema are listed in Table 74-4,[239–258] as reviewed recently by Lee-Chiong and Matthay.[258] Some are associated with this clinical syndrome only after an overdose. Pulmonary edema is the pattern of injury most closely associated with heroin overdose. Smoking of crack cocaine can be associated with acute respiratory illness including direct thermal injury to airways and air leak syndromes. It is also associated with subacute syndromes including pulmonary edema, "crack lung" (dyspnea, hypoxia, diffuse alveolar damage, alveolar hemorrhage), interstitial pneumonitis, and BOOP.[259–260] Cannabis smoking can be associated with chronic bronchitis or emphysematous changes with secondary pneumothorax.[261] For both crack cocaine and cannabis, the tendency for air leak is likely related to deep inhalation with the Valsalva maneuver to increase drug absorption. Intravenous drug abuse with methylphenidate and methadone have been associated with the development of panlobular emphysema, possibly related to injected talc.[262–265] While the incidence of venous thromboembolism and pulmonary embolism is relatively low in childhood, oral contraceptives[266] and the antipsychotic drugs clozapine and olanzapine[267] are sometimes used in children and are associated with increased risk.

SUMMARY

Lung injury caused by pharmacologic agents is recognized increasingly as a significant clinical problem. Lung disease caused by cytotoxic agents is particularly troublesome, and survivors of childhood cancer should be followed carefully for chronic pulmonary toxicity. Precise information about risk factors, including genetic predisposition, is required to bolster predictive capabilities for patients using these drugs. Additional information is needed about the mechanisms of injury in order to develop more specific interventions. Finally, more sensitive and widely available diagnostic and monitoring approaches are important if early intervention is to be of value.

Suggested Reading

Dimopoulou I, Bamias A, Lyberopoulos P, et al. Pulmonary toxicity from novel antineoplastic agents. *Ann Oncol.* 2006;17:372–379.

Kano Y, Shiohara T. The variable clinical picture of drug-induced hypersensitivity syndrome/drug rash with eosinophilia and systemic symptoms in relation to the eliciting drug. *Immunol Allergy Clin North Am.* 2009;29:481–501.

Liles A, Blatt J, Morris D, et al. Monitoring pulmonary complications in long-term childhood cancer survivors: guidelines for the primary care physician. *Cleve Clin J Med.* 2008;75:531–539.

Masson MJ, Collins LA, Pohl LR. The role of cytokines in the mechanism of adverse drug reactions. In: Uetrecht J, ed. *Adverse Drug Reactions, Handbook of Experimental Pharmacology.* Berlin: Springer-Verlag Berlin Heidelberg; 2010:195–231.

Rajpurkar M, Warrier I, Chitlur M, et al. Pulmonary embolism—experience at a single children's hospital. *Thromb Res.* 2007;119:699–703.

References

The complete reference list is available online at www.expertconsult.com

75 DISORDERS OF THE RESPIRATORY TRACT CAUSED BY TRAUMA

Matias Bruzoni, MD, and Thomas M. Krummel, MD

GENERAL CONSIDERATIONS

Traumatic thoracic injury in infants and children is uncommon, usually secondary to blunt mechanisms, and often managed nonoperatively. Penetrating injuries such as stab and gunshot wounds are fortunately rare, usually require some sort of operative intervention, and result in increased morbidity and mortality.[1-5]

More than 75% of pediatric blunt chest trauma is caused by automobile accidents. The rest result from sports injuries, battered-child syndrome, and falls from heights.[6] Children involved in automobile accidents tend to be pedestrians instead of occupants of the vehicles. The complete spectrum of chest trauma has been recorded, including pneumothorax, hemothorax, destruction of integrity of the chest wall and diaphragm, thoracic visceral damage, and combined thoracoabdominal injuries. The mortality rate from thoracic trauma has been reported to be approximately 26% and can be as high as 33% when penetrating injuries are involved.[7-9] Thoracic trauma is frequently associated with head, abdominal, and spine trauma, making the mortality rate higher in this combined scenario.

Pediatric deaths may occur in the prehospital setting and are secondary to hemorrhagic shock or cardiopulmonary arrest related to a tension pneumothorax or cardiac tamponade. This mortality and morbidity rate can be improved if the patient is transferred to a tertiary-level pediatric trauma center and managed within "the golden hour" described by the Advanced Trauma Life Support (ATLS) guidelines.

Most blunt thoracic injuries in children can be managed without operative intervention. This often involves significant respiratory support including analgesia, assisted ventilation, and aggressive physiotherapy. As in adults, the significance of thoracic trauma results from the concomitant pulmonary, cardiac, and systemic dysfunction that follows. Because of chest wall resiliency in the pediatric age group, profound physiologic aberrations can occur with trauma that does not fracture or penetrate. Respiratory and circulatory dysfunction secondary to chest injury is frequently complicated by blood loss and hypotension. Hypotension from hemorrhage can usually be managed through intelligent, arithmetic-specific volume replacement; algorithmic therapy is monitored, informed, and refined by serial determination of blood pressures, hematocrit, central venous pressure, blood gases, and, if necessary, blood volume. Restoration of the normal cardiopulmonary function fundamentally depends on a clean airway, intact chest and diaphragm, and unrestricted cardiopulmonary dynamics. In most instances, these therapeutic goals can be accomplished by maneuvers other than thoracotomy. The primary and secondary survey recommended by the ATLS guidelines are mandatory in pediatric trauma as well. If the patient is hemodynamically stable, chest high-resolution computed tomography (c-HRCT) should be considered as a routine measure to search for undetected injuries that may significantly alter the clinical approach. Significant mechanism predicts serious injury.

The long-term outcome of thoracic trauma in children has not been well studied. A single European study addressed the 5-year outcome of thoracic trauma in children; they concluded that most injuries resolve without significant late sequelae.[10]

FEATURES OF THE PEDIATRIC THORAX

The thorax of a child is different from that of an adult from both an anatomic and a physiologic point of view. The pediatric chest is more rounded, with less developed musculature. This characteristic, together with a more flexible and elastic rib cage, results in a very compliant chest. The ribs and sternum of a child can thus support a significant amount of blunt force without fracture. Deformability is such that the anterior and posterior curvatures of the ribs can contact each other without fracture. Therefore, blunt injury to the chest presents a diagnostic challenge because obvious external signs of injury may be minor, chest radiographs may be normal, and yet the visceral structures still may have sustained serious injury.

Additionally, the mediastinum is relatively mobile and thus less susceptible to the rapid acceleration and deceleration forces commonly experienced in blunt trauma. Increased medistinum mobility, together with the absence of pre-existing vascular disease in children, make injuries to the mediastinum and great vessels less frequent than in adults. On the other hand, conditions such as tension pneumothorax or hemothorax are very poorly tolerated and must be recognized and addressed emergently.

The physiologic compensation to trauma is different in children when compared with adults; the cardiovascular and pulmonary reserves are much greater in adults. Tachycardia may be the only compensatory mechanism in children who present with hypovolemic shock; hypotension will only occur in the very late stage, just before cardiac arrest. Massive gastric distention can seriously affect the pulmonary reserve, which is a very common finding in pediatric trauma. Prompt insertion of a nasogastric tube is recommended since many children will develop gastric distension following any type of trauma caused by orophagia.

STERNAL FRACTURES

Fractures of the sternum in infancy and childhood follow high-compression crush injuries and are usually associated with other thoracic and orthopedic injuries. Interestingly, one series has reported sternal fractures as the result of surprisingly minor trauma. The most common injury identified in this report was an isolated anterior cortical fracture.[11]

On physical examination, there is local tenderness, ecchymosis, and sometimes a peculiar concavity or paradoxical respiratory movement, but the sternal segments usually are well aligned, without much displacement. Dyspnea, cyanosis, tachycardia (or arrhythmia), and hypotension may be evidence of an underlying contusion of the heart.

Children with traumatic injury of the sternum should be admitted to the intensive care unit given the increased risk for arrhythmias. Cardiac tamponade and blunt myocardial damage must be ruled out by various studies, including serial electrocardiography, echocardiography, and careful monitoring of venous blood pressure. If the bony deformity is minimal, appropriate posture will suffice. Markedly displaced fragments are reduced under general anesthesia by closed or open technique in order to prevent a traumatic pectus excavatum. Violent paradoxical respirations can be controlled by assisted mechanical respiration through an endotracheal tube, or rarely, by operative fixation of rib fragments.

RIB FRACTURES AND FLAIL CHEST

Rib fractures are unusual in children because of the extreme flexibility of the osseous and cartilaginous framework of the thorax. The upper ribs are protected by the scapula and related muscles, and the lower ribs are quite resilient. As such, rib fractures are present in only about 3% of children admitted with thoracic injury.[12] Predictably, children with more than one rib fracture are more likely to have sustained multisystem trauma;[13] crush and direct-blow injuries are the usual etiologic factors. Multiple fractures of the middle ribs are almost diagnostic of battered-child syndrome.

Multiple rib fractures, resulting in destruction of the integrity of the thoracic skeleton, can cause the paradoxic "flail chest" motion (Fig. 75-1). The unsupported

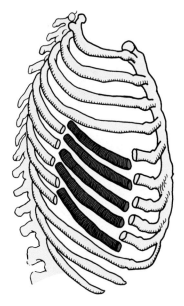

Fractured ribs

FIGURE 75-1. An illustration of five ribs broken in two places, with loss of chest wall stability and resultant paradoxical or "flail chest" wall.

area of the chest moves inward with inspiration and outward with expiration; these paradoxical respiratory excursions inexorably lead to dyspnea (Fig. 75-2). The explosive expiration of coughing is dissipated and made ineffectual by the paradoxical movement and intercostal pain. In effect, the ideal preparation for acute respiratory distress syndrome—airway obstruction, atelectasis, and pneumonia—has been established.

The clinical picture includes local pain that is aggravated by motion. Tenderness is elicited by pressure applied directly over the fracture or elsewhere on the same rib. The fracture site may be edematous and ecchymotic. The clinical manifestations may range from these minimal findings with simple, restricted fractures to the severest form of ventilatory distress with a flail chest and lung injury. Chest radiographs demonstrate the extent and displacement of the fractures and hint at underlying visceral damage.

Treatment of uncomplicated fractures requires pain control to allow unrestricted respiration. Displacement

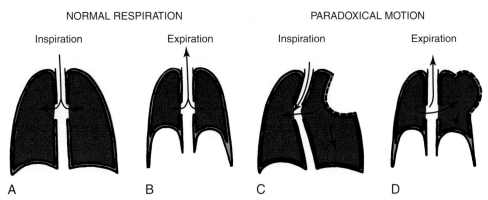

NORMAL RESPIRATION

Inspiration   Expiration

PARADOXICAL MOTION

Inspiration   Expiration

A   B   C   D

FIGURE 75-2. **A-D,** Diagram of the action of a normal chest compared with that of a "flail chest" during phases of the respiratory cycle.

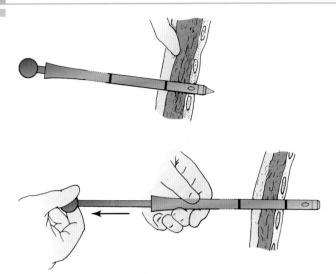

FIGURE 75-3. The trocar technique of chest tube insertion.

requires no therapy. With severe fractures, alleviation of pain and restoration of cough are important and can be provided by analgesics, physiotherapy, and intermittent positive-pressure breathing. Thoracentesis and insertion of thoracostomy tubes should be done promptly for pneumothorax and hemothorax (Figs. 75-3), and shock should be managed by appropriate replacement therapy and oxygen.

Paradoxical respiratory excursions with flail chest must be promptly brought under control, sometimes requiring mechanical positive pressure ventilation to help prevent respiratory distress syndrome, which may be the morbid pulmonary complication. In some cases, a thoracic epidural may be useful to provide appropriate analgesia and achieve effective ventilation. Immediate fixation is rarely indicated.

■ TRACHEOSTOMY IN CHEST WALL INJURY

Controlled mechanical respiration through an endotracheal tube is an essential component for respiratory insufficiency in the setting of thoracic trauma. In spite of vigorous therapy, secretions may be troublesome; they are managed using intermittent tracheal suctioning or bronchoscopy. There is evidence that tracheostomy in children could be avoided by long-term intubation in many cases.[14-15] However, long-term intubation itself has become the most important indication for tracheostomy, since it becomes useful in providing an avenue for the control of profuse secretions, diminution of ventilatory dead space, and control of an obstructed airway (Fig. 75-4). Mechanical respiration can be applied and maintained through the tracheotomy for an extended period.

During the first year of life, tracheostomy is a particularly morbid operation; pneumomediastinum, pneumothorax, and tracheal stenosis are well known complications.[15] Secretions may be difficult to aspirate, and the small tracheostomy tube easily becomes plugged; distal infection, often with staphylococci, is poorly handled by such young patients, and withdrawal of the tracheostomy tube can be a precarious and unpredictable endeavor. Nevertheless, even in this age group, and certainly later, tracheostomy can be lifesaving in specific instances of chest trauma.

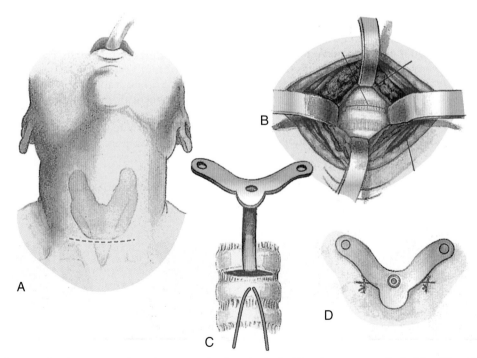

FIGURE 75-4. Techniques of tracheostomy performed over an oral endotracheal tube. Note the transverse skin incision **(A)** and the suture on the lower tracheal flaps to facilitate subsequent tube changes **(C). B,** The anatomy of the area. **D,** The tube in place.

The decision for tracheostomy in cases of chest injury can often be made if there is (1) a mechanically obstructed airway that cannot be managed more conservatively and (2) flail chest. The unstable, paradoxical chest wall movement can be controlled for long periods by assisted positive pressure respirations through a short, uncuffed Silastic tracheostomy tube.

TRAUMATIC PNEUMOTHORAX

Pneumothorax is one of the most common consequences of thoracic trauma and is identified in approximately 12.5% to 50% of chest trauma patients admitted to hospital.[16] Pneumothorax is potentially fatal and requires specific maneuvers to prevent or reverse a malignant chain of events.

The creation of a tension pneumothorax requires a valvular mechanism through which the amount of air entering the pleural space exceeds the amount escaping it. The positive intrapleural pressure is initially dissipated by a mediastinal shift, which compresses the opposite lung in the presence of ipsilateral pulmonary collapse and angulation of the great vessels entering and leaving the heart. Intrapleural pressure can be increased by traumatic hemothorax, and respiratory exchange and cardiac output are thus critically diminished.

In addition to chest wall and lung trauma, the etiologic possibilities include rupture of the esophagus, pulmonary cyst, emphysematous lobe, and postoperative bronchial fistula. These latter sources of tension pneumothorax almost always require thoracotomy for control.

The clinical findings may include external evidence of a wound, tachypnea, dyspnea, cyanosis with hyperresonance, absence of breath sounds, and dislocation of the trachea and apical cardiac impulse. The hemithoraces may be asymmetric, with the involved side appearing larger and hyperresonant.

A confirmatory radiograph is comforting, but often there is insufficient time in this thoracic emergency. Chest tube insertion is indicated for a tension pneumothorax or simple pneumothorax. Prompt relief and pulmonary expansion can be anticipated if the source of the intrapleural air has been controlled. A traumatic valvular defect in the chest wall can be occluded. If the pulmonary air leak persists or recurs, the possibility of tension

pneumothorax is circumvented by the insertion of one or more intercostal tubes connected to water-seal drainage with low suction. Most instances of traumatic tension pneumothorax require tube drainage for permanent decompression, although needle aspiration is indispensable for emergency management. Stubborn bronchopleural fistulas that continue to remain widely patent despite adequate intercostal tube deflation may need thoracotomy and repair versus resection of the affected lung segment.

An open, sucking pneumothorax into which atmospheric air has direct, unimpeded entrance and exit is a second equally urgent thoracic emergency. This pathology is almost always caused by a large traumatic wound. Ingress of air during inspiration and egress during expiration produce an extreme degree of paradoxical respiration and mediastinal flutter, which is partially regulated by the size of the chest wall defect in comparison with the circumference of the trachea. If a considerable segment of chest wall is open, more air is exchanged at this site than through the trachea, because the pressures are similar. Inspiration collapses the ipsilateral lung and drives its alveolar air into the opposite side. During expiration, the air returns across the carina. In addition, the mediastinum becomes a widely swinging pendulum that compresses the uninjured lung on inspiration and the injured lung during expiration (Fig. 75-5). Obviously, under these circumstances, little effective ventilation takes place because of the tremendous increase in the pulmonary dead space and the decrease in tidal exchange. A totally ineffective cough completes the clinical picture.

The diagnosis is readily made by inspection of the thoracic wound and the peculiar sibilant sound of air rushing in and coming out of the wound.

Emergency management of this critical situation is prompt occlusion of the chest wall defect by sterile dressings (Fig. 75-6) and measures to prevent conversion of this open pneumothorax into an equally threatening tension pneumothorax that can occur if the underlying visceral pleura has been injured. Pleural decompression by closed intercostal tube drainage is essential (see Fig. 75-6). A different technique consists of wound closure with an occlusive dressing that is sealed on three sides and acts as a one-way valve allowing air to escape from the pleural space on expiration but sealing and preventing further air

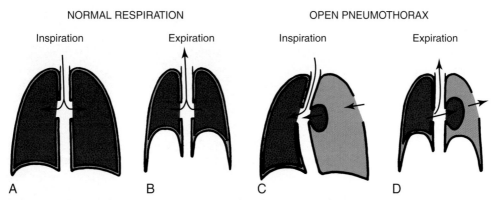

NORMAL RESPIRATION   OPEN PNEUMOTHORAX

Inspiration   Expiration   Inspiration   Expiration

A   B   C   D

FIGURE 75-5. **A-D,** Changes in the normal respiratory pattern brought about by an open, sucking thoracic wall injury.

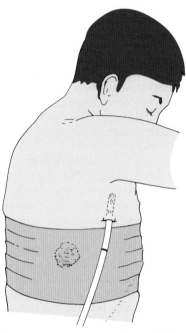

FIGURE 75-6. A temporary occlusive chest wall dressing applied to a sucking wound with underwater intercostal chest tube drainage. Once the period of emergency is over, operative débridement and closure of the chest wound is necessary.

entry on inspiration. After systemic stabilization, more formal surgical débridement, reconstruction, and closure of the chest wound can be done in the operating room.

Subcutaneous emphysema usually results from injury to the pulmonary ventilatory system (Fig. 75-7). The possibility of gastrointestinal tract injury must not be overlooked.

HEMOTHORAX

Blood in the pleural cavity is perhaps the most common sequela of thoracic trauma, regardless of type. Depending on the speed of the hemorrhage, it can be life-threatening.

Bleeding sources are abundant, with either systemic (high-pressure) or pulmonary (low-pressure) sources. Systemic bleeding usually originates in the chest wall from the intercostal branches. Hemorrhage from pulmonary vessels is usually self-limiting unless major tributaries have been transected. It is important to note that a child can accumulate about 40% of his or her blood volume in the chest.

The immediate findings are those of blood loss compounded by respiratory distress. The trachea and apical impulse may be dislocated, the percussion note is dull, and the breath sounds are indistinct. The actual diagnosis is confirmed by thoracentesis if time allows after adequate radiographic studies.

Management of hemothorax is prompt, continuous, and total evacuation of air and blood with a large-bore chest tube. Most often, evacuation of blood will obliterate the pleural space, and pleural aposition will tamponade parenchymal bleeding. A simple formula to define the need for urgent thoracotomy is a bloody chest tube output of more than 1 mL/kg/min with associated hemodynamic instability despite rigorous resuscitation. The surgeon's common sense is crucial in this setting, and if one suspects either persistent or voluminous bleeding, an operation should be performed.

Clotting, loculation, and infection may supervene despite vigorous initial therapy. Retained hemothorax can eventually result in empyema. Publications in the adult setting suggest early thoracoscopy and drainage of the retained hemothorax in order to avoid late infections.[17] Unevacuated intrapleural blood eventually clots and can become organized fibrous tissue (fibrothorax). With the development of a fibrothorax, the changes in cardiorespiratory dynamics become chronic as the lung becomes incarcerated and the chest wall is immobilized. Empyema from secondary contamination is always a threat when the pleural space is filled with blood. A small number of patients eventually require thoracotomy and decortication.

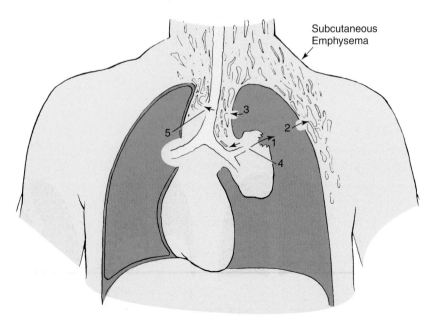

FIGURE 75-7. Subcutaneous emphysema resulting from an injury to the pulmonary system.

TRACHEOBRONCHIAL TRAUMA

Rupture of the trachea or bronchus in infants and children is usually preceded by a severe compression injury of the chest, a sharp blow to the anterior part of the neck, or penetrating injuries. These injuries always represent a diagnostic and therapeutic challenge. Discontinuity of a major airway is characterized by intrathoracic tension phenomena. When the leak is massive, unilateral or even bilateral pneumothorax is present, compromising not only respiratory function but also venous return.

Proximal upper airway lesions often present with pneumomediastinum with cervical or more extensive subcutaneous emphysema, followed by bilateral pneumothorax. This is caused by the intramediastinal location of the trachea, directing any air leak to this space, which is in continuity with the neck compartments. When the distal airway is involved, the air leak opens easily into either pleural space causing tension pneumothorax and a persistent air leak. Hemoptysis might also be present. Upper rib fractures are usually present on the involved side but certainly are not constant in children with partial tracheal or bronchial transection.

Conventional chest radiographs will show pneumomediastinum, pneumothorax, and subcutaneous emphysema. Air tracheobronchogram can suggest the diagnosis in the presence of a compatible clinical picture. Spiral computed tomography of the thorax and the neck may allow better visualization of complete or major disruptions, but bronchoscopic demonstration of the rupture is diagnostic.[18–20] The diagnosis may not be suspected in the acute phase of smaller bronchial transections but becomes obvious when late stricture with distal atelectasis and chronic pneumonitis is related retrospectively to a history of fairly severe chest trauma.

The initial management of bronchial rupture consists of maintenance of a patent airway and decompression of the pleura and mediastinum by one or more thoracostomy tubes connected to closed drainage suction. Emergency bronchoscopy and immediate repair of the defect are preferred to a course of delayed recognition and repair because morbidity can thus be circumvented. Operative repair requires thoracotomy, usually primary repair, and reinforcement with either a pleural or muscular flap.

Severe lacerations of the trachea can be immeasurably helped by bypassing the glottis with an artificial airway during the acute phase while preparing the patient for emergency tracheal repair. Smaller tears may heal spontaneously with tracheostomy alone; others result in stricture and require operative repair.

PULMONARY COMPRESSION INJURY (TRAUMATIC ASPHYXIA)

Explosive blasts compress a child's flexible ribs, sternum, and cartilages against the lungs with a sudden, violent increase in intra-alveolar pressure. These injuries are associated with not only pulmonary but also hepatic and cardiac contusions.[21] Alveolar disruption, interstitial emphysema, and pneumothorax may follow if the glottis is closed when the compression occurs. Distribution of this force to the great valveless veins of the mediastinum and jugular system leads to venous distention; extravasation of blood; purplish edema of the head, neck, and upper extremities; and possible central nervous system changes caused by intracerebral edema and petechial hemorrhages (traumatic asphyxia). The pulmonary contusion is represented pathologically by edema, hemorrhage, and atelectasis.

Clinically, there may be dyspnea, cough, chest pain, hemoptysis, hypoxia, hypercarbia, and mental confusion. The face and the neck can be grotesquely swollen, with crepitus and submucosal and subconjunctival hemorrhage. There is no need for evidence of external trauma or fractured ribs in a child, and accordingly, the indication for chest radiograph is merely the possible history of a blast, acceleration (fall), or deceleration (automobile) injury. Unilateral or bilateral pulmonary hematoma, hemothorax, pneumothorax, and pneumomediastinum can be encountered.

There is a high risk of airway compromise associated with this type of injury, and rapid establishment of a definitive airway is vital. With mild injuries, the subcutaneous emphysema and purplish hue gradually and spontaneously disappear over several days. Patients with more serious blast injuries are treated initially for anoxia and hypotension, and attention is then directed to the wet lung, atelectasis, and pleural complications. Rapid progression of the mediastinal and subcutaneous emphysema indicates a serious disruption of the trachea, bronchi, or lungs and may require intercostal tube drainage or even thoracotomy.

POSTTRAUMATIC ATELECTASIS

With pulmonary contusion from any source, production of tracheobronchial secretions is stimulated, but elimination may be impeded by airway obstruction, pain, and depression of cough. The addition of hemorrhage to these accumulated secretions produces atelectasis in the damaged lung and inevitable infection, a syndrome aptly called *wet lung*.

The clinical findings are dyspnea and cyanosis, an incessant, unproductive cough with wheezing and audible rattling, and gross rhonchi and rales. Chest radiographs show varying degrees of unilateral and bilateral atelectasis.

The syndrome demands vigorous treatment. Useful approaches are frequent postural changes, insistence on coughing, oxygen, humidification, antimicrobials, mechanical ventilation, diuretics, intravenous colloid, cautious hydration, and controlling amounts of depressant drugs. If a child with chest trauma will not cough, tracheal suctioning is instituted. Failure of this step should be followed in quick succession by endotracheal tube insertion or tracheostomy, and bronchoscopy.

The acute respiratory distress syndrome (ARDS) that occurs after critical illness, or trauma with congestion, edema, hemorrhage, pneumonia, and pulmonary fibrosis is rarely encountered in pediatric practice. A series reviewed 60 pediatric patients with ARDS and showed a mortality of approximately 60%. However, only 1 patient in the series presented with ARDS caused by thoracic trauma[22] (see Chapter 39 for more details).

CARDIAC TRAUMA

Though rare, cardiac wounds should be suspected after penetration of any part of the chest, lower part of the neck, or upper part of the abdomen. The possibility of heart injury also exists in the presence of blunt trauma to the anterior or left hemithorax with laceration by fractured sternum or ribs, or severe compression between the sternum and the vertebral column. The spectrum of blunt cardiac injury ranges from myocardial contusion to anatomic disruption such as valve dysfunction or myocardial rupture. The clinical manifestations of a myocardial contusion are arrhythmia, hypotension, and, in severe cases, aneurysms from myocardial wall weakness. Blood loss with perforation varies between exsanguination and minimal bleeding, with or without acute cardiac tamponade. Tamponade usually follows trauma to the myocardium when both pleura are intact; the hemopericardium cannot decompress. The resulting increase in intrapericardial pressure constricts the heart and great veins, and the venous return and the cardiac output are critically impaired.

The physical findings with acute tamponade can be classic. The veins of the neck and upper extremity may be distended. The heart sounds are distant and perhaps inaudible. The systolic pressure is depressed, the pulse pressure is narrow, and the venous pressure is elevated. However, the classic symptoms of distended neck veins, a raised central venous pressure, and pulsus paradoxus are not often evident in children with tamponade. The diagnosis is confirmed with echocardiogram or during the thoracic phase of the Focused Assesment with Sonography in Trauma (FAST) exam.

This condition is imminently life-threatening and requires emergent intervention. With a suggestive clinical picture, emergency needle aspiration of the pericardial sac through a subxiphoid approach should be performed, in addition to systemic resuscitation, while the operating room is being prepared. Aspiration of small amounts of blood can restore cardiopulmonary dynamics (Fig. 75-8).

Nonpenetrating trauma can produce various degrees of myocardial contusions ranging from a small area of edema to a ruptured chamber. The chest pain and tachycardia may be difficult to evaluate without evidence of cardiac failure. Serial electrocardiograms are recommended to monitor these patients (Fig. 75-9). When persistent arrhythmias or hypotension occur, an echocardiogram should be obtained for further workup.[23] Physicians attending an acutely injured child must be prepared to institute prompt external cardiac massage (i.e., internal cardiac massage or cardiac defibrillation). Penetrating trauma may injure myocardial chambers or coronary arteries and may require closure of the myocardial chambers or even coronary revascularization.

TRAUMATIC RUPTURE OF THE THORACIC AORTA

Thoracic aorta rupture is very uncommon. In a series published from Children's National Medical Center in Washington D.C., only 0.14% of the pediatric traumas treated over a period of 6 years presented with thoracic aorta injuries.[24] Aortic transection typically occurs at the level of the ligamentum arteriosum, just before takeoff of the left subclavian artery, and usually is caused by strong acceleration/deceleration forces. Mediastinal widening on routine chest radiography with a distorted aortic contour is the most significant initial diagnostic study. Even though thoracic aortography is the procedure of choice in hemodynamically stable patients, computed tomography angiogram is becoming widely accepted in many trauma centers as the gold standard. Many injuries of this type are associated with life-threatening injuries in other organs such as the abdomen and head. Treatment consists of aortic repair, usually requiring cardiopulmonary bypass, though endovascular techniques are showing promising results in the adult population.[25] There are some case reports in children with good short-term outcomes.[26-28] Long-term results of this approach are not yet available.

INJURIES TO THE ESOPHAGUS

Esophageal injury is more commonly associated with penetrating trauma. In this scenario, the cervical esophagus is commonly injured, usually associated with upper airway or vascular injuries as well. Blunt abdominal trauma or violent, forceful vomiting may cause a sudden increase in gastric pressure and thus create a tear in the wall of the distal esophagus. However, the most common cause of esophageal injury is iatrogenic during instrumentation of the esophagus, such as that seen in dilatations for esophageal strictures or during endoscopic removal of foreign bodies. Esophageal rupture can also follow ingestion of caustic agents. Perforation of the esophagus in the pediatric age group can also occur in the delivery room from extreme positive pressure resuscitation or aspiration with a stiff catheter. Finally, spontaneous rupture proximal to an esophageal web has been described.

Clinically, fever, hypotension, and chest and neck pain demonstrate the presence of mediastinitis. Pneumomediastinum, tension pneumothorax, subcutaneous emphysema, and hematemesis may be encountered.

Plain chest radiographs followed by a contrast esophagram will usually demonstrate the esophageal defect. Sometimes c-HRCT with a water-soluble oral contrast study will help in the diagnosis as well as localize the site and the size of the leak.

The fundamental principles of management in esophageal perforation include adequate pleural space drainage, intravenous antibiotics, and maintenance of adequate nutrition.[29] The operative therapy varies with the *cause*, the *location of the perforation*, and the *time interval* between the perforation and presentation. Many surgical maneuvers have been described. Given its anatomic location, the mid-esophagus is approached via the right chest, whereas the lower esophagus is approached via the left chest. Thoracic esophageal peforation that is recognized early (<48 hours) can be treated with primary repair and muscle or pleural flap reinforcement.

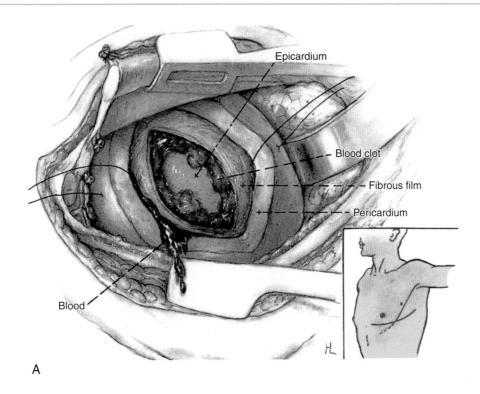

Epicardium

Blood clot

Fibrous film

Pericardium

Blood

A

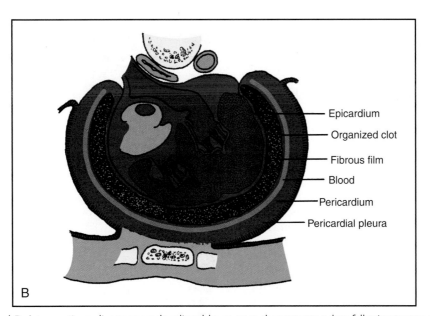

Epicardium

Organized clot

Fibrous film

Blood

Pericardium

Pericardial pleura

B

FIGURE 75-8. A and **B,** A traumatic cardiac tamponade relieved by an open thoracotomy 5 days following trauma and after two partially relieving pericardiocenteses.

If the tissues are very inflamed and cannot hold sutures, resection with proximal diversion and staged reconstruction is recommended. Alternatively, placement of an esophageal T-tube to create a controlled fistula is a viable option and avoids the high morbidity of resection and diversion.[30]

Modern technology and improvements in thoracoscopic and endoscopic techniques have allowed a minimally invasive approach to these lesions. Primary thoracoscopic repair and placement of esophageal stents or endoscopic clipping have been described with good short-term outcomes.[31,32] Cervical perforations usually can be managed with drainage alone because they are more likely to be contained by the surrounding tissues. Stable patients with contained thoracic esophageal perforations who present several days after the perforation occurred can be managed nonoperatively. This includes cessation of oral intake, broad-spectrum antimicrobials, and parenteral nutritional support. The overall health status of the patient, extent of associated injuries, and underlying esophageal pathologic findings are the critical determinants of successful therapy.

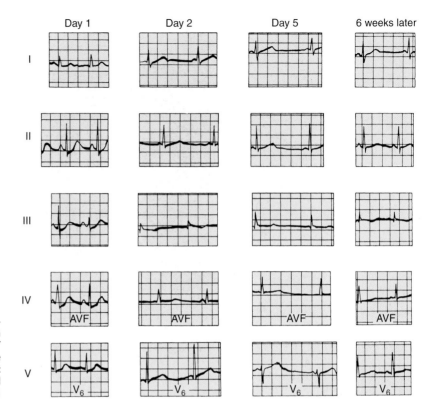

FIGURE 75-9. An electrocardiogram of a 15-year-old boy admitted for blunt chest wall trauma after an automobile accident. Note the progressive ST and T changes with marked depression immediately after the accident. There was an improvement in the ST segment and a flattening of the T waves on day 2 and a reversal to normal in later tracings. (Courtesy of Dr. C. McCue.)

TRAUMATIC BLUNT RUPTURE OF THE DIAPHRAGM

Traumatic injury of the diaphragm is often caused by penetrating thoracic or abdominal trauma; however, severe thoracic blunt force can also result in rupture. It is much more common on the left (90%) than on the right. Suggested explanations for this phenomenon include an increased strength of the right hemidiaphragm, the presence of the liver, and a weakness of the left hemidiaphragm at points of embryonic fusion.[33] Most of these injuries are small and will not declare themselves until later during the hospital course. The initial clinical presentation is very nonspecific; significant cardiorespiratory dysfunction may complicate the early stages. Many significant injuries in other organ systems may confuse the early diagnosis. If the rupture is not initially diagnosed, intestinal obstruction may be the leading symptom at the time of late diagnosis.

The most significant study to arouse suspicion is routine chest radiography, which will frequently show an abnormal diaphragmatic contour (Fig. 75-10). Placement of a nasogastric tube can sometimes show gastric herniation into the chest. Initially, the herniation may not be present or suspected. Serial radiographs are important to determine later herniation. A contrast swallow of Gastrografin or barium will help confirm the presence of stomach or intestine in the hemithorax. Computed tomography can be helpful in the diagnosis, mainly when there is evidence of an acute hernia. Its sensitivity and specificity is low for small diaphragmatic injuries. While magnetic resonance imaging (MRI) shows exquisite details of most the diaphragm, it is not recommended given its impracticality in the acute setting. In patients with high suspicion for

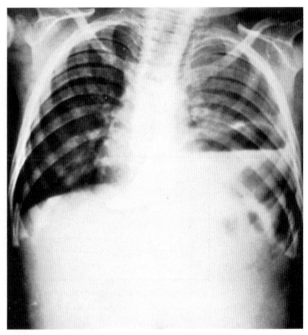

FIGURE 75-10. A blunt traumatic rupture of the left hemidiaphragm that went unrecognized. Death occurred 1 hour later from acute gastric dilation of the intrathoracic stomach (same physiologic effects as tension pneumothorax).

traumatic diaphragmatic rupture, exploratory laparoscopy or thoracoscopy play an important role and should be strongly considered.[34–35]

Acute traumatic diaphragmatic injuries are treated by surgical reduction of the herniated organs, and closure of the diaphragmatic defect (Fig. 75-11). It can

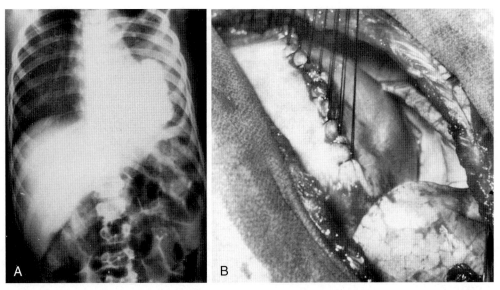

FIGURE 75-11. A blunt traumatic rupture of the left hemidiaphragm with barium swallow **(A)** confirmation and final closure **(B)** at operation.

be approached via either the chest or the abdomen, but most trauma surgeons recommend the abdominal approach given the high rate of associated abdominal injuries.

THORACOABDOMINAL INJURIES

In infants and children, combined injury to the thorax and abdomen, including diaphragm rupture, is usually preceded by a violent traffic accident or other form of sudden, jolting impact. Splenic and hepatic lacerations commonly occur with minimal external evidence of injury and need not be associated with fractured ribs or soft-tissue mutilation.

The clinical signs of upper abdominal tenderness, rigidity, and rebound tenderness almost uniformly accompany lower chest trauma and are explained by the abdominal distribution of the intercostal nerves. Therefore, peritoneal irritation, of itself, is not conclusive evidence of a combined or abdominal injury.

Careful repeated examinations correlated with laboratory data are necessary for the diagnosis of intra-abdominal perforation or hemorrhage in the presence of chest trauma.

Diaphragm rupture can occur with minimal soft-tissue injury, and there may be chest pain, dyspnea, and hypotension. On inspection, the involved chest wall lags during inspiration, and percussion can be dull or hyperresonant. Chest radiographs may not show fractured ribs but almost invariably demonstrate abnormality or absence of the diaphragmatic shadow on the affected side. There is usually mediastinal shift to the right, because in 90% of cases the posterolateral left leaf of the diaphragm is torn in a radial manner. At times, a spontaneous pneumoperitoneum is seen.

The preliminary management of combined thoracoabdominal injuries must include establishing an adequate airway and circulation, gastric decompression, and evaluation and control of other injuries. Intra-abdominal hemorrhage and perforation with thoracic and abdominal soiling is an obvious indication for immediate exploration. Ideally, exploration should be undertaken as soon as systemic stabilization has been achieved.

References

The complete reference list is available online at www.expertconsult.com

76 SUDDEN INFANT DEATH SYNDROME AND APPARENT LIFE-THREATENING EVENTS

JAMES S. KEMP, MD, JENNIFER M.S. SUCRE, MD, AND BRADLEY T. THACH, MD

Infants experiencing an apparent life-threatening event (ALTE) and premature infants with apnea may later die suddenly and unexpectedly, with a diagnosis of sudden infant death syndrome (SIDS). However, because about 80% of victims who died suddenly and unexpectedly were born at term and were never known to be apneic until they died, discussing ALTE, apnea of prematurity (AOP), and SIDS together has become controversial, particularly when the issue of apnea monitoring is raised.

Since the late 1980s, there has been a marked decrease in deaths attributed to SIDS—nearly 40% or more in many countries[1] (Fig. 76-1). The straightforward reason for this decrease is that changes in sleep practices[1] have led to a marked reduction in infants dying during sleep. Through experiments based on death scene and epidemiologic data, much progress has been made in understanding the physiologic bases for the greater risk of sudden death of infants in the prone position on softer, warmer beds[2] (Table 76-1).

Whether or not increased risk is sufficient to justify apnea monitoring,[22,23] premature infants and those experiencing ALTE do die unexpectedly more often. In this chapter, we will discuss ALTE, AOP, and SIDS as separate entities, but we will point out common physiologic and epidemiologic characteristics. We will focus on possible mechanisms for sudden and unexpected deaths that deserve investigation during a time when sleep practices can continue to reduce risk for death.

▆ APPARENT LIFE-THREATENING EVENTS IN INFANTS AND APNEA IN PREMATURE INFANTS

Apparent Life-Threatening Events

Definitions
An apparent life-threatening event is defined as "an episode that is frightening to the observer" and has one or more of the following characteristics: (1) apnea, usually central (less commonly obstructive); (2) color change, usually to blue or pale (less often to red and plethoric); (3) sudden limpness; (4) choking or gagging.

Apnea of infancy, by definition idiopathic or unexplained, is a type of ALTE because it frightens parents. Infants are beyond term postconceptional age when apnea is first noted. The components of an ALTE are usually present, except perhaps choking or gagging. (In our experience, caretakers will often describe gasping, also.)

The definitions of ALTE and apnea of infancy have remained standard for the past 20 years.[22]

▆ APPARENT LIFE-THREATENING EVENTS AND RECOMMENDATIONS FOR HOME CARDIORESPIRATORY MONITORING

The American Academy of Pediatrics' (AAP) last review and guidelines for the use of home monitors was published in 2003.[22] The AAP recommends monitoring in two specific circumstances: (1) It "may be warranted" in selected premature infants until "43 weeks postmenstrual age," or until "extreme episodes" of apnea, bradycardia, and hypoxemia stop; (2) infants who are usually supported at home by mechanical ventilation through a tracheotomy should be monitored.

Routine monitoring is not recommended by the AAP for infants with an ALTE or among siblings of SIDS victims. In a list of instructions, the AAP states: (1) "Home cardiorespiratory monitoring should not be prescribed to prevent SIDS"; (2) "Parents should be advised that ... monitoring has not been proven to prevent sudden unexpected deaths...."[22]

The AAP's recommendations reflect an accurate interpretation of published reports but also reflect compromises that are believed by some to be too generous toward[23] or too restrictive of monitoring. One expert,[24] apparently in disagreement, has written that "[p]atients with ALTE represent perhaps the group in which the indication for monitoring is least ambiguous, not as much with regard to SIDS prevention...," but to understand the cause of unexplained apnea. In our opinion, approaches to monitoring that are dogmatic, either pro or con, and not sympathetic to parents' concerns, should not be the norm.

Thus, although it is the official recommendation of the AAP that ALTE patients not be monitored, this recommendation remains controversial, and home monitoring appears to be a common practice. A review of the practical aspects of home monitoring has recently been published. The review emphasizes that if a monitor is prescribed, it is also critical to provide information about safe sleep practices.[25]

▆ EVALUATION OF AN INFANT WITH AN APPARENT LIFE-THREATENING EVENT

A clinical approach to the differential diagnosis is suggested by Box 76-1.[26-36] In the next section, we will discuss in more detail gastroesophageal reflux (GER) and upper airway protective reflexes that may cause an infant to have an ALTE.[12]

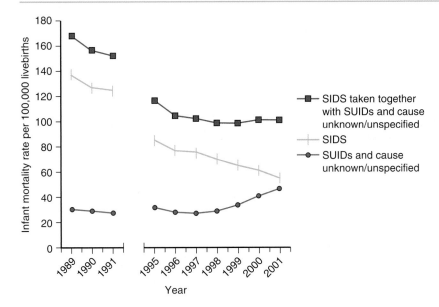

FIGURE 76-1. Mortality rates for three causes, United States, 1989-2001. SIDS deaths decreased after the Back-to-Sleep campaign. Deaths attributed to SIDS continued to decrease after 1998, but decreases in death rates caused by SIDS and related causes leveled off. No birth/death-linked data sets are available for 1992-1994. (From Shapiro-Mendoza CK, Tomashek KM, Anderson RN, et al. Recent trends in sudden, unexpected infant deaths: more evidence supporting a change in classification or reporting. *Am J Epidemiol.* 2006;163:762-769.)

TABLE 76-1 WELL-ESTABLISHED AND NEWER EPIDEMIOLGIC RISK FACTORS FOR SIDS AFTER REDUCTIONS IN SIDS RATES

Established epidemiologic characteristics and risk factors for SIDS[9] and the possible effects of reductions in SIDS rates caused by changes in sleep practices

CHARACTERISTIC OR RISK FACTOR	AFTER SLEEP POSITION INTERVENTION
Preterm birth <37 weeks	Still significant[7,9,76,]
Male sex	Still significant[8]
African-American race	Probably more important
Maternal parity more than two	Still significant[6] but less[7]
Late or no prenatal care	Less significant[3]
Mother <20 years of age	Still significant[8]
Smoking during pregnancy	More important[8]
Never breastfed	Significance less[9]
Upper respiratory infection	Significance less[3]
Winter peak	Results variable, sometimes absent[4] or less[10]
Age at death (89% >2 but <23 weeks)[4]	Little change,[10] older,[11] younger[12]

Newer Risk Factors for Sudden Unexpected Death Identified or Becoming More Significant After Interventions to Promote Back Sleeping

Side sleeping[13,14]
Soft bedding
Not using a pacifier [15]
Bed sharing[14,16,17]
Being inexperienced sleeping prone[17-19]
Head covered during sleep [17,20,21]
Out-of-home child care

BOX 76-1 SELECTED CAUSES IN THE DIFFERENTIAL DIAGNOSIS OF AN APPARENT LIFE-THREATENING EVENT

Respiratory syncytial virus, pertussis
Sepsis with apnea
Syndromes compromising the upper airway (e.g., Pierre Robin sequence)
Breath-holding spells
Seizures
Intracranial hemorrhages (e.g., caused by vascular malformations, child abuse, vitamin K deficiency)
Exaggerated laryngeal chemoreflex with or without gastroesophageal reflux
Drugs (e.g., phenothiazines, over-the-counter cold remedies)*
Tachyarrhythmias (e.g., Wolfe-Parkinson-White syndrome, prolonged QT syndrome)
Inborn errors of metabolism (e.g., MCAD deficiencies)
Hypoventilation during bed sharing or because nose and mouth become covered with bedding

*Pitetti RD, Whitman E, Zaylor A. Accidental and non-accidental poisonings as a cause of apparent life-threatening events in infants. *Pediatrics.* 2008;122:e359-e362.

The approach to infants with an ALTE will be influenced by one's understanding of the association between ALTE and eventual sudden death. Among infants with ALTEs requiring repeated resuscitation, 13% died in one series,[26] and in other studies, 7% to 9% of SIDS infants had a history of an ALTE.[27] Though representing a minority of infants dying, these percentages are not trivial and are comparable to other high-risk problems,

such as the percentage of children dying from asthma who have a history of respiratory failure.[28] This may not make home monitoring mandatory but reminds us that infants experiencing an ALTE are at a measurable risk of suddenly dying that far exceeds that of their age peers.

The clinical approach to an ALTE should, of course, be based on one's assessment of the validity of the caregivers' observations; "benign physiological events in babies may sometimes cause an overreaction by parents, particularly those who are anxious, are attention-seeking, or suffer a personality disorder."[29,30] On the other hand, one's approach should also be informed by the knowledge that 89% of infants with documented prolonged apnea, bradycardia, and marked hypoxemia when subsequently hospitalized for an ALTE had appeared well in the emergency department (Fig. 76-2)[31]

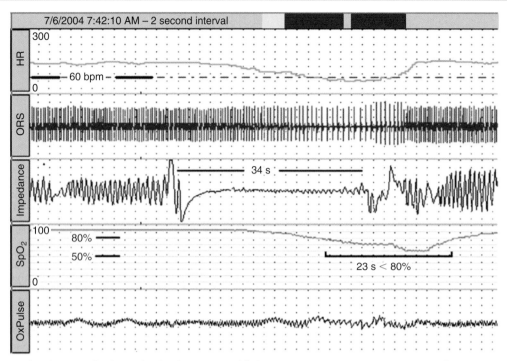

FIGURE 76-2. Recording from an infant hospitalized with an apparent life-threatening event. Representative example of the most common event classified as an extreme event. Note the 34-second central apnea with the associated desaturation below the level of 80%. The apparent small respiratory movements on the impedance channel during the apnea correspond to cardiogenic artifacts. *HR*, Heart rate; *QRS*, QRS wave of the electrocardiogram; *impedance*, respiratory movements detected by transthoracic impedance; *oxypulse*, plethysmographic wave obtained from the pulse oximeter. (From Al-Kindy HA, Gelinas J, Hatsakis G, et al. Risk factors for extreme events in infants hospitalized for apparent life-threatening events. *J Pediatr*. 2009;154:322-327.)

To begin to allay parental concern and to observe and monitor the infant, hospital admission for 2 to 3 days is often indicated after an ALTE.[30-32] The history and physical are critical in beginning to understand an ALTE, and the attending physician supervising the evaluation should make every effort to obtain the history himself or herself, including the duration of the event, time of day, adequacy of lighting, infant's position within his or her surroundings, and whether the episode began while awake or asleep. The infant's color, tone, and the need for and type of resuscitation must be noted. Was blood or pink froth coming from the infant's mouth or nose? The appropriateness of the caregivers' concern should be noted. Family history of seizures, sudden death, or serious illness with coma among young people must be ascertained. Was the infant in the early stages of a respiratory illness, or was he or she having coughing paroxysms? (It is surprising how often typical pertussis will evolve in infants presenting with an ALTE!)

Physical examination should focus on muscle tone, alertness, evidence of bruising or scalp swelling or disuse of extremities, and fundoscopic evidence of retinal hemorrhages. Evidence of stridor, stertor, chest wall retractions, poor skin perfusion, and cardiac murmurs or dysrhythmias should be sought. Infants younger than 2 months of age should be considered at risk for bacteremic sepsis when they present with apnea or hypotonia and should be treated accordingly (see Box 76-1).

Initial laboratory evaluation should include measurement of hemoglobin and white blood cell count with differential cell count; culture of blood and urine; nasal swabs for respiratory syncytial virus (RSV) and pertussis; a chest radiograph; and serum glucose, sodium, potassium, chloride, and bicarbonate. The child should be admitted to a unit where cardiorespiratory monitoring is available so that abnormalities in cardiac or respiratory rate can be detected in recorded data. If the infant continues to be limp or if apnea recurs, one should measure arterial blood gases, serum lactate, and ammonia, as well as screening the urine for abnormal levels of amino and organic acids and drugs.[33] In children who continue to appear ill or who have altered mental status with no other cause detected, video electroencephalography (EEG) should be conducted and imaging of the central nervous system (CNS) by computed tomography or, preferably, magnetic resonance imaging, should be performed.[34]

The positive predictive value of any series of tests in identifying a cause for ALTEs cannot be calculated in the absence of protocols for evaluation that are followed consistently,[32] and patient identification often depends on the degree of parental concern. Not surprisingly, between 16% and 50% of ALTE cases[32,35,36] remain unexplained, and by default such idiopathic ALTEs are attributed to apnea of infancy.

A recent study of 243 children systematically examined the *de facto* approach used to evaluate ALTE in a busy teaching hospital. A retrospective evaluation was done of tests ordered at clinicians' discretion, without a specific protocol. Of over 3700 tests performed, 17.7% of them were abnormal or positive, and one third of the positive results contributed to making a diagnosis that might explain an ALTE. Of the 32 types of tests done

3700 times, some were diagnostic only when the history and physical were suggestive (e.g., EEG, swabs for respiratory pathogens, and metabolic screening). When the history and physical did not suggest a diagnosis, only urinalysis with culture, CNS imaging, chest radiography, esophageal pH probe, and two-channel cardiorespirogram were deemed possibly useful in establishing an explanation for the ALTE.[32] Apropos of our discussion of GER and apnea later in the chapter, the authors cautioned us about concluding that there was a causal association when, for example, 27 of 33 ALTE infants with a negative history and physical examination had an abnormal pH probe.

A POTENTIAL MECHANISM FOR APPARENT LIFE-THREATENING EVENTS AFTER GASTROESOPHAGEAL REFLUX OR RESPIRATORY SYNCYTIAL VIRUS INFECTION

We will discuss laryngeal chemoreflex apnea (LCRA) at length because it may be a mechanism of life-threatening apnea in many conditions. Furthermore, we want to emphasize that what is usually pathologic when considering GER and an ALTE is the severity of the reflex apnea, not the reflux *per se*.[37]

Because it can be prolonged and fatal, LCRA has continued to interest many investigators.[37-42] Given the ubiquity of GER in young infants[43] and its vague link to apnea, a reflex such as LCRA elicited during GER that also may cause breathing to stop is of obvious potential importance. In fact, the inability to modulate LCRA has been proposed as an important mechanism for sudden death in the prone position.[38]

RELEVANT EPIDEMIOLOGY AND PHYSIOLOGY OF GASTROESOPHAGEAL REFLUX

The role of GER in infant apnea is, of course, controversial, although in recent series, 28% to 40% of ALTEs have been attributed to it.[32,34] For more than 30 years, GER has been linked to ALTE in published reports.[44] Many pediatric pulmonologists, in particular, seem convinced that GER frequently causes apnea in premature infants,[45] whereas their gastroenterologist colleagues have concluded that "In the majority of infants with apnea or apparent life-threatening events GER is not the cause."[46]

Acid reflux is common even in normal infants.[43] Vandenplas and colleagues used the pH probe to study 509 normal healthy infants younger than 12 months of age. Infants treated for GER were excluded from their study. Among healthy neonates without apnea or undue irritability, the 95th percentile extended to 13% of recording time with the pH less than 4 in the distal esophagus, and, at 1 year, 8% of the time. The average of the 95th percentile for reflux index for each of the first 12 months of life was 10%. Vandenplas and coworkers believe that acid "reflux is a phenomenon occurring to some extent in every human being."[43]

Gastroesophageal reflux is common and ALTEs relatively rare, and there are few data linking duration of acid reflux to frequency of apnea. Nevertheless, the authors of this chapter believe that reflex apnea may be elicited during GER in susceptible infants,[47] particularly when reflux reaches the pharynx, and this apnea may put these infants at risk for an ALTE if not sudden death.[47-49]

It is not necessary, however, for refluxed fluid to be acidic to elicit LCRA. Furthermore, the usefulness of conventional esophageal pH monitoring in identifying GER in infants is questionable.[50] Among preterm infants fed every 2, 3, or 4 hours, the pH in the stomach approximately 2 hours after feedings was >4, the pH threshold for detecting reflux into the esophagus. In all infants, gastric pH was <4 for only 24.5% of the time (range, 0.6% to 69.1%). The percentage of time with gastric pH >4 may be even higher in asymptomatic older term infants. A pH-independent technique for diagnosing fluid reflux into the esophagus and pharynx has, therefore, been developed (Fig. 76-3).[51,52] Using this technique in 19 preterm infants studied for 6 hours, Peter and colleagues showed that apnea was no more common during reflux than during "reflux-free epochs" (see Fig. 76-3).[53] The time interval used to analyze for a temporal link was 20 seconds. Although reflux reached the pharynx in the majority of episodes (345 of 524, 65.8%), apnea occurring within 20 seconds of reflux into the pharynx was no more common than during "reflux-free epochs." The preterm subjects had very frequent apnea of longer than 4 seconds, on average approximately 20 apnea episodes per hour. Thus, in infants having frequent apnea, the temporal link of apnea with GER, even into the pharynx, is unclear. However, their findings were somewhat inconclusive because reflux to the pharynx was more likely to occur within 20 seconds before apnea than within 20 seconds after, a sequence that would support a causal role.

The situation in term infants with less frequent apnea may be different. Among 22 term infants studied using the same technique, apnea was six times more likely to occur during GER than when GER was not occurring.[51] Again, the majority of reflux episodes extended to the pharynx (71.4%). During the 6-hour recordings, apnea was relatively infrequent in the term infants (1.2 per hour versus nearly 20 per hour among preterm subjects).[53]

To summarize these two studies using pH-independent methods to detect reflux, apnea temporally associated with reflux is common among term infants having relatively infrequent and brief apneic episodes. Among preterm infants having frequent apnea, the temporal link with GER is much less clear. It seems clear that acid reflux, *per se*, does not explain apnea.[54] Future studies using simultaneous intraluminal impedance and pH monitoring might clarify the impact of reflux from the stomach.[55]

Finally, there seems to be no obvious mechanism for reflux to elicit apnea, if it extends only to the distal esophagus. There are no known receptors modulating respiration in the distal esophagus. As described later, the most potent reflexes are elicited only if the refluxed liquid passes the supraesophageal sphincter, which is rare with passive reflux.

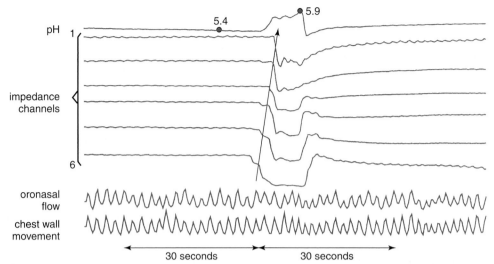

FIGURE 76-3. Sequential changes in electrical impedance between pairs were recorded for six electrodes positioned every 1.5 cm within a catheter from the pharynx to the gastric cardia. During normal swallowing, impedance changes sequentially from the pharynx toward the stomach. During reflux, shown here, the sequence of impedance changes is reversed, beginning in the stomach and extending proximally to the pharynx (channel 1). In this figure, pH increases in the esophagus during nonacid reflux. The pH probe is at the level of impedance channel 5. (From Wenzl TG, Schenke S, Peschgens T, et al. Association of apnea and nonacid gastroesophageal reflux in infants. Investigations with intraluminal impedance technique. *Pediatr Pulmonol.* 2001;31:144-149.)

CHARACTERISTICS OF LARYNGEAL CHEMOREFLEX APNEA

In experimental animals, prolonged apnea, bradycardia, and marked increases in central venous and arterial blood pressure are caused by electrical stimulation of unmyelinated nerve fibers arising in the laryngeal epithelium and traveling in the superior laryngeal nerve (Fig. 76-4). These unencapsulated nerve endings giving rise to afferent signals are most numerous in the mucosal epithelium of the epiglottis, aryepiglottic folds, and interarytenoid space.[56] Laryngeal chemoreception afferents function as irritant receptors, water receptors, and C fibers.[37] Water receptors respond to either reduced osmolarity or reduced chloride ion concentration. C fibers giving rise to LCRA are stimulated by noxious agents (e.g., ammonium, capsaicin, H^+ ions). Any liquid in contact with the laryngeal mucosa will trigger a more or less brisk LCRA. The sequence of response after single-fiber stimulation of these nerves is dramatic and is most marked in younger animals (e.g., piglets, lambs, puppies). Apnea beginning within 0.25 seconds of the stimulus may last 20 to 90 seconds and may be fatal in the laboratory.[40,41]

In young animals, LCRA is very robust in that water applied to the larynx in minute quantities almost always elicits prolonged apnea with bradycardia (76 of 76 trials in puppies, 29 of 30 in piglets). The chloride concentration in fluids contacting laryngeal nerves seems critical in eliciting the reflex.[41] Apnea is more pronounced with water as a stimulus than normal saline. Cow's milk and dog's milk, each low in chloride, will elicit prolonged apnea when applied to the larynx of puppies, piglets, and lambs. If even small quantities of water or milk (e.g., 0.2 mL) remain on the larynx and are not removed by swallowing, the associated apnea has often been fatal in experimental animals.[40] Thus, LCRA could cause an ALTE if elicited in humans.

Human infants attempt to clear fluid that elicits LCRA by laryngeal closure and swallowing during a central apnea (see Fig. 76-4).[39] After the central apnea, any breaths attempted are obstructed so long as upper airway closure persists. When swallowing presumably clears the fluid, the upper airway is opened with a return to eupneic breathing. The LCR sequence in more mature infants and experimental animals does not involve prolonged apnea, and is as follows: cough, swallowing, arousal if asleep. The cough-swallow-arousal sequence is much less common when elicited during sleep in immature subjects.[57]

As in experimental animals, among human preterm infants water is more potent than normal saline in eliciting severe LCRA. In infants, should swallowing be delayed or fail to occur, the apneic phase of the laryngeal chemoreflex can be prolonged, extending over 20 seconds and causing hypoxemia.[39,48] The duration of the apneic phase of the LCR seems to be inversely proportional to postnatal age.[41] Taken together, these findings suggest that in immature subjects airway protection from aspiration takes precedence over ventilation in some circumstances when even small quantities of fluids (~0.1 mL), including water, come in contact with the larynx.

With maturation in older infants and older experimental animals, apnea occurs as part of the laryngeal chemoreflex, but it is shorter than in preterm infants and newborn animals. Maturation is associated with reduction in central respiratory inhibition. Cough and arousal from sleep are also more likely to occur among mature subjects when water, acid, or milk comes in contact with the larynx.[56] Nevertheless, in susceptible infants, delays in maturational influences could put them at risk for prolonged apnea as part of the laryngeal chemoreflex.[42]

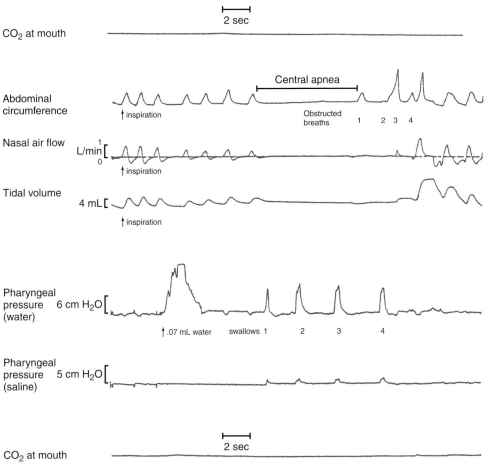

FIGURE 76-4. Sequence of response representing laryngeal chemoreflex apnea in an infant. Upward deflections on pharyngeal pressure tracing reflect swallows. Application of less than 0.1 mL of water onto the larynx leads to swallows and central apnea, followed by obstructive apnea and restoration of eupnea after water has been cleared by swallows. (From Davies AM, Koenig JS, Thach BT. Upper airway chemoreflex responses to saline and water in pre-term infants. *J Appl Physiol.* 1988;64:1412-1420.)

SOME RISK FACTOR FOR SIDS AND ALTE MAY BE EXPLAINED BY LCRA

Laryngeal Chemoreflex Apnea and Nicotine Exposure

Prenatal and postnatal exposure to cigarette smoke consistently and powerfully increases risk for sudden unexpected infant death.[58,59] Lambs exposed to intravenous nicotine from birth, compared with controls, had longer bradycardias and LCRA (8 to 14 seconds longer) when 1 mL of water was placed on their larynx. Some nicotine-exposed lambs "developed ... a sudden loss of muscle tone and were unresponsive to external stimuli."[60] This series of events resembles the definition of an ALTE.

Laryngeal Chemoreflex Apnea and Respiratory Syncytial Virus Infections

Acute infection with RSV has been associated with apnea, particularly among prone infants.[61,62] Evidence of a recent RSV infection also markedly increases the risk for SIDS among prone infants.[63] When studied in detail in a premature infant and a term infant, each experiencing apnea while infected with RSV, the spontaneous apneic events resemble LCRA (Fig. 76-5).[64] Duration of apnea in the RSV-infected infants was often longer than 30 seconds. Apnea was first central and then obstructed (i.e., mixed) and was usually terminated after a series of swallows, less often with a cough. Upper airway secretions, which are increased during acute RSV infection, might elicit prolonged LCRA unless cleared efficiently by swallowing.

In addition to provoking more secretions, other aspects of infection with RSV could prolong LCRA. Inflammatory cytokines (i.e., interleukins IL-1β, IL-6) produced during the infection but acting within the CNS prolong LCRA.[65]

Summary

The laryngeal chemoreflex is robust, and the apnea produced is profound, particularly in developmentally susceptible subjects. LCRA may help explain many types of ALTE. Reflux of acid to the larynx may elicit LCRA, but milk, water, and nonacid secretions are quite capable of eliciting profound apnea. The link between GER, which is common, and apnea, which is rare, may best be understood by asking why some infants have pathologic LCRA.

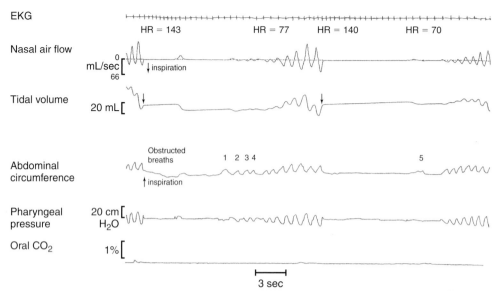

FIGURE 76-5. Spontaneous mixed apnea, resembling laryngeal chemoreflex apnea, in a preterm neonate infected with RSV at 37 weeks postconception. The assumption is that fluid secretions from the infected nasopharynx drained onto the larynx *(arrow, tidal volume tracing)*. The secretions elicited central and obstructive apnea *(1 to 4 on abdominal circumference tracing)*, followed by swallows *(pharyngeal pressure signal)*. The swallows cleared the secretions, and after a second period of central apnea, eupnea was restored. *HR*, heart rate (beats/min). (From Pickens DL, Schefft GL, Storch GA, et al. Characterization of prolonged apneic episodes associated with respiratory syncytial virus infection. *Pediatr Pulmonol.* 1989;6:195-201.)

APNEA IN PREMATURE INFANTS

Definition and Differential Diagnosis

During their initial hospitalization, 50% to 100% of premature infants born weighing less than 1500 g will require mechanical or pharmacologic interventions because of apnea.[66,67] AOP is defined as cessation of air flow for 10 to 20 seconds or longer. Shorter pauses in respiration associated with decreases in $SpO_2\%$ (e.g., to <90%) or in heart rate (e.g., to <100 beats/min) also are seen as important episodes of apnea in most neonatal intensive care units (NICUs). However, if apnea is <10 seconds, there is little consensus about the amount of reduction in $SpO_2\%$ that is worrisome.[66,68]

Other possibilities in the differential diagnosis of AOP besides immaturity of ventilatory control include intracranial hemorrhage, sedation crossing the placenta, sepsis with or without meningitis, heat or cold stress,[69] patent ductus arteriosus, hypoglycemia, electrolyte abnormalities (particularly hyponatremia), anemia, necrotizing enterocolitis, feeding-related apnea,[70] heart block or heart failure lowering cerebral perfusion, and excessive sedation given to the infant directly.

Most apnea among premature infants is "idiopathic" and attributed to immaturity of ventilatory control.

HYPOTHESES FOR PATHOGENESIS OF APNEA OF PREMATURITY

Ventilatory control among premature infants is sufficiently unstable that apnea, even prolonged, is provoked by problems (e.g., hyponatremia, heart failure) that would not be sufficient explanations beyond term postmenstrual age (PMA). Thus, the primary instability of ventilatory pattern and drive among premature infants, even when they are "well," is important.[71]

It is simplistic to state that most apnea among premature infants is central, although most episodes can be prevented with stimulants whose primary action is central. Indeed, it is probable that the majority of apneic events in premature infants have both obstructive and central components (i.e., they are mixed[72]). Furthermore, it seems likely that all three types of apnea described in preterm infants (i.e., central, obstructive, and mixed) occur when the frequency of output from the respiratory controller is at a low ebb, "suggesting that all three patterns had one common underlying mechanism."[71]

There is little recent published work that describes the prevalence of the various types of apnea or the impact of sleep state, or that explores critically the continued relevance of what has become "cribside" dogma.[73] Moreover, clinical rules have often been based on few observations; for example, the dogma that apnea is much more common in active than in quiet sleep is based on studies done on nine term infants.[74] With many smaller and more premature infants surviving, since the introduction of artificial surfactant nearly 20 years ago, these dicta need to be re-explored.

It was observed in the 1980s that the majority of central apneic episodes were either preceded or followed by evidence of upper airway obstruction (Fig. 76-6).[75,76] During apnea in premature infants, respiratory effort often continues, or resumes, before air flow returns, with phasic contraction of the diaphragm (electromyogram) associated with generation of progressively more negative intrathoracic pressures (P_{esoph}). Near the end of a typical mixed apnea, genioglossus contraction (submental electromyogram) opens the airway, and flow resumes.[77] It was thus recognized that apneic episodes in premature neonates could also appear on recordings to be bradycardia with desaturation, because impedance chest movement monitors would correctly indicate that respiratory efforts continued.

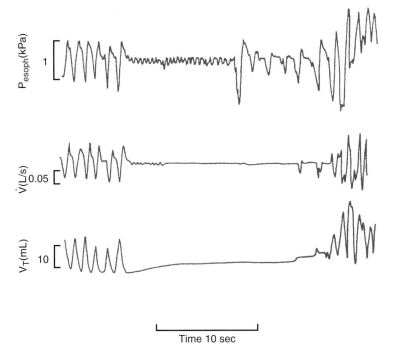

FIGURE 76-6. Spontaneous apnea in a premature infant. Esophageal pressure tracing with cardiogenic artifact demonstrates first central apnea, then respiratory efforts. Flow and volume tracings show that the first four or five efforts after central apnea are obstructed. Such mixed apneas are the most common type of apnea of prematurity. *Pesoph*, intrathoracic pressure; *VT*, tidal volume; $\dot{V}$, air flow. (From Milner AD, Greenough A. The role of the upper airway in neonatal apnea. *Semin Neonatol*. 2004;9:213-220.)

During quiet sleep, premature neonates with frequent apnea are less able than nonapneic controls to compensate for progressive increases in upper airway resistance. Neonates with apnea have much shorter and weaker inspiratory efforts in response to end-expiratory occlusion. Premature neonates with apnea also have a higher $Paco_2$ (~9 mm Hg higher) and a much flatter ventilatory response to breathing 4% CO_2 (V_E/min/kg) compared with controls.[78,79] In addition, infants in general have a flatter CO_2 response when breathing progressively more hypoxic gas mixtures.[80]

A series of explanations for the most common type of apnea among premature infants—mixed apnea—can be constructed from the following classic studies:

1. Upper airway obstruction, for which the infant has shorter and weaker "load compensation," is preceded by brief central apnea, or leads to longer central apnea.
2. Infants with a lower minute volume response to increasing CO_2 become progressively more hypercarbic and hypoxemic.
3. The development of hypoxemia further blunts CO_2 response, and the increasing CO_2 makes the activities of the diaphragm and genioglossus asynchronous,[81] perpetuating the cycle of obstructive and central (i.e., mixed) apneas.

The following other "classic" studies from the mid-1980s suggested additional physiologic mechanisms to explain why premature infants might be more at risk for mixed apnea and its complications during active sleep:

1. The inspiratory "load" for which premature infants are unable to "compensate" is caused by upper airway narrowing,[73,74] which usually occurs at the pharynx.[72]
2. Loss of intercostal tone[82] during active sleep would increase wasted "distortional" work[83] during the paradoxical breathing caused by pharyngeal airway narrowing.[72,84]

3. Loss of intercostal tone would also diminish functional residual capacity and thus worsen hypoxemia during compromised breathing.[82]

Furthermore, LCRA may also play a role in AOP. Swallowing interrupts LCRA. Premature infants swallow more frequently during apnea than during eupneic breathing. This suggests that exaggerated LCRA, such as that caused by spontaneous pooling of saliva, may explain some apneic episodes.[85] LCRA is, in fact, mixed apnea, and is similar to the most frequent type of AOP.

Although it may be simplistic to describe AOP as "primarily central," inadequate responses to upper airway obstruction do reflect a significant "central immaturity" among premature infants. Other evidence of the "central immaturity" of younger infants is the marked increase in periodic breathing, particularly during active sleep.[74] After the onset of periodic breathing, transient upper airway obstruction at the pharynx is common during the first inspiratory effort after the apneic pause. Thus, excessive periodic breathing, which is considered pathognomonic for "central immaturity" of respiratory control, frequently has both central and obstructive (i.e., mixed) apneic components.

During epochs of periodic breathing, preterm infants have decreases in SpO_2 % and are widely believed to be more susceptible to prolonged apneas. Their susceptibility to periodic breathing may be enhanced by the fact that their $PaCO_2$ during eupneic breathing may be only 1.3 mm Hg above their apneic threshold.[86] Thus any ventilatory overshoot after a periodic apnea makes preterm infants particularly vulnerable to resuming apnea. In this regard, evidence from lambs made to have periodic breathing suggests that increases in lung volume wrought by adding CPAP served to reduce the overshoot, or "loop gain," after a periodic apnea, followed by shortened epochs of periodic breathing.[87]

Premature infants also have more active sleep than quiet sleep, with the attendant irregularity in tidal volume (V_T) and ventilatory frequency (V_f), and increase in apnea. In the episodes of apnea when obstruction is not found (<50%), irregularities in respiratory pattern (i.e., V_f, V_T, periodic breathing) often explain a propensity for apnea that is "primarily central."

THE NATURAL HISTORY OF APNEA OF PREMATURITY

The natural history of AOP is unclear because interventions to treat it, and thus alter its natural history, have been tried ever since it was first described. Apneic pauses longer than 5 seconds are common on the first day of life among premature infants without respiratory distress syndrome and can increase to 25 per day by the third day.[88] One large study describing the incidence and age of cessation of apnea[73] showed that nearly all premature infants stopped having apnea of "clinical significance" by 40 weeks PMA. However, this study of more than 25,000 infants from the early 1980s included only 19 infants born before 28 weeks PMA (0.08%). By contrast, during a 5-year period (1989 to 1994), one NICU discharged 457 infants born at 24 to 28 weeks PMA.[67] All infants enrolled in the latter study were treated because all had apnea lasting longer than 20 seconds. In general, infants born earlier had apnea and bradycardia events that persisted until an older PMA (Fig. 76-7). In the study by Eichenwald and colleagues,[67] apnea was diagnosed when chest wall movement was not detected by impedance monitoring. The last events to disappear with maturation were bradycardia episodes without associated central

apnea. As noted earlier and as recognized by Eichenwald and coworkers, the explanation may be that obstructive apneic episodes with bradycardia continued until the age that the bradycardia episodes ceased. More recent studies using transthoracic impedance but incorporating motion-artifact resistant oximetry have led to similarly plausible speculations.[89] Finally, evidence for a persistent propensity for undetected mixed apneas is also suggested by detailed descriptions of maturation of upper airway–stabilizing mechanisms.[90] There seems to be a growth- and age-dependent threshold for improvement in upper airway stability beginning at about 36 weeks PMA.

One group of preterm infants whose ventilatory and general "autonomic instability" may not be appreciated are so-called *late preterm* infants, born at 33 or 34 to 37 weeks PMA. Most attention in diagnosing and treating apnea of prematurity is directed to infants born < 32 or < 28 weeks PMA.[67,91,92] However, compared to term infants in the CHIME study (Collaborative Home Infant Monitoring Evaluation),[93] late preterm infants had a relative risk > 5 for "extreme" apnea lasting longer than 30 seconds or bradycardia. (see Fig 76-2). Furthermore, late preterm infants frequently return to hospital with, for example, excessive periodic breathing, hypoxemia, and apnea at 40 weeks PMA or older,[94] and clinicians often seem surprised at the severity of their ventilatory instability.

THERAPIES FOR APNEA OF PREMATURITY AND MONITORING PREMATURE INFANTS AT HOME

The first-line treatment for AOP remains methylxanthines,[95] with approximately 75% of premature infants responding. Caffeine has replaced theophylline as the methylxanthine of choice because it is as effective and less likely than theophylline to cause tachycardia or poor feeding.[96]

Pulmonologists should also know that much recent enthusiasm has developed for the early introduction of caffeine for premature infants weighing 500 to 1250 grams, even before apnea of prematurity necessitates increased ventilatory support. It is not clear why, but subjects started on caffeine within the first 10 days of life in a randomized, controlled trial involving 2006 infants had a shorter need for supplemental O_2 and CPAP[97] and less neurodevelopmental disability at 18 to 21 months post-term corrected age.[98] Caffeine was begun before chronic lung disease had developed, and continued until apnea, if it developed, had resolved. It is not clear how caffeine given more or less prophylactically might reduce the incidence of chronic lung disease.[99,100] Although it reduces apnea frequency and, presumably, the associated hypoxemia, whether these effects on ventilatory stability provide the explanation for caffeine's apparent impact on neurodevelopmental outcome were not addressed in the large randomized trial.[99]

Infants who fail to respond to methylxanthines will often respond to nasal continuous positive airway pressure (NCPAP) or nasal intermittent positive pressure ventilation.[101] However, concerns about toxicity from

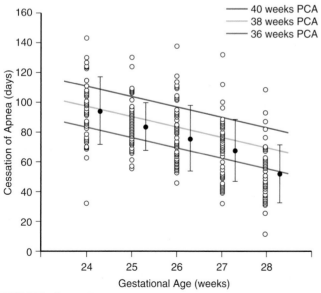

FIGURE 76-7. Infants born at earlier gestational ages, on average, have their last apneic event on a later postnatal day, even when corrected for postmenstrual age. Day of life is shown on the y-axis. Open circles, individuals born at corresponding gestational age, are shown on the x-axis. Closed circles show mean postnatal age (± SD) for the last apneic episode at corresponding gestational age. (From Eichenwald EC, Abimbola A, Stark AR. Apnea frequently persists beyond term gestation in infants delivered at 24 to 28 weeks. *Pediatrics.* 1997;100:354-359.)

high-dose methylxanthines and mucosal injury from NCPAP have led to widespread enthusiasm for early use of high-flow nasal cannulas. High-flow nasal cannulas use adequately warmed and humidified air to deliver distending pressures comparable to NCPAP and are often used at flow rates of 2.5 L/min or more.[102] These catheters have been shown to be as effective as NCPAP in reducing apnea, bradycardia, and episodes of desaturation. High-flow cannulas appear to stave off intubation both by stabilizing respiratory mechanics and treating AOP.

Potential explanations for the efficacy of high-flow therapy in treating AOP have not been evaluated empirically, despite its frequent use for this purpose.[103] However, it seems plausible that distending pressures from the high-flow catheters might mitigate the obstructive component of a typical preterm's mixed apnea (see Fig 76-6). Also, continued flow *per se* might stimulate laryngeal flow receptors[37] and, in effect, feed forward to stimulate continued respiratory effort.[104]

Another older intervention for apnea, blood transfusion, remains controversial.[105] Two recent studies have analyzed AOP as a secondary outcome of restrictive versus liberal transfusion thresholds in studies designed to assess the effect on rates of severe CNS injury (intracranial hemorrhage, periventricular leukomalacia). One study showed no differences in the prevalence of AOP if the hemoglobin was allowed to go as low as 6.8 g/dL versus no lower than 9.0 g/dL.[106] A second study confirmed how very likely preterm infants weighing 500 to 1300 g are to have AOP (98 of 100 subjects). However, the group (n = 51) whose hematocrit was kept 8% to 10% higher were less likely to have more than 1 apneic event per day. The higher and lower hematocrit groups had similar rates of significant CNS complications, however.[107] A recent review[108] admonishes against allowing the hemoglobin to remain < 7.5 gm/dl even in older, more stable preterm infants.

Pediatric pulmonologists who are not based in NICUs should be reminded that premature infants are at a much greater risk for serious apnea after general anesthesia.[109] After anesthesia, increased frequency of apnea and bradycardia can continue to beyond 46 weeks PMA, particularly among infants who required prolonged ventilatory support just after birth, or who have significant residual lung injury. Pulmonologists should be aware of the policies of local pediatric anesthesiologists with respect to perioperative monitoring, even for semielective surgery such as herniorrhaphy. A recent systematic review[110] from Copenhagen emphasized that "Grade 1 evidence (randomized, controlled trial) exists for recommending regional vs. general anesthesia when possible, and for the efficacy of prophylactic caffeine (10 mg/kg IV) on the day of surgery for preterm infants <44 weeks PMA." The Danish authors recommend at least 12 hours of nurse-supervised, postanesthesia monitoring using ECG and oximetry for all preterm infants <46 weeks PMA; infants 46 to 60 weeks PMA with a hematocrit <30%, and those 46 to 60 weeks PMA with "co-morbidities" including chronic lung disease, apnea at home, or CNS abnormalities. Six hours of recovery room monitoring is otherwise recommended for preterm infants 46 to 60 weeks PMA.[110]

Monitoring Premature Infants at Home

In a large multicenter study[111] of neonates born at less than 34 weeks PMA and discharged home at 34 to 38 weeks PMA, 11% (1588 newborns) used apnea monitors at home. Among over 20 NICUs in the study, the range of percentage of monitor use was 0% to 57%. Infants with a history of apnea and those receiving methylxanthines were more likely to be prescribed monitors. Those on monitors were not sent home earlier or later.

Other studies evaluating compliance with apnea monitor use suggest high rates of compliance among infants with AOP, particularly during the first month at home.[112] Abuses because of self-interest among those prescribing monitors not withstanding,[23,113] the promise or potential of monitors, when used to prevent deaths among "nursery graduates," should not be discounted. Infants born at 24 to 36 weeks PMA are from 2.1 to 3.3 times as likely to die of SIDS as infants born at more than 37 weeks PMA.[5]

The issue of monitor use is quite complex, however. In their review of more than 37,000 deaths and 3.8 million linked births, Malloy and Hoffman[5] showed that, depending on the estimated gestational age, the age of SIDS deaths among premature infants was, on average, 44.2 weeks to 47.8 weeks PMA (range, 32 to 85 weeks). On the basis of these data and those of the CHIMES study,[93] wherein "extreme" apneic spells among premature infants "disappeared once the infants were 43 weeks post-conceptional age," one editorial writer declared that the usefulness of prescribing monitors to detect extreme apneic spells and to prevent sudden death among premature infants and the "physiological basis for such a practice are more in doubt than ever."[23] However, because infants who have died were certainly apneic at least once, another possible scenario is that the time course of dangerous apnea activity among those premature infants dying is different from those having apnea and not dying. The vexing problem remains whether it is possible to select candidates who will benefit most from monitoring.

For the time being, we are in agreement with the AAP recommendations for monitoring premature infants having apnea until they are 43 weeks PMA.[22,24] Because the average time course until cessation of apnea among those infants dying must be different from that for the premature infants in the CHIMES study, monitoring infants past 43 weeks PMA who have frequent apnea lasting longer than 20 seconds, especially with reductions in heart rate, also seems prudent.

▬ SUDDEN INFANT DEATH SYNDROME: NEW EXPLANATIONS WITHIN A NEW DEFINITION

Triple-Risk Model and New Infant Variables

The definition for SIDS during the first 20 years after the syndrome was recognized was "the sudden death of an infant or young child, which is unexpected by history, and in which a thorough postmortem examination fails to demonstrate an adequate cause of death."[114]

Because of the recognition of risk factors related to sleep practices, the definition was broadened in 1991 to "the sudden death of an infant under one year of age which remains unexplained after a thorough case investigation, including performance of a complete autopsy, *examination of the death scene,* and review of the clinical history."[115,116] For a complete discussion of issues surrounding the definition of SIDS,[117] categorization when investigations are incomplete, and the importance of alternative definitions with subtle changes in emphasis, the reader can refer to reviews by Krous and co-workers and by Rognum.[116,118]

Over the past several years, there has been renewed interest in citing postmortem evidence for an infectious cause that might reduce the number of sudden infant deaths left unexplained. Though more systematic approaches have demonstrated higher isolation rates of bacteria, viruses, or *Pneumocystis jirovecii (carinii)* in infants at autopsy,[119] evidence is lacking linking the infections to tissue injury causing organ failure, or death because of collapse of life-sustaining reflexes.

In this regard, it is important to recall that the "SIDS era" arose from the recognition in the late 1960s that most sudden infant deaths occurred without sufficient pathologic findings to explain them.[120,121] Explanations were lacking beyond otitis media or mild interstitial pneumonia found at autopsy. This fundamental insight led to much research into reflexes, ventilatory control, and brain stem neurochemistry to clarify what was defined as "unexplained" by conventional histopathology.

While serving to stimulate new thinking about why infants die, the definitions just cited have led to nosologic uncertainty. Accepting an explanation for some deaths from a group defined because they "remain unexplained" presents an obvious conundrum. For example, once empirical data became available[122–126] that suggested how infants diagnosed as having died from SIDS might have subtly suffocated while facedown on soft bedding, it was claimed that these deaths were not caused by SIDS (a mystery) as they were originally diagnosed, but were, in fact, caused by suffocation (Fig. 76-8).[127] The diagnostic shifting described[128] is understandable in the context of a definition that, while useful in stimulating research, assured a nosologic conundrum if progress was made and some of the deaths became explicable.

A framework that, in our opinion, has stood the test of time as a way to study sudden unexpected infant deaths is the triple-risk model (Fig. 76-9).[129] Susceptible infants at a vulnerable physiologic and developmental stage are exposed to more-or-less potent environmental stressors that lead to death. In a given infant or group of infants, the relative importance of each influence may vary. Investigations into sleep practices over the past 20 years have increased the understanding of exogenous stressors.[130,131] Some would argue that these deaths should not be categorized as SIDS because they have had partial, new explanations,[124] even though the triple-risk model for SIDS encompasses them perfectly. This is also likely to be the case, and the conundrum, as more inborn

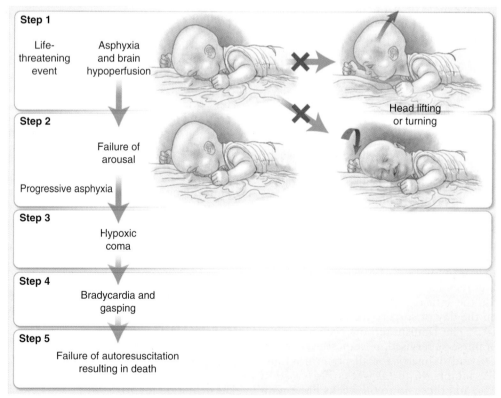

FIGURE 76-8. Five steps in the putative terminal respiratory pathway associated with sudden infant death syndrome. Death results from one or more failures in protective mechanisms against a life-threatening event during sleep in the vulnerable infant during a critical period. In particular, infants who are unaccustomed to prone sleep are at an 18-fold increased risk for sudden death when placed prone. (From Kinney HC, Thach BT. The sudden infant death syndrome. *N Engl J Med.* 2009;361:795-805.)

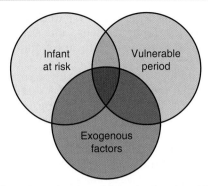

FIGURE 76-9. The triple-risk model was developed to address the problem of SIDS. It emphasizes the likelihood that most deaths have several partial explanations, within a causal sequence. It remains relevant when death scene investigations have caused diagnostic shifting among the diagnoses of SIDS, unexpected suffocation, and cause of death undetermined. (From Filiano JJ, Kinney HC. A perspective on neuropathologic findings in victims of the sudden infant death syndrome. The triple risk model. *Biol Neonate.* 1994;65:194-197.)

metabolic defects[132,133] and developmental anomalies[134,135] are identified that explain, at least partially, the previously inexplicable.

MULTIFACTORIAL EXPLANATIONS, NOT A SINGLE CAUSE

Although theoretically problematic, practical approaches to understanding related types of sudden unexpected infant deaths are possible under the rubric of SIDS. It is essential, however, to realize that there is little to be gained by an exclusionary definition of "true SIDS."[116,118]

Within the triple-risk model, for a given infant it is more helpful to think of a causal sequence. For example (see Fig 76-9),[129] we might consider a hypothetical infant with a sluggish arousal response to sleep environment threats while prone[136] who comes to lie prone on bedding that covers the nose and mouth.[18,137,138] The infant also has a respiratory infection[63] and is at a vulnerable age when the skills at gaining access to fresh air are poor.[134] Perhaps the infant has come to lie in the prone position for the first time, without the requisite learned skills to be safe prone.[18,136,139,140] In a given infant, each of these variables could be critical antecedents before autoresuscitation failure and sudden death (see Fig 76-9). Moreover, amelioration of one or more of the eight risk factors present in this example would reduce the risk for death. The success of supine sleep interventions in many countries suggests that the prone position is critical at several junctures in a hypothetical causal sequence, at least among infants sleeping alone.[138,141–143]

NEWER APPROACHES TO PATHOLOGY OF SUDDEN INFANT DEATH SYNDROME

By definition, conventional gross or microscopic necropsy materials do not explain a SIDS death. Consequently, studies of its pathology have usually described subtle quantitative abnormalities in groups of SIDS victims that distinguish them from controls dying of identified causes.[118,144,145] Alternatively, investigators relying on novel techniques that have been developed since SIDS was defined have studied lethal mechanisms that work quickly and do not yield abnormalities visible with light microscopy (e.g., autoradiography of neuroligands or markers for apoptosis, or analysis of gene polymorphisms seen more frequently among some children dying suddenly and unexpectedly). Studies of specimens from SIDS victims using the newest techniques have attempted to piece together its pathophysiology, rather than attempting to describe findings that are, by consensus, sufficient to explain death.

Thus, in general, when infants die suddenly and unexpectedly, perhaps 1 in 6 of the deaths will be explained by any postmortem findings or tests done on autopsy specimens. However, when infants die without forewarning in the first week of life (SUEND, or sudden, unexpected early neonatal death), conventional postmortem investigations may more often yield diagnostic findings. In a study from London, there were 55 SUENDs from 1996 to 2005. Over half (58%) were explained by autopsy, primarily by congenital heart disease, acute infections, and fatty acid oxidation deficiencies.[146]

Epidemiologic findings have always influenced studies of SIDS pathology. In particular, it has been recognized for the past 25 years that many deaths diagnosed as SIDS have involved sleep practices that increase the risk for death.[141] For this reason, pathogenetic models based on dysfunctional responses to stressors arising from sleep practices will be the focus of our review of newer approaches to pathology. In these models, the ultrastructural uniqueness of SIDS victims could cause abnormalities of ventilation, ventilatory control, or airway protection.

Programmed Cell Death Within the Central Nervous System

In earlier studies, markers of apoptosis, triggered presumably by CNS hypoxia within the previous 48 hours, have been demonstrated in 80% of 29 SIDS victims, and 0 controls.[147] The markers were in the brain stem or "hypoxia-sensitive subregions of the hippocampus," or both locations. A more recent study of three markers of apoptosis in 67 SIDS cases compared with 25 age-matched controls showed an association in SIDS between increased expression of markers of apoptosis and history of cigarette smoke exposure, bed-sharing, and prone sleeping position.[148] In the brainstem, markers of DNA fragmentation (by TUNEL assay) were found in the dorsal, rather than ventral, nuclei. Dorsal nuclei involved included those serving the spinal trigeminal tract, vestibular function of the eighth cranial nerve, and dorsal column nuclei (gracile and cuneate). These nuclei relay kinesthetic sensory data to the thalamus and play a role in controlling orientation. Involvement of these nuclei may be relevant to sleep practices that cause hypercapnic hypoxia because, as the authors speculate, environmental risk factors may contribute to damage of nuclei involved in head, neck, and body positioning (eighth nerve and DCN), and facial sensation (fifth nerve) may be altered, so that "suffocation may occur."

Neural Receptors and Sudden Infant Death Syndrome

Extensive investigations using carefully chosen controls seem to have established that specific receptors within the CNS are reduced in number among SIDS victims. These receptors are needed for the excitatory function of serotonergic networks within the brain stem, across sleep and wake cycles. A less well-known body of work, discussed briefly later, suggests that airway inflammation causing peripheral chemoreceptor dysfunction could also lead to SIDS.

During the past 25 years, Kinney and colleagues[129] have compared the brain stems of SIDS victims to brain stems from infants dying acutely from a known cause, or from chronic diseases causing hypoxia. Their approaches show that attempts to explain abnormal function, rather than only histologic neuropathology, are critical to understanding SIDS. Highlights of their work, for our purposes, can be summarized as follows:

1. These authors believe that structures in the human brain stem are "anatomically homologous" to chemosensitive areas in animals,[149] and two SIDS victims they studied had hypoplasia of the arcuate nucleus, a prime "candidate" site for human brain stem chemosensitivity.

2. SIDS victims have less functional activity of receptors binding radiolabeled cholinergic transmitters within the arcuate nucleus *in vitro,* compared with acute and chronic controls.[150]

3. Serotonin binding by serotonin receptors in the brain stems of SIDS victims compared with controls is reduced not only in the arcuate nucleus, but also in four other brain stem structures derived from the embryonic "rhombic lip" and the intermediate reticular zone.[132] In SIDS, it appears that the abnormal receptor binding patterns in the arcuate nucleus and other nuclei of the medullary serotonergic system are different than in infants who died of hypoxia of known etiology. This suggests that hypoxia alone does not cause the aberrant serotonin binding patterns in SIDS infants, but that other genetic or environmental exposures during development unique to SIDS are responsible for the aberrant patterns.[151]

4. The differences they describe occur within a serotonergic neural network involved with arousal, respiratory patterns, thermoregulation, chemoreception, and upper airway patency.[152] These findings are particularly relevant to asphyxia and hypercarbia that might occur but not be sensed by infants dying prone or supine with their nose and mouth covered.

5. There is a growing body of evidence that the medullary serotonergic system has neurons that are present as early as 7 weeks postconception, and that the nuclei composing the system are fully developed by 20 weeks.[151] The activity of receptors binding serotonin seems to be developmentally regulated, at least between 35 and 70 weeks after conception.[132]

6. The serotonergic neurons and receptors of this system are vulnerable to *in utero* exposure to nicotine and alcohol, with markedly decreased serotonin binding in the arcuate nucleus in babies who were exposed.[153] Studies in baboons showed that isolated exposure to nicotine altered patterns of serotonin binding in the raphe nucleus, and that this altered binding was associated with autonomic changes in the fetuses.[154]

In recent and likely related work, Livolsi and colleagues have shown that the hearts of 19 SIDS victims had overexpression of cardiac muscarinic receptors. Their erythrocytes also had more acetylcholinesterase, perhaps as a peripheral compensatory mechanism for increased cardiac parasympathetic tone.[155] And in the *in utero* nicotine exposure model mentioned earlier[154] that caused abnormalities in brainstem serotonergic systems, the young baboons had marked increases in their high-frequency heart rate variability, suggesting an abnormality in parasympathetic tone. It is plausible that these findings in SIDS victims and baboons suggest a link among *in utero* nicotine exposure, altered serotonergic receptor binding in the raphe nucleus of the medulla, and vulnerability to sudden cardiac death.

It is also interesting to speculate about neural mechanisms for the very high risk of dying when infants who usually sleep supine are placed prone for the first time[18] (see Fig 76-8). It is possible that infants who are usually placed prone learn to lift and turn their heads in order to gain access to fresh air. The cerebellum may have a role in learning this unconscious motor choreography. Some neurons in the cerebellum are known to respond to changes between real and anticipated sensory input and to modulate motor activity to respond to a changed environment with an unconscious change in motor activity.[139] Delayed cerebellar "motor learning" might be explained by brainstem findings implicating the medullary serotonergic system, which has multiple links to the cerebellum, including the inferior olivary nucleus.

In any event, it seems apparent, with respect to key receptor networks, that SIDS victims have the substrate for underlying susceptibilities that change with development. Taken together, these findings complete a triple-risk model (see Fig. 76-9) that might include exogenous stressors within the sleep environment.

Others have addressed the availability of serotonin to its receptors within the brain stems of SIDS victims. Polymorphisms occur in the promoter region for a gene controlling the reuptake of serotonin within the CNS. The number of repeats within the promoter region determines promoter activity. The majority of humans have either 14 or 16 repetitive elements—the S or L promoter alleles, respectively. In studies from Japan by Narita and coworkers,[156] genomic DNA in frontal cortex samples from SIDS victims (n = 27) was more likely to have 18 or 20 repetitive elements (n = 3, 11.1%) within the promoter alleles than was genomic DNA taken from peripheral blood of controls (n = 115, 0.9%). The effect of this promoter region difference on serotonin activity within the CNS is unclear, however. A recent study that looked for the L allele in 179 SIDS cases in the United States compared with 139 controls showed no association between the L allele and SIDS cases.[157] The authors of the U.S. study point out that the L allele and SIDS phenotype have not shown the same association as in Japan. They also note that of the gene polymorphisms possibly linked with

SIDS risk, no single gene has been shown to have a strong and consistent association with SIDS phenotype, suggesting that "multiple genes are likely to contribute to the pathogenesis of SIDS pathophysiology." Studies that analyze and compare the entire genome may be more useful at identifying clusters of gene polymorphisms that contribute to SIDS risk, although the small size of most SIDS databases do not permit genomewide association studies.[157]

Cutz and colleagues have studied the role of peripheral chemoreceptors arising in the lung. Their studies offer one explanation using neurochemical receptors for a classic finding,[158,159] namely, the association of SIDS deaths with findings of nonlethal airways inflammation.[63,159] Cutz and coworkers have shown marked increases in numbers of inflammatory cells in the airway epithelia and alveolar septa of SIDS victims.[159] The model developed by Cutz and coworkers also rests on another apparently consistent finding in SIDS victims, namely greater numbers of pulmonary neuroendocrine cells (PNECs) and larger neuroendocrine bodies (NEBs)[160] found in the intrapulmonary airways, near branchpoints.

PNECs and NEBs are composed of clusters of cells[161,162] containing serotonin and peptide neurotransmitters (e.g., bombesin, calcitonin, enkephalin, and others). They are detected using scanning electron microscopy near nerve endings whose afferent fibers ultimately reach the CNS via the vagus.[163] The primary function of PNECs and NEBs is theorized to be as sensors of airway hypoxia during the first months of extrauterine life. In animals, airway hypoxia leads to local secretion of serotonin by NEBs, presumably the beginning of a message to the CNS that local gas exchange has been compromised.

The models based on the work by Cutz and colleagues postulate that the peripheral hypoxia-sensing function of PNECs and NEBs may be a critical complement to carotid body chemoreception. Receptors within inflamed and tobacco smoke–exposed airways may have blunted responses to hypoxia during a time in infancy when carotid body sensitivity is downregulated. Their model, though complex, is based on increasing empirical evidence, especially findings showing increases in PNECs and NEBs in SIDS victims,[160,161] whose airways are more likely to be exposed to cigarette smoke and to be infected. Again, the findings of Cutz and coworkers are consistent with the tenets of the triple-risk model: hypoxia caused by sleep environment plus developmental downregulation of carotid body chemosensitivity plus susceptibility due to PNECs and NEBs dysfunction caused by known risk factors for SIDS (infection and smoke exposure).[58,63]

Fatty Acid Oxidation Deficiencies and the Contribution of Genetic Diseases of Metabolism to Sudden Infant Death Syndrome

The last two topics in our discussion of new pathology do not primarily involve respiration. However, a pulmonologist dealing with the sudden death of an infant will need a working familiarity with them.

Under the wide umbrella of SIDS, and related causes of death, there has been much recent interest in heritable diseases affecting energy metabolism.[116] It is not clear whether the diseases are similar to SIDS in that they can be lethal in 2 hours or less in previously healthy infants, or whether the age of death from inherited metabolic disease overlaps classic SIDS ages (peak rate at 3 months, 95% of deaths by age 6 months).[4]

The epidemiologic features of sudden deaths caused by inborn errors of energy metabolism are not well established. Furthermore, although techniques such as tandem mass spectroscopy can be used on neonatal blood spots to screen for many inborn errors, the ratios of false-positive to true-positive may be 8:1 or greater. It is unclear whether the public health commitment exists to address with new parents the problems of false-positive tests, or unpredictable prognosis of many diseases.[164] Nevertheless, it is certain that some deaths once called SIDS, or attributed to parental neglect, can be explained by deranged energy metabolism. We will discuss two important examples.

During significant fasting, beta oxidation of fatty acids occurs in mitochondria to provide energy substrates as alternatives to dietary sources of energy. There are 11 proteins controlling the 20 steps leading to beta oxidation, and, ultimately, the tricarboxylic acid cycle and the flavoprotein electron transport cycle.[133] Disorders may disrupt any step in the process, from substrate uptake to actual beta oxidation, and have their primary effects on the liver, the CNS, or the heart. The disorders are manifest during fasting, either very shortly after birth, or, in particular, associated with anorexia caused by a viral illness.

The most well-known defects are those causing pediatric cardiomyopathies. Newborns need the relevant enzyme, VLCAD (very long chain acyl-CoA dehydrogenase) to meet the extreme demands on their heart during the transition to extrauterine life. Infants with VLCAD deficiency may die suddenly but usually present in heart failure with a cardiomyopathy that is often familial and that responds to low-fat diets and avoidance of fasting.[165]

Altogether, recognized disorders of fatty acid beta oxidation may be more common (1:10,000 live births) than phenylketonuria (1:15,000). The most common inborn error of beta oxidation is a deficiency in medium-chain acyl-CoA dehydrogenase (MCAD). After periods of inadequate oral intake, infants present with hypoglycemia, neonatal apnea, and, in as many as one third of cases, sudden death.[166] However, their most frequent presentation is profound encephalopathy with cerebral edema, hypoketotic hypoglycemia, elevation of liver transaminases, and hyperammonemia. Because MCAD deficiency was not recognized until the early 1980s, it is probable, in retrospect, that some cases of Reye's syndrome were crises occurring in children with MCAD deficiency.[133,167]

It is also probable that infants with MCAD deficiency have been included in series of infants diagnosed as having died of SIDS.[168,169] For one large series of SIDS deaths in Maryland, the authors suggest that as many as 5% actually died of fatty acid oxidation disorders, although the very high frequency in this series of an otherwise very rare disorder (carnitine uptake deficiency) is not explained. Details about age at death, sleep practices, and prevalence of other SIDS risk factors have not been provided in the largest published series of infants with beta-oxidation defects, although there may be some age overlap with SIDS.[168] Two of three infants with MCAD or VLCAD deficiencies from Oregon died within the first 48 hours of life, and two of three were sharing a bed when found dead.[170]

The most common genetic defect leading to MCAD deficiency is homozygous A985G (A to G replacement at nucleotide 985). However, genetic testing after death may either underestimate or overestimate MCAD deficiency as a cause: Affected compound heterozygotes with only one A985G allele have been described. Alternatively, the infants' demise, particularly in the absence of fasting, could have been associated with a "coincidental" abnormality in MCAD.[171-173]

Improved postmortem approaches to the diagnosis of MCAD deficiency, once dependent on first identifying hepatic steatosis and then performing tissue culture analyses, have been made affordable by the availability of tandem mass spectroscopy. The protocol used in Oregon involves creating acyl-carnitine profiles using tandem mass spectroscopy on blood spots from postmortem cardiac puncture.[170] Markedly abnormal profiles of acyl-carnitine–fatty acid compounds (e.g., abnormal levels of octanoyl-carnitine [C8]) suggest deranged beta oxidation for some period before death. Such findings are very suggestive of death caused by MCAD and related disorders.[173] Infants dying suddenly and unexpectedly with a family history of a similar death, dying after fasting, or whose autopsy shows hepatic steatosis should most certainly be evaluated using acyl-carnitine profiles from tandem mass spectroscopy. In St. Louis, the medical examiner orders this test on all children who die unexpectedly before reaching 5 years of age.

In Oregon, from 1996 through 2002, deaths caused by disorders of beta oxidation occurred in an estimated 1.3 per 100,000 live births and constituted 1.2% of deaths occurring suddenly and unexpectedly among infants younger than 1 year of age. A retrospective study in North Carolina looked for hepatic steatosis in 220 consecutive deaths diagnosed as SIDS. Of the 16 infants with hepatic steatosis, 2 had known mutations that cause disordered fatty acid oxidation.[174]

To understand whether these deaths fit within the context of established SIDS epidemiology (see Table 76-1),[170] future reports on these types of deaths should emphasize how the infants compare to other infants dying, for example, with problematic sleep practices, in terms of age at death, birth weight, history of maternal smoking, and other factors known to be associated with higher risk for sudden death.

Prolonged Electrocardiogram QT Intervals and Lethal Cardiac Arrhythmias

In Italy, Schwartz and colleagues have been the most consistent proponents of the theory that cardiac arrhythmias can be lethal in SIDS victims with normal cardiac autopsy results. Arguments against this theory were as difficult to envision as were even partial proofs in empirical, population-based studies. Nevertheless, by recording more than 33,000 electrocardiograms on days 3 or 4 of life, Schwartz and colleagues[175] reported that the mean corrected QT (QT_C) interval was longer in the 24 infants eventually dying of SIDS (435 ± 45 versus 400 ± 20 msec) than in the survivors. None of the thousands of survivors had QT_C intervals greater than 440 msec, but 12 of 24 SIDS victims did. The prolonged QT_C interval is believed to be fatal because of an associated malignant arrhythmia (torsade de pointes).

In 2001, Ackerman and co-workers[176] showed that 2 of 93 infants diagnosed as SIDS in Arkansas had mutations causing cardiac sodium channel dysfunction, as compared with none of 400 controls. The mutation in the SCN5A sodium channel they studied is estimated to cause up to 10% of cases of long QT_C interval syndrome. Continued investigation of sodium channelopathies over the past decade have demonstrated the breadth and the complexity of their involvement in SUID.[177] For example, although unlikely alone to explain the increased risk of African-American infants for SIDS, "alleleic expression imbalance" of a single mutation causing a sodium channelopathy has been demonstrated in some African-American SIDS victims.[178] And a mutation in dystrophin-associated protein in the heart that has been linked to SIDS, alpha-1-Syntrophin, has also been shown using *in vitro* systems to cause an "abnormal biophysical phenotype" in myocardial cell sodium channels.[179]

The theories of Schwartz and coworkers now seem well established as causes for a small percentage of deaths (~2% to 5%) that might meet the criteria for SIDS. The impact of potent SIDS risk factors (e.g., prone sleep, maternal smoking) on the risk for lethal outcomes in infants who are homozygous or even heterozygous[178] for mutations in, for example, cardiac sodium channels, has not been calculated, so it is not yet possible to use this information to understand how it fits into the classic epidemiology of sudden death in infancy. Will infants with MCAD deficiency or SCN5A mutations be outliers in terms of age, or will their risk of dying be relatively unaffected by sleep practices?

Also, it is becoming less clear where the pathologic investigation of SIDS or other sudden unexpected infant death should stop,[116,180] as more causes for sudden death are discovered that were not known when SIDS was defined. Should molecular genetic mechanisms be pursued in all deaths? Alternatively, should they only be considered when there is a family history of SIDS, or only when sleep practices are not clearly implicated?[181,182] Or might, for example, exposure to hypoxia (described later in the chapter) and arising from the sleep environment place infants with mutations causing channelopathies at even greater risk for lethal dysrhythmias, according to the Triple Risk Model?

CURRENT UNDERSTANDING BASED ON INVESTIGATIONS OF THE SCENE AND CIRCUMSTANCES OF SUDDEN INFANT DEATH

After discussing high-technology tools, it is important to remember that major reductions in rates of sudden infant death in many countries have followed from low-tech observations and rigorous epidemiology.[1] For example, in 1978, Beal called attention to the probable importance of sleep position when infants die at night.[183] Her scene observations were viewed as unimportant[184] for more than 10 years, until there was widespread acceptance of the risk from prone positioning on soft bedding.

One type of sudden unexpected death for which scene investigations have always been crucial is infanticide. The perceived importance of infanticide as a frequent cause of death has waxed and waned. Dramatic series of cases[113] remind us that infanticide, with or without antecedent Munchausen syndrome by proxy, cannot be ignored. Gross and, occasionally, microscopic autopsy findings are of obvious importance when diagnosing nonaccidental trauma as a cause of death. However, it is less clear by autopsy how to prove intentional but subtle suffocation (e.g., using a pillow). Southall and coworkers[185] used covert video surveillance in the hospital to document that 30 of 39 very high-risk infants were subjected to intentional suffocation. Twelve had siblings who had died suddenly and unexpectedly. Although bloody froth about the nose and mouth is common among SIDS victims, 11 of 38 subjects in Southall's study had a history of an ALTE associated with frank bleeding from the nose and mouth, compared with none of 46 controls.

Two recent studies compared the presence of alveolar hemosiderin-laden macrophages (AHLMs) as evidence for pulmonary hemorrhage in cases of SIDS, suffocation,[186] and sudden unexpected infant deaths when nonaccidental injuries were suspected. AHLMs were more likely to be present in deaths associated with direct or circumstantial evidence for nonaccidental injuries.[187] Nevertheless, in this study, two thirds of infants with significant numbers of AHLM had no historical or postmortem evidence to suggest nonaccidental injury.

It seems probable that the percentage of sudden unexpected infant deaths that will be proven to be intentional will increase as the overall number of sudden deaths declines. Before the Back-to-Sleep campaign in the United States, based on serial cross-checks of data from social and law enforcement agencies, it was estimated that about 5% of SIDS deaths were likely to be caused by maltreatment.[188] Certainly, both multiple deaths within families, after genetic causes have been ruled out, and simultaneous deaths of twins should raise cautious suspicion. Nevertheless, the best evidence suggests that foul play is unlikely in the vast majority of second-infant deaths within a family.[189,190]

■■■ SLEEP PRACTICES AND THE DECLINE IN RATES OF SUDDEN INFANT DEATH SYNDROME—THE CHANGING EPIDEMIOLOGY

Success Story for Epidemiology

Supine sleep was recommended routinely in pediatric textbooks until the twentieth century.[191] However, in developed countries by the late twentieth century, 40% to 80% of infants were placed prone.[59]

In 1978, Beal and Blundell published findings emphasizing the position in which the infant was found at the time of death.[183] They carried out home visits and death scene investigations for the 35 to 40 deaths per year in South Australia. Seventy-five percent of victims were found prone, and more than half of all victims were facedown. Beal's findings triggered case-control studies in Australia and New Zealand, where in the mid-1980s the rates of SIDS were among the highest in the world. For example, in New Zealand the rate was 3.5 per 1000 births, and it was more than 6 per 1000 in the southern (Otago) district.[191,192]

In the New Zealand Cot Death Study, carried out from November 1987 through October 1990, the sleep practices and circumstances of death were reported for 485 SIDS victims and 1800 controls. The study emphasized four variables that increased risk that were also believed to be "modifiable"[193]: prone sleeping by infant (odds ratio, 3.70), maternal smoking, bed sharing, and never having been breastfed. Similar results that also implicated prone sleep were obtained in case-control studies in Australia and England.[194,195] Furthermore, several items of bedding were identified in these case-control studies that increased risk for dying among prone infants: sheepskins,[6] mattresses filled with bark and other natural fibers,[196] and duvets or comforters.[197] Subsequent interventions[3,195,198] in New Zealand, England, and Australia to reduce the prevalence of prone sleeping (from ~40% to <5%) were followed by reductions of 50% or more in deaths diagnosed as SIDS. Case-control studies in Seattle[199] and Chicago[200] have confirmed that prone sleep position and soft bedding[149] increase risk among infants in the United States.[201] The number of deaths attributed to SIDS fell in the United States after the Back-to-Sleep campaign (1994; see Fig. 76-1), although no postintervention case-control studies have been published. Unfortunately, as discussed later in the chapter, the number of sudden deaths during sleep has leveled off and may be increasing.

A formal argument has been substantiated that prone sleeping, or some factors strongly linked to prone sleeping, are part of a causal pathway for more than half of SIDS.[143] The findings of increased risk associated with prone sleep have been reproducible,[59] the odds ratios were large, and the temporal sequence (prone before death) is correct; there appears to be a dose effect, and reducing prone prevalence has reduced SIDS rates. Although the reduction in SIDS rates is a "success story" based largely in epidemiology, the mechanisms giving the prone position "biologic plausibility" as a cause for SIDS have been vigorously debated.[130,202,203] Before resuming our discussion of mechanisms, however, we will briefly call to mind "classic" SIDS epidemiology (before Back-to-Sleep) and how avoiding the prone position has changed the epidemiology of sudden unexpected infant deaths.

■■■ EPIDEMIOLOGY OF SUDDEN INFANT DEATH SYNDROME BEFORE AND AFTER BACK-TO-SLEEP INTERVENTIONS

As it was defined even before the current emphasis on knowledge of the circumstances of death,[116,117,151] infants dying of SIDS were often ill, but not ominously.[27] Their dispositions may have been placid, but their development was not worrisome. Complete autopsies showed groups of infants with minor abnormalities, but, by definition, nothing *per se* that would explain death.

Those who sought to solve the mystery of SIDS, the most common diagnosis when infants died beyond the neonatal period, were reminded that their hypothesis must deal with and account for certain epidemiologic realities. For the United States, these epidemiologic variables were defined by the National Institute of Child Health and Human Development Collaborative study (see Table 76-1).

The epidemiology of SIDS and sudden unexpected infant deaths has changed after successful sleep position interventions and because of the diagnostic shifting that has occurred with greater knowledge of the circumstances of death (see Table 76-1).[128]

◼◼ THE IMPACT OF SCENE INVESTIGATIONS ON THE UNDERSTANDING OF SUDDEN DEATH AND DIAGNOSTIC SHIFTING

During the first 20 years after SIDS was recognized, the definition and most of the research into its causes did not consider where the infant died. And an unexplained "cause of death," SIDS, was the official designation, even though the death scene was sparsely described, if at all. Nevertheless, the epidemiologic success story leading to SIDS reduction was based on careful descriptions of what was near the infant and how the infant was lying. Much of this information was collected before and around the time of the introduction of a new definition for SIDS that required a death scene investigation.

However, it is not clear, even now, that the majority of sudden unexpected infant deaths in the U.S. are diagnosed after a careful scene investigation.[204] It is also disappointing that reports used to set intervention agendas in high-risk populations did not include direct observations of the death scene or scene data on all deaths.[205,206] Nevertheless, sleep practices that increase risk and can be modified are still evident today in more than 80% of deaths.[141,207]

When the rubric for SIDS was introduced in 1973, "most of the deaths previously assigned strangulation or suffocation diagnoses ... were called SIDS."[208] Beginning in 1973, and for most of the 20 years thereafter, in the absence of information about how an infant was found, the majority of postneonatal deaths were considered unexplained and diagnosed as SIDS. However, by the early 1990s, as many as 56% of deaths diagnosed as SIDS were shown to have occurred prone and facedown on soft bedding, or with the head covered.[137,183] New hypothetical models suggested that thermal stress would be greater for those prone infants using soft bedding and comforters.[202,209] Furthermore, physiologic death scene re-creations showed that subtle but profound suffocation could have occurred in the infant's microenvironment within the death scene,[123,131,201,210,211] as the infant depleted the air near its nose of O_2 and enriched it with CO_2. Without scene information, deaths with negative medical histories and autopsies met the criteria used for SIDS before 1991.

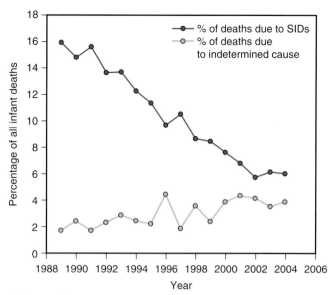

FIGURE 76-10. Increase in deaths about which there is more uncertainty about cause, as more scene data have become available in one state (California). Percentages of all infant deaths caused by SIDS *(closed circles)* and ill-defined or unspecified causes *(open circles)* are shown. (From Chang RK, Keens TG, Rodriguez S, et al. Sudden infant death syndrome: changing epidemiologic patterns in California 1989-2004. *J Pediatr.* 2008;153:498-502.)

The addition of scene data and the appreciation of the potential for thermal stress and lethal rebreathing have led to diagnostic shifting: Very similar deaths that had been called unexplained (SIDS) before death scene data became available are increasingly diagnosed as accidental suffocation positional asphyxia, or undetermined (Fig. 76-10).[128,212,213] This evolution in designation of manner and cause of death reflects the increase in information available to forensics teams. The prevalence of risks created within the sleep environment, especially for prone infants, is also more broadly realized.

Thus it seems likely, though still controversial, that compared to the early 1990s, fewer deaths will be designated as unexplained and SIDS, not because of arbitrary decisions, but because "previously unsuspected sleeping accidents are now being detected."[128]

In particular, diagnostic shifting has arisen from the investigation of deaths when asphyxia might play a partial role, whether accidental, caused by a sleep practice, or much less often, intentional. When asphyxia is a possibility, a modification of the Triple Risk Model (see Fig 76-9) that considers SIDS versus suffocation within interacting spectra of severity of environmental threat and infant vulnerabilities can provide a template for discussion between pathologists and physiologists who study the sleep environment of small infants (Fig. 76-11)[212,214]

Physiology Related to Sleep Position That May Make Infants More Vulnerable

Infants at increased risk for SIDS have been postulated and shown to have abnormal arousal, hypoxic drive, and airway protective reflexes, among other physiologic aberrations.[215,216] These abnormalities are reviewed later in the chapter and in light of the risk associated with prone sleep position.

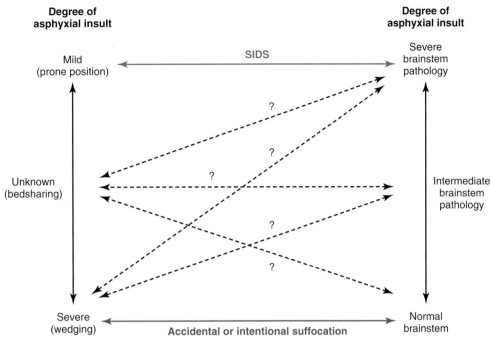

FIGURE 76-11. SIDS is conceptualized as a disorder of protective asphyxial challenge responses in which the vulnerable infant, due to brainstem pathology in neuronal networks that mediate responses to asphyxia, is compromised, and even mild asphyxial challenge causes death. At the other end of the spectrum, the asphyxial challenge is so severe that all infants, with or without underlying brainstem pathology, die. (From Randall BB, Wadee SA, Sens MA, et al. A practical classification schema incorporating consideration of possible asphyxia in cases of sudden unexpected infant death. *Forensic Sci Med Pathol.* 2009;5:254-260.)

ABNORMAL AROUSAL AND THE IMPACT OF SLEEP POSITION

Arousal during sleep is defined as full awakenings with eyes opened, or as a change to a different sleep stage by electroencephalogram (EEG) criteria, or by a constellation of EEG, electromyographic, and air flow changes. Arousal may be cortical as evidenced by obvious changes in EEG frequency, or imputed (subcortical arousal) from changes in autonomic measurements (e.g., changes in heart rate) or suppression of EEG sleep spindles.[217,218] Arousal has been assessed experimentally in response to airway obstruction[219-221] and central apnea,[219] breathing hypercarbic[222] or hypoxic[223] gas mixtures, laryngeal stimulation with fluid,[57] sound,[225] and jets of air hitting the face.[226] Changes in sleep state or awakening "may produce a fundamental change in the nature of the ventilatory response to a respiratory stimulus."[57] Arousal is often associated with the termination of obstructive apnea[221] and is the probable cause, at some level, of sleep fragmentation leading to daytime sleepiness with obstructive sleep apnea.[224]

Infants and adults exposed to external threats to their airways will often change their sleep state and awaken.[134,227] However, arousal is not always apparently needed. Infants sleeping facedown[228] and premature infants with central apnea[229] may also change position or resume breathing without awakening or showing changes in their cortical EEG.[219,229,230] These alternative strategies would preserve sleep while presumably ending the threat to ventilation.

Infants at greater statistical risk for SIDS compared with controls may have diminished arousal to breathing hypoxic and hypercarbic gases[216,222] and longer obstructive

apnea before arousal and resumption of eupneic breathing.[231] Infants at 8 weeks of age deprived of sleep by having their naps delayed, as may be the case when infants transition to daycare,[140] will have more spontaneous obstructive apneas during sleep, and the arousal threshold to white noise will be increased.[232] Cigarette smoke exposure *in utero*, which markedly increases the risk for SIDS, is also associated with higher auditory arousal thresholds during non–rapid eye movement sleep.[233] Consistent with the notion that thermal stress is a mechanism for SIDS, higher ambient temperature ($28°$ C versus $24°$ C) increases the arousal threshold to sound in infants about 3 months of age.[234] To summarize, then, in response to sound stimuli and air jets applied to the face, arousal from sleep is both altered and more difficult to elicit among sleep-deprived infants, prone-sleeping term and premature infants,[235] and prone infants with obstructive apnea.[226,231]

Although arousal may be essential to ending some threats to ventilation during sleep in infants (see Fig. 76-8), the reliability of arousal from sleep in interrupting threats due to sleep in risky environments is uncertain. For example, infants dying beneath bedclothes have often pulled them over their face, or moved beneath them.[20] Although these infants died while unobserved, it is conceivable that they suffocated while awake and not asleep, and that arousal played little role, except possibly to cause the awakening that got them into trouble in the first place. It has also been shown that the normal arousal sequence to having the nose and mouth covered—sigh, startle, arm thrashing, head lift, and turn—can actually worsen the infant's predicament within the sleep microenvironment, by pulling bedclothes farther over the head or by placing the infant facedown into soft bedding.[122,134]

Arousal deficits also do not appear to explain gender differences in susceptibility to SIDS. Male infants are at greater risk for dying suddenly and unexpectedly, but their arousal thresholds to air jets are the same as for females at 2 to 3 months of age, and actually is lower at 2 to 4 weeks.[230] Thus, a consistent finding when infants die suddenly and unexpectedly, male preponderance seems not to be explained by deficient arousal but may be explained by too brisk arousal. In this regard, it should be pointed out that arousal may foster excessive ventilatory compensation for transient underventilation. An "increased loop gain" in response to airway obstruction has been shown to increase respiratory pattern instability, and sustain rather than interrupt obstructive events.[87,236,237] Finally, as discussed above, infants may gain access to fresh air and end the threat to effective ventilation by subtle head (nose and mouth) repositioning without apparent awakening or EEG changes.[228]

In any event, whether or not an infant arouses to compromised ventilation, and how much ventilation is improved or further compromised as a result of movements or changes in breathing pattern during an arousal, may together define a developmental vulnerability for specific infants exposed to threats within their sleep environment.

ABNORMALITIES IN VENTILATORY RESPONSE AND THREATS WITHIN THE SLEEP ENVIRONMENT

In addition to blunted arousal, infants at particular risk for SIDS may have blunted ventilatory responses. Minute volume increases while breathing hypercarbic or hypoxic air are, in part, developmentally regulated,[238,239] and the increases are less in some high-risk infants than in controls.[78,79,223] In a hypercarbic environment, preterm infants at 35 to 37 weeks PMA have less respiratory drive ($P_{0.1}/P_{imax}$) in response to airway occlusion while prone compared to supine.[240] The ventilatory responses of normal infants may be less when prone than when supine.[241] Sleep environments that lead to trapping of exhaled air and creation of relatively hypoxic and CO_2-rich environments would be of particular relevance in this regard. As noted earlier, those areas in the brain stem with diminished cholinergic and serotonergic receptor activity among SIDS victims may be chemosensitive areas, particularly for changes in CO_2 and pH.

Thus, lines of investigation within respiratory physiology and neuropathology have merged to provide insight into mechanisms pertinent to epidemiologic studies implicating prone sleep position.

SOFT BEDDING AS AN EFFECT MODIFIER: PHYSIOLOGIC IMPLICATIONS

Arousal and ventilatory responses to challenges may be less in prone than in supine sleeping infants. What gives rise to the "challenge" that must be responded to is suggested by studies of factors within the sleep environment that increase risk in the prone position.

It has been known for 45 years, for example, that soft bedding use increases risk for "cot death."[242] Items of bedding that dramatically increase risk when used by prone infants have been shown using quantitative criteria[201] to be much softer than items not associated with increased prone risk. Soft, natural-fiber mattresses[196] and sheepskins[192,196] are not associated with increased risk of sudden unexpected death among supine infants. However, in Australia, for example, sleeping prone on a mattress filled with natural fibers increased risk by 20-fold.[196]

Items of bedding sharing similar physical properties[201] (e.g., soft, with porous covers) have been identified in other case series and case-control studies of sudden, unexpected infant deaths.[197,200] The bedding includes polystyrene bead–filled cushions,[124] comforters or duvets, pillows,[137] and various forms of "ordinary bedding."[211]

Anywhere from 20% to 70% of infants[18,19,242] dying suddenly and unexpectedly will be both prone and facedown when found (see Fig. 76-8). Using soft bedding increases the risk that an infant dying will be found facedown into the underlying bedding.[137] It has been possible to show with mechanical and animal models, and human infants that assuming the prone and facedown position on items of soft bedding can markedly increase CO_2 concentration and decrease O_2 concentration near the face of an infant (Figs. 76-12 and 76-13). This environment can be lethal in experimental animals and has been shown to cause hypercarbia and hypoxemia in living infants.[243]

Waters and colleagues[122] have also shown that this scenario occurs spontaneously. In a study done using home

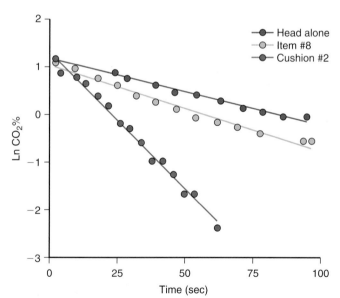

FIGURE 76-12. Results from studies done to quantify the rate of disappearance of exhaled CO_2. The mechanical model included the head from an infant mannequin, a syringe filled with 5% CO_2 attached to the mannequin's "airway" used to simulate ventilation, and an infrared CO_2 analyzer. The steepest line reflects the mannequin being ventilated without nose or mouth encumbered; the other two are with nose and mouth covered by soft "ordinary" bedding from death scene investigations. The rate constant for the time course of CO_2 dispersal correlates with the ability of the sleep environment to be asphyxiating. (From Kemp JS, Thach BT. Quantifying the potential of infant bedding to limit CO2 dispersal and factors affecting rebreathing in bedding. *J Appl Physiol.* 1995;78:740-745.)

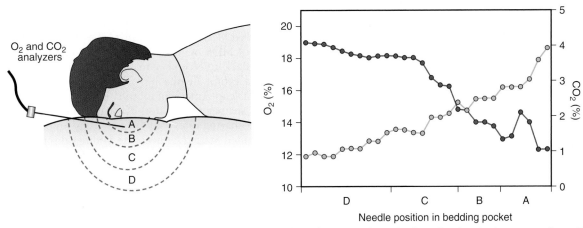

FIGURE 76-13. Inspired O_2 and CO_2 sampled at four different distances from the nose and mouth of an infant breathing into a comforter. The graph demonstrates the gradients of O_2 depletion and CO_2 accumulation. It is likely that hypoxemia is the more serious acute threat to vulnerable infants. (From Patel AL, Harris K, Thach BT. Inspired CO2 and O2 in sleeping infants rebreathing from bedding. Relevance for sudden infant death syndrome. *J Appl Physiol.* 2001;91:2537-2545.)

recordings of SpO_2, transcutaneous Pco_2, respiratory effort, and videos, they showed that an infant sleeping prone, without adults present, assumed the facedown position on a mattress pad. Although the infant escaped this position, her $PtcCO_2$ increased from 50 to 87 mm Hg. The danger of such a scenario would be obvious for an otherwise healthy infant with blunted responses to hypoxemia or CO_2 concentration, or inefficient airway-protective behaviors.

In addition to preventing the ingress of fresh air, soft bedding, particularly comforters (duvets), provides much thermal insulation and has the potential to cause thermal stress.[197,202] The thermal stress theory as a mechanism for prone death has been discussed in detail elsewhere.[130] Increases in thermal insulation around infants (quantified in tog units) are associated with increased risk of sudden death in some studies, particularly if an infant is prone and has a respiratory illness such as RSV infection.[63] Infants who are prone with the forehead covered have about 20% less surface for heat radiation than supine infants.[130]

The mechanism proposed in deaths caused by thermal stress is not heat stroke with multiorgan injury.[130,203] Rather, an abnormality in cardiorespiratory pattern may be elicited by their response to thermal stress and is suggested by preliminary studies in newborns. In experimental animals, increasing core temperature prolongs LCRA,[244] and there seems to be an interactive effect of hyperthermia and cigarette smoking in further prolonging the apneic phase of the LCR.[245]

What the mechanism or resultant cardiorespiratory abnormality caused by thermal stress is, particularly beyond the first month of life, is a question of great interest. Infants do seem to be able to thermoregulate when exposed to environments that had been presumed to cause thermal stress,[2,246] and success with Back-to-Sleep occurred without reduction in thermal stress.[3,197,198] Furthermore, analysis of data from New Zealand, based on hypothetical models of SIDS infants' thermal environment, has shown that "Too little thermal insulation for the lower critical temperature was associated with an increased risk of SIDS...."[247]

SHARING BEDS, RACIAL DISPARITIES, AND CONTINUED HIGH RATES OF SUDDEN UNEXPECTED INFANT DEATHS

Among infants sleeping alone in cribs, staying supine and keeping their heads from being covered by blankets should lead to further reductions in sudden death during sleep. Sharing an adult sleep surface, however, has been and remains a factor that increases risks for sudden death.* In some multivariate analyses, risks associated with bed sharing have been "clouded" and rendered statistically insignificant by very high rates (~ 90%)[250] of maternal cigarette smoking among infants dying while sharing a bed. More recent studies,[14,16,200] while noting an increased risk for infant death while sharing a bed if the mother smokes, have also found sharing a bed to be an important independent risk factor for sudden death, particularly among the youngest infants (odds ratio [OR] 2.4 to 4.1). Infants younger than 1 week of age are not typically included in studies of SIDS or SUID, perhaps because their deaths are quite frequently explained by postmortem investigations. Indeed, a recent case series from London, UK, of 55 sudden unexpected deaths in the first week of life revealed a plausible cause of death in 58%. However, of those whose death remained unexplained, 21of 23 involved "co-sleeping of an infant with an adult."[146]

In addition to increased risk for suffocation,[251] there is other evidence emerging that might explain increased risk for sudden and unexpected death among infants sharing an adult bed.

Careful studies of infants in their homes[2] comparing bed-sharing infants to those room sharing but on a separate crib ("cot") have shown that infants sharing a bed are exposed to an increased relative thermal stress (Fig. 76-14), "requiring more vasodilatation to maintain core temperature." Baddock and colleagues also found that bed-sharing infants were more likely to sleep on their sides and less likely to be found supine, and much more likely to have their heads covered,[252] both factors that increase SIDS risk dramatically. Infants who bed-shared also awoke more

---

*References 14, 16, 27, 200, 242, and 248 through 250.

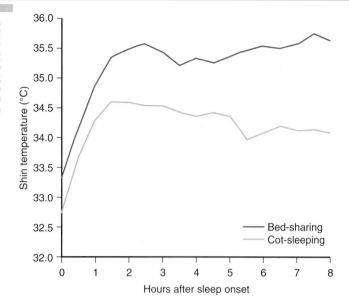

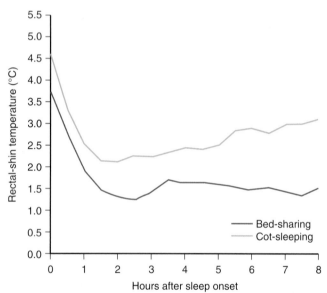

FIGURE 76-14. This figure shows that skin temperature, measured on the shin, was higher in infants who were bed-sharing. This led to a narrower gradient between core (rectal) and skin temperature over which thermal regulation occurred among bed-sharing infants. (From Baddock SA, Galand BC, Bekers MGS, et al. Bed-sharing and the infant's thermal environment in the home setting. *Arch Dis Child.* 2004;86:1111-1116.)

often. If they also had more spontaneous arousals, particularly with their heads covered, they might be more likely to experience the ventilatory instability discussed earlier in the chapter associated with desaturations and a dysfunctional arousal that did not gain access to fresh air.

In the United States, there are disparities in the rates of sudden unexpected infant deaths among African-American infants. African-American infants do sleep prone twice as often as other infants.[253] Thus, interventions to reduce racial disparities in SIDS should continue to foster supine sleep. Nevertheless, reducing rates of prone sleeping among African-American infants may have only a small effect on disparities because of high rates of bed sharing among African-American infants.[142] Supine sleep has never been shown to be protective while sharing a bed.[59] As an example, in New Zealand, among

Maori infants, 29% of whom shared beds in a case-control study,[254] dramatic reductions in rates of prone sleeping occurred (43% to <5%) with little impact on the Maoris' rates of SIDS or infant mortality.[255] In the United States, since Back-to-Sleep began, rates of SIDS and sudden unexpected infant deaths have decreased among both white and African-American infants, but the rate of fall has been much steeper among non–African-American infants.

Bed-sharing rates may be increasing among all infants in the United States.[256] Given the findings discussed, one must consider whether bed sharing, either to enhance nurturing behaviors or to foster breastfeeding, can be done safely.[257] It is not clear that it can. Sleep arrangements for infants who are bed sharing are softer[258] and much more likely to be associated with suffocation deaths.[251] In Norway, recommendations to increase rates of breastfeeding that included bed sharing were followed by an increase in the rate of bed sharing in sudden deaths from 2% to 34%.[12] All these findings raise the question of whether the impact of Back-to-Sleep, which may not "work" during bedsharing, has been blunted by persistently high or increased rates of bedsharing, particularly among infants at the highest risk for dying. In Canada, bed sharing has been officially discouraged,[259] and the AAP has developed a similar recommendation.

◼ SUMMARY

It was estimated in 1967 that in industrialized countries 25,000 infants per year died suddenly and unexpectedly.[120] Most children who died suddenly and unexpectedly then and now do not have pathologic findings to explain their demise and, after 1967, their deaths were diagnosed as SIDS.[208] A triple-risk model can be used to explore explanations for sudden death: Infant susceptibility, developmental vulnerability, and exogenous stressors of varying magnitude. Abnormalities in ventilatory control or reflexes, and in behavioral or minute volume responses can usually be implicated. These abnormalities may be nonlethal when most infants sleep supine on their own sleep surface. Newer approaches to the pathology of cardiorespiratory control, lethal inherited dysrhythmias and energy metabolism, and continued emphasis on safe sleeping practices should lead to further reductions in the number of infants dying suddenly and unexpectedly each year.

Suggested Reading

Darnall RA, Ariagno RL, Kinney HC. The late preterm infant and the control of breathing, sleep, and brainstem development. *Clin Perinatol.* 2006;33:883–914.

Dwyer T, Ponsonby A-L. Sudden infant death syndrome and prone sleep position. *Ann Epidemiol.* 2009;19:245–249.

Kemp JS, Thach BT. Rebreathing of exhaled air. In: Byard RW, Krous HF, eds. *Sudden Infant Death Syndrome—Problems, Progress and Possibilities.* London: Edward Arnold; 2001:138–155.

Kinney HC, Thach BT. The sudden infant death syndrome. *N Engl J Med.* 2009;361:795–805.

Poets CF. Apnea of prematurity: What can observational studies tell us about pathophysiology? *Sleep Med.* 2010;11:701–707.

Reix P, St Hilaire M, Praud J-P. Laryngeal sensitivity in the neonatal period: from bench to bedside. *Pediatr Pulmonol.* 2007;42:674–682.

Tester DJ, Ackerman MJ. Cardiomyopathic and channelopathic causes of sudden unexplained death in infants and children. *Annu Rev Med.* 2009;60:69–84.

References

The complete reference list is available online at www.expertconsult.com

77 DISORDERS OF BREATHING DURING SLEEP

David Gozal, MD, and Leila Kheirandish-Gozal, MD

◼ BASIC MECHANISMS AND ARCHITECTURE OF NORMAL SLEEP

Neural Circuitry of Sleep and Waking

Sleep is a global and dynamically regulated state. The control mechanisms of sleep are manifested at every level of biologic organization, from genes and intracellular mechanisms to networks of cell populations, and to all central neuronal systems at the organismal level, including those that control movement, arousal, autonomic functions, behavior, and cognition. In mammals, sleep states can be readily differentiated into two major types, namely rapid eye movement (REM) and non–rapid eye movement (NREM) sleep. These two distinctive sleep states are defined in terms of their electroencephalographic (EEG) and electromyographic (EMG) characteristics. NREM sleep involves high-voltage, low-frequency "synchronized" wave activity with relatively preserved skeletal muscle tonic activity, whereas REM sleep is characterized by wakelike high-frequency, low-amplitude "desynchronized" activity in the EEG along with a typical attenuation of skeletal muscle tonic activity (i.e., REM atonia). Bursts of 12- to 14-Hz sleep spindles are characteristic of NREM sleep in adults and children, although such bursts may also occur during REM sleep; maximal development of phasic spindle activity emerges after approximately 16 weeks postnatally.

The neural sites underlying the onset, maintenance, and function of NREM and REM sleep continue to be the object of intensive research; however, sufficient insights are now available to link certain breathing patterns with the neural properties and activity patterns of state-related regulatory structures. Areas within the basal forebrain, including regions within the preoptic region, have long been implicated in initiating NREM sleep, with local stimulation eliciting the typical NREM sleep state and lesion studies resulting in pronounced loss of sleep. Single-cell studies assessing the discharge patterns of neurons within these neural regions conclusively demonstrate the existence of neurons that selectively fire with the onset of NREM sleep in this area. Certain features of NREM sleep, such as the large synchronous slow waves (delta waves) and bursts of 12- to 14-Hz sleep spindles, are critically dependent on the integrity of the thalamocortical circuitry, even if these characteristic neural activity patterns can be generated under certain pharmacologic conditions, such as subsequent to atropine administration during waking states. Furthermore, recent work has implicated adenosine and its cognate receptors as an important mechanism of NREM sleep regulation, such that this neurotransmitter is currently believed to regulate metabolic and recovery aspects of NREM sleep within the basal forebrain and thalamocortical regions.[1,2]

It should also be stressed that thermoregulatory areas of the anterior hypothalamus closely interact with sleep-associated regions in the brain and dictate the generation of close relationships between warming, discharge of thermoregulatory neurons, and induction of sleep. Indeed, higher temperatures, whether externally applied or through localized warming of hypothalamic structures, will lead to increased sleepiness and NREM sleep duration.

Since the principal physiologic characteristics of REM sleep persist even after separation of the forebrain from the pons, it has been suggested that mechanisms underlying this unique sleep state lie caudal to the diencephalon within specific and spatially restricted brain stem regions such as the locus coeruleus and several pontine nuclei; notably, areas within the dorsal lateral pons have been particularly implicated in eliciting some of the characteristics of REM sleep state. For example, the atonia of REM sleep can be abolished by lesions in the dorsal pons ventral to the locus coeruleus, and phasic somatic events can be terminated by lesions in the pedunculopontine tegmentum. Certain phasic elements (e.g., the variation of sympathetic and parasympathetic outflow during REM sleep) are dependent on the integrity of vestibular nuclei, while phasic eye movements, a hallmark of REM sleep, will persist even in the presence of lesions in the vestibular sites. A number of brain stem regions, namely the dorsal and caudal raphe, locus coeruleus, and ventral medullary surface, show declines in neural activity during REM sleep; however, most of the brain will manifest substantial increases in neural cell activity and glucose consumption during REM sleep, sometimes exceeding levels seen during wakefulness. Brain regions that decrease their discharge patterns during REM sleep play important roles in blood pressure regulation; however, it is unclear whether the state-related cell patterns in these regions bear a relationship to blood pressure control (and indirectly to breathing patterns) during REM sleep.

◼ DEVELOPMENTAL ASPECTS OF SLEEP

Sleep state organization undergoes rapid development during the first 6 months of life. Neonates and young infants spend a disproportionate amount of time in REM sleep; indeed infants exhibit REM sleep at sleep onset, an event that is considered abnormal in the adult. NREM sleep (also termed *quiet sleep*) is poorly developed in newborns, since the slow oscillatory EEG patterns that define this state are not as readily apparent during early postnatal life and may manifest as intermittent slow and faster EEG patterns (e.g., tracé alternans). However, the relative amount of quiet sleep increases during the first 3 months of life, with K-complexes and sleep spindles becoming increasingly evident. Therefore, scoring of sleep using adult criteria is not applicable before 3 to 6 months of age, and a more simplistic categorization of sleep states into awake, quiet sleep, active sleep (equivalent to REM sleep), and indeterminate sleep is normally used during the first year of life.[3–9] The total duration of sleep decreases relative to the 24-hour period, the relative proportion of NREM sleep increases, and that of REM sleep decreases with advancing age. At 1 year of age, children will typically require 12 to 13 hours of sleep primarily during the night, with one or two naps during the day. At this age, well-defined NREM sleep alternates with REM sleep, the latter accounting for 30% of total sleep time in recurring 90-minute cycles very similar to those found in the adult. At approximately 2 years of age, the relative proportion of REM sleep will stabilize at approximately 20% to 25% of total sleep time and will remain somewhat constant until old age, despite gradual reductions in total sleep duration with advancing age. NREM sleep acquires its maximal expression in duration and depth during the first decade of life. Indeed, the depth of sleep in childhood is quite remarkable considering how difficult it is to arouse a child during the first cycle of slow-wave sleep. During the second decade of life, slow-wave sleep gradually decreases by approximately 40%, continuing its gradual decline until old age. It is during slow-wave sleep that growth hormone is secreted in large amounts, and thus either sleep deprivation or disorders of sleep may interfere with the secretion and regulation of growth hormone, with potential and rather immediate clinical consequences.[10]

RESPIRATORY CONTROL MECHANISMS

Our understanding of respiratory control has undergone multiple evolutionary waves in the last century. Obviously, breathing is an important and vital function. Nevertheless, despite the critical functions of respiration, it is undeniable that the respiratory control system undergoes substantial maturation during the first few years of life. There is no doubt that the relative uncertainty about the anatomic and functional aspects pertaining to the neural respiratory pathways, the complexities of neuronal firing activities, the multitude of neurotransmitters within each brain stem nucleus, and the frequently nucleus-dependent opposing roles played by these neurotransmitters in respiratory function can be quite overwhelming and difficult to comprehend. Despite such problems, the field of respiratory control has evolved tremendously in recent years, and we are now witnessing the initial discovery of several of the genes that control the development and maturation of multiple neurally controlled respiratory functions.[11]

THE RESPIRATORY RHYTHM GENERATOR

The putative neural center responsible for generation of respiratory rhythmic activity has now been identified,[12] and specific markers such as neurokinin and opioid receptors in these neurons have yielded estimates that this uniquely important neural center is a cluster of 150 to 200 neurons in the brain stem region designated as *Pre-Botzinger complex*.[13] This small number of rhythmically firing neurons appears both necessary and sufficient to generate most of the complex normal respiratory behaviors that we know such as eupnea, sigh, and gasping.[14–16] The development of several elegant models ranging from highly reductionistic (brain stem slice) to less reductionistic approaches (whole brain stem–heart-lung preparation) will undoubtedly permit extensive characterization of the network configuration responses, the functional neurotransmitters involved in generation of respiratory rhythm, and permit a thorough understanding of the electrophysiologic properties of these unique cells both during development as well as during disease. Several genes, such as *PHOX2A*, *HOX* paralogs, and HOX-regulating genes *MAFB* (formerly *Kreisler [mouse] maf-related leucine zipper homolog*) and *EGR2* (formerly *Krox20*), have been identified as important players in the embryonic generation of respiratory centers and their intrinsic connectivities.[17,18] These and other yet unknown genes that regulate the ontogeny of brain stem development may provide initial insights into the regulation of the initial phases involved in the normal and abnormal formation of the respiratory network.

SLEEP AND BREATHING DURING DEVELOPMENT

The cyclic activity of respiratory rhythm generation is further modulated by suprapontine sites that include important efferent projections to areas mediating the sleep-wake cycle, thermoregulation, and circadian rhythm rhythmicity. Respiratory control areas also receive afferent inputs from central and peripheral chemoreceptors and from other receptors within the respiratory pump (upper airways, chest wall, and lungs). During fetal life, breathing is discontinuous and coincides with REM-like sleep. After birth, respiratory rhythm is established as a continuous activity to maintain cellular O_2 and CO_2 homeostasis. Respiratory pattern instability during sleep is typically present during early life such that short apneic episodes lasting less than 5 seconds are extremely common in preterm neonates, and their frequency is reduced in full-term newborns. These episodes occur predominantly during REM sleep as a result of the greater respiratory instability in this state. Several developmental differences between the neonate and the adult respiratory systems may further account for the emergence of sleep-associated disruption of normal gas exchange in early postnatal life, and include the following:

- Neonates have greater difficulty switching from the nasal to the oral route of breathing, and the majority of younger neonates can be considered as obligatory or near-obligatory nasal breathers.
- In neonates, reflexes originating in the upper airway (laryngeal chemoreflex) are potentiated and can induce profound apnea and bradycardia. This respiratory depressant component of the laryngeal chemoreflex decreases with maturation, such that prolonged apnea induced by stimulation of the laryngeal chemoreflex is more prominent in preterm than in full-term neonates.[19]

- The chest wall compliance is increased in neonates, thereby requiring dynamic, rather than passive, maintenance of the functional residual capacity of the lungs. Furthermore, neonates have "barrel-shaped" rib cages, and the rib cage contribution to tidal breathing is smaller than in older children and adults. Thus, any condition whereby the ability to maintain functional residual capacity is compromised, as in REM sleep, will lead to increased susceptibility.
- Paradoxical breathing (i.e., asynchronous or out-of-phase motion of the chest and abdomen), especially during REM sleep, is common in newborns because of uncoordinated interactions between chest and abdominal respiratory musculature. The duration of paradoxical breathing during sleep decreases as postnatal age increases. Paradoxical breathing is rare or absent after 3 years of age.[20]
- The respiratory rate is high in the neonatal period and decreases during infancy and early childhood. Respiratory rate decreases exponentially with increasing body weight and parallels changes in overall metabolic rates. Notably, respiratory rate is higher during REM sleep than it is in NREM sleep.
- Apneas of short duration (<10 seconds) are extremely common during the early period of life. Apneic episodes are more frequent in REM sleep than during NREM sleep. Apneic episodes are mostly central, and they decrease in number with advancing postnatal age. Obstructive and mixed apneic episodes are more frequently seen in preterm than in full-term neonates, possibly reflecting developmental changes in pharyngeal, laryngeal, and central airway collapsibility.
- Periodic breathing, defined as three episodes of apnea lasting longer than 3 seconds and separated by continued respiration over a period of 20 seconds or less, is a common respiratory pattern in preterm neonates and may also be highly prevalent in full-term newborns.[21,22] However, periodic breathing decreases in frequency during the first year of life and usually is not considered to be of any specific pathologic significance. Notwithstanding such considerations, environmental variables such as sleep state transitions, arousals, hypoxia, and hyperthermia can enhance the frequency and magnitude of periodic breathing in newborns, and ultimately lead to destabilization of cardiorespiratory homeostasis.
- Apneic episodes during sleep in neonates are associated with a decrease in heart rate, particularly during NREM sleep. The presence of hypoxemia will enhance this reflex bradycardia during apnea.
- Arousal from sleep is thought to be a major determinant for termination of apnea, and therefore arousal deficits have been implicated in the pathophysiology of sudden infant death syndrome (SIDS). However, fewer than 10% of apneic episodes are terminated by a full-fledged EEG arousal in neonates. Autonomic arousals are nevertheless quite frequent during the period surrounding the termination of an apneic event. Moreover, while hypercapnia is a potent stimulus of arousal, hypoxia, and particularly rapidly developing hypoxia, is much less effective in inducing arousal. Finally, prone position, sleep deprivation, and prenatal-postnatal exposure to cigarette smoking are all accompanied by decreased arousability in neonates.
- Healthy full-term newborns will usually maintain oxyhemoglobin saturation values of 92% to 100% during sleep in the first 4 weeks of life. Arterial blood O_2 levels are lowest during the first week of life and increase during the next 1 to 3 months, such that all newborns will have values of 97% to 100% after 2 months of age. Basal values for arterial CO_2 tension during sleep are generally between 36 and 42 mm Hg in newborns and infants.

As delineated earlier in the chapter, the implications of REM sleep on breathing are substantial, and, as discussed later, the loss of muscle tone during REM sleep is particularly important to the upper airway muscles and airway patency. An important aspect of breathing control is the close interaction of breathing and blood pressure regulation. The respiratory system, using primarily somatic musculature, exerts substantial influence on moment-to-moment blood pressure; conversely, transient elevation of blood pressure can inhibit breathing efforts, while lowering of blood pressure can increase them. The interactions between the systems can be observed readily in breathing influences on heart rate (a classic example being respiratory sinus arrhythmia). Inspiratory efforts normally are associated with accelerated heart rate and expiratory efforts with deceleration, the result of reflex activity from pulmonary afferents and vagal outflow; the resulting coupling between breathing and heart rate is particularly prominent during NREM sleep, and measures of the interaction can provide a useful indication of state.[23] In addition, phasic activity during REM sleep induces substantial parasympathetic and sympathetic outflow, resulting in larger but typically slower variation in heart rate. Plots of cardiac beat-to-beat intervals demonstrate the substantial influences exerted normally during each state, with NREM sleep exerting a highly cyclic effect on heart rate variation and REM sleep showing a lesser extent of modulation by breathing but larger, slower sources of variation. Waking shows a large variation in heart rate changes; typically very active periods are accompanied by high heart rates with little variation. The cyclic nature of cardiac rate variation has led to a variety of procedures to measure the sympathetic and parasympathetic influences. Particular syndromes exert unique patterns of respiration-related variation; for example, children with congenital central hypoventilation syndrome (CCHS) show a relative absence of variation of respiratory modulation of heart rate, and infants who later succumb to SIDS also show reduced variation to breathing.

CENTRAL CHEMORECEPTORS AND THEIR DEVELOPMENT

The chemoreflexes exert powerful influences over breathing as well as cardiac and vascular control. Chemoreflex physiology is complex, and the exact molecular mechanisms by which the chemoreflexes are activated remain unclear. The traditional and classic theory formulated during the late 1950s proposed that the central chemoreceptors were located in the ventrolateral medullary surface of the brain stem and responded to hypercapnia and pH changes, whereas the peripheral chemoreceptors were located in the carotid bodies and primarily responded to changes in blood O_2 tension. While this concept has now evolved (see later in the chapter), it is worthwhile to mention that hypercapnia (particularly transient changes in CO_2 tension above the apneic threshold) can also activate the peripheral chemoreceptors, and it may account for as much as one third of peripheral chemoreceptor activity. Activation of either central or peripheral chemoreflexes exerts powerful effects on sympathetic activity in both health and disease and may be an important contributor to pathophysiology of obstructive sleep apnea (OSA).

MULTIPLICITY OF CENTRAL CHEMOSENSITIVE CENTERS

A critically important advance in the field of respiratory control involved discarding the classic concept of central chemosensitive sites as being located in restricted areas of the ventral medullary surface. Indeed, several lines of evidence have now clearly established that neurons showing intrinsic chemosensitive properties (i.e., the ability to sense changes in extracellular pH and contribute to the ventilatory response) are diffusely located in the central nervous system, and that regions such as the posterior hypothalamus, cerebellum, locus coeruleus, raphe, and multiple nuclei within the brain stem all contribute to the well-characterized hypercapnic ventilatory response.[24–26] Why is this important? One reason is that in these patients the phenotypic manifestations of conditions such as central alveolar hypoventilation, particularly when occurring secondary to other disorders (e.g., myelomeningocele, tumors, stroke), are not adequately explained by either the location or the magnitude of the brain lesions. Second, it is very possible that the normal developmental processes of the ventilatory response to elevations of CO_2 are not only important to long-term stability of the homeostatic system but may be even more important to the preservation of respiratory stability during respiratory transients, particularly during sleep. Conditions such as apparent life-threatening events or even SIDS may originate from dysfunctional development of either the respiratory rhythm controllers or, alternatively, that of the neural networks underlying hypoxic and hypercapnic chemosensitivities as well as those mediating arousal from sleep.[27,28]

The neurotransmitters involved in the intrinsic sensory pathways associated with central chemoreception are currently unknown. The presence of cholinergic muscarinic receptors in those brain stem areas traditionally associated with CO_2 chemosensitivity appears to play a major role in the neuronal excitation associated with the enhanced ventilatory response to hypercapnia, although additional neurotransmitters are also clearly involved. It must be emphasized that the central CO_2 chemosensory mechanisms may not be fully functional or mature at birth. Indeed, animal models in various species show that hypercapnic ventilatory responses will increase with advancing age. Hypercapnia elicits a relatively sustained ventilatory increase in term infants that is almost entirely caused by an increase in tidal volume without consistent change in respiratory frequency. In contrast, the ventilatory response to hypercapnia in premature infants is attenuated and can even

become inhibitory at higher concentrations of inhaled CO_2, with CO_2 overall respiratory responses increasing with postconceptional age. In preterm neonates, the ventilatory increase to hypercapnia is accompanied by a progressive increase in expiratory duration and a consequent reduction in frequency over time, both of which appear to be associated with diaphragmatic recruitment during expiration (respiratory braking or grunting). This unique mechanism appears to preserve a high end-expiratory lung volume such as to optimize gas exchange and promote respiratory stability. Little is known about the development of central chemoreceptor function beyond infancy. In awake prepubertal children, there appears to be an enhanced ventilatory response to hypercapnia compared with adults, and these differences may underlie differences in metabolic rate.[29] Similarly, significant developmental differences in CO_2 responses emerge when the CO_2 stimulus is presented in either a step (sudden increase) or ramp (slow progressive increase) fashion.[30] These findings in older children suggest that at some time during transition from infancy to childhood and on to adulthood, major changes occur in the relative contributions and integration of peripheral and central chemoreceptor activity. The cascades of genes, receptors, and neurotransmitters that mediate these developmental changes are unknown at the present time. Similarly, the elements involved in the integrated coordination of the developmental changes at the level of the carotid body, neural transmission, or central nervous system remain unclear.

PERIPHERAL CHEMOREFLEXES

The ventilatory responses related to changes in blood O_2 levels are a complex interaction of a variety of peripheral and central responses. Nevertheless, the rapidity of the peripheral chemoreceptor responses to blood oxygenation changes allows for assessment of the initial stimulatory effect elicited by activation of these peripherally located chemosensory cells, of which the most important are glomus cells within the carotid bodies. Peripheral chemoreceptor activity is typically assessed by monitoring the fast transient increase in minute ventilation after inhalation of gases containing low concentrations of O_2. Isocapnic hypoxic responses (over a period of 2 to 3 minutes) or five tidal breaths of pure N_2 are among the strategies that have been used.[31–33] Alternatively, the ventilatory decline subsequent to inhalation of 100% O_2 is also considered as a reliable indicator of peripheral chemoreceptor gain (Dejours test). However, it is important to indicate that the ventilatory decrease to acute hyperoxia is ultimately followed by an increase in ventilation that is centrally mediated.[34] More sophisticated paradigms using random alternations of N_2 and O_2 in a computerized setting have recently permitted the development of reproducible and consistent findings in infants and children suspected to be at risk for chemoreceptor dysfunction.[35–38] Independent of the test selected, substantial attention to sleep state is required when assessing respiratory chemoreceptor drive in infants and in the interpretation of such tests, such that these tests are best reserved for specialized laboratories in which specific normative values have been developed, and therefore allow for more reliable clinical assessment of individual patients presenting with symptoms suggestive of chemosensory dysfunction.

A typical phenomenon associated with more sustained exposure to hypoxic gas mixtures consists in the emergence of a relative ventilatory decline after 5 to 6 minutes of hypoxic exposure. This hypoxic ventilatory decline has also been termed *hypoxic ventilatory roll-off*. This phenomenon is particularly prominent during infancy, such that with sustained hypoxia in neonates there is a well-characterized increase in breathing followed by a reduction in ventilation that will usually reach levels below normoxic breathing. In more mature children and in adults, the reduction in ventilation will usually reach levels that are below peak but still higher than the ventilation measured during baseline room air breathing. A study of premature neonates showed that this biphasic response will persist into the second month of postnatal life, but this only represented a postconceptional age of about 35 weeks.[39] Even term neonates may retain the biphasic response characteristic for at least 2 months when tested with normal bedding at room temperature of 24° C during NREM sleep. In addition, very small preterm neonates may show only a decrease in ventilation with hypoxia. The apparent differences between preterm and term neonates may be partially accounted for by developmental status in relation to postnatal age; indeed, premature but not term lambs or piglets also exhibit an attenuated hypercapnic response. Thus, prematurity and factors delaying normal maturation emerge as important contributors to the attenuated hypercapnic and hypoxic responses in newborns.

Studies suggest that a relatively high ventilatory drive exists during wakefulness in children, and that this drive decreases during adolescence and stabilizes during adulthood; the reason for this transition is currently unknown. Marcus and colleagues[29] studied hypercapnic and hypoxic ventilatory responses in a group of subjects 4 to 49 years of age and found significant correlations between both the awake hypercapnic and hypoxic ventilatory responses when corrected for age and body size.

▰ THE UPPER AIRWAY

Upper Airway Control

Since both snoring and OSA are opposite ends of a spectrum of increased upper airway resistance, it is important to review the anatomic and physiologic mechanisms that underlie the maintenance of upper airway patency during sleep.[40] The upper airway comprises the nose, pharynx, larynx, and extrathoracic trachea, and is designed for vocalization, ingestion, airway protection, and respiration. Maintenance of a rigid and patent upper airway is mandatory for achieving adequate respiration and is the result of a balance between forces that promote airway closure and dilatation. Thus, the inherent collapsibility of the pharynx predisposes to impaired respiration when the regulation of the pharyngeal muscles is impaired, such as may occur during sleep.

Anatomically, it is clear that a smaller cross-sectional area of the upper airway is associated with decreased ability to maintain upper airway patency, and in adults the upper airway behaves as predicted by the Starling resistor model, a model that has been well characterized in biologic systems. This model describes the major determinants of air flow in terms of the mechanical properties of collapsible tubes and predicts that, under conditions of flow limitation, maximal inspiratory flow will be determined by the pressure changes upstream (nasal) to a collapsible site of the upper airway, and flow will be independent of downstream (tracheal) pressure generated by the diaphragm. Collapse occurs when the pressure surrounding the collapsible segment of the upper airway becomes greater than the pressure within the collapsible segment of the airway. Pressures at which collapse of the airway occurs have been termed *critical closing pressure (P_{crit})*.[41,42] In normal subjects with low upstream resistance, pressures downstream never approach P_{crit} and air flow is not limited. This model explains why snoring and obstructive apnea worsen during a common cold (increased nasal upstream resistance). Marcus and colleagues[43] further demonstrated the validity of this model in children and found that the upper airway collapsibility in children is reduced compared with the adult. Notably, and as predicted by the Starling model, the collapsible segment of the upper airway in children displayed less negative (higher and thus more collapsible) pressures in children with OSA. It follows that components that affect the upstream segment pressures or increase P_{crit} will be of major consequence to the ability to maintain airway patency. The contribution of the various anatomic nasopharyngeal structures to P_{crit} and the interactions between these structures that will lead to upper airway patency or obstruction during sleep are thus of clear importance in increasing our understanding of the pathophysiology of childhood OSA.

Although the overall ventilatory drive appears to be normal in children with OSA, it is possible that central augmentation of upper airway neuromotor function is abnormal. During sleep, upper airway tone is diminished even though the same structural factors are present during wake and sleep, and OSA occurs only during sleep. It is unknown whether children with OSA become obstructed because of a relatively larger decrease in airway tone during sleep in comparison to controls, or whether the decrease in tone is similar but subjects with OSA have an increased structural load. The upper airway muscles are accessory muscles of respiration and, as such, are activated by stimuli such as hypoxemia, hypercapnia, and upper airway subatmospheric pressure. Previous studies have shown that, when upper airway muscle function is decreased or absent, as in postmortem preparations, the airway is prone to collapse.[44] Conversely, stimulation of the upper airway muscles with hypercapnia[45,46] or electrical stimulation[47] results in decreased collapsibility. These studies confirm that the tendency of the upper airway to collapse is inversely related to the level of activity of the upper airway dilator muscles. Therefore, increased upper airway neuromotor tone may be one way that patients can compensate for a narrow upper airway. Indeed, this has been shown in adults. Mezzanotte and colleagues demonstrated that adult patients with OSA compensated for their narrow upper airway during wakefulness by increasing their upper airway muscle tone.[48] This compensatory mechanism was lost during sleep.[49] Recent studies in children have shown that children with OSA have greater genioglossal EMG activity during the awake state than control children and a greater decline in EMG activity during sleep onset.[50] Furthermore, upper airway dynamic responses are decreased in children with OSA but appear to recover after treatment. Thus, pharyngeal airway neuromotor responses are present in normal children and serve as a compensatory response for a relatively narrow upper airway compared with adults. However, this compensatory neuromotor response is lacking in children with OSA, probably as a result of habituation to chronic respiratory abnormalities during sleep, mechanical damage to the upper airway, or genetically determined differences in these upper airway protective reflexes.[51-53]

Ventilatory control in patients with OSA is the subject of intense study. In adults with OSA, it is suggested that there is a high-gain ventilatory control system that results in ventilatory instability and apnea.[54] However, studies in children have shown overall normal ventilatory responses to hypoxia and hypercapnia during wakefulness and during sleep when using standard tests.[29,30,55] Indeed, ventilatory responses to re-breathing hyperoxic hypercapnia were measured in 20 children and adolescents with OSA, and the mean slopes of the hypercapnic response were similar to those measured in age- and sex-matched controls.[56] Furthermore, no differences were found in the slopes calculated from plotting minute ventilation against O_2 saturation during isocapnic hypoxia. Nevertheless, other investigators have found some degree of blunting in central chemosensitivity of children with OSA undergoing surgery.[57,58] Despite such findings, central chemosensitivity during sleep was similar in children with OSA and matched controls. However, arousal to acutely induced hypercapnia was blunted during sleep in children with OSA, suggesting that subtle alterations in the central chemosensitive-arousal network have occurred in these patients. These subtle changes have been further substantiated by examination of the ventilatory responses to repetitive hypercapnic challenges during wakefulness, whereby reciprocal changes in respiratory frequency and tidal volume do occur.[59] In the study by Gozal and colleagues,[60] repeated CO_2 challenges were given in the early morning to children with OSA who were hypercapnic (as a result of obstructive alveolar hypoventilation) during sleep. These children showed a respiratory response to the CO_2 challenge but did not show the same adaptive changes in respiratory pattern that would be anticipated over the course of several CO_2 challenges as elicited from children without OSA. However, when children with OSA were studied later in the day (i.e., a few hours after awakening and resolution of sleep-associated alveolar hypoventilation) or after treatment of OSA, a similar respiratory pattern to that seen in controls emerged, suggesting that such deficits may be related to habituation to nocturnal hypercapnia. Additional evidence in support of this comes from Marcus and colleagues,[29] who found an inverse correlation between the duration of hypercapnia during the night and the awake hypercapnic ventilatory responses. In addition, children with OSA demonstrate impaired arousal responses to inspiratory loads during REM and non-REM sleep compared with control children.[61] This arousal threshold was particularly high during REM sleep, a time when most obstructive apneic

events occur, and suggests that neuromotor influences play a key role. The absence or delayed arousal in children during an obstructive respiratory event and the presumed lack of ventilatory compensation to upper airway loading may contribute to the development of the prolonged periods of obstructive alveolar hypoventilation that uniquely characterize OSA in children. Furthermore, diminished laryngeal reflexes to mechanoreceptor and chemoreceptor stimulation with reduced afferent inputs into central neural regions underlying inspiratory inputs could be present. For example, chemoreceptor stimuli such as increased $Paco_2$ or decreased Pao_2 stimulate the airway dilating muscles in a preferential mode; that is, upper airway musculature is more stimulated than the diaphragm.[62] This preferential recruitment tends to correct an imbalance of forces acting on the airway and therefore maintain airway patency. Similarly, stimuli resulting from suction pressures in the nose, pharynx, or larynx rapidly stimulate the activity of upper airway dilators, and this effect is also preferential to the upper airway, causing some degree of diaphragmatic inhibition and thus compensating for increase in upstream resistance. The function of these upper airway receptors in children with adenotonsillar hypertrophy with and without OSA is currently unknown.

While dynamic factors such as those just discussed have been implicated in the pathophysiology of upper airway obstruction during sleep in children, we should not omit the contribution of either anatomic elements or genetic factors to this complex equation. In otherwise normal children, Arens and colleagues have shown that the mandibular dimensions of children with OSA are similar to those of controls.[63] However, regional analysis of the upper airway using magnetic resonance imaging techniques further suggested that the upper airway in children with OSA is most restricted where adenoids and tonsils overlap.[64,65] Furthermore, the upper airway is narrowed throughout the initial two thirds of its length in pediatric patients with OSA, and this narrowing is not in a discrete region adjacent to either the adenoids or tonsils, but rather emerges in a continuous fashion along both lymphadenoid structures.[64,65] It should be emphasized that, contrary to the previous conceptual framework whereby the higher prevalence of OSA in children during the period from 2 to 8 years of age was attributed to the increased growth rate of lymphadenoid tissue within the upper airway compared with other upper airway structures,[66,67] recent evidence refutes this concept and shows that all tissues within the upper airway including adenoids and tonsils grow proportionally and thus that stimuli leading to enhanced proliferation of lymphadenoid tissue within the airway are probably implicated in the pathophysiology of OSA.[68,69] In fact, recent evidence has further indicated that the extent of lymphadenoid proliferation is not confined to the adenoids and tonsils, and in fact encompasses the full length of the upper airway including the nose and sinuses, suggesting that OSA is a diffuse disease of the upper airway. [70]

Upper Airway Dysfunction

In infancy, abnormalities that reduce the patency of the upper airway are frequently associated with OSA. The upper airway has decreased muscle tone, there is high nasal resistance, and the chest wall is highly compliant. The exact prevalence of OSA in infants is not well documented because most epidemiologic studies have concentrated on older children. However, OSA has been shown to occur in as many as 10% of infants, is more frequent in preterm infants, and is associated with hypoxemia. OSA occurs more frequently in male infants than in females, and this may be attributable to sex-related differences in the anatomy of the upper airway or to a protective role of female hormones. The main risk factors for OSA in this age group include: (1) craniofacial abnormalities (e.g., micrognathia, cleft palate, Pierre Robin syndrome, Treacher Collins syndrome, choanal atresia, mucopolysaccharidoses, Down syndrome); (2) soft tissue infiltration, which may result from infection, inflammation, laryngomalacia, subglottic stenosis, and adenotonsillar hypertrophy. Indeed, the last mentioned has been found to contribute significantly to the generation of OSA in infants younger than 1 year of age[71,72]; and (3) neurologic disorders that induce pharyngeal hypotonia such as Arnold-Chiari malformation, cerebral palsy, and poliomyelitis. Although the anatomic site of obstruction in infants is widely believed to be the retroglossal region,[73] recent evidence using magnetic resonance imaging and airway manometry suggests that upper airway obstruction with clinically significant OSA occurs in the retropalatal region 80% of the time and in the retroglossal region only 20% of the time.[74] Other influences may alter breathing characteristics and predispose infants to OSA, including upper airway reflexes such as the laryngeal chemoreflex. This unique defense reflex that aims to prevent aspiration of food is enhanced by upper airway infection. Indeed, respiratory syncytial virus infection, which potentiates the laryngeal chemoreflex, has also been shown to facilitate the occurrence of both central and obstructive apneic episodes.[75] Similarly, prenatal exposure to maternal smoking, which potentiates the laryngeal chemoreflex, also increases the frequency of OSA in infants.[76,77]

To determine the region of maximal airway narrowing in children with OSA, the static pressure/area relationships of the passive pharynx were endoscopically measured in 14 children with OSA and 13 normal children under general anesthesia with complete paralysis.[78,79] The minimum cross-sectional area was found to be at the level of the adenoid and the soft palate. Thus, children with OSA closed their airways at the level of enlarged tonsils and adenoids at low positive pressures, whereas normal children required subatmospheric pressures to induce upper airway closure. The cross-sectional area of the narrowest segment was significantly smaller in children with OSA, and particularly involved the retropalatal and retroglossal segments, such that it becomes clear that anatomic factors, both congenital and acquired, play a significant role in the pathogenesis of pediatric OSA.[80,81] Furthermore, as mentioned earlier, airway narrowing in children with OSA occurs along the upper two thirds of the airway and is maximal where the adenoids and tonsils overlap.[65,82]

In summary, several potential mechanisms have been identified in the maintenance of upper airway patency during sleep and wakefulness. Each of these mechanisms or a combination thereof probably plays a role in the causation of respiratory compromise in the normal child during sleep and in children with clinical problems that predispose to OSA. A systematic approach to identification and modification of these mechanisms may lead to improved therapeutic approaches and reduction of unnecessary morbidities in these patients.

APNEA

Central Apnea or Hypoventilation Syndromes

Unrelated to upper airway obstruction, insufficient central respiratory drive can also be a cause of hypoventilation. The presence of a hypoventilation syndrome is suggested by the medical history as well as examination of the patient during wakefulness and sleep. All disorders that could explain the hypoventilation must be excluded, and to confirm the diagnosis, a polysomnographic evaluation, including measurements of tidal volume, should be conducted. The measurement of spontaneous resting tidal volumes and noninvasive blood gas values across all sleep states should be sufficient to establish the presence and severity of alveolar hypoventilation. The most important objective is the inability to increase respiratory frequency, tidal volume, or both, regardless of the severity of the progressive asphyxia that occurs.

CONGENITAL CENTRAL HYPOVENTILATION SYNDROME

Central hypoventilation syndrome (CHS) can be primary (congenital CHS [CCHS] and late-onset CHS) or secondary (Box 77-1). Primary CCHS is a rare entity, with approximately 500 cases worldwide. It was originally described in 1970 by Mellins and colleagues[83] and is traditionally defined as the idiopathic failure of automatic control of breathing.[83,84] CCHS is a life-threatening disorder primarily manifesting as sleep-associated respiratory insufficiency and markedly impaired ventilatory responses to hypercapnia and hypoxemia.[85] Ventilation is most severely affected during quiet sleep, a state during which automatic neural control is predominant. Abnormal respiratory patterns also occur during active

---

BOX 77-1 CAUSES OF CENTRAL HYPOVENTILATION IN CHILDREN

Primary
Congenital (congenital central hypoventilation syndrome [CCHS]/Ondine's curse)
Late-onset central hypoventilation syndrome (CHS)
Idiopathic hypothalamic dysfunction
Arnold-Chiari malformation

Secondary
Trauma
Infection
Tumor
Central nervous system infarct
Asphyxia
Increased intracranial pressure
Metabolic

sleep and even during wakefulness, though to a milder degree. The spectrum of disease in CCHS cases is wide, ranging from relatively mild hypoventilation during quiet sleep with fairly good alveolar ventilation during wakefulness, to complete apnea during sleep with severe hypoventilation during waking. Progress in the recognition and clinical management of CCHS patients has revealed the presence of broader structural and functional impairments of the autonomic nervous system.[86-88] In particular, Hirschsprung's disease[86] and tumors of autonomic neural crest derivatives such as neuroblastoma, ganglioneuroblastoma, and ganglioneuroma,[89,90] are noted in 20% and in 5% to 10% of CCHS patients, respectively. In recent years, four major clinically relevant advances have developed with respect to the pathophysiology and treatment of CCHS: (1) the identification of the putative gene underlying CCHS; (2) the functional assessment of neural structures in patients with CCHS to provide insights into the respiratory and autonomic disturbances that characterize the syndrome; (3) the successful transition of many patients to noninvasive mechanical ventilatory support; and (4) the publication of a consensus statement on the diagnosis and management of this condition.[91]

A genetic origin has been hypothesized for CCHS because of (1) its early manifestation in the newborn period; (2) published reports of familial recurrence of CCHS, including one case each of monozygotic female twins, female siblings, and male-female half-siblings[92,93]; and (3) its association with Hirschsprung's disease, an autosomal-recessive disorder of neural crest origin.[94] Furthermore, a genetic segregation analysis among families of 50 probands with CCHS also indicated that CCHS was consistent with familial transmission.[95] Importantly, vertical transmission of CCHS has been reported, and among infants born to women with CCHS without Hirschsprung's disease.[96,97] The association of CCHS and Hirschsprung's disease suggested that both disorders may be related to abnormal development and/or migration of the neural crest cells; indeed, mutations of genes (e.g., the *RET* proto-oncogene) that are involved in neural crest development and/or migration have been found in patients with Hirschsprung's disease.[98-100] The putative gene, *paired-like homeobox 2B (PHOX2B)*, underlying CCHS was described in 2003 by Amiel and colleagues in France.[101] The *PHOX2B* gene mutation, consisting primarily of polyalanine expansions, manifests an autosomal-dominant mode of inheritance and *de novo* mutations at the first generation. This gene is critical for autonomic nervous system embryologic development, and *PHOX2B−/−* mice die *in utero* with absent autonomic nervous system circuits because the neurons either fail to form or degenerate.[102-105] Furthermore, selective stimulation of *PHOX2B* neurons in specific regions of the brainstem elicits the anticipated respiratory and cardiovascular responses,[106-108] and targeted disruption of *PHOX2B* in brainstem neurons leads to alterations in Task2 potassium channels, which are believed to be the main effectors in central chemoception.[109] Accordingly, heterozygous mutations of *PHOX2B* may account for several combined or isolated disorders of autonomic nervous system development, namely late-onset CHS,[110] Hirschsprung's disease,[111] and tumors of the sympathetic nervous system

such as neuroblastoma.[112] The identification of *PHOX2B* mutations in most patients with CCHS is an important landmark in the pursuit of the pathophysiologic mechanisms of this condition. Furthermore, the finding of *de novo PHOX2B* polyalanine expansion in the majority of patients with CCHS allows for genetic counseling in a disease with an unexpected autosomal-dominant mode of inheritance. Future research into the genetic basis of CCHS may improve our understanding of early breathing control disturbances such as SIDS. The prevalence of SIDS is high in CCHS families, suggesting that these two disorders may share developmental breathing control abnormalities.[113]

Taken together, the genetic data strongly suggest a diffuse alteration in autonomic nervous system function in patients with CCHS. This concept includes major disruption of multiple brain regions underlying autonomic functions, in particular those sites mediating respiratory and cardiovascular regulation, as evidenced from recent studies using functional magnetic resonance imaging approaches.[114-120] Decreased heart rate beat-to-beat variability is consistently found in Holter recordings, and the circadian patterning of such variability further suggests an imbalance in sympathetic/parasympathetic regulation in patients with CCHS.[121-124] As additional testament to such an assumption, alterations in blood pressure regulation during simple daily maneuvers or during sleep further support the presence of predominantly vagal dysfunction with signs of vagal withdrawal and baroreflex failure, and relative preservation of the cardiac and vascular sympathetic function.[125-127] In addition, the frequent neuro-ocular findings in children with CCHS[128] and the marked reduction in the size of arterial chemoreceptors, carotid bodies, and neuroepithelial bodies with decreased staining for tyrosine hydroxylase and serotonin[129] can all be construed as evidence for a more diffuse autonomic nervous system involvement. Putative models aiming to dissect the specific contributions of the various components of cardiorespiratory control have been recently proposed and provide a comprehensive and structured approach to the evaluation of patients with CCHS.[130]

Diagnosis and Clinical Management

The clinical presentation of CCHS varies greatly depending on the severity of the disorder. Some infants will not breathe at birth and will require assisted ventilation in the newborn nursery. Such infants may mature to a pattern of adequate breathing during wakefulness over time. However, apnea or hypoventilation will persist during sleep. The apparent improvement over the first few months of life most likely results from normal maturation of the respiratory system and does not represent a true change in the severity of the disorder.[131] Other infants may present at a later age with cyanosis, edema, and signs of right-sided heart failure and may be mistaken for patients with cyanotic congenital heart disease. However, cardiac catheterization reveals only pulmonary hypertension. Infants with even less severe CCHS may present with tachycardia, diaphoresis, and/or cyanosis during sleep, and others may present with unexplained apnea or an apparent life-threatening event. Thus, the wide spectrum of severity in clinical manifestations determines the age at which recognition of CCHS takes place. Increased awareness of this unusual clinical entity and a comprehensive evaluation of every patient are critical for early diagnosis and appropriate intervention.

Although other symptoms indicative of brain stem or autonomic nervous system dysfunction may be present, the criteria for diagnosis of CCHS usually include: (1) persistent evidence of sleep hypoventilation ($Paco_2$ >60 mm Hg), particularly during quiet sleep (best achieved by overnight polysomnography); (2) presentation of symptoms during the first year of life; and (3) absence of cardiac, pulmonary, or neuromuscular dysfunction that could explain the hypoventilation.[84,91] Hypercapnic ventilatory challenges are an important component for the diagnosis of CCHS. Steady-state or re-breathing incremental CO_2 challenges are similarly valid and will usually reveal an absent or near-absent response. Confounding variables, including asphyxia, infection, trauma, tumor, and infarction, must be distinguished from CCHS by appropriate assessments. Specific guidelines regarding the use of genetic testing for CCHS and other diagnostic considerations have now become available and should be implemented.[91] Identification of mutations in genes such as *RET, HASH, BDNF, GDNF,* and the endothelin gene family may be helpful, but assessment of *PHOX2B* gene mutations in the context of clinical manifestations supporting central alveolar hypoventilation should support the diagnosis of CCHS.[91,132,133]

CCHS is a lifelong condition and, depending on the severity of clinical manifestations, patients may require ventilatory support while asleep or as much as 24 hours a day. As such, a multidisciplinary approach to provide for comprehensive care and support of every child is needed. Treatment should aim to ensure adequate ventilation when the patient is unable to achieve adequate gas exchange while breathing spontaneously. Because CCHS does not resolve spontaneously, chronic ventilatory support is required, such as positive pressure ventilation, bilevel positive airway pressure, or negative pressure ventilation. The majority of children with CCHS use positive pressure ventilation through a permanent tracheotomy, although successful transition to noninvasive ventilation has now been extensively reported,[84] with a trend toward earlier intervention (sometimes even during infancy) and more widespread transition to noninvasive ventilation (typically mask ventilation).[134-140] Several families have opted to use negative pressure ventilation. Daytime diaphragm pacing in children with CCHS who exhibit 24-hour mechanical ventilation dependency provides greater mobility compared with mechanical ventilation. Thus, potential candidates for diaphragm pacing will be ambulatory patients who require ventilatory support 24 hours per day by means of tracheotomy and do not exhibit significant ventilator-related lung damage. Diaphragm pacer settings must provide adequate alveolar ventilation and oxygenation during rest as well as during daily activities such as exercise. Major disadvantages of diaphragm pacing include cost, discomfort associated with surgical implantation, and potential need for repeated surgical revisions due to pacer malfunction.[141,142] Despite such potential limitations, parental reports of their experience are favorable in the vast majority. Recent development of a quadripolar electrode offers several advantages, which primarily include greater durations of pacer support at diminished risk of phrenic nerve damage and diaphragmatic fatigue, and optimization of pacing requirements during exercise.[143,144]

SECONDARY CENTRAL HYPOVENTILATION SYNDROMES

Patients with myelomeningocele and/or Arnold-Chiari type II malformation frequently exhibit sleep-disordered breathing, and such respiratory control disturbances are frequently suspected as causative mechanisms in the sudden unexpected deaths that occur in this population. Moderate or severe breathing disturbances occur in approximately 20% of cases.[145,146] The largest proportion of patients exhibit central apnea, while others show obstructed breathing; patients with obstruction are seldom helped by surgical intervention for tonsillectomy, suggesting that the primary dysfunction is of neural origin. The possible damage to vermis cerebelli structures from foramen magnum herniation in Chiari type II malformation has the potential to interfere with both blood pressure and breathing regulation, particularly under extreme challenges of hypotension or prolonged apnea. Compression of ventral neural surfaces is also a concern. The presence of thoracic or thoracolumbar myelomeningocele or the addition of severe brain stem malformations has been shown to enhance the potential for sleep-disordered breathing. Support for affected patients with Chiari II syndrome must consider the needs for recovery from pronounced hypotension during sleep, the overall respiratory disturbances that are present, and the surgical interventions required for decompression of neural structures. As such, a multidisciplinary approach is necessary to yield optimal outcomes.[147]

Patients with Prader-Willi syndrome (PWS) present a unique combination of sleep- and breathing-related manifestations. Excessive daytime sleepiness and increased frequency of REM sleep periods occurs in some PWS patients, while others show disturbances in circadian rhythmicity with a tendency for multiple microsleep periods. In addition, the combination of obesity and hypotonia favors the occurrence of OSA. Patients with PWS also display significant alterations in central and peripheral elements of respiratory control that, though not immediately related to the obesity, can be severely affected by the mechanical consequences of increased adiposity that ultimately lead to ventilatory failure. A unique and almost universal feature of these patients is the absence of ventilatory responses to peripheral chemoreceptor stimulation; this deficiency leads to abnormal arousal patterns during sleep.[148-151] When untreated, obesity progressively reduces central chemosensitivity as well, with the latter being ameliorated by growth hormone therapy and increased muscle mass.[152,153] However, it is important to emphasize that sudden death cases have been reported worldwide in children with PWS receiving growth hormone therapy, and that the mechanisms of such adverse outcomes remain unclear.

A condition termed *late-onset central hypoventilation* has been observed in some children. Although an underlying congenital brain stem abnormality is probable, significant hypoventilation becomes evident only as a consequence of an intercurrent illness such as pneumonia, with the development of severe obesity, or as a consequence of cor pulmonale. In addition, a recognizable entity consisting of hypothalamic dysfunction and late onset of central hypoventilation is now well established, and may or may not be associated with *PHOX2B* mutations.[154-158] Alveolar hypoventilation can also develop in a child with previously normal control of breathing subsequent to an event resulting in brain stem injury, such as severe asphyxia, encephalitis, and infectious encephalopathies.

APNEA OF PREMATURITY

Apnea in newborns has been defined as a pause in breathing of longer than 20 seconds or an apneic event of shorter than 20 seconds associated with either bradycardia or cyanosis. Recurrent episodes of apnea are common in preterm neonates, and the incidence and severity increases with earlier gestational age. Reduced respiratory drive and impaired pulmonary function caused by lung immaturity, as well as a variety of mechanical variables impinging on respiratory mechanics, predispose the premature neonate to apnea and hypoventilation which, in turn, may precipitate oxyhemoglobin desaturation and/or bradycardia. Although they can occur spontaneously and be attributable to prematurity alone, such events can also be provoked or worsened if there is some additional insult such as infection, underlying hypoxemia, hyperthermia, or any evolving intracranial pathology. Although most apneic events are self-resolving and do not prompt medical recognition or intervention, apneic events associated with hypoxemia and reflex bradycardia may require active resuscitative efforts.

Idiopathic apnea of prematurity (AOP) is a common, albeit often unsuspected problem in the clinical setting[159] and appears to be primarily caused by immaturity of the neonate's neurologic and respiratory systems. The preterm neonate breathes irregularly during sleep and, in comparison to both the full-term neonate and the adult, there is much greater breath-to-breath variability. Both central and obstructive apneic episodes are frequently reported in preterm neonates, although the most common form is mixed apnea. Mixed apnea typically accounts for more than half of all clinically relevant apneic episodes, followed in decreasing frequency by central and obstructive apnea. By definition, there are no obstructions in central apnea, although some reports have suggested that the central airways will frequently close during the course of central apnea, with a rule of thumb indicating that such airway occlusion will more likely occur with increased duration of such events.[160-163] Thus, these apneic events have also been termed *silent obstruction* because of the lack of respiratory effort. AOP generally resolves by about 36 to 40 weeks postconceptional age. However, in the most premature infants (24 to 28 weeks gestation), apnea may frequently persist beyond 40 weeks postconceptional age, finally resolving at 43 to 44 weeks postconceptional age.[164,165] Beyond this time, the incidence

of cardiorespiratory events in preterm neonates does not appear to markedly exceed that of term newborns.

Pathophysiology

Immaturity of central respiratory control of the various ventilatory muscles is a key factor in the pathogenesis of AOP. The breathing pattern is more disorganized during REM sleep, which is the predominant mode of sleep in preterm neonates. Indeed, apneic episodes are more common, longer, and more frequently associated with profound bradycardia during active or REM sleep than during quiet or NREM sleep.[166,167] Although the pathogenesis of AOP has not been fully delineated, it is related to both neurologic and cardiorespiratory immaturity.[168,169] In particular, preterm neonates have an altered response to increased CO_2 in that they respond by diminished rather than increased inspiratory effort.[170,171] This unique response of respiratory timing during hypercapnic exposure is associated with prolongation of expiratory duration.[172,173] Animal models have revealed that this prolongation of expiration associated with hypercapnia is centrally mediated at the brain stem level.[174] Furthermore, the inhibitory neurotransmitter γ-aminobutyric acid (GABA) appears to be implicated.[175,176] It is well known that premature neonates exhibit a biphasic ventilatory response to a decrease in inspired O_2 concentration. Initially, there is a rapid increase in minute ventilation caused by peripheral chemoreceptor stimulation; this is followed by a decline in ventilation to baseline or below. The decrease in ventilation, also termed *hypoxic ventilatory depression*,[177,178] may persist for several weeks postnatally. Several theories have been postulated to explain hypoxic ventilatory depression, including a decrease in $Paco_2$ secondary to the initial hyperventilation and accompanying decrease in cerebral blood flow, a decrease in metabolic rate with hypoxia, hypoxia-mediated central depression of ventilation, and activation of receptors such as GABA-ergic, adenosinergic, and/or platelet-derived growth factor β receptors.[179-181]

There has been speculation that the hypoxic ventilatory depression may predispose preterm neonates to additional episodes of apnea. In other words, neonates experiencing more apneic episodes would have less initial increase in ventilation and subsequent greater depression of ventilation in response to hypoxia. However, this speculation has been challenged by Nock and colleagues,[182] who documented increased initial ventilation but attenuated ventilatory depression during the hypoxic challenge in premature neonates who developed more frequent and severe apnea. The speculation is that neonates with more severe and/or prolonged apnea have greater peripheral chemoreceptor sensitivity and possibly increased central respiratory network gain caused by the repetitive periods of intermittent hypoxia,[183] and that it is the resultant instability of respiratory control that may predispose preterm neonates to additional apneic episodes.[181]

The site of obstruction during either mixed or obstructive apneic events in the upper airways is mostly within the pharynx; however, it may also occur at the level of the larynx, and possibly at both sites. The mechanisms by which apnea may occur may be initiated by sleep-related decrease of pharyngeal airway dilation.[184-187]

Integration of pharyngeal muscle function is reduced during sleep, resulting in collapse and subsequent apnea in susceptible infants. In addition, the airway may be compromised by postural changes, although spontaneous obstructive apnea in the absence of a positional problem is probably uncommon. Reflexes originating in the upper airway may alter the pattern of respiration and play a role in the initiation and termination of apnea episodes.[188] Stimulation of the laryngeal mucosa, by either chemical or mechanical stimuli, may induce reflex inhibition of breathing and apnea in humans and animals, and it is mediated through activation of the superior laryngeal nerve. There seems to be a maturational change in reflex-induced apnea[74] because chemical stimulation of the larynx in newborn piglets causes respiratory arrest, which is not seen in older piglets. Preterm neonates have an exaggerated laryngeal inhibitory reflex, which may elicit prolonged apnea in response to instilling saline in the oropharynx, to gastroesophageal reflux (GER), or during the course of respiratory syncytial virus infection.[189–192]

Diagnosis

Although apnea typically results from immaturity of the respiratory control system, it also may constitute the presenting sign of other unrelated diseases or pathophysiologic states frequently affecting preterm neonates.[193] Thus, AOP is diagnosed after a thorough evaluation has been conducted and other potential influences have been excluded (Box 77-2). Particular caution must also be exercised when attributing apnea to GER.[194,195] Indeed, despite the frequent coexistence of apnea and GER in preterm neonates, investigations into the timing of reflux in relation to apneic events do not support a common temporal association.[196–198] Although physiologic experiments in animal models reveal that reflux of gastric contents to the larynx induces reflex apnea, there is no clear evidence that treatment of GER will affect frequency of apnea in most preterm neonates. Therefore, diagnosis of sleep-disordered breathing secondary to GER is not simple and can be easily missed or overinterpreted during polygraphic recordings. On the other hand, even the presence of GER as shown by esophageal pH monitoring or other techniques in an infant with polygraphically proven apnea does not necessarily demonstrate that GER is the cause of the respiratory disturbance during sleep. Hence, simultaneous recording of sleep measures and of esophageal pH and impedance is usually necessary to allow detection of tentative associations between GER and apnea, and it may allow for formulation of more effective management of both GER and resultant apnea and bradycardia in these infants.[199–203]

Notably, hypoventilation, O_2 desaturation, frank apnea, and bradycardia have also been documented during nutritive sucking and ascribed to the immaturity of the normal mechanisms that coordinate breathing, sucking, and swallowing. In the normal healthy infant, as fluid enters the pharynx or larynx, breathing ceases. This normal response protects the airway and prevents aspiration. However, this protective reflex is excessive in some infants because of the immaturity of the nervous system, resulting in prolonged apnea. With advancing maturation, feeding-related episodes of apnea become less frequent and eventually disappear.[203,204]

Treatment

Treatment is usually with pharmacologic therapy or continuous positive airway pressure (CPAP) ventilation, although other measures are important, such as placing the infant with the head in the midline and the neck in the neutral position to minimize upper airway obstruction. Methylxanthines have been the mainstay of pharmacologic treatment of AOP.[205] Both theophylline and caffeine citrate are effective, possibly through multiple physiologic and pharmacologic mechanisms of action. A probable major mechanism of action for xanthine therapy is through competitive antagonism of adenosine receptors because adenosine acts as an inhibitory neuroregulator in the central nervous system.

It is important to rule out systemic conditions (sepsis), seizure disorders, and GER before instituting methylxanthine therapy because these agents have been known to lower the seizure threshold and to decrease muscle tone of the esophageal sphincter.[206] Methylxanthines stimulate the central nervous system and rapidly decrease the frequency of all types of apnea. Xanthine therapy has been shown to increase minute ventilation, improve CO_2 sensitivity, decrease hypoxic depression of breathing, enhance diaphragmatic activity, and decrease periodic breathing. REM sleep may also be acutely decreased even if long-term therapy with xanthines does not seem to alter overall sleep architecture.[207] Caffeine has some advantages over theophylline because it is considered to be more effective in stimulating the central nervous and respiratory systems. In addition, because caffeine has a higher therapeutic index, central nervous system toxicity is not as problematic. A Cochrane review on the use of methylxanthines concluded that both theophylline and caffeine are effective in reducing the frequency and severity of apneic episodes, and are also of value in reducing the need for mechanical ventilation in preterm neonates with AOP.[208] Elimination of methylxanthines is prolonged in infants in comparison with children or adults, and it is particularly prolonged in preterm neonates. The metabolic pathways for the elimination of theophylline are underdeveloped in the premature neonate, and thus serum measurement of theophylline should be monitored whenever aminophylline or theophylline is used. Caffeine levels are less critical but should also be followed at least during the beginning of treatment.

BOX 77-2 CONDITIONS ASSOCIATED WITH APNEA IN INFANTS

Prematurity
Infection
Impaired oxygenation
Central nervous system problems (intracranial hemorrhage, asphyxic episode, malformation of the brain)
Gastroesophageal reflux
Metabolic disorders (hypoglycemia, electrolyte imbalance, fatty acid disorders, metabolic acidosis)
Temperature instability (hyperthermia, hypothermia)
Drugs (e.g., narcotics, anticonvulsants)

The decision to discontinue xanthine therapy is largely empiric, although it should be encouraged at least 1 to 2 weeks before discharge; this is especially relevant for caffeine with its longer half-life. Toxic levels may produce tachycardia, cardiac dysrhythmias, feeding intolerance, diuresis, and, infrequently, seizures, although these side effects are less commonly seen with caffeine at the usual therapeutic doses. However, recent concerns about potential long-term side effects of methylxanthines on the neurodevelopmental outcomes of low–birth weight infants have led to an increased interest in alternate methods of treating AOP.[208,209]

Role of Continuous Positive Airway Pressure

Among the nonpharmacologic strategies widely used in the treatment of apnea, CPAP is relatively safe and effective. Nasal CPAP (NCPAP) has also been shown to be effective in AOP,[210,211] with a therapeutic range usually within 3 to 6 cm H_2O. Since longer episodes of apnea frequently involve an obstructive component, CPAP seems to be effective through its effect in splinting the upper airway with positive pressure and decreasing the risk of pharyngeal or laryngeal obstruction. CPAP is also probably beneficial in AOP by increasing functional residual capacity and thereby improving oxygenation. Studies have also compared NCPAP to nasal intermittent positive pressure ventilation (NIPPV) in the treatment of AOP and found that NIPPV is potentially a beneficial treatment for AOP, particularly when apnea is frequent or severe.[212] NIPPV seems to reduce the frequency of apneic episodes more effectively than NCPAP.[213,214] Nonetheless, additional safety and efficacy data are required before recommending NIPPV as standard therapy for apnea. In addition, high-flow nasal cannula therapy has recently been suggested as an equivalent treatment modality to NCPAP while enhancing mobility of the infant for parents and caretakers.[215,216] Despite these noninvasive treatment options, endotracheal intubation and artificial ventilation may be needed for severe or refractory episodes.

The effect of supplemental O_2 on cardiorespiratory events and sleep architecture in premature neonates has also been explored; studies show that AOP and periodic breathing resolve when O_2 concentration is increased to a threshold level.[217,218] Rigatto and colleagues further reported that inhalation of 100% O_2 is associated with a decrease in periodic breathing and an increase in minute ventilation.[219] In fact, a modest increase in inspired O_2 concentration decreased apnea and periodicity in preterm neonates, not via an increase in alveolar ventilation but through a decrease in breath-to-breath variability instead.[220] Simakajornboon and colleagues have further demonstrated that in otherwise healthy premature neonates, unsuspected adverse cardiorespiratory events, including apnea and bradycardia, occur very frequently.[221] Moreover, administration of low-flow supplemental O_2 improves respiratory stability, as shown by a decrease in the frequency of respiratory and bradycardic events, a reduction in periodic breathing density, and an increase in overall O_2 saturation without adverse effects on alveolar ventilation. In addition, supplemental O_2

administration modified sleep architecture by increasing NREM sleep density and reciprocal decreases in REM sleep density. Of interest, initial studies using nonrandom mechanical stimulation may prove to be an alternative therapeutic intervention in the future.[222]

As mentioned earlier in the chapter, AOP generally resolves by 36 to 40 weeks postconceptional age, and beyond 43 to 44 weeks postconceptional age the incidence of cardiorespiratory events in preterm neonates is similar to that of term newborns. Thus, the majority of preterm neonates will have their AOP resolved by the time they are ready for home discharge.[223] In this context, a retrospective review of patient records by Darnall and colleagues[224] to determine the minimum apnea-free observation period before discharge suggested that 8 apnea-free days was probably safe. However, close monitoring in the neonatal intensive care unit (NICU) is essential because several reports have highlighted the observation that clinically significant apneas with resultant bradycardia and/or desaturation go unnoticed in the majority of cases.[225-227]

The clinical significance and long-term consequences of persistent apnea, bradycardia, or desaturation remain a subject of considerable debate. Although it is reasonable to be concerned about episodes that cause prolonged anoxia and acidosis, such events are unlikely to occur as a result of AOP in the closely monitored environment of modern NICUs. Attempts to quantify any prognostic risk that may be attributable to AOP have produced conflicting results. Because idiopathic apnea is most often seen in high-risk preterm neonates, separating the global consequences of premature birth from the specific effects of AOP has proven difficult. Premature newborns often have many problems during their stay in the NICU, and many of these conditions—particularly periventricular leukomalacia and intraventricular hemorrhage—may contribute to poor neurodevelopmental outcomes. Additionally, only a few studies have assessed improvement in long-term outcome as a result of treating AOP, and these studies have been confounded by the same problems. Reports of long-term follow-up of at-risk infants have attempted to address this issue.[228,229] In preterm infants followed to early school age, variables that predicted poor neurodevelopmental outcomes included AOP; however, these are by no means uniform findings, and thus additional studies will be necessary. For example, there is some initial evidence that caffeine may actually be beneficial to neurodevelopmental outcomes under certain circumstances.[230] It is also possible that the recurrent hypoxia accompanying AOP is a detrimental contributor to neurobehavioral outcome. Evidence to this effect has begun to emerge, whereby retinopathy of prematurity appears to be associated with the intermittent hypoxia of AOP.[231]

■■ OBSTRUCTIVE SLEEP APNEA

The spectrum of sleep-disordered breathing, which includes OSA and upper airway resistance syndrome, occurs in children of all ages, from neonates to adolescents. OSA is characterized by repeated events of partial or complete upper airway obstruction during sleep, resulting in disruption of normal gas exchange and sleep patterns (Figs. 77-1 to 77-5).[232] Nighttime symptoms and signs

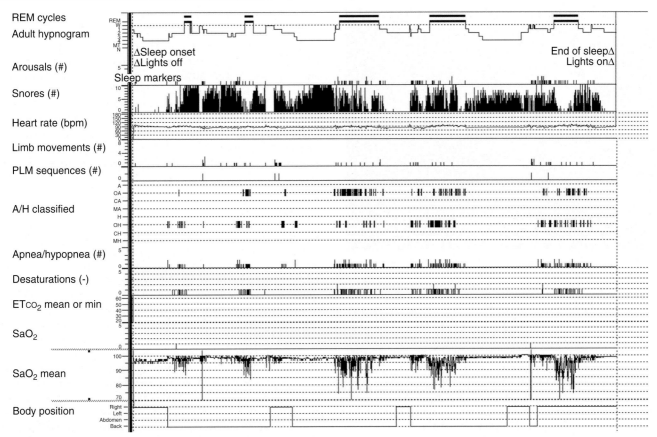

FIGURE 77-1. Overnight trends in several polysomnographic measures in a 7-year-old child with moderately severe obstructive sleep apnea. Note REM sleep clustering of respiratory events. *A*, apnea; *H*, hypopnea.

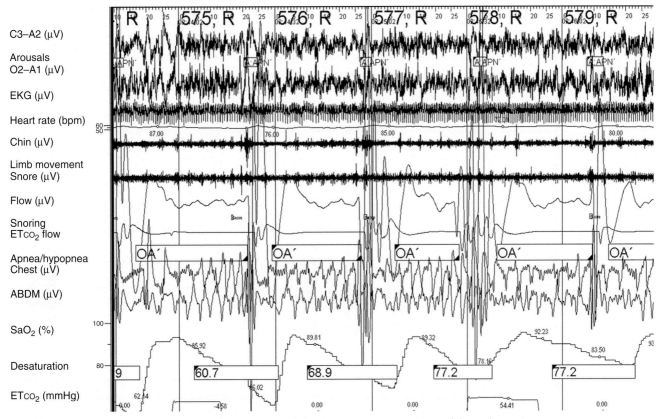

FIGURE 77-2. Polygraphic tracing in a child with REM-associated obstructive apneic events. *ABDM*, abdominal excursion.

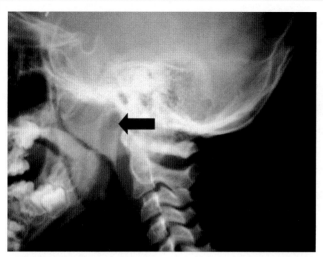

FIGURE 77-3. Lateral roentgenogram of the neck in a child with enlarged adenoid tissue and obstructive sleep apnea.

include snoring, paradoxical chest and abdomen motion, retractions, witnessed apnea, snorting episodes, difficulty breathing, cyanosis, sweating, and disturbed sleep. Daytime symptoms can include mouth breathing, difficulty to wake up, moodiness, nasal obstruction, daytime sleepiness, hyperactivity, and cognitive problems, with severe cases of OSA associated with cor pulmonale, failure to thrive, developmental delay, or even death. This complex and relatively frequent disorder is only now being recognized as a major public health problem, despite

being initially described more than a century ago[233] and rediscovered in children in 1976 by Guilleminault and colleagues.[234] It is clear that the classic clinical syndrome of OSA in children is a distinct disorder from the condition that occurs in adults, in particular with respect to gender distribution, clinical manifestations, polysomnographic findings, and treatment approaches.[235,236] As discussed earlier in the chapter, childhood OSA is frequently diagnosed in association with adenotonsillar hypertrophy and is also common in children with craniofacial abnormalities and neurologic disorders affecting upper airway patency.

Epidemiology

Obstructive sleep apnea occurs in all pediatric age groups including infancy. Accurate prevalence information is only now emerging in infants, and suggests that habitual snoring and mild sleep-disordered breathing are frequent even during infancy, and that the risk for OSA is exacerbated by cigarette smoking exposures and reduced by breast feeding.[237-239] OSA is particularly common in young children (preschool and early school years), with a peak prevalence around 2 to 8 years, and subsequent declines in frequency,[240] possibly related to reductions in viral loads associated with adenotonsillar lymphoid tissue proliferation.[241-244] Habitual snoring during sleep, the hallmark indicator of increased upper airway resistance, is an extremely frequent occurrence and affects as many as 27% of children.[245-252] While the exact clinical

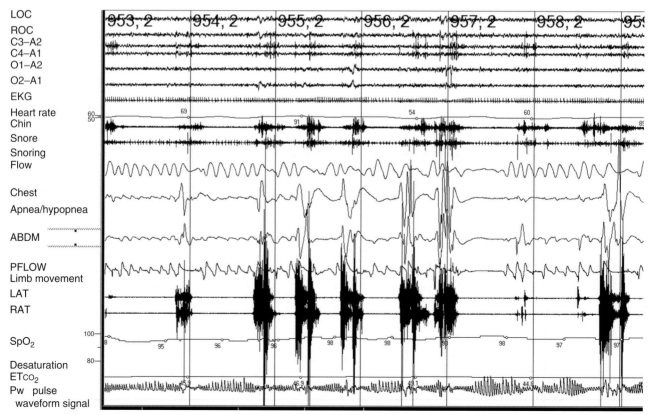

FIGURE 77-4. Bruxism in a child with mild sleep-disordered breathing. *ABDM*, abdominal excursion; *LAT*, left anterior fibialis EMG; *LOC*, left oculogram; *PFLOW*, nasal pressure–derived flow; *RAT*, right anterior fibialis EMG; *ROC*, right oculogram.

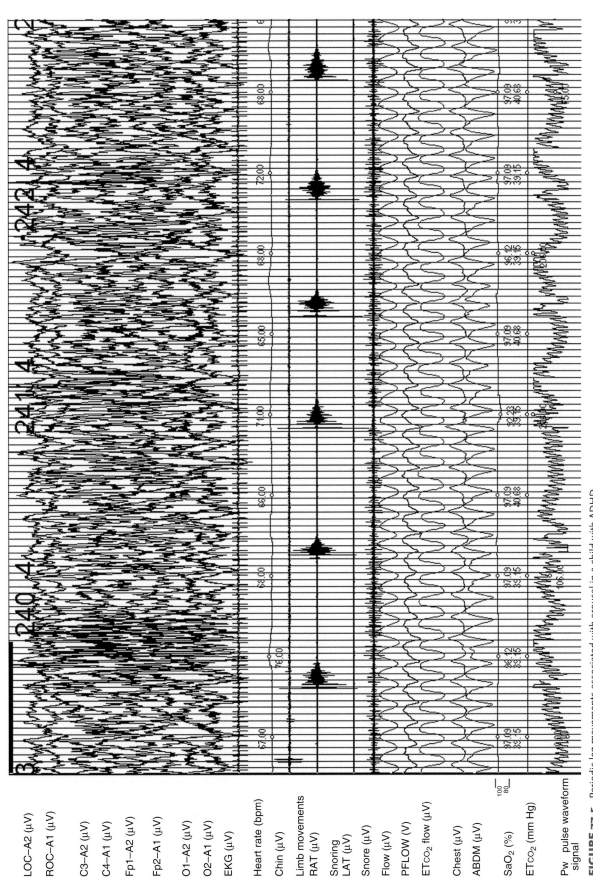

LOC–A2 (µV)
ROC–A1 (µV)
C3–A2 (µV)
C4–A1 (µV)
Fp1–A2 (µV)
Fp2–A1 (µV)
O1–A2 (µV)
O2–A1 (µV)
EKG (µV)
Heart rate (bpm)
Chin (µV)
Limb movements
RAT (µV)
Snoring
LAT (µV)
Snore (µV)
Flow (µV)
PFLOW (V)
ETco₂ flow (µV)
Chest (µV)
ABDM (µV)
SaO₂ (%)
ETco₂ (mm Hg)
Pw pulse waveform
signal

FIGURE 77-5. Periodic leg movements associated with arousal in a child with ADHD.

polysomnographically defined thresholds associated with morbidity in snoring children are only now being defined, the diagnosis of OSA based on consensus criteria[253] is currently estimated to affect approximately 2% to 3% of young children.[254] Thus, the ratio between habitual snoring and OSA is between 4:1 and 6:1, and accurate identification of habitually snoring children who have OSA is particularly challenging, considering that clinical history and physical examination are poor predictors of disease.[255] Although simple questionnaire-based,[256,257] overnight oximetry,[258] or biologically based[259,260] screening tools are being developed, they are either unreliable,[256,258] have not been validated,[257] or are not yet available for widespread use.[259,260] Thus, despite the objections to its widespread implementation and current prominent underuse,[261-263] the overnight polygraphic recording remains the only currently validated and accurate approach to unequivocally establishing whether or not a snoring child has OSA.

Pathophysiology

The pathophysiology of childhood OSA remains relatively poorly understood. As discussed earlier, OSA occurs when the upper airway collapses during inspiration. Such collapse is a dynamic process that involves interaction between sleep state, pressure-flow airway mechanics, and respiratory drive. When resistance to inspiratory flow increases or when activation of the pharyngeal dilator muscle decreases, negative inspiratory pressure may collapse the airway.[44] Both functional and anatomic variables may tilt the balance toward airway collapse. Indeed, it has been determined that the site of upper airway closure in children with OSA is at the level of the tonsils and adenoids, whereas in normal children it is at the level of the soft palate.[78] The size of the tonsils and adenoids increases from birth to approximately 12 years of age, with the greatest increase being in the first few years of life, albeit proportionately to the growth of other upper airway structures.[40] However, lymphadenoid tissue will grow especially large in children who are exposed to cigarette smoking,[264,265] children with allergic rhinitis,[266,267] children with asthma,[268-271] and, obviously, children who are exposed to a variety of upper airway respiratory infections, particularly viruses.[242-244]

Although childhood OSA is associated with adenotonsillar hypertrophy, it is not caused by large tonsils and adenoids alone. Several lines of evidence suggest that OSA is the combined result of structural and neuromuscular variables within the upper airway. Indeed, patients with OSA do not obstruct their upper airway during wakefulness, and thus structural factors alone cannot be fully responsible for this condition. In addition, several studies have failed to show a definitive correlation between upper airway adenotonsillar size and OSA, even if it accounts for a great proportion of the variance in the prediction of upper airway dysfunction during sleep. Furthermore, a small percentage of nonobese children with adenotonsillar hypertrophy but no other known risk factors for OSA are not cured by surgical removal of tonsils and adenoids. Finally, Guilleminault and colleagues reported a cohort of children whose OSA temporarily resolved after surgery but in whom OSA recurred during adolescence.[272,273]

Thus, it appears that childhood OSA is a dynamic process resulting from a combination of structural and neuromotor abnormalities rather than from structural abnormalities alone. These predisposing factors occur as part of a spectrum: In some children (e.g., those with craniofacial anomalies), structural abnormalities predominate, whereas in others (e.g., those with cerebral palsy), neuromuscular factors predominate. In otherwise healthy children with adenotonsillar hypertrophy, neuromuscular abnormalities are probably subtle.

Conditions Associated with Obstructive Sleep Apnea

Obstructive sleep apnea also occurs in children with upper airway narrowing caused by craniofacial anomalies, or those with neuromuscular abnormalities such as hypotonia (e.g., muscular dystrophy) or muscular lack of coordination (e.g., cerebral palsy). In addition to craniofacial anomalies and abnormalities of the central nervous system, altered soft tissue size may result from infection of the airways, allergy, supraglottic edema, adenotonsillar hypertrophy, mucopolysaccharide storage disease, laryngomalacia, subglottic stenosis, neck tumor, or hypothyroidism. In recent years, the epidemic increase in obesity seems to be leading to substantial changes in the cross-sectional demographic and anthropometric characteristics of the children being referred for evaluation of OSA. Indeed, while fewer than 15% of all children were obese (i.e., >95th percentile for body mass index adjusted for age and gender) in the early 1990s, more than 50% met the criteria for obesity in the last 2 years at our sleep center.[274] Genetic factors also play a role in the pathophysiology of OSA, as demonstrated by studies of family cohorts.[275,276] It is unclear whether the influence stems from the modulating effect of genetic factors on ventilatory drive, anatomic features, or both. Ethnicity is also important, with OSA occurring more commonly in African Americans.[251,275] Box 77-3 lists the major conditions associated with OSA in children.

BOX 77-3 CONDITIONS ASSOCIATED WITH OBSTRUCTIVE SLEEP APNEA IN CHILDREN

Adenotonsillar hypertrophy
Obesity
African-American race
Allergic rhinitis
Asthma
Micrognathia
Down syndrome
Craniofacial syndromes (e.g., Treacher Collins syndrome, midfacial hypoplasia, Crouzon's syndrome, Apert's syndrome, Pierre Robin sequence)
Achondroplasia
Mucopolysaccharidoses
Macroglossia
Sickle cell disease
Myelomeningocele
Cerebral palsy
Neuromuscular disorders (Duchenne's muscular dystrophy, spinal muscular atrophy)
Cleft palate repair and velopharyngeal flap
Foreign body

Clinical Evaluation and Diagnosis of Obstructive Sleep Apnea

It is clear that several potential mechanisms, including those genetically determined, are involved in the maintenance of upper airway patency during sleep and wakefulness. Each of these mechanisms or a combination thereof can, therefore, be implicated in the causation of respiratory compromise during sleep in the otherwise normal child with enlarged tonsils or adenoids, as well as in those children with clinical problems that predispose to OSA. The clinical presentation of a child with OSA syndrome is usually very nonspecific, requiring increased awareness on the part of the primary care professional because the current number of children being referred for evaluation of sleep-disordered breathing may in fact represent only the tip of the iceberg. A thorough history should include detailed information pertaining to the sleep environment (Box 77-4). In the otherwise normal child, the principal parental complaint will be snoring during sleep. Nevertheless, even when the diagnostic interview is conducted by a sleep specialist, the accuracy of OSA prediction based on history alone is poor, such that an overnight polysomnographic evaluation is required as the more definitive diagnostic tool. The routine clinical evaluation of a snoring child is usually not likely to demonstrate significant and obvious findings. Attention should be directed to the size of the tonsils,[277,278] with careful documentation of their position and relative intrusion into the retropalatal space. In addition, the presence of allergic rhinitis, nasal polyps, nasal septum deviation, or any other condition likely to increase nasal air flow resistance should be sought. The relative size (i.e., micrognathia) and positioning of the mandible (e.g., retrognathia) should also be documented when present. Body habitus, particularly the presence of obesity, and associated signs of complications such as acanthosis nigricans should be noted. Finally, attention should be paid to blood pressure values and to the presence of auscultatory findings suggestive of increased pulmonary arterial pressures.

Polysomnography

An overnight polysomnographic evaluation is, at least presently, the only definitive diagnostic approach for OSA.[232,279,280] The American Academy of Pediatrics has published a consensus statement outlining the requirements for pediatric polysomnography.[253] Box 77-5 shows the currently recommended channels usually used in the laboratory evaluation of snoring children. Available reference values in children are clearly lower than the thresholds defined for adults.[281-289] While the reasons are not completely understood, the relative resistance of the upper airway of children to collapse may underscore that complete obstructive events are less likely and that prolonged periods of heightened upper airway resistance associated with alveolar hypoventilation (also termed *obstructive hypoventilation*) are more readily apparent in children.[290] It should also be mentioned that, unlike adults, children with OSA often will not develop EEG arousals following obstructive apneas,[291,292] and, as a result, sleep architecture is relatively preserved in children with OSA.[293] This reduced propensity to manifest arousals (based on the 3-second EEG criteria developed for adults) has led to the assumption that excessive daytime sleepiness, the cardinal symptom of OSA syndrome in adults, is an uncommon feature in children with OSA. Indeed, in parental surveys, only 7% of parents indicated that excessive sleepiness was a problem.[255] Furthermore, more objective measurement of excessive daytime sleepiness using the multiple sleep

---

BOX 77-4 PERTINENT CLINICAL FINDINGS IN PEDIATRIC OBSTRUCTIVE SLEEP APNEA

During Sleep
Habitual snoring
Difficulty breathing during sleep with snorting episodes
Restless sleep and frequent awakenings
Excessive sweating
Night terrors
Enuresis
Breathing pauses reported by parents

During Daytime
Mouth breathing and limited nasal air flow
Chronic rhinorrhea
Adenoidal facies
Recurrent ear infections
Difficulty swallowing
Pectus excavatum
Retrognathia
Enlarged neck circumference
Truncal obesity
Frequent visits to primary care physician for respiratory-related symptoms

Sequelae
Neurobehavioral deficits (poor school performance, learning deficits, aggressive behavior, moodiness, shyness, and social withdrawal)
ADHD-like behaviors
Depression and low self-esteem
Excessive daytime sleepiness
Systemic hypertension
Left ventricular hypertrophy
Pulmonary hypertension and cor pulmonale
Failure to thrive
Reduced quality of life

BOX 77-5 USUAL POLYSOMNOGRAPHIC MONTAGE IN CHILDREN EVALUATED FOR SUSPECTED SLEEP-DISORDERED BREATHING*

Electroencephalogram: minimum two channels (central and occipital leads); usually four to eight channels
Chin EMG
Anterior tibial EMG, left and right
Electro-oculogram, left and right
Electrocardiogram
Pulse oximeter and pulse waveform
Oronasal air flow thermistor
Nasal pressure catheter†
End-tidal capnography and waveform
Chest and abdominal respiratory inductance plethysmography
Body position sensor
Tracheal sound sensor or microphone
Time-synchronized video

*In younger children, consider transcutaneous CO_2 tension measurements.
†Esophageal catheters are used in some laboratories instead of nasal pressure catheters to assess respiratory effort.

latency test in snoring children revealed that, although linear relationships existed between the severity of OSA (as measured by the obstructive apnea-hypopnea index) and the mean sleep latency measured during the multiple sleep latency test, manifest excessive daytime sleepiness occurred in only 13% of children.[294] However, excessive daytime sleepiness is very likely to occur in obese children with OSA[295] and has prompted the delineation of two distinct phenotypes in pediatric OSA.[296] More elaborate examination of the patterns of arousal among snoring children further showed that as respiratory-related arousals increase in frequency with increasing OSA disease severity, the opposite phenomenon occurs (i.e., decreases in spontaneous arousal index),[297] suggesting a very powerful attempt by these children to preserve sleep homeostasis. On the basis of the mutual interdependencies of these two types of arousal, a model was developed that allows for sensitive assessment of the resulting sleep pressure derived from disrupted sleep using polysomnographic data.[297] This approach has thus far permitted assessment of the independent contribution of sleep fragmentation to neurobehavioral morbidity in snoring children.[298] Thus, more subtle manifestations of arousal may be present in children, even if apnea-related EEG arousals are less common in children than in adults. For example, subcortical arousals, as demonstrated by movement, or autonomic changes, occur frequently in children.[299,300] It is also possible that subtle disturbances in sleep architecture are present that go undetected by routine polysomnography but are detectable through spectral analysis of EEG frequency domains,[301] and they may contribute to neurobehavioral and autonomic complications of OSA (see later in the chapter).

As mentioned earlier in the chapter, the role of ambulatory sleep studies, whether abbreviated (home video, sound recordings, or nocturnal oximetry) is now being intensively explored, along with exploration of biomarkers.[259,260,302–307]

Short-Term and Long-Term Morbidity of Obstructive Sleep Apnea

One of the major drives to treat any medical condition is the prevention of morbidity and mortality. Indeed, the consequences of untreated OSA in young children can be serious.

Early reports of children with severe OSA were often associated with failure to thrive, although currently only a minority of children with OSA will present with this problem, most probably because of earlier recognition and referral for evaluation and treatment. The mechanisms mediating reductions in growth velocity most likely represent a combination of increased energy expenditure during sleep,[308,309] and disruption of the growth hormone and insulin-like growth factor and binding proteins.[310,311] Tonsillectomy and adenoidectomy (T&A) and complete resolution of OSA in children with failure to thrive will result in catch-up growth and will also increase height and weight velocities, even in children with normal growth and OSA. Interestingly, even obese children with OSA will demonstrate weight gain following surgery.[312]

Frequent O_2 desaturations during sleep are common in children with OSA. Elevation of pulmonary arterial pressure caused by hypoxia-induced pulmonary vasoconstriction is a serious consequence of OSA in children and can lead to cor pulmonale. While pulmonary hypertension is probably more frequent than predicted from clinical assessment, the exact prevalence of this complication is unknown.[313–316] In addition, while treatment of OSA will result in normalization of pulmonary arterial pressures,[317] it remains unclear whether untreated OSA will result in persistent vascular remodeling of the pulmonary circulation. Indeed, evidence from animal models exposed to hypoxia for a short period of time during early postnatal life reveals that pulmonary hypertension is increased when exposed to hypoxia later in infancy, suggesting that some remodeling may have occurred.[318] Furthermore, intermittent hypoxia may also affect left ventricular function through both direct and indirect effects on myocardial contractility.[319] In the context of OSA, systemic hypertension has emerged as a major cardiovascular consequence in adult patients. Although the pathophysiologic mechanisms of such elevation in arterial tension are still under intense investigation, it appears that intermittent hypoxemia is the major contributor to this serious consequence of OSA, with lesser roles being played by sleep fragmentation and episodic hypercapnia. It is now thought that intermittent hypoxia during the night will lead to increased sympathetic neural activity, and that the latter will be sustained and induce changes in baroreceptor function leading to hypertension.[320] While the data pertaining to pediatric patients are still scant, increased surges in sympathetic activity have been reported in children with OSA,[321,322] and elevation of arterial blood pressure will occur.[323–325] It is also probable that episodic nocturnal hypoxia will induce changes in the physical properties of resistance vessels and contribute to the overall elevation of blood pressure.[326,327] Furthermore, preliminary evidence suggests that OSA-induced disruption of baroreceptor function may not resolve after treatment and in fact may be lifelong.[328–330] Thus, early childhood perturbations may lead to lifelong consequences, or, in other words, certain types of adult cardiovascular disease may represent, at least in part, sequelae from *a priori* "unrelated events" during childhood. Therefore, early identification of children with alterations of baroreceptor and autonomic nervous system function in the context of pediatric OSA may lead to detection of a population that is potentially at risk for ultimate development of hypertension and its cardiovascular-associated morbidity. More recent studies have further uncovered that pediatric OSA is associated with a systemic inflammatory response, leads to excessive catecholaminergic release, indicative of increased sympathetic activity, and promotes the occurrence of endothelial dysfunction, the latter being palliated by the intrinsic recruitment of endothelial progenitor cells.[331–344] However, accurate assessment of the long-term implications of the cardiovascular morbidity found in pediatric OSA has yet to be systematically pursued.

It is likely that similar mechanisms induced by OSA, particularly in the presence of concurrent obesity, will promote the development of dyslipidemia and insulin resistance, and also potentiate hepatic injury.[345–348]

Another potentially very serious consequence of intermittent hypoxia may involve its long-term deleterious effects on neuronal and intellectual functions. Reports of decreased intellectual function in children with tonsillar and adenoidal hypertrophy date back to 1889, when Hill reported on "some causes of backwardness and stupidity in children."[349] Schooling problems have been repeatedly reported in case series of children with OSA, and in fact may underlie more extensive behavioral disturbances such as restlessness, aggressive behavior, excessive daytime sleepiness, and poor test performances.[350–363] Moreover, habitual snoring in the absence of OSA has also been demonstrated to be associated with neurocognitive deficits, and therefore even mild disturbances in breathing patterns during sleep may change regional brain responses during attention tasks.[364,365]

There is increasing evidence to support an association between OSA and attention deficit–hyperactivity disorder (ADHD) in children, particularly with the hyperactive-impulsive subtype.[366] Several subjective studies have documented that children with habitual snoring and with OSA often have problems with attention and behavior similar to those observed in children with ADHD. In addition, several survey studies encompassing almost 8000 children have documented daytime sleepiness, hyperactivity, and aggressive behavior in children who snored. In a recent study from our laboratory, both subjective and objective sleep measures were obtained and showed that objectively measured sleep and respiratory disturbances are relatively frequent among children with ADHD, albeit not as frequent as anticipated from parental reports.[247] In this study, the prevalence of OSA in a cohort of children with ADHD, verified by neuropsychological testing, did not seem to differ from the prevalence found in the general population. However, an unusually high frequency of OSA was found among children with mild-to-moderate increases in hyperactivity, as opposed to those children with true ADHD. This suggests that while OSA can induce significant behavioral effects manifesting as increased hyperactivity and inattention, it will not overlap with true clinical ADHD when the latter is assessed by more objective tools than just parental perception.[247] Therefore, a careful sleep history should be taken in a child who presents with parental complaints of hyperactivity and does not meet the diagnostic criteria of ADHD after undergoing a thorough evaluation, , and, if snoring is present, an overnight polysomnographic evaluation should be performed.

The mechanism(s) by which OSA may contribute to hyperactivity remain unknown. It is possible that both the sleep fragmentation and episodic hypoxia that characterize OSA lead to alterations within the neurochemical substrate of the prefrontal cortex, with resultant executive dysfunction.[367,368] Notwithstanding these considerations, sleep disturbances are frequently reported by parents of ADHD children, even when snoring is excluded. According to the available literature, the comorbidity of OSA and ADHD could be shared by a substantial number of hyperactive children, and in fact, it has been suggested that as many as 25% of children with a diagnosis of ADHD may actually have OSA.[354] However, such rather extensive overlap may be less prominent than previously estimated if medication status and psychiatric comorbidity are accounted for in the analysis.

Inverse relationships between memory, learning, and OSA have also been documented. In addition, improvements in learning and behavior have been reported subsequent to treatment for OSA in children,[351,369–371] suggesting that the neurocognitive deficits are at least partially reversible. In a large cohort of first graders whose academic performance was in the lowest (10th) percentile of their class, a six- to nine-fold increase in the expected incidence of OSA was found. More important, however, is that a significant improvement in school grades following T&A and resolution of OSA occurred in these children.[351] Since the optimal learning potential for these children is unknown, it is possible that long-term residual deficits may occur even after treatment. Indeed, children who snored frequently and loudly during their early childhood were at greater risk for poor academic performance in later years, well after snoring had resolved.[372] These findings suggest, therefore, that even if a component of the OSA-induced learning deficits is reversible, there may be a long-lasting residual deficit in learning capability, and that the latter may represent a "learning debt"; in other words, the decreased learning capacity during OSA may have led to such a delay in learned skills that recuperation is only possible with additional teaching assistance. Alternatively, the processes underlying the learning deficit during OSA may have irreversibly altered the performance characteristics of the neuronal circuitry responsible for learning particular skills.

As mentioned earlier in the chapter, overt excessive daytime sleepiness is not immediately apparent in children with OSA, yet morbidity that could be construed as related to sleepiness is indeed detectable in children with OSA. Recent studies clearly support a role for sleepiness (measured as sleep pressure) in the cognitive and behavioral disturbances occurring in children with OSA.[298]

In animal models, we found that intermittent hypoxia during sleep is associated with significant increases in neuronal cell loss and adverse effects on spatial memory tasks in the absence of significant sleep fragmentation or deprivation. Furthermore, when this model was applied to developing rodents, a unique period of neuronal susceptibility to episodic hypoxia during sleep emerged and coincides with the ages at which OSA prevalence peaks in children.[373–375] Since this age coincides with that of a critical period for brain development, it is possible that during a critical time for brain development, delayed diagnosis and treatment of OSA will impose a greater burden on vulnerable brain structures and ultimately hamper the overall neurocognitive potential of children with OSA. Adverse effects of sleep-disordered breathing on quality of life,[376,377] mood,[377] enuresis,[370–380] and health-related costs,[381,382] further buttress the extensive and multifactorial impact of this condition.

In summary, it is becoming increasingly clear that OSA in children can have adverse effects on somatic growth; can induce cardiovascular and metabolic alterations such as pulmonary hypertension, systemic hypertension, insulin resistance, and hyperlipidemia; and can lead to substantial neurobehavioral deficits, some of which may not be reversible if treatment is delayed. Based on our current understanding of the morbidity affecting pediatric OSA, it is imperative to direct future efforts toward an improved definition of the spectrum of OSA-induced syndrome, such as to provide more accurate guidelines for treatment.

Treatment of Obstructive Sleep Apnea

Tonsillectomy and adenoidectomy is usually the first line of treatment for pediatric OSA, and a recent meta-analysis on the efficacy of T&A suggested a relatively high immediate curative rate of surgery for OSA in children.[383] Since OSA is the conglomerate result of the relative size and structure of the upper airway components, rather than the absolute size of the adenotonsillar tissue, both tonsils and adenoids should be removed, even when one or the other seems to be the primary culprit. Although the majority of children will have improvement in the severity of OSA, cure may actually occur in a smaller proportion than previously estimated, particularly in children with more severe OSA, in those who are obese, and in those with a positive family history of OSA or asthma.[72,384-388]

Children with OSA are at risk for respiratory compromise postoperatively as a result of upper airway edema, increased secretions, respiratory depression secondary to analgesic and anesthetic agents, and postobstructive pulmonary edema. A high risk for such complications is particularly encountered among children younger than 3 years of age, those with severe OSA, and those with additional medical conditions such as craniofacial syndromes; these patients should not undergo outpatient surgery, and cardiorespiratory monitoring should be performed for at least 24 hours postoperatively to ensure their stability.[389-393] Postoperative polysomnographic evaluation 10 to 12 weeks after surgery is probably needed in most patients.[388] However, it should definitely be recommended for patients with additional risk factors to ensure that additional interventions are not required.[388]

Additional treatment options are available for the management of OSA in children either before T&A, for those children who do not respond to T&A, or for the small minority in whom T&A is contraindicated. NCPAP has been reported to be both effective and well tolerated in hundreds of infants and older children, with only minor side effects (similar to those seen in adults) such as nasal symptoms and skin breakdown.[394-402] Younger children may develop central apneas or alveolar hypoventilation at higher pressure levels, presumably caused by activation of the Hering-Breuer reflex by stimulating pulmonary stretch receptors. However, this can be remedied by the use of bilevel positive airway pressure ventilation with a backup rate. Supplemental O_2 results in improved arterial O_2 saturation in children with OSA without worsening the degree of obstruction. However, since O_2 does not address many of the pathophysiologic features associated with the symptoms of OSA, it should be reserved as a temporary palliative measure preceding T&A, and it clearly should not be used as a first-line treatment. Furthermore, supplemental O_2 should never be used without monitoring the potential resultant changes in P_{CO_2} because some patients with OSA can develop unpredictable and potentially life-threatening hypercapnia when breathing supplemental O_2.[403,404]

Uvulopharyngopalatoplasty has not been systematically evaluated in children. It has been found to be useful in patients with upper airway hypotonia (i.e., those with Down syndrome or cerebral palsy). Craniofacial reconstructive procedures are reserved for some children with craniofacial anomalies. Other procedures such as tongue wedge resection, epiglottoplasty, mandibular advancement, and lingual tonsillectomy may occasionally be indicated. With the advent of CPAP, tracheostomy is now rarely required. Although pharmacologic agents are not usually useful in frank OSA, recent work has demonstrated that intranasal steroids[405-407] and oral leukotriene receptor modifiers may have a role in the clinical management of symptomatic children with either primary or secondary (after T&A) upper airway resistance syndrome.[408-410]

References

The complete reference list is available online at www.expertconsult.com

INDEX

Note: Page numbers followed by *b* indicate boxes, *f* indicate figures and *t* indicate tables.